# Comprehensive Handbook of Psychopathology

## THIRD EDITION

# Comprehensive Handbook of Psychopathology

## THIRD EDITION

### Edited by

## Patricia B. Sutker

*Department of Veterans Affairs Medical Center and*
*Tulane University School of Medicine*
*New Orleans, Louisiana*

### and

## Henry E. Adams

*University of Georgia*
*Athens, Georgia*

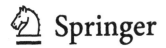 Springer

**Library of Congress Cataloging-in-Publication Data**

Comprehensive handbook of psychopathology/edited by Henry E. Adams and Patricia
B. Sutker.—3rd ed.
    p.   cm
   Includes bibliographical references and index.
   ISBN 978-1-4757-7526-6         ISBN 978-0-306-47377-7 (eBook)
   DOI 10.1007/978-0-306-47377-7
     1. Psychology, Pathological—Handbooks, manuals, etc.  I. Adams, Henry E., 1931–  II.
Sutker, Patricia B.

RC454 .C636 2000
616.89—dc21

                                                      00-046622

9 8 7 6 5 4 3          SPIN DY1160

springeronline.com

To our spouses, June and Chris, for their patience
and support during this project,
to our children, Kim Eddy, Karen, and Kim,
and to our delightful grandchildren—
all have made our lives wonderful.

# Contributors

**Henry E. Adams**
Department of Psychology
University of Georgia
Athens, Georgia 30602-3013

**Albert N. Allain, Jr.**
Veteran Affairs Medical Center
New Orleans, Louisiana 70146

**Arthur I. Alterman**
University of Pennsylvania School of Medicine
 and Veteran Affairs Medical Center
Philadelphia, Pennsylvania 19104

**Steven C. Ames**
Nicotine Research Center
Mayo Clinic
Rochester, Minnesota 55905

**David H. Barlow**
Center for Anxiety and Related Disorders
Boston University
Boston, Massachusettes 02215-2002

**Jessica L. Bar**
Department of Psychology
Boston University
Boston, Massachusettes 02215

**Deborah C. Beidel**
Maryland Center for Anxiety Disorders
Department of Psychology
University of Maryland
College Park, Maryland 20742

**Jeffrey A. Bernat**
Department of Psychology
University of Georgia
Athens, Georgia 30602-3013

**Richard R. Bootzin**
Department of Psychology
University of Arizona
Tucson, Arizona 85712

**Robert F. Bornstein**
Department of Psychology
Gettysburg College
Gettysburg, Pennsylvania 17325-1486

**Phillip J. Brantley**
Pennington Biomedical Research Center
Louisiana State University
Baton Rouge, Louisiana 70805

**Sandra A. Brown**
University of California, San Diego
 and VA San Diego Healthcare System
San Diego, California 92161-0002

**Rachel M. Burr**
Department of Psychology
University of Missouri-Columbia
Columbia, Missouri 65211

**James N. Butcher**
Department of Psychology
University of Minnesota
Minneapolis, Minnesota 55455

**Earl A. Burch**
William Jennings Bryan Dorn Veterans Hospital
Columbia, South Carolina 29201

**Juesta M. Caddell**
Research Triangle Institute
Research Triangle Park, North Carolina 27709

**Robert C. Carson**
Department of Psychology
Duke University
Durham, North Carolina 27708-0085

**Laura L. Carstensen**
Department of Psychology
Stanford University
Stanford, California 94305

**Steven A. Castellon**
Department of Psychiatry and Biobehavioral
    Sciences
UCLA School of Medicine
Los Angeles, California 90024

**Patricia J. Deldin**
Department of Psychology
Harvard University
Cambridge, Massachusetts 02138

**Joel Dillon**
Department of Psychology
University of North Carolina at Charlotte
Charlotte, North Carolina 28233

**Sara Dolan**
Department of Psychology
University of Iowa
Iowa City, Iowa 52242-1316

**Melanie P. Duckworth**
Department of Psychology
University of Houston
Houston, Texas 77204-5321

**Lori Ebert**
Research Triangle Institute
Research Triangle Park, North Carolina 27709

**John A. Fairbank**
Department of Psychiatry and Human Services
Duke University Medical Center
Durham, North Carolina 27719

**Sarah A. Feigon**
Department of Psychology
Emory University
Atlanta, Georgia 30322

**Jane E. Fisher**
Department of Psychology
University of Nevada-Reno
Reno, Nevada 89557

**Don C. Fowles**
Department of Psychology
University of Iowa
Iowa City, Iowa 52242-2914

**Peter L. Franzen**
Department of Psychology
University of Arizona
Tucson, Arizona 85712

**Paul J. Frick**
Department of Psychology
University of New Orleans
New Orleans, Louisiana 70148

**Sol L. Garfield**
Department of Psychology
Washington University
St. Louis, Missouri 63130

**Richard L. Gibson**
Mississippi State Hospital
Whitfield, Mississippi 39193

**Yuki Hadeishi**
Department of Psychology
Emory University
Atlanta, Georgia 30322

**William C. Heindel**
Department of Psychology
Brown University
Providence, Rhode Island 02912

**Nancy Heiser**
Maryland Center of Anxiety Disorders
Department of Psychology
University of Maryland
College Park, Maryland 20742

**Charles H. Hinkin**
Department of Psychiatry and Biobehavioral
    Sciences
UCLA School of Medicine
Los Angeles, California 90024

**Tony Iezzi**
London Health Sciences Center
London, Ontario N6B 1B8
Canada

**Carolyn Ivens-Tyndal**
Department of Psychology
University of Houston
Houston, Texas 77036

**John F. Kihlstrom**
Department of Psychology
University of California
Berkeley, California 94720-1650

**Tracy F. Kuo**
Department of Psychology
Stanford University
Stanford, California 94305

**Derek H. Loewy**
Department of Psychology
Stanford University
Stanford, California 94305

**Kristen Luscher**
Department of Psychology
University of Georgia
Athens, Georgia 30602-3013

**Brendan A. Maher**
Department of Psychology
Harvard University
Cambridge, Massachusetts 02138

**Victor J. Malatesta**
300 E. Lancaster Avenue, Suite 207
Wynnewood, Pennsylvania 19096-2139

**Rachel Manber**
Department of Psychology
Stanford University
Stanford, California 94305

**Corby Martin**
Pennington Biomedical Research Center
Louisiana State University
Baton Rouge, Louisiana 70803

**Richard D. McAnulty**
Department of Psychology
University of North Carolina at Charlotte
Charlotte, North Carolina 28223

**James R. McKay**
University of Pennsylvania School of Medicine
and Veterans Affair Medical Center
Philadelphia, Pennsylvania 19104

**A. Thomas McLellan**
University of Pennsylvania School of Medicine
and Veterans Affairs Medical Center
Phildelphia, Pennsylvania 19104

**Michael B. Miller**
Department of Psychology
University of Missouri-Columbia
Columbia, Missouri 65211

**Christa Minks-Brown**
Department of Psychology
University of Missouri-Columbia
Columbia, Missouri 65211

**Ricardo F. Muñoz**
Department of Psychiatry
University of California
San Francisco, California 94143

**Peter E. Nathan**
Department of Psychology
University of Iowa
Iowa City, Iowa 52242-1316

**Charles P. O'Brien**
University of Pennsylvania School of Medicine
and Veterans Affairs Medical Center
Phildelphia, Pennsylvania 19104

**Ronald M. Rapee**
Department of Psychology
Macquarie University
Sidney, New South Wales 2109
Australia

**Lynn P. Rehm**
Department of Psychology
University of Houston
Houston, Texas 77036

**Soo Hyun Rhee**
Institute for Behavioral Genetics
University of Colorado at Boulder
Boulder, Colorado 80309-0447

**David P. Salmon**
Department of Neurosciences
University of California, San Diego
San Diego, California 92093-0948

**Charles A. Sanislow**
Department of Psychiatry
Yale University School of Medicine
New Haven, Connecticut 06250-8098

**Paul Satz**
Department of Psychiatry and Biobehavioral
   Sciences
UCLA School of Medicine
Los Angeles, California 90024

**Franz Schneider**
Department of Psychiatry
Harvard Medical School
Boston, Massachusetts 02115

**Persephanie Silverthorn**
Department of Psychology
University of New Orleans
New Orleans, Louisiana 70148

**Anne Helene Skinstad**
College of Education
University of Iowa
Iowa City, Iowa 52242-1316

**Monique A. M. Smeets**
Pennington Biomedical Research Center
Louisiana State University
Baton Rouge, Louisiana 70803

**Melinda A. Stanley**
University of Texas—Houston Science Center
Houston, Texas 77030

**Patricia B. Sutker**
Department of Neuropsychiatry and
   Anesthesiology
Texas Tech University Health Sciences Center
Lubbock, Texas 79430 and Tulane University
   School of Medicine
New Orleans, Louisiana 70146

**Susan F. Tapert**
University of California, San Diego
   and VA San Diego Healthcare System
San Diego, California 92161-0002

**Susan R. Tate**
Veterans Affairs Medical Center
   and San Diego Healthcare System
San Diego, California 92161-0002

**Timothy J. Trull**
Department of Psychology
University of Missouri-Columbia
Columbia, Missouri 65211

**Jean Tsai**
Department of Psychology
Stanford University
Stanford, California 94305

**Samuel M. Turner**
Maryland Center for Anxiety Studies
Department of Psychology
University of Maryland
College Park, Maryland 20742

**J. David Useda**
Department of Psychology
University of Missouri-Columbia
Columbia, Missouri 65211

**Kelly Vitousek**
Department of Psychology
University of Hawaii
Honolulu, Hawaii 96822

**Alisha L. Wagner**
Department of Psychology
University of Houston
Houston, Texas 77036

**Irwin D. Waldman**
Department of Psychology
Emory University
Atlanta, Georgia 30322

**Thomas A. Widiger**
Department of Psychology
University of Kentucky
Lexington, Kentucky 40506-0044

**Donald A. Williamson**
Pennington Biomedical Research Center
Louisiana State University
Baton Rouge, Louisiana 70803

**Antonette M. Zeiss**
VA Palo Alto Health Care System
Palo Alto, California 94304

**Nancy Zucker**
Pennington Biomedical Research Center
Louisiana State University
Baton Rouge, Louisiana 70803

# Preface

The purpose of this handbook, originally published in 1984, was to provide a comprehensive review of current clinical descriptions, research , and theories of psychopathology. Descriptive psychopathology is a field that forms the foundation of clinical practice and research in clinical psychology, psychiatry, psychiatric social work, psychiatric nursing, and allied professions in mental health. Since the 1st edition, the editors have devised and updated a handbook to cover both general and specific topics in psychopathology that would be useful to researchers, practitioners, and graduate or other advanced students in the mental health and behavioral medicine professions. To implement this plan, we have very carefully chosen colleagues whom we respect for their expertise in particular fields. These authors include both clinicians and researchers who have outstanding national reputations, as well as more junior behavioral scientists and clinicians who, in our opinion, will achieve similar recognition in the future. The excellent chapters in this book lead us to believe that we have chosen wisely. We would like to express our appreciation to these authors for their outstanding contributions and cooperation.

This 3rd edition of the handbook was updated to include the most recent changes in the official diagnostic manual, the American Psychiatric Association *Diagnostic and Statistical Manual of Mental Disorders*, 4th ed. (DSM-IV), and two chapters were added to address schizophrenia, a topic of resurgent interest. The remaining chapters have been revised to reflect recent changes in research and theories. The authors were asked to provide a comprehensive overview of their topics rather than focusing on their own research or theoretical biases. Furthermore, emphasis has been placed on clinical description, research, and theoretical implications, rather than remedial or therapeutic procedures, although these topics are discussed briefly in some chapters.

The volume is divided into six major parts. Part 1 is an overview of various theoretical and methodological issues in psychopathology. In Part 2, the traditional areas of abnormal behavior, including the neurotic and psychotic disorders, are discussed. In Part 3, the personality disorders are described, reflecting the increased attention to these disorders. Part 4 covers the disorders associated with social and situational problems, and Part 5 focuses on disorders linked to physical trauma and medical illness. Parts 4 and 5 could have also been labeled Behavioral Medicine 1 and 2 because they include topics in behavioral medicine and health psychology. Part 6 describes disorders arising in specific life stages.

The editors express appreciation to Jay Allen and Garnett Stokes, Heads of the Department of Psychology at the University of Georgia, John Church, Director, and the Psychology staff of the Veterans Affairs Medical Center in New Orleans, other administrators, faculty, and graduate students at the University of Georgia, and Alan D. Kaye and

Randolph B. Schiffer, Chairmen of the Departments of Anesthesiology and Neuropsychiatry and Behavioral Science at Texas Tech University Health Sciences Center, whose cooperation and support made this project possible. We also thank Albert N. Allain, Jr., whose diligence kept this project together, and Mariclaire Cloutier, our sponsoring editor at Kluwer Academic/Plenum Publishers, who has offered ongoing encouragement during this effort. Additionally, the courtesy of publishers and authors who gave permission to include copyright material in this volume is acknowledged gratefully.

# Contents

# PART I

# Issues in Psychopathology

# CHAPTER 1

# The Classification of Abnormal Behavior: An Overview

## Henry E. Adams, Kristen A. Luscher, and Jeffrey A. Bernat

## Introduction

From the beginnings of life, as organisms attempt to understand their environment, they seek to organize a vast array of incoming stimuli. The recognition of similarities and the ordering of objects into sets on the basis of their relationships are primordial classificatory abilities that begin at a crude level but grow ever more discriminating as the organism matures. Even before the advent of *Homo sapiens*, classification ability must have been a component of fitness in biological evolution (Sokal, 1974). The acquisition of language by humans is clearly the most sophisticated example of this classificatory phenomenon in nature, for it is through learning words that we can select, evaluate, and categorize much of the information that bombards us in everyday life. In short, for human beings, words are classification; a sound or combination of sounds (or its representation in print) communicates a specific meaning (Davies, 1970). Because we possess this type of communication, we can discriminate a multitude of stimuli into categories that allow us to process, store, and act

Henry E. Adams, Kristen A. Luscher, and Jeffrey A. Bernat • Department of Psychology, University of Georgia, Athens, Georgia 30602-3013.

*Comprehensive Handbook of Psychopathology* (Third Edition), edited by Patricia B. Sutker and Henry E. Adams. Kluwer Academic/Plenum Publishers, New York, 2001.

on additional information at a level that no other organism can approach.

In the same way that lay persons use these categories to group concepts in an organized and common language, scientists, too, must have a means of communicating with each other. Their language requires even greater clarity and precision if knowledge is to be enhanced. Scientific classification systems use their own common language to organize and integrate data in a particular field and to work toward the goal of developing scientific principles and laws. It should be clear, then, that a science can develop only so far as it can classify the information in its field (Adams, 1981). Sartorius (1988) (p.14) highlighted the importance of classification when he stated that

no other intellectual act is of equal importance: if our classification of things and people in the world around us were to collapse, the world would cease to exist as a coherent and organized environment and would become a nebulous agglomeration of rubbish—matter, people, and things out of place.

The early stage in the development of a classification system should be guided by naturalistic and experimental observations rather than theoretical postures, despite the claims of some psychologists (Follette & Houts, 1996). In this way, scientific verification of theories and hypotheses generates the facts that can then be integrated into the development of an increasingly sophisticated classification scheme (Adams, Doster, & Calhoun, 1977). Unfortunately, in the study of abnormal behavior, the trend has long been to place the cart before the horse. Early efforts in the field have followed the medical model, which views abnormal behavior as a form of illness; specific symptoms are aggregated into patterns of clinical syndromes. Identifying these syndromes is termed *diagnosis*, which is defined as the use of specific taxonomic schemes or classification systems to identify illness. Other classification systems have been proposed, but these, too, have been based on theoretical concepts of the nature of abnormal behavior, such as trait theory (McLemore & Benjamin, 1979) and behaviorism (Bandura, 1968). Defining aberrant behavior on the basis of questionable theoretical beliefs has led to much confusion in the development of adequate classification systems. Furthermore, the self-fulfilling prophecies inherent in this type of approach have made it next to impossible to determine which of the competing theories best explains these disorders (Wakefield, 1998).

The goal of any system designed to classify behavior is that the assignment of an individual or a response pattern to allocation on a dimension or certain category permits useful statements about the behavior based on membership in that category. Classification should imply further information about the individual or the behavior, including prediction in terms of social interaction, response to treatment, and future behavior (Quay & Werry, 1979).

It should be noted that the classification of individuals, particularly the type that involves the diagnosis of deviant behavior, is considered questionable by some mental health professionals. For instance, Rogers (1951) stated that categorizing people is unnatural, arbitrary, and unnecessary. In his view, abnormal behavior is caused by certain ways of perceiving one's present circumstances; thus, only the person knows the complete dynamics of his or her own perceptions and behavior. Further, Rogers felt that classifying interferes with treatment by hampering communication between the therapist and the client. Thomas Szasz, one of the more vocal opponents of classification, bluntly stated that "classifiers should be classified, people should not be" (Szasz, 1961, p. 37). Indeed, he felt that the doctor–patient relationship fostered by the traditional medical model—in which a "sick" person is classified according to his or her particular "illness"—fosters an inappropriate dependency on the part of the person seeking treatment, who is supposed to be learning to be more responsible

and independent in psychotherapy, not merely having a disease "cured."

Similar arguments against classification have involved the assumption that each individual or each response pattern is unique, and therefore classification is rendered meaningless. However, a science searches for common elements in events to integrate them into a conceptual scheme, and psychology is no exception (Adams et al., 1977). Its classification schemes are conceptual models that seek commonalities in responses or individuals. It is true that the uniqueness of each individual cannot be accounted for in a conceptual model of classification, because the classification of abnormal behavior implies the categorization of maladaptive responses for future use in predicting proper treatment protocols. For example, a physician classifies a person who has a serious heart condition with regard to the type of ailment and the seriousness of the disease; the classification is based on a complaint, and for all practical purposes, the uniqueness of the individual is set aside until the maladaptive response is remedied.

The justification of a particular model of classification is determined by how accurately the model facilitates the prediction, control, and understanding of the response. If there are not common elements in behavioral patterns, then these goals cannot be accomplished. This is not to say that the uniqueness of the individual is irrelevant—far from it! Recognizing the individuality of each human being has been a cornerstone of medicine throughout history. However, little can be done for the individual without referring to general principles. It is these principles that allow a diagnosis, and as Cawley (1983) stated,

The diagnostic statement represents the point of contact between the experience of the individual patient and the relevant collective knowledge and its organization. The diagnosis is the link which enables the individual to benefit from what is already known, and also allows the assimilation of the individual's data into the collective store. (p. 773)

It must be noted, too, that the debate over classifying abnormal behavior is scientific and has political overtones as well. Much of the criticism of the medical model has resulted from competition between various mental health professions (Schacht & Nathan, 1977), a competition in which psychiatry has remained dominant. The medical model has been used to justify the preeminent role of physicians in treating mental disorders; if people exhibiting abnormal behavior are "ill," then they require treatment by a medical doctor. Current trends in society—that seem to label any persistent, maladaptive behavior a "disease"—indicate that the public is implicitly endorsing the medical model. As the cost of health care rises and competition among service providers increases, these issues are likely to take on increasing importance. Consider, for instance, the professional implications of the latest revision of the American Psychiatric Association's *Diagnostic and Statistical Manual*, which changed the label of Axis III from "physical disorders" to "other medical disorders" (Widiger, Frances, Pincus, & Davis, 1990), indicating that the medical model continues to have an overarching presence.

In summary, the primary purpose of classification is to develop a means of communication among scientists and/or clinicians for the purpose of scientific research. Other purposes served by classification include information retrieval, description, and prediction (Blashfield & Draguns, 1976). In the initial stages, classification should not attempt to explain a phenomenon, but only to identify and describe it (Adams et al., 1977). Historically, classification attempts in psychopathology have evolved out of the observations of clinicians working with individuals who exhibited daily aberrant behavior, so that the immediate requirements have seldom permitted systematic investigation. The clinician begins by noticing the regularity with which certain characteristics occur together and conceptualizing them as a diagnostic entity. These various entities then gain some degree of consensual validation, particularly in the clinical setting, and subsequently become codified into a classification system (Quay & Werry, 1979). This process does not occur in a political vacuum, however, and can be influenced by conceptual as well as empirical considerations. This chapter provides an overview of the principles of classification of abnormal behavior, normative behavior, a definition of abnormal behavior, the relationship between measurement and classification, evaluation and models of classification, and current classification systems used in the study of abnormal psychology.

## Principles of Classification

A classification scheme attempts to divide natural phenomena into mutually exclusive as well as exhaustive subsets. As mentioned previously, the first purpose of classifying is to permit accurate

communication that will allow developing, explaining, predicting, or controlling the events that constitute a particular phenomenon. To accomplish this goal, certain rules must be followed regarding the development of a conceptual scheme for classification. When psychologists attempt to classify their observations, they must keep in mind the conceptual nature of their efforts—for example, the idea of concept formation, which in reality is simply a model of natural events that simplifies the complex phenomena under study.

Because classification systems are first and foremost communication devices, it is vital that the characteristics defining a category be clearly detailed and described. The scientific or data language is the basic prerequisite for any classification scheme, and complex concepts need to be operationally defined so that measurement of the attributes of a particular category is possible (Bergmann, 1957). In the initial stages of developing a classification system, it is probably best to begin with what has been called *alpha taxonomy* or *lower order categories* (Bruner, Goodnow, & Austin, 1965; Kety, 1965; Mayr, 1952; Plutchik, 1968; Robins, 1966; Stengel, 1959). In essence, the construction of an alpha taxonomy requires a thorough description of the observable attributes of a phenomenon within a specific set. It should be demonstrated that the pattern exists with a cluster of covarying characteristics that are consistent over time and can be observed by various methods. As many subsets as possible should be constructed, so that all aspects of the phenomenon being classified may be included. The reliability of these subsets is greatly affected by the degree of care taken in specifying the definable aspects of the subsets and by how mutually exclusive they are.

Another important aspect of developing classification schemes is the unit used to assign an event to a given category or subcategory. Unfortunately, in the area of abnormal behavior, these units have tended to be abstract (e.g., personality structures, traits, or defense mechanisms rather than observations). An example is the first two editions of the American Psychiatric Association's (APA, 1952, 1968) *Diagnostic and Statistical Manual*, which were saturated with psychoanalytic terms and concepts. This problem has since been largely eliminated in subsequent versions. Classification units should be simple, capable of being observed, and amenable to measurement techniques. It will be argued that the appropriate units for classifying abnormal behavior are responses and their parameters. Furthermore, categories and subcategories of an adequate classification scheme of abnormal behavior should consist of response patterns or dimension of response patterns rather than individual persons as units of measurement. The advantage to this approach can be seen, for example, in using the more response-specific phrase *person with alcohol dependence* rather than labeling the person as *alcoholic* with its sweeping implications.

Ideally, the defining properties of subsets should establish which properties at what values are necessary prerequisites for membership in that particular class. It should be noted that when categories require only some group of attributes in some value, therefore allowing the same attribute to cause a phenomenon to be classified in more than one subset, then the categories are said to be *disjunctive*. Disjunctive categories can cause confusion about the way an event should be classified, and ultimately, problems of lower reliability, redundant categories, and decreased ability to identify specific etiologies and treatments may result. For example, if an individual exhibits depressed mood and depressed mood is a defining characteristic for a number of categories (e.g., schizoaffective disorder, dysthymic disorder, and major depressive disorder), the person could be given any of these diagnoses. The disjunctive categories in DSM-III (APA, 1980) led to considerable overlap in symptomatology (Kass, Skodol, Charles, Spitzer, & Williams, 1985; Pfohl, Coryell, Zimmerman, & Stangl, 1986; Widiger, Trull, Hurt, Clarkin, & Frances, 1987). The DSM-III-R and DSM-IV(APA, 1987, 1994) attempted to reduce the problems inherent in disjunctive categories by deleting some of the overlapping items. For instance, idealization/devaluation was deleted from narcissistic personality disorder and angry outbursts/tantrums deleted from histrionic personality disorder because these were not central features and both items overlapped borderline personality disorder. This was an attempt to pursue more *conjunctive* categories, in which rules specify the intrinsic attributes and specific levels thereof necessary for a phenomenon to qualify for membership in a particular class or category. However, there are still considerable problems in the DSM-IV because it typically uses such terminology as the patient has to exhibit "six to ten of the following symptoms," a method that ensures disjunctive categories.

Conjunctive categories are one alternative to the problems inherent when disjunctive categories are used. In this case, the absence of one or more attributes or a change in value of the attribute(s) would disqualify the phenomenon from membership. The end result is more homogeneous categories, which allows more precise scientific communication. Another benefit of this type of category is that borderline cases are clearly specified. For these reasons, conjunctive categories should be most useful scientifically. Unfortunately, they can be quite difficult to obtain. It appears that most naturally occurring categories (e.g., furniture, birds, or fruit) tend to be rather fuzzy sets with heterogeneous membership, overlapping boundaries, and many borderline cases (Mervis & Rosch, 1981; Wittgenstein, 1953). Natural categories are characterized by a set of correlated features that are imperfectly related to category membership (i.e., the defining features are not singly necessary). Some members of the category possess all of the defining features, but many—if not most—do not (Wittgenstein, 1953). Indeed, in the sciences of biology, zoology, and archaeology, the criteria tend to be polythetic (requiring only a specified number of a larger set of items, as in the DSM-IV) rather than nomothetic (requiring that all items are present).

In the field of abnormal behavior, growing awareness of the difficulties in striving for homogeneous syndromes with distinct boundaries led to major revisions in the DSM-III, III-R, and IV (APA, 1980, 1987, 1994). As Widiger, Frances, Spitzer, and Williams (1988) noted, the nomothetic nature of many of the DSM-III and III-R's criteria sets were overly restrictive, whereas the adoption of polythetic criteria for all disorders in DSM-III-R (and IV) improved reliability by not requiring the presence of every item in every disorder for making a diagnosis. Reliability was further improved by deleting some overlapping items, though this can become problematic if it cuts too big a swath through the essential features of related conditions. Many of the personality disorders, for example, inherently correlate with each other and necessarily share overlapping behaviors or characteristics. Thus, it is realistic to acknowledge this at a basic level. Consider social withdrawal, which is shared by avoidant, schizoid, and schizotypal personality disorders. Deleting this feature from one or two of these categories would improve differentiation but would virtually eliminate clinical usefulness.

It can be seen, then, that there are advantages and disadvantages to both disjunctive and conjunctive categories. Although the ideal scientific approach would be conjunctive, the reality of nature as well as practical considerations are moving the field toward polythetic and somewhat disjunctive criteria to emphasize the validity of categories (Spitzer & Williams, 1980). As noted before, however, efforts are continuing to work toward eliminating nonessential overlap to arrive at more homogeneous categories (as required in a conjunctive approach).

Another important principle of classification is the requirement to use a single classifying principle. Classification schemes dealing with human behavior have the option of sorting behaviors according to observed behavior, the cause of behavior patterns (etiology), development over time (prognosis), or response to treatment. Although ideally there should be classification schemes for all of these parameters of human behavior, initially they should be independent to avoid conceptual contamination. The descriptive classification of behavior, for example, should not include the causes of a particular behavior pattern as part of its defining factors.

In the early stages of a psychological science, behavior, etiology, and response to treatment should be classified independently, and a specific type of behavior should be related to a specific etiology on the basis of empirical facts or research. This results in a higher order of classification, termed *beta taxonomy* by Bruner et al. (1965), and through this approach the relational categories can then be empirically related to a particular treatment approach. A good example of this type of development is the identification of syphilis, which was followed by the demonstration that it is caused by spirochetes, and then by the development of penicillin to treat the disorder.

If an empirical relationship among behavior, etiology, prognosis, and response to treatment can be established, then a more scientific classification system results. On the other hand, if this approach is not adopted, and behavior, as well as the presumed causes of the behavior, is used in classification, then criterion contamination results. One good way to reduce criterion contamination is by using a multiaxial system that classifies behavior on one axis, etiological factors on a second axis, and so forth.

In summary, several principles of classification are important, including the use of adequate terminology or data language, simple classification units, conjunctive categories (as far as possible),

and a single classification principle. Inadequate terminology, overly disjunctive categories, and preconceived notions about etiology that influence the development of a classification system will result in difficulties in the system's reliability and validity.

## Defining Abnormal Behavior

Attempts to define abnormal, deviant, disordered, or psychopathological behavior in psychology have largely been disastrous, although this process is necessary to develop a classification system. Any number of attempts ranging from statistical to theoretical positions have been made; all cause more confusion than clarification. One possible solution to this problem is Wakefield's (1992a,b) notion of "harmful dysfunction," which is similar to the definition used by the DSM-IV.

A definition of abnormal behavior should be quite distinct from models or theories of behavior or abnormal behavior, contrary to the claims of Follette and Houts (1996). A definition of abnormal behavior is used to identify the domain (i.e., what it is) that theories or models attempt to explain (i.e., the causes or mechanisms of the disorder). Abnormal behavior defined in terms of a theory or causal model eliminates the possibility of empirically evaluating the theory or contrasting it with other explanations or theories of the behavior. If abnormal behavior is "mental illness," then by definition only a medical model is an appropriate explanation. Other definitions such as a "learned habit" or "residual deviance" cause similar problems. To avoid tautology, universal, plausible, "atheoretical" definitions and diagnostic criteria were important goals of individuals who devised the recent diagnostic and statistical manuals (i.e., DSM-III, DSM-III-R, and DSM-IV) (APA, 1980, 1987, 1994; Spitzer & Williams, 1983; Wakefield, 1992a,b).

Wakefield's analysis of the concept of disorder is one possible solution to this problem. He states, "a disorder exists when the failure of a person's internal mechanisms to perform their functions, as designed by nature, impinges harmfully on the person's well-being, as defined by social values and meaning" (Wakefield, 1992a, p.373). The "harmful dysfunction" notion is similar to the definition of disorder used by the DSM-IV. It requires two necessary conditions for a diagnosis of a disorder: "dysfunction" and "negative consequences." This definition addresses a number of vexing problems in defining abnormal behavior. We shall address a few of them.

## Mental Disorders: Scientific Concepts or Value Judgments?

It is true that many forms of abnormal behavior are normative concepts based on value judgments. Most mental disorders are negative conditions that justify social concerns, but defining them in terms of pure value judgments allows classifying many socially disapproved behaviors as disorders when they clearly are not. Incarcerated Soviet dissidents, "childhood masturbation disorder," *drapetomania* (slaves running away from their masters), or other socially deviant behavior, which violated social norms of the time or a particular culture, are clearly not disorders. In spite of Houts and Follette's (1998) claim that abnormal behavior is, first and foremost, a social judgment, this cannot and should not be the case because this means that disorders can become a method of social control associated with repression of unpopular behavior, as was done in Russia. Recent controversies about "self-defeating personalities" (Caplan, 1988) and homosexuality (Bayer & Spitzer, 1982) clearly illustrate this problem.

Similarly, if disorder is defined as a "dysfunction" in purely scientific terms, there are serious limitations. For example, a person in our culture who hears voices that others do not is assumed to have a disorder of cognitive processing. But, what about prophets, saints, and holy men who hear voices in other cultures or subcultures. Are they suffering from mental disorders? The point is that some internal malfunctions do not cause harm to the individual nor do they cause harm to others. Thus, to consider the dysfunction a mental disorder it must be harmful to the individual or society. A hybrid definition where the behavior represents both a dysfunction (i.e., a scientific concept) and harm (i.e., a value concept) is necessary to label a condition as a mental disorder. Both components are necessary, and neither is sufficient alone.

## Mental Disorders: External Behavior or Internal Mechanisms

Two frequent criticisms of Wakefield's concept of internal mechanisms are that the notion is both "mentalistic" (a term that drives strict behaviorists crazy) and biological. Most psychologists would agree that what goes on inside a person is important. However, important scientific methods and procedures must be considered when dealing with "unobservable" events. Operational definitions and similar procedures have facilitated the cognitive revolution in psychology, which is interested, primarily, in unobservable events. Not even the most radical behaviorist would deny the importance of internal mechanisms insofar as they are addressed scientifically. Consider, for example, the topics of memory, information processing, and similar areas of important recent cognitive research. Are we to dismiss these advances as mentalistic? The criticism of internal mechanisms as biological or genetic is also nonsensical. Few cognitive psychologists who deal constantly with internal mechanisms would label their explanations of these mechanisms as biological or genetic. Internal mechanisms can be created by environmental events and learning, as well as by biological factors. Internal does not necessarily mean biological. A person with a memory disorder may not exhibit obvious behavior that indicates this problem, and a "fine-grained analysis with all neuropsychological tests" may be necessary to detect the problem. Further, the memory deficit may be psychological or biological. There are numerous other examples.

On occasions, labeling a person as "disordered" when the problem resides in the environment is a mistake. For example, the loss of loved ones will cause people to look like they are depressed, but when a suitable time has passed, they again appear normal. The point is that a depressive disorder resides in the person and is due to the disruption of a normal mechanism, such as the emotional response system. This does not mean that environmental events cannot cause disruption of internal events. They can and do. Posttraumatic stress disorder is one such example. There are numerous other conditions caused by a malignant environment or an interaction of a malignant environment and biological predispositions.

Internal dysfunctions must be demonstrated by careful evaluation of environmental events, behavior, and internal functions. This process is called *case formulation*. Not all abnormal behavior is a disorder. This distinction is important legally (e.g., is the individual innocent because of mental disorder?) and socially (is oversensitivity to a Black person due to a politically repressive environment or a disorder such as "paranoia"?).

### Disorders: Mental or Medical?

A widespread controversy involves the medical model of mental illness as a "disease." Interestingly, definitions of disease or illness have the same conceptual difficulties in disentangling a scientific or neutral definition from value statements as definitions of abnormal behavior. All disorders are usually undesirable and harmful according to social values, but disorders are more than just values. They are failures of internal mechanisms that maintain coping behavior as well as psychological and physiological adjustment. The general concept of disorder applies to both mental and physical conditions, whereas the notion of internal mechanism refers to both physical structures and functioning as well as mental structures and functioning such as memory, perception, and other psychological systems that we shall discuss later. In the former case, the disorder is labeled a physical disorder, and in the latter case a mental disorder. The former involves the physiological response systems, and the latter the psychological response systems.

The overlap of the two types of disorders causes confusion among lay people as well as professionals. For example, cancer can cause severe depression, but it should be a "mental disorder" only if the physical illness has caused a dysfunction of the internal psychological mechanisms that control emotional behavior. If that is the case, then the individual has both a physical and mental disorder. The reverse can also occur. A mental disorder, such as alcohol abuse, can cause a physical disorder (i.e., liver damage). Physical and mental disorders can occur together or separately, but it is important to understand that they are different conditions. The relationship of the two conditions has instigated the growth and development of behavioral medicine and health psychology.

### Mental Disorders: What Are Dysfunctions?

A dysfunction is a failure of some mechanism to perform its natural function as designed by nature. For example, the natural function of the heart is to pump blood; the natural function of perception is to convey information about the environment; the natural function of emotions is to avoid harm and enhance pleasure. A mechanism may have other characteristics as well, such as the heart producing sounds. However, pumping blood is the natural function of the heart even though it has other characteristics, such as sounds, which may be helpful in diagnosing heart conditions.

The clause "as designed by nature" is the evolutionary explanation of the structure, existence, and activity of the organ or mechanism. In other words, mechanisms that contributed to the organism's coping and reproductive success over successive generations increased in frequency or were "naturally selected" and exist in today's organism (Buss, 1999). This evolutionary explanation is bound to cause criticism; however, determining how these organs and mechanisms came to be is not central to this notion. The fact that such organs and mechanisms exist is sufficient.

The major difficulty is that we know a great deal about physiological mechanisms and structures because of the basic research into normal functioning conducted by biological scientists. This is the basis of modern medicine, which uses the basic research to understand physical disorders and treatment. Physicians know what normal physiological functioning is and usually they can quickly spot a deviation from this normalcy. Psychology, on the other hand, is in a great state of ignorance regarding the causes of normal psychological functioning or its related mechanisms. To make matters worse, psychological practitioners are typically ignorant of basic research in psychology and fail to use the wealth of basic research available to them in clinical problems. As a group, clinical psychologists, particularly private practitioners, have disowned basic research, which has stifled advancements in applying basic knowledge.

## Normal Behavior and Psychopathology

A major question that has plagued the field of abnormal behavior is, what are the criteria for abnormal behavior (or psychopathology, mental illness, or a similar term)? Perhaps a clue to the answer can be seen in the medical profession, that can diagnose physical illness or disease fairly accurately. In the history of developing successful

**Table 1. Response Systems in the Behavior Classification System**

| Response Systems | Definition | Response Categories | Examples of Variations as Diagnosed by DSM-II and DSM-III |
|---|---|---|---|
| Emotional | Activity of tissues and organs innervated by the autonomic nervous system that is associated with specific behavior patterns and subjective experience of an individual | Anxiety Euphoria/ dysphoria Anger/affection | DSM-II—Anxiety neuroses, phobic neuroses, depressive neuroses, explosive personality DSM-III—Affective disorders, anxiety disorders, impulse disorders (anger), anxiety disorders of childhood or adolescence, intermittent explosive disorder |
| Sensory/ perceptual | Activities involving detection, discrimination, and recognition of environmental stimuli | Visual Auditory Gustatory Vestibular Visceral Olfactory Kinesthetic Cutaneous | DSM-II—Hysterical neuroses, conversion type (sensory) DSM-III—Somatoform disorders (sensory) |
| Cognitive | Behaviors involving the processing of information | Information selection Information retrieval Conceptualization Reasoning | DSM-II—Hysterical neuroses, dissociative type; depersonalization neuroses; obsessive-compulsive neuroses (obsessions); hypochondriacal neuroses DSM-III—Dissociative disorders |
| Motor | Activity of the muscles and glands involved in physical activities but exclusive of the meaning or content of those activities | Oculomotor Facial Throat Head Limb Trunk | DSM-II—Hysterial neuroses, conversion type (motor); obsessive-compulsive neuroses (motor rituals); tic; psychomotor disorders; speech disorders DSM-III—Obsessive-compulsive disorders (motor rituals); speech disorders; stereotyped movement disorders |
| Biological needs | Behaviors associated with basic body needs arising from specific biochemical conditions or unusually strong peripheral stimulation that can impair the well-being or health of the individual if not satisfied | Hunger Thirst Elimination Sex Sleep Respiration Harm avoidance | DMS-II—Neurasthenic neuroses; asthenic personality; sexual deviations; disorders of sleep; feeding disturbances; enuresis; encopresis DSM-III—Psychosexual dysfunctions; paraphilias; other sexual disorders; sleep disorders; eating disorders; enuresis; encopresis |
| Acquired biological needs | Acquired physical dependencies (intake of substances into the body that change the biochemistry of the physiological systems so that the presence of these substances is required to avoid physiological or psychological distress) | | DSM-II—Alcoholism, drug dependence DSM-III—Substance use disorders |

**Table 1.** (*Continued*)

| Response Systems | Definition | Response Categories | Examples of Variations as Diagnosed by DSM-II and DSM-III |
|---|---|---|---|
| Social | Reciprocal actions of two or more individuals | Aggression/ submission Dependency/ independency Altruism/ selfishness Conformity/ deviations | DSM-II and DSM-III—Personality disorders in adults and children |
| Complex variations | Functional interaction of two or more response systems | | DSM-II and DSM-III—Mental retardation (functional); schizophrenia; paranoid states; pervasive developmental disorders, including infantile autism; major affective disorders |

*Source: Abnormal Psychology* (p. 54) by H. E. Adams, 1981, Dubuque, IA: William C. Brown. Copyright 1981 by William C. Brown, Company Publishers. Reprinted by permission.

diagnostic procedures in medicine, a primary prerequisite has been a fairly precise knowledge of what constitutes normal anatomy and physiological functioning. In other words, before physicians can diagnose illness or disease, they must know the population parameters of "normal" biological functioning. The fact that an understanding of normal behavior is a prerequisite to identify and investigate abnormal behavior seems to have been all but ignored in developing classification systems for abnormal behavior. A classification scheme of normal behavior must be developed, and normative data must be obtained before one can empirically establish what constitutes deviant, abnormal, or unusual behavior.

Adams et al. (1977) developed such a preliminary scheme for classifying normal behavior. This taxonomy is organized around the notion of response systems, as may be seen in Table 1. The taxonomy is based on the assumption that various types of observable responses (behavior) can be grouped into categories that represent fairly homogeneous independent response systems. In this sense, it is similar to normal physiological systems or the taxonomy used by biologists, with such categories as the cardiovascular, gastrointestinal, nervous, and musculoskeletal. Although it can be argued that the response systems proposed by Adams et al. are not independent of each other and that they interact, resulting in somewhat arbitrary

divisions, note that the taxonomies of biological functioning and anatomy are also interrelated. Studying the interrelationships of biological systems, as well as the systems themselves, has proved useful to biological scientists and should provide similar knowledge to psychological scientists, so that they too can attempt to organize behavior into subsystems of responses.

Because the psychological response system of Adams et al. (1977) is based on units of behavior or responses, some professionals may assume that it is a classification system based on the theoretical position of behaviorism. This was not the aim of this scheme, and the assumption that the primitive units of observation in psychology are responses or response patterns does not imply a behavioral orientation. Most mental health professionals, including humanists, behaviorists, psychodynamic theorists, and those who are biologically oriented, would agree that the study of human beings begins with the observation of their behavior. The implications and explanations of that observed behavior constitute the various theoretical orientations. It is imperative that an adequate classification system precede the development of these theories. Although the temporal order is often confused in actual practice, the sequence of the development of a science involves classification, then measurement, and then theories as a basic prerequisite for knowledge.

Once there is some idea of the parameters of normal behavior and the way it varies as a function of age, sex, cultural groups, and similar features, then the question of what constitutes abnormal behavior can be more appropriately addressed (Costello, 1980; Lefkowitz & Burton, 1978). Essentially, psychopathology can be defined by two methods: the class model and the multivariate, dimensional, or quantitative model.

The *multivariate model* assumes that all behavior can be placed on a continuum; one example would be intelligence. When some behaviors, such as depression and anxiety, become so exaggerated that their intensity is exhibited by only a small fraction of the population, then psychopathology may be demarcated. In this sense, a disorder such as depression or anxiety is diagnosed in the same way as hypertension in medical classification. When these responses reach a certain frequency, intensity, and duration, they are labeled pathological. Note that to use this criterion, it is necessary to have the population parameters or, in less suitable situations, clinical knowledge of the attribute and to make some judgment about where the limits should be, a judgment that is somewhat arbitrary. Selecting the appropriate limits can be aided by knowledge of the consequences of the extremes of behavior. It is also necessary to know the environmental aspects and other related circumstances of these behaviors (stimulus parameters) to make such a decision. The loss of a loved one, for example, is typically assessed with an increase in depression of high intensity, but of limited duration. Epidemiological inquiry and the notion of prevalence are the key concepts in this approach, although it is important to keep in mind Costello's (1980) warning that merely because behavior patterns are frequent does not mean that they are normal or acceptable. For example, posttraumatic stress disorder is a frequent, albeit arguably "abnormal," response to traumatic events. The dimensional approach to classification is the essence of this method, which assumes that a particular aberrant response is dimensional (i.e., everyone has the characteristic to some degree).

In addition, establishing that a particular behavioral pattern is deviant or statistically rare is only the first step in developing a classification scheme for psychopathology (Adams, 1981; Costello, 1980). The second step is to demonstrate that these behavior patterns are clinically significant and cause objective or subjective distress to the individual or to others (see Wakefield, 1992a,b). Two general criteria can be used in arriving at this decision. The first has been called the *criterion of labeled deviance*. Under this criterion, deviant behavior or psychopathology is defined by behavior patterns that violate social norms. This criterion varies as a function of local conventions and changes from society to society, from time to time, and even from place to place. An example of this relativity is homosexuality. In DSM-I and DSM-II, homosexuality was considered a form of mental illness. In DSM-III-R and IV, however, it is not. For example, homosexuality is barely referenced at all in DSM-III-R and IV, where "persistent and marked distress about sexual orientation" is cited as an example under the category "sexual disorders not otherwise specified."

The second criterion is the *criterion of adjustment*. This criterion is based on how well individuals cope with their environments and is, within limits, independent of culture, because it is keyed only to the satisfaction of one's biological and/or social needs and one's ability to survive. These two criteria can conflict with each other; for instance, hardworking executives may meet all the deviance criteria of normality but would qualify as abnormal in terms of the adjustment criterion if their hard work has caused a potentially life-threatening stress disorder. Another case would be a young man whose draft resistance during the war in Vietnam qualified him as deviant in terms of social norms but who, alive and well in Canada, is normal by the adjustment criterion. Therefore, it is obvious that what is perceived as normal behavior may depend on which criterion is used, and it should be clear that these criteria differ. However, it is also apparent that when an individual satisfies both criteria, the label of psychopathology is greatly enhanced. The validity of these judgments of abnormality must be established by research efforts.

Another approach to classification is the *class* or *qualitative difference model*, which assumes that some psychopathological disorders do not occur in the normal population. For example, some disease processes (e.g., cancer or syphilis) do not vary in degree in all people, even in a mild form. Such diseases are either present or absent. Because it is difficult to conceive of any response— even a loosening of associations—that does not occur at some time to some extent in most people, the classification categories and subcategories in psychopathology must refer to a constellation of responses that are functionally related, so that they have simultaneous and/or consecutive variation within a given subset of the population. Even though each response may occur in some form in the normal population, these responses do not co-vary in the same manner as in the deviant subset, or they may be independent of one another.

Note that this type of classification scheme requires careful determination of the relationship of the constellation of responses. A good example is schizophrenia. Earlier definitions of schizophrenia required that the individual exhibit the fundamental symptoms of altered associations, altered affect, ambivalence, and autism. At one time or another, all of us have demonstrated any or all of these responses to some degree. However, it is doubtful that the four symptoms covary together in the normal population, and this covariation permits us to use the label of schizophrenia and to assume that it does not occur in the normal population.

According to this approach, if it is assumed that there is such a phenomenon known as schizophrenia that does not occur in the normal population, then such a phenomenon needs to be demonstrated or verified before it can be used as a classificatory concept. This prerequisite is often neglected, and the hypothesis that there is a pathological condition known as schizophrenia is transformed into the fact that an entity known as schizophrenia exists. This is known as the process of *reification*. The question as to whether there is such a phenomenon as schizophrenia has received scant attention, and as a number of theorists have noted, the phenomenon of schizophrenia may well be a figment of psychologists' and psychiatrists' imaginations (Laing, 1960; Sarbin, 1967; Szasz, 1966). Carson (1996 and in this book) has been particularly critical of the DSM-IV and its tendency toward an Aristotelian mode of thought. Further, there are even those who feel that it is unimportant whether such entities exist. Kendell (1983) found the "truth value" of classificatory schemata irrelevant and emphasized instead their heuristic value. He stated that "diagnostic terms are no more than convenient labels for arbitrary groupings of clinical phenomena" and that these are "concepts justified only by their usefulness" (p. 51).

The point is that deviant behavior should be assumed dimensional, something we all have to some degree—like blood pressure—unless otherwise demonstrated. To verify that a disorder is categorical (i.e., limited to some people but not others), it must be demonstrated by research evidence. In a recent development, Meehl and his colleagues (Meehl & Golden, 1982, Waller & Meehl, 1998) described taxometric procedures that can determine if a classification category is typological (i.e., class or latent class, taxonic) or dimensional/continuous. The procedure is too complicated to describe in detail here, but it is obviously a method that should resolve many classification controversies in the argument about whether a disorder is a category or a dimensional variable. This procedure has the potential to revolutionize classification if it is used.

In summary, adequate knowledge of normal behavior and behavioral norms are necessary prerequisites for establishing a reliable and valid classification system for psychopathology. Then, either the class or quantitative methods can be used to establish categories of psychopathology.

### Classification and Measurement

In the initial stages of developing a classification system, observations comprise a classification scheme. If the categories or subcategories are adequately defined, then the next step in the process is measuring the attributes. Measurement is the technological implementation of a classification scheme; in psychology, it involves assessing behavior or response patterns. Which response should be measured is determined by the definition of the particular category or subcategory, and measurement involves operationally defining the category so that the presence or absence of the attribute or its magnitude and duration can be determined.

Several points are relevant to measuring both normal and abnormal behavior for diagnostic purposes. On a practical level, clinicians should devise a standardized psychological examination similar to the physical examination administered by physicians. This examination should inspect an individual's response systems and include a specific examination of the person's emotions, sensory-perceptual processes, cognitive processes, motor behavior, biological needs, acquired biological needs (addictions), and social behavior. This exam could be conducted by a standardized interview or, in some cases, by rapid screening tests to determine if a more thorough examination of a particular aspect of the individual's behavior is indicated. Omnibus personality inventories, such as the Minnesota Multiphasic Personality Inventory-II (MMPI-2) and problem checklists have been used for similar purposes or as screening devices. Unfortunately, these are not satisfactory because they fail to detect problems that are obvious by simple observation (e.g., obesity, tics, or substance abuse), give few clues to more precise assessment, are often cumbersome methods of determining the obvious (e.g., whether someone is hallucinating), and are based on theoretical propositions (e.g., trait theories) that can impede an objective evaluation of the problem.

Furthermore, the psychological exam should indicate what particular aspect of the individual's behavior is aberrant, not whether the individual is aberrant. Such a screening procedure should lead to specific tests or examinations for specific problem behaviors. Thus, if it were suspected that an individual was demonstrating a thought disorder, a more thorough examination of information processing could be conducted, perhaps by means of the situations or tests used in research programs such as that by Shakow (1977). On the other hand, if there were no indication that the individual was experiencing sexual problems, then it would be foolish and an invasion of privacy to conduct an extensive examination of the individual's sexual orientation and behavior. For the practicing clinician concerned with a variety of diagnostic problems, there is a serious need to organize and develop a series of different tests to evaluate different disorders and a need for some type of standardized psychological examination.

The procedure for diagnosing specific problems should attempt to assess all three channels of behavior: cognitive, behavioral, and physiological. Adequate assessment should include the individual's subjective report (both self-monitoring and self-reporting), behavioral observation or behavioral analogue tests, and when possible, physiological indexes, such as those used in assessing aberrant sexual behavior (Tollison & Adams, 1979). Even though they are crude and imperfect, behavioral avoidance tests that are used to detect phobic behavior are an example of the way specific disorders should be evaluated. In this procedure, an individual is placed in an appropriate situation where a subjective report, observation of

approach or avoidance behavior, and psychophysiological indexes of autonomic arousal can all be obtained. Similar experimental procedures already present in the literature could be modified and adapted to detect and evaluate other specific disorders.

Because of the appeal of rapid screening devices and the influence of personality and trait theory, the role of stimulus variables and the environmental context of behavior has traditionally been ignored. Typically, every individual in an assessment situation is exposed to a standard set of stimuli (e.g., test items or ink blots), and it has been assumed that behavior exhibited in this situation allows predicting behavior in other situations. Unfortunately, this assumption has proven questionable. The constructive controversy, elicited by the work of Mischel (1968, 1973) on situationalism versus trait approaches to behavior, has indicated the naivete of that assumption and clearly has shown that situational or stimulus factors must be considered in assessing behavior. That situations often determine behavior is obvious to even the casual observer; it is not difficult to imagine oneself as aggressive with Pee-Wee Herman and being extremely considerate of Clint Eastwood's "Dirty Harry."

Therefore, to make meaningful observations and inferences, one must consider two aspects of stimulus variables. First, the intensity of the stimulus must be varied, and then the change in response must be observed. For example, a phobic individual may exhibit fear upon entering a room containing a caged snake. Even a normal individual may exhibit the same response if the intensity is increased by requiring the person to handle the snake. Second, the variation in stimulus situations is also crucial. A person with a snake phobia may show little anxiety in New York City but may be greatly handicapped on an overgrown, rocky hillside. An interesting implication of the situational-versus-trait argument has been suggested by Adams (1981) and Marrioto and Paul (1975): Individuals who do not vary their behavior as situations change, and thus appear to be more "trait like," may be more psychologically disturbed than people who have the more common pattern of varying their behavior as a function of stimulus situations. In any case, a basic factor in adequate assessment is that stimulus factors (the independent variables) must be manipulated if one is to observe changes in responses (the dependent variables).

Thus, adequate measurement for assessment involves a stimulus-organism-response-consequences (S-O-R-C) approach. The stimulus content and intensity can be varied as independent variables, whereas responses can be viewed as dependent variables. The organismic variable, which includes age, sex, activity levels, and so forth, can be viewed as modulating variables, which may directly influence the S–R relationship. The consequences of behavior are, strictly speaking, more relevant to etiological classification because consequences give a clue to the development and maintenance of a behavior pattern. Perhaps, at this stage of the game, consequences should not be considered in assigning behavior patterns to classification categories because confusion of the occurrence of a disorder with its cause results in a self-fulfilling prophecy. Currently, it seems that the more we know, the more we learn how rare are complete and specific associations between a disorder's etiology, symptomatology, and consequences (Cawley, 1983). On the other hand, if it has been empirically demonstrated that a particular behavior is a direct function of a certain consequence of the behavior, then it is legitimate to use it as a classification attribute.

A similar argument can be made with respect to personality traits, often used to classify types of behavior disorders. This is not usually advisable except in classifying dysfunctions of social behavior or personality disorders. For example, people with obsessive-compulsive personality traits may or may not demonstrate compulsive rituals, such as hand washing. Therefore, this personality type should not be used as an attribute for classifying behavior in a category of obsessive-compulsive disorders. This type of trait is an extraclassificatory correlate of behavior and is not an intrinsic attribute of the behavior disorder. Consequently, it should not be used to classify a behavior pattern. If it is used in this way, it often leads to a great deal of confusion.

There are a number of parametric issues that must be addressed when devising suitable measuring instruments for classification purposes, including reliability, validity, demand characteristics, and similar issues. These are important and complex issues that cannot be adequately addressed in the limited space of this chapter. For further information in these areas, the reader is referred to more relevant references and textbooks (e.g., Anastasi & Urbina, 1997).

## Evaluation and Methods of Classification

Classification research for the development of classification schemes requires a framework for describing the approach to and evaluating classification schemes. In evaluation, there are four major aspects that are very important in producing a reliable and valid classification system (Skinner, 1981):

1. The classification system should be reliable and consistent from user to user (interrater agreement) and within the same user over different time periods (stability).
2. The system should describe the domains of behaviors it encompasses. This aspect of a classification system always involves a trade-off between the extent of coverage and the precision of measurement. A good example of broad coverage is the series of APA *Diagnostic and Statistic Manuals* that include behavioral disorders and organic conditions, as well as numerous mental disorders.
3. The system should have descriptive validity, which is the degree to which the categories within it are homogenous with respect to their relative attributes (e.g., symptoms, personality constructs, biographical data, and other defining attributes of the categories).
4. The system should have predictive and clinical validity, which addresses the question of whether classification predicts other variables and whether the predicted variables are clinically significant, respectively.

As a framework for clinical research, the three-states paradigm described by Skinner (1981), evolving from the work of Loevinger (1957), is a useful model and is shown in Figure 1. The theoretical formulation should lead to hypotheses that are open to empirical evaluation so that the classification system can be shown capable of scientific evaluation. As Popper (1972) has noted, a scientific theory is only useful if it suggests repudiation rather than truth. Thus, a classification system should include a precise definition of each type of functional relationship among the various subtypes (i.e., a nomological network), a method of explicating the development and etiology of the disorders, a description of the prognosis, the appropriate treatment interventions, and a discussion of the population for which the classification oc-

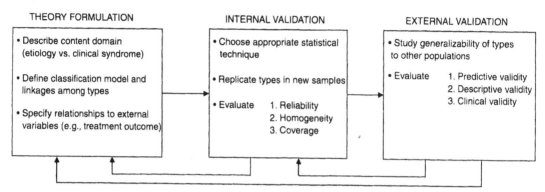

**Figure 1.** Framework for classification research. (From Toward the integration of classification theory and methods by H. A. Skinner, 1981, *Journal of Abnormal Psychology, 90*, 70. Copyright 1981 by the American Psychological Association. Reprinted by permission.)

curs. Irrefutable theories and classification systems that cannot be evaluated are of little value to the scientific clinician.

The content domain should describe clearly the variables on which the classification is based. In other words, is the individual or the behavior placed in a category on the basis of clinical symptoms (aberrant behavior), the course of the disorder, its etiology, or some combination of these variables? The two major competing classification variables are behavior and etiology. However, any system that uses both variables to classify a disorder hopelessly confounds the issue of whether a certain etiological factor causes a specific type of deviant behavior. There is considerable argument that the use of etiology as a method of classifying behavior is premature and that the description of behavior is most appropriate for the current state of the science (Zigler & Phillips, 1961).

The validity of this argument has been recognized in DSM-III, III-R, and IV, which reversed the trend toward classification by etiology in favor of more descriptive, observational notions. Klerman, Vaillant, Spitzer, and Michels (1984) clearly indicated the reasons for the reversal, stating that the reliance on descriptive rather than etiological criteria "represents a strategic mode of dealing with the frustrating reality that, for most of the disorders we treat, there is only limited evidence for their etiologies." The obvious solution would be to construct one classification system for abnormal behavior and a second for etiology, in accordance with Hempel's (1965) view of logical empiricism, which holds that we can claim to

understand concepts scientifically only if we are able (1) to describe them and (2) to explain or predict them through general laws and theories. An example of etiological classification is Zubin and Spring's (1977) description of six approaches to the classification of schizophrenia: the ecological, developmental, learning, genetic, internal, and neurophysiological models. Their variables are categories of etiology and are similar to the classification system described by Hebb (1966) and shown in Table 2.

When using two classification systems, it is possible to demonstrate by research that a specific behavior type is associated with specific kinds of etiology. This type of research leads to refinements in classification systems. As a matter of fact, a multiaxial system—similar to that introduced in DSM-III, in which the clinical syndrome is diagnosed separately from its etiology—would be one possible step toward that end (Essen-Moller, 1973). Nevertheless, it must be emphasized that scientific documentation rather than theoretical speculation is the only method by which a classification scheme can use both etiology and behavior (or symptoms) in a classification system.

There are basically three types of structural models that can be used to develop a classification system. The first is the hierarchical model that classifies individuals into subsets that are themselves successively classified into groups at a higher level in the hierarchy (see Fig. 2). One example is schizophrenia, which in the figure is subdivided into acute or chronic types and then further subdivided into various subtypes, like

### Table 2. Classes of Causal Factors in Human Behavior

| No. | Class | Source, Mode of Action, etc. |
|---|---|---|
| I | Genetic | Physiological properties of the fertilized ovum |
| II | Chemical, prenatal | Nutritive or toxic influence in the uterine environment |
| III | Chemical, postnatal | Nutritive or toxic influence: food, water, oxygen, drugs, etc. |
| IV | Sensory, constant | Pre- and postnatal experience normally inevitable for all members of the species |
| V | Sensory, variable | Experience that varies from one member of the species to another |
| VI | Traumatic | Physical events tending to destroy cells: an "abnormal" class of events to which an animal might conceivably never be exposed, unlike Factors I to V |

*Source: A Textbook of Psychology* (p. 109) by D. O. Hebb, 1966, Philadelphia: Saunders. Copyright 1966 by W. B. Saunders Company. Adapted by permission.

hebephrenic (disorganized), catatonic, and paranoid, where each category is distinct from other subcategories but all share characteristics at higher levels. For instance, all subsets of schizophrenia would include the defining attributes of schizophrenia, such as disorders of cognition. Another example is the four-tiered system of Foulds and Bedford (1975), which begins with neurosis and personality disorders and progresses up the hierarchy to depression, mania, and paranoia; schizophrenia; and organic brain syndromes. These classes are ordered in terms of increasing severity and assume that a person with symptoms of a given class necessarily has the symptoms of all of the lower classes in the hierarchy.

Another approach is to use categorical systems, which assume that individuals can be classified into discrete classes that are seen as internally coherent but distinct from each other. This was the primary approach adopted in DSM-III, DSM-III-R, and DSM-IV. An example of this type is the cluster analysis depicted in Figure 3.

The third method is the dimensional system, which orders individuals along axes in a multidimensional scale. This has been the most common method employed in personality research, perhaps because the literature in this area has failed to establish any sharp boundaries between personality styles or between adaptive and maladaptive traits (Eysenck, Wakefield, & Friedman,

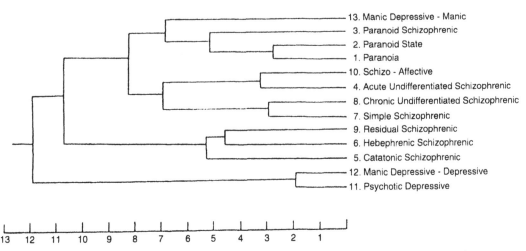

**Figure 2.** Hierarchical model of classification. Hierarchical solution of 13 psychotic prototypes. (From *Applied multivariate analysis* by J. E. Overall and C. J. Klett (p. 196), 1972, New York: McGraw-Hill. Copyright 1972 by the McGraw-Hill Book Company. Reprinted by permission.)

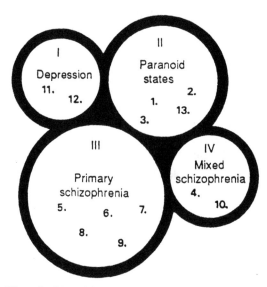

**Figure 3.** Categorial or cluster model. Distinct clusters solution of 13 psychotic prototyes. (From *Applied multivariate analysis* by J. E. Overall and C. J. Klett (p. 196), 1972, New York: McGraw-Hill. Copyright 1972 by the McGraw-Hill Book Company. Reprinted by permission.)

1983). An example of this approach is the three-dimensional model of DSM-III personality disorders developed by Widiger et al. (1987), which identified these disorders along the dimensions of social involvement, assertiveness, and acting-out behavior (see Fig. 4). A more recent alternative is the translation of the DSM-IV personality disorders along the dimensions of the five-factor model of personality (Widiger, Trull, Clarkin, Sanderson, & Costa, 1994).

Dimensional models provide more flexible, specific, and comprehensive information, whereas categorical models tend to be Procrustean, to lose information, and to result in many classificatory dilemmas for borderline cases (Kendell, 1975; Strauss, 1975). If one accepts these advantages, however, one is still confronted with the difficult question of which dimensions to choose in defining these disorders. Figure 4 demonstrates one option. Still another dimensional approach is the circumplex, a circular model in which disorders that appear across from each other are considered opposites, whereas disorders that are next to each

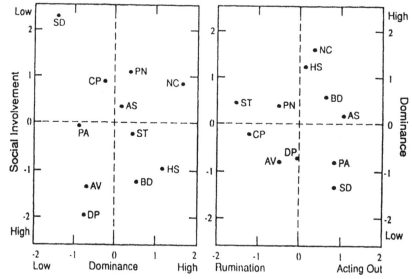

**Figure 4.** A three-dimensional model of classification of DSM-III personality disordrs. Placement of DSM-III personality disorders along three dimensions. Numbers along axes are stimulus coordinates. SD = schizoid; CP = compulsive; PN = paranoid; NC = narcissitic; AS = antisocial; PA = passive-aggressive; AV = avoidant; DP = dependent; ST = schizotypal; HS = histrionic; and BD = borderline. (From A Multidimensional Scaling of the DSM-III Personality Disorders by Widiger et al., 1987, *Archives of General Psychiatry, 44,* 560. Copyright 1987 by the American Psychiatric Association. Reprinted by permission.)

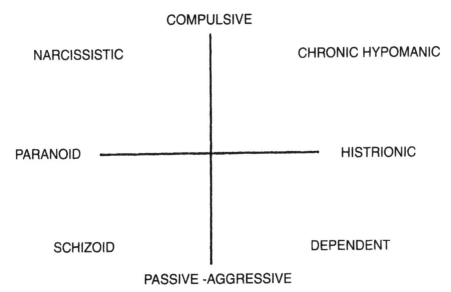

**Figure 5.** Wiggins' circumplex of personality disorders. (From *Circumplex models of interpersonal behavior in clinical psychology* by J. Wiggins (p. 208), 1982. In P. Kendall and J. Butcher (Eds.), *Handbook of research methods in clinical psychology.* New York: Wiley. Copyright 1982 by the American Medical Association. Reprinted by permission.)

other are considered similar. An example of a circumplex for personality disorders proposed by Wiggins (1982) is depicted in Figure 5.

Cantor, Smith, French, and Mezzich (1980) objected to the traditional view of classification, which places attributes in distinct categories on the basis of necessary and sufficient defining features. They further discussed how the classical view assumes a particular relationship between categories. For example, if two categories have a subset relationship, the defining features of the more abstract category are included or nested in those of the subset. To illustrate, the defining features of schizophrenia are also included in the subset of paranoid schizophrenia. Thus, in a categorization system, according to the classic view, the features of any higher level category should occur in every subset of that category. Cantor and her colleagues pointed out that there are a number of difficulties with this approach. They claimed that the classical view suffers from a failure to specify defining features for most categories, the existence of borderline cases, the heterogeneity of the members of a category with respect to their features, the variation among category members with respect to their typicality and ease of categorization, and less than perfect nesting of a general category's features among its subsets.

What Cantor et al. suggested as a solution to these problems is *prototype categorization*, where an ideal type is specified in terms of its features, but it is assumed that the features in most cases need only be similar, not necessarily identical. Attributes need only be correlated with category membership and need not be necessary and sufficient. In other words, if there are four features of a category such as histrionic personality disorder, an individual could have two, three, or four of the features and still be labeled histrionic. Thus, the features are not defining but correlational. This type of approach, as Cantor and her colleagues mentioned, eliminates the existence of borderline cases and causes heterogeneity of categories. It does not require perfect nesting of a general category's features in the subset, and, they claimed, prototypes make sense of variations in typicality. This point was expanded upon by Schwartz and Wiggins (1987), who stated that by depicting the perfect case, the "ideal types" permit us to pinpoint in specific terms the areas that require further inquiry. For any given disorder, deviations from the pure case—the ideal case—should spur the clinician to focus on these omissions (or additions) as indicative of the uniqueness of the individual within the framework of the general disorder. In short, framed in terms of ideal types, the clinician's inquiry is given shape and direction in a heuristic manner, without regard to a truth value, in a practical effort to understand a person's problems.

This lack of truth or falsity, however, makes prototypes (or ideal types) problematic from a scientific point of view, because it may violate Popper's (1972) doctrine of the ability to falsify a hypothesis. Furthermore, the fact that the criticisms by Cantor et al. (1980) of the traditional view (existence of borderline cases, inability to specify defining features, the heterogeneity of the members of a category, and less than perfect nesting of a general category's features) are in themselves the criteria used to evaluate classification systems that further violate Popper's doctrine. Schwartz and Wiggins (1987) disputed this criticism, stating that the ideal type guides the clinician to particular beliefs about an individual that are themselves falsifiable with respect to that particular patient. In essence, however, advocates of this approach are abandoning the logical empiricism that has guided science for more than 100 years in favor of practical considerations. This approach aggravates the situation described by Birley (1975), who maintained that psychiatry is already littered with a mixture of irrefutable theories, including classification systems, that explain a great deal and refutable theories that explain very little.

More complex models of classification may solve the problem that some behavioral disorders differ in kind and others in degree from normal behavior. The multiaxial diagnostic system, for example, is a hybrid model that allows evaluating an individual in terms of several different domains. Each of the domains is assessed quasi-independently of the others, but together they represent a more comprehensive evaluation than when an evaluation is limited to one mental disorder (Williams, 1985). The use of various domains permits a class-quantitative structure in which quantitative dimensions are superimposed on qualitative categories (Mezzich, 1979). For example, Axes I and II of the DSM-IV allow differentiations on qualitative dimensions, whereas Axes IV and V (which indicate severity of psychosocial stressors and global assessment of functioning) are quantitative.

Another interesting approach is the Radex that integrates dimensions and spheroids (Degerman, 1972). An example is the vector model of disease

described by Sneath (1975): Disease states are represented by a swarm of points around the origin (which represents health) in dimensional space. As people become ill, they move away from the origin; the length of the vector (or the distance from the origin) indicates a symptom's severity, and the direction of the vector indicates the type of disease.

In terms of the internal validation (see Fig. 1) of a classification scheme, some decision should be made about the appropriate statistical techniques, usually such multivariate statistical methods as factor or cluster analysis. If the disorder is assumed to be categorical, then Meehl's taxonomic methods should be used to establish this fact empirically. There are a number of other methods that can be used, but as Skinner (1981) indicated, there is no real way of evaluating which statistical procedure is more appropriate. Indeed, few would disagree that thus far factor analysis and discriminant functions have yielded few new insights. However, Zubin (1984) reminded us that statistical treatment lies in the realm of verification rather than discovery and that therefore statistics are still important to scientists. In any case, internal validation would also involve replicating the types in other samples of the population and evaluating the reliability, the homogeneity, and the coverage of the system. External validation in this framework would involve studies of the generalizability of types to the overall population, the predictive validity of the categories, the descriptive or content validity of the disorders, and the clinical usefulness of the system.

## Current Classification Systems

There has been a variety of attempts to devise a classification system for abnormal behavior, from several different theoretical viewpoints. This section is a brief overview of a behavioral approach, a psychometric approach, and the psychiatric approach, as evidenced by the developmental history of the DSM-IV.

### A Social Learning Taxonomy

Albert Bandura (1968) delineated a social learning model for classifying psychological dysfunctions as an alternative to the medical or disease model. In essence, a social learning taxonomy of psychopathology observes the interaction between behavioral predispositions (subject variables) and stimulus events. An analysis of this type, according to Bandura, can help to explain the acquisition and maintenance of deviant response patterns and to guide therapeutic processes. His taxonomic scheme treats mediating events as intervening variables, which are related to manipulable stimulus variables and their response sequences by well-defined laws. Abnormal behavior is seen as the learning of maladaptive behavioral response patterns that can be directly modified by the stimulus variables that affect both the mediating and terminal behavior. In this type of theoretical orientation, no underlying pathology needs to be modified or removed; the behavior itself is changed.

In this view, the conditions that maintain deviant behavior are a function of the environmental contingencies of which the individual is a part. A social learning taxonomy then, necessarily "highlights the reciprocal relationship between stimulus events and behavioral variables" (Bandura, 1968, p. 298). The taxonomic scheme that Bandura proposed for abnormal behavior is based on six distinct patterns of deviant behavior: (1) behavioral deficits, (2) defective stimulus control of behavior, (3) inappropriate stimulus control of behavior, (4) defective or inappropriate incentive systems, (5) aversive behavioral repertoires, and (6) aversive self-reinforcing systems. Each of these will be discussed briefly.

**Behavioral Deficits.** Some persons are considered maladjusted because of a lack of the requisite skills for coping effectively with the social, academic, and vocational demands of their environment. These individuals receive insufficient rewards and may receive punishment because of their deficits. Inadequate modeling and insufficient or poorly managed reinforcements are likely to produce behavioral deficits. Individuals who have poor social skills (personality disorders) may be viewed as examples of this disorder.

**Defective Stimulus Control of Behavior.** Individuals may possess adequate repertoires of responses that enable them to receive positive reinforcement from the environment, but they may behave inappropriately and go unreinforced because of an inability to discriminate among important stimuli. Defective stimulus control is due to faulty social training or to a breakdown of previously established discriminative behavior.

Schizophrenic behavior, such as failure to respond to social cues, may be an example of this disorder. **Inappropriate Stimulus Control of Behavior.** Maladaptive responses may arise from formerly innocuous and inappropriate stimuli that have acquired the capacity to elicit highly intense emotional reactions. This category involves autonomic reactivity and the physiological response. Disorders are reflected in a wide variety of somatic complaints, including muscular tension, anxiety, phobia, insomnia, fatigue, gastrointestinal disorders, and cardiovascular disturbances. Control of the previously innocuous stimuli is brought about through aversive and vicarious classical conditioning.

**Defective or Inappropriate Incentive Systems.** Maladaptive behavior may be due in large part to the fact that certain potentially harmful or culturally prohibited stimuli have very strong positive reinforcing functions for the individual. Sexual deviations, such as fetishism and transvestism, are examples of these maladaptive patterns. Various types of drug abuse and their reinforcing pharmacological aspects are other examples. These response patterns are learned through reinforcement and modeling.

**Aversive Behavioral Repertoires.** In this category, an individual engages in behavior that generates aversive consequences to others. Individuals in this category include children who are very aggressive, annoying, or attention seeking; children who show clinging dependence; and adolescents or adults who engage in antisocial activities or other forms of socially disruptive behavior. Aversive behavioral patterns are learned patterns of response to stress, frustration, and other forms of emotional arousal, originating from the observation of adult and peer models who provide the developing child with ample opportunities to observe their frustration reactions in different stimulus situations (Bandura, 1968, p. 322). Bandura's modeling experiment with a "Bobo" doll and children imitating aggression are examples of this type of behavioral repertoire (Bandura & Ross, 1963).

**Aversive Self-Reinforcing Systems.** In contrast to the external reinforcing stimuli highlighted previously, this group implies self-administered reinforcers. Self-reinforcement may be contingent upon performance that is indicative of personal merit or achievement. Self-administered positive and negative stimuli are powerful incentives for learning and are effective reinforcers in maintaining behavior in humans. A good example of this type of disorder is depression.

Although Bandura's taxonomic schemata demonstrated the strong influence of social learning upon behavior, a major problem with this approach is that a person's psychopathology may be classified on the basis of behavior (behavioral deficits), etiology (defective stimulus control), or inferred states (aversive self-reinforcing systems). To further aggravate this problem, a given "individual's learning history may have produced deficient behavioral responses, avoidant response patterns under inappropriate stimulus control, and a powerful aversive self-reinforcement system" (Bandura, 1968, p. 334). Thus, this system violates the principle of a single classification variable and hopelessly confuses the issue of an empirical determination of the cause or causes of a given behavior pattern. Is compulsive hand washing a response pattern caused by social learning? Research has not been able to establish definitely the etiological components of this behavior; therefore, should they be established by definition?

A very serious problem is that social learning theory is theoretical. Consequently, such a system biases any attempt to test social learning theory against competing explanations. A circular argument always occurs when a specific theory of behavior is evaluated by measurement procedures developed from that theory. Systems of classification and their concomitant measurement procedures must be independent of specific theories of behavior to allow an objective evaluation of competing theories.

## Interpersonal Diagnosis

McLemore and Benjamin (1979) proposed an interpersonal behavior taxonomy, based on their contention that useful aspects of psychiatric diagnostic schemata are psychosocial and that most diagnoses of "functional mental disorders" are made on the basis of observed interpersonal behavior. Interpersonal is described as what "one person does, overtly or covertly, in relation to another person who, in some sense, is the object of this behavior" (Leary, 1957, p. 4). McLemore and Benjamin claim that interpersonal taxonomy would be more useful in understanding and treating psychological difficulties and that it may also help to identify constructive factors in human development, thereby enhancing efforts to prevent the appearance of behavior disorders.

The concept of interpersonal diagnosis was developed by Timothy Leary in 1957. This interpersonal system concerned itself with "the impact one person has or makes with others" and allows for the "interaction of psychological pressures among the different levels of personality." Benjamin (1974) expanded this idea to develop a clinical classification model of social behavior known as the *structural analysis of social behavior* (SASB). In this circumplex type of analysis, three diamonds are used to express interpersonal, self, and intrapsychic (or introjected other to self) quadrants (Fig. 6). Horizontal axes on all three diamonds concern love–hate affiliations, and a vertical axis outlines interdependence with maximum independence at the top. An advantage of this model is that it has been tested with certain types of circumplex analysis, factor analysis, and autocorrelational methods, and fairly high reliabilities have been demonstrated. An interpersonal nosology is emphasized by McLemore and Benjamin to ameliorate the complicated business of how one person (the therapist) is best advised to behave toward another person (the client) to improve the latter's life (via successful psychotherapy). It allows assessing interpersonal functioning, with an additional provision that interpersonal experiences may be internalized. A more complete discussion and appropriate references can be found in Benjamin (1996).

The major assumption of this approach is that personality traits are substrates that cause all normal or abnormal behavior. Thus, personality (interpersonal interaction) is human psychology, and aberrant behavior reflects an aberrant personality. McLemore and Benjamin agree with Szasz (1966) that only social and interpersonal behavior is diagnosed and classified. The social category is seen as a window through which to view the other domains of human functioning. Other processes that affect or derive from social behavior are critical, and McLemore and Benjamin (1979) believe that the "object of one's social behavior may be oneself." They further state that social behavior "regardless of its causes or correlates" is more accessible to the psychologists' (or psychotherapist's) interventions (pp. 25–26).

There are serious questions about the validity of these assumptions. It is not at all clear that conditions such as tics, stuttering, phobias, compulsive rituals, obesity, and sleep disorders can be viewed as disorders of interpersonal relations or maladaptive styles of interacting. Even though a number of conditions, such as the personality disorders, may

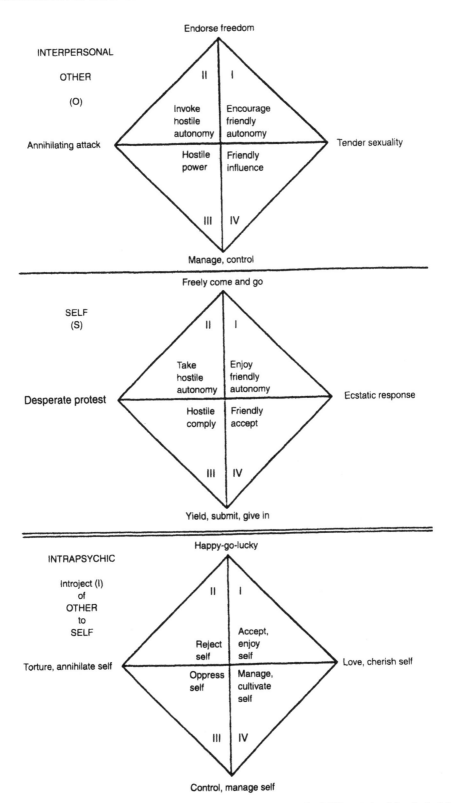

**Figure 6.** Benjamin's structural analysis of social behavior. (From Structural analysis of differentiation failure by L. S. Benjamin, 1979, *Psychiatry, 42*, 4. Copyright 1979 by the William Alanson White Psychiatric Foundation. Reprinted by permission.)

reflect aberrant interpersonal interactions, the assumption that all psychopathology is similarly based is certainly open to debate. This assumption is the primary difficulty with this system, although other criticisms have been voiced as well, such as those regarding the use of terms like introjection.

### Psychiatric Approaches

**The American Psychiatric Association's *Diagnostic and Statistical Manual of Mental Disorders* (DSM-III, DSM-III-R, and IV).** The first two editions of the American Psychiatric Association's (1952, 1968) classification scheme were uniformly unsatisfactory and subject to valid theoretical and practical criticism. Begelman (1976) summarized a number of published articles and derived a fairly comprehensive list of criticisms.

In response to these criticisms and concurrent with resurgent emphasis on the medical foundations of psychiatry, a third edition of the Diagnostic and Statistical Manual was published in 1980. DSM-III had a more complex system than previous editions, encompassing twice as many separate diagnostic descriptions as DSM-II. It was developed to reflect the current state of knowledge regarding mental disorders by (1) allowing clear and brief professional communication to facilitate inquiry, (2) providing a guide to current differentiated treatments, (3) providing information concerning likely outcomes with and without treatment, (4) reflecting the current level of knowledge of etiology and pathophysiology, and (5) meeting the needs of practitioners and administrators in a wide variety of settings (Schacht & Nathan, 1977).

DSM-III corrected many problems inherent in DSM-II. First, DSM-III was not heavily influenced by any given theoretical position except the assumption that aberrant behavior is an illness. Second, it adopted a more operational language and required that specific criteria be met before an individual was diagnosed. This latter aspect led to more homogeneous categories and helped reduce disjunctive categories.

The attempt to develop an empirical classification was continued with the development of the DSM IV. In essence, thirteen workgroups, each chaired by a member of the task force whose members were appointed by the Board of Trustees of the American Psychiatric Association, reviewed the data on various subgroups of disorders to modify the criteria of DSM III and III-R, if necessary, or to develop new criteria for each type of disorder. These empirical reviews were intended to resolve issues of criteria and clinical controversies by a comprehensive overview of the relevant research by a scholar who was, hopefully, neutral on these issues. We think it is fair to say that this produced some good and useful review but did not resolve many of the controversies because there are many "gaps" in the literature and because of the more fundamental problem of the assumptions made by this classification model, as vociferously and frequently discussed by Robert Carson (Carson, 1996). Nevertheless, the culmination of these literature reviews and data reanalyses was the DSM-IV sourcebooks. These books presented the major diagnostic issues, as well as options for dealing with them, and encouraged critical and constructive comments. The next stage was to perform focused field trials to determine the reliability/validity of the revised criteria and to address some of the issues raised by the literature reviews. A DSM-IV draft criteria was then published to invite reviews and comments which led to the publication of the DSM-IV. It has to be admitted that a great deal of work and thought went into the final version. Although certainly not perfect nor acceptable to some, this classification system is much better than our earlier efforts.

The major innovation introduced in DSM-III, III-R, and IV's psychiatric diagnostic classification is the use of five dimensions or axes, which are designed for planning treatment and predicting outcome, as well as in categorizing and classifying (Schacht & Nathan, 1977). Some minor modifications in the multiaxial system were implemented in the 1987 revision (DSM-III-R) and in DSM-IV. These axes will be described as covered in the DSM-IV.

**Axis I: Clinical Disorders and Other Conditions That May Be a Focus of Clinical Attention.** This axis is used to designate behavioral patterns associated with such abnormal states as schizophrenia, bipolar affective disorder, or dysthymic disorder. It covers all of the psychological disorders except the personality disorders and mental retardation. An individual may have more than one of these disorders and all should be reported. The principal reason for the visit should be labeled as the "Principal Diagnosis."

**Axis II: Personality Disorders and Mental Retardation.** This axis was used in the DSM-III to designate specific developmental disorders, such as learning disabilities in children and adolescents, as well as personality disorders in adults. In DSM-III-R, mental retardation was removed from Axis I to Axis II at the suggestion of Kendell (1983) and others who felt that the changes to Axis II would better distinguish "lifelong and stable handicaps" and restrict them to a single axis. In the DSM-IV, developmental disorders have been placed on Axis I, and Axis II is reserved for personality disorders and mental retardation. This change was an improvement.

A major difficulty with Axis II is low reliability and much overlap or comorbidity among the categories. Recently, two very innovative studies of the classification of personality disorders were conducted by Westen and Shedler (1999a,b). They noted that the assessment of personality disorders has relied almost exclusively on self-report inventories and assessed DSM-IV categories and criteria, which limits their utility in making meaningful revisions of these criteria. They devised an assessment tool, the Shedler–Westen Assessment Procedure or the SWAP-200, where the clinicians rated their patients on 200 items. These items included descriptions such as "has an exaggerated sense of self-importance," "seeks to be the center of attention," "tends to feel helpless, powerless, or at the mercy of forces outside his/her control," and a number of similar items from a variety of clinical sources. A Q-sort technique was used in which the statements (i.e., items) were printed on separate index cards. The clinician then sorted the cards into eight categories where the first category (assigned a value of "0") contained statements judged irrelevant or inapplicable to the patient and the last category (assigned a value of "7") contained statements that were highly relevant or applicable to the individual. The Q-sort technique required that the clinician assign a specific number of statements to each category. For example, with the Swap-200, the clinicians must place eight items into category 7 (i.e., the most relevant items), ten items into category 6 (i.e., the next most relevant items), and so on until all items have been exhausted and assigned to specific categories. Clinicians then rated a hypothetical prototypical patient who exhibited a histrionic personality disorder, which allowed the development of a *diagnostic prototype* (see Cantor et al., 1980). Then they rated actual patients with specific personality disorders. A composite description of the patients could then be developed. The correlation between the composite description and the diagnostic prototype yielded a personality disorder score (ten disorders currently in Axis II, four disorders in the appendix or previous versions of the DSM, and a prototype of a healthy, functioning person). The personality score obtained indicated how closely the patient "matched" the diagnostic protocol for each personality disorder. Their results show high divergence and discrimination in a variety of criteria.

Using this methodology, Westen and Shedler (1999b) developed an empirical classification system of personality disorder taxonomy. Their analysis found eleven naturally occurring diagnostic categories, some of which resemble current DSM-IV personality categories, whereas others do not. In some cases, the DSM-IV categories place dissimilar cases in the same categories and in other cases made diagnostic distinctions when none actually existed. The empirically derived system is more faithful to the clinical data and eliminated much of the comorbidity in their categories. Thus, the system proposed by Westen and Shedler eliminates much of the difficulty resulting from comorbidity that plagues the current classification system for personality disorders proposed by the DSM-IV. These are the categories that resulted from the classification system proposed by Westen and Shedler:

1. Dysphoric personality disorder
   Subtypes
   A. Avoidant
   B. Dysphoric (essentially a high functioning neurotic)
   C. Emotionally dysregulated (similar to the borderline personality disorder)
   D. Dependent masochistic
   E. Dysphoric: Hostile-external (similar to passive-aggressive personality disorder)
2. Antisocial personality disorder
3. Schizoid personality disorder
4. Paranoid personality disorder
5. Obsessional personality disorder
6. Histrionic personality disorder
7. Narcissistic personality disorder

These important studies conducted by Westen and Shedler have great relevance for developing a more adequate classification system and should be extended to Axis I disorders to determine if the methodology generalizes to this set of disorders. It is an important wedding of basic research and clinical activity.

**Axis III: General Medical Conditions.** This axis provides a way for clinicians to indicate any current physical conditions that they consider relevant to understanding or treating patients. Although Kendell (1983) urged that this axis be revised to include "all etiological factors, both proven and suspected, to purge the first two axes of all etiological implications" (p. 87), it was not revised for DSM-III-R or IV. Inclusion of this axis in no way implies that clinicians are expected to evaluate their patients physically, for most mental health practitioners (including psychiatrists) do not conduct physical examinations or make physical diagnoses. Nonetheless, a verbal screening for notable physical problems should be included as part of any clinician's comprehensive evaluation (Williams, 1985).

**Axis IV: Psychosocial and Environmental Problems.** This axis is for reporting psychosocial and environmental problems that may affect the diagnosis, treatment, and prognosis of the disorder. This axis changed considerably from the DSM-III and III-R and allows the examiner to note the presence of psychosocial stressors (e.g., poverty) that have contributed to the development or exacerbation of the disorder.

**Axis V: Global Assessment of Functioning.** This axis had the largest revision in DSM-III-R. In DSM-III, it was labeled "highest level of adaptive functioning in the past year" and used a seven-point scale to assess adaptive functioning in terms of social relationships, occupational performance, and use of leisure time. The primary use of this scale was considered its potential prognostic validity, and DSM-III-R expanded the clinician's ability to judge this area by specifying that the individual be assessed for current functioning as well as level of functioning during the past year. Comparing the two ratings is said to reflect both the current need for treatment and the degree of deviation from the individual's premorbid functioning. In the DSM-IV, the patient is rated on a scale that gives the clinician's judgment of the overall level of function from 0–100. However the GAF may reflect current functioning, functioning at discharge, or functioning in the past (i.e., GAF = 75 (past year) and GAF = 85 (current). Thus, a DSM-IV diagnosis might look like this: Axis I = 305.00, alcohol abuse; Axis II = 301.6 Dependent Personality Disorder; Axis IV = Unemployed; Axis V = 65 (current).

The choice of these five axes was made after careful consideration. Williams (1985) noted that the committee sought to make the system comprehensive yet practical enough for routine clinical use. This limited the number of axes that could be included, although various authors have proposed separate axes for such areas as intelligence (Rutter, Shaffer, & Shepherd, 1975), substance abuse (Treece, 1982), family factors (Fleck, 1983), and response to treatment (Schacht & Nathan, 1977).

It is apparent that, despite its flaws, the DSM-IV and its successors represent a decided improvement over previous efforts. This system came about in response to the resurgence of the neo-Kraepelian movement in psychiatry—and hence continues to overemphasize the medical model—but at least criteria now exist that can be operationally evaluated. It is hoped that the heuristic value of the DSM series will lead to continued advancement in classifying abnormal behavior.

## Summary

Tremendous progress in classifying abnormal behavior has been made in the past 25 years. With the advent of DSM-III and its multiaxial system, along with the purging of psychodynamic theory from classification in favor of operational definitions, we now have a much improved classification scheme. Nonetheless, there is still room for improvement within that system, including a more open-minded evaluation of the feasibility of the medical model, as opposed to a classification system based on classification theory and models, and more empirically based decision making. The latter is expected to occur as the literature base expands, and perhaps future systems will be revolutionary not so much for their changes but for their demonstrations of the validity of earlier schemata.

In addition to new classification systems, the atmosphere regarding classification and the ensuing dialogues concerning methods, principles, and models of classification are very positive indications that we will have a better understanding of classification schemes in the future. We are also likely to continue proceeding toward more accurate classification based on truly scientific principles of behavior.

## References

Adams, H. E. (1981). *Abnormal psychology*. Dubuque, IA: William C. Brown.

Adams, H. E., Doster, J. A., & Calhoun, K. S. (1977). A

psychologically based system of response classification. In A. R. Ciminero, K. S. Calhoun, & H. E. Adams (Eds.) *Handbook of behavioral assessment*. New York: Wiley.

American Psychiatric Association. (1952). *Diagnostic and statistical manual of mental disorders*. Washington, DC: Author.

American Psychiatric Association. (1968). *Diagnostic and statistical manual of mental disorders* (2nd ed.). Washington, DC: Author.

American Psychiatric Association. (1980). *Diagnostic and statistical manual of mental disorders* (3rd ed.). Washington, DC: Author.

American Psychiatric Association. (1987). *Diagnostic and statistical manual of mental disorders* (3rd ed., rev.). Washington, DC: Author.

American Psychiatric Association. (1994). *Diagnostic and statistical manual of mental disorders* (4th ed.). Washington, DC: Author.

Anastasi, A., & Urbina, S. (1997). *Psychological testing* (7th ed.). Upper Saddle River, NJ: Prentice-Hall.

Bandura, A. (1968). A social learning interpretation of psychological dysfunctions. In P. London & P. Rosenhan (Eds.), *Foundations of abnormal psychology* (pp. 293–344). New York: Holt, Rinehart & Winston.

Bandura, A., & Ross, S. A. (1963). Transmission of aggression through imitation of aggressive models. *Journal of Abnormal and Social Psychology, 66*, 3–11.

Bayer, R., & Spitzer, R. L. (1982). Edited correspondence on the status of homosexuality in DSM-III. *Journal of the History of the Behavioral Sciences, 18*, 35–52.

Begelman, D. A. (1976). Behavioral classification. In M. Hersen & A. E. Bellack (Eds.), *Behavioral assessment: A practical handbook* (pp. 23–48). New York: Pergamon.

Benjamin, L. S. (1974). Structural analysis of social behavior. *Psychological Review, 81*, 392–425.

Benjamin, L. S. (1996). *Interpersonal diagnosis and treatment of personality disorders* (2nd ed.). New York: Guilford.

Bergmann, G. (1957). *Philosophy of science*. Madison: University of Wisconsin Press.

Birley, J. L. T. (1975). The history of psychiatry as the history of an art. *British Journal of Psychiatry, 127*, 393–400.

Blashfield, R., & Draguns, J. (1976). Evaluative criteria for psychiatric classification. *Journal of Abnormal Psychology, 85*, 140–150.

Bruner, J. W., Goodnow, J. J., & Austin, G. A. (1965). *A study of thinking*. New York: Science Editions.

Buss, D. M. (1999). *Evolutionary psychology: The new science of mind*. Boston, MA: Allyn & Bacon.

Cantor, N., Smith, E. E., French, R. D., & Mezzich, J. (1980). Psychiatric diagnoses as prototype categorization. *Journal of Abnormal Psychology, 89*, 181–193.

Caplan, P. J. (1988). The psychiatric association's failure to meet its own standards: The dangers of self-defeating personality disorder as a category. *Journal of Nervous and Mental Disease, 168*, 178–182.

Carson, R. C. (1996). Aristotle, Galileo, and the DSM taxonomy: The case of schizophrenia. *Journal of Consulting and Clinical Psychology, 64*, 1133–1139.

Cawley, R. H. (1983). Psychiatric diagnosis: What we need. *Psychiatric Annals, 13*, 772–782.

Costello, C. G. (1980). Childhood depression: Three basic but questionable assumptions in the Lefkowitz and Burton critique. *Psychological Bulletin, 87*, 185–190.

Davies, (1970). *The American Heritage dictionary of the English language*. New York: Dell.

Degerman, R. L. (1972). The geometric representation of some simple structure. In R. N. Shepard, A. K. Romney, & S. B. Nerlove (Eds.), *Multidimensional scaling* (Vol. 1, pp. 27–34). New York: Seminar Press.

Essen-Moller, E. (1973). Standard lists of threefold for mental disorders. *Acta Psychiatrica Scandinavica, 49*, 198–212.

Eysenck, H. J., Wakefield, J. A., & Friedman, A. (1983). Diagnosis and clinical assessment: The DSM-III. *Annual Review of Psychology, 34*, 167–193.

Follette, W. C., & Houts, A. C. (1996) Models of scientific progress and the role of theory in taxonomic development. *Journal of Consulting and Clinical Psychology, 64*, 1120–1132.

Fleck, S. (1983). A holistic approach to family typology and the axes of DSM-III. *Archives of General Psychiatry, 40*, 901–906.

Foulds, G. A., & Bedford, A. (1975). Hierarchies of classes of personal illness. *Psychosomatic Medicine, 5*, 181–192.

Hebb, D. O. (1966). *A textbook of psychology*. Philadelphia: Saunders.

Hempel, C. G. (1965). *Aspects of scientific explanation and other essays in the philosophy of science*. New York: Free Press.

Houts, A. C., & Follette, W. C. (1998) Mentalism, mechanism, and medical analogues: Reply to Wakefield (1998). *Journal of Consulting and Clinical Psychology, 66*, 853–855.

Kass, F., Skodol, A. E., Charles, E., Spitzer, R. L., & Williams, J. B. W. (1985). Scaled ratings of DSM-III personality disorders. *American Journal of Psychiatry, 142*, 627–630.

Kendell, R. E. (1975). *The role of diagnosis in psychiatry*. Oxford, England: Blackwell Scientific.

Kendell, R. E. (1983). DSM-III: A major advance in psychiatric nosology. In R. Spitzer, J. Williams, & A. Skodol (Eds.), *International perspectives on DSM-III* (pp. 122–139). Washington, DC: American Psychiatric Association.

Kety, S. S. (1965). Problems in psychiatric nosology from the viewpoint of the biological sciences. In M. M. Katz, J. O. Cole, & W. E. Barton (Eds.), *The role and method of classification in psychiatry and psychopathology* (pp. 36–63). Chevy Chase, MD: National Institute of Mental Health.

Klerman, G. L., Vaillant, G. E., Spitzer, R. L., & Mechels, R. (1984). A debate on DSM-III. *American Journal of Psychiatry, 141*, 539–553.

Laing, R. D. (1960). *The divided self: A study of sanity and madness*. Chicago: Quadrangle.

Leary, T. (1957). *Interpersonal diagnosis of personality: A functional theory and methodology for personality evaluation*. New York: Ronald.

Lefkowitz, M. M., & Burton, N. (1978). Childhood depression: A critique of the concept. *Psychological Bulletin, 85*, 716–726.

Loevinger, J. (1957). Objective tests as instruments of psychological theory. *Psychological Reports, 3*, 635–694.

Marrioto, M. J., & Paul, G. L. (1975). Persons versus situations in the real life functioning of chronic institutionalized mental patients. *Journal of Abnormal Psychology, 84*, 483–493.

Mayr, E. (1952). Concepts of classification and nomenclature in higher organisms and microorganisms. *Annals of the New York Academy of Science, 56*, 391–397.

McLemore, C. W., & Benjamin, L. S. (1979). Whatever happened to interpersonal diagnosis? A psychosocial alternative to DSM-III. *American Psychologist, 34*, 17–34.

Meehl, P. E., & Golden, R. R. (1982) Taxometric methods. In P. Kendall & J. Butcher (Eds.), *Handbook of research methods in clinical psychology* (pp. 127–181). New York: Wiley.

Mervis, C., & Rosch, E. (1981). Categorization of natural objects. *Annual Review of Psychology, 32,* 89–115.

Mezzich, J. E. (1979). Patterns and issues in multiaxial psychiatric diagnosis. *Psychological Medicine, 9,* 125–137.

Millon, T. (1981). *Disorders of personality, DSM-III: Axis II.* New York: Wiley.

Mischel, W. (1968). *Personality and assessment.* New York: Wiley.

Mischel, W. (1973). Toward a cognitive social learning reconceptualization of personality. *Psychological Review, 80,* 252–283.

Overall, J. E., & Klett, C. J. (1972). *Applied multivariate analysis.* New York: McGraw-Hill.

Pfohl, B., Coryell, W., Zimmerman, M., & Stangl, P. (1986). DSM-III personality disorders: Diagnostic overlap and internal consistency of individual DSM-III criteria. *Comprehensive Psychiatry, 27,* 21–34.

Plutchik, R. (1968). *Foundations of experimental research.* New York: Harper & Row.

Popper, K. R. (1972). *The logic of scientific discovery.* London: Hutchinson.

Quay, H. C., & Werry, J. S. (1979). *Psychopathological disorders of childhood.* New York: Wiley.

Robins, L. L. (1966). A historical review of classification of behavior disorders and one current perspective. In L. D. Eron (Ed.), *The classification of behavior disorders* (pp. 44–58). Chicago: Aldine.

Rogers, C. R. (1951). *Client-centered therapy.* Boston: Houghton Mifflin.

Rutter, M., & Shaffer, D. (1980). DSM-III: A step forward or back in the classification of child psychiatric disorders? *Journal of the American Academy of Child Psychiatry, 19,* 371–394.

Rutter, M., Shaffer, D., & Shepherd, M. (1975). *A multi-axial classification of child psychiatric disorders: An evaluation of a proposal.* Geneva: World Health Organization.

Sarbin, T. R. (1967). On the futility of the proposition that some people can be labeled "mentally ill." *Journal of Consulting Psychology, 31,* 447–453.

Sartorius, N. (1988). International perspectives of psychiatric classification. *British Journal of Psychiatry, 152* (Suppl. 1), 9–14.

Schacht, T. E., & Nathan, P. E. (1977). But is it good for the psychologists? Appraisal and status of DSM-III. *American Psychologist, 32,* 1017–1025.

Schwartz, A. S., & Wiggins, O. P. (1987). Diagnosis and ideal types: A contribution to psychiatric classification. *Comprehensive Psychiatry, 28,* 277–291.

Shakow, D. (1977). Segmental set: The adoptive process in schizophrenia. *American Psychologist, 32,* 129–139.

Skinner, H. A. (1981). Toward the integration of classification theory and methods. *Journal of Abnormal Psychology, 90,* 68–87.

Sneath, P. H. E. (1975). A vector model of disease for teaching and diagnosis. *Medical Hypothesis, 1,* 12–22.

Sokal, R. R. (1974). Classification: Purposes, principles, progress, prospects. *Science, 185,* 1115–1123.

Spitzer, R. L., & Williams, J. B. W. (1980). Classification of mental disorders in DSM-III. In H. Kaplan, A. Freedman, & B. Sadock (Eds.), *Comprehensive textbook of psychiatry* (3rd ed., pp. 374–402). Baltimore: Williams & Wilkins.

Stengel, E. (1959). Classification of mental disorders. *Bulletin of the World Health Organization, 21,* 601–663.

Strauss, S. (1975). A comprehensive approach to psychiatric diagnosis. *American Journal of Psychiatry, 132,* 1193–1197.

Szasz, T. S. (1961). *The myth of mental illness: Foundations of a theory of personal conduct.* New York: Hoeber Medical Division, Harper & Row.

Szasz, T. S. (1966). The psychiatric classification of behavior: A strategy of personal constraint. In L. D. Eron (Ed.), *The classification of behavior disorders* (pp. 37–51). Chicago: Aldine.

Tollison, C. D., & Adams, H. E. (1979). *Sexual disorders: Theory, research, and treatment.* New York: Gardner.

Treece, C. (1982). DSM-III as a research tool. *American Journal of Psychiatry, 139,* 577–583.

Wakefield, J. C. (1992a). The concept of mental disorder: On the boundary between biological facts and social values. *American Psychologist, 47,* 373–388.

Wakefield, J. C. (1992b). Disorder as harmful dysfunction: A conceptual critique of DSM-IIIR's definition of mental disorder. *Psychological Review, 99,* 232–247.

Wakefield, J. C. (1998). The DSM's theory neutral nosology is scientifically progressive: Response to Follette and Houts (1996). *Journal of Consulting and Clinical Psychology, 66,* 846–852.

Waller, N. G. & Meehl, P.E. (1998). *Multivariate taxometric procedures.* Thousand Oaks, CA: Sage.

Westen, D., & Shedler, J. (1999a). Revising and assessing Axis II (Part 1): Developing a clinically and empirically valid assessment method. *American Journal of Psychiatry, 156,* 258–272.

Westen, D., & Shedler, J. (1999b). Revising and assessing Axis II (Part 2): Developing a clinically and empirically valid assessment method. *American Journal of Psychiatry, 156,* 273–285.

Widiger, T. A., Frances, A. J., Pincus, H. A., & Davis, W. W. (1990). DSM-IV literature reviews: Rationale, process, and limitations. *Journal of Psychopathology and Behavioral Assessment, 12,* 189–202.

Widiger, T. A., Frances, A. J., Spitzer, R. L., & Williams, J. B. W. (1988). The DSM-III-R personality disorders: An overview. *American Journal of Psychiatry, 145,* 786–795.

Widiger, T. A., Trull, T., Hurt, S., Clarkin, J., & Frances, A. J. (1987). A multidimensional scaling of the DSM-III personality disorders. *Archives of General Psychiatry, 44,* 557–563.

Widiger, T. A., Trull, T. J., Clarkin, J. F., Sanderson, C., & Costa, P. J. (1994). A description of the DSM-III-R and DSM-IV personality disorders with the five-factor model of personality. In P. J. Costa & T. A. Widiger (Eds.), *Personality disorders and the five-factor model of personality* (pp. 41–56). Washington, DC: American Psychological Association.

Wiggins, J. (1982). Circumplex models of interpersonal behavior in clinical psychology. In P. Kendall & J. Butcher (Eds.), *Handbook of research methods in clinical psychology* (pp. 183–220). New York: Wiley.

Williams, J. B. W. (1985). The multiaxial system of DSM-III: Where did it come from and where should it go? *Archives of General Psychiatry, 42,* 175–186.

Wittgenstein, L. (1953). *Philosophical investigations.* Oxford, England: Blackwell Scientific.

Zigler, E., & Phillips, L. (1961). Psychiatric diagnoses and symptomatology. *Journal of Abnormal and Social Psychology, 63,* 69–75.

Zimmerman, M. (1988). Why are we rushing to publish DSM-IV? *Archives of General Psychiatry, 45,* 1135–1138.

Zubin, J. (1984). Commentary. *Integrative Psychiatry, 2,* 52–54.

Zubin, J., & Spring, B. (1977). Vulnerability: A new view of schizophrenia. *Journal of Abnormal Psychology, 86,* 103–126.

# CHAPTER 2

# Methodological Issues in Clinical Diagnosis

## Sol L. Garfield

## Introduction

Clinical appraisal and diagnosis in health-related disciplines are clearly of great importance. No one seriously advocates providing treatment before some kind of diagnostic appraisal has been made to guide the treatment. Furthermore, particularly in the medical specialty of psychiatry, as new knowledge has been secured and new theories developed, diagnoses and diagnostic approaches have been modified, new diagnoses added, and old ones discarded. In some instances the descriptive symptomatic patterns of the disorder is little changed, but its official clinical diagnosis or categorization is changed as a result of newer conceptualizations and points of view. Such developments have occurred with particular frequency in the period from 1980 to 1994 with official publication of three new *Diagnostic and Statistical Manuals of Mental Disorders* by the American Psychiatric Association (1980, 1987, 1994).

Therefore, clinical diagnoses are not invariant, and problems in this area have been topics of discussion and controversy over the years. Disagreements have stemmed from differences in disciplinary orientation, theoretical considerations,

and interpretations of research data concerning the reliability and validity of clinical diagnosis. The issues generated are complex and have important research and practical implications for the entire field of psychopathology. Consequently, methodological problems in this area are not mere academic concerns but directly affect all professional disciplines in the area of psychopathology and, thus, the actual treatment and disposition of those individuals whose difficulties are considered psychopathological. Furthermore, although official systems of diagnosis or nosology may show significant changes over time, the basic methodological issues involved remain very much the same and require careful consideration in evaluating any formalized classification system.

## Clinical Diagnosis: Some Possible Meanings

Before discussing some of the methodological problems and issues in clinical diagnosis, it is important to discuss briefly the possible meanings or interpretations attached to this term. Traditionally, clinical diagnosis has referred to discovering, describing, and designating a specific illness or disease. Deriving from the field of medicine, it has been closely identified with medical conceptions of disease entities. The Funk & Wagnalls *New College Standard Dictionary* (1950) gives the following as the first definition for the word diagnosis: "The art or act of discriminating between

Sol L. Garfield • Department of Psychology, Washington University, St. Louis, Missouri 63130.

*Comprehensive Handbook of Psychopathology* (Third Edition), edited by Patricia B. Sutker and Henry E. Adams. Kluwer Academic / Plenum Publishers, New York, 2001.

diseases and distinguishing them by their characteristics." Websters Unabridged Dictionary (1979) defines diagnosis as "the act or process of deciding the nature of a diseased condition by examination."

Thus, diagnosis has been based on the disease entity concept used in medicine. Within this orientation, clinical diagnosis is of great importance, for appropriate treatment depends on the correct diagnosis. Medicine, based on scientific advances in such basic areas as biochemistry, genetics, microbiology, and comparable advances in instrumentation and equipment, has used the disease entity model with success. Many illnesses have been identified in terms of symptomatology, course of illness, prognosis, and possible causes. Treatments for a number of these illnesses subsequently have been discovered or developed. Consequently, the correct clinical diagnosis may lead to the selection and administration of an appropriate and effective treatment.

Psychiatry, the branch of medicine concerned with psychopathology, has modeled itself after the practices of the parent field. Various neurologists and psychiatrists during the latter part of the nineteenth century and thereafter identified specific mental illnesses which they discovered or described, for example, general paresis, Korsakoff's syndrome, and Alzheimer's disease. This process has been relatively more successful in organic or neurological disorders where both the symptomatology and the course of the disorder can be more successfully described and the etiology more clearly ascertained. This, however, has not kept psychiatrists from describing and designating forms of mental illness which do not always fit the disease entity model successfully. Since the time that catatonia and hebephrenia were identified as separate types of mental illness more than 100 years ago, numerous designations and classifications have been devised by psychiatrists, individually or in organized groups (Zilboorg & Henry, 1941). Some categories, particularly those with a known etiology or course, have withstood the test of time. Others, however, have appeared on the diagnostic stage for an interval of time, and have then disappeared or were replaced. Dementia praecox, conceived by Kraepelin to incorporate the separate diagnoses of catatonia, hebephrenia, and paranoia, has given way to schizophrenia. The latter, in turn, has undergone several modifications and transformations, and questions are still raised

about its diagnostic classification (Carson, 1996; Carson & Sanislow, 1993). In the latest revision of the official diagnostic manual of the American Psychiatric Association (1994), DSM-IV, thirteen new diagnoses were added, and eight were deleted.

In addition to changes in nosologies and designations of disease over time, different classifications or diagnostic schemes were promulgated during the same period. Thus, diagnostic schemes and specific diagnostic terms in psychiatry reflect the views of individuals and also of committees or groups of individuals who participated in the diagnostic classification process. For such reasons, both individual and group values and interests may influence the diagnostic system formally adopted at a given time. This point is mentioned to emphasize that the creation and adoption of a diagnostic system is not a result of scientific research *per se*. In more recent times, even economic considerations deriving from third-party payments have played a possible role in retaining or adding selected diagnoses.

In any event, diagnoses or diagnostic labels have been used in psychiatry, in conformance with medical views concerning illness and disease, to designate various types of psychopathology or deviant behavior. Because the care and treatment of disturbed individuals was gradually entrusted to the medical profession, such individuals also tended to be viewed as mentally ill, and their deviant behaviors, thoughts, and moods were considered symptoms of mental illness. This has had a number of important theoretical, practical, and research implications. Although our primary concern in this chapter is with methodological issues and problems, it is worth commenting here on some of the broader implications of using clinical diagnosis in the mental health field.

Clearly, accurate diagnosis of illness or disease is an important prerequisite for selecting the most efficacious treatment. In severe illness, incorrect diagnosis may have serious consequences, including death. As medical science has advanced and as greater knowledge of disease has been accumulated, more effective diagnostic and treatment procedures have also been developed. The net result has been improved medical service. Thus, the concept of disease has worked well in medicine. However, when applied to psychiatry and psychopathology, the results have not been quite as successful.

One obvious problem with psychiatric diagnostic systems is the difficulty in deciding what is mental illness and what is not. For example, in the DSM II diagnostic system of the American Psychiatric Association (American Psychiatric Association, 1968), homosexuality was at first included as a mental disorder and then later was excluded. In DSM III, many new diagnostic categories were added, including such new disorders as pathological gambling and developmental reading disorders. In fact, the number of officially diagnosable disorders has increased markedly over the years. For example, DSM-I, published in 1952, listed slightly more than 100 disorders (American Psychiatric Association). DSM-II, published in 1968, contained more than 180 distinct psychiatric disorders, DSM-III in 1980 included more than 260 disorders (Kazdin, 1986), and both DSM-III-R (1987) and DSM IV (1994) have more; DSM-IV leads with 357 disorders. This large increase in the number of specific mental disorders reflects changes in characterizing, delineating, and approaching the formal listing of types of psychopathology and is not an epidemic of new and strange disorders.

At present, it is difficult to know if the increase in the currently available psychiatric diagnoses facilities the process of diagnosis and subsequent treatment or if the diagnostic task has become more complicated and overly cumbersome. The slim diagnostic manuals of DSM I and DSM II have been replaced by the heavier tomes of DSM III, DSM III-R, and DSM IV. DSM-I consisted of 130 small pages, and DSM-II had 134 similar pages. However, the three most recent diagnostic manuals have increased noticeably; DSM-IV is far and away the largest with 886 pages. In a rather humorous publication, Blashfield and Fuller (1996) used regression estimates based on data from past editions of the DSM to make predictions about DSM V. On the basis of their analysis, DSM V will have 390 disorders and the estimated number of pages is 1026. It is still not clear if bigger is better. Guze (1995) in reviewing DSM-IV was both "impressed by and worried about the phenomenal growth in the number of diagnoses now recommended ... (because) few of the hundreds of diagnoses have been satisfactorily validated" (p. 1228).

In any event, it is apparent that there are difficulties in deciding what are diagnosable mental disorders and that such decisions have important social consequences. There is still some stigma associated with being mentally ill, but sometimes there also are more positive effects—for example, individuals may be provided treatment and avoid punishment. In a previous publication, for example, I raised some question about the appropriateness of listing "pathological gambling" as a mental disorder in DSM-III and mentioned that it had been used by a defense counsel on behalf of a defendant in a federal court trial (Garfield, 1986). However, in this case, the jury did not consider this defense acceptable and found the defendant guilty of kidnapping and auto theft. This may have been noted by those involved in preparing DSM-III-R because the following cautionary statement is contained in the introduction to DSM-III-R:

It is to be understood that inclusion here, for clinical and research purposes, of a diagnostic category such as Pathological Gambling or Pedophilia does not imply that the condition meets legal or other nonmedical criteria for what constitutes mental disease, mental disorder, or mental disability. (American Psychiatric Association, 1987, p. *XXIX*).

This statement is also included in the introduction to DSM-IV (p. *XXVII*).

Apart from such issues, there is the fact that the diagnostic categories or disorders included in conventional diagnostic systems are not really comparable. On the one hand, as already mentioned, there are neurological or organic brain disorders that more clearly resemble what is usually termed illness in other fields of medicine. However, at the same time, there are a variety of other designated disorders that are quite different. Schizophrenia, for example, has been considered a major form of mental illness for many years. However, whether it is one disease or many or whether it is caused primarily by genetic, biological, or psychosocial factors, or by all three, is still not known. One critical review even states that schizophrenia is not a valid object of scientific inquiry and casts doubt on the reliability, construct validity, predictive validity, and "aetiological specificity of the schizophrenia diagnosis" (Bentall, Jackson, & Pilgrim, 1988, p. 303). The less severe forms of psychological disturbance are even more difficult to equate with medical conceptions of illness. For example, phobias, compulsions, anxieties, and similar problems are less like illnesses and more like variations from normative behaviors. In such behaviors or disorders, the distinction between discrete disorders or illnesses and behavioral patterns that can be viewed as more extreme variations on a continuum of normal behaviors becomes rather blurred. The DSMs, however, are based on a categorical system rather than on a continuous or dimensional one.

Therefore, there are different bases for the definition and classification of the different diagnostic categories. Some are based on known etiologies, some are organically caused, and some can be diagnosed systematically and reliably. Others are somewhat diffuse diagnoses in which the cause, course, and symptom pattern of the illness is cloaked in ambiguity. This is another way of saying that some may resemble traditional types of disease entities, but that others do not. Although clinical diagnosis has traditionally referred to medical conceptions of disease, the apparent difficulties in applying such conceptions to many of the problems of psychopathology encountered in clinical work has led to dissatisfaction with such diagnostic systems, particularly by psychologists (Adams, 1952; Carson, 1997; Eysenck, 1986; Follette & Houts, 1996; Garfield, 1974, 1986). Some of these difficulties will be discussed later. Other attempts to appraise psychological disorders, however, can be mentioned briefly at this point.

Individuals with psychodynamic or interpersonal orientations have been more concerned with ideographic means of personality appraisal or diagnosis. Traditional psychiatric categories of diagnosis were viewed as too broad and of relatively little help in understanding the individual's problems and in planning a program of treatment. The focus was on appraising the personality dynamics of the individual client with an emphasis on unconscious conflicts and defenses rather than on the diagnostic label that might be attached to the client. However, relatively less emphasis recently on psychoanalytic theory and increased emphasis on biological factors in psychiatry may also have played a role in the recent changes.

Various other schemes have been developed, but they have not received wide clinical usage (Adams & Cassidy, 1993). For example, attempts to apply factor analysis to the results of psychological tests and rating scales have been made to identify more refined and reliable categories of psychopathology. The Inpatient Multidimensional Psychiatric Scale (Lorr, Klett, McNair, & Lasky, 1966) is one illustration of such an approach. Twelve specific syndromes were identified by factor analysis that reflected specific patterns of disturbance such as Excitement, Paranoid Projection, Perceptual Distortion, and Motor Disturbance. Al-

though this scale was used in the past in research on chemotherapy, it has not been used much for regular clinical diagnosis. Nevertheless, such measures allow for dimensional studies of psychopathology that could provide more information than a categorical system like that used in psychiatric diagnosis.

Similarly, related statistical approaches such as cluster analysis have also been used to classify or designate types of psychopathology. However, much of this research has been criticized as mainly descriptive in approach. "Too often, a clustering algorithm has been applied to a convenient data set as an end in itself. Few attempts have been made to determine whether the derived types have prognostic value with respect to treatment outcome or to integrate the types with previous research" (Skinner, 1986). Lorr (1986) also reports in a review that cluster analytic studies do not consistently offer support for the existing psychiatric diagnostic categories.

Reference can also be made to the activities of clinical psychologists in diagnosis. Because of the primacy of psychiatry in diagnosing and treating psychopathology and disordered behavior, clinical psychologists who worked in medical installations, tended to follow the conventional diagnostic nosology. Most clinical staff conferences tended to center around discussions of the "correct" diagnosis. In some settings, the clinical director made the official diagnosis (diagnosis by authority). In other settings, the final diagnosis was reached by majority vote (diagnosis by democratic methods). I have no research data to report on which procedure was more efficacious.

However, with the expansion of the field in the post-World War II era and with the creation of nonmedically dominated clinical centers, dissatisfaction with psychiatric diagnosis on the part of a number of psychologists was apparent. Many psychologists preferred to use the term, assessment, rather than diagnosis, and to focus on the problems, strengths, and deficiencies of the client or patient, rather than on bestowing a diagnostic label. This is a broader concept than the more traditional psychiatric diagnostic concept and is not tied to a disease model. Thus, the terms diagnostic appraisal or assessment tended to be favored over the term, diagnosis. In a survey reported a few years after the publication of DSM-III, only a small number of psychologists reported a preference for using DSM-III over other methods of diagnosis (Smith & Kraft, 1983). However, in recent years, with third party payments usually tied to formal psychiatric diagnoses, there has been much less criticism from practicing clinical psychologists. There has also been a noticeable increase in the forms of psychotherapy developed for specific psychiatric diagnostic groups, and psychologists have played a leading role in this development (Chambles & Hollon, 1998; Garfield, 1998).

Thus, as noted, the term, diagnosis, may be used in somewhat different ways and with somewhat different meanings even though it has been traditionally associated with medicine and conceptions of disease. In the past, psychologists have favored a broader conception of assessment in which both the strengths and weaknesses of the individual evaluated were emphasized and less emphasis was placed on psychiatric diagnosis. However, relative improvements in recent diagnostic manuals and the importance of diagnosis for third-party payers has changed the situation for at least a number of clinical psychologists.

## Reliability and Validity of Clinical Diagnosis

As indicated, clinical diagnosis usually results in a specific categorization or label. After the patient has been appraised, the clinician offers a diagnosis (e.g., schizophrenia, paranoid type). If the diagnosis reflects a specific disease process that is known and understood, there is a reasonable probability that most diagnosticians might agree on the correct diagnosis. However, if the diagnostic category lacks preciseness and covers a moderate variety of behaviors, the reliability of the diagnosis may be impaired. This is of some importance for both practice and research. For example, if a specific treatment is indicated for a given disorder, a misdiagnosis may lead to improper treatment. In research investigations, unreliable diagnoses for the subjects studied may lead to unreliable or invalid results. Thus, the reliability of the diagnosis is of some consequence; most of the research in the past has not secured high agreement among psychiatrists who provided diagnoses on the same group of subjects (Ash, 1949; Beck, Ward, Mendelson, Mock, & Erbaugh, 1962; Blashfield, 1973; Hunt, Wittson, & Hunt, 1953; Kreitman, 1961; Kuriansky, Demingk, & Gurland, 1974; Malamud,

1946; Spitzer & Fleiss, 1974). Although several of these studies have flaws, they do illustrate the problem of the lack of reliability in psychiatric diagnosis. The percentage of agreement between two psychiatrists for specific subtype diagnosis, excluding organic brain syndromes, varied from 6 to 57% in one study (Schmidt & Fonda, 1956). In a study of three psychiatrists who worked in the same hospital with comparable groups of patients, one of the psychiatrists diagnosed two-thirds of his patients as schizophrenic, compared with 22 and 29% by the other two psychiatrists (Pasamanick, Dinitz, & Lefton, 1959). Anyone who has worked for a time in a psychiatric hospital has had the opportunity to observe the diagnostic preferences and biases of other staff members.

Other examples of the possible unreliability of psychiatric diagnosis can be found in differences in proportions or distribution of diagnoses over time and in different countries or geographic locations. Kramer (1965), for example, collected data that showed large variations over time in first admission rates to state mental hospitals in the United States for different diagnoses. The rates of schizophrenic admissions were 17.2, 22.0, and 25.3 per 100,000 for the years 1940, 1950, and 1960, respectively. The 1960 rate of admission for patients diagnosed as schizophrenic exceeded the 1940 rate by 47%. The rates of affective psychosis, on the other hand, showed a steady decline from 11.2 to 9.5 to 7.4 for the same periods, or a decline of 33.9%. Does this represent a real increase in rates of admission for schizophrenia and a real decrease in such rates for affective psychosis, or does this reflect inconsistency in applying diagnostic criteria? Similar questions can be raised concerning other diagnoses for which large differences in rates of admission are observed. "The large increases in the rates for the psychoneuroses, personality disorders, and alcoholic addictions raise questions as to whether they represent true increases in rates of admission for these diagnostic groups or differences in diagnostic fads and criteria or other factors that lead mental hospital psychiatrists to place nonpsychotic diagnoses on increasing numbers of patients" (Kramer, 1965, pp. 104–105).

It is reasonably clear from the kinds of data mentioned before, as well as from studies comparing psychiatric diagnoses obtained in different countries, that unreliability in diagnosis has constituted a problem of some importance. It is certainly a serious problem for research on psychopathology. If there is limited reliability for the diagnostic groups studied, the results secured for any investigation may lack stability, and replication and generalization of results will be difficult. Clinically, lack of reliability may lead to incorrect diagnosis and treatment. As a result of faulty diagnosis, individuals may be socially stigmatized or inappropriately institutionalized. Thus, reliability of diagnosis is not merely an academic issue, even though our concern here with methodological issues may pertain more directly to problems of research in psychopathology.

Although the reliability of clinical diagnosis is important, there is also the matter of the validity of the diagnoses secured. Reliability, although necessary, does not guarantee validity. As emphasized in a critical review, "Even if the reliability of schizophrenia could be assured, therefore, the validity of the concept would require further demonstration" (Bentall, Jackson, & Pilgrim, 1988, p. 306). The importance of the validity of clinical diagnoses in psychiatry, however, has not received very much research attention, perhaps because of the difficulties in securing adequate criteria for evaluative purposes. How does one decide if a diagnosis of anxiety disorder or schizophrenia is valid? In essence, in evaluating disorders without physical components or clearly known etiologies, one must rely on clinical judgments or psychological tests, which in turn have been based largely on clinical judgments. In the absence of some standard or accepted criteria against which to evaluate clinical diagnoses, the process of validation is difficult and thus somewhat neglected. Reliability, by contrast, is much easier to appraise and has received increased attention in the preparation of DSM-IV.

Nevertheless, the problem of validity remains. It may not be viewed as of great importance when there are no treatments of proven worth or preventive strategies for different diagnostic categories. However, where different and effective treatments or methods of prevention are available, the validity of differential diagnosis becomes important. It is, however, always significant for studies of particular types of disorders and may be particularly so for certain types of research.

One kind of research in which the validity of clinical diagnoses is of great importance is that conducted with subjects at high risk for schizophrenia. Although the problem of low reliability

of psychiatric diagnoses can be overcome with competent and specially trained diagnosticians who are provided with accurate and detailed information and with structured interview guidelines, the matter of validity is more complex and difficult. Nevertheless, "For high-risk researchers, the issue of the predictive validity of the diagnoses of schizophrenia is of central importance" (Hanson, Gotterman, & Meehl, 1977, p. 576).

## The Recent DSMs-III, III-R, AND IV

As already noted, there has been considerable activity in recent years in forming new psychiatric diagnostic systems. Three revised diagnostic manuals have been published in just 14 years. Furthermore, these manuals were considerably larger than their predecessors, and the approach and methods for producing them differed in important ways. These new diagnostic manuals manifest a definite sensitivity to the criticisms made of the older systems. The authors have been particularly sensitive to issues of definition and reliability, and the new diagnostic systems have stimulated a considerable amount of research (McReynolds, 1989; Millon & Klerman, 1986; Sutker & Adams, 1993). Some of these studies are reviewed here briefly, mainly to illustrate methodological issues.

In many respects, DSM-III was a radical departure from its predecessors. Its authors attempted to avoid any theoretical partisanship or controversies, and they also attempted to emphasize operational criteria and descriptive psychopathology. "These criteria are based, for the most part, on manifest descriptive psychopathology, rather than inferences or criteria from presumed causation or etiology, whether this causation be psychodynamic, social, or biological. The exception to this is the category of organic disorders whose etiology is established as caused by central nervous system pathology" (Klerman, 1986, p. 5). However, this distinction for organic disorders was omitted in DSM-IV. "The term 'organic mental disorders' has been eliminated from DSM-IV because it implies that the other disorders in the manual do not have an 'organic' component" (American Psychiatric Association, 1994, p. 776). This change appears to reflect political-guild issues more than diagnostic ones (Follette & Houts, 1996), and I will say no more about it here.

Although some have criticized the deliberate

avoidance of a theoretical approach to diagnosis (Follette & Houts, 1996; Skinner, 1986), the authors of DSM-III, as well as DSM-III-R and IV, emphasized the need for accurate description and reliability of diagnosis and even carried out reliability studies, particularly for DSM-IV. Let us now turn to some studies of reliability and related issues.

In one study, twenty psychiatrists made independent diagnoses on twenty-four actual case histories of childhood psychiatric disorders (Cantwell, Russell, Mattison, & Will, 1979). The average agreement of these clinicians with the authors' consensus on the expected DSM-III diagnosis was just less than 50%. In another report on this study, the average agreement between the psychiatrists on their most common diagnosis (they were allowed more than one) was 57% for DSM-II and 54% for DSM-III (Mattison, Cantwell, Russell, & Will, 1979). Interrater agreement for DSM-III reached 80% for only four of the twenty-four cases; the best results were obtained for diagnoses of mental retardation. Noteworthy disagreement was noted in both systems for anxiety disorders, complex cases, and in the subtypes of depression.

The lack of agreement among the different diagnostic systems and the fact that they tend to select different samples of subjects for the same diagnostic category has also been noted by others (Endicott, Nee, Fleiss, Cohen, Williams, & Simon, 1982; Fenton, Mosher, & Matthews, 1981). In the study by Endicott et al. (1982) of diagnostic criteria for schizophrenia, six well-known systems were used to evaluate newly admitted patients including the Research Diagnostic Criteria (RDC) (Spitzer, Endicott, & Robins, 1975), the Feighner Criteria (Feighner, Robins, Guze, Woodruff, Winokur, & Munoz, 1972), and DSM-III. "The most salient finding of the study is that the systems vary greatly in the rates at which they make the diagnosis of schizophrenia" (Endicott et al., 1982, p. 888). The percentage of cases diagnosed as cases with schizophrenia ranged from 3.6 to 26%, a sevenfold difference, although most systems showed acceptable rater reliability. "The disparity illustrates the degree of difficulty associated with the diagnosis of schizophrenia and in the concept of schizophrenia ..." (Endicott et al., p. 888).

A somewhat similar study of forty-six cases of schizophrenia was reported by Klein (1982) who compared seven diagnostic systems including most of those evaluated by Endicott et al. (1982).

These patients had to have a hospital diagnosis of schizophrenia based on DSM-II, a score of four or more on the New Haven Schizophrenic Index (Astrachan et al., 1972), and be under age 56 with no evidence of organic brain damage, toxic psychosis, drug abuse, and the like. The DSM-III correlated .89 with the Feighner Criteria and .84 with the RDC, diagnostic systems which were models for it. However, its correlations with the remaining four scales were considerably lower. Use of the DSM-III led to diagnosis of 28% of the sample as cases of schizophrenia; the range was 24 to 63% for the other diagnostic systems. Furthermore, only nine of the forty-four patients were diagnosed by all seven systems as either cases of schizophrenia (N = 3) or as not such cases (N = 6).

Somewhat comparable findings were reported in a more recent study (Hill et al., 1996). "The aim of this study was to determine the extent to which diagnoses of schizophrenia from forensic sources can be seen to meet formal diagnostic criteria through use of both a structured undiagnostic approach and a multidiagnostic chart review based on case histories" (p. 534). Each of the eighty-three subjects had a recorded diagnosis of schizophrenia at coronal autopsy. Thirty one percent did not meet the criteria for any of the five diagnostic systems, 68.7% met criteria for at least one system, and 20.5% met the criteria for all five diagnostic systems. Agreement ranged from 42.2% for the Feighner criteria to 63.9% for DSM-III-R.

Although it seems reasonably clear that DSM-III, DSM-III-R, and DSM-IV are more precise in their delineation of many mental disorders than was true of DSM-II and that the reliability of diagnosis has been enhanced in many instances, some important problems remain. The lack of comparability of diagnostic systems has already been noted, and this clearly presents problems for both research and practice. If everyone adhered to one diagnostic system exclusively, then perhaps this problem would be less serious. However, when new official systems are introduced within a period as brief as seven years, the comparability and meaningfulness of clinical diagnosis becomes more problematic. DSM-IV, for example, was being prepared while research studies on DSM-III-R were still underway. Thus, although the DSM-IV Task Force profited from the research and data sets resulting from DSM-III, it could have learned more by awaiting additional research based on DSM-III-R.

In the introductory section of the DSM-III-R manual, it is stated that the American Psychiatric Association decided in 1983 to work on a revision of DSM-III for several reasons. Data from new studies were inconsistent with some of the diagnostic criteria. "In addition, despite extensive field testing of the DSM-III diagnostic criteria before their official adoption, experience with them since their publication had revealed, as expected, many instances in which the criteria were not entirely clear, were inconsistent across categories, or were even contradictory" (American Psychiatric Association, 1987, p. *XVII*). Therefore, a thorough review was instituted, and the required modifications were made. Although the revised DSM-III essentially follows the same overall scheme and rationale as the original, some modifications were made and comparisons of the two diagnostic systems have been reported. Some examples of the problems encountered follow.

One study attempted to evaluate the reliability, sensitivity, and specificity of DSM-III and DSM-III-R criteria for the category of autism in relation to each other and to the clinical diagnoses made (Volkmar, Bregman, Cohen, & Cicchetti, 1988). The subjects were fifty-two individuals diagnosed as autistic and sixty-two considered developmentally disordered but not autistic. The reliability of the specific criteria tended to be high. The DSM-III criteria were judged more specific but less sensitive than the DSM-III-R criteria. As a result, the investigators concluded that the diagnostic concept of autism has been greatly broadened in the revised system.

In the light of the preceding paragraph, it is of interest to list the changes made for autistic disorder in DSM-IV:

*Autistic Disorder.* The DSM-III-R defining features (impaired social interaction, communication, and stereotyped patterns of behavior) are retained in DSM-IV, but the individual items and the overall diagnostic algorithm have been modified to (1) improve clinical utility by reducing the number of items from 16 to 12 and by increasing the clarity of individual items; (2) increase compatibility with the ICD-10 Diagnostic Criteria for Research; and (3) narrow the definition of caseness so that it conforms more closely with clinical judgment, DSM-III, and ICD-10. In addition an "age of onset" requirement (before age 3 years in DSM-IV), which had been dropped in DSM-III-R, has been reinstated to conform to clinical usage and to increase the homogeneity of this category. (American Psychiatric Association, 1994, p. 774)

Another problem in clinical diagnosis is illustrated in a study of the differential diagnosis of attention deficit disorder (ADD) and conduct disorder using conditional probabilities (Milich, Widiger, & Landau, 1987). Although these two disorders are considered separate disorders, there has been a substantial overlap in symptoms. Using a standardized interview designed to represent the diagnostic criteria contained in DSM-III, seventy-six boys referred to a psychiatric outpatient clinic were evaluated and the conditional probabilities and base rates of the symptoms for both disorders were ascertained. The results indicated that the symptom with the highest covariation with the specific disorder was not always the most useful in diagnosis. Furthermore, some symptoms are most useful as inclusion criteria, whereas some are most useful as exclusion criteria. The authors also point out that the interview used was based on DSM-III and that the application of different diagnostic criteria could change the pattern of results obtained. This, of course, is always a problem when diagnostic criteria are revised and new systems instituted. A final important point made by these investigators is that the symptom criteria offered for ADD in DSM-III-R are weighted equally "whereas the results of the present study suggest that some symptoms are more effective inclusion criteria than others. In addition, the DSM-III-R offers only inclusion criteria and makes no attempt to use symptoms as exclusion criteria" (Milich, Widiger, & Landau, 1987, p. 766).

Because of space limitations, only a few other studies can be mentioned. The introduction of many new diagnoses obviously created many new potential problems, among them, estimating the incidence of specific disorders. For example, "In the years since 1980, bulimia has gone from being virtually unknown to being described by some medical investigators as a 'major public health problem' (Pope, Hudson, & Yurgelun-Todd, 1984) and being designated by one prominent nonmedical leader of contemporary female opinion as a disorder of 'epidemic proportions'" (Ben-Tovin, 1988, p. 1000). This author also states that "The use of DSM-III-R seems likely to lead to a dramatic decline in the diagnosis and prevalence of bulimia" (Ben-Tovin, 1988, p. 1002).

Somewhat comparable comparisons have been reported by others. In one study of the definitions of schizophrenia for 532 inpatients treated and reevaluated 15 years later, the use of DSM-III-R reduced the number of patients diagnosed with schizophrenia by 10%. However, the DSM-III diagnosed patients included and excluded by DSM-III-R did not differ in terms of demographic, premorbid, or long-term outcome characteristics. The authors of this report emphasized that in the absence of improved validity, frequent changes in diagnostic systems were likely to impede research progress (Fenton, McGlashan, & Heinssen, 1988). Zimmerman (1988) also expressed his doubts that new changes in such a short time would actually improve the practice of psychiatry.

A number of clinical researchers have published various critiques of some of the diagnostic categories listed in the new classification systems. Aronson (1987) stated that the definition of panic attack in DSM-III lacks precision and that the overlap with other disorders raises questions about what is a distinct psychiatric disorder. Leavitt and Tsuang (1988) reviewed the literature on schizoaffective disorder and concluded that "Until there is greater agreement on the criteria for and the meaning of schizoaffective disorder, reports on treatment results will not be generalizable" (p. 935). In DSM-IV, the criteria set for schizoaffective disorder "has been changed to focus on an uninterrupted episode of illness rather than on the lifetime pattern of symptoms" (American Psychiatric Association, 1994, p. 779).

Obviously, there are significant differences in validity and reliability of diagnosis among diagnostic categories. In recent years, some of the personality diagnoses such as narcissistic personality disorder or borderline personality disorder have been popularized by several psychoanalytically oriented clinicians and, in part due to this, have been included as distinct disorders in the official nomenclature. Although a *definite* diagnosis of a *borderline* condition has always seemed rather illogical to me, apparently it is no problem to many people. However, as some have noted, the category of borderline personality disorder has been used to include a variety of pathological behaviors. "Exhibiting almost all of the clinical attributes known to descriptive psychopathology, borderline conditions lend themselves to a simplistic, if not perverse, form of diagnostic logic, that is, patients who display a potpourri of clinical indices, especially where symptomatic relationships are unclear or seem inconsistent, must perforce be borderlines" (Millon, 1988).

The use of a multiaxial system has also led to an increase in what has been termed "comorbidity," having two or more concurrent diagnoses. Axis I

in DSM-IV, Clinical Disorders, contains most of the more traditional psychiatric diagnoses, whereas Axis II includes only Personality Disorders and Mental Retardation. In DSM-III, it was originally stated that "This separation ensures that consideration is given to the possible presence of disorders that are frequently overlooked when attention is directed to the usually more florid Axis I disorder" (American Psychiatric Association, 1980, p. 23). However, it appears that personality disorders are diagnosed quite frequently as either a primary diagnosis or as a secondary diagnosis. In a recent critical appraisal of the use of the terms of *comorbidity* or *comorbid* in psychopathology research, Lilienfeld, Waldman, & Israel (1994) indicated the growth in their use. After appearing only twice in 1986, "the number of journal abstracts or titles containing these terms increased to 21 in 1987, 43 in 1988, 97 in 1989, 147 in 1990, 192 in 1991, 191 in 1992, and 243 in 1993" (Lilienfeld et al., 1994, p. 71). This trend raises some question concerning the use of traditional views of medical diagnosis in psychopathology and "implicitly assumes a categorical model of diagnosis that may be inappropriate for personality disorders ..." (Lilienfeld et al., 1994, p. 79).

In a study of more than 200 adults at risk of AIDS, multiple diagnoses of personality disorder were recorded for most individuals with any DSM-III-R Axis II diagnosis. Almost half of the subjects with a diagnosis in one personality cluster also had a concurrent diagnosis in another cluster (Jacobsberg, Francis, & Perry, 1995). A study of the comorbidity of alcoholism and personality disorders in a clinical population of 366 patients also obtained comparable findings. There was extensive overlap between Axis I disorders and personality disorders, as well as among personality disorders themselves (Morgenstern, Langenbucher, Lubouvie, & Miller, 1997). In another study of 118 gay men conducted to investigate the stability of personality disorder, it was reported that diagnoses of personality disorders had low stability over a 2-year period (Johnson et al., 1997). A study of seventy-eight adult outpatients with attention deficit hyperactive disorder evaluated by standard tests showed high comorbidity with current depressive disorder, antisocial personality disorder, and alcohol and drug abuse dependence (Downey, Stanton, Pomerleau, & Giordani, 1997). In a sample of 716 opioid abusers, psychiatric comorbidity was documented in 47% of the sample based on a

DSM-III-R diagnostic assessment. Such comorbidity was especially noted for personality and mood disorders for both sexes (Brooner, King, Kidorf, Schmidt, & Bigelow, 1997). There have been additional studies published on this issue, but there is no need to review them here. As Robins (1994) commented, "When standardized interviews demonstrate that a single patient qualifies for an unreasonable number of diagnoses, that should motivate the field to rethink this proliferation of categories" (p. 94).

Thus, the categorical delineation of psychiatric disorders presents problems for meaningful diagnosis. Dumont (1984), for example, feels strongly that psychiatry errs in attempting to divide all abnormal behavior into discrete illness categories. He believes that labels such as "hyperactivity" and "learning disorders" for children "are a capricious and arbitrary drawing of lines through a spectrum of behavioral, intellectual, emotional, and social disabilities" (Dumont, 1984, p. 326). Marmor (1983) in discussing systems thinking in psychiatry also emphasizes "that the growing tendency to think in terms of distinct and sharply demarcated phenomenological entities, as exemplified in DSM-III, deserves some skeptical evaluation despite its usefulness pragmatically" (p. 834). Although categorization may be simpler to handle than a dimensional approach, a combination of the two suggested by Lorr (1986) and by McReynolds (1989) may be more meaningful in the long run and provide more information as well as potentially greater predictive power. Others also suggest that the use of both psychometric and fixed diagnostic criteria could lead to a better and more valid definition of schizophrenia (Moldin, Gottesman, & Erlenmeyer-Kimling, 1987). However, despite such criticisms, as well as others (Carson, 1996, 1997; Follette & Houts, 1996; Millon, 1991; Sarbin, 1997), the neo-Kraepelinian model has continued to be used.

## Research Issues and Problems

As already mentioned, problems pertaining to the reliability and validity of diagnosis are of definite importance for research in psychopathology. Research results based on inadequately diagnosed patients are of dubious value. However, there are other considerations that are equally important. One frequent and serious problem pertains to the specific sample of subjects or patients used in particular research investigations. Investigators generally can never study all individuals who supposedly manifest a particular form or type of psychopathology. Rather, they must usually settle for a much smaller number of cases that purportedly represent or typify the disorder under investigation. A variety of sampling problems may be encountered in this process, and it is worth examining some of these problems.

### Sampling Problems

As indicated, investigators usually can study only small samples of the population they are interested in evaluating. An immediate critical issue is how well the sample selected for study actually represents the population or group it supposedly represents. How typical, for example, is a sample of thirty or fifty patients diagnosed as cases of schizophrenia in a state hospital in New Jersey, of *all* "schizophrenics" or of those in other types of settings? How far can one generalize from the findings obtained with this specific sample? Ostensibly, at least, findings obtained from a particular sample representative of a given category of disorder presumably have relevance for other comparable samples. The problem, therefore, is how does one define both the sample studied and the other samples of the population or diagnostic group to which the results are supposedly applicable?

Unfortunately, there are no true standard reference measures which can be used to define a particular clinical group of subjects, and the terms used for clinical diagnosis leave much to be desired. Consequently, it is exceedingly important to select the sample with great care and to provide as much useful descriptive information as possible concerning the sample. However, some published studies fail to provide adequate descriptive data for their samples. Such items as age, length of hospitalization, frequency of hospitalization, marital status, work history, previous treatments, family resources, education, intelligence, type of psychiatric ward or institutional setting, maintenance on medications, and the like, are all potentially important variables which may influence test performance, treatment outcome, duration of improvement, and similar variables. It should be apparent that significant variation on some or many of these variables between studies limits the reliability of the results secured and the drawing of conclusions that may have broad applicability.

The problems mentioned are particularly apparent when samples of modest size are drawn from institutional settings that vary widely in a number of dimensions. Patients in university or private hospitals generally are quite different from those in state or VA psychiatric hospitals, and generalizations from one setting do not necessarily fit other settings, even though the patients may all carry an official diagnosis of schizophrenia. For example, in a previous study of prognostic scales used in research on schizophrenic patients, we were unable to obtain an adequate number of "reactive" or good prognosis patients in the state hospital where we were conducting our study and had to secure patients from a city hospital that had fewer chronic patients (Garfield & Sundland, 1966).

Although sample size is of some importance because small-scale studies are more prone to produce findings limited in reliability, size, alone, is not a sufficient criterion. The selection of subjects and sample specifications are clearly of prime importance. If one is studying or comparing selected types of disordered behavior, the criteria used in selecting subjects should be explicit, and the procedures used should be those for which the reliability and validity are known or available and which meet commonly accepted standards. Particularly where studies are conducted of groups based largely on psychiatric diagnosis, it is essential to state clearly how the diagnoses were derived and that other supporting selection criteria be used. One large recent study examined the extent to which diagnostic instruments for assessing axis II personality disorders diverge from clinical diagnostic procedures. "Whereas current instruments rely primarily on direct questions derived from DSM-IV, clinicians of every theoretical persuasion found direct questions useful for assessing axis I disorders but only marginally so for axis II" (Westen, 1997, p. 895). Axis II diagnoses were made by "listening to patients describe interpersonal interactions and observing their behavior with the interviewer. In contrast to findings with current research instruments, most patients with personality disorders in clinical practice receive only one axis II diagnosis" (Westen, 1997, p. 895).

Diagnoses based on old records and provided by different psychiatrists also do not constitute a sound or reliable basis for subject selection. Diagnostic criteria and nomenclature change over the years, and it is a difficult task to compare and equate diagnoses based on different diagnostic schemes, as several studies have indicated (Fenton, Mosher, & Matthews, 1981; Goldstein & Anthony, 1988; Hill et al., 1996; Klein, 1982; Rutherford, Alterman, Cassiola, & Snider, 1995).

Another problem is the randomization of subject selection. For example, were the subjects selected at random from a previously selected pool of available subjects or were they selected because they were not on drugs, happened to be available to the investigator, were in a special ward, were judged to be cooperative, or in some other manner were really not "typical subjects?" Some studies use moderately complex tasks that necessitate some screening or selection of subjects to comply with the demands of the investigation. Such research compliance leads to a rather selected sample of subjects. The Vigotsky Test of conceptual thinking was at times used as a diagnostic test for schizophrenia, although even non-college-educated normal subjects could not perform satisfactorily on it (Garfield, 1974). Clearly, such selectivity can bias the results and limit the extent to which generalized statements can be made.

Selection of subjects on the basis of a single scale may also not be adequate, particularly if they are then considered to represent a particular diagnostic group. For example, not all subjects who score at 70 or higher on a scale of the MMPI may resemble groups diagnosed on other criteria as schizophrenic, depressed, etc. College students who obtain such scores may or may not be clinically depressed, psychotic, etc., and therefore comparisons with actual clinical populations may not be warranted.

It is clearly desirable to use more than one procedure or method for establishing the diagnosis of the subjects to be used in any research study in which the diagnosis is considered a significant variable. Psychiatric or clinical diagnosis should be supplemented by other criteria such as scores on appropriate tests or standardized rating scales. In depression, for example, scores on the MMPI, the Hamilton Rating Scale (1960), and the Beck Depression Inventory (1972) could be, and should be, used in addition to clinical diagnosis. Other instruments that were developed to aid in obtaining more reliable diagnoses are the Schedule for Affective Disorders and Schizophrenia (SADS) (Endicott & Spitzer, 1978) and the Research Diagnostic Criteria (Spitzer, Endicott, & Robins, 1975).

The former is a structured interview guide with rating scales relevant to the specific diagnostic categories, whereas the latter provides criteria whereby investigators can select relatively homogeneous groups of subjects who meet specified criteria of diagnosis. Although the Research Diagnostic Criteria were used to obtain more precise diagnostic designations, as noted earlier, such diagnostic criteria tended to be quite selective and to leave a significant number of patients undiagnosed. In the NIMH Treatment of Depression Collaborative Research Program, uniform inclusion criteria, including a diagnosis of Major Depressive Disorder based on the Research Diagnostic Criteria and a score of 14 or greater on a modified seventeen-item Hamilton Rating Scale for Depression were used "and uniform exclusion criteria were used across sites" (Elkin, 1994, p. 116). Data were also obtained on a number of patient clinical, demographic, and personality variables that might be related to eventual outcome.

With the advent of DSM-III-R, a new structured interview for use with the new diagnostic system was developed with somewhat separate forms for diagnosing psychiatric inpatients, outpatients, and nonpatients (Spitzer, Williams, & Gibbon, 1987). Although highly structured like most interview schedules of this type, a number of open-ended questions are used. Other more specialized interview schedules have also been developed (McReynolds, 1989).

Various experimental or laboratory tests of thought disorder and communication have also been used in studies of patients with schizophrenia. However, none of these have attained any general recognition as diagnostic measures. On the other hand, investigators do believe that the use of psychometric data along with fixed diagnostic criteria can lead to a more valid definition of schizophrenia (Moldin, Gottesman, & Erlenmeyer-Kimling, 1987).

In addition, clinical diagnoses for research purposes should be based on diagnoses from two or more clinicians with a reasonably high indication of reliability between them. In a study on the use of many raters to increase the validity of judges, groups of one to ten judges rated a patient's mood from speech samples taken at various times during psychotherapy (Horowitz, Inouye, & Siegelman, 1979). These ratings were averaged and then correlated with an objective measure of anxiety. The correlations increased noticeably, up to a theoretical asymptote, as the number of judges increased. Thus, using five or six judges will tend to increase both the reliability and validity of ratings.

If such procedures are followed, there is greater assurance of the reliability of diagnosis, and there are several external or operational reference points in defining the samples used. To be sure, extra effort is required to carry out such procedures and, to a certain extent, such procedures might reduce the size of potential samples and raise new issues of selectivity and limited generalizability. However, the samples would be more clearly defined, and the dangers of relying exclusively on somewhat haphazard means of classification would be lessened. In the long run, the conflicting results obtained with the use of diffuse, unclear, and unreliable diagnostic categorization might lessen.

Another issue involves the possible selectivity of a patient sample to match it with an available control group. For example, if the control group has an average IQ of 98, an average educational attainment of tenth grade, or is composed primarily of ward attendants, a subject sample selected to match them on one or more of these variables may be a highly selective and unrepresentative sample of the patient group they are supposed to represent. They are not patients typical of a particular diagnostic group, and broad generalizations to other more randomly selected groups would not be justified. For example, in my previous study of hospitalized patients diagnosed as schizophrenic, very different patterns of performance on the Wechsler–Bellevue Scale were obtained for patients who differed in education and IQ (Garfield, 1949). The most striking difference was noted on the arithmetic subtest for individuals who differed in educational levels. Schizophrenics from the lowest educational group performed at their lowest level on this subtest, whereas the group with some college education obtained its highest score on this subtest. Furthermore, comparisons of samples of schizophrenic patients studied in different investigations, who differed noticeably in mean IQ, also revealed significant differences on test patterns among these samples (Garfield, 1949). In other words, there were as many significant differences among the various samples of patients as there were between a given sample and a normal group of control subjects.

The selection and specification of subjects used in research on clinical diagnosis is thus a matter of primary importance, and would-be investigators, as well as those who read the research reports, should give careful attention to the issues discussed in the preceding paragraphs. In the final analysis, the results can be no better than the type and representativeness of the subjects used.

## Proper Control Groups

Another problem frequently encountered in research reports involves the appropriateness of the control groups used. Although we are more sophisticated about such matters now than in the past, problems of appropriate controls are still evident. Obviously, a group of patients that has been hospitalized for some time should not usually be compared with a group of apparently normal college students, but comparisons like this have been made.

The problem becomes especially significant when a particular investigation focuses on differential clinical diagnosis or on the specification and appraisal of patterns of test performance or other diagnostic indicators for a specific category of patients. If the results of the study are to have any clinical significance in the practical sense, then the experimental group must be compared to other clinical groups with which they would normally be compared in the actual clinical situation. For example, comparisons of test performance or other measures of a sample of patients with a diagnosis of schizophrenia should be made with other clinical groups normally seen in that type of clinical situation and in approximately the usual proportions. In any clinical or hospital setting where a clinical diagnosis is sought, the problem is rarely one of comparing the given patient to a normal population. Rather, the issue is one of differential diagnosis and appraisal in which a number of specific diagnostic questions, such as the following may be raised: Is there any suggestion of psychotic disturbance or of possible brain damage? How serious is the thought disturbance or depression manifested by the patient? In trying to reach answers to such questions, clinicians must consider and compare the patterns of various types of psychopathology. They do not simply compare or contrast the patient's performance to the performance of nonpathological or normally adjusted individuals.

Thus, in studying a diagnostic pattern for possible use in clinical diagnosis, the investigator should compare the results of the particular clinical group of interest with those of other diagnostic groups that are usually encountered in practice and from whom the aforementioned group is to be compared or differentiated. For clinical diagnosis, it is efficacious to have a control group made up of the proper mix of the other diagnostic groups that are normally encountered in the particular setting or of several groups representing the types of disorders that are most frequently confused with the group under study.

As emphasized earlier, the investigator should provide adequate information on all groups of subjects, indicating how they were selected and from what subpopulation they were drawn. For example, if a control group of thirty patients was selected for comparison with the group under study, why and how were these particular subjects selected, and from what number of comparable subjects were they drawn? If they were the only ones who had certain data or test scores available, what were the reasons for this particular state of affairs? How selective is the group, and how representative is it of supposedly similar subjects? Selective bias may greatly impair the kinds of conclusions that may be drawn and the extent to which the findings may be generalized.

It should be stressed that whatever control groups are used, they should be comparable in the variables of importance for a particular investigation. Where cognitive tests are used, the groups should show some comparability in level of ability, education, and age, because these may affect performance. Obviously, however, if one's particular focus is the diagnosis of mental retardation, such comparability may not be necessary or meaningful. Length of institutionalization, medications, type of ward, degree of cooperation, and other such attributes may also be important variables.

In essence, therefore, considerable attention should be given to selecting adequate and appropriate control groups in research on clinical diagnosis. Although this is particularly relevant to differential diagnosis and related problems, the issue of appropriate control groups also applies to experimental or theoretical studies of psychopathology. Numerous studies of various psychological functions in schizophrenic subjects have compared the latter quite frequently with normal controls. This may have value at a certain stage of investigation, but it has limited value if one is interested in ascertaining or demonstrating particular patterns of response or thought in patients with this specific clinical disorder. The investigator is actually trying to discover or demonstrate response patterns that characterize a particular pathological group. Whether the patterns obtained are distinctive of the particular type of pathology in question can be demonstrated only if the performance of the pathological group is compared with other pathological groups of comparable severity. In this particular instance, other psychotic groups would be the most adequate control group.

Although many of the points stressed in this section may appear obvious, they have been overlooked and continue to be disregarded by investigators in psychopathology. For example, a recent study of borderline personality disorder, with several positive features, also exhibited some of the deficiencies previously discussed (Nurnberg, Hurt, Feldman, & Suh, 1988). Patients for this study were selected from consecutive admissions to a twenty-three bed adult inpatient unit of a university teaching hospital. The criteria used specified an age range of 16 to 45, "no evidence or history of organic mental disorder, neurologic disorder, substantial concurrent medical illness, mental retardation, or alcohol or drug addiction as a primary diagnosis; no DSM-III-R diagnosis of schizophrenia, major affective disorder, paranoid disorder, or schizoaffective disorder; and an independent clinical diagnosis of borderline personality disorder by the treatment team" (p. 1280). All patients also were rated independently before discharge by the senior investigator to confirm the diagnosis of borderline personality disorder according to DSM-III, an appropriate score on the Diagnostic Interview for Borderline Patients (Gunderson, Kolb, & Austin, 1981), and the absence of exclusion criteria. In this way seventeen patients (ten women and seven men) ages 17 to 35 years were selected.

Let us now evaluate what has been presented thus far about this study. A number of inclusive and exclusionary criteria have been specified to obtain what might be viewed as clear or "pure" cases of borderline personality disorder. The procedures and age and sex of the subjects have been clearly indicated so that an attempt at replication is possible. However, no data are provided on how many patients were evaluated, how many were rejected for not meeting study criteria, and the educational or socioeconomic status of the sample selected. In other words, is this group highly selective, for example, 17 out 1,000, or is such a group

easily obtained from newly admitted inpatients? There is also no information on the reliability of the diagnosis.

So much for the experimental group. The control group with which it was compared consisted of twenty subjects (twelve women and eight men) selected from the hospital staff. These individuals were subjected to the same exclusion criteria that were used for the patients. In addition, they had to have no previous or present psychiatric treatment and be free from emotional disturbance or an acute major life event change within the past year. They ranged in age from 18 to 40 years. Again there is no information on the size of the group from which this control sample was selected or on educational and social class indexes.

The two groups were compared on the basis of a seventeen-item criteria instrument. By using the five best items, it was found that the presence of any two was a good predictor of borderline personality disorder in the patient group but produced a false negative rate of 30% in the controls. However, the use of four out of the best five predictors reduced diagnostic errors significantly.

As already pointed out, the use of a normal group or in this case, a rather selective normal control group, greatly increases the possibility of obtaining significant differences. Comparisons need to be made with other comparable diagnostic groups and attempts at cross-validation would be required if the criteria are to have diagnostic utility in the clinical situation. This is particularly true because many patients have more than one diagnosis (Wolf, Schubert, Patterson, Grande, et al., 1988) and as pointed out earlier, the rate of comorbidity is especially high for personality disorders.

## Clinical Versus Statistical Significance

In a number of articles, significant correlations or differences at the .05 level of significance are reported with little concern shown over the number of significance tests performed. Although it should be apparent that the interpretation of the significant findings obtained is directly related to the number of statistical tests performed, this stricture is not always observed. If thirty-five comparisons or correlations are performed and two are at the .05 level of significance, it seems clear that the results obtained are so close to a chance occurrence that little should be made of them.

Similarly, post hoc analyses are sometimes

treated as if explicit hypotheses were being tested. Obviously, considerations enter into such analyses that differ when a specific hypothesis, stated in advance of the investigation, is being tested. Although these matters are rather basic in experimental design and statistical analysis, the lessons on these topics are either not learned well or are quickly forgotten. When the investigators emphasize significant findings that they have not predicted in advance and that are noted after the investigation has been completed, they essentially are capitalizing on chance occurrences. For the results to be taken seriously, they should be replicated on a new sample of subjects.

A related issue involves the practical or clinical significance of findings that are significant statistically at the .05 or even at the .001 level of significance. It appears from numerous reports that researchers have been led to worship at the shrine of statistical significance. Very likely, this may result from the emphasis individuals place on obtaining "positive" results and the fear of not being able to reject the null hypothesis. Many investigators appear content, and some even euphoric, at obtaining "positive results" at the .05 level of significance, regardless of whether the results appear to have potential diagnostic use. Of all the limitations the present writer has encountered in reviewing journal manuscripts, the emphasis on statistical significance and the disregard of practical psychological significance is probably the most frequent.

Clearly, researchers must examine their data to see if the results obtained are due to chance. A statistical test of the differences obtained between selected clinical groups or of the correlations obtained on certain measures and designated criteria for specific diagnostic categories is a necessary procedure for estimating the influence of chance on the results. No criticism of this procedure is intended here. However, one should recognize that for clinical research this represents only the first of the necessary procedures for appraising the results obtained. Such a statistical test informs us of the probability that our results may be explained by chance occurrences. If our results are significant at the .05 level, the interpretation should be that there are only five chances in a hundred that the results obtained may be attributed to chance. The findings, of course, could be due to chance, but the odds are against it. However, all one can reasonably conclude from such findings is that they do not appear to be due to chance, and that if the study

were repeated, we might expect comparable findings. This, of course, does not guarantee that the new findings will be comparable to those in the original study, for conflicting findings are by no means uncommon in studies of psychopathology. However, whether the results obtained have any potential clinical usefulness cannot be determined by these statistical tests alone. Other appraisals must be made.

Some factors that influence statistical results also need to be considered. Statistical tests are very much influenced by the size of the samples used and by their variability. Large samples are generally less influenced by selective and chance variables than very small samples. Thus, findings that are small may be statistically significant in the former instance, whereas they would fail to attain significance with smaller samples. For example, with samples of around thirty subjects, correlations have to be in the neighborhood of .35 or so to reach significance. In contrast to this, with a sample of several hundred subjects, a much lower correlation, in the neighborhood of .10, may be statistically significant, although the amount of predicted variance in the scores has no practical significance. For example, in a study that I conducted of 855 clinical psychologists, a correlation of .086 was obtained between career satisfaction and satisfaction with the American Psychological Association (Garfield & Kurtz, 1976). This correlation was significant at the .01 level. However, such a correlation is clearly a "low correlation" and has little or no practical significance.

Thus, besides the level of significance, we must also consider the size of the sample and the actual amount of variance accounted for by the correlation coefficient if we are to interpret the findings in terms of their utility. Moderately high correlations that are not statistically significant have little value and are unreliable.

Similarly, low variability within groups of subjects generally increases the probability of securing statistically significant differences. However, though small standard deviations increase the possibility of useful discrimination between different clinical groups, the actual utility of the measures or comparisons used requires further analysis of the actual data obtained.

Although there have been some discussions of the difference between clinical and statistical significance in the published literature, the importance of this topic has received attention only recently (Jacobson & Revenstorf, 1988; Jacobson & Truax, 1991; Kazdin, 1994; Lambert & Hill, 1994). Many investigators appear content to rest on their statistical laurels and manifest little concern about the practical value of their results. However, there are several aspects of the research data which should be examined for their potential clinical significance. For example, regardless of the mathematical procedures used to test hypotheses within a statistical model, it is also important to know how much of the variance is accounted for by the particular variables studied. For practical as well as theoretical purposes this is an important consideration, but it is frequently omitted in the discussion of results. In the case of correlational data, simply squaring the coefficient of correlation provides an estimate of the amount of variance accounted for by the particular set of correlates. With other methods of analysis, the implications may not be as readily apparent, but it is equally important to provide an estimate of the variance accounted for by the experimental manipulation.

The importance of such analyses can be illustrated briefly here. In the report of the activities and preferences of a sample of 855 clinical psychologists (Garfield & Kurtz, 1976), numerous findings at the .01 level of significance or better were obtained. Some may have been the result of the numerous comparisons made, but the sample size was very likely of some importance. Consequently, correlations of .10 which were highly significant statistically were judged of little practical importance because they accounted for only 1% of the variance. In another study of more than 1000 clients in a number of community mental health centers, several correlations of around .10 were reported as highly significant, even though they were obviously of little significance clinically or socially (Sue, McKinney, Allen, & Hall, 1974). For example, the correlation between diagnosis and premature termination was .10, and this was significant at the .001 level of confidence. However, by itself, such a significant finding accounts for a negligible amount of the variance. Particularly where large samples are used, authors should feel obligated to stress the implications of their findings in terms of the variance accounted for by the variables under study.

In addition to estimating the amount of variance accounted for by the variables studied, other analyses can also be performed. The means and standard deviations for the clinical samples studied are of potential value to other clinicians and investigators. Consequently, they should be reported, and the extent of overlap of the distributions also should be stated clearly. Also of value for clinical diagnosis are the numbers of subjects who would be correctly diagnosed by the diagnostic procedures evaluated and those who would be misdiagnosed—that is, data on false positives and false negatives. Such data are clearly important in evaluating any diagnostic procedures, but they are not always obtained or provided. It should be apparent that a particular diagnostic technique may differentiate two or more clinical groups at the .05 level of significance but yet produce so many false positives or negatives that it has very limited clinical utility. For such reasons, it is important that investigators analyze their data in terms of clinically relevant diagnostic considerations and present their analyses clearly.

## Base Rates

Another related problem in research on clinical diagnosis concerns the old issue of base rates. Although this important matter was raised some years ago and is not an unfamiliar topic in either the areas of diagnostic assessment or psychotherapy (Gathercole, 1968; Meehl & Rosen, 1955; McNair, Lorr, & Callahan, 1963; Milich, Widiger, & Landau, 1987), a number of studies seemingly have disregarded it even when it was clearly relevant. Consequently, base rates are worth some discussion.

I can begin by referring to an earlier experience of mine. Working as a clinical psychologist in a VA Hospital more than 50 years ago, I collected psychological test data on a moderate sized sample of patients who had been referred for psychological evaluation. I compared my diagnostic impressions based on test data with the clinical diagnoses made at the staff conferences on these patients and, among other things, noted that my diagnosis of schizophrenia agreed with the staff diagnosis in 67% of the cases. On the whole, I was not displeased with this degree of agreement. I prepared an article on this study and submitted it to the Branch Chief Psychologist for his evaluation. The Branch Chief, David Shakow, returned it to me with his comments. He particularly raised the issue of how my diagnosis of schizophrenia compared with the rates of such admissions to the hospital, and suggested that I secure the base rates for diagnoses of schizophrenia in my hospital for comparison. I reluctantly carried out a survey of hospital admissions for a specific period and discovered to my surprise that the number of patients officially diagnosed as cases of schizophrenia was just about 67%. In other words, my diagnostic work did not exceed the base rate for diagnoses of schizophrenia, and automatically diagnosing every admitted patient as a schizophrenic would have been as accurate as the diagnoses derived from my psychological test evaluation. Needless to say, this was a sobering experience which has remained rather vivid in my memory.

The matter of base rates, thus, is a factor that must be considered in evaluating certain kinds of research on clinical diagnosis. To be worthwhile clinically, diagnostic procedures must clearly exceed the base rates for a particular disorder. Otherwise, one may be wasting time and effort. Attention to such matters, along with attention to false positives and negatives indicates the potential difficulties in using diagnostic procedures for disorders where the incidence is very high, or where it is very low, as in the case of suicide. In the latter instance, a diagnostic or predictive measure must be extremely effective in discriminating the cases being evaluated if it is to be clinically useful.

Thus, for specific kinds of problems pertaining to differential diagnosis or prediction, it is essential for the researcher to provide data on the base rates for the disorders of interest and to clearly show the advantages as well as disadvantages for the procedures being evaluated.

### Inadequate Data Presentation

In this section, I discuss some of the deficiencies noted in some research reports on clinical diagnosis. These include such problems as not providing basic information on the measures used, necessary information on important variables that might influence results, how diagnoses were secured, how the subjects were selected, and similar aspects. The examples discussed will illustrate the kinds of problems encountered when such information is not included in the report.

At present, when a large number of patients, both inpatients and outpatients, are receiving medication of various kinds, it is extremely important to provide this information in the research report. If the medications used have any potency, they are bound to influence the behavior and mental functioning of the subjects studied. The taking of medication must be clearly mentioned, and also the medication used, the dosages, and in many cases, the duration of medication should also be specified. If part of a group of subjects is on medication and part not on medication, there are clearly problems in mixing the results of these two subgroups and treating them as one relatively homogeneous group. In a related fashion, comparing a clinical group of subjects receiving medication with a control group which is not must obviously limit the kinds of conclusions that can be drawn from such comparisons. If one is attempting to compare the effects of drugs on two groups of comparable patients, then, of course, the previous comparison would be feasible, providing that a placebo was used with the control group. However, if the comparison is done to compare the mental functioning, behavior, or personality characteristics of a given diagnostic group with some other group, then such a comparison would provide results that were contaminated by the influence of the medication.

Another more common problem involves the lack of adequate information presented on the particular techniques or methods of appraisal used in the research study. This is of particular importance when the procedures used are not standardized or have been constructed by the investigators for their specific research without adequate preliminary reliability or validity studies. It is the responsibility of investigators to describe clearly the procedures and techniques they have used in their study so that others may fully understand what has taken place and be able to attempt replications of the study. Readers of such reports should also evaluate the adequacy of the research before attempting to apply it to their own clinical or research work.

With the pressures for publication and the corresponding desire to use journal space efficaciously, it is understandable that editors want manuscripts to be as brief and concise as possible. Nevertheless, this does not mean that significant information about a research project should be omitted. For example, when relatively unknown tests or rating scales are used, the investigator should describe them in sufficient detail so that the reader clearly understands the techniques used and can appraise their suitability for the samples and the problem under investigation. This is not an infrequent occurrence. Lambert and Hill (1994) stated,

"The proliferation of outcome measures (a sizable portion of which were unstandardized scales) is overwhelming if not disheartening" (p. 74). The investigator should also provide pertinent data concerning the reliability and validity of the procedures used in these instances as well. Because the value of the results obtained in any research study depends on the adequacy of the measures used, such information is essential.

A final point concerns inadequate or apparently biased citing of the relevant research literature. I cannot recall seeing any discussion of this topic in presentations of research on either clinical diagnosis or treatment. Perhaps it is assumed that all investigators are aware of the need to review carefully the existing research on the topic under investigation. Nevertheless, this issue is mentioned in critiques of research reports or reviews of research (Garfield, 1977, 1978). The issue is of some importance where there is conflicting literature on a specific topic and investigators refer primarily to those published reports that support their findings or position and omit mention of findings that fail to do so. Such a practice violates accepted standards of scholarship, misleads uninformed readers of the research reports, and may tend to perpetuate the use of fallible diagnostic techniques.

## Cross-Validation

One of the concerns about much past research, not limited to clinical diagnosis alone, has been the large number of conflicting findings in the literature and the difficulty in replicating published findings. This has become such a frequent occurrence in research in clinical psychology that many review articles tend to present a summary of the number of positive and negative studies on a given topic (e.g., Garfield, 1994; Luborsky, Singer, & Luborsky, 1975). If more than half of the studies are favorable to a given proposition, then that view may be judged to have some support, even where the studies may vary greatly in quality. This is a rather risky means of drawing conclusions about some technique or finding. If a particular clinical treatment for schizophrenia, for example, is found helpful in eight investigations and harmful in four, should we conclude that overall the treatment is helpful? The fact that we have such conflicting findings should make us suspect some possible limitations in the research reported and to withhold judgment until we are able to explain the discrepant findings.

Most likely, the discrepancies among research reports are due to subject variables, sample size, and variations in diagnostic and treatment procedures, as well as to chance variables. Because of the kinds of problems already mentioned concerning variations in assigning clinical diagnoses, in selecting subject samples, in the kind of settings used, and in the procedures used, the findings from any single investigation are probably best viewed as suggestive. Although attempted replications by other investigators in different settings are essential for appraising the value of any investigation, there is one procedure that most researchers could use to improve the reliability of their findings—and I am surprised that it is not used more frequently. This is simply to secure enough subjects in the experimental and control groups so that all groups can be randomly divided into two subgroups. The study is then conducted so that one set of subgroups serves as the initial group and the second set serves as an attempt at cross-validation. This is a relatively straightforward procedure which has been used in some past studies, but relatively infrequently (Garfield & Wolpin, 1963; Lorr, Katz, & Rubenstein, 1958; Sullivan, Miller, & Smelser, 1958).

In the study by Sullivan et al. (1958), two cross-validations were carried out on MMPI profiles of patients who terminated prematurely from psychotherapy; the results of the cross-validation attempts were clearly very important for the final conclusions drawn. Significant differences between premature terminators and those who continued in therapy were found for several MMPI Scales for *each* of the several groups of subjects investigated. However, *none* of the scales that differentiated the two groups under study in one sample showed a consistent pattern. For each separate appraisal, different scales were found significant in their differentiation. Consequently, the findings secured in the first appraisal were not supported in the subsequent cross-validations, and the final conclusions reached were different from what they would have been if the cross-validations had not been attempted. This old but well-conducted study clearly illustrates the importance and the necessity of cross-validation.

Although attempted replications or cross-validations by other investigators are also required to evaluate fully the significance and utility of findings reported in any single investigation, the procedure suggested above is useful for increasing the potential value of single studies.

## Problems in Validating Tests and Scales for Clinical Diagnosis

Traditionally, the clinical diagnosis of a patient was made by a clinician, usually a physician, on the basis of a personal interview, some type of case history, and perhaps also a physical or neurological examination. As medicine developed, a variety of diagnostic procedures were developed such as X rays, blood tests, etc., which greatly facilitated the accuracy of the diagnosis made by the clinician. In psychopathology, similar attempts to increase the accuracy of diagnosis have been made. For psychologists, the main techniques have been psychological tests and rating scales. Essentially, these have been attempts to objectify clinical observation and to provide a more systematic appraisal of the psychological functioning of the patient as an aid to diagnosis.

There are potential advantages in using such instruments compared with clinical judgment alone. The former can be administered in a standard fashion, normative data can be secured, scoring and interpretation are potentially more objective, and comparisons of comparable samples of subjects are facilitated. Nevertheless, despite these potential advantages, psychological tests and rating scales developed for evaluating psychopathology for clinical diagnosis have been seriously limited by problems in the validation process.

Although a number of psychologists and psychopathologists have been critical of the reliability and validity of psychiatric diagnoses and have attempted to develop better diagnostic techniques, nevertheless, they have frequently relied on them as a basis for validating their own diagnostic procedures. Using a fallible criterion for the purpose of validation is bound to produce difficulties. In the present instance, there is also evidence of what appears to be circular or faulty reasoning. The initial premise is that clinical diagnoses have serious limitations. Consequently, more effective techniques need to be developed. To validate these potentially more effective techniques, clinical diagnoses will be used as the criteria of validity. If there is reasonable agreement between the tests and clinical diagnoses, then the tests themselves can be considered valid. If this procedure doesn't make good sense to you, the reader, then you are comprehending it correctly. It should be apparent that it is difficult to improve diagnostic procedures if inadequate criteria of validity are used.

The issue mentioned here has constituted a serious problem in the attempt to develop tests and scales to improve clinical diagnosis. The real issue ultimately goes back to the adequacy of the diagnostic system being followed. Where syndromes or categories of illness can be clearly described, where the focus is on physical factors or observable behavior, and where there is relatively little overlap with competing diagnostic categories, the chances of devising diagnostic techniques that will increase the efficacy of clinical diagnosis is enhanced. If the categories themselves are vague and unreliable, it is difficult to see how tests and scales can be adequately validated unless only very "clear-cut" cases are used. In such instances, of course, the procedures will apply only to selected cases.

The reliability and validity of diagnoses also have implications for treatments developed for specific disorders. To the extent that psychotherapy manuals are currently geared to psychiatric diagnoses, the importance of variability among patients is minimized (Garfield, 1996). "With diagnostic categories being the focus of our outcome research, little concern is given to the unique determinants/dynamics that may be relevant to our interventions (see Clarkin & Kendall, 1992)" (Goldfried & Wolfe, 1998, p. 145).

## Clinical Diagnosis: Some Concluding Comments

It is readily apparent that any research on diagnostic groups (e.g., schizophrenia or bipolar disorder) can be no better than the validity or meaningfulness of the diagnoses obtained and used. This problem has plagued research in this area for many years. On the one hand, systematic and reliable classification of subjects facilitates research and the accumulation of potentially meaningful data about types of psychopathology. On the other hand, if the classification scheme used for such research is beset with problems of clarity, reliability, and validity, the results based on such classification are bound to be limited in their usefulness. An unreliable and loose scheme is bound to produce unreliable and variable results. The most highly quantified data and the most exacting statistical analyses cannot provide worthwhile conclusions if the assumptions or foundation upon which they are based are weak.

In line with suggestions discussed earlier, investigators need to specify and describe their research subjects in ways that give more meaning to the diagnostic categories studied. In cases diagnosed as schizophrenia, for example, the patients should also be described in terms of other related measures such as the process-reactive continuum, good or poor premorbids, the MMPI, IQ, factored scales such as those developed by Lorr et al. (1966), and the like. Major symptoms of the subjects should also be described and rated on reliable scales. To treat schizophrenia as a single category or disorder is to court trouble.

Unless we pay attention to the important issues involved and try for as much specification as possible of the disorders we are studying, our research efforts will tend to produce conflicting and disappointing results, and clinical practice will be the loser. We can learn from our past deficiencies and, hopefully, strive to improve the quality of our investigative efforts. I acknowledge that considerable effort and thought have gone into the planning and completion of DSM-IV, and in many ways it represents a considered attempt at improving the diagnostic nomenclature. However, DSM-IV, as indicated previously, has problems deriving from its categorical diagnostic system, and decisions concerning diagnoses have been reached on other than scientific or critical clinical study. As Meehl (1995) has suggested, "Further research of diagnostic systems should be based on taxometric analyses rather than on committed decisions based on clinical impressions and nontaxometric research" (p. 266). I would add, also, that frequent changes in official diagnostic systems create additional problems for research and should be avoided as much as possible and limited to those disorders that clearly need rather immediate revision or removal.

# References

Adams, H. B. (1952). "Mental illness" or interpersonal behavior? *American Psychologist, 19,* 191–197.

Adams, H. E., & Cassidy, J. E. (1993). The classification of abnormal behavior. In P. B. Sutker & H. E. Adams (Eds.), *Comprehensive handbook of psychopathology* (2nd ed.) (pp. 3–25). New York: Plenum Press.

American Psychiatric Association. (1952). *Diagnostic and statistical manual of mental disorders.* Washington, DC: Author.

American Psychiatric Association. (1968). *Diagnostic and statistical manual of mental disorders* (2nd ed.). Washington, DC: Author.

American Psychiatric Association. (1980). *Diagnostic and statistical manual of mental disorders* (3rd ed.). Washington, DC: Author.

American Psychiatric Association. (1987). *Diagnostic and statistical manual of mental disorders* (3rd ed., rev.). Washington, DC: Author.

American Psychiatric Association. (1994). *Diagnostic and statistical manual of mental disorders* (4th ed.). Washington, DC: Author.

Aronson, T. A. (1987). Is panic disorder a distinct diagnostic entity? A critical review of the borders of a syndrome. *Journal of Nervous and Mental Disease, 175,* 584–594.

Ash, P. (1949). The reliability of psychiatric diagnosis. *Journal of Abnormal and Social Psychology, 44,* 272–276.

Astrachan, B. M., et al. (1972). A checklist for the diagnosis of schizophrenia. *British Journal of Psychiatry, 121,* 529–539.

Beck, A. T. (1972). *Depression: Causes and treatment.* Philadelphia: University of Pennsylvania Press.

Beck, A. T., Ward, C. H., Mendelson, M., Mock, J. E., & Erbaugh, J. K. (1962). Reliability of psychiatric diagnoses: 2. A study of consistency of clinical judgments and ratings. *American Journal of Psychiatry, 119,* 351–357.

Bentall, R. P., Jackson, H. F., & Pilgrim, D. (1988). Abandoning the concept of "schizophrenia": Some implications of validity arguments for psychological research into psychotic phenomena. *British Journal of Clinical Psychology, 27,* 303–324.

Ben-Tovin, D. I. (1988). DSM-III, draft DSM-III-R, and the diagnosis and prevalence of bulimia in Australia. *American Journal of Psychiatry, 145,* 1000–1002.

Blashfield, R. K. (1973). An evaluation of the DSM-II classification of schizophrenia as a nomenclature. *Journal of Abnormal Psychology, 82,* 382–389.

Blashfield, R. K., & Fuller, K. (1996). Predicting the DSM-V. *Journal of Nervous and Mental Disease, 184,* 4–7.

Brooner, R. K., King, V. L., Kidorf, M., Schmidt, Jr., C. W., & Bigelow, G. E. (1997). Psychiatric and substance use comorbidity among treatment seeking opioid abusers. *Archives of General Psychiatry, 54,* 71–80.

Cantwell, D. P., Russel, A. T., Mattison, R., & Will, L. (1979). A comparison of DSM-II and DSM-III in the diagnosis of childhood psychiatric disorders. I. Agreement with expected diagnosis. *Archives of General Psychiatry, 36,* 1208–1213.

Carson, R. C. (1996). Aristotle, Galileo, and the *DSM* taxonomy: The case of schizophrenia. *Journal of Consulting and Clinical Psychology, 64,* 1133–1139.

Carson, R. C. (1997). Costly compromises: A critique of the *Diagnostic and Statistical Manual of Mental Disorders.* In S. Fisher & R. P. Greenberg (Eds.), *From placebo to panacea: Putting psychiatric drugs to the test* (pp. 98–112). New York: Wiley.

Carson, R. C., & Sanislow III, C. A. (1993). The schizophrenias. In P. B. Suther & H. E. Adams (Eds.), *Comprehensive handbook of psychopathology* (2nd ed.) (pp. 295–333) New York: Plenum Press.

Chambles, D. L., & Hollon, S. D. (1998). Defining empirically supported therapies. *Journal of Consulting and Clinical Psychology, 66,* 7–18.

Clarkin, J. R., & Kendall, P. D. (1992). Comorbidity and treatment planning: Summary and future directions. *Journal of Consulting and Clinical Psychology, 66,* 904–908.

Downey, K. K., Stelson, F. W., Pomerleau, O. F., & Giordani, B. (1997). Adult attention deficit hyperactivity disorder:

Psychological test profiles in a clinical population. *Journal of Nervous and Mental Disease, 185,* 32–38.

Dumont, M. P. (1984). The nonspecificity of mental illness. *American Journal of Orthopsychiatry, 54,* 326–334.

Endicott, J., Nee, J., Fleiss, J., Cohen, J., Williams, J. B. W., & Simon, R. (1982). Diagnostic criteria for schizophrenia. Reliabilities and agreement between systems. *Archives of General Psychiatry, 39,* 884–889.

Endicott, J., & Spitzer, R. L. (1978). A diagnostic interview: The schedule of affective disorders and schizophrenia. *Archives of General Psychiatry, 35,* 837–844.

Eysenck, J. H. (1986). A critique of contemporary classification and diagnosis. In T. Millon & G. L. Klerman (Eds.), *Contemporary directions in psychopathology. Toward the DSM-IV* (pp. 73–98). New York: Guilford.

Feighner, J. P., Robins, E., Guze, S. B., Woodruff, R. A., Winokur, G., & Munoz, R. (1972). Diagnostic criteria for use in psychiatric research. *Archives of General Psychiatry, 26,* 57–63.

Fenton, W. S., McGlashan, T. H., & Heinssen, R. K. (1988). A comparison of DSM-III and DSM-III-R schizophrenia. *American Journal of Psychiatry, 145,* 1446–1449.

Fenton, W. S., Mosher, L. R., & Mathews, S. M. (1981). Diagnosis of schizophrenia: A critical review of current diagnostic systems. *Schizophrenia Bulletin, 7,* 452–476.

Follette, W. C., & Houts, A. C. (1996). Models of scientific progress and the role of theory in taxonomy development: A case study of the *DSM. Journal of Consulting and Clinical Psychology, 64,* 1120–1132.

Frances, A. J., Widiger, T. A., & Pincus, H. A. (1989). *Archives of General Psychiatry, 46,* 373–375.

*Funk & Wagnalls New College Standard Dictionary.* New York: 1950.

Garfield, S. L. (1949). An evaluation of Wechsler–Bellevue patterns in schizophrenia. *Journal of Consulting Psychology, 13,* 279–287.

Garfield, S. L. (1974). *Clinical psychology. The study of personality and behavior.* Chicago: Aldine.

Garfield, S. L. (1977). Further comments on "dropping out of treatment": A reply to Baekeland and Lundwall. *Psychological Bulletin, 84,* 306–308.

Garfield, S. L. (1978). Research on client variables in psychotherapy. In S. L. Garfield & A. E. Bergin (Eds.), *Handbook of psychotherapy and behavior change* (2nd ed.) (pp. 191–232). New York: Wiley.

Garfield, S. L. (1986). Problems in diagnostic classification. In T. Millon & G. L. Klerman (Eds.), *Contemporary directions in psychopathology. Toward the DSM-IV* (pp. 99–114). New York: Guilford.

Garfield, S. L. (1994). Research on client variables in psychotherapy. In A. E. Bergin & S. L. Garfield (Eds.), *Handbook of psychotherapy and behavior change* (4th ed.) (pp. 190–228). New York: Wiley.

Garfield, S. L. (1996). Some problems associated with "validated" forms of psychotherapy. *Clinical Psychology: Science and Practice, 3,* 218–229.

Garfield, S. L. (1998). Some comments on empirically supported treatments. *Journal of Consulting and Clinical Psychology, 66,* 121–125.

Garfield, S. L., & Kurtz, R. (1976). Clinical psychologists in the 1970s. *American Psychologist, 31,* 1–9.

Garfield, S. L., & Sundland, D. M. (1966). Prognostic scales in schizophrenia. *Journal of Consulting Psychology, 30,* 18–24.

Garfield, S. L., & Wolpin, M. (1963). Expectations regarding psychotherapy. *Journal of Nervous and Mental Disease, 137,* 353–362.

Gathercole, C. E. (1968). *Assessment in clinical psychology.* Baltimore: Penguin.

Goldfried, M. R., & Wolfe, B. E. (1998). Toward a more clinically valid approach to therapy research. *Journal of Consulting and Clinical Psychology, 66,* 143–150.

Goldstein, W. N., & Anthony, R. N. (1988). The diagnosis of depression and the DSMs. *American Journal of Psychotherapy, 42,* 180–196.

Gunderson, J. G., Kolb, J. E., & Austin, V. (1981). The diagnostic interview for borderline patients. *American Journal of Psychiatry, 138,* 896–903.

Guze, S. B. (1995) (Review of *DSM-IV*, no title). *American Journal of Psychiatry, 152*(8), 1228.

Hamilton, M. A. (1960). A rating scale for depression. *Journal of Neurology, Neurosurgery, and Psychiatry, 23,* 56–61.

Hanson, D. R., Gottesman, I. I., & Meehl, P. E. (1977). Genetic theories and the validation of psychiatric diagnoses: Implications for the study of children of schizophrenics. *Journal of Abnormal Psychology, 86,* 575–588.

Hill, C., Keks, N., Roberts, S., Opeskin, K., Dean, B., Mackinnon, A., & Copolov, D. (1996). Problems of diagnosis in postmortem brain studies of schizophrenia. *American Journal of Psychiatry, 153,* 533–537.

Horowitz, L. M., Inouye, D., & Siegelman, E. Y. (1979). On averaging judges' ratings to increase their correlation with an external criterion. *Journal of Consulting and Clinical Psychology, 47,* 453–458.

Hunt, W. A., Wittson, C. L., & Hunt, E. B. (1953). A theoretical and practical analysis of the diagnostic process. In P. H. Hoch and J. Zubin (Eds.), *Current problems in psychiatric diagnosis.* New York: Grune & Stratton.

Jacobsberg, L., Francis, A., & Perry, S. (1995). Axis II diagnoses among volunteers for HIV testing and counseling. *American Journal of Psychiatry, 152,* 1222–1224.

Jacobson, N. S., & Revenstorf, D. (1988). Statistics for assessing the clinical significance of psychotherapy techniques: Issues, problems, and new developments. *Behavioral Assessment, 10,* 133–145.

Jacobson, N. S., & Truax (1991). Clinical significance: A statistical approach to defining meaningful change in psychotherapy research. *Journal of Consulting and Clinical Psychology, 59,* 12–19.

Johnson, J. G., Williams, J. B. W., Goetz, R. R., Rabkin, G., Lipsitz, J. D., & Remien, R. H. (1997). Stability and change in personality disorder symptomatology: Findings from a longitudinal study of HIV+ and HIV− men. *Journal of Abnormal Psychology, 106,* 154–158.

Kazdin, A. E. (1986). The evaluation of psychotherapy: Research design and methodology. In S. L. Garfield & A. E. Bergin (Eds.), *Handbook of psychotherapy and behavior change* (3rd ed.) (pp. 23–68). New York: Wiley.

Kazdin, A. E. (1994). Methodology, design, and evaluation in psychotherapy research. In A. E. Bergin & S. L. Garfield (Eds.), *Handbook of psychotherapy and behavior change* (4th ed.) (pp. 19–71). New York: Wiley.

Klein, D. N. (1982). Relation between current diagnostic criteria for schizophrenia and the dimensions of premorbid adjustment, paranoid symptomatology, and chronicity. *Journal of Abnormal Psychology, 91,* 319–325.

Klerman, G. L. (1986). Historical perspectives on contemporary schools of psychopathology. In T. Millon & G. L. Klerman (Eds.), *Contemporary directions in psychopathology. Toward the DSM-IV* (pp. 3–28). New York: Guilford.

Kramer, M. (1965). Classification of mental disorders for epidemiologic and medical care purposes: Current status, problems and needs. In M. M. Katz, J. O. Cole, & W. E. Barton (Eds.), *The role and methodology of classification in psychiatry and psychopathology.* Chevy Chase, MD.: National Institute of Mental Health, U.S. Department of Health, Education and Welfare. Public Health Service Publication No. 1584.

Kreitman, N. (1961). The reliability of psychiatric diagnosis. *Journal of Mental Science, 107,* 876–886.

Kuriansky, J. B., Deming, W. E., & Gurland, B. J. (1974). On trends in the diagnosis of schizophrenia. *American Journal of Psychiatry, 131,* 402–408.

Lambert, M. J., & Hill, C. A. (1994). Assessing psychotherapy outcomes and processes. In A. E. Bergin & S. L. Garfield (Eds.), *Handbook of psychotherapy and behavior change* (4th ed.) (pp. 72–113). New York: Wiley.

Leavitt, J. J., & Tsuong, M. T. (1988). The heterogeneity of schizoaffective disorder: Implications for treatment. *American Journal of Psychiatry, 145,* 926–936.

Lick, J. (1973). Statistical vs. clinical significance in research on the outcome of psychotherapy. *International Journal of Mental Health, 22,* 26–37.

Lilienfield, S. O., Waldman, I. D., & Israel, A. C. (1994). A critical examination of the use of the term and concept of *comorbidity* in psychopathology research. *Clinical Psychology: Science and Practice, 1,* 71–83.

Lorr, M. (1986). Classifying psychotics: Dimensional and categorical approaches. In T. Millon & G. L. Klerman (Eds.), *Contemporary directions in psychopathology. Toward the DSM-IV* (pp. 331–346). New York: Guilford.

Lorr, M., Katz, M. M., & Rubenstein, E. A. (1958). The prediction of length of stay in psychotherapy. *Journal of Consulting Psychology, 22,* 321–327.

Lorr, M., Klett, J. J., McNair, D. M., & Lasky, J. J. (1966). *Inpatient Multidimensional Psychiatric Scale, 1966 Revision.* Palo Alto, CA: Consulting Psychologists Press.

Luborsky, L., Singer, B., & Luborsky, L. (1975). Comparative studies of psychotherapy: Is it true that "Everyone has won and all must have prizes"? *Archives of General Psychiatry, 32,* 995–1008.

Malamud, D. I. (1946). Objective measurement of clinical status in psychopathological research. *Psychological Bulletin, 43,* 240–258.

Marmor, J. (1983). Systems thinking in psychiatry: Some theoretical and clinical implications. *American Journal of Psychiatry, 140,* 833–838.

Mattison, R., Cantwell, D. P., Russel, A. T., & Will, L. (1979). A comparison of DSM-II and DSM-III in the diagnosis of childhood psychiatric disorders. II. Interrater agreement. *Archives of General Psychiatry, 36,* 1217–1222.

McNair, D. M., Lorr, M., & Callahan, D. M. (1963). Patient and therapist influences on quitting psychotherapy. *Journal of Consulting Psychology, 27,* 10–17.

McReynolds, P. (1989). Diagnosis and clinical assessment: Current status and major issues. In M. R. Rosenzweig & L. W. Porter (Eds.), *Annual Review of Psychology, 40,* 83–108.

Meehl, P. E. (1995). Bootstrap taxometrics. Solving the classification problem in psychopathology. *American Psychologist, 50,* 266–275.

Meehl, P. E., & Rosen, A. (1955). Antecedent probability and the efficiency of psychometric signs, patterns, or cutting scores. *Psychological Bulletin, 52,* 194–216.

Milich, R., Widiger, T. A., & Landau, S. (1987). Differential diagnosis of attention deficit and conduct disorders using conditional probabilities. *Journal of Consulting and Clinical Psychology, 55,* 762–767.

Millon, T. (1988). Falling short of the borderline [Review of *The borderline patient: Emerging concepts in diagnosis, psychodynamics, and treatment,* Vols. 1 and 2]. *Contemporary Psychology, 33,* 902–903.

Millon, T. (1991). Classification in psychopathology: Rationale, alternatives, and standards. *Journal of Abnormal Psychology, 100,* 245–261.

Millon, T. & Klerman, G. L. (1986). *Contemporary directions in psychopathology: Toward the DSM-IV.* New York: Guilford.

Moldin, S. O., Gottesman, I. I., & Erlenmeyer-Kimling, L. (1987). Searching for the psychometric boundaries of schizophrenia: Evidence from the New York high-risk study. *Journal of Abnormal Psychology, 96,* 354–363.

Morgenstern, J., Langenbucher, J., Labouvie, E., & Miller, K. J. (1997). The comorbidity of alcoholism and personality disorders in a clinical population: Prevalence and relation to alcohol typology variables. *Journal of Abnormal Psychology, 106,* 74–84.

Nurnberg, H. G., Hurt, S. W., Feldman, A., & Suh, R. (1988). Evaluation of diagnostic criteria in borderline personality disorder. *American Journal of Psychiatry, 145,* 1280–1284.

Overall, J. R., & Hollister, L. E. (1979). Comparative evaluation of research diagnostic criteria for schizophrenia. *Archives of General Psychiatry, 36,* 1198–1205.

Pasamanick, B., Dinitz, S., & Lefton, H. (1959). Psychiatric orientation and its relation to diagnosis and treatment in a mental hospital. *American Journal of Psychiatry, 116,* 127–132.

Pope, H. G., Jr., Hudson, J. I., Yurgelun-Todd, D. (1984). Anorexia nervosa and bulimia among 300 suburban women shoppers. *American Journal of Psychiatry, 141,* 292–294.

Robins, L. N. (1994). How recognizing "comorbidities" in psychopathology may lead to an improved research nosology. *Clinical Psychology: Science and Practice, 1,* 93–95.

Rutherford, M. J., Alterman, A. I., Cassiola, J. S., & Snider, E. C. (1995). Gender differences in diagnosing antisocial personality disorder in methadone patients. *American Journal of Psychiatry, 152,* 1309–1316.

Sarbin, T. R. (1997). On the futility of psychiatric diagnostic manuals (DSMs) and the return of personal agency. *Applied and Preventive Psychology, 6,* 233–243.

Schmidt, H. D., & Fonda, C. P. (1956). The reliability of psychiatric diagnosis: A new look. *Journal of Abnormal and Social Psychology, 52,* 262–267.

Skinner, H. A. (1986). Construct validation approach to psychiatric classification. In T. Millon & G. L. Klerman (Eds.), *Contemporary directions in psychopathology. Toward the DSM-IV* (pp. 307–330). New York: Guilford.

Smith, D. & Kraft, W. A. (1983). DSM-III: Do psychologists really want an alternative? *American Psychologist, 38,* 777–785.

Spitzer, R. L., Endicott, J., & Robins, E. (1975). Research diagnostic criteria (RDC). *Psychopharmacology Bulletin, 11,* 22–24.

Spitzer, R. L., & Fleiss, J. L. (1974). A reanalysis of the

reliability of psychiatric diagnosis. *British Journal of Psychiatry, 125,* 341–347.

Spitzer, R. L., Williams, J. B. W., & Gibbon, M. (1987). *Instruction manual for the Structured Clinical Interview for DSM-III-R (SCID, 4/1/87 Revised).* New York: New York State Psychiatric Institute.

Sue, S., McKinney, H., Allen, D., & Hall, J. (1974). Delivery of community mental health services to black and white clients. *Journal of Consulting and Clinical Psychology, 42,* 794–801.

Sullivan, P. L., Miller, C., & Smelser, W. (1958). Factors in length of stay and progress in psychotherapy. *Journal of Consulting Psychology, 22,* 1–9.

Sutker, P. B. & Adams, H. E. (Eds.). (1993). *Comprehensive handbook of psychopathology* (2nd ed.). New York: Plenum Press.

Volkmar, F. R., Bregman, J., Cohen, D. J., & Cicchetti, D. V. (1988). DSM-III and DSM-III-R diagnoses of autism. *American Journal of Psychiatry, 145,* 1404–1408.

Westen, D. (1997). Divergences between clinical and research methods for assessing personality disorders: Implications for research and the evolution of Axis II. *American Journal of Psychiatry, 154,* 895–903.

Widiger, T. A., Frances, A. J., Pincus, H. A., & Davis, W. W. (1990). DSM-IV literature reviews: Rationale, process, and limitations. *Journal of Psychopathology and Behavioral Assessment, 12,* 189–202.

Wolf, A. W., Schubert, D. S., Patterson, M. B., Grande, T. P., Brocco, K. J., & Pendleton, L. (1988). Associations among major psychiatric diagnoses. *Journal of Consulting and Clinical Psychology, 56,* 292–294.

Zilboorg, G., & Henry, G. W. (1941). *A history of medical psychology.* New York: W.W. Norton.

Zimmerman, M. (1988). Why are we rushing to publish DSM-IV? *Archives of General Psychiatry, 45,* 1135–1138.

# CHAPTER 3

# Behavior Genetic Approaches to the Study of Psychopathology

## Soo Hyun Rhee, Sarah A. Feigon, Jessica L. Bar, Yukiharu Hadeishi, and Irwin D. Waldman

## Introduction

Psychopathologists have long been interested in the etiology of mental disorders. The earliest rudimentary attempts at classifying mental disorders were accompanied by similar efforts at divining their causes. Along with classification, treatment, developmental course, and outcome, etiology forms one of the cornerstones of psychopathological research. There are many approaches for investigating the underlying causes of a disorder. These include examining a broad class of biological variables such as psychophysiological, neurotransmitter, and hormonal activity, as well as social variables such as parental behavior, social class, peer group influences, and the effects of growing up in a particular neighborhood. Behavior genetic methods for investigating the etiology of a disorder represent a useful, complementary alternative to these other approaches. These methods that include family, adoption, and twin designs are particularly useful for disentangling genetic and

environmental influences on a disorder or its symptoms. As such, they have certain advantages over the other approaches mentioned, particularly that the distinction between genetic and environmental influences is typically "cleaner" than that between biological and social influences, for example. Nonetheless, as we will discuss at the end of this chapter, the most powerful inferences regarding etiology may come from combining behavior genetic methods with these other approaches to investigating etiology.

The past 15 years has seen a dramatic increase in the number of behavior genetic studies of psychopathology, the sample size in such studies, and the sophistication of the analytic methods used to infer genetic and environmental influences. It was not that long ago that the evidence for genetic and environmental influences on most psychiatric disorders came from a handful of studies using small, clinically referred samples. The first major shift came with the Scandinavian adoption studies of schizophrenia, affective disorder, alcoholism, and criminality. These studies employed national registries of both adoptions and mental disorders to recruit large samples of nonreferred adoptees and their adoptive (and often times biological) parents. Although the sample sizes in these studies were quite large, the statistical methods used were still fairly rudimentary and relied primarily on the simple comparison of parent–offspring concordances or correlations to infer genetic and environmental causes. Following from these adoption studies in

Soo Hyun Rhee • Institute for Behavioral Genetics, University of Colorado at Boulder, Boulder, Colorado 80309-0447. Jessica L. Bar • Department of Psychology, Boston University, Boston, Massachusetts 02215. Sarah A. Feigon, Yukiharu Hadeishi, and Irwin D. Waldman • Department of Psychology, Emory University, Atlanta, Georgia 30322.

*Comprehensive Handbook of Psychopathology* (Third Edition), edited by Patricia B. Sutker and Henry E. Adams. Kluwer Academic / Plenum Publishers, New York, 2001.

the 1970s and early 1980s came large twin studies of the major mental disorders, using more sophisticated biometric model-fitting methods that allowed statistical contrast of alternative etiological models for their fit to the observed correlations. In some studies, such analyses included correlations from many different familial relationships and combined data from many different samples to infer genetic and environmental influences while examining cross-sample heterogeneity (e.g., McGue, Gottesman, & Rao, 1985). Indeed, behavior genetic studies of psychopathology have increased sufficiently in number, sample size, and methodological sophistication that now a sufficient number of them permit meta-analyses for a number of disorders, including alcoholism (Heath et al., 1996), aggression (Miles & Carey, 1997), and antisocial behavior (Rhee & Waldman, 1998).

In this chapter, we will give a brief presentation of behavior genetic methods, focusing especially on twin designs, because twin studies have certain advantages over family and adoption designs. We will then summarize the results of recent behavior genetic studies for a number of the major mental disorders, including schizophrenia and schizophrenia spectrum disorders, mood and anxiety disorders, including childhood internalizing disorders, and childhood externalizing disorders. For a number of disorders, we will also review multivariate behavior genetic studies that are especially useful for illuminating comorbidity among disorders. We will conclude by highlighting some new approaches and future directions in behavior genetic studies of psychopathology. These will include approaches for examining whether genetic and environmental influences differ throughout the range of symptoms from those at the disordered extreme, the inclusion of specific environmental variables and putative endophenotypic variables within behavior genetic models, and the examination of genotype–environment interactions and correlations. In addition, although the focus of this chapter is on quantitative genetic studies, we will briefly discuss the promise of molecular genetic studies of psychopathology in the final section.

## The Use of Twin Data for Drawing Inferences Regarding Genetic and Environmental Influences

Although family and adoption studies are part of the armamentarium of behavior genetic methods,

twin studies have become the design of choice in contemporary behavior genetic studies. Family studies are useful for examining whether and to what extent the causes of disorders are familial or nonfamilial but cannot resolve whether this familiality is genetic or environmental in origin. Adoption and twin studies are required to disentangle genetic and environmental sources of familial aggregation of disorders. Twin studies have a number of advantages over adoption studies, however. These include greater accessibility and representativeness of samples to the general population, thus yielding greater generalizability of findings; contemporaneous measurement of relatives who are the same versus different ages (i.e., twin pairs versus adoptees and their biological and adoptive parents), which permits using the same rather than different measures; and greater statistical power due to both larger sample sizes and greater genetic similarity between relatives. In addition, it often is difficult if not impossible to assess disorders in the biological parents of adoptees, and the assessment of psychopathology in their adoptive parents frequently is based on retrospective reports. These factors make twin studies the more powerful, less problematic, and hence more popular behavior genetic design.

A brief description of the use of data from twins to estimate genetic and environmental influences on symptoms of a disorder may be helpful before reviewing the results of behavior genetic studies of psychopathology. Behavior geneticists typically are interested in disentangling three sets of influences that may cause individual differences or variation in a given trait. First, heritability, or $h^2$, refers to the proportion of variance in the trait that is due to genetic differences among individuals in the population. Second, shared environmental influences, or $c^2$, refer to the proportion of variance in the trait that is due to environmental influences that family members experience in common and which increase their similarity for the trait. Third, nonshared environmental influences, or $e^2$, refer to the proportion of variance in the trait that is due to environmental influences that are experienced uniquely by family members and which decrease their similarity for the trait.

To estimate these influences, twin studies rely on the fact that monozygotic (MZ) twins are identical genetically, whereas fraternal or dizygotic (DZ) twins, just like non-twin siblings, on average, are only 50% similar genetically. It also is assumed that MZ twins are no more similar than

DZ twins for the *trait-relevant* aspects of the shared environment; that is, that environmental influences on the trait of interest are shared in common between members of fraternal twin pairs to the same extent that they are shared between members of identical twin pairs (this is known as the *equal environments assumption*). Given these assumptions, the correlation between identical twins comprises heritability and shared environmental influences (i.e., $r_{MZ} = h^2 + c^2$), because these are the two sets of influences that can contribute to identical twins' similarity for the trait. In contrast, the correlation between fraternal twins comprises one-half of heritability and shared environmental influences [i.e., $r_{DZ} = (1/2h^2) + c^2$], reflecting the smaller degree of genetic similarity between fraternal twins. Algebraic manipulation of the two equations for twin similarity allows one to estimate $h^2$, $c^2$, and $e^2$ [viz., $h^2 = 2(r_{MZ} - r_{DZ})$, $c^2 = 2r_{DZ} - r_{MZ}$, $e_2 = 1 - r_{MZ}$].

Although estimating these influences by using the twin correlations can be done simply by hand, contemporary behavior geneticists use biometric model-fitting analytic methods that can incorporate additional information on familial relationships (e.g., correlations between non-twin siblings or parents and their children), provide statistical tests of the adequacy of these three influences (viz., $h^2$, $c^2$, and $e^2$) in accounting for the observed familial correlations, and test alternative models for the causal influences underlying the trait (e.g.,

a model including genetic and nonshared environmental influences versus a model that also includes shared environmental influences). In the path diagram in Figure 1, we present a comprehensive biometric model for the genetic and environmental influences on symptoms of a disorder for two twins. This path diagram shows the basic biometric model (Neale & Cardon, 1992) for estimating additive and dominance genetic influences, shared and nonshared environmental influences, and the direct influence of one twin's behavior problems on the co-twin's behavior problems. Note that there are now two types of genetic influences, dominance and additive genetic influences, which are summed to arrive at an estimate of broad-sense heritability, or $h^2$. Although this path model represents the full set of potential causes on twins' behavior problems, there is not enough information in the conventional twin study design to estimate all five of these parameters simultaneously. Consequently, contemporary twin studies present and contrast the results of a series of restricted models (i.e., models that contain a subset of all potential causes) to find the most parsimonious model that fits the data well.

In the path diagram in Figure 1, D represents dominance genetic influences, A represents additive genetic influences, C represents shared environmental influences, E represents nonshared environmental influences, and i represents the direct

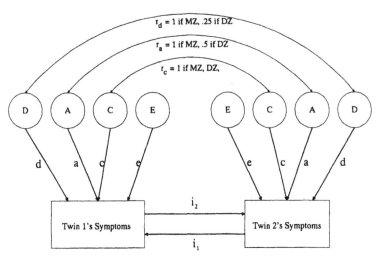

**Figure 1.** Path model for univariate behavior genetic analyses of a disorder. D = dominance genetic influences, A = additive genetic influences, C = shared environmental influences, E = nonshared environmental influences, and i = direct influence of one twin's symptoms on the co-twin's symptoms.

influence of one twin or sibling's behavior problems on the co-twin or co-sibling's behavior problems. The circles that contain these capital letters represent these latent causal genetic and environmental variables, whereas the corresponding lower case letters (viz., $d$, $a$, $c$, $e$, and $i$) represent the magnitude of these influences (i.e., the parameter estimates, which are regression coefficients) on each twin or sibling's behavior problems. The squares of these parameter estimates (viz., $d^2$, $a^2$, $c^2$, and $e^2$) represent the variance components corresponding to dominance and additive genetic influences and shared and nonshared environmental influences. The three correlations in the model— $r_d$, $r_a$, and $r_c$—represent the similarity of particular causal influences between twins. For example, MZ and DZ twins are both correlated 1.0 for shared environmental influences (viz., $r_c$) consistent with the equal environments assumption. In contrast, MZ twins are correlated 1.0 for both dominance and additive genetic influences (viz., $r_d$ and $r_a$), whereas DZ twins are correlated .25 and .5 for dominance and additive genetic influences, respectively, consistent with their average level of genetic similarity.

Programs such as LISREL and MX (Jöreskog & Sörbom, 1999; Neale, Boker, Xie, & Maes, 1999) can iteratively fit such models to twin correlations (or variances and covariances) to provide the best estimates of the parameters; that is, parameter estimates that minimize the difference between the twin correlations implied by the model and those observed in the data. The fit of the model to the data is summarized by a $\chi^2$ statistic, that allows statistical testing of both the fit of a given model and the comparative fit of alternative models. This property often results in restricted models— models that contain only a subset of the parameters in the full model (e.g., only $a$ and $e$)—that provide an adequate fit to the data. In addition, although we presented the biometric model as it applies to data from twins, the model also can include siblings. This model is equally applicable to adoption study data on biologically related and adoptive siblings and can be extended to analyze data from biologically related and adoptive parent–offspring pairs.

These models and analyses also can be extended to examine genetic and environmental influences on the overlap or covariation between different disorders or symptom dimensions. A recent trend in behavior genetic analyses has been to extend the investigation of genetic and environmental influences on traits considered singly to the case of multiple traits considered conjointly (Neale & Cardon, 1992). Multivariate behavior genetic analyses seek to explain the covariation among different traits by examining the common genetic and environmental influences. As suggested in the following sections that present the results of multivariate behavior genetic analyses, such analyses can shed considerable light on the classification of psychopathology and the nature of comorbidity. Most published multivariate behavior genetic studies of psychopathology have focused on testing whether the overlap among multiple disorders is due to genetic versus environmental influences and on estimating the magnitude of the genetic and environmental contributions to covariation among the symptoms of those disorders. Multivariate behavior genetic analyses can also be used in a more confirmatory manner to test specific hypotheses relevant to the classification and etiology of psychopathology. For example, one could test the alternative hypotheses that all genetic or environmental influences act individually on the anxiety disorders without contributing to their comorbidity, that the only genetic or environmental influences on specific and social phobias are those that also influence generalized anxiety disorder (GAD), or that the only genetic or environmental influences on specific and social phobias are completely independent of GAD. In addition, different specific alternative hypotheses can be tested for the genetic and shared and nonshared environmental influences. Conducting multivariate behavior genetic analyses in this hypothesis-driven fashion should ensure that their results are even more informative for resolving issues in classifying psychopathology.

A few brief examples should illustrate a number of the hypotheses that can be addressed using multivariate behavior genetic analytic methods. Shown in Figure 2 is a particular type of multivariate behavior genetic model, known as a Cholesky decomposition, which has been used most frequently in multivariate behavior genetic analyses of psychopathology. In this model, one first extracts the genetic and shared and nonshared environmental influences that specific and social phobia share in common with GAD (represented by factors $A_1$, $C_1$, and $E_1$, respectively), then the genetic, and shared, and nonshared environmental influences that social phobia shares in common

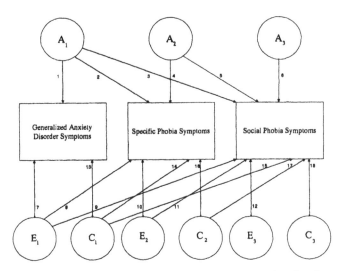

**Figure 2.** Cholesky decomposition of symptoms of three anxiety disorders.

with specific phobia that are not shared with GAD (represented by factors $A_2$, $C_2$, and $E_2$, respectively), and finally the genetic and shared and nonshared environmental influences that are unique to social phobia (represented by factors $A_3$, $C_3$, and $E_3$, respectively). Although most often used in an exploratory fashion, this model can be used to test a number of substantively driven hypotheses regarding classification and comorbidity among anxiety disorders. As suggested before, one can test whether the only genetic influences on specific and social phobia are those that also influence GAD by testing whether one can drop paths 4–6 from the model without a decrement in fit and do the same for the nonshared environmental and shared environmental influences by dropping paths 10–12 and 16–18, respectively, and testing the change in model fit. One can also test the alternative hypothesis that the only genetic or environmental influences on specific and social phobia are completely independent of GAD by assessing the fit of the model if one drops paths 1–3, 7–9, and 13–15 for the common genetic, nonshared, and shared environmental influence factors, respectively.

Two more restrictive multivariate behavior genetic models, the independent and common pathway models, are shown in Figures 3 and 4. (These models also include symptoms of Panic Disorder to show how they would be extended to reflect four anxiety disorders). The independent pathway

model differs from the Cholesky decomposition in that for each etiological influence (viz., genetic and shared and nonshared environmental influences), there is a single common factor that underlies symptom covariation and a unique factor that is specific to each symptom dimension. The fact that there is only a single common factor for each etiological influence, rather than multiple factors for each etiological influence in the Cholesky decomposition model, means that the independent pathway model places greater constraints on the possible explanations of comorbidity among disorders than the Cholesky decomposition model. For example, the independent pathway model would provide a bad fit to the data if there were common genetic influences on GAD and Panic Disorder, and on specific and social phobia, that did not overlap each other, whereas a Cholesky decomposition model could fit these data quite well. The common pathway model is still more restrictive because it posits that symptoms of all four anxiety disorders reflect a common anxiety disorders factor that has a single set of underlying genetic and shared and nonshared environmental influences and residual genetic and environmental influences that are unique to the symptoms of each of the four disorders. Thus, the common pathway model places very strong constraints on explanations of comorbidity because the comorbidity between two disorders depends solely on their loadings on the latent anxiety disorders factor and the

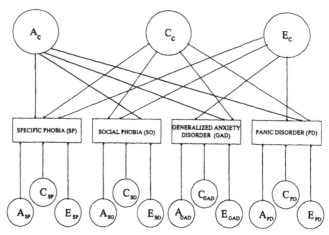

**Figure 3.** Multivariate genetic analysis of symptoms of four anxiety disorders—independent pathway model.

single set of genetic and shared and nonshared environmental influences that underlie it. Viewed another way, comparisons among these multivariate behavior genetic models provide a strong basis for contrasting competing models for the comorbidity among disorders.

## Schizophrenia

Schizophrenia is a relatively common mental disorder that has a life-time prevalence of approximately 1% in the general population (Kleinman,

1988; Thakker & Ward, 1998). The disorder has been defined in various ways since it was first described by Bleuler and Kraepelin in the early 1900s (Kraepelin, 1904; Andreasen & Carpenter, 1993). At present, the most widely used definition of schizophrenia comes from the 4th edition of the *Diagnostic and Statistical Manual of Mental Disorders* (DSM-IV, 1994). According to the DSM-IV, schizophrenia is defined by the presence of two or more of the following symptoms for a significant portion of time during a 1-month period: delusions, hallucinations, disorganized speech, grossly disorganized or catatonic behavior, or neg-

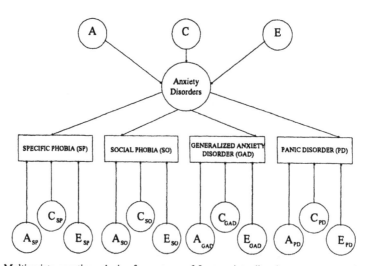

**Figure 4.** Multivariate genetic analysis of symptoms of four anxiety disorders—common pathway model.

ative symptoms, that is, affective flattening, alogia, or avolition. Research has found that this complex mental disorder is associated with a wide variety of both genetic and environmental risk factors (Cannon, Kaprio, Lonnqvist, Huttunen, & Koskenvuo, 1998; for reviews, see Van Os & Marcelis, 1998; McGuffin & Owen, 1996; Syvalahti, 1994; and Egan & Weinberger, 1997). Several different quantitative genetic models have been proposed to describe the etiology of schizophrenia (e.g., Slater, 1958; Elston, Namboodiri, Spence, & Rainer, 1978; Kidd & Cavalli-Sforza, 1973; Matthysse & Kidd, 1976; Gottesman & Shields, 1967). Behavioral genetic techniques can be used to determine the relative contribution of genetic and environmental influences on the development of schizophrenia.

One of the first things that behavioral geneticists noted in their study of schizophrenia is that the disorder tends to aggregate in families. Indeed, Kraepelin himself emphasized the importance of familial factors in his description of dementia praecox (Kraepelin, 1904). Family studies have indicated that the lifetime prevalence of schizophrenia in close relatives of schizophrenic patients is much higher than the population base rate of 1% noted before. Eight to ten percent of full siblings and 12 to 15% of the offspring of schizophrenic patients will be diagnosed as schizophrenic at some point during their lifetimes (Gottesman, 1993). Although these findings suggest that genetic factors may be involved in the etiology of schizophrenia, it is not possible to differentiate between genetic or environmental influences using data from family studies. These influences can be distinguished by using twin studies, many of which have been conducted over the years.

The twin study of schizophrenia conducted by Franz Kallmann is one of the largest twin studies of schizophrenia. As of 1950, Kallmann had registered a total of 953 schizophrenic index twin cases (Kallmann, 1950; Shields, Gottesman, & Slater, 1967). Four years before this, Kallmann published a more detailed report on 691 twin pairs which has received a great deal of scientific scrutiny over the years (Kallmann, 1946; see Jackson, 1960, and Rosenthal, 1962, for criticisms of Kallmann, 1946). Some of the criticisms that have been leveled against Kallmann's 1946 report have been addressed in subsequent reanalyses of Kallmann's original data (Kety, 1958; Shields et al., 1967). According to Shields et al.'s relatively conserva-

tive reanalysis of Kallmann's data, 50% of his MZ twins had both received definite diagnoses of schizophrenia, whereas only 6% of DZ twins were concordant for schizophrenia. It must be noted that these pairwise concordance rates may be artificially inflated due to the manner in which the schizophrenic co-twins were ascertained (see Shields et al., 1967, for practical reasons and Smith, 1974, for statistical reasons why this may be so). Indeed, the concordance rates reported by other investigators tend to be lower than Kallmann's concordance rates (Farmer, McGuffin, & Gottesman, 1987; Kendler & Robinette, 1983; Moskalenko & Gindilis, 1981; Onstad, Skre, Torgersen, & Kringlen, 1991; Torrey, 1992; for reviews, see Gottesman, 1996; Portin & Alanen, 1997; Pulver et al., 1996; Tsuang, 1998; Van Os & Marcelis, 1998). Nevertheless, the concordance rates in MZ twins are higher than concordance rates for DZ twins in every twin study of schizophrenia conducted to date, thus providing strong evidence for the contention that genetic factors contribute to the development of this disorder. In addition, the fact that the concordance rate for MZ twins is far less than 100% suggests that nongenetic (i.e., environmental) factors play an important role in the etiology of schizophrenia.

One difficulty with the early twin studies reviewed before is that most of them used pairwise concordances to summarize the similarity between MZ and DZ twins. Probandwise concordances are superior to pairwise concordances in several ways (McGue, 1992). These include (1) characterizing risk for disorder at the level of the individual, rather than at the level of the twin pair, thus facilitating the comparison of risk to a twin with the risks to other types of relatives; (2) the similarity of probandwise concordances to concordances among other relatives (e.g., parents and their offspring) and to the prevalence of the disorder, whereas pairwise concordances have no direct analogue for non-twin relative pairs and are not directly comparable to the prevalence of the disorder. This renders the interpretation of pairwise concordances and the comparison of twin and non-twin resemblance difficult at best; (3) a clear and useful statistical basis for the interpretation of probandwise concordances (viz., the probability that a twin will be affected given that their co-twin is affected), which is lacking for pairwise concordances; and (4) valid estimation of the magnitude of twin resemblance under both complete and incomplete ascertainment, and hence comparability across studies regardless of the thoroughness of ascertainment. In contrast, sample pairwise concordance rates vary as a function of the thoroughness of ascertainment and thus are not comparable across studies unless the studies have similar levels of ascertainment. In addition, Heath (personal communication, 1994) has pointed out that the analysis of tetrachoric correlations estimated from MZ and DZ concordances and population base rates yield more valid inferences regarding the magnitude of genetic and environmental influences than the concordances themselves, given that the interpretation of concordances and their differences depend heavily on the base rate of the disorder.

Other behavioral genetic studies have provided insight into the question of whether a single gene or multiple genes are responsible for the increased liability to develop schizophrenia. For example, a twin study conducted by Kendler and Robinette (1983) compared the single-locus, two-allele model of the transmission of schizophrenia with the polygenic, multifactorial threshold model (Falconer, 1965; Smith, 1974). The single locus, two-allele model assumes that schizophrenia is due to the effects of a single gene of major effect and that one allele confers a heightened risk for schizophrenia, whereas the other does not (Elston et al., 1978; Kruger, 1973; Slater, 1958). The multifactorial polygenic threshold model, on the other hand, posits that there are multiple genes each of which confers a small degree of risk of developing schizophrenia. According to the multifactorial threshold model, schizophrenia develops when the total liability toward schizophrenia due to the combined genetic and environmental risk factors exceeds a certain threshold. Kendler and Robinette (1983) were able to show that results for schizophrenia in their twin registry were not compatible with a fully penetrant, single-locus, two-allele model of schizophrenia with no phenocopies, nor were they compatible with the more flexible, generalized single-locus model developed by Kidd and Cavalli-Sforza (1973) that allows for incomplete penetrance and the presence of phenocopies. In contrast, their results were consistent with the multifactorial threshold model of the inheritance of schizophrenia. As Kendler and Robinette note, this superiority of the polygenic model to monogenic models is consistent with a more extensive model-fitting study conducted by

O'Rourke, Gottesman, Suarez, Rice, and Reich (1982). Making an assumption of polygenic transmission of schizophrenia allows behavioral geneticists to estimate the broad heritability of schizophrenia (Falconer, 1965). In the Kendler and Robinette study, for example, the estimated $h^2 = .91 \pm 0.16\%$. This value for $h^2$ is within the range obtained from other twin studies. Values for broadsense heritability estimated from the concordance rates obtained in six studies cited in Gottesman's review of twin studies of schizophrenia (1991) vary between .52 and .92.

Adoption studies provide another way of disentangling genetic and environmental influences. If the incidence of schizophrenia in the adopted-away offspring of schizophrenic individuals raised by normal parents is higher than that of the adopted-away offspring of nonschizophrenic individuals, this provides strong evidence that genetic influences are involved in the etiology of schizophrenia. Indeed, this has been the case across schizophrenia adoption studies. For example, in the Danish Adoption Study, Kendler, Gruenberg, and Kinney (1994) compared the prevalence of DSM-III diagnoses of schizophrenia in the relatives of schizophrenic and control adoptees. The first-degree biological relatives of schizophrenic adoptees showed an increased risk for schizophrenia compared with the relatives of control adoptees (7.9% vs. 0.9%). This was also true if all interviewed biological relatives were taken into consideration (3.3% vs. 0.3%). The difference in prevalence was larger if the entire schizophrenia spectrum of disorders was considered (23.7% vs. 4.7% in first-degree relatives and 13.0% vs. 3.0% in all interviewed biological relatives).

Another useful method for disentangling genetic and environmental influences on schizophrenia is to compare the rates of schizophrenia in the offspring of MZ twins discordant for schizophrenia. If schizophrenia is primarily due to environmental factors, one would predict that the prevalence of schizophrenia should be considerably higher in the offspring of the schizophrenic twin than in the offspring of the nonschizophrenic co-twin. In contrast, to the extent that schizophrenia is genetically influenced, rates of schizophrenia will be equally high in both sets of offspring. The results of studies using this method are varied. In a follow-up study of Fischer's (1971) Danish twin sample, Gottesman and Bertelsen (1989) found no difference between the prevalence of schizophrenia in the offspring of schizophrenic (16.8%, N = 47) and nonschizophrenic co-twins (17.4%, N = 24). The rates of schizophrenia in both sets of offspring are well above the prevalence in European populations, which is approximately 1% (Kleinman, 1988; Thakker & Ward, 1998). In a somewhat smaller study using the Norwegian national twin sample, Kringlen and Cramer (1989) found that, whereas 17.9% of the children of schizophrenic twins were later diagnosed with schizophrenia, only 4.4% of the children of nonschizophrenic twins developed schizophrenia. Although this difference does not quite reach statistical significance at the .05 level, the trend for the children of schizophrenic twins who have higher rates of schizophrenia does imply that familial environmental factors may significantly influence the development of schizophrenia in addition to genetic influences.

Considering the results of the disparate behavior genetic designs reviewed before, the overwhelming majority of the evidence indicates that genetic influences play a substantial role in the development of schizophrenia. Indeed, behavioral geneticists have progressed from asking the question of whether genetic factors are important in the etiology of schizophrenia to the question of which model of genetic transmission most accurately describes the inheritance of this disorder (Kendler and Robinette, 1983; McGue, Gottesman, & Rao, 1985; O'Rourke et al., 1982). In general, results of these model-fitting studies favor the multifactorial polygenic threshold model over other models of genetic transmission.

## SCHIZOPHRENIA SPECTRUM DISORDERS

As reviewed before, strong evidence exists that schizophrenia is a familial disorder and that genetic influences are involved in the clustering of schizophrenia in families. The liability to schizophrenia seems to be manifested in families not only through the occurrence of the classical disorder, but through other related phenotypes as well. That is, the predisposition to schizophrenia may be expressed in a number of different ways, including schizophrenia-like personality traits and cognitive dysfunctions, personality disorders, and possibly some other nonschizophrenic psychoses. Disorders that occur more frequently in the bio-

logical relatives of schizophrenic individuals than in the biological relatives of nonschizophrenic individuals are called schizophrenia spectrum disorders. Disagreement exists as to the exact composition of this spectrum, however. An accurate description of its boundaries is necessary so that researchers can determine which phenotypes reflect susceptibility to schizophrenia and thus which phenotypes should be included in genetic research on schizophrenia. Examining how the various spectrum disorders aggregate in families can also provide information about the mode of genetic transmission of the liability.

The notion of a *spectrum* of schizophrenic disorders first arose nearly a hundred years ago, when psychiatrists and practitioners began to notice an excess of eccentric personality and character traits among the relatives of their patients with schizophrenia (e.g., Bleuler, 1911/1950; Kraepelin 1909–1913/1971). This less severe, nonpsychotic, familial syndrome was characterized by social anxiety, aloofness, limited emotional response, and odd or disordered thinking. Thus, Bleuler reasoned that schizophrenia might manifest itself in alternate forms and coined the term *latent schizophrenia*, which he applied to individuals who evidenced affective flattening, social withdrawal, and related characteristics, in the absence of psychotic symptoms. He noted that such a dimensional construct might be important for studies of the hereditary basis of schizophrenia.

The first systematic family study involving the schizophrenia spectrum was conducted at Kraepelin's Psychiatric Institute in 1916 (Rudin, 1916). Researchers noticed increased rates of schizophrenia and also of other potentially related psychotic disorders in the siblings of schizophrenic probands. The first behavior genetic study of schizophrenic spectrum disorders was conducted in 1941 in Sweden, when Essen-Moller decided to count twins who had mental disorders with schizophrenic features concordant with their schizophrenic co-twins (Essen-Moller, 1941). Essen-Moller noted the existence of schizophrenia-like personality traits in the schizophrenics' co-twins and found concordance rates of 64% for MZ pairs and 15% for DZ pairs. Early twin studies conducted in England and Japan found similar concordance rates (65% vs. 14% and 59% vs. 15%, respectively; Inouye, 1972; Slater, 1953). In addition, both studies found an excess of traits such as aloofness, lack of feeling, and suspiciousness in the unaffected MZ co-twins and first-degree relatives of schizophrenic probands.

The study of schizophrenia spectrum disorders gained momentum in 1963 when Kety and his colleagues began the first large-scale adoption study of schizophrenia in Denmark (Kety, Rosenthal, Wender, & Schulsinger, 1968). The Danish Adoption Study was composed of a series of studies designed to gather information about which disorders occurred more frequently among the biological relatives of schizophrenic adoptees than among the biological relatives of control adoptees. In the first, or Copenhagen, sample, Kety looked at hospital records and conducted personal interviews with the biological and adoptive relatives of schizophrenic adoptees (Kety et al., 1968; Kety, Rosenthal, Wender, Schulsinger, & Jacobsen, 1975). Rates of latent schizophrenia—a DSM-II (American Psychiatric Association, 1968) disorder based on Bleuler's construct—were significantly elevated in the biological relatives of schizophrenic probands (14.8%) compared to those of control adoptees (0.9%). Rates were low and equal in the adoptive relatives of both the schizophrenic and nonschizophrenic adoptees. These findings provided empirical support for a schizophrenic-like, nonpsychotic disorder found in the relatives of individuals with schizophrenia. Moreover, the use of an adoption design provided support for Bleuler's idea that latent schizophrenia was related to schizophrenia itself through genetic factors. In 1975, Kety began gathering information for adoptees who lived throughout the rest of Denmark. The findings gathered from this Provincial sample replicated those of the Copenhagen sample (Kety, Rosenthal, Wender, Schulsinger, & Jacobsen, 1978). When both samples were combined to form a National sample, the rates of latent schizophrenia in the biological relatives of schizophrenic probands was 10.8%, whereas the corresponding rates in the biological relatives of control probands was 1.7% (Kety et al., 1994).

The results of Kety's studies were used to develop empirically based diagnostic criteria for DSM-III schizophrenia spectrum disorders (American Psychiatric Association, 1980; Spitzer, Endicott, & Gibbon, 1979). These included the diagnosis of "schizotypal personality disorder" (SPD), an operationalization of the schizophrenic-like, nonpsychotic syndrome of latent schizophrenia. (The term "schizotypal" was chosen because it means "like schizophrenia.") These criteria were later reapplied blindly to the same samples, and

Kety's original results based on global diagnoses were confirmed. For example, DSM-III schizotypal personality disorder was found in 13.6% of the biological relatives of schizophrenic adoptees in the Copenhagen sample, versus 2.0% of the biological relatives of control adoptees (Kendler, Gruenberg, & Strauss, 1981). The application of DSM-III criteria to the relatives of probands in the National sample resulted in rates of schizophrenia spectrum disorders (defined as schizophrenia; schizoaffective disorder, mainly schizophrenic subtype; and schizotypal and paranoid personality disorders) of 23.7% in the first-degree biological relatives of adoptees with DSM-III schizophrenia and 4.7% in the first-degree biological relatives of controls (Kendler et al., 1994). Lowing, Mirsky, and Pereira (1983) found that 15.4% of the adopted-away offspring of schizophrenic mothers in the sample had DSM-III SPD, compared with 7.7% of the adopted-away offspring of controls.

The Danish Adoption Study was the first to provide empirical evidence for the increased prevalence of a less severe, nonpsychotic, genetically related form of schizophrenia. Subsequent family, twin, and adoption studies have confirmed the presence of SPD in the families of schizophrenic individuals (Baron, Gruen, Rainer, et al., 1985; Frangos, Athanassenas, Tsitourides, Katsanou, & Alexandrakou, 1985; Gershon et al., 1988; Kendler, McGuire, Gruenberg, O'Hare, et al., 1993). Kendler & Gardner (1997) found that odds ratios (OR) for SPD in the first-degree biological relatives of schizophrenic probands were homogeneous across three independent family studies and computed a common OR estimate of 5.0 for SPD. Higher rates of schizophrenia were also found among the relatives of probands with SPD, compared with the relatives of psychiatric and normal controls (Baron, Gruen, Anis, & Lord, 1985; Battaglia et al., 1991; Lenzenweger & Loranger, 1989; Schulz et al., 1986; Siever et al., 1990). Researchers now seek to further clarify the nature of SPD by determining its heritable components, that is, which of the components of SPD are seen more frequently in the biological relatives of individuals with schizophrenia and which are affected by genetic influences common to schizophrenia. It appears that SPD may be a heterogeneous category, that is, only part of the disorder defined by DSM-IV (American Psychiatric Association, 1994) may be heritable. In particular, family, twin, and adoption studies suggest that, among schizotypal criteria, only eccentricity, affective constriction, and excessive social anxiety are genetically related to schizophrenia (Torgersen, 1994).

Analyses of interviews of the biological relatives of schizophrenic probands from the Danish Adoption Study found that these relatives were more likely to describe themselves as having been withdrawn or antisocial as children (Ingraham, 1995; Kendler, Gruenberg, & Strauss, 1982). Three traits were observed more frequently among the biological relatives of schizophrenic probands: suspiciousness, flat affect, and withdrawn behavior. Psychotic-like features (e.g., cognitive and perceptual distortions) were not observed. Subsequent twin studies have replicated these findings. In a series of studies conducted with the Norwegian Twin Registry, Torgersen found a higher frequency of SPD among MZ co-twins of probands with SPD compared with DZ co-twins (33% vs. 4%), as well as increased rates of SPD in the MZ co-twins of schizophrenics compared with DZ co-twins (20% vs. 14.8%) (Torgersen, 1984; Torgersen, Onstad, Skre, Edvardsen, & Kringlen, 1993). Personal interviews showed that feelings of isolation, social anxiety, and inadequacy were common among the co-twins of schizophrenic probands and that inappropriate affect and odd speech and behavior also were common among first-degree relatives. Psychotic-like phenomena were absent once again. Torgersen et al. (1993) concluded that schizotypal features were genetically transmitted but that the only heritable aspects of SPD were the affect-constricted and eccentric features. Further evidence that the negative symptom criteria of SPD may be heritable independently of the positive symptom criteria comes from Kendler, Ochs, Gorman, and Hewitt's (1991) factor analysis of schizotypal symptoms in normal MZ twins. The authors' factor analyses revealed two independent dimensions of schizotypy, one related to the social withdrawal and deficit symptoms, the other related to the positive, or psychotic-like, symptoms. Thus findings from behavior genetic studies of SPD seem to consistently point to the negative symptom criteria of SPD as those responsible for its familial association with, and genetic relatedness to, schizophrenia. Negative symptoms may be a more direct reflection, or true manifestation, of the underlying schizophrenic genotype—an interpretation consistent with Bleuler's early descriptions.

Evidence that supports the inclusion of DSM-IV disorders other than SPD in the schizophrenia spectrum is less consistent. Elevated rates of paranoid personality disorder (PPD) were found in the biological relatives of schizophrenic adoptees, compared to controls in the Copenhagen sample of the Danish Adoption Study (6% vs. 1%; Kendler, Masterson, Ungaro, & Davis, 1984). In contrast, Lowing et al. (1983) did not find a higher frequency of PPD in the adopted-away offspring of schizophrenic, compared to control parents, but did find increased rates of schizoid personality disorder (10% vs. 3%). The relationships between these personality disorders and schizophrenia may be an artifact, however. Both PPD and schizoid personality disorder are defined by a subset of SPD criteria; thus diagnoses of either may be coextensive with a diagnosis of SPD (Parnas et al., 1993). The literature on psychotic disorders is also inconsistent. Several family studies have found higher rates of schizoaffective disorder among the relatives of schizophrenic than among control probands (Gershon et al., 1988; Maier, Hallmayer, Minges, & Lichtermann, 1990; Kendler, McGuire, Gruenberg, Spellman, et al., 1993). Some evidence for a familial relationship between nonaffective psychoses and schizophrenia also exists, and studies found increased rates of schizophreniform disorder, delusional disorder, and/or atypical psychosis in the families of schizophrenic versus control probands (Baron, Gruen, Rainer, et al., 1985; Gershon et al., 1988; Kendler, Gruenberg, & Tsuang, 1985; Kendler, McGuire, Gruenberg, Spellman, et al., 1993; Maier et al., 1990). Kendler and Gardner (1997) computed a common OR estimate of 4.0 for "other non-affective psychoses" across three independent family studies. These included the DSM-III/DSM-III-R (American Psychiatric Association, 1987) categories of schizophreniform disorder, schizoaffective disorder, delusional disorder, and atypical psychosis (psychosis not otherwise specified).

In sum, the boundaries of the schizophrenia spectrum extend from schizophrenia-like personality traits such as poor social functioning, odd thoughts and behavior, and suspiciousness at one end, to the full-blown disorder of classical schizophrenia at the other. Included within these boundaries are the DSM-IV disorders of SPD, possibly PPD, and probably several other nonschizophrenic psychotic disorders (Kendler & Gruenberg, 1984). Many family studies have been conducted to establish that a familial association exists between these disorders and schizophrenia, but fewer twin and adoption studies have been conducted to investigate the role that genetic influences play in their etiology. As stated earlier, different models exist to explain the genetic transmission of the liability to schizophrenia. For example, some researchers believe that a single major gene specific to schizophrenia exists, and that this liability will be expressed in alternative phenotypes, depending upon the presence or absence of other genetic potentiators and environmental stressors (Meehl, 1962). An influential alternative model is the multifactorial polygenic threshold model (Gottesman & Shields, 1982). According to this view, there is no single gene primarily responsible for the liability to schizophrenia. Rather, a large number of vulnerability genes and environmental influences exist that contribute to an individual's liability, and a liability threshold must be surpassed for an individual to manifest the disorder. Thus, different disorder phenotypes will be expressed by surpassing successively higher severity thresholds. Mixed models combine features of both of them. For example, a single major gene may operate in some families in addition to the polygenic effects that may be primarily responsible for the genetic liability to schizophrenia (Morton & MacLean, 1974). Alternatively, several genes may be necessary but not sufficient to trigger vulnerability (Gottesman, 1991). A better understanding through twin and adoption studies of the way spectrum disorders are genetically related to schizophrenia, combined with knowledge about the way these disorders aggregate in families, will help researchers decide which, if any, of these models may be correct. Knowledge of the genetic model underlying schizophrenia and the schizophrenia spectrum disorders can help significantly in guiding molecular genetic studies of these disorders.

# MOOD AND ANXIETY DISORDERS

The results of recent twin studies of mood and anxiety disorder symptoms across the life span suggest some differences in the etiology of these symptoms in childhood versus adulthood. Only a few twin studies hav been conducted with children and adolescents, so we will begin with a review of the more extensive adult findings. In the final section of the chapter, we discuss the potential theoretical implications of discrepancies between the child and adult findings concerning mood and anxiety disorder symptoms in terms of genotype-environment correlation. In this section, we will review univariate findings (concerning the etiology of a single symptom dimension) before discussing multivariate findings (concerning common etiological influences acting on two or more different symptom dimensions) for mood and anxiety disorders.

## Univariate Studies of Mood and Anxiety Disorder Symptoms

**Adults.** Kendler, Heath, Martin, & Eaves (1986) examined the causes of individual differences in anxiety and depressive symptoms in adults recruited from a large, nationwide twin registry in Australia. Symptoms of anxiety and depression were assessed by using a self-report questionnaire, the Delusions-Symptoms-States Inventory (DSSI). The authors found that a model including only genetic and nonshared environmental influences provided a satisfactory fit to the observed data, and the heritability for most symptoms ranged from .33 to .46. Several studies have been based on assessments of DSM-III, DSM-III-R, or DSM-IV affective disorders. In a sample of adult female twins recruited from a large population-based twin registry in Virginia, Kendler and colleagues (1992b) found that liability to major depression was moderately heritable ($h^2 = .20$ to $.45$), and the remainder of the variance in liability was once again attributable to nonshared environmental influences. The authors later conducted analyses on follow-up data from the same sample that allowed them to control for unreliability of measurement and obtained an increased heritability estimate of around 70% for major depression (Kendler et al., 1993b). This suggests that a sizable proportion of the nonshared environmental influences in the earlier study was due to measurement error rather than specific environmental risk factors. Kendler et al. (1994) extended these findings to twins and to non-twin relatives recruited from the American Association of Retired Persons as well as the Virginia Twin Registry and found that additive genetic influences explained 30–37% of the variance in symptoms, with no evidence for shared environmental influences.

Consistent with these results from unselected samples, McGuffin, Katz, Watkins, and Rutherford (1996) obtained moderate estimates of the heritability for unipolar depression by using a variety of diagnostic criteria in a selected sample of hospitalized adult probands and their co-twins, where $h^2$ ranged from .48 to .75. Once again, the authors found no evidence for shared environmental influences. The higher heritability obtained in the McGuffin et al. study may be due to sampling characteristics because hospitalized probands are more likely to be severely ill than individuals who manifest depressive symptoms in an unselected sample.

Kendler et al. (1996) were interested in determining whether various alternative manifestations of depression would show different etiologies. They performed a latent class analysis of the DSM-III-R symptoms of major depression in a population-based sample of female twins. The analysis yielded three classes of clinically significant depressive symptoms, which were termed "severe typical depression" (distinguished by frequent weight loss and decreased appetite rather than weight gain and increased appetite, insomnia rather than hypersomnia, and frequent co-occurrence of anxiety and panic), "mild typical depression" (characterized by similar but less severe symptoms than "severe typical depression"), and "atypical depression" (characterized by frequent hypersomnia, increased appetite, and weight gain, associated with co-occurring bulimia). They found that among twins concordant for major depression, concordance for the specific subtype was more common than would be predicted by chance. The concordance for specific subtype of depression was also greater in monozygotic than in dizygotic twins, suggesting a genetic basis for the observed patterns of symptoms. They concluded that depression is not etiologically homogeneous but may consist of subtypes that have differing etiologies.

Finally, several studies examined the causes of affective illness defined broadly (including both depressive disorders and bipolar disorders). McGuffin and Katz (1989) reanalyzed twin data previously reported by Bertelsen, Harvald, and Hauge (1977) and obtained a high heritability of .86, with a very modest contribution of environmental influences ($c^2 = .07$; $e^2 = .07$). Kendler, Pedersen, Neale, and Mathé (1995) assessed genetic and environmental influences on affective illness (defined using DSM-III-R diagnostic criteria as either major depression [with or without history of mania] or bipolar illness) in a combined hospital-ascertained and population-based (i.e., unselected) Swedish

sample. The hospital-ascertained sample was combined with the unselected sample to increase the number of participants with rare diagnoses such as bipolar illness without sacrificing the greater generalizability afforded by including nonreferred participants (Kendler et al., 1995). The authors did not find that the estimated heritability of affective illness (either bipolar or unipolar illness) differed between the hospital-ascertained and population-ascertained samples. They found that liability to major depression (with or without mania) was attributable primarily to genetic influences ($h^2 = .60$) and the remaining liability variance was attributable to nonshared environmental influences and measurement error. Potential explanations for the higher heritability found in this study, compared with the results obtained by Kendler et al. (1992b), include the older average age of subjects in the Swedish study, the use of questionnaire versus interview-based assessment, and possible population heterogeneity in the variance component estimates. Liability to bipolar illness was more highly heritable ($h^2 = .79$) than liability to major depression, and liability to affective illness (defined as either bipolar or unipolar illness) was intermediate in heritability ($h^2 = .64$), the remaining liability variance in all cases was attributable solely to nonshared environmental influences and measurement error.

Univariate behavior genetic findings for anxiety disorders suggest a pattern of causal influences similar to those found for depression. Several large-scale behavior genetic studies of anxiety disorders in adults have been conducted using DSM-III or DSM-III-R diagnostic criteria. Kendler, Neale, Kessler, Heath, & Eaves (1992a), using data from the same Virginia-based, adult female sample described before, conducted model-fitting analyses on liability to DSM-III generalized anxiety disorder and reported that the best fitting model included additive genetic and nonshared environmental influences, and about 30% of the variance in liability was attributable to additive genetic influences. The same authors (Kendler et al., 1993a) conducted univariate analyses of liability to DSM-III-R panic disorder in women from the same twin sample. Results were similar to those for generalized anxiety disorder, that is, a model including additive genetic and nonshared environmental influences provided the best fit to the data for most definitions of panic disorder, and genetic influences accounted for about 30% of the variance in liability. In the case of phobias, Kendler et al. (1992d) reported that liability to any phobia (agoraphobia, social phobia, animal phobia, or situational phobia) in women drawn from the Virginia population-based sample was attributable solely to additive genetic and nonshared environmental influences, and the heritability was .32. The only phobia subtype for which shared environmental influences contributed significantly to liability was situational phobias (e.g., phobias of tunnels, bridges, and airplanes). No significant heritable influences were found for this phobia subtype. Shared environmental influences, it was estimated, accounted for 27% of the variance in liability to situational phobias, and the remaining variance was attributable solely to nonshared environmental influences. Heritabilities were moderate (and similar) for agoraphobia ($h^2$ = .39), social phobia ($h^2$ = .32), and animal phobias ($h^2$ = .32).

Univariate behavior genetic analyses have suggested that both depression and anxiety are moderately heritable in adults. Expressed differently, these findings suggest that nonshared environmental influences account for at least half of the variance in symptoms of anxiety and depression in adults. Bear in mind, however, that part of the nonshared environmental portion of the variance represents measurement errors; therefore, when estimates are corrected for unreliability of measurement, heritability estimates may increase somewhat (e.g., Kendler et al., 1993b). Still, environmental influences almost always account for a significant portion (usually at least a third) of the population variance in symptoms of these disorders, even after correction for measurement error. There is little evidence, however, that shared environmental influences are an important source of variation in adults' symptoms.

**Children and Adolescents.** There have been several univariate twin studies of depressive symptoms in childhood. Eley and Stevenson (1997; see Eley, 1997) obtained evidence for a small-to-moderate effect of shared environmental influences (accounting for about 20% of the variance) as well as additive genetic influences (accounting for about a third of the variance) in children's self-reported depressive symptoms. Thapar and McGuffin (1994) found that the presence of shared environmental influences on depressive symptoms depended upon the age of the children. In younger children (age 8–11), variation in symptoms

was attributable predominantly to shared environmental influences ($c^2$ = .77), whereas in adolescents (ages 11–16), shared environmental influences could be dropped from the model, and additive genetic influences, it was found, accounted for the majority (70–80%) of the variance in symptoms. Eaves et al. (1997) also found modest shared environmental influences (as well as moderate genetic influences) on depressive symptoms, but only when children's self-report was used ($h^2$ = .15–.16; $c^2$ = .14–.26). When parent report was used, depressive symptoms in children were highly heritable, and there was no evidence for shared environmental influences ($h^2$ = .54–.66). Finally, Rende, Plomin, Reiss, & Hetherington (1993) found shared environmental influences for extreme depression scores in adolescents ($c^2$ = .44) and no significant genetic influence on extreme scores. In contrast, these authors found genetic influences, but not shared environmental influences, for individual differences in the normal range of depressive symptoms ($h^2$ = .34).

With regard to anxiety symptoms, Thapar and McGuffin (1995) reported that variation in parent ratings of children's anxiety symptoms (using the Revised Children's Manifest Anxiety Scale) could be accounted for by additive genetic and nonshared environmental influences, and that the heritability was .59. In contrast, when child report was used, additive genetic influences could be dropped from the model, and shared environmental influences accounted for 55% of the variance. Topolski et al. (1997) reported that shared environmental influences, but not additive genetic influences, substantially influenced liability to DSM-III-R separation anxiety disorder (SAD) in children ages 8–16 using children's self-report ($c^2$ = .40). For overanxious disorder (OAD, a DSM-III-R diagnosis that corresponds to DSM-IV GAD), on the other hand, they found that shared environmental influences could be dropped from the model without a significant reduction in fit, whereas additive genetic influences, it was estimated, contributed moderately to the variance in liability ($h^2$ = .37).

The finding of shared environmental influences on children's anxiety symptoms is not limited to self-report data, however. Slutske et al. (1996) reported that genetic and shared environmental influences each accounted for roughly half of the variance ($h^2$ = .52; $c^2$ = .38) in lifetime DSM-IV SAD symptoms in adolescent girls using mother report. Similarly, Feigon et al. (1997a) found moderate genetic and shared environmental influences on parent-rated DSM-III-R SAD symptoms among nonreferred Australian twin children ages 4–18 ($h^2 = .46$; $c^2 = .22$). The same authors (Feigon et al., 1997b) also found moderate shared environmental, as well as genetic, influences on DSM-III-R avoidant disorder symptoms ($h^2 = .41$; $c^2 = .52$) and somatic complaints ($h^2 = .45$; $c^2 = .37$) in children. Eley and Stevenson (1997) found that shared environmental influences accounted for about a third of the variance in children's anxiety symptoms using several self-report scales, and about 10% of the variance was due to genetic influences. Feigon and Waldman (1998) obtained similar estimates of genetic and environmental influences on mother reports of SAD symptoms ($h^2 = .58$; $c^2 = .27$) and GAD symptoms ($h^2 = .36$; $c^2 = .35$) but did not find any shared environmental influences on social phobia symptoms ($h^2 = .67$) in twins aged 5–18 recruited from the Georgia Twin Registry. The authors also found significant etiological heterogeneity due to sex in the case of SAD and evidence for shared environmental influences on girls' but not boys' symptoms. Genetic influences on SAD symptoms were greater in boys than girls ($h^2 = .83$ and .49, respectively).

In contrast to other findings that support a substantial shared environmental contribution to children's anxiety symptoms, Eaves et al. (1997) did not find evidence for shared environmental influences on symptoms of either DSM-III-R SAD or OAD in children ages 8–16. In their sample, additive genetic influences, it was estimated, accounted for about 75% of the variance in SAD symptoms for girls ages 8–16 when parent report was used, but there was no substantial familial correlation among boys. When child report was used, the heritability estimates were modest in boys ($h^2 = .19$) and girls ($h^2 = .31$), but there was still no evidence for shared environmental influences in either sex. For OAD, they found moderate additive genetic influences in both boys and girls ($h^2 = .30–.66$). Surprisingly, in contrast to the results for SAD and OAD, shared environmental influences were moderate on a self-report, composite measure of global anxiety symptoms in boys ($c^2 = .33$).

In contrast to the failure to find appreciable shared environmental influences on mood and anxiety, disorder symptoms in adults, the results from several twin studies suggest that shared envi-

ronmental influences, as well as additive genetic influences and nonshared environmental influences, contribute moderately to anxiety and mood symptoms in children (collectively termed the childhood internalizing disorders). The finding of shared environmental influences on children's internalizing symptoms is not entirely consistent, however, with heterogeneity across diagnostic categories, parent versus child informant, and variables such as age and sex (see Feigon, Waldman, Levy, & Hay, 1997b; Feigon & Waldman, 1998). An important caveat is also that rater effects, such as the tendency for parents to contrast their DZ twins when rating their characteristics, may lead to biased heritability and shared environmental influence estimates in children and adolescents. In future studies, these methodological issues and discrepant findings will need to be addressed by using models that incorporate information from multiple raters. With respect to the generalizability of the findings reviewed, it is worth nothing that few studies of anxiety and mood disorders in children have employed DSM diagnoses based upon strict diagnostic criteria (although most of the studies reported here assessed DSM-III or DSM-III-R symptoms), and most have been based on self- or parent-report questionnaires rather than on diagnostic interviews (exceptions are the studies by Eaves et al., 1997, and Topolski et al., 1997, in which assessments were both interview- and questionnaire-based).

## Multivariate Behavior Genetic Studies of Mood and Anxiety Disorder Symptoms

Most multivariate behavior genetic contributions to the classification of mood and anxiety disorders have been based on three general approaches: (1) split an existing diagnostic category into subtypes and examine differences in the causes of the resulting subtypes; (2) look for common causes that cut across the symptoms of several diagnostic categories, using multivariate behavior genetic methods; or (3) combine the first two approaches (i.e., break down a given diagnostic category into clusters of symptoms and then examine their common causes) to determine whether the etiologies of various symptom clusters may be partially overlapping and partially independent.

One example of the splitting approach is the

study by Kendler et al. (1996; see earlier), who reported that genetic and environmental influences on various subtypes of depressive illness appeared to have different etiologies. Research with adults suggests that genes may act in a nonspecific way to confer risk for a variety of mood and anxiety syndromes, and the particular syndrome manifested depends either on the degree of genetic risk (e.g., as indexed by number of ill relatives) or on individual-specific, nonshared environmental influences. On the other hand, a few studies (reviewed later) suggest that the mood and anxiety syndromes are etiologically heterogeneous, and different sets of genes and/or environmental risk factors influence different patterns of symptoms within a diagnostic grouping. In this way, behavior genetic research can contribute to the development of an etiologically based classification of psychopathological syndromes. Following, we review multivariate behavior genetic studies that have contributed to our understanding of the boundaries between different mood and anxiety disorders by examining their common and unique causes.

**Adults.** Kendler et al. (1992c) reported that additive genetic influences largely explained the observed covariation of symptoms of GAD and major depression in women and were entirely shared between the two disorders; nonshared environmental influences accounted for the remaining unique liability variance for these disorders. The finding of a common genetic factor for GAD and major depression (with no unique genetic influences) was replicated by Roy, Neale, Pedersen, Mathé, and Kendler (1995) in an extension to a mixed male and female adult sample. Kendler et al. (1993c) also found that the observed covariation of major depression and phobia symptoms in women was largely attributable to additive genetic influences and that nonshared environmental influences contributed to the unique variance in liability to each of the two disorders. When the same authors investigated sources of overlap among phobias (agoraphobia, social phobia, animal phobia, and situational phobia; Kendler et al., 1992d), they found that the familial aggregation of these phobias in women could be explained by common genetic and nonshared environmental influences and that additional unique genetic and nonshared environmental influences contributed to the variance in liability to each of the specific subtypes of phobia. For most of the phobias (except animal

phobia), however, the common nonshared environmental factor contributed a greater share of the liability variance than the common genetic factor. Using the same Virginia-based twin sample, Kendler et al. (1995) examined the causes of comorbidity among panic disorder, phobias, GAD, major depression, alcoholism, and bulimia nervosa in women. They reported that the genetic influences responsible for the overlap between major depression and GAD in female twins appeared to be distinct from the genetic influences responsible for the overlap between panic disorder and phobias. Based on the finding of more than one shared genetic factor, the authors speculated that the anxiety disorders may be etiologically heterogeneous. Although provocative, this hypothesis seems hard to reconcile with the earlier findings by this group on common genetic influences on depression and phobias (Kendler et al., 1993c).

Additional evidence for a genetic basis to the overlap of anxiety and depressive symptoms comes from studies using the Australian National Health and Medical Research Council twin Registry, a nationwide, volunteer registry. Jardine, Martin, and Henderson (1984) found that genetic influences accounted for about 50–60% of the observed covariance between Neuroticism (a personality dimension associated with risk for mood and anxiety disorders), symptoms of anxiety, and symptoms of depression, and that the remaining covariation was attributable to nonshared environmental influences and/or measurement error. Kendler, Heath, Martin, and Eaves (1987) reanalyzed the same data (focusing on anxiety and depressive symptoms but not Neuroticism), and concluded that common genetic influences largely-explained the covariance between anxiety symptoms and depressive symptoms, and that nonshared environmental influences primarily contributed to the unique variance in anxiety and depressive symptoms.

The relationship between unipolar affective disorder and bipolar affective disorder has also been examined using twin data. Kendler, Pedersen, Neale, and Mathé (1995) reported that their data were consistent with a multiple threshold model in which the two forms of affective disorder are alternative manifestations of a single continuum of liability, rather than separate phenomena with distinct causes, and that bipolar disorder represents a more severe point on the continuum. Karkowski and Kendler (1997) analyzed data from the Virginia-based female twin sample described earlier and reported that the data supported the conceptualization of unipolar and bipolar affective disorder as points of differing severity along the same continuum of illness (i.e., the two disorders have common causes). The application of the multiple threshold model to the bipolar-unipolar distinction is also consistent with two other pieces of data: (1) epidemiological studies showing that bipolar disorder occurs much less frequently in the population than unipolar depressive disorder, and (2) family studies showing a higher rate of affective disorders in the relatives of bipolar versus unipolar probands (Tsuang & Faraone, 1996). Both the greater familial loading of affective disorders in bipolar patients compared to unipolar patients and the lower population prevalence of bipolar compared to unipolar disorder are consistent with a model in which bipolar disorder is only manifest when a higher threshold of liability (resulting from a high degree of genetic and/or environmental risk) is surpassed.

Evidence from multivariate behavior genetic analyses in adult twin samples suggests that familial causes contribute substantially to the diagnostic overlap (or symptom covariation) among the anxiety and depressive disorders. In addition, the results of these studies suggest that the familial causes underlying the covariation among anxiety and depressive symptoms in adults are largely or entirely genetic. Now we review the results of the few multivariate behavior genetic studies of mood and anxiety disorders in children and adolescents to examine the extent to which the causes of comorbidity are similar to those found in adults.

**Children and Adolescents.** In contrast to the growing body of data on genetic and environmental influences on the covariation between anxiety and depressive symptoms in adults, very few multivariate behavior genetic studies of similar disorders or symptoms have been conducted with children and adolescents. Recently, two multivariate behavior genetic studies examined the causes of covariation among symptoms of various internalizing disorders in children. Eley and Stevenson (1997; see Eley, 1997) found that genetic influences accounted for 80% of the covariation between children's reports of anxiety and depressive symptoms and that shared environmental influences explained the remaining 20% of the covariation. Feigon et al. (1997b) examined the causes of covariation among three different types of anxiety disorder symptoms (separation anxiety symp-

toms, avoidant disorder symptoms, and somatic complaints) and found that the covariation among the three types of symptoms was largely attributable to common environmental influences (primarily common shared environmental influences). There was no evidence for common genetic influences on symptom covariation, that is, genetic influences contributed only to the variance that was unique to each of the three types of symptoms.

Thus, studies obtained evidence for common shared environmental influences on symptom overlap, although the magnitude of these influences differed greatly between the two studies. An obvious difference, of course, is the finding of substantial common genetic influences on symptom overlap in Eley and Stevenson's but not Feigon et al.'s study. Several differences in design may have contributed to the differences in the findings of these two studies. One difference is that Eley and Stevenson (1997) were interested in the causes of covariation between anxiety and depressive symptoms, whereas Feigon et al.'s (1997b) study was concerned with the causes of covariation among various types of anxiety symptoms. A second difference is that Feigon et al. used parent ratings of symptoms and Eley and Stevenson used child self-report measures. Both studies, however, support the notion that familial causes (whether genetic or shared environmental) are likely to be most important in accounting for the overlap among anxiety and depression disorders in children, as well as in adults. Additional data from new twin samples are needed to clarify the causal mechanisms that underlie comorbidity between anxiety and depressive disorders in children and adolescents.

# CHILDHOOD DISRUPTIVE BEHAVIOR DISORDERS

In this section, behavior genetic studies that examined childhood externalizing disorders (i.e., the disruptive behavior disorders attention deficit hyperactivity disorder [ADHD], oppositional defiant disorder [ODD], and conduct disorder [CD]) will be reviewed. ADHD is characterized by symptoms of inattention, hyperactivity, and impulsivity. Although the distinction between inattention, hyperactivity, and impulsivity, on the one hand, and aggression and conduct problems, on the other, was at one time controversial (see Barkley, 1982; Rutter, 1983), recent reviews and studies (e.g., Hinshaw, 1987; Loney & Milich, 1982) have provided ample support for their discriminant validity. The essential feature of ODD is defiant, hostile behavior toward authority (e.g., parents and teachers), whereas the essential feature of CD is serious violation of age-appropriate norms and rules. In a review of studies that examined the relationship between ODD and CD, Loeber, Lahey, and Thomas (1991) concluded that ODD and CD are developmentally related but clearly distinct and that there are unique covarying groups of ODD and CD symptoms.

## Univariate Behavior Genetic Studies of Childhood Disruptive Behavior Disorders

**ADHD.** The largest family studies of ADHD were conducted by Biederman and his colleagues (e.g., Biederman et al., 1986; Biederman, Faraone, Keenan, Knee, & Tsuang, 1990; Biederman et al., 1992). In general, they found that the first-degree relatives of ADHD probands are at significantly higher risk of ADHD than the first-degree relatives of controls. The risk of ADHD for the relatives of probands increases further when ADHD in the probands is accompanied by CD (Faraone, Biederman, Keenan, & Tsuang, 1991; Faraone, Biederman, Jetton, & Tsuang, 1997).

Adoption studies of ADHD provide evidence that the familiality in ADHD can be attributed largely to genetic influences. Biological parents of hyperactive children are more likely to have been hyperactive themselves as children or to show signs of attentional problems (e.g., slower mean reaction times) than the adoptive parents of hyperactive children (Alberts-Corush, Firestone, & Goodman, 1986; Cantwell, 1975; Morrison & Stewart, 1971). A history of psychiatric problems in their biological parents is also related to increased rates of hyperactivity or ADHD in adoptees (Cadoret & Stewart, 1991; Cunningham, Cadoret, Loftus, & Edwards, 1975).

Goodman and Stevenson (1989) conducted the first large twin study (102 MZ and 111 same-sex DZ twin pairs) of ADHD symptoms and reported heritability estimates that ranged from 32 to 42% ($c^2$ = 12 to 28%; $e^2$ = 40 to 46%) for measures of inattention and 42 to 100% ($c^2$ = 0 to 27%; $e^2$ = 0 to 58%) for measures of hyperactivity. Gilger, Pennington, and DeFries (1992) assessed ADHD

in eighty-one MZ and fifty-two DZ twin pairs using the Diagnostic Interview for Children and Adolescents and found that the probandwise concordance rates were significantly different for MZ (81%) and DZ (29%) twin pairs. Waldman, Rhee, Hay, and Levy (1998) examined DSM-III-R ADHD symptoms in a large population-based twin sample (1034 MZ pairs, 1009 DZ pairs, and 345 sibling pairs) and found that ADHD was influenced mostly by genetics ($h^2$ = .90; $e^2$ = .10).

Edelbrock, Rende, Plomin, and Thompson (1995) examined Child Behavior Checklist (CBCL) attentional problems in ninety-nine MZ and eighty-two DZ twin pairs and found evidence of significant genetic influences but no shared environmental influences ($h^2$ = .66; $e^2$ = .34). Schmitz, Fulker, and Mrazek (1995) and Gjone, Stevenson, and Sundet (1996) also examined CBCL attentional problems in larger samples and found similar results (Schmitz et al., 1995: $h^2$ = .65; $e^2$ = .35 in 66 MZ and 137 DZ twin pairs; Gjone et al., 1996: $h^2$ = .73 to .79; $e^2$ = .21 to .27 in 526 MZ and 389 DZ pairs).

Several studies examined the heritability of extreme levels of activity and inattention (labeled $h^2_g$, following DeFries & Fulker, 1988). Stevenson (1992) examined several measures of inattention and hyperactivity and reported varying levels of $h^2_g$ for inattention (.25 to .76) and for hyperactivity (.16 to .75). Gillis, Gilger, Pennington, and DeFries (1992) and Rhee, Waldman, Hay, and Levy (1999) reported higher $h^2_g$ levels for ADHD symptoms ($h^2_g$ = .98 and .99, respectively). Gjone, Stevenson, and Sundet (1996) reported $h^2_g$ for attention problems by symptom severity and found that $h^2_g$ did not increase as severity increased ($h^2_g$ = .82 for ≥ 0 SD above the mean, $h^2_g$ = .88 for ≥ 0.5 SD above the mean, $h^2_g$ = .86 for ≥ 1.0 SD above the mean, and $h^2_g$ = .77 for ≥ 1.5 SD above the mean).

If the MZ correlation is more than twice the DZ correlation, the presence of nonadditive genetic influences and of contrast effects is a possibility. In some twin studies of ADHD, the DZ correlation was very low or even negative (e.g., Nadder, Silberg, Eaves, Maes, & Meyer, 1998; Silberg et al., 1996; Thapar, Hervas, & McGuffin, 1995). One explanation for extremely low DZ correlations (viz., near-zero or slightly negative) is a contrast effect, that is, raters exaggerating the difference between DZ twin pairs. Another explanation is sibling interaction, where one twin's ADHD level has a direct opposite effect on the other twin's ADHD level. When data from only one rater is used, it is not possible to distinguish between a contrast effect and sibling interaction. Several researchers have examined alternative models testing for the presence of sibling interaction/contrast effects.

Thapar et al. (1995) compared a model positing that hyperactivity is caused by additive genetic influences and nonshared environmental influences (an AE model) to a model which also included a sibling interaction/contrast effect (an AE-B model). The AE-B model ($h^2 = .88$; b = $-.24$) fit significantly better than the AE model, and Thapar et al. interpreted these results as evidence for sibling interaction. Silberg et al. (1996) examined hyperactivity in four groups of children (older boys, older girls, younger boys, younger girls), and also found that an AE-B model was the best fitting model in all four groups ($h^2 = .67$ to .70; $e^2 = .25$ to .32; b = $-.22$ to $-.08$). Nadder et al. (1998) compared models including and excluding the sibling interaction/contrast effect for ADHD symptoms. The AE-B model was the best fitting model, the heritability estimate was 58 to 61%, the nonshared environment estimate was 39 to 42%, and a sibling interaction/contrast effect was $-.13$ to $-.18$, but this model did not fit significantly better than an ADE-B model.

Eaves et al. (1997) examined the issue of possible rater bias by testing for the presence of sibling interaction/contrast effects and by comparing the results of parent and teacher reports of ADHD symptoms. For parent reports, the AE-B model fit better than a model including dominance genetic influences (the ADE model); the heritability estimates after removing contrast effects ranged from .55 to .82, and the magnitude of nonshared environmental influences ranged from .18 to .45 (the magnitude of rater contrast effects ranged from $-.09$ to $-.24$). For teacher reports, the AE model was the best fitting model ($h^2 = .54$ to .62; $e^2 = .38$ to .46), and there was no evidence of significant contrast effects. Because contrast effects were present in parent reports but not in teacher reports, Eaves et al.'s results suggest that the very low DZ correlations are caused by contrast effects rather than sibling interaction. In another recent paper that examined hyperactivity in this sample, Simonoff et al. (1998) were also able to show that such findings are due to rater contrast effects rather than direct sibling interaction because

mother ratings show a contrast effect, whereas teacher ratings show a different form of bias that can be due to either twin confusion (difficulty attributing behavior to the correct child) or to correlated errors.

In the most recent version of the DSM (DSM-IV; American Psychiatric Association, 1994), there are three subtypes of ADHD: predominantly inattentive type, predominantly hyperactive-impulsive type, and the combined type. These three subtypes are based on surpassing the diagnostic thresholds on one or both of the inattention and hyperactivity-impulsivity symptom dimensions underlying DSM-IV ADHD. This is a significant change from the DSM-III-R (American Psychiatric Association, 1987), where ADHD symptoms were viewed as one dimension and a diagnosis of ADHD was given if $\geq 8$ out of 14 symptoms (of inattention, hyperactivity, or impulsivity) were present. This change was based in part on factor analytic evidence that the symptoms of ADHD load on two separate dimensions (inattention-disorganization and hyperactivity-impulsivity; e.g., Lahey et al., 1988; Pelham, Gnagy, Greenslade, & Milich, 1992), as well as on evidence that there are significant differences between children with symptoms of inattention only (e.g., greater academic difficulty; Edelbrock, Costello, & Kessler, 1984) and children with symptoms of both inattention and hyperactivity (e.g., poor peer relationships; Lahey, Schaughency, Strauss, & Frame, 1984).

Given the evidence supporting the distinctiveness of two separate ADHD symptoms dimensions, it is important to examine potential heterogeneity in the etiology of inattention and hyperactivity-impulsivity symptoms. Goodman & Stevenson (1989) calculated separate heritability estimates for inattention and hyperactivity and found lower heritabilities for inattention (32 to 42%) than for hyperactivity (42 to 100%). Unfortunately, inattention and hyperactivity were assessed by using different methods (laboratory measures for inattention and parent or teacher ratings for hyperactivity) and make these results difficult to interpret.

More recently, Sherman, Iacono, and McGue (1997) conducted a behavior genetic study that examined inattention and hyperactivity-impulsivity symptoms separately. A different pattern of results was found for teacher and mother reports. For teachers, the best fitting model for inattention was the ACE model ($h^2 = .39$, $c^2 = .39$, and $e^2 = .22$), whereas for hyperactivity-impulsivity, the AE model provided the best fit ($h^2 = .69$; $e^2 = .31$). For mother reports, the AE model was the best fitting for both inattention ($h^2 = .69$; $e^2 = .31$) and for hyperactivity-impulsivity ($h^2 = .91$; $e^2 = .09$). Sherman et al. also conducted bivariate genetic analyses to examine the magnitude of genetic influences on the co-variation between inattention and hyperactivity-impulsivity symptoms. The covariation between inattention and hyperactivity-impulsivity symptoms was due to genetic influences, shared environmental influences, and nonshared environmental influences ($h^2 = .33$; $c^2 = .45$; $e^2 = .22$) for teacher reports, but there was no evidence of shared environmental influences for mother reports ($h^2 = .86$; $e^2 = .14$). Heath et al. (1996) also examined inattention and hyperactivity separately but reported similar heritability estimates for inattention ($h^2 = .88$; $e^2 = .12$) and for hyperactivity ($h^2 = .89$; $e^2 = .11$) and found a moderate genetic correlation ($r_g = .52$) between inattention and hyperactivity. Waldman, Elder, Levy, and Hay (1996) reported slightly higher heritability levels for hyperactivity-impulsivity ($h^2 = .88$ to $.92$; $e^2 = .08$ to $.12$) than for inattention ($h^2 = .81$ to $.83$; $e^2 = .17$ to $.19$), and a higher genetic correlation ($r_g = .8$) between inattention and hyperactivity-impulsivity.

**ODD and CD.** Compared to the number of studies that examined ADHD and the symptoms of inattention, hyperactivity, and impulsivity, there are fewer behavior genetic studies that have examined ODD or CD symptoms. Many studies have examined related antisocial behavior constructs in children and adolescents such as delinquency (e.g., Rowe, 1983) or aggression (e.g., van den Oord, Verhulst, & Boomsma, 1996), but given the evidence that behavior genetic studies examining different operationalizations of antisocial behavior (e.g., DSM CD diagnostic criteria versus aggression) result in significantly different results (Rhee & Waldman, 1998), the present review will be limited to studies that examined ODD or CD symptoms assessed via DSM criteria.

Several studies examined ODD and CD symptoms as a composite variable, and their results vary. Simonoff et al. (1995) found little evidence of shared environmental influences on ODD/CD ($h^2 = .40$ to $.73$; $c^2 = .00$ to $.03$, $e^2 = .27$ to $.60$). Similarly, Nadder et al. (1998) found that an AE model with no contrast effects was the best fitting model for ODD/CD symptoms ($h^2 = .53$ to $.65$; $e^2 = .35$ to $.47$). In contrast, Silberg et al. (1996)

examined a composite variable of ODD and CD symptoms in four groups of children (i.e., older and younger boys and girls) and found that the ACE model was the best fitting ($h^2 = .25$ to $.66$; $c^2 = .04$ to $.42$; $e^2 = .29$ to $.33$) because it fit significantly better than a model, including sibling interaction/contrast effects.

Several studies conducted behavior genetic studies that examined ODD symptoms without confounding CD symptoms. Eaves et al. (1997) examined mother, father, and child interview data and found that the AE model was the best fitting across informants but that heritability was higher for parent reports ($h^2 = .49$ to $.65$; $e^2 = .36$ to $.51$) than for child reports ($h^2 = .21$ to $.23$; $e^2 = .77$ to $.79$). They found no evidence of sibling interaction/contrast effects. Willcutt, Shyu, Green, and Pennington (1995) found that ODD symptoms were moderately heritable ($h^2 = .55$; $e^2 = .45$), and Waldman, Rhee, Levy, and Hay (1998) found evidence of substantial additive genetic influences ($h^2 = .85$) and minimal shared environmental influences ($c^2 = .01$; $e^2 = .14$) on ODD symptoms.

Studies that examined CD symptoms separately also reported varying results. Willcutt et al. (1995) and Waldman et al. (1998) found similar results for the etiology of CD symptoms, including moderate genetic, shared, and nonshared environmental influences (Willcutt et al., 1995: $h^2 = .34$ to $.38$; $c^2 = .29$ to $.38$; $e^2 = .24$ to $.37$; Waldman et al., 1998: $h^2 = .51$; $c^2 = .34$; $e^2 = .14$), whereas Lyons et al. (1995) reported a lower magnitude of genetic influences ($h^2 = .07$; $c^2 = .31$; $e^2 = .62$). In contrast, Slutske et al. (1997) found no evidence for shared environmental influences on retrospective reports of CD symptoms during childhood or adolescence ($h^2 = .71$; $c^2 = .00$; $e^2 = .29$). Eaves et al. (1997) found different results for mother and father reports of CD symptoms. For mothers' interview data, there was evidence of substantial additive genetic influences ($h^2 = .69$; $e^2 = .31$) and no shared environmental influences for both sexes, whereas for fathers' interview data, the ACE model fit best for both sexes ($h^2 = .27$ to $.58$; $c^2 = .09$ to $.37$; $e^2 = .33$ to $.36$). Eaves et al. found no evidence of sibling interaction/contrast effects across informant and sex.

Several adoption studies (Cadoret, Cain, & Crowe, 1983; Cloninger, Sigvardsson, Bohman, & von Knorring, 1982; Mednick, Gabrielli, & Hutchings, 1983) showed evidence of genotype–environment interaction in criminality. These studies found that adoptees with criminality in both their biological and adoptive parents are more likely to be criminal themselves than those with criminality in either their biological or adoptive parents. Unfortunately, similar studies examining ODD and CD are not available. Future adoption studies should examine genotype–environment interaction in ODD and CD given the evidence suggesting that childhood externalizing behavior and adulthood criminality are substantially related (e.g., Pulkkinen & Pitkänen, 1993; Robins, 1966).

## Multivariate Behavior Genetic Studies of Childhood Disruptive Behavior Disorders

Numerous studies have documented a significant overlap between ADHD, ODD, and CD in both clinical and nonreferred samples. Biederman, Newcorn, and Sprich's (1991) review found that ADHD and CD co-occur in 30 to 50% of children and ADHD and ODD co-occur in a least 35% of children and that this result is consistent across both clinical and epidemiological samples. The considerable phenotypic overlap among these disorders suggests that the disorders share common etiological influences. Several behavior genetic studies have examined the etiology of the overlap among ADHD, ODD, and CD by using multivariate behavior genetic analytic methods.

Nadder et al. (1998) conducted bivariate behavior genetic analyses to examine the covariation between ADHD and ODD/CD symptoms. The best fitting model was an AE-B model that included common additive genetic, nonshared environmental, and contrast effects explaining the covariation between ADHD and ODD/CD symptoms. The genetic correlation between ADHD and ODD/CD symptoms was .50, and the correlation for nonshared environmental influences was .39.

Silberg et al. (1996) also used bivariate behavior genetic analyses to study to covariation between hyperactivity and ODD/CD symptoms. For both younger (8 to 11 years old) and older (12 to 16-year-old) children, the covariation between hyperactivity and ODD/CD symptoms was due predominantly to common genetic influences and small to moderate common nonshared environmental influences. A model that posited a single genetic factor for conduct problems and hyperactivity fit best for the younger children ($r_g = 1.00$; $r_e = .07$ to .08), whereas a model that included common

and specific genetic influences for hyperactivity and ODD/CD fit best for the older children ($r_g = .46$ to .58; $r_e = .23$ to .32).

Willcutt et al. (1995) conducted bivariate behavior genetic analyses for the pairwise combinations of ADHD, ODD, and CD symptoms. They found substantial common genetic influences on the covariation between ADD and ODD symptoms (bivariate $h^2_g = .56$ to .87), but statistically nonsignificant common genetic influences on the covariation between ADD and CD (bivariate $h^2_g = .16$ to .26) and the covariation between ODD and CD (bivariate $h^2_g = .21$ to .22).

Waldman et al. (1998) took a different approach to examine the etiology of the covariation among ADHD, ODD, and CD symptoms simultaneously and conducted a Cholesky decomposition to test whether there are specific genetic and environmental influences on childhood antisocial behavior (i.e., ODD and CD symptoms) that are unique compared to those on ADHD. Waldman et al. found evidence for common additive genetic influences on ADHD, ODD, and CD, a distinct set of common additive genetic influences that affect only ODD and CD, and additive genetic influences on specific only to CD. The only shared environmental influences were common to ODD and CD. The correlations for the additive genetic influences among ADHD, ODD, and CD symptoms were all high ($r_{ADHD.ODD} = .73$; $r_{ADHD.CD} = .82$; $r_{ODD.CD} = .79$), and the correlation for the common shared environmental influences between ODD and CD was 1. The covariance between ADHD and ODD and between ADHD and CD was mostly due to additive genetic influences (93% of the covariance was due to additive genetic influences and 7% to nonshared environmental influences). In contrast, the covariance between ODD and CD was due to additive genetic influences (79%), shared environmental influences (9%), and nonshared environmental influences (12%).

## Conclusions Regarding Behavior Genetic Studies of Childhood Disruptive Behavior Disorders

Despite heterogeneity in the results of the behavior genetic studies of childhood externalizing disorders, several general conclusions can be drawn. First, both ADHD symptoms in the general population and extreme levels of ADHD in selected populations are highly heritable, and there is little evidence of shared environmental influences. Several researchers have found near-zero or slightly negative DZ correlations that suggest the presence of sibling interaction (siblings influencing each other's traits in an opposite direction) or contrast effects (raters exaggerating the difference between twins), rather than nonadditive genetic influences (Thapar et al., 1995; Silberg et al., 1996; Eaves et al., 1997; Nadder et al., 1998; Simonoff et al., 1988). In their comparison of results across multiple informants, Eaves et al. (1997) and Simonoff et al. (1998) provided evidence that the very low DZ correlations for ADHD are most likely the result of rater contrast effects rather than sibling interaction. Most researchers who have conducted behavior genetic studies of ADHD have examined ADHD symptoms as a single dimension rather than examining inattention and hyperactive-impulsive symptoms separately. Given the evidence regarding the classification of ADHD symptoms, more behavior genetic studies examining the etiology of inattention and hyperactivity-impulsivity as two separate dimensions need to be conducted.

The results of behavior genetic studies that examined ODD symptoms separately resemble those for ADHD, and there is substantial additive genetic influences and little evidence of shared environmental influences (Willcutt et al., 1995; Eaves et al., 1997; Waldman et al., 1998). The results for CD symptoms are less consistent, but unlike the results of studies that examined ADHD or ODD symptoms, most researchers found significant shared environmental influences on CD (Willcutt et al., 1995; Eaves et al., 1997; Waldman et al., 1998). All researchers who tested for the presence of contrast effects on ODD or CD symptoms did not find evidence of them (Silberg et al., 1996; Eaves et al., 1997; Nadder et al., 1998). The differing results for genetic and environmental influences on ODD and CD symptoms emphasize the distinctiveness of their etiologies and the importance of examining ODD and CD symptoms separately in future behavior genetic studies.

Several researchers conducted multivariate behavior genetic analyses to examine the etiology of the overlap among ADHD, ODD, and CD (Nadder et al., 1998; Silberg et al., 1996; Waldman et al., 1998; Willcutt et al., 1995). In general, these studies found substantial overlap between the genetic influences on ADHD and the genetic influences on ODD and CD. Given that these genetic correlations are not equal to 1, however, there is also evidence of genetic influences that act specifically on ADHD, ODD, and CD symptoms.

# FUTURE DIRECTIONS

## Genetic and Environmental Influences on Normal Range Variation and on the Disordered Extreme

An emerging topic in behavior genetic studies of psychopathology is whether genetic and environmental influences are similar across the range of symptoms as for the disordered extreme, or whether the etiology of normal range variation in the trait(s) relevant to a disorder is the same as the etiology of the disorder itself. Behavior genetic methods are beginning to be used to test contrasting models of psychopathology that regard disorders as merely the extreme of normal functioning, as opposed to categorically distinct entities. Several behavior genetic techniques have been developed to address this issue, and each of those techniques does so slightly differently. For example, one can use a multiple regression approach to test whether the genetic and environmental influences on symptoms of a disorder increase or decrease with increasing symptom levels. One can also use model fitting techniques to test whether the magnitude of genetic and environmental influences—and the best fitting etiological model—for symptoms of a disorder are the same as those on the diagnosis. The most commonly used method to address such questions is a regression-based method (DeFries & Fulker, 1988) which tests whether the heritability of the extreme condition (i.e., $h^2_g$), often a diagnosis, differs from the heritability of normal range variation of symptoms in the population (i.e., $h^2$). Unfortunately, the test of $h^2_g - h^2$ tends to be very low in statistical power, as pointed out by the authors (DeFries & Fulker, 1988), and thus may suggest that the etiology of normal range variation in symptoms is the same as that of the disordered extreme, even in the presence of sizable differences in the two heritabilities. Hopefully, researchers will begin to use a diversity of behavior genetic methods to address the differential etiology issue. Thus, although there is considerable interest in the use of behavior genetic methods to address such questions, a number of technical problems and conceptual issues in these analyses need to be resolved before they yield clear answers to the classificatory issues raised before.

## Inclusion of Specific Environmental and Endophenotypic Variables in Behavior Genetic Models

Standard behavior genetic analyses represent genetic and environmental influences as unspecified, anonymous, or "black box" variables (Kendler, 1993). Kendler (1993) notes that the statistical power to detect shared environmental influences is low in such standard models, whereas incorporating specified environmental variables within a behavior genetic model increases the power to detect such influences if they are present. Accordingly, behavior genetic research has begun to incorporate specific environmental measures to detect the effects of these variables against a background of multiple genetic and environmental influences. Perhaps the most widely cited example of this approach is one that is relevant to the etiology of depression and anxiety disorders in adults. The results of standard behavior genetic analyses of twin data, reviewed earlier, typically have not suggested any significant role for shared environmental influences in the etiology of adults' mood and anxiety disorder symptoms. Kendler, Neale, Kessler, Heath, and Eaves (1992e) demonstrated a statistically significant effect of childhood parental loss (i.e., separation or death) on liability to DSM-III-R major depression, GAD, phobias, and panic disorder in adult females, against a background of other (anonymous) genetic and environmental risk factors. Nonetheless, the estimated relative magnitude of this influence in explaining variation in liability to mood and anxiety disorders in adulthood was small (accounting for 4.9% of the variance in liability to panic disorder, 2.9% of the variance in liability to phobias, 2.5% of the variance in liability to GAD, and 1.6% of the variance in liability to major depression in the population of women studied).

Thus, this study represents a specific example of a more general research design, namely, including specific, putative causal mechanisms within multivariate behavior genetic models. This extended behavior genetic design is appropriate for including many different types of putative causal variables (e.g., perinatal birth complications, measures of executive functions, psychopathological measures, specific family and/or neighborhood environmental variables) within behavior genetic models. Findings from these studies can establish whether the relationship of such putative causal variables to the disorder is due primarily to common genetic or common environmental influences. These analyses can be useful for testing whether these putative causal variables represent *endophenotypes* that may be closer to the underlying genetic and environmental influences than the disorders themselves. Thus, another way to view such analyses is that they can help elaborate the specific causal mechanisms for a disorder that are captured by the broad and abstract genetic and environmental variance components that emerge from behavior genetic analyses. Another putative causal mechanism that may be included in behavior genetic models is specific candidate genes that are hypothesized to play some causal role in a disorder. With this in mind, we briefly discuss burgeoning molecular genetic studies of psychopathology in the next section.

## Molecular Genetic Studies of Psychopathology

Molecular genetic studies of most major forms of psychopathology have become a major area of contemporary etiological research. Approaches to finding genes that underlie psychiatric disorders have included both association studies of the role of specific candidate genes, as well as genome scans of anonymous DNA markers by using linkage analysis. Generally speaking, such studies have produced mixed findings for almost all psychiatric disorders; some studies report exciting positive findings, and others report failures to replicate. There are many reasons for these mixed findings and failures to replicate, but one of these deserves special attention, in our opinion. Molecular genetic analyses of psychiatric disorders might be more successful if continuous symptom dimensions or related traits are analyzed either along with, or instead of, the categorical disorder phenotype (viz., the diagnosis).

Consider the case of the genetics of schizophrenia as a specific example. Recent results suggest that linkage analyses based on more specific phenotypic indicators than the schizophrenia diagnosis alone may be more successful than a search for linkage among individuals diagnosed with schizophrenia but with disparate syndromes and symptoms. For example, Brzustowicz et al. (1997) hypothesized that different aspects of the schizophrenic phenotype may be influenced by different genes. Their evaluation of genetic markers on the short arm of chromosome 6 revealed no evidence for linkage by using categorical schizophrenia diagnostic definitions (i.e., narrow, broad, and very broad). Examining linkage for positive symptom, negative symptom, and general psychopathology symptom scales, however, yielded significant evidence for linkage for the positive symptom scale only (empirical $p < .05$). The specificity of these results suggests that the positive and negative dimensions of schizophrenia may have different susceptibility loci, in which case schizotypy may be genetically related to schizophrenia through a common diathesis pertaining to negative symptoms. Similarly, Serretti, Macciardi, and Smeraldi (1998) hypothesized that the influence of dopamine D2 receptor gene (DRD2) variants should be analyzed at the symptom dimension, rather than syndrome, level. They based their reasoning on the results of a previous study that found a stronger association between DRD2 and schizophrenia in those subjects without negative symptoms (Arinami et al., 1996). Serretti et al. (1998) identified four factors of psychotic symptoms. Subjects with the S311C variant of DRD2 presented with higher scores on the Disorganization factor than those without this particular variant. Moreover, none of the other factors (Excitement, Depression, Delusion) was associated with the S311C variant. These results also suggest that different aspects of the schizophrenic phenotype may be influenced by different underlying genetic vulnerabilities.

The results of multivariate behavior genetic studies of disorders also have important implications for molecular genetic studies of those disorders. It is important to know, for example, whether candidate genes that influence one disorder (e.g., ADHD) also influence other related disorders (e.g., ODD and CD). Multivariate behavior genetic analyses of such disorders can help guide molecular genetic research by determining to what extent the substantial phenotypic overlap among them is due to common genetic influences compared with common environmental influences. Multivariate behavior genetic analyses also can suggest whether all of the genetic influences on these disorders are shared in common or whether each of the disorders exhibits genetic influences that are unique compared to those on the others. If the latter is true, a search for candidate genes that influence ODD and CD uniquely would be fruitful, whereas if the former is true, one would need merely to search for candidate genes for ADHD to find those that also influence childhood antisocial behavior.

## Examination of Genotype–Environment Interactions and Correlations

**Genotype–Environment Interaction—The Contingent Contributions of Genes and Environments to Disorder.** Despite the importance of genotype–environment interactions to many theories of the development and etiology of psychopathology, genotype–environment interaction has received relatively little attention in recent behavior genetic studies of psychopathology. There are a number of reasons for investigating genotype–environment interactions for psychopathology. First, although the vast majority of behavior genetic studies of psychopathology implicitly assume that genetic and environmental influences on the liability to a disorder act additively and independently, this is not necessarily the case. Individuals' genetic predispositions for a disorder may be actualized to a greater or lesser extent in different environments, and certain environmental risk factors may contribute to vulnerability to disorder only in individuals who are genetically predisposed. Second, many developmental psychopathologists have emphasized the point that, at least in theory, genetic and environmental influences on a trait are population-specific. This suggests that the heritability of a disorder may be high in one population and low in another or that shared environmental influences may be important in some populations or environments (e.g., in extreme circumstances of poverty or abuse) but not in others (e.g., in the majority of rearing environments.).

We used the term ''at least in theory'' above because most advocates of the population-specificity of genetic and environmental influences have proposed this in the absence of any research to support it. Indeed, the consistency of heritability estimates across studies varies considerably for different disorders. In the area of childhood disruptive behavior disorders, for example, the heritability of ADHD is estimated consistently in the .6–.9 range, whereas estimates of the heritability of CD are much more variable. Although this may simply reflect methodological differences in behavior genetic studies of ADHD and CD (e.g., more similar operationalizations, measures, and informants across studies for ADHD than for CD), it also may indicate that CD is a more sensitive phenotype than ADHD, in the sense that the causes of CD may differ appreciably, depending on the characteristics of the population and environment in which it is being studied. Needless to say, this is a highly speculative notion that awaits targeted investigations of genotype–environment interaction for support or refutation.

One final point regarding genotype–environment interaction concerns the behavior genetic designs in which it has traditionally been examined. Most investigations of genotype–environment interaction have been conducted within the context of adoption study designs rather than twin study designs. Adoption studies have provided intriguing findings regarding genotype–environment interaction for a number of disorders, such as the findings for criminality and antisocial behavior mentioned before. Nonetheless, adoption studies have a number of limitations, such as relatively small and unrepresentative samples that are not characteristic of large, contemporary twin studies. Consequently, it would be beneficial for behavior geneticists to examine different types of genotype–environment interactions for a variety of disorders within the context of large twin studies. Twin researchers could expand on their examination of differences in genetic and environmental influences as a function of sex and age to include a multitude of environmental moderator variables. These variables could include perinatal complications, family environmental variables such as socioeconomic status and parental supervision and monitoring, and neighborhood characteristics such as income disparity and crime rates. The inclusion of such variables in twin studies of psychopathology will paint a more complete picture of the degree to which genetic and environmental influences vary across populations and environmental contexts, rather than treating this merely as a theoretical possibility. Such studies also will increase our understanding of the specific ways in which genetic and environmental influences combine in determining individuals' liability to psychopathology.

### Genotype–Environment Correlation—Possible Theoretical Implications of the Decline of Shared Environmental Influences with Age.

The finding of a decreasing impact of shared environmental influences or an increasing impact of genetic influences on symptoms of psychopathology (e.g., anxiety and depression) during development may support Scarr and McCartney's (1983) hypothesis that maturation is associated with an increase in *active genotype–environment correlation* and a corresponding decrease in *passive genotype–environment correlation*. *Genotype–environment correlation* refers to the tendency for individuals' genetic propensities for a trait or disorder to be associated with their environmental exposures or experiences that also influence the trait or disorder. There are three types of genotype–environment correlation: *passive, reactive,* and *active. Passive* genotype–environment correlation refers to the tendency for children in intact biological families to experience a rearing environment that is correlated with their genetically influenced characteristics, because they are genetically related to their parents and siblings who provide that environment. *Reactive* genotype–environment correlation refers to the tendency for individuals to elicit certain responses from others in their environment based (in part) on their genetically influenced characteristics. *Active* genotype–environment correlation refers to the tendency of individuals to choose or construct (Plomin, 1994) environments that are consistent with their genetically influenced characteristics. Note that genotype–environment correlations are not necessarily positive; they can also be negative. For example, individuals may elicit or choose environments that help to *counteract* their genetic propensities (Plomin, 1994). Note also that genotype–environment correlation refers to the tendency to experience or seek out certain characteristics based partly on one's genetic predispositions and also to the fact that both the genetic predispositions and the environments *influence* the trait or disorder being studied.

The notion of genotype–environment correlation also suggests that the environment does not act entirely independently from heritable influences (Plomin, 1994). Social supports and life events (both known to be associated with the level of depressive symptoms in adults) are examples of environmental variables that may be differentially experienced by adults based in part on their genetically predisposed characteristics and result in genetic "mediation" of an environmental influence on symptoms of depression. Multivariate studies have been conducted to test for genetic mediation of the relationships of both social supports and life events to depression. Neiderhiser, Plomin, Lichtenstein, Pedersen, and McClearn (1992) found evidence for partial genetic mediation of the relationship between life events and depressive symptoms. Similarly, in the case of social supports, Bergeman, Plomin, Pedersen, and McClearn (1991) found that the relationship of social support to depressed mood and life satisfaction was mediated in part genetically. Kessler et al. (1992) replicated this finding for the relationship between social support and depression (see Plomin, 1994, for a thorough review of this topic).

To the degree that genotype–environment correlation is involved in the etiology of a particular trait, it is expected that measures of the trait-relevant environment experienced by an individual will show genetic influences. Scarr and McCartney's (1983) hypothesis concerning "genotype → environment effects" sought to address several puzzling findings for a variety of traits: (1) over the course of childhood and adolescence, the similarity of MZ twins increases, whereas that of DZ twins decreases; (2) a similar divergence in similarity occurs between biological and adopted siblings, and there is a greater decrease in similarity among adopted siblings; (3) MZ twins reared apart are unexpectedly similar to one another and show a level of similarity for most traits that is greater than that of DZ twins reared together and that is often almost as high as that of MZ twins reared together. Scarr and McCartney proposed that all of these findings could be explained by an age-graded increase in the magnitude of active genotype–environment correlation and a concomitant decrease in the magnitude of passive genotype–environment correlation. This would explain the relative decline in similarity between DZ twins and adoptive siblings because an increase in active genotype–environment correlation would lead DZ twins (whose genetic relatedness is less than that of MZ twins) and adoptive siblings (who are unrelated genetically) to select increasingly disparate environmental experiences than MZ twins (who are genetically identical).

Based on the prediction of a divergence with age between the MZ and DZ twin correlations, the Scarr–McCartney hypothesis posits that heritability should increase with age, whereas the magnitude of shared environmental influences should decrease with age, a prediction that receives some support from findings for childhood and adolescent anxiety and depression. Feigon et al. (1997) were interested in directly testing the

expected age-related changes in heritability and shared environmental influences in analyses of data on DSM-III-R separation anxiety disorder (SAD) symptoms in children. This hypothesis was tested by modeling age moderation of the genetic and environmental estimates using multiple regression methods. Indeed, Feigon et al. (1997) found that the magnitude of genetic influences on DSM-III-R SAD symptoms in children increased with age. This finding was consistent with the results reported before by Thapar and McGuffin (1994; see also Thapar & McGuffin, 1996), who found that age moderated the heritability for depressive symptoms in children and adolescents, such that the magnitude of genetic influences was greater in older than in younger children, but the magnitude of shared environmental influences was lower in older than in younger children. An increase in the relative magnitude of genetic influences with age also has been observed for childhood fears (Rose & Ditto, 1983). It has been hypothesized that this increase is due in part to the increasing role of active genotype–environment correlation across development proposed by Scarr and McCartney (1983). For the case of fears, Stevenson et al. (1992) proposed that active genotype–environment correlation may take the form of avoidance of fear-provoking situations. Such avoidance would be expected to increase as the child ages because of a decrease in forced exposures to feared situations which were previously imposed by parents. The increased ability of the child to avoid fear-provoking situations might thus result in the loss of opportunities for habituation, thus allowing greater expression of the genetic liability to be fearful.

Although the increase in active genotype–environment correlation is a compelling explanation for these findings, it is important to consider that changes in the magnitude of heritability with age is also consistent with other hypotheses. These include an increase in genetic variance due to the age-specific activation of genes that influence risk for the disorder, as well as a decrease in the experience of disorder-relevant environmental risk factors.

## Summary

In this chapter, we have reviewed the behavior genetic literature for a number of the major forms of child and adult psychopathology, including schizophrenia, schizophrenia spectrum disorders, and schizotypal personality; affective and anxiety disorders in both children and adults; and the childhood disruptive disorders ADHD, ODD, and CD. Unfortunately, space limitations precluded our review of behavior genetic research on other important disorders, such as autism, substance abuse and dependence, and personality disorders. We also provided background material on the statistical methods used in contemporary twin studies to conduct univariate and multivariate behavior genetic analyses, as well as a brief discussion of some exciting new and future directions in behavior genetic studies of psychopathology. The latter included genetic and environmental influences on normal range variation and on the disordered extreme, the inclusion of specific environmental and endophenotypic variables in behavior genetic models, molecular genetic studies of psychopathology, and the examination of genotype-environment interaction and correlation. These future directions will facilitate the progression of behavior genetic studies of psychopathology beyond the simple estimation of broad, abstract genetic and environmental variance components for a single disorder to the examination of more complex models for the specific etiological mechanisms that underlie disorders and their overlap.

# References

Alberts-Corush, J., Firestone, P., & Goodman, J. T. (1986). Attention and impulsivity characteristics of the biological and adoptive parents of hyperactive and normal control children. *American Journal of Orthopsychiatry, 56*, 413–423.

American Psychiatric Association. (1968). *Diagnostic and statistical manual of mental disorders* (2nd ed.). Washington, DC: Author.

American Psychiatric Association. (1980). *Diagnostic and statistical manual of mental disorders* (3rd ed.). Washington, DC: Author.

American Psychiatric Association. (1987). *Diagnostic and statistical manual of mental disorders* (3rd ed., rev.). Washington, DC: Author.

American Psychiatric Association. (1994). *Diagnostic and statistical manual of mental disorders* (4th ed.). Washington, DC: Author.

Andreasen, N. C., & Carpenter, W. T., Jr. (1993). Diagnosis and classification of schizophrenia. *Schizophrenia Bulletin, 19*(2), 199–214.

Arinami, T., Itokawa, M., Aoki, J., Shibuya, H., Ookubo, Y., Iwawaki, A., Ota, K., Shimizu, H., Hamaguchi, H., & Toru, M. (1996). Further association study on dopamine D2 receptor variant S311C in schizophrenia and affective disorders. *American Journal of Medical Genetics, 67*, 133–138.

Barkley, R. A. (1982). Guidelines for defining hyperactivity in children: Attention deficit disorder with hyperactivity. In B. B. Lahey & A. E. Kazdin (Eds.), *Advances in clinical psychology* (Vol. 5, pp. 137–180). New York: Plenum Press.

Baron, M., Gruen, R., Asnis, L., & Lord, S. (1985). Familial transmission of schizotypal and borderline personality disorders. *American Journal of Psychiatry, 142*, 927–934.

Baron, M., Gruen, R., Rainer, J. D., Kane, J., Asnis, L., & Lord, A. (1985). A family study of schizophrenia and normal control probands: Implications for the spectrum concept of schizophrenia. *American Journal of Psychiatry, 142*, 447–455.

Battaglia, M., Gasperini, M., Sciuto, G., Scherillo, P., Diaferia, G., & Bellodi, L. (1991). Morbidity risk for psychiatric disorders in the families of schizotypal subjects. *Schizophrenia Bulletin, 17*, 659–668.

Bergeman, C. S., Plomin, R., Pedersen, N. L., McClearn, G. E., & Nesselroade, J. R. (1990). Genetic and environmental influences on social support: The Swedish Adoption/Twin Study of Aging. *Journal of Gerontology, 45*, 101–106.

Bergeman, C. S., Plomin, R., Pedersen, N. L., & McClearn, G. E. (1991). Genetic mediation of the relationship between social support and psychological well-being. *Psychology and Aging, 6*, 640–646.

Bertelsen, A., Harvald, B., & Hauge, M. (1977). A Danish twin study of manic-depressive disorders. *British Journal of Psychiatry, 130*, 330–351.

Biederman, J., Faraone, S. V., Keenan, K., Benjamin, J., Krifcher, B., Moore, C., Sprich-Buckminster, S., Ugaglia, K., Jellinek, M. S., Steingard, R., Spencer, T., Norman, D., Kolodny, R., Kraus, I., Perrin, J., Keller, M. B., & Tsuang, M. T. (1992). Further evidence for family-genetic risk factors in attention deficit hyperactivity disorder: Patterns of comorbidity in probands and relatives in psychiatrically and pediatrically referred samples. *Archives of General Psychiatry, 49*, 728–738.

Biederman, J., Faraone, S. V., Keenan, K., Knee, D., & Tsuang, M. T. (1990). Family genetic and psychosocial risk factors in DSM-III attention deficit disorder. *Journal of the American Academy of Child and Adolescent Psychiatry, 29*, 526–533.

Biederman, J., Munir, K., Knee, D., Habelow, W., Armentano, M., Autor, S., Hoge, S. K., & Waternaux, C. (1986). A family study of patients with attention deficit disorder and normal controls. *Journal of Psychiatry Research, 20*, 263–274.

Biederman, J., Newcorn, J., & Sprich, S. (1991). Comorbidity of attention deficit hyperactivity disorder with conduct, depressive, anxiety, and other disorders. *American Journal of Psychiatry, 148*, 564–577.

Bleuler, E. (1950). *Dementia praecox or the group of schizophrenias.* (J. Zinkin, Trans.). New York: International Universities Press. (Original work published 1911).

Brzustowicz, L. M., Honer, E. G., Chow, E. W. C., Hogan, J., Hodgkinson, K., & Bassett, A. S. (1997). Use of a quantitative trait to map a locus associated with severity of positive symptoms in familial schizophrenia to chromosome 6p. *American Journal of Human Genetics, 61*, 1388–1396.

Cadoret, R. J., Cain, C. A., & Crowe, R. R. (1983). Evidence for gene-environment interaction in the development of adolescent antisocial behavior. *Behavior Genetics, 13*, 301–310.

Cadoret, R. J., & Stewart, M. A. (1991). An adoption study of attention deficit/hyperactivity/aggression and their relationship to adult antisocial personality. *Comprehensive Psychiatry, 32*, 73–82.

Cannon, T. D., Kaprio, J., Lonnqvist, J., Huttunen, M., & Koskenvuo, M. (1998). The genetic epidemiology of schizophrenia in a Finnish twin cohort: A population-based modeling study. *Archives of General Psychiatry, 55*, 67–74.

Cantwell, D. (1975). Genetic studies of hyperactive children: Psychiatric illness in biologic and adopting parents. In R. Fieve, D. Rosenthal, & H. Brill (Eds.), *Genetic research in psychiatry* (pp. 273–280). Baltimore: Johns Hopkins University Press.

Cloninger, C. R., Sigvardsson, S., Bohman, M., & von Knorring, A.-L. (1982). Predisposition to petty criminality in Swedish adoptees. II. Cross-fostering analysis of gene-environment interaction. *Archives of General Psychiatry, 39*, 1242–1247.

Cunningham, L., Cadoret, R. J., Loftus, R., & Edwards, J. E. (1975). Studies of adoptees from psychiatrically disturbed biological parents: Psychiatric conditions in childhood and adolescence. *British Journal of Psychiatry, 126*, 534–549.

DeFries, J. C., & Fulker, D. W. (1988). Multiple regression analysis of twin data: Etiology of deviant scores versus individual differences. *Acta Geneticae Medicae et Gemellologiae, 37*, 205–216.

Eaves, L. J., Silberg, J. L., Meyer, J. M., Maes, H. H., Simonoff, E., Pickles, A., Rutter, M., Neale, M. C., Reynolds, C. A., Erikson, M. T., Heath, A. C., Loeber, R., Truett, K. R., & Hewitt, J. K. (1997). Genetics and developmental psychopathology: 2. The main effects of genes and environment on behavioral problems in the Virginia Twin Study of Adolescent Behavioral Development. *Journal of Child Psychology and Psychiatry and Allied Disciplines, 38*, 965–980.

Edelbrock, C., Costello, A. J., & Kessler, M. D. (1984). Empirical corroboration of the attention deficit disorder. *Journal of the American Academy of Child Psychiatry, 23*, 285–290.

Edelbrock, C., Rende, R., Plomin, R., & Thompson, L. A. (1995). A twin study of competence and problem behavior in childhood and early adolescence. *Journal of Child Psychology and Psychiatry and Allied Disciplines, 36*, 775–785.

Egan, M. F., & Weinberger, D. R. (1997). Neurobiology of schizophrenia. *Current Opinion in Neurobiology, 7*, 701–706.

Eley, T. C. (1997). General genes: A new theme in developmental psychopathology. *Current Directions in Psychological Science, 6*(4), 90–95.

Eley, T. C., & Stevenson, J. (1997). Using genetic analyses to clarify the distinction between depressive and anxious symptoms in children and adolescents. Manuscript submitted for publication.

Elston, R. C., Namboodiri, K. K., Spence, M. A., & Rainer, J. D. (1978). A genetic study of schizophrenia pedigrees. II. One-locus hypotheses. *Neuropsychobiology, 4*(4), 193–206.

Essen-Moller, E. (1941). Psychiatrische untersuchungen an einer serie von zwillingen. *Acta Psychiatrica et Neurologica Scandinavica, Supplement 23.*

Falconer, D. S. (1965). The inheritance of liability to certain diseases, estimated from the incidence among relatives. *Annals of Human Genetics, 29*, 51–71.

Faraone, S. V., Biederman, J., Jetton, J. G., & Tsuang, M. T. (1997). Attention deficit disorder and conduct disorder: Longitudinal evidence for a familial subtype. *Psychological Medicine, 27*, 291–300.

Faraone, S. V., Biederman, J., Keenan, K., & Tsuang, M. T. (1991). Separation of DSM-III attention deficit disorder and conduct disorder: Evidence from a family-genetic study of American child psychiatric patients. *Psychological Medicine, 21*, 109–121.

Farmer, A. E., McGuffin, P., & Gottesman, I. I. (1987). Twin concordance for DSM-III schizophrenia: Scrutinizing the validity of the definition. *Archives of General Psychiatry, 44*, 634–641.

Feigon, S. A., & Waldman, I. D. (1998, June). Genetic and environmental influences on childhood anxiety disorder symptoms and their moderation by age and sex. Paper presented at the *Annual Meeting of the Behavior Genetics Association*, Stockholm, Sweden.

Feigon, S. A., Waldman, I. D., Levy, F., & Hay, D. A. (1997a). Genetic and environmental influences on separation anxiety disorder symptoms and their moderation by age and sex. Manuscript submitted for publication.

Feigon, S. A., Waldman, I. D., Levy, F., & Hay, D. A. (1997b). Genetic and environmental influences on various anxiety disorder symptoms in children: Same environments, different genes? Paper presented at the *Annual Meeting of the Behavior Genetics Association*, Toronto, Canada.

Fischer, M. (1971). Psychoses in the offspring of schizophrenic monozygotic twins and their normal co-twins. *British Journal of Psychiatry, 118*, 43–52.

Frangos, E., Athanassenas, G., Tsitourides, S., Katsanou, N., & Alexandrakou, P. (1985). Prevalence of DSM-III schizophrenia among the first-degree relatives of schizophrenic probands. *Acta Psychiatrica Scandinavica, 72*, 382–386.

Gershon, E. S., DeLisi, L. E., Hamovit, J., Nurnberger, J. I., Maxwell, M. D., Schreiber, J., Dauphinais, D., Dingman, C. W., & Guroff, J. J. (1988). A controlled family study of chronic psychoses. *Archives of General Psychiatry, 45*, 328–336.

Gilger, J. W., Pennington, B. F., & DeFries, J. C. (1992). A twin study of the etiology of comorbidity: Attention deficit hyperactivity disorder and dyslexia. *Journal of the American Academy of Child and Adolescent Psychiatry, 31*, 343–348.

Gillis, J. J., Gilger, J. W., Pennington, B. F., & DeFries, J. C. (1992). Attention deficit disorder in reading-disabled twins: Evidence for a genetic etiology. *Journal of Abnormal Child Psychology, 20*, 303–315.

Gjone, H., Stevenson, J., & Sundet, J. M. (1996). Genetic influence on parent-reported attention-related problems in a Norwegian general population twin sample. *Journal of the American Academy of Child and Adolescent Psychiatry, 35*, 588–596.

Goodman, R., & Stevenson, J. (1989). A twin study of hyperactivity—II. The aetiological role of genes, family relationships and perinatal adversity. *Journal of Child Psychology and Psychiatry, 30*, 691–709.

Gottesman, I. I. (1993). Origins of schizophrenia: Past and prologue. In R. Plomin & G. E. McClearn (Eds.), *Nature, nurture and psychology*. Washington, DC: American Psychological Association.

Gottesman, I. I. (1991). *Schizophrenia genesis: The origins of madness*. San Francisco: W.H. Freeman.

Gottesman, I. I. (1996). Blind men and elephants: Genetic and other perspectives on schizophrenia. In L. L. Hall (Ed.), *Genetics and mental illness* (pp. 51–57). New York: Plenum Press.

Gottesman, I. I., & Bertelsen, A. (1989). Confirming unexpressed genotypes for schizophrenia: Risks in the offspring of Fischer's Danish identical and fraternal twins. *Archives of General Psychiatry, 46*, 867–872.

Gottesman, I. I., & Shields, J. (1967). A polygenic theory of schizophrenia. *Proceedings of the National Academy of Sciences in the United States of America, 58*, 199–205.

Gottesman, I. I., & Shields, J. (1982). *Schizophrenia, the epigenetic puzzle.* New York: Cambridge University Press.

Heath, A. C., Hudziak, J. Reich, W., Madden, P. A. F., Slutske, W. S., Bierut, L., & Bucholz, K. K. (1996). The inheritance of hyperactivity and inattention in girls: Results from the Missouri Twin Study. *Behavior Genetics, 26*, 587–588.

Hinshaw, S. P. (1987). On the distinction between attentional deficits/hyperactivity and conduct problems/aggression in child psychopathology. *Psychological Bulletin, 101*, 443–463.

Ingraham, L. J. (1995). Family-genetic research and schizotypal personality. In A. Raine, T. Lencz, & S. A. Mednick (Eds.), *Schizotypal personality* (pp. 19–42). Cambridge: Cambridge University Press.

Inouye, E. (1972). Monozygotic twins with schizophrenia reared apart in infancy. *Japanese Journal of Human Genetics, 16*, 182–190.

Jackson, D. D. (1960). A critique of the literature on the genetics of schizophrenia. In D. D. Jackson (Ed.), *The etiology of schizophrenia* (pp. 37–87). New York: Basic Books.

Jardine, R., Martin, N. G., & Henderson, A. S. (1984). Genetic covariation between neuroticism and the symptoms of anxiety and depression. *Genetic Epidemiology, 1*, 89–107.

Jöreskog, K. G., & Sörbom, D. (1999). *LISREL 8.3: User's Reference Guide.* Chicago, IL: Scientific Software International.

Kallman, F. J. (1946). The genetic theory of schizophrenia: An analysis of 691 schizophrenic twin index families. *American Journal of Psychiatry, 103*, 309–322.

Kallmann, F. J. (1950). The genetics of psychosis: An analysis of 1,232 twin index families. In *Congres international de psychiatre, rapports VI psychiatrie sociale* (pp. 1–27). Paris: Hermann.

Karkowski, L. M., & Kendler, K. S. (1997). An examination of the genetic relationship between bipolar and unipolar illness in an epidemiological sample. *Psychiatric Genetics, 7*(4), 159–163.

Kendler, K. S. (1993). Twin studies of psychiatric illness: Current status and future directions. *Archives of General Psychiatry, 50*, 905–915.

Kendler, K. S., Eaves, L. J., Walters, E. E., Neale, M. C., Heath, A. C., & Kessler, R. C. (1996). The identification and validation of distinct depressive syndromes in a population-based sample of female twins. *Archives of General Psychiatry, 53*, 391–399.

Kendler, K. S., & Gardner, C. O. (1997). The risk for psychiatric disorders in relatives of schizophrenic and control probands: A comparison of three independent studies. *Psychological Medicine, 27*, 411–419.

Kendler, K. S., & Gruenberg, A. M. (1984). An independent analysis of the Danish adoption study of schizophrenia. VI. The relationship between psychiatric disorders as defined by DSM-III in the relatives and adoptees. *Archives of General Psychiatry, 41*, 555–564.

Kendler, K. S., Gruenberg, A. M., & Kinney, D. K. (1994). Independent diagnoses of adoptees and relatives as defined by DSM-III in the provincial and national samples of the Danish Adoption Study of Schizophrenia. *Archives of General Psychiatry, 51*, 456–468.

Kendler, K. S., Gruenberg, A. M., & Strauss, J. S. (1981). An independent analysis of the Copenhagen sample of the Danish adoption study of schizophrenia. II. The relationship between schizotypal personality disorder and schizophrenia. *Archives of General Psychiatry, 38*, 982–984.

Kendler, K. S., Gruenberg, A. M., & Strauss, J. S. (1982). An independent analysis of the Copenhagen sample of the Danish adoption study of schizophrenia. V. The relationship between childhood social withdrawal and adult schizophrenia. *Archives of General Psychiatry, 39*, 1257–1261.

Kendler, K. S., Gruenberg, A. M., & Tsuang, M. T. (1985). Psychiatric illness in first-degree relatives of schizophrenic and surgical control patients: A family study using DSM-III criteria. *Archives of General Psychiatry, 42*, 770–779.

Kendler, K. S., Heath, A., Martin, N. G., & Eaves, L. J. (1986). Symptoms of anxiety and depression in a volunteer twin population: The etiologic role of genetic and environmental factors. *Archives of General Psychiatry, 43*, 213–221.

Kendler, K. S., Heath, A., Martin, N. G., & Eaves, L. J. (1987). Symptoms of anxiety and symptoms of depression: Same genes, different environments? *Archives of General Psychiatry, 44*, 451–457.

Kendler, K. S., Masterson, C. C., Ungaro, R., & Davis, K. L. (1984). A family history study of schizophrenia-related personality disorders. *American Journal of Psychiatry, 141*, 424–427.

Kendler, K. S., McGuire, M., Gruenberg, A. M., Spellman, M., O'Hare, A., & Walsh, D. (1993). The Roscommon Family Study. II: The risk of nonschizophrenic nonaffective psychoses in relatives. *Archives of General Psychiatry, 50*, 645–652.

Kendler, K. S., McGuire, M., Gruenberg, A. M., O'Hare, A., Spellman, M., & Walsh, D. (1993). The Roscommon Family Study. III: Schizophrenia-related personality disorders in relatives. *Archives of General Psychiatry, 50*, 781–788.

Kendler, K. S., Neale, M. C., Kessler, R. C., Heath, A. C., & Eaves, L. J. (1992a). Generalized anxiety disorder in women: A population-based twin study. *Archives of General Psychiatry, 49*, 267–272.

Kendler, K. S., Neale, M. C., Kessler, R. C., Heath, A. C., & Eaves, L. J. (1992b). A population-based twin study of major depression in women: The impact of varying definitions of illness. *Archives of General Psychiatry, 49*, 257–266.

Kendler, K. S., Neale, M. C., Kessler, R. C., Heath, A. C., & Eaves, L. J. (1992c). Major depression and generalized anxiety disorder: Same genes, (partly) different environments? *Archives of General Psychiatry, 49*, 716–722.

Kendler, K. S., Neale, M. C., Kessler, R. C., Heath, A. C., & Eaves, L. J. (1992d). The genetic epidemiology of phobias in women: The interrelationship of agoraphobia, situational phobia, and simple phobia. *Archives of General Psychiatry, 49*, 273–281.

Kendler, K. S., Neale, M. C., Kessler, R. C., Heath, A. C., & Eaves, L. J. (1992e). Childhood parental loss and adult psychopathology in women: A twin study perspective. *Archives of General Psychiatry, 49*, 109–116.

Kendler, K. S., Neale, M. C., Kessler, R. C., Heath, A. C., & Eaves, L. J. (1993a). Panic disorder in women: A population-based twin study. *Psychological Medicine, 23*, 397–406.

Kendler, K. S., Neale, M. C., Kessler, R. C., Heath, A. C., & Eaves, L. J. (1993b). The lifetime history of major depression in women: Reliability of diagnosis and heritability. *Archives of General Psychiatry, 50*, 863–870.

Kendler, K. S., Neale, M. C., Kessler, R. C., Heath, A. C., & Eaves, L. J. (1993c). Major depression and phobias: The genetic and environmental sources of comorbidity. *Psychological Medicine, 23,* 361–371.

Kendler, K. S., Ochs, A. L., Gorman, A. M., & Hewitt, J. K. (1991). The structure of schizotypy: A pilot multitrait twin study. *Psychiatry Research, 36,* 19–36.

Kendler, K. S., Pedersen, N. L., Neale, M. C., & Mathé, A. A. (1995). A pilot Swedish twin study of affective illness including hospital- and population-ascertained subsamples: Results of model fitting. *Behavior Genetics, 23,* 217–232.

Kendler, K. K., & Robinette, C. D. (1983). Schizophrenia in the National Academy of Sciences-National Research Council Twin Registry: A 16-year update. *American Journal of Psychiatry, 140,* 1551–1563.

Kendler, K. S., Walters, E. E., Neale, M. C., Kessler, R. C., Heath, A. C., & Eaves, L. J. (1995). The structure of the genetic and environmental risk factors for six major psychiatric disorders in women: Phobia, generalized anxiety disorder, panic disorder, bulimia, major depression, and alcoholism. *Archives of General Psychiatry, 52,* 374–383.

Kendler, K. S., Walters, E. E., Truett, K. R., Heath, A. C., Neale, M. C., Martin, N. G., & Eaves, L. J. (1994). Sources of individual differences in depressive symptoms: Analysis of two samples of twins and their families. *American Journal of Psychiatry, 151,* 1605–1614.

Kessler, R. C., Kendler, K. S., Heath, A., Neale, M. C., & Eaves, L. J. (1992). Social support, depressed mood, and adjustment to stress: A genetic epidemiologic investigation. *Journal of Personality and Social Psychology, 62,* 257–272.

Kety, S. S. (1959). Biochemical theories of schizophrenia: Part I of a two-part critical review of current theories and of the evidence used to support them. *Science, 129,* 1528–1532.

Kety, S. S., Rosenthal, D., Wender, P. H., & Schulsinger, F. (1968). The types and prevalence of mental illness in the biological and adoptive families of adopted schizophrenics. *Journal of Psychiatric Research, 6,* 345–362.

Kety, S. S., Rosenthal, D., Wender, P. H., Schulsinger, F., & Jacobsen, B. (1975). Mental illness in the biological and adoptive families of adopted individuals who have become schizophrenic: A preliminary report based on psychiatric interviews. In R. Fieve, D. Rosenthal, & H. Brill (Eds.), *Genetic research in psychiatry* (pp. 147–165). Baltimore: Johns Hopkins University Press.

Kety, S. S., Rosenthal, D., Wender, P. H., Schulsinger, F., & Jacobsen, B. (1978). The biological and adoptive families of adopted individuals who became schizophrenic: Prevalence of mental illness and other characteristics. In L. C. Wynne, R. L. Cromwell, & S. Matthysse (Eds.), *The nature of schizophrenia* (pp. 25–37). New York: Wiley.

Kety, S. S., Wender, P. H., Jacobsen, B., Ingraham, L. J., Jansson, L., Faber, B., & Kinney, D. K. (1994). Mental illness in the biological and adoptive relatives of schizophrenic adoptees. *Archives of General Psychiatry, 51,* 442–455.

Kidd, K. K., & Cavalli-Sforza, L. L. (1973). An analysis of the genetics of schizophrenia. *Social Biology, 20,* 254–265.

Kleinman, A. (1988). *Rethinking psychiatry: From cultural category to personal experience.* New York: The Free Press.

Kraepelin, E. (1904). *Clinical psychiatry: A textbook for students and physicians.* New York: Macmillan.

Kraepelin, E. (1971). *Dementia praecox and paraphrenia* (R. M. Barclay, Trans.; G. M. Robertson, Ed.). Huntington, NY: Krieger. (Original work published 1909–1913).

Kringlen, E., & Cramer, G. (1989). Offspring of monozygotic twins discordant for schizophrenia. *Archives of General Psychiatry, 46,* 867–872.

Kruger, J. (1973). Zur Unterscheidung zwischen multifaktoriellem Erbgang mit Schwellenwerteffekt und einfachem diallelen Erbgang. [Discrimination between multifactorial inheritance with threshold effect and two-allele single-locus hypothesis]. *Humangenetik, 17*(3), 181–252.

Lahey, B. B., Pelham, W. E., Schaughency, E. A., Atkins, M. S., Murphy, H. A., Hynd, G., Russo, M., Hartdagen, S., & Lorys-Vernon, A. (1988). Dimensions and types of attention deficit disorder. *Journal of the American Academy of Child and Adolescent Psychiatry, 27,* 330–335.

Lahey, B. B., Schaughency, E. A., Strauss, C. C., & Frame, C. L. (1984). Are attention deficit disorders with and without hyperactivity similar or dissimilar disorders? *Journal of the American Academy of Child Psychiatry, 23,* 302–309.

Lenzenweger, M. F., & Loranger, A. W. (1989). Detection of familial schizophrenia using a psychometric measure of schizotypy. *Archives of General Psychiatry, 46,* 902–907.

Loeber, R., Lahey, B. B., & Thomas, C. (1991). Diagnostic conundrum of oppositional defiant disorder and conduct disorder. *Journal of Abnormal Psychology, 100,* 379–390.

Loney, J., & Milich, R. (1982). Hyperactivity, inattention, and aggression in clinical practice. In M. Wolraich & D. K. Routh (Eds.), *Advances in developmental and behavioral pediatrics* (Vol. 3, pp. 113–147). Greenwich, CT: JAI Press.

Lowing, P. A., Mirsky, A. F., & Pereira, R. (1983). The inheritance of schizophrenia spectrum disorders: A reanalysis of the Danish Adoptee Study data. *American Journal of Psychiatry, 140,* 1167–1171.

Lyons, M. J., True, W. R., Eisen, S. A., Goldberg, J., Meyer, J. M., Faraone, S. V., Eaves, L. J., & Tsuang, M. T. (1995). Differential heritability of adult and juvenile antisocial traits. *Archives of General Psychiatry, 52,* 906–915.

Maier, W., Hallmayer, J., Minges, J., & Lichtermann, D. (1990). Affective and schizoaffective disorders: Similarities and differences. In A. Marneros & M. T. Tsuang (Eds.), *Morbid risks in relatives of affective, schizoaffective, and schizophrenic patients—Results of a family study* (pp. 201–207). New York: Springer Verlag.

Matthysse, S. W., & Kidd, K. K. (1976). Estimating the genetic contribution to schizophrenia. *American Journal of Psychiatry, 133,* 185–191.

McGue, M. (1992). When assessing twin concordance, use the probandwise not the pairwise rate. *Schizophrenia Bulletin, 18,* 171–176.

McGue, M., Gottesman, I. I., & Rao, D. C. (1985). Resolving genetic models for the transmission of schizophrenia. *Genetic Epidemiology, 2*(1), 99–110.

McGuffin, P., & Katz, R. (1989). The genetics of depression and manic-depressive illness. *British Journal of Psychiatry, 155,* 294–304.

McGuffin, P., Katz, R., Watkins, S., & Rutherford, J. (1996). A hospital-based twin register of the heritability of DSM-IV unipolar depression. *Archives of General Psychiatry, 53,* 129–136.

McGuffin, P., & Owen, M. J. (1996). Molecular genetic studies of schizophrenia. *Cold Spring Harbor Symposium on Quantitative Biology, 61,* 815–822.

Mednick, S. A., Gabrielli, W. F., & Hutchings, B. (1983). Genetic influences in criminal behavior: Evidence from an adoption cohort. In K. T. Van Dusen & S. A. Mednick (Eds.),

*Prospective studies of crime and delinquency* (pp. 39–56). Boston: Kluwer-Nijhof.

Meehl, P. E. (1962). Schizotaxia, schizotypy, schizophrenia. *American Psychologist, 17,* 827–838.

Miles, D. R., & Carey, G. (1997). Genetic and environmental architecture of human aggression. *Journal of Personality and Social Psychology, 72,* 207–217.

Morrison, J. R., & Stewart, M. A. (1971). A family study of the hyperactive child syndrome. *Biological Psychiatry, 3,* 189–195.

Morton, N. E., & MacLean, C. J. (1974). Analysis of family resemblance. III. Complex segregation of quantitative traits. *American Journal of Human Genetics, 26,* 489–503.

Moskalenko, V. D., & Gindilis, V. M. (1981). [Concordance in twins and the component partition of phenotypic variance in schizophrenia]. *Tsitologiia I Genetika, 15*(5), 70–72.

Nadder, T. S., Silberg, J. L., Eaves, L. J., Maes, H. H., & Meyer, J. M. (1998). Genetic effects on ADHD symptomatology: Results from a telephone survey. *Behavior Genetics, 28,* 83–99.

Neale, M. C., & Cardon, L. R. (1992). *Methodology for genetic studies of twins and families.* Dordrecht, The Netherlands: Kluwer Academic Publishers.

Neale, M. C., Boker, S. M., Xie, G., & Maes, H. H. (1999). *Mx: Statistical modeling, 5th edition.* Richmond: Virginia Commonwealth University Department of Psychiatry.

Neiderhiser, J. M., Plomin, R., Lichtenstein, P., Pedersen, N. L., & McClearn, G. E. (1992). The influence of life events on depressive symptoms over time [abstract]. *Behavior Genetics, 22,* 740.

Onstad, S., Skre, I., Torgersen, S., & Kringlen, E. (1991). Twin concordance for DSM-III-R schizophrenia. *Acta Psychiatrica et Neurologica Scandinavica, 83,* 395–401.

O'Rourke, D. H., Gottesman, I. I., Suarez, B. K., Rice, J., & Reich, T. (1982). Refutation of the general single locus model for the etiology of schizophrenia. *American Journal of Human Genetics, 34,* 630–649.

Parnas, J., Cannon, T. D., Jacobsen, B., Schulsinger, H., Schulsinger, F., & Mednick, S. A. (1993). Lifetime DSM-III-R diagnostic outcomes in offspring of schizophrenic mothers: Results from the Copenhagen high-risk study. *Archives of General Psychiatry, 50,* 707–714.

Pelham, W. E., Gnagy, E. M., Greenslade, K. E., & Milich, R. (1992). Teacher ratings of DSM-III-R symptoms of the disruptive behavior disorders. *Journal of the American Academy of Child and Adolescent Psychiatry, 31,* 210–218.

Plomin, R. (1994). *Genetics and experience: The interplay between nature and nurture.* Thousand Oaks, CA: Sage.

Plomin, R., Lichtenstein, P., Pedersen, N. L., McClearn, G. E., & Nesselroade, J. R. (1990). Genetic influence on life events during the last half of the life span. *Psychology of Aging, 5,* 25–30.

Portin, P., & Alanen, Y. O. (1997). A critical review of genetic studies of schizophrenia. I. Epidemiological and brain studies. *Acta Psychiatrica et Neurologica Scandinavica, 95,* 1–5.

Pulkkinen, L., & Pitkänen, T. (1993). Continuities in aggressive behavior from childhood to adulthood. *Aggressive Behavior, 19,* 249–263.

Pulver, A. E., Wolyniec, P. S., Housman, D., Kazazian, H. H., Antonarakis, S. E., Nestadt, G., Lasseter, V. K., McGrath, J. A., Dombroski, B., Karayiorgou, M., Ton, C., Blouin, J.-L., & Kempf, L. (1996). The Johns Hopkins University collaborative schizophrenia study: An epidemiologic-genetic approach to test the heterogeneity hypothesis and identify schizophrenia susceptibility genes. *Cold Spring Harbor Symposia on Quantitative Biology, 61,* 797–814.

Rende, R. D., Plomin, R., Reiss, D., & Hetherington, E. M. (1993). Genetic and environmental influences on depressive symptomatology in adolescence: Individual differences and extreme scores. *Journal of Child Psychology and Psychiatry and Allied Disciplines, 34,* 1387–1398.

Rhee, S. H., & Waldman, I. D. (1998). Genetic and environmental influences on antisocial behavior: A meta-analysis of twin and adoption studies. Manuscript submitted for publication.

Rhee, S. H., Waldman, I. D., Hay, D. A., & Levy, F. (in press). Sex differences in genetic and environmental influences on DSM-III-R attention-deficit hyperactivity disorder (ADHD). *Journal of Abnormal Psychology.*

Robins, L. N. (1966). *Deviant children grown up.* Baltimore: Williams & Wilkins.

Rose, R. J., & Ditto, W. B. (1983). A developmental-genetic analysis of common fears from early adolescence to early adulthood. *Child Development, 54,* 361–368.

Rosenthal, D. (1962). Sex distribution and the severity of illness among samples of schizophrenic twins. *Journal of Psychiatric Research, 1,* 26–36.

Rowe, D. C. (1983). Biometrical genetic models of self-reported delinquent behavior: A twin study. *Behavior Genetics, 13,* 473–489.

Roy, M. A., Neale, M. C., Pedersen, N. L., Mathé, A. A., & Kendler, K. S. (1995). A twin study of generalized anxiety disorder and major depression. *Psychological Medicine, 25,* 1037–1049.

Rudin, E. (1916). *Zur vererbung und neuentstehung der dementia praecox.* Berlin and New York: Springer Verlag.

Rutter, M. (1983). Behavioral studies: Questions and findings on the concept of a distinctive syndrome. In M. Rutter (Ed.), *Developmental neuropsychiatry* (pp. 259–279). New York: Guilford.

Scarr, S., & McCartney, K. (1983). How people make their own environments: A theory of genotype → environment effects. *Child Development, 54,* 424–435.

Schmitz, S., Fulker, D. W., & Mrazek, D. A. (1995). Problem behavior in early and middle childhood: An initial behavior genetic analysis. *Journal of Child Psychology and Psychiatry, 36,* 1443–1458.

Schulz, M. P., Schulz, S. C., Goldberg, S. C., Ettigi, P., Resnick, R. J., & Friedel, R. O. (1986). Diagnoses of the relatives of schizotypal outpatients. *Journal of Nervous and Mental Disease, 174,* 457–463.

Serretti, A., Macciardi, F., & Smeraldi, E. (1998). Dopamine receptor D2 Ser/Cys311 variant associated with disorganized symptomatology of schizophrenia. *Schizophrenia Research, 34,* 207–210.

Sherman, D. K., Iacono, W. G., & McGue, M. K. (1997). Attention-deficit hyperactivity disorder dimensions: A twin study of inattention and impulsivity-hyperactivity. *Journal of the American Academy of Child and Adolescent Psychiatry, 36,* 745–753.

Shields, J., Gottesman, I. I., & Slater, E. (1967). Kallmann's 1946 schizophrenic twin study in the light of new information. *Acta Psychiatrica et Neurologica Scandinavica, 43,* 385–396.

Siever, L. J., Silverman, J. M., Horvath, T. B., & Klar, H. M.

(1990). Increased morbid risk for schizophrenia-related disorders in relatives of schotypal personality disordered patients. *Archives of General Psychiatry, 47,* 634–640.

Silberg, J., Rutter, M., Meyer, J., Maes, H., Hewitt, J., Simonoff, E., Pickles, A., Loeber, R., & Eaves, L. (1996). Genetic and environmental influences on the covariation between hyperactivity and conduct disturbance in juvenile twins. *Journal of Child Psychology and Psychiatry and Allied Disciplines, 37,* 803–816.

Simonoff, E., Pickles, A., Hervas, A., Silberg, J. L., Rutter, M., & Eaves, L. (1998). Genetic influences on childhood hyperactivity: Contrast effects imply parental rating bias, not sibling interaction. *Psychological Medicine, 28,* 825–837.

Simonoff, E., Pickles, A., Hewitt, J., Silberg, J., Rutter, M., Loeber, R., Meyer, J., Neale, M., & Eaves, L. (1995). Multiple raters of disruptive child behavior: Using a genetic strategy to examine shared views and bias. *Behavior Genetics, 25,* 311–326.

Slater, E. (1958). The monogenic theory of schizophrenia. *Acta Genetica et Statistica Medica, 8,* 50–56.

Slutske, W. S., Heath, A. C., Bucholz, K. K., Madden, P. A. F., Bierut, L., & Reich, W. (1996, June). Lifetime history of separation anxiety disorder and the risk for alcoholism: A study of female adolescent twins and their parents. Paper presented at the meeting of the Behavior Genetics Association, Pittsburgh, PA.

Slutske, W. S., Heath, A. C., Dinwiddie, S. H., Madden, P. A. F., Bucholz, K. K., Dunne, M. P., Statham, D. J., & Martin, N. G. (1997). Modeling genetic and environmental influences in the etiology of conduct disorder: A study of 2,682 adult twin pairs. *Journal of Abnormal Psychology, 106,* 266–279.

Smith, C. (1974). Concordance in twins: Methods and interpretation. *American Journal of Human Genetics, 26,* 454–466.

Spitzer, R. L., Endicott, J., & Gibbon, M. (1979). Crossing the border into borderline personality and borderline schizophrenia. *Archives of General Psychiatry, 36,* 17–24.

Stevenson, J. (1992). Evidence for a genetic etiology in hyperactivity in children. *Behavior Genetics, 22,* 337–344.

Stevenson, J., Batten, N., & Cherner, M. (1992). Fears and fearfulness in children and adolescents: A genetic analysis of twin data. *Journal of Child Psychology and Psychiatry, 33,* 977–985.

Syvalahti, E. K. G. (1994). I. The theory of schizophrenia, biological factors in schizophrenia: Structural and functional aspects. *British Journal of Psychiatry, 164*(Suppl. 23), 9–14.

Thakker, J., & Ward, T. (1998). Culture and classification: The cross-cultural application of the DSM-IV. *Clinical Psychology Review, 18,* 501–529.

Thapar, A., Hervas, A., & McGuffin, P. (1995). Childhood hyperactivity scores are highly heritable and show sibling competition effects: Twin study evidence. *Behavior Genetics, 25,* 537–544.

Thapar, A., & McGuffin, P. (1994). A twin study of depressive symptoms in childhood. *British Journal of Psychiatry, 165,* 259–265.

Thapar, A., & McGuffin, P. (1995). Are anxiety symptoms in childhood heritable? *Journal of Child Psychology and Psychiatry, 36,* 439–447.

Thapar, A., & McGuffin, P. (1996). The genetic etiology of childhood depressive symptoms: A developmental perspective. *Development and Psychopathology, 8,* 751–760.

Topolski, T. D., Hewitt, J. K., Eaves, L. J., Silberg, J. L., Meyer, J. M., Rutter, M., Pickles, A., & Simonoff, E. (1997). Genetic and environmental influences on child reports of manifest anxiety and symptoms of separation anxiety and overanxious disorders: A community-based twin study. *Behavior Genetics, 27,* 15–28.

Torgersen, S. (1984). Genetic and nosological aspects of schizotypal and borderline personality disorders. A twin study. *Archives of General Psychiatry, 41,* 546–554.

Torgersen, S. (1994). Genetics in borderline conditions. *Acta Psychiatrica Scandinavica, 89*(Suppl. 379), 19–25.

Torgersen, S., Onstad, S., Skre, I., Edvardsen, J., & Kringlen, E. (1993). "True" schizotypal personality disorder: A study of co-twins and relatives of schizophrenic probands. *American Journal of Psychiatry, 150,* 1661–1667.

Torrey, E. F. (1992). Are we overestimating the genetic contribution to schizophrenia? *Schizophrenia Bulletin, 18*(2), 159–170.

Tsuang, M. T. (1998). Recent advances in genetic research on schizophrenia. *Journal of Biomedical Science, 5*(1), 28–30.

Tsuang, M. T., & Faraone, S. V. (1996). The inheritance of mood disorders. In L. L. Hall (Ed.), *Genetics and mental illness: Evolving issues for research and society* (Chap. 5, pp. 79–109). New York: Plenum Press.

van den Oord, E. J. C. G., Verhulst, F. C., & Boomsma, D. I. (1996). A genetic study of maternal and paternal ratings of problem behaviors in 3-year-old twins. *Journal of Abnormal Psychology, 105,* 349–357.

Van Os, J., & Marcelis, M. (1998). The ecogenetics of schizophrenia: A review. *Schizophrenia Research, 32,* 127–135.

Waldman, I. D., Elder, R. W., Levy, F., & Hay, D. A. (1996). Competing models for the underlying structure of the attention deficit disorders: Confirmatory factor analyses and multivariate genetic analyses in an Australian twin sample. *Behavior Genetics, 26* 602.

Waldman, I. D., Rhee, S. H., Levy, F., & Hay, D. A. (1998). Causes of the overlap among symptoms of attention deficit hyperactivity disorder, oppositional defiant disorder, and conduct disorder. Manuscript submitted for publication.

Willcutt, E. G., Shyu, V., Green, P., & Pennington, B. F. (1995, April). A twin study of the comorbidity of the disruptive behavior disorders of childhood. Paper presented at the *Annual Meeting of the Society for Research in Child Development.* Indianapolis, IN.

# CHAPTER 4

# Biological Variables in Psychopathology: A Psychobiological Perspective

## Don C. Fowles

## Introduction

The purpose of this chapter is to advocate a psychobiological approach to theories of psychopathology—appealing especially to psychologists to adopt a more biological perspective. Even though, happily, in recent years acceptance of biological influences on psychopathology has increased considerably among psychologists, many still give little more than lip service, and training in neuroscience is seldom part of a clinical curriculum. As a result, clinical psychologists tend to be cut off from various biopsychological disciplines that have obvious relevance to understanding behavior and psychopathology.

Foremost among these, the field of behavior genetics provides ample demonstrations of the influence of genetic differences on behavior. Additionally, behavior genetics provides perhaps the greatest justification for the study of personality differences that are so important in the clinic. A second, and more clinical, area that cannot be ignored is psychopharmacology and the related

Don C. Fowles • Department of Psychology, University of Iowa, Iowa City, Iowa 52246-2914.

*Comprehensive Handbook of Psychopathology* (Third Edition), edited by Patricia B. Sutker and Henry E. Adams. Kluwer Academic/Plenum Publishers, New York, 2001.

discipline of behavioral pharmacology. Even though the situation is not as simple as one drug, one diagnosis, undeniably there is some specificity involved in the use of drugs to treat psychopathological disorders: the different classes of drugs have different effects, and there is some specificity of the efficacy of the pharmacological treatment as a function of patient diagnosis. This drug-to-diagnosis matching is not well understood, and drug effects often cut across diagnostic boundaries. Nevertheless, the effects of these drugs must be understood if we are to have a comprehensive and adequate theory of psychopathology. Indeed, one of the most important potential advantages of adopting a psychobiological perspective is to develop a theoretical bridge between the effects of pharmacological treatment on neuroregulators, on the one hand, and the behavioral phenomena that constitute the disorder, on the other hand.

This theoretical bridge is an appropriate contribution for psychologists to make to the understanding of psychopathology because they are in a position to develop expertise in both behavioral theories and theories of brain–behavior relationships. Doing so will require mastery of such areas of study as behavioral neuroscience, behavioral pharmacology, and behavioral endocrinology. The rapid growth of knowledge in these fields is increasing our knowledge of neuroregulators and providing a better understanding of brain–behavior relationships. Although now it is difficult to span the theoretical gulf seamlessly between clinical phenomena and the concepts of these fields, attempts can be made and such an integration ultimately will contribute to our understanding of psychopathology.

Just as many psychologists have tended to minimize biology, many psychiatrists have tended to minimize psychological influences. The zeitgeist in psychiatry has so emphasized biological, especially genetic, factors—and this view has so pervaded the mass media—that the importance of environmental influences also needs to be stressed. Both clinical psychology and psychiatry can benefit from a psychobiological approach.

In part, the gulf between psychology and psychiatry is enhanced by uncritical use of the disease model. For example, some members of both professions tend to conclude that biological variables are important in psychopathology as support for the so-called medical or disease model. That conclusion is fundamentally flawed: biology is not a disease. Within-species genetic variation is entirely natural and affects virtually every aspect, at least to some degree, of brain structure and function (Rutter & Plomin, 1997). Whatever merit there may be to a disease model, it must rest on more than the demonstration of a genetic influence on behavior or on the finding that behavior has a biological substrate. In fact, there have been recent challenges to the uncritical application of the disease model that may help to move the two disciplines closer together. These will be discussed here.

## Compatibility of Biology and Psychology

Several important trends have served to underscore the need for more complex theories of psychopathology and to blur the distinction between biological and environmental influences. These trends include (1) clear demonstrations of environmental effects on brain structure and even gene manifestation, (2) the documentation of pervasive comorbidity in psychiatric disorders, and (3) evidence that both pharmacological treatments and genetic influences on psychopathology may be better understood as affecting temperament rather than discrete diseases.

## Environmental Effects on Brain Structure

In the traditional biological approach to psychopathology, genes determine brain structure, which, in turn, creates a vulnerability or predisposition to psychopathology. In recent years, however, a burgeoning literature points to experience-dependent changes in brain structure even in adults (e.g., Garraghty, Churchill, & Banks, 1998), dramatically blurring the distinction between biological-genetic and environmental influences. Kolb & Whishaw (1998) describe the evolution of this literature from the early reports of increased cortical mass for animals raised in "enriched" environments to current documentation that numerous types of experience produce major increases in the number of synaptic connections in species ranging from fruit flies to humans. The increased synaptic connections are promoted especially through the growth of dendrites (representing up to 95% of the receptor surface on which synaptic connections are formed) and of surrounding tissue that provides support for the increased metabolic demands of the enlarged neurons. These changes reflect an increase in the functional capacity of neural systems that have been stimulated by environmental conditions.

Along the same lines, Depue, Collins, and Luciana (1996) apply evidence for experiential effects on brain structure to the development of what Depue calls the Behavioral Facilitation System or BFS (described in more detail later), which responds to reward incentive stimuli. These authors argue that during sensitive periods in brain development, characterized by widespread overproduction of cortical synapses, the presence or absence of environmental stimulation greatly influences a process of "pruning back" these synaptic connections, that is, these transient synaptic connections are preserved on a long-term basis with relevant environmental experiences but otherwise are lost (pruned back). Further, two assumptions underscore a self-maintaining property of these environmental effects: an individual who has a strong BFS is said to have a lower threshold for responding to incentive cues and also will engage in greater exploration of the environment in search of rewarding stimulation. Both processes increase the environmental stimulation of the BFS, tending to maintain or strengthen synaptic connections in the Dopamine (DA) pathways. This focus on experiential effects on the strength of the BFS is important because, as will be seen later, the BFS is a motivational system that has clear relevance to theories of temperament and psychopathology.

Kandel (1998) addresses the implications of these environmental influences on brain structure for psychiatry. Although the basic genetic material is fixed (except mutations) and is passed on from generation to generation, the *expression* of a gene is highly subject to regulation. Hormones, stress, learning, and social interaction all produce changes in patterns of neuronal connections by influencing gene expression. Thus, all functions of the brain are susceptible to social influences. Consistent with this perspective, Kandel suggests that successful psychotherapy (or behavior therapy) produces alterations in gene expression and brain structure that may be similar to or synergistic with those produced by pharmacotherapy. Evidence in support of this expectation was provided in an imaging study of obsessive-compulsive disorder (OCD) in which both types of treatment produced changes in brain structure.

It should be clear from these examples that dichotomies between psychological and biological influences are inappropriate. Experience and behavior affect gene expression and brain structure, and reciprocally genes and brain structure affect behavior and experience. There should be no conflict between these perspectives but rather an effort to sort out the processes involved and their complex interactions.

## Comorbidity

Mineka, Watson, and Clark (1998) note that DSM-III (American Psychiatric Association, 1980) that embraces a neo-Kraepelinian belief in discrete mental disorders incorporated extensive exclusionary criteria to minimize diagnoses of more than one disorder. In response to criticism of that approach, DSM-III-R (American Psychiatric Association, 1987) greatly reduced these exclusionary criteria. On the basis of research conducted both before and after DSM-III-R, the pervasiveness of comorbidity has been well-documented (e.g., Clark, Watson, and Reynolds, 1995; Hinshaw, 1987; Maser & Cloninger, 1990; Meltzer, 1984; Mineka et al., 1998; Procci, 1989).

This comorbidity challenges the discrete disease model, inasmuch as the rates of comorbidity are too high to be assimilated by the chance occur-

rence of two independent diseases. Rather, comorbidity is more easily compatible with etiological models that hypothesize multiple biological and environmental influences that may involve some common elements of different disorders as we currently conceptualize them. As the discrete disease model becomes less and less tenable, the gap between psychologists and psychiatrists should narrow.

## Genetic Vulnerability, Pharmacological Treatment, and Temperament

Kendler, Neale, Kessler, Heath, & Eaves (1992) found that the data from a large twin study fit a model in which Generalized Anxiety Disorder (GAD) and Major Depression shared a common genetic vulnerability, and environmental factors determined whether anxiety or depression dominated the clinical picture. Also of interest, the authors suggest that the genes act largely by predisposing to *general distress*—a concept entirely consistent with concepts of temperament and the notion that dimensions of temperament contribute to the risk of psychopathology. Thus, a genetic study has challenged the older notion that these two common disorders are discrete diseases that have different underlying genetic etiologies, suggesting instead that more temperament-like processes are involved and that environmental influences determine which disorder develops. Along the same lines, Ely (1997) found a substantial common genetic influence for the Aggression and Delinquency scales of the Child Behavior Checklist (Achenbach, 1991) in Swedish twins aged 8–9 and, more surprisingly, cited other data for a major common genetic influence on aggression and depression among adolescents.

In a major paper championing the integration of genetic and environmental influences on psychopathology, Rutter (1997) notes that even large heritability estimates do not preclude large changes as a result of environmental effects. For example, both height and antisocial-criminal behavior show high heritabilities, yet the height of London schoolboys increased 12 cm during the first 50 years of the twentieth century, and crime rates increased fivefold during the last 50 years in most industrialized countries—both changes are attributable to environmental influences. Rutter (1997; Rutter & Plomin, 1997) concludes that the literature suggests a shift from a focus on genetic causes of a discrete categorical disorder to a focus on polygenetic contributions to the various dimensional risk factors (among which are temperament) involved in the multifactorial origins of psychopathology. Further, the behavior genetics literature has documented the ubiquity of environmental influences, leading to the conclusion that it is nature *and* nurture, not nature *or* nurture (Owen & McGuffin, 1997; Rutter & Plomin, 1997). There is no incompatibility between genetic and environmental approaches.

A similar emphasis on the fundamental relevance of temperament to psychopathology can be seen in the popular book *Listening to Prozac* (Kramer, 1993). (Prozac is a selective serotonin reuptake inhibitor, thereby increasing the activity of the neurotransmitter serotonin.) Kramer, a psychiatrist, discusses the implications of the drug's apparent success in altering personality and temperament in ways that patients find desirable. In contrast to earlier antidepressants, Prozac produced fewer unwanted negative effects (so-called "side effects"), allowing it to become very popular with his patients because of its effects on their *personalities*.

Kramer struggles with the realization that he was practicing "cosmetic psychopharmacology" (pp. 15, 184). Further, Prozac, along with many other psychotropic medications, is useful in a wide range of disorders (p. 45)—thereby undermining the simple one drug, one diagnosis disease model. Kramer concludes that medications do not treat specific illnesses but rather alter neurochemical systems (p. 45) and that Prozac's effects point to the importance of biological temperament (p. 182). Finally, Kramer embraces a "functional theory of psychopathology." He suggests that neurotransmitters (and medication) relate to such behavioral dimensions/functions as anxiety, aggression, and the ability to anticipate future pleasure in activities (p. 183), not to complex entities such as personality or mental illness. Consequently, progress in treating mental illness cannot be separated from progress in altering temperament (p. 184).

Thus, results from the two cornerstones of biological psychiatry—genetics and psychopharmacology—point to the importance of personality, temperament, and such behavioral dimensions as anxiety-proneness, aggressiveness, and sensitivity to reward incentive stimuli. These concepts could hardly be more compatible with psychology, suggesting that a rapprochement between psychological and biological approaches to psychopathology is in sight. With this conclusion, it is now time to turn to examples of the use of a motivational theory to understand psychopathology.

## Appetitive and Aversive Motivation

A comprehensive review of biological approaches to psychopathology is beyond the scope of a single chapter. Consequently, selected topics are reviewed to illustrate various points of articulation between biology and psychopathology. Specifically, the constructs of appetitive and aversive motivation are employed to illustrate a theoretical framework in which biological and psychological approaches to understanding psychopathology may be integrated (Fowles, 1988, 1992b, 1994).

In the attempt to formulate a psychobiological theory of psychopathology, motivational constructs borrowed from animal learning literature prove particularly useful for several reasons. First, their origin in research with nonhumans makes it possible to examine the contribution of neurotransmitter systems, which then relate directly to pharmacological and other biological theories of psychopathology. Second, the overlap between the concepts of motivation and emotion is sufficiently great that it is plausible to apply motivational constructs to what have traditionally been viewed as emotional disorders. Third, because these motivational constructs derive from the animal learning tradition, they necessarily emphasize environmental influences and have clear implications for behavior. Fourth, in the particular theoretical approach employed here, cognitive/information processing plays a large role, making this approach not at all incompatible with cognitive approaches to psychopathology. Thus, motivational constructs provide a theoretical bridge between biological concepts and the emotional and behavioral features that define psychopathology.

The constructs in question are hypothesized antagonistic appetitive and aversive motivational systems (e.g., Gray, 1975, 1987; Mackintosh, 1974). The primary function of these systems is to influence the probability of a behavioral response. The appetitive system activates behavior in response to cues indicating response-contingent positive outcomes, whereas the aversive system inhibits behavior in response to cues indicating response-contingent negative outcomes. In conflict situations, in which cues indicate both positive and negative outcomes, the appetitive and aversive systems oppose each other, and the probability of the response is determined by the relative strengths of the output from these reciprocally antagonistic systems. In addition to the behavioral consequences of activity in these motivational systems, both systems have affective components, as well: positively hedonic for the appetitive system and negatively hedonic for the aversive system.

For the present purposes, it is convenient to focus on Gray's (e.g., 1976, 1979, 1982, 1987; McNaughton & Gray, 1999) portrayal of the appetitive and aversive motivational systems, in part because Gray has also dealt with topics that are relevant to a biological approach to psychopathology. Gray calls the aversive motivational system the Behavioral Inhibition System or BIS, underscoring its effect on behavior. This author (Fowles, 1980) suggested *Behavioral Activation System* or BAS as a parallel name for the appetitive system, and Gray prefers to call it the *Behavioral Approach System* (also BAS); both names similarly call attention to the behavioral effect of this system. To understand the functions of the BAS and BIS and their interaction, it is necessary to consider four basic paradigms.

The first paradigm is a simple reward paradigm with 100% reinforcement, in which the organism learns to respond to obtain a reward. In this situation, conditioned stimuli associated with reward (Rew-CSs) exert their control over behavior via the BAS, that is, the BAS activates reward-seeking behavior in response to Rew-CSs.

This simple reward-learning situation can be transformed into an approach–avoidance conflict by introducing response-contingent punishment, once the rewarded response has been established. The introduction of punishment (in addition to the reward) results in reducing the rate or probability of responding (passive avoidance). Passive avoidance in the conflict situation is attributed to the inhibition of the approach response by the BIS in response to conditioned stimuli for punishment (Pun-CSs). Thus, it can be seen that, in this conflict situation, the BAS and the BIS act in opposition to each other: the BAS tends to activate approach behavior in response to Rew-CSs, and the BIS tends to inhibit these responses in the face of Pun-CSs. Whether an approach response will occur depends on which of these mutually antagonistic

systems is dominant—an outcome that, in turn, is influenced by the relative strength of the Rew-CS and Pun-CS inputs.

A similar mutual antagonism between the two systems is found in extinction: the nonoccurrence of an expected reward produces frustration, the functional equivalent of punishment. Stimuli in extinction become conditioned stimuli for frustrative nonreward, which activate the BIS and subsequently inhibit the approach response. As the nonreward CSs (nonRew-CSs) increase in strength over extinction trials, BIS activity increases and eventually becomes strong enough to inhibit the approach response. This brief description shows that the approach–avoidance conflict and the extinction paradigms are similar in many respects; the major difference is in the source of the aversive unconditioned stimulus (UCS)—whether it is an externally applied punishment or the nonoccurrence of an expected reward.

The fourth paradigm is the one-way, active-avoidance task, in which a conditioned stimulus is presented for several seconds before the onset of a shock. The animal receives the shock if it does nothing, but if it makes a response during the CS that takes it out of the compartment, it can avoid the shock altogether. The avoidance response is maintained by the nonoccurrence of an expected punishment, the functional equivalent of a reward. Consequently, the avoidance response is activated by the BAS in response to conditioned stimuli for relieving nonpunishment (nonPun-CSs), that is, the active-avoidance response is comparable to responses in a reward-learning situation. A paradigm traditionally viewed as involving anxiety in response to the threat of shock is viewed, in this model, as primarily involving the activation of behavior under the control of positive incentive motivation. Note that this conclusion implicates the appetitive motivational system in the response to stressful events. When faced with a threat of punishment, activation of the BAS may lead one to *actively cope*—that is, attempt to find a successful active-avoidance response. Alternatively, dominance of the BIS will inhibit responding (passive coping or inactivity).

Several aspects of the analysis of the four paradigms in terms of the two motivational systems require comment. First, the crucial variable is what happens to behavior. If behavior is activated, the BAS is involved; if behavior is inhibited, the BIS is involved. Second, Gray offered four terms to refer to the emotional or motivational state induced by each of these CSs. The two aversive motivational states are called "frustration" (for nonRew-CSs) and "fear or anxiety" (for Pun-CSs). The two appetitive motivational states are called "hope" (for Rew-CSs) and "relief" (for nonPun-CSs). Frustration and anxiety involve the same underlying motivational state; the difference between them is a matter of labeling based on the external stimulus conditions. Similarly, hope and relief involve a single motivational state; the differences again are attributable to the circumstances that induced that state. Third, in contrast to earlier S–R learning theories, this model incorporates an *expectancy* concept that allows the theory to account for the effects of the *non*occurrence of rewards and punishments.

Gray (1987, pp. 294–313) summarized his view of the neurophysiological substrate of the BIS that has been the focus of much of his own work. The BIS centers on the septohippocampal system (SHS), especially the control of hippocampal theta activity (5–12 Hz in the rat) by a pacemaker in the medial septal area, but includes the closely related Papez loop, noradrenergic pathways that ascend from the locus coeruleus to the SHS, serotonergic pathways that ascend from the raphe nuclei to the SHS, and neocortical structures (entorhinal, prefrontal, and cingulate cortex) that have two-way communication with the SHS. The SHS functions as a comparator, comparing actual with expected stimuli. When there is a mismatch (i.e., novelty) or when signals of punishment or nonreward are encountered, the SHS shifts to the control mode, in which it activates the (behaviorally inhibiting) outputs of the BIS. To fulfill this comparator function, the SHS must have access to information about current sensory events, past environmental regularities that allow predicting events, the next intended motor programs or plans, and information about the past consequences of such motor programs (Gray, 1987, pp. 293–294). Thus, the operation of the BIS involves extensive *information processing* that requires input from many higher level functions.

Gray has not been as concerned with the neural basis of the BAS, but he does suggest (e.g., Gray, 1987, pp. 308–309) that DA pathways are involved. Specifically, there is consistent evidence that the mesolimbic DA pathway that ascends from the A10 nucleus in the ventral tegmental area to the nucleus accumbens and the ventral striatum

plays a key role in incentive motivation. Consequently, it is likely that this pathway plays a central role in the BAS. As will be seen later, the mesolimbic DA system has been implicated in theories of both drug abuse and of the affective disorders. In both instances, the mesolimbic DA system is presumed to activate behavior in response to (reward) incentive cues—a function quite consistent with serving as the neurophysiological substrate for Gray's BAS. Thus, there is consistent support for the hypothesis that the mesolimbic DA system is involved in activating behavior in response to cues for reward. It should also be noted that Gray's BAS overlaps substantially with Depue's BFS (mentioned before and described more fully later), in both behavioral functions and underlying neurochemical pathways (Fowles, 1994).

Gray includes a third major system in his theoretical framework—the *fight/flight system*. This system is said to mediate the behavioral effects of *un*conditioned punishment and nonreward that result in escape and defensive aggression. The major pathways in the fight/flight system are the amygdala, the ventromedial nucleus of the hypothalamus, and the central gray of the midbrain (Gray, 1987, pp. 324). The ventromedial nucleus exerts tonic inhibitory control over the central gray, which is the "ultimate executive organ for either flight or defensive attack" (p. 324). In response to unconditioned punishment and unconditioned frustrative nonreward stimuli, the amygdala sends inhibitory signals to the ventromedial nucleus, thereby disinhibiting the central gray and the fight/flight response. Interestingly, the SHS sends excitatory signals to the ventromedial nucleus that intensify inhibition of the central gray in response to novel or threatening stimuli. Whether passive avoidance or fight/flight occurs in response to these stimuli depends on the relative strength of the inputs from the SHS and the amygdala.

To the extent that the material just presented identifies major motivational systems that play a central role in both emotional response and the regulation of behavior, it should be possible to identify their contribution to most major forms of psychopathology, as attempted by Fowles (1992b, 1994). This contribution may be direct or indirect. Direct effects include either *quantitative* individual differences in the strength of one of these systems inherently relevant to psychopathology (e.g., a weak but functioning BIS tends to produce BAS dominant or impulsive behavior) or a *qualitative* breakdown of function (e.g., an absence of BIS control over the BAS will lead to the unrestrained appetitive behavior seen in mania). Indirect effects occur when the primary source of the psychopathology is not found in one of the motivational systems—for example, schizophrenia—but where individual differences in the activity of the BAS and BIS affect the symptom pattern.

## Anxiety Disorders

### Competing Conceptualizations of Anxiety

In a number of papers published in the 1970s, Gray (e.g., 1976, 1978, 1979) proposed a "neuropsychological theory of anxiety" that draws on the motivational constructs described before. This early work can best be viewed as an attempt to understand, in terms of the constructs of learning theory, the common behavioral effects of those pharmacological agents that clinically reduce anxiety. Among these are alcohol, barbiturates, and minor tranquilizers.

Gray (1977) reviewed the extensive literature on the behavioral effects of antianxiety drugs, and he (1979) summarized the conclusions from that review. The studies reviewed pointed to reduced effectiveness of the BIS in inhibiting behavior in response to PUN-CSs and nonREW-CSs. With respect to the paradigms described before, the antianxiety drugs disinhibit behavior in the passive-avoidance situation, and they increase resistance to extinction following continuous reinforcement. Rates of response are also reliably increased under fixed-interval, fixed-ratio, and differential reinforcement of low-rate (DRL) schedules. The common feature of these three schedules is that an event signals that the animal's responses will not be rewarded for a period of time, thereby serving as a nonREW-CS. On the other hand, the antianxiety drugs do not affect responses that are viewed as primarily mediated by the BAS (e.g., simple reward learning and one-way active avoidance) or the fight/flight system. This specific effect of antianxiety drugs on the BIS, combined with the aversive quality of the stimuli that activate the BIS (i.e., cues for punishment and frustrative nonreward) make a strong case for Gray's conclusion that the BIS represents an anxiety system. Thus,

Gray's work provides a behavioral construct (the BIS) that is centrally involved in anxiety and that provides a link to biological treatments.

In recent years, however, a burgeoning literature has emphasized the importance of the *amygdala* for developing conditioned fear (e.g., LeDoux, 1995, 1996, pp. 157–174). More specifically, the lateral nucleus of the amygdala receives input (CSs from fear conditioning), and the central nucleus of the amygdala generates output for the fear response (e.g., freezing, autonomic nervous system responses, stress hormone release, etc.). The work of Davis (e.g., 1992) on the ability of CSs from fear conditioning to potentiate the startle response inspired Lang and his colleagues (e.g., Lang, Bradley, & Cuthbert, 1990) to develop the fear-potentiated startle paradigm with human subjects. This paradigm stimulated hundreds of studies and underscored the importance of the amygdala in fear and anxiety.

Noting the popularity of this work on the amygdala and the view of many that the amygdala rather than the SHS is centrally involved in anxiety, Gray and McNaughton (1998) attributed the differences between the SHS/BIS theory and the amygdala/startle theory to different starting points. Gray begins with the assumption that anxiolytic drugs affect anxiety and this path leads to the SHS. LeDoux and Davis begin with the assumption that responses to the CS in a classical aversive conditioning paradigm define anxiety and follow a path to the amygdala.

In a summary and revision of Gray's theory, McNaughton and Gray (2000) include the amygdala in an expanded and somewhat more complex BIS that provides, to some degree, an integration of the two approaches to understanding anxiety. McNaughton and Gray employ Blanchard's (e.g. Blanchard & Blanchard, 1990; Blanchard, Griebel, Henrie, & Blanchard, 1997) distinction between fear-related versus anxiety-related behaviors. *Fear-related* behaviors are those associated with the *fight/flight* response when a predator or an impending punishment is *present*. In contrast, *anxiety-related* behaviors are associated with *exploration or approach* in an approach–avoidance conflict, when a predator/punishment may or may not be present, that is, *fear* involves simple avoidance without conflict, whereas *anxiety* involves approach and goal conflict.

In this view, the SHS codes anxiety, whereas the amygdala mediates the fear that underlies both active and passive avoidance tendencies, controls behavioral avoidance consequent on anxiety, and increases arousal and autonomic responding. The SHS and its control of theta in the hippocampus is still the most important neural component of the BIS/anxiety system, and the amygdala is more obviously related to fear and fight/flight. However, the two structures are viewed as interacting in many situations as part of the BIS, and the amygdala contributes especially to passive avoidance in response to output from the SHS.

To summarize, the different perspectives offered by the septohippocampal and the amygdala literatures have not been fully reconciled, but some suggestions can be made. First, the cornerstone of Gray's theory of anxiety is the effects of anxiolytic drugs, whereas the amygdala/startle literature is tied strongly to immediate fear stimuli such as the CS in classical conditioning paradigms. Second, in the revised theory, the BIS is tied to approach–avoidance (goal) conflict. Anxiety derived from activity of the BIS involves *approach* to a source of danger, whereas the fight/flight system and *fear* involve *avoidance* of a source of danger. The amygdala is centrally involved in fear and fight/flight. Third, activity in the central nucleus of the amygdala produces an increase in autonomic and central nervous system *arousal*, whereas activity in the SHS involves more *information processing* and is more cognitive.

### Application to Anxiety Disorders

In an interesting extrapolation to psychopathology, McNaughton and Gray attribute GAD to excessive output from the SHS. Underscoring the information processing aspects of the SHS, they describe GAD as primarily a *cognitive disorder* that involves an excessive perception of threat and a subsequent suppression of approach and excessive avoidance of threat. In contrast, the fight/flight system (which has a greater involvement of the amygdala/fear system) mediates panic attacks (Gray, 1987, p. 366).

Gray's BIS theory readily accounts for the association between anxiety, on the one hand, and such characteristics as shyness, social withdrawal, sensitivity to punishments, a tendency to be easily discouraged, and a failure to develop active means of coping with situations, on the other hand—a dimension of internalizing disorders identified in

multivariate studies of children (Achenbach & McConaughy, 1997; Quay, 1986). These are the characteristics to be expected in an individual in whom the balance between the BIS and the BAS has shifted heavily toward dominance of the BIS. The more reactive BIS would generate anxiety in situations that are only moderately threatening. On the assumption that other people dispense both rewards and punishments, much social interaction can be seen as involving an approach–avoidance conflict. The dominance of the BIS over the BAS would, in this case, result in passive avoidance (shyness and social withdrawal). Similarly, the dominance of passive avoidance in conflict situations would impede the development of active coping skills. Finally, the dominance of the BIS in extinction situations would produce more rapid extinction that is manifested as a tendency to become easily discouraged and to give up when pursuing goals. Therefore, this cluster of characteristics can be seen as a consequence of a temperament in which the BIS is strongly dominant.

To more clearly assess application to anxiety disorders, it is useful to consider Barlow's (1988) theoretical analysis. Barlow distinguishes between two types of anxiety, which he calls anxiety and fear. More completely, anxiety is termed *anxious apprehension*, whereas fear is an *alarm reaction*. Anxious apprehension refers to a process of anticipatory anxiety that helps to prepare the organism to cope with the challenges and stresses of everyday life, and this process (in extreme form) underlies GAD. At pathological levels, anxious apprehension is said to consist of a diffuse cognitive-affective structure that has the following components: (1) negative affect, (2) high arousal, (3) perceptions of helplessness or uncontrollability of future events, and (4) "worry" or the allocation of attention to negatively valenced self-evaluative concerns and/or the autonomic correlates of the arousal itself.

Although Barlow's (1988) "anxiety" and Gray's BIS are not identical, there is enough overlap to argue that similar constructs are involved (Fowles, 1992a). Barlow's emphasis on preparation for stresses and challenges is entirely consistent with the role of the BIS in approach–avoidance conflict situations and situations involving frustration (failure) and with Gray's (1987, p. 263) comment that it prepares the organism for vigorous activity. Both anxiety systems, it is assumed, produce an increase in arousal. Barlow's emphasis on "worry" can be seen in Gray's (1982, p. 13) comment that the BIS allocates attention to "the maximum possible analysis of current environmental stimuli, especially novel ones" and his (1987, p. 263) description of the BIS as the "stop, look, and listen" system. Further, the conclusion, cited before from McNaughton and Gray (1999), that excessive output from the SHS is involved in the etiology of GAD underscores the similarity of Barlow's anxiety systems and Gray's BIS. Because the BIS is responding to potential threats (including uncertain threats in the form of novelty), it is reasonable to see that this vigilant anticipation and appraisal of threats involve worry. More recently, Barlow and Durand (1995, p. 157) comment that the BIS "seems heavily involved in anxiety" and agree that "Gray's thinking is very close to" Barlow's (1988) theory of anxiety and anxiety disorders. Overall, then, the two theoretical constructs share enough features that it can be proposed that Gray's behavioral inhibition system is involved in the etiology of GAD.

Returning to Barlow's (1988) theory, fear is modeled on Cannon's fight or flight response and is seen as a massive alarm reaction to potentially life-threatening situations. Panic attacks are viewed as alarm reactions, albeit *false alarms* in the sense that they are not based on objectively life-threatening situations. Panic attacks seen in the clinic include a fear of dying or losing control, as well as acute anxiety accompanied by somatic symptoms.

Citing evidence that false alarm panics are common in the population, Barlow suggests that they may serve as *un*conditioned stimuli for classical conditioning, leading to further conditioned panic attacks, which Barlow calls *learned alarms*. Because patients with Panic Disorder focus strongly on their internal physiological cues, both Barlow (1988) and Mineka (1985) suggest that interoceptive conditioning is involved, in which internal physiological cues become conditioned stimuli for panic attacks. What brings patients with Panic Disorder to the clinic, however, is not just the occurrence of panic attacks, but rather their anxiety over possible future uncued panic attacks. Whereas many individuals are not disabled by learned and/or unlearned panic attacks, Barlow suggests that those who become *anxiously apprehensive* about future attacks are disabled and seek treatment, that is, the same process of anxiety seen in GAD is proposed as a core feature of Panic Disorder. This line of reasoning is supported by the finding that patients with Panic Disorder almost always also meet the criteria for GAD.

Both Barlow's alarm reaction and Gray's fight/ flight system are modeled after Cannon's fight or flight response. Further, Barlow (Barlow and Durand, 1995, p. 157) cites Gray's fight/flight system as the basis for panic attacks and, as noted above, Gray (1987) relates the fight/flight system to panic attacks. Consequently, panic disorder can be seen as a strong response in Gray's fight/flight system combined with higher levels of activation of the BIS (producing worry and anxious apprehension). That is, Gray's motivational theory describes neurobehavioral systems that are involved in the major anxiety disorders.

Finally, the perception that alarm reactions and/ or negative events are neither predictable nor controllable is a risk factor for anxious apprehension in Barlow's theory (see also Mineka, 1985). This perception can be seen as related to the expectancies of response-contingent reward or relieving nonpunishment associated with activation of the BAS. Positive expectancies reduce the perceived threats of frustrative nonreward (failure) and punishment and, thereby, reduce input to the BIS, whereas activation of the BAS has a direct inhibitory effect on the BIS. In contrast, negative expectations will have the opposite effects.

## Substance Abuse

Major aspects of the literature on substance abuse fit particularly well with the motivational model. Although at one time it was argued that drug abuse could be attributed to physiological dependence *per se* (Jaffe, 1980; Leshner, 1997), there has been a substantial move toward the view that "abuse of reinforcers" conveys the essence of drug abuse, either through the termination of distress or dysphoria (negative reinforcement) or through the induction of pleasure or euphoria (positive reinforcement) (Baker, 1988; Wise, 1988).

The present discussion focuses on positive reinforcement as a mechanism underlying substance abuse. Such a mechanism suggests the involvement of Gray's BAS. It will be recalled that the BAS responds to cues for rewards, activates behavior, generates a positive emotional state, and is associated with the DA pathways that project from the ventral tegmental area to the limbic system (the mesolimbic DA system).

The contribution of appetitive motivation is particularly clear in the case of stimulant drugs (e.g., cocaine, amphetamines) and opioids (e.g., heroin, morphine). Conditioned incentive stimuli (environmental stimuli previously associated with the consumption of these drugs) generate appetitive motivational states and energize drug-seeking behavior (Stewart, de Witt, & Eikelboom, 1984). These conditioned incentive stimuli, it is also believed, contribute to relapse (Stewart et al., 1984)—that is, former addicts often relapse in the presence of cues previously associated with drug consumption.

Wise (1988) adopts a similar position but emphasizes that positive reinforcers elicit forward locomotion. Additionally, the ability to induce "psychomotor activation" is a common mechanism that underlies almost all drugs of abuse—not only stimulants and opioids, but also alcohol, barbiturates, benzodiazepines, cannabis, and others. This description of the common mechanism in Wise's theory of drug abuse as response to rewards and activating behavior is quite similar to the behavioral functions of Gray's BAS (and Depue's BFS).

A consensus has emerged concerning the neurochemical mechanisms that mediate the addicting effects of many drugs of abuse: these mechanisms involve the mesolimbic and mesocortical DA pathways (Koob & Le Moal, 1997; Leshner, 1997; Stewart et al., 1984; Wise, 1988; Wise & Rompre, 1989; Wise & Bozarth, 1987). Leshner (1997, p. 46) asserts that "Virtually all drugs of abuse have common effects, either directly or indirectly, on ... the mesolimbic *reward* system.... Activation of this system appears to be a common element in what keeps drug users taking drugs ... all addictive substances affect this circuit." Thus, the construct of appetitive motivation occupies a central position in the current literature on substance abuse, and the neurochemical substrate for these drug effects is the DA pathways associated with the BAS.

It is reasonable to further suggest that drug-seeking and drug-consuming behavior reflect the outcome of an approach–avoidance conflict, in which the BAS responds to the immediate positive reinforcing properties of the drugs, whereas the BIS responds to the much delayed negative consequences of drug consumption (e.g., loss of job and friends, legal problems, withdrawal distress, social disapproval, etc.). This conflict model explains

why a temperament of impulsivity/disinhibition is a strong risk factor for substance abuse (Sher & Trull, 1994). A dominance of the BAS over the BIS would produce both an impulsive temperament and a bias toward the positively reinforcing effects of drugs of abuse over the delayed negative consequences. Therefore, to the extent that this approach–avoidance conflict model applies, appetitive and aversive motivational constructs are particularly useful to understanding substance abuse.

# Affective Disorders

Much theorizing about affective disorders implicates concepts similar or identical to Gray's BAS. Almost all theories of depression implicate a loss of appetitive motivation, and Depue's theory of bipolar affective disorder parallels the BAS at both the behavioral and neurochemical levels.

## Appetitive and Aversive Motivation in Depression

The constructs of appetitive and aversive motivation are central to behavioral theories of depression. Depression is viewed as associated with the activation of aversive motivation and/or a disruption of appetitive motivation, and the greater emphasis is on the disruption of appetitive motivation. Indeed, disruption of appetitive motivation is a common feature of almost all behavioral theories of depression (e.g., Eastman, 1976). Similarly, in the cognitive theories of Beck (e.g., 1974, 1983, 1984) and Abramson and her colleagues (Abramson, Seligman, and Teasdale, 1978; Abramson, Metalsky, & Alloy, 1989), the depressed patient is seen as having developed expectations that reward-seeking will be ineffective (hopelessness). Bereavement, the prototype for reactive depressions, causes a reduction in, or absence of, both rewards and cues for rewards. A primary anhedonia—an inability to experience pleasure or to respond to rewards—is postulated by the more biological approaches (Davidson, 1994; Henriques, Glowacki, & Davidson, 1994; Klein, 1974). In still other theories, activation of aversive motivation is said to disrupt or inhibit appetitive motivation (e.g., Eastman, 1976; Ferster, 1973).

Note that in many of these theories aversive motivation is relevant to depression primarily insofar as it inhibits or disrupts appetitive motivation, because the loss of appetitive motivation is what distinguishes depression from anxiety. This view is supported by findings based on self-report inventories, in which high negative affect is associated with both anxiety and depression, but only depression is associated with the absence of positive affect (Mineka et al., 1998). Taking a more cognitive approach, Clark, Beck, & Stewart (1990) found that anxious patients expressed more fear of punishment in the form of thoughts of anticipated harm and danger, whereas depressed patients showed more concern about an inability to obtain rewards as indicated by hopelessness and more negative thoughts involving loss and past failure. The depressed patients expressed certainty (a "knowing" mode) about these events, whereas the anxious patients were apprehensive about what might happen (a "questioning" mode).

The application of Gray's theory organizes these theoretical approaches along the following lines. In the *extinction model*, any event that interferes with reward-seeking behavior (e.g., loss events, failures, or disabilities) places the person on extinction, initially creating negative affect (frustrative nonreward) as a result of disconfirmed positive expectations. To the extent that this interference is perceived as enduring—either by an evaluation of the initial event or resulting from experience with continued trials—expectancies change in the direction of seeing one's behavior as ineffective (hopelessness as proposed by the cognitive theories). As these expectancies change in a negative direction from helplessness (uncertainty) to hopelessness (certainty), the aversive motivational reaction diminishes (there are no longer positive expectations to be frustrated) and is replaced by the failure to activate appetitive motivation. In the *approach–avoidance conflict model*, reward motivation is blocked by aversive motivation in the form of fears of response-contingent punishment for making the appetitive response itself or for failure to perform successfully. If the person is strongly tempted to make the appetitive response, the aversive state of fear or anxiety will predominate. However, if the person comes to feel that the cost of such responding is unacceptably high and gives up, then hopelessness will prevail, appetitive behavior will be abandoned (a dominance of passive avoidance), and the anxiety will diminish (there is no threat in the absence of a response). In one well-documented phenomenon,

anxiety disorders precede major depression rather than the reverse (Mineka et al., 1998); this is interpreted in this context as an anxiety-induced shift from approach–avoidance conflict to a dominance of passive avoidance and the accompanying hopelessness. In the *uncontrollable punishment model* (e.g., an abused child, a battered wife, or a humiliated employee), avoidance responses are unsuccessful, leading to a state of hopelessness. In this case, however, aversive motivation will continue to be strong because of the continuing threat of punishment. Not infrequently, uncontrollable punishment will be mixed with one of the other models. For example, a young widow with several children, little education, and few financial resources may be exposed to numerous threats of punishment, as well as with the loss of rewards previously associated with her husband.

It is also important to note that the reciprocal antagonism between the appetitive and aversive motivational systems means that they are not completely independent. Activation of either system will tend to inhibit the other to some extent, and inactivation of either system will tend to disinhibit the other. Thus, even with a depression whose primary etiology involves inactivating appetitive motivation, there may be an increase in aversive motivation as well (e.g., Klein, 1974). Consequently, aversive motivation may increase as a primary etiological factor and also as a secondary consequence of the disruption of appetitive motivation that contributes to the common finding that anxiety is frequently seen in depression (Mineka et al., 1998). The amount of aversive motivation will depend on the strength of the person's aversive motivational system (disinhibiting a weak system will not result in much anxiety) and on the strength of the environmental cues for punishment and frustrative nonreward.

## Mania

The genetic contribution to mania is strong (e.g., Gershon, 1990; Katz and McGuffin, 1993; Owen & McGuffin, 1997; Rutter & Plomin, 1997), underscoring the need to consider biological factors. Mania appears to fit nicely into the theoretical framework that employs appetitive and aversive motivational systems, as seen in Depue's attempt to specify a biological substrate for mania within a neurobehavioral framework.

With respect to motivational systems, the symptoms of mania suggest that appetitive motivation is activated noncontingently, unrestrained by the BIS. These symptoms include an elevated, expansive mood, an increase in motor activity, engaging in activities with a high potential for painful consequences that is not recognized, and inflated self-esteem and overconfidence. The manic strongly seeks rewards (i.e., behavioral activation) in an unrestrained manner, confidently expects to achieve them due to insensitivity to the risks of punishment and frustrative nonreward, and enjoys a positive mood and high self-esteem in anticipation of attaining those rewards. Activation of the BAS in Gray's model should produce this covariation of behavioral activation, reward-seeking behavior, and positive mood. The breakdown of restraint of the BAS by the BIS would result in lack of awareness of potential risks and a minimal impact of actual failures. The strength of the activation of the BAS seen in mania suggests that the primary problem is excessive activation of the BAS, as opposed to simple lack of restraint by the BIS, but it is difficult to be certain. This author has suggested elsewhere (Fowles, 1988) that the irritability that arises when the manic is thwarted (Tyrer & Shopsin, 1982) could represent a response to frustration that violates social norms as a result of the lack of control by the BIS.

Depue and his colleagues (Depue, Arbisi, Spoont, Leon, & Ainsworth, 1989; Depue & Iacono, 1989; Depue, Krauss, & Spoont, 1987) proposed a neurobiological theory of bipolar affective disorder that bears many similarities to the perspective adopted here. Also consistent with the theme of this chapter, Depue and Iacono emphasize the importance of placing neurobiological hypotheses within a neurobehavioral framework that allows relating neurochemical deficits to the behaviors critical for diagnosis. At the level of a behavioral theory, the behavioral facilitation system (BFS) described by these authors is strikingly similar to the BAS. The BFS facilitates behavior via activation of locomotor activity and reward-incentive motivation, just as the BAS does. Similarly, Depue and Iacono conclude that the mesolimbic DA system is critically involved in the BFS, especially the projections of the A10 DA cell group in the ventral tegmental area to the nucleus accumbens (mesolimbic DA pathway) and the prefrontal cortex (mesocortical DA pathway).

Depue (Depue et al., 1987; Depue & Iacono, 1989) describe mania as exhibiting high levels of

the multiple manifestations of activity in the BFS: high motor activity (hyperactivity, rapid and pressured speech, and expressive facies), high incentive reward activation (excessive interest and pleasure, desire for excitement), a positive mood (elation, euphoria), high nonspecific arousal (manifested in changes in appetite, energy level, need for sleep, thought, attention, and sensory vividness), and cognitive changes (increased optimism and feelings of self-worth). Bipolar depression represents the opposite of mania, an absence of activity in the BFS (e.g., retardation—an absence of motor activity, anhedonia—no interest or pleasure, etc.). (See also Healy, 1989; Silverstone, 1985; and Wilner 1985, pp. 147–192, for dopamine involvement in mania.)

Depue et al. (1987) propose that the fundamental deficit in bipolar disorder is a failure to regulate the BFS (trait *variability*), which is different from the trait *level* of the strength of the BFS. Individual differences in the strength of the BFS (trait level) will affect the severity of manic episodes when regulation fails. A strong unregulated BFS will more often reach clinical severity for mania, and the manic component will be prominent. In contrast, a weak unregulated BFS is much less likely to result in a clear manic syndrome—producing a clinical picture of unipolar depression, even though the underlying etiology is the same as for bipolar disorder. This model is one of the few that can account for the appearance of unipolar depression among the relatives of bipolar probands, as is found in the genetics literature (e.g., Nurnberger & Gershon, 1992). This account explains the partial effectiveness of the traditional antipsychotic medications in treating mania because these drugs block dopaminergic activity in the mesolimbic and mesocortical pathways (see later). In this theory, the drugs would not address the problem of dysregulation, but they would weaken the BAS and thereby reduce manic behavior.

To summarize, Depue's theory of the etiology of bipolar disorder invokes an appetitive motivational system almost identical to the BAS. A failure of regulation of this system is the primary etiological factor that allows it to swing from excessive activation in mania and an absence of activation in bipolar depression (and some unipolar depressions). Implicating the mesolimbic and mesocortical dopamine pathways as central to this motivational system parallels Wise's concept of psychomotor activation in response to reward in substance abuse, as well as Gray's own suggestion for the BAS. Thus, the role of dopamine pathways for this appetitive motivational system is strongly documented. The dopamine projections from the ventral tegmental area to the nucleus accumbens are cited by all authors, whereas those to the prefrontal cortex are not always mentioned.

## Psychopathy

The modern usage of the term psychopathy dates from Cleckley's (e.g., 1964) clinical descriptions. Two of the features, impulsivity and an absence of anxiety, have been the object of motivational hypotheses. Lykken (1957) demonstrated poor electrodermal conditioning and/or rapid extinction using electric shock as the unconditioned stimulus and proposed that the electrodermal hyporeactivity reflected low fear in anticipation of punishment. Further, he showed that, in a "mental maze" task, psychopaths failed to avoid a punished incorrect alternative as well as controls. Poor performance on this passive avoidance task (an analog impulsivity task) was also attributed to poor fear conditioning.

Both findings have been conceptually replicated many times. After replicating the poor conditioning, Hare introduced a "countdown" to punishment task that also reliably shows electrodermal hyporeactivity in psychopaths in the few seconds before the delivery of punishment. All reviewers have found that electrodermal hyporeactivity in anticipation of punishment is a reliable finding (e.g., Fowles, 1993; Hare, 1978, 1998; Siddle & Trasler, 1981; Zahn, 1986). Similarly, the passive avoidance deficit has been demonstrated many times in psychopaths (e.g., Newman & Kosson, 1986; Newman, Patterson, & Kosson, 1987; Newman, Patterson, Howland, & Nichols, 1991; Newman, Widom, & Nathan, 1985; Schachter & Latane, 1964; Schmauk, 1970; Siegel, 1978) and in conduct disordered children who are low in anxiety (Frick, 1998).

Recent interpretations of Lykken's low fear hypothesis have employed Gray's model to propose that psychopaths have a weak BIS and a normal (or strong) BAS (e.g., Fowles, 1980, 1993; Frick, 1998; Gray, 1970, 1976; Lykken, 1995; Trasler, 1978). This hypothesis accounts for the disinhibitory psychopathology and lack of anxiety seen in psychopaths clinically—both central components

of the BIS. Normal reward learning and active avoidance of punishment is consistent with a normal (or strong) BAS.

In contrast to the electrodermal data, heart rate responses in paradigms that involve punishment do not show hyporeactivity in psychopaths and may even be larger than in controls (Hare, 1978, 1998). To account for this directional fractionation of electrodermal and cardiovascular reactivity, Fowles (1980, 1993) proposed that electrodermal activity in response to threats of punishment may reflect BIS activity, whereas heart rate more strongly reflects somatic activity and activation of the BAS.

Alternative biological hypotheses are also prominent in the literature. For example, Hare (1998) reviews an extensive literature that suggests a broader range of neurobiological anomalies than can be subsumed under the low fear hypothesis. In a similar vein, Patrick and Lang (1999) propose that, in addition to a primary fear deficit, psychopaths show a deficit in higher information processing systems that interact with motivational systems. Resolving these issues is beyond the scope of this chapter, but it is clear that (1) Gray's motivational concepts have been prominent in theories of the deficit associated with psychopathy and (2) alternative theories also refer to neurobiological processes.

## Schizophrenia

Two lines of research on schizophrenia provide much of the impetus for biological approaches to psychopathology: the importance of genetic influences in schizophrenia and the efficacy of neuroleptic drugs in ameliorating symptoms. Positive evidence on both counts supports the view that biology must be incorporated into theories of schizophrenia. Thus, schizophrenia provides clear support for the thesis that biological variables are important in psychopathology.

The case for applying motivational constructs to schizophrenia is less clear than in most other disorders because the central features of schizophrenia do not reflect too much or too little of the motivational systems discussed here. Nevertheless, it is reasonable to expect that such fundamental motivational systems might play an important role in modifying the clinical picture in schizophrenia and, for that reason, might account for some of the considerable heterogeneity in schizophrenia. Adopting this perspective, Fowles (1992b, 1994) proposed that individual differences in the strength of motivational systems constitute part of the genetic contribution to schizophrenia. The following is a brief summary of that effort.

## Genetic Contributions

The massive literature on the genetics of schizophrenia can be assimilated into a multifactorial polygenic model but cannot be made to fit a single-major-locus model with high penetrance (Faraone & Tsuang 1985; Gottesman, 1991; Moldin & Gottesman, 1997; Risch, 1990). There is no clear evidence against a simple multifactorial polygenic model, but Gottesman (e.g., 1991) notes the possibility of a mixed model. This model includes a small number of mostly genetic cases (a few single rare genes with high penetrance), a small number of cases due primarily to environmental factors, and a large number of cases falling within one of two polygenic models (one simply polygenic, the other a specific major gene of small effect embedded in a polygenic etiology). Thus, the vast majority of cases involve a polygenic etiology.

Heterogeneity in schizophrenia in the form of a chronic versus an episodic course is, at least as a first approximation, easy to conceptualize in a polygenic model. In the polygenic model with a threshold at which total liability produces symptoms of schizophrenia, a chronic course will (on average) be associated with greater genetic liability because there is an inverse relationship between the amount of genetic liability and the amount of environmental liability needed to reach threshold (Gottesman & Shields, 1982, pp. 63–69, 220–221). At high genetic loading, most environments will bring total liability above the threshold, making a chronic course likely. As the genetic loading decreases and more stressful environments are required to reach the threshold for symptom onset, the probability of encountering such environments diminishes, and an episodic course is more likely.

The polygenic model articulated by Gottesman includes environmental influences in the multifactorial etiology of schizophrenia (*general* environmental liability) and thus falls within the diathesis-stress model in which genetic vulnerability and environmental stress combine to produce an episode of schizophrenia. Additionally, the polygenic model includes both *specific* and *general* genetic

liability. Specific genetic liability increases the risk of schizophrenia *per se*. The sources of general genetic liability have not been specified other than to indicate that they have nothing to do with schizophrenia *per se*. Presumably, they represent *modifiers* or *potentiators* of the specific liability— that is, they are *nonspecific* contributors to etiology. As such, they are not part of the schizophrenia spectrum and will segregate independently of schizophrenia in family studies.

Fowles (1992b) proposed that the general genetic liability includes factors relevant to the stress component in the diathesis-stress model. Two broad categories of such factors are obvious. First, some genetically influenced characteristics may increase stress indirectly by making the environment objectively more stressful. For example, low IQ contributes to educational and occupational disadvantages, and temperament factors may interfere with one's ability to reach an adequate social and occupational adjustment (e.g., such behavioral deficit traits as anhedonia, shyness, social withdrawal, etc.). Second, any factor that increases stress reactivity will directly increase sensitivity to stressful environments (see Gottesman & Moldin, 1998). This second group of influences is especially relevant to motivational theories.

Because the BIS is an anxiety system and it has been suggested that it contributes to GAD, a genetic contribution to the BIS is an obvious potential contributor to general genetic liability. The BAS, with its accompanying positive affect, is less obvious but nonetheless also relevant. First, as noted before, the BAS is involved in many aspects of actively coping with threats. Consequently, it is likely to be activated strongly in stressful situations. Additionally, the finding that dopaminergic activity is increased during stressful events (Brier, Wolkowitz, & Pickar, 1991; Gray, 1987, p. 337; Healey, 1989) implicates the BAS in stress responses. This train of thought suggests that there might be two dimensions of arousal associated with heterogeneity in schizophrenia: (1) BAS activation involving *behavioral activation*, dopaminergic activity, and (sometimes) positive affect; and (2) BIS activation involving *behavioral inhibition* and aversive arousal (anxiety).

## The Dopamine Hypothesis

The second major development in biological approaches to schizophrenia was the demonstration of at least some therapeutic benefit from neuroleptics or antipsychotic drugs in treating schizophrenia and the determination that it is positive rather than negative symptoms (see later for this distinction) that respond to these drugs (e.g., Buckley & Meltzer, 1995; Crow, 1980; Weinberger & Lipska, 1995; Wirshing, Marder, Van Putten, & Ames, 1995). The therapeutic efficacy of antipsychotic drugs can be attributed to their ability to block DA receptors (e.g., Grace & Moore, 1998; Haracz, 1982; Losonczy, Davidson, & Davis, 1987; Snyder, 1978; Weinberger & Lipska, 1995). This suggests that DA pathways are important in schizophrenia and leads to the dopamine hypothesis of schizophrenia (Snyder, 1978). Much debate has centered on whether an increased sensitivity to dopamine might be a *primary* etiological factor in schizophrenia. At present, it appears more likely that dopamine makes a *secondary* contribution by interacting with some other primary deficit that makes the person sensitive to dopaminergic activity (e.g., Healy, 1989; Liddle, Carpenter, & Crow, 1993; Weinberger & Lipska, 1995).

Regardless of the eventual explanation, these findings concerning DA must be incorporated into a theory of schizophrenia. To bridge the theoretical gulf between neuroregulator effects and behavior, two questions must be answered: What are the behavioral implications of activity in the DA pathways? What do DA-related behaviors have to do with the behavioral phenomena of schizophrenia? If it is true that the mesolimbic (and mesocortical) DA pathways are involved in the BAS (activation of behavior in response to cues for reward and relieving nonpunishment with an accompanying positive hedonic tone), it is likely that antipsychotic drugs reduce activity in this system. From this perspective, one of the major behavioral effects of these drugs would be to reduce the responsiveness of the BAS. As expected from this hypothesis, patients treated with antipsychotic drugs show reduced positive affect and reduced sensitivity to rewards—that is, pharmacologically induced anhedonia (Harrow, Yonan, Sands, & Marengo, 1994; Healy, 1989; Sommers, 1985) that involves a range of negative symptoms (e.g., lack of emotional reactivity, lack of goal-directedness, reduced or retarded speech, diminished social and vocational initiative, etc.).

## Positive and Negative Symptoms

Strauss, Carpenter, & Bartko (1974) introduced the distinction between positive and negative symptoms, promoting awareness of an important aspect of heterogeneity in schizophrenia. Carpenter (1992; Liddle, Carpenter, & Crow, 1993) emphasized the challenge of this distinction to the conceptualization of schizophrenia. Positive symptoms are the presence of abnormal functioning, such as hallucinations and delusions, whereas negative symptoms reflect an inadequacy of normal functioning, such as affective flattening, poverty of speech, and social withdrawal (Sommers, 1985). Crow (1980, 1985) proposed a Type I dimension of schizophrenia characterized by prominent positive symptoms, responsiveness to antipsychotics, an acute onset, an episodic course, and good premorbid adjustment. Because of the role of DA in positive symptoms, Crow suggested that the Type I dimension is due to a neurochemical imbalance that involves dopamine. In contrast, Crow's Type II dimension involves prominent negative symptoms, a chronic course, an insidious onset, poor premorbid adjustment, intellectual deterioration, and a poor response to antipsychotics (Crow, 1985).

Early studies of the activity-withdrawal dimension in schizophrenia (based on ratings of ward behavior among hospitalized schizophrenics) are relevant to understanding negative symptoms. Active schizophrenics are characterized as restless, loud, overtalkative, overactive, and as having many friends and interests; withdrawn patients showed an absence of these features. Withdrawal has been related to chronicity, poor premorbid adjustment, negative symptoms, anhedonia, and high levels of (purportedly cortical) arousal as measured by skin potential and two perceptual measures (Depue, 1976; Venables, 1963a,b, 1967; Venables & Wing, 1962).

The activity-withdrawal dimension is important in this context because the balance between the BAS and BIS should influence the degree of activity versus withdrawal. This perspective suggests that negative-symptom, withdrawn patients show a dominance of passive avoidance due to high BIS activity and, quite likely, a deficiency in BAS activity. The low BAS activity could be due to a temperament-based weak BAS or to depression from a variety of sources (genetic factors, life events, demoralization, institutionalism, etc.).

Assuming that negative-symptom patients are BIS-dominant, the high arousal is presumably aversive arousal and mediates the stress response in the diathesis-stress model. If so, one would expect that anxiolytic drugs would be of some benefit in treating a subset of schizophrenic patients. In a review of pharmacological treatment, Wolkowitz and Pickar (1991) found that 30–50% of schizophrenic patients show favorable response to benzodiazepines and that this response is predicted by a range of symptoms including negative symptoms, core psychotic symptoms, and negative affect symptoms (see Fowles, 1994, for a more complete description). These findings are consistent with the notion that BIS activation may contribute to a wide range of symptoms.

At the other end of the activity-withdrawal dimension, the active behavior, interest in rewarding activities, and dominance of positive rather than negative symptoms among active schizophrenics all point to a contribution to liability from activation of the BAS. These patients have features of mania (Klein, 1982), further indicating BAS activation. Similarly, the good premorbid adjustment (extraverted behavior) and the contribution of dopamine to positive symptoms in Crow's Type I dimension suggest a BAS contribution to liability.

### The Schizoaffective Continuum

Although our diagnostic system treats schizophrenia and the affective disorders as unrelated diseases, there is a continuum from schizophrenia to affective disorders, patients with schizoaffective symptoms outnumber those with purely schizophrenic or purely affective symptoms (Kendell, 1982). Crow (1998, p. 502) concludes that "no objective genetic boundaries can be drawn" between predominantly affective and predominantly schizophrenic patients. The theoretical challenge of the schizoaffective disorders is well recognized (e.g., Baron & Gruen, 1991; Crow, 1986, 1991; Kendell, 1982; Meltzer, 1984; Taylor, 1992; Taylor, Berenbaum, Jampala, & Cloninger, 1993).

In schizoaffective disorder with manic symptoms, the DA theory of schizophrenia combined with Depue's DA theory of mania points to the obvious possibility that some vulnerability to schizophrenia (a primary schizophrenia deficit) combines with the high level of BAS-based DA activity in mania to produce schizophrenic symptoms. The continuum from schizophrenia to mania reflects the relative contributions of specific genetic liability for schizophrenia and the BAS-based general liability. A relatively large liability for schizophrenia requires only a modest amount

of BAS-DA activation and thus frequently would present as schizoaffective mania, mainly the schizophrenic subtype. In contrast, a more moderate liability for schizophrenia requires a strong BAS activation (more clearly a manic episode) to reach the threshold for symptom production, thereby presenting as the schizoaffective manic, mainly the manic subtype. Intermediate cases would show a more or less equal manifestation of schizophrenic and manic symptoms. Thus, the dopamine theories of schizophrenia and mania offer an explanation for the fusion of the boundaries of schizophrenia and the affective disorders. It should be noted that Braden (1984) proposed a very similar model.

In schizoaffective disorder with depressive symptoms, a similar suggestion can be made for a nonspecific contribution of depression to general liability for schizophrenia. Assuming that depression usually involves aversive arousal (from BIS activation), depression can be seen to fit the proposal cited before that aversive arousal contributes to the appearance of schizophrenic symptoms and a negative symptom pattern. Moreover, the hopelessness associated with depression will depress reward-seeking behavior and especially promote the anhedonic features of the negative symptoms. In support of this perspective, the symptoms of depression so overlap with the negative symptom pattern in schizophrenia that it is difficult to distinguish between the two (Sommers, 1985).

### Summary

Application of the motivational concepts of appetitive and aversive motivational systems to schizophrenia offers a theoretical framework for potentially understanding aspects of heterogeneity in schizophrenia. Both the BAS and BIS are involved in contributions to general liability to schizophrenia—both through responses to stressful environments and through adding to genetic liability. In this view, the BIS contributes passive avoidance and aversive arousal in the negative symptom syndrome in response to aversive environments and is involved in the schizoaffective continuum with depression. The BAS is involved in DA activity (and positive symptoms) during attempts to cope with stress, with the effects of antipsychotic medications on DA and the subsequent anhedonia, with the schizoaffective continuum with mania, and (when inactive during depression) with the anhedonia in the negative symptom syndrome.

## Final Comment

There are many biological theories of psychopathology, but motivational approaches have the advantages of being embedded in an overall theory of behavior, of inherently involving systems that respond to environmental influences, and of articulating with underlying neurobiological systems. The purpose of this chapter is to advocate a psychobiological approach. A motivational approach was used to illustrate how such an approach can integrate clinical features of disorders with genetic hypotheses, pharmacological treatments, and neurobiological systems. Whether or not the specifics of the suggestions offered here withstand the test of time and further research, it is hoped that the general approach illustrates the importance and attractiveness of adopting a psychobiological perspective.

## References

Abramson, L. Y., Seligman, M. E. P., & Teasdale, J. D. (1978). Learned helplessness in humans: Critique and reformulation. *Journal of Abnormal Psychology, 87,* 49–74.

Abramson, L. Y., Metalsky, G. I., & Alloy, L. B. (1989). Hopelessness depression: A theory-based subtype of depression. *Psychological Review, 96,* 358–372.

Achenbach, T. M. (1991). *Manual for the Child Behavior Checklist and 1991 profile.* Burlington: University of Vermont, Department of Psychology.

Achenbach, T. M., & McConaughy, S. H. (1997). *Empirically based assessment of child and adolescent psychopathology: Practical applications* (2nd ed.). Thousand Oaks, CA: Sage.

American Psychiatric Association. (1980). *Diagnostic and statistical manual of mental disorders* (3rd ed.). Washington, DC: Author.

American Psychiatric Association. (1987). *Diagnostic and statistical manual of mental disorders* (3rd ed., rev.). Washington, DC: Author.

Baker, T. B. (1988). Models of addiction: Introduction to the special issue. *Journal of Abnormal Psychology, 97,* 115–117.

Barlow, D. H. (1988). *Anxiety and its disorders.* New York: Guilford.

Barlow, D. H., & Durand, V. M. (1995). *Abnormal psychology: An integrative approach.* Pacific Grove, CA: Brooks/Cole.

Baron, M., & Gruen, R. S. (1991). Schizophrenia and affective disorder: Are they genetically linked? *British Journal of Psychiatry, 159,* 267–270.

Beck, A. T. (1974). The development of depression: A cognitive model. In R. J. Friedman & M. M. Katz (Eds.), *The psychology of depression* (pp. 3–27). Washington, DC: Winston & Sons.

Beck, A. T. (1983). Cognitive therapy of depression: New perspectives. In P. J. Clayton & J. E. Barrett (Eds.), *Treatment of depression: Old controversies and new approaches* (pp. 265–284). New York: Raven Press.

Beck, A. T. (1984). Cognition and therapy. *Archives of General Psychiatry, 41,* 1112–1114.

Blanchard, R. J., & Blanchard, DC (1990). Anti-predator defense as models of animal fear and anxiety. In P. F. Brain, S. Parmigiani, R. J. Blanchard, & D. Mainardi (Eds.), *Fear and defense* (pp. 89–108). Chur. Harwood Academic.

Blanchard, R. J., Griebel, G., Henrie, J. A., & Blanchard, DC (1997). Differentiation of anxiolytic and panicolytic drugs by effects on rat and mouse defense test batteries. *Neuroscience and Biobehavioral Reviews, 21,* 783–789.

Braden, W. (1984). Vulnerability and schizoaffective psychosis: A two-factor model. *Schizophrenia Bulletin, 10,* 71–86.

Brier, A., Wolkowitz, O. M., & Pickar, D. (1991). Stress and schizophrenia. In C. A. Tamminga & S. C. Schulz (Eds.), *Advances in neuropsychiatry and psychopharmacology: Vol. 1. Schizophrenia research* (pp. 141–152). New York: Raven Press.

Buckley, P. F., & Meltzer, H. Y. (1995). Treatment of schizophrenia. In A. F. Schatzberg & C. B. Nemeroff (Eds.), *Textbook of psychopharmacology* (2nd ed., pp. 615–639). Washington, DC: American Psychiatric Press.

Carpenter, W. T., Jr. (1992). The negative symptom challenge. *Archives of General Psychiatry, 49,* 236–237.

Clark, D. A., Beck, A. T., & Stewart, B. (1990). Cognitive specificity and positive-negative affectivity: Complementary or contradictory views on anxiety and depression? *Journal of Abnormal Psychology, 99,* 148–155.

Clark, L. A., Watson, D., & Reynolds, S. (1995). Diagnosis and classification of psychopathology: Challenges to the current system and future directions. *Annual Review of Psychology, 46,* 121–153.

Cleckley, H. (1964). *The mask of sanity* (4th ed.). St. Louis: Mosby.

Cole, J. O. (1964). Phenothiazine treatment in acute schizophrenia. *Archives of General Psychiatry, 10,* 246–261.

Crow, T. (1980). Molecular pathology of schizophrenia: More than one disease process? *British Medical Journal, 280,* 66–68.

Crow, T. J. (1985). The two-syndrome concept: Origins and current status. *Schizophrenia Bulletin, 11,* 471–486.

Crow, T. J. (1986). The continuum of psychosis and its implications for the structure of the gene. *British Journal of Psychiatry, 149,* 419–429.

Crow, T. J. (1991). The search for the psychosis gene. *British Journal of Psychiatry, 158,* 611–614.

Crow, T. J. (1998). From Kraepelin to Kretschmer leavened by Schneider. *Archives of General Psychiatry, 55,* 502–504.

Davidson, R. J. (1994). Asymmetric brain function, affective style, and psychopathology: The role of early experience and plasticity. *Development and Psychopathology, 6,* 741–758.

Davis, M. (1992). The role of the amygdala in fear-potentiated startle: Implications for animal models of anxiety. *Trends in Pharmacological Science, 13,* 35–41.

Depue, R. A. (1976). An activity-withdrawal distinction in schizophrenia: Behavioral, clinical brain damage, and neurophysiological correlates. *Journal of Abnormal Psychology, 85,* 174–185.

Depue, R. A., Arbisi, P., Spoont, M. R., Leon, A., & Ainsworth, B. (1989). Dopamine functioning in the Behavioral Facilitation System and seasonal variation in behavior: Normal population and clinical studies. In N. Rosenthal & M. Blehar (Eds.), *Seasonal affective disorder* (pp. 230–259). New York: Guilford.

Depue, R. A., Krauss, S. P., & Spoont, M. R. (1987). A two dimensional threshold model of seasonal bipolar affective disorder. In D. Magnusson & A. Ohman (Eds.), *Psychopathology: An interactional perspective* (pp. 95–123). New York: Academic Press.

Depue, R. A., & Iacono, W. G. (1988). Neurobehavioral aspects of affective disorders. *Annual Review of Psychology, 40,* 457–492.

Eastman, C. (1976). Behavioral formulations of depression. *Psychological Review, 83,* 277–291.

Ely, T. C. (1997). General genes: A new theme in developmental psychopathology. *Current Directions in Psychological Science, 6,* 90–95.

Faraone, S. V., & Tsuang, M. T. (1985). Quantitative models of the genetic transmission of schizophrenia. *Psychological Bulletin, 98,* 41–66.

Ferster, C. B. (1973). A functional analysis of depression. *American Psychologist, 28,* 857–870.

Fowles, D. C. (1980). The three arousal model: Implications of Gray's two-factor learning theory for heart rate, electrodermal activity, and psychopathy. *Psychophysiology, 17,* 87–104.

Fowles, D. C. (1988). Psychophysiology and psychopathology: A motivational approach. *Psychophysiology, 25,* 373–391.

Fowles, D. (1992a). Motivational approach to anxiety disorders. In D. G. Forgays, T. Sosnowski, & K. Wrzesniewski (Eds.), *Anxiety: Recent developments in cognitive, psychophysiological, and health research* (pp. 181–192). Washington/Philadelphia/London: Hemisphere.

Fowles, D. (1992b). Schizophrenia: Diathesis-stress revisited. *Annual Review of Psychology, 43,* 303–336.

Fowles, D. (1993). Electrodermal activity and antisocial behavior: Empirical findings and theoretical issues. In J.-C. Roy, W. Boucsein, D. Fowles, & J. Gruzelier (Eds.), *Progress in electrodermal research* (pp. 223–237). London: Plenum Press.

Fowles, D. (1994). A motivational theory of psychopathology. In W. Spaulding (Ed.), *Nebraska Symposium on Motivation: Integrated views of motivation and emotion* (Vol. 41) (pp. 181–238). Lincoln: University of Nebraska Press.

Frick, P. J. (1998). Callous-unemotional traits and conduct problems: Applying the two-factor model of psychopathy to children. In D. J. Cooke, A. E. Forth, & R. D. Hare (Eds.), *Psychopathy: Theory, research and implications for society* (pp. 161–187). Dordrecht, Netherlands: Kluwer Academic.

Garraghty, P. E., Churchill, J. D., & Banks, M. K. (1998). Adult neural plasticity: Similarities between two paradigms. *Current Directions in Psychological Science, 7,* 87–91.

Gershon, E. S. (1990). Genetics. In F. K. Goodwin & K. R. Jamison (Eds.), *Manic-depressive illness* (pp. 373–401). New York: Oxford University Press.

Gottesman, I. I. (1991). *Schizophrenia genesis.* New York: W.H. Freeman.

Gottesman, I. I., & Moldin, S. O. (1998). Genotypes, genes, genesis, and pathogenesis in schizophrenia. In M. F. Lenzenweger & R. H. Dworkin (Eds.), *Origins and development of schizophrenia* (pp. 5–26). Washington, DC: American Psychological Association.

Gottesman, I. I., & Shields, J. (1982). *Schizophrenia: The epigenetic puzzle.* New York: Cambridge University Press.

Grace, A. A., & Moore, H. (1998). Regulation of information flow in the nucleus accumbens: A model for the pathophysiology of schizophrenia. In M. F. Lenzenweger & R. H. Dworkin (Eds.), *Origins and development of schizophrenia* (pp. 123–157). Washington, DC: American Psychological Association.

Gray, J. A. (1970). The psychophysiological basis of intraversion-extraversion. *Behavior Research and Therapy, 8,* 249–266.

Gray, J. A. (1975). *Elements of a two-process theory of learning.* New York: Academic Press.

Gray, J. A. (1976). The behavioural inhibition system: A possible substrate for anxiety. In M. P. Feldman & A. Broadhurst (Eds.), *Theoretical and experimental bases of the behaviour therapies* (pp. 3–41). London: Wiley.

Gray, J. A. (1977). Drug effects on fear and frustration: Possible limbic site of action of minor tranquilizers. In L. L. Iversen, S. D. Iversen, & S. H. Snyder (Eds.), *Handbook of psychopharmacology: Vol. 8. Drugs, neurotransmitters, and behavior* (pp. 433–529). New York: Plenum Press.

Gray, J. A. (1978). The neuropsychology of anxiety. *British Journal of Psychology, 69,* 417–434.

Gray, J. A. (1979). A neuropsychological theory of anxiety. In C. E. Izard (Ed.), *Emotions in personality and psychopathology* (pp. 303–335). New York: Plenum Press.

Gray, J. A. (1982). *The neuropsychology of anxiety: An enquiry into the functions of the septo-hippocampal system.* Oxford: Oxford University Press.

Gray, J. A. (1987). *The psychology of fear and stress* (2nd ed.). Cambridge, England: Cambridge University Press.

Gray, J. A., & McNaughton, N. (1998, January). What's where in the neuropsychology of anxiety. Paper presented at a *Workshop on Arousal and Anxiety,* sponsored by NIMH, Rockville, MD.

Haracz, J. L. (1982). The dopamine hypothesis: An overview of studies with schizophrenic patients. *Schizophrenia Bulletin, 8,* 438–469.

Hare, R. D. (1978). Electrodermal and cardiovascular correlates of psychopathy. In R. D. Hare & D. Schalling (Eds.), *Psychopathic behavior: Approaches to research* (pp. 107–144). New York: Wiley.

Hare, R. D. (1998). Psychopathy, affect and behavior. In D. J. Cooke, A. E. Forth, & R. D. Hare (Eds.), *Psychopathy: Theory, research and implications for society* (pp. 105–137). Dordrecht, Netherlands: Kluwer Academic.

Harrow, M., Yonan, C. A., Sands, J. R., & Marengo, J. (1994). Depression in schizophrenia: Are neuroleptics, akinesia, or anhedonia involved? *Schizophrenia Bulletin, 20,* 327–338.

Healy, D. (1989). Neuroleptics and psychic indifference: A review. *Journal of the Royal Society of Medicine, 82,* 615–619.

Henriques, J. B., Glowacki, J. M., & Davidson, R. (1994). Reward fails to alter response bias in depression. *Journal of Abnormal Psychology, 103,* 460–466.

Hinshaw, S. P. (1987). On the distinction between attentional deficits/ hyperactivity and conduct problems/aggression in child psychopathology. *Psychological Bulletin, 101,* 443–463.

Jaffe, J. H. (1980). Drug addiction and drug abuse. In A. S. Gilman, L. Goodman, & A. Gilman (Eds.), *The pharmacological basis of therapeutics* (6th ed., pp. 535–584). New York: Macmillan.

Kandel, E. R. (1998). A new intellectual framework for psychiatry. *American Journal of Psychiatry, 155,* 457–469.

Katz, R., & McGuffin, P. (1993). The genetics of affective disorders. In L. J. Chapman, J. P. Chapman, & D. Fowles (Eds.), *Progress in experimental personality and psychopathology research: Vol. 16* (pp. 200–221). New York: Springer Publishing.

Kendell, R. E. (1982). The choice of diagnostic criteria for biological research. *Archives of General Psychiatry, 39*, 1334–1339.

Kendler, K. S., Neale, M. C., Kessler, R. C., Heath, A. C., & Eaves, L. J. (1992). Major depression and generalized anxiety disorder: Same genes, (partly) different environments. *Archives of General Psychiatry, 49*, 716–722.

Klein, D. F. (1974). Endogenomorphic depression: A conceptual and terminological revision. *Archives of General Psychiatry, 31*, 447–454.

Klein, D. N. (1982). Activity-withdrawal in the differential diagnosis of schizophrenia and mania. *Journal of Abnormal Psychology, 91*, 157–164.

Kolb, B., & Whishaw, I. Q. (1998). Brain plasticity and behavior. *Annual Review of Psychology, 49*, 43–64.

Koob, George F., & Le Moal, Michel. (1997). Drug abuse: Hedonic homeostatic dysregulation. *Science, 278*, 52–58.

Kramer, Peter D. (1993). *Listening to Prozac.* New York: Penguin.

Lang, P. J., Bradley, M. M., & Cuthbert, B. N. (1990). Emotion, attention and the startle reflex. *Psychological Review, 97*, 377–395.

LeDoux, Joseph E. (1995). Emotion: Clues from the brain. *Annual Review of Psychology, 46*, 209–235.

LeDoux, Joseph E. (1996). *The emotional brain: The mysterious underpinnings of emotional life.* New York: Simon & Schuster.

Leshner, Alan I. (1997). Addiction is a brain disease, and it matters. *Science, 278*, 45–47.

Liddle, P., Carpenter, W. T., & Crow, T. (1993). Syndromes of schizophrenia: Classic literature (editorial). *British Journal of Psychiatry, 165*, 721–727.

Losonczy, M. F., Davidson, M., & Davis, K. L. (1987). The dopamine hypothesis of schizophrenia. In H. Y. Meltzer (Ed.), *Psychopharmacology: The third generation of progress* (pp. 715–726). New York: Raven Press.

Lykken, D. T. (1957). A study of anxiety in the sociopathic personality. *Journal of Abnormal Psychology, 55*, 6–10.

Mackintosh, N. J. (1974). *The psychology of animal learning.* New York: Academic Press.

Maser, J. D., & Cloninger, C. R. (1990). Comorbidity of anxiety and mood disorders: Introduction and overview. In J. D. Maser & C. R. Cloninger (Eds.), *Comorbidity of mood and anxiety disorders* (pp. 3–12). Washington, DC: American Psychiatric Press.

McNaughton, N., & Gray, J. A. (2000). Anxiolytic action on the behavioral inhibition system implies multiple types of arousal contribute to anxiety. *Journal of Affective Disorders, 61*, 161–176.

Meltzer, H. Y. 1984. Schizoaffective disorder; Editor's introduction. *Schizophrenia Bulletin, 10*, 11–13.

Mineka, S. (1985). Animal models of anxiety-based disorders: Their usefulness and limitations. In A.H. Tuma & J. D. Maser (Eds.), *Anxiety and anxiety disorders* (pp. 199–244). Hillsdale, NJ: Erlbaum.

Mineka, S., Watson, D., & Clark, L. A. (1998). Comorbidity of anxiety and unipolar mood disorders. *Annual Review of Psychology, 49*, 377–412.

Moldin, S. O., & Gottesman, I. I. (1997). At issue: Genes, experience, and chance in schizophrenia—positioning for the 21st century. *Schizophrenia Bulletin, 23*, 547–561.

Newman, J. P., & Kosson, D. S. (1986). Passive avoidance learning in psychopathic and nonpsychopathic offenders. *Journal of Abnormal Psychology, 95*, 252–256.

Newman, J. P., Patterson, C. M., Howland, E. W., & Nichols, S. L. (1990). Passive avoidance in psychopaths: The effects of reward. *Personality and Individual Differences, 11*, 1101–1114.

Newman, J. P., Patterson, C. M., & Kosson, D. S. (1987). Response perseveration in psychopaths. *Journal of Abnormal Psychology, 96*, 145–148.

Newman, J. P., Widom, C. S., & Nathan, S. (1985). Passive-avoidance in syndromes of disinhibition: Psychopathy and extraversion. *Journal of Personality and Social Psychology, 48*, 1316–1327.

Nurnberger, J. I., Jr., & Gershon, E. S. (1992). Genetics. In E. S. Paykel (Ed.), *Handbook of affective disorders* (pp. 131–148). New York: Guilford.

Owen, M. J., & McGuffin, P. (1997). Genes and psychiatry (editorial). *British Journal of Psychiatry, 171*, 201–202.

Patrick, C. J., & Lang, A. R. (1999). Psychopathic traits and intoxicated states: Affective concomitants and conceptual links. In M. Dawson and A. Schell (eds.), *Startle modification: Implications for neuroscience, cognitive science, and clinical science* (pp. 209–230). New York: Cambridge University Press.

Paykel, E. S. (1982). Life events and early environment. In E. S. Paykel (Ed.), *Handbook of affective disorders* (pp. 146–161). New York: Guilford.

Procci, W. R. 1989. Psychotic disorders not elsewhere classified. In H. I. Kaplan and B. J. Sadock, Eds., *Comprehensive textbook of psychiatry/V* (pp. 830–842). Baltimore: Williams & Williams.

Quay, H. C. (1986). Classification. In H. C. Quay & J. S. Werry (Eds.), *Psychopathological disorders of childhood* (3rd ed., pp. 1–34). New York: Wiley.

Risch, N. 1990. Genetic linkage and complex diseases, with special reference to psychiatric disorders. *Genetic Epidemiology, 7*, 3–16.

Rutter, M. L. (1997). Nature-nurture integration. The example of antisocial behavior. *American Psychologist, 52*, 390–398.

Rutter, M., & Plomin, R. (1997). Opportunities for psychiatry from genetic findings. *British Journal of Psychiatry, 171*, 209–219.

Schachter, S., & Latane, B. (1964). Crime, cognition, and the autonomic nervous system. In M. R. Jones (Ed.), *Nebraska Symposium on Motivation* (Vol. 12), (pp. 221–273). Lincoln, NE: University of Nebraska Press.

Schmauk, F. J. (1970). Punishment, arousal, and avoidance learning in sociopaths. *Journal of Abnormal Psychology, 76*, 325–335.

Sher, K. J., & Trull, T. J. (1994). Personality and disinhibitory psychopathology: Alcoholism and antisocial personality disorder. *Journal of Abnormal Psychology, 103*, 92–102.

Siddle, D. A. T., & Trasler, G. (1981). The psychophysiology of psychopathic behaviour. In M. J. Christie & P. G. Mellett (Eds.), *Foundations of psychosomatics.* London: Wiley.

Siegel, R. A. (1978). Probability of punishment and suppression of behavior in psychopathic and non-psychopathic offenders. *Journal of Abnormal Psychology, 87*, 514–522.

Silverstone, T. (1985). Dopamine in manic depressive illness. *Journal of Affective Disorders, 8*, 225–231.

Snyder, S. H. (1978). Dopamine and schizophrenia. In L. C. Wynne et al. (Eds.), *The nature of schizophrenia* (pp. 87–94). New York: Wiley.

Sommers, A. A. (1985). "Negative symptoms": Conceptual and methodological problems. *Schizophrenia Bulletin, 11,* 364–379.

Stewart, J., de Witt, H., & Eikelboom, R. (1984). Role of unconditioned and conditioned drug effects in the self-administration of opiates and stimulants. *Psychological Review, 91,* 251–268.

Strauss, J., Carpenter, W. T., Jr., & Bartko, J. (1974). The diagnosis and understanding of schizophrenia: Part III. Speculations on the processes that underlie schizophrenic symptoms and signs. *Schizophrenia Bulletin, 1* (Experimental Issue #11), 61–69.

Taylor, M. A. (1992). Are schizophrenia and affective disorder related? A selective review of the literature. *American Journal of Psychiatry, 149,* 22–32.

Taylor, M. A., Berenbaum, S. A., Jampala, V. C., & Cloninger, C. R. (1993). Are schizophrenia and affective disorder related? Preliminary data from a family study. *American Journal of Psychiatry, 150,* 278–285.

Tellegen, A. (1985). Structures of mood and personality and their relevance to assessing anxiety, with an emphasis on self-report. In A. H. Tuma & J. D. Maser (Eds.), *Anxiety and the anxiety disorders* (pp. 681–706). Hillsdale, NJ: Erlbaum.

Trasler, G. (1978). Relations between psychopathy and persistent criminality—methodological and theoretical issues. In R. D. Hare & D. Schalling (Eds.), *Psychopathic behavior: Approaches to research* (pp. 273–298). New York: Wiley.

Tyrer, S., & Shopsin, B. (1982). Symptoms and assessment of mania. In E. S. Paykel (Ed.), *Handbook of affective disorders* (pp. 12–23). New York: Guilford.

Venables, P. H. (1963a). The relationship between level of skin potential and fusion of paired light flashes in schizophrenic and normal subjects. *Journal of Psychiatric Research, 1,* 279–287.

Venables, P. H. (1963b). Selectivity of attention, withdrawal, and cortical activation. *Archives of General Psychiatry, 9,* 74–78.

Venables, P. H. (1967). The relation of two flash and two click thresholds to withdrawal in paranoid and non-paranoid schizophrenics. *British Journal of Social and Clinical Psychology, 6,* 60–62.

Venables, P. H., & Wing, J. K. (1962). Level of arousal and the subclassification of schizophrenia. *Archives of General Psychiatry, 7,* 114–119.

Ventura, J., Nuechterlein, K. H., Lukoff, D., & Hardesty, J. P. (1989). A prospective study of stressful life events and schizophrenic relapse. *Journal of Abnormal Psychology, 98,* 407–411.

Weinberger, D. R., & Lipska, B. K. (1995). Cortical maldevelopment, antipsychotic drugs, and schizophrenia: A search for common ground. *Schizophrenia Research, 16,* 87–110.

Wirshing, W. C., Marder, S. R., Van Putten, T., & Ames, D. (1995). Acute treatment of schizophrenia. In F. E. Bloom & D. J. Kupfer (Eds.), *Psychopharmacology: The fourth generation of progress* (pp. 1259–1266). New York: Raven Press.

Wise, R. A. (1988). The neurobiology of craving: Implications for the understanding and treatment of addiction. *Journal of Abnormal Psychology, 97,* 118–132.

Wise, R. A., & Bozarth, M. A. (1987). A psychomotor stimulant theory of addiction. *Psychological Review, 94,* 469–492.

Wise, R. A., & Rompre, P.-P. (1989). Brain dopamine and reward. *Annual Review of Psychology, 40,* 191–225.

Wolkowitz, O. M., & Pickar, D. (1991). Benzodiazepines in the treatment of schizophrenia: A review and reappraisal. *American Journal of Psychiatry, 148,* 714–726.

Zahn, T. P. (1986). Psychophysiological approaches to psychopathology. In M. G. H. Coles, S. W. Porges, & E. Donchin (Eds.), *Psychophysiology: Systems, processes, and applications* (Vol. 1) (pp. 508–610). New York: Guilford.

# CHAPTER 5

# Culture, Ethnicity, and Psychopathology

## Jeanne L. Tsai, James N. Butcher, Ricardo F. Muñoz, and Kelly Vitousek

For decades, transcultural psychiatrists, cross-cultural psychologists, clinical psychologists, medical anthropologists, and others have been interested in answering the following questions: Are mental disorders that are observed in Western cultural contexts also seen in other cultural contexts? Does culture influence the expression and meaning of symptoms? Are there disorders that exist only in specific cultural contexts? Does the social and psychological impact of mental illness vary across cultural contexts? And how should clinicians treat individuals of cultural backgrounds different from their own?

Scientists and clinicians have been very interested in answering these questions for several reasons. Cultural studies of psychopathology distinguish among aspects of mental illness that generalize across cultures, that are culture-specific, and that are unique to the individual. These studies advance our knowledge about human disease and dysfunction. Most studies in psychology and psychiatry have focused primarily on White populations of European descent and assume that what is true for White European samples is true for other cultural groups. However, cross-cultural studies have demonstrated that this is not the case. For instance, cross-cultural studies of depression have revealed that feelings of guilt and self-reproach are more frequently associated with depression in Western than in non-Western cultural contexts (Sartorius, Jablensky, Gulbinat, & Ernberg, 1980). Thus, these symptoms may not be universal aspects of depression.

Cultural studies of psychopathology are also important because they elucidate the subjective experience or meaning of mental illness. For example, Estroff (1989) argues that the disorganizing symptoms of schizophrenia may be experienced more negatively in cultures that view the self as stable than in cultures that view the self as dynamic. Understanding cultural influences on psychopathological processes and the meanings of mental illness is critical for accurately diagnosing and effectively treating culturally diverse clinical populations. This becomes increasingly urgent as our society becomes more global and multicultural.

Jeanne L. Tsai • Department of Psychology, Stanford University, Stanford, California 94305.    James N. Butcher • Department of Psychology, University of Minnesota, Minneapolis, Minnesota 55455-0344.    Ricardo F. Muñoz • Department of Psychiatry, University of California, San Francisco, California 94143.    Kelly Vitousek • Department of Psychology, University of Hawaii, Honolulu, Hawaii 96822.

*Comprehensive Handbook of Psychopathology* (Third Edition), edited by Patricia B. Sutker and Henry E. Adams. Kluwer Academic / Plenum Publishers, New York, 2001.

## Defining "Culture," "Ethnicity," and "Psychopathology"

*Culture* has been defined in a variety of ways. Anthony Marsella, a leading expert in cross-cultural psychology, provides one of the most comprehensive definitions:

At an external level, culture is represented in various artifacts, architectural and expressive forms, institutions, and role and behavioral patterns. But culture is also represented internally, in the values, attitudes, beliefs, cognitive styles, and patterns of consciousness of an individual. As such, it is the primary mediator or filter for interacting with the world; it is the lens by which we experience and define reality and orient ourselves to others, the unknown, and to our subjective experience. (Marsella, 1987, p. 381)

*Ethnicity* is the "culture" of a specific ethnic group or the segment of a larger society that views itself and is viewed by others as different from the majority culture in language, religion, customs, beliefs, values, physical characteristics, and/or ancestral homeland. Members of an ethnic group "participate in shared activities built around their (real or mythical) common origin and culture" (Yinger, 1986, p. 22). In this chapter, the term "culture" subsumes "ethnicity."

In general, cross-cultural studies of psychopathology have operationalized "culture" poorly. Most studies use national status as a proxy for culture and race as a proxy for ethnicity. As a result, these studies overlook the tremendous variation within national and racial groups and the similarity among national and racial groups in values, beliefs, and other cultural variables that may influence aspects of psychopathology. Few investigators explicitly identify or measure the cultural variables that presumably explain differences between cultural groups.

*Psychopathology* is the study of abnormal behavior (Davison & Neale, 1994). However, even in Western clinical psychology and psychiatry, it is difficult to define what constitutes "abnormal" behavior. Davison & Neale (1994) propose that "abnormal behavior" is statistically infrequent, violates cultural or societal norms, creates personal distress and suffering, impairs the individual functionally, and is an unexpected response to environmental cues. In general, cross-cultural studies of psychopathology have relied on Western classification systems such as the *Diagnostic and Statistical Manual of Mental Disorders*, 4th edition (DSM-IV) (American Psychiatric Association, 1994) or the International Classification of Diseases (ICD-10) (World Health Organization, 1992) to define abnormal behavior. The problems with this approach will be discussed later in the chapter.

## Theoretical Perspectives

Scholars differ in the degree to which they believe that abnormal behavior is similar across cultural contexts. Traditionally, theoretical perspectives were cast as either "culture-specific" or "universal." Culture-specific perspectives maintain that because cultures define what is "normal" and "abnormal" and because cultures change over time, what constitutes "abnormal behavior" can be defined only by members of a particular cultural group at a particular time in history (Draguns, 1977). Thus, abnormal behavior is culturally relative. Most proponents of culture-specific approaches endorse the use of "emic" methods, or tools and instruments that are specific to the culture of interest, to study the cultural aspects of psychopathology.

Universal perspectives, however, view particular behaviors as "abnormal," regardless of cultural context and historical time. According to this perspective, Western conceptions of abnormal behavior are applicable to other cultural contexts. Proponents of universal perspectives use "etic" methods, or tools and instruments that presumably can be applied in different cultural contexts and, therefore, allow cross-cultural comparisons. The tools and instruments used in "etic" studies are typically developed in Western cultural contexts and translated into the language of the culture of study (Segall, Lonner, & Berry, 1998).

Most current views of psychopathology rarely assume either the "culture-specific" or the "universal" stances in their extreme forms. Instead, current perspectives acknowledge that both cultural similarities and cultural differences exist. However, they vary in what they consider the defining aspect of mental illness, which influences the degree to which they hypothesize cultural variation in mental illness.

### Cultural Idioms of Distress

One prevailing viewpoint, the *cultural idioms of distress* perspective, posited by Arthur Kleinman, Byron Good, Janis Jenkins (1991) and other medical anthropologists, suggests that mental illness cannot be separated from its sociocultural context. As stated by Draguns (1982), a particular symptom only becomes an indicator of distress in its "transaction with the environment." From this standpoint, what matters is not whether specific symptoms exist across cultures, but whether the *meaning* and *subjective experience* of and the *social response* to these symptoms are similar across cultures (Jenkins, Kleinman, & Good, 1991; Krause, 1989).

## Biomedical Approach

In contrast, the *biomedical* perspective, shared primarily by mainstream psychiatrists and psychologists, views the cause of mental disorders as physical dysfunction, such as biochemical or anatomical defects (Rosenhan & Seligman, 1989, p. 47). From this standpoint, internal *symptoms* are the defining aspects of mental illness. Culture may influence the content of specific symptoms (e.g., the religious content of hallucinations) and patients' beliefs about the origins of mental illness (e.g., spiritual vs. biological causes), but the core symptoms of a specific disorder and their impact on psychological functioning are assumed to be similar across cultures.

## Variation Across Different Types of Mental Disorders

Marsella (1987) offers a slightly different perspective that accounts for variation among mental disorders. He proposes that the least cultural variation occurs in mental disorders that are the most biologically based, such as severe neurological disease, and the most cultural variation occurs in mental disorders that most closely resemble "normal" behavior (and therefore, are presumably the least biologically based). Thus, he classifies disorders in the following way (from the least to the most culturally variable): severe neurological disease, minor neurological disease, functional psychotic disorders, neurotic disorders, and minor transient states. According to Marsella (1987), disorders such as schizophrenia would vary less across cultures than unipolar depression or general anxiety disorder. Although this perspective appears to explain much of the current empirical findings, it is limited by our incomplete knowledge of the "biological" aspects of various mental

disorders. Thus, it is unclear whether specific neurotic disorders such as depression are indeed less biological than psychotic disorders such as schizophrenia.

Findings from the empirical literature do not entirely confirm or disconfirm any of these theoretical perspectives. Instead, empirical findings support different aspects of each theoretical perspective. Before turning to the empirical literature on culture and psychopathology, we discuss one of the most challenging issues in the cross-cultural study of psychopathology—assessment.

## Assessing Psychopathology Across Cultures

To study mental illness across cultures, one must first be able to identify and then classify mental illness in different cultural contexts (see later section for assessment in clinical treatment). This is one of the most challenging aspects of studying psychopathology across cultures. The most widely used nosological systems were developed in Europe (ICD-9) and North America (DSM-IV) and have been criticized for their Western cultural assumptions (Fabrega, 1989). These systems are fraught with shortcomings, even when applied in Western settings. Low reliability, poor validity, and high rates of comorbidity (i.e., the co-occurrence of presumably distinct disorders) are of highest concern (Butcher, 1982; Clark, Watson, & Reynolds, 1995; Krueger, Caspi, Moffitt, & Silva, 1998).

Additional challenges arise when these systems are used with non-Western cultural and ethnic groups. First, because these systems rely primarily on clinical diagnosis, they may obscure cultural differences and/or similarities in specific symptoms. Thus, cultural differences in prevalence rates of clinical depression, for example, may belie cultural differences in the specific symptoms of depression, such as depressed mood, loss of energy, and sleep problems. Second, behavior that is defined as "abnormal" by these Western classification systems may fall well within the realm of normal behavior in other cultural contexts. In Puerto Rico, for instance, dissociative states are considered normal aspects of religious and spiritual practices, whereas in many Western contexts, they are considered symptoms of mental illness (Lewis-Fernandez, 1998). Third, abnormal behaviors in non-Western cultural contexts may be excluded in these classification systems. In an attempt to address this last issue, DSM-IV (American Psychiatric Association, 1994) includes an appendix that lists "culture-bound syndromes," or disorders that occur in specific cultural settings only. For example, "koro" is a disorder primarily found in parts of Southern Asia (Taiwan, Indonesia, Malayasia, Borneo, and Southern China) in which males harbor an "obsessive fear that their penises will withdraw into their abdomens." More recently, specific disorders found primarily in Western cultures have also been considered "culturally bound." They include "anorexia nervosa," in which individuals (typically females) have an obsessive concern with their weight, and "multiple personality disorder," in which one person is thought to have multiple personalities that assume control over that person's behavior (Takahashi, 1990).

Although the inclusion of "culturally bound syndromes" into the DSM-IV has been hailed as a major step toward acknowledging the influence of culture on psychopathology, it has also encountered much criticism (Hughes, 1998). This debate will be discussed at greater length later in the chapter. Despite these problems, Western classification systems are widely used in cultural studies of psychopathology due to the lack of alternative non-Western classification systems.

Researchers have employed different methods for assessing psychopathology across cultures. These include self-report inventories (e.g., rating scales, personality instruments) and interview schedules (e.g, structured vs. open-ended).

## Self-Report Inventories

Most self-report inventories of psychopathology were developed in Western cultural contexts. These are often translated into another language and adapted in ways that increase their cultural relevance for use in non-Western cultural contexts. These instruments include the Beck Depression Inventory, which has been translated for use with Chinese, Vietnamese, Latino, Hmong and other cultural groups and the Minnesota Multiphasic Personality Inventory (MMPI), which has been translated more than 150 times, validated in numerous cross-cultural settings, and used in more than 46 countries. Recently, the MMPI was revised to assess a broader range of problems, to contain more contemporary items, and to include norms that are more appropriate for cross-cultural comparisons (Butcher, Dahlstrom, Graham, Tellegen, & Kaemmer, 1989). This version of the MMPI, the MMPI-2 (for adults), has already been translated into more than 26 languages. The MMPI-A (for adolescents) has also been translated into more than a dozen languages.

**The Issue of Equivalence.** The main problem with using Western instruments to assess psychopathology in other cultural contexts is their *equivalence* (i.e., the extent to which a word, concept, scale, or norm structure can be considered relevant and applicable to cultural groups other than those for which the instrument was developed) (Marsella, 1987). For example, *linguistic equivalence* is achieved when a specific term is the same across languages. Tanaka-Matusmi and Marsella (1976) demonstrated the lack of linguistic equivalence between the words "depression" and "yuutsu" (the Japanese translation of "depression") by having Americans and Japanese list words that they associated with the terms. Whereas Americans associated depression with being "blue," "sad," "down," in "despair," and "dejected," Japanese associated depression with the "mountains," "rain," "storms," and the "dark." *Conceptual equivalence* is achieved when constructs assume the same meaning across cultures. An example of the lack of conceptual equivalence also comes from American-Japanese comparisons: "dependency" in American culture is considered a negative attribute; in Japan, it is the cultural ideal for interpersonal relationships (Doi, 1973). Other forms of equivalence are *psychometric* and *psychological equivalence*, which demonstrate that the psychometric properties of translated instruments are similar and that the items assume the same significance and meaning across languages respectively (Butcher, Coelho, & Tsai, in press).

Various techniques have been proposed to establish instrument equivalence. Extensive research on the MMPI-2 has shown that equivalence can be achieved by following specific procedures (Butcher, 1996). These include (1) having independent investigators translate English versions of an instrument into the language of interest; (2) combining these independent translations into one version, based on decisions by a committee of cultural and linguistic experts; (3) conducting a series of translations and back-translations until all item wordings are accurate; (4) administering the original and translated versions of the instrument to bilinguals to ensure that their responses are captured similarly by both versions; and (5) using methods such as item response theory, factor analysis, and norm development to assess the conceptual equivalence of the scale.

For some investigators, however, these techniques for ensuring equivalence are not at all sufficient. They argue that regardless of the lengths taken to establish equivalence, instruments developed in Western culture are replete with Western cultural assumptions and exclude non-Western processes and phenomena. These investigators prefer emically derived instruments. Unfortunately, truly emic instruments are rare. The Hispanic Stress Inventory (Cervantes, Salgado de Snyder, & Padilla, 1991) and a number of African-American instruments (Jones, 1996) are among the few that exist.

### Interviews

Interviews have also been used to assess psychopathology across cultural contexts. Structured clinical interviews such as the Diagnostic Interview Schedule (Robins, Helzer, Croughan, & Ratcliff, 1981) and the Present State Examination (Wing, Cooper, & Sartorius, 1974) have been used widely in cross-cultural studies of mental illness. For example, the latter was used in the World Health Organization's study of schizophrenia across cultures (Jablensky, 1989). Issues of equivalence apply here because these interview schedules were developed in Western cultural contexts. Ethnographic interviews are more open-ended and presumably allow respondents to reveal their cultural conceptions of mental illness. Therefore, they are considered more emic in nature. For example, Krause (1989) conducted ethnographic interviews with ten Punjabi men and women of diverse ages to examine "sinking heart," a syndrome of heart distress that has been compared to Western conceptions of depression, Type A behavior, and stress. Krause asked her respondents questions about the causality, symptomatology, treatment, and consequences of "sinking heart," but also encouraged them to talk about what they considered the important aspects of this illness. Based on her interviews, Krause concluded that although Western conceptions of depression, Type A behavior, and stress overlap with "sinking heart," they do not capture its more subtle physical, cultural, and emotional aspects. For example, "sinking heart" experiences are related to problems in individuals' emotional, sexual, and marital relationships and to conflicts in honor and morality (Krause, 1989).

The primary criticism of ethnographic interviews is that, compared to self-report questionnaires, they are more time- and labor-intensive. As a result, they can be conducted only with small samples. In addition, they are more idiographic (specific to each individual) and do not lend themselves to nomothetic (group) comparisons. Often the lack of standardization in interview format also makes comparisons across ethnographic studies extremely challenging. Thus, critics often question the generalizability of findings from ethnographic interviews.

### Multimethod Approaches

The most convincing studies of psychopathology across cultures are those that employ multiple methods and therefore incorporate the strengths of each method. For example, Guarnaccia studied "ataques de nervios" using both ethnographic (Guarnaccia, DeLaCancela, & Carrillo, 1989) and epidemiological methods (Guarnaccia, 1993). From his comprehensive study of four cases of "ataques de nervios," Guarnaccia was able to identify the most meaningful aspect of "ataques de nervios," i.e., their relationship to upsetting or frightening events in the family sphere. In his larger scale epidemiological study, Guarnaccia was able to assess whether these findings generalized to a larger population. He also administered the Diagnostic Interview Schedule/Disaster Supplement (Robins & Smith, 1983) to this population to examine how "ataques de nervios" related to Western psychiatric disorders. Guarnaccia (1993) found that the descriptions of "ataques de nervios" revealed in his case studies generalized to a larger Puerto Rican population. In addition, he found that although the majority of Puerto Ricans who reported an "ataque" also suffered from symptoms of depression and anxiety, "ataque de nervios" could not be easily mapped onto either of these psychiatric disorders. Thus, by using multiple methods, Guarnaccia was able to examine the meaning of "ataque de nervios," its generalizability across cultural subgroups, and its relationship to Western psychiatric disorders.

# Central Questions Regarding Culture and Psychopathology

Researchers have used the methods described previously to answer some of the central questions about culture and psychopathology: Are mental disorders observed in Western contexts seen in other cultural contexts? Does culture influence the expression and meaning of symptoms? Do "culturally bound" syndromes exist? Does the social and psychological impact of mental illness vary across cultural contexts? And how should clinicians treat individuals of cultural backgrounds different from their own? Significantly more empirical research has been conducted on the occurrence and presentation of mental illness (the first four questions) than on the impact and treatment of mental illness (the last two questions). In the next section, we review some of this research.

### Are Mental Disorders Observed in Western Contexts Seen in Other Cultural Contexts?

Emil Kraeplin, the principal founder of psychiatric nosology, was one of the first scholars interested in the occurrence and expression of mental illness across cultures. He hypothesized that cultural differences in incidence and prevalence rates of mental disorders across cultures existed and were related to differences in social conditions and ethnocultural characteristics (e.g., values). Furthermore, he believed that examining such differences would advance our understanding of pathological processes (Jilek, 1995):

If the characteristics of a people are manifested in its religion and its customs, in its intellectual and artistic achievements, in its political acts and its historical development, then they will also find expression in the frequency and clinical formation of its mental disorders, especially those that emerge from internal conditions. ("Voelkerpsychologie," Kraeplin, 1904, p. 437, as cited in Jilek, 1995)

Kraeplin journeyed to Java to collect data to support his hypothesis. He concluded that several disorders that were prevalent in Europe were absent in Java and that the expressions of affective and schizophrenic disorders were somewhat different in Java from those in the United States.

Although he was unable to test this hypothesis directly or in other cultures, investigators since his time have (Jilek, 1995). Most of the existing research on psychopathology across cultures has focused on schizophrenia (and related psychotic disorders), depression (and related affective disorders), anxiety, and substance abuse and dependence.

Investigations of the occurrence of specific mental disorders across cultures are epidemiological. Typically, they use Western classification systems to diagnose mental disorders and then compare the total number of cases of a particular disorder within a specific period (i.e., prevalence) across cultures. A few studies examine the number of *new* cases of a particular disorder within a specific period (i.e., incidence) across cultures, but these studies are relatively rare.

**Schizophrenia.** The term "schizophrenia" has been used to describe a cluster of symptoms that include delusions; hallucinations; disorganized thought, speech, and/or behavior; restrictions in emotional experience and expression; and lack of goal-directed behavior (American Psychiatric Association, 1994). There is strong evidence of a genetic and biological component in schizophrenia. However, this genetic vulnerability is expressed only under stressful environmental conditions (Gottesman & Moldin, 1997; Gottesman & Bertelsen, 1989). Most of the empirical findings suggest that schizophrenia occurs across cultural contexts at similar annual incidence and lifetime prevalence rates.

The WHO Program of Cross-Cultural Research on Schizophrenia is the most comprehensive of cross-cultural studies of schizophrenia. Conducted from 1967–1986, this research program was comprised of three studies that sampled more than eighteen psychiatric centers in Africa, Asia, Europe, and Latin and North America. More than 3,000 patients were assessed using a standard clinical interview (Present State Examination) and then were reassessed 1, 2, and/or 5 years after the initial screening (Jablensky, 1989). The psychiatric centers included were divided into those that represented "developing" (e.g., Nigeria, India, Taiwan) and those that represented "developed" (e.g., United States, United Kingdom) countries. Across cultural contexts, the lifetime prevalence rate of schizophrenia was a little more than 1% of the population (Jablensky, 1989). Moreover, when schizophrenia was conservatively defined, its annual incidence rates did not statistically differ among the cultures sampled and ranged from 0.7 to 1.4 per 10,000 persons across cultures (Jablensky, 1989). The external correlates of schizophrenia were also similar across cultural groups. Males showed an earlier onset of symptoms than females across the cultural groups; Cetingok, Chu, & Park (1990) found similar sex differences in their study of schizophrenia in Turkish and European-American samples. Schizophrenia was also associated with other cerebral and physical diseases across cultures (Jablensky, 1989). These findings suggest that the core aspects of schizophrenia are minimally shaped by culture.

Exceptions to the WHO findings, however, have been observed. For example, higher incidence rates of schizophrenia were found among British Afro-Caribbean immigrant groups (for review, see Jarvis, 1998). Schizophrenia occurs six to eight times more frequently among British Afro-Caribbean immigrant groups than in the native White British population. Several studies suggest that these differences are not due to misdiagnosis (Jarvis, 1998). Therefore, Jarvis (1998) argues that schizophrenia is not biologically based and, instead, results from environmental stresses such as migration, broken family structure, socioeconomic disadvantage, and racism. Future research must assess whether this is the case.

**Affective Disorders.** There are several types of affective disorders, but unipolar and bipolar depression are the most distinct. Unipolar depression refers to a constellation of affective and vegetative symptoms that include depressed mood, loss of interest and pleasure in activities, fatigue, agitated movement, sleep problems, and changes in appetite and weight. Other symptoms associated with unipolar depression in Western contexts include feelings of worthlessness and thoughts of death. Bipolar depression describes manic symptoms such as grandiosity, flight of ideas, pressured speech, and irritability; often these manic states are interrupted by episodes of unipolar depression. Unlike unipolar depression, there is evidence that bipolar disorder has a strong genetic component (Egeland, 1994). The bulk of the research findings suggest that unipolar and bipolar depression occur across cultures, but at varying prevalence rates.

*Bipolar Depression.* Epidemiological studies conducted in the United States did not find ethnic differences in lifetime prevalence rates of bipolar depression. For example, in the Epidemiological Catchment Area Study (ECA) of 18,000+ adults in five U.S. communities, lifetime prevalence rates of one type of bipolar disorder for White American, African-American, and Hispanic groups were 0.8, 1.0, and 0.7%, respectively (Weissman et al., 1991). Moreover, there were no significant sex differences in lifetime prevalence rates of bipolar depression across the three ethnic groups. More recently, findings from the National Comorbidity Survey (NCS) (Kessler et al., 1994), a study of psychiatric disorders in a national probability sample of 8,090 respondents including African-American, White American, and Hispanic groups, also suggest that prevalence rates of bipolar depression do not differ by ethnicity or sex.

*Unipolar Depression.* Lifetime prevalence rates of unipolar depression, however, differ among ethnic and cultural groups. For example, in the ECA study, lifetime prevalence rates of unipolar depression were higher for White Americans (5.1%) than for African-Americans (3.1%) and Hispanics (4.4%). Moreover, prevalence rates were higher for women than for men (Weissman et al., 1991) across the three ethnic groups. Findings from the NCS also suggest that African-Americans have significantly lower prevalence rates of depressive disorders than White Americans, even after controlling for differences in income and education. Contrary to the ECA findings, Hispanic groups in the NCS study had significantly higher rates of unipolar depression than non-Hispanic White Americans and African-Americans (Kessler et al., 1994). There are a variety of possible explanations for the discrepancy in findings between the ECA and NCS studies. For instance, the stresses and life circumstances encountered by Hispanic groups may have increased during the two periods. It is also possible that the studies included Hispanic samples that varied in their generational status, acculturation levels, and specific Hispanic heritage (e.g., Cuban vs. Puerto Rican).

In fact, differences in prevalence rates have been found among specific Hispanic groups. For instance, Moscicki et al. (1987) analyzed the Hispanic Health and Nutrition Examination Survey (H-HANES) data and found that the prevalence rates for unipolar depression (in parentheses) varied for Cuban males (1.4%), Cuban females (2.9%), Mexican males (1.0%), Mexican females (3.6%), Puerto Rican males (3.4%), and Puerto Rican females (7.4%). Within the same subgroup, differences were reported based on the length of the stay in the United States and the generational level. In a study of Mexican immigrants and Mexican-Americans in California, Vega and colleagues (1998) found that unipolar depression levels were lowest for recent immigrants (3.2%), were higher for those who had been in the United States thirteen years or more (7.9%), and were highest for those born in the United States (14.4%). The rates of the last group did not differ significantly from those reported for the entire NCS sample (17.2%).

Although the NCS and ECA studies did not include a significant number of Asian-Americans to allow for statistically powerful analyses, findings from other studies demonstrate differences between White and Asian-American prevalence rates of depression. In a study of 1,747 Chinese-Americans in Los Angeles, Takeuchi and colleagues (1998) found that the lifetime prevalence of depression was 6.9%, which was higher than that for White Americans in the ECA study. Other studies also found higher levels of depressive symptomatology among Asian-Americans compared to White Americans. In a San Francisco community sample, Ying (1988) found that Chinese-Americans had higher levels of depressive symptoms as measured by the Center for Epidemiological Studies-Depression Scale (CES-D) than White American community samples. Asian-American college students also reported *higher* levels of depressive symptoms than their White American counterparts (as measured by the Zung Self-Rating Depression Scale [Fugita & Crittenden, 1990] and the Beck Depression Inventory [Okazaki, 1997]). However, because these studies examined reported levels of depressive symptomatology as measured by rating scales, it is unclear whether the groups would have differed in rates of diagnosable clinical depression.

Prevalence rates of unipolar depression also differ across cultures (Jenkins, 1991). For instance, lifetime prevalence rates of unipolar depression are lower in Asian countries than in Western countries. The Taiwan Psychiatric Epidemiological Project found that prevalence rates of depression in Taiwanese samples were significantly lower than those of White Americans in the ECA study (1.14% in Taiwan, compared with 4.9% in ECA) (Hwu et al., 1986). Recent evidence, however, suggests that the magnitude of this Western-Asian cultural difference may be decreasing (Nakane et al., 1991). A variety of explanations have been proposed to explain these cultural differences in prevalence rates of depression. For instance, some propose that because Asian cultures place a greater emphasis on family and other social relationships than Western cultures, the occurrence of depression is rare. Others, however, argue that depressive symptoms occur at similar rates in Asian and Western cultures, but because mental illness is severely stigmatized in Asian cultures, depressive symptoms are rarely diagnosed as such (Kleinman, 1986).

**Anxiety Disorders.** Anxiety disorders are generally characterized by excessive worry and apprehension about the future (Castillo, 1998). Specific anxiety disorders include obsessive-compulsive disorder, panic disorder, simple phobias, and post-traumatic stress disorder. Compared to schizophrenia and depression, we know little about the way culture influences anxiety disorders (Draguns, 1994; Guarnnaccia, 1997). This may be due to the rare occurrence of "pure" anxiety disorders. Because anxiety often co-occurs with other disorders such as depression (Sartorius et al., 1996), it may be obscured by these other disorders.

In general, findings from epidemiological studies suggest that groups that are under significant stress have higher prevalence rates of anxiety disorders. The ECA study (Robins & Regier, 1991) found that generalized anxiety disorder was more common among females than males, among individuals of lower income than of higher income, and among African-Americans than White Americans when panic and depression were excluded (Blazer et al., 1991). In a separate analysis of the Los Angeles ECA data, however, Karno and colleagues (1989) found that Mexican-Americans had *lower* rates of generalized anxiety disorder than White Americans. The Mexican American Prevalence and Services Survey (MAPSS) (Vega et al., 1998) found further differences in prevalence rates for anxiety disorder among specific Mexican-American groups. The lowest rates of "any anxiety disorder" were found for recent Mexican immigrants (7.6%); a higher rate was found for immigrants who lived in the United States for 13 years or more (17.1%), and the highest rate was found for U.S.-born Mexicans (24.1%), which was similar to the rate for the entire NCS sample (25.0%). Vega and colleagues (1998) propose that traditional aspects of Mexican culture may protect individuals from these disorders.

Although the NCS study also found sex differences in rates of generalized anxiety disorder, none of the ethnic differences found in the ECA study emerged. Although there are many possible explanations for the discrepancy in findings between the ECA and NCS studies, it is possible that levels of stress among ethnic groups were less similar during the ECA study than during the NCS study. This possibility is consistent with findings that prevalence rates of depression and related disorders are increasing across the world (Klerman, 1993).

Ethnic differences were also found in prevalence rates of specific anxiety disorders. In the ECA study, African-Americans demonstrated nearly twice the rate of simple phobia and agoraphobia than White Americans (Eaton, Dryman, & Weissman, 1991). In a separate analysis of the Los Angeles ECA data, American-born Mexicans had higher rates of simple phobia and agoraphobia than White Americans or immigrant Mexican-Americans (Karno and colleagues, 1989). These findings were not replicated in the NCS study. In both the ECA and NCS studies, ethnic differences were not found for panic disorder; however, across ethnic groups, females demonstrated higher rates of panic disorder than males. Differences in rates of obsessive-compulsive disorder were also found among ethnic American populations in the ECA study. Specifically, rates of obsessive-compulsive disorder were highest among White American females and lowest among Hispanic males (Karno & Golding, 1991).

Although Asian-Americans were not included in either the ECA or NCS studies, other studies (Okazaki, 1997; Uba, 1994; Ying, 1988) suggest that they have higher levels of anxiety symptoms than White Americans, especially those related to social concerns. Because these findings were based on levels of symptomatology, it is unclear whether White and Asian-American groups would differ in prevalence rates of diagnosable anxiety disorders. Regardless, these differences have been attributed to higher levels of acculturative stress and language difficulties among Asian-American populations, although no studies have assessed whether this is in fact the case (Al-Issa & Oudji, 1998).

Very little is known across cultures about prevalence and incidence rates of most types of anxiety, except obsessive-compulsive disorder. Lifetime prevalence rates of obsessive-compulsive disorder are similar across a number of Western and non-Western countries, including Taiwan, Uganda, Puerto Rico, Greece, Italy, New Zealand, Korea, and Hong Kong, and range from 1 to 3% (Weissman et al., 1994; Staley & Wand, 1995).

In summary, cultural and ethnic variation have been found in prevalence rates of general anxiety disorder and specific phobias. These differences have been attributed to cultural and ethnic differences in life circumstances and stress. Prevalence rates for disorders such as panic disorder and obsessive-compulsive disorder, however, demonstrate few cultural and ethnic differences. Because relatively few studies have examined the prevalence rates of anxiety disorders across cultural and ethnic groups, more studies are needed before more definitive statements can be made.

**Substance Abuse and Dependence.** Substance abuse refers to the overuse of alcohol and/or drugs that results in harmful physical, social, legal, or interpersonal consequences; substance dependence is marked by continued use of alcohol or other drugs, despite these consequences. The WHO has argued that an individual's cultural context must be considered when diagnosing an alcohol problem. For a drinking problem to exist, individuals must drink more than is considered acceptable by their culture, must drink during times that are not culturally acceptable, and must drink to the extent that their health and social relationships are harmed (WHO, 1975). Obviously, these criteria can be applied to other substances as well. Like anxiety, there is relatively little cross-cultural work on substance abuse and dependence. In part, this may be because alcoholism and other forms of substance abuse have been considered actual diseases only in the past few decades (Bennett, Janca, Grant, & Sartorius, 1993; Caetano, 1989). Therefore, we expect to see more cross-cultural work on alcoholism and substance abuse and dependence in the near future.

Ethnic differences in rates of alcohol consumption have been found. However, these studies received much criticism (Trimble, 1991). Within the United States, Native Americans have the highest alcohol consumption rate, followed by White Americans, African-Americans, and Hispanic-Americans (Baxter, Hinson, Wall & McKee, 1998). Among Native American tribes, there is considerable variation in alcohol consumption: May (1982) found that whereas a minority of Navajo (30%) reported drinking during the last year, a majority of Ojibwa (84%) reported drinking during the last year. White Americans tend to use more non-alcoholic recreational drugs than other ethnic groups, except inhalants and cocaine (Baxter, Hinson, Wall & McKee, 1998). Weatherspoon, Danko, and Johnson (1994) found that Koreans living in Korea drink more than Chinese living in Taiwan; however, these differences did not carry over to Korean-Americans and Chinese-Americans living in Hawaii. Across cultural groups, men engage in greater substance use than women (Baxter, Hinson, Wall & McKee, 1998).

It is unclear whether cultural and ethnic differences in consumption rates of alcohol and other substances translate into different prevalence rates for substance abuse and dependence (Trimble, 1991). Evidence from cross-cultural studies of alcohol consumption suggests they do not. Cultures that have the most severe alcohol-related problems actually have the lowest rates of alcohol consumption (Al-Issa, 1995). Cockerham, Kunz, & Lueschen (1989) found that whereas for Americans, alcohol use was associated with depression, for West Germans (who have higher levels of alcohol consumption), it was not. Thus, it appears that cultural attitudes and norms regarding drinking influence the occurrence of alcoholism. Grant and Harford (1995) also found that within the United States, the relationship between alcohol abuse and depression was stronger for females and African-Americans than for males and non-African-American groups. Thus, drinking may also be a form of coping with life stress.

Interestingly, for some Hispanic groups, alcohol consumption is not related to acculturative stress. For example, Caetano (1994) found that the more acculturated to mainstream American culture Hispanic women were, the more they engaged in drinking. However, these higher alcohol consumption rates were related to more positive associations with drinking rather than to higher levels of acculturative stress (Cervantes et al., 1991). Specifically, American-born Mexicans associated drinking with social pleasure, assertiveness, elevated mood, decreased tension, and disinhibition (Caetano, 1994; Cervantes et al., 1991; Gilbert, 1991). These findings suggest that for Mexican groups, acculturating to American cultural norms may render alcoholism more culturally and socially acceptable behavior. The MAPSS figures (Vega et al., 1998) support this prediction: Rates of alcohol dependence were lowest for recent immigrants (8.6%), higher for immigrants residing in

the United States for 13 years or more (10.4%), and highest for U.S.-born Mexican-Americans (18.0%). The latter rates were most similar to the NCS U.S. National sample (15.1%).

In summary, most major mental disorders occur across cultures. Cases of schizophrenia, depression, anxiety, and substance abuse have been found in a variety of cultural and ethnic contexts. The prevalence rates of these disorders, however, vary among cultural and ethnic groups. Consistent with Marsella (1987), the prevalence rates of disorders that are more neurologically based (i.e., schizophrenia and bipolar depression) vary less than those that are less neurologically based (i.e., unipolar depression and generalized anxiety). These different prevalence rates may stem from a variety of sources. They may reflect greater exposure to life stress for some groups than others. Interestingly, several studies (Vega et al., 1998; Ying et al., 2000) have found that groups presumed to be under greater environmental stress (e.g., minority groups and recent immigrants) do *not* demonstrate higher rates of affective disorders. Another possibility is that cultures vary in how syntonic or dystonic specific disorders are with particular cultural values and beliefs. For example, the emphasis placed on interpersonal relationships in many Asian and Latino cultures may serve as a buffer against depression and explain why Mexican and Taiwanese nationals demonstrate lower levels of depression than their American counterparts. Yet another possible explanation is that the expression and meaning of symptoms related to major mental disorders may be culturally shaped. As a result, these symptoms may not be easily classified by Western diagnostic systems. We discuss these latter two possibilities next.

## Does Culture Influence the Expression of Symptoms?

Both the biomedical and cultural idioms of distress perspectives acknowledge that culture may influence the expression of symptoms. For example, culture may influence the frequency with which specific symptoms are expressed. Biomedical perspectives view cultural differences in symptoms as peripheral aspects of universal syndromes. Cultural idioms of distress perspectives, however, view such differences as evidence that the disorders themselves are distinct.

**Schizophrenia.** Findings from the WHO study revealed interesting cultural variation in schizophrenic symptoms. Although schizophrenic patients of "developed" and "developing" countries reported having their thoughts stopped, taken away, "read" by alien agents, and "broadcast" publicly, the relative frequency of other symptoms varied across cultures. In "developed" countries, patients were more likely to manifest depressive affect, whereas in "developing" countries, patients were more likely to experience visual hallucinations (Jablensky, 1989). The latter findings were consistent with those of Ndetei and Vadher (1984), which suggest that auditory and visual hallucinations were more common in African, West Indian, and Asian schizophrenic groups than in English (i.e., from England) schizophrenic groups.

Despite the fact that the WHO study is the most widely cited cross-cultural study of schizophrenia, critics argue that the differences between "developed" and "developing" countries in the WHO study are at most speculative (Edgerton & Cohen, 1994). These critics argue that the WHO study did not measure specific cultural variables, wrongly assumed that countries within the "developing" and "developed" groups were more similar than different, and did not provide any compelling explanations for the cultural differences found (Edgerton & Cohen, 1994). More recent studies have provided clearer cultural explanations for cultural differences in symptomatology. For example, Tateyama, Asai, Hashimoto, Bartels, and Kasper (1998) compared schizophrenic patients (according to ICD-9 criteria) in Tokyo, Vienna, and Tubingen matched by sex, duration of illness, and mean age at onset and on admission. They found that across the three cities, similar percentages of patients reported having delusions (89.5%, 91.1%, and 87.3%, respectively). Furthermore, there were no cultural differences in the frequency of delusions of persecution/injury or of grandeur. City differences emerged in delusions of "belittlement" (e.g., being dead, feeling guilty or sinful), which were attributed to cultural differences in religion. Specifically, non-Christian Tokyo patients reported fewer delusions regarding guilt and sin than patients from European cities who were more influenced by Christianity. Not surprisingly, the specific religious figures in the delusions were culture-specific: whereas patients of European descent spoke of "Jesus Christ" or "The Father of Europe," Tokyo patients spoke of "Shakyamuni" or "Nichiren."

Furthermore, when Tateyama, Asai, Hashimoto, Bartels, and Kasper (1998) used a different classification scheme to decompose delusions of persecution/injury, Tokyo patients reported "being slandered by surrounding people" more than Europeans. The authors interpreted this difference as reflecting a greater desire for social approval in Japanese than in Western cultures. In a similar vein, Phillips, West, and Wang (1996) observed that Chinese schizophrenic patients (according to DSM criteria) are more likely to manifest "erotomania," the delusion of being loved by another person from afar, than Western patients. They also attribute these differences to cultural factors: in general, Chinese may be more concerned with social approval and have greater restrictions on sexual expression than Westerners.

Other studies conducted before the WHO study proposed that cultural values and beliefs influenced the expression of schizophrenia. For example, Opler and Singer (1956) predicted that Irish and Italian patients would differ in their schizophrenic symptoms because of cultural differences in their expression of emotion and views of sex, and in which parent assumed the dominant role in the home. Their findings supported their predictions for a male sample and were subsequently replicated in a female sample by Fantl and Schiro (1959). For example, consistent with notions that Italians accept more emotional expression and impulsiveness than the Irish, these researchers found greater behavioral problems such as impulsiveness, open rebellion and physical assault among Italian patients than Irish patients. Unfortunately, these studies relied primarily on diagnoses that were not based on standard classification criteria; therefore, it is unclear whether members of the cultural groups would be diagnosed similarly according to ICD or DSM criteria. However, Enright and Jaekle (1961) compared Japanese and Filipino patients in Hawaii who were diagnosed with "schizophrenic reaction, paranoid type" according to DSM criteria and also found ethnic differences in symptomatology that were consistent with cultural differences in emotional expression and control. Filipino patients were more expressive, less restrained, and exerted more primary than secondary control compared to Japanese patients.

**Affective Disorders.** Cultural differences in the expression of bipolar disorder have been documented. For example, Mukherjee and colleagues

(1983) found that African-American and Hispanic patients with bipolar disorder manifested more auditory hallucinations than White patients. As a result, they were more frequently misdiagnosed with schizophrenia than White patients. Most research, however, has focused on cultural expressions of unipolar depression.

As with schizophrenia, the WHO conducted a study in the 1970s to examine whether the symptoms of unipolar depression varied cross-culturally (Sartorius, Jablensky, Gulbinat, & Ernberg, 1980). This study examined unipolar depression in 573 patients from Canada, Iran, Japan, and Switzerland, using the WHO Standardized Assessment of Depressive Disorders (SADD). Across sites, depressive patients demonstrated a "core" profile of depressive symptoms that included sadness, joylessness, anxiety and tension, lack of energy, loss of interest, inability to concentrate, and feelings of worthlessness. Beiser, Cargo, & Woodbury (1994) also found evidence of a core constellation of depressive symptoms in a community sample of 1348 Southeast Asian refugees and 319 Canadians. Participants completed questionnaires that contained items assessing depression, anxiety, and somatization, as well as items that tapped into culture-specific idioms of distress. Using grade-of-membership analysis, Beiser et al. (1994) found that for both Southeast Asians and Canadians, items loaded into three distinct categories: Major Depression, Depression with Panic, and Subclinical Depression.

Other evidence in support of the universality of depressive symptoms comes from studies of "culturally bound syndromes." Increasingly, researchers find that syndromes that were previously considered "culturally bound" resemble depressive disorders. For example, "dhat syndrome" in Indian culture, marked by the belief that semen is being lost, was initially regarded by Wig in 1960 as a culturally bound syndrome; however, recent work suggests that it is strongly associated with depressed mood, fatigue, and the DSM-III-R diagnosis of depression (Mumford, 1996). Similarly, "hwa-byung," considered a "Korean folk illness" marked by multiple somatic and psychological symptoms, is also strongly associated with DSM-III diagnoses of major depression (Lin et al., 1992).

Cultural variation has been found in the frequency of specific depressive symptoms, however. For example, the WHO study found that feelings of guilt and self-reproach were more frequently reported in Western countries than in non-Western countries (Sartorius et al., 1980). As in schizophrenia, the lower frequency of guilt-related symptoms has been attributed to cultural differences in religious traditions. Hamdi, Amin, and Abou-Saleh (1997)'s findings were consistent with those of the WHO study. Although the general disorder of endogenous depression exists in Arab culture, the loss of libido, a distinct quality of depressed mood, and feelings of guilt are less common in Arab than in Western cultures. Again, these differences may be related to different religious and cultural traditions among the ethnocultural groups.

Other differences have been found between members of Asian and Western cultures. Members of Asian cultures have been described as "somatizing" their depressive symptoms more than members of Western cultures (Kleinman, 1986). This may be particularly true for Chinese samples. Ying and colleagues (2000) found that compared to Chinese Americans, Chinese who lived in Taiwan reported more somatic symptoms of depression (as assessed by the Center for Epidemiological Studies Depression Scale), despite no differences between the two groups in overall levels of depressive symptoms. Various hypotheses were posited to explain this cultural difference. Compared to their Western counterparts, Asians have been described as using more somatic terms to describe their emotional states (Tung, 1994), as believing that somatic complaints are a more culturally appropriate way to present their distress (Kleinman, 1986), and as suffering from a disorder (i.e., neurasthenia) that is distinct from depression (Ying et al., under review). Some recent evidence, however, suggests that Asian-Americans may not somatize more than White Americans. For example, Zhang, Snowden, and Sue (1998) found that Asian-Americans and White Americans in the ECA data for the Los Angeles community reported similar levels of somatic discomfort.

**Anxiety Disorders.** Cultural differences in the expression of anxiety have been documented. For instance, although posttraumatic stress disorder (PTSD) can be diagnosed in American populations and Southeast Asian refugees (Carlson & Rosser-Hogan, 1994), clinicians and researchers have found higher levels of dissociation among Southeast Asian refugees with PTSD (Carlson & Rosser-Hogan, 1994; Guarnaccia, 1997; Kirmayer, 1996). This may be due to the greater cultural acceptance of dissociative states in Southeast

Asian culture (Lewis-Fernandez, 1998). Similarly, among many African-American populations, isolated sleep paralysis is associated with anxiety. In some cases, these cultural expressions of anxiety were misinterpreted as psychotic symptoms and diagnosed as such (Friedman et al., 1994; Williams & Chambless, 1994).

Most studies have focused on the way culture influences the causes and content of anxiety, which may be related to specific cultural norms and values. For instance, the emphasis on interpersonal harmony and appropriate social behavior in many Asian cultures may result in distinct social triggers of anxiety. In Japan, allocentricism, issues of amae (i.e., dependence), the denial of the self, and the importance of harmonious interpersonal relationships (Russell, 1989) result in the existence of "taijin kyofusho." "Taijin kyofusho" is marked by fear that one's body is displeasing or offensive to others, fear of eye-to-eye confrontation, fear of giving off an offensive odor, and fear of having unpleasant facial expressions (Tanaka-Matsumi, 1979). Although "taijin kyofusho" has been compared to social phobia in the United States, the two disorders involve considerably different fears. Whereas social phobia is a fear of strangers and people, "taijin kyofusho" is a fear that one might not be acceptable to others (Russell, 1989). Moreover, many of the fears of social phobics are different from those harbored by sufferers of "taijin kyofusho" (Russell, 1989). Cultural differences also occur in the content of specific obsessions and compulsions. For example, in many cultural contexts, the content of obsessions and compulsions is related to the dominant religion (Al-Issa & Oudji, 1998).

**Substance Abuse and Dependence.** Almost no studies have examined how the expression of alcoholism and other forms of substance abuse vary across cultures. Studies are needed to fill this gap in the literature.

In summary, cultural values and beliefs, views of emotion, concerns about social relationships, and religious traditions appear to influence the expression of symptoms associated with major mental disorders.

## Does Culture Influence the Meaning of Mental Illness?

Most of the research reviewed until now was conducted using translated Western instruments and classification systems by investigators who view mental illness from a biomedical perspective. Proponents of cultural idioms of distress perspectives argue that mental illness cannot be separated from the cultural context in which it occurs. The cultural context may shape the meaning and subjective experience of mental illness, which may influence its prognosis.

**Schizophrenia.** Even though schizophrenic symptoms are similar across cultures, evidence suggests that the meaning that cultural and ethnic groups attach to these symptoms may differ. For example, Jenkins (1997) asked schizophrenic and depressed Latino and European-Americans who lived in Los Angeles to describe their "life situations." She found that European-Americans, particularly those with schizophrenia, were more likely to characterize their life situations in terms of mental illness than Latinos. Latinos, on the other hand, particularly those with schizophrenia, were more likely to describe their life situations in terms of "nervios," or nerves. "Nervios" is a culturally acceptable way of describing emotional distress in Latino cultures that imparts sympathy onto the suffering person (Jenkins, 1997). Thus, because Latino culture may view mental illness more sympathetically, Latinos who suffer from mental illness may be less alienated from their society and therefore, demonstrate better prognoses than their European-American counterparts. Similarly, based on interview data with schizophrenic patients and their families in Sri Lanka, Waxler (1979) found that the social and clinical outcome of Sri Lankan patients 5 years after their first hospital admission was better than that of schizophrenic patients in Denmark and Russia. Waxler attributes these findings to differences across the cultures in the meanings of deviance and mental illness. Deviance and mental illness are more culturally accepted in Sri Lanka than in Denmark or Russia.

Other studies suggest that individuals with schizophrenia also do better (e.g., are hospitalized less often) in cultures that view the self as dynamic and that afford individuals opportunities to move easily between reality and fantasy (Corin, 1990; Estroff, 1989). Presumably, these cultures give individuals with schizophrenia a "way of being" that promotes their mental health (Corin, 1990).

**Affective Disorders.** Most research on the cultural meaning of affective illness has focused on unipolar depression. Findings from these studies suggest that the cultural context shapes the way specific depressive symptoms are understood. For example, although "dhat syndrome" in India resembles depression, it exists in a cultural context that views semen as the vital source of male physical and mental energy (Mumford, 1996).

Ying (1988) provides additional evidence that cultural contexts influence conceptions of depression. She found that for a Chinese-American community sample, somatic and affective symptoms of depression were inseparable constructs, whereas for a White American community, they were distinct constructs. The mixing of somatic and affective symptoms is consistent with Chinese notions that the mind and body are one. Similarly, Ying et al. (2000) found that affective and somatic symptoms were inseparable for Chinese college students who lived in Taiwan; however, they were separable factors for Chinese-Americans who lived in the United States. Thus, although depressive symptoms themselves may not be invariant across cultures, how they are viewed and how they relate to each other may.

**Anxiety Disorders.** Cultural idioms of distress perspectives argue that anxiety symptoms are shaped by the cultural contexts in which they occur. Thus, because cultures differ in the events that trigger anxiety, the meanings of anxiety may vary across cultures. For example, Guarnaccia (1993) found that although "ataque de nervios" resembles depressive and anxious symptoms, it is defined by its triggering event—upsetting or frightening events in the family sphere. Russell (1989) and Tanaka-Matsumi (1979) argue that "taijin kyofusho" is unique to Japanese contexts because it can be understood only in terms of Japanese values and norms. Malgady, Rogler, and Cortes (1996) demonstrate that Puerto Rican adults use cultural idioms of anger (e.g., aggression and assertiveness) to express their depression and anxiety, suggesting that the cultural meanings of depression and anxiety may be different from those of European-American adults.

**Substance Abuse and Dependence.** Variation among cultures in the meaning of alcohol and substance use may influence consumption rates. For instance, Caetano (1989) found that although African-American, Hispanic, and White American adults in the United States (controlling for differences in income and education) agreed that alcoholism is a disease, the first two groups were more likely than White Americans to view alcoholics as morally weak. These findings are consistent with the ethnic patterns in alcohol consumption described earlier. Sigelman and colleagues

(1992) found that Native American schoolchildren were less likely to see alcoholism as serious, saw alcoholics as less responsible for their problems, and viewed alcoholism as a disease more than Hispanic or White American children. These findings are consistent with Pedigo's (1983) assertions that alcohol and substance use and abuse have cultural meanings for Native Americans that render them more culturally acceptable in Native American culture than in White American culture. For instance, Native Americans are more likely to view individuals holistically and therefore to be more accepting and less critical of problem drinking than members of other cultural groups. Furthermore, in some Native American groups, drinking and other forms of substance use are often viewed as ways of coping with past and present stresses. In all likelihood, this explains why alcohol consumption rates are higher in Native American groups than in other ethnic groups in the United States. In other cultural contexts, the use of alcohol and other substances in spiritual and religious ceremonies may also influence the cultural meaning of alcohol and substance consumption.

In summary, cultures vary in their views of mental illness, tolerance of deviant behavior, and conceptions of emotion, the self, and the mind–body relationship. These cultural differences shape the meaning of and social response to mental illness and may influence the course of mental illness.

### Do "Culture-Bound" Syndromes Exist?

Throughout this chapter, we referred to "culture-bound syndromes," or syndromes that are found only in one culture. By definition, culture-bound syndromes are more than variants of "universal" disorders and are determined by the specific beliefs and practices of a particular culture (Ahktar, 1988). Originally, "culture-bound" syndromes were limited to syndromes observed in non-Western cultures, but more recent modifications of the term acknowledge that certain syndromes may occur only in Western cultures. Among these is multiple personality disorder (MPD). Although MPD is extremely rare in the United States, in Japan, it is virtually nonexistent. Takahashi (1990) found that among all inpatients in a Japanese hospital from 1983–1988, not one diagnosis of MPD was made, based on DSM-III and DSM-III-R criteria. Takahashi argues that MPD is inconsistent with Japanese cultural norms.

In such a culture where one's thinking, or identity in the sense of western cultures, is altered to fulfil society's needs, the need for an individual to develop a psychiatric disorder such as MPD might not be very strong. (Takahashi, 1990, p. 59)

Heated debate exists regarding whether culture-bound syndromes actually exist. The DSM-IV acknowledged the existence of such disorders by including a list of culture-bound syndromes as an appendix. However, recent evidence suggests that many syndromes that were previously considered "culture-bound" are variations of depression and anxiety (Mumford, 1996). Thus, many critics of the DSM-IV argue that the term "culture-bound syndrome" assumes that culture is a secondary process and exists only in extreme forms, when in fact, culture influences all aspects of mental illness (Guarnaccia, 1993). Whether or not one views a specific syndrome as "culturally bound" may depend largely upon what one considers the defining aspect of mental illness. If one focuses only on symptoms, many syndromes that were traditionally considered "culturally bound" could be considered cultural manifestations of depression and anxiety. However, if one focuses on cultural meanings, then to some degree, all syndromes are "culturally bound."

### Does Culture Influence the Social and Psychological Impact of Mental Illness?

Compared to work on the incidence and prevalence of mental illness across cultures, little research has examined how the personal and social impact of mental illness varies across cultures. This is somewhat surprising, given that societal and community responses to mental illness may have the greatest influence on prognosis and may vary the most across cultures. In the WHO study described earlier, Jablensky and colleagues (1989) found that patients from "developing" countries had better outcomes 2 and 5 years after the initial onset of schizophrenia than patients from "developed" countries. It is possible that this finding reflects cultural variation in the social and personal impact of schizophrenia. Although a variety of cultural factors might influence the personal and social consequences of mental illness, we highlight three: (1) the value of social relationships, (2) views of mental illness, and (3) views of the self.

The extent to which cultures value social relationships and therefore provide social support to individuals with mental illness may influence psy-chiatric outcome (Lefley, 1990). For example, having strong family ties reduces the risk of schizophrenic relapse (Birchwood, Cochrane, MacMillan, Copestake, Kucharska, & Cariss, 1992). Therefore, schizophrenia may have a better prognosis in cultures that place greater emphasis on the family unit. In addition, family interaction styles may vary across cultures and may also affect prognosis. In schizophrenia, for example, levels of expressed emotion in the family have been correlated with poor patient prognosis (Brown, Birley, & Wing, 1972). "Expressed emotion" is comprised of three components: criticism, emotional overinvolvement, and hostility. Although expressed emotion exists across cultures (e.g., Japan, India, England, Brazil, and Mexico), levels of expressed emotion vary across cultures. For example, compared to American households of schizophrenic patients, Japanese (Mino, Tanaka, Inoue, Tsuda, Babazono, & Aoyama, 1995) and Indian (Wig et al., 1987) households demonstrated less, whereas Portuguese-speaking Brazilian households demonstrated more expressed emotion (Martins, de Lemos, & Bebbington, 1992).

These differences can be further broken down into the specific components of expressed emotion. Greater levels of expressed emotion in the Brazilian households than in American households were due to greater levels of emotional over-involvement in Brazilian than in American households (Martins, de Lemos, & Bebbington, 1992). Compared to British and Anglo-American families, Mexican families demonstrate less criticism (Jenkins, 1991). Moreover, the content of expressed emotion differs across cultures. Jenkins (1991) found that critical Mexican family members were less likely to make negative character attributions about schizophrenic patients' behavior than Anglo-Americans; instead, they were more critical of disruptive or disrespectful behavior toward the family (Jenkins, 1991). These differences may explain why schizophrenic patients who lived in "developing" countries improved more than those who lived in "developed" or industrialized countries.

The impact of mental disorder in a particular cultural context may depend on the way that culture views mental illness and those afflicted with mental illness. According to social labeling theory (Waxler, 1979), the way a society responds to patients influences their prognosis. This theory suggests that patients have better prognoses in societies that expect them to recover from mental affliction and return to normalcy rapidly than in societies that view mental illness as a permanent condition and that ostracize and stigmatize patients. For example, in Spanish, the mentally afflicted are described as having "nervios," a term that elicits sympathy in Mexican culture. In contrast, in English, mental illness connotes biological defects intrinsic to the individual (Jenkins, 1991). Social labeling theory predicts that the mentally ill have better prognoses in Mexican culture than in mainstream European-American culture.

Few studies examined whether the psychological impact of mental disorders generalizes across cultures. For instance, the impact of mental illness on one's self concept may depend on cultural views of the self. For example, Estroff (1989) and Fabrega (1989) argue that in cultures that value independence and view the self as a stable, context-independent entity, disorders that disorganize or fragment the self (e.g., schizophrenia) may have greater personal consequences than in cultures that view the self as a fluid, dynamic entity. Moreover, the latter cultures may be more accepting of mentally ill individuals' dependence on caretakers (Lin & Kleinman, 1988; Lefley, 1990). The impact of mental illness on psychological processes such as cognition and emotion may also vary across cultures. Unfortunately, few studies have examined this possibility. For instance, several empirical studies demonstrated that depression alters various aspects of emotional processing. Depressed individuals are less sensitive to both positive and negative emotional cues than nondepressed individuals (Wexler et al., 1994). Depression also alters the behavioral and physiological aspects of emotional response. However, these studies have been conducted primarily on European-American samples. No studies have examined whether the psychological impact of depression generalizes to other cultural contexts. Thus, significantly more research is needed to examine the cultural factors that influence the social and psychological impact of mental illness. Such studies may reveal whether and why the prognosis of specific mental disorders may be better or worse across cultural contexts.

## How Do We Consider Culture in Diagnosis and Treatment?

Cultural variation (or the lack of cultural variation) in the occurrence and course of mental illness and in the presentation of psychiatric symptoms all have implications for treatment. Most importantly, they highlight aspects of psychotherapy and other psychiatric treatments that may require modification to be effective with different cultural groups. Given that individuals vary in the extent to which they demonstrate culturally normative behavior and that there is considerable variability in empirically based knowledge about cultural influences on psychopathology, clinicians should use clinical recommendations judiciously. These recommendations should lead to culture-related hypotheses about client dysfunction that require additional data specific to the client (and to the specific form of distress) for support. Because cultural considerations become more salient when working with individuals of cultural backgrounds different from one's own, the next section will discuss diagnosis and treatment in multicultural settings such as the United States.

**Cultural Patterns of Service Utilization.** Ethnic groups in the United States vary in their rates of mental health service utilization. These rates may reflect cultural attitudes toward mental health treatment. For example, compared to White Americans, Asian-Americans tend to "underutilize" services (Sue et al., 1991). Asian-Americans tend to seek help from family members, medical services (Western and Asian), and community services before using mental health services. As a result, Asian-Americans may enter mental health treatment with little optimism about their recovery which may interfere with treatment outcome. Clinicians may have to consider these attitudes toward treatment when formulating a treatment plan. In addition, because Asian-Americans use mental health services as a last resort, those who enter mental health settings tend to be the most severely distressed. Thus, clinicians may have to provide more acute care to these individuals. Similar issues may arise for members of other cultural and ethnic groups.

**Cultural Diagnosis.** Although culture may shape the experience and expression of distress, this may vary across individuals. Individuals within cultural groups vary in the extent to which they endorse the values, norms, and beliefs of their cultural group and the meanings of their cultural identity (Tsai, Ying, & Lee, 2000). In diagnosis, understanding an individual's cultural orientation will help clinicians assess how an individual's expressions of distress are culturally shaped, as well as prevent errors of misdiagnosis (Dana,

1998). For example, although African-American and Hispanic clients with affective disorders often report more delusions and hallucinations than their White American counterparts, this may not hold for a specific African-American or Hispanic individual. It is possible that under specific circumstances, one's cultural heritage is less relevant to one's symptoms than other influences, such as one's socioeconomic status. Therefore, a critical aspect of diagnosis, especially with patients of different cultural backgrounds, is assessing the patients' cultural history, cultural identity and orientation, and subjective experience of culture (Dana, 1998).

**Therapist and Client Interactions.** The current DSM-IV contains guidelines for conducting a "cultural formulation," or assessing how cultural factors influence a client's psychology (American Psychiatric Association, 1994). These guidelines also emphasize the importance of assessing the cultural aspects of the therapist–client relationship. Cultures vary in their emphasis on and expectations of interpersonal relationships. Clinicians' ability to establish rapport with clients of different cultural backgrounds may hinge on their knowledge of the clients' cultural expectations for the therapist–client relationship. In some cases, this rapport is critical. For example, an overwhelming majority of Asian-American patients discontinue mental health treatment after the first session. These drop-out rates, however, are significantly reduced when the therapist has the same ethnocultural background as the client (Sue et al., 1991). Similarly, Takeuchi, Sue, and Yeh (1995) found that in Los Angeles, Asian-American, African-American, and Mexican-American patients were more likely to continue in mental health programs if the programs were oriented toward their specific ethnic heritage.

Culture may influence different aspects of the clinician–patient interaction. First, culture may influence nonverbal communication (e.g., interpersonal space, body movement, paralanguage, eye contact). For example, in Asian cultural groups, clinicians are considered authority figures, and therefore, clients may avert their gaze as an expression of deference and respect. This behavior is a culturally appropriate response, rather than an indication of abnormal interpersonal behavior. Second, culture may influence expectations of therapist credibility (e.g., expertise and trustworthiness). Certain groups may explicitly inquire

about clinicians' credentials or may require demonstration of clinical expertise before engaging in treatment. Again, this may be considered a culturally appropriate response rather than an anomalous response to treatment. Third, culture may influence expectations of the therapist–client relationship. For example, whereas some cultural groups may expect a formal interaction style between clinician and client, other cultural groups may expect an informal interactional style (Sue & Sue, 1990). In these cases, patients may expect clinicians to share personal information as a way of demonstrating their trustworthiness. Finally, cultural groups may vary in their exposure to and experience with mental health services; therefore, patients may require explicit education about the process of and regulations related to treatment.

**Cultural Adaptations of Treatment.** The most popular treatments for mental disorders in psychiatric settings were developed for use with mainstream European-American populations. Many clinicians have recommended ways of adapting Western treatments for culturally diverse populations. We discuss a few of these adaptations here.

Many Western treatments must be adapted for culturally diverse populations because their basic cultural assumptions may not apply to non-Western cultural groups. For example, Randall (1994) argues that the concepts of time and self that underlie cognitive therapy stem from a Western European cultural tradition that may differ for ethnic clients. Minority clients from cultures in which time is less salient and concepts of the self are more sociocentric than in Western cultures may not do as well in cognitive therapy. Randall (1994) proposes changes to traditional forms of cognitive therapy that may make it more relevant for one such cultural group, African-American women. Even in medication treatments, research has demonstrated that "standard" dosages of psychotropic medications must be modified when administered to specific ethnic groups. For example, Lin, Poland, and Lesser (1986) found that Asian-American patients often require only half of the standard "European-American" dosage of psychotropic medications.

Other adaptations include greater involvement of the family in treatment. In cultures that emphasize familialism, treating the individual without the family may be counterproductive and culturally inappropriate. In addition, when working with members of different cultural groups, clinicians often must employ interpreters. In these cases, culturally sensitive nonverbal communication is even more critical in developing rapport with the client. Moreover, clinicians must develop a positive working relationship with the interpreter before obtaining rapport with the client. Finally, Western forms of treatment may have to work in collaboration with non-Western forms of treatment. Patients may be using traditional medicines or seeking the help of traditional healers while they are seeking treatment in Western psychiatric settings.

In summary, when working with individuals of cultural backgrounds different from one's own, it becomes imperative that clinicians entertain hypotheses that account for cultural differences at all stages of diagnosis and treatment. The extent to which cultural considerations should be included in diagnosis and treatment, however, depends on the specific individual.

## Future Research Directions in Cross-Cultural Psychopathology

During the past few decades, significant advances have been made in studying psychopathology across cultures. However, after reviewing the literature, what becomes even more apparent is the dire need for future research. Thus far, we have reviewed studies that provide some answers to basic questions about psychopathology across cultures. Next, we discuss issues that must be addressed in future research to advance our understanding and treatment of psychopathology across cultures.

### Methodological Issues

To gain a more comprehensive understanding of cultural influences on psychopathology, future empirical studies must use more sophisticated measures of culture, employ multiple methods of assessment, and integrate qualitative and quantitative research methods.

**More Sophisticated Measurement of Cultural Variables.** A common critique of cross-cultural studies of psychopathology is their poor measurement of cultural variables. Most studies assume that individuals who reside in specific countries also represent the cultural values and beliefs associated with that country. For example, in epidemiological studies of mental disorders across countries, national differences in incidence and prevalence rates are attributed to cultural factors. Only by explicitly measuring cultural factors can we determine whether national differences are indeed due to culture. Thus, future studies of the incidence and prevalence of mental disorders across cultures or of cultural influences on symptom expression should explicitly measure the cultural variables of interest and then examine how they relate to the occurrence and expression of psychopathology. These cultural variables include individualism–collectivism, cultural orientation/acculturation, and views of mental illness.

**Multiple Methods of Assessment.** Most cross-cultural studies of psychopathology rely on self-report data. Although self-report data are invaluable, they are also vulnerable to a number of biases, including self-presentation biases, unreliability, and contextual demands. Self-report data become even less reliable when collected across cultures. Given that the symptoms of mental disorder span various domains—cognitive, behavioral, and physiological—our assessments of psychopathology should reflect such variation. Thus, future studies should include physiological and behavioral assessments.

Examples of research that attempts to integrate physiological and cultural aspects of psychopathology are studies of the "psychobiology of ethnicity" (Lin, Poland, & Nakasaki, 1993). These studies have found ethnic differences in responses to psychotropic medications. Hispanic patients require less antidepressant medication and report more side effects at lower dosages than White patients (Marcos & Cancro, 1982; Mendoza, Smith, Poland, Lin, & Strickland, 1991). African-Americans respond better and more rapidly to tricyclic antidepressants than Whites (Lawson, 1986; Silver et al., 1993). Although studies have attempted to disentangle cultural (Smith, Lin, & Mendoza, 1993) and biological influences (Silver, Poland, & Lin, 1993) on responses to medication, more research is needed.

**Integration of Qualitative and Quantitative Methods.** A variety of methods has been used to study cultural variation in psychopathology, ranging from smaller scale ethnographic interviews to larger scale epidemiological studies. Each method has its advantages and disadvantages. Therefore, multiple methods should be used. This may be particularly important if specific cultural groups respond more to one method than another. For instance, cultural groups that value personal contact may respond in more truthful and thoughtful ways during an interview than they would to a questionnaire, whereas cultural groups that are concerned with self-presentation may be more likely to respond truthfully to a questionnaire than to an interviewer. Thus, converging findings from studies that employ multiple research methods will allow a comprehensive understanding of the way culture shapes psychopathology.

## Conceptual Issues

Future studies must address the following conceptual issues to advance our understanding of psychopathology across cultural contexts.

**Cultural Differences in Response Styles or Psychopathology?** Cultural differences exist in participants' responses to assessment instruments. For example, cultural differences exist in using standard rating scales in questionnaires and interview schedules. Compared to members of European-American culture, members of Asian cultures have been described as using the middle of rating scales (Chen, Lee, & Stevenson, 1995), whereas members of Latino cultures have been described as using the extreme ends of the scale. Thus, cultural differences in the reported intensity of specific symptoms may reflect culturally normative response styles rather than true differences in symptomology.

Cultural groups may also vary in their responses to particular treatment modalities. For instance, work by Hall and colleagues (1994) showed that for English-speaking, White smokers, adding a mood management component to a smoking cessation group intervention substantially increases quit rates for smokers with a history of major depression. However, Muñoz and colleagues (1997) found that this treatment was not effective with a Spanish-speaking group because they did not attend the group interventions. When Muñoz and colleagues (1997) conducted their intervention through the mail, the treatment was as effective for Spanish speakers as the group intervention was for English-speaking White Americans. Cultural groups may also respond more to specific instruments than others. For example, Vietnamese women reported fewer depressive symptoms on the Diagnostic Interview Schedule than on the Edinburgh Postnatal Depression Scale or the General Health Questionnaire-30 (Matthey, Barnett, & Elliott, 1997).

It should be noted that although cultural differences in responses to questionnaires may exist, relationships across variables may still hold across cultural groups. For example, Spanish-speaking respondents scored much higher than English-speaking respondents on the Personal Beliefs Inventory (PBI), a self-report measure of what Albert Ellis termed "irrational beliefs" related to depression. In particular, Spanish speakers endorsed items regarding the desirability of being loved ("Everyone needs the love and approval of those persons who are important to them,") and of being accepted by friends and family ("What others think of you is most important") more than English speakers. In Albert Ellis' individualistic New York culture, high endorsement of these items was culturally inappropriate; however, in collectivistic Latino culture, high endorsement of these items was culturally desirable. Regardless, for both cultural groups, scores on the PBI were positively correlated with depression (Muñoz, 1986).

**Do Mental Disorders Impair Psychological Functioning Similarly Across Cultures?** Previous studies of psychopathology across cultures have focused on cultural variation in incidence rates and symptom presentation. This work has advanced our knowledge of the existence of mental disorders across cultures. The next step in cultural studies of psychopathology is to examine the impact of such disorders on "basic" psychological processes related to emotion, memory, and cognition. Such studies will elucidate whether the mechanisms that underlie specific symptoms are the same across cultures.

**Are the Clinical Recommendations Regarding the Treatment of Clients of Different Cultural Backgrounds Effective?** Volumes of clinical recommendations regarding the assessment and treatment of clients of different cultural backgrounds have been written (Sue & Sue, 1990; Tseng & Streltzer, 1997; Pedersen et al., 1996). In this chapter, we reviewed only a few recommendations. Unfortunately, we know very little about the way clinicians implement these clinical recommendations and whether they are actually effective (Dana, 1998). Clearly, such knowledge would shape our future clinical interventions. Therefore, empirical studies of the implementation and effectiveness of culturally sensitive treatments are needed.

## Conclusion

In this chapter, we examined cultural influences on various aspects of psychopathology—assessment, incidence and prevalence rates, symptom expression, meaning, prognosis, and treatment. Our review illustrates what we know and what we still have to learn about the cultural shaping of mental illness. We look forward to future research that will advance our understanding of human processes and also enhance our ability to treat and live with mental illness across cultures.

## References

Akhtar, S. (1988). Four culture-bound psychiatric syndromes in India. *International Journal of Social Psychiatry, 34*, 70–74.

Al-Issa, I. (1995). Culture and mental illness in an international perspective. In I. Al-Issa (Ed.), *Handbook of culture and mental illness: An international perspective* (pp. 3–49). Madison, CT: International Universities Press.

Al-Issa, I., & Oudji, S. (1998). Culture and anxiety disorders. In S. S. Kazarian & D. Evans (Eds.), *Cultural clinical psychology: Theory, research, and practice* (pp. 127–151). New York: Oxford University Press.

American Psychiatric Association. (1994). *Diagnostic and statistical manual of mental disorders* (4th ed.). Washington, DC: Author.

Baxter, B., Hinson, R. E., Wall, A., & McKee, S. A. (1998). Incorporating culture into the treatment of alcohol abuse and dependence. In S. S. Kazarian & D. R. Evans (Eds), *Cultural clinical psychology: Theory, research, and practice* (pp. 215–245). New York: Oxford University Press.

Beiser, M., Cargo, M., & Woodbury, M. A. (1994). A comparison of psychiatric disorder in different cultures: Depressive typologies in Southeast Asian refugees and resident Canadians. *International Journal of Methods in Psychiatric Research, 4*, 157–172.

Bennett, L. A., Janca, A., Grant, B. F., & Sartorius, N. (1993). Boundaries between normal and pathological drinking: A cross-cultural comparison. *Alcohol Health and World, 17*, 190–195.

Birchwood, M., Cochrane, R., Macmillan, F., Copestake, S., et al. (1992). The influence of ethnicity and family structure on relapse in first-episode schizophrenia: A comparison of Asian, Afro-Caribbean, and White patients. *British Journal of Psychiatry, 161*, 783–790.

Blazer, D., Hughes, D., George, L. K., Swartz, M., & Boyer, R. (1991). Generalized anxiety disorder. In L. N. Robins & D. A. Regier (Eds.), *Psychiatric disorders in America: The Epidemiological Catchment Study* (pp. 180–203). New York: The Free Press.

Brown, G., Birley, J. L. Y., & Wing, J. (1972). Influence of family life on the course of schizophrenic disorders: A replication. *British Journal of Psychiatry, 121*, 241–258.

Butcher, J. N. (1982). Cross-cultural research methods in clinical psychology. In P. Kendall & J. N. Butcher (Eds.), *Handbook of research methods in clinical psychology* (pp. 273–310). New York: Wiley.

Butcher, J. N. (1996). *International adaptations of the MMPI-2*. Minneapolis: University of Minnesota.

Butcher, J. N., Coelho, S., & Tsai, J. L. (in press). International adaptations of the Minnesota Multiphasic Personality Inventory and the MMPI-2. In P. F. Merenda, R. K. Hambleton, & C. D. Spielberger (Eds.), *Adapting educational and psychological tests for cross-cultural assessment*. Mahwah, NJ: Erlbaum.

Butcher, J. N., Dahlstrom, W. G., Graham, J. R., Tellegen, A. M., & Kaemmer, B. (1989). *MMPI-2: Manual for administration and scoring*. Minneapolis: University of Minnesota Press.

Caetano, R. (1989). Concepts of alcoholism among Whites, Blacks, and Hispanics in the United States. *Journal of Studies on Alcohol, 50*, 580–582.

Caetano, R. (1994). Drinking and alcohol-related problems among minority women. *Alcohol Health and Research World, 18*, 233–241.

Carlson, E. B., & Rosser-Hogan, R. (1994). Cross-cultural responses to trauma: A study of traumatic experiences and posttraumatic symptoms in Cambodian refugees. *Journal of Traumatic Stress, 7*, 43–58.

Castillo, R. J. (1998). *Meanings of madness*. Pacific Grove, CA: Brooks/Cole.

Cervantes, R., Gilbert, M. J., Salgado de Snyder, S. N., & Padilla, A. M. (1991). Psychosocial and cognitive correlates of alcohol use in younger adult immigrant and U.S. born Hispanics. *The International Journal of the Addictions, 25*, 687–708.

Cetingok, M., Chu, C. C., & Park, D. B. (1990). The effect of culture on the sex differences in schizophrenia. *The International Journal of Social Psychiatry, 36*, 272–279.

Chen, C., Lee, S. Y., & Stevenson, H. W. (1995). Response style and cross-cultural comparison of rating scales among East Asian and North American students. *Psychological Science, 6*, 170–175.

Clark, L. A., Watson, D., & Reynolds, S. (1995). Diagnosis and classification of psychopathology: Challenges to the current system and future directions. *Annual Review of Psychology, 46*, 121–153.

Cockerham, W. C., Kunz, G., & Lueschen, G. (1989). Alcohol use and psychological distress: A comparison of Americans and West Germans. *The International Journal of the Addictions, 24*, 951–961.

Corin, E. E. (1990). Facts and meanings in psychiatry. An anthropological approach to the lifeworld of schizophrenics. *Culture, Medicine, and Psychiatry, 14*, 153–188.

Dana, R. H. (1998) (Ed.). *Understanding cultural identity in intervention and assessment*. Thousand Oaks, CA: Sage.

Davison, G. C., & Neale, J. M. (1994). *Abnormal psychology* (6th ed.). New York: Wiley.

Doi, T. (1973). *The anatomy of dependence*. Translated by John Bester. (1st ed.). New York: Harper & Row.

Draguns, J. (1977). Problems of defining and comparing abnormal behavior across cultures. *Annals of the New York Academy of Sciences, 285,* 66–679.

Draguns, J. (1982). Methodology in cross-cultural psychopathology. In Al-Issa (Ed.). *Culture and psychopathology.* Baltimore: University Park Press.

Draguns, J. G. (1994). Pathological and clinical aspects. In L. Adler and U. P. Gielen (Eds.), *Cross-cultural topics in psychology* (pp. 165–177). Westport, CT: Praeger/Greenwood.

Eaton, W. W., Dryman, A., & Weissman, M. (1991). Panic and phobia. In L. N. Robins & D. A. Regier (Eds.), *Psychiatric disorders in America: The Epidemiological Catchment Study* (pp. 155–179). New York: The Free Press.

Edgerton, R. B., & Cohen, A. (1994). Culture and schizophrenia: The DOSMD challenge. *British Journal of Psychiatry, 164,* 222–231.

Egeland, J. A. (1994). An epidemiologic and genetic study of affective disorders among the Old Order Amish. In D. F. Papolos & H. M. Lachman (Eds.), *Genetic studies in affective disorders: Overview of basic methods, current directions, and critical research issues* (pp. 70–90). New York: Wiley.

Enright, J. B., & Jaeckle, W. R. (1961). Ethnic differences in psychopathology. *Social Process, 25,* 71–77.

Estroff, S. E. (1989). Self, identity, and subjective experiences of schizophrenia: In search of the subject. *Schizophrenia Bulletin, 15,* 189–196.

Fabrega, H. (1989). Cultural relativism and psychiatric illness. *Journal of Nervous and Mental Disease, 177,* 415–425.

Fabrega, H. (1989). The self and schizophrenia: A cultural perspective. *Schizophrenia Bulletin, 15,* 277–290.

Fantl, B., & Schiro, J. (1959). Cultural variables in the behaviour patterns and symptom formation of 15 Irish and 15 Italian female schizophrenics. *International Journal of Social Psychiatry, 4,* 245–253.

Friedman, S., Paradis, C. M., & Hatch, M. L. (1994). Issues of misdiagnosis in panic disorder with agoraphobia. In S. Friedman (Ed.), *Anxiety disorders in African-Americans* (pp. 128–146). New York: Springer Publishing.

Fugita, S. S., & Crittenden, K. S. (1990). Towards culture- and population-specific norms for self-reported depressive symptomology. *International Journal of Social Psychiatry, 36,* 83–92.

Gilbert, M. J. (1991). Acculturation and changes in drinking patterns among Mexican-American women: Implications for prevention. *Alcohol Health and World, 15,* 234–238.

Gottesman, I., & Moldin, S. (1997). Schizophrenia genetics at the millennium: Cautious optimism. *Clinical Genetics, 52,* 404–407.

Gottesman, I., & Bertelsen, (1989). Confirming unexpressed genotypes for schizophrenia. *Archives of General Psychiatry, 46,* 867–872.

Grant, B. F., & Harford, T. C. (1995). Comorbidity between DSM-IV alcohol use disorders and major depression: Results of a national survey. *Drug and Alcohol Dependence, 39,* 197–206.

Guarnaccia, P. J. (1993). Ataques de nervios in Puerto Rico: Culture-bound syndrome or popular illness? *Medical Anthropology, 15,* 157–170.

Guarnaccia, P. J. (1997). A cross-cultural perspective on anxiety disorders. In S. Friedman (Eds.), *Cultural issues in the treatment of anxiety.* New York: Guilford.

Guarnaccia, P. J., DeLaCancela, V., & Carrillo, E. (1989). The multiple meanings of ataques de nervios in the Latino community. *Medical Anthropology, 11,* 47–62.

Hall, S. M., Muñoz, R. F., & Reus, V. (1994). Cognitive-behavioral intervention increases abstinence rates for depressive-history smokers. *Journal of Clinical and Consulting Psychology, 62,* 141–146.

Hamdi, E., Amin, Y., & Abou-Saleh, M. T. (1997). Problems in validating endogenous depression in the Arab culture by contemporary diagnostic criteria. *Journal of Affective Disorders, 44,* 131–143.

Hughes, C. C. (1998). The glossary of "culture-bound syndromes" in DSM-IV: A critique. *Transcultural Psychiatry, 35,* 413–421.

Hwu, H. G., Yeh, E. K., Chang, L. Y., & Yeh, Y. L. (1986). Chinese Diagnostic Interview Schedule. II. A validity study estimation of lifetime prevalence. *Acta Psychiatrica Scandinavica, 73,* 348–357.

Jablensky, A. (1989). Epidemiology and cross-cultural aspects of schizophrenia. *Psychiatric Annals, 19,* 516–524.

Jarvis, E. (1998). Schizophrenia in British immigrants: Recent findings, issues, and implications. *Transcultural Psychiatry, 35,* 39–74.

Jenkins, J. H. (1991). Anthropology, expressed emotion, and schizophrenia. *Ethos, 19,* 387–431.

Jenkins, J. H. (1997). Subjective experience of persistent schizophrenia and depression among U.S. Latinos and Euro-Americans. *British Journal of Psychiatry, 171,* 20–25.

Jenkins, J. H., Kleinman, A., & Good, B. J. (1991). Cross-cultural studies of depression. In J. Becker & A. Kleinman (Eds.), *Psychosocial aspects of depression* (pp. 67–99). Hillsdale, NJ: Erlbaum.

Jilek, W. G. (1995). Emil Kraepelin and comparative socio-cultural psychiatry. *European Archives of Psychiatry and Clinical Neuroscience, 245,* 231–238.

Jones, R. L. (Ed.). (1996). *Handbook of tests and measurements for Black populations* (Vols. 1–2). Hampton, VA: Cobb & Henry.

Karno, M., & Golding, J. M. (1991). Obsessive-compulsive disorder. In L. N. Robins & D. A. Regier (Eds.). *Psychiatric disorders in America: The Epidemiologic Catchment Area Study* (pp. 204–219). New York: Free Press.

Karno, M., Golding, J. M., Burnam, M., Hough, R. L., et al. (1989). Anxiety disorders among Mexican-Americans and non-Hispanic Whites in Los Angeles. *Journal of Nervous and Mental Disease, 177,* 202–209.

Kessler, R. C., McGonagle, K. A., Zhao, S., Nelson, C. B., Hughes, M., Eshleman, S., Wittchen, H. U., & Kendler, K. S. (1994). Lifetime and 12-month prevalence of DSM-III-R psychiatric disorders in the United States. *Archives of General Psychiatry, 51,* 8–19.

Kirmayer, L. (1996). Confusion of the senses: Implications of ethnocultural variations in somatoform and dissociative disorders for PTSD. In A. J. Marsella, M. J. Friedman, E. T. Gernty, & R. M. Scurfield (Eds.), *Ethnocultural aspects of PTSD: Issues, research, and clinical applications.* Washington, DC: American Psychological Association.

Kleinman, A. (1986). *Social origins of distress and disease: Depression, neurasthenia, and pain in modern China.* New Haven, CT: Yale University Press.

Klerman, G. L. (1993). The postwar generation and depression. In A. Abdu'l-Missagh, H. Ghadirian, & E. Lehmann (Eds.), *Environment and psychopathology* (pp. 73–86). New York: Springer Publishing.

Krause, I. B. (1989). Sinking heart: A Punjabi communication of distress. *Social Science Medicine, 29,* 563–575.

Krueger, R. F., Caspi, A., Moffitt, T. E., & Silva, P. A. (1998). The structure and stability of common mental disorders (DSM-III-R): A longitudinal-epidemiological study. *Journal of Abnormal Psychology, 107,* 216–227.

Lawson, W. B. (1986). Racial and ethnic factors in psychiatric research. *Hospital and Community Psychiatry, 37,* 50–54.

Lefley, H. P. (1990). Culture and chronic mental illness. *Hospital and Community Psychiatry, 41,* 277–286.

Lewis-Fernandez, R. (1998). A cultural critique of the DSM-IV dissociative disorders section. *Transcultural Psychiatry, 35,* 387–400.

Lin, K. M., & Kleinman, A. M. (1988). Psychopathology and clinical course of schizophrenia: A cross-cultural perspective. *Schizophrenia Bulletin, 14,* 555–567.

Lin, K. M., Lau, J. K., Yamamoto, J., Sheng, Y. P., Kim, H. S., Cho, K. H., & Nakasaki, G. (1992). Hwa-byung: A community study of Korean Americans. *Journal of Nervous and Mental Disease, 180,* 386–391.

Lin, K. M., Poland, R. E., & Lesser, I. M. (1986). Ethnicity and psychopharmacology. *Culture, Medicine, and Psychiatry, 10,* 151–165.

Lin, K. M., Poland, R. E., & Nakasaki, G. (Eds.). (1993). *Psychopharmacology and psychobiology of ethnicity.* Washington, DC: American Psychiatric Press.

Malgady, R. G., Rogler, L. H., & Cortes, D. E. (1996). Cultural expression of psychiatric symptoms: Idioms of anger among Puerto Ricans. *Psychological Assessment, 8,* 265–268.

Manson, S. M. (1995). Culture and major depression: Current challenges in the diagnosis of mood disorders. *Cultural Psychiatry, 18,* 487–501.

Marcos, L. R., & Cancro, R. (1982). Pharmacotherapy of Hispanic depressed patients: Clinical observations. *American Journal of Psychotherapy, 36,* 505–512.

Marsella, A. (1987). The measurement of depressive experience and disorder across cultures. In A. Marsella, R. M. Hirschfeld, & M. M. Katz (Eds.), *The measurement of depression* (pp. 376–397). New York: Guilford.

Martins, C., de Lemos, A. I., & Bebbington, P. E. (1992). A Portuguese/Brazilian study of expressed emotion. *Social Psychiatry and Psychiatric Epidemiology, 27,* 22–27.

Matthey, S., Barnett, B. E. W., & Elliott, A. (1997). Vietnamese and Arabic women's responses to the Diagnostic Interview Schedule (depression) and self-report questionnaires: Cause for concern. *Australian and New Zealand Journal of Psychiatry, 31,* 360–369.

May, P. A. (1982). Substance abuse and American Indians: Prevalence and susceptibility. *The International Journal of the Addictions, 17,* 1185–1209.

Mendoza, R., Smith, M. W., Poland, R. E., Lin, K. M., & Strickland, T. L. (1991). Ethnic psychopharmacology: The Hispanic and Native American perspective. *Psychopharmacology Bulletin, 27,* 449–461.

Mino, Y., Tanaka, S., Inoue, S., Tsuda, T., Babazono, A., & Aoyama, H. (1995). Expressed emotion components in families of schizophrenic patients in Japan. *International Journal of Mental Health, 24*(2), 38–49.

Moscicki, E. K., Rae, D. S., Regier, D. A., & Locke, B. Z. (1987). The Hispanic Health and Nutrition Examination Survey: Depression among Mexican-Americans, Cuban-Americans, and Puerto Ricans. In M. Gaviria & J. D. Arana (Eds.), *Health and behavior: Research agenda for Hispanics* (pp. 145–159). Chicago: University of Illinois.

Mukherjee, S., Shukla, S., Woodle, J., et al. (1983). Misdiagnosis of schizophrenia in bipolar patients: A multiethnic comparison. *American Journal of Psychiatry, 140,* 1571–1574.

Mumford, D. B. (1996). The "Dhat syndrome": A culturally determined symptom of depression? *Acta Psychiatrica Scandinavica, 94,* 163–167.

Muñoz, R. F. (1986). Opportunities for prevention among Hispanics. In R. L. Hough, P. Gongla, V. Brown, & S. Goldston (Eds.), *Psychiatric epidemiology and primary prevention: The possibilities* (pp. 109–129). Los Angeles: University of California Neuropsychiatric Institute.

Muñoz, R. F., Marín, B. V., Posner, S. F., and Pérez-Stable, E. J. (1997). Mood management mail intervention increases abstinence rates for Spanish-speaking Latino smokers. *American Journal of Community Psychology, 25,* 325–343.

Nakane, Y., Ohta, Y., Radford, M., Yan, H., et al. (1991). Comparative study of affective disorders in three Asian countries: II. Differences in prevalence rates and symptom presentation. *Acta Psychiatrica Scandinavica, 84,* 313–319.

Ndetei, D. M., & Vadher, A. (1984). A comparative cross-cultural study of the frequencies of hallucination in schizophrenia. *Acta Psychiatrica Scandinavica, 70,* 545–549.

Neff, J. A., & Hoppe, S. K. (1992). Acculturation and drinking patterns among U.S. Anglos, Blacks, and Mexican-Americans. *Alcohol and Alcoholism, 27,* 293–308.

Okazaki, S. (1997). Sources of ethnic differences between Asian-American and White American college students on measures of depression and social anxiety. *Journal of Abnormal Psychology, 106,* 52–60.

Opler, M. K., & Singer, J. L. (1956). Ethnic differences in behavior and psychopathology: Italian and Irish. *International Journal of Social Psychiatry, 2,* 11–23.

Pedersen, P. B., Draguns, J. G., Lonner, W. J., & Trimble, J. E. (Eds.). (1996). *Counseling across cultures* (4th ed.). Thousand Oaks, CA: Sage.

Pedigo, J. (1983). Finding the "meaning" of Native American substance abuse: Implications for community prevention. *The Personnel and Guidance Journal, 61,* 273–277.

Phillips, M. R., West, C. L., & Wang, R. (1996). Erotomanic symptoms in 42 Chinese schizophrenic patients. *British Journal of Psychiatry, 169,* 501–508.

Randall, E. J. (1994). Cultural relativism in cognitive therapy with disadvantaged African-American women. *Journal of Cognitive Psychotherapy: An International Quarterly, 8,* 195–207.

Robins, L. N., Helzer, J. E., Croughan, J. L., & Ratcliff, K. S. (1981). National Institute of Mental Health Diagnostic Interview Schedule: Its history, characteristics, and validity. *Archives of General Psychiatry, 38,* 381–189.

Robins, L. N., & Regier, D. A. (1991). *Psychiatric disorders in America. The Epidemiological Catchment Area Study.* New York: Free Press.

Robbins, L., & Smith, E. (1983). *The Diagnostic Interview Schedule Disaster Supplement.* St. Louis, MO: Washington University School of Medicine.

Rosenhan, D., & Seligman, M. (1989). *Abnormal psychology* (2nd ed.). New York: W.W. Norton.

Russell, J. G. (1989). Anxiety disorders in Japan: A review of the Japanese literature on Shinkeishitsu and Taijinkyofusho. *Culture, Medicine, and Psychiatry, 13,* 391–403.

Sartorius, N., Jablensky, A., Gulbinat, W., & Ernberg, G. (1980). WHO Collaborative Study: Assessment of depressive disorders. *Psychological Medicine, 10,* 739–79.

Sartorius, N., Ustun, T. B., Lecrubier, Y., & Wittchen, H. U. (1996). Depression comorbid with anxiety: Results for the

WHO study on psychological disorders in primary health care. *British Journal of Psychiatry, 168*(Suppl. 30), 38–43.

Segall, M., Lonner, W., & Berry, J. (1998). Cross-cultural psychology as a scholarly discipline: On the flowering of culture in behavioral research. *American Psychologist, 53,* 1101–1110.

Sigelman, C., Didjurgis, T., Marshall, B., Vargas, F., & Stewart, A. (1992). Views of problem drinking among Native American, Hispanic, and Anglo children. *Child Psychiatry and Human Development, 22,* 265–276.

Silver, B., Poland, R. E., & Lin, K. E. (1993). Ethnicity and the pharmacology of tricyclic antidepressants. In K. M. Lin, R. E. Poland, & G. Nakasaki (Eds.), *Psychopharmacology and psychobiology of ethnicity* (pp. 61–89). Washington, DC: American Psychiatric Press.

Smith, M., Lin, K. M., & Mendoza, R. (1993). "Nonbiological" issues affecting psychopharmacotherapy: Cultural considerations. In K. M. Lin, R. E. Poland, & G. Nakasaki (Eds.), *Psychopharmacology and psychobiology of ethnicity* (pp. 37–58). Washington, DC: American Psychiatric Press.

Staley, D., & Wand, R. R. (1995). Obsessive-compulsive disorder: A review of the cross-cultural epidemiological literature. *Transcultural Psychiatric Research Review, 32,* 103–136.

Sue, D. W., & Sue, D. (1990). *Counseling the culturally different: Theory and practice* (2nd ed.). New York: Wiley.

Sue, S., Fujino, D. C., Hu, L., Takeuchi, D. T., et al. (1991). Community mental health services for ethnic minority groups: A test of the cultural responsiveness hypothesis. *Journal of Consulting and Clinical Psychology, 59,* 533–540.

Takahashi, Y. (1990). Is multiple personality disorder really rare in Japan? *Dissociation: the official journal of the International Society for the Study of Multiple Personality and Dissociation, 3,* 57–59.

Takeuchi, D. T., Chung, R., Lin, K. M., Shen, H., Kurasaki, K., Chun, C. A., & Sue, S. (1998). Lifetime and twelve-month prevalence rates of major depressive episodes and dysthymia among Chinese Americans in Los Angeles. *American Journal of Psychiatry, 155,* 1407–1414.

Takeuchi, D. T., Sue, S., & Yeh, M. (1995). Return rates and outcomes from ethnicity-specific mental health programs in Los Angeles. *American Journal of Public Health, 85,* 638–643.

Tanaka-Matsumi, J., & Marsella, A. (1976). Cross-cultural variation in the phenomenological experience of depression: Word association. *Journal of Cross-Cultural Psychology, 7,* 379–396.

Tanaka-Matsumi, J. (1979). Taijin Kyofusho: Diagnostic and cultural issues in Japanese psychiatry. *Culture, Medicine, and Psychiatry, 3,* 231–245.

Tateyama, M., Asai, M., Hashimoto, M., Bartels, M., & Kasper, S. (1998). Transcultural study of schizophrenic delusions. *Psychopathology, 31,* 59–68.

Trimble, J. E. (1991). Ethnic specification, validation prospects, and the future of drug use research. *The International Journal of the Addictions, 25,* 149–170.

Tsai, J. L., Ying, Y. W., & Lee, P. A. (2000). The meaning of "being Chinese" and "being American": Variation among Chinese American young adults. *Journal of Cross-Cultural Psychology, 31,* 302–322.

Tseng, W. S., & Streltzer, J. (1997). *Culture and psychopathology: A guide to clinical assessment.* New York: Brunner/Mazel.

Tung, M. (1994). Symbolic meanings of the body in Chinese culture and "somatization." *Culture, Medicine, and Psychiatry, 18,* 483–492.

Uba, L. (1994). *Asian-Americans: Personality patterns, identity, and mental health.* New York: Guilford.

Vega, W. A., Kolody, B., Aguilar-Gaxiola, S., Alderete, E., et al. (1998). Lifetime prevalence of DSM-III-R psychiatric disorders among urban and rural Mexican-Americans in California. *Archives of General Psychiatry, 55,* 771–778.

Waxler, N. E. (1979). Is outcome for schizophrenia better in nonindustrial societies? The case of Sri Lanka. *Journal of Nervous and Mental Disease, 167,* 144–158.

Weatherspoon, A. J., Danko, G. P., & Johnson, R. C. (1994). Alcohol consumption and use norms among Chinese-Americans and Korean-Americans. *Journal of Studies on Alcohol, 55,* 203–206.

Weissman, M. M., Bland, R. C., Canino, G. J., Greenwald, S., Hwu, H., Lee, C. K., Newman, S. C., Oakley-Browne, M. A., Rubio-Stipel, M., Wickreamaratne, P. J., Wittchen, H., & Hey, E. (1994). The cross-national epidemiology of obsessive-compulsive disorder. *Journal of Clinical Psychiatry, 55*(Suppl.), 5–10.

Weissman, M., Livingston Bruce, M., Leaf, P. J., Florio, L. P., & Holzer, C. (1991). Affective disorders. In L. N. Robins & D. A. Regier (Eds.), *Psychiatric disorders in America: The Epidemiological Catchment Study* (pp. 53–80). New York: The Free Press.

Wexler, B. E., Levenson, L., Warrenberg, S., & Price, L. (1994). Decreased perceptual sensitivity to emotion-evoking stimuli in depression. *Psychiatry Research, 51,* 127–138.

Wig, N. N. (1960). Problems of mental health in India. *Journal of the Clinical Society of the Medical College, 17,* 48.

Wig, N. N., Menon, D. K., Bedi, H., Ghosh, A., et al. (1987). Expressed emotion and schizophrenia in North India: I. Cross-cultural transfer of ratings of relatives' expressed emotion. *British Journal of Psychiatry, 151,* 156–160.

Williams, K. E., & Chambless, D. (1994). The results of exposure-based treatment of agoraphobia. In S. Friedman (Ed.), *Anxiety disorders in African-Americans* (pp. 149–165). New York: Springer Publishing.

Wing, J. K., Cooper, J. E., & Sartorius, N. (1974). *Measurement and classification of psychiatric symptoms: An instruction manual for the PSE and Catego program.* Cambridge: Cambridge University Press.

World Health Organization. (1975). *A manual on drug dependence.* Geneva: Author.

World Health Organization. (1992). *The ICD-10 classification of mental and behavioral disorders: Clinical descriptions and diagnostic guidelines.* Geneva: Author.

Ying, Y. W. (1988). Depressive symptomatology among Chinese-Americans as measured by the CES-D. *Journal of Clinical Psychology, 44,* 739–746.

Ying, Y. W., Lee, P. A., Tsai, J. L., Yeh, Y., & Huang, J. (2000). The concept of depression in Chinese American college students. *Cultural Diversity and Ethnic Minority Psychology, 6*(2), 183–195.

Yinger, J. M. (1986). Intersecting strands in the theorization of race and ethnic relations. In J. Rex & D. Mason (Eds.), *Theories of race and ethnic relations* (pp. 20–41). Cambridge: Cambridge University Press.

Zhang, A. Y., Snowden, L. R., & Sue, S. (1998). Differences between Asian and White Americans' help seeking and utilization patterns in the Los Angeles area. *Journal of Community Psychology, 26,* 317–326.

# PART II

# Neurotic and Psychotic Disorders

# CHAPTER 6

# Generalized Anxiety Disorders, Panic Disorders, and Phobias

## Ronald M. Rapee and David H. Barlow

## Introduction

Anxiety disorders encompass what is probably the most diverse group of psychopathological problems. Included among the anxiety disorders are such behaviors as repetitive hand washing, ritualizing, unexpected and apparently inexplicable bursts of panic, and an inability to eat or drink in front of other people. Anxiety disorders include a wide array of features, and the intensity of the disorders can also vary tremendously. They can range from relatively "normal" features such as worrying about bills to extremely debilitating problems such as a total inability to leave home. Yet, this seemingly diverse group of disorders all share a single, basic, common feature—anxiety. All of the seemingly bizarre thoughts, feelings, and behaviors in these disorders center around and are motivated by feelings of fear and anxiety.

This chapter will examine four of the major anxiety disorders: generalized anxiety disorder, panic disorder (including agoraphobia), social phobia, and specific phobia. Because these disorders share the basic feature of anxiety, there are a number of other commonalities among them, such as similar symptomatology, similar cognitive styles, and similar treatment options and response. However, each disorder also has a number of unique features, perhaps best summarized by the specific focus of the anxious response. Thus, we will examine both the similarities and, in particular, the differences among these four disorders. Each section will be similarly organized and will cover the definition of the disorder, clinical features, maintaining factors, and treatment. Naturally, with such a broad topic and limited space, this chapter will simply provide a broad overview of the disorders.

## Generalized Anxiety Disorder

### Diagnosis

In many ways, generalized anxiety disorder (GAD) can be considered the basic anxiety disorder. It can be thought of almost as an expression of "pure" high trait anxiety. By definition, GAD is not characterized primarily by a focus on any specific situation or object. Rather, the central characteristic of GAD is what many people would see as the fundamental feature of anxiety: worry. According to DSM-IV (American Psychiatric Association, 1994), a diagnosis of GAD requires a report of excessive worry over a number of events or activities, more days than not, over at least 6 months. In addition, the person must report difficulty controlling the worry and must also experi-

Ronald M. Rapee • Department of Psychology, Macquarie University, Sydney, New South Wales 2109, Australia. David H. Barlow • Center for Anxiety and Related Disorders, Boston University, Boston, Massachusetts 02215-2002.

*Comprehensive Handbook of Psychopathology* (Third Edition), edited by Patricia B. Sutker and Henry E. Adams. Kluwer Academic/Plenum Publishers, New York, 2001.

ence three out of a list of six symptoms. The symptoms are related mainly to various features of excessive arousal. However, these symptoms are probably not a particularly important defining characteristic of GAD because many subjects with other anxiety disorders report a number of the same symptoms (Barlow, Blanchard, Vermilyea, Vermilyea, & DiNardo, 1986). Thus, it seems that chronic worry is the best distinguishing characteristic of GAD. Of course, worry about specific areas is naturally present in all of the anxiety disorders; however, DSM-IV specifies that the source of worry must not be another Axis I disorder. For example, if someone met criteria for a diagnosis of social phobia, then worry about social situations would not count toward a diagnosis of GAD.

The exclusion of worry about other diagnoses is essential to distinguish GAD from other anxiety disorders, but this feature makes the diagnosis of GAD sometimes difficult. In addition, the overlap between many of the features of GAD and other anxiety disorders also adds to this difficulty (Brown, Barlow, & Liebowitz, 1994). For these reasons, agreement among raters regarding a diagnosis of GAD in an individual (measured by the kappa statistic) is generally the lowest for GAD of any of the anxiety disorders (kappas between .27 and .57) (DiNardo, Moras, Barlow, Rapee, & Brown, 1993; Mannuzza et al., 1989; Wittchen, Kessler, Zhao, & Abelson, 1995). It should be noted that these studies have all used DSM-III-R criteria, and studies using DSM-IV are still awaited.

## Clinical Features

**Epidemiology.** Probably because of the "normality" of GAD, it is difficult to obtain estimates of its prevalence and incidence because such estimates are likely to be very dependent on minor definitional differences. Nevertheless, several studies in recent years have indicated that GAD is one of the more prevalent disorders; it is diagnosed at around 3% of the population over a given 12-month period and around 5% across the lifetime (Kessler et al., 1994). Similar figures are reported in children (Fergusson, Horwood, & Lynskey, 1993). Interestingly, despite its prevalence, it is one of the least common anxiety disorders presenting to mental health practitioners and accounts for around 10% of anxiety disorder patients (Barlow, 1988). GAD is found commonly,

however, among patients in general medical practice (Brawman-Mintzer & Lydiard, 1996).

**Sex Distribution.** As with most of the other anxiety disorders, GAD is more common in females. However, GAD has a more equal sex distribution than some of the other disorders; most populations of GAD contain around 60% females (Anderson, Noyes, & Crowe, 1984; Rapee, 1985).

**Onset.** Most studies report that GAD generally begins around the midteens to early 20s (Anderson et al., 1984; Barlow et al., 1986; Rapee, 1985). However, calculation of a mean age of onset for this order is probably fairly meaningless because a large number of GAD patients report experiencing symptoms all of their lives. This indication of a lifelong existence for GAD is consistent with some growing speculation that GAD should actually be considered a lifelong psychological trait or personality disorder (Rapee, 1991). If this is so, then an average age of onset really does not provide any useful information.

Along similar lines, GAD patients generally describe the onset of their disorder as gradual and insidious (Anderson et al., 1984; Rapee, 1985). This evidence is also consistent with a personality orientation in GAD. Thus, we may describe GAD as a general characteristic of an individual that perhaps becomes more severe at some point in the person's life. Alternately, the disorder itself may not become more intense, but it may be that one of a number of reasons eventually leads the individual to decide to do something about the problem. For example, a change in life circumstances may cause people's usual behaviors to interfere with their lives.

**Worry.** Because worry is the central characteristic in GAD, these individuals will present as "chronic worriers." But what do they worry about? One study that examined this question categorized the worries reported by twenty-two GAD patients during clinical intake interviews into common spheres (Sanderson & Barlow, 1990). The researchers came up with four major spheres in the following descending order of importance: family, finances, work, and personal illness. In addition, 91% of the patients reported "worrying excessively about minor things," compared to 40% of subjects with other anxiety disorders.

A second study asked nineteen GAD patients and twenty-six nonanxious controls to record three instances of "significant" worry during a 3-week period (Craske, Rapee, Jackel, & Barlow,

1989). GAD subjects worried most about illness, second most about family, and least about finances. This seemed to be a slightly different pattern from that of the controls, who worried most about work and least about illness. Thus, although the worries reported by GAD patients cover very normal areas, the relative weight that these individuals give to these spheres may be somewhat different from that given by nonanxious subjects.

Another important difference emerged in the study comparing the worries of GADs and nonanxious controls (Craske, Rapee, et al., 1989) (note that this study was based on DSM-III-R criteria). The GAD subjects reported that their worries were significantly less controllable than the normals' worries and, similarly, that they were less able than the normals to stop or prevent their worrying. This uncontrollability aspect of chronic worrying was also reported in a college sample (Borkovec, Robinson, Pruzinsky, & DePree, 1983). It has been suggested that a general sense of uncontrollability is a fundamental characteristic of anxiety disorders (Barlow, 1988), and this quality may be the most distressing to persons with GAD and most responsible for making GAD into a "disorder." Recognizing this crucial role of uncontrollability, this feature is now included as a diagnostic criterion in the DSM-IV.

### Etiology and Maintenance

**Genetic and Familial Factors.** Family studies of GAD indicated that these patients were more likely to have a first-degree relative with GAD than subjects with panic disorder or no anxiety disorder (Noyes, Clarkson, Crowe, Yates, & Mc-Chesney, 1987). Of course, family studies are influenced by both genetic and environmental factors. Twin studies demonstrated a moderate genetic influence in GAD; around 30% of the variance was attributable to genetic factors (Kendler et al., 1992a, 1995). Importantly, the genetic influence for any anxiety disorder is not likely to be specific. Rather, it is more likely that genetic factors influence the development of a general neurotic syndrome, and individual environmental factors are more important in the emergence of specific features of GAD (Andrews, 1996; Kendler et al., 1995).

**Psychological Factors.** Given the fact that a tendency to worry excessively is one of the main defining features of GAD, there has been a wealth of research during the past few years to better understand this phenomenon (Borkovec, Shadick, & Hopkins, 1991). According to Borkovec and colleagues (1991), worry serves as a type of avoidance purpose and allows individuals to engage in excessive conceptual and semantic thinking, but avoid imagery and emotional processing. Therefore, worrying does not allow habituation, and this lack of habituation helps to maintain the anxiety experienced by people with GAD. The fact that worry is largely semantic and also uses up many resources in working memory has been demonstrated by several studies (e.g. Borkovec & Inz, 1990; Eysenck, 1985; Rapee, 1993a).

A related direction of research has focused on examining the way in which people with GAD process information (MacLeod, 1996; Mathews, Mackintosh, & Fulcher, 1997). In one of the earliest studies, Butler and Mathews (1983) found that GAD subjects were more likely than normal controls to interpret ambiguous events as threatening. In addition, the GAD subjects believed that there was a higher likelihood that threatening events would happen to themselves, but they did not believe there was a higher likelihood that threatening events would happen to someone else. Thus, in line with suggestions by Beck (Beck & Emery, 1985), anxious individuals have a tendency to see themselves in particular danger in the world.

There is also considerable evidence to suggest that persons with GAD have an attentional bias toward threatening cues. In other words, potentially threatening stimuli in the environment grab the attention of persons with GAD more easily and quickly than that of nonanxious people. This would suggest that such individuals are constantly scanning the environment (not necessarily consciously) for any signs of possible danger (Mathews et al., 1997). For example, one study demonstrated that anxious subjects were faster than controls in detecting a dot on a computer screen when it was immediately preceded by a threatening word in the same part of the screen, but were slower than controls in detecting the dot when the threatening word was in a different part of the screen (MacLeod, Mathews, & Tata, 1986).

For memory, the results have been somewhat less clear, and indeed it looks as though there may be little memory bias in people with GAD (MacLeod, 1996). For example, one of the earliest studies found a trend whereby GAD subjects actually recalled *fewer* threatening words than normal controls (Mogg, Mathews, & Weinman, 1987). The authors suggested that once persons with GAD have detected a threat, they may cognitively avoid this information, leading to decreased memory. In a later study, no significant difference in memory for threatening words was found between GAD subjects and controls using a controlled memory task (i.e., one that requires attentional processes), but using a more automatic task, GAD subjects did have better memory for threatening words, perhaps suggesting that the information had been extensively processed (Mathews, Mogg, May, & Eysenck, 1989).

In summary, it seems that persons with GAD (and probably all individuals who are high in trait anxiety) are characterized by a tendency to interpret ambiguous information as threatening and to pay excessive attention to potential threats. Once they detect a threat, people with GAD elaborate the possibilities extensively in working memory, thereby reducing habituation. The crucial question, of course, is whether these processes are causal or are simply a consequence of anxiety. Research being conducted in several laboratories that is aimed at training people to shift their attention will help to answer this question during the coming years (MacLeod, 1996; Mathews et al., 1997).

**Neurobiological Factors.** There is little research into the biological factors associated with GAD specifically, although a large body of work has examined the role of biological factors in anxiety generally. The majority of the biochemical work has centered on the role of the benzodiazepine receptor complex (Insel, Ninan, Aloi, Jimerson, Skolnick, & Paul, 1984). Discovery of a specific brain receptor for the benzodiazepines (Squires & Braestrup, 1977) led to speculation that there must be a naturally occurring neurotransmitter that uses this receptor and therefore may be involved in producing anxiety. A number of chemicals were examined with this role in mind, and the research is still continuing.

A specific anxiety neurotransmitter has proven difficult to identify, but some researchers have attempted to examine the interaction between various neurotransmitter systems and neuroanatomical sites. The main research of this type has been conducted by Jeffrey Gray (e.g., 1982; Gray & McNaughton, 1996), who has been involved in a systematic course of research examining the neuropsychology of anxiety. Although Gray's model is very involved, it centers largely around the septohippocampal system, which (according to Gray) acts as a type of comparator, comparing actual with expected stimuli. The system "turns on" (i.e., anxiety) when there is a mismatch between actual and expected stimuli or when the expected stimuli are aversive. Gray does not really apply his model to specific anxiety disorders, but it could be suggested that GAD involves some type of dysfunction in the septohippocampal system.

Whether one is specifying neurotransmitter systems or neuroanatomical pathways, it is clear that biological correlates of anxiety cannot be isolated to one neurotransmitter or one pathway. Any useful neurobiological model of anxiety will have to be very comprehensive (for a review, see Barlow, 1988, in press). Currently, Gray's model most closely approaches this characteristic.

Another interesting neurobiological process recently discovered in individuals with GAD is a distinct lack of autonomic reactivity, or what has come to be called "autonomic inflexibility" (Borkovec, 1994; Hoehn-Saric et al., 1989; Thayer, Friedman, & Borkovec, 1996). Interestingly, this process seems directly associated with the cognitive process of worry described before. Further investigations revealed that this psychophysiological characteristic is mediated by low vagal tone resulting in a high unstable heart rate and decreased heart rate reactivity, among other responses (Thayer et al., 1996). In fact, a similar relationship was noted by several researchers such as Kagan (Kagan et al., 1990) who observed autonomic inflexibility in behaviorally inhibited children. Borkovec (1994) relates autonomic inflexibility in GAD patients to the fact that the stimuli feared by these patients are not produced by external environmental stressors but are internally generated thoughts about potential future events. Thus, these individuals are caught up in a perpetual state of scanning for danger (Mathews, 1990). Sapolsky (1992) studying free ranging baboons in Africa observed a similar process in his baboons who were subject to chronic stress. He suggests that this process, if chronic, leads to hippocampal lesions. Brain imaging is beginning to confirm the generality of these observations in patients with anxiety disorders (Barlow & Durand, 1999). These findings supported the substantial change in the symptoms that comprise the somatic criteria for DSM-IV definitions of GAD (Barlow & Wincze, in press). Several studies demonstrated the construct validity of these changes suggesting that symptoms of motor tension and vigilance and scanning are more strongly correlated with measures of GAD (e.g., the Penn State Worry Questionnaire) than symptoms that reflect autonomic hyperactivity (Brown, Martin, & Barlow, 1995). More recent structural equation modeling has demonstrated the unique and important contribution of autonomic inflexibility to generalized anxiety disorder in the context of all anxiety and mood disorders (Brown, Chorpita, & Barlow, 1998).

## Treatment

**Psychological Techniques.** Psychological treatment of anxiety disorders has involved broadly similar techniques, where only the specific content differs. The main techniques used include relaxation, cognitive restructuring, and exposure. For GAD, most successful treatments used a combination of relaxation and cognitive restructuring because the seeming lack of response to external cues has made *in vivo* exposure seem inappropriate. However, it is certainly possible to use exposure to subtle cues (such as being late or making mistakes) with GADs, and more comprehensive programs have included this technique (Barlow & Rapee, 1991). Additional strategies were also included in some packages including time management, assertiveness training, and problem solving (Barlow & Rapee, 1991). In general, cognitive behavioral treatment packages for GAD produce moderate to large improvements in anxiety symptoms and related problems such as depression (Chambless & Gillis, 1993; Gould, Otto, Pollack, & Yap, 1997; Harvey & Rapee, 1995). In a quantitative analysis of twenty-two controlled trials of cognitive behavior therapy for GAD, Gould et al. (1997) found that the best cognitive behavioral treatments resulted in a reduction in anxiety that was 0.9 standard deviations greater than that produced by control conditions. Furthermore, several studies showed that cognitive behavior therapy is more effective than other supposedly active treatments. For example, cognitive behavior therapy is more effective in reducing GAD than analytic psychotherapy (Durham et al., 1994), nondirective counseling (Blowers et al., 1987; Borkovec & Costello, 1993), and treatment with diazepam (Power et al., 1989, 1990). Perhaps even more important is the demonstration that the effects of treatments last for up to one year and that this maintenance is greater than that achieved with

medication (Chambless & Gillis, 1993; Gould et al., 1997). Despite these impressive results, treatment effects for GAD are not quite as large as for some of the other anxiety disorders, and the area will benefit from further development. One potential innovation involves exposure to the actual behavior of worrying (Craske, Barlow, & O'Leary, 1992). In this program, the uncontrollable process of worry itself is the principal source of chronic anxiety, rather than the rapidly changing content. Treatment involves regaining a sense of control of this out-of-control, anxiety-driven process. Evaluation of this strategy is continuing (Barlow, in press).

**Pharmacological Treatment.** Medication has also proven generally effective in treating GAD, although the effects have not been quite as strong as for cognitive behavior therapy (Gould et al., 1997). The most widely used drugs have been benzodiazepines, and the average effect size improvement is around 0.7 (Gould et al., 1997). However, despite the fact that the benzodiazepines produce good short-term changes, they tend to result in relatively rapid tolerance, and the effects decrease within a few weeks (Rickels, Downing, Schweizer, & Hassman, 1993). Other medications such as buspirone and the tricyclics produce a slower response that tends to last for a longer period. In one study that compared the tricyclic drug imipramine with the benzodiazepine diazepam, diazepam produced a significantly greater reduction in anxiety during the first two weeks but was no better than placebo from three weeks on (Rickels et al., 1993). In contrast, imipramine showed significantly greater effects than placebo from week 4 until the end of the trial (week 8). Despite these promising results with medication, the major limitation of this form of treatment is the tendency for subjects to relapse after administration of the drug stops (Schweizer & Rickels, 1996; Tyrer, Owen, & Dawling, 1983). As Schweizer and Rickels (1996) point out, the fact that GAD is a chronic disorder that begins at an early age, provides major problems for drug therapy.

## Panic Disorder

### Diagnosis

In its original conceptualization, agoraphobia was seen as a fear of external situations such as a marketplace (Westphal, 1871). Consequently, much attention has been focused on the phobic (behavioral) aspects of agoraphobia over the years. Before the publication of DSM-III (APA, 1980), panic attacks were largely ignored, although panic disorder existed under a wide range of names (including anxiety neurosis, neurocirculatory asthenia, effort syndrome, soldier's heart, irritable heart, etc.; see Barlow, 1988).

With the publication of the DSM-III-R (APA, 1987) it was officially acknowledged that agoraphobia and panic attacks were most often manifestations of the same disorder (panic disorder with agoraphobia). With publication of the DSM-IV, it was officially recognized that panic attacks could occur across a number of anxiety disorders. According to the DSM-IV, a panic attack involves a discrete period of fear or anxiety accompanied by a number of physiological and cognitive symptoms. There is some discussion about the actual number of symptoms necessary to constitute a panic attack: DSM-IV requires four or more symptoms at the same time. However, it has been found that patients themselves do not distinguish attacks with more than four symptoms from attacks with less than four (Rapee, Craske, & Barlow, 1990). A diagnosis of panic disorder requires that the individual experience recurrent panic attacks and worries about the next possible panic attack or consequences of the attack for at least 1 month. Importantly, for making a diagnosis of panic disorder, the individual must experience attacks that are unexpected or appear to be "out of the blue." In addition to the attacks, these individuals may display a range of phobic avoidance from no avoidance at all (panic disorder without agoraphobia) to being almost totally housebound (panic disorder with extensive agoraphobic avoidance).

Panic disorder is a very recognizable disorder, and studies of diagnostic reliability have generally indicated good agreement among raters; kappas range from .72 to .81 (DiNardo et al., 1993; Mannuzza et al., 1989). Generally, agreement is slightly better for subjects with more extensive avoidance (agoraphobia) than for those with less avoidance (panic disorder).

## Clinical Features

**Epidemiology.** One of the original epidemiological studies found that agoraphobia occurs in 0.6% of the population (Agras, Sylvester, & Oliveau, 1969). More recently, the National Comorbidity Survey reported a lifetime prevalence of 3.5% (Kessler et al., 1994). The reason for the discrepancy between these studies is more likely attributable to the interviewing techniques and criteria than to any increase in the prevalence of agoraphobia.

Though panic disorder is less prevalent than several other anxiety disorders, it is the most common anxiety disorder presenting to anxiety disorder clinics and is one of the most common disorders in any outpatient facility (Barlow, 1988). This is an indication of the tremendous distress and interference that panic attacks can cause in an individual's life (Norton et al., 1996).

**Sex Distribution.** By far, the majority of panic disorder sufferers are female. This ratio varies, however, depending on the degree of avoidance. Subjects with more extensive avoidance comprise a higher proportion of females (around 75% to 90%), whereas subjects with less avoidance comprise a slightly lower proportion of females (around 60% to 75%; Barlow et al., 1985; Craske & Barlow, 1988; Rapee & Murrell, 1988). The reasons for this sex difference are not clear but may reflect either a real difference in fear levels or a difference in reporting and presentation that is attributable to cultural influences.

**Onset.** Panic attacks most commonly begin around the middle to late 20s (Anderson et al., 1984; Rapee, 1985; Thorpe & Burns, 1983). In most cases, the onset is sudden and unexpected (Anderson et al., 1984; Rapee, 1985), and most individuals can clearly recall their first panic attack (Rapee, 1985). Despite the fact that most patients will report that the panic attacks are different from anything they have experienced before, several studies show that many patients may have a somewhat somatic or even hypochondriacal focus before their panic attacks begin (Ehlers, 1993; Fava, Grandi, & Canestrari, 1988; Schmidt, Lerew, & Jackson, 1997a).

**Cognitive Symptoms.** Panic disorder is characterized by a specific type of cognitive focus. Specifically, a number of studies demonstrated that panic disorder cognitions center around thoughts of dramatic and immediate threats such as death or insanity (Hibbert, 1984; Ottaviani & Beck, 1987; Rapee, 1985). For example, Hibbert (1984) found that compared to individuals with GAD, subjects with panic disorder were more likely to experience thoughts related to physical, psychological, or social disaster. Similarly, some studies showed that people with panic disorder are more likely than others to interpret ambiguous situations as indicating physical danger (Harvey, Richards, Dziadosz, & Swindell, 1993; McNally & Foa, 1987).

**Somatic Symptoms.** As mentioned before, panic disorder patients are very somatically focused and typically report a large number of somatic symptoms (Barlow et al., 1985; King, Margraf, Ehlers, & Maddock, 1986). In fact, studies find that panic disorder subjects report more somatic symptoms than subjects with almost any other anxiety disorder (Anderson et al., 1984; Barlow et al., 1985; Hibbert, 1984). When the specific patterns of symptoms are compared, it has been found that panic disorder subjects report more symptoms related to the respiratory and cardiovascular systems during their panic attacks than GAD patients during their high levels of anxiety (Anderson et al., 1984; Hoehn-Saric, 1982; Rapee, 1985). Most studies have found no differences in the somatic symptoms, nor the frequency of panic attacks, between extensive and minimal avoiders (Barlow et al., 1985; Craske, Sanderson, & Barlow, 1987; Rapee & Murrell, 1988). Interestingly, some studies demonstrated a relationship between cognitive and somatic symptoms in panic disorder such that certain types of somatic symptoms were more likely to be found together with specific cognitive symptoms (e.g., palpitations, chest pain, and thoughts of a heart attack) (Lelliot & Bass, 1990).

**Behavioral Features.** Typically, panic disorder is associated with avoidance of a large number of external situations, although there is large individual variation in the extent of avoidance. Some commonly avoided situations include shopping malls, driving, theaters, being alone, and going far from home. Although it has often been assumed that individuals diagnosed with panic disorder without agoraphobia do not avoid; clinical observation in fact suggests that these individuals avoid a large number of subtle situations that produce somatic sensations (e.g., saunas, aerobic exercise, or inflating balloons) (Rapee, Craske, & Barlow, 1994).

### Etiology and Maintenance

**Genetic and Familial Factors.** A series of early studies conducted by a group of researchers in Iowa indicated that panic disorder subjects were more likely to have first-degree relatives with panic disorder (or agoraphobia) than nonanxious controls or subjects with other anxiety disorders (Noyes, Crowe, Harris, Hamra, McChesney, & Chaudhry, 1986). Such data have often been cited as evidence for a genetic basis to panic disorder (Pauls, Bucher, Crowe, & Noyes, 1980), but methodology of this type cannot distinguish genetic from environmental factors. At least one study demonstrated greater concordance for panic disorder among monozygotic twins than dizygotic twins (Kendler et al., 1995). Thus, there is some evidence of a role for genetic factors in panic disorder. However, as discussed earlier, it is most likely that any genetic factors are general to all of the anxiety disorders.

**Environmental Factors.** A number of uncontrolled trials have suggested that agoraphobic avoidance (and thus probably the first panic attack) is preceded by a major life event in a majority of subjects (Klein, 1964; Roth, 1959; Thorpe & Burns, 1983). Controlled retrospective trials, however, have not been completely consistent. One study found that panic disorder subjects reported a greater number of stressors during the year before onset of their symptoms compared with normal controls (Faravelli, 1985). Similarly, more symptoms were reported by one group of agoraphobics in the year before onset of the disorder compared with another group of agoraphobics in a year not immediately before onset (Pollard, Pollard, & Corn, 1989). However, other studies have not found a greater number of stressors reported by panic disorder subjects compared with individuals with other anxiety disorders (de Loof, Zandbergen, Lousberg, & Griez, 1989; Hibbert, 1984; Rapee, Litwin, & Barlow, 1990). Simply experiencing a stressor may not be the important factor: Two studies found that panic disorder subjects report a greater impact of stressors than normal controls (Rapee et al., 1990; Roy-Byrne, Geraci, & Uhde, 1986) but not more than individuals with other anxiety disorders (Rapee et al., 1990). Of course, these results may have been influenced by retrospective distortion, and final decisions will have to await prospective studies.

**Psychological Factors.** Despite certain specific differences, most psychological models of panic disorder see the central problem as the individuals' fear of their own physical sensations (e.g., Barlow, 1988; Clark & Ehlers, 1993; Rapee, 1993b). In this way, panic disorder is seen as almost a phobic disorder, and the feared (phobic) stimuli are internal (somatic symptoms) rather than external. Basically, these models suggest that somatic symptoms are experienced for a number of possible reasons such as normal activities (e.g., exercise), hyperventilation, or normal bodily fluctuations. Individuals with panic disorder are especially likely to notice any such symptoms because they are hypervigilant for bodily sensations (Schmidt, Lerew, & Trakowski, 1997b). In other words, such individuals constantly scan their bodies (not necessarily consciously) for any possible internal danger, in much the same way that persons with GAD scan the environment for potential external danger. Thus, whenever a physical symptom occurs, those with panic disorder will notice it far more quickly and efficiently than other people, in turn triggering panic.

A large amount of research supports these psychological models of panic attacks. We can briefly mention only some of this research; the reader is encouraged to consult more detailed reviews (e.g., Barlow, 1988; Clark & Ehlers, 1993; McNally, 1990).

As mentioned earlier, questionnaire studies have shown that individuals with panic disorder are more likely than those with GAD to have thoughts related to dramatic outcomes such as death or insanity (Hibbert, 1984; Rapee, 1985). Related studies demonstrated that individuals with panic disorder find that these catastrophic outcomes have high emotional salience and preferentially allocate attentional resources to them (Asmundson, Sandler, Wilson, & Walker, 1992; Hope, Rapee, Heimberg, & Dombeck, 1990).

It has also been shown that individuals with panic disorder experience greater anxiety when they undergo procedures that produce bodily sensations such as breathing carbon dioxide and hyperventilating than subjects with other anxiety disorders (Holt & Andrews, 1989; Liebowitz et al., 1985; Rapee, Brown, Antony, & Barlow, 1992). Further, for people with panic disorder, simply believing that their heart rates have increased is sufficient to produce considerable anxiety regardless of any actual change in their heart rates (Ehlers, Margraf, Roth, Taylor, & Birbaumer, 1988). Importantly, several studies demonstrated the role of psychological factors in these procedures by showing that the degree of anxiety in response to physical sensations can be altered by manipulating various psychological parameters (Rapee, 1995a).

Putting these two areas of research together, it has been found that when individuals with panic disorder are given part of an ambiguous sentence relating to physical sensations, they are more likely than normal controls to complete the sentence with catastrophic outcomes (Clark & Ehlers, 1993). Similarly, using a questionnaire measure, people with panic disorder report misinterpreting their physical sensations as indicators of extreme catastrophe (Clark et al., 1997). However, some recent research has questioned whether, at an automatic level, people with panic disorder associate somatic sensations with threat to a greater extent than nonclinical controls (Schniering & Rapee, 1997). Finally, some recent research has begun to indicate that a tendency to interpret somatic sensations as a sign of threat may actually precede the first panic attack (Ehlers, 1995; Maller & Reiss, 1992; Schmidt, Lerew, & Jackson, 1997a). Such a finding suggests that this cognitive style may cause the development of panic disorder.

There has been considerably less research examining reasons for agoraphobic avoidance. First, many studies failed to demonstrate differences between people with panic disorder who do not avoid external situations and those with extensive avoidance (agoraphobia) on several parameters to do with the actual panic attack, such as the frequency of attacks or the location of the first attack. Differences have been found in the mental association between attacks and external situations. Subjects who show more extensive avoidance report a greater expectancy of experiencing a panic attack in particular situations (Craske, Rapee, & Barlow, 1988; de Jong & Bouman, 1995; Rapee & Murrell, 1988; Whittal & Goetsch, 1997). In addition, marked avoiders also score higher on measures of social anxiety and lower on assertiveness and extraversion than minimal avoiders (Chambless, 1985; de Jong, & Bouman, 1995; Rapee & Murrell, 1988; Whittal & Goetsch, 1997).

**Biological Factors.** There is a long history of research into biological aspects of panic disorder. Most of the evidence in humans has come from biological challenge procedures and pharmacological treatment and manipulation studies. More recently, evidence has accumulated from neuroimaging studies of people with panic attacks (Bourin, Baker, & Bradwejn, 1998; Klein, 1993; Krystal, Niehoff, Deutsch, & Charney, 1996; Nutt & Lawson, 1992).

A large number of chemical substances, it has

been found, produce panic attacks in individuals with panic disorder (Bourin et al., 1998; Rapee, 1995a). These substances include sodium lactate (Liebowitz et al., 1985), carbon dioxide (Gorman, Papp, & Coplan, 1994), yohimbine (Gurguis & Uhde, 1990), flumazenil (Nutt, Glue, Lawson, & Wilson, 1990), and caffeine (Charney, Heninger, & Jatlow, 1985). Yohimbine is a relatively specific alpha-2-adrenergic receptor antagonist that, by blocking the alpha-adrenergic autoreceptors in the locus coeruleus, results in increased levels of norepinephrine in the central nervous system (CNS). The fact that this substance can produce panic attacks provides evidence for the role of increased firing of the locus coeruleus in panic (Goddard & Charney, 1997; Krystal et al., 1996). However, it must be remembered that the response to biological challenge procedures is also markedly influenced by psychological factors (Rapee, 1995a). Other research provided evidence for the importance of serotonin in panic attacks (Evans, 1990; Krystal et al., 1996). Pharmacologically, it has been found that drugs that block panic attacks affect both the noradrenergic and serotonergic systems (Krystal et al., 1996). Obviously, locating the biological basis of any disorder in one or two broad neurochemical systems is too simplistic. Recently, some researchers have begun to develop more extensive and detailed models of panic disorder. One example described a model in terms of both neurochemistry and brain structures, centering on the amygdala and all of its afferent and efferent pathways, including the noradrenergic system (Goddard & Charney, 1997).

Many of the biological challenge substances have also been linked to panic attacks through their putative action on the central medullary carbon dioxide ($CO_2$) chemoreceptor (Gorman, Liebowitz, Fyer, & Stein, 1989; Klein, 1993). Specifically, it has been suggested that the $CO_2$ receptors of individuals with panic disorder have greater sensitivity. Anatomically, it has been found that the $CO_2$ chemoreceptors in the medulla and the norepinephrine receptors of the locus coeruleus are closely linked (Gorman et al., 1989). A recent model of the neurobiology of panic disorder has argued that the main pathology in people with panic disorder is hypersensitivity of their central $CO_2$ chemoreceptors (Klein, 1993). These receptors act as a suffocation alarm mechanism, and this alarm fires in people with panic disorder earlier than it should. Therefore, people with panic dis-

order will frequently experience breathlessness as their respiratory mechanisms try to keep their $CO_2$ levels lower and even a relatively minor increase in $CO_2$ can trigger a suffocation alarm (panic attack).

## Treatment

**Psychological Treatments.** During the past 10 years, there has been extensive evaluation of the psychological treatment of panic disorder, with and without extensive agoraphobic avoidance. This evaluation has overwhelmingly demonstrated that cognitive behavioral packages are extremely successful in managing panic disorder (Barlow, 1997; Margraf, Barlow, Clark, & Telch, 1993). In general, following treatment, around 80% of participants are free of panic attacks and 60–70% of those who exhibit severe avoidance behavior are markedly improved in their degree of avoidance. In addition, relatively good results can also be obtained from very brief interventions (four sessions) (Craske, Maidenberg, & Bystritsky, 1995) and even from treatments offered in a self-help format (Hecker, Losee, Fritzler, & Fink, 1996). More importantly, treatment results continue for up to two years (Barlow, 1997). However, there are still considerable improvements to be made. Despite the fact that cognitive behavioral treatments produce excellent results with respect to panic attacks and very good results with respect to agoraphobic avoidance, the overall individual picture is far from perfect. Recent longitudinal follow-up of individuals who completed a cognitive behavioral program for panic disorder has shown that more than 50% do not meet criteria for high end state functioning and/or continue to seek treatment during the following two years (Brown & Barlow, 1995).

Several studies also demonstrated that cognitive behavioral treatment packages result in greater and longer lasting improvements than medication (Barlow, 1997). One large study demonstrated that 90% of patients treated with cognitive therapy were free of panic attacks at the end of treatment (85% at 1 year follow-up) compared with 55% treated with imipramine (60% at follow-up) (Clark et al., 1994). In a recent multicenter comparison, 56% of people treated with cognitive behavior therapy alone were considered "treatment responders" compared with 49% of those treated with imipramine alone and 67% of those treated with a combination of CBT and imipramine. At 12-month follow-up, these figures were 92%, 75%, and 63%, respectively, among those who completed treatment (Barlow, Gorman, Shear, & Woods, 1998). The surprising tendency for those treated with a combination of cognitive behavior therapy and medication to show slightly worse outcome at follow-up has been demonstrated elsewhere (Otto, Pollack, & Sabatino, 1996) and requires further investigation.

**Pharmacological Treatment.** In one of the earliest studies in this area, Klein and Fink (1962) found that imipramine, a tricyclic antidepressant, blocked "spontaneous" panic attacks but did not affect more chronic or anticipatory anxiety. Since that time, a number of studies have been conducted indicating the value of tricyclics and monoamine oxidase inhibitors (MAOIs) in reducing panic attacks (van Balkom et al., 1997). These results, together with the early work by Klein, led to the suggestion that panic attacks were specifically affected by the tricyclics and MAOIs, whereas the benzodiazepines were more effective for anticipatory anxiety (Liebowitz & Klein, 1981). More recently, however, this simple formula has been challenged by the finding that many benzodiazepines are effective in reducing panic attacks when given in large enough doses (Ballenger et al., 1988; Noyes et al., 1984). Recent interest has begun to focus more closely on the selective serotonin re-uptake inhibitors as the treatment of choice for panic disorder. Controlled treatment outcome studies are currently still few, but preliminary data suggest that the effects are at least as good as the tricyclics and with fewer side effects (Sheehan & Harnett-Sheehan, 1996).

# Social Phobia

## Diagnosis

Social phobia was first identified in the DSM system with the publication of DSM-III, although it had been described clinically by a number of authors well before this time (e.g., Marks, 1969; Shaw, 1979). Social phobia is described as a fear and/or avoidance of situations involving the possibility of scrutiny by others (APA, 1994; Marks, 1969). It is diagnosed reliably and demonstrates good diagnostic agreement between clinicians based on DSM-III-R criteria (DiNardo et al., 1989, kappa = .79; Mannuzza et al., 1989, kappa = .68).

In addition to research into social phobia as a clinical disorder, there has been extensive investigation for many years into the nature of social anxiety in nonclinical populations (Buss, 1980; Zimbardo, 1986). This extensive literature is likely to have major relevance for the clinical disorder of social phobia because some researchers have noted that the two lie along a continuum of severity (Rapee, 1995b; Turner, Beidel, & Larkin, 1986). Thus, much can be learned about the clinical disorder, social phobia, by examining research into social anxiety in nonclinical populations.

## Clinical Features

**Epidemiology.** Social anxiety and reports of shyness in general populations are particularly common; they occur in around 40% of college students (Pilkonis & Zimbardo, 1979). In addition, social anxiety is a common accompaniment of all of the anxiety disorders (Rapee et al., 1988). Based on DSM-III-R criteria, social phobia has a lifetime prevalence of 13.3% in the general adult population (Kessler et al., 1994) and a point prevalence of around 2–4% in adolescents (Fergusson et al., 1993; Verhulst, van der Ende, Ferdinand, & Kasius, 1997).

**Sex Distribution.** Both epidemiological and questionnaire studies of the general population reported higher levels of social anxiety and social phobia in females than males (Lovibond & Rapee, 1993; Schneier et al., 1992; Verhulst et al., 1997). Yet, clinical studies regularly report a relatively equal gender distribution or even a preponderance of males (Heimberg et al., 1990; Turner, Beidel, Cooley, Woody, & Messer; 1994). It is likely that Western cultural factors result in greater interference from social avoidance for males than for females, and result in a greater proportion of socially anxious males who seek treatment (Rapee, 1995b).

**Onset.** Studies reported signs of onset for social phobia that range from early (Rapee et al., 1988; Thyer et al., 1985; Turner, Beidel, Dancu, & Keys, 1986) to late adolescence (Amies et al., 1983), and the most common consensus is that social phobia begins, on average, in late childhood or early adolescence (Turner & Beidel, 1989). Nevertheless, extreme shyness and social reticence can be seen by the time a child is 2 or 3 years of age (Kagan, Snidman, Arcus, & Reznick, 1994), and many people report shyness for as long as they can recall. As with GAD, the onset is generally gradual, and clinically, many social phobics report that they cannot specifically remember the beginning of their symptoms. However, there are certainly some social phobics who report specific traumatic experiences before the onset of their disorder (Ost, 1987). It may be that these latter individuals are more likely to develop a fear of a few circumscribed situations rather than a broad range of situations (designated as "generalized social phobia" in the DSM-IV).

**Somatic Symptoms.** People with social phobia report experiencing a number of somatic symptoms, including palpitations, sweating, tension, nausea, and blurred vision (Amies et al., 1983; Barlow et al., 1986; Heimberg, Dodge, & Becker, 1987; Liebowitz et al., 1985). Nevertheless, people with social phobia report greater concern over those symptoms that are visible to others such as trembling, shaking, blushing, twitching, and sweating (Alden & Wallace, 1995; McEwan & Devins, 1983). Physiological measures generally support these reports by demonstrating that social phobics have greater increases in physiological activity than normal controls when confronting social situations (Borkovec et al., 1974; Turner, Beidel, & Larkin, 1986). Interestingly, however, some research has shown that people with social phobia overestimate the degree of visibility of their symptoms (McEwan & Devins, 1983; Mulkens, de Jong, & Bögels, 1997).

**Cognitive Symptoms.** In terms of broad assessment, social phobics report more negative thoughts and less positive thoughts than nonanxious controls before and during a social interaction (Cacioppo, Glass, & Merluzzi, 1979; Heimberg, Acerra, & Holstein, 1985; Turner, Beidel, & Larkin, 1986). More specifically, Hartman (1984) found that the thoughts of social phobics fell into four factor analytically derived categories: general physiological discomfort and social inadequacy, concern with others' awareness of distress, fear of negative evaluation, and perceptions of autonomic arousal.

A number of studies showed that the thoughts and beliefs entertained by social phobics about their own appearance or performance are generally not accurate. More specifically, people with social phobia, it has been found, rate their own performance significantly worse than that performance is rated by independent judges, despite the fact that they can rate other people's performance

accurately (Rapee & Lim, 1992; Stopa & Clark, 1993). Similarly, people with social phobia see themselves as less attractive than others (Montgomery, Haemmerlie, & Edwards, 1991), even though their attractiveness is not rated any differently by independent observers (Jones, Briggs, & Smith, 1986).

**Behavioral Features.** By definition, social phobics fear or avoid situations in which scrutiny by others is possible. The more common situations include parties, meeting members of the opposite sex, public speaking, lecture halls, using the telephone, and public transport (Amies et al., 1983; Rapee et al., 1988; Turner, Beidel, Dancu, & Keys, 1986). In addition, there is a subgroup of social phobics who fear specific activities such as eating, drinking, or writing in public (Mattick & Peters, 1989; Turner, Beidel, Dancu, & Keys, 1986). More than 90% of social phobics fear more than one social situation (Mattick, Peters, & Clarke, 1989; Turner, Beidel, Dancu, & Keys, 1986) demonstrating that it is seldom a monosymptomatic phobia.

It is often assumed that social phobia is a relatively nondistressing problem, probably due to the continuum with social anxiety. However, this is not necessarily the case, and the consequences of social phobia can be extreme and varied (Rapee, 1995b). On average, social phobics rate at an intermediate level of severity when compared to other anxiety disorders (Marks, 1969; Turner, McCann, Beidel, & Mezzich, 1986). This average, however, is made up of individuals that range from those who only fear speaking in front of large crowds to those who are virtually housebound and are almost as distressed as the most severe agoraphobic. Some research has shown that on various measures, people with social phobia are actually more debilitated than people with panic disorder (Norton et al., 1996). Clinically, it is often found that social phobics are engaged in occupations that are considerably below the level of their qualifications and many people with social phobia have little social support, long-term partners, and financial independence (Schneier et al., 1992). Further, social phobia, probably more than any other anxiety disorder, is often associated with excessive alcohol consumption (Amies et al., 1983; Heimberg et al., 1987; Turner, Beidel, Dancu, & Keys, 1986).

A more controversial issue is whether people with social phobia lack social skills. Empirical findings relating to the social performance of social phobics has been mixed (Rapee, 1995b). Some studies have shown clear differences between social phobics and nonclinical subjects on overall performance (Twentyman & McFall, 1975; Stopa & Clark, 1993), but others have failed to show a difference (Burgio, Glass, & Merluzzi, 1981; Rapee & Lim, 1992). It may be that the nature of the situation is important in determining whether a difference in performance will be detected; some studies have shown differences between groups on some tasks but not others (Beidel, Turner, & Dancu, 1985; Pilkonis, 1977). It is most likely that people with social phobia do not actually have a deficit of skills but rather their social performance may be affected by both their degree of anxiety and the parameters of the situation (Rapee & Heimberg, 1997).

## Etiology and Maintenance

**Genetic and Familial Factors.** As for the other anxiety disorders, family studies showed a higher concordance for social phobia among the first-degree relatives of people with the disorder (Reich & Yates, 1988). In contrast, twin studies typically demonstrated that most of the genetic variance is consistent with the importance of a general neurotic syndrome. However, there has also been some suggestion of the possibility of a specific genetic loading for social phobia (Kendler et al., 1992b). These findings have been supported by a wealth of studies demonstrating a genetic influence in nonclinically shy populations (Hudson & Rapee, 2000). In general, these studies supported the importance of both genetic factors and nonshared environmental variables in the development of shyness. Finally, one adoption study supported the importance of both genetic and family variables in shyness and sociability (Daniels & Plomin, 1985).

**Family Factors.** Parental factors have been suggested as potentially important in producing social anxiety (Allaman, Joyce, & Crandell, 1972; Bruch, 1989). In an early study, Parker (1979) found that social phobics perceived their parents as overprotective and low in emotional support compared to a nonanxious control group. Several studies have now replicated these results (Arrindell, Emmelkamp, Monsma, & Brilman, 1983; Bruch & Heimberg, 1994). Further, in some research, social phobics report that their parents isolated them

from social experiences, overemphasized the opinions of others, and deemphasized socializing with others as a family (Bruch & Heimberg, 1994; Bruch, Heimberg, Burger, & Collins, 1989). Of course, the main problem with all of these studies is that they utilize retrospective self-report, and as such, it is impossible to know how much of the results are due to reporting (or recall) biases caused by the disorder (Hudson & Rapee, 2000). A few studies demonstrated similar findings in children with social fears, but data are still sparse (Hudson & Rapee, 2000). More importantly, some observational research is now beginning to show that mothers of children with any anxiety disorders (including social phobia) show overintrusive behaviors in a laboratory situation compared with mothers of nonclinical children (Hudson & Rapee, 1998). Of course, determining the causality of any of these effects is extremely difficult.

**Psychological Factors.** Several models of social phobia have argued that the central problem in social phobia is the belief by individuals that they cannot measure up to the audiences' expectations of them (Clark & Wells, 1995; Rapee & Heimberg, 1997; Schlenker & Leary, 1982). As a result, individuals believe that audiences will evaluate them negatively, despite the fact that people with social phobia do not hold unrealistic expectations for their own performance—nor do they believe that the audiences hold an excessively high standard for them (Alden, Bieling, & Wallace, 1994; Wallace & Alden, 1995).

An important factor in these models is the role of self-focused attention. People with social phobia pay excessive attention to their own outward appearance (often referred to as public self-consciousness) (Hope, Gansler, & Heimberg, 1989; Woody, 1996) and hold negative images of their appearance when in social situations (Hackman, Surawy, & Clark, 1998). According to Rapee and Heimberg (1997), a negative mental image is likely to be very important in producing anxiety in social phobics, but is not necessarily veridical. In fact, based on the research described earlier, people with social phobia frequently see themselves as less capable than they are viewed by others.

In addition to an attentional focus onto their own appearance, people with social phobia are likely to preferentially allocate attentional resources to external indicators of negative evaluation (Asmundson & Stein, 1994; Mattia, Heimberg,

& Hope, 1993; McNeil et al., 1995). In one *in vivo* study, socially anxious individuals were more accurate at detecting indicators of negative evaluation from their audiences (e.g., frowns) while giving a speech than low anxious subjects (Veljaca & Rapee, 1998). As a result, people with social phobia will attend less to the task at hand, possibly resulting in poorer performance (Heimberg, Acerra, & Holstein, 1985).

People with social phobia are likely to hold strong expectations of negative evaluation by others and to interpret ambiguous social information negatively (Amir, Foa, & Coles, 1998). In addition, the consequences of negative evaluation by others are seen to be especially dire by people with social phobia (Foa, Franklin, Perry, & Herbert, 1996; Lucock & Salkovskis, 1988; Poulton & Andrews, 1994). In addition, change in the fear of negative evaluation or in the perceived consequences of negative evaluation is a very strong predictor of treatment response (Foa et al., 1996; Mattick & Peters, 1988).

**Biological Factors.** Research into central biochemical factors associated with social phobia has not been as extensive as that for panic disorder, and many studies provided mixed findings (Nicholas & Tancer, 1995; Potts, Book, & Davidson, 1996). The most consistent results implicated serotonin in the pathogenesis of social phobia (Jefferson, 1996; Potts et al., 1996). The most obvious evidence came from treatment with serotonin-reducing agents (see later). However, because many of these drugs also affect other neurotransmitter systems, based on this evidence, the neurobiology of social phobia cannot be narrowed down to a single neurotransmitter system (Nickell & Uhde, 1995). Other evidence has included challenges with fenfluramine, a serotonin agonist, and brain imaging studies.

Based on the large number of symptoms reported by social phobics that are mediated by the sympathetic nervous system and the beneficial effects of beta-blockade on performance anxiety, there is some suggestion that social phobics may have elevated peripheral sympathetic activity (Levin, Schneier, & Liebowitz, 1989; Stein, Tancer, & Uhde, 1992). However, socially anxious individuals and controls do not differ in catecholamine response to social stimuli (Dimsdale, Hartley, Ruskin, Greenblatt, & LaBrie, 1984; Levin et al., 1989), and infusions of epinephrine do not pro-

voke excessive reports of anxiety in people with social phobia (Papp et al., 1988).

### Treatment

**Psychological Techniques.** A number of studies demonstrated the value of cognitive behavioral treatment packages for reducing social phobia, compared with wait list and with a credible placebo treatment (Beidel & Turner, 1998; Feske & Chambless, 1995; Heimberg & Juster, 1995; Taylor, 1996). In addition, follow-up assessment indicated that in most studies continued improvement is seen following the end of treatment (Taylor, 1996).

In terms of specific techniques, *in vivo* exposure is generally considered an essential component of successful treatment (Butler, 1989; Beidel & Turner, 1998). Role-playing within a group treatment has also been found useful (Heimberg et al., 1990), perhaps simply as a more structured form of exposure. As mentioned earlier, there is some question whether social phobics actually lack social skills or whether their anxiety simply interferes with performance. Thus, the specific inclusion of social skills training is questioned (Heimberg, 1989), and more research will be required to ascertain when it is necessary and how it works. Nevertheless, some treatment packages have focused on this technique as a major component of treatment (Turner et al., 1994). Cognitive restructuring (aimed especially at the fear of negative evaluation) is considered essential by some researchers (e.g., Butler, 1989; Mattick et al., 1989), though some studies have questioned its unique contribution (Feske & Chambless, 1995).

Finally, a large, recent multicenter trial compared group cognitive behavioral therapy with phenelzine in treating social phobia (Heimberg et al., 1998). Phenelzine resulted in a more rapid effect. However, at the end of treatment, both active treatments resulted in similar effects that were considerably greater than that of placebo. However, at follow-up, the cognitive behavior therapy condition maintained greater gains than phenelzine (Liebowitz et al., 1999).

**Pharmacological Treatments.** Although a considerable literature suggests that beta-blockers are effective in reducing performance anxiety (Gorman & Gorman, 1987) that is related to social anxiety, these results have generally been observed in subjects without extreme levels of performance anxiety. Furthermore, any significant results are confined to performance involving motor activity, which suggests that beta-blockers may work mainly for nonclinical subjects by improving performance rather than reducing anxiety (Barlow, 1988). More recent studies that examined the effectiveness of beta-blockers for social phobia have shown minimal effects compared with placebo (Turner, Beidel, & Jacob, 1994). The major medications that have been tested for treating social phobia are the MAOIs. In general, studies demonstrated good results with these medications (Potts & Davidson, 1995). Unfortunately, their potentially dangerous side effects mean that they must be used together with severe dietary restrictions. More recently, reversible MAOIs were developed that do not require dietary restrictions and are considerably safer. Early data with these medications show some positive effects, but not all results have been positive (Potts & Davidson, 1995). Several studies also demonstrated positive effects from the serotonin specific reuptake inhibitors (SSRIs) (Potts & Davidson, 1995). At this stage, studies are still relatively few and have included small numbers; further research is required.

# Specific Phobias

The DSM diagnosis of specific phobia refers to a heterogeneous collection of fears and/or avoidance of a broad range of specific objects or situations. Recent attempts to make sense of the heterogeneity centered on trying to identify subgroups of specific phobias that share characteristics. Thus, some researchers distinguished blood and injury fears from other phobias because of the unique physiological response accompanying the former (Ost, Sterner, & Lindahl, 1984; Page, 1994; Thyer, Himle, & Curtis, 1985). Similarly, factor-analytic studies of agoraphobics' fears often identify a claustrophobia factor (Hamann & Mavissakalian, 1988), suggesting that claustrophobia may have much in common with agoraphobic fears. In a recent factor analysis, three subtypes of fears were identified: situational phobias, animal phobias, and mutilation phobias (Fredrikson, Annas, Fischer, & Wik, 1996). Based on these considerations, the DSM-IV has distinguished four subtypes of specific phobia: animal fears, natural environment fears, blood-injection-injury fears, and situational

fears (e.g., flying, small spaces). However, despite the implication of independence among fears, at least one study showed that people with one specific phobia are likely to be comorbid for other specific phobias (Hofmann, Lehman, & Barlow, 1997), calling into question the "specificity" of specific phobias (Harvey & Rapee, in press).

Not surprisingly, given their heterogeneity, specific phobias show varied diagnostic reliability estimates among studies. Mannuzza et al. (1989) found a kappa of .29, whereas DiNardo et al. (1993) found a kappa of .82. It should be noted that studies to date have used DSM-III-R criteria in which subtypes of specific phobias were not distinguished. It remains to be seen whether the specification of subtypes in DSM-IV improves the diagnostic reliability.

## Clinical Features

**Epidemiology.** Mild fears of specific objects or situations are extremely common in the general population (Agras et al., 1969; King et al., 1989). Fears that are considered clinically severe are still relatively common compared to the other anxiety disorders. The National Comorbidity survey found a lifetime prevalence for specific phobias of approximately 11% in adults (Kessler et al., 1994) and the 6-month prevalence in adolescents was around 5% according to self-report (Fergusson et al., 1993; Verhulst et al., 1997).

Despite the common occurrence of specific phobias in the community, this problem rarely provides the impetus for presentation to treatment centers (Merkelbach, de Jong, Muris, & van den Hout, 1996). This is possibly partly because specific phobic stimuli can often be avoided by most people with little interference in their lives and most people with specific phobia have few difficulties outside of the immediate phobic situation (Harvey & Rapee, in press).

**Sex Distribution and Age of Onset.** Both mild fears in the general population and specific clinical phobias are considerably more common in females than in males (Fredrikson et al., 1996; Kessler et al., 1994). Estimates of the proportion of females in clinical populations generally range around 75 to 95% (Barlow et al., 1985; McNally & Steketee, 1985; Ost, 1987; Thyer, Parrish, et al., 1985). Differences in the proportion of females among the various specific phobia subtypes have been reported (Fredrikson et al., 1996; Ost, 1987).

Age of onset is generally quite early in specific phobia and averages around the early to middle teens (Ost, 1987; Thyer, Parrish, et al., 1985). However, an average age of onset for specific phobia ignores the heterogeneity of the disorder. In fact, consistent differences are found among the ages of onset for different types of specific phobias. Claustrophobia usually begins around the early to middle 20s, an age closer to panic disorder (Ost, 1987), whereas blood/injury and animal phobias typically begin in childhood (Ost, 1987; Thyer, Himle, & Curtis, 1985).

**Cognitive Symptoms.** Studies of cognitive symptoms in specific phobics have not been very common, possibly because it has been assumed that any thoughts would naturally be related to the phobic object and because thoughts have not usually been considered etiologically important. Nevertheless, a few studies have asked specific phobics about their thoughts when confronting phobic stimuli and found that, although the majority are primarily concerned with harm in the immediate situation, a number engage in other types of thoughts such as concerns over their own sensations (Last & Blanchard, 1982; McNally & Steketee, 1985; Thorpe & Salkovskis, 1995). Other research showed that phobic fear and avoidance is mediated either by beliefs over the ability to complete a particular action (self efficacy) (Williams & Watson, 1985) or by beliefs relating to the likelihood and consequences of danger in the situation (Menzies & Clarke, 1995a).

**Somatic Symptoms.** When specific phobics are not confronting their feared object, they experience the least severe and debilitating anxiety disorder (Barlow et al., 1985; Turner, McCann, et al., 1986), generally demonstrating relatively normal levels of trait anxiety. Such subjective reports are supported by physiological assessment, which also demonstrates that specific phobics in chronic arousal are not different from normal controls (Lader & Mathews, 1968).

When confronting their feared situations, specific phobics report a number of common anxiety-related somatic symptoms, including palpitations, trembling, and sweating (Rachman, Levitt, & Lopatka, 1988). Physiologically, many studies demonstrated increases in indexes of arousal in specific phobics upon exposure to their feared cues (Cook, Melamed, Cuthbert, McNeil, & Lang, 1988; Ost, 1987), although results are not always consistent, and desynchrony between response

systems has commonly been noted (Sartory, Rachman, & Grey, 1977). In one careful and detailed study, ten animal phobic females were scored on a series of measures (e.g., state anxiety, blood pressure, epinephrine, and cortisol) during *in vivo* exposure sessions (Nesse, Curtis, Thyer, McCann, Huber-Smith, & Knopf, 1985). Most measures showed marked increases during exposure compared to control periods, although the measure of subjective units of discomfort evidenced the most consistent increase.

As mentioned before, many blood and injury phobics are characterized by a unique physiological response to their feared cues (Ost et al., 1984; Page, 1994; Thyer, Himle, & Curtis, 1985). Page (1994) argued that there may be two subtypes of blood/injury phobia. One group shows the usual sympathetic reaction to blood/injury cues described before. The other group shows an initial increase in heart rate and blood pressure followed by a dramatic drop in these measures, often leading to fainting. Associated with this different physiological reaction, many blood/injury phobics report a feeling of disgust on exposure to their feared cues, distinct from the more usual reports of fear found with other phobias (Tolin, Lohr, Sawchuk, & Lee, 1997). In fact, several types of phobias are characterized more strongly by the emotion of disgust rather than fear, and it is possible that this is an alternate method of subtyping phobias (Matchett & Davey, 1991).

## Etiology and Maintenance

**Genetic and Familial Factors.** First-degree relatives of people with specific phobias are more likely themselves to have a specific phobia providing evidence for the importance of either genetic or environmental family factors in the disorder (Fyer et al., 1990). More specifically, a few twin studies demonstrated a genetic involvement in specific phobias but the importance of environmental factors was also shown by these studies (Kendler et al., 1992; Torgersen, 1979).

The nature of the genetic influence has not been demonstrated, and it is likely that some of the genetic involvement is mediated via the general neurotic aspects of other anxiety disorders. However, some authors have argued for the possibility that specific phobias represent the emergence of specific, innate fears (Menzies & Clarke, 1995b). The fact that certain normal fears emerge innately at specific periods of developmental history has been clearly demonstrated (e.g., Berenthal, Campos, & Barrett, 1984). Therefore, it has been suggested that some individuals simply have a greater degree of these innate fears constitutionally or that normal fears are not extinguished for certain reasons (Menzies & Clarke, 1995b). Evidence for this approach has come from interview studies of adults and children with specific phobias in which a majority of subjects reported having the phobia for as long as they could remember (Menzies & Clarke, 1993a,b), but these reports have been criticized by many as reflecting overly narrow views of associative learning (Mineka & Zinbarg, 1996; Barlow, in press).

**Environmental Factors.** Since the demonstration by Watson and Rayner (1920) that a fear of white, furry objects could be produced in a child, conditioning theories of phobias have abounded (e.g., Mowrer, 1939). More specifically, it has been suggested that phobic concerns could be acquired through three basic methods: verbal information, vicarious learning, and direct conditioning (Rachman, 1977). Support for this suggestion has come from studies that asked specific phobics to state retrospectively what they consider the cause of their disorder. Most of these studies find a large proportion of subjects reporting that their phobias began suddenly following a conditioning episode (including an unexpected burst of fear), whereas a smaller proportion report seeing a traumatic event or hearing about the dangers of the object or situation (Merkelbach et al., 1996). However, some authors pointed out that the method of collecting these data has often been flawed because subjects are forced into one response and are often not given the opportunity to state that they have always had the fear (Barlow, 1988; Menzies & Clarke, 1995b). Studies in which this alternative was given to subjects showed a considerably smaller number reporting acquisition via the three main pathways (Menzies and Clarke, 1993a,b), although these studies are subject to the strong criticisms alluded to before.

**Preparedness.** Many objects that are in the subject's immediate environment when traumatic events occur do not acquire fearful properties. Subsequently, phobias are usually found in response to a limited set of all of the possible cues in the world. Observations such as these led Seligman (1971) to propose that certain stimuli are biologically "prepared" to become associated with danger. According to Seligman, these prepared stimuli can acquire fearful properties after a single traumatic pairing and, once conditioned, are extremely difficult to extinguish. The types of stimuli that possess prepared properties are those that have ecological validity (such as heights or snakes), as opposed to more modern dangers (such as guns or electrical outlets). Although Seligman's theory makes considerable intuitive sense and there has been considerable laboratory support for his predictions (Cook & Mineka, 1989; Ohman, 1994, 1996), studies that examined the preparedness hypothesis have had mixed results (McNally, 1987). The only one of Seligman's predictions that has found consistent laboratory support has been the difficulty in extinguishing responses to prepared stimuli, and this phenomenon could find alternate explanations (McNally, 1987; Bond & Siddle, 1996).

Combining cognitive data with the concept of preparedness, some interesting data have shown that fearful subjects are more likely to believe that aversive experiences are associated with phobic stimuli than with nonphobic stimuli (de Jong, Merkelbach, Arntz, & Nijman, 1992; Tomarken, Sutton & Mineka, 1995). In the typical paradigm, subjects are shown slides of fear-relevant images (e.g., snakes) and fear-irrelevant images (e.g., flowers) and are given random outcomes that are either aversive (e.g., electric shock) or nonaversive (e.g., nothing). Even though there is no relationship between slides and outcomes, subjects are more likely to perceive an association between fear-relevant slides and aversive outcomes, and this effect is stronger for highly fearful subjects. This may suggest that the preparedness phenomenon is mediated by biases in the way stimulus information is processed. However, some research has shown that these biased perceptions can be demonstrated before any experience the subject has with slides or outcomes (de Jong, 1993; Honeybourne, Matchett, & Davey, 1993; McNally & Heatherton, 1993), suggesting that the effect is based on preexperimental expectancies and not biased processing (Davey, 1992). More recently, some research has demonstrated that both preexperimental expectancies and experience play a role in the covariation phenomenon, indicating a possible role for both expectancy and processing bias in the effect (Kennedy, Rapee, & Mazurski, 1997).

## Treatment

There is widespread agreement that the treatment of choice for phobic fear and avoidance is *in vivo* exposure (Barlow, 1988; Marks, 1981). Some evidence has even suggested that excellent gains can be achieved through a single session of intensive exposure (Arntz & Lavy, 1993; Ost 1996). Some attempts have been made to match the reported mode of acquisition or individual differences to specific types of treatment (Jerremalm et al., 1986; Ost et al., 1982), but these have provided mixed success. Further, the addition of cognitive restructuring, relaxation, or drug treatment has generally not provided increased gains over basic exposure (Barlow, 1988). The one exception may be blood and injury phobia for which the addition of applied tension improved gains, especially for some subjects (Ost, Fellenius, & Sterner, 1991; Page, 1994).

Few studies have tested psychopharmacology in treating specific phobias (Harvey & Rapee, in press). Some research has shown minimal, short-term effects from using benzodiazepines and beta-blockers (Bernadt, Silverstone, & Singleton, 1980; Campos, Solyom, & Koelink, 1984), but improvements did not generalize or last.

## Conclusions

We discovered much in the past decade about the nature of anxiety. We also devised new psychological and pharmacological treatments that are effective in varying degrees for anxiety disorders. Nevertheless, we are only beginning to understand the riddle of anxiety. As Freud (1917) noted, the solution to this riddle "must cast a flood of light upon our whole mental life" (p. 401).

Current interest is beginning to focus on improved understanding of the origins and development of anxiety and anxiety disorders. This will allow the development of early intervention and prevention programs so that the life course of people with anxiety disorders and the subtle but extensive interference that these disorders cause can be reduced from an early age. Most importantly, we should develop a deeper understanding of the meaning and purpose of anxiety and the very nature of emotion. It is only by thoroughly understanding the nature of normal and pathological emotion that we will be able to cope effectively with anxiety disorders, which are the most common psychological disorders known to humans.

## References

Agras, S., Sylvester, D., & Oliveau, D. (1969). The epidemiology of common fears and phobias. *Comprehensive Psychiatry, 10*, 151–156.

Alden, L. E., Bieling, P. J., & Wallace, S. T. (1994). Perfectionism in an interpersonal context: A self-regulation analysis of dysphoria and social anxiety. *Cognitive Therapy and Research, 18*, 297–316.

Alden, L. E., & Wallace, S. T. (1995). Social phobia and social appraisal in successful and unsuccessful social interactions. *Behaviour Research and Therapy, 33*, 497–506.

Allaman, J. D., Joyce, C. S., & Crandell, V. C. (1972). The antecedents of social desirability response tendencies of children and young adults. *Child Development, 43*, 1135–1160.

American Psychiatric Association. (1987). *Diagnostic and statistical manual of mental disorders* (3rd ed., rev.). Washington, DC: Author.

American Psychiatric Association. (1994). *Diagnostic and statistical manual of mental disorders* (4th ed.). Washington, DC: Author.

Amies, P. L., Gelder, M. G., & Shaw, P. M. (1983). Social phobia: A comparative clinical study. *British Journal of Psychiatry, 142*, 174–179.

Amir, N., Foa, E. B., & Coles, M. E. (1998). Negative interpretation bias in social phobia. *Behaviour Research and Therapy, 36*, 945–958.

Anderson, D. J., Noyes, R., Jr., & Crowe, R. R. (1984). A comparison of panic disorder and generalized anxiety disorder. *American Journal of Psychiatry, 141*, 572–575.

Andrews, G. (1996). Comorbidity in neurotic disorders: The similarities are more important than the differences. In R. M. Rapee (Ed.), *Current controversies in the anxiety disorders* (pp. 3–20). New York: Guilford.

Arntz, A., & Lavey, E. (1993). Does stimulus elaboration potentiate exposure in-vivo treatment? Two forms of one-session treatment of spider phobia. *Behavioural Psychotherapy, 21*, 1–12.

Arrindell, W. A., Emmelkamp, P. M. G., Monsma, A., & Brilman, E. (1983). The role of perceived parental rearing practices in the aetiology of phobic disorders: A controlled study. *British Journal of Psychiatry, 143*, 183–187.

Asmundson, G. J., Sandler, L. S., Wilson, K. G., & Walker, J. R. (1992). Selective attention toward physical threat in patients with panic disorder. *Journal of Anxiety Disorders, 6*, 295–303.

Asmundson, G. J. G., & Stein, M. B. (1994). Selective processing of social threat in patients with generalized social phobia: Evaluation using a dot-probe paradigm. *Journal of Anxiety Disorders, 8*, 107–117.

Ballenger, J. C., Burrows, G. D., DuPont, R. L., Jr., Lesser, I. M., Noyes, R., Jr., Pecknold, J. C., Rifkin, A., & Swinson, R. P. (1988). Alprazolam in panic disorder and agoraphobia: Results from a multicenter trial. I. Efficacy in short-term treatment. *Archives of General Psychiatry, 45*, 413–422.

Barlow, D. H. (1988). *Anxiety and its disorders: The nature and treatment of anxiety and panic.* New York: Guilford.

Barlow, D. H. (in press). *Anxiety and its disorders: The nature and treatment of anxiety and panic.* New York: Guilford.

Barlow, D. H. (1997). Cognitive-behavioral therapy for panic disorder: Current status. *Journal of Clinical Psychiatry, 58* (Suppl. 2), 32–36.

Barlow, D. H., & Durand, V. M. (1999). Abnormal psychology: An integrative approach (2nd ed.). Pacific Grove, CA: Brooks/Cole.

Barlow, D. H., & Rapee, R. M. (1991). *Mastering stress: A lifestyle approach.* Dallas, TX: American Health.

Barlow, D. H., & Wincze, J. (1998). DSM-IV and beyond: What is generalized anxiety disorder? *Acta Psychiatrica Scandinavica, 98*(393), 23–29.

Barlow, D. H., Blanchard, E. B., Vermilyea, J. A., Vermilyea, B. B., & DiNardo, P. A. (1986). Generalized anxiety and generalized anxiety disorder: Description and reconceptualization. *American Journal of Psychiatry, 143,* 40–44.

Barlow, D. H., Gorman, J. M., Shear, M. K., & Woods, S. W. (1998). Cognitive-behavioral treatment vs imipramine and their combination for panic disorder: Primary outcome results. Unpublished manuscript.

Barlow, D. H., Vermilyea, J., Blanchard, E. B., Vermilyea, B. B., DiNardo, P. A., & Cerny, J. A. (1985). The phenomenon of panic. *Journal of Abnormal Psychology, 94,* 320–328.

Beck, A. T., & Emery, G. (1985). *Anxiety disorders and phobias: A cognitive perspective.* New York: Basic Books.

Beidel, D. C., & Turner, S. M. (1998). *Shy children, phobic adults: Nature and treatment of social phobia.* Washington, DC: American Psychological Association.

Beidel, D. C., Turner, S. M., & Dancu, C. V. (1985). Physiological, cognitive and behavioral aspects of social anxiety. *Behaviour Research and Therapy, 23,* 109–117.

Berenthal, B. I., Campos, J. J., & Barrett, K. C. (1984). Self-produced locomotion: An organizer of emotional, cognitive, and social development in infancy. In E. R. Harmon (Ed.), *Continuities and discontinuities in development* (pp. 175–210). New York: Plenum Press.

Bernadt, M. W., Silverstone, T., & Singelton, W. (1980). Behavioural and subjective effects of beta-adrenergic blockade in phobic subjects. *British Journal of Psychiatry, 137,* 452–457.

Blowers, C., Cobb, J., & Mathews, A. (1987). Generalized anxiety: A controlled treatment study. *Behaviour Research and Therapy, 25,* 493–502.

Bond, N. W., & Siddle, D. A. T. (1996). The preparedness account of social phobia: Some data and alternative explanations. In R. M. Rapee (Ed.), *Current controversies in the anxiety disorders* (pp. 291–314). New York: Guilford.

Borkovec, T. D. (1994). The nature, functions, and origins of worry. In G. C. Daley & F. Tallis (Eds.), *Worrying: Perspectives on theory, assessment and treatment.* Wiley series in clinical psychology (pp. 5–33). Chichester, England: Wiley.

Borkovec, T. D., & Costello, E. (1993). Efficacy of applied relaxation and cognitive-behavioral therapy in the treatment of generalized anxiety disorder. *Journal of Consulting and Clinical Psychology, 61,* 611–619.

Borkovec, T. D., & Inz, J. (1990). The nature of worry in generalized anxiety disorder: A predominance of thought activity. *Behaviour Research and Therapy, 28,* 153–158.

Borkovec, T. D., Robinson, E., Pruzinsky, T., & DePree, J. A. (1983). Preliminary exploration of worry: Some characteristics and processes. *Behaviour Research and Therapy, 212,* 9–16.

Borkovec, T. D., Shadick, R. N., & Hopkins, M. (1991). The nature of normal and pathological worry. In R. M. Rapee & D. H. Barlow (Eds.), *Chronic anxiety: Generalised anxiety disorder and mixed anxiety-depression* (pp. 29–51). New York: Guilford.

Borkovec, T. D., Stone, N. M., O'Brien, G. T., & Kaloupek, D. G. (1974). Evaluation of a clinically relevant target behavior for analog outcome research. *Behavior Therapy, 5,* 503–513.

Bourin, M., Baker, G. B., & Bradwejn, J. (1998). Neurobiology of panic disorder. *Journal of Psychosomatic Research, 44,* 163–180.

Brawman-Mintzer, O., & Lydiard, R. B. (1996). Generalized anxiety disorder: Issues in epidemiology. *Journal of Clinical Psychiatry, 57*(Suppl. 7), 3–8.

Brown, T. A., & Barlow, D. H. (1995). Long-term outcome in cognitive-behavioral treatment of panic disorder: Clinical predictors and alternative strategies for assessment. *Journal of Consulting and Clinical Psychology, 63,* 754–765.

Brown, T. A., Barlow, D. H., & Liebowitz, M. R. (1994). The empirical basis of generalized anxiety disorder. *American Journal of Psychiatry, 151,* 1272–1280.

Brown, T. A., Marten, P. A., & Barlow, D. H. (1995). Discriminant validity of the symptoms comprising the DSM-III-R and DSM-IV associated symptom criterion of generalized anxiety disorder. *Journal of Anxiety Disorders, 9,* 317–238.

Brown, T. A., Chorpita, B. F., & Barlow, D. H. (1998). Structural relationships among dimensions of the *DSM-IV* anxiety and mood disorders and dimensions of negative affect, positive affect, and autonomic arousal. *Journal of Abnormal Psychology, 107,* 179–192.

Bruch, M. A. (1989). Familial and developmental antecedents of social phobia: Issues and findings. *Clinical Psychology Review, 9,* 37–48.

Bruch, M. A., & Heimberg, R. G. (1994). Differences in perceptions of parental and personal characteristics between generalized and nongeneralized social phobics. *Journal of Anxiety Disorders, 8,* 155–168.

Bruch, M. A., Heimberg, R. G., Berger, P., & Collins, T. M. (1989). Social phobia and perceptions of early parental and personal characteristics. *Anxiety Research, 2,* 57–65.

Burgio, K. L., Glass, C. R., & Merluzzi, T. V. (1981). The effects of social anxiety and videotape performance feedback on cognitions and self-evaluations. *Behavioral Counselling Quarterly, 1,* 288–301.

Buss, A. H. (1980). *Self-consciousness and social anxiety.* San Francisco: W.H. Freeman.

Butler, G. (1989). Issues in the application of cognitive and behavioral strategies to the treatment of social phobia. *Clinical Psychology Review, 9,* 91–106.

Butler, G., & Mathews, A. (1983). Cognitive processes in anxiety. *Advances in Behavior Research and Therapy, 5,* 51–62.

Cacioppo, J. T., Glass, C. R., & Merluzzi, T. V. (1979). Self-statements and self evaluations: A cognitive-response analysis of heterosocial anxiety. *Cognitive Therapy and Research, 3,* 249–262.

Campos, P. E., Solyom, L., & Koelink, A. (1984). The effects of timolol maleate on subjective and physiological components of air travel phobia. *Canadian Journal of Psychiatry, 29,* 570–574.

Chambless, D. L. (1985). The relationship of severity of agoraphobia to associated psychopathology. *Behaviour Research and Therapy, 23,* 305–310.

Chambless, D. L., & Gillis, M. M. (1993). Cognitive therapy of anxiety disorders. *Journal of Consulting and Clinical Psychology, 61,* 248–260.

Charney, D. S., Heninger, G. R., & Jatlow, P. I. (1985). Increased anxiogenic effects of caffeine in panic disorders. *Archives of General Psychiatry, 42,* 233–243.

Clark, D. M., & Ehlers, A. (1993). An overview of the cognitive theory and treatment of panic disorder. *Applied and Preventive Psychology, 2,* 131–139.

Clark, D. M., Salkovskis, P. M., Hackmann, A., Middleton, H., Anastasiades, P., & Gelder, M. (1994). A comparison of cognitive therapy, applied relaxation and imipramine in the treatment of panic disorder. *British Journal of Psychiatry, 164,* 759–769.

Clark, D. M., Salkovskis, P. M., Ost, L., Breitholtz, E., Koehler, K. A., Westling, B. E., Jeavons, A., & Gelder, M. (1997). Misinterpretation of body sensations in panic disorder. *Journal of Consulting and Clinical Psychology, 65,* 203–213.

Clark, D. M., & Wells, A. (1995). A cognitive model of social phobia. In R. G. Heimberg, M. R. Liebowitz, D. A. Hope, & F. R. Schneier (Eds.), *Social phobia: Diagnosis, assessment, and treatment* (pp. 69–93). New York: Guilford.

Cook, E. W., III, Melamed, B. G., Cuthbert, B. N., McNeil, D. W., & Lang, P. J. (1988). Emotional imagery and the differential diagnosis of anxiety. *Journal of Consulting and Clinical Psychology, 56,* 734–740.

Cook, M., & Mineka, S. (1989). Observational conditioning of fear to fear-relevant versus fear-irrelevant stimuli in Rhesus monkies. *Journal of Abnormal Psychology, 98,* 448–459.

Craske, M. G., & Barlow, D. H. (1988). A review of the relationship between panic and avoidance. *Clinical Psychology Review, 8,* 667–685.

Craske, M. G., Barlow, D. H., & O'Leary, T. (1992). *Mastery of your anxiety and worry: Client workbook.* San Antonio, TX: Graywind/The Psychological Corporation.

Craske, M. G., Maidenberg, E., & Bystritsky, A. (1995). Brief cognitive-behavioral versus non-directive therapy for panic disorder. *Journal of Behavior Therapy and Experimental Psychiatry, 26,* 113–120.

Craske, M. G., Rapee, R. M., & Barlow, D. H. (1988). The significance of panic-expectancy for individual patterns of avoidance. *Behavior Therapy, 19,* 577–592.

Craske, M. G., Rapee, R. M., Jackel, L., & Barlow, D. H. (1989). Qualitative dimensions of worry in DSM-III-R generalized anxiety disorder subjects and nonanxious controls. *Behaviour Research and Therapy, 27,* 397–402.

Craske, M. G., Sanderson, W. C., & Barlow, D. H. (1987). The relationships among panic, fear and avoidance. *Journal of Anxiety Disorders, 1,* 153–160.

Daniels, D., & Plomin, R. (1985). Origins of individual differences in infant shyness. *Developmental Psychology, 21,* 118–121.

Davey, G. C. L. (1992). An expectancy model of laboratory preparedness effects. *Journal of Experimental Psychology: General, 121,* 24–40.

de Jong, G. M., & Bouman, T. K. (1995). Panic disorder: A baseline period. Predictability of agoraphobic avoidance behavior. *Journal of Anxiety Disorders, 9,* 185–199.

de Jong, P. J. (1993). Covariation bias in phobia: Mere resistance to preexperimental expectancies? *Behavior Therapy, 24,* 447–545.

de Jong, P. J., Merkelbach, H., Arntz, A., & Nijman, H. (1992). Covariation detection in treated and untreated spider phobics. *Journal of Abnormal Psychology, 101,* 724–727.

de Loof, C., Zandbergen, J., Lousberg, H., Pols, H., & Griez, E. (1989). The role of life events in the onset of panic disorder. *Behaviour Research and Therapy, 27,* 461–463.

Dimsdale, J. E., Hartley, H., Ruskin, J., Greenblatt, D. J., & LaBrie, R. (1984). Effect of beta blockade on plasma catecholamines during psychological and exercise stress. *American Journal of Cardiology, 54,* 182–185.

DiNardo, P., Moras, K., Barlow, D. H. Rapee, R. M., & Brown, T. A. (1993). Reliability of DSM-III-R anxiety disorder categories using the Anxiety Disorders Interview Schedule-Revised (ADIS-R). *Archives of General Psychiatry, 50,* 251–256.

Durham, R. C., Murphy, T., Allan, T., Richard, K., Treliving, L. R., & Fenton, G. W. (1994). Cognitive therapy, analytic psychotherapy, and anxiety management training for generalised anxiety disorder. *British Journal of Psychiatry, 165,* 315–323.

Ehlers, A. (1993). Somatic symptoms and panic attacks: A retrospective study of learning experiences. *Behaviour Research and Therapy, 31,* 269–278.

Ehlers, A. (1995). A 1-year prospective study of panic attacks: Clinical course and factors associated with maintenance. *Journal of Abnormal Psychology, 104,* 164–172.

Ehlers, A., Margraf, J., Roth, W. T., Taylor, C. B., & Birbaumer, N. (1988). Anxiety induced by false heart rate feedback in patients with panic disorder. *Behaviour Research and Therapy, 26,* 1–12.

Evans, L. (1990). Serotonin and panic. In N. McNaughton & J. G. Andrews (Eds.), *Anxiety.* Dunedin, New Zealand: Otago University Press.

Eysenck, M. W. (1985). Anxiety and cognitive task performance. *Personality and Individual Differences, 6,* 579–586.

Faravelli, C. (1985). Life events preceding the onset of panic disorder. *Journal of Affective Disorders, 9,* 103–105.

Fava, G. A., Grandi, S., & Canestrari, R. (1988). Prodromal symptoms in panic disorder with agoraphobia. *American Journal of Psychiatry, 145,* 1564–1567.

Fergusson, D. M., Horwood, L. J., & Lynskey, M. T. (1993). Prevalence and comorbidity of DSM-III-R diagnoses in a birth cohort of 15 year olds. *Journal of the American Academy of Child and Adolescent Psychiatry, 32,* 1127–1134.

Feske, U., & Chambless, D. L. (1995). Cognitive behavioral versus exposure only treatment for social phobia: A meta-analysis. *Behavior Therapy, 26,* 695–720.

Foa, E. B., Franklin, M. E., Perry, K. J., & Herbert, J. D. (1996). Cognitive biases in social phobia. *Journal of Abnormal Psychology, 105,* 433–439.

Fredrikson, M., Annas, P., Fischer, H. & Wik, G. (1996). Gender and age differences in the prevalence of specific fears and phobias. *Behaviour Research and Therapy, 34,* 33–39.

Freud, S. (1963). Introductory lectures on psycho-analysis: Lecture 25. Anxiety. In S. Strachey (Ed. and Trans.), *The standard edition of the complete psychological works of Sigmund Freud,* Vol. 16. London: Hogarth Press. (Original work published 1917).

Fyer, A. J., Mannuzza, S., Gallops, M. S., & Martin, L. Y. (1990). Familial transmission of simple phobia and fears: A preliminary report. *Archives of General Psychiatry, 47,* 252–256.

Goddard, A. W., & Charney, D. S. (1997). Toward and integrated neurobiology of panic disorder. *Journal of Clinical Psychiatry, 58*(Suppl. 2), 4–11.

Gorman, J. M., & Gorman, L. K. (1987). Drug treatment of social phobia. *Journal of Affective Disorders, 13*, 183–192.

Gorman, J. M., Liebowitz, M. R., Fyer, A. J., & Stein, J. (1989). A neuroanatomical hypothesis for panic disorder. *American Journal of Psychiatry, 146*, 148–161.

Gorman, J. M., Papp, L. A., & Coplan, J. D. (1994). Anxiogenic effects of $CO_2$ and hyperventilation in patients with panic disorder. *American Journal of Psychiatry, 151*, 547–553.

Gould, R. A., Otto, M. W., Pollack, M. H., & Yap, L. (1997). Cognitive behavioral and pharmacological treatment of generalized anxiety disorder: A preliminary meta-analysis. *Behavior Therapy, 28*, 285–305.

Gray, J. A. (1982). *The neuropsychology of anxiety: An inquiry into the functions of the septo-hippocampal system.* Oxford: Clarendon.

Gray, J. A., & McNaughton, N. (1996). The neuropsychology of anxiety: Reprise. In D. A. Hope (Ed.), *Perspectives on anxiety, panic and fear* (The 43rd Annual Nebraska Symposium on Motivation) (pp. 61–134). Lincoln: University of Nebraska Press.

Gurguis, G. N. M., & Uhde, T. W. (1990). Plasma 3-methoxy-4-hydroxyphenylethylene glycol (MHPG) and growth hormone responses to yohimbine in panic disorder patients and normal controls. *Psychoneuroendocrinology, 15*, 217–224.

Hackmann, A., Surawy, C., & Clark, D. M. (1998). Seeing yourself though others' eyes: A study of spontaneously occurring images in social phobia. *Behavioural and Cognitive Psychotherapy, 26*, 3–12.

Hamann, M. S., & Mavissakalian, M. (1988). Discrete dimensions in agoraphobia: A factor analytic study. *British Journal of Clinical Psychology, 27*, 137–144.

Hartman, L. M. (1984). Cognitive components of social anxiety. *Journal of Clinical Psychology, 40*, 137–139.

Harvey, A. G., & Rapee, R. M. (1995). Cognitive-behavior therapy for generalized anxiety disorder. *The Psychiatric Clinics of North America, 18*, 859–870.

Harvey, A. G., & Rapee, R. M. (in press). Specific phobias. In D. J. Stein & E. Hollander (Eds.), *Textbook of anxiety disorders.* Washington, DC: American Psychiatric Press.

Harvey, J. M., Richards, J. C., Dziadosz, T., & Swindell, A. (1993). Misinterpretation of ambiguous stimuli in panic disorder. *Cognitive Therapy and Research, 17*, 235–248.

Hecker, J. E., Losee, M. C., Fritzler, B. K., & Fink, C. M. (1996). Self-directed versus therapist-directed cognitive behavioral treatment for panic disorder. *Journal of Anxiety Disorders, 10*, 253–265.

Heimberg, R. G. (1989). Cognitive and behavioral treatments for social phobia: A critical analysis. *Clinical Psychology Review, 9*, 187–228.

Heimberg, R. G., Acerra, M. C., & Holstein, A. (1985). Partner similarity mediates interpersonal anxiety. *Cognitive Therapy and Research, 9*, 443–453.

Heimberg, R. G., Dodge, C. S., & Becker, R. E. (1987). Social phobia. In L. Michelson & M. Ascher (Eds.), *Cognitive behavioral assessment and treatment of anxiety disorders.* New York: Guilford.

Heimberg, R. G., Dodge, C. S., Hope, D. A., Kennedy, C. R., Zollo, L. J., & Becker, P. E. (1990). Cognitive behavioral treatment of social phobia: Comparison to a credible placebo control. *Cognitive Therapy and Research, 14*, 1–23.

Heimberg, R. G., & Juster, H. R. (1995). Cognitive-behavioral treatments: Literature review. In R. G. Heimberg, M. R. Liebowitz, D. A. Hope, & F. R. Schneier (Eds.), *Social phobia: Diagnosis, assessment, and treatment.* New York: Guilford.

Heimberg, R. G., Liebowitz, M. R., Hope, D. A., Schneier, F. R., Holt, C. S., Welkowitz, L., Juster, H. R., Campeas, R., Bruch, M. A., Cloitre, M., Fallon, B., & Klein, D. F. (1998). Cognitive-behavioral group therapy versus phenelzine in social phobia: 12-week outcome. *Archives of General Psychiatry, 55*, 1133–1141.

Hibbert, G. A. (1984). Ideational components of anxiety: Their origin and content. *British Journal of Psychiatry, 144*, 618–624.

Hoehn-Saric, R. (1982). Comparison of generalized anxiety disorder with panic disorder patients. *Psychopharmacology Bulletin, 18*, 104–108.

Hoehn-Saric, R., McLeod, D. R., & Zimmerli, W. D. (1989). Somatic manifestations in women with generalized anxiety disorder: Psychophysiological responses to psychological stress. *Archives of General Psychiatry, 46*, 1113–1119.

Hofmann, S. G., Lehman, C. L., & Barlow, D. H. (1997). How specific are specific phobias? *Journal of Behavior Therapy and Experimental Psychiatry, 28*, 233–240.

Holt, P. E., & Andrews, G. (1989). Provocation of panic: A comparison on three elements of the panic reaction in four anxiety disorders. *Behaviour Research and Therapy, 27*, 253–261.

Honeybourne, C., Matchett, G., & Davey, G. C. L. (1993). Expectancy models of laboratory preparedness effects: A UCS-expectancy bias in phylogenetic and ontogenetic fear-relevant stimuli. *Behavior Therapy, 24*, 253–264.

Hope, D. A., Gansler, D. A., & Heimberg, R. G. (1989). Attentional focus and attributions in social phobia: Implications from social psychology. *Clinical Psychology Review, 9*, 49–60.

Hope, D. A., Rapee, R. M., Heimberg, R. G., & Dombeck, M. J. (1990). Representations of the self in social phobia: Vulnerability to social threat. *Cognitive Therapy and Research, 14*, 177–189.

Hudson, J. L., & Rapee, R. M. (1998). Parent-child interactions and anxiety. Paper presented at the *World Congress of Cognitive and Behavioural Therapies,* Acapulco, Mexico, July.

Hudson, J. L., & Rapee, R. M. (2000). The origins of social phobia. *Behavior Modification, 24*, 102–129.

Insel, T. R., Ninan, P. T., Aloi, J., Jimerson, D. C., Skolnick, P., & Paul, S. M. (1984). A benzodiazepine receptor-mediated model of anxiety. *Archives of General Psychiatry, 41*, 741–750.

Jefferson, J. W. (1996). Social phobia: Everyone's disorder? *Journal of Clinical Psychiatry, 57*(Suppl. 6), 28–32.

Jerremalm, A., Jansson, L., & Ost, L. G. (1986). Cognitive and physiological reactivity and the effects of different behavioral methods in the treatment of social phobia. *Behaviour Research and Therapy, 24*, 171–180.

Jones, W. H., Briggs, S. R., & Smith, T. G. (1986). Shyness: Conceptualization and measurement. *Journal of Personality and Social Psychology, 51*, 629–639.

Kagan, J., Gibbons, J. L., Johnson, M. O., Reznick, J. S., & Snidman, N. (1990). A temperamental disposition to the state of uncertainty. In J. E. Rolf & A. S. Masten (Eds.), *Risk and protective factors in the development of psychopathology* (pp. 164–178). New York: Cambridge University Press.

Kagan, J., Snidman, N., Arcus, D., & Reznick, J. S. (1994).

*Galen's prophecy: Temperament in human nature.* New York: Basic Books.

Kendler, K. S., Neale, M. C., Kessler, R. C., Heath, A. C., & Eaves, L. J. (1992a). Generalized anxiety disorder in women: A population-based twin study. *Archives of General Psychiatry, 49,* 267–272.

Kendler, K. S., Neale, M. C., Kessler, R. C., Heath, A. C., & Eaves, L. J. (1992b). The genetic epidemiology of phobias in women: The interrelationship of agoraphobia, social phobia, situational phobia, and simple phobia. *Archives of General Psychiatry, 49,* 273–281.

Kendler, K. S., Walters, E. E., Neale, M. C., Kessler, R. C., Heath, A. C., & Eaves, L. J. (1995). The structure of the genetic and environmental risk factors for six major psychiatric disorders in women: Phobia, generalized anxiety disorder, panic disorder, bulimia, major depression, and alcoholism. *Archives of General Psychiatry, 52,* 374–383.

Kennedy, S. J., Rapee, R. M., & Mazurski, E. J. (1997). Covariation bias for phylogenetic versus ontogenetic fear-relevant stimuli. *Behaviour Research and Therapy, 35,* 415–422.

Kessler, R. C., McGonagle, K. A., Zhao, S., Nelson, C. B., Hughes, M., Eshleman, S., Wittchen, H., & Kendler, K. S. (1994). Lifetime and 12-month prevalence of DSM-III-R psychiatric disorders in the United States: Results from the national comorbidity survey. *Archives of General Psychiatry, 51,* 8–19.

King, N. J., Ollier, K., Iacuone, R., Schuster, S., Bays, K., Gullone, E., & Ollendick, T. H. (1989). Fears of children and adolescents: A cross-sectional Australian study using the Revised-Fear Survey Schedule for Children. *Journal of Child Psychology and Psychiatry, 30,* 775–784.

King, R., Margraf, J., Ehlers, A., & Maddock, R. J. (1986). Panic disorder—overlap with symptoms of somatization disorder. In I. Hand & H. U. Wittchen (Eds.), *Panic and phobias.* Berlin: Springer Verlag.

Klein, D. F. (1964). Delineation of two drug-responsive anxiety syndromes. *Psychopharmacologia, 5,* 397–408.

Klein, D. F. (1993). False suffocation alarms, spontaneous panics, and related conditions: An integrative hypothesis. *Archives of General Psychiatry, 50,* 306–317.

Klein, D. F., & Fink, M. (1962). Psychiatric reaction patterns to imipramine. *American Journal of Psychiatry, 119,* 432–438.

Krystal, J. H., Niehoff Deutsch, D., & Charney, D. S. (1996). The biological basis of panic disorder. *Journal of Clinical Psychiatry, 57*(Suppl. 10), 23–31.

Lader, M. H., & Mathews, A. M. (1968). A physiological model of phobic anxiety and desensitization. *Behaviour Research and Therapy, 6,* 411–421.

Last, C. G., & Blanchard, E. B. (1982). Classification of phobics versus fearful nonphobics: Procedural and theoretical issues. *Behavioral Assessment, 4,* 195–210.

Lelliot, P., & Bass, C. (1990). Symptom specificity in patients with panic. *British Journal of Psychiatry, 157,* 593–597.

Levin, A. P., Schneier, F. R., & Liebowitz, M. R. (1989). Social phobia: Biology and pharmacology. *Clinical Psychology Review, 9,* 129–140.

Liebowitz, M. R., Heimberg, R. G., Schneier, F. R., Hope, D. A., Davies, S., Holt, C. S., Goetz, D., Juster, H. R., Lin, S-L., Bruch, M. A., Marshall, R., & Klein, D. F. (1999). Cognitive-behavioral group therapy versus phenelzine in social phobia: Long-term outcome. *Depression and Anxiety, 10,* 89–98.

Liebowitz, M. R., & Klein, D. F. (1981). Differential diagnosis and treatment of panic attacks and phobic states. *Annual Review of Medicine, 32,* 583–599.

Liebowitz, M. R., Fyer, A. J., Gorman, J. M., Dillon, D., Davies, S. O., Stein, J., Cohen, B., & Klein, D. F. (1985). Specificity of lactate infusions in social phobia versus panic disorders. *American Journal of Psychiatry, 142,* 947–950.

Lovibond, P. F., & Rapee, R. M. (1993). The representation of feared outcomes. *Behavior Research and Therapy, 31,* 595–608.

Lucock, M. P., & Salkovskis, P. M. (1988). Cognitive factors in social anxiety and its treatment. *Behaviour Research and Therapy, 26,* 297–302.

MacLeod, C. (1996). Anxiety and cognitive processes. In I. G. Sarason, G. P. Pierce, & B. R. Sarason (Eds.), *Cognitive interference: Theories, methods, and findings* (pp. 47–76). Mahwah, NJ: Erlbaum.

MacLeod, C., Mathews, A., & Tata, P. (1986). Attentional bias in emotional disorders. *Journal of Abnormal Psychology, 95,* 15–20.

Maller, R. G., & Reiss, S. (1992). Anxiety sensitivity in 1984 and panic attacks in 1987. *Journal of Anxiety Disorders, 6,* 241–247.

Manuzza, S., Fyer, A. J., Martin, L. M., Gallops, M. S., Endicott, J., Gorman, J., Liebowitz, M. R., & Klein, D. F. (1989). Reliability of anxiety assessment: I. Diagnostic agreement. *Archives of General Psychiatry, 46,* 1093–1101.

Margraf, J., Barlow, D. H., Clark, D. M., & Telch, M. J. (1993). Psychological treatment of panic: Work in progress on outcome, active ingredients, and follow-up. *Behaviour Research and Therapy, 31,* 1–8.

Marks, I. M. (1969). *Fears and phobias.* London: Heineman.

Marks, I. M. (1981). New developments in psychological treatments of phobias. In M. Mavissakalian & D. H. Barlow (Eds.), *Phobia psychological and pharmacological treatment.* New York: Guilford.

Matchett, G., & Davey, G. C. L. (1991). A test of a disease-avoidance model of animal phobias. *Behaviour Research and Therapy, 29,* 91–94.

Mathews, A. (1990). Why worry? The cognitive function of anxiety. *Behaviour Research and Therapy, 28,* 455–468.

Mathews, A., Mackintosh, B., & Fulcher, E. P. (1997). Cognitive biases in anxiety and attention to threat. *Trends in Cognitive Sciences, 1,* 340–345.

Mathews, A., Mogg, K., May, J., & Eysenck, M. W. (1989). Implicit and explicit memory biases in anxiety. *Journal of Abnormal Psychology, 98,* 236–240.

Mattia, J. I., Heimberg, R. G., & Hope, D. A. (1993). The revised Stroop color-naming task in social phobics. *Behaviour Research and Therapy, 31,* 305–313.

Mattick, R. P., & Peters, L. (1988). Treatment of severe social phobia: Effects of guided exposure with and without cognitive restructuring. *Journal of Consulting and Clinical Psychology, 56,* 251–260.

Mattick, R. P., Peters, L., & Clarke, J. C. (1989). Exposure and cognitive restructuring for social phobia: A controlled study. *Behavior Therapy, 20,* 3–24.

McEwan, K. L., & Devins, G. M. (1983). Is increased arousal in social anxiety noticed by others? *Journal of Abnormal Psychology, 92,* 417–421.

McNally, R. J. (1987). Preparedness and phobias: A review. *Psychological Bulletin, 101,* 283–303.

McNally, R. J. (1990). Psychological approaches to panic disorder: A review. *Psychological Bulletin, 108,* 403–419.

McNally, R. J., & Foa, E. B. (1987). Cognition and agoraphobia: Bias in the interpretation of threat. *Cognitive Therapy and Research, 11,* 567–581.

McNally, R. J., & Heatherton, T. F. (1993). Are covariation biases attributable to a priori expectancy biases ? *Behaviour Research and Therapy, 31,* 653–658.

McNally, R. J., & Steketee, G. S. (1985). The etiology and maintenance of severe animal phobias. *Behaviour Research and Therapy, 23,* 431–435.

McNeil, D. W., Ries, B. J., Taylor, L. J., Boone, M. L., Carter, L. E., Turk, C. L., & Lewin, M. R. (1995). Comparison of social phobia subtypes using Stroop tests. *Journal of Anxiety Disorders, 9,* 47–57.

Menzies, R. G., & Clarke, J. C. (1993a). The etiology of fear of heights and its relationship to severity and individual response patterns. *Behaviour Research and Therapy, 31,* 355–365.

Menzies, R. G., & Clarke, J. C. (1993b). The etiology of childhood water phobia. *Behaviour Research and Therapy, 31,* 499–501.

Menzies, R. G., & Clarke, J. C. (1995a). Danger expectancies and insight in acrophobia. *Behaviour Research and Therapy, 33,* 215–222.

Menzies, R. G., & Clarke, J. C. (1995b). The etiology of phobias: A nonassociative account. *Clinical Psychology Review, 15,* 23–48.

Merckelbach, H., de Jong, P., Muris, P., & van den Hout, M. A. (1996). The etiology of specific phobias: A review. *Clinical Psychology Review, 16,* 337–361.

Mineka, S., & Zinbarg, R. E. (1996). Conditioning and ethological models of anxiety disorders: Stress-in-dynamic context anxiety models. In D. A. Hope (Ed.), *Perspectives on anxiety, panic and fear* (The 43rd Annual Nebraska Symposium on Motivation) (pp. 135–210). Lincoln: University of Nebraska Press.

Mogg, K., Mathews, A., & Weinman, J. (1987). Memory bias in clinical anxiety. *Journal of Abnormal Psychology, 96,* 94–98.

Montgomery, R. L., Haemmerlie, F. M., & Edwards, M. (1991). Social, personal, and interpersonal deficits in socially anxious people. *Journal of Social Behavior and Personality, 6,* 859–872.

Mowrer, O. H. (1939). A stimulus-response analysis of anxiety and its role as a reinforcing agent. *Psychological Review, 46,* 553–565.

Mulkens, S., De Jong, P. J., & Bögels, S. M. (1997). High blushing propensity: Fearful preoccupation or facial coloration? *Personality and Individual Differences, 22,* 817–824.

Nesse, R. M., Curtis, G. C., Thyer, B. A., McCann, D. S., Huber-Smith, M. J., & Knopf, R. F. (1985). Endocrine and cardiovascular responses during phobic anxiety. *Psychosomatic Medicine, 47,* 320–332.

Nicholas, L. M., & Tancer, M. E. (1995). Neurobiological studies of social phobia. *Psychiatric Annals, 25,* 564–569.

Nickell, P. V., & Uhde, T. W. (1995). Neurobiology of social phobia. In R. G. Heimberg, M. R. Liebowitz, D. A. Hope, & F. R. Schneier (Eds.), *Social phobia: Diagnosis, assessment, and treatment.* New York: Guilford.

Norton, G. R., McLeod, L., Guertin, J., Hewitt, P. L., Walker, J. R., & Stein, M. B. (1996). Panic disorder or social phobia: Which is worse? *Behaviour Research and Therapy, 34,* 273–276.

Noyes, R., Jr., Anderson, D. J., Clancy, J., Crowe, R. R., Slymen, D. J., Ghoneim, M. M., & Hinrichs, J. V. (1984).

Diazepam and propranolol in panic disorder and agoraphobia. *Archives of General Psychiatry, 41,* 287–292.

Noyes, R., Jr., Clarkson, C., Crowe, R. R., Yates, W. R., & McChesney, C. M. (1987). A family study of generalized anxiety disorder. *American Journal of Psychiatry, 141,* 1019–1024.

Noyes, R., Jr., Crowe, R. R., Harris, E. L., Hamra, B. J., McChesney, C. M., & Chaudhry, D. R. (1986). Relationship between panic disorder and agoraphobia: A family study. *Archives of General Psychiatry, 43,* 227–232.

Nutt, D. J., Glue, P., Lawson, C., & Wilson, S. (1990). Flumazenil provocation of panic attacks: Evidence for altered benzodiazepine receptor sensitivity in panic disorder. *Archives of General Psychiatry, 47,* 917–925.

Nutt, D. J., & Lawson, C. (1992). Panic attacks: A neurochemical overview of models and mechanisms. *British Journal of Psychiatry, 160,* 165–178.

Ohman, A. (1994). Fear and anxiety as emotional phenomena: Clinical phenomenology, evolutionary perspectives, and information processing mechanisms. In M. Lewis & J. M. Haviland (Eds.), *Handbook of emotions.* New York: Guilford Press.

Ohman, A. (1996). Preferential preattentive processing of threat in anxiety: Preparedness and attentional biases. In R. M. Rapee (Ed.), *Current controversies in the anxiety disorders* (pp. 253–290). New York: Guilford.

Ost, L. G. (1987). Age of onset in different phobias. *Journal of Psychology, 96,* 223–229.

Ost, L. G. (1996). One session group treatment of spider phobia. *Behaviour Research and Therapy, 34,* 707–715.

Ost, L. G., Fellenius, J., & Sterner, U. (1991). Applied tension, exposure in vivo, and tension only in the treatment of blood injury phobia. *Behaviour Research and Therapy, 29,* 561–574.

Ost, L. G., Johansson, J., & Jerremalm, A. (1982). Individual response patterns and the effects of different behavioral methods in the treatment of claustrophobia. *Behaviour Research and Therapy, 20,* 445–460.

Ost, L. G., Sterner, U. S., & Lindahl, I. L. (1984). Physiological responses in blood phobics. *Behaviour Research and Therapy, 22,* 109–117.

Ottaviani, R., & Beck, A. T. (1987). Cognitive aspects of panic disorder. *Journal of Anxiety Disorders, 1,* 15–28.

Otto, M. W., Pollack, M. H., & Sabatino, S. A. (1996). Maintenance of remission following cognitive behavior therapy for panic disorder: Possible deleterious effects of concurrent medication. *Behavior Therapy, 27,* 473–482.

Page, A. C. (1994). Blood-injury phobia. *Clinical Psychology Review, 14,* 443–461.

Papp, L. A., Gorman, J. M., Liebowitz, M. R., Fyer, A. J., Cohen, B., & Klein, D. F. (1988). Epinephrine infusions in patients with social phobia. *American Journal of Psychiatry, 145,* 733–736.

Parker, G. (1979). Reported parental characteristics of agoraphobics and social phobics. *British Journal of Psychiatry, 135,* 550–560.

Pauls, D. L., Bucher, K. D., Crowe, R. R., & Noyes, R., Jr. (1980). A genetic study of panic disorder pedigrees. *American Journal of Human Genetics, 32,* 639–644.

Pilkonis, P. A. (1977). The behavioral consequences of shyness. *Journal of Personality, 45,* 596–611.

Pilkonis, P. A., & Zimbardo, P. G. (1979). The person and social dynamics of shyness. In C. E. Izard (Ed.), *Emotions in personality and psychopathology.* New York: Plenum Press.

Pollard, C. A., Pollard, H. J., & Corn, K. J. (1989). Panic onset and major events in the lives of agoraphobics: A test of contiguity. *Journal of Abnormal Psychology, 98,* 318–321.

Potts, N. L. S., Book, S., & Davidson, J. R. T. (1996). The neurobiology of social phobia. *International Clinical Psychopharmacology, 11*(Suppl. 3), 43–48.

Potts, N. L. S., & Davidson, J. R. T. (1995). Pharmacological treatments: Literature review. In R. G. Heimberg, M. R. Liebowitz, D. A. Hope, & F. R. Schneier (Eds.), *Social phobia: Diagnosis, assessment, and treatment.* New York: Guilford.

Poulton, R. G., & Andrews, G. (1994). Appraisal of danger and proximity in social phobics. *Behaviour Research and Therapy, 32,* 639–642.

Power, K. G., Jerrom, D. W. A., Simpson, R. J., Mitchell, M. J., & Swanson, V. (1989). A controlled comparison of cognitive-behaviour therapy, diazepam, and placebo in the management of generalized anxiety. *Behavioural Psychotherapy, 17,* 1–14.

Power, K. G., Simpson, R. J., Swanson, V., Wallace, L. A., Feistner, A. T. C., & Sharp, D. (1990). A controlled comparison of cognitive-behaviour therapy, diazepam, and placebo, alone and in combination, for the treatment of generalised anxiety disorder. *Journal of Anxiety Disorders, 4,* 267–292.

Rachman, S. (1977). The conditioning theory of fear acquisition: A critical examination. *Behaviour Research and Therapy, 15,* 375–387.

Rachman, S., Levitt, K., & Lopatka, C. (1988). Experimental analyses of panic-III. Claustrophobia subjects. *Behaviour Research and Therapy, 26,* 41–52.

Rapee, R. (1985). Distinctions between panic disorder and generalized anxiety disorder: Clinical presentation. *Australian and New Zealand Journal of Psychiatry, 19,* 227–232.

Rapee, R. M. (1991). Generalized anxiety disorder: A review of clinical features and theoretical concepts. *Clinical Psychology Review, 11,* 419–440.

Rapee, R. M. (1993a). The utilisation of working memory by worry. *Behaviour Research and Therapy, 31,* 617–620.

Rapee, R. M. (1993b). Psychological factors in panic disorder. *Advances in Behaviour Research and Therapy, 15,* 85–102.

Rapee, R. M. (1995a). Psychological factors influencing the affective response to biological challenge procedures in panic disorder. *Journal of Anxiety Disorders, 9,* 59–74.

Rapee, R. M. (1995b). Descriptive psychopathology of social phobia. In R. G. Heimberg, M. R. Liebowitz, D. A. Hope, & F. R. Schneier (Eds.), *Social phobia: Diagnosis, assessment, and treatment* (pp. 41–66). New York: Guilford.

Rapee, R. M., Brown, T. A., Antony, M. M., & Barlow, D. H. (1992). Response to hyperventilation and inhalation of 5.5% carbon dioxide-enriched air across the DSM-III-R anxiety disorders. *Journal of Abnormal Psychology, 101,* 538–552.

Rapee, R. M., Craske, M. G., & Barlow, D. H. (1990). Subject described features of panic attacks using self monitoring. *Journal of Anxiety Disorders, 4,* 171–181.

Rapee, R. M., Craske, M. G., & Barlow, D. H. (1994). Assessment instrument for panic disorder that includes fear of sensation-producing activities: The Albany Panic and Phobia Questionnaire. *Anxiety, 1,* 114–122.

Rapee, R. M., & Heimberg, R. G. (1997). A cognitive-behavioral model of anxiety in social phobia. *Behaviour Research and Therapy, 35,* 741–756.

Rapee, R. M., & Lim, L. (1992). Discrepancy between self and observer ratings of performance in social phobics. *Journal of Abnormal Psychology, 101,* 727–731.

Rapee, R. M., Litwin, E. M., & Barlow, D. H. (1990). Life events in panic disorder: A comparison study. *American Journal of Psychiatry, 147,* 640–644.

Rapee, R. M., & Murrell, E. (1988). Predictors of agoraphobic avoidance. *Journal of Anxiety Disorders, 2,* 203–217.

Rapee, R. M., Sanderson, W. C., & Barlow, D. H. (1988). Social phobia features across the DSM-III-R anxiety disorders. *Journal of Psychopathology and Behavioral Assessment, 10,* 287–299.

Reich, J., & Yates, W. (1988). Family history of psychiatric disorders in social phobia. *Comprehensive Psychiatry, 29,* 72–75.

Rickels, K., Downing, R., Schweizer, E., & Hassman, H. (1993). Antidepressants for the treatment of generalized anxiety disorder: A placebo-controlled comparison of imipramine, trazodone, and diazepam. *Archives of General Psychiatry, 50,* 884–895.

Roth, M. (1959). The phobic anxiety-depersonalization syndrome. *Proceedings of the Royal Society of Medicine, 52,* 587–596.

Roy-Byrne, P. P., Geraci, M., & Uhde, T. W. (1986). Life events and the onset of panic disorder. *American Journal of Psychiatry, 143,* 1424–1427.

Sanderson, W. C., & Barlow, D. H. (1990). A description of patients diagnosed with DSM-III-revised generalized anxiety disorder. *Journal of Nervous and Mental Disease, 178,* 588–591.

Sapolsky, R. M. (1992). *Stress, the aging brain, and the mechanisms of neuron death.* Cambridge: MIT Press.

Sartory, G., Rachman, S., & Grey, S. (1977). An investigation of the relation between reported fear and heart rate. *Behaviour Research and Therapy, 15,* 435–438.

Schlenker, B. R., & Leary, M. R. (1982). Social anxiety and self-presentation: A conceptualization and model. *Psychological Bulletin, 92,* 641–669.

Schmidt, N. B., Lerew, D. R., & Jackson, R. J. (1997a). The role of anxiety sensitivity in the pathogenesis of panic: Prospective evaluation of spontaneous panic attacks during acute stress. *Journal of Abnormal Psychology, 106,* 355–364.

Schmidt, N. B., Lerew, D. R., & Trakowski, J. H. (1997b). Body vigilance in panic disorder: Evaluating attention to bodily perturbations. *Journal of Consulting and Clinical Psychology, 65,* 214–220.

Schneier, F. R., Johnson, J., Hornig, C. D., Liebowitz, M. R., & Weissman, M. M. (1992). Social phobia: Comorbidity and morbidity in an epidemiologic sample. *Archives of General Psychiatry, 49,* 282–288.

Schniering, C. A., & Rapee, R. M. (1997). A test of the cognitive model of panic: Primed lexical decision in panic disorder. *Journal of Anxiety Disorders, 11,* 557–571.

Schweizer, E., & Rickels, K. (1996). The long-term management of generalized anxiety disorder: Issues and dilemmas. *Journal of Clinical Psychiatry, 57*(Suppl. 7), 9–12.

Seligman, M. E. P. (1971). Phobias and preparedness. *Behavior Therapy, 2,* 307–320.

Shaw, P. M. (1979). A comparison of three behaviour therapies in the treatment of social phobia. *British Journal of Psychiatry, 134,* 620–623.

Sheehan, D. V., & Harnett-Sheehan, K. (1996). The role of SSRIs in panic disorder. *Journal of Clinical Psychiatry, 57*(Suppl. 10), 51–58.

Squires, R. F., & Braestrup, C. (1977). Benzodiazepine receptors in rat brain. *Nature, 226,* 732–734.

Stein, M. B., Tancer, M. E., & Uhde, T. W. (1992). Heart rate and plasma norepinephrine responsivity to orthostatic challenge in anxiety disorders. *Archives of General Psychiatry, 49*, 311–317.

Stopa, L. & Clark, D. M. (1993). Cognitive processes in social phobia. *Behaviour Research and Therapy, 31*, 255–267.

Taylor, S. (1996). Meta-analysis of cognitive-behavioral treatment for social phobia. *Journal of Behavior Therapy and Experimental Psychiatry, 27*, 1–9.

Thayer, J. F., Friedman, B. H., & Borkovec, T. D. (1996). Autonomic characteristics of generalized anxiety disorder and worry. *Biological Psychiatry, 39*, 255–266.

Thorpe, G. L., & Burns, L. E. (1983). *The agoraphobic syndrome: Behavioural approaches to evaluation and treatment.* New York: Wiley.

Thorpe, S. J., & Salkovskis, P. M. (1995). Phobic beliefs: Do cognitive factors play a role in specific phobias. *Behaviour Research and Therapy, 33*, 805–816.

Thyer, B. A., Himle, J., & Curtis, G. C. (1985). Blood-injury-illness phobia: A review. *Journal of Clinical Psychology, 41*, 451–459.

Thyer, B. A., Parrish, R. T., Curtis, G. C., Nesse, R. M., & Cameron, O. G. (1985). Ages of onset of DSM-111 anxiety disorders. *Comprehensive Psychiatry, 26*, 113–122.

Tolin, D. F., Lohr, J. M., Sawchuk, C. N., & Lee, T. C. (1997). Disgust and disgust sensitivity in blood-injection-injury and spider phobia. *Behaviour Research and Therapy, 35*, 949–953.

Tomarken, A. J., Sutton, S. K., & Mineka, S. (1995). Fear-relevant illusory correlations: What types of associations promote judgemental bias? *Journal of Abnormal Psychology, 104*, 312–326.

Torgersen, S. (1979). The nature and origin of common phobic fears. *British Journal of Psychiatry, 134*, 343–351.

Turner, S. M., & Beidel, D. C. (1989). Social phobia: Clinical syndrome, diagnosis, and comorbidity. *Clinical Psychology Review, 9*, 3–18.

Turner, S. M., Beidel, D. C., Cooley, M. R., Woody, S. R., & Messer, S. C. (1994). A milticomponent behavioral treatment for social phobia: Social effectiveness therapy. *Behaviour Research and Therapy, 32*, 381–390.

Turner, S. M., Beidel, D. C., Dancu, C. V., & Keys, D. J. (1986). Psychopathology of social phobia and comparison to avoidant personality disorder. *Journal of Abnormal Psychology, 95*, 389–394.

Turner, S. M., Beidel, D. C., & Jacob, R. G. (1994). Social phobia: A comparison of behavior therapy and atenolol. *Journal of Consulting and Clinical Psychology, 54*, 523–527.

Turner, S. M., Beidel, D. C., & Larkin, K. T. (1986). Situational determinants of social anxiety in clinic and nonclinic samples: Physiological and cognitive correlates. *Journal of Consulting and Clinical Psychology, 54*, 523–527.

Turner, S. M., McCann, B. S., Beidel, D. C., & Mezzich, J. E. (1986). DSM-III classification of the anxiety disorders: A psychometric study. *Journal of Abnormal Psychology, 95*, 168–172.

Twentyman, C. T., & McFall, R. M. (1975). Behavioral training of social skills in shy males. *Journal of Consulting and Clinical Psychology, 43*, 384–395.

Tyrer, P., Owen, R., & Dawling, S. (1983, June 25). Gradual withdrawal of diazepam after long-term therapy. *Lancet*, 1402–1406.

van Balkom, A. J. L. M., Bakker, A., Spinhoven, P., Blaauw, B. M. J. W., Smeenk, S., & Ruesink, B. (1997). A meta-analysis of the treatment of panic disorder with or without agoraphobia: A comparison of psychopharmacological, cognitive-behavioral, and combination treatments. *Journal of Nervous and Mental Disease, 185*, 510–516.

Veljaca, K., & Rapee, R. M. (1998). Detection of negative and positive audience behaviours by socially anxious subjects. *Behaviour Research and Therapy, 36*, 311–321.

Verhulst, F. C., van der Ende, J., Ferdinand, R. F., & Kasius, M. C. (1997). The prevalence of DSM-III-R diagnoses in a national sample of Dutch adolescents. *Archives of General Psychiatry, 54*, 329–336.

Wallace, S. T., & Alden, L. E. (1995). Social anxiety and standard setting following social success or failure. *Cognitive Therapy and Research, 19*, 613–631.

Watson, J. B., & Rayner, R. (1920). Conditioned emotional reactions. *Journal of Experimental Psychology, 3*, 1–14.

Westphal, C. (1871). Die agoraphobie: Eine neuropathische erscheinung. *Archiv für Psychiatric und Neruenkrankheit, 3*, 138–161.

Whittal, M. L., & Goetsch, V. L. (1997). The impact of panic expectancy and social demand on agoraphobia avoidance. *Behaviour Research and Therapy, 35*, 813–821.

Williams, S. L., & Watson, N. (1985). Perceived danger and perceived self-efficacy as cognitive determinants of acrophobic behavior. *Behavior Therapy, 16*, 136–146.

Wittchen, H-U., Kessler, R. C., Zhao, S., & Abelson, J. (1995). Reliability and clinical validity of UM-CIDI DSM-III-R generalized anxiety disorder. *Journal of Psychiatric Research, 29*, 95–110.

Woody, S. R. (1996). Effects of focus of attention on anxiety levels and social performance of individuals with social phobia. *Journal of Abnormal Psychology, 105*, 61–69.

Zimbardo, P. G. (1986). The Stanford shyness project. In W. H. Jones, J. M. Cheek, & S. R. Briggs (Eds.), *Shyness: Perspectives on research and treatment.* New York: Plenum Press.

# CHAPTER 7

# Obsessive-Compulsive Disorder

## Samuel M. Turner, Deborah C. Beidel, Melinda A. Stanley, and Nancy Heiser

## Introduction

The past two decades were characterized by enormous advancement in understanding the nature of mental illness. In particular, findings from basic neuroscience raised the possibility of eventually unraveling the pathophysiology of mental disorders. Similarly, cognitive theories have taken on increasing prominence in explanations for maladaptive psychological functioning. With respect to the anxiety disorders in general, and obsessive-compulsive disorder in particular, there has been a virtual explosion of research since the introduction of DSM-III in 1980; much of which is biological and cognitive. In this chapter, we will discuss the syndrome of OCD, which has remained remarkably consistent during the many decades since its description. Specifically, we will describe the syndrome and its manifestation, discuss diagnosis and the emerging literature on the comorbidity of OCD and other disorders, as well as the concept of OCD Spectrum Disorder. We will devote considerable time to discussing and evaluating findings

from biological and cognitive research with respect to the impact these findings have had in furthering our understanding of the nature and phenomenology of OCD.

## Diagnosis and Phenomenology

### Diagnosis of the Disorder

Obsessive-compulsive disorder (OCD) is one of the most severe and chronic of the anxiety disorders delineated in the current psychiatric nomenclature (American Psychiatric Association [APA], 1994). It is characterized by the presence of obsessions or compulsions, although the majority of patients report both types of symptoms (Foa & Kozak, 1995). An *obsession* is any recurrent, intrusive thought, image, or urge that is unwanted but cannot be controlled. Obsessions differ from the excessive preoccupation with real-life worries that characterizes generalized anxiety disorder (GAD) in content, form, resistance, and precipitating stimuli (Turner, Beidel, & Stanley, 1992). Patients with the two disorders are also easily distinguishable based on core clinical features (Brown, Moras, Zinbarg, & Barlow, 1993). The most common types of obsessions involve themes of contamination, dirt or illness (e.g., fearing that one will contract or transmit a specific disease, such as cancer or HIV, or a more general, vague fear of not being clean enough), and pathological doubting (e.g., that some action has not been performed adequately and will consequently result in harm to

Samuel M. Turner, Deborah C. Beidel, and Nancy Heiser • Maryland Center for Anxiety Disorders, Department of Psychology, University of Maryland, College Park, Maryland 20742. Melinda A. Stanley • University of Texas—Houston Science Center, Houston, Texas 77030.

*Comprehensive Handbook of Psychopathology* (Third Edition), edited by Patricia B. Sutker and Henry E. Adams. Kluwer Academic/Plenum Publishers, New York, 2001.

self and/or others) (Rasmussen & Eisen, 1994). Other common themes include the need for symmetry or orderliness, somatic concerns, and aggressive, sexual, or religious ideation. Generally, patients try to suppress or ignore the thoughts, and diagnostic criteria require that patients realize that the obsessions are products of their own minds (APA, 1994).

A *compulsion* is any purposeful, repetitive behavior or mental activity that is performed in a ritualistic or stereotypical way, generally with the goal of reducing anxiety associated with obsessive ideation. As such, compulsions can be conceptualized as escape or avoidance mechanisms, although it should be noted that not all conceptualizations of the disorder include a central role for anxiety (Antony, Downie, & Swinson, 1998). The most frequently reported compulsive behaviors include repetitive washing (e.g., handwashing, showering, house cleaning) and checking (e.g., of locks, appliances, numerical figures, or mathematical calculations) (Rasmussen & Eisen, 1994). These classes of behaviors generally are associated, respectively, with obsessive thoughts of contamination and excessive doubting (Baer, 1994; Rachman & Hodgson, 1980). Other common types of compulsions include repeating rituals (e.g., getting up and down from a chair repeatedly, going in and out of doorways), ordering/arranging behaviors, and hoarding. Cognitive compulsions (e.g., mental counting or repetition of certain words, phrases, or images) also occur frequently and generally serve the same function as behavioral rituals (Foa & Kozak, 1995). However, mental rituals often go unnoticed by inexperienced clinicians. To differentiate obsessions from cognitive compulsions, it is essential to determine the function of the mental activity. If the function is to reduce discomfort about an obsessive thought, characterization of the cognition as a compulsion should be considered.

To diagnose OCD, patients must acknowledge at some point that the symptoms are/were excessive and unreasonable. However, diagnostic criteria call for specification of *poor insight* when the patient fails to recognize the irrationality of the thoughts or behaviors at the time of diagnosis (APA, 1994). Patients in this subgroup also are often classified as exhibiting *overvalued ideation* (OVI). Although early clinical data indicated that OVI was associated with poor response to behavioral treatment (Foa, 1979), more recent studies

addressing this issue have not been consistent (Kozak & Foa, 1994). This literature is difficult to interpret, however, given that patients with OCD exhibit a wide range of insight and fixity of beliefs (Eisen & Rasmussen, 1993; Foa & Kozak, 1995) that make categorization into OVI and non-OVI subgroups challenging at best. Moreover, until recently, no psychometrically sound measure of OVI was available. Due to the lack of well-standardized assessment tools, it has been difficult to interpret and integrate findings across studies. However, preliminary data on a new measure created by Eisen and colleagues show promise in this regard (Eisen et al., 1998). The Brown Assessment of Beliefs Scale is a seven-item clinician-rated scale that assesses degree of delusionality in OCD and other psychiatric disorders. Initial psychometric data suggested strong interrater agreement, internal consistency, convergent and divergent validity, and sensitivity to change (Eisen et al., 1998). As such, this measure should provide a solid tool for further investigation into the role of overvalued ideation in OCD.

As with other psychiatric disorders, to diagnose OCD, the symptoms need to create significant distress and/or interfere with functioning. Numerous studies have documented that patients with OCD experience significant disruption in social and family relationships, impaired work performance, and decreased quality of life (Antony, Roth, Swinson, Huta, & Devins, 1998; Calvocoressi et al., 1995; Hollander et al., 1997; Koran, Thienemann, & Davenport, 1996). Economic costs of the disorder are also high due to inappropriate treatments, unemployment, absenteeism from work, and increased use of welfare or family support (Hollander et al., 1997; Steketee, Grayson, & Foa, 1987). In these instances, OCD should be considered a severe psychiatric disorder that has pervasive and serious impact on the individual and society.

## Symptom Subtypes

Given the wide variety of symptom patterns that may be present in OCD, a number of attempts have been made to subclassify the disorder to enhance understanding of its pathophysiology and treatment. Most often, attempts to identify subtypes have been based on the predominant type of rituals reported by the patient. In these schemes, subgroups of patients always include (but are not limited to) those with predominant washing and checking rituals. As noted earlier, these types of rituals are the most commonly reported by clinic patients (Rasmussen & Eisen, 1994). As such, it is not surprising that much of the evidence that supports the utility of behavioral treatment for OCD has been obtained largely with patients who can be classified as "washers" or "checkers" (Ball, Baer, & Otto, 1996). Studies of the potential utility of subclassifying OCD in this manner have indicated a variety of differences in demographic and clinical variables for patients classified as "washers" and "checkers." For example, patients in these two subgroups differ in age of onset and gender distribution (Khanna & Mukherjee, 1992; Minichiello, Baer, Jenike, & Holland, 1990), frequency of personality disorders (Horesh, Dolberg, Kirschenbaum-Aviner, & Kotler, 1997), triggers for obsessional fears, and retrospective reports of parental style (Steketee, Grayson, & Foa, 1985). These data suggest the potential utility of a symptom classification scheme to enhance understanding and treatment of OCD.

Recent factor analyses of OCD symptoms in larger groups of patients suggested three or four major subgroups of symptoms. Baer (1994) reported an analysis of symptoms in 107 patients that yielded three factors characterized by symmetry/hoarding (symmetry and saving obsessions, and ordering, hoarding, repeating, and counting rituals), contamination/cleaning, and pure obsessions (aggressive, sexual, and religious obsessions). Leckman and colleagues (Leckman et al., 1997) reported four factors in two independent samples of more than 300 patients with OCD. These factors included obsessions/checking (aggressive, sexual, religious, and somatic obsessions and checking rituals), symmetry/ordering (including also repeating and counting compulsions), cleanliness/washing, and hoarding. Overlap in the factor structures of these two reports is evident, although no data yet have addressed the utility of subclassifying patients according to these broader subgroups of symptoms. In fact, despite evidence of meaningful differences between washers and checkers, the general utility of classifying patients according to symptom subtypes has been questioned, given that symptom clusters generally are not mutually exclusive and constellations of symptoms may change over time (Baer, 1994; Rettew, Swedo, Leonard, Lenane, & Rapoport, 1992).

Other subclassification schemes have also been suggested, the most viable of them probably is

based on coexistent diagnoses. In particular, coexistent Tourette's syndrome or chronic tic disorder in OCD has been associated with differential obsessive-compulsive symptom profiles (Baer, 1994; Leckman et al., 1997), gender distribution (George et al., 1993; Zohar et al., 1997), age of onset for OCD and neurochemical findings (Leonard et al., 1992), and treatment response (McDougle, Goodman, Leckman, Barr, Heninger, & Price, 1993). This literature taken together supports the potential utility of subclassifying patients with OCD who also have a chronic tic disorder to enhance clinical understanding and treatment of patients. Similarly, patients with some coexistent personality disorders or features have unique patterns of OCD symptoms (Baer, 1994; Stanley, Turner, & Borden, 1990) and differential treatment response (McDougle, Goodman, Leckman, Lee, Heninger, & Price, 1994). This literature is less well developed, however, and requires further study.

Possibly of even more heuristic value are subclassification schemes based on function rather than content of symptoms. Such systems allow subclassification of patients regardless of specific symptom constellations that may vary over time. Mavissakalian (1979) proposed such a system that included four forms of obsessive-compulsive symptoms: (1) obsessions only, (2) obsessions plus anxiety-reducing compulsions, (3) obsessions plus anxiety-increasing compulsions, and (4) compulsions independent of anxiety and/or obsessions. Although this type of system holds some promise for treatment refinement (Mavissakalian, 1979), very little relevant empirical work has addressed the utility of functional classification schemes. In the context of a DSM-IV field trial, Foa and Kozak (1995) examined the usefulness of subcategories of OCD including *predominantly obsessions, predominantly compulsions,* and *mixed obsessions and compulsions.* Results revealed that more than 90% of patients reported both obsessive and compulsive symptoms, although based on interview data, clinicians categorized 30% of patients with predominantly obsessions, 21% with predominantly compulsions, and 49% with mixed obsessions and compulsions. Significant differences in the frequency of various specific symptoms occurred across these subgroups, although data overall were equivocal with regard to the utility of this type of classification.

In summary, numerous models have been proposed for subclassifying OCD. To date, the most promising of these involve subgroups based on the presence or absence of co-occurring chronic tic disorders and the predominant type of symptom reported; the majority of data here address differences between patients with primary washing or checking compulsions.

## Comorbidity, Differential Diagnosis, and the Obsessive-Compulsive Spectrum Disorders

OCD is frequently accompanied by increased levels of anxiety and depression; estimates of coexistent disorders range from 42–83% (Antony et al., 1998). Despite these high rates of overlap with other disorders, the diagnosis of OCD can be made quite reliably, particularly when behavioral compulsions are present (Brown, 1998). Key differential diagnostic issues still are relevant, however, and these will be reviewed briefly here.

Generally, the differentiation of OCD from other anxiety disorders is fairly straightforward. First, although there is clearly overlap between obsessional thinking and worry, as already noted, the diagnostic differentiation of OCD and GAD can be made reliably (Brown et al., 1993). In differentiating these disorders, it is of note that obsessions generally are associated with a greater degree of resistance and increased perceptions of unacceptability than worry (Turner et al., 1992). Obsessions are also less likely to be precipitated by and focused on circumstances of daily living (Turner et al., 1992). Even when GAD is diagnosed in patients with principal OCD, it is associated with more frequent worries about daily life events (Abramowitz & Foa, 1998). Moreover, although repetitive checking may be present in GAD, rituals that accompany OCD are usually more pervasive and intrusive.

Differentiation of OCD and other disorders with more focal fears (e.g., specific phobia, social phobia, specific subtype) is usually not difficult because any obsessional ideation that accompanies these syndromes revolves around a single fear. Ritualistic behavior also typically does not accompany fears with a more specific focus. The distinction between OCD and specific phobias of illness, however, can be slightly more complicated because fears of contamination/illness are the most prevalent form of obsessions generally reported (Brown, 1998). In these cases, differentia-

tion can be relatively straightforward if rituals accompany the fear. In addition, specific phobias of illness involve more focused health-related fears than the pervasive concerns usually evident in OCD.

Differentiating OCD and depression is also an important issue, given the high rates of comorbidity between these conditions. Although figures vary across studies, as many as one-third of patients with OCD also meet criteria for coexistent depression or dysthymia (Antony et al., 1998a). In these cases, it can be important for treatment planning to identify which disorder is considered principal. Generally, the principal disorder is assumed to be that with the earlier onset (Turner & Beidel, 1988). Using this criterion, OCD more often is considered the principal diagnosis when both disorders are present (Antony et al., 1998a). There is support, however, for the notion that all anxiety and affective disorders share a similar biological pathophysiology, although environmental factors shape symptom expression (Kendler, Heath, Martin, & Eaves, 1987).

Of more recent interest in the literature, however, are issues concerning the relationship between OCD and a wide range of other psychiatric and neuropsychiatric disorders that, it is hypothesized, comprise a group of disorders known as the obsessive-compulsive spectrum disorders (Hollander, 1993; McElroy, Phillips, & Keck, 1994). Disorders proposed as members of this spectrum include the somatoform disorders (e.g., body dysmorphic disorder, hypochondriasis), eating disorders (e.g., anorexia nervosa, bulimia nervosa, and binge-eating disorder), impulse control disorders (e.g., trichotillomania, pathological gambling) and related symptoms (skin picking, nail biting, and compulsive buying), and movement disorders (e.g., Tourette's disorder, Sydenham's chorea). These disorders, it has been hypothesized, share common phenomenological features, patterns of comorbidity, family history, clinical course, treatment response, and neurobiological mechanism with OCD.

The proposed concept of obsessive-compulsive spectrum disorders has generated much controversy in the field. In particular, some authors have argued that this classification scheme is vague, overinclusive, and characterized by a lack of clear inclusion and exclusion criteria (Rasmussen, 1994). Other authors have argued that the spectrum disorders are part of an even broader class of affective disorders (McElroy, Hudson, & Pope, 1992). Subclassification schemes have also been proposed, and some include disorders of altered risk assessment, incompleteness/habit spectrum disorders, and psychotic spectrum disorders (Pigott, L'Heureux, Dubbert, Bernstein, & Murphy, 1994). Another perspective suggests that disorders along the obsessive-compulsive spectrum vary across a continuum of compulsivity versus impulsivity (Hollander & Cohen, 1996). In this scheme, compulsive disorders, it is proposed, reflect excessive harm avoidance and risk aversion, whereas impulsive disorders are characterized by minimization of harm and risk.

Empirical literature addressing the potential overlap between OCD and the other proposed spectrum disorders is limited at present. Nevertheless, in some cases, the apparent overlap is more striking than in others. It has been suggested that those disorders that would be classified along the compulsive end of the spectrum (e.g., the somatoform and eating disorders) are more similar to OCD than those proposed that fall along the impulsive end (e.g., impulse control disorders) (Goldsmith, Shapira, Phillips, & McElroy, 1998). The extant literature supports this notion, at least in part because of striking phenomenological similarities between OCD and body dysmorphic disorder (BDD), hypochondriasis, and eating disorders. In particular, preoccupations with perceived physical defects, serious disease, and food or body weight that are present in BDD, hypochondriasis, and eating disorders, respectively, strongly resemble the obsessions that occur in OCD. In addition, ritualistic behavior generally accompanies these other syndromes. For example, patients with BDD frequently check their appearance in the mirror, seek reassurance about the imagined physical defect, and perform excessive grooming behaviors. Patients with hypochondriasis often repetitively check physical symptoms, request medical treatment, and seek reassurance regarding health. Individuals with eating disorders also regularly report repetitive behaviors surrounding eating behaviors. In addition to these striking phenomenological similarities, there is some evidence that these disorders respond to pharmacological interventions (e.g., serotonergic reuptake inhibitors) and behavioral treatments (exposure and response prevention) that are the treatments of choice for OCD (Goldsmith et al., 1998).

Despite these areas of overlap between OCD and those spectrum disorders proposed, potentially important differences in these conditions are also evident. For example, both BDD and hypochondriasis generally are associated with greater levels of impaired insight than is typically seen in OCD. Additionally, bulimia nervosa and binge eating disorder are associated with more frequent impulsive behaviors than OCD. Finally, there is some evidence that hypochondrias and eating disorders also respond to nonserotonergic antidepressants that have not demonstrated efficacy in OCD (Goldsmith et al., 1998). Nevertheless, the possibility that these disorders are related in some way to OCD deserves additional empirical attention.

In the case of those disorders proposed that lie along the impulsive end of the spectrum, it is our opinion that differences among these disorders in phenomenology, neurobiology, and treatment far outweigh any similarities. The impulse control disorders (ICDs; e.g., pathological gambling, kleptomania, trichotillomania) and possible ICDs (e.g., nail biting, repetitive self-mutilation, skin picking) are characterized by repetitive behaviors over which patients report no control. These behaviors often, it is reported, have an anxiety-relieving function, and it is in these domains that there is some overlap with OCD. Other data also have suggested overlap between the ICDs and OCD in family history and treatment response (Goldsmith et al., 1998).

Despite these areas of overlap, other phenomenological, neurobiological, and treatment data suggest important differences between OCD and ICDs. The majority of literature in this area has addressed the potential overlap between OCD and trichotillomania (TM), a disorder characterized by repetitive hair pulling. In a review of this literature, Stanley and Cohen (1999) summarized areas of similarity and dissimilarity between these conditions. One major phenomenological difference included the fact that obsessional thoughts usually do not accompany repetitive hair pulling, although this type of cognitive activity is central to the diagnosis of OCD. In addition, hair pulling occurs in response not just to anxiety, but also to a variety of affective states, and the behavior frequently produces feelings of pleasure that are not characteristic of OCD. Moreover, sensory stimuli (e.g., itching, burning) are important precipitators of hair pulling, although these have no central role in OCD. Neurobiological and neuropsychological correlates of OCD and TM are also different, although the literature addressing these issues in TM is still somewhat limited. Finally, pharmacological treatment data for TM do not provide a consistent picture of the efficacy of serotonergic reuptake inhibitors, and the modes of behavioral treatment for TM (habit reversal training) and OCD (exposure and response prevention) are quite different. In summary, the range of important differences between these two syndromes calls into question the utility of combining them under a single spectrum of obsessive-compulsive-related disorders. However, Stanley and Cohen (1999) highlighted the notion that some subtypes of TM may reflect more overlap with OCD and further suggested that any appearance of association between these disorders may result from the heightened states of negative affect that accompany each. These hypotheses require further study.

Overall, the notion of an obsessive-compulsive spectrum of disorders continues to generate controversy in the field. Difficulties in assessing the utility of this scheme reflect in part the fact that there are not yet any established criteria for membership in this family of disorders. Furthermore, the amount of literature that has provided direct comparisons between patients with OCD and those with proposed related disorders remains limited.

## Epidemiology

The now well-known Epidemiological Catchment Area (ECA) survey conducted during the early 1980s indicated lifetime prevalence rates for OCD of 1.9 to 3.3% in five U.S. communities and an overall rate of 2.5% (Karno, Golding, Sorenson, & Burnam, 1988). These rates were much higher than any previous estimates and were confirmed by similar epidemiological, albeit smaller scale, surveys conducted at approximately the same time in the United States and Canada (Bland, Orn, & Newman, 1988; Henderson & Pollard, 1988). In all of these studies, however, interviews were conducted by lay interviewers, and it is notable that prevalence estimates were considerably lower in surveys using clinician interviewers (Faravelli, Degl'Innocenti, & Giardinelli, 1989; Nestadt, Samuels, Romanoski, Folstein, & McHugh, 1994). In fact, a more recent study confirmed that prevalence rates for OCD within a single sample were indeed lower when clinicians, rather than lay interviewers, conducted diagnostic interviews (Stein, Forde, Anderson, & Walker, 1997). Issues

such as lay interviewers' inexperience in establishing and labeling psychiatric symptoms and difficulty in estimating degree of dysfunction and distress are particularly relevant in this regard (Stein et al., 1997).

The limitations of the ECA study are well known and have been discussed in detail elsewhere (Beidel & Turner, 1991; McNally, 1994). The most striking of these, however, are the aforementioned potential for overdiagnosis due to use of lay interviewers and diagnostic structured interview tools that do not allow for follow-up questions to clarify patient reports. Of even more concern are recent data suggesting poor temporal stability of OCD diagnoses for a subset of ECA survey participants who were reassessed 12 months after the initial interview (Nelson & Rice, 1997). Taken together, these data call into question prevalence rates based on the ECA survey. It is unfortunate that the only subsequent large epidemiological survey conducted in the United States, the National Comorbidity Survey, failed to assess the prevalence of OCD (Kessler et al., 1994). As a result, the true prevalence of this disorder is now uncertain.

At least partly due to general difficulties in estimating prevalence rates, data are mixed with regard to the impact of ethnicity on the prevalence of OCD. Across all five ECA sites, figures indicated that lifetime OCD was significantly less prevalent among Black respondents than non-Hispanic White respondents (Karno et al., 1988). Data from the Los Angeles site alone indicated no difference in prevalence rates for OCD among Mexican-Americans and non-Hispanic Whites (Karno et al., 1989). When ECA data were compared with surveys that used similar methodology in Canada, Puerto Rico, Germany, Taiwan, Korea, Hong Kong, and New Zealand, relatively consistent prevalence figures emerged (1.9–2.5%), except Taiwan where the prevalence of OCD was only 0.7% (Weissman et al., 1994). In a more recent survey of more than 800 residents of Baltimore, OCD tended to be more prevalent among Whites (2.1%) than non-Whites (0.8%) (Nestadt et al., 1994). Clinical data also routinely show a greater prevalence of OCD among Whites than non-Whites (e.g., Antony et al., 1998a). It is not clear, however, that interview questions are always sensitive to ethnic differences in the experience or description of relevant symptoms. It is known, for example, that members of various minority groups tend to focus on somatic complaints in descriptions of anxiety-related symptoms and often present for assistance to medical rather than psychiatric clinics (Friedman, Hatch, Paradis, Popkin, & Shalita, 1993). Other sociocultural variables, including religious background, can also significantly impact the presentation and assessment of OCD symptoms (Okasha, Saad, Khalil, Seif El Dawla, & Yehia, 1994). Thus, more research using culturally sensitive diagnostic tools is needed to ascertain the impact of ethnicity on prevalence rates of OCD.

Epidemiological data generally have indicated that community prevalence rates are slightly higher for women than men (Henderson & Pollard, 1988; Karno et al., 1988; Weissman et al., 1994). However, data from the ECA survey indicated that gender effects were eliminated when other demographic variables were controlled statistically (Karno et al., 1988). Nevertheless, consistent gender differences have been demonstrated in the prevalence of specific obsessive-compulsive symptoms. In particular, women are significantly more likely than men to report washing and cleaning rituals (Khanna & Mukherjee, 1992; Minichiello et al., 1990), and there is some suggestion that men report more frequent sexual obsessions (Antony et al., 1998a). These findings further support the potential role of sociocultural variables in the presentation of OCD.

Gender differences have also been noted in the onset of OCD. Although the disorder most often begins between late adolescence and early adulthood, onset is earlier for males than females (Rasmussen & Eisen, 1990). Retrospective data have suggested that later onset for women may result from the appearance of initial symptoms during pregnancy or after childbirth (Neziroglu, Anemone, & Yaryura-Tobias, 1992; Sichel, Cohen, Dimmock, & Rosenbaum, 1993). However, these findings simply may reflect the notion that OCD often has its onset after a period of significant life stress, although data addressing this issue are almost uniformly collected retrospectively and produce questionable conclusions. Although few longitudinal studies have been conducted, the course of OCD is generally chronic and unremitting without treatment.

## Biological Contributions

In 1985, Turner, Beidel, and Nathan reviewed the available data that addressed biological factors in OCD. Included in the review were genetic and family studies, neurophysiological and neuropsychological studies, neuroanatomical studies, and biochemical and pharmacological studies. Turner et al. (1985) concluded that although biological factors correlated with OCD from the evidence available then, it did not appear that the disorder was strictly a biological abnormality. Rather, the most parsimonious explanation was that there might be a biological predisposition that leaves the individual more vulnerable to the development of OCD, perhaps from psychological and/or environmental stress. One important limitation of the studies reviewed in 1985 was that there were few data that directly assessed brain function, and inferences had to be made from indirect measures such as blood or plasma neurochemistry. During the past 15 years, advances in scientific and medical technology offer heretofore unavailable opportunities to directly assess brain structures and functions. In this section, the biological basis of OCD will be examined using biochemical and neuropharmacological studies, neuropsychological assessment, structural and functional neuroanatomy literature, and psychosurgery follow-up studies.

### Biochemistry and Neuropharmacology

Although they are an indirect assessment of brain function, data from biochemical challenge studies and pharmacological treatment outcome studies suggest that the orbital and cingulate cortex may be potential neuroanatomical sites of dysfunction in OCD. Data that address the neurochemistry of OCD have been collected under three conditions: steady-state assessment in untreated patients and comparisons to normal controls, pharmacological challenge studies in untreated patients, and changes in neurochemistry after pharmacological treatment. Each of these categories is discussed here.
**Biochemistry.** Initially, cerebral spinal fluid (CSF) studies of adult patients with OCD primarily assessed serotonin levels and activity, but the findings were inconsistent (e.g., Thoren, Asberg, Bertilsson, Mellstrom, Sjoqvist, & Traskman, 1980; Yaryura-Tobias, Neziroglu, & Bergman, 1976). Whereas some studies found higher levels of serotonin among OCD patients, others reported reduced levels. More recently, a broader range of substances has been investigated. For example, Swedo et al. (1992) examined eight different neurochemicals and their various combinations and found only a few significant differences between

patients with OCD and normal control subjects including a significant negative correlation between 5-HIAA concentration and one of eight baseline OCD severity ratings (whereas three of eight correlations were significant after 5 weeks of treatment with clomipramine). Before treatment, the concentration of arginine vasopressin (a stress-responsive neurohormone) was negatively correlated with OCD symptoms, whereas corticotropin releasing hormone (another stress-responsive neurohormone) did not differentiate the two groups. The authors concluded that arginine vasopressin might be related to OCD symptom severity whereas 5-HIAA might be associated with treatment response. However, as discussed in greater detail in the functional neuroanatomy section, the only comparison group used consisted of normal controls. Thus, it is unclear if the negative correlation is specific to OCD or whether it is present in other disordered mood states. Using similar methodology, Altemus et al. (1992) reported that those with OCD had significantly higher levels of arginine vasopressin and corticotropin releasing hormone compared to normal controls, similar to the findings of Swedo et al. (1992). However, in contrast to that study, Altemus et al. (1992) did not find a relationship between arginine vasopressin and any clinical rating of OCD. Corticotropin releasing factor level, on the other hand, was significantly related to scores on the Yale–Brown Obsessive-Compulsive scale but not with several other ratings of OCD. Thus, like the earlier studies that assessed serotonin, the relationship of these neurohormones to OCD is unclear.

Another CSF neuropeptide, somatostatin, has also been the subject of investigation (Altemus et al., 1993). As noted by these authors, when somatostatin is administered centrally to animals, it delays extinction of various behaviors or produces stereotyped behaviors that appear topographically similar to OCD rituals. When compared to those without a disorder, drug-free adult outpatients with OCD had higher levels of CSF somatostatin, a finding that is consistent with an earlier study of children with OCD (Kruesi et al., 1990). As Altemus et al. (1993) noted, the functional importance of the high somatostatin levels for patients with OCD is not known. What is known is that animal studies indicate an association of increased somatostatin with increased repetitive behaviors and that following pharmacotherapy with antidepressants, reductions occur in both OCD behav-

iors and somatostatin across multiple brain regions. However, the specificity of this decrease in somatostatin for reduction of OCD symptomatology is unclear (i.e., change also might occur in behaviors unrelated to OCD).

In contrast to assessment consisting solely of resting levels, a second series of studies used neuroendocrine challenge tests, most of which assessed serotonin (5-HT) function. These studies also produced inconsistent findings. Some reported increased 5-HT mediated responses after administering various pharmacological agents, whereas others reported normal or decreased responses (e.g., Fineberg et al., 1994; Fineberg, Roberts, Montgomery, & Cowen, 1997; Hewlett et al., 1992; Hollander et al., 1992; Lopez-Ibor et al., 1994; Lucey et al., 1992). As noted by Fineberg et al. (1997), these conflicting results indicate that 5-HT mediated neuroendocrine responses are inconsistent and probably do not play an important role in the pathophysiology of OCD.

**Neuropharmacology.** Numerous studies that date back to the late 1970s examined the response of various neurochemicals after treatment with selective serotonin reuptake inhibitors (SSRIs). A review of this extensive literature is beyond the scope of this chapter, and the interested reader is referred to Blier and de Montigny (1998). Two studies are presented here for illustration. In an early study, treatment with clomipramine produced decreases in platelet serotonin concentration and an increase in standing plasma norepinephrine (Flament, Rapoport, Murphy, Berg, & Lake, 1987). More recently, patients treated with fluvoxamine had a normalized plasma prolactin response to d-fenfluramine (a pharmacological challenge agent), in contrast to the abnormal (decreased) response before treatment (Monteleone, Catapano, Bortolotti, & Maj, 1997). Overall, this literature suggests that treatment with SSRIs may result in "normalization" of neurohormonal and neuroendocrine responses and that these changes are evident in areas of the brain that have been previously associated with dysfunction. For example, SSRIs enhance 5-HT release in the orbitofrontal cortex, but this enhanced release occurs only after a period of prolonged drug administration (e.g., after 8 weeks for paroxetine; Blier & de Montigny, 1998). These authors noted that because this neurochemical change in brain function occurs only after several weeks of pharmacotherapy, it is theoretically very important. It suggests that the mechanism of drug action is not simply by blocking serotonin re-uptake at the level of the individual synapse (which occurs almost immediately after drug ingestion). If this were the important mechanism of action, there should be an immediate decrease in OCD symptoms from taking the medication. Rather, the delayed onset of the clinical change is correlated with the time necessary to produce desensitization of the 5-HT terminals in the orbitofrontal cortex (Blier & de Montigny, 1998). Potentially, this is a very important finding in understanding brain pathology, but further studies are needed to verify this hypothesis.

In summarizing the literature on biochemistry and neuropharmacology, one of the most important limitations is that there are few studies that have used clinical control groups in addition to those without a psychiatric disorder. Thus, it is impossible to associate neurochemical changes specifically with OCD. For example, patients with anorexia nervosa show the same increased disregulation in arginine vasopressin as that of patients with OCD. Similarly, the positive correlation between arginine vasopressin and the dopamine metabolite HVA found in patients with OCD is also found in patients with schizophrenia (Altemus et al., 1992). Similarities in neurochemistry across individuals with diverse types of disorders suggest that reported significant differences between patients with OCD and normal controls may reflect a general stress response rather than the pathophysiology of a specific disorder.

## Neuropsychology

It is beyond the scope of this chapter to review all of the individual tests that have assessed cognitive functioning in OCD patients. Therefore, the discussion will be restricted to four general categories: general intellectual functioning, an "underinclusive" thinking style, frontal lobe impairment, and memory (Tallis, 1997). With respect to general intellectual functioning, some early studies reported above average intellect among patients with OCD. However, more recent studies have not supported these early findings. Furthermore, a few studies reported lower IQ scores in those with OCD (see Tallis, 1997 for a review). However, it is important to note that performance deficits usually occur on subtests that are timed, making it difficult to disentangle specific cognitive processing deficits from nonneurological influences on process-

ing speed such as obsessional slowness or meticulousness (see limitations section later).

Neuropsychological assessment has also addressed the concept of underinclusion, defined as the inability to organize and integrate experiences. As discussed by Tallis (1997), it has been hypothesized that the formal characteristics of obsessional thinking result in an inability to organize experiences, thus leading to an overdefinition of categorical boundaries. Thus, those with OCD are expected to be too exclusive in their classification strategies and thereby produce too many categories. Most data in support of this hypothesis come from studies of "anacastic personalities" or those with obsessive-compulsive personality disorder. Only one study that consisted of seven patients reported support for underinclusiveness in patients with a DSM-III diagnosis of OCD (Persons & Foa, 1984). As Tallis (1997) noted, the relationship of underinclusion to OCD etiology or symptomatology is unclear. Thus, although it might represent a particular cognitive style, it is unclear how underinclusiveness represents a biological abnormality.

A third type of neuropsychological testing assesses frontal lobe function and includes tests of abstract thinking, visual attention, response inhibition, and shifting of mental set (Tallis, 1997). Only in this latter category (i.e., shifting of mental set or the ability to choose an alternative strategy when the first is no longer effective) have there been consistent reports of differences between those with OCD and normal controls. However, these tests usually are timed, and again, the differences must be interpreted cautiously (see later).

Neuropsychological assessment has also addressed memory (also known as mnestic) deficits, but again there is little consistency with respect to outcome. For example, Purcell and her colleagues (Purcell, Maruff, Kyrios, & Pantelis, 1998), using an extensive test battery, reported that patients with OCD had deficits only in spatial working memory, spatial recognition, and motor initiation and execution, particularly when there was increasing task difficulty. These differences were not affected by medication, clinical severity, or general levels of anxiety and depression. The deficits reflect an inability to develop a strategy to meet task demands and were similar to, but less severe than, those found in individuals with documented focal frontal lobe lesions. Interestingly, PET studies assessing brain activation for this type of task in normal subjects implicated the dorso-lateral frontal cortex, an area identified as a possible site for psychosurgery for intractable OCD (Owen, Evans, & Petrides, 1996). Overall, Purcell et al. (1998) concluded that the pattern of cognitive deficits exhibited by OCD patients suggests a syndrome of frontal-subcortical dysfunction. However, another recent study that used a similar sample of adults with OCD found differences in cognitive processing that reflected involvement of the anterior cingulate but not the dorsolateral prefontal circuit (Schmidtke, Schorb, Winkelmann, & Hohagen, 1998). Thus, these two recent studies using similar patient samples report very different results and illustrate the inconsistency in findings across the literature.

Tallis (1997) succinctly reviewed the neuropsychological assessment literature and reached a number of conclusions. First, some studies have not identified cognitive deficits in patients with OCD; however, those data are often discounted in favor of studies that show positive differences. Second, appropriate control groups are not always used, and when they are, deficits are apparent only when patients with OCD and normal controls are compared. Few differences emerge when other types of anxiety disorder patients constituted the control group. This suggests that differences found in comparison to normal control subjects reflect anxiety or general distress, rather than deficits specific to OCD. Third, Tallis (1997) argued that group differences based on timed tests should be discounted because "obsessional slowness" might also result from nonneurological factors such as intrusive cognitions or indecisiveness. When time penalties were excluded from analyses, performance differences between OCD patients and normal controls were substantially reduced (e.g., Christiansen, Kim, Dyksen, & Hoover, 1992). Fourth, memory deficits were most commonly documented, particularly memory related to visual and visuospatial functioning, and suggest basal ganglia involvement. Even if one hypothesizes that the checking behaviors in patients with OCD result from memory deficits, it does not explain why those who feel compelled to check do so selectively (e.g., locks, doorknobs or electrical appliances; Tallis, 1997). Furthermore, there is no documented relationship between memory deficit severity and clinical symptom severity in OCD patients, again suggesting that these deficits may be a correlate of, but not the cause of, OCD.

In summary, it is clear that some patients with OCD sometimes exhibit cognitive deficits. However, there is no consistent pattern of results, although deficits or abnormalities in frontal-striatal functioning are the most commonly implicated. Few studies have used clinical control groups, and thus it is unclear if reported deficits are specific to OCD or merely reflect an abnormal mood state. Furthermore, neuropsychological assessment does not indicate whether these deficits result from neuroanatomical structural or functional abnormalities. We now turn our attention to these studies.

## Neuroanatomy

In this section, we will examine the long-term follow-up of psychosurgery for OCD patients in an attempt to understand neuroanatomical contributions to OCD. In addition, the results from recent sophisticated neuroimaging techniques will be presented.

**Psychosurgery.** One of the earliest associations between OCD and brain function is the use of psychosurgery to ameliorate intractable symptoms. Although not developed specifically for OCD, psychosurgery for this disorder has its roots in the initial prefrontal leukotomies first introduced by Moniz in the mid-1930s. Four different surgical procedures have been most commonly used: anterior cingulotomy, subcaudate tractotomy, limbic leukotomy, and anterior capsulotomy. The different operating procedures, their neuroanatomical basis, their effectiveness, and potential side effects are reviewed in detail by Chiocca and Martuza (1990). Briefly, anterior cingulotomy interrupts fibers in the cingulate bundle. This area is part of the Papez circuit which theoretically is linked to anxiety but not specific OCD symptoms. Anterior cingulotomy results in few side effects, and the treatment success rate is approximately 50%. A different surgical procedure, limbic leukotomy, with an 89% success rate, combines the production of lesions to the bilateral cingulate area (as in anterior cingulotomy) with lesions to the orbitomedial frontal areas. Neurons in these latter areas are believed critical in the formation of specific OCD symptoms (as opposed to general anxiety). The other two procedures, subcaudate tractotomy and anterior capsulotomy, have improvement rates that range from 50–70%, lower than for limbic leukotomy. Furthermore, as noted by Chiocca and Martuza (1990), these latter two procedures were more likely than either anterior cingulotomy or limbic leukotomy to result in negative "personality changes" such as increased aggressiveness, lack of inhibition, hypomania, irritability, outspokenness, and emotional shallowness.

Several studies have reported long-term followup of patients treated with psychosurgery. Sachdev, Hay, and Cummig (1992) reported 10-year follow-up data for twenty-six patients who had surgical lesions involving the cingulate area, the bilateral orbitomedial cortex, or their combination. Consistent with the results presented by Chiocca and Martuza (1990), the cingulate lesion alone group was less improved at follow-up compared to those who had orbitomedial or combined cingulate and orbitomedial lesions. Again, this may suggest that cingulate lesion target sites are associated with general anxiety but not with specific OCD symptoms. In another follow-up study, Irle and her colleagues (Irle, Exner, Thielen, Weniger, & Ruther, 1998) evaluated sixteen patients who had received leukotomies during the 1970s. Patients had either ventromedial frontal lesions, ventral striatum plus ventromedial frontal lesions, or dorsally extended lesions (to isolate the precallosal part of the cingular gyrus) plus ventromedial frontal lesions. Those with frontostriatal lesions (i.e., subjects in one of the first two groups) were the most improved. Interestingly, those with OCD plus obsessive-compulsive personality disorder were the least improved. A substantial percentage of those with ventral striatum lesions developed substance abuse postoperatively, which led the authors to suggest that this area may be associated with addictive behaviors, although this suggestion involves a good deal of circular logic.

As noted by Sachdev et al. (1992), recent MRI scans of some of the surgical sites indicated that the original lesions missed their mark (e.g., the cingulate bundle). Similarly, among their followup sample, Jenike and Baer (1992) also reported MRI confirmation that not all of the original lesions were precisely placed. Although now MRI confirmation of the surgical site is obtained before initiating surgery, conclusions based on the currently available follow-up data must be interpreted cautiously. For example, is the procedure itself ineffective or are the lower success rates the result of inaccurate lesion placement? Obviously, controlled trials are not appropriate, but MRI technology will allow more accurate placement and in the future, help clarify this issue. Second, although

individuals may improve, the follow-up studies do not allow for a determination of the patients' final clinical status, that is, evaluation of improvement is based on percentage change on the Yale–Brown Obsessive Compulsive Inventory (Y-BOCS), but actual scale scores are not presented. Therefore, the findings are difficult to interpret because mere reporting of change scores does not allow determining whether the patient is still symptomatic. Relatedly, improvement ratings from the current long-term follow-up studies are based on changes in pre- and posttreatment scores, primarily using the Y-BOCS. However, many of the pretreatment ratings were made retrospectively and therefore are subject to all of the biases of this form of assessment. Third, there is indication of a circular argument in the conclusions that are drawn from these findings. For example, if a lesion at a particular site results in a decrease in activity, is that concrete evidence that this is the site of the disorder? There is evidence, for example, that those who have had psychosurgery have lower IQ scores and lower scores on the Wisconsin Card Sorting Test than those who have not undergone the procedure (Irle et al., 1998). In this case, psychosurgery results in a decrement in a broad range of purposeful behaviors and abilities, not just a decrease in OCD symptoms. A final issue that must be noted is that these surgical procedures typically are performed on only the most intractable cases, patients who do not respond to any other form of therapy. This suggests that these patients have the most complicated form of OCD and findings from this group do not necessarily represent the pathology of all patients with this disorder.

**Structural Neuroanatomy.** Structural imaging studies primarily use computerized tomography (CT) or magnetic resonance imaging (MRI). Compared to CT, MRI produces enhanced spatial resolution, better distinction between gray and white matter and greater visualization of neuroanatomic structures (Saxena et al., 1998). For example, three CT studies (Behar et al., 1984; Insel et al., 1983; Luxenberg et al., 1988) were negative for the presence of anatomical lesions, although Luxenberg et al. (1988) reported atrophy at the head of the caudate nucleus. However, MRI studies (Garber et al., 1989; Kellner et al., 1991) reported that the caudate nucleus of OCD patients appeared normal. Breiter et al. (1994) reported retrocallosal white matter abnormalities in six patients with OCD. Scarone et al. (1992) reported increased right caudate volume in twenty treated patients with OCD, whereas Robinson et al. (1995) reported bilateral reduced mean caudate volumes using a sample of twenty-six patients with OCD. Aylward et al. (1996) examined caudate nucleus and putamen volumes of twenty-four adults with OCD and twenty-one control subjects using MRI. There were no differences between those with OCD and normal controls in any of the areas assessed. Finally, using the more powerful short echo $^1$H magnetic resonance spectroscopy ($^1$H-MRS), Bartha et al. (1998) did not find reduced caudate volumes. There was evidence, however, of lower $N$-acetylaspartate levels (a brain metabolite whose decline might indicate a decrease in neuronal density) in the left corpus striatum, suggesting reduced neuronal density in this region, but the significance of this finding is unclear. As noted by Insel (1992) and Trivedi (1996), the results of CT and MRI studies do not consistently document structural brain abnormalities in patients with OCD who did not have a concurrent neurological disorder (Insel, 1992). Methodological variations across studies, variations in illness chronicity, and prior psychotropic medication use may contribute to the inconclusive data (Rosenberg & Keshavan, 1998). Because of the overall lack of positive findings, researchers have turned their attention to the possibility of abnormalities in neuroanatomical function, as opposed to structure.

**Functional Neuroanatomy.** In contrast to the lack of consistent findings using structural imaging techniques, there is a growing consistent literature on functional imaging. Functional imaging techniques use either single photon emission computed tomography (SPECT), positron emission tomography (PET), or functional MRI. SPECT and PET use trace amounts of ligands that are "labeled" with radiation-emitting isotopes that measure cerebral metabolism or cerebral blood flow (Saxena et al., 1998). This material is injected into the blood stream, and the PET or SPECT scanners detect the radiation that the isotopes emit, thereby quantifying their concentration in various brain regions. Because SPECT uses single photon emitters and the PET isotopes emit positrons and two gamma protons (i.e., PET uses a double rather than a single signal; see Saxena et al., 1998), PET has higher spatial resolution than SPECT. With respect to the activity being measured, in nonstarvation conditions, cerebral glucose is a highly sensitive indicator of cerebral function, and cerebral blood flow is highly correlated with glucose metabolism (Saxena et al., 1998). As with the biochemical and neuropharmacological studies, functional imaging assessments are usually conducted under one of three sets of conditions: symptomatic patients in a resting state, symptomatic patients under challenge conditions, and symptomatically improved patients (after treatment). With these caveats and conditions in mind, the results of functional imaging studies are examined here.

The majority of studies examined symptomatic patient samples under resting conditions. The series of studies by Baxter and his colleagues illustrate this approach. Baxter et al. (1987, 1988, 1989) assessed cerebral glucose metabolic rates in patients with OCD. Specific sample characteristics differed slightly across the three studies, but the results were fairly consistent. Those with OCD had increased F-fluorodeoxyglucose uptake (indicative of elevated metabolic rates) in the overall cerebral hemispheres, heads of the caudate nuclei, orbital gyri, and ratio of orbital gyrus relative to the ipsilateral hemisphere. Other studies reported increased perfusion in the prefrontal cortex and cingulate (Machlin et al., 1991) and increased normalized regional glucose metabolism in the right orbitofrontal cortex and left anterior frontal cortex (Nordahl et al., 1989). Rubin et al. (1992) reported elevated uptake in the dorsal parietal cortex, the left posterofrontal cortex, and the orbitofrontal cortex, whereas Swedo et al. (1989) reported decreased uptake in the head of the caudate nuclei and increased metabolic rates in the right prefrontal and left anterior cingulate regions. Furthermore, in this latter study, there was a significant relationship between metabolic activity and both state and trait measures of OCD and anxiety. As illustrated before and noted by Trivedi (1996), taken together, the results of resting studies suggest abnormal activity in the orbitofrontal cortex, anterior cingulate, and caudate nuclei.

A second functional imaging strategy assessed symptomatic OCD patients under challenge conditions. For example, Zohar and his colleagues (Zohar et al., 1989) assessed 10 OCD patients at rest, when exposed to actual "contamination," and during imaginal flooding. Compared to resting, there was increased regional cerebral blood flow (rCBF) only in the temporal region after imaginal flooding, whereas there was a decrease in rCBF across a wide cortical area, including the temporal lobes, during *in vivo* exposure. Why these two forms of exposure, which are functionally equivalent with respect to treatment effects, should produce such different types of brain activity is unclear. Similarly, McGuire et al. (1994) used brief exposures to contaminants and found the urge to perform rituals increased rCBF in the orbitofrontal cortex, neostriatum, globus pallidus, and thalamus. Feelings of anxiety were related to increases in rCBF in the hippocampus and the posterior cingulate. Rauch et al. (1994) reported that, compared to resting, exposure to individually tailored stimuli resulted in increased rCBF in the right caudate nucleus, left anterior cingulate cortex, and the bilateral orbitofrontal cortex.

In addition to psychological challenges, pharmacological challenges such as *meta*-chlorophenylpiperazine (*m*-CPP) challenge have been used. Usually, *m*-CPP increases symptoms in OCD patients. In addition to confirming increases in OC symptoms, Hollander et al. (1991) reported an increase in rCBF, particularly in the frontal lobes following *m*-CPP challenge. In contrast, a study by Pian and his colleagues (Pian, Westenberg, Den Boer, De Bruin, & van Rijk, 1998) compared patients with OCD to healthy controls. In this case, *m*-CPP did not induce or exacerbate OC symptoms. In addition, rather than an increase in rCBF, there was a decrease in rCBF across various brain regions, including the cerebellum and whole brain, and in the frontal cortex, caudate nucleus, putamen, and thalamus. Thus, although the psychological challenge studies implicate the orbitofrontal cortex, anterior cingulate, striatum, and thalamus (Trivedi, 1996), the results of pharmacological challenges do not implicate any one particular area.

Finally, assessing patients with OCD after successful pharmacological or behavioral treatment, or optimally, pre- and post treatment, provides another approach to functional brain imaging studies. Studies that assess patients treated with MAOIs or SSRIs indicate that remediation of OCD symptoms also results in decreased regional cerebral blood flow or cerebral metabolism in the caudate nuclei, orbitofrontal cortex, medialfrontal cortex, cingulate cortex, thalamus, caudate nucleus, posterofrontal and dorsal parietal regions, right lateral temporal, and left posterior

thalamic regions (Baxter et al., 1988, 1992; Benkefalt et al., 1990; Hoehn-Saric et al., 1991; Perani et al., 1995; Rubin et al., 1995; Swedo et al., 1992; Trivedi, 1996). Similarly, PET scans of patients who successfully completed behavior therapy (flooding and response prevention) also indicated bilateral decreases in caudate glucose metabolic rates (Baxter et al., 1992). In addition, decreases were significantly greater in those who had a good, as opposed to a poor response (Schwartz, Stoessel, Baxter, Martin, & Phelps, 1996). Furthermore, when the patients from these latter two studies were combined, there were pretreatment significant correlations in glucose metabolic rates among the right orbital gyri, head of the caudate nucleus, and thalamus. At posttreatment, these correlation coefficients were no longer significant. The significance of this finding is that in samples of normal controls and patients with untreated unipolar depression, brain activity in these regions is not correlated. The fact that there is such a correlation among untreated patients with OCD "suggests that 'coupling' of activity among elements in this cortico-striato-thalamic circuit may be related to the expression of OCD symptoms" (Schwartz et al., 1996, p. 112). Using a different approach, Aylward et al. (1996) conducted a quantitative meta-analysis of the functional neuroimaging literature. The results indicated no consistent abnormalities of the caudate nucleus. These authors concluded that although theories of OCD suggest a dysfunction of the caudate nucleus, structural and functional MRI studies currently do not support this hypothesis. Trivedi (1996) concluded that, despite some discrepancies, the results of functional imaging studies implicate dysfunction in the prefrontal cortex, cingulate, and basal ganglia and that these neurocircuitry loops are hyperactive in OCD. Inconsistencies may be due to the use of different technologies, scanning environments, or methods for analyzing and comparing regions.

Insel (1992) also noted a number of other methodological and theoretical caveats that must be considered when interpreting these data. First, many of the studies use small sample sizes and make multiple comparisons, thereby increasing the experimental error rate. Second, there is the issue of anatomical ambiguity. For example, the orbitofrontal cortex is often defined somewhat differently by different investigators and although some of the areas represent contiguous regions topographically, they also represent areas that are "cyboarchitecturally and functionally distinct" (Insel, 1992, p. 740). Furthermore, again there is the issue of epiphenomenon versus causality, that is, abnormality does not equal causality. Increases in metabolic activity in some areas of the brain may be compensating for decreased function in other areas, as is the case for neurodegenerative disorders (Insel, 1992).

In addition to these limitations, a close perusal of this literature requires even further consideration of these outcomes. In all of the studies mentioned, those with OCD were compared to individuals without a psychiatric disorder or in one case, patients with untreated mood disorders. Thus, an alternative interpretation for the findings is that the increased blood flow or glucose metabolism is not specific to OCD but may be the result of any type of psychological disorder, and in particular, an anxiety disorder. In a recent SPET (single photon emission tomography) study, Lucey et al. (1997) examined cerebral blood flow in patients with OCD, panic disorder with agoraphobia, posttraumatic stress disorder (PTSD), and normal controls. Those with OCD or PTSD had significantly higher rCBF but only in the bilateral superior frontal cortex and the right caudate nuclei. Whole brain blood flow correlated positively with anxiety but not with any specific disorder. These authors suggested that the similarities in blood flow between the OCD and PTSD groups were consistent with the shared cognitive symptomatology of these two groups (obsessive thinking, intrusive imagery). Another hypothesis is that they could represent groups with the most severe anxiety symptoms. Consistent with the latter hypothesis, because increased whole brain activity did not differ among the three anxiety groups, the most parsimonious explanation is that increased rCBF in certain brain regions is common across all of the anxiety groups. Thus, some elevations in brain activity reflect abnormal mood state and not necessarily a particular disorder. Only when appropriate comparison groups are used can conclusions about disorder specificity be made. Finally, it is important to remember that despite these sophisticated approaches, PET and SPECT basically assess ongoing biochemical activity in the brain, not the cause of a disorder (Baxter et al., 1988). Thus, the data from functional neuroimaging studies merely identify sites of abnormal cerebral activity and do not identify etiology.

## A Neurodevelopmental Model of Obsessive-Compulsive Disorder?

Rosenberg and Keshavan (1998) recently tried to draw together these various literatures into a neurodevelopmental model of OCD. First, they noted that several lines of evidence suggest that OCD may result from a neurodevelopmental rather than a degenerative process: (1) a number of cases of OCD begin in childhood; (2) there is a similarity between many OCD rituals and "developmentally normal" childhood rituals; and (3) neurological soft signs present at the onset of the disorder do not show any exacerbation, even when OCD symptoms progress and increase in severity. Second, as noted from the data presented earlier, if there is a region of the brain involved in OCD, it is probably part of the ventral prefrontal cortical region (VPFC). Recall that this region has been identified from psychosurgery (e.g., Jenike & Baer, 1992) and functional neuroimaging studies (e.g., Baxter et al., 1988), as well as treatment response studies (e.g., Baxter et al., 1992). This zone is also connected to limbic structures in the cingulate and anterior lobes (Rosenberg & Keshavan, 1998). Importantly, developmental brain morphology studies indicate that there is substantial maturation in the brain cortex from birth up to about 20 years of age. To test their hypothesis, Rosenberg and Keshavan (1998) conducted an MRI study of twenty-one treatment-naive pediatric outpatients with OCD and twenty-one normal control subjects. Those with OCD had significantly larger anterior cingulate volumes than normal control subjects but did not have differences in posterior cingulate, dorsolateral prefrontal cortex, amygdala, hippocampal, superior temporal gyral, or whole temporal lobe volumes. Additionally, there was a significant positive correlation between anterior cingulate volume and severity of obsessional, but not compulsive symptoms. Furthermore, there was a trend ($p = .055$) for a significant correlation between age and cingulate volumes among the control patients ($r = .45$), but not among the patients with OCD ($r = -.12$). Rosenberg and Keshavan (1998) suggested that the lack of correlation between age and anterior cingulate volumes in patients with OCD may represent a delay in the normal neuronal "pruning" process (i.e., the normal developmental reduction in the number of neuronal circuits), leading to larger caudate volumes and more neuronal circuits. Because these circuits are involved in regulating purposive behaviors, abnormality in these circuits (as evidenced by dysplasia) could manifest itself clinically as an inability to regulate behavior or conversely, the production of excessive behaviors such as excessive washing or checking behaviors.

Although this is an interesting model, as the authors noted, it is not without its limitations. First, again the study is based on a small number of patients, and it is one of the few studies to date with a pediatric population. As illustrated throughout this chapter, initial positive findings are often followed by negative findings. Second, the relationship between age and anterior cingulate volume was a statistically significant trend but did not meet the traditional criterion for significance. One or two additional subjects could substantially affect the correlation coefficient. Thus, replicative studies are necessary before one can draw firm conclusions. Third, more sophisticated neuroimaging techniques such as PET are necessary to delineate the relationship more clearly between developmental neurochemical changes in serotonin and the neurobehavioral and functional neuroanatomic development in OCD (Rosenberg & Keshavan, 1998).

## PANDAS

If there are no structural brain abnormalities, then what might cause abnormal brain functioning? Recently, there has been increased speculation that at least some children who develop obsessive-compulsive disorder may do so in response to an external pathogen (in this case β-hemolytic streptococcal infection). Studies of Sydenham's chorea, childhood onset OCD, and Tourette's syndrome isolated a subgroup of children with either OCD or Tourette's who had a symptom course marked by abrupt, dramatic exacerbations which were temporally related to β-hemolytic streptococcal infection (Swedo et al., 1997). Additional studies then identified a group of children whose first onset of OCD occurred after streptococcal infection. This group was identified by the term PANDAS (pediatric autoimmune neuropsychiatric disorders associated with streptococcal infections; for a review, see Swedo et al., 1998). Several studies (Murphy et al. 1997; Swedo et al., 1997) identified an antigen marker (D8/17) which appears more frequently in children with PANDAS

or Sydenham's chorea compared to normal controls. Importantly, those with PANDAS did not have Sydenham's chorea, thus leading the authors to suggest that these two disorders may share a similar poststreptococcal autoimmunity. Although these findings are intriguing, it is important to recognize that even if PANDAS is associated with one form of OCD, it apparently accounts for only a small percentage of childhood OCD cases. For example, beginning by soliciting 270 children who had a sudden onset of symptomatology, fifty (18.5%) had PANDAS. However, even among that fifty, only ten (20%) had OCD only, whereas 16% had tics alone and the remainder of the sample (64%) had subclinical OCD and tics or OCD and tics. Therefore, this means that only 3% of those originally identified by this abrupt onset symptom picture had "classic" OCD. Furthermore, because the rate of streptococcal infection decreases dramatically after puberty, this explanation would not account for onsets of OCD that occur during adolescence and adulthood.

### Summary of Biological Contributions

In summary, the conclusions that could be drawn from the current literature are remarkably similar to those drawn by Turner et al. (1985). In short, much of the current evidence regarding altered brain functioning in patients with OCD is conflictual. Although some data suggest that the ventral prefrontal cortical region is the most likely area that is involved, the evidence is far from overwhelming. As presented earlier, Tallis (1997) noted that a number of neuropsychological investigations have not found differences in those with OCD, but these negative studies are often discounted in favor of those finding group differences. Similarly, Aylward et al. (1996) did not find any consistent abnormalities of the caudate nucleus when meta-analytic procedures were used to analyze the available data. They noted that, although there might be a theoretical basis suggesting a dysfunction of the caudate nucleus, structural and functional MRI studies do not provide empirical support. The issue of a theoretical basis is important because in many instances, it appears that the biological assessment studies are not grounded in any theory explaining why abnormalities might be expected. Rather, much of the data generated appear to have been collected because of the availability of technology or procedures rather than a clear theory-driven research program.

Another major issue is that even if specific abnormalities are identified, do these abnormalities represent activity specific to OCD, or do they merely reflect a general stress response? Certainly, the few studies that used clinical comparison groups did not identify any abnormalities specific to OCD. Furthermore, none of these data necessarily indicate a biological etiology for this disorder and, except for Rosenberg and Keshavan (1998) and perhaps Swedo et al. (1997), no one has yet addressed the question of what produces the altered or abnormal brain function. Even if the D8/17 antigen plays a role, PANDAS accounts for only a few cases of those who meet diagnostic criteria for OCD. In conclusion, it is clear that all of the data presented are fully consistent with the alternative proposal that these data represent epiphenomena, or correlates of this disorder and although biological structures and functions might be altered as a result of the disorder, the current database indicates that it is premature to refer to OCD as a neuropsychiatric disorder.

## Cognitive Contributions

A second major development during the past 20 years was the emergence of cognitive theory as a theoretical explanation for anxiety disorders (Beck, Emery, & Greenberg, 1985). Just as there is no one behavioral theory, there are different cognitive conceptions of anxiety. However, the basic premise of all approaches is that emotional disorders develop from distorted and maladaptive thought processes and that treatment of anxiety states requires altering these dysfunctional thought processes. In many ways, the development of an effective treatment approach for OCD is one of the real success stories of this century. Although OCD had been a clearly identified syndrome for at least a century (e.g., Rachman, 1985), it remained the most retractable nonpsychotic mental disorder until the 1970s. During this decade, Victor Meyer described the successful treatment of OCD at Middlesex Hospital in London, relying on strategies rooted in the two-factor theory of learning (Mowrer, 1939) and findings from basic laboratory studies of avoidance learning. The success of this treatment approach, which has come to be known as response prevention and exposure (flooding), has been well documented and is considered the

standard psychological treatment at this time (Stanley & Turner, 1995).

It has been said that during the past 20 years or so, psychology has undergone a cognitive revolution, and the influence of cognitive approaches have heavily influenced clinical theorizing and treatment. Actually, it is somewhat surprising that it took so long for cognitive theories regarding OCD to develop because a major part of the phenomena of OCD is cognitive (i.e., obsessions). One explanation for the failure of cognitive theorists to address OCD might be the success of behavioral treatments. However, despite that success, clearly not all of those who suffer from OCD benefit from the treatment, and clearly there are major gaps in current behavioral conceptions of the disorder. One of the primary deficiencies of behavioral explanations of OCD is reliance on the equipotentiality principle, that is, all stimuli have the equal potential to be conditioned and capable of instigating the OCD syndrome. There is considerable evidence that this is not the case because certain types of stimuli are much more likely to serve this role than others. Salkovskis (1985) discussed these issues and concluded that behavioral theory was inadequate to account for the OCD syndrome, and although his critique of behavioral outcome data led him to a conclusion different from most others, it seems clear that there are major deficiencies in current behavioral theory regarding the nature of OCD. Although several theorists have proposed cognitive conceptualizations (e.g., Carr, 1974; McFall & Wollersheim, 1979), Salkoviskis provided the most elaborate cognitive explanation, maintaining that treatment derived from this model should improve outcome for those suffering from OCD. We will examine this theory and then turn to an evaluation of treatment derived from this model.

As noted, Salkovskis (1985, 1996) proposed the most comprehensive cognitive theory of OCD, which begins with the premise that intrusive thoughts are everyday occurrences, experienced by almost everyone. In some individuals, the intrusive thoughts activate preexisting cognitive schemata, which in turn, evaluate the intrusive thoughts in a negative light (e.g., it is bad to have a thought about killing my spouse). In addition to appraising the thought as "bad," individuals believe that they have the "pivotal power" to bring about or prevent the negative consequences (i.e., killing the spouse). These beliefs and cognitive schemata generate distress that leads to efforts to

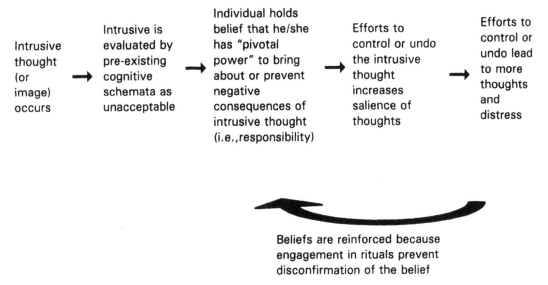

**Figure 1.** Salkovskis' cognitive model of OCD.

control or undo the thoughts (i.e., avoidance and ritualistic behavior) thereby (1) increasing their salience and frequency and (2) creating emotional distress. The theory also postulates a feedback loop; beliefs about "pivotal power" (i.e., responsibility) actually are reinforced because the rituals designed to eliminate the thoughts prevent disconfirmation of the responsibility beliefs. The theory is based on several basic assumptions to which we now turn our attention (see Fig. 1).

**Everyday Intrusive Thoughts.** The first, and perhaps the most crucial, premise is that obsessional thoughts are commonplace and are experienced by everyone; those with and without OCD. However, important questions surround the content and frequency of intrusive thoughts in individuals without OCD (or any type of emotional distress). In the earliest study that assessed form and content, Rachman and DeSilva (1978) reported that those without OCD endorse the presence of intrusive thoughts and that the intrusions are similar in form to abnormal obsessions. This basic conclusion has been consistently cited as evidence that normals and obsessional patients do not differ in experiencing intrusive cognitive phenomena. However, there are a number of questions regarding the nature of the data generated in this seminal study. For example, the sample was not random, and although the individuals were described as "normal people," no diagnostic interviews were conducted to screen out the presence

of psychological disorders. It is well known that samples of unselected participants often include those who suffer from numerous disorders. In this study, participants were given a list of intrusive thoughts and were asked (1) to indicate if they had experienced these thoughts and impulses, (2) how frequently they had the thoughts, and (3) whether they could be easily dismissed. However, it does not appear that these terms were further operationalized. Eighty percent of the respondents endorsed having either thoughts or images in the past month; 66% of that group reported that the thoughts occurred ten times per month or less. Stated differently, only 20% of this nonclinical sample reported intrusive thoughts as often as once per day. Similarly, only 9% of those reporting intrusive images reported their occurrence as often as once per day. Thus, although the form and content of these intrusive cognitive phenomena were endorsed by individuals who ostensibly did not have OCD, the frequency was substantially less than that found in those with the disorder.

It appears that as the results of this study have been cited in subsequent years, there has been a "drift" in the manner in which the outcome has been described. Rachman and DeSilva's (1976) outcome has been cited as evidence that "repetitive, intrusive thoughts" are common in normal populations, but considering the questions raised above, this conclusion might be premature. Indeed, recent studies (e.g., England & Dickerson,

1988; Freeston, Ladouceur, Thibodeau, & Gagnon, 1991, 1992) that are cited as supportive of the "normal, everyday" occurrence of intrusive thoughts actually do not examine the frequency with which these thoughts occur. For example, England and Dickerson (1988) described intrusions as repetitive, spontaneous thoughts and asked undergraduate students to identify the most memorable intrusive thought experienced in the past 2 weeks. However, no data were reported regarding the actual frequency of the identified thought and the instructions did not request the students to identify their most repetitive thought, only the most memorable one. Similarly, the studies by Freeston et al. (1991, 1992) also defined cognitive intrusions as repetitive phenomena. Yet, the data presented indicate that over a 1-month period, the frequency of "repetitive thoughts" averaged 4.5 occurrences. Thus, in this case, repetitive means one intrusive thought per week, which is far less than the definition of repetitive necessary for a diagnosis of OCD. Therefore, even if those without a disorder sometimes experience cognitive phenomena resembling the form and content of obsessions, the frequency and distress are substantially less. The issue of cognitive intrusions among those without OCD remains very much open and in our judgment, extant data call into question this critical component of the Salkovskis theory.

**Evaluation of the Intrusive Thoughts as "Bad" Using Preexisting Cognitive Schemata.** If one accepts the premise that cognitive intrusions are common in the general population, it is possible that what differentiates those with OCD is their negative evaluation of the thoughts, as Salkovskis theorizes. However, what is not clear from existing cognitive explanations is why some individuals apply negative evaluations, whereas others do not. Put another way, why is it that some people have "OCD schemata" and some do not? This is an issue for all of cognitive theory of emotional disorders and the premise seems to be that the cognitive schemata are preexisting and dormant and are activated by the intrusive thoughts. Cognitive theorists have argued that such schemata are not "hard wired" but have failed to clearly articulate their origins.

**Schemata May Include the Belief That One Has the "Pivotal Power" to Bring About or Prevent Negative Consequences.** Within the cognitive framework, the negative automatic

thoughts are related to ideas of personal responsibility to produce OCD. The appraisal of personal responsibility is what produces OCD, rather than anxiety or depression. Again, as with the etiology of the cognitive schemata, the cognitive theorists are silent on the origins of this pivotal power belief. Despite this uncertainty about their origins, the issue of responsibility has received considerable attention in recent years, and studies have been conducted using both clinical and nonclinical samples.

With respect to clinical samples, Lopatka and Rachman (1995) examined how exposure to different levels of responsibility affected urges to check and the level of discomfort, using a within-subject design. Subjects were asked to encounter their most feared event. In the low responsibility condition, the subject was informed that the experimenter would take complete responsibility for any untoward event, would make any necessary reparations, and signed a statement to that effect. In the high responsibility condition, the patient had to sign a statement assuming full responsibility for any untoward event that occurred. Following this manipulation, the level of perceived responsibility was rated on a verbal analogue scale ranging from 0 to 100. Those in the low condition averaged 16.47 on the rating scale versus 90.17 for the high condition, suggesting that the manipulation was successful. When compared to the control condition, decreased feelings of responsibility were associated with decreased anxiety and urges to check. However, increased feelings of responsibility (over the control condition) did not produce statistically higher levels of anxiety and urges to check. Interestingly, the authors noted that the strong influence of reduced responsibility on decreased compulsive checking may not be replicable for compulsive cleaners. Interestingly, a similar conclusion was drawn by Rheaume, Ladouceur, Freeston, and Letarte (1995).

In another study of responsibility and OCD, Shafran (1997) used a modified between-subject design and manipulated the level of responsibility through the presence/absence of the experimenter when the subject was exposed to a feared stimulus. In the absence of the investigator, responsibility for the perceived threat while engaged in an exposure task was rated higher (60.9 on a scale of 0–100) than when the participant was in the presence of the experimenter (44.54). This difference, though statistically significant, did not produce the magnitude of same group differences as the Lopatka and Rachman (1995) study, and it is not clear why the mere presence of the experimenter would be sufficient to change beliefs about responsibility. Those with trichotillomania or tics, for example, can often control their repetitive behavior when in the presence of others, but it would be difficult to accept that the reason for the control is that they turn over "responsibility" for their tics/hair pulling to others. Nevertheless, subjects in the high responsibility condition reported significantly more discomfort/anxiety, were more fearful that the consequences would happen, and had a significantly higher urge to perform the compulsion. However, there were no significant differences in ratings of responsibility for their thoughts or ratings of control over the threat. Furthermore, the correlation between perceived responsibility and the urge to neutralize was $r = .42$ for the high responsibility condition and $r = .38$ for the low responsibility condition. Although not tested statistically, it is unlikely that these correlations are significantly different. Finally, this study did not find differences in responsibility based on type of compulsion; however, subsample sizes consisted of fourteen checkers and eight cleaners, and thus, there may have been insufficient power to determine group differences.

Most of the studies of responsibility have used nonclinical (i.e., undergraduate student) populations. Ladouceur et al. (1995) randomly assigned participants to high and low responsibility conditions and had them perform a sound recognition task. In a replicative sample, a manual classification task was used. In the high responsibility condition, subjects were told that their responses were very important because they would be used by an insurance company (experiment one) or a pharmaceutical company (replicative sample) and could significantly impact the health and safety of others. In both tasks, the manipulation was judged successful. Those in the high responsibility group reported more anxiety during the tasks. However, only in the manual classification task did participants also check more often and report more preoccupation with errors. One problem with the interpretation of this study is that the authors did not discuss why the manipulation was successful in one instance but not the other. Thus, the results must be considered equivocal.

In a similar study, Ladouceur et al. (1997) noted that Salkovskis' definition of responsibility includes both the constructs of pivotal power and potential negative consequences. Therefore, in an effort to examine the influence of these two variables more closely, the authors created four combinations of perceived influence and negative consequences. Then, each group engaged in a sorting task. In the high negative consequences, high influence condition, subjects were told that their role was crucial to the project's success and their results would be decisive and directly influential. In the high influence only condition, subjects were told that they were part of a small sample and their results would directly influence the project but that consequences would be minimal. In the high negative consequences only condition, subjects were told that there were high negative consequences but their direct influence was minimal because 2000 people were included in the sample. Subjects in the fourth condition were told that they were part of a large group and the consequences were minimal. The manipulation was successful in that the four groups varied significantly in the independent variable ratings of perceived influence and negative consequences. Only when there were both high levels of perceived influence and negative consequences did the subjects perceive themselves as more responsible, endorse more doubt, and were more preoccupied with errors, suggesting that both variables (influence and negative consequences) were necessary for an inflated sense of responsibility.

Two other studies directly attempted to assess the responsibility definition put forth by cognitive theorists. Rheaume et al. (1995) examined Salkovskis' definition (responsibility is the belief that one possesses pivotal power to provoke or prevent subjective crucial negative outcomes). Using fourteen situations relevant to OCD patients and nonclinical samples, participants rated possible negative outcomes in terms of severity, probability, personal influence, pivotal influence, and responsibility. Ratings of personal influence and pivotal influence were highly correlated with ratings of responsibility, whereas correlations of ratings of severity and probability of outcome were only weakly and moderately correlated, respectively. The findings were generally replicated in a second sample and may be interpreted to indicate that the definition of responsibility may be reduced to whether or not individuals perceive that they have the power to control the events.

In the strongest study that examined the relationship of responsibility to OCD, Rachman and his colleagues (Rachman, Thordarson, Shafran, & Woody, 1995) developed a reliable self-report scale (the Responsibility Appraisal Questionnaire; RAQ). Unlike previous investigations, care was taken to develop a responsibility scale that was free of OCD-related items. Thus, the scale assessed five content areas: responsibility for property damage, responsibility for physical harm to others, responsibility in social contexts, positive outlook for responsibility, and thought-action fusion (TAF). The results indicated that only the TAF subscale was associated with measures of responsibility. When RAQ scores of those with high levels of obsessionality were compared to the rest of the sample, again only scores on the TAF subscale differentiated the groups. As noted by these authors, the results indicate that the original view of inflated responsibility in OCD patients requires revision. Feelings of broad overresponsibility were not substantiated. In fact, in contrast to cognitive theories, these authors noted that there does not appear to be a unitary factor of responsibility. The inflated responsibility associated with obsessions is situation-specific, idiosyncratically connected primarily to checking behaviors, and does not preclude that an individual with OCD may easily accept other forms of responsibility.

**Belief in Pivotal Power Leads to Efforts to Control or Undo the Thoughts and Creates Emotional Distress.** Returning to the tenets of cognitive theory, one of the loopholes in the cognitive explanation of OCD is that if individuals believe that they have the power of prevention, why should the mere thought of such an event elicit such negative distress and produce rituals? Why do reassuring thoughts counteract the negative thought? In other words, why does the negative thought, coupled with a belief in personal power to prevent the event, still result in the levels of distress commonly seen in OCD patients? According to O'Kearny (1998), the Salkovskis theory needs some revision because it disregards Rachman's (1993) thought-action fusion concept as a component of responsibility. With respect to the latter, those with OCD consider thinking about an unacceptable behavior as the equivalent of carrying it out. Those with OCD often describe feeling that thinking about the behavior is the same as actually committing the behavior and that the feelings of responsibility extend to having the thoughts in addition to actually committing the act. Simply

put, those with OCD often confuse having the thought about an abhorrent behavior with actually carrying out the behavior and are distressed by the occurrence of the thought. According to O'Kearny (1998), it is only if this thought-action fusion is included will cognitive theories provide an appropriate cognitive explanation of OCD.

**Efforts to Control or Undo Increase the Salience of Thoughts and Result in More Thoughts and Distress.** A comprehensive review of this aspect of the theory is beyond the scope of this chapter but is provided by O'Kearny (1998). As one example, laboratory studies of the paradoxical effects of controlling or suppressing thoughts reveals that there is an increased frequency of a thought when an attempt is made to suppress it. However, subjects in these studies do not report volitional disturbances or compulsions. To summarize this discussion, cognitive theory, like every other theory of OCD, must account for the apparent failure of the patient's ability to neutralize the intrusive thought as evidenced by the repetitious and compulsive qualities of the behavior. Cognitive theory fails to do so because it does not recognize the importance of self-doubt and ambivalence. By focusing exclusively on cognitions, it fails to recognize the affective and motivational bases of the disorder. The premise of all cognitive theories (including Salkovskis') is that initial intrusive thoughts are emotionally neutral but, as noted by O'Kearny (1998), the content almost always has to do with harm happening to another or oneself. O'Kearny (1998) identified the absence of an account of affect as a major deficiency of the theory. In short, this argument returns, once again, to the age-old argument of the prominence of cognition versus affect.

One recent study provides support for the notion that any theory of OCD will need to account for the variable of affect. Scarrbelotti, Duck, and Dickerson (1995) examined the impact of extraversion, neuroticism, psychoticism, and responsibility in predicting discomfort from obsessions and compulsions. The results indicated that, among undergraduate students, the more emotionally labile (i.e., neurotic) and responsible a person is, the more likely that person is to be distressed by obsessions and compulsions. These findings point to characteristics of the individual outside of the cognitive dimensions that are apparently important. Although this study does not determine whether emotionality or cognition "came first," it is clear that affect, in addition to cognition, is necessary to explain the distress experienced by those with obsessions and compulsions and attempts to foster a purely cognitive explanation are likely to fall short.

## Treatment Based on Cognitive Theories

We mentioned earlier that treatments based on a behavioral conception have resulted in remarkably positive outcomes. In recent years, positive outcomes for cognitive strategies have been reported but supportive empirical data often are lacking. Several authors (Freeston, Rheaume, & Ladouceur, 1996; van Oppen & Arntz, 1984) described how traditional cognitive strategies such as disputing catastrophic and responsibility beliefs by examining their rational basis or by using behavioral experiments could be used to treat OCD. Similarly, Shafran and Somers (1998) described two cases of "cognitive intervention" for adolescents with OCD. The therapist explained to the patient that attempting to suppress thoughts often led to an increase in thoughts, just as trying not to think of a "white bear" produced images of a white bear. It was reported that patients understood the connection to their own attempts to suppress their intrusive obsessions and that being provided with an alternative, benign explanation for the significance of intrusive thoughts resulted in "marked" or "excellent" improvement (not further defined), although it appears that in at least one of the cases, behavioral interventions also were used.

There are few studies where the effectiveness of cognitive therapy for OCD has been examined empirically. In the earliest studies, Emmelkamp and his colleagues (Emmelkamp, Visser, & Hoekstra, 1988; Emmelkamp & Beens, 1991) compared Rational Emotive Therapy (RET) with self-controlled exposure *in vivo*. Furthermore, in the 1991 study, all subjects later received exposure *in vivo*. The results indicated that both interventions produced improvement in self-report measures of affect and OCD symptoms. Improvement was maintained at a 6-month follow-up, and there were no significant differences between the groups. However, inasmuch as RET includes behavioral procedures, it is impossible to untangle exactly what the effective components were.

More recent studies attempted to apply cognitive interventions that do not include behavioral procedures such as exposure. Ladouceur and his colleagues (Ladouceur, Leger, Rheaume, & Dube, 1996) used a multiple baseline design to evaluate "pure" cognitive therapy (e.g., identification and correction of automatic thoughts and development of adequate perceptions or responsibility) to treat four OCD patients with checking rituals. No exposure or response prevention procedures were used. Up to thirty-two treatment sessions were used and at posttreatment, Y-BOCS scores were decreased by 52–100%, and gains were maintained at 12-month follow-up for two of the four patients. The other two had some relapse, although only one required additional treatment in the form of traditional behavior therapy. Jones and Menzies (1998) treated eleven patients with washing/contamination rituals using a procedure called danger ideation reduction therapy (DIRT), which was directed solely at decreasing danger-related expectancies and did not include behavioral procedures. Compared to a wait list control group, those treated with DIRT had significant decreases in several self-report inventories of affect and OCD symptoms, although examination of actual raw scores revealed that the changes were quite minimal in clinical significance. In the only large, randomized trial, seventy-one patients were randomized to either cognitive therapy or self-controlled exposure *in vivo* (van Oppen, de Haan, van Balkom, Spinhoven, et al., 1995). Both groups evidenced significant improvement. Finally, two recent reviews (James & Blackburn, 1995; Sica, 1998) and one meta-analysis (van Balkom et al., 1994) all suggest that it is premature to draw conclusions about the efficacy of cognitive interventions (without the inclusion of behavioral procedures) for treating OCD. Thus, although there is much enthusiasm for using cognitive interventions to treat OCD, at the present time empirical data are lacking.

In summary, it was noted in the biological section of this chapter that patients with OCD do not appear to have basic cognitive deficits. In this section, cognitive theories of OCD were examined and the cognitive phenomena that are part of this disorder were highlighted. Interest in the cognitive aspects of this disorder has resulted in the creation of an Obsessive Compulsive Cognitions Working Group (1997). Although their concept is not a cognitive theory, this group has put forth the following conceptualization regarding cognitive phenomena. First, there are three levels of cognitions: intrusions, appraisals, and assumptions or beliefs. Appraisals are involved in perceiving threat, and different levels of assumptions interact with one another and influence the contents and processes of appraisal. Thus, appraisals are defined in part from one's beliefs. Second, there are seven belief domains relevant to OCD: inflated responsibility, overimportance of thoughts, beliefs about the importance of controlling thoughts, overestimation of threat, intolerance of uncertainty, perfectionism, and fixity of beliefs (overvalued ideation). Like the cognitive theories that have been proposed, this statement of cognitive phenomena does not explain the etiology of the disorder. However, it does provide the basis for a series of testable hypotheses that might further understanding of this disorder. Furthermore, although there is widespread acceptance that cognitive interventions alone are useful for OCD, to date few controlled, randomized group trials have examined this issue. Thus, final conclusions on the usefulness of these procedures, either alone or in combination with traditional behavioral procedures, await further investigation.

## Conclusions

Descriptions of OCD have remained remarkably consistent throughout the years with very little variation in the various iterations of the DSM. Indeed, as discussed here, there have been no significant empirical findings to alter the basic way in which OCD has been defined since its description in DSM-III. However, recent studies have raised important questions in need of further study, and some of these were discussed. These include the concept of overvalued ideation, the possible importance of symptom subtyping, and the issue of subclassification schemes. Studies that address these issues could reveal information important for the way we think about the psychopathology of the condition as well as for the way treatment is conceptualized.

The issue of comorbidity of mental disorders is critical for the field because the presence of high overlap of symptoms and syndromes raises interesting questions regarding the nature of mental disorders but also the adequacy of our current diagnostic system of categorical disorders. Overlapping anxiety symptoms and syndromes are commonplace among the anxiety disorders, including OCD. Of particular interest in OCD is the controversial concept of OCD Spectrum Disorder,

the suggestion that a number of disorders share the basic ingredient of obsessionality. Although the relationship between OCD and many of the disorders discussed in this regard seems less than compelling, its relationship to others (e.g., Tourette's Syndrome, Somatoform Disorders) rests on a stronger empirical foundation. Here, too, however, despite symptom similarly, important differences exist. Hence, based on the current empirical literature, it is somewhat premature to think of OCD as a spectrum of disorders.

The past two decades have been marked by a resurgence of interest in the biology of mental illness. Similarly, within psychology, cognitive approaches to understanding and treating emotional disorders have been prominent. With respect to biology, there has been intense study, but to date there has been no clear delineation of the pathophysiology of the disorder. At this juncture, the findings are disparate and do not cohere meaningfully or provide insight into possible biological mechanisms of OCD. The most consistent findings are that serotonin plays some role and the portion of the brain most likely involved is the orbitofrontal cortex. Yet, even findings in these areas are not consistent, and there is no clear indication as to whether serotonin is involved in the etiology of OCD or whether the noted anomalies are secondary effects of some other disordered system. Similar conclusions pertain to abnormalities of the orbitofrontal cortex. In our view, one reason for the lack of progress in this area is that much of the research has taken place outside the context of cohesive biological theories. Much of the research has emerged from the availability of new technology (e.g., PET) or as the result of sweeping attempts to find relevant biological variables. Our understanding of the basic biological underpinnings of OCD are not likely to be revealed until more systematic theory-driven studies are conducted.

Cognitive research in OCD has been very similar to biological research. That is to say, very little has been based on cognitive theory rooted in basic cognitive science. The only cognitive explanation of OCD that approaches the formality of a theory is that of Sakovskis. As was discussed here, this explanation falls short of providing a full explanation of OCD, and there is a lack of unequivocal empirical support for its basic premises. Furthermore, there is no evidence that treatments that embody cognitive principles improve outcome above that of response prevention and flooding (James & Blackburn, 1995; Sica, 1998).

Overall, we must conclude that recent biological and cognitive research have not significantly improved our understanding of the phenomenology, etiology, or treatment of OCD. Although it is true that pharmacological treatment using selective serotonin inhibitors produces positive treatment outcomes in OCD, it is not more effective than response prevention and flooding, and it has a considerably higher relapse rate. Thus, response prevention and flooding remain the treatment of choice for OCD (Stanley & Turner, 1995).

# References

Abramowitz, J. S., & Foa, E. B. (1998). Worries and obsessions in individuals with obsessive-compulsive disorder with and without comorbid generalized anxiety disorder. *Behaviour Research and Therapy, 36,* 695–700.

Altemus, M., Pigott, T., Kalogeras, K. T., Demitrack, M., Dubbert, B., Murphy, D. L., & Gold, P. W. (1992). Abnormalities in the regulation of vasopressin and corticotropin releasing factor secretion in obsessive-compulsive disorder. *Archives of General Psychiatry, 49,* 9–20.

Altemus, M., Piggott, T., L'Heureux, F., Davis, C. L., Rubinow, D. R., Murphy, D. L., & Gold, P. W. (1993). CSF somatostatin in obsessive-compulsive disorder. *American Journal of Psychiatry, 150,* 460–464.

American Psychiatric Association. (1994). *Diagnostic and statistical manual of mental disorders* (4th ed.). Washington, DC: Author.

Antony, M. M., Downie, F., & Swinson, R. P. (1998a). Diagnostic issues and epidemiology in obsessive-compulsive disorder. In R. P. Swinson, M. M. Antony, S. Rachman, & M. A. Richter (Eds.), *Obsessive-compulsive disorder: Theory, research, and treatment* (pp. 3–32). New York: Guilford.

Antony, M. M., Roth, D., Swinson, R. P., Huta, V., & Devins, G. M. (1998b). Illness intrusiveness in individuals with panic disorder, obsessive compulsive disorder, or social phobia. *Journal of Nervous and Mental Disease, 186,* 193–197.

Aylward, E. H., Harris, G. J., Hoehn-Saric, R., Barta, P. E., Machlin, S. R., & Pearlson, G. D. (1996). Normal caudate nucleus in obsessive-compulsive disorder assessed by quantitative neuroimaging. *Archives of General Psychiatry, 53,* 577–584.

Baer, L. (1994). Factor analysis of symptom subtypes of obsessive compulsive disorder and their relation to personality and tic disorders. *Journal of Clinical Psychiatry, 55,* 18–23.

Ball, S. G., Baer, L., & Otto, M. W. (1996). Symptom subtypes of obsessive-compulsive disorder in behavioral treatment studies: A quantitative review. *Behaviour Research and Therapy, 34,* 47–51.

Bartha, R., Stein, M. B., Williamson, P. C., Drost, D. J., Neufeld, R. W. J., Carr, T. J., Canaran, G., Densmore, M., Anderson, G., & Razzaque Siddiqui, A. (1998). A short echo $^1$H spectroscopy and volumetric MRI study of the corpus

striatum in patients with obsessive-compulsive disorder and comparison subjects. *American Journal of Psychiatry, 155,* 1584–1591.

Baxter, L. R., Jr., Phelps, M. E., Mazziotta, J. C., Guze, B. H., Schwartz, J. M., & Selin, C. E. (1987). Local cerebral glucose metabolic rates in obsessive-compulsive disorder: A comparison with rates in unipolar depression and in normal controls. *Archives of General Psychiatry, 44,* 211–218.

Baxter, L. R., Jr., Schwartz, J. M., Mazziotta, J. C., Phelps, M. E., Pahl, J. J., Guze, B. H., & Fairbanks, L. (1988). Cerebral glucose metabolic rates in non-depressed patients with obsessive-compulsive disorder. *American Journal of Psychiatry, 145,* 1560–1563.

Baxter, L. R., Jr., Schwartz, J. M., Phelps, M. E., Mazziotta, J. C., Guze, B. H., Selin, C. E., Gerner, R. H., & Sumida, R. M. (1989). Reduction of prefrontal cortex glucose metabolism common to three types of depression. *Archives of General Psychiatry, 46,* 253–260.

Baxter, L. R., Schwartz, J. M., Bergman, K. S., Szuba, M. P., Guze, B. H., Maziotta, J. C., Akazraju, A., Selin, C. E., Ferng, H.-K., Munford, P., & Phelps, M. E. (1992). Caudate glucose metabolic rate changes with both drug and behavior therapy for obsessive-compulsive disorder. *Archives of General Psychiatry, 49,* 681–689.

Beck, A. T., Emery, G., & Greenberg, R. L. (1985). *Anxiety disorders and phobias: A cognitive perspective.* New York: Basic Books.

Behar, D., Rapoport, J. L., Berg, C. J., Denckla, M. B., Mann, L., Cox, C., Fedio, P., Zahn, T., & Wolfman, M. G. (1994). Computerized tomography and neuropsychological test measures in adolescents with obsessive-compulsive disorder. *American Journal of Psychiatry, 141,* 363–369.

Beidel, D. C., & Turner, S. M. (1991). Anxiety disorders. In M. Hersen & S. M. Turner (Eds.), *Adult psychopathology and diagnosis,* 2nd ed. (pp. 226–278). New York: Wiley.

Benkefalt, C., Nordahl, T. E., Semple, W. E., King, A. C., Murphy, D. L., & Cohen, R. M. (1990). Local cerebral glucose metabolic rates in obsessive-compulsive disorder: Patients treated with clomipramine. *Archives of General Psychiatry, 47,* 840–848.

Bland, R. C., Orn, H., & Newman, S. C. (1988). Lifetime prevalence of psychiatric disorders in Edmonton. *Acta Psychiatrica Scandinavica, 77,* 24–32.

Blier, P., & de Montigny, C. (1998). Possible serotonergic mechanisms underlying the antidepressant and anti-obsessive-compulsive disorder responses. *Society of Biological Psychiatry, 44,* 313–323.

Breiter, H. C., Filipek, P. A., Kennedy, D. N., Baer, L., Pticher, D. A., Olivares, M. J., Rensha, W. P. F., & Caviness, V. S. (1994). Retrocallosal white matter abnormalities in patients with obsessive-compulsive disorder [letter]. *Archives of General Psychiatry, 51,* 663–664.

Brown, T. A. (1998). The relationship between obsessive-compulsive disorder and other anxiety-based disorders. In R. P. Swinson, M. M. Antony, S. Rachman & M. A. Richter (Eds.), *Obsessive-compulsive disorder: Theory, research, and treatment* (pp. 207–226). New York: Guilford.

Brown, T. A., Moras, K., Zinbarg, R. E., & Barlow, D. H. (1993). Diagnostic and symptom distinguishability of generalized anxiety disorder and obsessive-compulsive disorder. *Behavior Therapy, 24,* 227–240.

Calvocoressi, L., Lewis, B., Harris, M., Trufan, S. J., Goodman, W. K., McDougle, C. J., & Price, L. H. (1995). Family accommodation in obsessive-compulsive disorder. *American Journal of Psychiatry, 152*, 441–443.

Carr, A. T. (1974). Compulsive neurosis: A review of the literature. *Psychological Bulletin, 81*, 311–318.

Chiocca, E. A., & Martuza, R. L. (1990). Neurosurgical therapy of obsessive-compulsive disorder. In M. A. Jenike, L. Baer, & W. E. Minichiello (Eds.), *Obsessive-compulsive disorders* (pp. 283–294). Chicago: Year Book Medical.

Christiansen, K., Kim, S. W., Dyksen, M. W., & Hoover, K. M. (1992). Neuropsychological performance in obsessive-compulsive disorder. *Biological Psychiatry, 31*, 4–18.

Eisen, J. L., Phillips, K. A., Baer, L., Beer, D. A., Atala, K. D., & Rasmussen, S. A. (1998). The Brown Assessment of Beliefs Scale: Reliability and validity. *American Journal of Psychiatry, 155*, 102–108.

Eisen, J. L., & Rasmussen, S. A. (1993). Obsessive compulsive disorder with psychotic features. *Journal of Clinical Psychiatry, 54*, 373–379.

Emmelkamp, P. M. G., Visser, S., & Hoekstra, R. J. (1998). Cognitive therapy versus exposure in vivo in the treatment of obsessive-compulsives. *Cognitive Therapy and Research, 12*, 103–114.

Emmelkamp, P. M. G., & Beens, H. (1991). Cognitive therapy with obsessive-compulsive disorder: A comparative evaluation. *Behavior Research and Therapy, 29*, 291–300.

England, S. L., & Dickerson, M. (1988). Intrusive thoughts: Unpleasantness not the major cause of uncontrollability. *Behaviour Research and Therapy, 26*, 279–282.

Faravelli, C., Degl'Innocenti, B. G., & Giardinelli, L. (1989). Epidemiology of anxiety disorders in Florence. *Acta Psychiatrica Scandinavica, 79*, 308–312.

Fineberg, N. A., Cowen, P. J., Kirk, J. W., & Montgomery, S. A. (1994). Neuroendocrine responses to intravenous L-tryptophan in obsessive-compulsive disorder. *Journal of Affective Disorders, 32*, 97–104.

Fineberg, N. A., Roberts, A., Montgomery, S. A., & Cowen, P. J. (1997). Brain 5-HT function in obsessive-compulsive disorder. *British Journal of Psychiatry, 171*, 280–282.

Flament, M. F., Rapoport, J. L., Murphy, D. L., Berg, C. J., & Lake, R. (1987). Biochemical changes during clomipramine treatment of childhood obsessive-compulsive disorder. *Archives of General Psychiatry, 44*, 219–225.

Foa, E. B. (1979). Failures in treating obsessive-compulsives. *Behaviour Research and Therapy, 17*, 169–176.

Foa, E. B., & Kozak, M. J. (1995). DSM-IV field trial: Obsessive compulsive disorder. *American Journal of Psychiatry, 152*, 90–96.

Freeston, M. H., Ladouceur, R., Thibodeau, N., & Gagnon, F. (1991). Cognitive intrusions in a non-clinical population. I. Response style, subjective experience, and appraisal. *Behaviour Research and Therapy, 29*, 585–597.

Freeston, M. H., Ladouceur, R., Thibodeau, N., & Gagnon, F. (1992). Cognitive intrusions in a non-clinical population. II. Associations with depressive, anxious, and compulsive symptoms. *Behaviour Research and Therapy, 30*, 263–271.

Freeston, M. H., Rheaume, J., & Ladouceur, R. T. (1996). Correcting faulty appraisals of obsessional thoughts. *Behaviour Research and Therapy, 34*, 433–446.

Friedman, S., Hatch, M., Paradis, C. M., Popkin, M., & Shalita, A. R. (1993). Obsessive compulsive disorder in two black ethnic groups: Incidence in an urban dermatology clinic. *Journal of Anxiety Disorders, 7*, 343–348.

Garber, H. J., Ananth, J. V., Chiu, L. C., Griswold, V. J., &

Oldendorf, W. (1989). Nuclear magnetic resonance study of obsessive-compulsive disorder. *American Journal of Psychiatry, 146*, 1001–1005.

George, M. S., Trimble, M. R., Ring, H. A., Sallee, F. R., & Robertson, M. M. (1993). Obsessions in obsessive-compulsive disorder with and without Gilles de la Tourette's syndrome. *American Journal of Psychiatry, 150*, 93–97.

Goldsmith, T., Shapira, N. A., Phillips, K. A., & McElroy, S. L. (1998). Conceptual foundations of obsessive-compulsive spectrum disorders. In R. P. Swinson, M. M. Antony, S. Rachman, & M. A. Richter (Eds.), *Obsessive-compulsive disorder* (pp. 397–425). New York: Guilford.

Henderson, J. G., & Pollard, C. A. (1988). Three types of obsessive compulsive disorder in a community sample. *Journal of Clinical Psychology, 44*, 747–752.

Hewlett, W. A., Vinogarov, S., Martin, K., Berman, S., & Csernansky, J. G. (1992). Fenfluramine stimulation of prolactin on obsessive-compulsive disorder. *Psychiatry Research, 42*, 81–92.

Hoehn-Saric, R., Pearlson, G. D., Harris, G. L., Machlin, S. R., & Camargo, E. E. (1991). Effects of fluoxetine on regional cerebral blood flow in obsessive-compulsive patients. *American Journal of Psychiatry, 148*, 1243–1245.

Hollander, E. (Ed.). (1993). *Obsessive-compulsive-related disorders*. Washington, DC: American Psychiatric Press.

Hollander, E., & Cohen, L. J. (1996). Psychobiology and psychopharmacology of compulsive spectrum disorders. In J. Oldham, E. Hollander, & A. E. Skodol (Eds.), *Impulsivity and compulsivity* (pp. 167–195). Washington, DC: American Psychiatric Press.

Hollander, E., DeCaria, C. M., Nitescu, A., Gilly, R., Suckow, R. F., Cooper, T. B., Gorman, J. M., Klein, D. F., & Liebowitz, M. R. (1992). Serotonergic function in obsessive-compulsive disorder: Behavioural and neuroendocrine responses to oral *m*-chlorophenylpiperazine and fenfluramine in patients and health volunteers. *Archives of General Psychiatry, 49*, 21–28.

Hollander, E., DeCarla, C. M., Saoud, J. B., et al. (1991). M-CPP activated regional cerebral blood flow in obsessive-compulsive disorder [abstract]. *Biological Psychiatry, 29*, 170A.

Hollander, E., Stein, D. J., Kwon, J. H., Rowland, C., Wong, C., Broatch, J., & Himelein, C. (1997). Psychosocial function and economic costs of obsessive-compulsive disorder. *CNS Spectrums, 2*, 16–25.

Horesh, N., Dolberg, O. T., Kirschenbaum-Aviner, N., & Kotler, M. (1997). Personality differences between obsessive-compulsive disorder subtypes: Washers versus checkers. *Psychiatry Research, 71*, 197–200.

Insel, T. R. (1992). Toward a neuroanatomy of obsessive-compulsive disorder. *Archives of General Psychiatry, 49*, 739–744.

Insel, T. R., Donnelly, E. F., Lalakea, M. L., Alterman, I. S., & Murphy, D. L. (1983). Neurological and neuropsychological studies of patients with obsessive-compulsive disorder. *Biological Psychiatry, 8*, 741–751.

Irle, E., Exner, C., Thielen, K., Weniger, G., & Ruther, E. (1998). Obsessive-compulsive disorder and ventromedial frontal lesions: Clinical and neuropsychological findings. *American Journal of Psychiatry, 155*, 255–263.

James, I. A., & Blackburn, I. M. (1995). Cognitive therapy with obsessive-compulsive disorder. *British Journal of Psychiatry, 166*, 444–450.

Jenike, M. A., & Baer, L. (1992). Psychosurgical treatment of obsessive-compulsive disorder. *Archives of General Psychiatry, 49,* 583–584 (letter).

Jones, M. K., & Menzies, R. G. (1998). Danger ideation reduction therapy (DIRT) for obsessive-compulsive washers. A controlled trial. *Behaviour Research and Therapy, 36,* 959–970.

Karno, M., Golding, J. M., Burnam, M. A., Hough, R. L., Escobar, J. I. Wells, K. M., & Boyer, R. (1989). Anxiety disorders among Mexican Americans and non-Hispanic whites in Los Angeles. *The Journal of Nervous and Mental Disease, 177,* 202–209.

Karno, M., Golding, J. M., Sorenson, S. B., & Burnam, A. (1988). The epidemiology of obsessive-compulsive disorder in five US communities. *Archives of General Psychiatry, 45,* 1094–1099.

Kellner, C. H., Jolley, R. R., Holgate, R. C., Austin, L., Lydiard, R. B., Laraia, M., & Ballenger, J. C. (1991). Brain MRI in obsessive-compulsive disorder. *Psychiatry Research, 36,* 45–49.

Kendler, K. S., Heath, A. C., Martin, N. G., & Eaves, L. J. (1987). Symptoms of anxiety and symptoms of depression: Same genes, different environments? *Archives of General Psychiatry, 44,* 451–457.

Kessler, R. G., McGonagle, K. A., Zhao, S., Nelson, C. B., Hughes, M., Eshleman, S., Wittchen, H.-U., & Kendler, K. S. (1994). Lifetime and 12-month prevalence of DSM-III-R psychiatric disorders in the United States: Results from the National Comorbidity Survey. *Archives of General Psychiatry, 51,* 8–19.

Khanna, S., & Mukherjee, D. (1992). Checkers and washers: Valid subtypes of obsessive-compulsive disorder. *Psychopathology, 25,* 283–288.

Koran, L. M., Thienemann, M. L., & Davenport, R. (1996). Quality of life for patients with obsessive-compulsive disorder. *American Journal of Psychiatry, 153,* 783–788.

Kozak, M. J., & Foa, E. B. (1994). Obsessions, overvalued ideas, and delusions in obsessive-compulsive disorder. *Behaviour Research and Therapy, 32,* 343–353.

Kruesi, M. J. P., Swedo. S., Leonard, H., Rubinow, D. R., & Rapoport, J. L. (1990). CSF somatostatin in childhood psychiatric disorders: A preliminary investigation. *Psychiatric Research, 33,* 277–284.

Ladouceur, R., Rheaume, J., Freeston, M. H., Aublet, F., Jean, K., Lachance, S., Lnglois, F., & De Pokomandy-Morin, K. (1995). Experimental manipulations of responsibility: An analogue test for models of obsessive-compulsive disorder. *Behavior Research and Therapy, 33,* 937–946.

Ladouceur, R., Leger, E., Rheaume, J., & Dube, D. (1996). Correction of inflated responsibility in the treatment of obsessive-compulsive disorder. *Behaviour Research and Therapy, 34,* 767–774.

Ladouceur, R., Rheaume, J., & Aublet, F. (1997). Excessive responsibility in obsessional concerns: A fine grained experimental analysis. *Behaviour Research and Therapy, 35,* 423–427.

Leckman, J. F., Grice, D. E., Boardman, J., Zhang, H., Vitale, A., Bondi, C., Alsobrook, J., Peterson, B. S., Cohen, D. J., Rasmussen, S. A., Goodman, W. K., McDougle, C. J., & Pauls, D. L. (1997). Symptoms of obsessive-compulsive disorder. *American Journal of Psychiatry, 154,* 911–917.

Leonard, H. L., Lenane, M. C., Swedo, S. E., Rettew, D. C., Gershon, E. S., & Rapoport, J. L. (1992). Tics and Tourette's disorder: A 2- to 7-year follow-up of 54 obsessive-compulsive children. *American Journal of Psychiatry, 149,* 1244–1251.

Lopatka, C., & Rachman, S. J. (1995). Perceived responsibility and compulsive checking: An experimental analysis. *Behaviour Research and Therapy, 33,* 673–684.

Lopez-Ibor, J. J., Sias, J., & Vinas, R. (1994). Obsessive-compulsive disorder and in depression. In S. A. Montgomery & T. H. Corn (Eds.), *Psychopharmacology of depression* (pp. 185–217). Oxford: Oxford University Press.

Lucey, J. V., Costa, D. C., Adshead, G., Deahl, M., Busatto, G., Gacinovic, S., Travis, M., Pilowsky, L., Ell, P. J., Marks, I. M., & Kerwin, R. W. (1997). Brain blood flow in anxiety disorders. *British Journal of Psychiatry, 171,* 346–350.

Lucey, J. V., O'Keane, V., Butcher, G., Clare, A. W., & Dinan, T. G. (1992). Cortisol and prolactin responses to *d*-fenfluramine in non-depressed patients with obsessive-compulsive disorder: A comparison with depressed and healthy controls. *British Journal of Psychiatry, 161,* 517–521.

Luxenberg, J. S., Swedo, S. E., Flament, M. F., Friedland, R. P., Rapoport, J., & Rapoport, S. I. (1988). Neuroanatomical abnormalities in obsessive-compulsive disorder detected with quantitative X-ray computed tomography. *American Journal of Psychiatry, 145,* 1089–1093.

Machlin, S. R., Harris, G. J., Pearlson, G. D., Hoehn-Saric, R., Jeffery, P., & Camargo, E. E. (1991). Elevated medial-frontal cerebral blood flow in obsessive-compulsive patients: A SPECT study. *American Journal of Psychiatry, 148,* 1240–1242.

Mavissakalian, M. R. (1979). Functional classification of obsessive-compulsive phenomena. *Journal of Behavioral Assessment, 1,* 271–279.

McDougle, C., Goodman, W., Leckman, J., Barr, L. C., Heninger, G. R., & Price, L. H. (1993). The efficacy of fluvoxamine in obsessive-compulsive disorder: Effects of comorbid chronic tic disorder. *Journal of Clinical Psychopharmacology, 13,* 354–358.

McDougle, C., Goodman, W., Leckman, J., Lee, N., Heninger, G., & Price, L. (1994). Haloperidol addition in fluvoxamine-refractory obsessive-compulsive disorder: A double-blind, placebo-controlled study in patients with and without tics. *Archives of General Psychiatry, 51,* 302–308.

McElroy, S. L., Hudson, J. I., & Pope, H. G. (1992). The DSM-III-R impulse control disorders not elsewhere classified: Clinical characteristics and relationship to other psychiatric disorders. *American Journal of Psychiatry, 149,* 318–327.

McElroy, S. L., Phillips, K. A., & Keck, P. E. (1994). Obsessive-compulsive spectrum disorder. *Journal of Clinical Psychiatry, 55,* 33–51.

McFall, M. E., & Wollersheim, J. P. (1979). Obsessive-compulsive neurosis: A cognitive-behavioral formulation and approach to treatment. *Cognitive Therapy and Research, 3,* 333–348.

McGuire, P. K., Bench, C. J., Frith, C. D., Marks, I. M., Frackowiak, R. S., & Dolan, R. J. (1994). Functional anatomy of obsessive-compulsive phenomena. *British Journal of Psychiatry, 164,* 459–468.

McNally, R. J. (1994). *Panic disorder: A critical analysis.* New York: Guilford.

Minichiello, W. E., Baer, L., Jenike, M. A., & Holland, A. (1990). Age of onset of major subtypes of obsessive-compulsive disorder. *Journal of Anxiety Disorders, 4,* 147–150.

Monteleone, P., Catapano, F., Bortolotti, F., & Maj, M. (1997). Plasma prolactin response to *d*-fenfluramine in obsessive-compulsive patients before and after fluvoxamine treatment. *Society of Biological Psychiatry, 42,* 175–180.

Mowrer, O. (1939). A stimulus-response analysis of anxiety and its role as a reinforcing agent. *Psychological Review, 46,* 553–565.

Murphy, T. K., Goodman, W. K., Fudge, M. W., Williams, R. C., Jr., Ayoub, E. M., Dalal, M., Lewis, M. H., & Zabriskie, J. B. (1997). B lymphocyte antigen D8/17: A peripheral marker for childhood-onset obsessive-compulsive disorder and Tourette's syndrome? *American Journal of Psychiatry, 154,* 402–407.

Nelson, E., & Rice, J. (1997). Stability of diagnosis of obsessive-compulsive disorder in the Epidemiologic Catchment Area study. *American Journal of Psychiatry, 154,* 826–831.

Nestadt, G., Samuels, J. F., Romanoski, A. J., Folstein, M. F., & McHugh, P. R. (1994). Obsessions and compulsions in the community. *Acta Psychiatrica Scandinavica, 89,* 219–224.

Neziroglu, F., Anemone, R., & Yaryura-Tobias, J. A. (1992). Onset of obsessive-compulsive disorder in pregnancy. *American Journal of Psychiatry, 149,* 947–950.

Nordahl, T. E., Benkelfat, C., Semple, W. E., Gross, M., King, A. C., & Cohen, R. M. (1989). Cerebral glucose metabolic rates in obsessive-compulsive disorder. *Neuropsychopharmacology, 2,* 23–28.

Obsessive Compulsive Cognitions Working Group. (1997). Cognitive assessment of obsessive-compulsive disorder. *Behaviour Research and Therapy, 35,* 667–681.

Okasha, A., Saad, A., Khalil, A. H., Seif El Dawla, A., & Yehia, N. (1994). Phenomenology of obsessive-compulsive disorder: A transcultural study. *Comprehensive Psychiatry, 35,* 191–197.

O'Kearny, R. O. (1998). Responsibility appraisals and obsessive-compulsive disorder: A critique of Salkovskis's cognitive theory. *Australian Journal of Psychology, 50,* 43–47.

Owen, A. M., Eans, A. C., & Petrides, M. (1996). Evidence for a two-stage model of spatial working memory processing within the lateral frontal cortex: A positron emission tomography study. *Cerebral Cortex, 6,* 31–38.

Perani, D., Colombo, C., Bressi, S., Bonfanti, A., Grassi, F., Scarone, S., Belladi, L., Smeraldi, E., & Fazio, F. (1995). [$^{18}$F]FDG PET study in obsessive-compulsive disorder: A clinical/metabolic correlation study after treatment. *British Journal of Psychiatry, 38,* 244–250.

Persons, J., & Foa, E. (1984). Processing of fearful and neutral information by obsessive compulsives. *Behaviour Research and Therapy, 22,* 259–265.

Pian, K. L., Westenberg, H. G. M., den Boer, J. A., DeBruin, W. I., & van Rijk, P. P. (1998). Effects of *meta*-chlorophenyl-piperazine on cerebral blood flow in obsessive-compulsive disorder and controls. *Society of Biological Psychiatry, 44,* 367–370.

Pigott, T. A., L'Heureux, F., Dubbert, B., Bernstein, S., & Murphy, D. L. (1994). Obsessive compulsive disorder: Comorbid conditions. *Journal of Clinical Psychiatry, 55,* 15–27.

Purcell, R., Maruff, P., Kyrios, M., & Pantelis, C. (1998). Cognitive deficits in obsessive-compulsive disorder on tests of frontal-striatal functions. *Society of Biological Psychiatry, 43,* 348–357.

Rachman, S. J. (1985). An overview of clinical research issues in obsessive-compulsive disorders. In M. Mavissakalian, S. M. Turner, & L. Michelson (Eds.), *Obsessive-compulsive disorder: Psychological and pharmacological treatment* (pp. 1–47). New York: Plenum Press.

Rachman, S. J. (1993). Obsessions, responsibility and guilt. *Behaviour Research and Therapy, 31,* 149–154.

Rachman, S., & de Silva, P. (1978). Abnormal and normal obsessions. *Behaviour Research and Therapy, 14,* 223–248.

Rachman, S. J., & Hodgson, R. J. (1980). *Obsessions and compulsions.* Englewood Cliffs, NJ: Prentice-Hall.

Rachman, S., Thordarson, D. S., Shafran, R., & Woody, S. R. (1995). Perceived responsibility: Structure and significance. *Behaviour Research and Therapy, 33,* 779–784.

Rasmussen, S. A. (1994). Obsessive compulsive spectrum disorders [commentary]. *Journal of Clinical Psychiatry, 55,* 89–91.

Rasmussen, S. A., & Eisen, J. L. (1990). The epidemiology of obsessive compulsive disorder. *Journal of Clinical Psychiatry, 51,* 20–23.

Rasmussen, S. A., & Eisen, J. L. (1994). The epidemiology and differential diagnosis of obsessive compulsive disorder. *Journal of Clinical Psychiatry, 55,* 5–14.

Rauch, S. L., Jenike, M. A., Alpert, N. M., Baer, L., Breiter, H. C., Savage, C. R., & Fischman, A. J. (1994). Regional cerebral blood flow measured during symptom provocation in obsessive-compulsive disorder using oxygen 15-labeled carbon dioxide and positron emission tomography. *Archives of General Psychiatry, 51,* 62–70.

Rettew, D. C., Swedo, S. E., Leonard, H. L., Lenane, M. C., & Rapoport, J. L. (1992). Obsessions and compulsions across time in 79 children and adolescents with obsessive-compulsive disorder. *Journal of the American Academy of Child and Adolescent Psychiatry, 31,* 1050–1056.

Rheaume, J., Freeston, M. H., Dugas, M. J., Letarte, H., & Ladouceur, R. (1995). Perfectionism, responsibility obsessive-compulsive symptoms. *Behaviour Research and Therapy, 33,* 785–794.

Rheaume, J., Ladouceur, R., Freeston, M. H., & Letarte, H. (1995). Inflated responsibility in obsessive-compulsive disorder: Validation of an operational definition. *Behaviour Research and Therapy, 33,* 159–169.

Robinson, D., Wu, H., Munne, R. A., Ashtari, M., Alvir, J. M., Lerner, G., Koreen, A., Cole, K., & Bogarts, B. (1995). Reduced caudate nucleus volume in obsessive-compulsive disorder. *Archives of General Psychiatry, 52,* 393–398.

Rosenberg, D. R., & Keshavan, M. S. (1998). Toward a neurodevelopmental model of obsessive-compulsive disorder. *Biological Psychiatry, 43,* 623–640.

Rubin, R. T., Ananth, J., Villanueva-Meyer, J., Trajmar, P. G., & Mena, I. (1995). Regional $^{133}$xenon cerebral blood flow and cerebral $^{99m}$Tc-HMPAO uptake in patients with obsessive-compulsive disorder before and after treatment. *Biological Psychiatry, 38,* 429–437.

Rubin, R. T., Villanueva-Meyer, J., Ananth, J., Trajmar, P. G., & Mena, I. (1992). Regional xenon 133 cerebral blood flow and cerebral technetium 99$^m$ HMPAO uptake in unmedicated patients with obsessive-compulsive disorder and matched normal control subjects. *Archives of General Psychiatry, 49,* 695–702.

Sachdev, P., Hay, P., & Cumming, S. (1992). Psychosurgical treatment of obsessive-compulsive disorder (letter). *Archives of General Psychiatry, 49,* 582–583.

Salkovskis, P. M. (1985). Obsessional-compulsive symptoms: A cognitive-behavioral analysis. *Behaviour Research and Therapy, 25,* 571–583.

Salkovskis, P. (1996). Cognitive-behavioural approaches to the understanding of obsessional problems. In R. M. Rapee (Ed.), *Current controversies in the anxiety disorders* (pp. 103–133). New York: Guilford.

Saxena, S., Brody, A. L., Schwartz, J. M., & Baxter, L. R. (1998). Neuroimaging and frontal-subcortical circuitry in obsessive-compulsive disorder. *British Journal of Psychiatry* (Supplement), *35*, 26–37.

Scarone, S., Colombo, C., Livian, S., Abbruzzese, M., Ronchi, P., & Lacatelli, M. (1992). Increased right caudate nucleus size in obsessive compulsive disorder: Detection with magnetic resonance imaging. *Psychiatry Research, 45,* 115–121.

Scarrbelotti, M. B., Duck, J. M., & Dickerson, M. M. (1995). Individual differences in obsessive-compulsive behaviour: The role of the Eysenckian dimensions and appraisals of responsibility. *Personal and Individual Differences, 18,* 413–421.

Schmidtke, K., Schorb, A., Winkelmann, G., & Hohagen, F. (1998). Cognitive frontal lobe dysfunction in obsessive-compulsive disorder. *Society of Biological Psychology, 43,* 666–673.

Schwartz, J. M., Stoessel, P. W., Baxter, L. R., Martin, K. M., & Phelps, M. E. (1996). Systematic changes in cerebral glucose metabolic rate after successful behavior modification treatment of obsessive-compulsive disorder. *Archives of General Psychiatry, 53,* 109–113.

Shafran, R. (1997). The manipulation of responsibility in obsessive-compulsive disorder. *British Journal of Clinical Psychology, 36,* 397–407.

Shafran, R., & Somers, J. (1998). Treating adolescent obsessive-compulsive disorder: Applications of the cognitive theory. *Behaviour Research and Therapy, 36,* 93–97.

Sica, C. (1998). Efficacy of cognitive and behavioral therapy in the treatment of obsessive-compulsive disorders: A review. *Acta Compartamentalia, 6,* 173–192.

Sichel, D. A., Cohen, L. S., Dimmock, J. A., & Rosenbaum, J. F. (1993). Postpartum obsessive compulsive disorder: A case series. *Journal of Clinical Psychiatry, 54,* 156–159.

Stanley, M. A., & Cohen, L. J. (1999). Trichotillomania and obsessive-compulsive disorder. In D. Stein, G. Christenson, & E. Hollander (Eds.), *Trichotillomania: New developments* (pp. 225–261). Washington, DC: American Psychiatric Association Press.

Stanley, M. A., & Turner, S. M. (1995). Current status of pharmacological and behavioral treatment of obsessive-compulsive disorder. *Behavior Therapy, 26,* 163–186.

Stanley, M. A., Turner, S. M., & Borden, J. W. (1990). Schizotypal features in obsessive-compulsive disorder. *Comprehensive Psychiatry, 31,* 511–518.

Stein, M. B., Forde, D. R., Anderson, G., & Walker, J. R. (1997). Obsessive-compulsive disorder in the community: An epidemiologic survey with clinical reappraisal. *American Journal of Psychiatry, 154,* 1120–1126.

Steketee, G. S., Grayson, J. B., & Foa, E. B. (1985). Obsessive-compulsive disorder: Differences between washers and checkers. *Behaviour Research and Therapy, 23,* 197–201.

Steketee, G. S., Grayson, J. B., & Foa, E. B. (1987). A comparison of characteristics of obsessive-compulsive disorder and other anxiety disorders. *Journal of Anxiety Disorders, 1,* 325–335.

Swedo, S. E., Leonard, H. L., Garvey, M., Mittleman, B., Allen, A. J., Perlmutter, S., Dow, S., Zamkoff, J., Dubbert, B. K., & Lougee, L. (1998). Pediatric autoimmune neuropsychiatric disorders associated with streptococcal infections: Clinical description of the first 50 cases. *American Journal of Psychiatry, 155,* 264–271.

Swedo, S. E., Leonard, H. L., Kruesi, M. J. P., Rettew, D. C., Listwak, S. J., Berrettini, W., Stipetic, M., Hamberger, S., Gold, P. W., Potter, W. Z., & Rapoport, J. L. (1992). Cerebrospinal fluid neurochemistry in children and adolescents with obsessive-compulsive disorder. *Archives of General Psychiatry, 49,* 29–36.

Swedo, S. E., Leonard, H. L., Mittleman, B. B., Allen, A. J., Rapoport, J. L., Dow, S. P., Banter, M. E., Chapman, F., & Zabriskie, J. (1997). Identification of children with pediatric autoimmune neuropsychiatric disorders associated with streptococcal infections by a marker associated with rheumatic fever. *American Journal of Psychiatry, 154,* 110–112.

Swedo, S. E., Schapiro, M. B., Grady, C. L., Cheslow, D. L., Leonard, H. L., Kumar, A., Friedland, R., Rapoport, S. I., & Rapoport, J. L. (1989). Cerebral glucose metabolism in childhood-onset obsessive-compulsive disorder. *Archives of General Psychiatry, 46,* 518–523.

Swedo, S. E., Pietrini, P., Leonard, H. L., Schapiro, M. B., Rettew, D. C., Goldberger, E. L., Rapoport, S. I., Rapoport, J. L., & Grady, C. L. (1992). Cerebral glucose metabolism in childhood-onset obsessive-compulsive disorder. *Archives of General Psychiatry, 49,* 690–694.

Tallis, F. (1997). The neuropsychology of obsessive-compulsive disorder: A review and consideration of clinical implications. *British Journal of Clinical Psychology, 36,* 3–20.

Thoren, P., Asberg, M., Bertilsson, L., Mellstrom, B., Sjoqvist, F., & Traskman, L. (1980). Clomipramine treatment of obsessive-compulsive disorder. II: Biochemical aspects. *Archives of General Psychiatry, 37,* 1289–1294.

Trivedi, M. H. (1996). Functional neuroanatomy of obsessive-compulsive disorder. *Journal of Clinical Psychiatry, 57* (Suppl. 8), 26–35.

Turner, S. M., & Beidel, D. C. (1988). *Treating obsessive compulsive disorder.* New York: Pergamon Press.

Turner, S. M., Beidel, D. C., & Nathan, R. S. (1985). Biological factors in obsessive-compulsive disorders. *Psychological Bulletin, 97,* 430–450.

Turner, S. M., Beidel, D. C., & Stanley, M. A. (1992). Are obsessional thoughts and worry different cognitive phenomena? *Clinical Psychology Review, 12,* 257–270.

van Balkom, A. J. L. M., van Oppen, P., Vermeulen, A. W. A., van Dyck, R., Nauta, M. C. E., & Vorst, H. C. M. (1994). A meta-analysis on the treatment of obsessive-compulsive disorder: A comparison of antidepressants, behavior, and cognitive therapy. *Clinical Psychology Review, 14,* 359–381.

van Oppen, P., & Arntz, A. (1994). Cognitive therapy for obsessive-compulsive disorder. *Behaviour Research and Therapy, 32,* 79–87.

van Oppen, P., De Haan, E., Van Balkom, A. J. L. M., Spinhoven, P., Hoogduin, K., & Van Dyck, R. (1995). Cognitive therapy and exposure in vivo in the treatment of obsessive compulsive disorder. *Behavior Research and Therapy, 33,* 379–390.

Weissman, M. M., Bland, R. C., Canino, G. J., Greenwald, S., Hwu, H.-G., Lee, C. K., Newman, S. C., Oakley-Browne, M. A., Rubio-Stipec, M., Wickramaratne, P. J., Wittchen, H.-U., & Yeh, E.-K. (1994). The cross national epidemiology of obsessive compulsive disorder. *Journal of Clinical Psychiatry, 55,* 5–10.

Yaryura-Tobias, J. A., Neziroglu, F., & Bergman, L. (1976). Chlorimipramine for obsessive-compulsive neurosis: An organic approach. *Current Therapeutic Research, 20,* 541–548.

Zohar, J., Insel, T. R., Berman, K. F., Foa, E. B., Hill, J. L., & Weinberger, D. R. (1989). Anxiety and cerebral blood flow during behavioral challenge: Dissociation of central from peripheral and subjective measures. *Archives of General Psychiatry, 46,* 505–510.

Zohar, A. H., Pauls, D. L., Ratzoni, G., Apter, A., Dycian, A., Binder, M., King, R., Leckman, J. F., Kron, S., & Cohen, D. J. (1997). Obsessive-compulsive disorder with and without tics in an epidemiological sample of adolescents. *American Journal of Psychiatry, 154,* 274–276.

# CHAPTER 8

# Posttraumatic Stress Disorder

## John A. Fairbank, Lori Ebert, and Juesta M. Caddell

## Traumatic Experiences

In the field of mental health, the word "trauma" generally connotes a wide range of intensely stressful experiences that involve exposure to levels of danger and fear that exceed normal capacity to cope (Brett, 1993; Kleber & Brom, 1992; van der Hart, Brown, & van der Kolk, 1995). In the DSM-III (American Psychiatric Association, 1980) and DSM-III-R (American Psychiatric Association, 1987), the American Psychiatric Association (APA) defined trauma as an event that is "outside the range of usual human experience" and likely to "evoke significant symptoms of distress in most people." The DSM-III/III-R definitions of trauma were based on the notion that most people exposed to catastrophic, but presumably uncommon, events such as rape, war, torture, or natural disaster would be likely to show signs and symptoms of serious psychological distress. However, subsequent research on the prevalence of exposure to potentially traumatic events in the general population showed that exposure to such events is much more common than assumed. Indeed, a majority of adults experiences at least one potentially traumatic event over the course of a lifetime (Breslau, Davis, Andreski, & Peterson,

John A. Fairbank • Department of Psychiatry and Human Services, Duke University Medical Center, Durham, North Carolina 27719. Lori Ebert and Juesta M. Caddell • Research Triangle Institute, Research Triangle Park, North Carolina 27709.

*Comprehensive Handbook of Psychopathology* (Third Edition), edited by Patricia B. Sutker and Henry E. Adams. Kluwer Academic/Plenum Publishers, New York, 2001.

1991; Kessler, Sonnega, Bromet, Hughes, & Nelson, 1995). Furthermore, research clearly shows that the majority of persons exposed to such experiences does not develop significant symptoms of psychological distress or impairments in their everyday functioning. Clearly, the DSM-III/III-R conceptualization of trauma as an unusual rare event that would elicit extreme distress in most people begged reconsideration.

## Current Diagnostic Criteria for Posttraumatic Stress Disorder

With the publication of the 4th edition of the DSM (DSM-IV; APA, 1994), the concept of trauma evolved from focusing on uncommon, highly adverse, external events to describing the specific characteristics of a traumatic event, including the individual's psychological response to the event regardless of whether the event is rare or common. Specifically, the DSM-IV definition of a traumatic event has two criteria: the first is that a person "experienced, witnessed or was confronted with an event or events that involved actual or threatened death or serious injury, or a threat to the physical integrity of self or others," and the second is that "the person's response involved intense fear, helplessness, or horror" (APA, 1994, pp. 427–428).

Although exposure to a stressful event is an indispensable condition, exposure alone is insufficient for determining whether the experience is traumatic. In DSM-IV, the critical determinant is the person's cognitive and affective reactivity to an event. Therefore, if an event, such as a motor vehicle accident, involves "actual or threatened death or serious injury ... to self or others" (APA, 1994, p. 427) and also elicits severe and incapacitating psychological distress such as "intense fear, helplessness, or horror" (APA, 1994, p. 428), the experience is traumatic. Studies of extreme situations have shown that in some individuals exposed to the most severe events, serious psychopathology develops, including but not limited to posttraumatic stress disorder (PTSD) (Dohrenwend, 1998). Indeed, traumatic experiences can lead to the development of several different disorders, including major depression, specific phobias, panic disorder, disorders of extreme stress not otherwise specified (DESNOS), personality disorders such as borderline personality disorder, and a range of physical symptoms, as well as PTSD (Foa, Keane, & Friedman, in press; Hyams, Wignall, & Roswell, 1996). Although it is important to understand the range of potential syndromes and disorders associated with traumatic experiences, the focus of this chapter is to review and synthesize the epidemiologic and clinical research that examines the nature, assessment, and treatment of PTSD, specifically.

The symptoms that characterize PTSD include distressing thoughts, feelings, and images that recapitulate the traumatic event, avoidance of stimuli associated with the event, emotional numbing of responsiveness, and a collection of symptoms that represent a persistent increase in stress and arousal (Keane, Weathers, & Foa, in press). The duration of the disturbance is longer than one month and "causes clinically significant distress or impairment in occupational, social, and other areas of functioning" (APA, 1994).

Specifically, PTSD is characterized by reexperiencing symptoms that include (1) recurrent and intrusive distressing recollections of the event, (2) recurrent distressing dreams of the event, (3) acting or feeling as if the event were recurring, (4) intense psychological distress at exposure to cues that symbolize the event, and (5) physiological reactivity to reminders of the experience. PTSD also involves persistent avoidance of stimuli associated with the trauma and numbing of general responsiveness. Symptoms of avoidance and emotional numbing can include (1) efforts to avoid thoughts, feelings, or conversations about the event; (2) efforts to avoid activities, places or people associated with the trauma; (3) an inability to recall important details of the trauma; (4) a

markedly diminished interest in formerly important activities; (5) a feeling of detachment or estrangement from other people; (6) a restricted range of affect; and (7) a sense of a shortened future. Symptoms of arousal that were not present before the traumatic event are also a component of the PTSD symptom profile. PTSD arousal symptoms can include (1) insomnia, (2) irritability or anger outbursts, (3) difficulty concentrating, (4) hypervigilance, and (5) an exaggerated and distressing startle response.

## Epidemiology

Epidemiology is the study of patterns and correlates of disease onset and course in human populations. Psychiatric epidemiology includes studies of the prevalence of psychiatric disorders (i.e, how many people have specific disorders), the distribution of disorders among subgroups of populations, the relationship of a particular disorder to other disorders, and factors that affect the onset and course of a disorder. In the following sections, we review findings addressing (1) the frequency of exposure to potentially traumatic events, (2) the prevalence of PTSD, (3) putative risk factors for PTSD, and (4) the comorbidity of PTSD with other mental and physical health problems.

### Exposure to Traumatic Events

Posttraumatic stress disorder is unusual in the psychiatric nosology in that it ascribes etiological significance to a particular type of life experience—exposure to a traumatic event. Although such experiences were once considered rare (i.e., "outside the range of normal human experience;" see DSM III-R, APA, 1987), epidemiologic studies conducted in the United States suggest that the majority of Americans will experience a potentially traumatic event at least once in their lives. In the National Comorbidity Study (NCS; Kessler et al., 1995), a survey interview of psychiatric disorder administered to a probability sample of persons aged 15 to 54 years in the noninstitutionalized civilian population living in the 48 contiguous United States and the first nationally representative general population survey to assess traumatic stressor exposure and PTSD, 60.7% of men and 51.2% of women reported exposure to a potentially traumatic event. Moreover, most NCS participants who indicated that they had experienced one potential trauma reported experiencing two or more types of trauma. In the NCS, which used DSM-III-R criteria for trauma exposure and PTSD, the most frequently identified types of trauma were witnessing someone being badly injured or killed (35.6% of men and 14.5% of women); involvement in a fire, flood, or natural disaster (18.9% of men and 15.2% of women); and involvement in a life-threatening accident (25% of men and 13.8% of women). Using a DSM-IV definition of traumatic events, a recent survey found that the unexpected death of a loved one was the most frequently reported trauma in a random sample of 18- to 45-year-old Detroit residents (Breslau et al., 1998).

Research suggests that the types of potentially traumatic events men and women experience may differ. For example, in the NCS (Kessler et al., 1995), men were more likely than women to report witnessing injury or death, involvement in a natural disaster or life-threatening accident, involvement in a physical attack, and combat exposure. Women were more likely to report having experienced rape, sexual molestation, and childhood physical abuse. Consistent with these results, findings from a national survey of adult women in the United States, the National Women's Study (NWS; Resnick, Kilpatrick, Dansky, Saunders, & Best, 1993), indicated that 12.7% of participants had experienced a completed rape, 14.3% had experienced molestation or attempted sexual assault, and 10.3% had been physically assaulted. Nearly 30% of rapes reported in the NWS occurred before age 11, and approximately two-thirds occurred before age 18.

Epidemiologic studies have identified various risk factors for exposure to potentially traumatic events. As suggested by findings from the NCS (Kessler et al., 1995) and substantiated by a sizable body of research (e.g., Breslau et al., 1998; Kilpatrick, Resnick, Saunders, & Best, 1998), past exposure to potentially traumatic events confers increased risk of future exposure to such events. In a prospective epidemiologic study of 21- to 30-year-old members of a health maintenance organization, persons who had a history of traumatic stressor exposure at baseline were nearly twice as likely to report an additional trauma during the 3-year follow-up (Breslau, Davis, & Andreski, 1995). Exposure to traumatic stressors also varies with age, socioeconomic status, psychiatric his-

tory, substance use, personality characteristics, family history of psychiatric disorder and substance use problems, and geographic location (Adler et al., 1994; Breslau et al., 1991; Breslau et al., 1995; Breslau et al., 1998; Bromet, Sonnega, & Kessler, 1998; Norris, 1992). For example, a 1993 report by the International Federation of Red Cross and Red Crescent Societies found that in the period from 1967 to 1991, disasters affected people in developing countries as compared with developed countries at a ratio of more than 150 to 1 (International Federation of Red Cross and Red Crescent Societies, 1993).

Epidemiologic studies also have examined the prevalence of exposure to potentially traumatic events among children and adolescents; the majority of these studies assessed physical victimization, sexual victimization, or exposure to community violence. A telephone survey of a nationally representative sample of 2000 10- to 16-year-old children found that more than 40% reported at least one experience that could be categorized as violent victimization (Boney-McCoy & Finkelhor, 1995). Consistent with these findings, Kilpatrick, Saunders, and Resnick (1998) estimated the lifetime prevalence of exposure to sexual assault, physical assault, and witnessing violence as 8%, 17%, and 39%, respectively, in a national sample of 12- to 17-year-old adolescents. In addition, a number of school surveys evaluated rates of exposure to community violence. In one sample of more than 500 Black elementary and middle school students in Chicago, 30% said they had witnessed a stabbing, and 26% reported that they had seen someone being shot (Bell & Jenkins, 1993). Another survey of 2248 students in the sixth to eighth and tenth grades in an urban public school system found that 41% reported witnessing a stabbing or shooting in the past year (Schwab-Stone et al., 1995). Another survey of 3735 high school students in six schools in Ohio and Colorado found relatively high rates of exposure to violence within the past year that varied by size and location of the school (Singer, Anglin, Song, & Lunghofer, 1995). Among male adolescents, 3% to 22% reported being beaten or mugged in their own neighborhoods, 3% to 33% reported being shot at or shot, and 6% to 16% reported being attacked with a knife. Reported rates of most types of victimization were lower for adolescent females than males; however, more females reported sexual abuse or assault. Although a number of studies reported PTSD prevalence estimates among youths exposed to specific types of traumatic events, we were unable to identify any general population studies of PTSD prevalence among children and adolescents in the scientific literature. Thus, the remainder of this review of the epidemiology of PTSD focuses on PTSD in adults.

## Prevalence of PTSD

Epidemiologic studies conducted over the past two decades provided empirical information about the prevalence of PTSD in the general population and among individuals who have been exposed to specific types of potentially traumatic events. This research indicates that most individuals who are exposed to a potential trauma do not develop PTSD. However, this research also suggests that the likelihood of developing PTSD following traumatic stressor exposure varies with the type of trauma experienced. Additional factors that affect people's risk of developing PTSD following traumatic stressor exposure are discussed in a subsequent section.

Estimates of the lifetime prevalence of PTSD from surveys of the general adult population in the United States have ranged from 1.0% to 12.3%. The two earliest community studies of the prevalence of PTSD were carried out as part of the Epidemiologic Catchment Area (ECA) program. Using DSM-III criteria as operationalized in the Diagnostic Interview Schedule (DIS; Robins, Helzer, Cottler, & Golding, 1988), these studies reported lifetime prevalence estimates for PTSD of 1.0% in metropolitan St. Louis (Helzer, Robins, & McEvoy, 1987) and 1.3% in the Piedmont region of North Carolina (Davidson, Hughes, Blazer, & George, 1991). More recent surveys have found substantially higher rates of PTSD in the general population. The NCS, which also used a version of the DIS to assess PTSD, estimated a lifetime prevalence of DSM-III-R PTSD of 7.8% among persons ages 15 to 54 in the United States (Kessler et al., 1995); the estimated current (30-day) prevalence of PTSD in the NCS was 2.8%. Using the DIS-IV(Robins, Cottler, Bucholz, & Compton, 1995), Breslau et al. (1998) estimated the conditional risk of PTSD following exposure to any traumatic stressor at 9.2% in their Detroit sample. It has been postulated that a number of factors account for variations in PTSD prevalence estimates in these and other studies, including differ-

ences in (1) diagnostic criteria, (2) the measurement approach used to ascertain exposure and assess PTSD, and (3) the demographic characteristics and representativeness of the study populations (e.g., Acierno, Kilpatrick, & Resnick, 1999; Kessler et al., 1995).

The risk of developing PTSD following exposure to a potentially traumatic event also varies with the nature of the exposure. In the NCS, the trauma most likely to be associated with PTSD was rape; 65% of men and 45.9% of women who identified rape as their most upsetting trauma developed PTSD. In contrast, among NCS respondents who identified a natural disaster or fire as their most upsetting trauma, only 3.7% of men and 5.4% of women met lifetime diagnostic criteria for PTSD. In addition to rape, other most upsetting traumas associated with a comparatively high risk of PTSD in the NCS were combat exposure, childhood neglect, and childhood physical abuse among men (probabilities of lifetime PTSD were 38.8%, 23.9%, and 22.3%, respectively) and sexual molestation, physical attack, being threatened with a weapon, and childhood physical abuse among women (probabilities of lifetime PTSD of 26.5%, 21.3%, 32.6%, and 48.5%, respectively). Consistent with these findings, in the NWS (Resnick et al., 1993), women who had experienced interpersonal violence (i.e., physical assault, sexual assault, or the homicide of a close friend or relative) were more than twice as likely to meet criteria for lifetime (25.8%) and current (9.4%) PTSD than women who reported noncrime stressors only. (PTSD rates in this subgroup were 9.7% lifetime and 3.4% current). Similarly, Breslau et al. (1998) found that among the men and women in their sample who reported exposure to a potential trauma, the highest conditional risk of PTSD (21.9%) was associated with the experience of assaultive violence.

Epidemiologic studies of PTSD often have assessed at-risk groups of individuals who have experienced a specific type of trauma, such as veterans of armed conflicts (Goldberg, True, Eisen, & Henderson, 1990; Kulka et al., 1990; Solomon, Weisenberg, Schwarzwald, & Mikulciner, 1987; Sutker, Uddo, Brailey, & Allain, 1993), internally displaced persons and refugees (Sack et al., 1995; Steel, Silove, Bird, McGorry, & Mohan, 1999), and victims of a range of criminal acts, including sexual assault (Saunders, Kilpatrick, Hanson, Resnick, & Walker, 1999), terrorist attacks (Abenhaim, Dab, & Salmi, 1999; North et al., 1999), and torture (Basoglu et al., 1997). Although it was largely through observing the postwar experiences of soldiers engaged in combat that the syndrome known as PTSD was recognized, PTSD was not broadly or systematically studied among war veterans until the Vietnam War. Study of PTSD among Vietnam veterans was facilitated by publication of DSM-III (APA, 1980) that included PTSD as a diagnostic category defined by specific behavioral criteria. To date, the most comprehensive examination of the prevalence of PTSD among Vietnam veterans comes from the 1989 National Vietnam Veterans Readjustment Study (NVVRS; Kulka et al., 1990), a congressionally mandated, community epidemiologic study of the prevalence of PTSD and other postwar psychological problems among veterans who served in the Vietnam theater of operations. Findings from the NVVRS indicated that 15.2% of men and 8.5% of women who served in Vietnam had "current" PTSD (i.e., met DSM-III-R criteria for PTSD during the 6 months before the study interview). By contrast, the current PTSD prevalence among a matched (for age and race/ethnicity) sample of military veterans who did not serve in Vietnam was 2.5% among men and 1.1% among women; for nonveterans, current PTSD prevalence was 1.2% among men and 0.3% among women. The NVVRS reported lifetime PTSD prevalence rates among Vietnam veterans of 30.9% for men and 26.9% for women. Findings from other major epidemiologic studies of the prevalence of PTSD among Vietnam veterans are generally consistent with these results. Estimates of current PTSD prevalence from the majority of these studies lie within the 95% confidence interval of the NVVRS estimates (13.0–17.4%). More recent studies evaluated PTSD prevalence among military personnel who served in the Persian Gulf War (Operation Desert Shield/Storm; ODS). Estimates of current PTSD prevalence rates among ODS veterans varied across studies and ranged from 4 to 19%; however, studies generally found higher rates of PTSD among ODS veterans than among military personnel who served during the same time period but were not deployed to the Persian Gulf (Perconte, Wilson, Pontius, Dietrick, & Spiro, 1993; Southwick et al., 1993, 1995; Sutker et al., 1993; Wolfe, Brown, & Kelley, 1993).

During the past decade, the prevalence of PTSD associated with forms of interpersonal violence

other than combat also has been evaluated. In the NCS (Kessler et al., 1995), sexual assault (i.e., rape) was associated with comparatively high rates of PTSD, as found in other studies (Kilpatrick, Saunders, Vernonen, Best, & Von, 1987; Resnick et al., 1993; Rothbaum, Foa, Riggs, Murdock, & Walsh, 1992). Whereas sexual assaults were strongly associated with PTSD for both men and women in the NCS, only 1.8% of men who reported a physical attack as their most upsetting trauma developed PTSD, compared with 21.3% of women. Research indicates that, in general, rates of PTSD in women following physical assault are relatively high and in many cases comparable to those observed among women sexual assault survivors (Kilpatrick et al., 1987; Norris, 1992; Resnick et al., 1993). Sexual victimization in childhood is also associated with PTSD in *adult* women. For example, in the NWS, women who were raped before age 18 were four times more likely to meet criteria for PTSD at the time of the study interview than women who were not raped as children or adolescents (Saunders et al., 1999).

McFarlane and Potts (1999) noted that the field of traumatic stress research largely evolved from the study of victims of three types of potentially traumatic events: war, interpersonal violence and related crimes, and disasters. Studies of the prevalence of PTSD among survivors of a variety of natural and technological disasters have been conducted in the United States and other countries, including several developing countries. Not surprisingly, research suggests that rates of PTSD among disaster survivors vary with the population and the type of disaster. The 1972 Buffalo Creek dam collapse and flood is one of the most widely studied natural disasters in the United States (Grace, Green, Lindy, & Leonard, 1993; Green, Lindy, Grace, & Leonard, 1992; Green & Lindy, 1994). Green and colleagues found that, as long as 14 years after this disaster, 25% of a sample of survivors followed longitudinally met criteria for a current diagnosis of PTSD. Although high, this estimate represents a decrease from the 44% current PTSD prevalence estimated 2 years after the flood. Comparatively high rates of PTSD were also reported among survivors of other natural and technological disasters, including a tornado (59%; Madakasira & O'Brien, 1987) and an industrial accident (71–80%; Weisaeth, 1989) both in the U.S., a cyclone in Fiji (Fairley, Langeluddecke, & Tennant, 1986), and earthquakes in Armenia (67%;

Goenjian et al., 1994) and Mexico (32%; Conyer, Sepulveda, Medina, Caraveo, & De La Fuente, 1987). However, other investigators reported considerably lower rates of PTSD among disaster survivors. For example, Canino, Bravo, Rubio-Stipec, and Woodberry (1990) reported PTSD prevalence rates of approximately 5% among survivors of a mud slide and flood in Puerto Rico that killed 800 people. Similarly, Shore, Vollmer, and Tatum (1989) reported PTSD prevalence rates of 4.5% for men and 3% for women in a large sample of survivors of the Mt. St. Helens volcanic eruption. Consistent with these findings, Norris (1992), in an epidemiological study of 1000 residents of four southeastern cities in the U.S., estimated that the rate of PTSD in disaster-exposed individuals was between 5 and 6%. The variability in PTSD prevalence rates among studies of disaster survivors suggests consideration of the dimensions of exposure (e.g., whether the individual was seriously injured or perceived a significant threat to personal safety) within classes of potentially traumatic stressors, an issue further addressed in the next section on risk factors for PTSD.

## Risk Factors for PTSD

Epidemiologic studies are empirical sources of information about risk factors for PTSD—preexposure factors, exposure characteristics, and postexposure factors that are believed to be related to the probability of an individual developing PTSD following exposure to a potentially traumatic event. A small number of general population studies have examined risk factors for PTSD. General population studies have focused primarily on the role of preexposure factors in the development of PTSD. Studies also examined risk factors for PTSD among individuals exposed to specific types of stressors. The most consistently reported preexposure risk factors for PTSD among individuals who experienced a potential trauma include female gender, preexisting psychiatric disorder, family history of psychopathology, and prior exposure to trauma including abuse in childhood (Breslau et al., 1991, 1998; Bromet et al., 1998; Kilpatrick et al., 1998). Within classes of potentially traumatic stressors, characteristics of the stressor exposure also influence risk for developing PTSD (e.g., Kilpatrick et al., 1989; Winfield, George, Swartz, & Blazer, 1990; Shore, Tatum, & Vollmer, 1986). Postexposure factors, including

postexposure social support and exposure to other potentially traumatic events, also affect the risk for PTSD.

Epidemiologic studies in the United States have generally found higher rates of PTSD in women than in men (Breslau et al., 1991, 1998; Kessler et al., 1995). These findings for PTSD are consistent with gender differences reported for other anxiety disorders and major depression. This gender difference is not due to higher overall rates of exposure to potentially traumatic events among women. Data from community surveys indicate that men are more likely than women to be exposed to potential traumas (Breslau et al., 1991; Kessler et al., 1995). At the same time, the types of potential traumas that men and women experience may differ. For example, studies consistently find that women are more likely than men to experience sexual victimization (Breslau et al., 1991; Kessler et al., 1995; Norris, 1992). Differences in the types of traumas to which men and women are exposed may partially account for gender differences in the rates of PTSD. However, in both the Detroit Area Survey of Trauma (Breslau et al., 1998) and the NCS (Kessler et al., 1995), the probability of PTSD among respondents reporting exposure to a potential trauma was two to four times higher in women than men, even after statistically adjusting for gender differences in the distribution of trauma types. Note that these findings do not rule out the possibility that gender differences in the characteristics of stressors experienced within broad categories of trauma types may contribute to the higher rates of PTSD observed among women. (See Saxe & Wolfe, 1999, for a detailed discussion of gender and PTSD.)

Among both men and women, preexisting psychiatric disorder and a family history of psychiatric disorder are associated with increased risk for PTSD following exposure to a potentially traumatic event (Breslau et al., 1991; Bromet et al., 1998; King, King, Foy, & Gudanowski, 1996; Sack et al., 1994). In the NCS, preexisting anxiety disorder and preexisting affective disorder were associated with PTSD in men and women, respectively, even after statistically adjusting for the nature of the index trauma (Bromet et al., 1998). Consistent with these findings, in Breslau et al.'s (1991) sample of urban young adults, the probability of developing PTSD among individuals reporting exposure to a potential trauma was more than twofold for those with a preexisting anxiety disorder or preexisting major depression. With respect to family history, Breslau et al. found that the risk of developing PTSD from exposure to a potential trauma was significantly higher among individuals who reported a family history of anxiety, depression, psychosis, or antisocial behavior. (A family history of substance abuse did not increase vulnerability to PTSD in this sample.)

In addition to conferring increased risk for future exposure on such events, past exposure to potentially traumatic events elevates the risk of developing PTSD upon exposure to a subsequent trauma. In the NWS, for example, women who reported exposure to multiple potentially traumatic events were more likely to receive a PTSD diagnosis than women who reported only a single exposure (Kilpatrick et al., 1998). Findings from several studies conducted with military veterans suggest that prior physical or sexual abuse, including abuse in childhood, is a risk factor for developing PTSD following military service in a war zone (Engel et al., 1993; Fontana, Schwartz, & Rosenheck, 1997; King et al., 1996).

Research indicates that the number and type of stressor exposures and also the specific characteristics of the exposure can influence the risk of developing PTSD. Subjective characteristics of stressor exposures (e.g., perceived life threat) as well as objective characteristics of the stressor (e.g., experienced injury) have been considered, and both influence the development of PTSD. Studies conducted with Vietnam veterans were among the first to consider multiple aspects of exposure to a particular type of stressor rather than simply measuring exposure as a dichotomous variable. Indeed, these studies have repeatedly found associations between risk of PTSD and the degree and nature of war zone stressor exposure (King, King, Foy, Keane, & Fairbank, 1999; Kulka et al., 1990). Evidence for an association between stressor characteristics and PTSD prevalence rates are not limited, however, to studies of war zone stressor exposure. In the NWS (Resnick et al., 1993), for example, the rate of lifetime PTSD among the women who reported assaults that involved both perceived life threat and injury (45.2%) was more than double that observed among assault survivors who reported neither perceived life threat nor injury (19%). In studying individuals exposed to the Mount St. Helens volcano eruption, Shore et al. (1986) found a strong association between proximity to the mountain and the effects

of exposure. Among males, first-year postdisaster onset rates for the three stress-related disorders evaluated (of which PTSD was one) were 0.9% in nonexposed controls, 2.5% in the low exposure group, and 11.1% in the high exposure group. Onset rates for females in these groups were 1.9, 5.6, and 20.9%, respectively.

Compared with research on preexposure factors and exposure characteristics, relatively few studies examined the role of postexposure factors in the development of PTSD. In one study L. King, D. King, Fairbank, & Adams (1998) used structural equation modeling to assess the contribution of postexposure factors to the development of PTSD in Vietnam veterans. Among the postexposure factors examined, postwar functional social support and stressful life events had direct effects on PTSD in both genders, as did structural social support for men. In this study, functional support was operationalized in terms of veterans' perceptions of the availability of emotional and instrumental support. Structural support was operationalized by a measure of the size and complexity of the veterans's social network. The impact on current PTSD of what King et al. (1998) referred to as "resilience factors" (e.g., hardiness) was also evaluated in this study. Consistent with these results, Fontana & Rosenheck (1994) found that homecoming experiences along with war zone stressor exposures were key correlates of PTSD among Vietnam veterans. Findings from a small number of studies suggest that social reactions that followed exposure to interpersonal violence may also affect the development of posttraumatic symptoms in civilian populations (e.g., Astin, Lawrence, & Foy, 1993; Zoellner, Foa, & Brigidi, 1999).

## Comorbidity

Another key component of the epidemiology of PTSD is its pattern of occurrence with other psychiatric and physical conditions, or *comorbidities*. Both general population studies and studies of individuals exposed to particular traumas indicate that the experience of other psychiatric disorders is common among individuals with PTSD. For example, in the St. Louis ECA study, almost 80% of persons with PTSD had a previous or concurrent psychiatric disorder, compared to about one-third of persons with no posttraumatic symptoms (Helzer et al., 1987). Similarly, in Breslau et al.'s

(1991) urban young adult sample, 83% of participants with lifetime PTSD had at least one other lifetime psychiatric disorder. In interpreting these and other findings addressing the psychiatric comorbidity of PTSD, however, it is worth noting that such results may in part be an artifact that reflects similarities in the diagnostic criteria for PTSD and other anxiety or depressive disorders. Further, as suggested by Acierno et al. (1999, p. 62) in reviewing research on crime-related PTSD, "large relative risk estimates may be a function of exposure to traumatic events, rather than PTSD *per se*" and thus may indicate of the potentially broad-reaching effects of traumatic life experiences.

In the NCS, the most extensive study of psychiatric comorbidities conducted to date, lifetime comorbidity between PTSD and the other DSM-III-R disorders was 88% for men and 79% for women (Kessler et al., 1995). In contrast, 46% of women and 55% of men with disorders other than PTSD had lifetime histories of another psychiatric disorder. The disorders most prevalent among men with lifetime histories of PTSD were alcohol abuse or dependence (51.9%), major depression (47.9%), conduct disorder (43.3%), and drug abuse or dependence (34.5%). The disorders most prevalent among women with lifetime PTSD were major depression (48.5%), simple phobia (29.0%), social phobia (28.4%), and alcohol abuse/dependence (27.9%). In Breslau et al.'s (1991) young adult sample, the two most prevalent disorders among individuals with lifetime PTSD were major depression (36.6%) and alcohol abuse or dependence (31.2%). Note, however, that comorbidity rates in both of these studies refer to lifetime disorder rather than current disorder and therefore do not necessarily imply the simultaneous occurrence of PTSD with other psychiatric disorders.

High rates of psychiatric comorbidity have been also found in studies of PTSD among individuals who experienced specific types of trauma. In the NVVRS, Kulka et al. (1990) found that virtually all Vietnam veterans with PTSD had met the criteria for one or more other psychiatric disorders at some time during their lives (three-quarters if alcohol disorders are excluded). Moreover, half of the veterans with PTSD met criteria for another current psychiatric disorder. In men with PTSD, the most frequent diagnostic comorbid disorders were alcohol abuse or dependence (75% lifetime, 20% current), generalized anxiety disorder (44%

lifetime, 20% current), and major depression (20% lifetime, 16% current). Among women veterans with PTSD, the most frequent disorders were major depression (42% lifetime, 23% current), generalized anxiety disorder (38% lifetime, 20% current), and dysthymic disorder (33% lifetime). Consistent with these findings for women military veterans, a study of criminal victimization among women community residents (Boudreaux, Kilpatrick, Resnick, Best, & Saunders, 1998) also found that women with current PTSD were more likely than women without PTSD to meet criteria for the following disorders: major depression (32% vs. 4%), obsessive-compulsive disorder (27% vs. 3%), agoraphobia (18% vs. 1%), and social phobia (18% vs. 4%).

Epidemiologic studies also examined the temporal order of PTSD in relation to other psychiatric disorders that are highly comorbid with PTSD. In the NCS (Kessler et al., 1995), the absence of a PTSD assessment for all traumas experienced precluded an unequivocal determination of how often comorbid PTSD was a primary disorder (in the sense of having an earlier onset than other psychiatric disorders). By placing upper and lower bounds on this figure, however, Kessler et al. estimated that PTSD was primary with respect to all other disorders between 29% and 51% of the time among men and between 41% and 58% of the time among women. In a community sample of 801 women (Breslau, Davis, Peterson, & Schulz, 1997), PTSD was associated with an increased risk for first-episode onset of major depression and alcohol abuse or dependence (but not any anxiety disorder). Exposure to a potentially traumatic event also was associated with an increased risk of alcohol abuse or dependence in this sample. In Breslau et al.'s sample of young adults, PTSD was associated with an increased risk of subsequent drug abuse or dependence, whereas exposure to a potential trauma in the absence of PTSD did not increase risk for drug use disorders (Chilcoat & Breslau, 1998).

In addition to studies of psychiatric comorbidity, there is a growing body of research on the physical health comorbidities and life adjustment problems associated with PTSD. Correlates of PTSD identified in the empirical literature include more somatic complaints, poorer health status, increased use of health services, and higher rates of cardiovascular symptoms, neurological symptoms, gastrointestinal symptoms, and other physical symptoms of known and unknown etiology (Beckham et al., 1998; Boscarino & Chang, 1999; Holen, 1991; Kulka et al., 1990; Long, Chamberlain, & Vincent, 1992; McFarlane, Atchison, Rafalowicz, & Papay, 1994; Schnurr & Spiro, 1999; Shalev, Bleich, & Ursano, 1990). Research also has shown a greater frequency of adverse health practices (e.g., smoking, alcohol use) among persons with PTSD (Beckham, 1999; Beckham et al., 1997; Schnurr & Spiro, 1999). Although the impact of PTSD on functioning has not been well-studied, a few studies found evidence of impaired functioning (e.g., more physical limitations, a greater likelihood of not being employed) among individuals with PTSD (Fairbank, Ebert, Zarkin, & Johnson, 1999; Zatzick et al., 1997a,b).

## Assessment

During the past decade, the literature devoted to the clinical assessment of PTSD advanced considerably. Of particular note is the increase in attention to the development of assessment tools for use with noncombatants and even more specifically with survivors of specific civilian traumas (e.g., tools developed specifically for use with rape survivors, crime victims, etc.), the increase in the number of tools available for use with children, as well as the progress that has been made toward understanding the neurobiological factors that may contribute to the development and maintenance of PTSD. However, because there is still no one absolute diagnostic measure of PTSD, state-of-the-art and comprehensive assessment of PTSD uses a multiaxial, multimodal approach (Caddell & Drabman, 1993; Keane, Wolfe, & Taylor, 1987; Litz et al., 1992; Newman, Kaloupek, & Keane, 1996; Schlenger, Fairbank, Jordan, & Caddell, 1997). The term *multiaxial* denotes that multiple sources of information are used in the assessment process (e.g., clinical interview, collateral report, self-report inventories). To capture the nature and extent of dysfunction more fully, a multimodal approach is used to access selected response modalities that have demonstrated utility in measuring the anxiety construct and specifically PTSD (e.g., overt behavioral responses, subjective responses, physiological responses, cognitive/neuropsychological status) (Barlow & Wolfe, 1981; Keane, Wolfe, & Taylor, 1987; King, Hamilton, & Ollendick, 1988; Lang, 1977; Newman, Kaloupek, & Keane, 1996). The ultimate goals of this compre-

hensive assessment of PTSD are to identify signs and symptoms of the disorder, as well as comorbid disorders; to determine factors that have contributed to the development of the disorder, as well as factors that maintain current symptoms; to gain an understanding of an individual's functional status; and to establish a baseline against which to gauge treatment gains. The use of a multiaxial, multimodal assessment protocol allows the determination of a DSM-IV diagnosis, as well as further functional analysis, to specify the behavioral, cognitive, and physiological excesses and deficits displayed by an individual who meets diagnostic criteria.

Generally, the multiaxial, multimodal assessment approach should be used to gather converging data to indicate the presence of clinically significant symptoms of PTSD. The possibility of monetary compensation for PTSD makes the issue of assessment validity a paramount concern for clinicians who conduct PTSD evaluations. Every effort should be made to ensure that multiple data corroborate the diagnostic impression. Additionally, when assessing for PTSD, it is most important to remember that symptoms of PTSD show considerable overlap with other diagnostic categories. Consequently, the diagnostician must strive to determine that symptoms are manifest in response to experiencing a traumatic event and that the current level of functioning represents a change, compared to functioning before the traumatic experience. Furthermore, the clinical evaluator should be aware that the symptom picture presented can vary as a function of the amount of time that elapsed since the trauma. The clinician should also be sensitive to the differences in the symptom picture and the response to trauma displayed by various racial and cultural groups, as well as those displayed in response to different types of traumas (e.g., repeated sexual abuse vs. a single automobile accident). Finally, when assessing children, the evaluator should make every effort to tailor the selection and use of assessment tools to the developmental level of the child being assessed (Caddell & Drabman, 1993; Ollendick & Hersen, 1984).

Practical considerations may dictate using a more streamlined approach to assessing PTSD. Likewise, a comprehensive assessment battery that uses the full array of available tools may not be required in all situations. Nonetheless, numerous components are available to choose from in selecting an assessment protocol to meet the requirements of a specific context, and using the most comprehensive assessment battery possible is generally recommended in any given situation. It is beyond the scope of the current chapter to review in any detail the large number of relevant assessment tools that have been developed and refined in the last decade, but we present information to introduce the reader to the following types or categories of assessments that can be used in a PTSD assessment battery: structured clinical interviews, self-report psychometric rating scales, clinician rating scales, psychophysiological assessment, and neurobiological and neuropsychological assessments. For a more complete treatment of the broad range of issues surrounding the assessment of PTSD, we refer the reader to several other excellent sources that address these issues and describe specific assessment instruments in more detail (Friedman, 2000; Newman et al., 1996; Stamm, 1996; Weathers & Keane, 1999; Wilson & Keane, 1997).

## Structured Clinical Interviews

There is no definitive diagnostic tool available for making any psychiatric diagnosis, but the clinical interview currently stands as the linchpin of a multiaxial, multimodal assessment protocol. With a goal of improving diagnostic validity and reliability, a number of structured and semistructured clinical interviews have been developed to assess psychological and psychiatric problems. The *Structured Clinical Interview for DSM-IV* (SCID; First, Spitzer, Williams, & Gibbon, 1996) was designed for use by trained clinicians to assess signs and symptoms of both Axis I and Axis II disorders. The interview is divided into modules that assess the presence of major categories of disorders and also assess specific diagnoses within each category. The format of the interview is such that the diagnostic criteria are presented concurrently with the stem questions to assess the presence of each DSM diagnostic criterion. However, the stem questions are not intended to be used in the absence of further probing by the clinician.

The original PTSD module of the SCID was developed for use in the National Vietnam Veterans Readjustment Study (NVVRS; Kulka et al., 1990); consequently, considerable data have been collected regarding the reliability and the validity of the PTSD module in a veteran population. In the

NVVRS, interrater reliability for the DSM-III version of the PTSD module was .933 (kappa coefficient). Additionally, the correspondence in PTSD diagnosis between the SCID and other measures of PTSD (e.g., Mississippi Scale for Combat-Related PTSD, the Keane et al. MMPI-PTSD subscale) was high. As the diagnostic criteria for PTSD (and other psychiatric disorders) have been revised, subsequent versions of the SCID have been revised to correspond to current nosological specifications.

As researchers and clinicians have gained a better understanding of the complexities of PTSD and its co-occurrence with other psychiatric disorders, recognition of the importance of the capacity to assess comorbid disorders has been commensurate. Instruments such as the SCID that assess the full spectrum of Axis I and Axis II diagnoses offer a decided advantage in this regard. However, the same concerns about ensuring reliable and valid diagnosis apply to assessing these comorbid conditions. Fortunately, the SCID has been fairly rigorously tested across the diagnostic spectrum. For example, the SCID has been shown reliable when distinguishing major depressive disorder from generalized anxiety disorder (Riskind, Beck, Berchick, Brown, & Steer, 1987).

In child and adolescent assessment, the Diagnostic Interview for Children and Adolescents—Revised (DICA-R; Nader, 1997) offers an approach similar to that of the SCID; that is, the instrument assesses several DSM-IV disorders, including PTSD. A four-point rating scale of symptom frequency is part of this assessment. Examination of the reliability of the PTSD module has indicated good interrater reliability; however, validity studies of the PTSD module of the DICA-R revealed variable sensitivity and specificity (Friedman, 2000).

Several interviews have been designed that are narrower in focus; that is, they were developed for assessing PTSD exclusively. One notable example of this type of interview is the Clinician Administered PTSD Scale (CAPS; Blake, Weathers, Nagy, Kaloupek, Gusman, Charney, & Keane, 1995; Blake, Weathers, Nagy, Kaloupek, Klauminzer, Charney, & Keane, 1990). The CAPS was designed to address the shortcomings of previously developed structured interviews for diagnosing PTSD. The CAPS is a comprehensive interview that (1) uses behavioral referents for symptoms when feasible; (2) assesses all DSM-IV criteria, as well as a selected sample of relevant associated features; (3) provides separate intensity and frequency ratings of symptoms; (4) specifically establishes that the time frame for symptom occurrence is consistent with diagnostic criteria; and (5) determines both current and lifetime symptoms. Additionally, the CAPS provides ratings of global functioning and of the impact of PTSD symptoms on relevant areas of life functioning. Evaluations of reliability and validity indicate strong psychometric performance. Initial examinations of interrater reliability were quite good (at the symptom level, $r$ ranges from .92 to .99, and there is perfect agreement at the diagnostic level), and subsequent examinations of test–retest reliability for PTSD were .89 (Weathers, Blake et al., 1997). Weathers, Blake et al. (1997) also found a coefficient alpha of .89, and compared to a SCID PTSD diagnosis, they obtained a sensitivity of .91, a specificity of .86, and a kappa of .77. Additionally, the CAPS has shown strong correlation with other psychometric measures of PTSD, including the Mississippi Scale and the PK Scale of the MMPI (Weathers and Keane, 1999). Recent additions to the CAPS include changes to accommodate DSM-IV symptom revisions, as well as additional questions to assess trauma exposure in more detail.

A version of the CAPS for use with children has also been developed—the CAPS-C (Nader, Kriegler, Blake, Pynoos, Newman, & Weathers, 1996). This instrument is based on DSM-IV diagnostic criteria but also includes the assessment of additional symptoms/features that have been documented in children. Assessment of academic and social functioning are also included in the CAPS-C. This relatively new instrument has not yet reached full psychometric maturity but shows promise, particularly given the full range of symptoms and functional variables that are assessed. There is some indication, however, that the length and the demand of completing the rating scales may be problematic for younger children (Nader, 1997).

In this section, we have provided only a brief introduction to the types of clinical interviews and approaches now available for assessing PTSD, as well as examples of some of the more notable of these interviews. Other choices of clinical interviews that are currently available are delineated and reviewed more extensively in other sources (Friedman, 2000; Newman et al., 1996; Stamm, 1996; Weathers & Keane, 1999; Wilson & Keane, 1996).

## Assessments of Trauma History

Because the hallmark symptom of PTSD is exposure to a traumatic event, it is crucial that any assessment of PTSD determine that exposure has occurred. Researchers and clinicians have not yet reached a consensus regarding how best to identify and characterize events that meet the diagnostic criteria for traumatic event exposure as specified in DSM-IV. Approaches to developing instruments to assess the nature and level of exposure to trauma have focused variously on identifying the type of event, characterizing the degree or level of exposure, defining characteristics of the events that are purportedly related to poorer outcome, and determining the subjective response of an individual to an event. Currently, DSM specifies that a traumatic event is defined both by the objective characteristics of an event and the subjective response to that event. At present, however, there are few published instruments designed to assess trauma history that assess both the objective characteristics and the subjective reaction to the event. Additionally, it should be noted that more formalized and quantitative assessments of trauma histories are at times incorporated into clinical interviews (e.g., the CAPS). To provide a flavor of the type of instruments available for use as "stand-alone" trauma assessments, we review here two widely used instruments that represent different approaches to trauma assessment: (1) the Potential Stressful Events Interview that assesses exposure to a broad array of potentially traumatic events and is designed to provide an assessment that corresponds with the DSM-IV definition of a traumatic event and (2) the Combat Exposure Scale that is limited to assessing combat-related traumatic events and does not attempt to provide results that correspond to the current DSM conceptualization of traumatic events. For a more complete treatment of instruments that assess trauma history, we refer the reader to Friedman (2000), Newman et al. (1996), Stamm (1996), and Weathers & Keane (1999).

The Potential Stressful Events Interview (PSEI; Falsetti, Resnick, Kilpatrick & Freedy, 1994) was developed initially for use in the DSM-IV PTSD field trial. This interview gathers information on exposure to low magnitude stressors and high magnitude stressors, as well as objective and subjective information on high magnitude stressors. The interview inquires about experiencing a broad array of potential traumatic events using well-crafted and direct language. This instrument is used quite widely, but currently there is no reliability or validity information published on it. Additionally, the detail obtained by using this instrument requires considerable time and effort that may prove prohibitive in some situations. In an effort to address the issue of burden, researchers have developed a brief self-report instrument that is based on the PSEI—the Trauma Assessment for Adults (TAA; Resnick, Best, Freedy, Kilpatrick, & Falsetti, 1993). Using the TAA may be more feasible when time availability for gathering information is a primary consideration—such as community epidemiologic studies (Schlenger, Fairbank, Jordan, & Caddell, 1996).

One of the most rigorously tested measures of combat exposure is the *Combat Exposure Scale* (CES; Keane, Fairbank, Caddell, Zimering, Taylor, & Mora, 1989). The CES was partly derived from Figley's (1978) combat scale, and additional items were constructed by PTSD content experts. Individuals who complete the scale rate items that describe various types of combat-related experiences on a Likert scale, and ratings are totaled to yield a range of possible scores between 0 and 41. Items are weighted in determining the total score based on the severity of the combat experience described by the item. This scale has demonstrated good internal consistency (coefficient alpha = .85), high test–retest reliability ($r = .97$), and some concurrence with measures of PTSD. Although this scale was developed initially for use with Vietnam veterans, item content is not exclusive to Vietnam combat experiences, and it has been adapted for use with veterans of the Persian Gulf War, as well as soldiers who served in Somalia and Bosnia (Friedman, 2000). Note that this measure does not have validity indicators, thus highlighting the importance of corroborating results obtained with other sources of information.

## Self-Report Psychometric Rating Scales

Attention in the field of PTSD assessment has turned from developing purely descriptive measures to designing instruments that have sound psychometric properties and acceptable diagnostic accuracy (Litz et al., 1992). During the past decade, researchers have worked to advance the psychometric maturity of self-report instruments, and particular advances have been made in assessing noncombat trauma and trauma in children. The sheer number of self-report instruments that were developed in the past decade is truly astounding. This proliferation of assessment tools is generally positive, but it does create some concern because assessment protocols used across clinical settings and research studies are rarely uniform, and many of the tools currently available are still in their infancy with regard to assessing their psychometric properties (Weathers & Keane, 1999). Because it is not possible to provide even a cursory overview of all these instruments within this chapter, a selected set of illustrative instruments that are widely used with adults and were developed with adherence to sound psychometric methods will be reviewed here. Other existing sources can be consulted for more exhaustive reviews of self-report instruments, including those designed for use with children and adolescents (Friedman, 2000; Stamm, 1996).

The instruments that assess PTSD symptoms and functioning can be classified according to whether they use a DSM framework. Additionally, there are a number of self-report measures available that are designed to assess associated features or other areas of functioning that are relevant for trauma survivors.

**Measures Focusing on Assessing DSM PTSD Criteria.** The PTSD Checklist (PCL) was developed at the National Center for PTSD as a tool for validating the CAPS (Weathers, Litz, Herman, Huska, & Keane, 1993). This seventeen-item scale uses a five-point Likert rating (1 = not at all, 5 = extremely) of DSM-IV PTSD symptoms. There is a generic civilian version and a generic military version for use when a specific traumatic event has not been identified. There also is a specific stressor version for which the respondent provides symptom ratings in relation to a specific event that has been identified by taking a trauma history. Examinations of the psychometric properties of the PCL indicated that it has performed very well in veteran populations (Weathers, Litz et al., 1997). Although the PCL was strongly correlated with other psychometric measures of PTSD (e.g., the MS Scale, the PK Scale), most impressive is its performance compared to the SCID. Using a cut score of 50, the PCL produced a sensitivity of .82, a specificity of .83, and a kappa of .64. The bulk of the research that examined the utility of the PCL was with veteran populations, but it is important to note that the PCL has shown promise as a measure of PTSD symptoms in other traumatized populations (Blanchard, Jones-Alexander, Buckley, & Forneris, 1996; Cordova et al., 1995).

The Davidson Trauma Scale (DTS; Davidson, 1996) is another DSM-based self-report measure of PTSD. This scale also includes seventeen items, indicative of DSM symptoms, that are rated using a Likert scale in terms of frequency (0 = not at all, 4 = every day) and severity (0 = not at all distressing, 4 = extremely distressing) during the past week. The respondent must specifically identify a "most disturbing" traumatic event that then serves as the anchor event for symptom ratings. The DTS provides a continuous measure of PTSD symptoms, and in addition the DTS manual provides information for converting these scores to a PTSD diagnosis. The DTS has shown good correspondence with CAPS diagnosis and correlates strongly with the Impact of Event Scale (IES; Horowitz, Wilner, & Alvarez, 1979) and other measures of trauma symptoms. It also has shown good test–retest reliability—.86 at 1 week. Another potential advantage of the DTS is that it is sensitive to symptom improvement. However, note that limiting the symptom ratings to the past week does not permit assessment of the 1-month symptom duration criteria for diagnosing PTSD that is specified in DSM-IV.

**Measures That Assess PTSD from a Non-DSM Framework.** The *Minnesota Multiphasic Personality Inventory* (MMPI; Hathaway & McKinley, 1967) has long been a standard of personality assessment. Two subscales to assess PTSD in a veteran population were developed from the existing clinical scales of the MMPI: the Keane MMPI-PTSD subscale (PK; Keane, Malloy, & Fairbank, 1984), and the Schlenger and Kulka PTSD subscale (Kulka et al., 1990) derived from the MMPI-2. Both of these subscales were empirically derived and therefore are not as susceptible to problems related to the face validity of items as other instruments that will be reviewed. Additionally, the validity scales of the MMPI can be used to determine whether a biased response style was used in endorsing items on the subscale. Both subscales have performed well in diagnostic accuracy, but their utility has been established largely with a veteran population. Koretsky and Peck (1990), however, found that the PK subscale could

accurately identify cases of PTSD that result from nonmilitary trauma. Note, however, that the performance of the PK subscale varied across studies and consequently, establishing optimal cut scores for specific populations is recommended (Lyons & Keane, 1992; Newman et al., 1996). Differences in performance highlight the importance of using these MMPI scales primarily as corroborative measures within a more comprehensive assessment battery.

The Mississippi Scale for Combat-Related PTSD (MS Scale; Keane, Caddell, & Taylor, 1988) was developed to provide a psychometrically sound quantitative self-report measure of combat-related PTSD that can be administered easily. This scale includes thirty-five items that represent selected behavioral manifestations of some of the DSM-III PTSD diagnostic criteria, selected associated features of PTSD, and items describing functional deficits commonly observed in traumatized veterans. Subjects rate each item on a five-point Likert scale. Suggested cutoffs for total scores (sum of item ratings) were determined for both clinical and community-based non-help-seeking Vietnam veteran populations. Total scores possible range from 35 to 175, and higher scores indicate the endorsement of more PTSD symptomatology. To maximize diagnostic accuracy, sensitivity, and specificity, a cutoff of 107 was suggested to distinguish PTSD patients from non-PTSD patients in a hospital sample (Keane et al., 1988) and another score of 89 to distinguish patients from nonpatients in a community population (Kulka et al., 1990). However, note that subsequent analyses of the NVVRS data indicate that a cutoff score of 95 may be more appropriate for distinguishing cases from noncases in a community sample. The relatively high face validity of the MS Scale can be problematic in some situations, though, such as when secondary gain is an important issue.

Several versions of the Mississippi Scale were developed, including a version for civilians, various abbreviated versions, and a Spouse/Partner version. Although relatively little work has focused on instruments designed to systematically collect data from collateral sources to assist with patient diagnosis, the Spouse/Partner version of the Mississippi Scale is an attempt to address this need (MS Scale-S/P; Caddell, Fairbank, Schlenger, Jordan, & Weiss, 1991). This instrument was initially developed for use in the NVVRS. Although further refinement and testing are required, initial tests of psychometric properties indicate adequate internal consistency (alpha = .937 for S/Ps of male veterans and .864 for S/Ps of female veterans) and good correspondence between the MS Scale-S/P and other indicators of PTSD. This instrument clearly requires further validation, but it shows promise as a quantitative tool to corroborate patient self-reports.

The Impact of Event Scale (IES; Horowitz et al., 1979) is one of the most widely used self-report scales designed for assessing trauma-related symptoms. Two of the advantages of this instrument are that it is applicable to veteran and civilian populations and that considerable work has been done with standardization samples that include women. When completing the IES, individuals identify a stressful event and then rate items pertaining to intrusion and avoidance of that event. Although the IES is primarily focused on assessing avoidance and intrusive symptomatology, it has recently been revised to assess manifestations of other symptoms in the PTSD diagnostic construct—most specifically symptoms of hyperarousal (Weiss & Marmar, 1997). The IES has acceptable reliability but does not offer scores that indicate clinically significant symptoms of PTSD. Furthermore, the IES offers no guidelines for having the subject identify stressful events that would be classified as traumatic by DSM-IV standards. Still, this instrument can be quite useful as a research tool and as a clinical tool to help delineate the major response that an individual manifests to trauma (intrusion, avoidance, or a combination), thereby assisting in developing relevant treatment strategies.

**Non-PTSD Self-Report Instruments Relevant to Trauma Populations.** Other more generic self-report instruments have also been employed with PTSD populations to assess non-PTSD psychological constructs that may be of interest when attempting to characterize the functioning of trauma populations. Because trauma survivors often display deficits across multiple domains of life functioning as well as comorbid symptoms beyond classic PTSD symptoms, the astute clinician and researcher will consider using the variety of other well-established instruments available to further define patient/subject functioning.

For example, the State-Trait Anxiety Inventory (STAI; Spielberger, Gorsuch, & Lushene, 1970), the Beck Depression Inventory (BDI; Beck, Ward, Mendelson, Mock, & Erbaugh, 1961), and the State-Trait Anger Scale/T-Anger (Spielberger, 1988) have been used with PTSD patients (Chemtob, Hamadam, Roitblat, Muraoka, & Pelowski, 1991; Keane, Fairbank et al., 1985; Riley, Treiber, & Woods, 1989). In a comparison of Vietnam veterans with PTSD to well-adjusted Vietnam veteran and to noncombat veterans with other nonpsychotic psychiatric disorders, veterans with PTSD scored consistently higher on the STAI and BDI than the comparison groups (Fairbank, Keane, & Malloy, 1983). Additionally, veterans with PTSD scored higher on the Trait scale of the State-Trait Anger Scales than relevant comparison groups (Chemtob et al., 1991; Riley et al., 1989). Therefore, these instruments may be useful for assessing generic symptoms of anger, anxiety, and depression that are often associated with PTSD.

The Dissociative Experiences Scale (DES; Carlson & Putnam, 1993) is an example of a measure that attempts to capture and characterize one particular associated feature often seen in trauma survivors—dissociation. Although understanding the level and phenomenology of dissociation is not necessary for making a diagnostic determination of PTSD, obtaining such information can be invaluable in treatment planning and in research studies. The DES is a twenty-eight-item measure of the frequency of experiences that represent differing levels of dissociation. A large body of research has been conducted on this scale, and it has shown excellent psychometric properties.

The few instruments described represent only a small subset of the large number of well-researched instruments that are available. Consequently, clinicians and researchers have the opportunity to tailor their selection of instruments to address the issues that are of the most interest or importance in any given context.

## Psychophysiological Assessments

The psychophysiological measurement of anxiety is a particularly attractive assessment strategy in that it offers a potentially more objective measure of the anxiety construct and the symptomatology of anxiety disorders. As used in this context, the phrase "more objective measure" does not necessarily imply a more accurate or more fundamental measure, but rather a measure not solely dependent on the individual's subjective perceptions and less easily subject to direct manipulation by the individual. Psychophysiological techniques have been used to assess a variety of anxiety disorders, including PTSD. Typically, PTSD symptoms have been measured by presenting trauma-related stimuli and comparison stimuli while measuring the three modalities of response most relevant to anxiety: physiological response, behavioral avoidance, and subjective response. Physiological measures of PTSD have included heart rate, skin conductance, and electromyogram (EMG). Subjective response is usually measured by some self-report rating of arousal, such as the Subjective Units of Distress Scale (SUDS). Typically, the behavioral response is measured as a function of the subject terminating the assessment or avoiding the trauma-related stimuli.

Numerous studies using a variety of stimulus presentation methods (imaginal, auditory, visual) demonstrated that veterans with PTSD respond with increased arousal to combat-related stimuli, compared to control stimuli, and likewise respond with more arousal to combat-related stimuli than relevant control groups (Blanchard & Buckley, 1999; Blanchard, Kolb, Pallmeyer, & Gerardi, 1982; Malloy, Fairbank, & Keane, 1983; Pitman, Orr, Forgue, de Jong, & Claiborne, 1987). Indeed, the vast majority of physiological assessments of trauma survivors have been conducted with veterans. However, a burgeoning literature exists that examines psychophysiological response in other trauma populations, particularly motor vehicle accident victims and survivors of sexual assault. Overall, these studies indicate a pattern of response among nonveteran populations similar to that documented in veterans; that is, individuals with PTSD display more reactivity in response to trauma-relevant stimuli than control subjects, although this trend is not as clear or strong among sexual assault survivors (Blanchard & Buckley, 1999). Additionally, physiological measurement used as a within-subject measure of progress in treatment has shown promise with both veteran and nonveteran populations (Boudewyns and Hyer, 1990; Fairbank & Keane, 1982; Keane & Kaloupek, 1982; McCaffrey & Fairbank, 1985; Rychtarik, Silverman, van Landingham, & Prue, 1984). Nonetheless, psychophysiological measures are still used primarily within a more comprehensive assessment battery as a corroborative measure for determining a PTSD diagnosis.

To refine and streamline physiological assessment procedures, Blanchard and Buckley (1999) recommend dropping EMG and temperature from most psychophysiological batteries, and generally believe that heart rate and electrodermal activity provide the most significant results. Additionally, there is interest in using psychophysiological measures to better characterize treatment prognosis, although efforts in this area are relatively new and require considerably more research to refine (Blanchard & Buckley, 1999).

## Neurobiological and Neuropsychological Assessment

Considerable progress has been made in the last decade in documenting and understanding the potential neurobiological underpinnings of PTSD. Although this approach may eventually provide more objective and biological tests for diagnosing PTSD, at this point that literature is still focused on elucidating the potential relationships of neurobiology to symptom development and presentation rather than on using neurobiological methods as diagnostic tools. Consequently, we will not review or present the findings from neurobiological research (see Bremner, Southwick, & Charney, 1999 for an overview of these findings to date). Likewise, research that focuses on the use of neuropsychological testing to characterize cognitive and behavioral deficits and excesses in trauma patients is also in its early phases compared with other areas of trauma research. Neuropsychology does not yet offer diagnostic tools to assist in making PTSD diagnosis, nor does it currently offer definitive assessment strategies to define the neurocognitive concomitants of PTSD. Still, neuropsychological assessment can be of considerable clinical utility now (Knight, 1997). As one example, standardized neuropsychological testing can shed light on aspects of a patient's cognitive functioning that could interfere with maximum treatment benefit (e.g., memory deficits or abstraction difficulties could prove problematic when using cognitive behavioral treatment strategies) (Knight, 1997). Gaining a fuller understanding of this type of functional factor through neuropsychological testing could be invaluable in treatment planning.

## Approaches to Treating PTSD

Psychosocial and neurobiological models of PTSD have influenced the development of clinical interventions for this disorder (Fairbank, Friedman, & Basoglu, in press; Southwick & Friedman, in press). Among the main approaches to treating PTSD that are conceptually linked to these models are cognitive behavioral therapy (CBT), psychodynamic therapy, pharmacotherapy, and eye movement desensitization and reprocessing (EMDR). Other approaches used to address the psychological sequelae of potentially traumatic experiences are family and marital therapy, supportive psychotherapy, inpatient and milieu therapy, professional and self-help group therapies, hypnotherapy, pastoral counseling, and interventions based on community psychology and public health models of prevention (e.g., education, debriefing, crisis counseling, early intervention).

This section provides a selective overview of interventions that have been used, separately and in combination, to treat people with PTSD. Emphasis is placed on summarizing the results of treatment outcome studies for those interventions that have been evaluated empirically.

## Cognitive-Behavioral Therapy for PTSD

Early behavioral conceptual models of PTSD were largely based on the two-factor learning theory of psychopathology originally proposed by Mowrer (Keane, Zimering, & Caddell, 1985). As applied to PTSD, two-factor conditioning models posit that fear and other aversive emotions are learned through association via mechanisms of classical conditioning (Fairbank & Nicholson, 1987). Such fear conditioning is the first factor in the acquisition of aversive emotions characteristic of PTSD. The second factor involves principles of instrumental conditioning in that persons with PTSD will learn to escape from and to avoid cues that stimulate aversive emotions. Through the process of fear conditioning, neutral cues associated with a traumatic (or otherwise aversive) event acquire the capacity subsequently to evoke a conditioned emotional (fearful) response in the absence of the aversive stimulus. First described by Pavlov and associates, this psychological mechanism, it is posited, preserves information about exposure to previous threats to promote future survival.

More recent conceptual models have emphasized the role of cognitive factors in developing and maintaining PTSD symptoms (Brewin, Dalgleish, & Joseph, 1996; Chemtob, Roitblatt, Hamada, Carlson, & Twentyman, 1988; Foa, Steketee, & Rothbaum, 1989; Lang, 1977; Resick & Schnicke, 1993). Information processing theory has been proposed as an explanation of the ways in

which information associated with traumatic experiences is encoded and recalled in memory (Foa & Kozak, 1986; Foa, Rothbaum, & Molnar, 1995; Foa et al., 1989). Foa et al. (1989), for example, offered a model based upon the concept of a fear structure, which they describe as a network in memory that includes three types of information: (1) information about the feared stimulus situation; (2) information about verbal, physiological, and overt behavioral responses; and (3) interpretive information about the meaning of the stimulus and the response elements of the structure (Foa et al., 1989, p. 166). Foa and colleagues proposed that during periods of extreme distress, information processing is interrupted, and traumatic memories are consequently fragmented and disorganized. Nevertheless, persons with PTSD are assumed to have an attentional bias toward threat cues (Foa, Feske, Murdock, Kozak, & McCarthy, 1991) that is hypothesized to account for the reexperiencing phenomenon of PTSD. Foa and her colleagues (Foa et al., 1995) proposed that treatment should be based upon activating and correcting information in fear structures by prolonged exposure (PE) to traumatic stimuli and cognitive restructuring, respectively. According to Foa and colleagues, exposure within and across trials is an opportunity to integrate traumatic memories with the individual's existing conceptualization of safety versus danger. Foa and colleagues further hypothesize that this exposure can result in organizing trauma memory. The information processing model has yielded a productive, theoretically grounded approach to research into the clinical efficacy of cognitive-behavioral therapy (CBT) for PTSD.

CBT approaches to treating PTSD include exposure therapy, cognitive therapy, cognitive processing therapy, stress inoculation training, systematic desensitization, assertiveness training, and biofeedback and relaxation training (Friedman, 2000). To date, exposure therapy is the most rigorously evaluated intervention for PTSD (Friedman, 2000; Rothbaum, Meadows, Resick, & Foy, in press). Exposure treatment methods involve confronting fearful stimuli associated with the traumatic memories within the context of a stable therapeutic relationship (Fairbank & Nicholson, 1987). The process of exposure therapy for PTSD involves having the patient experience the arousal associated with the traumatic event through imagery or *in vivo* exposure exercises and intentionally maintaining the arousal until it diminishes.

Exposure therapy has been used to treat PTSD symptoms associated with combat, sexual assault, and motor vehicle accidents. Exposure therapy has been applied in treating adults, adolescents, and children who experienced traumatic events. For example, four controlled clinical trials of the efficacy of exposure therapy for combat-related PTSD in Vietnam veterans reported generally positive findings (Boudewyns & Hyer, 1990; Cooper & Clum, 1989; Glynn et al., 1999; Keane, Fairbank, & Zimering, 1989). Two randomly controlled studies of exposure therapy for female sexual assault survivors also found that exposure therapy is efficacious in reducing PTSD symptoms (Foa et al., 1991, in press).

Resick and Schnicke (1992) reported improvements in the PTSD symptoms of rape survivors using a particular form of CBT—cognitive processing therapy. The authors state that this treatment includes education about PTSD symptoms, exposure, and cognitive therapy. Instead of using *in vivo* imagery, the exposure component involved having participants write and read a detailed account of the rape. Safety, trust, power, esteem, and intimacy were beliefs addressed in cognitive therapy. Treatment was administered in a group format during 12 weekly sessions and was compared to a waiting-list control. Treatment subjects improved significantly from pretreatment to posttreatment in depression and PTSD measures and maintained these gains at the six-month follow-up. The waiting-list group did not significantly improve.

Another frequently reported behavioral approach to treating PTSD involves teaching patients specific coping skills for reducing or managing PTSD symptoms and/or alternative responses to fear and anxiety. Specific interventions applicable to PTSD include relaxation training, anger management training, thought stopping, assertiveness training, self-dialogue, problem-solving skills training, and relapse prevention (Friedman, 2000). An example of this approach is Kilpatrick and Veronen's (1983) stress inoculation training (SIT) procedure for treating rape victims. Directed at the acquisition and application of coping skills, the SIT package includes Jacobsonian relaxation, diaphragmatic breathing, role playing, cognitive modeling, thought stopping, and guided self-dialogue. Patients are given homework assignments that require them to practice each coping skill.

The effectiveness of SIT was examined in four controlled studies (Foa et al., 1991, in press; Resick, Jordan, Girelli, Hutter, & Marhoefer-Dvorak, 1988). In one of these studies, Foa et al. (1991) reported findings of the comparative efficacy of SIT and PE for treating rape-related PTSD from a randomized trial. Specifically, these investigators compared the effectiveness of a wait-less control group and three interventions—prolonged exposure (PE), SIT, and supportive counseling (SC). PE consisted of both *in vivo* exposure exercises and imaginal exposure, SIT consisted of a modified version of Kilpatrick and Veronen's (1983) multi-intervention package, and SC consisted of a form of problem-oriented counseling where the counselors played a supportive role in the patients recovery; no instructions for exposure or stress management were included in the SC regimen. Wait-list clients were randomly assigned to one of the three treatments following a 5-week period. Treatment consisted of nine twice-weekly individual sessions conducted by a female therapist. Indicators of general psychological distress and PTSD reexperiencing, avoidance, and arousal symptoms were collected at intake, at completion of treatment, and at follow-up (mean = 3.5 months posttreatment). Only SIT produced significantly more improvement than wait list in PTSD symptoms at termination, but PE produced superior outcome at follow-up. Patients in the SIT and supportive counseling conditions showed little improvement of symptoms between termination and follow-up, whereas patients in the PE group that received *in vivo* and imaginal exposure continued to improve. The authors interpreted these findings as suggesting that (1) SIT procedures produce immediate relief in PTSD symptoms because they are aimed at the acquisition of anxiety management skills but show decreased effectiveness over time as performance compliance erodes and (2) PE shows less of an effect than SIT in the short term (a function of temporary increased levels of arousal induced by repetitive exposure to traumatic memories) but greater effectiveness over the long term, because therapeutic exposure is thought to lead to permanent change in the rape memory, thus producing durable gains.

## Psychodynamic Therapy

Horowitz et al. (1973, 1986; Horowitz & Kaltreider, 1980) present a psychodynamic formulation of stress response syndromes characterized by two psychological states; one is typified by intrusive experiences, the other by denial and numbing. Psychodynamic interventions for PTSD tend to focus on tailoring treatment to symptoms and context and thus vary depending on whether the patient is experiencing intrusive or avoidance symptoms. When intrusive symptoms predominate, the immediate goal of treatment is to bring those symptoms under control. Mild intrusive symptoms may respond to social and informational "reassurances" in the form of relevant educational presentations and debriefing groups (DeWitt, 1990). As symptoms become more severe, more individual and intensive approaches are necessary, and "covering" techniques (i.e., reducing exposure) such as supportive measures and stress management approaches are appropriate.

When avoidance symptoms predominate, interventions are aimed at removing blocks to processing and encouraging encounter with the event. As noted by DeWitt (1990), an important aspect of brief dynamic therapy is the concept of *dosing*, in which the person is encouraged to approach ideas and feelings at tolerable levels for reasonable time periods, turning away and then returning to the traumatic memories until they become more manageable. At this stage, "uncovering" techniques (i.e., increasing exposure) such as psychodrama and imagery are recommended. Once intrusive and avoidance systems are within manageable limits, the full meaning of the event can be explored and worked through. Since its introduction more than two decades ago, Horowitz's brief phase-oriented approach to treating stress response syndromes has evolved into one of the most frequently employed clinical interventions for PTSD (Fairbank & Nicholson, 1987; Marmar & Freeman, 1988).

Two uncontrolled evaluations of this approach reported findings that provide modest support (Horowitz, Marmar, Weiss, DeWitt, & Rosenbaum, 1984; Lindy, Green, Grace, Titchener, 1983). A randomly controlled trial condition (Brom, Kleber, & Defares, 1989) found a significant reduction in PTSD symptoms among patients who completed a course of brief dynamic psychotherapy compared to patients assigned to a wait-list control. Brom et al. (1989) also reported that the efficacy of brief dynamic psychotherapy compared favorably with two behaviorally oriented exposure-based treatment conditions: trauma focused desensitization and exposure in imagination

via hypnotherapy. Interestingly, these investigators reported that patients in the two exposure interventions showed superior reductions at posttreatment and follow-up assessment on intrusive symptoms, whereas patients who received brief dynamic psychotherapy showed the best improvement in avoidance symptoms.

## Pharmacological Approaches

A substantial body of research demonstrated abnormalities in psychobiological systems and function in persons with PTSD (Friedman, Charney, & Deutch, 1995). The strongest evidence shows alteration of adrenergic and hypothalamic-pituitary-adrenocortical (HPA) mechanisms, elevated physiological reactivity, and sleep disturbances (Bremner, Southwick, & Charney, 1999; Friedman, Davidson, Mellman, & Southwick, in press). Many medications have been used to treat specific PTSD symptoms, separately or in combination with psychotherapy. Pharmacological treatments for PTSD have included antidepressants, such as selective serotonin re-uptake inhibitors (SSRIs), tricyclic antidepressants (TCAs), and monoamine oxidase inhibitors (MAOIs). Other drugs evaluated for their efficacy against specific PTSD symptoms are inhibitors of adrenergic activity, including propranolol and clonidine; benzodiazepines, such as alprazolam (though the patients must be thoroughly evaluated for the potential for substance abuse); and antimanic drugs, including carbamazepine and lithium carbonate (Silver, Sandberg, & Hales, 1990). Among drugs applied to the treatment of PTSD, the most widely studied and most widely prescribed are antidepressants. Antidepressants are the only drugs that have been tested for PTSD outcome efficacy under double-blind experimental conditions.

Several randomized clinical trials examined the efficacy of SSRIs (fluoxetine and sertraline) for reducing symptoms of PTSD (Brady et al., 1998; Davidson et al., 1997; van der Kolk et al., 1994). A majority of the studies found that SSRI treatments led to more improvement in PTSD symptoms than a placebo. Several studies of the PTSD efficacy of older antidepressants (MAOIs and TCAs) reported significant effects (e.g., Davidson et al., 1990; Frank et al., 1988), whereas other double-blind comparisons of antidepressants and placebo have reported no differences in PTSD treatment efficacy (Reist et al. 1989; Shestatsky et al., 1988).

Although findings on the outcome efficacy of TCA and MAOI antidepressant medications for PTSD are mixed, evidence from clinical trials indicates that the SSRI antidepressants are currently the most efficacious drug treatment for PTSD (Friedman et al., in press).

## Eye Movement Desensitization and Reprocessing (EMDR)

Eye movement desensitization and reprocessing (EMDR) is a relatively new treatment for PTSD in which patients are asked to focus attention on certain distressing aspects of the relevant traumatic memory while simultaneously following the movements of the clinicians' finger in front of their visual fields (Chemtob, Tolin, van der Kolk, & Pitman, in press; Shapiro, 1995). More specifically, the patient is instructed to select (1) a disturbing image associated with the memory, (2) a negative cognition associated with the memory, and (3) associated bodily sensations, and to try to keep these in mind during the eye movement procedure. The procedure is then repeated until the distress surrounding the memory decreases and until more adaptive cognitions develop regarding the experience. In addition, the eye movement procedure is used for installing new adaptive behaviors, coping strategies, and alternative positive cognitions.

In randomly controlled trials, EMDR has been shown to have greater efficacy for treating PTSD than no treatment (wait-list control), standard care, and some active treatments. However, such empirical support for the efficacy of the overall process does not necessarily imply support for the idea that the eye movement component is critical to the clinical effects. In fact, randomized dismantling studies to date have provided little support for the postulated role of the eye movements. More specific identification of the beneficial components of EMDR will require additional dismantling studies of sufficiently rigorous design (Chemtob et al., in press).

## Crisis Counseling

Crisis counseling is a supportive intervention that provides traumatized individuals with a forum to express feelings about the event within a nonjudgmental environment. Crisis counseling is frequently provided to victims of violent crimes, such as rape or sexual assault, as well as to survivors of natural and manmade disasters (Kilpatrick & Veronen, 1983; Sowder, 1985). General characteristics of crisis counseling are (1) it is time limited and issues oriented, (2) the counselor responds to the crisis request of the victim, (3) the counselor responds to the crisis-related problems and not to other problems, and (4) the counselor takes an active role in initiating follow-up contacts (Burgess & Holmstrom, 1974; Kilpatrick & Veronen, 1983). This approach is often carried out by peer counselors who offer support, information, and empathy to the victim. Hartsough and Myers (1985) emphasized that providing crisis counseling to victims can be stressful for the provider, and they outlined a training program for providers to minimize these effects.

## Family Considerations

In addition to the effects of PTSD on those who have the disorder, PTSD also affects family members and others (Danieli, 1998). For example, studies of the families of Holocaust survivors (Bergman & Jucovy, 1982; Danieli, 1985; Solomon, 1998; Yehuda et al., 1998), survivors of the atomic bombing of Japan during World War II (Tatara, 1998), refugees and internally displaced persons (Kinzie, Boehnlein, & Sack, 1998; Rousseau & Drapeau, 1998), and veterans of armed conflicts (Rosenheck & Nathan, 1985; Rosenheck & Fontana, 1998) demonstrated transgenerational effects on the children of survivors. Rosenheck and colleagues (Rosenheck & Nathan, 1985; Rosenheck & Fontana, 1998) similarly described a process they called "secondary traumatization" among some children of combat veterans, in which the child develops symptoms that mirror those of the veteran father. Davidson, Smith, and Kudler (1989) found that children of veterans with PTSD were at increased risk of developing psychiatric or behavioral problems, particularly hyperactivity/attention-deficit problems.

Findings with clinical studies of veterans with PTSD suggest important impacts on family relationships. Solomon, Mikulincer, Fried, and Wosner (1987) showed that levels of family cohesion and expressiveness were inversely related to the severity of PTSD symptomatology among Israeli veterans who suffered combat stress reactions. Verbosky and Ryan (1988) found increased levels of stress among wives of veterans with PTSD.

Roberts, Penk, Gearing, Robinowitz, Dolan, and Patterson (1982) found more difficulties in the areas of intimacy and sociability among Vietnam veterans with PTSD, whereas Carroll, Rueger, Foy, and Donahoe (1985) reported that Vietnam veterans with PTSD admitted more global relationship problems, problems with self-disclosure and expressiveness, and physical aggression toward their partners than non-PTSD help-seeking Vietnam veterans.

Findings from the NVVRS community sample confirm many of these clinical and research observations. Reporting on findings from interviews with the spouses/partners of a national sample of Vietnam veterans, Jordan et al. (in press) described markedly elevated levels of problems in marital and family adjustment, parenting skills, violent behaviors, and child behavior in families of male Vietnam veterans with PTSD.

Results of these early investigations reveal the need for a comprehensive treatment plan to take account of the individuals patient's family situation and the needs of the patient's family members. For example, Figley (1988) outlined a five-phased approach to the treatment of PTSD in families that emphasized developing a shared understanding of the problem and the joint development and acceptance by the family of a "healing theory" (see Figley, 1983).

### Community-Level Interventions

Clinical or therapeutic interventions for PTSD focus on the cure or care of the individual patient. Community psychology and public health interventions for PTSD focus on preventing and controlling exposure to traumatic stress and ultimately on the psychological sequelae of such exposures in the community. Integrated clinical and community strategies are needed to address the complex matrix of issues involved in providing appropriate and potentially effective PTSD prevention and treatment services to populations that have been exposed to traumatic events or are at risk of such exposures. The area of youth violence prevention is a good example of an evolving comprehensive approach based on community and clinical treatment models. Currently a repertoire of violence prevention strategies exists that operate at different levels of intervention (community programs, school programs, peer training programs, family interventions, individual treatment).

## Summary and Conclusions

PTSD is an anxiety disorder that occurs in some individuals who were exposed to traumatic events. Traumatic events are defined in the DSM-IV as experiences that (1) "involve actual or threatened death or serious injury, or a threat to the physical integrity of oneself or others" and (2) produce feelings of "intense fear, helplessness, or horror" (American Psychiatric Association, 1994, pp. 427–428). PTSD is characterized by three kinds of symptoms: reexperiencing symptoms, avoidance and numbing symptoms, and symptoms of increased arousal. The best available estimates suggest a lifetime prevalence of PTSD in the general adult population of the United States between 7 and 12% (Breslau et al., 1991, 1998; Kessler at al., 1995). At the same time, epidemiologic studies in the United States indicate that more than half of the population is likely to be exposed to potentially traumatic events at some time in their lives. Taken together these findings suggest that most people exposed to potentially traumatic events will not develop PTSD. Thus, researchers have attempted to identify risk factors that affect the likelihood of developing PTSD following exposure to such events.

The bulk of the research evidence to date is consistent with an etiologic model of PTSD that posits a role for preexposure factors (potentially including biological, psychological, and sociocultural factors), a role for characteristics of the stressor, and a role for postexposure variables. The most frequently identified preexposure risk factors for PTSD include female gender, preexisting psychiatric disorder, prior exposure to trauma, and a family history of psychopathology. The nature and characteristics of the stressor exposure are another important determinant of the likelihood of developing PTSD, and some stressors such as rape or those that involve both perceived life threat and injury are associated with comparatively high rates of PTSD. The role of postexposure factors in the development of PTSD has not been as well studied; however, postexposure social support and conflict are potential moderators. Although epidemiologic studies have provided valuable information about risk factors for PTSD and trauma exposure, additional research is required to improve our understanding of the relationships among these variables and the processes through which they affect the development and *course* of PTSD.

Studies consistently find that the experience of other psychiatric disorders is common among individuals with PTSD. The most frequent comorbid disorders are major depression, substance abuse disorders, and other anxiety disorders. However, data from general population studies typically pertain to lifetime disorder rather than current comorbidity. Additional research is needed to determine the extent to which psychiatric comorbidities among individuals with PTSD are (1) artifactual, reflecting overlapping diagnostic criteria; (2) exacerbations of preexisting pathology; (3) part of an overall syndrome of response to traumatic events, including reactions to PTSD symptoms; or (4) independent disorders.

The PTSD assessment literature has burgeoned considerably during the past decade. Of particular note are the advances in the development of (1) measures for nonveteran populations and children and (2) instruments designed to obtain a comprehensive trauma history. Additionally, the utility of psychophysiological measures to assess PTSD has been demonstrated with some nonveteran populations, and researchers have refined their understanding of the response channels that are most beneficial to include in psychophysiological batteries. Although the literature on neuropsychological testing is not as mature, such testing can serve as a useful adjunct for treatment planning in PTSD. Despite these considerable advances, state-of-the-art assessment of PTSD should continue to use multiple assessment strategies and sources of data to confirm or rule out a diagnosis of PTSD as well as to assess for other comorbidities and other indicators of functional status. Future efforts focusing on further elucidating the neurobiological underpinnings of PTSD have the potential to produce more objective and biological diagnostic measures of PTSD.

Findings from randomly controlled trials provide strong evidence that cognitive behavioral therapy (CBT), antidepressant pharmacological agents, and EMDR are efficacious treatments for PTSD. Much more research is needed, however, to clarify the active components of treatment for PTSD. At present, the science of PTSD treatment and trauma prevention has yet to determine which types and levels of treatment are most effective for which populations of trauma survivors. We still lack essential information on the relative effectiveness of the various approaches to PTSD treatment in different communities, cultures, and political, economic and religious traditions, and systems.

# References

Abenhaim, L., Dab, W., & Salmi, L. (1992). Study of civilian victims of terrorist attacks. *Journal of Clinical Epidemiology*, 103–109.

Acierno, R., Kilpatrick, D. G., & Resnick, H. S. (1999). Posttraumatic stress disorder in adults relative to criminal victimization: Prevalence, risk factors, and comorbidity. In P. A. Saigh & J. D. Bremner (Eds.), *Posttraumatic stress disorder: A comprehensive text* (pp. 44–68). Boston: Allyn & Bacon.

Adler, N. E., Boyce, T., Chesney, M. A., Cohen, S., Folkman, S., Kahn, R. L., & Syme, S. L. (1994). Socioeconomic status and health. *American Psychologist, 49*, 15–24.

American Psychiatric Association. (1980). *Diagnostic and statistical manual of mental disorder* (3rd ed.) Washington, DC: Author.

American Psychiatric Association. (1987). *Diagnostic and statistical manual of mental disorders* (3rd ed., rev.). Washington, DC: Author.

American Psychiatric Association. (1994). *Diagnostic and statistical manual of mental disorders* (4th ed.). Washington DC: Author.

Astin, M. A., Lawrence, K. J., & Foy, D. W. (1993). Posttraumatic stress disorder among battered women: Risk and resiliency factors. *Violence and Victims, 8*, 17–28.

Barlow, D. H., & Wolfe, B. E. (1981). Behavioral approaches to anxiety disorders: A report on the NIMH-SUNY Albany research conference. *Journal of Consulting and Clinical Psychology, 49*, 448–454.

Basoglu, M., Mineka, S., Parker, M., Aker, T., Livanou, M., & Gok, S. (1997). Psychological preparedness for trauma as a protective factor in survivors of torture. *Psychological Medicine, 27*, 1421–1433.

Beck, A. T., Ward, C. H., Mendelson, M., Mock, J., & Erbaugh, J. (1961). An inventory for measuring depression. *Archives of General Psychiatry, 4*, 561–571.

Beckham, J. C. (1999). Smoking and anxiety in combat veterans with posttraumatic stress disorder: A review. *Journal of Psychoactive Drugs, 31*, 103–110.

Beckham, J., Kirby, A. C., Feldman, M. E., Hertzberg, M. A., Moore, S. D., Crawford, A. L., Davidson, J. R. T., & Fairbank, J. A. (1997). Prevalence and correlates of heavy smoking in Vietnam veterans with chronic posttraumatic stress disorder. *Addictive Behavior, 22*, 637–647.

Beckham, J. C., Moore, S. D., Feldman, M. E., Hertzberg, M. A., Kirby, A. C., & Fairbank, J. A. (1998). Health status, somatization, and severity of posttraumatic stress disorder in Vietnam veterans with posttraumatic stress disorder. *American Journal of Psychiatry, 155*, 1565–1569.

Bell, C. B., & Jenkins, E. (1993). Community violence and children on Chicago's south side. *Psychiatry, 56*, 46–54.

Bergman, M. S., & Jucovy, M. C. (Eds.). (1982). *Generation of the Holocaust.* New York: Basic Books.

Blake, D. D., Weathers, F. W., Nagy, L. M., Kaloupek, D. G., Gusman, F. D., Charney, D. S., & Keane, T. M. (1995). The development of a clinician-administered PTSD scale. *Journal of Traumatic Stress, 8*, 75–90.

Blake, D. D., Weathers, F. W., Nagy, L. M., Kaloupek, D. G., Klauminzer, G., Charney, D. S., & Keane, T. M. (1990). A clinician rating scale for assessing current and lifetime PTSD: The CAPS-1. *Behavior Therapist, 13*, 187–188.

Blanchard, E. B., & Buckley, T. C. (1999). Psychophysiological assessment of posttraumatic stress disorder. In P. A. Saigh & J. D. Bremner (Eds.), *Posttraumatic stress disorder: A comprehensive text* (pp. 248–266). Boston: Allyn & Bacon.

Blanchard, E. B., Jones-Alexander, J., Buckley, T. C., & Forneris, C. A. (1996). Psychometric properties of the PTSD Checklist (PCL). *Behavior Research and Therapy, 34*, 669–673.

Blanchard, E. B., Kolb, L. C., Pallmeyer, T. P., & Gerardi, R. J. (1982). The development of a psychophysiological assessment procedure for post-traumatic stress disorder in Vietnam veterans. *Psychiatric Quarterly, 4*, 220–229.

Bloom, B. L. (1979). Prevention of mental disorders: Recent advances in theory and practice. *Community Mental Health Journal, 16*, 179–191.

Boney-McCoy, S., & Finkelhor, D. (1995). Psychosocial sequelae of violent victimization in a national youth sample. *Journal of Consulting and Clinical Psychology, 63*, 726–736.

Boscarino, J. A., & Chang, J. (1999). Electrocardiogram abnormalities among men with stress-related psychiatric disorders: Implications for coronary heart disease and clinical research. *Annals of Behavioral Medicine, 21*, 227–234.

Boudewyns, P. A., & Hyer, L. (1990). Physiological response to combat memories and preliminary treatment outcome in Vietnam veteran PTSD patients with direct therapeutic exposure. *Behavior Therapy, 21*, 63–87.

Boudewyns, P. A., & Hyer, L. (1990). Physiological response to combat memories and preliminary treatment outcome in Vietnam veterans PTSD patients treated with direct therapeutic exposure. *Behavior Therapy, 21*, 63–87.

Boudreaux, E., Kilpatrick, D. G., Resnick, H. S., Best, C. L., & Saunders, B. E. (1998). Criminal victimization, posttraumatic stress disorder, and comorbid psychopathology among a community sample of women. *Journal of Traumatic Stress, 11*, 665–678.

Brady, D. G., & Farfel, G. (1998). The sertraline PTSD study group. Double-blind multicenter comparison of sertraline and placebo in post-traumatic stress disorder. *American College of Neuropsychopharmacology Abstracts, 37th Annual Meeting*, Kona, Hawaii.

Bremner, J. D., Southwick, S. M., & Charney, D. S. (1999). The neurobiology of posttraumatic stress disorder: An integration of animal and human research. In P. A. Saigh & J. D. Bremner (Eds.), *Posttraumatic stress disorder: A comprehensive text* (pp. 103–143). Boston: Allyn & Bacon.

Breslau, N., Davis, G. C., & Andreski, P. (1995). Risk factors for PTSD-related traumatic events: A prospective analysis. *American Journal of Psychiatry, 152*, 529–535.

Breslau, N., Davis, G. C., Andreski, P., & Peterson, E. L. (1991). Traumatic events and posttraumatic stress disorder in an urban population of young adults. *Archives of General Psychiatry, 48*, 216–222.

Breslau, N., Davis, G. C., Peterson, E. L., & Schultz, L. R. (1997). Psychiatric sequela of posttraumatic stress disorder in women. *Archives of General Psychiatry, 54*, 81–87.

Breslau, N., Kessler, R. C., Chilcoat, H. D., Schultz, L. R., Davis, G. C., & Andreski, P. (1998). Traumatic and post-traumatic stress disorder in the community: The 1996 Detroit Area Survey of Trauma. *Archives of General Psychiatry, 55*, 626–631.

Brett, E. A. (1993). Psychoanalytic contributions to a theory of traumatic stress. In J. P. Wilson & B. Raphael (Eds.), *International handbook of traumatic stress syndromes* (pp. 61–68). New York: Plenum.

Brewin, C. R., Dalgleish, T., & Joseph, S. A. (1996). A dual representation theory of posttraumatic stress disorder. *Psychological Review, 103*, 670–686.

Brom, D., Kleber, R. J., & Defares, P. B. (1989). Brief psychotherapy for posttraumatic stress disorders. *Journal of Consulting and Clinical Psychology, 57*, 607–612.

Bromet, E., Sonnega, A., & Kessler, R. C. (1998). Risk factors for DSM-III-R posttraumatic stress disorder: Findings from the National Comorbidity Study. *American Journal of Epidemiology, 147*, 353–361.

Brown, P. C. (1984). Legacies of a war: Treatment considerations with Vietnam veterans and their families. *Social Work*, 372–379.

Burgess, A. W., & Holstrom, L. L. (1974). *Rape: Victims of crisis*. Bowie, MD: Robert J. Brady.

Caddell, J. M., & Drabman, R. S. (1993). Post-traumatic stress disorder in children. In R. T. Ammerman & M. Hersen (Eds.), *Handbook of behavior therapy with children and adults: A longitudinal perspective* (pp. 219–235). Boston: Allyn & Bacon.

Caddell, J. M., Fairbank, J. A., Schlenger, W. E., Jordan, B. K., & Weiss, D. S. (1991, August). Psychometric properties of a spouse/partner version of the Mississippi Scale for Combat-related PTSD. Paper presented at *American Psychological Association Annual Convention*, San Francisco.

Canino, G., Bravo, M., Rubio-Stipec, M., & Woodberry, M. (1990). The impact of disaster on mental health: Prospective and retrospective analyses. *International Journal of Mental Health, 19*, 51–69.

Caplan, G. (1964). *Principles of preventive psychiatry*. New York: Basic Books.

Carlson, E. B., & Putnam, F. W. (1993, March). An update on the Dissociative Experiences Scale. *Dissociation, 6*(1), 16–27.

Caroll, E. M., Rueger, D. B., Foy, D. W., & Donahue, C. P., Jr. (1985). Vietnam combat veterans with posttraumatic stress disorder: Analysis of marital and cohabitating adjustment. *Journal of Abnormal Psychology, 94*, 329–337.

Chemtob, C. M., Hamada, R. S., Roitblat, H. L., Muraoka, M. Y., & Pelowski, S. R. (1991). Anger, impulsivity, and anger control in combat-related PTSD. Unpublished manuscript.

Chemtob, C. M., Tolin, D. F., van der Kolk, B. A., & Pitman, R. K. (in press). Eye Movement Desensitization and Reprocessing (EMDR). In E. B. Foa, T. M. Keane, & M. J. Friedman (Eds.), *Effective treatments for PTSD: Practice guidelines from the International Society for Traumatic Stress Studies*. New York: Guilford.

Chemtob, C., Roitblatt, H. L., Hamada, R. S., Carlson, J. G., & Twentyman, C. T. (1988). A cognitive action theory of post-traumatic stress disorder. *Journal of Anxiety Disorders, 2*, 253–275.

Chilcoat, H. D., & Breslau. N. (1998). Posttraumatic stress disorder and drug disorders: Testing causal pathways. *Archives of General Psychiatry, 55*, 913–917.

Conyer, R. C., Sepulveda, A. J., Medina, M. M. E., Caraveo, J., & De La Fuente, J. R. (1987). Prevalencia del sindrome de estres posttraumatic en la poblacion sobreviviente a un desastre natural. *Salud Publica Mexicana, 29,* 406–411.

Cooper, N. A., & Clum, G. A. (1989). Imaginal flooding as a supplementary treatment for PTSD in combat veterans: A controlled study. *Behavior Therapy, 3,* 381–391.

Cordova, M. J., Andrykowski, M. A., Kenady, D. E., McGrath, P. C., Sloan, D. A., & Redd, W. H. (1995). Frequency and correlates of posttraumatic-stress-disorder-like-symptoms after treatment for breast cancer. *Journal of Consulting and Clinical Psychology, 63,* 981–986.

Danieli, Y. (1985). The treatment and prevention of long-term effects and intergenerational transmission of victimization: A lesson from Holocaust survivors and their children. In C. R. Figley (Ed.), *Trauma and its wake.* New York: Brunner/Mazel.

Danieli, Y. (Ed.). (1998). *International handbook of multigenerational legacies of trauma.* New York: Plenum Press.

Davidson, J. (1996). *Davidson Trauma Scale [Manual].* Toronto, Ontario, Canada: Multi-Health Systems.

Davidson, J. R. T., Hughes, D., Blazer, D. G., & George, L. K. (1991). Posttraumatic stress disorder in the community: An epidemiological study. *Psychological Medicine, 21,* 713–721.

Davidson, J., Kudler, H., Smith, R., Mahorney, S. L., Lipper, S., Hammett, E., Saunders, W. B., & Cavenar, J. O. (1990). Treatment of posttraumatic stress disorder with amitriptyline and placebo. *Archives of General Psychiatry, 47,* 259–266.

Davidson, J., Smith, R., & Kudler, H. (1989). Familial psychiatric illness in chronic posttraumatic stress disorder. *Comprehensive Psychiatry, 30,* 339–345.

Davidson, J., Landburg, P. D., Pearlstein, T., et al. (1997). Double-blind comparison of sertraline and placebo in patients with posttraumatic stress disorder (PTSD). *American College of Neuropsychopharmacology Abstracts, 36th Annual Meeting,* Kamuela, Hawaii.

DeWitt, K. N. (1990). Psychological interventions for responses to stressful life events. *California Psychologist, 22,* 4, 8.

Dohrenwend, B. P. (1998). A psychosocial perspective on the past and future of psychiatric epidemiology. *American Journal of Epidemiology, 147,* 222–231.

Engel, C. C., Engel, A. L., Campbell, S. J., McFall, M. E., Russo, J., & Katon, W. (1993). Posttraumatic stress disorder symptoms and precombat sexual and physical abuse in Desert Storm veterans. *Journal of Nervous and Mental Disease, 181,* 683–688.

Fairbank, J. A., Ebert, L., Zarkin, G. A., & Johnson, C. (November, 1999). The Economic Costs of Posttraumatic Stress Disorder: Analyses of Labor Market Variables. Paper presented at the *Annual Meeting of the International Society for Traumatic Stress Studies,* Miami, FL.

Fairbank, J. A., & Keane, T. M. (1982). Flooding for combat-related stress disorders: Assessment of anxiety reduction across traumatic memories. *Behavior Therapy, 13,* 499–510.

Fairbank, J. A., Keane, T. M., & Malloy, P. M. (1983). Some preliminary data on the psychological characteristics of Vietnam veterans with posttraumatic stress disorders. *Journal of Clinical Psychology, 43,* 44–55.

Fairbank, J. A., Friedman, M. J., & Basoglu, M. (in press). Psychosocial models. In E. Gerrity, T. M. Keane, & F. Tuma (Eds.), *The mental health consequences of torture and related violence and trauma.* New York: Plenum Press.

Fairbank, J. A., Friedman, M. J., & Southwick, S. (in press). Veterans of armed conflicts. In E. Gerrity, T. M. Keane, and F. Tuma (Eds.), *The mental health consequences of torture and related violence and trauma.* New York: Plenum Press.

Fairbank, J. A., & Nicholson, R. A. (1987). Theoretical and empirical issues in the treatment of post-traumatic stress disorder in Vietnam veterans. *Journal of Clinical Psychology, 43,* 44–55.

Fairley, M., Langeluddeck, P., & Tennant, C. (1986). Psychological and physical morbidity in the aftermath of a cyclone. *Psychological Medicine, 16,* 671–676.

Falsetti, S. A., Renick, H. S., Kilpatrick, D. G., & Freedy, J. R. (1994). A review of the Potential Stressful Events Interview: A comprehensive assessment instrument of high and low magnitude stressors. *Behavior Therapist, 17,* 66–67.

Figley, C. R. (Ed.). (1978). *Stress disorders among Vietnam veterans: Theory, research, and treatment.* New York: Brunner/Mazel.

Figley, C. R. (1983). Catastrophe: An overview of family reactions. In C. R. Figley & H. I. McCubbin (Eds.), *Stress and the family:* Vol. II. *Coping with catastrophe* (pp. 3–20). New York: Brunner/Mazel.

Figley, C. R. (1988). A five-phase treatment of post-traumatic stress disorder in families. *Journal of Traumatic Stress, 1,* 127–141.

First, M. B., Spitzer, R. L., Williams, J. B. W., & Gibbon, M. (1996). *Structured clinical interview for DSM-IV.* New York: New York State Psychiatric Institute, Biometrics Research.

Foa, F. B., Keane, T. M., & Friedman, M. J. (in press). Introduction to the practice guidelines for the treatment of PTSD. In E. B. Foa, T. M. Keane, & M. J. Friedman (Eds.), *Effective treatments for PTSD: Practice guidelines from the International Society for Traumatic Stress Studies.* New York: Guilford.

Foa, E. B., Dancu, C. V., Hembree, E. A., Jaycox, L. H., Meadows, E. A., & Street, G. P. (in press). The efficacy of exposure therapy, stress inoculation training and their combination in ameliorating PTSD for female victims of assault. *Journal of Consulting and Clinical Psychology, 63,* 948–955.

Foa, E. B., & Kozak, M. J. (1986). Emotional processing of fear: Exposure to corrective information. *Psychological Bulletin, 99,* 20–35.

Foa, E. B., Feske, U., Murdock, T. B., Kozak, M. J., & McCarthy, P. R. (1991). Processing of threat-related information in rape victims. *Journal of Abnormal Psychology, 100*(2), 156–162.

Foa, E. B., Rothbaum, B. O., & Molnar, C. (1995). Cognitive-behavioral therapy of post-traumatic stress disorder. *Journal of Traumatic Stress, 8,* 675–690.

Foa, E. B., Steketee, G., & Rothbaum, B. O. (1989). Behavioral/cognitive conceptualizations of post-traumatic stress disorder. *Behavior Therapy, 20,* 155–176.

Fontana, A., & Rosenheck, R. (1994). Posttraumatic stress disorder among Vietnam theater veterans: A causal model of the etiology in a community sample. *Journal of Nervous and Mental Disease, 182,* 677–684.

Fontana, A., Schwartz, L. S., & Rosenheck, R. (1997). Posttraumatic stress disorder among female Vietnam veterans: A causal model of etiology. *American Journal of Public Health, 87,* 169–175.

Frank, J. B., Kosten, T. R., Giller, E. L., & Dan, E. (1988). A randomized clinical trial of phenelzine and imipramine for posttraumatic stress disorder. *American Journal of Psychiatry, 145,* 1289–1291.

Friedman, M. J., Charney, D. S., & Deutch, A. Y. (Eds.). (1995). *Neurobiological and clinical consequences of stress: From normal adaptation to post-traumatic stress disorder.* Philadelphia: Lippincott-Raven.

Friedman, M. J. (2000). *Post traumatic stress disorder: The latest assessment and treatment strategies.* Kansas City, MO: Compact Clinicals.

Friedman, M. J., Davidson, J. R. T., Mellman, T. A., & Southwick, S. M. (in press). Pharmacotherapy for PTSD. In E. B. Foa, T. M. Keane, & M. J. Friedman (Eds.), *Effective treatments for PTSD: Practice guidelines from the International Society for Traumatic Stress Studies.* New York: Guilford.

Glynn, S. M., Eth, S., Randolph, E. T., Foy, D. W., Urbatis, M., Boxer, L., Paz, G. B., Leong, G. B., Firman, G., Salk, J. D., Katzman, J. W., & Crothers, J. (1999). A test of behavioral family therapy to augment exposure for combat-related PTSD. *Journal of Consulting and Clinical Psychology, 67,* 243–251.

Goenjian, A. K., Najarian, L. M., Pynoos, R. S., Steinberg, A. M., Petrosian, P., Setrakyan, S., & Fairbanks, L. A. (1994). Posttraumatic stress reactions after single and double trauma. *Acta Psychiatrica Scandinavica, 90,* 214–221.

Goldberg, J., True, W. R., Eisen, S. A., & Henderson, W. C. (1990) A twin study of the effects of the Vietnam war on posttraumatic stress disorder. *Journal of American Medical Association, 263,* 1227–1232.

Grace, M. C., Green, B. L., Lindy, J. D., & Leonard, A. C. (1993). The Buffalo Creek disaster: A 14-year follow-up. In J. P. Wilson & B. Raphael, (Eds.), *International handbook of traumatic stress syndromes* (pp. 441–449). New York: Plenum Press.

Green, B. L., & Lindy, J. D. (1994). Posttraumatic stress disorder in victims of disaster. *Psychiatric Clinics of North America, 17*(2), 301–309.

Green, B. L., Lindy, J. D., Grace, M. C., & Leonard, A. C. (1992). Chronic posttraumatic stress disorder and diagnostic comorbidity in a disaster sample. *Journal of Nervous and Mental Disease, 180,* 760–766.

Hartsough, D. M., & Myers, D. G. (1985). Disaster work and mental health: Prevention and control of stress among workers. Rockville, MD: National Institute of Mental Health.

Hathaway, S. R., & McKinley, J. C. (1967). *Minnesota Multiphasic Personality Inventory: Manual for administration and scoring.* New York: Psychological Corporation.

Helzer, J. E., Robins, L. N., & McEvoy, L. (1987). Posttraumatic stress disorder in the general population: Findings of the Epidemiologic Catchment Area survey. *New England Journal of Medicine, 317,* 1630–1634.

Holen, A. (1991). A longitudinal study of the occurrence and persistence of posttraumatic health problems in disaster. *Stress Medicine, 7,* 11–17.

Horowitz, M. J. (1973). Phase oriented treatment of stress response syndromes. *American Journal of Psychotherapy, 27,* 506–515.

Horowitz, M. J. (1986). Stress-response syndromes: A review of posttraumatic and adjustment disorders. *Hospital and Community Psychiatry, 37,* 241–249.

Horowitz, M. J., & Kaltreider, N. B. (1980). Brief psychotherapy of stress response syndromes. In T. B. Karasu & L. Bellak (Eds.), *Specialized techniques in individual psychotherapy.* New York: Brunner/Mazel.

Horowitz, M. J., Wilner, N., & Alvarez, W. (1979). Impact of Event Scale: A measure of subjective stress. *Psychosomatic Medicine, 41,* 209–218.

Horowitz, M. J., Marmar, C., Weiss, D. D., DeWiss, K. N., & Rosenbaum, R. (1984). Brief psychotherapy of bereavement reactions. *Archives of General Psychiatry, 41,* 438–448.

Hyams, K. C, Wignall, F. S., & Roswell, R. (1996). War syndromes and their evaluation: From the U.S. Civil War to the Persian Gulf War. *Annals of Internal Medicine, 125,* 398–405.

International Federation of Red Cross and Red Crescent Societies. (1993). *World disaster report.* Dordrecht, The Netherlands: Martinus Nijhoff.

Jordan, B. K., Marmar, C. R., Fairbank, J. A., Schlenger, W. E., Kulka, R. A., Hough, R. L., & Weiss, D. (in press). Problems in families of male Vietnam veterans with post-traumatic stress disorder (PTSD). *Journal of Consulting and Clinical Psychology.*

Keane, T. M., Fairbank, J. A., Caddell, J. M., Zimering, R. T., & Bender, M. E. (1985). A behavioral approach to assessing and treating posttraumatic stress disorder in Vietnam veterans. In C. R. Figley (Ed.), *Trauma and its wake: The study and treatment of posttraumatic stress disorder.* New York: Brunner/Mazel.

Keane, T. M., Caddell, J. M., & Taylor, K. L. (1988). Mississippi Scale for combat-related posttraumatic stress disorder: Three studies in reliability and validity. *Journal of Consulting and Clinical Psychology, 56,* 85–90.

Keane, T. M., Fairbank, J. A., Caddell, J. M., & Zimering, R. T. (1989). Implosive (flooding) therapy reduces symptoms of PTSD in Vietnam combat veterans. *Behavior Therapy, 20,* 245–260.

Keane, T. M., Fairbank, J. A., Caddell, J. M., Zimering, R. T., Taylor, K. L., & Mora, C. A. (1989). Clinical evaluation of a measure to assess combat exposure. *Psychological Assessment, 1,* 53–55.

Keane, T. M., & Kaloupek, D. G. (1982). Imaginal flooding in the treatment of a posttraumatic disorder. *Journal of Consulting and Clinical Psychology, 50,* 138–140.

Keane, T. M., Malloy, P. F., & Fairbank, J. A. (1984). Empirical development of an MMPI subscale for the assessment of combat-related posttraumatic stress disorders. *Journal of Consulting and Clinical Psychology, 52,* 888–891.

Keane, T. M., Wolfe, J., & Taylor, K. L. (1987). Post-traumatic stress disorder: Evidence for diagnostic validity and methods of psychological assessment. *Journal of Clinical Psychology, 43,* 32–43.

Keane, T. M., Weathers, F. W., & Foa, E. B. (in press). Assessment and diagnosis of posttraumatic stress disorder. In E. B. Foa, T. M. Keane, & M. J. Friedman (Eds.), *Effective treatments for PTSD: Practice guidelines from the International Society for Traumatic Stress Studies.* New York: Guilford.

Keane, T. M., Zimering, R. T., & Caddell, J. M. (1985). A behavioral formulation of posttraumatic stress disorder in Vietnam veterans. *Behavior Therapist, 8,* 9–12.

Kessler, R. C., Sonnega, A., Bromet, E., Hughes, M., & Nelson, C. B. (1995). Posttraumatic stress disorder in the National Comorbidity Survey. *Archives of General Psychiatry, 52,*1048–1060.

Kilpatrick, D. G., Resnick, H. S., Saunders, B. E., & Best, C. L. (1998). Rape, other violence against women, and posttraumatic stress disorder: Critical issues in assessing the adversity-stress-psychopathology relationship. In B. P.

Dohrenwend (Ed.), *Adversity, stress, and psychopathology* (pp. 161–176). New York: Oxford University Press.

Kilpatrick, D. G., Saunders, B. E., Amick-Mullan, A., Best, C., Veronen, L. J., & Resnick, H. S. (1989). Victim and crime factors associated with the development of crime-related post-traumatic stress disorder. *Behavior Therapy, 20*, 199–214.

Kilpatrick, D. G., Saunders, B. E., Veronen, L. J., Best, C. L., & Von, J. M. (1987). Criminal victimization lifetime prevalence, reporting to police, and psychological impact. *Crime and Delinquency, 33*, 479–489.

Kilpatrick, D. G., Saunders, B. E., & Resnick, H. S. (1998 March). Violence history and comorbidity among a national sample of adolescents. Lake George Research Conference on Posttraumatic Stress Disorder Program, Bolton Landing, New York.

Kilpatrick, D. G., & Veronen, L. J. (1983). Treatment for rape-related problems: Crisis intervention is not enough. In L. H. Cohen, W. L. Claiborn, & G. A. Specter (Eds.), *Crisis intervention*. New York: Human Sciences Press.

King, D. W., King, L. A., Foy, D. W., & Gudanowski, D. M. (1996). Prewar factors in combat-related posttraumatic stress disorder: Structural equation modeling with a national sample of male and female Vietnam veterans. *Journal of Abnormal Psychology, 104*, 184–196.

King, D. W., King, L. A., Foy, D. W., Keane, T. M., & Fairbank, J. A. (1999). Posttraumatic stress disorder in a national sample of female and male Vietnam veterans: Risk factors, war-zone stressors, and resilience-recovery variables. *Journal of Abnormal Psychology, 108*, 164–170.

King, L. A., King, D., Fairbank, J. A., Keane, T. M., & Adams, G. A. (1998). Resilience/recovery factors in posttraumatic stress disorder among female and male Vietnam veterans: Hardiness, postwar social support, and additional stressful life events. *Journal of Personality and Social Psychology, 74*, 420–434.

King, N. J., Hamilton, D. I., & Ollendick, T. H. (1988). *Children's phobias: A behavioral perspective*. New York: Wiley.

Kinzie, J. D., Boehnlein, J. K., & Sack, W. H. (1998). The effects of massive trauma on Cambodian parents and children. In Y. Danieli (Ed.), *International handbook of multi-generational legacies of trauma* (pp. 69–83). New York: Plenum Press.

Kleber, R. J., & Brom, D. (1992). *Coping with trauma: Theory, prevention and treatment*. Amsterdam: Swets & Zeitlinger.

Knight, J. A. (1997). Neuropsychological assessment in posttraumatic stress disorder. In J. P. Watson & T. M. Keane (Eds.), *Assessing psychological trauma and PTSD*. New York: Guilford.

Koretzky, M. B., & Peck, A. H. (1990). Validation and cross-validation of the PTSD subscale of the MMPI with civilian trauma victims. *Journal of Clinical Psychology, 46*, 297–300.

Kulka, R. A., Schlenger, W. E., Fairbank, J. A., Hough, R. L., Jordan, B. K., Marmar, C. R., & Weiss, D. (1990). *Trauma and the Vietnam War generation: Report of findings from the National Vietnam Veterans Readjustment Study*. New York: Brunner/Mazel.

Lang, P. J. (1977). The psychophysiology of anxiety. In H. Akiskal (Ed.), *Psychiatric diagnosis: Exploration of biological criteria*. New York: Spectrum.

Lang, P. J. (1977). Imagery in therapy: An information processing analysis of fear. *Behavior Therapy, 8*, 862–886.

Lindy, J. D., Green, B. L., Grace, M., & Titchener, J. (1983).

Psychotherapy with survivors of the Beverly Hills supper club fire. *American Journal of Psychotherapy, 37*, 593–610.

Litz, B. T., Penk, W. E., Gerardi, R. J., & Keane, T. M. (1992). The assessment of post-traumatic stress disorder. In P. A. Saigh (Ed.), *Post-traumatic stress disorder: A behavioral approach to assessment and treatment* (pp. 50–84). New York: Pergamon Press.

Long, N., Chamberlain, K., & Vincent, C. (1992). The health and mental health of New Zealand Vietnam war veterans with posttraumatic stress disorder. *New Zealand Medical Journal, 105*, 417–419.

Lyons, J., & Keane, T. (1992). Keane PTSD scale: MMPI and MMPI-2 update. *Journal of Traumatic Stress, 5*, 111–117.

Madakasira, S., & O'Brien, K. F. (1987). Acute posttraumatic stress disorders in victims of natural disaster. *Journal of Nervous and Mental Disease, 175*, 286–288.

Malloy, P. F., Fairbank, J. A., & Keane, T. M. (1983). Validation of a multimethod assessment of PTSD in Vietnam veterans. *Journal of Consulting and Clinical Psychology, 51*, 488–494.

Marmar, C. R., & Freeman, M. (1988). Brief dynamic psychotherapy of posttraumatic stress disorders: Management of narcissistic regression. *Journal of Traumatic Stress, 1*, 323–337.

McCaffrey, R. J., & Fairbank, J. A. (1985). Posttraumatic stress disorder associated with transportation accidents: Two case studies. *Behavior Therapy, 16*, 406–416.

McFarlane, A. C., Atchison, M., Rafalowicz, E., & Papay, P. (1994). Physical symptoms in post-traumatic stress disorder. *Journal of Psychosomatic Research, 38*, 715–726.

McFarlane, A. C., & Potts, N. (1999). Posttraumatic stress disorder: Prevalence and risk factors relative to disasters. In P. A. Saigh & J. D. Bremner (Eds.), *Posttraumatic stress disorder: A comprehensive text* (pp. 92–102). Boston: Allyn & Bacon.

Nader, K. O. (1997). Assessing traumatic experiences in children. In J. P. Wilson & T. M. Keane (Eds.), *Assessing psychological trauma and PTSD* (pp. 291–348). London: Guilford.

Nader, K. O., Kriegler, J. A., Blake, D. D., Pynoos, R. S., Newman, E., & Weather, F. (1996). *Clinician Administered PTSD Scale, Child and Adolescent Version (CAPS-C)*. White River Junction, VT: National Center for PTSD.

Newman, E., Kaloupek, D. G., & Keane, T. M. (1996). Assessment of posttraumatic stress disorder in clinical and research settings. In B. A. van Der Kolk, A. C. McFarlane, & L. Weisaeth (Eds.), *Traumatic stress: The effects of overwhelming experiences on mind, body, and society* (pp. 242–275). New York: Guilford.

Norris, F. H. (1992). Epidemiology of trauma: Frequency and impact of potentially traumatic events on different demographic events. *Journal of Consulting and Clinical Psychology, 60*, 409–418.

North, C. S., Nixon, S. J., Shariat, S., Mallonee, S., McMillen, J. C., Spitznagel, E. L., & Smith, E. M. (1999). Psychiatric disorders among survivors of the Oklahoma City bombing. *Journal of American Medical Association, 282*, 755–762.

Ollendick, T. M., & Hersen, M. (1984). *Child behavioral assessment*. New York: Pergamon Press.

Perconte, S. T., Wilson, A. T., Pontius, E. B., Dietrick, A. L., & Spiro, K. J. (1993). Psychological and war stress symptoms among deployed and non-deployed reservists following the Persian Gulf War. *Military Medicine, 158*, 516–521.

Pitman, W. E., Orr, S. P., Forgue, D. F., de Jong, J. B., &

Claiborne, J. M. (1987). Psychophysiologic assessment of post-traumatic stress disorder in Vietnam combat veterans. *Archives of General Psychiatry, 44,* 970–975.

Reist, C., Kauffmann, C. D., Haier, R. J., Sangdahl, C., DeMet, E. M., Chicz-DeMet, A., & Nelson, J. N. (1989). A controlled trial of desipramine in 18 men with posttraumatic stress disorder. *American Journal of Psychiatry, 146,* 513–516.

Resick, P. A., & Schnicke, M. K. (1993). *Cognitive processing therapy for rape victims: A treatment manual.* Newbury Park: Sage.

Resick, P. A., & Schnicke, M. K. (1992). Cognitive processing therapy for sexual assault victims. *Journal of Consulting and Clinical Psychology, 60,* 748–756.

Resick, P. A., & Schnicke, M. K. (Eds.). (1993). *Cognitive processing therapy for rape victims.* Newbury Park, CA: Sage.

Resick, P. A., Jordan, C. G., Girelli, S. A., Hutter, C. K., & Marhoefer-Dvorak, S. (1988). A comparative outcome study of behavioral group therapy for sexual assault victims. *Behavior Therapy, 19,* 385–401.

Resnick, H. S., Best. C. L., Freedy, J. R., Kilpatrick, D. G., & Falsetti, S. A. (1993). *Trauma assessment for adults.* Unpublished interview protocol, Crime Victims Research and Treatment Center, Department of Psychiatry, Medical University of South Carolina, Charleston, SC.

Resnick, H. S., Kilpatrick, D. G., Dansky, B. S., Saunders, B. E., & Best, C. L. (1993). Prevalence of civilian trauma and posttraumatic stress disorder in a representative national sample of women. *Journal of Consulting and Clinical Psychology, 61,* 984–991.

Riley, W. T., Treiber, F. A., & Woods, M.G. (1989). Anger and hostility in depression. *Journal of Nervous and Mental Disease, 177,* 668–674.

Riskind, J. H., Beck, A. T., Berchick, R. J., Brown, G., & Steer, R. A. (1987). Reliability of DSM-III diagnosis for major depression and generalized anxiety disorder using the Structured Clinical Interview for DSM-III. *Archives of General Psychiatry, 44,* 817–820.

Roberts, W. R., Penk, W. E., Gearing, M. L., Robinowitz, R., Dolan, M. P., & Patterson, E. T. (1982). Interpersonal problems of Vietnam combat veterans with symptoms of posttraumatic stress disorder. *Journal of Abnormal Psychology, 91,* 444–450.

Robins, L., Cottler, L., Bucholz, K., & Compton, W. (1995). *Diagnostic Interview Schedule for DSM-IV (DIS-IV).* St. Louis, MO: Washington University, School of Medicine, Department of Psychiatry.

Robins, L. N., Helzer, J. E., Cottler, L. B., & Goldring, E. (1988). *The Diagnostic Interview Schedule, Version IIIR.* St. Louis, MO: Washington University School of Medicine.

Rosenheck, R., & Nathan, P. (1985). Secondary traumatization in children of Vietnam veterans. *Hospital and Community Psychiatry, 36,* 538–539.

Rosenheck, R. A. & Fontana, A. (1998). Warrior fathers and warrior sons: Intergenerational aspects of trauma. In Y. Danieli (Ed.), *International handbook of multigenerational legacies of trauma* (pp. 69–83). New York: Plenum Press.

Rothbaum, B. O., Foa, E. B., Riggs, D. S., Murdock, T., & Walsh, W. (1992). A prospective examination of posttraumatic stress disorder in rape victims. *Journal of Traumatic Stress, 5,* 455–475.

Rothbaum, B. O., Meadows, E. A., Resick, R., & Foy, D. W. (in press). Cognitive-behavioral treatment. In E. B. Foa, T. M. Keane, & M. J. Friedman (Eds.), *Effective treatments for PTSD: Practice guidelines from the International Society for Traumatic Stress Studies.* New York: Guilford.

Rousseau, C., & Drapeau, A. (1998). The impact of culture on the transmission of trauma: Refugee's stories and silence embodied in their children's lives. In Y. Danieli (Ed.), *International handbook of multigenerational legacies of trauma* (pp. 465–486). New York: Plenum Press.

Rychtarik, R. G., Silverman, W. K., van Landingham, W. P., & Prue, D. M. (1984). Treatment of an incest victim with implosive therapy: A case study. *Behavior Therapy, 15,* 410–420.

Sack, W. H., Clarke, G. N., Kinney, R., Belestos, G., Chanrithy, H., & Seeley, J. (1995). The Khmer Adolescent Project II: Functional capacities in two generations of Cambodian refugees. *Journal of Nervous and Mental Disease, 183,* 177–181.

Sack, W. H., McSharry, S., Clarke, G. N., Kinney, R., Seeley, J., & Lewinsohn, P. (1994). The Khmer Adolescent Project I. Epidemiological findings in two generations of Cambodian refugees. *Journal of Nervous and Mental Disease, 182,* 387–395.

Saunders, B. E., Kilpatrick, D. G., Hanson, R. F., Resnick, H. S., & Walker, E. (1999). Prevalence, case characteristics, and long-term psychological correlates of child rape among women: A national survey. *Child Maltreatment, 4,* 187–200.

Saxe, G., & Wolfe, J. (1999). Gender and posttraumatic stress disorder. In P. Saigh & D. Bremner (Eds.), *Posttraumatic stress disorder: A comprehensive text* (pp. 160–179). Boston: Allyn & Bacon.

Schlenger, W. E., Fairbank, J. A., Jordan, B. K., & Caddell, J. M. (1997). Epidemiological methods for assessing trauma and posttraumatic stress disorder. In J. P. Wilson & T. M. Keane (Eds.), *Assessing psychological trauma and PTSD.* New York: Guilford.

Schnurr, P. P., & Spiro, A. (1999). Combat exposure, posttraumatic stress disorder symptoms, and health behaviors as predictors of self-reported physical health status in older veterans. *Journal of Nervous and Mental Disease, 187,* 353–359.

Schwab-Stone, M. E., Ayers, T. S., Kasprow, W., Voyce, C., Barone, C., Shriver, T., & Weissberg, R. P. (1995). No safe haven: A study of violence exposure in an urban community. *Journal of the American Academy of Child and Adolescent Psychiatry, 34,* 1343–1352.

Shalev, A., Bleich, A., & Ursano, R. J. (1990). Posttraumatic stress disorder: Somatic comorbidity and effort tolerance. *Psychosomatics, 31,* 197–203.

Shestatsky, M., Greenberg, D., & Lerer, B. (1988). A controlled trial of phenelzine in posttraumatic stress disorder. *Psychiatry Research, 24*(2), 149–155.

Shapiro, F. (1995). *Eye movement desensitization and reprocessing: Basic principles, protocols, and procedures.* New York: Guilford.

Shore, J. H., Tatum, E., & Vollmer, W. M. (1986). Psychiatric reactions to disaster: The Mt. St. Helen's experience. *American Journal of Psychiatry, 143,* 590–595.

Shore, J. H., Vollmer, W. M., & Tatum, E. L. (1989). Community patterns of posttraumatic stress disorders. *Journal of Nervous and Mental Disease, 177,* 681–685.

Silver, J. M., Sandberg, D. P., & Hales, R. E. (1990). New approaches in the pharmacotherapy of posttraumatic stress disorder. *Journal of Clinical Psychiatry, 51,* 33–38.

Singer, M. I., Anglin, T. M., Song, L. Y., & Lunghofer, L. (1995). Adolescents' exposure to violence and associated symptoms of psychological trauma. *Journal of the American Medical Association, 273,* 477–482.

Solomon, Z., Weisenberg, M., Schwarzwald, J., & Mikulincer, M. (1987). Posttraumatic stress disorder among frontline soldiers with combat stress reaction: 1982 Israeli experience. *American Journal of Psychiatry, 144,* 448–454.

Solomon, Z., Mikulincer, M., Fried, B., & Wosner, Y. (1987). Family characteristics and posttraumatic stress disorder: A follow-up of Israeli combat stress reaction casualties. *Family Process, 26,* 383–394.

Solomon, Z. (1998). Transgenerational effects of the Holocaust: The Israeli research perspective. In Y. Danieli (Ed.), *International handbook of multigenerational legacies of trauma* (pp. 141–146). New York: Plenum Press.

Southwick, S., & Friedman, M. J. (in press). Neurobiological models of posttraumatic stress disorder. In E. Gerrity, T. Keane, & F. Tunna (Eds.), *The mental health consequences of torture.* New York: Kluwer Academic/Plenum.

Southwick, S. M., Morgan, C. A., III, Darnell, A., Bremner, D., Nicolaou, A. L., Nagy, L. M., & Charney, D. S. (1995). Trauma-related symptoms in veterans of Operation Desert Storm: A 2-year follow-up. *American Journal of Psychiatry, 152,* 1150–1155.

Southwick, S. M., Morgan, A., Nagy, L. M., Bremner, D., Nicolaou, A. L., Johnson, D. R., Rosenheck, R., & Charney, D. S. (1993). Trauma-related symptoms in veterans of Operation Desert Storm: A preliminary report. *American Journal of Psychiatry, 150,* 1524–1528.

Sowder, B. J. (1985). *Disasters and mental health: Selected contemporary perspectives.* Rockville, MD: National Institute of Mental Health.

Spielberger, C. D. (1988). *State-trait anger expression inventory: Research edition professional manual.* Odessa, FL: Psychological Assessment Resources.

Spielberger, C. D., Gorsuch, R. L., & Lushene, R. E. (1970). *Manual for the State-Trait Anxiety Inventory (self-evaluation questionnaire).* Palo Alto, CA: Consulting Psychologists Press.

Stamm, B. H. (Ed.). (1996). *Measurement of stress, trauma, and adaptation* (pp. 317–322). Lutherville, MD: Sidran Press.

Steel, Z., Silove, D. M., Bird, K., McGorry, P. D., & Mohan, P. (1999). Pathways from war trauma to posttraumatic stress symptoms among Tamil asylum seekers, refugees, and immigrants. *Journal of Traumatic Stress, 12,* 421–435.

Sutker, P. B., Uddo, M., Brailey, K., & Allain, A. N., Jr. (1993). War-zone trauma and stress-related symptoms in Operation Desert Shield/Storm (ODS) returnees. *Journal of Social Issues, 49,* 33–49.

Tatara, M. (1998). The second generation of Hibakusha, atomic bomb survivors. In Y. Danieli (Ed.), *International handbook of multigenerational legacies of trauma* (pp. 69–83). New York: Plenum Press.

Van der Hart, O., Brown, P., & van der Kolk, B. A. (1995). Pierre Janet's treatment of post-traumatic stress. In G. S. Everly & J. M. Lating (Eds.), *Psychotraumatology: Key papers and core concepts in post-traumatic stress* (pp. 195–210). New York: Plenum Press.

Van der Kolk, B. A., Dryfuss, D., Michaels, M., et al. (1994). Fluoxetine in post-traumatic stress disorder. *Journal of Clinical Psychiatry, 55,* 517–522.

Verbosky, S. J., & Ryan, D. A. (1988). Female partners of Vietnam veterans: Stress by proximity. *Issues in Mental Health Nursing, 9,* 95–105.

Weathers, F. W., Blake, D. D., Krinsley, K. E., Haddad, W., Huska, J. A., & Keane, T. M. (1997). Reliability and validity of the Clinician-Administered PTSD Scale. Manuscript submitted for publication.

Weathers, F. W., & Keane, T. M. (1999). Psychological assessment of traumatized adults. In P. A. Saigh & J. D. Bremner (Eds.), *Posttraumatic stress disorder: A comprehensive text* (pp. 219–247). Boston: Allyn & Bacon.

Weathers, F. W., Litz, B. T., Herman, D. S., Huska, J. A., & Keane, T. M. (1993, October). *The PTSD Checklist (PCL): Reliability, validity, and diagnostic utility.* Paper presented at the *Annual Meeting of the International Society for Traumatic Stress Studies,* San Antonio, CA.

Weathers, F. W., Litz, B. T., Herman, D. S., King, D. W., King, L. A., Keane, T. M., & Huska, J. A. (1997). Three studies on the psychometric properties of the PTSD Checklist (PCL). Manuscript submitted for publication.

Weisaeth, L. (1989). The stressors and post-traumatic stress syndrome after an industrial disaster. *Acta Psychiatrica Scandinavica, 80,* 25–37.

Weiss, D. S., & Marmar, C. R. (1997). The Impact of Event Scale-Revised. In J. P. Wilson & T. M. Keane (Eds.), *Assessing psychological trauma and PTSD.* New York: Plenum Press.

Wilson, J. P., & Keane, T. M. (1997). *Assessing psychological trauma and PTSD.* New York: Guilford.

Winfield, I., George, L. K., Swartz, M., & Blazer, D. G. (1990). Sexual assault and psychiatric disorders among a community sample of women. *American Journal of Psychiatry, 147,* 335–341.

Wolfe, J., Brown, P. J., & Kelley, J. M. (1993). Reassessing war stress: Exposure and the Persian Gulf War. *Journal of Social Issues, 49,* 15–31.

Yehuda, R., Schmeidler, J., Elkin, A., Wilson, S., Siever, L. J., Binder-Brynes, K. L., Wainberg, M., & Aferiot, D. (1998). Phenomenology and psychobiology of the intergenerational response to trauma. In Y. Danieli (Ed.), *International handbook of multigenerational legacies of trauma* (pp. 639–655). New York: Plenum Press.

Zatzick, D. F., Marmar, C. R., Weiss, D. S., Browner, W. S., Metzler, T. J., Golding, J. M., Stewart, A., Schlenger, W. E., & Wells, K. (1997a). Posttraumatic stress disorder and functioning and quality of life outcomes in a nationally representative sample of male Vietnam veterans. *American Journal of Psychiatry, 154,* 1690–1695.

Zatzick, D. F., Weiss, D. S., Marmar, C. R., Metzler, T. J., Wells, K., Golding, J. M., Stewart, A., Schlenger, W. E., & Browner, W. S. (1997b). Posttraumatic stress disorder and functioning and quality of life outcomes in female Vietnam veterans. *Military Medicine, 162,* 661–665.

Zoellner, L. A., Foa, E. B., & Brigidi, B. D. (1999). Interpersonal friction and PTSD in female victims of sexual and nonsexual assault. *Journal of Traumatic Stress, 124,* 689–700.

# CHAPTER 9

# Somatoform and Factitious Disorders

Tony Iezzi, Melanie P. Duckworth, and Henry E. Adams

## Introduction

Although somatoform and factitious disorders have been recognized throughout the years and have received considerably more empirical attention during the last 10 years, these disorders continue to represent categories of psychiatric disturbances that are highly misunderstood. This is not surprising for a number of reasons. The empirical database for these disorders continues to be inadequate and largely dated. This group of disorders still relies heavily on an either/or (e.g., organic versus psychogenic) conceptualization of psychopathology. The diagnosis of some of these disorders is largely by exclusion and based more on a collection of symptoms rather than signs. The symptom cutoffs or thresholds that indicate the presence or absence of a disorder are somewhat arbitrary. The etiology and symptomatology are sometimes treated as the same. Still, despite these problems, these disorders continue to fascinate researchers, clinicians, and laypersons alike.

Tony Iezzi • London Health Sciences Center, Victoria Hospital, London, Ontario N6B 1B8, Canada. Melanie P. Duckworth • Department of Psychology, University of Houston, Houston, Texas 77204-5321. Henry E. Adams • Department of Psychology, University of Georgia, Athens, Georgia 30602-3013.

*Comprehensive Handbook of Psychopathology* (Third Edition), edited by Patricia B. Sutker and Henry E. Adams. Kluwer Academic / Plenum Publishers, New York, 2001.

According to the 4th edition of the *Diagnostic and Statistical Manual of Mental Disorders* (DSM-IV; American Psychiatric Association [APA], 1994), somatoform disorders are characterized by physical symptoms that suggest a general medical condition but are not fully explained by a general medical condition, by the direct effects of a substance, or by another mental disorder. To be considered a somatoform disorder, these physical symptoms need to cause significant emotional distress and impairment in social, occupational, or other areas of functioning. The somatoform disorders section of the DSM-IV include somatization disorder, undifferentiated somatoform disorder, conversion disorder, pain disorder, hypochondriasis, body dysmorphic disorder, and somatoform disorder not otherwise specified.

Unlike somatoform disorders, where physical symptoms, it is believed, occur unintentionally, factitious disorders are characterized by physical or psychological symptoms that are intentionally induced or feigned. In contrast to malingering, where the presumed goal is to accomplish an externally recognizable objective (e.g., obtaining financial compensation or avoiding unpleasant tasks), the presumed goal of factitious behavior is to assume the "sick role." Factitious disorders in DSM-IV (APA, 1994) are subcategorized as factitious disorder with predominantly psychological signs and symptoms, factitious disorder with predominantly physical signs and symptoms, and factitious disorder with combined psychological and physical signs and symptoms. Clinical descriptions, diagnostic requirements, theoretical issues, and relevant research pertaining to the identification and management of individual somatoform and factitious disorders are reviewed in the following sections.

## Somatoform Disorders

### Somatization Disorder

Broadly defined, somatization is a term that covers a broad range of physical symptoms that occur in the absence of organic pathology or the amplification of bodily sensations that accompany physical conditions beyond those that can be explained by organic pathology (Barsky & Klerman, 1983; Ford, 1986; Katon, 1982; Kellner, 1985; Lipowski, 1988). Somatization has also been defined as a bodily or somatic expression of psychic distress (Barsky & Klerman, 1983; Ford, 1986; Katon, 1982; Kellner, 1985; Lipowski, 1988). In other words, patients who ought to be complaining of problems in daily living often focus on bodily sensations and seek a medical cure for these problems. For example, it is easier for these patients to say to a physician "my back hurts" than it is to say "I want to die because my life has no meaning."

The history of somatization disorder is intimately tied to the history of hysteria. Although the origins of somatization can be attributed to Sydenham in 1682 and Sims in 1799 (Lipowski, 1988), it was not until 1856 that Paul Briquet published his oft-quoted classical study on hysteria that somatization was more firmly established (Lipowski, 1988; Mai & Merskey, 1980, 1981; Nemiah, 1985). Briquet's work is contained in a 700-page compendium that describes and categorizes symptoms of 430 patients seen during a 10-year period. Except for a handful of patients, most of the cases he studied were women. According to Briquet's conceptualization, hysteria resulted from stress or stimuli that affect the central nervous system of susceptible individuals, causing a plethora of physical symptoms. He conceptualized this syndrome as a form of hysteria, but it is clear from some of his descriptions that he also captured elements of conversion reactions.

In 1909, Briquet's work was followed by Thomas Saville's study of 500 hysterical patients (Nemiah, 1985). Adopting Briquet's methodology and con-

ceptualization, Saville came to similar conclusions about hysteria. The term somatization was first used by Steckel (1943), who defined somatization as a bodily disorder that arises out of a deep-seated neurosis and as a disease of the conscious. Purtell, Robins, and Cohen (1951) later rediscovered the ideas of Briquet and Saville, but their study also emphasized the dramatic, vague, and exaggerated manner in which these patients described their symptoms.

The study of somatization culminated in extensive phenomenological studies conducted by Guze and his colleagues at Washington University in St. Louis (Arkonac & Guze, 1963; Cloninger & Guze, 1970; Gatfield & Guze, 1962; Guze, 1983; Guze, Kloninger, Martin, & Clayton, 1986; Guze, Tuason, Gatfield, Stewart, & Picken, 1962; Guze, Wolfgram, McKinney, & Cantwell, 1967; Guze, Woodruff, & Clayton, 1971a,b; Perley & Guze, 1962; Woerner & Guze, 1968). These studies were aimed at defining relatively distinct psychiatric disturbances in terms of characteristics, phenomenology, natural history, prognosis, treatment response, and family history. The emergence of somatization disorder was primarily out of a controversy in the mid-1960s between Samuel Guze and Elliot Slater, then the editor of the British Journal of Psychiatry. Guze's work on hysteria was seriously questioned by Slater and Glithero's (1965) classical study. As Guze (1983) stated, it was because of Slater's influence and in an attempt to reduce confusion surrounding hysteria, that he renamed hysteria after Briquet. In 1971, hysteria became known as Briquet's syndrome (Guze et al., 1971a). Over the years, Guze and his associates and others were able to demonstrate that Briquet's syndrome had excellent diagnostic stability (Perley & Guze, 1962), a high degree of reliability (Spitzer, Endicott, & Robins, 1978), and good validity (Guze, 1975). Briquet's syndrome was conceived as a polysymptomatic syndrome that begins early in life, occurs primarily in women, and is associated with marital problems, poor work history, teenage delinquency, alcohol problems, and sociopathy in first-degree relatives (Guze, 1983).

**Diagnosis.** As a diagnostic entity, somatization disorder is a fairly recent addition to the DSM nomenclature and was intended as a simplified version of Briquet's syndrome. Somatization disorder was officially recognized in DSM-III (APA, 1980) and was also included in DSM-III-R (APA,

1987) with some minor changes. Before DSM-III, the criteria for Briquet's syndrome required at least twenty-five of sixty physical symptoms without clear organic explanation from at least nine out of ten symptom groups (Perley & Guze, 1962). It should be emphasized that the number of symptoms required for somatization disorder had been established arbitrarily rather than empirically. In an attempt to be nonsexist, DSM-III-R required the presence of at least thirteen physical symptoms for both men and women; in DSM-III, the diagnosis of somatization disorder required twelve physical symptoms for men and fourteen physical symptoms for women. The DSM-IV (APA, 1994) requires eight physical symptoms to diagnose somatization disorder. The current diagnostic criteria for somatization disorder are listed in Table 1.

The criteria for somatization disorder proposed in DSM-IV have fared well in DSM field trials. Yutzy et al. (1995) examined the concordance between the proposed diagnostic criteria for DSM-IV somatization disorder and DSM-III-R, DSM-III, Perley–Guze, and the International Classification of Diseases-10 (ICD-10) criteria in 353 female patients recruited from five sites; recruitment procedures were designed to maximize sociocultural, ethnic, and geographic diversity. The ICD-10 criteria agreed poorly with all other diagnostic sets including DSM-IV, which is consistent with other work (Rief & Hiller, 1998). Yutzy et al. (1995) found that the DSM-IV criteria were an accurate and simpler method for diagnosing somatization disorder and had excellent concordance with DSM-III-R criteria. The authors reported that the DSM-IV criteria did not require special expertise in administration. Of note, no racial differences were observed as a result of any of the criteria sets used. However, the determination of which criteria are best in diagnosing somatization disorder depends on the specificity and sensitivity of the criteria (Bucholz, Dinwiddle, Reich, Shayka, & Cloninger, 1993). Sensitivity is defined by the proportion of true cases correctly classified, and specificity is defined by the proportion of true noncases classified. Bucholz et al. (1993) compared the sensitivity, specificity, and positive predictive value (proportion of test positives who are truly positive) of DSM-IV criteria, a DSM-III-R seven-item symptom screen, and Swartz, Blazer, George, and Landerman's (1986) eleven-item screen. The authors found that no one set of criteria was clearly superior and that selection criteria should be based

## Table 1. DSM-IV Criteria for Somatization Disorder

A. A history of many physical complaints beginning before age 30 years that occur over a period of several years and result in treatment being sought or significant impairment in social, occupational, or other important areas of functioning.

B. Each of the following criteria must have been met, with individual symptoms occurring at any time during the course of the disturbance:

  (1) *four pain symptoms*: a history of pain related to at least four extremities, chest, rectum, during menstruation, during sexual intercourse, or during urination)

  (2) *two gastrointestinal symptoms*: a history of at least two gastrointestinal symptoms other than pain (e.g., nausea, bloating, vomiting other than during pregnancy, diarrhea, or intolerance of several different foods)

  (3) *one sexual symptom*: a history of at least one sexual or reproductive symptom other than pain (e.g., sexual indifference, erectile or ejaculatory dysfunction, irregular menses, excessive menstrual bleeding, vomiting throughout pregnancy)

  (4) *one pseudoneurological symptom*: a history of at least one symptom or deficit suggesting a neurological condition not limited to balance, paralysis or localized weakness, difficulty swallowing or lump in throat, aphonia, urinary retention, hallucinations, loss of touch or pain sensation, double vision, blindness, deafness, seizures; dissociative symptoms such as amnesia; or loss of consciousness other than fainting)

C. Either (1) or (2)

  (1) after appropriate investigation, each of the symptoms in Criterion B cannot be fully explained by a known general medical condition or the direct effects of a substance (e.g., a drug of abuse, a medication)

  (2) when there is a related general medical condition, the physical complaints or resulting social or occupational impairment are in excess of what would be expected from the history, physical examination, or laboratory findings

D. The symptoms are not intentionally produced or feigned (as in Factitious Disorder or Malingering)

*Source*: American Psychiatric Association. (1994) *Diagnostic and Statistical Manual of Mental Disorders*, 4th ed. (pp. 449–450). Washington, DC: Author. Reprinted by permission.

on the intended application. For example, the results indicated that DSM-IV criteria for somatization disorder had almost perfect specificity and the highest predictive value of all screening sets, but sensitivity calculations yielded 33 to 50% missed cases.

**Clinical Description.** A somatizing patient may present with many symptoms referred to any body part or organ system, and these symptoms may indicate any type of disease entity, but none of the physical symptoms of somatization disorder are pathognomonic. The clinician working with somatizers needs to be aware that multiple physical symptoms, in and of themselves, do not imply psychopathology. Furthermore, the diagnosis of somatization does not preclude the patient from experiencing true pathological conditions. For example, the co-occurrence of somatization and a medical disorder has been noted in the following conditions: cardiovascular disease (Bass & Wade, 1984), chronic fatigue syndrome (Manu, Lane, & Matthews, 1989), and fibromyalgia (Walker, Keegan, Gardner, Sullivan, Katon, & Bernstein, 1997).

Pain is by far the most common complaint of somatizers, especially pain involving the back, neck, head, pelvis, abdomen, and diffuse muscle aches (Ford, 1986; Iezzi, Stokes, Adams, Pilon, & Ault, 1994; Katon, Ries, & Kleinman, 1984a; Lipowski, 1988). Complaints of fatigue, shortness of breath, dizziness, and palpitations are also common. The presentation of symptoms is often elaborate, involving obsessively detailed symptom descriptions, but the chronology itself can be very vague.

Nemiah (1985) presents a thorough description of behaviors observed in the somatizer. He noted that somatizers are often exhibitionistic, particularly in terms of overly made-up or overdressed women. These individuals tend to be more revealing of their bodies in session and during physical examinations than necessary. Somatizers display an excessive preoccupation with themselves at the expense of others and, though this is not apparent at first, are highly dependent individuals. They demonstrate a wide range of affect that at times can be bewildering to the clinician. These patients are often perceived as flirtatious and seductive, but evaluation of sexual functioning frequently finds that they are tolerant at best, if not indifferent, toward sex. Somatizers are especially skilled at manipulating family, friends, and the health care system to meet their needs. They are prone to

suicide attempts but rarely follow through successfully.

Somatizers frequently have a history of multiple hospitalizations and surgeries. These patients represent a major source of health care utilization (Miranda, Perez-Stable, Munoz, Hargreaves, & Henke, 1991). An estimated 50% of ambulatory health care costs in the United States has been attributed to somatizers (Barsky & Klerman, 1983; Kellner, 1985). In 1980, the per capita expenditure of health care costs for hospital services was $543 for the average consumer, whereas it was $4,700 for somatizing patients (Smith, Monson, & Ray, 1986a). Interestingly enough, despite the multiple symptom presentation of somatizers, somatization disorder is not associated with increased mortality (Coryell, 1981).

In addition to multiple somatic symptoms, somatizers also present with a diversity of psychological and psychosocial complaints. Depression and anxiety are prominent features in somatizers. Although patients with somatization disorder appear heterogeneous, they all share one essential feature: a predominant pattern of somatic, rather than cognitive, response to emotional arousal (Lipowski, 1988). Barsky, Wyshak, and Klerman (1986) went even further in stating that somatic symptoms represent a final common pathway through which emotional disturbances, psychiatric disorders, and pathophysiological processes all express themselves and cause the patient to seek medical care.

Psychosocially, somatizers come from inconsistent, unreliable, and emotionally unsupportive family environments (Mai & Merskey, 1980). Physical and sexual trauma are common among somatizers (Kinzl, Traweger, & Biebl, 1995; Leserman, Zhiming, Drossman, Toomey, Nachman, & Glogau, 1997; McCauley et al., 1997; Walker, Keegan, Gardner, Sullivan, Bernstein, & Katon, 1997). Marital discord, separation, and divorce are also frequently observed. Because of their incapacitating symptomatology, somatizers often have poor occupational histories. Interpersonally, relationships with somatizers tend to be shallow and chaotic.

**Epidemiology and Demographics.** The estimated prevalence of somatization ranges from relatively uncommon (Fabrega, Mezzich, Jacob, & Ulrich, 1988; Swartz et al., 1986) to very common (Barsky & Klerman, 1983; Kellner, 1985). It has been estimated that 20 to 84% of patients seen by primary care physicians suffer from idiopathic somatic complaints (Barsky & Klerman, 1983; Kellner, 1985). The prevalence of somatization tends to be higher in primary care facilities (Barsky & Klerman, 1983; Kellner, 1985; Kirmayer & Robbins, 1991, 1996) than in psychiatric facilities (Fabrega et al., 1988). Several studies have examined prevalence rates of somatization disorder in the community at large. Prevalence estimates of somatization disorder in the community ranged from 0.06 to 0.6% (Blazer et al., 1985; Escobar, Burnam, Karno, Forsythe, & Golding, 1987; Robins et al., 1984; Swartz et al., 1986).

DSM-IV (APA, 1994) states that the prevalence of somatization disorder is 0.2 to 2% among women and less than 0.2% in men. In the Epidemiological Catchment Area Study (Robins & Regier, 1991), somatization disorder was most prevalent among African-American women (0.8%) followed by African-American men (0.4%); however, race is not a mediating variable in somatization disorder (Swartz, Landerman, Blazer, & George, 1989; Yutzy et al., 1995). Using DSM-III-R criteria for somatization disorder, Kroenke and Spitzer (1998) examined gender differences in the reporting of physical symptoms. One thousand patients from four primary care sites were evaluated with the Primary Care Evaluation of Mental Disorders Interview. After controlling for depressive and anxiety disorders, age, race, education, and medical comorbidity, results revealed that twelve out of thirteen physical symptoms were more commonly reported by women (odds ratio ranged from 1.5 to 2.5), and the reporting differences were statistically significant for ten of the thirteen physical symptoms. The authors concluded that increased symptom reporting in women may be a generic phenomenon rather than about specific symptoms, that medically unexplained symptoms are more common in women, and that the effect of gender on symptom reporting is independent of psychiatric comorbidity.

The notion used to be generally held that somatization was more common in non-Western cultures, but this view is no longer held (Kirmayer & Young, 1998). Although the prevalence and specific features of somatization may vary across cultures, the presentation of somatic symptoms as an expression of emotional distress is worldwide. In a cross-cultural study of somatization disorder, consecutive primary care patients (N = 25, 916) were screened using the General Health Questionnaire, and a stratified sample of 5438 patients was interviewed with the Composite International Diagnostic Interview (Gureje, Simon, Ustun, & Goldberg, 1997). Patients were recruited from fourteen countries: Turkey, Greece, India, Germany, Netherlands, Nigeria, United Kingdom, Japan, France, Brazil, Chile, United States, China, and Italy. Across all cultures, somatization was a common problem in primary care settings and was associated with significant health problems and functional disability. Thus, the prevalence of somatization disorder depends much on the clinical setting, patient sample, and definition of somatization used.

Somatization disorder is reportedly more common in individuals from lower socioeconomic status, lower educational level, and rural background (Barsky & Klerman, 1983; Escobar, Rubio-Stipec, Canino, & Karno, 1989; Swartz et al., 1986). Although Swartz and his associates (1986) found an increased rate of somatization disorder in rural areas, in another study they found an increased prevalence of somatization disorder in urban areas (Swartz et al., 1989). Thus, the role of rural versus urban background in somatization disorder remains to be clarified. The age of onset of somatization disorder is usually in early childhood and adolescence (Campo & Fritsch, 1994; Garralda, 1996; Kriechman, 1987; Livingston & Martin-Cannici, 1985; Terre & Ghiselli, 1997). By definition, somatization disorder has to occur before the age of 30.

**Etiological Formulations.** Somatizers are a physically and psychiatrically heterogeneous group. The diversity in the clinical manifestations of somatizers suggests multifactorial etiology. Dominant etiological factors in one patient may be fleeting or minor in another patient. The predisposing factors in somatization disorder are likely to include genetic, neuropsychological, neurophysiological, and psychophysiological, developmental learning, personality trait, and sociocultural formulations.

*Genetic.* Guze and his associates have been instrumental in proposing a multifactorial model of disease transmission in somatization disorder (Cloninger, Reich, & Guze, 1975a,b; Guze, 1983; Reich, Cloninger, & Guze, 1975). According to their model, hysteria (i.e., somatization disorder) and sociopathy cluster in the same families. Hysteria in women is believed to be a more prevalent and less deviant form of the same process that causes sociopathy in women. Based on their research, hysterics and sociopaths mate assortatively, thereby increasing the observed similarities among relatives, but this familial clustering does not completely depend on assortative mating. Other studies have noted an increased prevalence of 20% of somatization disorder in first-degree relatives of index cases (Cloninger & Guze, 1970; Guze, Cloninger, Martin, & Clayton, 1986; Woerner & Guze, 1968) and an increased rate of marital problems, poor occupational history, social dysfunction, teenage delinquencies, alcohol problems, and sociopathy in first-degree relatives of patients (Guze et al., 1971b). Adoption studies yielded similar findings (Bohman, Cloninger, Von Knorring, & Sigvardsson, 1984; Cloninger, Sigvardsson, Von Knorring, & Bohman, 1984; Sigvardsson, Von Knorring, Bohman, & Cloninger, 1984). Although the pattern of findings from these studies is very impressive, it is very unlikely that genetics alone accounts for somatization disorder.

*Psychodynamic.* Psychoanalysts view somatization as a form of symbolic communication, defense mechanism, and conflict resolution (Kellner, 1990). Somatization is a process whereby the body translates mental stress into physical expressions that have symbolic value (Steckel, 1943). The process of somatization also represents primitive defense mechanisms, like denial and repression, against undesirable wishes or urges. Finally, as a means to resolve conflict, somatizers blame their failures on their bodily symptoms or focus on their symptoms to avoid intolerable situations. As intuitive as the psychodynamic conceptualization of somatization is, it remains extremely difficult to test or validate.

*Neuropsychological, Neurophysiological, and Psychophysiological.* A number of studies propose a neuropsychological, neurophysiological, psychophysiological formulation of somatization disorder (Flor-Henry, Fromm-Auch, Tapper, & Schopflocher, 1981; Gordon, Kraiuhin, Meares, & Howson, 1986; James et al., 1987; Wickramasekera, 1989). Comprehensive neuropsychological examination, auditory evoked-response potentials, and cerebral blood flow studies of patients with somatization disorder demonstrated that these individuals display excessive distractibility, an inability to habituate to repetitive stimuli, and cognitive functioning characterized as concrete, partial, and circumstantial. These findings are associated with bilateral frontal and right hemisphere dysfunction. Another study examined the laterality of symptoms in sixty-one patients with depressive, anxiety, and somatoform disorders (Min & Lee, 1997). The authors found that somatic complaints, especially pain, together with other somatic complaints, occurred more often on the left side of the body. They concluded that the right hemisphere of the brain is more involved in somatization symptom formation than the left hemisphere; however, causal statements about the relationship between symptom formation and brain hemisphere cannot be made. Most recently, Wickramasekera (1989) developed a high-risk model of threat perception that identifies three major risk factors for developing somatization. He found that patients who have high hypnotic ability, low hypnotic ability, or who are high on social desirability are most prone to developing somatization and other psychophysiological disorders. Chronic pain subjects high on one or more of these risk factors evidenced higher skin conductance in response to cognitive threat (mental arithmetic; Wickramasekera, Pope, & Kolm, 1996). These studies, however, need to be replicated with more sensitive designs and larger samples sizes to determine the stability of these results.

*Personality Trait.* Personality characteristics, like the tendency to amplify bodily sensations, to focus excessively on physical symptoms, and to misinterpret physical symptoms may predispose individuals to somatization (Barsky & Klerman, 1983). Somatization may also reflect a form of "neuroticism" (Lipowski, 1988). Somatizers score high on measures of neuroticism such as self-consciousness, vulnerability to stress, low self-esteem, anxiety, depression, and hostility. Somatization has also been associated with negative affectivity (Kirmayer, Robbins, & Paris, 1994; Rief & Hiller, 1998; Watson & Pennebaker, 1989). The tendency to misinterpret bodily sensations or to overreact to minor bodily sensations as disabling has been interpreted as an enduring personality trait. The term alexithymia (Sifneos, 1973) also describes a personality trait that is apparently common among individuals with psychosomatic disorders. Patients with alexithymia have difficulties expressing affect, their fantasies tend to be devoid of feelings and emotions, and their thinking is characterized primarily by concrete operations rather than abstract operations. Although Shipko (1982) reported a positive relationship between somatization and alexithymia, it is unclear whether alexithymia is really a manifestation of an emotional state, a cognitive style, or a form of repression and denial (Kellner, 1990). More recent data suggests that somatization and alexithymia are independent of each other (Bach & Bach, 1995; Bach, Bach, & Zwann, 1996).

*Developmental Learning.* Childhood experiences that involve exposure to models with frequent complaints of pain play an instrumental role in childhood somatization (Kellner, 1990; Lipowski, 1988). Children who learn early that being ill or complaining of symptoms is likely to be rewarded with attention and sympathy or to lead to avoidance of conflict and responsibilities will be predisposed toward somatization as a coping style (Campo & Fritsch, 1994; Craig, Drake, Mills, & Boardman, 1994; Garralda, 1996). Later, as adults, these individuals maintain their behavior because of secondary gain and social reinforcement. The relationship between pain behavior and role models has received support in children with recurrent abdominal pain (Walker, Garber, & Zeman, 1991), headache (Deubner, 1977), and low back pain (Rickard, 1988). Family environment has also been implicated in the development of somatization. Sherry, McGuire, Mellins, Salmonson, Wallace, and Nepom (1991) found two predominant abnormal family milieus present in 100 children with musculoskeletal pain. One family environment could best be described as cohesive, stable, organized but intolerant of separation and individuation. The second predominant family milieu was characterized as chaotic, emotionally unsupportive, and highly conflictual. In a healthy sample of 933 subjects, ages ranging from 6–16, an examination of the relationship between family environment and physical health complaints indicated that disorganized and less cohesive family environments were associated with more health complaints (Terre & Ghiselli, 1997). In a two-year longitudinal study, parental lack of care was the best predictor of adult somatization (Craig, Boardman, Mills, Daly-Jones, & Drake, 1993). Finally, Livingston, Witt, and Smith (1995) found that parental somatization, substance abuse, and antisocial symptoms predicted children's somatization. In addition, children of adults with DSM-III-R somatization disorder had 11.7 times more emergency room visits and missed 8.8 times more school than children of adults with few unexplained somatic symptoms.

*Sociocultural.* Sociocultural aspects of somatization have received considerable attention (Brodsky, 1984; Goldberg & Bridges, 1988; Katon, Kleinman, & Rosen, 1982; Kirmayer & Young, 1998). As noted earlier, somatization is a worldwide phenomenon. Sociocultural aspects of somatization may really reflect differences in the way individuals somatize rather than psychologize their distress as a coping response (Goldberg & Bridges, 1988). In other cultures (e.g., Ayurveda or Chinese), the distinction between body and mind is usually not made (Kirmayer & Young, 1998). Especially within the Western culture, somatization and psychologization tend to be seen as mutually exclusive response styles. However, even Western societies are increasing their rates of somatization, despite the greater quality of medical care (Gureje, Simon, et al., 1997; Kirmayer & Young, 1998). It will be interesting to observe whether, with the advent of managed care in Western societies, the frequency and expression of somatization will change.

**Somatization and Associated Psychopathology.** Given the heterogeneous nature of somatization disorder, the process of somatization is associated with a spectrum of affective, personality, and thought disorders. In a large community study (N = 11,519), 24.6% of respondents experienced the co-occurrence of somatization disorder and depression (Boyd et al., 1984). From this same study, individuals with somatization disorder also had a 96.5% chance of having panic disorder and a 27.3% risk of having agoraphobia. In examining 100 consecutive somatizing patients, Katon, Ries, and Kleinman (1984b) noted that somatizers were more likely to suffer from depression (48%), personality disorder (37%), psychogenic pain disorder (11%), psychophysiological illness (9%), and panic disorder (4%) than a nonsomatizing group referred for psychiatric consultation. Sixty-one percent of females and 33% of males in a sample of fifty-five panic disorder cases displayed somatization (Katon, 1982).

The prevalence of somatization disorder in the presence of other DSM-IV Axis I and Axis II disorders has been documented in the context of epidemiological studies, as well as in studies of primary care facilities. Brown, Golding, and Smith (1990) calculated lifetime prevalence rates for comorbid disorders in 119 DSM-III-R somatization patients referred to primary care physicians. The most prevalent comorbid diagnoses were major depression (54.6%), generalized anxiety disorder (33.6%), phobic disorders (31.1%), panic disorder (26.0%), and alcohol abuse/dependence (21.0%).

In a study by Sheehan and Sheehan (1982), 71%

of patients with agoraphobia met the criteria for Briquet's syndrome. The results of Orenstein's (1989) examination of 188 consecutive female psychiatric patients indicated that Briquet's syndrome was associated with a lifetime history of major depression (81%) and a lifetime history of spontaneous panic attacks (69%). Orenstein commented that his results were consistent with a shared diathesis hypothesis underlying some cases of major depression, panic disorder, agoraphobia, and Briquet's syndrome. Moreover, Briquet's syndrome may represent the most extreme expression of a proclivity for physical and psychological syndromes to aggregate.

As part of a large epidemiological study of psychiatric disorders in a community sample of 3783 participants, 77.7% of the sixteen participants with somatization disorder met another concurrent psychiatric diagnosis, compared to 9.7% of patients with a dual diagnosis who did not have somatization disorder (Swartz et al., 1986). The most frequent concurrent diagnoses with somatization disorder included simple phobia (70%), major depression (65%), agoraphobia (64%), obsessive-compulsive disorder (52%), panic disorder (42%), schizophrenia (38%), atypical bipolar disorder (35%), social phobia (30%), alcohol abuse and dependence (17% each), and dysthymia (16%). Whether somatization disorder produces other psychiatric disorders is not known, but as Swartz et al. (1986) noted, by definition, individuals who endorse a plethora of symptoms to yield a diagnosis of somatization disorder are also more likely to endorse other physical and psychological symptoms at a high rate.

Liskow and his associates found a lifetime prevalence of depression in 87%, panic disorder in 45%, and phobic disorder in 39% of seventy-eight women diagnosed with somatization disorder (Liskow, Othmer, Penick, DeSouza, & Gabrielli, 1986). In addition, the prevalence of other psychiatric disturbances was considerable and included the following: obsessive-compulsive disorder (27%), schizophrenia (27%), drug dependence (23%) and drug abuse (17%), and antisocial personality disorder (17%). Using a genetic-epidemiological approach to examine the comorbidity of panic and somatization disorder, 159 outpatients with DSM-III-R panic disorder and seventy-six surgical controls were screened for the lifetime presence of DSM-III-R somatization (Battalgia, Bernadeschi, Politi, Bertella, & Bellodi, 1995).

The investigators found that 23% of women and 5% of men with panic disorder also had somatization disorder at one time. The authors also concluded that panic disorder and somatization disorder may coexist without sharing a common genetic diathesis and that the DSM-IV criteria for somatization disorder are simpler than the DSM-III-R criteria. Along similar lines, in a DSM-IV posttraumatic stress disorder field trial involving 395 traumatized subjects, a strong relationship was evidenced among reports of posttraumatic stress disorder, dissociation, and somatization (van der Kolk, Pelcovitz, Roth, Mandel, McFarlane, & Herman, 1996).

The relationship of histrionic personality disorder and antisocial personality disorder to somatization disorder (Lilienfeld, 1992; Lilienfeld, Van Valkenburg, Larntz, & Akiskal, 1986), as well as the relationship between hysteroid and obsessive features and Briquet's syndrome, has been similarly documented (Kaminsky & Slavney, 1983). Hudziak, Boffeli, Kriesman, Battaglia, Stanger, and Guze (1996) conducted a multisite study that examined the relationship of borderline personality to Briquet's syndrome (hysteria), somatization disorder, antisocial personality disorder, and substance abuse disorders in eighty-seven women (seventy-five from St. Louis and twelve from Milan) who met DSM-III-R borderline personality disorder. Patients were further examined with the DSM-III-R Checklist and the Perley–Guze Hysteria Checklist. Results indicated that every patient had at least one additional DSM diagnosis and patients from St. Louis and Milan averaged five and four additional diagnoses, respectively. Eighty-four percent of the St. Louis sample met criteria for somatization disorder, Briquet's syndrome, antisocial personality disorder, and substance abuse disorders. Patterns of comorbidity included major depression (87%), generalized anxiety disorder (55%), and panic disorder (51%). Two other studies looked at the prevalence of personality disorders and somatization disorder. Rost, Akins, Brown, and Smith (1992) evaluated thirteen personality disorders with the Structured Clinical Interview in ninety-four subjects with DSM-III-R somatization disorder from multiple primary care settings. The data indicated that 23.4% of somatization disorder cases had one personality disorder and 37.2% had two or more personality disorders. The four most common personality disorders included avoidance (26.7%), paranoia (21.3%), self-defeating (19.1%), obsessive-compulsive (17.1%), and, interestingly enough, histrionic personality disorder (12.8%) and antisocial personality disorder (7.4%). In a small British sample, twenty-five women with somatization disorder were compared to a control group (clinical patients but without somatization disorder) of 25 women using the Personality Assessment Schedule (Stern, Murphy, & Bass, 1993). The prevalence of personality disorders among the somatization disorder group was 72%, compared to 36% in the control group.

In sum, physical and psychological symptoms are common and often co-occur in the same individual. Although considerable data support somatization disorder, there should be concerns when a clinical condition overlaps with many other DSM-IV disorders. Somatization disorder is associated with so many things that it runs the risk of having little discriminatory clinical value.

**Prognosis and Treatment.** Somatization disorder is a condition with a poor prognosis. The disorder runs a fluctuating course with periodic exacerbations during stressful episodes, but as noted earlier, somatization disorder is not associated with a higher mortality rate than that of the general population (Coryell, 1981). Briquet stated that hysteria was one of the most difficult illnesses to cure (Mai & Merskey, 1980). He reported that one-quarter of hysterics never recover. More dramatically, young girls with hysteria before the age of 12 or 13 were condemned to a lifetime of suffering; if the onset of hysteria occurred after 25 years of age, then the prognosis was more favorable. In another study, only 31% of patients with somatization disorder fully recovered in 15-year follow-up assessments (Coryell & Norton, 1981). Guze and his colleagues noted that 80 to 90% of their cases retained the diagnosis of hysteria 6 to 8 years later (Guze et al., 1986; Perley & Guze, 1962).

Unlike other psychiatric conditions, there is no definitive therapy for all somatizers. From a medical viewpoint, in many respects, the best treatment is no treatment at all. Medical management focuses on early diagnosis and conservative treatment to reduce iatrogenic effects from invasive diagnostics and surgical interventions. A study by Smith, Monson, and Ray (1986b) demonstrated the cost-effectiveness of noninvasive, supportive long-term care of somatization disorder patients by focusing largely on containing their health care utilization. Thirty-eight patients with somatiza-

tion disorder were randomly assigned either to a treatment group (i.e., instructing primary care physicians to see patients in a supportive manner, perform brief physical examinations, and avoid unnecessary hospitalizations) or to a no-treatment control group, and the two groups crossed over 8 months later. The investigators found a 40 to 53% decrease in health care charges for the treatment condition.

Much of the general discussion around treating somatization disorder is geared toward physicians in primary care, because they are most likely to see psychiatric disorders, somatizing or not (Lipowski, 1988). Unfortunately, general practitioners are not equipped to handle this type of patient on their own, and somatizers often refuse psychiatric referral. Reducing the physical distance between the physician's office and the mental health professional by relocating the mental health professional in the physician's office or right next door does much to increase the follow-through on psychological evaluation and possible treatment (Wickramasekera, 1989). The aim of treatment for somatizers is to help them cope with their symptoms, not to cure them. Given the chronic nature of somatization disorder, a rehabilitative approach that consists of comprehensive medical, psychiatric, and psychosocial evaluation and treatment with adequate follow-up to prevent relapses is well suited to somatization disorder.

Psychiatric and psychological management typically has consisted of ego-supportive techniques and has been beneficial in treating somatizers (Kellner, 1990). Several studies described the utility of inpatient and outpatient group therapy with somatization disorder (Abbey & Lipowski, 1987; Bass & Benjamin, 1993; Levine, Brooks, Irving, & Fishman, 1994). Group treatment has consisted of different combinations of therapeutic approaches with varying emphasis on support therapy, problem-solving skills, improving interpersonal relationships, occupational and vocational rehabilitation, physiotherapy, and cognitive-behavioral techniques. However, these studies are generally descriptive instead of evaluative, they are usually uncontrolled studies with poor methodology and small sample sizes, and they tend to lack objective outcome measures.

More recently, Kasher, Rost, Cohen, Anderson, and Smith (1995) conducted a randomized controlled clinical trial of group therapy for seventy somatization disorder patients. The patients assigned to the treatment condition were required to attend eight group meetings lasting 2 hours each; these group meetings were held every 2 weeks. Groups of four to six patients were involved in a number of exercises designed to increase peer support, increase communications about coping with physical problems, develop strategies to express emotions more openly, and increase personal risk-taking. The experimental group experienced better physical and mental health in the year following group treatment. The experimental condition also resulted in a 52% net saving in health charges. Employing Kellner's definition for somatization disorder rather than the stricter DSM-IV definition, Lidbeck (1997) assigned fifty somatization disordered subjects either to a treatment condition or to a waiting-list control condition. Using a cognitive-behavioral treatment approach (e.g., stress management, relaxation training, and cognitive restructuring), subjects met for eight, 3-hour meetings. At 6 months follow-up, the treatment group evidenced modest improvement with respect to physical illness, somatic preoccupation, hypochondriasis, and medication usage. Although these two studies of group treatment for somatization disorder (Kasher et al., 1995; Lidbeck, 1997) suffer from a number of threats to internal validity (e.g., small samples sizes, less restrictive definition of somatization disorder, and patients only from primary care facilities), the utility of group treatment for somatization disorder is still worth pursuing. Pharmacotherapy should be avoided whenever possible with somatizers, but judicious use of antidepressants and anxiolytics is helpful (Kellner, 1990; Lipowski, 1988).

**Undifferentiated Somatoform Disorder**

Undifferentiated somatoform disorder was apparently created to capture a sizable proportion of patients with multiple, chronic, physical symptomatology similar to somatization disorder, but do not meet the eight physical-symptom requirement. This diagnosis is given to persons with one or several medically unsupported physical complaints that are of at least 6-months duration and are not due to the effects of a substance (APA, 1994). The symptom or symptoms have to cause clinically significant distress in a number of functional domains. The diagnosis of undifferentiated somatoform disorder is precluded if physical symptoms occur in the course of another mental disorder and if the symptom are intentionally produced or feigned (APA, 1994). Undifferentiated somatoform disorder, when compared to somatization disorder, is apparently less disabling and has a more variable course. Nonetheless, it is likely that undifferentiated somatoform disorder has a putative etiology similar to that of somatization disorder.

However, the utility of undifferentiated somatoform disorder as a diagnostic category is questionable. It is a relatively recent addition to the DSM (APA, 1987), difficult to use in a clinical setting, possibly overly inclusive (one unexplained symptom is enough for a diagnosis), and lacks validity data (Kroenke et al., 1997; Kroenke, Spitzer, deGruy, & Swindle, 1998). A number of investigators attempted a more systematic approach to somatic presentations that do not meet a formal diagnosis of somatization disorder. In two earlier studies, Escobar and his colleagues (Escobar et al., 1987, 1989) demonstrated the utility of the Somatic Symptom Index (SSI 4,6) as an abridged version of the somatization construct. The SSI consisted of four symptoms for men and six for women. Most recently, Escobar, Waitzkin, Silver, Gara, and Holman (1998) examined abridged somatization in primary care. Using the Composite International Diagnostic Interview (CIDI), 1456 patients were recruited from a university-affiliated outpatient clinic. The CIDI probed for symptoms of somatization, hypochondriasis, generalized anxiety, panic, agoraphobia, simple phobia, dysthymia, and major depression. The sample included four ethnic groups: U.S.-born non-Latinos (whites), U.S. born Latinos, Mexican immigrants, and Central American immigrants. The investigators found that one-fifth of the total sample met a diagnosis of abridged somatization and that somatizers had higher levels of psychiatric comorbidity and functional disability than non-somatizers. In addition, the authors found evidence for a new series of abridged somatization subtypes based upon the number of organ body systems involved ("simple" versus "polymorphous"), the type of body system involved (seven-organ system cluster, two distinct three-symptom clusters, and three single-organ system subtypes-genitourinary, cardiorespiratory, and headache), and discrete (one-third of the sample with abridged somatization did not meet criteria for any other psychiatric disorder) versus comorbid (two-thirds of the sample with abridged somatization met criteria for other lifetime psychiatric disorders). Preliminary data on 108 psychiatric inpatients demonstrated that three unexplained symptoms for men and five for women out of thirty-three DSM-IV somatization symptoms were equivalent to Escobar SSI 4,6 (Rief, Heuser, Mayrhuber, Stelzer, Hiller, & Fichter, 1996).

Other ways of conceptualizing subthreshold somatization disorder have been put forward by other researchers. Robbins, Kirmayer, and Hemami (1997) used latent variable models to test "functional syndromes" in 686 primary care patients. Symptom items were derived from the National Institute of Mental Health Diagnostic Interview Schedule and were made to approximate diagnoses of fibromyalgia syndrome, chronic fatigue syndrome, and irritable bowel syndrome. Three models were tested for goodness of fit: the first model assumes that all forms of functional symptoms may be traced to a single underlying construct of somatic distress; the second model tests whether functional symptoms common to fibromyalgia, chronic fatigue, and irritable bowel can be subsumed under the physical symptoms for depression and anxiety; and the third model tests the convergent validity of these syndromes as discrete from one another and from depression and anxiety. The data indicated that patients with functional symptoms (multiple medically unexplained somatic symptoms) should be categorized in two groups: one group with distress across multiple-organ systems often associated with another psychiatric disorder; the second group with concerns limited to a single-organ system.

Finally, Kroenke and his colleagues (Kroenke et al., 1997, 1998) proposed multisomatoform disorder as an alternative to undifferentiated somatoform disorder. The authors defined multisomatoform disorder as three or more currently bothersome unexplained physical symptoms (from a fifteen-item symptom checklist) that are present more often than not for at least 2 years (Kroneke et al; 1997). Kroenke et al. (1998) then used data from the Primary Care Evaluation of Mental Disorders (PRIME-MD, N = 1000) and Somatization in Primary Care Studies (N = 258) to determine the optimal threshold of a fifteen-item checklist and to determine the concordance between multisomatoform disorder and somatization disorder. The optimal threshold for pursuing a diagnosis of multisomatoform disorder was seven or greater. The majority of multisomatoform disorder patients (88%) met a diagnosis of either full somatization disorder or abridged somatization disorder. The authors also found that multisomatoform disorder was intermediate between abridged and full somatization disorder in functional impairment, psychiatric comorbidity, family dysfunction, and health care utilization and charges. The other advantage of the multisomatoform disorder diagnosis is that it takes less time to administer than Escobar's SSI 4,6 and Rief's SSI 3,5.

In sum, undifferentiated somatoform disorder is likely to continue being problematic in its application, but the number of persons subsumed under such a label necessitates continued efforts toward improving its diagnostic usefulness. Other subthreshold versions of somatization disorder have been developed, and their utility is more promising. Among them, multisomatoform disorder is most promising; this diagnostic category affords greater specificity in defining physical symptom requirements.

## Conversion Disorder

Given the popularity of conversion disorder, it is surprising that little research work was done on this topic during the past 10 years. Conversion disorder remains an elusive entity, even though conversion phenomena have been described throughout the medical literature since antiquity. It has engendered much controversy as to its very existence (Chodoff, 1974; Engel, 1970; Ford & Folks, 1985; Lewis, 1974; Slater, 1965; Whitlock, 1967); a great deal of the confusion is due to changing diagnostic criteria and terminology and to the interchangeable use of diagnostic terms throughout the years. The ubiquitous term hysteria has often been used to refer to conversion hysteria, hysterical personality, somatization disorder, or some combination of all three (Chodoff, 1974; Chodoff & Lyons, 1958; Guze et al., 1971a; Kendell, 1972; Purtell et al., 1951). Note that on occasion these terms will be used interchangeably in this chapter so as to be consistent with the terminology in cited studies, although we do not feel that these terms are in fact interchangeable.

Although conversion phenomena were brought to the forefront by Freud (1956), the concept was originally put forward by the Egyptians. The term was derived from the Greek word hustera, meaning "uterus," because the ancient Egyptians and Greeks attributed a number of physical symptoms in women to the "wandering of the uterus" (Jones, 1980). In the seventeenth century, the concept of conversion was further developed by Sydenham, who emphasized that hysterical phenomena could mimic almost all known physical diseases (Nemiah, 1985). In 1856, a French physician, Paul Briquet, published a comprehensive monograph on 430 clinical cases (Mai & Merskey, 1980, 1981). Although Briquet's investigation attempted to provide a clearer and more systematic definition of hysteria than previously achieved, his work ultimately provided more support for somatization disorder than conversion disorder.

Around the same time, Jean Martin Charcot was credited with some of the seminal ideas regarding hysteria (Jones, 1980). Charcot's contributions included the view that hysteria was a special type of consciousness, whereby individuals actually experienced the lack of physical functioning because they were highly suggestible. Charcot went on to postulate that conversion symptoms were attributable to an inherited degenerative process of the nervous system. He also became famous for his theatrical use of hypnosis, and, in fact, he indicated that hypnotizability was pathognomonic for the condition of hysteria. Pierre Janet, a student of Charcot, extended the theoretical formulations of hysteria to include a description of dissociative phenomena. A dissociated system represents a system of ideas and functions that, although no longer available to consciousness, could continue to be active and exert sensory and motor effects via unconscious mechanisms (Nemiah, 1985).

Sigmund Freud (1956), who was also a student of Charcot for a brief period, used hypnosis with conversion patients to demonstrate that the recollection of past memories and experiences could alleviate conversion symptoms. Freud developed the theory of conservation of psychophysical energy, which proposed that emotions not expressed or discharged lead to physical symptoms. Freud added that affect associated with a traumatic event that could not be expressed because of moral or ethical concerns would be repressed and converted to a somatic-hysterical symptom that was symbolic of the original trauma in some way. The repression of affect later became known as la belle indifference, one of the mainstays of hysterical conversion. Freud also noted that repressed ideas, affects, and conflicts were often sexual.

**Diagnosis.** Diagnostic considerations and terminology used to capture conversion disorder var-

ied over time. In the first edition of the DSM (DSM-I; APA, 1952), conversion reactions were defined as functional symptoms in organs or systems that were believed to be mainly under voluntary control and due to impulses that cause anxiety. Conversion reactions were distinguished from "dissociative reactions," which referred to such phenomena as amnesias and fugue states. In the second edition of the DSM (DSM-II; APA, 1968), the term conversion reaction was changed to "hysterical neurosis," returning the term hysteria to the nomenclature. The qualifying descriptors of conversion and dissociative were also retained by the DSM-II and the diagnostic subtypes were known as "hysterical neurosis of conversion type" and "hysterical neurosis of dissociative type." La belle indifference, symbolism of symptoms, and secondary gain were considered essential features of hysterical neurosis of the conversion type.

In DSM-III (APA, 1980), hysterical neurosis of the conversion type became known as "conversion disorder" and was considered a subtype of the somatoform disorders; hysterical neurosis of the dissociative type was placed in a completely new category, the dissociative disorders. Much of the DSM-III description of conversion disorder was retained in DSM-III-R (APA, 1987) and DSM-IV (APA, 1994). DSM-IV criteria for conversion disorder are presented in Table 2. DSM-III-R diagnostic criteria for conversion disorder required that the clinician specify whether the conversion symptom represented a single episode or a recurrent phenomenon; this requirement has been dropped from the current edition of the DSM. Instead, now the DSM-IV requires the clinician to specify the type of symptom or deficit that characterizes the conversion (see Table 2).

**Clinical Description.** The manifestations of conversion are protean and may mimic many different known medical conditions. Conversion symptoms can be categorized according to four major subtypes (APA, 1994). Conversion disorder with motor symptom or deficit includes symptoms such as paralysis, paresis, impaired coordination, aphonia, difficulty in swallowing, or a lump in the throat (APA, 1994). Astasia-abasia is another classic example of a motor conversion (Nemiah, 1985). Individuals with astasia-abasia can be categorized by gross, irregular, pseudotaxic movements of the trunk, staggering and halting steps, and waving of the hands and arms. Like patients with pseudoseizures, these individuals often do not hurt them-

## Table 2. DSM-IV Criteria for Conversion Disorder

A. One or more symptoms or deficits affecting voluntary motor or sensory function that suggest a neurological or other general medical condition.

B. Psychological factors are judged to be associated with the symptom or deficit because the initiation or exacerbation of the symptom or deficit is preceded by conflicts or other stressors.

C. The symptom or deficit is not intentionally produced or feigned (as in Factitious Disorder or Malingering).

D. The symptom or deficit cannot, after appropriate investigations, be fully explained by a medical condition, or by the direct effects of a substance, or as a culturally sanctioned behavior or experience.

E. The symptom or deficit causes clinically significant distress or impairment in social, occupational, or other important areas of functioning or warrants medical evaluation.

F. The symptom or deficit is not limited to pain or sexual dysfunction, does not occur exclusively during the course of Somatization Disorder, and is not better accounted for by another mental disorder.

*Specify* type of symptom or deficit:

**With Motor Symptom or Deficit**
**With Sensory Symptom or Deficit**
**With Seizures or Convulsions**
**With Mixed Presentations**

*Source*: American Psychiatric Association. (1994). *Diagnostic and Statistical Manual of Mental Disorders*, 4th ed. (p. 457). Washington, DC: Author. Reprinted by permission.

selves when falling to the ground and may have complete control of the body while sitting. A second subtype of conversion disorder is characterized by some sensory symptom or deficit. Sensory disturbances usually come in the form of anesthesias and are experienced most frequently in the extremities. Glove anesthesia of the hands and sock anesthesia of the feet represent classic examples of sensory conversions. The sense organs for vision and audition can be used as sources of conversion. Seizures or convulsions with sensory or motor components represent a third subtype of conversion disorder. Pseudoseizures are characterized by wild, disorganized writhing of the body and arms and legs flailing with abandon. Unlike individuals with true seizures, this all occurs without the patients injuring themselves. In addition, individuals with pseudoseizures do not void or soil themselves. The final subtype of conversion disorder tends to be characterized by a mixed presentation of more than one of the previous subtypes.

**Epidemiology and Demographics.** Because of the almost ephemeral nature of conversion and the differences in defining the term, the reported prevalence of conversion disorder fluctuates from rare (Lewis, 1974; Slater, 1965; Whitlock, 1967) to ubiquitous (Engel, 1970). Prevalence rates for conversion vary as a function of clinical setting. Guze et al. (1971a) found that 24% of 500 psychiatric outpatients had a history of conversion symptoms. Engel (1970) estimated that 20 to 25% of patients admitted to general medical services will experience a conversion symptom at one time or another; however, Engel's estimate was not empirically based. Empirical investigations resulted in more likely estimates of conversion that suggest that the prevalence is between 5 and 14% of all consultations in a general medical setting (Folks, Ford, & Regan, 1984; McKegney, 1967; Stefansson, Messina, & Meyerowitz, 1976; Ziegler, Imboden, & Meyer, 1960). DSM-IV notes the prevalence of conversion disorder at 1–3% of outpatient referrals. The use of such different diagnostic terms as conversion and hysteria have surely confounded efforts to determine accurate prevalence estimates across different samples.

The distribution of conversion in men and women is equivocal. It is generally believed that conversion symptoms occur more frequently in women (Folks et al., 1984; Gatfield & Guze, 1962; Guze & Perley, 1963; Perley & Guze, 1962; Purtell et al., 1951; Raskin, Talbott, & Meyerson, 1966; Whitlock, 1967). Engel (1970) reported that conversion symptoms occur two or three times more frequently in women than in men. The DSM-IV (APA, 1994) reports a 2:1 to 10:1 ratio in favor of women. The typical patient with conversion reaction has been described as a woman less than 40 years old from a rural and/or impoverished environment (Folks et al., 1984). On the other hand, Chodoff (1974) contended that conversion reactions occur as frequently in men as women. In fact, men experience conversion more frequently than women in such settings as industry (Allodi, 1974) and the military (Carden & Schramel, 1966). Ziegler, Imboden, and Rogers (1963) commented that women may use conversion symptoms more than men because the feminine role inherently sanctions greater dependency and reliance on others, and more readily lends itself to a "sick role." Probably there is little sex difference in the prevalence of conversion. Differences reported in studies may reflect social and cultural influences on the expression and diagnosis of conversion instead of true sex differences.

The onset of conversion disorder is usually from late childhood to early adulthood (APA, 1994). The onset is typically acute and tends to resolve quickly, usually within 2 weeks. Factors associated with a good prognosis include acute onset, identifiable stress before hospitalization, and good premorbid functioning (Couprie, Wijdicks, Rooijmans, & van Gijn, 1995; Singh & Lee, 1997).

There has been considerable interest in examining conversion disorder in children and adolescents (Goodyer, 1981; Kriechman, 1987; Maloney, 1980; Siegel & Barthel, 1986; Spierings, Poels, Sijben, Gabreels, & Renier, 1990; Volkmar, Poll, & Lewis, 1984). The prevalence of conversion in children and adolescents has been estimated at approximately 5% (Maloney, 1980; Siegel & Barthel, 1986). However, an older study by Robins and O'Neal (1953) estimated that the prevalence of conversion reactions is as high as 17%. The presence of a family role model with similar physical symptoms, familial discord, early sexual trauma, and stress has been consistently found in children and adolescents with conversion symptoms (Goodyer, 1981; Kriechman, 1987; Volkmar et al., 1984). Spierings et al. (1990) conducted a 9-year retrospective study of eighty-four children between the ages of 6 and 17 who met DSM-III-R criteria for conversion disorder of various types (paresthesia, anesthesia, pseudoseizure, and loss of consciousness were the most common), and a number of noteworthy findings were revealed. They reported a 2.2:1 gender ratio for females, but below the age of 10 the ratio was even. Sixty-two percent of patients and 45% of family members had a history of significant organic disease. A personal model for the symptoms was observed in 29% of cases, suggesting a learning process. In general, studies of conversion in children and adolescents are particularly impressive and suggest possible genetic, environmental, and role-model influences in the expression of conversion disorder.

In 1896, Freud stated that conversion phenomena were rare in the lower class (Freud, 1956); however, today the reverse is true (Guze & Perley, 1963; Stefansson et al., 1976). Conversion reactions are observed more frequently in individuals who reside in rural areas and in less psychologically sophisticated populations (Folks et al., 1984). Patients from rural and uneducated backgrounds also tend to present to clinicians with more primitive, bizarre, and dramatic clinical presentations of conversion, whereas more educated and sophisticated patients tend to present with symptoms that more closely simulate physical disease (Engel, 1970; Jones, 1980).

**Etiological Formulations.** Conversion disorder has proven difficult to define, partly because most of the conceptual formulation for conversion disorder has come from the psychoanalytic literature. Many of the ideas put forward by psychoanalysts are too vague and elusive to be properly and scientifically evaluated. Over time, the literature has incorporated behavioral, sociological, and neurophysiological conceptualizations of conversion disorder.

*Psychoanalytic.* Although psychoanalytic formulations have undergone considerable revision over the years (Chodoff, 1974; Lazare, 1981; Lewis, 1974; Nemiah, 1985; Viederman, 1995), a series of papers on an integrated theory of conversion written in the late nineteenth century by Freud (1956) continues to influence thinking about conversion disorder. He stated that a conversion symptom is usually associated with a passive sexual seduction that typically occurs during the oedipal period. Due to sexual feelings and situations that arise around puberty, the childhood seduction is then followed by a resensitization of the early childhood episode. At puberty, sexual urges recall frightening affects and memory traces of an earlier sexual trauma. In an attempt to cope with this, repression (as a defense) leads to the conversion of sexual arousal into a somatic symptom. Freud added that the actual early childhood sexual trauma did not have to be real and that sexual fantasy alone could produce a conversion reaction.

Lazare (1981) theorized that conversion reactions can result from impulses other than sexual, for example, aggression and dependency. Engel (1970) stated that conversion may develop for several reasons: (1) to permit expression of a forbidden wish or impulse, (2) as a form of punishment for a forbidden need, (3) to remove oneself from an overwhelming threatening life situation, and (4) to allow gratification of dependency needs by assuming the sick role. In sum, a conversion symptom represents a compromise between the need to express ideas or feelings that are unconscious and the fear of expressing them (Viederman, 1995).

*Behavioral.* Conversion reactions can be conceptualized as behavioral excesses or deficits that follow a traumatic event or emotional state and are reinforced by particular outcomes (Mumford, 1978). A conversion symptom can be used to manipulate others, to get special attention, to receive special privileges, and to avoid unpleasant tasks or responsibilities. Use of a conversion symptom can also be reinforced and facilitated by a reduction in the intensity of a drive (Nemiah, 1985). For example, an initial episode of a conversion paralysis can result in a reduction of a painful emotional drive such as anxiety. This initial pairing of a stimulus and response can predispose an individual to using the same palliative response whenever anxiety occurs; consequently, responding to external stressors or pressures with a conversion reaction may represent a primary, although maladaptive, coping response. Others have conceptualized conversion symptoms as an adaptation to frustrating or stressful life experiences (Barr & Abernathy, 1977). The influence of role-modeling in the development of a conversion symptom in children and adolescents has been noted earlier (Spierings et al., 1990).

From a broader conceptual perspective, conversion reactions, it has been thought, result from cultural, social, and interpersonal influences (Celani, 1976). Individuals with conversion disorder learn to use their symptoms to communicate helplessness, thereby fostering an environment that reinforces helplessness and inhibits aggressive impulses. Thus, a patient's conversion disorder can be reinforced by the reactions of caretakers or families and by the formation of a conversion symptom in times of stress or conflict. Strangely enough, much of the behavioral formulation of conversion disorder has come from psychiatrists. As behaviorally oriented clinicians get more involved in assessing and treating conversion disorder, our understanding of conversion should increase substantially.

*Sociological.* A different approach to understanding conversion phenomena comes from the field of medical sociology. Mechanic (1962) and Parsons (1951) have been most responsible for increasing our understanding of illness behavior and the sick

role. Illness behavior can be defined by the ways in which symptoms are perceived, evaluated, and acted upon (Mechanic, 1962). In other words, the context in which symptoms occur and the way that they are perceived by the individual are extremely important. Once illness has been recognized and legitimized by the physician, then individuals can be relieved of their duties or responsibilities, and others in the "system" may be required to be considerate and supportive of the sick individual (Parsons, 1951). In assuming the sick role, the patient is obliged to cooperate with treatment and to withdraw from activities, even those that are considered enjoyable. Variations of this model of conversion have been proposed by other investigators (Ziegler & Imboden, 1962).

*Neurophysiological.* Neurophysiological formulations of conversion reactions have received considerable attention. The neurophysiological formulation for conversion suggests that conversion symptoms result from some form of damage or malfunction of the brain (Ludwig, 1972; Whitlock, 1967). Whitlock (1967) proposed a neurophysiological conceptualization of conversion in which conversion disorder is considered primarily a disorder of attention and vigilance. The lack of attention and concern (i.e., la belle indifference) on the part of the conversion patient is due to a "selective depression of awareness of a bodily function" brought on by corticofugal inhibition of afferent stimulation (Whitlock, 1967). The corticofugal inhibition of sensory stimulation occurs at the level of the brain stem reticular formation. Ludwig (1972) added that memory impairments observed in patients with hysteria were due to the same mechanism proposed by Whitlock (1967).

In an attempt to examine neurophysiologically based assumptions pertaining to attention and memory dysfunction, Bendefeldt, Miller, and Ludwig (1976) had seventeen hospitalized conversion hysterics complete a series of tasks under nonstress (supportive behavior on the part of the experimenter) and stress (unsupportive behavior on the part of the experimenter) conditions. Their study also included a control group of nonpsychotic patients. Overall, the results indicated that the conversion group had heightened suggestibility, greater field dependency, and greater impairment of recent memory, vigilance, and attention. The authors then used stepwise discriminant function analysis and were able to classify correctly fourteen subjects out of seventeen in the nonstress condition and sixteen subjects out of seventeen in the stress condition. However, the classification analysis should be questioned because the authors essentially had one subject per dependent variable. Despite this statistical weakness, their data does provide some interesting possibilities for a neurophysiological model of conversion disorder.

Studies that examined somatosensory average evoked responses substantiate the utility of a neurophysiological formulation of conversion disorder. In a study by Hernandez-Peon, Chavez-Ibarra, and Aguilar-Figueroa (1963), monitoring of somatosensory evoked responses from both the affected left upper extremity and the corresponding unaffected limb of a 15-year-old female patient with hysterical paralysis revealed an absence of evoked potentials during wakeful stimulation. However, during light central anesthesia (using a barbiturate), significant evoked potentials appeared following stimulation of the left upper extremity. Halliday (1968) found no appreciable differences between normal and anesthetic conditions in his analysis of somatosensory evoked potentials in a 40-year-old man with hysterical anesthesia of the left thumb and index finger. Levy and his associates confirmed the Hernandez-Peon et al. (1963) findings for low levels but not for high levels of sensory stimulation (Levy & Behrman, 1970; Levy & Mushin, 1973).

Another line of research supporting the neurophysiological formulation of conversion disorder came from studies that examined lateralization of symptoms in conversion hysterics. Bishop, Mobley, and Farr (1978), having conducted or in conducting a 10-year retrospective study of conversion reactions, reported that 70% of 430 patients with conversion neurosis, hysterical neurosis, hysterical personality, and psychophysiological CNS or musculoskeletal disorders had their symptoms on the left side of the body. Similar findings have been reported in other studies (Galin, Diamond, & Braff, 1977; Stern, 1977). These studies also suggest that the right cerebral hemisphere is particularly involved in modifying affective or motivational components of somatic symptoms.

**Conversion Disorder and Associated Psychopathology.** One reason that conversion disorder has questionable utility as a diagnostic entity is because this disorder often co-occurs with a variety of psychiatric disorders and personality styles. Although patients with conversion disorder

are generally considered more likely to have hysterical personality disorder, this relationship has fueled a great deal of controversy. Chodoff and Lyons (1958) stated that hysterical personality is a description of women by men and is basically a caricature of femininity. This stereotyping seemingly also holds for men. One group of authors suggested that hysterical personality disorder in men reflects a homosexual process, and if not a homosexual process, then these men are likely to have sexual problems and display "affectations" (Luisada, Peele, & Pittard, 1974). Kendell (1972) strongly stated that hysterical personality is a label used to describe a woman if the individual is perceived as difficult, demanding, and manipulative, whereas the same symptoms observed in a man will lead to the label of psychopathy.

The DSM-IV (APA, 1994) presentation of histrionic personality disorder includes the following traits: overly dramatic, incessant need for attention and reassurance, sensation seeking, reactions out of proportion to minor stimuli, irritability with outbursts of anger, shallowness, vanity, and proneness to manipulative suicidal gestures. Past studies have essentially used variations of the DSM-IV definition of histrionic personality disorder. A comprehensive review of studies of hysterical personality characteristics dating from 1949 to 1970 was conducted by Alacron (1973). Analysis of fourteen studies revealed a high degree of consensus for hysterical personality traits including emotional lability, dependency, excitability, egocentrism, and suggestibility. Alacron concluded that all patients with hysteria have some of the features of hysterical personality, whereas not all patients with hysterical personality will have typical features of hysteria.

The estimated percentage of the co-occurrence of conversion and hysterical personality has ranged from 5 to 50% (Lewis & Berman, 1965; Raskin et al., 1966; Stephens & Kamp, 1962). Ziegler et al. (1960) noted that less than half of their sample of 134 conversion patients had "hysterical character," which led the authors to conclude that the hysterical personality pattern was not a prerequisite for a conversion process. Barnert (1971) found that 7% of forty-six patients with conversion reactions exhibited a hysterical personality disorder. Of fifty patients with a DSM-III diagnosis of conversion disorder, only 6% of the cases had co-occurring histrionic personality disorder (Folks et al., 1984).

Given the difficulty in determining the validity of conversion disorder and the almost anecdotal definition of hysterical or histrionic personality, it is not surprising that determining the true co-occurrence of these two conditions is problematic. Although hysterical personality disorder may predispose individuals to conversion reactions, no single personality pattern characterizes individuals with conversion disorder.

Of greater interest is the relationship of depression and schizophrenia to conversion reactions. Ziegler et al. (1963) found rates of 29.9% for depression and 14.2% for schizophrenia in their conversion patient sample, and in another sample, prevalence rates of 17% for depression and 7% for schizophrenia were observed (Stephens & Kamp, 1962). Barnert (1971) reported overt depression in 33%, covert depression in 21%, and schizophrenia in 7% of patients diagnosed with conversion symptoms. Lewis and Berman (1965) observed that eight out of fifty-seven conversion patients evidenced schizophrenia or schizoid character. Roy (1980) found that 88% of fifty patients with hysterical conversion had depression and suggested that conversion symptoms may serve more as a "signal of distress" than anything else. Folks et al. (1984) indicated that 44% of their sample did not have any psychopathology other than conversion disorder but noted that 8% of their patients had depression and 29% had somatization disorder concurrent with conversion reactions.

Two studies by the same group of investigators (Kent, Tomasson, & Coryell, 1995; Tomasson, Kent, & Coryell, 1991) examined differences between conversion and somatization disorders. In the first study (Tomasson et al., 1991), the investigators reviewed charts of patients seen over a 2-year period at a large medical center. Cases were assessed for conversion disorder (N = 51) and somatization disorder (N = 65) using DSM-III criteria. Seventy-eight percent of the conversion disorder group and 95% of the somatization disorder group were women. Conversion disorder cases were overrepresented in the neurology services, whereas somatization patients tended to come from all units throughout the hospital. Age of onset occurred across the life span of the conversion group and tended to occur before 21 years of age in the somatization disorder group. The somatization disorder group tended to have a greater history of depression, attempted suicide, panic disorder, and divorce, suggesting that con-version disorder was less pathological than somatization disorder. The investigators then went on to follow the course and outcome of these patients during a 4-year period (Kent et al., 1995). Still using DSM-III criteria, the conversion disorder group (N = 32) and the somatization disorder group (N = 38) were given follow-up interviews by a rater blind to the baseline diagnosis. Patients in the conversion disorder group were less likely to be given the same diagnosis at follow-up than patients in the somatization disorder group. Interestingly, six cases in the conversion disorder group were given a diagnosis of somatization disorder at follow-up and four other cases in the conversion disorder group were eventually diagnosed with an organic condition. Follow-up comparisons of overall distress and impairment were made using the Symptom Checklist-90 and the Short-Form General Health Survey. Again, the somatization disorder group displayed higher levels of emotional turmoil and functional impairment relative to the conversion disorder group. These two studies are compromised by the retrospective nature of the design, as well as diagnoses based on chart review.

In one of the more rigorous studies of conversion reactions, Binzer, Andersen, and Kullgen (1997) examined thirty consecutive patients with conversion disorder, motor symptom subtype, and compared them to a control group with corresponding motor symptoms due to an organic lesion. All patients were assessed with the DSM-III-R diagnostic system, the Hamilton Depression Rating Scale, and a special life events schedule. The results indicated that the conversion group had a higher degree of psychopathology. Thirty-three percent of the conversion group had an Axis I diagnosis, and 50% had an Axis II diagnosis, compared to 10 and 17% of control group patients, respectively. The conversion group also had higher depression scores and special life events before the onset of conversion symptoms. A logistic regression analysis indicated that low education, the presence of a personality disorder, and depression were associated with increased risk of conversion disorder.

Clearly, further research is needed to determine whether conversion disorder represents a unitary diagnosis or should be considered more as part of another psychiatric condition. Conservatively, conversion reactions can be thought of as the "tip of the iceberg," suggesting the presence of other concurrent psychiatric disorders or serious medical disorders (Roy, 1980).

*La Belle Indifference.* The assumed sine qua non of conversion disorder is la belle indifference, or what is referred to as an indifference or lack of concern toward symptoms on the part of conversion patients. Chodoff (1974) noted that la belle indifference occurred as often as not in his sample of hysterics. He speculated that la belle indifference represented an example of the use of denial to defend against psychological stressors and not an indifference *per se.* Other studies reported la belle indifference in 30% (Stephens & Kamp, 1962), 41% (Raskin et al., 1966), and 54% (Barnert, 1971) of their respective samples.

One of the better studies that argued against the presence of la belle indifference in conversion hysteria was provided by Lader and Sartorius (1968). The authors compared a self-report of anxiety, psychiatrist ratings, and psychophysiology in a conversion hysteria group and an anxiety disorder group. The patients in the conversion hysteria group rated themselves as significantly more anxious than did the anxiety group, whereas the ratings of patients by examining psychiatrists were in the opposite direction, that is, psychiatrists rated conversion hysteria patients as less anxious than anxiety patients. As measured by galvanic skin response, patients in the conversion group (N = 10) displayed higher autonomic levels of arousal than the comparison anxiety group (N = 71) and a normal control group (N = 75). In another study, Meares and Horvath (1972) indicated that a group of seventeen patients who suffered from conversion could be separated on the basis of psychophysiological and biographical variables. One group, identified as "chronic hysterics," had more debilitating conversion symptoms, poor interpersonal and occupational coping skills, and longer histories of multiple medical complaints than a second group identified as "acute hysterics." In addition, the chronic hysterics displayed higher levels of heart rate, sweat gland, and muscle activity than the acute hysterics. On closer analysis of these two groups, the chronic hysterics label may be a misnomer; the profile obtained by chronic hysterics is more consistent with a somatization disorder profile.

Despite the long history, la belle indifference is not a reliable indicator or marker of conversion disorder. Conversion disorder patients are actually quite concerned about their symptoms, although this concern may not be readily apparent (Lewis & Berman, 1965). A true indifference to symptomatology or disability is usually indicative of central nervous system damage (Gould, Miller, Goldberg, & Benson, 1986).

**Organic Illness and Misdiagnosis.** Because of the implications for both treatment and prognosis, a discussion of organic illness and misdiagnosis of conversion disorder before the review of treatments and prognosis for conversion disorder is appropriate. The diagnosis of conversion disorder is not as simple as might be expected. There are two salient aspects to the relationship between organic illness and conversion symptoms that are vitally important in understanding the complexities of clinical diagnosis in conversion disorder (Lazare, 1981). First, there are a substantial number of patients whose initial diagnosis of conversion symptoms is changed to organic illness. Second, there is a high incidence of patients with conversion reactions and concomitant organic illness. Clinicians who ignore these two basic tenets will experience many problems in understanding and managing this group of patients.

Conversion reactions can occur in isolation, as part of another psychiatric disorder, or as part of a neurological disorder. The following studies strongly challenge the diagnostic utility of conversion hysteria. In a seminal piece of research, Slater and Glithero (1965) performed a 7- to 10-year follow-up of ninety-nine patients discharged from the National Hospital in London. Four patients who had committed suicide and eight patients who died from an organic illness were not included at follow-up. Of the seventy-three patients contacted at follow-up, 30% of the cases initially diagnosed with conversion symptoms had organic illnesses that accounted for the presenting problem. Of the thirty-two patients who did not have organic illnesses, only thirteen patients could be truly said to have been without pathology, whereas the rest suffered from schizophrenia, depression, and severe disability. Because an organic illness may appear asymptomatic or atypical at one phase of an illness, clinicians may be predisposed to misdiagnose bona fide medical disorders as "conversions" (Slater & Glithero, 1965). Moreover, an organic illness may produce behavioral disturbances (e.g., emotional lability, attention seeking, constant need for reassurance, and aggressiveness) that mimic psychiatric presentations.

Gatfield and Guze (1962) performed a 2.5- to

10-year follow-up of twenty-four patients who were discharged from neurological and neurosurgical wards with a diagnosis of conversion reaction. Five of twenty-five patients had neurological disease. Raskin et al. (1966) examined fifty patients referred from an inpatient and outpatient neurological service of two teaching hospitals; follow-up periods ranged from 6 to 12 months. Organic illness was found in seven patients. Whitlock (1967) noted that almost 64% of his sample showed evidence of an accompanying or preceding organic brain disorder, compared to 5% for a control group of persons diagnosed with depression and/or anxiety. Merskey and Buhrich (1975) observed a prevalence of 50% for organic cerebral disorders in conversion patients (N = 89). In a 10-year follow-up of forty male patients with conversion, a 25% false positive rate was obtained (Watson & Buranen, 1979). Watson and Buranen reported that symptoms most characteristic of the false positives were degenerative diseases and structural damage that affected the spinal cord, peripheral nerves, bones, muscles, and connective tissue. Roy (1980) found that 40% of his sample had organic brain disease, whereas Folks et al. (1984) noted a 17.7% rate of organicity in their sample of patients with conversion disorder. In another study, a remarkable 80% of thirty patients originally diagnosed with conversion hysteria had, it was eventually found, diagnosable medical disorders as an underlying cause (Gould et al., 1986). Couprie et al. (1995) reviewed medical records of patients admitted with conversion disorders other than pseudoseizures over a seven-year span. A total of fifty-six patients were identified and interviewed in person (N = 22) or by phone (N = 34). The median interval from the onset of symptom to interview was 4.5 years. Contrary to findings from earlier studies, Couprie and colleagues found that only two of the fifty-six patients later developed neurological conditions. These data are consistent with other data presented by Kent et al. (1995) in which only four out of thirty-two conversion disorder cases followed 4 years later had organic conditions. The smaller number of cases of conversion disorder eventually diagnosed as organic conditions in more recent studies might suggest better psychiatric and medical assessments.

As it is currently conceptualized, conversion disorder will likely become more of a rarity in the clinical setting. Clearly, many patients are diagnosed with conversion disorder who then develop significantly more serious medical or neurological disorders. Although no one has calculated the cost of the misdiagnosis of medical conditions, it is obvious that, if the error in diagnosis results in the deaths of patients (as some of the above studies suggest), then the price is extremely high. Consequently, it may be wise that the diagnosis of conversion disorder not be seen as an either-or decision between organic versus psychological symptomatology. However, if the diagnosis of conversion disorder is given, the clinician is well advised to carefully monitor ongoing symptomatology to ensure detection of an organic process.

**Treatment and Prognosis.** As Ford and Folks (1985) noted, a wide variety of treatment interventions have been suggested for conversion disorders. As they note, a plethora of therapies suggest that nothing is very effective and that most therapies help to some degree with conversion disorder. Treatment interventions have included psychoanalysis, supportive therapy, hypnosis, physical therapy, amobarbital interviewing, and behavior therapy. Concurrent mood or anxiety disorders associated with conversion disorder may also require pharmacological treatment. Direct confrontation of a patient's conversion symptom has no real benefit, and the interview should be carefully conducted so as to avoid a confrontational stance; otherwise, a confrontation is only likely to exacerbate the patient's defensiveness. A careful psychosocial evaluation and examination of possible precipitating life events and past history of psychological trauma should lead to an appropriate treatment intervention. Several case studies have demonstrated the utility of behavioral applications in treating conversion disorder (Barr & Abernathy, 1977; Fishbain et al., 1988).

It should be evident from the information in the prior section on organic illness and misdiagnosis of conversion disorder that the prognosis for conversion disorder is not encouraging. However, two studies reported favorable outcomes. Carter (1949) reported that 83% of ninety inpatients and outpatients were well or significantly improved at 4- to 6-year follow-up. Hafeiz (1980) found that there was an immediate favorable response to treatment in all of sixty-one psychiatric outpatients and only twelve patients had relapses at the end of 1 year. His treatment consisted of faradic stimulation, somlec (electro-sleeping machine), sodium amylobarbitone, and methylamphetamine. A good prognosis for conversion disorder is associated with an acute or recent onset of symptomatology, a definite identification of a precipitant, good premorbid health, and the absence of concurrent organic illness or a major psychiatric condition (Couprie et al., 1995; Lazare, 1981; Singh & Lee, 1997).

## Pain Disorder

Pain disorder was previously known as somatoform pain disorder in DSM-III-R and as psychogenic pain disorder in DSM-III. The essential feature of pain disorder in DSM-IV (APA, 1994) is a preoccupation with pain in one or more anatomical areas that is sufficiently severe to warrant clinical attention; that causes impairment in daily living; and psychological factors, it is judged, have a prominent role in the onset, exacerbation, and maintenance of pain. In addition, the pain is not intentionally produced or feigned and is not due to another affective or thought disorder or to dyspareunia. Unlike in the DSM-III-R, there is an attempt to identify subtypes of pain disorder in DSM-IV (APA, 1994) based on the predominant factors that characterize the etiology and maintenance of the pain: pain disorder associated with psychological factors, pain disorder associated with both a psychological and a general medical condition, and pain disorder associated with a general medical condition. In pain disorder associated with psychological factors, psychological factors, it is judged, have primary influence on the onset, exacerbation, and maintenance of the pain. A general medical condition plays little or no role in the etiology of pain in this subtype. In addition, this subtype cannot be diagnosed if the criteria for somatization disorder are met. As the name implies, both psychological factors and a general medical condition play an important role in the etiology of pain in the second subtype of pain disorder. The anatomical site or associated medical condition is coded on Axis III (e.g., diabetic neuropathy). In the third subtype of pain disorder, pain is due to a medical condition, is coded on Axis III, and is essentially not a mental disorder. In the first subtype of pain disorder, the duration of pain can be specified as acute if less than 6 months and chronic if longer than 6 months.

Nosologically, the history of pain disorder continues to be one of the least satisfactory of the somatoform disorders. Very few studies in the pain literature have ever used a DSM conceptualization. King and Strain (1992) noted that only five studies had used somatoform pain disorder based on DSM-III-R criteria. The difficulty with this category is inherent in the complicated and experiential nature of pain. Pain is a multifaceted experience characterized by affective, sensory, and evaluative components. Although pain can be simultaneously pathogenic and psychogenic, the correlation between the subjective report of pain and the physiological evidence of pain is relatively low. Other problems include the fact that the majority of chronic pain patients have pain in one or more areas, so that the majority of chronic pain patients would meet this first criterion (Fishbain, 1996). The remaining criteria for pain disorder are equally overinclusive, and most chronic pain patients report that pain interferes with social, occupational, and other domains of functioning and that psychological factors play a role in the etiology of pain. Chronic pain patients are bound to be affected physically and psychologically; however, they do not necessarily have to be psychiatrically disturbed (Iezzi, Adams, Stokes, Pilon, & Ault, 1992).

## Hypochondriasis

As early as 350 B.C., hypochondriasis sparked the imagination of the medical community and laypersons alike. Similar to conversion disorder, hypochondriasis has been described in the writings of the Hippocratic era (Nemiah, 1985). The word hypochondriasis is of Greek origin and is literally translated as "below the cartilage" (Kenyon, 1976). Hypochondriasis, it was speculated, was attributable to disturbances in bodily function, and mental changes were particularly associated with changes in the organs below the xiphoid process. Hypochondriasis was characterized by sharp belching, abdominal pains, flatulence, cold sweat, and sour eructations. Galen stated that hypochondriasis was a special form of melancholia and was the result of "black bile" (Nemiah, 1985). Galen's viewpoint was consistent with Greek humoral theories of disease and illness.

It was not until the seventeenth and eighteenth centuries that hypochondriasis became associated with a morbid preoccupation with one's body or state of health (Kenyon, 1965; Nemiah, 1985). During this era, hypochondriasis was variously described as a species of melancholy, "the spleen," "the vapors," and "the English malady" (Kenyon, 1965). Hypochondriasis was then thought of especially as a complaint of the English, and in

1733, Cheyne's treatise called "The English Malady" reviewed hypochondriasis within a cultural context (Kenyon, 1965; Nemiah, 1985). Moreover, Cheyne's treatise was also known for a detailed account of the author's own suffering.

Paradoxically, it was a layperson named Burton who wrote "The Anatomy of Melancholy" in 1651, which inspired the medical conceptualization of hypochondriasis (Kenyon, 1965; Nemiah, 1985). In addition, a theatrical representation performed and written in 1673 by Moliere in Le Malade Imaginaire captured the imagination of the public (Kenyon, 1965; Nemiah, 1985). In 1877, seventy essays outlining many references to personal experiences with hypochondriasis were written by Boswell during a 6-year period (Kenyon, 1965). During the next 150 years, because of Sydenham's influence, hypochondriasis was viewed as a male version of hysteria in women, and not surprisingly, the diagnostic terms were often used interchangeably (Fischer-Homberger, 1972).

By the early twentieth century, in a classic paper by Gillespie (1928), a strict definition of hypochondriasis was stated. Based on the review of thirteen cases, hypochondriasis was characterized by a variety of paresthesias, a thorough observation of bodily function, a firm conviction of illness or sickness, an inability to be reassured, and finally, a failure to respond to psychotherapy. It was not until the mid-1920s that hypochondriasis was listed as a diagnostic category in the American Psychiatric Association classification system (Nemiah, 1985).

**Diagnosis.** It is not presently clear whether hypochondriasis is a true independent, discrete, and cohesive diagnostic category. The scientific examination of hypochondriasis has been problematic for several reasons (Barsky & Klerman, 1983). First, hypochondriacal patients often present themselves to general medical settings rather than to psychiatric settings. Second, hypochondriasis tends to be a condition that falls between medicine and psychiatry. Third, the lack of clarity and knowledge about hypochondriasis reflects modern medicine's emphasis on disease rather than illness. On a positive note, there has been a significant increase in empirical attention to this topic in the last 10 years.

Despite their best intentions, internists and general practitioners are not equipped to handle these cases. Even among psychiatrists, who are more interested in hypochondriasis than internists and general practitioners, there has been some degree of controversy. For example, hypochondriasis was not included in DSM-I (APA, 1952). Hypochondriasis was first included in DSM-II and has remained the same until DSM-IV, but hypochondriasis was moved from the neurosis section in DSM-II to the somatoform section in DSM-III where it has remained. DSM-III-R added a 6-month duration requirement before the diagnosis of hypochondriasis could be given. DSM-IV (APA, 1994) includes the specifier "poor insight" when the person does not recognize that the concern of serious illness for most of the duration of a hypochondriacal symptom is exaggerated or unreasonable. Table 3 presents the DSM-IV (APA, 1994) criteria for hypochondriasis.

**Clinical Description.** Although not data based, Nemiah (1985) presents an excellent description of the clinical aspects of hypochondriasis. Hypo-

### Table 3. DSM-IV Criteria for Hypochondriasis Disorder

A. Preoccupation with fears of having, or the idea that one has, a serious disease based on the person's misinterpretation of bodily symptoms.

B. The preoccupation persists despite appropriate medical evaluation and reassurance.

C. The belief in Criteria A is not of delusional intensity (as in Delusional Disorder, Somatic Type) and is not restricted to a circumscribed concern about appearance (as in Body Dysmorphic Disorder).

D. The preoccupation causes clinically significant distress or impairment in social, occupational, or other important areas of functioning.

E. The duration of the disturbance is at least 6 months.

F. The preoccupation is not better accounted for by Generalized Anxiety Disorder, Obsessive-Compulsive Disorder, Panic Disorder, a Major Depressive Disorder, Separation Anxiety, or another Somatoform Disorder.

*Specify* if:

**With Poor Insight**: if, for most of the time during the current episode, the person does not recognize that the concern about having a serious illness is excessive or unreasonable

*Source*: American Psychiatric Association. (1994). *Diagnostic and Statistical Manual of Mental Disorders*, 4th ed. (p. 465). Washington, DC: Author. Reprinted by permission.

chondriacal symptoms are often diffuse and involve many areas of the body. As observed in Kenyon's (1964) study, the abdomen, viscera, chest, head, and neck are the areas most commonly affected. Patients commonly experience a general bodily sense of fatigue or malaise. A patient's symptoms typically arise from a heightened awareness of normal bodily functions (i.e., bowel movements or heartbeats). Patients with hypochondriacal concerns usually present their complaints at great length and may even exhibit what may look like pressured speech.

The clinical encounter with the hypochondriac can be characterized more as a monologue than as a dialogue. Hypochondriacal patients' thoughts and speech are entirely centered around their symptomatology, and any attempt by the clinician to discuss anything else is resisted. These patients are very well versed in medical terminology, which makes them more likely to try to manage their medical care instead of following the clinician's recommendations. Doctor–patient relationships tend to be difficult and rife with tension and hostility on both sides. Unlike patients with conversion disorder, who may show a lack of concern, hypochondriacal patients are very worried and anxious about their symptoms. Frequently, hypochondriacal patients present symptomatology that is out of proportion to the medical findings.

**Epidemiology and Demographics.** Although there are no prevalence figures for hypochondriasis in the general population, its prevalence in a medical practice, it has been estimated, ranges from 4 to 9% (APA, 1994). It has been estimated that from 60 to 80% of the normal population will experience, on average, at least one physical symptom in a given week (Kellner, 1985). Using a more restrictive definition, hypochondriasis, it has been noted, occurs in 3 to 14% of patients seen in medical settings (Kenyon, 1976). Using DSM-III-R diagnostic criteria, Barsky, Wyshak, Klerman, and Latham (1990) found that the 6-month prevalence rate of hypochondriasis falls between 4.2 and 6.3% in a tertiary academic medical setting. Based on a screening scale, the prevalence of hypochondriasis was 14% in a general medical clinic (Noyes, Kathol, Fisher, Phillips, Suelzer, & Holt, 1993). Hypochondriasis occurs equally among men and women (APA, 1994; Gureje, Ustun, & Simon, 1997). With respect to course, hypochondriacal symptoms tend to wax and wane over a long period of time.

Until recently, much of what was known about hypochondriasis was based on Kenyon's classic study of 1964. Kenyon reviewed case records of all patients who attended Bethlem Royal and Maudley hospitals during a 10-year period from 1951 to 1960. A total of 512 patients was identified and characterized as either primary (hypochondriasis was the only complaint) or secondary (hypochondriasis was secondary to a preexisting disorder) hypochondriacs. He classified somatic complaints according to the distribution of symptoms in different parts of the body, physiological systems affected, and whether symptoms were unilateral or bilateral. The areas most commonly reported to be of hypochondriacal focus were the head, neck, abdomen, and chest, in that order. Musculoskeletal, gastrointestinal, and central nervous system areas were the bodily systems most involved. Pain (e.g., headache, chest pain, backache, and abdominal pain), the most common symptom reported, occurred in approximately 70% of the entire sample. Seventy-three percent of the whole sample reported symptoms primarily on the left side of the body. No striking differences in age, sex, religion, social class, marital status or relevant clinical variables were found between primary hypochondriacs ($N = 301$) and secondary hypochondriacs ($N = 211$). Among 295 patients subsequently admitted for inpatient hospitalization, Kenyon found an absence of significant physical abnormality in 47% of these cases, and in approximately one-half of these cases, no precipitating factors were noted.

The onset of hypochondriasis, it is believed, occurs as early as childhood (Nemiah, 1985) or as late as senescence (Brink, Janakes, & Martinez, 1981), but more commonly by early adulthood (APA, 1994). Kenyon (1964) found that the overall peak age of incidence for hypochondriasis was 30 to 39 years of age; the peak for males was in the 30 to 39 age group, and the peak for females was in the 40 to 49 age group.

**Etiological Formulations.** A number of theories have been presented to explain hypochondriacal behavior. For years, the psychoanalytic formulation of hypochondriasis has been the predominant conceptual framework. More recently, the psychoanalytic conceptualization of hypochondriasis has been replaced with models that emphasize the influences of learning, cognition, and attitudes. *Psychoanalytic.* Freud was the earliest proponent of the theory that hypochondriasis was the result of sexual drives (Nemiah, 1985). He originally stated that the sexual libido, when withdrawn from external objects, would be redirected to the self in the form of narcissistic libido. Eventually, the narcissistic libido "overflows," and the resulting energy is transformed into physical symptoms. Brown and Vaillant (1981) conceptualized hypochondriasis as repressed hostility. These authors felt that the disorder arose from anger over having been disappointed, hurt, abandoned, or unloved; rather than openly complain, the individual displaces these thoughts and feelings onto the body. Other analysts thought that hypochondriasis occurred in individuals defending against very low self-esteem and against the experience of the self as worthless, inadequate, and defective (McCranie, 1979). According to this view, it is easier and more tolerable to feel that something is wrong with one's body than with oneself. In addition, pain and physical suffering in the hypochondriacal patient can be seen as an atonement, expiation, and deserved punishment for past wrongdoing and the sense that one is evil and sinful (Engel, 1959).

*Learning, Conditioning, and Cognitive-Behavioral.* It is well known that autonomic responses can be acquired by classical and operant conditioning (Kellner, 1985). Because of the fear of disease, repeated attention to and selective focus on parts of one's body may be enhanced. The resulting anxiety and concomitant physiological changes that lead to somatic symptoms (e.g., tachycardia or irritable bowel) can be conditioned via cues in the external environment, internal cues, and even thoughts about disease. Hypochondriasis can then be characterized by a vicious cycle of anxiety and somatic sensations leading to more anxiety, and with more frequent repetitions of this cycle, an overlearned pattern of behavior occurs in a rapid and predictable sequence (Kellner, 1985). Modeling influences have also been implicated in the development of hypochondriasis (Kreitman, Sainsbury, Pearce, & Costain, 1965). As a result of observing an illness model and assuming the sick role, the individual learns that sympathy, attention, and support for the patient can be received and unpleasant duties and obligations can be avoided.

More recently, a cognitive-behavioral formulation of hypochondriasis has been developed (Salkovskis & Warwick, 1986; Warwick, 1995; Warwick & Salkovskis, 1990). Salkovskis and Warwick proposed that the central feature of hypochon-

driasis is the occurrence of negative automatic thoughts resulting from the misinterpretation of innocuous physical symptoms and signs. These symptoms tend to be misinterpreted as indicators of illness. The typical reaction to this misinterpretation is anxiety that leads to cognitive changes that maintain the physical symptom. Information is consistently selected and attended to in ways that confirm a hypochondriacal concern. Bodily checking, avoidance, and reassurance seeking are examples of this selective attention. This model has yet to be empirically tested by other investigators.

*Perceptual and Cognitive Abnormalities.* A very interesting etiological formulation of hypochondriasis comes from the work of Barsky and Klerman (1983). They proposed that hypochondriasis results from perceptual and cognitive abnormalities. There are three major components to their formulation: that hypochondriacal patients amplify normal bodily sensory input, that these patients incorrectly assess and misinterpret somatic symptoms, and that they are innately predisposed to thinking and perceiving concretely rather than in emotional and subjective terms. Within this model, sensory input is magnified or altered by the degree of attention and arousal experienced. Anxiety that is paired with sensory input is misinterpreted, and negative meanings are attached to benign bodily sensations. The authors have provided considerable empirical work to support their model (Barsky & Wyshak, 1989, 1990; Barsky, Wyshak, & Klerman, 1990, 1991).

Various aspects of Barsky and Klerman's (1983) model have also been verified by other investigators. DSM-III-R-defined hypochondriasis patients, it was demonstrated, report more bodily sensations when not given instruction to attend to bodily sensations and consider themselves more sensitive to benign bodily sensations without being better able to discriminate two tactual bodily signals (Haenen, Schmidt, Schoemakers, & van den Hout, 1997). Gramling, Clawson, and McDonald (1996) assessed pain perception and stress reactivity in fifteen hypochondriacal female subjects versus fifteen control subjects. The hypochondriacal group displayed significant increases in heart rate during a cold pressor test, as well as a significant hand temperature drop and slower return to baseline for hand temperature during the recovery period, compared to the control group. Hypochondriacal patients also terminated the cold pressor task more frequently, left their foot in the cold bath water for a shorter period of time, and rated the cold pressor task as more unpleasant. MacLeod, Haynes, and Sensky (1998) compared three groups (anxious hypochondriacal, generally anxious, and nonanxious general practice attenders) on their propensity to give somatic, psychological, or normalizing attributions for common bodily sensations as measured by the Symptom Interpretation Questionnaire. The anxious hypochondriacal group gave more somatic attributions, whereas the generally anxious group tended to give more psychological and fewer normalizing attributions.

Ludwig's (1972) neurophysiological model of hysteria and hypochondriasis can also be invoked as support for Barsky and Klerman's etiological conceptualization of hypochondriasis. As noted earlier, Ludwig indicated that hypochondriasis was the flip side of hysteria. He noted that, whereas patients with hysteria have a separation or dissociation of attention from their symptoms, patients with hypochondriasis have their attention focused and locked onto their symptoms. He noted that hysterics tend to show a lack of concern about their symptoms, whereas hypochondriacs show an exaggerated sense of concern regarding their symptoms. In addition, he remarked that although hysterics did not appear to be motivated to obtain symptom relief, hypochondriacs spent most of their time looking for relief. Ludwig hypothesized that hypochondriasis results from reduced corticoreticular inhibition, which causes an increase in attention that is directed and locked onto a source of afferent stimulation. It is still early to tell, but Barsky and Klerman's (1983) etiological formulation of hypochondriasis appears promising.

*Hypochondriasis as a Constellation of Illness Attitudes and Behaviors.* Considerable interest in the overt attitudes, fears, and beliefs of the hypochondriacal patient has emerged (Barsky & Wyshak, 1989; Bianchi, 1971, 1973; Kellner, Abbott, Winslow, & Pathak, 1987; Pilowsky, 1967). Pilowsky (1967) administered a yes/no questionnaire to a group of hypochondriacs and to a group of psychiatric patients without hypochondriasis. He found that seventeen out of twenty questions significantly discriminated the two groups: four questions related to worry or fear of disease, two questions related to the experience of somatic symptoms, two questions related to the amount of attention paid to symptoms, two questions related to hypo-

chondriacal beliefs, and seven questions pertained to attitudes other than fears and beliefs about disease. The hypochondriacal group displayed more anxiety, fear of disease, and greater attention to symptoms than the comparison group.

In 1971, Bianchi used a structured general psychiatric and hypochondriasis interview with 235 psychiatric patients evaluated as part of a larger study that examined depression. Thirty subjects with disease phobia were found. This subgroup was compared to a nonhypochondriacal group composed of psychiatric inpatients. Cancer phobia (47%) and heart phobia (30%) were the most common conditions observed in the hypochondriacal group. This group was more prone to anxiety, obsessiveness, inhibition of anger, and lower self-esteem. In addition, this study was positive in demonstrating a relationship between hypochondriasis and a family history of disease; cancer and heart phobics tended to have more family members with histories of the respective disease.

In another study by Bianchi (1973), twenty-four historical, clinical, and experimental variables were examined in a principal-components analysis conducted on 118 psychiatric inpatients. Patients were included in the analysis if they had one or more physical symptoms, disease phobia, disease conviction, bodily preoccupation, and psychogenic pain. Bianchi identified eight factors; five factors reflected clinical aspects of hypochondriasis. Two patterns of disease phobia were particularly noted: one was identified as "programmed augmentation" that reflects the indirect influence of family illness on the patient's subsequent disease phobia; the second reflects current anxiety and depression associated with disease phobia and was identified as "current augmentation." The author also found evidence for another subgroup of patients who had marked paranoid feelings and delusions of disease. This last group's presentation is more consistent with a thought disorder than with a somatoform process.

Using DSM-III criteria of hypochondriasis, Kellner et al. (1987) administered illness attitude scales developed by Kellner to twenty-one patients with hypochondriasis matched with a group of patients from a family practice, a group of nonpatient employees, and a group of nonhypochondriacal psychiatric patients. Hypochondriacal patients reported significantly more fears of and false beliefs about disease, attended more to bodily sensations, had more fears about death, and had more distrust of a physician's judgments than all of the other groups. Interestingly enough, hypochondriacal subjects sought more medical treatment than the other subjects, but they did not take better precautions about their health.

In another study (Barsky & Wyshak, 1989), 177 outpatients at a general medical clinic underwent a comprehensive evaluation including descriptive questionnaires, the Whitley Index (a thirteen-item questionnaire developed by Pilowsky that focuses on hypochondriacal attitudes and beliefs), the somatization subscale from the Hopkins Symptom Checklist-90, and the hypochondriasis subscale of the Minnesota Multiphasic Personality Inventory. A five-item self-report questionnaire that examines a patient's propensity for amplification of symptoms and questionnaires that examine health-related variables and health care utilization were also used. Hypochondriasis was positively related to amplification of symptoms fears of aging and death, importance placed on health, sense of body vulnerability to illness and injury, and greater value placed on physical appearance. The authors performed a cluster analysis and found three discrete clusters of patients. One group was characterized by evaluating health very highly, being more concerned with their bodies, and feeling more vulnerable to disease. This group was significantly more hypochondriacal than the other cluster groups. A second, more stoic group of individuals was relatively disinterested in their health and appearance, was less concerned about death, did not feel particularly vulnerable to disease, and did very little to look after themselves. The final cluster group was moderately interested in health, had moderate concerns about disease, and engaged in relatively high levels of self-treatment. The authors concluded that hypochondriacal patients have an amplifying style that has widespread repercussions on health-related attitudes and concerns about their body and disease. Although hypochondriasis is typically conceptualized as heterogeneous, it is reasonable to assume that there is a subgroup of hypochondriacal patients with a fear of and preoccupation with disease that can be readily identified.

Although considerable emphasis has been placed on hypochondriasis as a diagnostic entity, worrying about illness is common. It can range from rational concerns or intermittent short-lived worries about illness to persistent, incapacitating fears. Transient or "normal" hypochondriasis is a common response to stressful life events (Idzorek, 1975). Patients who have recently experienced a real medical disease (e.g., cancer) may become very preoccupied and narrowly focused on normal aches and pains, which may lead to misinterpretation of these symptoms. The patient's anxiety in this situation is quite understandable and often can be alleviated with medical evaluation and reassurance. Hypochondriacal concerns also can be increased or triggered by intense study of disease. Transient hypochondriacal concerns are very common among medical students (Hunter, Lohrenz, & Schwartzman, 1964; Woods, Natterson, & Silverman, 1976). From 70% (Hunter et al., 1964) to 76% (Woods et al., 1976) of medical students in studies admitted to hypochondriacal concerns.

In another interesting study by Barsky and his associates, a group of transiently hypochondriacal patients was compared with a group of nonhypochondriacal medical patients and a group of DSM-III-R-diagnosed hypochondriacal patients (Barsky, Wyshak, & Klerman, 1990). All patients were recruited from a general medicine outpatient clinic. Patients who exceeded a predetermined cutoff score on a hypochondriasis self-report questionnaire but failed to meet a DSM-III-R diagnosis of hypochondriasis during a structured interview were included in the transient hypochondriacal group (N = 22). The transient hypochondriasis group was compared to a group of DSM-III-R-diagnosed hypochondriacs (N = 41) and a comparison group (N = 75) of patients who did not meet the hypochondriasis cutoff score nor met a diagnosis of hypochondriasis during the structured interview. All patients underwent structured interviews, self-report questionnaires, and cognitive and perceptual tests.

The results indicated that the transient hypochondriacal group evidenced significant decreases in hypochondriasis questionnaire scores during a 3-week period, had less psychiatric disorders, and had more medical morbidity than the DSM-III-R hypochondriacal group. In addition, the transient hypochondriacal group viewed their medical care more positively and were rated as less hypochondriacal by physician ratings. In contrast to the comparison group, the hypochondriacal group had more Axis I and Axis II disorders, reported higher levels of physical symptom amplification, and experienced more medical disorders. Using matching procedures and an analysis of covariance to control for medical morbidity, the differences in psychiatric comorbidity and amplification style were still present. The authors concluded that patients with personality disorders and a predisposition to somatic sensations were more prone to develop transient hypochondriasis.

Finally, Gureje, Ustun, et al. (1997) examined the construct of abridged hypochondriasis. The triad of disease conviction, associated emotional distress, and medical help-seeking behavior defined abridged hypochondriasis. In a fourteen-country study of primary care facilities, the authors found that persons with abridged hypochondriasis were significantly more psychologically impaired (General Health Questionnaire) and more likely to receive a diagnosis of generalized anxiety disorder and major depression than nonhypochondriacal patients. Patients with abridged hypochondriasis were perceived by physicians as having poorer physical health. These patients also rated themselves as functionally more impaired.

**Hypochondriasis and Associated Psychopathology.** Hypochondriacs are a heterogeneous group and require thorough assessment (Warwick, 1995). The problems of classifying and defining hypochondriasis are largely due to the overlap of this disorder with a wide spectrum of psychiatric disorders. Hypochondriasis has been associated with characterological types, affective disorders, and thought disorders.

Psychoanalysts have typically viewed the hypochondriac as displaying obsessive-compulsive traits, especially those of orderliness, obstinacy, and parsimoniousness (Kenyon, 1976). Narcissism also has been considered a prominent feature of hypochondriasis (Kenyon, 1976). Consistent with narcissism, hypochondriacal patients are described as egocentric and excessively concerned with their bodies at the expense of regard for others or objects in their natural environment. Other patients with hypochondriasis may present with passive-aggressive, passive-dependent, borderline, or paranoid personality features. Although these personality descriptions are interesting, there are no consistent data that demonstrate a personality pattern characteristic of hypochondriacs (Kellner, 1985; Kenyon, 1976; Ladee, 1966).

Hypochondriasis is most commonly associated with an affective disorder. In his 1964 study, Kenyon found that 12% of primary hypochondriacs and 82% of secondary hypochondriacs had coexisting affective disorders. Dividing affective disorders into depressive disorders and anxiety disorders, Kenyon determined that 44% of hospitalized primary hypochondriacs and 63% of the hospitalized secondary hypochondriacs experienced depression. Anxiety was present in 18% of patients in the primary hypochondriasis group and in 20% of patients in the secondary hypochondriasis group. These results led Kenyon to conclude that hypochondriasis is frequently part of another syndrome, usually an affective one. In an extensive review of 225 cases with hypochondriacal symptoms, Ladee (1966) determined that only three patients could not be included in a broader syndrome. Consequently, Ladee, like Kenyon, concluded that hypochondriasis does not exist as an entity in its own right. Other studies have also noted the relationship between hypochondriasis and depression and its associated morbidity (Kreitman et al., 1965; Lesse, 1968).

In contrast to Kenyon and Ladee's viewpoint, Pilowsky argued for the existence of both primary and secondary forms of hypochondriasis, distinguished by their associated features. By conducting psychiatric and physical evaluations of 147 patients, Pilowsky (1970) demonstrated that primary hypochondriacs had longer disease histories before referral for psychiatric treatment and reported more musculoskeletal and dermal symptoms, whereas patients with secondary hypochondriasis reported greater feelings of depersonalization, poor male sexual adjustment, and apprehensiveness of future disease. Pilowsky then concluded that the two groups could be differentiated in terms of variables other than the defining characteristics. However, as Kenyon (1976) noted, Pilowsky's results can be seriously questioned, because he performed all of the psychiatric and physical evaluations himself.

Barsky, Wyshak, and Klerman (1992) examined psychiatric comorbidity in forty-two DSM-III-R hypochondriacs. With a random sample of seventy-six outpatients as a comparison group, the authors noted that the hypochondriasis group had twice as many lifetime Axis I diagnoses, twice as many Diagnostic Interview Schedule symptoms, and three times as many personality disorders compared to the control group. Eighty-eight percent of the hypochondriasis group had one or more Axis I disorders (greatest for depressive and anxiety disorders). Of note, 20% of hypochondriacs had somatization disorder. The significant overlap between hypochondriasis and somatization disorder has been reported in other studies (Barsky, Wyshak, & Klerman, 1992; Kirmayer & Robbins, 1991; Noyes, Holt, Happel, Kathol, & Yagla, 1997; Noyes, Kathol, Fisher, Phillips, Suelzer, & Woodman, 1994a). Barsky, Barnett, and Cleary (1994) screened 1634 cases who attended a primary care clinic and identified 100 lifetime DSM-III-R panic disorder cases. Patients then completed a structured diagnostic interview and a battery of self-report measures. Physicians also completed a questionnaire about their respective patients. Twenty-five of the 100 panic disorder cases met a diagnosis of hypochondriasis. The comorbid group was compared to the remaining seventy-five "pure" panic disorder cases, a "pure" hypochondriac group (N = 51), and a fourth group of randomly selected medical outpatients without hypochondriasis or panic disorder (N = 96). Patients with pure panic disorder were less hypochondriacal, somatized less, were less disabled, were more satisfied with their medical care, and were rated by physicians as less help-rejecting and less demanding than the comorbid panic disorder and hypochondriasis group. Major depression and phobias were also more prevalent in the pure panic disorder group. Somatization disorder and generalized anxiety disorder were more prevalent in the comorbid group. The authors concluded that there is an overlap between panic disorder and hypochondriasis, but these two conditions are phenomenologically and functionally distinct and are viewed differently by physicians. Similar conclusions have been reported by other investigators (Bach, Nutzinger, & Hartl, 1996; Noyes et al., 1993). However, because of the significant overlap between hypochondriasis, somatization, and affective disorders (Barsky et al., 1992; Noyes et al, 1994a), the independence of hypochondriasis from other psychiatric conditions has to be questioned.

Hypochondriasis may present as part of a prodromal stage of a schizophrenic reaction (Kenyon, 1965). In a study by Lucas, Sainsbury, and Collins (1962), 71% of 405 unselected schizophrenic inpatients had delusions, and paranoid delusions were the most common type of delusion. Notably, 20% of 127 males and 21% of 161 females schizophrenic inpatients had hypochondriacal delusions. However, Kenyon (1976) suggested referring to these hypochondriacal delusions as somatic delusions to reduce confusion. Monosymptomatic hypochondriasis is a good example of this diagnostic confusion; it has been used to refer to delusions of parasitosis (the belief that one is being infested), delusions of bromosis (the belief that one is emitting an offensive odor), and dysmorphophobia (the belief that one is physically malformed or unattractive; Bishop, 1980). Dysmorphophobia will be discussed in another section of this chapter. Delusions of parasitosis or bromosis, however, reflect a thought disorder more than a true somatoform process. Delusions of parasitosis and delusions of bromosis have been associated with manic-depressive illness, folie à deux, schizophrenia, and organic brain diseases (Hopkinson, 1973; Pryse-Phillips, 1971). Monosymptomatic hypochondriasis is clearly not a run-of-the-mill hypochondriasis.

Although the clinical lore of hypochondriasis has always been colorful, a critical review of this area reveals that this disorder has a number of diagnostic weaknesses (Schmidt, 1994). There is an unsatisfactory distinction between a hypochondriacal attitude (which is usually based on a continuum) versus actual hypochondriasis (having it or not). This has introduced a type of hypochondriasis that can be transitory or acute, which is really quite different from hypochondriasis as a psychiatric disorder. Hypochondriasis conceptualized as primary or secondary is not useful. Pure or primary hypochondriasis can best be thought of as disease phobia and would best go under simple phobia in the anxiety disorders section of the DSM. Hypochondriasis, conceptualized in generic form, is so associated with other psychiatric conditions that it may be of little clinical use. Thus, it should be stricken from the somatoform disorders section.

**Treatment and Prognosis.** There are only a handful of treatment studies of hypochondriasis. The treatment outcome depends very much on the type of hypochondriasis. Treatment for a disease phobia can be easily implemented with a behavioral package (e.g., flooding, implosion, and thought stopping), but a strict behavioral approach will be less successful with monosymptomatic hypochondriasis. Kellner (1982) reported improvement in hypochondriacal patients at 2-year follow-up with techniques that included reassurance and explanations, multiple physical examinations, and suggestions. If depression or anxiety is present, then treatment of these conditions may lead to a resolution of hypochondriasis. Electroconvulsive therapy and leucotomy as options of last resort have been used to treat hypochondriasis but without much success (Kenyon, 1976).

In a test of the effectiveness of cognitive-behavioral intervention, Avia et al. (1996) assigned patients with hypochondriasis to either a cognitive-behavioral treatment condition (N = 9) or a waiting-list control condition (N = 8). The treatment, based on Barsky, Geringer, and Wool's (1988) treatment model, consisted of six 1½ hour sessions that largely covered discussions of inadequate and selective attention, muscle tension and bad breathing habits, environmental factors, stress and dysphoric mood, and explanations of somatic signals. Improvements were noted in decreasing fears, reducing dysphoric mood, as well-treated subjects noted an improvement in being more warm, open, and extroverted. Five subjects in the waiting group were also treated, and similar improvements were noted. However, the small sample size severely limits the strength of the conclusions in this study. In a better controlled study, Warwick, Clark, Cobb, and Salkovskis (1996) randomly assigned thirty-two hypochondriacs either to a cognitive-behavioral treatment group or to a waiting-list control group. Treatment consisted of sixteen individual sessions conducted during a 4-month period, followed by a 3-month reassessment. Treatment emphasized identifying and challenging misinterpretations of symptoms and signs, restructuring images, modifying dysfunctional assumptions, deliberate body focusing, response prevention for body checking, graded exposure to previously avoided illness-related situations, and prevention of reassurance seeking. Treatment was provided by the first author, who is also a psychiatrist. The waiting-list group waited for 4 months and then were given sixteen individual treatment sessions. The treatment group showed improvement in a number of dependent variables including, among others, disease conviction, need for reassurance, time spent worrying about health, health anxiety, and Beck Depression and Anxiety. The treatment group also showed significant improvements in therapist and assessor ratings of subjects. More recently, in a systematic, three-case analysis (Papageorgiou & Wells, 1998), attention training (Wells, 1990) was used to treat hypochondriasis, and early results appear very promising. This type of treatment consists of regular practice of selective attention, attention switching, and divided attention. The treatment is designed to teach patients how to "switch off" preservative self-focused processing. Clinical improvements were noted in self-report measures of anxiety, mood,

health, worry, and illness-related beliefs and behaviors. Most impressive was the finding that none of the three subjects met the criteria for DSM-III-R hypochondriasis at the end of treatment. Obviously, controlled outcome studies are required before embracing this technique to treat hypochondriasis.

The advent of specific serotonin re-uptake inhibitors has also been instrumental in improving hypochondriasis (Escobar, 1996; Fallon et al., 1996). Preliminary data suggest that fluoxetine may be beneficial in treating hypochondriasis. Future studies that integrate cognitive-behavioral treatment and pharmacotherapy will aid in managing hypochondriasis.

Hypochondriacal patients are generally best managed in medical rather than psychiatric settings (Barsky, 1996). In terms of prognosis, hypochondriasis is generally believed to be chronic with periodic remissions and exacerbations (Noyes, Kathol, Fisher, Phillips, Suelzer, & Woodman, 1994b). A better prognosis for hypochondriasis is reportedly associated with the concurrent presence of anxiety or depression, less serious personality disorder, acute onset of symptomatology, younger age, less secondary gain, absence of an organic process, shorter duration of illness, and less severe hypochondriasis at the time of assessment (Barsky, 1996; Noyes et al., 1994b).

### Body Dysmorphic Disorder.

Dysmorphophobia, originally conceptualized by Morselli in 1886, refers to a subjective feeling of ugliness or physical defect in a person of normal appearance (Andreasen & Bardach, 1977; De Leon, Bott, & Simpson, 1989; Thomas, 1984). It also includes individuals with a minimal physical defect who react out of proportion to this defect (Andreasen & Bardach, 1977; Thomas, 1984). Dysmorphophobia is a label that has largely been used in Europe (Hay, 1970a) but ignored in the United States (Nakdimen, 1977); it was originally introduced in the United States by Finkelstein (1963) and was neglected until Andreasen and Bardach (1977) brought it back into the psychiatric nomenclature.

Historically, dysmorphophobia was thought of as part of monosymptomatic hypochondriasis (Bishop, 1980). As discussed earlier, dysmorphophobia is not a hypochondriacal process. Hypochondriacs draw attention to themselves by saying they are not normal, whereas dysmorphophobics wish to appear normal but feel that other people notice that they are not normal (Hay, 1970a).

**Diagnosis.** In DSM-III (APA, 1980), dysmorphophobia was categorized as an atypical somatoform disorder in the somatoform disorders section. Dysmorphophobia as a term was replaced by "body dysmorphic disorder" in DSM-III-R. Because the disturbance did not involve true phobic avoidance, the term was considered a misnomer. Table 4 presents the DSM-IV (APA, 1994) diagnostic criteria for body dysmorphic disorder. DSM-III-R classified body dysmorphic disorder as delusional in the delusional disorders (somatic subtype) section. However, in DSM-IV, a diagnosis of delusional disorder, somatic type, can be added to body dysmorphic disorder if the individual's preoccupation with an imagined defect has delusional intensity. Even with this addition to DSM-IV, it is not clear whether body dysmorphic disorder and delusional disorder, somatic subtype, are really variants of the same disorder or are two different disorders.

**Clinical Description.** Although much of the early information on dysmorphic disorder was based on case studies, there has been a significant increase in systematic studies of body dysmorphic disorder. Research with these patients is difficult, because they are usually seen by cosmetic or plastic surgeons and dermatologists instead of mental health professionals. These patients also avoid reporting their concerns to others because of shame and embarrassment. Individuals with body dysmorphic disorder typically focus their attention on the face, ears, nose, hair, breasts, or geni-

talia (Andreasen & Bardach, 1977; De Leon et al., 1989; Thomas, 1984). Frequent complaints also include skin blemishes and facial wrinkles. Men tend to focus on genitals, height, excessive body hair, body build, and hair thinning, and women tend to focus on breasts, legs, hips, and weight (Perugi, Akiskal, Giannotti, Frare, Di Vaio, & Cassano, 1997; Phillips & Diaz, 1997). Individuals may focus on one body part or simultaneously focus on several body parts.

The current fad of patients who seek liposuction for excess cellulite in the thighs, buttocks, and abdomen, breast enhancement and reduction, rhinoplasty, lip enhancement, and hair growth treatments is a good example of how difficult it is to separate body dysmorphic disorder from normal body image concerns about physical appearance (Sarwer, Wadden, Pertschuk, & Whitaker, 1998). DSM-IV includes the clause "normal concerns about appearance" in the differential diagnosis section without defining what "normal" represents.

At its worst, body dysmorphic disorder is the belief that one is truly ugly, and at its best, that one is unattractive but could be made attractive if surgery is performed (Andreasen & Bardach, 1977). Little is known about the psychological status of patients who pursue cosmetic surgery (Sarwer et al., 1998), given the psychological profile of body dysmorphic disorder, but surgical patients who evidence body dysmorphic disorder are likely to be very dissatisfied following surgery and to engage in an adversarial relationship with surgeons (Phillips, McElroy, Keck, Hudson, & Pope, 1994). Alternatively, many individuals have accurate perceptions of their physical defect and will respond very favorably to corrective surgery (Hay & Heather, 1973). No relationship between the degree of deformity and the presence of psychological disturbances has been found (Hay, 1970b; Lacey & Birtchnell, 1984), but dysmorphophobics do tend to be less satisfied with their body images than others (Hardy, 1982).

Body dysmorphic disorder usually begins in adolescence and early adulthood (De Leon et al., 1989; Phillips, 1996; Rosen, 1995). At times, body dysmorphic disorder can occur spontaneously or can be precipitated by innocuous remarks (Hay, 1970a). Examples of seemingly innocuous remarks include, "You have such dark eyebrows" or "Your nose looks so much like daddy's." Other triggers include sexual and physical abuse, sexual

---

**Table 4. DSM-IV Criteria
for Body Dysmorphic Disorder**

A. Preoccupation with an imagined defect in appearance. If a slight physical anomaly is present, the person's concern is markedly excessive.

B. The preoccupation causes clinically significant distress or impairment in social, occupational, or other important areas of functioning.

C. The preoccupation is not better accounted for by another mental disorder (e.g., dissatisfaction with body shape and size in Anorexia Nervosa).

*Source*: American Psychiatric Association. (1994). *Diagnostic and Statistical Manual of Mental Disorders*, 4th ed. (p. 468). Washington, DC: Author. Reprinted by permission.

harassment, and physical injury and illness (Rosen, Reiter, & Orosan, 1995). Men will tend to camouflage with hats (Perugi et al., 1997), and women will tend to camouflage with makeup (Phillips & Diaz, 1997). These patients will often brood for many years before consulting a physician or plastic surgeon. Patients with body dysmorphic disorder tend to perceive their preoccupations as distressing, time-consuming, and difficult to resist. Often, these preoccupations become repetitive and ritualistic. Because feelings of ugliness are common but usually temporary in adolescence, it is not surprising that this disorder usually begins during this period. Typically by the third decade, these patients come into contact with physicians (Hay, 1970a). The course for body dysmorphic disorder is chronic and has a mean duration of illness of 16 years in one study (Phillips et al., 1994). In a subgroup of body dysmorphic disorder cases, patients can be highly avoidant of social situations and ultimately become housebound. Consistent with this, 75% of one sample of body dysmorphics was unmarried (Phillips et al., 1994).

**Epidemiology and Demographics.** The prevalence of body dysmorphic disorder continues to be uncertain. Estimates have varied from rare to 2% in clinical samples (Andreasen & Bardach, 1977; De Leon et al., 1989; Thomas, 1984). There is some controversy regarding the gender distribution for body dysmorphic disorder. Three studies reported that body dysmorphic disorder was more common in men (62% of fifty subjects, 62% of thirteen subjects, 58.6% of fifty-eight subjects, respectively; Hollender, Cohen, & Simeon, 1993; Neziroglu & Yaryura-Tobias, 1993; Perugi et al., 1997). Two other studies noted that body dysmorphic disorder was more common in women (72% of eighty-two subjects and 76% of fifty subjects, respectively; Rosen & Reiter, 1996; Veale, Boocock, et al., 1996). In the largest studied sample of persons with body dysmorphic disorder (N = 188), the gender ratio was essentially 1:1 (Phillips & Diaz, 1997). In the same study, men were as likely to seek nonpsychiatric medical and surgical care as women, but women were more likely to receive such care.

Body dysmorphic patients typically come from middle class environments (Andreasen & Bardach, 1977). Their intelligence is in the average or above average range, and insight into their preoccupations ranges from good to delusional (Hollender, Neville, Frenkel, Josephson, & Liebowitz, 1992; Phillips, Kim, & Hudson, 1995). Unlike many of those with other somatoform disorders, their health tends to be normal except for concern about their apparent physical defect (Andreasen & Bardach, 1977). Due to the increased importance that society places on physical appearance, the prevalence of body dysmorphic disorder is likely to increase.

**Body Dysmorphic Disorder and Associated Psychopathology.** It is often assumed that body dysmorphic disorder arises from another, more pervasive affective disorder (e.g. depression or anxiety), personality disorder (e.g., schizoid), or psychotic disorder (e.g., schizophrenia). Many of the earlier studies that examined dysmorphophobia and associated psychopathology came from the plastic surgery literature. Through a series of investigations, Edgerton, Jacobson, Meyer and their colleagues determined that the prevalence of psychiatric disturbances in women undergoing facelifts was 74%; enlargement of breasts, 80%; and rhinoplasty, 53% (Edgerton, Meyer, & Jacobson, 1961; Edgerton, Webb, Slaughter, & Meyer, 1964; Meyer, Jacobson, Edgerton, & Canter, 1960). All 100 men seeking cosmetic surgery were regarded as suffering from psychiatric disorders (Jacobson, Edgerton, Meyer, Canter, & Slaughter, 1960).

One of the most widely cited papers on dysmorphophobia (Andreasen & Bardach, 1977) was based largely on anecdotal impressions and two case studies. Hay's work (1970a,b) is among the few attempts to obtain a larger sample of dysmorphophobics and to include a comparison group. In one study, Hay (1970a) compared seventeen dysmorphophobic patients to an age- and gender-matched control group. All subjects completed a structured psychiatric interview and psychological test battery (Hysteroid-Obsessoid Questionnaire, Personal Illness Scales, punitive scale, vocabulary scale, and Eysenck's Personality Inventory). The clinical group complained of various physical defects concerning the penis, mouth, breasts, eyes, arms, and other miscellaneous body parts. Eleven patients with dysmorphophobia had personality disorders, five patients were schizophrenic, and one patient was depressed. Dysmorphophobics tended to be more obsessoid, introverted, intropunitive, sensitive, and insecure than the comparison group. In a second study, Hay (1970b) examined a total of forty-five dysmorphophobics with complaints about their noses. Using a similar control group and protocol as in his earlier investigation, Hay found less psychopathology in this second sample of dysmorphophobics. Still, he found that eighteen of the forty-five dysmorphophobics were diagnosed with a personality disorder, and one evidenced psychosis. The personality disorders noted in this study were similar to the prior study.

Connolly and Gibson (1978) performed a controlled follow-up study of eighty-six patients who underwent cosmetic rhinoplasty, compared to 101 patients who received reparative rhinoplasty for disease or injury. At 15-year follow-up assessment, 37% of the cosmetic surgery cases (as opposed to 9% of reparative cases) had "severe neurotic disorders." The authors also found that 7% of the cosmetic cases were schizophrenic, compared to 1% of the reparative cases. In a later study, twelve dysmorphophobic patients with dermatological symptoms were compared to eleven matched psoriatic patients and twelve matched controls (Hardy & Cotterill, 1982). Based on the Beck Depression Inventory and the Leyton Obsessional Inventory, the dysmorphophobics were more depressed than and as obsessional as the psoriatics. Both clinical groups were more depressed and obsessional than the control group. These authors concluded that dysmorphophobia was associated more with a depressed state than with an obsessional state.

More recent studies have found a strong association between body dysmorphic disorder and affective disorders. The prevalence of depression in body dysmorphic patients ranges from 68% (Hollender et al., 1993) to 80% (Phillips et al., 1994). Other studies have examined the prevalence of body dysmorphic disorder in patients with affective disorders. Brawman-Mintzer et al. (1995) compared rates of body dysmorphic disorder among patients with social phobia (N = 54), obsessive-compulsive disorder (N = 53), generalized anxiety disorder (N = 32), panic disorder (N = 47), major depression (N = −42), and a normal comparison subjects (N = 33). Body dysmorphic disorder was most prevalent in social phobia (11%) and obsessive-compulsive disorder (8%). The authors concluded that body dysmorphic disorder may share etiologic elements with both social phobia and obsessive-compulsive disorder. A cross-sectional, interview-based survey of fifty patients who met the DSM-IV diagnosis of body dysmorphic disorder revealed that patients were female (76%), primarily single or divorced (74%), and suffered from a mood disorder (26%), social phobia (16%), or obsessive-compulsive disorder (6%) (Veale, Boocock, et al., 1996). Personality disorders were present in 72% of cases; paranoid, avoidant, and obsessive-compulsive were the most common. Wilhelm, Otto, Zucker, and Pollack (1997) examined comorbidity rates among 165 outpatients who sought treatment for anxiety disorders. Following structured interviews, the authors identified eighty patients with panic disorder, forty patients with obsessive-compulsive disorder, twenty-five patients with social phobia, and twenty patients with generalized anxiety disorder. Overall, 6.7% of anxiety disordered patients met a diagnosis of body dysmorphic disorder, and the rate of body dysmorphic disorder was highest among patients with social phobia (12.0%). They also concluded that social phobia precedes the onset of body dysmorphic disorder.

The specific relationship between body dysmorphic disorder and obsessive-compulsive disorder has been examined in other reports (Phillips, McElroy, Hudson, & Pope, 1995; Simeon, Hollender, Stein, Cohen, & Aronowitz, 1995). In a DSM-IV field trial of 442 patients who met a diagnosis of obsessive-compulsive disorder, 12% met a comorbid diagnosis of body dysmorphic disorder (Simeon et al., 1995). This subsample had more anxious, impulsive, and schizotypal features than obsessive-compulsive disorder patients without body dysmorphic disorder. The comorbid group also had less insight into their condition, less insight associated with greater severity of illness, and more functional impairment. No differences between the two groups in demographic variables, obsessive-compulsive symptoms, or age of onset were noted. The authors concluded that, given the comorbidity between obsessive-compulsive disorder and body dysmorphic disorder and the similarities in age of onset, gender ratio, and clinical characteristics, the two disorders are strongly related and may be part of the same spectrum. In an excellent review article that examined the question whether body dysmorphic disorder is part of an obsessive-compulsive spectrum, affective spectrum, or both, Phillips et al. (1995) concluded that body dysmorphic disorder could be conceptualized more narrowly as an obsessive-compulsive spectrum disorder and more broadly as a form of affective spectrum disorder.

Phillips and colleagues have also been instrumental in trying to differentiate insight, overvalued ideation, and delusional thinking in body dysmorphic disorder (McElroy, Phillips, Keck, Hudson, & Pope, 1993). Fifty consecutive patients with possible or current histories of body dysmorphic disorder (DSM-III-R) underwent a Structured Clinical Interview and were divided into body dysmorphic disorder patients with somatic delusions (N = 26) and without somatic delusions (N = 24). Patients had a delusional preoccupation when they were, or ever had been, completely (100%) convinced that their supposed defect was real and that their perception of their defect was accurate and undistorted. Patients who stated that they might have a real defect or the their perception was probably accurate and who consistently retained some insight were thought to have overvalued ideas (twenty cases out of twenty-four body dysmorphic disorder without somatic delusions fit this description). As expected, patients with somatic delusions had a higher lifetime rate of DSM-III-R psychotic disorders than patients without somatic delusions. Interestingly, there were surprisingly few differences in other variables (e.g., demographics, comorbidity with other mood, anxiety, and substance use disorders, and selective response to serotonin re-uptake inhibitors). The authors concluded that a subgroup of patients with imagined physical defects may display a psychotic subtype of body dysmorphic disorder. In addition, the authors stated that insight into perceived body defects can range from overvalued ideation to delusional thinking and that within some cases, insight may fluctuate from one end of the continuum to the other (Phillips et al., 1993).

In sum, body dysmorphic disorder is associated with a number of other psychiatric conditions. However, the homogeneity of body dysmorphic disorder as a psychiatric condition remains equivocal, and much research will be needed before firm conclusions about body dysmorphic disorder can be drawn.

**Treatment.** Psychological treatment and pharmacological agents have been effective in treating body dysmorphic disorder. Earlier studies in the treatment of body dysmorphic disorder included psychodynamic approaches (Bloch & Glue, 1988; Philippopoulos, 1979) as well as behavioral approaches (Marks & Mishan, 1988; Neziroglu & Yaryura-Tobias, 1993), both of which appeared

promising. However, these are uncontrolled case studies that suffer from a number of methodological problems. Recent studies have yielded more impressive results. Rosen et al. (1995) randomly assigned fifty-four body dysmorphic disorder cases to a cognitive-behavior therapy group or a no-treatment control group. The treatment group received eight 2-hour sessions. Therapy focused on modifying intrusive thoughts of body dissatisfaction and overvalued thoughts about physical appearance, exposure to avoided body image situations, and eliminating body-checking. Symptoms of body dysmorphic disorder were significantly reduced in the treatment group, and the disorder was eliminated in 82% of cases at 2 weeks posttreatment and in 77% at the 18-week follow-up. Veale and associates (Veale, Gournay, et al., 1996) also evaluated cognitive-behavioral treatment of body dysmorphic disorder. Nineteen patients were randomly assigned to twelve sessions of cognitive-behavioral treatment (N = 9) or a waiting-list control condition (N = 10). The results indicated that subjects in the treatment condition experienced a 50% reduction in symptoms on the Yale–Brown Obsessive-Compulsive Scale at posttreatment. Follow-up data were not available.

MAO inhibitors (Jenike, 1984) and tricyclic antidepressants (Brotman & Jenike, 1984) were reportedly effective in treating body dysmorphic disorder. Consistent with the debate over dysmorphophobia as an overvalued idea versus a delusion, Riding and Munro (1975) advocated the use of pimozide, an antipsychotic agent, to treat body dysmorphic disorder. According to these authors, a positive response to pimozide was indicative of a delusional process, and a negative response was indicative of a disturbance rooted in personality. More recent pharmacological studies of body dysmorphic disorder emphasized the utility of serotonin re-uptake inhibitors (e.g., fluoxetine, paroxetine, and fluvoxamine). One retrospective study of 316 treatment trials on 130 patients noted clinical improvement in 42% of sixty-five serotonin re-uptake inhibitor trials in contrast to 30% of twenty-three trials with MAO inhibitors, 15% of forty-eight trials with nonserotonin re-uptake inhibitor tricyclics, and 3% of trials with neuroleptics (Phillips, 1995). In a clinical series by Phillips (1995), 70% of sixty-one serotonin re-uptake inhibitor trials demonstrated significant clinical improvement. In a retrospective study by Hollender et al. (1993), fifty patients were reviewed, and thirty-five cases were deemed much improved in serotonin re-uptake inhibitor trials. Eighteen cases on nonserotonin re-uptake inhibitor tricyclics evidenced no improvement at all. The preferential response of body dysmorphic disorder to serotonin re-uptake inhibitors is similar to the response of obsessive-compulsive disorder to serotonin re-uptake inhibitors, and this has added to the speculation that body dysmorphic disorder is part of the obsessive-compulsive spectrum (Hollender et al. 1992; Phillips, 1995). There is also the potential to augment serotonin re-uptake inhibitor trials with other medications (e.g., buspirone and pimozide) to enhance the treatment outcome, but controlled trials are needed (Phillips, 1995).

## Somatoform Disorder Not Otherwise Specified

Included in this wastebasket category of disorders are somatoform presentations that do not meet the criteria for any specific somatoform disorder. Table 5 presents DSM-IV (APA, 1994) examples of somatoform disorder not otherwise specified. No other information is presented about this category of disorders in the DSM-IV.

### Table 5. Somatoform Disorder Not Otherwise Specified

This category includes disorders with somatoform symptoms that do not meet the criteria for any specific Somatoform Disorder. Examples include

1. Pseudocyesis: a false belief of being pregnant that is associated with objective signs of pregnancy, which may include abdominal enlargement (although the umbilicus does not become everted), reduced menstrual flow, amenorrhea, subjective sensation of fetal movement, nausea, breast engorgement and secretions, and labor pains by the expected date of delivery. Endocrine changes may be present, but the syndrome cannot be explained by a general medical condition that causes endocrine changes (e.g., a hormone-secreting tumor).
2. A disorder involving nonpsychotic hypochondriacal symptoms of less than 6 months' duration.
3. A disorder involving unexplained physical complaints (e.g, fatigue or body weakness) of less than 6 months' duration that are not due to another mental disorder.

Source: American Psychiatric Association. (1994). *Diagnostic and Statistical Manual of Mental Disorders*, 4th ed. (pp. 468–469). Washington, DC: Author. Reprinted by permission.

## Factitious Disorders

If the somatoform disorders are replete with conceptual difficulties, diagnostic quandaries, and insufficient empirical data, these problems are even more prominent with factitious disorders. The existing literature is reviewed and diagnostic and clinical features are outlined along with information pertaining to etiology and treatment.

**Diagnosis and Clinical Description.** Factitious disorders are characterized by deliberate and apparently senseless simulation or feigning of psychological and/or physical illness. Unlike malingering, where there is recognized secondary gain, patients with factitious disorders undergo medical or psychiatric assessment and treatment for the primary purpose of assuming the sick role. Although their behavior is typically considered under voluntary control, these patients believe that it is in fact beyond their control and that their behavior feels quite compulsive. To support their claimed histories, these patients go to great lengths to produce symptomatology: engage in self-mutilating behaviors (e.g., picking away at a scab wound), self-inject bacteria to produce septicemia, contaminate urine samples with feces or blood, or manipulate thermometers (Feldman, Ford, & Reinhold, 1994). These patients are usually very colorful and dramatic in presentation; their self-reports tend to be extremely vague and inconsistent (bordering on pathological lying); they often are very knowledgeable about medical assessments and treatments; they are eager to undergo highly invasive, even life-threatening procedures; and they deny allegations and will eventually bolt out of the hospital against medical advice, only to start the whole process again at another hospital.

In DSM-IV (APA, 1994), there are two categories of factitious disorders presented: factitious disorder and factitious disorder not otherwise specified. Factitious disorder is also coded according to three subtypes: factitious disorder with predominantly psychological signs and symptoms, factitious disorder with predominantly physical signs and symptoms, and factitious disorder with combined psychological and physical signs and symp-

## Table 6. Factitious Disorder Not Otherwise Specified

This category includes disorders with factitious symptoms that do not meet the criteria for Factitious Disorder. An example is factitious by proxy: the intentional production or feigning of physical or psychological signs or symptoms in another person who is under the individual's care for the purpose of indirectly assuming the sick role (see. p. 725 for suggested research criteria).

*Source*: American Psychiatric Association. (1994). *Diagnostic and Statistical Manual of Mental Disorders*, 4th ed. (p. 475). Washington, DC: Author. Reprinted by permission.

toms. Table 6 includes DSM-IV diagnostic criteria for factitious disorder. Compared to DSM-III-R criteria for factitious disorder, there is one change of note in the DSM-IV criteria. Factitious disorder with combined psychological and physical signs and symptoms was categorized under factitious disorder, not otherwise specified, in DSM-III-R (APA, 1987).

The essential feature of factitious disorder with psychological signs and symptoms is simulation and feigning of mental illness. The range of psychopathology simulated may include hallucinations, delusions, depression and suicidal ideations, anxiety, and other bizarre behavior. Associated with the representation of depression is factitious bereavement, which represents a false claim of a recent death of someone significant under very dramatic circumstances (Sussman, 1989). Other types of factitious presentations with psychological signs and symptoms include factitious posttraumatic stress disorder associated with combat experiences (Lacoursiere, 1993; Lynn & Belza, 1984), factitious multiple personality (Toth & Baggaley, 1991), and factitious AIDS (Songer, 1995).

The detection of mental illness is a difficult task, and diagnosis is usually made after prolonged observation. Simulation of mental illness is suspected when a patient's symptoms become worse upon being observed or when new symptoms arise whenever discharge attempts are made (Sussman, 1989). Patients who participate in clinical trials of a new drug should be carefully evaluated for this disorder (Sussman, 1989). The iatrogenic effects of psychiatric care are probably not as life-threatening as those of medical care, but these patients are willing to take massive doses of potent psychotropics and undergo electroconvulsive therapy.

The term Munchausen's syndrome is perhaps the most enduring and widely used label for factitious disorder with physical signs and symptoms. The label was first used in a seminal paper by Richard Asher in 1951. The eponym was named after Baron Karl Friedrich Hieronymus Friehess von Munchausen, an eighteenth-century figure renowned for his tall tales of adventure in foreign lands. This fictional character became popular through the writings of Rudolf Raspe (Sakula, 1978). Asher (1951) noticed that a group of patients encountered in his work at a large-scale British hospital were characterized by far-reaching travels and dramatic and colorful recounting of personal medical histories that were, nonetheless, contrived. These cases often came in as medical emergencies and were categorized as acute abdominal type, hemorrhagic type, and neurological type. A multitude of scars all over their bodies (especially the abdominal area), truculent and irritable behavior while hospitalized, and multiple hospitalizations were commonly observed by Asher. Other terms used to describe these patients or their disorder include "hospital hoboes," "hospital vagrants," "hospital addiction," "peregrinating patients," "polysurgical addiction," "artifactual illness," and "S-H-A-F-T syndrome" (Sussman, 1989).

Asher's paper was followed by two review studies of Munchausen's syndrome (Ireland, Sapira, & Templeton, 1967; Spiro, 1968). Spiro (1968), in particular, was instrumental in asserting that Munchausen's syndrome was a misnomer, and he suggested the term chronic factitious illness as a replacement, which eventually became incorporated in the DSM-III. Nadelson (1979) agreed that the earlier term was a misnomer, noting that Baron Munchausen was not known for multiple hospital stays, nor did he submit himself to multiple invasive procedures or engage in self-destructive acts. Despite the change in label to factitious disorder, the term Munchausen's syndrome continues to remain popular. There are many case examples of factitious disorder with physical signs and symptoms in the literature: cancer (Feldman et al., 1994), septic arthritis of the right knee (Guziec, Lazarus, & Harding, 1994), hermaphrodism (Warren, Sutherland, & Lenz, 1994), hypoglycemia (Roy & Roy, 1995), penetrating chest wound due to sewing needles (Dixon & Abbey, 1995), and factitious quadriplegia (Feldman & Duval, 1997).

Except for a handful of case studies (Linde, 1996; Parker, 1993; Powell & Boast, 1993), there is very little formal information on factitious disorder with mixed psychological and physical signs and symptoms. One particular case is worth reporting because of its significant morbidity and cost (Powell & Boast, 1993). During a 12-year period, a subnormal man spent 6 years in institutions, 1300 days in psychiatric units, 556 days in prison, 354 days in medical care, leading the authors to refer to their case as "the million dollar man." Interestingly enough, the authors refer to their case as an example of Munchausen's syndrome. This illustrates the main problem with factitious disorder with physical signs and symptoms. In all practicality, most, if not all, cases of factitious disorder with physical signs and symptoms have a psychological component. At present, factitious disorder with mixed features is likely to represent a wastebasket category, including cases that do not fit neatly into other diagnostic categories.

Few data are available on the age of onset, prevalence, or family pattern of factitious disorder. Although factitious disorder has resulted in death (Feldman et al., 1994), the morbidity and mortality rates for factitious disorder are not known. The course of factitious disorder may be episodic or last a lifetime, and symptom experiences may vary in severity, chronicity, and resulting level of functional impairment. The Munchausen's syndrome version of factitious disorder (i.e., factitious disorder with physical signs and symptoms) is considered the most severe form and occurs in approximately 10% of all cases with factitious disorder (Eisendrath, 1989). Thirty-two of 343 patients referred to the National Institute for Allergy and Infectious Disease had factitious disorder (Aduan, Fauci, Dale, Herzberg, & Wolff, 1979). Sutherland and Rodin (1990) retrospectively reviewed 1288 case files consecutively referred to a psychiatric consultation service in a tertiary care hospital. A diagnosis of factitious disorder was made in ten (0.8%) of these cases; seven of the ten cases were females. Five (0.3%) of 1538 cases referred to a neurological unit had DSM-III-R factitious disorder, feigning neurological syndromes (Bauer & Boegner, 1996). They also concluded that all factitious disorder patients

displayed the characteristic features of self-discharge, aggressive behavior, pathological lying, and hospital wandering.

Through retrospective review of cases seen during a 9-year period in the consultation and liaison service of a large-scale medical hospital, Freyberger, Nordmeyer, Freyberger, and Nordmeyer (1994) identified seventy patients with factitious disorder, the largest sample of factitious disorder cases from a single setting. General characteristics of the sample were that it was primarily female (57%), unmarried (69%), the age of onset was in the early to midthirties, less than half the sample had elementary school education, but a substantial proportion (24%) of the sample worked in academic and professional settings. Pankratz (1981) surveyed the medical literature from 1968 to 1980 and attempted to tabulate the characteristics of patients with Munchausen's syndrome. Pankratz was able to document 104 adult cases and eleven child cases of Munchausen's syndrome. He found that males were twice as likely as females to have Munchausen's syndrome. The mean age for males was 39.9, and the mean age for females was 30.9. The age range varied from early childhood to 64 years of age. As with the somatoform disorders, pain was the most common complaint and was mentioned in 75% of the cases. The next most common complaint was bleeding, mentioned in 31% of cases. About one-quarter of all cases reported difficulties with the genitourinary system, and another one-quarter of the cases had cardiac difficulties. Ninety-five percent of patients surveyed had multiple hospitalizations, 77% did some "hospital shopping," and 61% had multiple surgeries. Leaving against medical advice occurred in 42% of the patients. Twenty-two percent of the cases were related to the medical profession in one capacity or another, a finding noted by other investigators (Aduan et al., 1979; Nadelson, 1979).

In another interesting study, Carney (1980) examined 35 patients, seen during a 10-year period, whose behavior gained them admittance to hospitals. Carney's sample consisted of nine males and twenty-six females whose mean age was 32.2 years. He divided his sample into "wandering" (N = 15) and "nonwandering" (N = 20) groups; however, the criteria used in assigning patients to wandering or nonwandering groups were not forwarded. Still, with this wandering/nonwandering variable, he obtained some revealing findings. Wanderers were more likely to be male and unemployed, changed employment more frequently, abused alcohol and drugs, were more motivated by external gains, had personal histories lasting more than 10 years, were socially more maladjusted, and achieved less than nonwanderers. Conversely, nonwanderers were more stable, had less dramatic and more subtle symptomatology, and were harder to detect as artifactual. These patients were also more likely to be socially conforming women who worked hard as nurses. Twenty-six of the thirty-five patients had sexual and marital problems. Carney's study demonstrates the extent of impairment that individuals with factitious disorder have across many areas of functioning. Furthermore, it shows that patients with factitious disorder are not homogeneous in presentation (Sutherland & Rodin, 1990).

**Factitious Disorder and Associated Psychopathology.** Persons diagnosed with factitious disorder with psychological signs and symptoms generally have concurrent diagnoses of borderline personality disorder (Sussman, 1989). Hay (1983) conducted a review of the literature on the simulation of psychosis and additionally provided a presentation of six cases for discussion purposes. He concluded that the simulation of schizophrenia is a prodromal phase of psychosis that occurs in deviant premorbid personalities. Pope, Jonas, and Jones (1982) were able to identify nine patients with factitious psychosis out of 219 patients admitted with a psychotic disorder. After conducting 4- to 7-year follow-ups, they concluded that these patients did not develop typical psychotic episodes. However, these persons had high psychiatric comorbidity and poor social outcomes due to the severity of underlying personality disorders. These investigators aptly stated that "acting crazy may bode more ill than being crazy."

The differential diagnosis of factitious disorder with psychological signs and symptoms typically involves organic mental syndromes (e.g., pseudodementia), personality disorders (e.g., antisocial personality disorder), and malingering. In organic mental syndromes, the behavior is usually consistent with medical evidence and neuropsychological findings that reflect an organic profile. Cases with factitious disorder have difficulty feigning corroborating organic findings or providing an organic neuropsychological profile. Unlike factitious disorder, true psychotic behavior does not change upon observation. Simulated mental illness by antisocial types is also likely to fluctuate

and to be noticed after prolonged observation in the hospital. In malingering, identifiable secondary gain is present, whereas in factitious disorder with psychological symptoms, assuming the role of a psychiatric patient is the main goal. However, this may be extremely difficult to identify in the clinical setting. Some investigators have argued that factitious disorder with psychological signs and symptoms should be considered under the provisional diagnosis section in future editions of the DSM, if not dropped altogether from the DSM due to subjectivity in interpreting criteria and poor reliability of this diagnostic subcategory (Rogers, Bagby, & Rector, 1989; Rogers, Bagby, & Vincent, 1994).

In diagnosing factitious disorder, any disorder in which physical symptoms are prominent should be considered part of the differential diagnosis (Sussman, 1989). As noted earlier, the possibility of factitious disorder in the presence of actual physical disease must always be explored. A good example of this was reported in a case whereby an organic brain disorder led to the development of Munchausen's (Lawrie, Goodwin, & Masterton, 1993). Factitious disorder with physical symptoms is differentiated from somatization disorder in that factitious patients are consciously producing physical symptomatology, are more willing to undergo multiple procedures, and display a more extreme course of hospitalizations than patients with somatization disorder. There is often a symbolic significance or temporal relationship between the symptoms displayed and the emotional conflicts experienced by persons with conversion disorder, which factitious disorder cases are not likely to exhibit. Hypochondriacs do not produce their symptoms voluntarily and are usually not willing to submit themselves to aggressive and invasive procedures.

Consideration of personality disorders is also essential in establishing a diagnosis of factitious disorder. Antisocial, borderline, histrionic, schizoid, and narcissistic personality disorders have been noted in factitious disorder with physical signs and symptoms (Bauer & Boegner, 1996; Freyberger et al., 1994; Sutherland & Rodin, 1990). Due to pathological lying, inability to form close relationships, hostile and aggressive behavior, and alcohol and drug abuse, factitious disorder cases can be mistaken for antisocial personality disorder. However, even when individuals with antisocial traits have physical symptomatology, they do not admit themselves for invasive procedures, nor do they spend most of their time in hospitals. Though the recounting of symptomatology by factitious cases may be done in a dramatic and histrionic fashion, these patients are actually quite withdrawn and bland on closer inspection. The differential between factitious disorder and borderline personality disorder is very difficult because of the similarly chaotic lifestyles, interpersonal problems, self-destructive behaviors, and the sense of entitlement that both groups evidence. One psychiatrist stated that Munchausen's syndrome should be considered a subgroup of the borderline character (Nadelson, 1979). Sussman (1989) similarly states that patients with factitious disorder should carry a diagnosis of borderline disorder on Axis II. As bizarre as the behavior of factitious disorder cases with physical symptoms is, they do not display any evidence of the marked thought disorder or prominent delusions of the schizophrenic. Malingerers can be differentiated from factitious disorder by the identification of secondary gain and their ability to terminate their symptomatology as soon as it is not profitable.

**Etiological Formulations.** Factitious disorder is multifactorially determined. Most of the discussion of the etiology of this disorder is based on psychodynamic theory (Folks, 1995; Nadelson, 1979; Pankratz, 1981; Spivak, Rodin, & Sutherland, 1994; Sussman, 1989). Common psychodynamic themes revolve around dependency, abandonment, masochism, and mastery. Many patients with Munchausen's syndrome have experienced some form of parental cruelty, neglect, or abandonment. Early experiences of this kind prevent the patient from developing an adequate sense of worth and independence. Often, the patients are hospitalized for a genuine medical concern in childhood or adolescence. Factitious disorder can be reflected in socially sanctioned behavior that allows a dependent person to receive care from a symbolic parental figure (e.g., a physician). The invitation of painful diagnostic procedures and medical interventions may reflect a need to suffer for past sins or to reduce guilt associated with unconscious sexual impulses or rage. Others have argued that patients with factitious disorder may have disturbances in the core self (Spivak et al., 1994), which would be consistent with the prominent association of factitious disorder with borderline personality disorder. Factitious disorder can be also used to gain mastery over parental figures

by fooling and frustrating them. In assuming the role of the patient and reliving the painful experience through multiple hospitalizations, the patient can seize control of the illness by terminating it voluntarily. A simpler explanation for factitious disorder is the powerful reward in the form of identity and recognition that the patient obtains in taking on the sick role.

A diathesis-stress model of factitious disorder has recently been presented (Trask & Sigmon, 1997). Early conditioning or traumatic experiences combined with biological predisposition lead the individual to develop factitious disorder. Trask and Sigmon (1997) reviewed fifty-six cases of Munchausen's syndrome from the literature and noted that 42% of cases had either traumatic events in childhood or prehospitalization stressors, and the majority of the remaining cases failed to provide enough information to determine the presence of early childhood traumas. However, there is very little data available to ascertain the value of this model. Regardless of theoretical orientation, the difficulty in understanding the etiology of factitious disorder is best captured in the following quote from Pankratz (1981):

It is difficult to construct one theory that can explain the self-destructiveness of injecting oneself with parrot feces, the grandiosity of claiming to be an oceanographic physicist working with Jacques Cousteau, the passivity of submitting to 48 lumbar punctures, the skill to stop breathing to unconsciousness, and the wanderlust for 423 admissions. (p. 74)

**Treatment.** Needless to say, there are no controlled comparative outcome studies of factitious disorder; consequently, most of what is known about treatment is based on anecdotal reports. Clearly, the most important facet in treating this disorder is early diagnosis. This allows prevention of harmful iatrogenic effects. Once the assessment is completed, the disposition consists of a referral for psychiatric care or confrontation by the medical team and support staff. Although psychiatric hospitalization is probably the first essential step with these patients, much of this depends on the way patients respond to confrontation. Some authors believe that confronting the patient with the "facts" in a noncondemning fashion is therapeutic (Nadelson, 1979; Reich & Gottfried, 1983), whereas others feel that confrontation can be harmful (Eisendrath, 1989). There is a general consensus that room searches and "unmasking ceremonies" should be avoided at all costs because this sets up an adversarial relationship and may provoke departure against medical advice (Sussman, 1989). Given the complexity of factitious disorder, it is not surprising that multimodal approaches (combined medical and psychiatric interventions) work best in managing factitious disorder. Folks (1995) reported that successfully managed case of factitious disorder share three common therapeutic approaches. He noted that it is important to reinforce healthy behaviors, emphasize the role of a primary therapist, and maintain a consistent relationship with a primary physician, regardless of the clinical outcome.

## Factitious Disorder Not Otherwise Specified.

In DSM-III-R, factitious disorder not otherwise specified was designed to capture factitious presentations that were not consistent with either factitious disorder with psychological symptoms or factitious disorder with physical symptoms. This is still the case. However, now DSM-IV suggests categorizing factitious disorder by proxy as factitious disorder not otherwise specified (APA, 1994). Factitious disorder by proxy is also listed in the DSM-IV section of criteria sets and axes provided for further studies. The research criteria for factitious disorder by proxy are listed in Table 7. The essential feature of this presentation is the deliberate production and simulation of psychological and physical signs or symptoms in another person who is under the perpetrator's care. Very often, the victim is a child, and a parent, usually the mother, intentionally fabricates or feigns symptoms in the child. The parent's aim is to have the child sub-

## Table 7. DSM-IV Research Criteria for Factitious Disorder by Proxy

A. Intentional production or feigning of physical or psychological signs or symptoms in another person who is under the individual's care.
B. The motivation for the perpetrator's behavior is to assume the sick role by proxy.
C. External incentives for the behavior (such as economic gain) are absent.
D. The behavior is not better accounted for by another mental disorder.

Source: American Psychiatric Association. (1994). *Diagnostic and Statistical Manual of Mental Disorders*, 4th ed. (p. 727). Washington, DC: Author. Reprinted by permission.

jected to a number of tests and invasive treatments; this behavior essentially constitutes a form of abuse.

Although there are a number of colorful case descriptions of factitious disorder by proxy (Feldman et al., 1994; Fisher, Mitchell, & Murdoch, 1993; Livingston, 1987; Sigal, Altmark, & Carmel, 1986), there is little actual data on factitious disorder by proxy. With a discussion of two cases, Meadow (1977) was first responsible for bringing attention to factitious disorder by proxy. Based on case reports and literature review, significant morbidity and mortality in factitious disorder by proxy have been noted (Jani, White, Rosenberg, & Miasami, 1992; Meadow, 1990; Ostfeld & Feldman, 1996; Rosenberg, 1987; Schreier & Libow, 1993; Taylor & Hyler, 1993). Multiple surgeries, impaired gastrointestinal functioning, joint and gait problems, brain damage, seizures, fevers, apnea, and bleeding, are common medical sequelae of factitious disorder by proxy. In her review of the literature, Rosenberg (1987) noted a 9% mortality rate. In a sample twenty-seven victims of repeated suffocations, Meadow (1990) noted that there was a 55% mortality rate in their siblings. Although there is little data on prevalence and gender breakdown of victims, perpetrators are usually mothers. Sometimes older siblings are coached into colluding with a parent in perpetrating factitious acts on younger children and sometimes victims, themselves, can play active roles in being victims of factitious acts (Sanders, 1995).

A number of explanations for the etiology of factitious disorder by proxy have been put forward. Psychodynamic theory suggests that the parental figure is using the child to act out transference issues against the physician (Feldman, Rosenquist, & Bond, 1997; Schreier & Libow, 1993). Schreier & Libow (1993) have come to view the mother as engaged in a sadomasochistic relationship with the physician, where the child serves as a way to control the symbolic parental figure, the physician or the hospital. Behaviorally, the perpetrator may be responding poorly to stress from parenting, marriage, social relationships, and other life demands, and factitious behavior may be a cry for help and attention (Rosenberg, 1987; Sanders, 1995; Schreier & Libow, 1993). From the perspective of family systems, factitious behavior may be due to enmeshment, marital dysfunction, and substance and sexual abuse (Feldman et al., 1994; Rosenberg, 1987).

There is little data on comorbidity in perpetrators of factitious disorder by proxy. Similar to the factitious disorder with psychological and physical signs and symptoms, the personality types of adults engaged in factitious behaviors by proxy tend to be borderline, histrionic, and narcissistic. In the only group study of factitious disorder by proxy (Bools, Neale, & Meadow, 1994), psychiatric histories were reported in forty-seven mothers with factitious disorder by proxy. Seventeen subjects were thought to have personality disorders, usually histrionic and borderline. Ten subjects had histories of substance abuse, twenty-six subjects had histories of self-harm, and nine subjects had criminal histories that were independent of convictions related to the children. Thirty-four subjects had histories of factitious disorder or somatoform disorder.

Although there is no specific effective treatment for factitious disorder by proxy, the ultimate goal of treatment is the safety of children (Folks, 1995). Meadows (1982) outlined a treatment plan that consists of separating the child from the parental figure; corroborating the details of the history and the temporal relationships among signs, symptoms, and the presence of the parental figure; thoroughly investigating the reliability of signs and symptoms; and psychiatric consultation. Video surveillance has been proposed to confirm factitious disorder by proxy (Foreman & Farsides, 1993), but this is controversial from ethical, medical, legal, and psychological perspectives (Feldman et al., 1994; Southall & Samuels, 1993). In the absence of consistent effective treatment of the perpetrator and a safe environment for the child, the separation of the child from the parental figure is the primary intervention (Feldman et al., 1997). When there is a high risk for reoffending, foster home placement needs to be considered (Feldman et al., 1997). Bools et al. (1994) reported that when children were returned to parental figures rated as having moderate to severe factitious disorder by proxy, illness was again fabricated 35% of the time. Some emphasis has been placed on education in early detection and management of potential cases of factitious disorder by proxy to reduce the overall cost to individuals, systems, and society (Jani et al., 1992; Ostfeld & Feldman, 1996).

An interesting variant of Munchausen by proxy syndrome is Munchausen by adult proxy syndrome, whereby the elicitation of symptomatology in an adult is produced by another adult (Sigal et al., 1986). Sigal et al. (1986) presented a fascinating case of a 34-year-old man who killed his wife with injections of gasoline during several years. Three years later, he repeated the process with a girlfriend who was threatening to leave him. After drugging her with flunitrazepam, he resorted to injections of gasoline in the neck, breast, and backside of his girlfriend's body. She eventually became a paraplegic, and he spent most of his time looking after her. He was apparently more interested in attention from the medical staff than he was in his girlfriend's health. He is now serving 46 years in jail for murdering his wife.

## Conclusion

This group of disorders is unquestionably one of the least understood of mental disorders. A great deal of research in some areas (e.g., somatization disorder, body dysmorphic disorder, and hypochondriasis disorder) has emerged. Yet, our understanding of this fascinating but complicated group of disorders has not improved much.

The database continues to be inadequate for many of the diagnostic entities present in this group. In part, this is related to the general observation that these patients are seen primarily by physicians and resist psychological evaluation and treatment. As more psychologists and other health care professionals find their way into medical settings, it is hoped that an increase in our understanding of these disorders will occur. In addition, the base rates of some of these disorders are so low that it may take many years before an adequate database can be established.

Though the database is not satisfactory, even more disturbing are the conceptual problems associated with these disorders. These conceptual problems are rampant in the DSM-IV section of somatoform and factitious disorders. The validity and reliability of the diagnostic entities are poor because these diagnostic categories overlap, are poorly defined, and are too simplistic. Many of these disorders do not have pathognomonic criteria. The diagnosis of these disorders is often based on exclusion; diagnosticians find themselves first establishing what the clinical presentation is not and then concluding what it might be. Such an approach is fertile ground for diagnostic inaccuracies. These disorders, as conceptualized, also require an organic versus psychogenic distinction.

This is an extremely difficult task to accomplish: What physical condition does not have a psychological component, and vice versa? Thus, inclusion criteria for these diagnostic categories should be conjunctive and should incorporate psychological criteria. Consistent with this approach, strict psychological versus organic etiological formulations do not take into full account the complexity of somatoform and factitious disorders. Integrated conceptual formulations are likely to lead to a better understanding of these interesting and frustrating disorders.

# References

Abbey, S. E., & Lipowski, Z. J. (1987). Comprehensive management of persistent somatization: An innovative in-patient program. *Psychotherapy and Psychosomatics*, 48, 110–115.

Aduan, R. P., Fauci, A. S., Dale, D. C., Herzberg, M. D., & Wolff, S. M. (1979). Factitious fever and self-induced infection: A report of 32 cases and review of the literature. *Annals of Internal Medicine*, 90, 230–242.

Alacron, R. D. (1973). Hysteria and hysterical personality: How come one without the other? *Psychiatric Quarterly*, 47, 258–275.

Allodi, F. A. (1974). Accident neurosis: Whatever happened to male hysteria? *Canadian Psychiatric Association Journal*, 19, 291–296.

American Psychiatric Association. (1952). *Diagnostic and statistical manual of mental disorders*. Washington, DC: Author.

American Psychiatric Association. (1968). *Diagnostic and statistical manual of mental disorders* (2nd ed.). Washington, DC: Author.

American Psychiatric Association. (1980). *Diagnostic and statistical manual of mental disorders* (3rd ed.). Washington, DC: Author.

American Psychiatric Association. (1987). *Diagnostic and statistical manual of mental disorders* (3rd ed., rev.). Washington, DC: Author.

American Psychiatric Association. (1994). *Diagnostic and statistical manual of mental disorders* (4th ed.). Washington, DC: Author.

Andreasen, N. C., & Bardach, J. (1977). Dysmorphophobia: Symptom or disease? *American Journal of Psychiatry*, 134, 673–676.

Arkonac, O., & Guze, S. B. (1963). A family study of hysteria. *New England Journal of Medicine*, 268, 239–242.

Asher, R. (1951). Munchausen's syndrome. *Lancet*, 1, 339–341.

Avia, M. D., Ruiz, M. A., Olivares, M. E., Crespo, M., Guisado, A. B., Sanchez, A., & Varela, A. (1996). The meaning of psychological symptoms: Effectiveness of a group intervention with hypochondriacal patients. *Behaviour Research and Therapy*, 34, 23–31.

Bach, M., & Bach, D. (1995). Predictive value of alexithymia: A prospective study in somatizing patients. *Psychotherapy and Psychosomatics*, 64, 43–48.

Bach, M., Bach, D., & de Zwann, M. (1996). Independency of alexithymia and somatization. *Psychosomatics*, 37, 451–458.

Bach, M., Nutzinger, D. O., & Hartl, L. (1996). Comorbidity of anxiety disorders and hypochondriasis: Considering different diagnostic systems. *Comprehensive Psychiatry*, 37, 62–67.

Barnert, C. (1971). Conversion reactions and psychophysiologic disorders: A comparative study. *Psychiatry in Medicine*, 2, 205–220.

Barr, R., & Abernathy, V. (1977). Conversion reaction: Differential diagnosis in the light of biofeedback research. *Journal of Nervous and Mental Disease*, 164, 287–292.

Barsky, A. J. (1996). Hypochondriasis: Medical management and psychiatric treatment. *Psychosomatics*, 37, 48–56.

Barsky, A. J., Barnett, M. C., & Cleary, P. D. (1994). Hypochondriasis and panic disorder. *Archives of General Psychiatry*, 51, 918–925.

Barsky, A. J., Geringer, E., & Wool, C. (1988). A cognitive-educational treatment for hypochondriasis. *General Hospital Psychiatry*, 10, 322–327.

Barsky, A. J., & Klerman, G. L. (1983). Overview: Hypochondriasis, bodily complaints and somatic styles. *American Journal of Psychiatry*, 140, 273–283.

Barsky, A. J., & Wyshak, G. (1989). Hypochondriasis and related health attitudes. *Psychosomatics*, 30, 412–420.

Barsky, A. J., & Wyshak, G. (1990). Hypochondriasis and somatosensory amplification. *British Journal of Psychiatry*, 157, 404–409.

Barsky, A. J., Wyshak, G., & Klerman, G. L. (1986). Hypochondriasis: An evaluation of the DSM-III criteria in medical outpatients. *Archives of General Psychiatry*, 43, 493–500.

Barsky, A. J., Wyshak, G., & Klerman, G. L. (1990). Transient hypochondriasis. *Archives of General Psychiatry*, 47, 746–752.

Barsky. A. J., Wyshak., G., & Klerman, G. L. (1991). The relationship between hypochondriasis and medical illness. *Archives of Internal Medicine*, 151, 84–88.

Barsky, A. J., Wyshak, G., & Klerman, G. L. (1992). Psychiatric comorbidity in DSM-III-R hypochondriasis. *Archives of General Psychiatry*, 49, 101–108.

Barsky, A. J., Wyshak, G., Klerman, G. L., & Latham, K. S. (1990). The prevalence of hypochondriasis in medical outpatients. *Social Psychiatry and Psychiatric Epidemiology*, 25, 89–94.

Bass, C., & Benjamin, S. (1993). The management of somatization. *British Journal of Psychiatry*, 162, 472–480.

Bass, C., & Wade, C. (1984). Chest pain with normal coronary arteries: A comparative study of psychiatric and social morbidity. *Psychological Medicine*, 14, 51–61.

Battaglia, M., Bernardeschi, L., Politi, E., Bertella, S., & Bellodi, L. (1995). Comorbidity of panic and somatization disorder: A genetic-epidemiological approach. *Comprehensive Psychiatry*, 36, 411–420.

Bauer, M., & Boegner, F. (1996). Neurological syndromes in factitious disorder. *Journal of Nervous and Mental Disease*, 184, 281–288.

Bendefeldt, F., Miller, L. L., & Ludwig, A. M. (1976). Cognitive performance in conversion hysteria. *Archives of Psychiatry*, 33, 1250–1254.

Bianchi, G. N. (1971). The origins of disease phobia. *Australia and New Zealand Journal of Psychiatry*, 5, 241–257.

Bianchi, G. N. (1973). Patterns of hypochondriasis: A principal components analysis. *British Journal of Psychiatry*, 12, 541–548.

Binzer, M., Andersen, P. M., & Kullgren, G. (1997). Clinical characteristics of patients with motor disability due to con version disorder: A prospective control group study. *Journal of Neurology, Neurosurgery, and Psychiatry, 63,* 83–88.

Bishop, E. R., Jr. (1980). Monosymptomatic hypochondriasis. *Psychosomatics, 21,* 731–747.

Bishop, E. R., Jr., Mobley, M. C., & Farr, W. F., Jr. (1978). Lateralization of conversion symptoms. *Comprehensive Psychiatry, 19,* 393–396.

Blazer, D., George, K., Landerman, R., Pennebaker, M., Melville, M. L., Woodbury, M., Manton, K. G., Jordan, K., & Locke, B. (1985). Psychiatric disorders: A rural/urban comparison. *Archives of General Psychiatry, 42,* 651–656.

Bloch, S., & Glue, P. (1988). Psychotherapy and dysmorphophobia: A case report. *British Journal of Psychiatry, 152,* 271–274.

Bohman, M., Cloninger, C. R., Von Knorring, A. L., & Sigvardsson, S. (1984). An adoption study of somatoform disorders. III. Cross-fostering analysis and genetic relationship to alcoholism and criminality. *Archives of General Psychiatry, 41,* 872–878.

Bools, C., Neale, B., & Meadow, R. (1994). Munchausen syndrome by proxy: A study of psychopathology. *Child Abuse and Neglect, 18,* 773–788.

Boyd, J. H., Burke, J. D., Jr., Gruenberg, E., Holzer, C. E., III, Rae, D. S., George, L. K., Karno, M., Stoltzman, R., McEvoy, L., & Nestadt, G. (1984). Exclusion criteria of DSM-III: A study of co-occurrence of hierarchy-free syndromes. *Archives of General Psychiatry, 41,* 983–989.

Brawman-Minzer, O., Lydiard, R. B., Phillips, K. A., Morton, A., Czepowicz, V., Emmanuel, N., Villareal, G., Johnson, M., & Ballenger, J. C. (1995). Body dysmorphic disorder in patients with anxiety disorders and major depression: A comorbidity study. *American Journal of Psychiatry, 152,* 1665–1667.

Brink, T. L., Janakes, C., & Martinez, N. (1981). Geriatric hypochondriasis: Situational factors. *Journal of the American Geriatric Society, 29,* 37–39.

Brodsky, C. M. (1984). Sociocultural and interpersonal influences on somatization. *Psychosomatics, 9,* 673–680.

Brotman, A. W., & Jenike, M. A. (1984). Monosymptomatic hypochondriasis treated with tricyclic antidepressants. *American Journal of Psychiatry, 141,* 1608–1609.

Brown, F. W., Golding, J. M., & Smith, G. R. (1990). Psychiatric comorbidity in primary care somatization disorder. *Psychosomatic Medicine, 52,* 445–551.

Brown, H. N., & Vaillant, G. E. (1981). Hypochondriasis. *Archives of Internal Medicine, 141,* 723–726.

Bucholz, K. K., Dinwiddle, S. H., Reich, T., Shayka, J. J., & Cloninger, C. R. (1993). Comparison of screening proposals for somatization disorder: Empirical analyses. *Comprehensive Psychiatry, 34,* 59–64.

Campo, J. V., & Fritch, S. L. (1994). Somatization in children and adolescents. *Journal of the American Academy in Child and Adolescent Psychiatry, 33,* 1223–1235.

Carden, N. L., & Schramel, D. J. (1966). Observations of conversion reactions seen in troops involved in the Vietnam conflict. *American Journal of Psychiatry, 123,* 21–31.

Carney, M. W. P. (1980). Artifactual illness to attract medical attention. *British Journal of Psychiatry, 136,* 542–547.

Carter, A. B. (1949). The prognosis of certain hysterical symptoms. *British Medical Journal, 1,* 1076–1079.

Celani, D. (1976). An interpersonal approach to hysteria. *American Journal of Psychiatry, 133,* 1412–1418.

Chodoff, P. (1974). The diagnosis of hysteria: An overview. *American Journal of Psychiatry, 131,* 1073–1078.

Chodoff, P., & Lyons, H. (1958). Hysteria, the hysterical personality and "hysterical" conversion. *American Journal of Psychiatry, 114,* 734–740.

Cloninger, C. R., & Guze, S. B. (1970). Psychiatric illness and female criminality: The role of sociopathy and hysteria in the antisocial woman. *American Journal of Psychiatry, 127,* 303–311.

Cloninger, C. R., Reich, T., & Guze, S. B. (1975a). The multifactorial model of disease transmission: II. Set differences in the familial transmission of sociopathy. *British Journal of Psychiatry, 127,* 11–22.

Cloninger, C. R., Reich, T., & Guze, S. B. (1975b). The multifactorial model of disease transmission: III. Familial relationship between sociopathy and hysteria. *British Journal of Psychiatry, 127,* 23–32.

Cloninger, R., Sigvardsson, S., Von Knorring, A. L., & Bohman, M. (1984). An adoption study of somatoform disorders: II. Identification of two discrete somatoform disorders. *Archives of General Psychiatry, 41,* 863–871.

Connolly, F. H., & Gibson, M. (1978). Dysmorphophobia: A long-term study. *British Journal of Psychiatry, 132,* 568–570.

Coryell, N. (1981). Diagnosis-specific mortality: Primary unipolar depression and Briquet's syndrome (somatization disorder). *Archives of General Psychiatry, 38,* 939–942.

Coryell, Q., & Norton, S. G. (1981). Briquet's syndrome and primary depression: Comparison of background and outcome. *Comprehensive Psychiatry, 22,* 249–256.

Couprie, W., Wijdicks, E. F. M., Rooijmans, H. G. M., & van Gijn, J. (1995). Outcome in conversion disorder: A follow-up study. *Journal of Neurology, Neurosurgery, and Psychiatry, 58,* 750–752.

Craig, T. K. J., Boardman, A. P., Mills, K., Daly-Jones, O., & Drake, H. (1993). The South London somatisation study I: Longitudinal course and the influence of early life experiences. *British Journal of Psychiatry, 163,* 579–588.

Craig, T. K. J., Drake, H., Mills, K., & Boardman, A. P. (1994). The South London somatisation study II: Influence of stressful events and secondary gain. *British Journal of Psychiatry, 165,* 248–258.

De Leon, J., Bott, A., & Simpson, G. M. (1989). Dysmorphophobia: Body dysmorphic disorder or delusional disorder, somatic subtype? *Comprehensive Psychiatry, 30,* 457–472.

Deubner, D. C. (1977). An epidemiologic study of migraine and headache in 10–20 year olds. *Headache, 17,* 173–180.

Dixon, D., & Abbey, S. (1995). Cupid's arrow: An unusual presentation of factitious disorder. *Psychosomatics, 36,* 502–504.

Edgerton, M. T., Meyer, E., & Jacobson, W. E. (1961). Augmentation mammoplasty: II. Further surgical and psychiatric evaluation. *Plastic and Reconstructive Surgery, 27,* 279–302.

Edgerton, M. T., Webb, W. L., Jr., Slaughter, R., & Meyer, E. (1964). Surgical results and psychosocial change following rhytidectomy: An evaluation of face-lifting. *Plastic and Reconstructive Surgery, 33,* 503–521.

Eisendrath, S. J. (1989). Factitious physical disorders: Treatment without confrontation. *Psychosomatics, 30,* 383–387.

Engel, G. E. (1959). "Psychogenic" pain and the pain-prone patient. *American Journal of Medicine, 16,* 899–918.

Engel, G. E. (1970). Conversion symptoms. In C. M. MacBryde (Ed.), *Signs and symptoms: Applied physiology and clinical interpretation* (pp. 650–658). Philadelphia: Lippincott.

Escobar, J. I. (1996). Pharmacological treatment of somatization/hypochondriasis. *Psychopharmacology Bulletin, 32,* 589–596.

Escobar, J. I., Burnam, M. A., Karno, M., Forsythe, A., & Golding, J. M. (1987). Somatization in the community. *Archives of General Psychiatry, 44,* 713–718.

Escobar, J. I., Rubio-Stipec, M., Canino, G., & Karno, M. (1989). Somatic symptom index (SSI): A new and abridged somatization construct. *Journal of Nervous and Mental Disease, 177,* 140–146.

Escobar, J. I., Waitzkin, H., Silver, R. C., Gara, M., & Holman, A. (1998). Abridged somatization: A study in primary care. *Psychosomatic Medicine, 60,* 466–472.

Fabrega, H., Jr., Mezzich, J., Jacob, R., & Ulrich, R. (1988). Somatoform disorder in a psychiatric setting: Systematic comparisons with depression and anxiety disorders. *Journal of Nervous and Mental Disease, 176,* 431–439.

Fallon, B. A., Schneier, F. R., Marshall, R., Campeas, R., Vermes, D., Goetz, D., & Liebowitz, M. R. (1996). The pharmacotherapy of hypochondriasis. *Psychopharmacology Bulletin, 32,* 607–611.

Feldman, M. D., & Duval, N. H. (1997). Factitious quadriplegia: A rare new case and literature review. *Psychosomatics, 38,* 76–80.

Feldman, M. D., Ford, C. V., & Reinhold, T. (1994). *Patient or pretender: Inside the strange world of factitious disorders.* New York: Wiley.

Feldman, M. D., Rosenquist, P. B., & Bond, J. P. (1997). Concurrent factitious disorder and factitious disorder by proxy. *General Hospital Psychiatry, 19,* 24–28.

Finkelstein, B. A. (1963). Dysmorphophobia. *Disorders of the Nervous System, 24,* 365–370.

Fishbain, D. A. (1996). Where have two DSM revisions taken us for the diagnosis of pain disorder in chronic pain patients? *American Journal of Psychiatry, 153,* 137–138.

Fishbain, D. A., Goldberg, M., Khalil, T. M., Asfour, S. S., Abdel-Moty, E., Meagher, B. R., Santana, R., Rosomoff, R. S., & Rosomoff, H. L. (1988). The utility of electromyographic biofeedback in the treatment of conversion paralysis. *American Journal of Psychiatry, 145,* 1572–1575.

Fischer-Homberger, E. (1972). Hypochondriasis of the eighteenth century—neurosis of the present century. *Bulletin in the History of Medicine, 46,* 391–401.

Fisher, G. C., Mitchell, I., & Murdoch, D. (1993). Munchausen's syndrome by proxy: The question of psychiatric illness in a child. *British Journal of Psychiatry, 162,* 701–703.

Flor-Henry, P., Fromm-Auch, D., Tapper, M., & Schopflocher, D. (1981). A neuropsychological study of the stable syndrome of hysteria. *Biologic Psychiatry, 16,* 601–626.

Folks, D. G. (1995). Munchausen's syndrome and other factitious disorders. *Neurologic Clinics, 13,* 267–281.

Folks, D. G., Ford, C. V., & Regan, W. M. (1984). Conversion symptoms in a general hospital. *Psychosomatics, 25,* 285–295.

Ford, C. V. (1986). The somatizing disorders. *Psychosomatics, 27,* 327–337.

Ford, C. V., & Folks, D. G. (1985). Conversion disorder: An overview. *Psychosomatics, 26,* 371–383.

Foreman, D. M., & Farsides, C. (1993). Ethical use of covert videotaping techniques in detecting Munchausen's syndrome by proxy. *British Journal of Psychiatry, 307,* 611–613.

Freud, S. (1956). Defense neuro-psychoses. Collected papers. London: Hogarth.

Freyberger, H., Nordmeyer, J. P., Freyberger, H. J., & Nordmeyer, J. (1994). Patients suffering from factitious disorders in the clinico-psychosomatic consultation liaison service: Psychodynamic processes, psychotherapeutic initial care and clinicointerdisciplinary cooperation. *Psychotherapy and Psychosomatics, 62,* 108–122.

Galin, D., Diamond, R., & Braff, D. (1977). Lateralization of conversion symptoms: More frequent on the left. *American Journal of Psychiatry, 134,* 578–580.

Garralda, M. E. (1996). Somatization in children. *Journal of Child Psychology and Psychiatry, 37,* 12–33.

Gatfield, P. D., & Guze, S. B. (1962). Prognosis and differential diagnosis of conversion reactions: A follow-up study. *Diseases of the Nervous System, 23,* 623–631.

Gillespie, R. O. (1928). Hypochondria: Its definition, nosology and psychopathology. *Guy's Hospital Report, 78,* 408–460.

Goldberg, D. P., & Bridges, K. (1988). Somatic presentations of psychiatric illness in primary care settings. *Journal of Psychosomatic Research, 32,* 137–144.

Goodyer, I. (1981). Hysterical conversion reactions in childhood. *Journal of Child Psychology and Psychiatry, 22,* 179–188.

Gordon, E., Kraiuhin, C., Meares, R., & Howson, A. (1986). Auditory evoked response potentials in somatization disorder. *Journal of Psychiatric Research, 20,* 237–248.

Gould, R., Miller, B. L., Goldberg, M. A., & Benson, D. F. (1986). The validity of hysterical signs and symptoms. *Journal of Nervous and Mental Disease, 174,* 593–597.

Gramling, S. E., Clawson, E. P., & McDonald, M. K. (1996). Perceptual and cognitive abnormality model of hypochondriasis: Amplification and physiological reactivity in women. *Psychosomatic Medicine, 58,* 423–431.

Gureje, O., Simon, G. E., Ustun, T. B., & Goldberg, D. B. (1997). Somatization in cross-cultural perspective: A World Health Organization study in primary care. *American Journal of Psychiatry, 154,* 989–995.

Gureje, O., Ustun, T. B., & Simon, G. E. (1997). The syndrome of hypochondriasis: A cross-national study in primary care. *Psychological Medicine, 27,* 1001–1010.

Guze, S. B. (1975). The validity and significance of the clinical diagnosis of hysteria (Briquet's syndrome). *American Journal of Psychiatry, 132,* 138–141.

Guze, S. B. (1983). Studies in hysteria. *Canadian Journal of Psychiatry, 28,* 434–437.

Guze, S. B., Cloninger, C. R., Martin, R. L., & Clayton, P. J. (1986). A follow-up and family study of Briquet's syndrome. *British Journal of Psychiatry, 149,* 17–23.

Guze, S. B., & Perley, J. J. (1963). Observation on the natural history of hysteria. *American Journal of Psychiatry, 119,* 960–965.

Guze, S. B., Tuason, V. B., Gatfield, P. D., Stewart, M. A., & Picken, B. (1962). Psychiatric illness and crime with particular reference to alcoholism: A study of 223 criminals. *Journal of Nervous and Mental Disease, 134,* 512–521.

Guze, S. B., Wolfgram, E. D., McKinney, J. K., & Cantwell, D. P. (1967). Psychiatric illness in the families of convicted criminals: A study of 519 first-degree relatives. *Disease of the Nervous System, 28,* 651–659.

Guze, S. B., Woodruff, R. A., & Clayton, P. J. (1971a). A study of conversion symptoms in psychiatric outpatients. *American Journal of Psychiatry, 128,* 643–646.

Guze, S. B., Woodruff, R. A., Jr., & Clayton, P. J. (1971b). Hysteria and antisocial behavior: Further evidence of an association. *American Journal of Psychiatry, 127,* 957–960.

Guziec, J., Lazarus, A., & Harding, J. J. (1994). Case of 29-year-old nurse with factitious disorder: The utility of psychiatric intervention on a general medical floor. *General Hospital Psychiatry, 16,* 47–53.

Haenen, M. A., Schmidt, A. J. M., Schoenmakers, M., & van den Hout, M. A. (1997). Tactual sensitivity in hypochondriasis. *Psychotherapy and Psychosomatics, 66,* 128–132.

Hafeiz, H. (1980). Hysterical conversion: A prognostic study. *British Journal of Psychiatry, 136,* 548–551.

Halliday, A. M. (1968). Computing techniques in neurological diagnosis. *British Medical Bulletin, 24,* 253–259.

Hardy, G. E. (1982). Body image disturbance in dysmorphophobia. *British Journal of Psychiatry, 141,* 181–185.

Hardy, G. E., & Cotterill, J. A. (1982). A study of depression and obsessionality in dysmorphophobic and psoriatic patients. *British Journal of Psychiatry, 140,* 19–22.

Hay, G. G. (1970a). Dysmorphophobia. *British Journal of Psychiatry, 116,* 399–406.

Hay, G. G. (1970b). Psychiatric aspects of cosmetic nasal operations. *British Journal of Psychiatry, 116,* 85–87.

Hay, G. G. (1983). Feigned psychosis—a review of the simulation of mental illness. *British Journal of Psychiatry, 143,* 8–10.

Hay, G. G., & Heather, B. B. (1973). Changes in psychometric test results following cosmetic nasal operations. *British Journal of Psychiatry, 122,* 89–90.

Hernandez-Peon, R., Chavez-Ibarra, G., & Aguilar-Figueroa, E. (1963). Somatic evoked potentials in one case of hysterical anaesthesia. *Electroencephalography and Clinical Neurophysiology, 15,* 889–892.

Hollender, E., Cohen, L. J., & Simeon, D. (1993). Body dysmorphic disorder. *Psychiatric Annals, 23,* 359–364.

Hollender, E., Neville, D., Frenkel, M., Josephson, S., & Liebowitz, M. R. (1992). Body dysmorphic disorder: Diagnostic issues and related disorders. *Psychosomatics, 33,* 156–165.

Hopkinson, G. (1973). The psychiatric syndrome of infestation. *Psychiatric Clinics, 6,* 330–345.

Hudziak, J. J., Boffeli, T. J., Kriesman, J. J., Battaglia, M. M., Stanger, C., & Guze, S. B. (1996). Clinical study of the relation of borderline personality disorder to Briquet's syndrome (hysteria), somatization disorder, antisocial personality disorder, and substance abuse disorders. *American Journal of Psychiatry, 153,* 1598–1606.

Hunter, R. C. A., Lohrenz, J. G., & Schwartzman, A. E. (1964). Nosophobia and hypochondriasis in medical students. *Journal of Nervous and Mental Disease, 139,* 147–152.

Idzorek, S. (1975). A functional classification of hypochondriasis with specific recommendations for treatment. *Southern Medical Journal, 68,* 1326–1332.

Iezzi, A., Adams, H. E., Stokes, G. S., Pilon, R. N., & Ault, L. C. (1992). An identification of low back pain groups using biobehavioral variables. *Journal of Occupational Rehabilitation, 2,* 19–33.

Iezzi, A., Stokes, G. S., Adams, H. E., Pilon, R. N., & Ault, L. C. (1994). Somatothymia in chronic pain patients. *Psychosomatics, 35,* 460–468.

Ireland, R., Sapira, J., & Templeton, B. (1967). Munchausen's syndrome. *American Journal of Medicine, 43,* 579–592.

Jacobson, W. E., Edgerton, M. T., Meyer, E., Canter, A., & Slaughter, R. (1960). Psychiatric evaluation of male patients seeking cosmetic surgery. *Plastic and Reconstructive Surgery, 26,* 350–371.

James, L., Singer, A., Zurynski, Y., Gordon, E., Kraiuhin, C., Harris, A., Howson, A., & Meares, R. (1987). Evoked response potentials and regional cerebral blood flow in somatization disorder. *Psychotherapy and Psychosomatics, 47,* 190–196.

Jani, S., White, M., Rosenberg, L. A., & Maisami, M. (1992). Munchausen syndrome by proxy. *International Journal of Psychiatry in Medicine, 22,* 343–349.

Jenike, M. A. (1984). A case report of successful treatment of dysmorphophobia with tranylcypromine. *American Journal of Psychiatry, 141,* 1463–1464.

Jones, M. M. (1980). Conversion reaction: Anachronism or evolutionary form? A review of the neurological, behavioral, and psychoanalytic literature. *Psychological Bulletin, 87,* 427–441.

Kaminsky, M. J., & Slavney, P. R. (1983). Hysterical and obsessional features in patients with Briquet's syndrome (somatization disorder). *Psychological Medicine, 13,* 111–120.

Kasher, T. M., Rost, K., Cohen, B., Anderson, M., & Smith, G. R. (1995). Enhancing the health of somatization disorder patients: Effectiveness of short-term group therapy. *Psychosomatics, 36,* 462–470.

Katon, W. (1982). Depression: Somatic symptoms and medical disorders in primary care. *Comprehensive Psychiatry, 23,* 274–287.

Katon, W. (1984). Panic disorder and somatization. *American Journal of Medicine, 77,* 101–106.

Katon, W., Kleinman, A., & Rosen, G. (1982). Depression and somatization: A review. Part I. *American Journal of Medicine, 72,* 127–135.

Katon, W., Ries, R. K., & Kleinman, A. (1984a). The prevalence of somatization in primary care. *Comprehensive Psychiatry, 25,* 208–215.

Katon, W., Ries, R. K., & Kleinman, A. (1984b). Part II: A prospective DSM-III study of 100 conservative somatization patients. *Comprehensive Psychiatry, 25,* 305–314.

Kellner, R. (1982). Psychotherapeutic strategies in hypochondriasis: A clinical study. *American Journal of Psychotherapy, 36,* 146–157.

Kellner, R. (1985). Functional somatic symptoms and hypochondriasis: A survey of empirical studies. *Archives of General Psychiatry, 42,* 821–833.

Kellner, R. (1990). Somatization. *Journal of Nervous and Mental Disease, 178,* 150–160.

Kellner, R., Abbott, P., Winslow, W. W., & Pathak, D. (1987). Fears, beliefs, and attitudes in DSM-III hypochondriasis. *Journal of Nervous and Mental Disease, 175,* 20–25.

Kendell, R. E. (1972). A new look at hysteria. *Medicine, 30,* 1780–1783.

Kent, D. A., Tomasson, K., & Coryell, W. (1995). Course and outcome of conversion and somatization disorders: A four-year follow-up. *Psychosomatics, 36,* 138–144.

Kenyon, F. E. (1964). Hypochondriasis: A clinical study. *British Journal of Psychiatry, 110,* 478–488.

Kenyon, F. E. (1965). Hypochondriasis: A survey of some historical, clinical and social aspects. *British Journal of Medical Psychology, 38,* 117–133.

Kenyon, F. E. (1976). Hypochondriacal states. *British Journal of Psychiatry, 129,* 1–14.

Kimball, C. P., & Blindt, K. (1982). Some thoughts on conversion. *Psychosomatics, 23,* 647–649.

King, S. A., & Strain, J. J. (1992). Revising the category of somatoform pain disorder. *Hospital and Community Psychiatry, 43*, 217–219.

Kinzl, J. F., Traweger, C., & Biebl, W. (1995). Family background and sexual abuse associated with somatization. *Psychotherapy and Psychosomatics, 64*, 82–87.

Kirmayer, L. J., & Robbins, J. M. (1991). Three forms of somatization in primary care: Prevalence, co-occurrence and sociodemographic characteristics. *Journal of Nervous and Mental Disease, 179*, 647–655.

Kirmayer, L. J., & Robbins, J. M. (1996). Patients who somatize in primary care: A longitudinal study of cognitive and social characteristics. *Psychological Medicine, 26*, 937–951.

Kirmayer, L. J., Robbins, J. M., & Paris, J. (1994). Somatoform disorders: Personality and social matrix of somatic distress. *Journal of Abnormal Psychology, 103*, 125–136.

Kirmayer, L. J., & Young, A. (1998). Culture and somatization: Clinical, epidemiological, and ethnographic perspectives. *Psychosomatic Medicine, 60*, 420–430.

Kreitman, N., Sainsbury, P., Pearce, K., & Costain, W. R. (1965). Hypochondriasis and depression in outpatients at a general hospital. *British Journal of Psychiatry, 3*, 607–615.

Kriechman, A. M. (1987). Siblings with somatoform disorders in childhood and adolescence. *Journal of the American Academy of Child and Adolescent Psychiatry, 26*, 226–231.

Kroenke, K., & Spitzer, R. J. (1998). Gender differences in the reporting of physical and somatoform symptoms. *Psychosomatic Medicine, 60*, 150–155.

Kroenke, K., Spitzer, R. J., deGruy, F. V., Hahn, S. R., Linzer, M., Williams, J. B., Brody, D., & Davies, M. (1997). Multisomatoform disorder: An alternative to undifferentiated somatoform disorder for the somatizing patient in primary care. *Archives of General Psychiatry, 54*, 352–358.

Kroenke, K., Spitzer, R. J., deGruy, F. W., & Swindle, R. (1998). A symptom checklist to screen for somatoform disorders in primary care. *Psychosomatics, 39*, 263–272.

Lacey, J. M., & Birtchnell, S. A. (1984). Body image and its disturbances. *Journal of Psychosomatic Research, 30*, 623–631.

Lacoursiere, R. B. (1993). Diverse motives for factitious posttraumatic stress disorder. *Journal of Traumatic Stress, 6*, 141–149.

Ladee, G. A. (1966). *Hypochondriacal syndromes*. New York: Elsevier.

Lader, M., & Sartorius, N. (1968). Anxiety in patients with hysterical conversion symptoms. *Journal of Neurology, Neurosurgery, and Psychiatry, 31*, 490–495.

Lawrie, S. M., Goodwin, G., & Masterton, G. (1993). Munchausen's syndrome and organic brain disorder. *British Journal of Psychiatry, 162*, 545–549.

Lazare, A. (1981). Current concepts in psychiatry. *New England Journal of Medicine, 305*, 745–748.

Leserman, J., Zhiming, L., Drossman, D. D., Toomey, T. C., Nachman, G., & Glogau, L. (1997). Impact of sexual and physical abuse dimensions on health status: Development of an abuse severity measure. *Psychosomatic Medicine, 59*, 152–160.

Lesse, S. (1968). Hypochondriasis and psychosomatic disorders masking depression. *American Journal of Psychotherapy, 21*, 607–620.

Levine, J. B., Brooks, J. D., Irving, K. K., & Fishman, G. G. (1994). Group therapy and the somatoform patient: An integration. *Psychotherapy, 30*, 625–634.

Levy, R., & Behrman, J. (1970). Clinical and laboratory notes: Cortical evoked responses in hysterical hemianaesthesia. *Electroencephalography and Clinical Neurophysiology, 29*, 400–402.

Levy, R., & Mushin, J. (1973). The somatosensory evoked response in patients with hysterical anaesthesia. *Journal of Psychosomatic Research, 17*, 81–84.

Lewis, W. C. (1974). Hysteria—the consultant's dilemma: Twentieth century demonology, pejorative epithet, or useful diagnosis? *Archives of General Psychiatry, 30*, 145–151.

Lewis, W. C., & Berman, M. (1965). Studies of conversion hysteria: Operational study of diagnosis. *Archives of General Psychiatry, 13*, 275–282.

Lidbeck, J. (1997). Group therapy for somatization disorders in general practice: Effectiveness of a short cognitive-behavioural treatment model. *Acta Psychiatrica Scandinavica, 96*, 14–24.

Lilienfeld, S. O. (1992). The association between antisocial personality and somatization disorders: A review and integration of theoretical models. *Clinical Psychology Review, 12*, 641–662.

Lilienfeld, S. O., Van Valkenburg, C., Larntz, K., & Akiskal, H. S. (1986). The relationship of histrionic personality disorder to antisocial personality and somatization disorders. *American Journal of Psychiatry, 143*, 718–722.

Linde, P. R. (1996). A bewitching case of factitious disorder in Zimbabwe. *General Hospital Psychiatry, 18*, 440–443.

Lipowski, Z. J. (1988). Somatization: The concept and its clinical application. *American Journal of Psychiatry, 145*, 1358–1368.

Liskow, B., Othmer, E., Penick, E. C., DeSouza, C., & Gabrielli, W. (1986). Is Briquet's Syndrome a heterogeneous disorder? *American Journal of Psychiatry, 143*, 626–629.

Livingston, R. (1987). Maternal somatization disorder and Munchausen Syndrome by proxy. *Psychosomatics, 28*, 213–217.

Livingston, R., & Martin-Cannici, C. (1985). Multiple somatic complaints and possible somatization disorder in prepubertal children. *Journal of the American Academy of Child Psychiatry, 24*, 603–607.

Livingston, R., Witt, A., & Smith, G. R. (1995). Families who somatize. *Developmental and Behavioral Pediatrics, 16*, 42–46.

Lucas, C. J., Sainsbury, P., & Collins, J. G. (1962). A social and clinical study of delusions in schizophrenia. *Journal of Mental Science, 108*, 747–758.

Ludwig, A. M. (1972). Hysteria: A neurobiological theory. *Archives of General Psychiatry, 27*, 771–777.

Luisada, P. V., Peele, R., & Pittard, E. A. (1974). The hysterical personality in men. *American Journal of Psychiatry, 131*, 518–522.

Lynn, E. J., & Belza, M. (1984). Factitious post-traumatic stress disorder: The veteran who never got to Vietnam. *Hospital and Community Psychiatry, 35*, 697–701.

MaCleod, A. K., Haynes, C., & Sensky, T. (1998). Attributions about common bodily complaints: Their associations with hypochondriasis and anxiety. *Psychological Medicine, 28*, 225–228.

Mai, F. M., & Merskey, H. (1980). Briquet's treatise on hysteria: A synopsis and commentary. *Archives of General Psychiatry, 37*, 1401–1405.

Mai, F. M., & Merskey, H. (1981). Briquet's concept of hysteria: A historical perspective. *Canadian Journal of Psychiatry, 26*, 57–63.

Maloney, J. J. (1980). Diagnosing hysterical conversion reactions in children. *Journal of Pediatrics, 97,* 1016–1020.

Manu, P., Lane, T. J., & Matthews, D. A. (1989). Somatization disorder in patients with chronic fatigue. *Psychosomatics, 30,* 388–395.

Marks, I., & Mishan, J. (1988). Dysmorphophobic avoidance with disturbed bodily perception. *British Journal of Psychiatry, 152,* 674–678.

McCauley, J., Kern, D. E., Kolodner, K., Dill, L., Schroeder, A. F., DeChant, H. K., Ryden, J., Derogatis, L. R., & Bass, E. B. (1997). Clinical characteristics of women with a history of childhood abuse: Unhealed wounds. *Journal of the American Medical Association, 277,* 1362–1368.

McCranie, E. J. (1979). Hypochondriacal neurosis. *Psychosomatics, 20,* 11–15.

McElroy, S. L., Phillips, K. A., Keck, P. E., Hudson, J. I., & Pope, H. G. (1993). Body dysmorphic disorder: Does it have a psychotic subtype? *Journal of Clinical Psychiatry, 54,* 389–395.

McKegney, F. P. (1967). The incidence and characteristics of patients with conversion reactions: I. A general hospital consultation service sample. *American Journal of Psychiatry, 124,* 542–545.

Meadow, R. (1977). Munchausen by proxy: The hinterland of child abuse. *Lancet, 2,* 343–345.

Meadow, R. (1982). Munchausen syndrome by proxy. *Archives of Disease in Childhood, 57,* 92–98.

Meadow, R. (1990). Suffocation: Recurrent apnea and sudden infant death. *Journal of Pediatrics, 117,* 351–358.

Meares, R., & Horvath, T. (1972). "Acute" and "chronic" hysteria. *British Journal of Psychiatry, 121,* 653–657.

Mechanic, D. (1962). The concept of illness behavior. *Journal of Chronic Diseases, 15,* 189–194.

Merskey, H., & Buhrich, N. A. (1975). Hysteria and organic brain disease. *British Journal of Medical Psychology, 48,* 359–366.

Meyer, E., Jacobson, W. E., Edgerton, M. T., & Canter, A. (1960). Motivational patterns in patients seeking elective plastic surgery: I. Women who seek rhinoplasty. *Psychosomatic Medicine, 3,* 193–203.

Min, S. K., & Lee, B. O. (1997). Laterality in somatization. *Psychosomatic Medicine, 59,* 236–240.

Miranda, J., Perez-Stable, E. J., Munoz, R. F., Hargreaves, W., & Henke, C. J. (1991). Somatization, psychiatric disorder, and stress in utilization of ambulatory medical services. *Health Psychology, 10,* 46–51.

Mumford, P. R. (1978). Conversion disorder. *Psychiatry Clinics of North America, 1,* 370–390.

Nadelson, T. (1979). The Munchausen spectrum: Borderline character features. *General Hospital Psychiatry, 1,* 11–17.

Nakdimen, A. (1977). A neglected reference. *American Journal of Psychiatry, 134,* 1313–1316.

Nemiah, J. C. (1985). Somatoform disorders. In H. I. Kaplan & B. J. Saddock (Eds.), *Comprehensive textbook of psychiatry,* 4th ed. (pp. 924–942). Baltimore, MD: Williams & Wilkins.

Neziroglu, F. A., & Yarura-Tobias, J. A. (1993). Exposure, response prevention, and cognitive therapy in the treatment of body dysmorphic disorder. *Behavior Therapy, 24,* 431–438.

Nickoloff, S. E., Neppe, V. M., & Ries, R. K. (1989). Factitious AIDS. *Psychosomatics, 30,* 342–345.

Noyes, R., Holt, C. S., Happel, R. C., Kathol, R. G., & Yagla, S. J. (1997). A family study of hypochondriasis. *Journal of Nervous and Mental Disease, 185,* 223–232.

Noyes, R., Kathol, R. G., Fisher, M. M., Phillips, B. M., Suelzer, M. T., & Holt, C. S. (1993). The validity of DSM-III-R hypochondriasis. *Archives of General Psychiatry, 50,* 961–970.

Noyes, R., Kathol, R. G., Fisher, M. M., Phillips, B. M., Suelzer, M. T., & Woodman, C. L. (1994a). Psychiatric comorbidity among patients with hypochondriasis. *General Hospital Psychiatry, 16,* 78–87.

Noyes, R., Kathol, R. G., Fisher, M. M., Phillips, B. M., Suelzer, M. T., & Woodman, C. L. (1994b). One-year follow-up of medical outpatients with hypochondriasis. *Psychosomatics, 35,* 533–545.

Orenstein, H. (1989). Briquet's syndrome in association with depression and panic: A reconceptualization of Briquet's Syndrome. *American Journal of Psychiatry, 146,* 334–338.

Ostfeld, B. M., & Feldman, M. D. (1996). Factitious disorder by proxy: Awareness among mental health practitioners. *General Hospital Psychiatry, 18,* 113–116.

Pankratz, L. (1981). A review of the Munchausen syndrome. *Clinical Psychology Review, 1,* 65–78.

Papageorgiou, C., & Wells, A. (1998). Effects of attention training on hypochondriasis: A brief case series. *Psychological Medicine, 28,* 193–200.

Parker, P. E. (1993). A case report of Munchausen Syndrome with mixed psychological features. *Psychosomatics, 34,* 360–364.

Parsons, T. (1951). Illness and the role of the physician: A sociological perspective. *American Journal of Orthopsychiatry, 21,* 452–460.

Perley, M. J., & Guze, S. B. (1962). Hysteria: The stability and usefulness of clinical criteria. *New England Journal of Medicine, 260,* 421–426.

Perugi, G., Akiskal, H. S., Giannotti, D., Frare, F., Di Vaio, S., & Cassano, G. B. (1997). Gender-related differences in body dysmorphic disorder (dysmorphophobia). *Journal of Mental and Nervous Disease, 185,* 578–582.

Philippopoulos, G. S. (1979). Analysis of a case of dysmorphophobia, psychopathology and psychodynamics. *Canadian Journal of Psychiatry, 24,* 397–401.

Phillips, K. A. (1995). Body dysmorphic disorder: Clinical features and drug treatment. *CNS Drugs, 3,* 30–40.

Phillips, K. A. (1996). Body dysmorphic disorder: Diagnosis and treatment of imagined ugliness. *Journal of Clinical Psychiatry, 57*(Suppl. 8), 61–65.

Phillips, K. A., & Diaz, S. F. (1997). Gender differences in body dysmorphic disorder. *Journal of Mental and Nervous Disease, 185,* 570–577.

Phillips, K. A., Kim. J. M., & Hudson, J. I. (1995). Body image in body dysmorphic disorder and eating disorders. *Psychiatric Clinics of North America, 18,* 317–333.

Phillips, K. A., McElroy, S. L., Hudson, J. I., & Pope, H. G. (1995). Body dysmorphic disorder: An obsessive-compulsive spectrum disorder, a form of affective spectrum disorder, or both? *Journal of Clinical Psychiatry, 56*(Suppl. 4), 41–51.

Phillips, K. A., McElroy, S. L., Keck, P. E., Pope, H. G., & Hudson, J. I. (1994). A comparison of delusional and non-delusional body dysmorphic disorder in 100 cases. *Psychopharmacology Bulletin, 30,* 179–186.

Pilowsky, I. (1967). Dimensions of hypochondriasis. *British Journal of Psychiatry, 113,* 89–93.

Pilowsky, I. (1970). Primary and secondary hypochondriasis. *Acta Psychiatrica Scandinavica, 46,* 273–285.

Pope, H. G., Jonas, J. M., & Jones, B. (1982). Factitious psychosis: Phenomenology, family history, and long-term outcome of nine patients. *American Journal of Psychiatry, 139,* 1480–1483.

Powell, R., & Boast, N. (1993). The million dollar man: Resource implications for chronic Munchausen's syndrome. *British Journal of Psychiatry, 162,* 253–256.

Pryse-Phillips, W. (1971). An olfactory reference syndrome. *Acta Psychiatrica Scandinavica, 47,* 484–509.

Purtell, J. J., Robins, E., & Cohen, M. E. (1951). Observations on clinical aspects of hysteria: A quantitative study of 50 hysteria patients and 156 control subjects. *Journal of the American Medical Association, 146,* 902–909.

Raskin, M., Talbott, J. A., & Meyerson, T. (1966). Diagnosis of conversion reactions. *Journal of the American Medical Association, 197,* 102–106.

Reich, P., & Gottfried, L. A. (1983). Factitious disorders in a teaching hospital. *Annals of Internal Medicine, 99,* 240–247.

Reich, T., Cloninger, C. R., & Guze, S. B. (1975). The multifactorial model of disease transmission: I. Description of the model and its use in psychiatry. *British Journal of Psychiatry, 127,* 1–10.

Rickard, K. (1988). The occurrence of maladaptive health-related conduct problems in children of chronic low back pain patients. *Journal of Behavioral Medicine, 11,* 107–115.

Riding, J., & Munro, A. (1975). Pimozide in the treatment of monosymptomatic hypochondriacal psychosis. *Acta Psychiatrica Scandinavica, 52,* 23–30.

Rief, W., Heuser, J., Mayrhuber, E., Stelzer, I., Hiller, W., & Fichter, M. M. (1996). The classification of multiple somatoform symptoms. *Journal of Nervous and Mental Disease, 184,* 680–687.

Rief, W., & Hiller, W. (1998). Somatization: Future perspectives on a common phenomenon. *Journal of Psychosomatic Research, 44,* 529–536.

Robbins, J. M., Kirmayer, L. J., & Hemami, S. (1997). Latent variable models of functional somatic distress. *Journal of Nervous and Mental Disease, 185,* 606–615.

Robins, E., & O'Neal, P. (1953). Clinical features of hysteria in children with a note on prognosis. *Nervous Child, 10,* 246–271.

Robins, L. N., Helzer, J. E., Weissman, M. M., Orvaschel, H., Gruenberg, E., Burke, J. D., Jr., & Regier, D. A. (1984). Lifetime prevalence of specific psychiatric disorders in three sites. *Archives of General Psychiatry, 41,* 949–958.

Robins, L. N., & Regier, D. (1991). *Psychiatric disorders in America: The epidemiologic catchment area study.* New York: The Free Press.

Rogers, R., Bagby, R. M., & Rector, N. (1989). Diagnostic legitimacy of factitious disorders with psychological symptoms. *American Journal of Psychiatry, 146,* 1312–1314.

Rogers, R., Bagby, R. M., & Vincent, A. (1994). Factitious disorders with predominantly psychological signs and symptoms: A conundrum for forensic experts. *Journal of Psychiatry and Law, 22,* 91–106.

Rosen, J. C. (1995). The nature of body dysmorphic disorder and treatment with cognitive behavior therapy. *Cognitive and Behavioral Practice, 2,* 142–166.

Rosen, J. C., & Reiter, J. (1996). Development of the body dysmorphic disorder examination. *Behaviour Research and Therapy, 34,* 755–766.

Rosen, J. C., Reiter, J., & Orosan, P. (1995). Cognitive-behavioral body image therapy for body dysmorphic dis-

order. *Journal of Consulting and Clinical Psychology, 63,* 263–269.

Rosenberg, D. (1987). Web of deceit: A literature review of Munchausen Syndrome by proxy. *Child Abuse and Neglect, 11,* 547–563.

Rost, K. M., Akins, R. N., Brown, F. W., & Smith, G. R. (1992). The comorbidity of DSM-III-R personality disorders in somatization disorder. *General Hospital Psychiatry, 14,* 322–326.

Roy, A. (1980). Hysteria. *Journal of Psychosomatic Research, 24,* 53–56.

Roy, M., & Roy, A. (1995). Factitious hypoglycemia: An 11-year follow-up. *Psychosomatics, 36,* 64–66.

Sakula, A. (1978). Munchausen: Fact and fiction. *Journal of the Royal College of Physicians, 12,* 286–292.

Salkovskis, P. M., & Warwick, H. M. C. (1986). Morbid preoccupations, health anxiety and reassurance: A cognitive-behavioural approach to hypochondriasis. *Behaviour Research and Therapy, 24,* 597–602.

Sanders, M. J. (1995). Symptom coaching: Factitious disorder by proxy with older children. *Clinical Psychology Review, 15,* 423–442.

Sarwer, D. B., Wadden, T. A., Pertschuk, M. J., & Whitaker, L. A. (1998). The psychology of cosmetic surgery: A review and reconceptualization. *Clinical Psychology Review, 18,* 1–22.

Schmidt, A. J. M. (1994). Bottlenecks in the diagnosis of hypochondriasis. *Comprehensive Psychiatry, 35,* 306–315.

Schreier, H. A., & Libow, J. A. (1993). Munchausen syndrome by proxy: Diagnosis and prevalence. *American Journal of Orthopsychiatry, 63,* 318–321.

Sheehan, D. V., & Sheehan, K. H. (1982). The classification of anxiety and hysterical states: Part I. Historical review and empirical delineation. *Journal of Clinical Psychopharmacology, 2,* 235–243.

Sherry, D. D., McGuire, T., Mellins, E., Salmonson, K., Wallace, C. A., & Nepom, B. (1991). Psychosomatic musculoskeletal pain in childhood: Clinical and psychological analyses of 100 children. *Pediatrics, 88,* 1093–1099.

Shipko, S. (1982). Alexithymia and somatization. *Psychotherapy and Psychosomatics, 37,* 193–201.

Siegel, M., & Barthel, R. P. (1986). Conversion disorders on a child psychiatry consultation service. *Psychosomatics, 27,* 201–204.

Sifneos, P. E. (1973). The prevalence of "alexithymic" characteristics in psychosomatic patients. *Psychotherapy and Psychosomatics, 22,* 255–262.

Sigal, M. D., Altmark, D., & Carmel, I. (1986). Munchausen syndrome by adult proxy: A perpetrator abusing two adults. *Journal of Nervous and Mental Disease, 174,* 696–698.

Sigvardsson, S., Von Knorring, A. L., Bohman, M., & Cloninger, C. R. (1984). An adoption study of somatoform disorders: I. The relationship of somatization to psychiatric disability. *Archives of General Psychiatry, 41,* 853–859.

Simeon, D., Hollender, E., Stein, D. J., Cohen, L., & Aronowitz, B. (1995). Body dysmorphic disorder in the DSM-IV field trial for obsessive-compulsive disorder. *American Journal of Psychiatry, 152,* 1207–1209.

Singh, S. P., & Lee, A. S. (1997). Conversion disorders in Nottingham: Alive, but not kicking. *Journal of Psychosomatic Research, 43,* 425–430.

Slater, E. (1965). Diagnosis of "hysteria." *British Medical Journal, 1,* 1395–1399.

Slater, E. T. O., & Glithero, E. (1965). A follow-up of patients diagnosed as suffering from "hysteria." *Journal of Psychosomatic Research, 9,* 9–13.

Smith, G. R., Monson, R. A., & Ray, D. C. (1986a). Patients with multiple unexplained symptoms. *Archives of Internal Medicine, 146,* 69–72.

Smith, G. R., Monson, R. A., & Ray, D. C. (1986b). Psychiatric consultation in somatization disorder. *New England Journal of Medicine, 314,* 1407–1413.

Songer, D. A. (1995). Factitious AIDS. A case report and literature review. *Psychosomatics, 36,* 406–411.

Southall, D. P., & Samuels, M. P. (1993). Ethical use of covert videotaping techniques in detecting Munchausen's syndrome by proxy: A response to Drs. Foreman and Samuels. *British Journal of Psychiatry, 307,* 613.

Spierings, C., Poels, P. J. E., Sijben, N., Gabreels, F. J. M., & Renier, W. O. (1990). Conversion disorders in childhood: A retrospective follow-up of 84 inpatients. *Developmental Medicine and Child Neurology, 32,* 865–871.

Spiro, H. R. (1968). Chronic factitious illness. *Archives of General Psychiatry, 18,* 569–579.

Spitzer, R. L., Endicott, J., & Robins, E. (1978). Research diagnostic criteria: Rationale and reliability. *Archives of General Psychiatry, 35,* 773–782.

Spivak, H., Rodin, G., & Sutherland, A. (1994). The psychology of factitious disorders: A reconsideration. *Psychosomatics, 35,* 25–34.

Steckel, W. (1943). *The interpretation of dreams.* New York: Liveright.

Stefansson, J. G., Messina, J. A., & Meyerowitz, S. (1976). Hysterical neurosis, conversion type: Clinical and epidemiological considerations. *Acta Psychiatrica Scandinavica, 53,* 119–138.

Stephens, J. H., & Kamp, M. (1962). On some aspects of hysteria: A clinical study. *Journal of Nervous and Mental Disease, 134,* 305–315.

Stern, D. B. (1977). Handedness and the lateral distribution of conversion reactions. *Journal of Nervous and Mental Disease, 164,* 122–128.

Stern, J., Murphy, M., & Bass, C. (1993). Personality disorders in patients with somatisation disorder: A controlled study. *British Journal of Psychiatry, 163,* 785–789.

Sussman, N. (1989). Factitious disorders. In H. I. Kaplan & B. J. Saddock (Eds.), *Comprehensive handbook of psychiatry,* 5th ed. (pp. 1136–1140). Baltimore: Williams & Wilkins.

Sutherland, A. J., & Rodin, G. M. (1990). Factitious disorders in a general hospital setting: Clinical features and a review of the literature. *Psychosomatics, 31,* 392–399.

Swartz, M., Blazer, D., George, L., & Landerman, R. (1986). Somatization disorder in a community population. *American Journal of Psychiatry, 143,* 1403–1408.

Swartz, M., Landerman, R., Blazer, D., & George, L. (1989). Somatization symptoms in the community: A rural/urban comparison. *Psychosomatics, 30,* 44–53.

Taylor, S., & Hyler, S. (1993). Update on factitious disorders. *International Journal of Psychiatry in Medicine, 23,* 81–94.

Terre, L., & Ghiselli, W. (1997). A developmental perspective on family risk factors in somatization. *Journal of Psychosomatic Research, 42,* 197–208.

Thomas, C. S. (1984). Dysmorphophobia: A question of definition. *British Journal of Psychiatry, 144,* 513–516.

Tomasson, K., Kent, D., & Coryell, W. (1991). Somatization and conversion disorders: Comorbidity and demographics at presentation. *Acta Psychiatrica Scandinavica, 36,* 138–144.

Toth, E. L., & Baggaley, A. (1991). Coexistence of Munchausen's syndrome and multiple personality disorder: Detailed report of a case and theoretical discussion. *Psychiatry, 54,* 176–183.

Trask, P. C., & Sigmon, S. T. (1997). Munchausen syndrome: A review and new conceptualization. *Clinical Psychology: Science and Practice, 4,* 346–358.

van der Kolk, B. A., Pelcovitz, D., Roth, S., Mandel, F. S., McFarlane, A., & Herman, J. L. (1996). Dissociation, somatization, and affect regulation: The complexity of adaptation to trauma. *American Journal of Psychiatry, 153,* 83–93.

Veale, D., Boocock, A., Gournay, K., Dryden, W., Shah, F., Willson, R., & Walburn, J. (1996). Body dysmorphic disorder: A survey of fifty cases. *British Journal of Psychiatry, 169,* 196–201.

Veale, D., Gournay, K., Dryden, W., Boocock, A., Shah, F., Willson, R., & Walburn, J. (1996). Body dysmorphic disorder: A cognitive-behavioural model and pilot randomised controlled trial. *Behaviour Research and Therapy, 34,* 717–729.

Viederman, M. (1995). Metaphor and meaning in conversion disorder: A brief active therapy. *Psychosomatic Medicine, 57,* 403–409.

Volkmar, F. R., Poll, J., & Lewis, M. (1984). Conversion reactions in childhood and adolescence. *Journal of the American Academy of Child Psychiatry, 23,* 424–430.

Walker, L. S., Garber, J., & Zeman, J. W. (1991). Somatic complaints in pediatric patients: A prospective study of the role of negative life events, child social and academic competence, and parental somatic symptoms. *Journal of Consulting and Clinical Psychology, 62,* 1213–1221.

Walker, E. A., Keegan, D., Gardner, G., Sullivan, M., Bernstein, D., & Katon, W. J. (1997). Psychosocial factors in fibromyalgia compared with rheumatoid arthritis: II. Sexual, physical, and emotional abuse and neglect. *Psychosomatic Medicine, 59,* 572–577.

Walker, E. A., Keegan, D., Gardner, G., Sullivan, M., Katon, W. J., & Bernstein, D. (1997). Psychosocial factors in fibromyalgia compared with rheumatoid arthritis: I. Psychiatric diagnoses and functional disability. *Psychosomatic Medicine, 59,* 565–571.

Warren, A., Sutherland, A. J., & Lenz, R. (1994). Factitious hermaphroditism. *Psychosomatics, 35,* 578–581.

Warwick, H. M. C. (1995). Assessment of hypochondriasis. *Behaviour Research and Therapy, 33,* 845–853.

Warwick, H. M. C., Clark, D. M., Cobb, A. M., & Salkovskis, P. M. (1996). A controlled trial of cognitive-behavioural treatment of hypochondriasis. *British Journal of Psychiatry, 169,* 189–195.

Warwick, H. M. C., & Salkovskis, P. M. (1990). Hypochondriasis. *Behaviour Research and Therapy, 28,* 105–117.

Watson, C. G., & Buranen, C. (1979). The frequency and identification of false positive conversion reactions. *Journal of Nervous and Mental Disease, 167,* 243–247.

Watson, D., & Pennebaker, J. W. (1989). Health complaints, stress, and distress: Exploring the central role of negative affectivity. *Psychology Review, 96,* 234–254.

Wells, A. (1990). Panic disorder in association with relaxation induced anxiety: An attentional training approach to treatment. *Behaviour Therapy, 21,* 273–280.

Whitlock, F. A. (1967). The aetiology of hysterical. *Acta Psychiatrica Scandinavica, 43,* 144–162.

Wickramasekera, I. (1989). Somatizers, the health care system, and collapsing the psychological distance that the somatizer has to travel for help. *Professional Psychology: Research and Practice, 20*, 105–111.

Wickramasekera, I., Pope, A. T., & Kolm, P. (1996). On the interaction of hypnotizability and negative affect in chronic pain: Implications for the somatization of trauma. *Journal of Nervous and Mental Disease, 184*, 628–635.

Wilhelm, S., Otto, M. W., Zucker, B. G., & Pollack, M. H. (1997). Prevalence of body dysmorphic disorder in patients with anxiety disorders. *Journal of Anxiety Disorders, 11*, 499–502.

Woerner, P. I., & Guze, S. B. (1968). A family and marital study of hysteria. *British Journal of Psychiatry, 114*, 161–168.

Woods, S. M., Natterson, J., & Silverman, J. (1976). Medical student's disease: Hypochondriasis in medical education. *Journal of Medical Education, 41*, 785–790.

Yutzy, S. H., Cloninger, R., Guze, S. B., Pribor, E. F., Martin, R. L., Kathol, R. G., Smith, G. R., & Strain, J. J. (1995). DSM-IV field trial: Testing a new proposal for somatization disorder. *American Journal of Psychiatry, 152*, 97–101.

Ziegler, F. J., & Imboden, J. B. (1962). Contemporary conversion reactions. II. A conception model. *Archives of General Psychiatry, 6*, 37–45.

Ziegler, F. J., Imboden, J. B., & Meyer, E. (1960). Contemporary conversion reactions: I. A clinical study. *American Journal of Psychiatry, 116*, 901–909.

Ziegler, F. J., Imboden, J. B., & Rodgers, D. A. (1963). Contemporary conversion reactions: III. Diagnostic considerations. *Journal of the American Medical Association, 186*, 91–95.

# CHAPTER 10

# Dissociative Disorders

## John F. Kihlstrom

## Introduction

In current diagnostic nosology, the category of dissociative disorders includes a wide variety of syndromes whose common core is an alteration in consciousness that affects memory and identity (American Psychiatric Association [APA], 1994). In *dissociative amnesia* (formerly, psychogenic amnesia), the patient suffers a loss of autobiographical memory for certain past experiences; in *dissociative fugue* (psychogenic fugue), the amnesia is much more extensive and covers the whole of the individual's past life; and it is coupled with a loss of personal identity and, often, physical movement to another location; in *dissociative identity disorder* (multiple personality disorder), a single individual appears to manifest two or more distinct identities; each personality alternates in control over conscious experience, thought, and action and is separated by some degree of amnesia from the other(s); in *depersonalization disorder*, the person believes that he or she has changed in some way, or is somehow unreal (in *derealization* the same beliefs are held about one's surroundings).

Impairments of memory and consciousness are often observed in the organic brain syndromes, but dissociative disorders are functional: they are attributable to instigating events or processes that do not result in insult, injury, or disease to the brain, and produce more impairment than would normally occur in the absence of this instigating event or process (Kihlstrom & Schacter, 2000). Dissociative disorders are rather rare, but for more than 100 years, these and related phenomena have been objects of fascination for clinicians and experimentalists alike (for other recent reviews, see Bremner & Marmar, 1998; Kihlstrom, Tataryn, & Hoyt, 1993; Klein & Doane, 1994; Lynn & Rhue, 1994; Michaelson & Ray, 1996; Ross, 1997; Spiegel, 1991, 1994).

Once considered exotic, in the 1990s, dissociative disorders have become the syndromes of the moment. In March 1999, a search of the PsycINFO database revealed forty entries on psychogenic or dissociative amnesia; twenty-eight of them (70%) had appeared since the prior edition of this chapter was completed in 1990; there was also a total of eight entries on psychogenic or dissociative fugue, five of which (63%) had appeared in that same period. Multiple personality, or dissociative identity disorder, the crown jewel of dissociative disorders, yielded 868 entries: more than half of these (485, or 56%) appeared since 1990, and 708 (82%) had appeared since the first edition of this handbook was published in 1984. Remarkably, however, little of this literature consists of quantitative clinical studies, much less experimental research. Thus, the enormous amount of clinical and popular interest in dissociative disorders has not yet translated into a substantial body of research.

John F. Kihlstrom • Department of Psychology, University of California, Berkeley, California 94720-1650.

*Comprehensive Handbook of Psychopathology* (Third Edition), edited by Patricia B. Sutker and Henry E. Adams. Kluwer Academic / Plenum Publishers, New York, 2001.

## The Evolution of a Concept

The term "dissociative disorder" is almost unique in the psychiatric nosology because the label also implies a specific mechanism, dissociation, to account for the disturbances observed. Other category labels, such as schizophrenia, anxiety disorders, and personality disorders carry no such surplus etiologic baggage. The origins of the idea of dissociation lie in a body of medical and scientific literature that emerged from 1775 to 1900 and represents what Ellenberger (1970) called the "First Dynamic Psychiatry." The first dynamic psychiatrists were interested in a wide spectrum of phenomena, including hypnosis and other forms of suggestion; spiritism (automatic writing, crystal-gazing); the "magnetic diseases" of catalepsy, lethargy, and somnambulism (so named because of their resemblance to certain phenomena of animal magnetism, a precursor of hypnosis); ambulatory automatisms (fugue); multiple personality; and hysterical anesthesias and paralyses. Each of these phenomena reflected the power of ideas to engender action, as well as a change in consciousness in which experience, thought, and action occurred outside of phenomenal awareness and voluntary control. The pathological forms, such as hysteria and multiple personality, were "dynamic illnesses," caused by a suggestion or idea whose origins lay in some psychological trauma whose nature was unknown to the victim. As a result of this trauma, certain experiences, thoughts, and actions become separated from the monitoring and controlling function of a central executive ego.

The dominant figure in the First Dynamic Psychiatry was Pierre Janet (1889, 1907), who identified the elementary structures of the mental system as "psychological automatisms." Each automatism represented a complex act, finely tuned to external (environmental) and internal (intrapsychic) circumstances, preceded by an idea, and accompanied by an emotion. According to Janet, the normal person's entire repertoire of elementary psychological automatisms was bound together into a single, united stream of consciousness, accessible to introspective phenomenal awareness and voluntary control. However, under certain circumstances, one or more automatisms could be split off from the rest, thus functioning outside of awareness, independent of voluntary control, or both—a condition which Janet labeled *desaggre-*

*gation*, translated into English as dissociation. The dissociation view of the unconscious, as distinct from the repression view elaborated by Freud and his followers, was endorsed by William James (1890/1980; Taylor, 1982, 1996), and promoted in America by Morton Prince and Boris Sidis, among others.

The dissociative conceptualization of consciousness was briefly popular, but the claims of the dissociation theorists were often overly broad, and their clinical and experimental studies often methodologically flawed. In the clinic, the Second Dynamic Psychiatry of Freud and his followers, with its emphasis on sex and aggression, dreams and repression, soon triumphed over the First. In the laboratory, the behaviorist revolution banished all reference to mental states, conscious or not, from the vocabulary of scientific discourse. After World War II, however, interest in consciousness—attention, primary memory, and imagery—was revived in the course of the cognitive revolution. The concept of dissociation and the dissociative disorders played a role in this revival, as indicated by Hilgard's (1977; see also Kihlstrom, 1992, 1998) "neodissociation" theory of divided consciousness.

Neodissociation theory assumes that the mind is organized as a system of mental structures that monitor and control experience, thought, and action in different domains. In principle, each of the structures can process inputs and outputs independently of the others, although under ordinary circumstances each structure is in communication with the others, and several different structures might compete for a single input or output channel. At the center of the system, yet another structure exercises executive functions of monitoring and control and provides the mental basis for the experience of phenomenal awareness and voluntary control. According to Hilgard, the operations of the central executive can be constrained, and the integration and organization of the individual control structures can be disrupted, producing a state of divided consciousness. For example, the lines of communication between two subordinate structures might be cut. The operations of each would be represented in phenomenal awareness and perceived as under voluntary control, but they would not be integrated with each other. Alternatively, the links between a subordinate structure and the executive might be cut. Under these circumstances, the operations of the subordinate would be isolated from phenomenal awareness and the experience of intentionality—a classic instance of dissociation.

Whereas both the classical dissociation theory of Janet (1889) and the neodissociation theory of Hilgard (1977; Kihlstrom, 1992) assume that the normal unity of consciousness is disrupted by an amnesia-like process, Woody and Bowers (1994) offered an alternative view that many mental and behavioral functions are performed unconsciously and automatically to begin with, by specialized cognitive modules. Thus, some degree of dissociation is the natural state. Rather than reflecting the imposition of an amnesic barrier, the phenomena of dissociation reflect the failure of these modules to be integrated at higher levels of the system (e.g., by executive control structures associated with the frontal lobes). Currently, the distinction between dissociated experience and dissociated control is debated chiefly in the literature on hypnosis (Kihlstrom, 1998; Kirsch & Lynn, 1998; Woody & Sadler, 1998), but the two competing formulations of neodissociation theory are clearly relevant to the dissociative disorders as well.

## The Evolution of a Diagnosis

Dissociative disorders have a somewhat checkered history in the *Diagnostic and Statistical Manual of Mental Disorders* (DSM) periodically published by the American Psychiatric Association (Kihlstrom, 1994). In the first edition of DSM (DSM-I; APA, 1952) dissociative syndromes were classified as Psychoneurotic Disorders, in which anxiety is either "directly felt and expressed or ... unconsciously and automatically controlled" by various defense mechanisms" (p. 32). Under this label, the dissociative syndromes included depersonalization, dissociated (multiple) personality, stupor, fugue, amnesia, dream states, and somnambulism. Precursors to DSM-I had grouped the dissociative and conversion disorders under the single rubric of "conversion hysteria," but the two subclasses were now distinguished—dissociation by personality disorganization; conversion by isolated symptoms of anesthesia, paralysis, and dyskinesia. (DSM-I also carried a special listing of somnambulism, but this apparently referred specifically to sleepwalking.) The DSM-I conceptualization of the dissociative disorders was heavily influenced by psychoanalytic theory, as evidenced by its reference to the discharge or deflection of repressed impulses.

In some respects, DSM-II (APA, 1968) reverted to pre-DSM practices. Here, Hysterical Neurosis, Dissociative Type, defined as an alteration in consciousness and identity, was joined by Hysterical Neurosis, Conversion Type, defined as a disorder of the special senses or the voluntary nervous system. Hysterical neurosis itself was characterized in psychoanalytic terms of the unconscious and automatic control of anxiety. However, explicit references to repression and the psychoanalytic theory of neurosis were absent from the description.

DSM-III (APA, 1980) and its revision, DSM-III-R (APA, 1987), abandoned both neurosis and hysteria as technical terms. The class of Dissociative Disorders included Psychogenic Amnesia, Psychogenic Fugue, Multiple Personality Disorder (MPD), and Depersonalization Disorder—as well as Atypical Dissociative Disorder. Conversion Disorder, by contrast, was grouped with Body Dismorphic Disorder, Hypochondriasis, Somatization Disorder, and Somatoform Pain Disorder, under the heading of Somatoform Disorders. DSM-III-R stated that the essential feature of the dissociative disorders was "a disturbance in the normally integrative functions of identity, memory, or consciousness ..." in the absence of brain insult, injury, or disease. In the case of Psychogenic Amnesia, the essential feature is, of course, loss of memory. Psychogenic Fugue added the assumption of a new identity, as well as physical relocation away from the customary home or workplace. Somewhat surprisingly, however, the DSM-III-R criterion for Multiple Personality Disorder specified only the alternating control of behavior by at least two distinct personalities, permitted making the diagnosis on the basis of personality fragments rather than complex, integrated structures, and made no reference to interpersonality amnesia. Thus, the DSM-III-R criterion was rather liberal because it diagnosed patients who formerly might qualify only for Atypical Dissociative Disorder as instances of full-blown MPD. This liberal diagnostic criterion may account for some of the increased reporting of MPD in the 1980s and 1990s.

This situation was corrected, to some degree, in DSM-IV (APA, 1994), which returned an explicit criterion of amnesia to the diagnostic criteria for Multiple Personality Disorder, which was also renamed Dissociative Identity Disorder (DID). Thus, it is not enough simply to find evidence of two or more "ego states" in the same person—a likely factor in the recent proliferation of the diagnosis. Some evidence of amnesia is also required, although the criterion does not specify interpersonality amnesia. Cases resembling DID, but without amnesia, are removed to the new category of "Dissociative Disorder Not Otherwise Specified" (DDNOS)—a category that also covers derealization in the absence of depersonalization and trance states such as *amok* and *latah*. DSM-IV also strengthens the emphasis, in diagnosing psychogenic fugue, on changes in personal identity, whether the loss of an old one or the assumption of a new one.

## Dissociative (Psychogenic) Amnesia

Dissociative amnesia, also known as limited functional amnesia (Schacter & Kihlstrom, 1999), entails a loss of personal memory that cannot be accounted for by ordinary forgetting or by brain insult, injury, or disease (for other reviews, see Arrigo & Pezdek, 1997; Kopelman, 1995, 1997; Loewenstein, 1996; Pratt, 1977; Kihlstrom & Schacter, 2000; Stengel, 1966). The amnesia is typically retrograde, in that it covers a period of time before the precipitating event, although Janet (1893) did describe an unusual case of *anterograde* psychogenic amnesia, in which memory before the trauma remained intact, but the patient showed an inability, reminiscent of that observed in the organic amnesic syndrome, to remember events that transpired *since* the traumatic event. Nemiah (1979) distinguished three forms of psychogenic amnesia, depending on its extent: localized, covering hours or weeks; systematized, covering only specific events and related material; and generalized, involving a transitory loss of memory for one's entire life—a condition that shades into psychogenic fugue.

Although dissociative amnesia, by definition, is not caused by brain insult, injury, or disease, the relationship between the syndrome and brain injury is better characterized as one of independence. Brain injury can occur without amnesia as one of its sequelae, and functional amnesia can occur in association with head injury (Treadwell, Cohen, & McCloskey, 1988). Although psycho-

genic amnesia has been the frequent subject of popular treatments, there has been very little research on the nature of the memory loss, its eliciting conditions, and the circumstances that lead to recovery of the lost memories (Kihlstrom & Schacter, 2000). Even Janet (1907) barely mentioned psychogenic amnesia outside of the context of somnambulism, fugue, and multiple personality. One important question for future research, especially in a forensic context, concerns the symptoms that differentiate organic and functional amnesias (Kopelman, 1995). Such information, in turn, would permit conclusions about the extent to which functional, psychogenic amnesias are misdiagnosed as organic amnesias, simply because they occur in temporal association with head injury.

## Dissociative (Psychogenic) Fugue

Somewhat more is known about psychogenic fugue, also called functional retrograde amnesia (for reviews see Kopelman, 1997; Loewenstein, 1996; Pratt, 1977; Kihlstrom & Schacter, 2000; Stengel, 1966). Fugue adds a loss of identity to the loss of personal memory observed in psychogenic amnesia and sometimes physical relocation (hence the name), to boot. Fugue is often associated with physical or mental trauma, depression, problems with the legal system, or some other personal difficulty (Eisen, 1989; Kaszniak, Nussbaum, Berren, & Santiago, 1988).

Fisher (1945; Fisher & Joseph, 1949) distinguished three types of fugues. In the classic instance, there is amnesia for personal history, accompanied by a change in identity and relocation to another domicile. Fugue may also entail amnesia accompanied by the simple loss, but no change, in personal identity. Finally, a reversion to an earlier period in one's own life may occur, with an amnesia for the interval between that earlier period and the present, but no change in identity. Clearly, the distinction between psychogenic fugue and psychogenic amnesia is difficult to make. One might say that fugues are simply very generalized amnesias, but the loss of identity that is pathognomic of fugue may be a qualitative difference.

The process of recovery from fugue is not well understood. Patients typically come to clinical attention when they become spontaneously aware of the situation or when they fail to respond appropriately to specific questions about their background when questioned by the police, potential employers, or others. Some patients experience a sudden awakening to their original identity; others experience a sudden awareness that they do not know who they are. Nevertheless, when the situation is resolved, the patient is typically left with an island of amnesia that covers the period of the fugue state itself.

Although many clinical reports of psychogenic fugue exist, apparently only a single case has been subjected to controlled, experimental analysis. Schacter, Wang, Tulving, and Friedman (1982) performed such an analysis on a case, P.N., whose condition was apparently precipitated by the death of his grandfather. The boundaries of the amnesia were explored by the "Crovitz–Robinson" technique (Crovitz & Shiffman, 1974; Robinson, 1976), in which common words are presented as cues for retrieving conceptually related autobiographical memories. When tested during the fugue state, 86% of the patient's memories were drawn from the period covered by the fugue—a stronger recency bias than is normally observed in such situations. Two weeks later, after the amnesia had remitted, fully 92% of the memories predated the amnesia (the lack of recency bias thus reflected an amnesia for the fugue itself). By contrast, when asked to identify pictures of famous people, the patient performed equally well during and after the amnesia. Such findings were interpreted by Schacter et al. (1982) as reflecting a selective impairment in episodic memory which spares semantic memory. However, it should be noted that semantic memory includes aspects of personal identity—one's name, birthdate, physical and psychosocial characteristics, the names of family members, etc., as well as impersonal world knowledge (Kihlstrom & Klein, 1994, 1997). Fugue impairs semantic memory for personal information, as well as episodic memory for personal experiences.

## Dissociative Identity (Multiple Personality) Disorder

Dissociative identity disorder (DID) takes the disruption of memory and identity observed in dissociative fugue one step further because there is an alternation of both memory and identity (for

recent reviews see Bliss, 1986; Putnam, 1989; Ross, 1997). When one ego state is in control of thought and action and is monitoring environmental events, memory is continuous within that ego state. However, when monitoring and control shift to another ego state, the new personality may have no access to memories of the activities and experiences of the other(s). However, some degree of cooperation is possible among ego states, when one has information or resources that the other one needs.

On the basis of their review of seventy-six named (mostly classic) cases, Taylor and Martin (1944) listed a number of features that distinguish the various ego states:

1. the "general quality" of the personality, as a whole;
2. propriety of behavior;
3. gender identity or erotosexual orientation;
4. age, handedness, or language differences; and
5. anesthesia in one or more sensory modalities, or paralysis in one or more limbs.

About two-thirds of the cases studied by Taylor and Martin were dual personalities, and about half of them showed a pattern of mutual or symmetrical amnesia. Of the remainder, most displayed only three personalities and a more complex pattern of asymmetrical amnesia. Ellenberger (1970) classified DID into three major categories: (1) successive multiple personalities, the usual case, with either symmetrical or asymmetrical amnesias (Ellenberger thought that "mutually cognizant" alter egos were infrequent); (2) simultaneous multiple personalities, very rare; and (3) personality clusters.

However, it is by no means a straightforward matter to discern which ego state, if any, is "primary." Following the example of Eve (Thigpen & Cleckley, 1954) and perhaps influenced by the psychoanalytic concept of the repression of conflict-laden ideas, drives, affects, and impulses, there is some tendency to identify the primary personality with the ego-state that displays the most conventional, socially desirable qualities. However, Taylor and Martin (1944) argued that there was no clear pattern of "normality" or "pathology" that distinguishes the primary personality from the alter egos; sometimes, a normally subconscious personality is better adjusted than a normally conscious one. In most cases, it may be convenient to assign the label "primary" to the ego state that is most frequently encountered or has the longest running identity. In the case of I.C. (Schacter, Kihlstrom, Canter Kihlstrom, & Berren, 1989), the pattern of memory deficit observed strongly suggested that the "primary" personality, defined in terms of frequency of encounter and degree of familiarity to other people, was actually an alter ego who first appeared when the patient was about 10 years old.*

## The History of DID

The formal history of DID reaches back more than 200 years to the very beginnings of modern medical literature (Carlson, 1981, 1989).† What might be called a "classic period" for the study of DID extended from about 1880 to 1920, as reflected in the well-known reports of Azam, Janet, Prince, Sidis, and others. Of the seventy-six named cases covered by Taylor and Martin (1944) in their exhaustive review of the published literature, fifty-one (67%) were first reported during this period, and the vast majority of the rest shortly before or after it. Almost two decades later, Sutcliffe and Jones (1962) added only a single acceptable case, the "Three Faces of Eve" (Thigpen & Cleckley, 1954).

Case reports of DID fell off rapidly in the half-

century following 1920, a trend that may be attributable in part to the triumph of Freud over Janet, and in part to increased diagnosis of schizophrenia. Then, they took a sharp upward turn beginning around 1970—a trend that may be attributable in large part to the publication of *Sybil* in the popular press (Schreiber, 1973).‡ A literal avalanche of case reports followed that appeared in both the popular and professional press (Boor, 1982; Greaves, 1980; Kihlstrom et al., 1993). For example, a mail survey of selected clinicians identified 100 cases currently or recently in treatment as of 1982 (Putnam, Guroff, Silberman, Barban, & Post, 1986).

In the 1970s alone, at least by a liberal count, more cases of DID were reported than in all of the time since Mary Reynolds. Ross (1997) wrote that between 1979 and 1991 he saw "about 80" (p. 256) cases of DID in his practice in Winnipeg, Manitoba, and that between 1991 and 1997 more than 500 cases had been admitted to a single dissociative disorder treatment unit in Dallas, Texas. As if that were not enough, there has been a dramatic increase in the number of alter egos manifested in the individual case. The vast majority of cases listed by Taylor and Martin (1944)—forty-eight, or 63%—presented dual personalities, and only one case presented as many as twelve alter egos. By contrast, the majority of new cases listed by Greaves (1980) and Boor (1982) had three or more personalities, and the cases registered by Putnam et al. (1986) presented 13.3. Ross (1997) reported an average of 15.7 alter egos in a series of 236 patients.

The degree to which some of these cases are iatrogenic, or simply misdiagnosed, remains to be seen (Fahy, 1988). It is worth remembering that even in the heyday of multiple personality, around the turn of the century, when clinicians were very alert to the possibility of new cases, very few were actually diagnosed: even Janet and Prince described only four cases each (Taylor & Martin, 1944). And despite hundreds of referrals, Thigpen and Cleckley (1984) saw only one other case after Eve.

---

*Although DID is usually considered a syndrome of adult psychopathology, the fact that alter egos may begin to appear in childhood suggests that it can be diagnosed and treated in children as well (Main & Morgan, 1996; Putnam, 1997).

†The best known of the earliest cases is Mary Reynolds, reported by Mitchill (1816; see Carlson, 1984). Ellenberger (1970) cited this case on the basis of secondary reports by S. W. Mitchell (1888) and others. However, he was unable to locate the primary reference, attributed to the *Medical Repository* of 1815. A diligent search of the library shelves by Dr. Malcolm Macmillan, now of Deakin University, Australia, turned up the primary reference in the 1816 volume (Mitchill, 1816), as correspondence dated that year. The 1816 and 1817 volumes were bound together, which may explain why Taylor and Martin (1944) provided the correct volume and page number, but dated the article 1817. Ellenberger also misspells Samuel Latham Mitchill's last name, and incorrectly identifies him with John Kearsley Mitchell, father of Silas Weir Mitchell (1888), who knew the Reynolds family and brought the case to the attention of William James (1890, pp. 359–363). I thank Dr. Macmillan for his kindness in sharing his detective work and refer readers to his important historical work on the relationship between Freud and Janet (e.g., Macmillan, 1996). For a further history of the Mary Reynolds case, see also Carlson (1981, 1984, 1989). For a history of another famous case, Miss Beauchamp, see Rosenzweig (1987, 1988).

‡This claim has been made by Putnam (1989), Borch-Jacobson (1997), and Acocella (1998), among others. (For a description of the impact of this case on a DID patient, see Atwood, 1978). Interestingly, Herbert Spiegel, a Columbia University psychiatrist and distinguished hypnosis researcher who examined Sybil and also occasionally served as her surrogate therapist, has expressed doubts that she was a genuine case of multiple personality (Borch-Jacobson, 1997).

## Laboratory Studies

In view of the virtual avalanche of cases reported in both the professional and popular press since 1973, it is especially surprising that so few cases have been subject to controlled experimental analysis employing laboratory procedures. During the classic period, Prince and Sidis reported a number of studies of perception, reasoning, free association, and psychophysiology (for a review, see Kihlstrom et al., 1993). Later, Osgood and Luria (1954) and Osgood, Luria, Jeans, and Smith (1976; see also Kroonenberg, 1985) reported on blind analyses of semantic differential protocols collected from various personalities. The recent revival of interest in DID has yielded a number of psychometric studies that employed both projective and objective instruments (for a review, see Kihlstrom et al., 1993), but experimental studies have been somewhat rarer.

A salient exception to this rule is the case of Jonah, a man with three (perhaps four) alter egos, studied by Ludwig and his associates (Brandsma & Ludwig, 1974; Ludwig, Brandsma, Wilbur, Bendfeldt, & Jameson, 1972). Each of the four principal alter egos was administered a battery of personality and intelligence tests (including the MMPI and the Gough Adjective Check List, and the WAIS), a number of learning and memory tasks (including paired-associate learning and prose memory), conditioning, and psychophysiological recordings (including electrodermal responses, EEG, and event-related potentials). Another study employed experiential time sampling to document state changes in a woman vulnerable to extremely rapid alterations of personality (Lowenstein, Hamilton, Alagna, Reid, & deVries, 1987). Schacter et al. (1989) used the "Crovitz–Robinson" technique to study I.C., a case of DID with a very extensive childhood amnesia, compared to a carefully matched control group. Unfortunately, these investigators were not able to study autobiographical memory in any of the alter egos, although such an experimental case study was recently reported by Bryant (1995).

Further experimental study of DID is warranted because, although this syndrome is defined in DSM-IV as a disorder of identity and the integration of self, it is also fundamentally a disorder of memory. In every dissociative disorder, patients are unable to recollect some or all of their past actions and experiences, and in DID, an interpersonality amnesia reflects the inability of one alter ego to consciously recall the activities and experiences of others. However, there is more to memory than what the individual can bring to awareness, and there is evidence that memory of these forgotten events may influence the patient's ongoing experience, thought, and action outside of conscious awareness. In fact, as indicated earlier, clinical observation of such influences were the reason for the notion of "dissociation" in the first place.

In modern terminology, dissociative disorders may involve a dissociation between two expressions of memory, explicit and implicit (Schacter, 1987). Explicit memory refers to the person's conscious, intentional recollection of some previous episode, most commonly reflected in recall and recognition. Implicit memory, or memory without awareness, is reflected in any change in the person's experience, thought, or action which is attributable to some prior episode of experience, but which cannot be accounted for by explicit memory for that event. Dissociations between explicit and implicit memory are a common feature of the "organic" amnesias associated with brain insult, injury, or disease (Shimamura, 1989) and are found in the "functional" amnesias associated with dissociative disorders as well (Kihlstrom & Schacter, 2000).

Although hints of implicit memory are found in some of the earliest cases of DID, the first formal demonstration along these lines was reported in the case of Jonah (Ludwig et al., 1972), who was completely unaware of his three other alter egos. To document the pattern of interpersonality amnesia apparent on clinical examination and history, Ludwig et al. conducted various studies of verbal learning, classical conditioning, transfer of training, and learning-to-learn. For example, Jonah could not recall paired associates learned by the other personalities; and although the others could recall items learned by Jonah, they could not recall items learned by each other. However, when one alter ego was asked to learn (rather than remember) a list of paired associates initially mastered by another, each showed considerable savings. Thus, there was transfer of information between personalities on the paired-associate learning test, but not on the paired-associate recall test.

The dissociation between explicit and implicit memory observed by Ludwig et al. (1972) was further explored by Nissen, Ross, Willingham, Mackenzie, and Schacter (1988), who performed a careful comparison between explicit and implicit memory in a single DID patient who had twenty-two different alter egos. On each test, items were presented to one alter ego, and memory for these items was tested in another; a total of eight personalities, each separated from the others by an amnesic boundary, were tested in the experiment. On two tests of explicit memory, cued recall and yes-no recognition, each ego state showed a dense amnesia for items presented to the others—in other words, there was no interpersonality transfer of explicit memory. The corresponding tests of implicit memory, however, yielded complex results: five tasks yielded some evidence of interpersonality transfer, but four others gave no evidence that implicit memory transferred between alter egos. Moreover, on some tasks there was less implicit memory between alter egos than within a single personality, indicating that even implicit memory sometimes failed to cross the amnesic barrier.

Recently, Eich and his colleagues reported a nomothetic comparison of explicit and implicit memory in nine DID patients (Eich, Macaulay, Loewenstein, & Dihle, 1997). As in Nissen et al.'s (1988) case study, free recall and cued recall tests of explicit memory yielded strong evidence of interpersonality amnesia that confirmed the clinical picture. However, a test of picture-fragment completion indicated that implicit memory was spared, but a test of word-stem completion did not. On the latter task, implicit memory was displayed only within, not between, alter egos. Eich et al. concluded that although tests of implicit memory could reveal transfer of information from one alter ego to another, "how much leakage occurs across personality states depends on the extent to which encoding and retrieval processes are susceptible to personality-specific factors" (p. 421). It would be tempting to conclude that implicit memory transfers across ego-state boundaries in DID, and explicit memory does not, but the actual pattern of results is somewhat more complex than this and remains to be clarified by further research.

A more recent development, reflecting the increased interest in biological processes in psychopathology generally, has been the use of brain-imaging techniques such as EEG frequency analysis and event-related potentials (for a review, see Kihlstrom et al., 1993). Putnam (1984) presented a preliminary report of a study of eleven DID patients and ten simulating controls that successfully distinguished the two groups on the basis of event-related potentials. Within subjects, genuine alter egos showed greater differences in amplitude and latency than simulated ones. Mathew, Jack, & West (1985) reported a shift in regional cerebral blood flow (toward the right temporal lobe) in one patient, but there have been no similar studies employing PET or fMRI technologies. Given the enormous amount of interest in dissociative identity disorder, it is remarkable that these intriguing findings have not been followed up by studies using more rigorous methodologies that might reveal the biological substrates of amnesia, fugue, and multiple personality.

## Sociocultural Influences

Some of the most difficult aspects of the current DID "epidemic" are the loosening of diagnostic criteria, the influence of popular culture (in the late nineteenth century, Stevenson's *Dr. Jekyll and Mr. Hyde*; in the late twentieth century, the cases of Eve and Sybil themselves) on patient and therapist alike, the investment that some clinicians seem to have in the syndrome, and the recent proliferation of cases with extremely large numbers of alter egos. Another troublesome aspect is the apparently common practice of eliciting alter egos through hypnosis, instead of observing them emerge spontaneously. Because the hypnotic interaction itself is highly suggestive, hypnosis affords an especially good opportunity to create alter egos out of whole cloth and for their nature to be shaped by the hypnotist's suggestions and other cues and demands contained in the hypnotic situation (Bowers & Farvolden, 1996; Frankel, 1994).

Drawing on his social–psychological analysis of hypnotic phenomena, Spanos (1986, 1994, 1996; but see Gleaves, 1996) offered an interpretation of dissociative identity disorder (and, by extension, the other dissociative disorders as well; see Spanos & Gottlieb, 1979) as a strategic social enactment in which an individual disavows responsibility for certain actions by attributing them to some "indwelling entity," "part," or "personality" other than the self (p. 36). Just as people learn the hypnotic role and then enact it under appropriate conditions, so people can learn to enact the role of multiple personalities—to create a social impression that is congruent with the diagnosis and that fulfills certain interpersonal goals. Just as the hypnotist abets this process by giving suggestions as to how the subject should behave, so clinicians explicitly and implicitly shape the behavior of their patients by encouraging then to adopt the role in the first place, providing them information about how to do so convincingly (for example, by displaying interpersonality amnesia), and then validating the performance by conferring a psychiatric diagnosis, and offering a particular form of therapy. Thus, the multiple personality is not so much a discovery as a creation—a creation on the part of both patient and therapist. Even so, the benefits for achieving the diagnosis—relief from interpersonal distress, mitigation of criminal responsibility, control of others, permission for untoward behavior—may be so powerful as to lead patients to "become convinced by their own enactments and come to believe that they possess multiple selves" (p. 47).

The influence of interpersonal, cultural, and historical factors on dissociative identity disorder can hardly be denied, but it is also something of a puzzle. The fact that the diagnosis experienced a golden age, waned after 1920, and showed a resurgence in the 1970s makes one wonder about the social conditions in which dissociative behaviors are expressed and corresponding diagnoses are made. This point has been made most forcefully by Kenny (1986), who provided an ethnographic analysis of dissociative identity disorder and related conditions. Analyzing the classic cases of Mary Reynolds, Ansel Bourne, Miss Beauchamp, B.C.A., Eve, and Sybil, Kenny (1986) argues that DID is a response to changing conditions in American culture. For example, Mary Reynolds' alter ego seems not so much an alternate to her normal state as a contradiction of it, a rebellion against her old self. Similarly, Ansel Bourne's fugue state may be interpreted as a symbolic representation of his self-perceived status as a "changed man" following his religious conversion. Miss Beauchamp rebelled against the limitations imposed on women in turn-of-the-century America and was used as a vehicle for Morton Prince's campaign against Freudian psychoanalysis. Kenney does not argue that most, or even many, cases of DID are fraudulent. He closes his book with an image of an intense and preoccupied Ansel Bourne, "trying—and failing—to remember something important" (1986, p. 188). Rather, his purpose is to understand how the definition and experience of self is shaped by the surrounding culture. There is no contradiction between excepting certain cases of dissocia-

tive disorder as genuine and understanding the sociocultural context in which they occur.

## Depersonalization and Derealization

In addition to the gross disruptions of autobiographical memory self-integration seen in psychogenic amnesia, fugue, and dissociative identity disorder, dissociative disorders include the experiences of depersonalization and derealization (Coons, 1996; Reed, 1979, 1988). As originally defined, it was thought that depersonalization and derealization co-occur. People experience themselves as totally different, and the world as strange and new. Later, they were construed as independent entities. Nemiah (1989) suggested that derealization is the more general case and depersonalization is a limited form in which only the experience of self is changed. Both depersonalization and derealization are frequently seen as symptoms of other syndromes, such as anxiety, depression, and obsession—for example, the phobic anxiety-depersonalization syndrome (Roth & Argyle, 1988). Depersonalization and derealization are nonspecific symptoms independent of other diagnoses (Brauer, Harrow, & Tucker, 1970; Fleiss, Gurland, & Goldberg, 1975), and are salient components in the "near-death experience" reported by those who have been rescued at the last moment from drownings, falls, and other kinds of accidents. However, depersonalization and derealization also constitute psychopathological syndromes in their own right.

As a primary diagnosis, the central feature of depersonalization disorder is a subjective awareness or feeling of change in oneself (depersonalization) or the world (derealization). This often occurs suddenly after awakening from sleep or after a frightening incident. The feeling puzzles the experiencers. The changed condition is perceived as unreal and as discontinuous with their previous ego states. The object of the experience, self (in depersonalization) or world (in derealization), is commonly described as isolated, lifeless, strange, and unfamiliar; oneself and others are perceived as "automatons," behaving mechanically without initiative or self-control. Although the feeling of depersonalization and derealization may be pleasant when self-induced by psychedelic drugs, in clinical cases it is unpleasant, even aversive: the victims often feel as if they were going insane, or dying. Throughout, however, the persons retain insight into what is happening: they remain aware of the contradictions between subjective experience and objective reality—it is only "as if" things were not real. Occasionally, the person will develop a delusional explanation about the experience (Kihlstrom & Hoyt, 1988), in which case both the puzzlement and the "as if" quality will disappear. Finally, depersonalization and derealization usually involve diminished emotional responsivity—a loss of interest in the outside world, of feelings for other people, and of anxiety or depression.

Mayer-Gross (1935) noted that depersonalization and derealization may occur with a host of other symptoms, including deja vu (in which the sense of having been in a place before coexists with the knowledge that this is not the case) and jamais vu (in which a situation is experienced as unfamiliar, despite the person's knowledge that it has been experienced many times before). In its totality, then, the experience of depersonalization is one of strangeness in oneself, in others, and of one's relationship to them. Viewed from the perspective of cognitive psychology, these syndromes represent failures of recognition—an inability to match current experience with past memories, something like what happens when one enters a familiar room whose furniture or paint scheme has been changed (Reed, 1979, 1988). Especially important here is the disruption of self-reference, which seems so crucial to the experience of recognition (Kihlstrom, 1997).

## Diagnosis and Assessment of Dissociation

The actual incidence and prevalence of dissociative disorders is hard to estimate. Dissociative disorders were excluded from the massive Epidemiological Catchment Area survey (Regier, Myers, Kramer, et al., 1984), presumably because appropriate diagnostic criteria were not provided by the standardized assessment instruments available at the time. This situation has now been corrected. Steinberg and her colleagues produced a version of the Structured Clinical Interview for DSM-IV Dissociative Disorders (SCID-D), which diagnoses these syndromes according to the rules of DSM-IV (Steinberg, 1996).

Several investigators have also developed questionnaire surveys of dissociative experiences that can be conveniently administered to large samples. The most popular of these is the Dissociative Experiences Scale (DES) of Bernstein and Putnam (1986; Carlson & Putnam, 1993) that holds promise as a diagnostic screening tool, locating high-scoring subjects who might be at risk for dissociative disorder (Carlson, Putnam, Ross, et al., 1993). For example, a doctoral dissertation by Angiulo (1994) found that college students who achieved extremely high scores on the DES were significantly more likely to qualify for a formal diagnosis of dissociative disorder (usually DDNOS) when subsequently administered the SCID-D. Of course, the DES and similar instruments can also be employed for research on normal personality structure and processes. For example, although the DES assesses levels of dissociation on a trait-like continuum from low to high, Waller and his colleagues (Waller, Putnam, & Carlson, 1996; Waller & Ross, 1997) employed taxometric techniques to argue that individuals who score high on the DES constitute a fairly discrete personality type.

Although instruments such as the SCID-D and the DES are intended to measure relatively stable trait-like dispositions toward dissociation, the Clinician-Administered Dissociative States Scale (CADSS; Bremner, Krystal, Putnam, Southwick, Marmar, Charney, & Mazure, 1998) was developed to measure episodic dissociative states and is suitable for measuring changes in symptoms. Examination of item content, however, indicates that the CADSS focuses on symptoms of depersonalization and derealization, not on the disruptions of memory and identity that lie at the heart of dissociative amnesia and fugue and dissociative identity disorder.

## Forensic Aspects of Dissociative Disorder

In addition to being a puzzle for clinicians and experimentalists, dissociative disorders have created substantial difficulties for the legal system. A victim who cannot remember the circumstances of a crime cannot offer valuable testimony that might lead to a conviction, and amnesic defendants cannot assist in their own defense. Moreover, the presence of amnesia for a criminal act may suggest that the crime was committed in an altered state of consciousness in which normal processes of monitoring and control were inoperative—thus potentially qualifying the defendant for the insanity defense. Unfortunately, the diagnosis of dissociative disorder is difficult to substantiate—even the structured clinical interview is susceptible to faking—and there is no way to tell for sure whether a particular suspect's claim of amnesia is genuine or simulated (Kopelman, 1995; Schacter, 1986a,b).

The legal problems associated with DID are especially severe, as illustrated by the case of Kenneth Bianchi, the "Hillside Strangler" (State v. Bianchi, No. 79-10116, Washington Superior Court, October 19, 1979).* Bianchi was charged, along with his cousin, in ten rape-murders in Los Angeles, and alone in two similar cases in Bellingham, Washington (Allison, 1984; Orne, Dinges, & Orne, 1984; Watkins, 1984). According to his defense, the crimes were perpetrated by an alter ego, "Steve Walker," a claim that was supported by evidence of high hypnotizability (a characteristic commonly associated with DID). However, the claim was undercut by other evidence suggesting that Bianchi had simulated hypnosis, and especially by inconsistencies in the self-presentation of the alter egos, psychological test evidence, and the lack of independent corroboration of the alter egos by people who knew him before he was arrested. Bianchi also had a great deal of background psychological knowledge, had practiced psychotherapy under a false name, and faked credentials (at one point in the proceedings he claimed that this was the work of a third alter ego, named "Billy"). Bianchi was convicted of eight counts of murder in the Hillside Strangler cases. Subsequently, he offered to testify against his cousin, who was also convicted.

danger and of psychogenic amnesia and fugue in victims of crime and disaster has already been noted, as has the apparent frequency with which amnesia and fugue are seen in cases of "war neurosis."[†] In particular, many authorities have noted an apparently strong relationship between DID and a history of childhood physical and sexual abuse. For example, Putnam et al. (1986) noted that fully 86% of their 100 recent cases presented a self-reported history of sexual abuse, 75% reported repeated physical abuse (68% reported both kinds of abuse), and 45% reported witnessing a violent death during childhood; only 3% of these cases had no history of significant childhood trauma. Reflecting a broad consensus among clinicians and researchers, Horevitz and Loewenstein (1994) characterized DID as "a traumatically induced developmental disorder of childhood" (p. 290).

At the same time, it must be underscored that this consensus is largely based on retrospective surveys of a sample of patients (and clinicians) whose representativeness of the population of DID is unknown. The definition of childhood trauma in these surveys is often very broad, includes extreme neglect and poverty as well as sexual and physical abuse, and there is rarely any quantification of the number of traumatic episodes, their severity, or their duration. The extent to which reports of childhood sexual abuse and other trauma may be biased by the patients' or clinicians' own intuitive theories of DID is unknown, but it is fairly certain that those who seek evidence of abuse and other trauma in childhood will be able to find it. Self-reported histories of childhood trauma, abuse, and neglect are rarely subject to independent verification, perhaps because since the earliest days of psychoanalysis, the

## Etiology of Dissociative Disorders

Stress, whether acute or chronic, is an extremely prominent feature in dissociative disorders—so much so that they are sometimes considered forms of posttraumatic stress disorder (PTSD; e.g., Putnam, 1985; Spiegel, 1984). The occurrence of depersonalization in response to life-threatening

[†]Even this evidence is ambiguous with respect to the traumatic etiology of dissociative disorder. For example, because depersonalization occurs in association with anxiety, the mere fact that disaster victims report increased levels of depersonalization (Cardena & Spiegel, 1993) cannot be taken as evidence that trauma causes any form of dissociative disorder. Similarly, biological factors such as concussive head injury and sleep deprivation cannot be ruled out in cases of war-related amnesia, and amnesia for crime may reflect intoxication (Piper, 1998; Pope, Hudson, Bodkin, & Oliva, 1998; Pope, Oliva, & Hudson, 1999). For a debate concerning the status of repressed or dissociated memories of trauma, see Scheflin and Brown (1996) and Piper (1997). For a critical analysis of the argument that traumatic memories are "special," see Shobe & Kihlstrom (1997).

*The Bianchi case was extensively documented in a two-hour *Frontline* documentary, "The Mind of a Murderer," broadcast on PBS in 1984.

causal link between trauma and dissociation is so intuitively appealing.

Even with independent corroboration of abuse histories, most studies in this area are retrospective and necessarily overestimate the strength of the relationship, if indeed any relationship exists at all between childhood trauma and adult dissociative disorder (Dawes, 1993; Kihlstrom, Eich, Sandbrand, & Tobias, 1997; Pope & Hudson, 1995). For this purpose, the gold standard is provided by prospective studies that condition subjects on the antecedents—e.g., taking representative groups of abused and nonabused children and following them into adulthood to determine who among them develops dissociative disorder.

In fact, authoritative reviews of prospective research failed to find evidence of any specific impact of child sexual abuse on adult personality and psychopathology (Kendall-Tackett, Williams, & Finkelhor, 1993; Nash, Mulsey, Sexton, et al., 1993). This is not to say that child sexual abuse is benign—it is only to say that there are currently no empirical grounds to accept the proposition that childhood sexual abuse causes or even increases the risk for later dissociative disorder. Prospective analyses of other kinds of trauma yield similar findings. For example, Holocaust survivors may show signs of PTSD, but dissociative amnesia is not a prominent feature of their profiles (Wagenaar & Groeneweg, 1990). At this point, the traumatic etiology for dissociative identity disorder and other dissociative disorders must be considered a hypothesis—not an established empirical fact that can inform prevention and treatment.

## Treatment of Dissociative Disorders

Other than dissociative identity disorder, little has been written about the treatment of dissociative disorders (Reid, 1989). Apparently, most cases of psychogenic amnesia and fugue resolve themselves spontaneously. Sometimes, patients recover their memories and identities unaided. In other cases, this process is prompted by contact with family and friends or by hints generated through free associations or dream reports. Many cases report that recovery was stimulated by the induction of hypnosis or sedation by intravenous barbiturates such as thiopental. However, these reports should be viewed against a background of experimental literature indicating that hypnosis has no special efficacy for the recovery of forgotten, repressed, or dissociated memories (Kihlstrom & Barnhardt, 1992; Kihlstrom & Eich, 1994). Moreover, no clinical or experimental study of barbiturate hypnosis has attempted independent corroboration of the ostensibly recovered memories (Piper, 1993).

Depersonalization symptoms are typically intermittent. But because episodes are often associated with acute mood disorder, drug treatment for anxiety and/or depression is often recommended. Presumably, benzodiazepines and other psychoactive drugs act on the anxiety and depression in which depersonalization and derealization occur, rather than directly on the feelings of unreality.

With respect to dissociative identity disorder, the traditional approach to the treatment of DID, initially popularized by Thigpen and Cleckley (1957), involves psychodynamic uncovering, abreaction, and working through of the trauma and other conflictual issues presumed to underlie the disorder, followed by an attempt at integrating the personalities into a single identity (Braun, 1986). The cooperation of each personality is required, entailing considerable effort directed toward developing therapeutic alliances. Hypnosis is often used, both for communicating with the personalities and for the integration, which is sometimes performed almost as a ceremony. Of course, psychotherapy does not necessarily stop with fusion. Additional time may be required to work through the insights achieved earlier in therapy, support the new fusion among the alter egos, and cope with the changes produced by integration.

Even though the modal therapy for DID is insight-oriented, there have been occasional attempts at cognitive-behavioral treatments (e.g., Kirsch & Barton, 1988). Regardless of treatment approach, there is a general consensus that the syndrome presents a number of specific challenges to treatment (Reid, 1989), including secondary gain (for the patient and for the therapist); countertransference reactions of anger, exasperation, aggression (as well as sexual attraction); suggestibility (especially where the evidence for DID is elicited by hypnosis, without independent corroboration), and the integration of confabulations and other distortions into memory.

As with the other dissociative disorders, there is little in the literature by way of systematic outcome studies (Reid, 1989; Ross, 1997). One exception is a report by Coons (1986) on twenty cases; another is the periodic updates by Kluft (e.g., 1988) on a large series of cases. Ross (1997) reported a two-year follow-up of fifty-four patients (from an original sample of 103); only twelve of these patients had achieved a therapeutic goal of stable integration, although the group as a whole reported diminished levels of dissociative experiences. Still, as Ross (1997) notes, "strictly speaking, there are no treatment outcome data for dissociative identity disorder in the literature" (p. 247). Given all the attention that DID has received since 1980, the fact that whole units, if not entire hospitals, have been developed for treating it, and the ensuing claims for out-of-pocket and third-party payment, this situation is remarkable and deplorable.

Most current treatments of DID are predicated on the notion that the syndrome is caused by childhood trauma such as sexual and physical abuse (Horevitz & Loewenstein, 1994; Ross, 1997). Thus, after the patient has been stabilized, Kluft (1993) recommends a focus on uncovering and resolving trauma and abandoning dissociative defenses. This recommendation would make no sense if there were not memories of trauma to be uncovered and dissociative defenses against such memories to be eliminated. However, as noted earlier, it is not at all clear that the origins of dissociative identity disorder lie in sexual abuse or any other form of childhood trauma. In the absence of convincing prospective evidence that DID has its origins in childhood trauma, such a postcentered focus seems premature at best and at worst raises the possibility that false memories of childhood sexual abuse may be constructed during the course of treatment.

## The Dissociative Spectrum

Dissociative disorders constitute only a portion of what was formerly described as "hysteria" (Kihlstrom, 1994). In his pioneering classificatory work, Janet was quite clear that the functional anesthesias, paralyses, and amnesias, including the amnesias of fugue and multiple personality, belonged together in a single class, distinct from phobias, obsessions and compulsions, and other subtypes of neurosis. Early diagnostic usage through DSM-II essentially honored Janet's principles. However, DSM-III and its revision, DSM-III-R,

abandoned hysteria and separated dissociative disorders from conversion disorders. Conversion disorders, in turn, were removed to the category of "Somatoform Disorders" along with somatization disorder (Briquet's syndrome), hypochondriasis, somatoform (psychogenic) pain disorder, body dysmorphic disorder (formerly known as dysmorphophobia), and the like (for reviews of the somatoform disorders, see Cloninger, 1996; Kihlstrom & Canter Kihlstrom, 1999). This separation persists in DSM-IV.

Put bluntly, this reclassification was, and remains, a mistake. It has long been known that conversion disorder, reflecting monosymptomatic disorders of the sensory-motor system, has nothing in common with Briquet's syndrome, hysterical personality, hypochondriasis, and the other somatoform disorders (Kihlstrom, 1992, 1994). They have much more in common with dissociative disorders. In both cases, events (in the current or past environment) have been registered and influence the patient's experience, thought, and action, even though the patient is not consciously aware of them.

The proper classification of conversion disorders, as essentially dissociative, is suggested by the pseudoneurological nature of their presenting symptoms and is further supported by closer psychological analysis of the paradoxes and contradictions in behavior observed in the classic cases described by Janet (1907). The functionally blind patient complains of being unable to see but correctly guesses how many fingers the examiner holds up before his eyes. Functionally deaf patients claim to be unable to hear but orient when their names are called from outside their fields of vision. In both cases, the patient's problem is in gaining conscious access to something that has been processed and registered in the sensory-perceptual system. But in the absence of conscious access, the percepts in question nevertheless influence the patient's experience, thought, and action outside of phenomenal awareness. The parallel to functional amnesia, where the patient complains of being unable to recollect past episodes but is nevertheless influenced by the unremembered events, is clear—at least to us. Just as functionally amnesic patients are not conscious of what they remember, functionally blind or deaf patients are not conscious of what they see or hear. This disruption of conscious awareness is the essence of dissociation.

By analogy with implicit memory, the paradoxes and contradictions in the behavior of conversion disorder patients may be labeled as expressions of "implicit perception" (Kihlstrom, 1996, 1999; Kihlstrom, Barnhardt, & Tataryn, 1992): they show the influence of events in the current environment without consciously perceiving these events.

Fundamentally, then, both dissociative and conversion disorders reflect a disruption of the normal functions of consciousness (Hilgard, 1977; Kihlstrom, 1984, 1992, 1994). These functions include (1) monitoring ourselves and our environment, permitting us to be aware of current events and to recollect the past, such that the world is accurately represented in phenomenal awareness; and (2) controlling ourselves, so that we have the experience of voluntarily initiating and terminating mental activities, at will, to achieve our personal goals and meet environmental demands. Accordingly, their essential unity should be reflected in our diagnostic nosology (for a similar suggestion, see Nemiah, 1989). Therefore, we suggest that henceforth the term "conversion disorder" be dropped from the diagnostic nosology as an inappropriate holdover from the days when psychoanalysis dominated our conception of the neuroses. Furthermore, the erstwhile conversion disorders should be removed from the somatoform category and regrouped with other dissociative disorders, forming three subcategories: (1) dissociative anesthesia, including psychogenic blindness, deafness, analgesia, and other functional disorders of sensation and perception; (2) dissociative paralysis, including psychogenic aphonia and other functional disorders of motor function; and (3) dissociative amnesia, including dissociative amnesia and fugue, dissociative identity, depersonalization and dissociation, and other functional disorders of memory and awareness.

ACKNOWLEDGMENT. Preparation of this chapter and the research that contributed to the point of view represented herein was supported in part by Grant #MH-35856 from the National Institute of Mental Health. I thank Douglas J. Tataryn and Irene P. Tobis (nee Hoyt) for the contributions to the version of this chapter published in the 2nd edition of this book (Kihlstrom et al., 1993). Some material from that chapter has been retained in the present edition, but a great deal of material had to be excluded for reasons of space. The interested reader is referred there for more comprehensive treatment of the literature before 1990.

# References

Acocella, J. (1998, April 6). The politics of hysteria. *The New Yorker*, 64–79.

Allison, R. B. (1984). Difficulties diagnosing the multiple personality syndrome in a death penalty case. *International Journal of Clinical and Experimental Hypnosis, 32*, 102–117.

American Psychiatric Association. (1952). *Diagnostic and statistical manual of mental disorders*. Washington, DC: Author.

American Psychiatric Association. (1968). *Diagnostic and statistical manual of mental disorders* (2nd ed.). Washington, DC: Author.

American Psychiatric Association. (1980). *Diagnostic and statistical manual of mental disorders* (3rd ed.). Washington, DC: Author.

American Psychiatric Association. (1987). *Diagnostic and statistical manual of mental disorders* (3rd ed., rev.). Washington, DC: Author.

American Psychiatric Association. (1994). *Diagnostic and statistical manual of mental disorders* (4th ed.). Washington, DC: Author.

Angiulo, M. J. (1994). Screening instruments for dissociative disorders: Their evaluation in a college population. Doctoral dissertation, University of Arizona. *Dissertation Abstracts International: Section A: The Humanities and Social Sciences, 55*, 507.

Arrigo, J. M., & Pezdek, K. (1997). Lessons from the study of psychogenic amnesia. *Current Directions in Psychological Science, 6*, 148–152.

Atwood, G. E. (1978). The impact of Sybil on a patient with multiple personality. *American Journal of Psychoanalysis, 38*, 277–279.

Bernstein, E. M., & Putnam, F. W. (1986). Development, reliability, and validity of a dissociation scale. *Journal of Nervous and Mental Disease, 174*, 727–735.

Bliss, E. L. (1986). *Multiple personality, allied disorders, and hypnosis*. New York: Oxford.

Boor, M. (1982). The multiple personality epidemic: Additional cases and inferences regarding diagnosis, etiology, dynamics, and treatment. *Journal of Nervous and Mental Disease, 170*, 302–304.

Borch-Jacobson, M. (1997, April 24). Sybil—The making of a disease: An interview with Dr. Herbert Spiegel. *New York Review of Books*, 60–64.

Bowers, K. S., & Farvolden, P. (1996). Revisiting a century-old Freudian slip—from suggestion disavowed to the truth repressed. *Psychological Bulletin, 119*, 355–380.

Brandsma, J. M., & Ludwig, A. M. (1974). A case of multiple personality: Diagnosis and therapy. *International Journal of Clinical and Experimental Hypnosis, 22*, 216–233.

Brauer, R., Harrow, M., & Tucker, G. J. (1970). Depersonalization phenomena in psychiatric patients. *British Journal of Psychiatry, 117*, 509–515.

Braun, B. G. (1986). *Treatment of multiple personality disorder*. Washington, DC: American Psychiatric Press.

Bremner, J. D., Krystal, J. H., Putnam, F. W., Sothwick, S. M., Marmar, C., Charney, D. S., & Mazure, C. M. (1998). Measurement of dissociative states with the Clinician-Administered Dissociative States Scale (CADSS). *Journal of Traumatic Stress, 11*, 125–136.

Bremner, J. D., & Marmar, C. R. (Eds.). (1998). *Trauma, memory, and dissociation.* Washington, DC: American Psychiatric Press.

Bryant, R. A. (1995). Autobiographical memory across personalities in dissociative identity disorder: A case report. *Journal of Abnormal Psychology, 104*, 625–631.

Cardena, E., & Spiegel, D. (1993). Dissociative reactions to the Bay Area Earthquake. *American Journal of Psychiatry, 150*, 474–478.

Carlson, E. T. (1981). The history of multiple personality in the United States: 1. The beginnings. *American Journal of Psychiatry, 183*, 666–668.

Carlson, E. T. (1984). The history of multiple personality in the United States: Mary Reynolds and her subsequent reputation. *Bulletin of the History of Medicine, 58*, 72–78.

Carlson, E. T. (1989). Multiple personality and hypnosis: The first one hundred years. *Journal of the History of the Behavioral Sciences, 25*, 315–322.

Carlson, E. B., & Putnam, F. W. (1993). An update on the Dissociative Experiences Scale. *Dissociation, 6*, 16–27.

Carlson, E. B., Putnam, F. W., Ross, C. A., Torem, M., Coons, P., Bowman, E. S., Chu, J., Dill, D. L., Loewenstein, R. J., & Braun, B. G. (1993). Predictive validity of the Dissociative Experiences Scale. *American Journal of Psychiatry, 150*, 1030–1036.

Cloninger, C. R. (1996). Somatization disorder. In T. A. Widiger, A. J. Frances, H. A. Pincus, R. Ross, M. B. First, and W. W. Davis (Eds.), *DSM-IV sourcebook* (Vol. 2, pp. 885–892). Washington, DC: American Psychiatric Association.

Coons, P. M. (1986). Treatment progress in 20 patients with multiple personality disorder. *Journal of Nervous and Mental Disease, 174*, 715–721.

Coons, P. M. (1996). Depersonalization and derealization. In L. K. Michaelson & W. J. Ray (Eds.), *Handbook of dissociation: Theoretical, empirical, and clinical perspectives* (pp. 291–306). New York: Plenum.

Coons, P. M., Milstein, V., & Marley, C. (1982). EEG studies of two multiple personalities and a control. *Archives of General Psychiatry, 39*, 823–825.

Crovitz, H. F., & Schiffman, H. (1974). Frequency of episodic memories as a function of their age. *Bulletin of the Psychonomic Society, 4*, 517–518.

Dawes, R. M. (1993). Prediction of the future versus an understanding of the past: A basic asymmetry. *American Journal of Psychology, 106*, 1–24.

Eich, E., Macaulay, D., Loewenstein, R. J., & Dihle, P. H. (1997). Memory, amnesia, and dissociative identity disorder. *Psychological Science, 8*, 417–422.

Eisen, M. R. (1989). Return of the repressed: Hypnoanalysis of a case of total amnesia. *International Journal of Clinical and Experimental Hypnosis, 37*, 107–119.

Ellenberger, H. F. (1970). *The discovery of the unconscious: The history and evolution of dynamic psychiatry.* New York: Basic Books.

Fahy, T. A. (1988). The diagnosis of multiple personality disorder: A critical review. *British Journal of Psychiatry, 153*, 597–606.

Fisher, C. (1945). Amnesic states in war neuroses: The psychogenesis of fugues. *Psychoanalytic Quarterly, 14*, 437–468.

Fisher, C., & Joseph, E. (1949). Fugue with loss of personal identity. *Psychoanalytic Quarterly, 18*, 480–493.

Fleiss, J. L., Gurland, B. J., & Goldberg, K. (1975). Independence of depersonalization-derealization. *Journal of Consulting and Clinical Psychology, 43*, 110–111.

Frankel, F. H. (1994). Dissociation in hysteria and hypnosis: A concept aggrandized. In S. J. Lynn & J. W. Rhue (Eds.), *Dissociation: Clinical and theoretical perspectives* (pp. 80–93). New York: Guilford.

Gershberg, F. B., & Shimamura, A. P. (1998). The neuropsychology of human learning and memory. In J. L. Martinez & R. P. Kesner (Eds.), *Neurobiology of learning and memory* (pp. 333–359). New York: Academic Press.

Gleaves, D. H. (1996). The sociocognitive model of multiple personality disorder: A reexamination of the evidence. *Psychological Bulletin, 120*, 42–59.

Greaves, G. B. (1980). Multiple personality 165 years after Mary Reynolds. *Journal of Nervous and Mental Disease, 168*, 577–596.

Hilgard, E. R. (1977). *Divided consciousness: Multiple controls in human thought and action.* New York: Wiley-Interscience.

Horevitz, R., & Loewenstein, R. J. (1994). The rational treatment of multiple personality disorder. In S. J. Lynn & J. W. Rhue (Eds.), *Dissociation: Clinical and theoretical perspectives* (pp. 289–316). New York: Guilford.

James, W. (1980). *Principles of psychology.* Cambridge, MA: Harvard University Press. (Originally published 1890).

Janet, P. (1889). [*Psychological automatisms.*] Paris: Alcan.

Janet, P. (1907). *The major symptoms of hysteria.* New York: Macmillan.

Kaszniak, A. W., Nussbaum, P. D., Berren, M. R., & Santiago, J. (1988). Amnesia as a consequence of male rape: A case report. *Journal of Abnormal Psychology, 97*, 100–104.

Kendall-Tackett, K. A., Williams, L. M., & Finkelhor, D. (1993). Impact of sexual abuse on children: A review and synthesis of recent empirical studies. *Psychological Bulletin, 113*, 164–180.

Kenny, M. G. (1986). *The passion of Ansel Bourne: Multiple personality in American culture.* Washington, DC: Smithsonian Institution Press.

Kihlstrom, J. F. (1984). Conscious, subconscious, unconscious: A cognitive perspective. In K. S. Bowers & D. Meichenbaum (Eds.), *The unconscious reconsidered* (pp. 149–211). New York: Wiley.

Kihlstrom, J. F. (1992). Dissociation and dissociations: A comment on consciousness and cognition. *Consciousness and Cognition, 1*, 47–53.

Kihlstrom, J. F. (1992). Dissociative and conversion disorders. In D. J. Stein & J. Young (Eds.), *Cognitive science and clinical disorders* (pp. 247–270). San Diego, CA: Academic Press.

Kihlstrom, J. F. (1994). One hundred years of hysteria. In S. J. Lynn & J. W. Rhue (Eds.), *Dissociation: Theoretical, clinical, and research perspectives* (pp. 365–394). New York: Guilford.

Kihlstrom, J. F. (1996). Perception without awareness of what is perceived, learning without awareness of what is learned. In M. Velmans (Ed.), *The science of consciousness: Psychological, neuropsychological, and clinical reviews* (pp. 23–46). London: Routledge.

Kihlstrom, J. F. (1997). Consciousness and me-ness. In J. Cohen & J. Schooler (Eds.), *Scientific approaches to the question of consciousness* (pp. 451–468). Mahwah, NJ: Erlbaum.

Kihlstrom, J. F. (1998). Exhumed memory. In S. J. Lynn & K. M. McConkey (Eds.), *Truth in memory* (pp. 3–31). New York: Guilford.

Kihlstrom, J. F. (1999). Conscious and unconscious cognition. In R. J. Sternberg (Ed.), *The nature of cognition* (pp. 173–204). Cambridge, MA: MIT Press.

Kihlstrom, J. F., & Barnhardt, T. R. (1992). The self-regulation of memory, for better or worse, with hypnosis and without. In D. Wegner & J. Pennebaker (Eds.), *Handbook of mental control* (pp. 17–54). Englewood Cliffs, NJ: Prentice-Hall.

Kihlstrom, J. F., & Canter Kihlstrom, L. (1999). Self, sickness, somatization, and systems of care. In R. J. Contrada & R. D. Ashmore (Eds.), *Self, social identity, and physical health: Interdisciplinary explorations* (pp. 23–42). New York: Oxford University Press.

Kihlstrom, J. F., & Eich, E. (1994). Altering states of consciousness. In D. Druckman & R. A. Bjork (Eds.), *Learning, remembering, and believing: Enhancing performance* (pp. 207–248). Washington, DC: National Academy Press.

Kihlstrom, J. F. & Hoyt, I. P. (1988). Hypnosis and the psychology of delusions. In T. F. Oltmanns & B. A. Maher (Eds.), *Delusional beliefs: Interdisciplinary perspectives* (pp. 66–109). New York: Wiley.

Kihlstrom, J. F., & Klein, S. B. (1994). The self as a knowledge structure. In R. S. Wyer & T. K. Srull (Eds.), *Handbook of social cognition* (Vol. 1, 2nd ed., pp. 153–208). Hillsdale, NJ: Erlbaum.

Kihlstrom, J. F., & Klein, S. B. (1997). Self-knowledge and self-awareness. In J. G. Snodgrass & R. L. Thompson (Eds.), *The self across psychology: Self-recognition, self-awareness, and the self-concept. Annals of the New York Academy of Sciences, 818,* 5–17.

Kihlstrom, J. F., & Schacter, D. L. (2000). Functional amnesia. In F. Boller & J. Grafman (Eds.), *Handbook of neuropsychology* (2nd ed., pp. 409–427). Amsterdam: Elsevier Science.

Kihlstrom, J. F., Barnhardt, T. M., & Tataryn, D. J. (1992). Implicit perception. In R. F. Bornstein & T. S. Pittman (Eds.), *Perception without awareness: Cognitive, clinical, and social perspectives* (pp. 17–54). New York: Guilford.

Kihlstrom, J. F., Tataryn, D. J., & Hoyt, I. P. (1993). Dissociative disorders. In P. J. Sutker & H. E. Adams (Eds.), *Comprehensive handbook of psychopathology* (2nd ed.). (pp. 203–234). New York: Plenum Press.

Kihlstrom, J. F., Eich, E., Sandbrand, D., & Tobias, B. A. (1997). Emotion and memory: Implications for self-report (with a critique of retrospective analyses). In A. Stone & J. Turkkan (Eds.), *The science of self-report: Implications for research and practice* (pp. 81–99). Mahwah, NJ: Erlbaum.

Kirsch, I., & Barton, R. D. (1988). Hypnosis in the treatment of multiple personality: A cognitive-behavioural approach. *British Journal of Experimental and Clinical Hypnosis, 5,* 131–137.

Kirsch, I., & Lynn, S. J. (1998). Dissociation theories of hypnosis. *Psychological Bulletin, 123,* 100–115.

Klein, R. M., & Doane, B. K. (1994). *Psychological concepts and dissociative disorders.* Hillsdale, NJ: Erlbaum.

Kluft, R. P. (1988). The postunification treatment of multiple personality disorder: First findings. *American Journal of Psychotherapy, 42,* 212–228.

Kluft, R. P. (1993). Basic principles in conducting the treatment

of multiple personality disorder. In R. P. Kluft & C. G. Fine (Eds.), *Clinical perspectives on multiple personality disorder* (pp. 53–73). Washington, DC: American Psychiatric Press.

Kopelman, M. D. (1995). The assessment of psychogenic amnesia. In A. D. Baddeley, B. A. Wilson, & F. N. Watts (Eds.), *Handbook of memory disorders* (pp. 427–448). Chichester, England: Wiley.

Kopelman, M. D. (1997). Anomalies of autobiographical memory: Retrograde amnesia, confabulation, delusional memory, psychogenic amnesia, and false memories. In J. D. Read & D. S. Lindsay (Eds.), *Recollections of trauma: Scientific evidence and clinical practice* (pp. 273–303). New York: Plenum Press.

Kroonenberg, P. M. (1985). Three-mode principal components: Analysis of semantic differential data: The case of a triple personality. *Applied Psychological Measurement, 9,* 83–94.

Loewenstein, R. J. (1996). Dissociative amnesia and dissociative fugue. In L. K. Michelson & W. J. Ray (Eds.), *Handbook of dissociation: Theoretical, empirical, and clinical perspectives* (pp. 307–336). New York: Plenum Press.

Lowenstein, R. J., Hamilton, J., Alagna, S., Reid, N., & deVries, M. (1987). Experiential sampling in the study of multiple personality disorder. *American Journal of Psychiatry, 144,* 19–24.

Ludwig, A. M., Brandsma, J. M., Wilbur, C. B., Bendfeldt, F., & Jameson, D. H. (1972). The objective study of a multiple personality: Or are four heads better than one? *Archives of General Psychiatry, 26,* 298–310.

Lynn, S. J., & Rhue, J. W. (Eds.). (1994). *Dissociation: Clinical and theoretical perspectives.* New York: Guilford.

Macmillan, M. (1996). *Freud evaluated: The completed arc.* Cambridge, MA: MIT Press.

Main, M., & Morgan, H. (1996). Disorganization and disorientation in infant strange situation behavior: Phenotypic resemblance to dissociative states. In L. K. Michaelson & W. J. Ray (Eds.), *Handbook of dissociation: Theoretical, empirical, and clinical perspectives* (pp. 107–138). New York: Plenum.

Mathew, R. J., Jack, R. A., & West, W. S. (1985). Regional cerebral blood flow in a patient with multiple personality. *American Journal of Psychiatry, 142,* 504–505.

Mayer-Gross, W. (1935). On depersonalization. *British Journal of Medical Psychology, 15,* 103–121.

Michaelson, L. J., & Ray, W. J. (Eds.). (1996). *Handbook of dissociation.* New York: Plenum Press.

Mitchill, S. L. (1816). A double consciousness, or a duality of person in the same individual [dated January 16, 1816]. *Medical Repository, 3,* 185–186.

Mitchell, S. W. (1888). Mary Reynolds: A case of double consciousness. *Transactions of the College of Physicians of Philadelphia, 10,* 366–389.

Nash, M. R., Hulsey, T. L., Sexton, M. C., Harralson, T. L., & Lambert, W. (1993). Long-term sequelae of childhood sexual abuse: Perceived family environment, psychopathology, and dissociation. *Journal of Consulting and Clinical Psychology, 61,* 276–283.

Nemiah, J. C. (1979). Dissociative amnesia: A clinical and theoretical reconsideration. In J. F. Kihlstrom & F. J. Evans (Eds.), *Functional disorders of memory* (pp. 303–324). Hillsdale, NJ: Erlbaum

Nemiah, J. C. (1989). Dissociative disorders (hysterical neuroses, dissociative type). In H. I. Kaplan & B. J. Sadock

(Eds.), *Comprehensive textbook of psychiatry* (Vol. 1, 5th ed., pp. 1028–1044). Baltimore: Williams & Wilkins.

Nissen, M. J., Ross, J. L., Willingham, D. B., Mackenzie, T. B., & Schacter, D. L. (1988). Memory and awareness in a patient with multiple personality disorder. *Brain and Cognition, 8,* 117–134.

Orne, M. T., Dinges, D. F., & Orne, E. C. (1984). On the differential diagnosis of multiple personality in the forensic context. *International Journal of Clinical and Experimental Hypnosis, 32,* 119–169.

Osgood, C. E., & Luria, Z. (1954). A blind analysis of a case of multiple personality using the semantic differential. *Journal of Abnormal and Social Psychology, 49,* 579–591.

Osgood, C. E., Luria, Z., Jeans, R. F., & Smith, S. W. (1976). The three faces of Evelyn: A case report. I. An independently validated case of multiple personality [by R. F. Jeans]. II. A blind analysis of another case of multiple personality using the semantic differential technique [by C. E. Osgood, Z. Luria, & S. W. Smith]. III. Reactions to the blind analysis [by R. F. Jeans]. IV. A postscript to "The three faces of Evelyn" [by Z. Luria & C. E. Osgood]. *Journal of Abnormal Psychology, 85,* 247–286.

Piper, A. (1993). "Truth serum" and "recovered memories" of sexual abuse: A review of the evidence. *Journal of Psychiatry and Law, 21,* 447–471.

Piper, A. (1997). What the science says—and doesn't say—about repressed memories: A critique of Scheflin and Brown. *Journal of Psychiatry and Law, 25,* 614–639.

Piper, A. (1998). Repressed memories from World War II: Nothing to forget. Examining Daron and Widener's (1997) claim to have discovered evidence for repression. *Professional Psychology: Research and Practice, 29,* 476–478.

Pope, H. G., & Hudson, J. I. (1995). Can individuals "repress" memories of childhood sexual abuse? An examination of the evidence. *Psychiatric Annals, 25,* 715–719.

Pope, H. G., Hudson, J. I., Bodkin, J. A., & Oliva, P. (1998). Questionable validity of "dissociative amnesia" in trauma victims: Evidence from prospective studies. *British Journal of Psychiatry, 172,* 210–215.

Pope, H. G., Oliva, P., & Hudson, J. I. (1999). The scientific status of repressed memories. In D. L. Faigman, D. H. Kaye, M. J. Saks, & J. Sanders (Eds.), *Modern scientific evidence: The law and science of expert testimony,* Vol. 1, Pocket part (pp. 115–155). St. Paul, MN: West.

Pratt, R. T. C. (1977). Psychogenic loss of memory. In C. W. M. Whitty & O. L. Zangwill (Eds.), *Amnesia* (2nd ed., pp. 224–232). London: Butterworth.

Putnam, F. W. (1984). The psychophysiologic investigation of multiple personality disorder: A review. *Psychiatric Clinics of North America, 7,* 31–39.

Putnam, F. W. (1985). Dissociation as a response to extreme trauma. In R. P. Kluft (Ed.), *Childhood antecedents of multiple personality* (pp. 65–97). Washington, DC: American Psychiatric Press.

Putnam, F. W. (1989). *Diagnosis and treatment of multiple personality disorder.* New York: Guilford.

Putnam, F. W. (1997). *Dissociation in children and adolescents: A developmental perspective.* New York: Guilford.

Putnam, F. W., Guroff, J. J., Silberman, E. K., Barban, L., & Post, R. M. (1986). The clinical phenomenology of multiple personality disorder: Review of 100 recent cases. *Journal of Clinical Psychiatry, 47,* 285–293.

Reed, G. (1979). Anomalies of recall and recognition. In J. F.

Kihlstrom & F. J. Evans (Eds.), *Functional disorders of memory* (pp. 1–28). Hillsdale, NJ: Erlbaum.

Reed, G. (1988). *The psychology of anomalous experience* (rev. ed.). Buffalo, NY: Prometheus.

Regier, D. A., Myers, J. K., Kramer, M., Robins, L. N., Blazer, D. G., Hough, R. L., Eaton, W. W., & Locke, B. Z. (1984). The NIMH Epidemiologic Catchment Area Program: Historical context, major objectives, and study population characteristics. *Archives of General Psychiatry, 41,* 934–941.

Reid, W. H. (1989). Dissociative disorders (Hysterical neuroses, dissociative type). In W. H. Reid (Ed.), *The treatment of psychiatric disorders: Revised for the DSM-III-R* (pp. 266–272). New York: Brunner/Mazel.

Robinson, J. A. (1976). Sampling autobiographical memory. *Cognitive Psychology, 8,* 578–595.

Rosenzweig, S. (1987). Sally Beauchamp's career: A psychoarcheological key to Morton Prince's classic case of multiple personality. *Genetic, Social, and General Psychology Monographs, 113,* 5–60.

Rosenzweig, S. (1988). The identity and idiodynamics of the multiple personality "Sally Beauchamp": A confirmatory supplement. *American Psychologist, 43,* 45–48.

Ross, C. A. (1997). *Dissociative identity disorder: Diagnosis, clinical features, and treatment of multiple personality.* New York: Wiley.

Roth, M., & Argyle, N. (1988). Anxiety, panic, and phobic disorders: An overview. *Journal of Psychiatric Research, 22*(Suppl. 1), 33–54.

Schacter, D. L. (1986a). Amnesia and crime: How much do we really know? *American Psychologist, 41,* 286–295.

Schacter, D. L. (1986b). On the relation between genuine and simulated amnesia. *Behavioral Sciences and the Law, 4,* 47–64.

Schacter, D. L. (1987). Implicit memory: History and current status. *Journal of Experimental Psychology: Learning, Memory, and Cognition, 13,* 501–518.

Schacter, D. L., & Kihlstrom, J. F. (1999). Functional amnesia. In F. Boller & J. Grafman (Eds.), *Handbook of neuropsychology* (2nd ed., pp. 407–427). Amsterdam: Elsevier Science.

Schacter, D. L., Kihlstrom, J. F., Canter Kihlstrom, L., & Berren, M. (1989). Autobiographical memory in a case of multiple personality disorder. *Journal of Abnormal Psychology, 98,* 508–514.

Schacter, D. L., Wang, P. L., Tulving, E., & Friedman, M. (1982). Functional retrograde amnesia: A quantitative case study. *Neuropsychologia, 20,* 523–532.

Scheflin, A. W., & Brown, D. (1996). Repressed memory or dissociative amnesia: What the science says. *Journal of Psychiatry and Law, 24,* 143–188.

Schreiber, F. L. (1973). *Sybil.* Chicago: Regnery.

Shimamura, A. P. (1993). Neuropsychological analyses of implicit memory: History, methodology, and theoretical interpretations. In P. Graf & M. E. J. Masson (Eds.), *Implicit memory: New directions in cognition, development, and neuropsychology* (pp. 265–285). Hillsdale, NJ: Erlbaum.

Shobe, K. K., & Kihlstrom, J. F. (1997). Is traumatic memory special? *Current Directions in Psychological Science, 6,* 70–74.

Silberman, E. K., Putnam, F. W., Weingartner, H., Braun, B. G., & Post, R. M. (1985). Dissociative states in multiple personality disorder: A quantitative study. *Psychiatry Research, 15,* 253–260.

Spanos, N. P. (1986). Hypnosis, nonvolitional responding and multiple personality. In B. Maher & W. Maher (Eds.), *Progress in experimental personality research*, Vol. 14 (pp. 1–62). New York: Academic Press.

Spanos, N. P. (1994). Multiple identity enactments and multiple personality disorder: A sociocognitive perspective. *Psychological Bulletin, 116*, 143–165.

Spanos, N. P. (1996). *Multiple identities and false memories: A sociocognitive perspective.* Washington, DC: American Psychological Association.

Spanos, N. P., & Gottlieb, J. (1979). Demonic possession, mesmerism, and hysteria: A social psychological perspective on their historical interrelations. *Journal of Abnormal Psychology, 88*, 527–546.

Spiegel, D. (1984). Multiple personality as a post-traumatic stress disorder. *Psychiatric Clinics of North America, 7*, 101–110.

Spiegel, D. (Ed.). (1991). Dissociative disorders. In A. Tasman & S. M. Goldfinger (Eds.), *American Psychiatric Press Review of Psychiatry*, Vol. 10 (pp. 143–280). Washington, DC: American Psychiatric Press.

Spiegel, D. (Ed.). (1994). *Dissociation: Culture, mind, and body.* Washington, DC: American Psychiatric Press.

Steinberg, M. J. (1996). The psychological assessment of dissociation. In L. K. Michaelson & W. J. Ray (Eds.), *Handbook of dissociation: Theoretical, empirical, and clinical perspectives* (pp. 251–268). New York: Plenum Press.

Stengel, E. (1966). Psychogenic loss of memory. In C. W. M. Whitty & O. L. Zangwill (Eds.), *Amnesia* (pp. 181–191). London: Butterworth.

Sutcliffe, J. P., & Jones, J. (1962). Personal identity, multiple personality, and hypnosis. *International Journal of Clinical and Experimental Hypnosis, 10*, 231–269.

Taylor, E. (1982). *William James on exceptional mental states: The 1896 Lowell Lectures.* New York: Scribner's.

Taylor, E. (1996). *William James on consciousness beyond the margin.* Princeton, NJ: Princeton University Press.

Taylor, W. S., & Martin, M. F. (1944). Multiple personality. *Journal of Abnormal and Social Psychology, 39*, 281–300.

Thigpen, C. H., & Cleckley, H. M. (1954). A case of multiple personality. *Journal of Abnormal and Social Psychology, 49*, 135–151.

Thigpen, C. H., & Cleckley, H. M. (1957). *The three faces of Eve.* New York: Popular Library.

Thigpen, C. H., & Cleckley, H. M. (1984). On the incidence of multiple personality disorder. *International Journal of Clinical and Experimental Hypnosis, 32*, 63–66.

Treadwell, M., McCloskey, M., Gordon, B., & Cohen, N. J. (1992). Landmark life events and the organization of memory: Evidence from functional retrograde amnesia. In S.-A. Christianson (Ed.), *Handbook of emotion and memory* (pp. 389–410). Hillsdale, NJ: Erlbaum.

Wagenaar, W. A., & Groeneweg, J. (1990). The memory of concentration camp survivors. *Applied Cognitive Psychology, 4*, 77–87.

Waller, N. G., Putnam, F. W., & Carlson, E. B. (1996). Types of dissociation and dissociative types: A taxometric analysis of dissociative experiences. *Psychological Methods, 1*, 300–321.

Waller, N. G., & Ross, C. (1997). The prevalence and biometric structure of pathological dissociation in the general population: Taxometric and behavior genetic findings. *Journal of Abnormal Psychology, 106*, 49–510.

Watkins, J. G. (1984). The Bianchi (L.A. hillside strangler) case: Sociopath or multiple personality? *International Journal of Clinical and Experimental Hypnosis, 32*, 67–101.

Woody, E. Z., & Sadler, P. (1998). On reintegrating dissociated theories: Commentary on Kirsch & Lynn (1998). *Psychological Bulletin, 123*, 192–197.

Woody, E. Z., & Bowers, K. S. (1994). A frontal assault on dissociated control. In S. J. Lynn & J. W. Rhue (Eds.), *Dissociation: Clinical and theoretical perspectives* (pp. 52–79). New York: Guilford.

# CHAPTER 11

# Mood Disorders: Unipolar and Bipolar

Lynn P. Rehm, Alisha L. Wagner, and Carolyn Ivens-Tyndal

## Diagnostic Distinctions and Clinical Phenomenology

### Unipolar–Bipolar Distinction

A historical review of the conceptualization, diagnosis, and categorization of psychopathology reveals a series of attempts to develop meaningful distinctions or subcategories to reduce the heterogeneity of affective disorders. Kraeplin (1921) subsumed most major forms of depression under the rubric of "manic-depressive illness," which he distinguished from dementia praecox (schizophrenia). This classification scheme prevailed for several decades and was reflected in the *Diagnostic and Statistical Manual of Mental Disorders*, 2nd edition (DSM-II; American Psychiatric Association [APA], 1968) which remained in use until 1980. Under this diagnostic approach, individuals with recurrent depressions and those with depressions plus manic episodes were both considered manic-depressive. Only involutional melancholia, psychotic-depressive reaction, and depressive neurosis were differentiated from manic-depressive illness, chiefly on the basis of recurrence of depressive episodes.

As early as 1957, Leonhard suggested that individuals with depressions plus manic episodes (bipolar) should be distinguished from persons with only recurrent depressive episodes (unipolar) on the basis of differences in various clinical dimensions. During the following three decades, studies of clinical, familial, genetic, pharmacological, and biological factors supported such a distinction, resulting in a reversal of the old classification and conceptual framework such that current theories, diagnostic schemes, and treatment strategies treat unipolar and bipolar affective disorders as distinct entities. Among specific distinctions, age of onset for bipolar disorder tends to be significantly earlier than for unipolar depressions (Angst et al., 1973; Burke, Burke, Regier, & Rae, 1990; Gershon, Dunner, & Goodwin, 1971; Perris, 1966), and genetic factors have a more important role in the occurrence of bipolar disorder than that of unipolar disorder (Allen, 1976). Differences in specific depressive-episode symptoms have been observed; unipolar depressives are more commonly characterized by agitated psychomotor activity (Beigel & Murphy, 1971; Bunney & Murphy, 1973; Kupfer et al., 1974), hyposomnia (Detre et al., 1972; Hartmann, 1968; Kupfer et al., 1972), somatic complaints (Beigel & Murphy, 1971), and anger at self and others (Beigel & Murphy, 1971), and depressed bipolar subjects are characterized by psychomotor retardation, hypersomnia, fewer

Lynn P. Rehm, Alisha L. Wagner, and Carolyn Ivens-Tyndal • Department of Psychology, University of Houston, Houston, Texas 77036.

*Comprehensive Handbook of Psychopathology* (Third Edition), edited by Patricia B. Sutker and Henry E. Adams. Kluwer Academic / Plenum Publishers, New York, 2001.

somatic complaints, and mild or no anger. Although these data support the unipolar–bipolar distinction at a number of levels and in a number of arenas, including clinical presentation of depressive symptoms, the current diagnostic system, DSM-IV (APA, 1994), distinguishes between unipolar and bipolar mood disorders solely on the basis of a history of mania. There is no attempt to differentiate bipolar from unipolar depressive states on any other grounds.

## Unipolar Depression Criteria

According to DSM-IV, criteria for a major depressive episode are (1) the presence of either depressed mood (in children or adolescents, depressed or irritable mood) or loss of interest or pleasure in all or most activities for a minimum of 2 weeks and (2) the presence of at least four criterion symptoms for a period of at least 2 weeks. The criterion symptoms include appetite disturbance; change in weight; sleep disturbance; psychomotor agitation or retardation; decreased energy; feelings of worthlessness or excessive or inappropriate guilt; difficulty with thinking, concentrating, or decision making; and recurrent thoughts of death or suicidal ideation or attempts. Symptoms must represent a change from previous functioning, be relatively persistent during the minimum 2-week period, and cause clinically significant distress or impairment in social, occupational, or other important areas of functioning.

Historically, a distinction has been made between depressions believed to be caused by some external event (termed reactive or exogenous) and those believed to be caused primarily by internal biological factors (termed endogenous). Endogenous depressions are believed to be more severe and to be characterized by prominent somatic symptoms. Because the identification of an external cause is unreliable and because the identification of internal causes in other cases is only inferred from the lack of an external cause, this distinction was not included in DSM-II. However, DSM-III (APA, 1980), DSM-III-R (APA, 1987), and DSM-IV substituted major depressive episode, melancholic type, as a subgroup of unipolar depression defined in terms of current symptoms rather than a putative cause. The specific symptoms include (1) the presence of either loss of pleasure in all or almost all activities or a lack of reactivity to usually pleasurable stimuli and

(2) three or more of the following symptoms: distinct quality of depressed mood (a different kind of feeling than, for example, what is experienced after the death of a loved one); a diurnal variation of mood with a depression worse in the morning; early morning awakening (at least 2 hours before the usual time); marked psychomotor retardation or agitation; significant anorexia or weight loss; and excessive or inappropriate guilt.

Dysthymia, referred to as "depressive neurosis" by previous diagnostic systems, is also a common unipolar depressive disorder. Symptoms are fewer and typically less severe than in major depressive episodes, but these symptoms generally cause clinically significant distress or impairment in social, occupational, or other important areas of functioning. The essential features of dysthymia are depressed mood (or irritable mood in children and adolescents) for most of the day during most days for at least 2 years (1 year for children and adolescents), and the presence of at least two of the criterion depressive symptoms described before as part of the unipolar diagnosis. As a stable and enduring disorder, dysthymia (along with cyclothymia, discussed later) was earlier considered among the personality disorders. Debate as to its status continues. The relationship between dysthymia and major depression is complex. The DSM system allows making both diagnoses simultaneously, sometimes referred to as double depression. In DSM-IV, sequence is also important. If the 2-year period begins with an episode of major depression, then the milder continuation is assumed to be part of the major depression, and the diagnosis is major depression in partial remission, not dysthymia.

A residual category of depressive disorder, not otherwise specified, is included in DSM-IV for disorders with depressive features that do not meet the criteria for any specific mood disorder, or for adjustment disorder with depressed mood. Examples of depressive disorder NOS include premenstrual dysphoric disorder; minor depressive disorder; recurrent brief depressive disorder; postpsychotic depressive disorder of Schizophrenia; and a Major Depressive Episode superimposed on Delusional Disorder, Psychotic Disorder NOS, or the active phase of Schizophrenia. Adjustment disorder with depressed mood is not classified as a mood disorder, despite the primary features of depressive symptoms, because adjustment disorders, it is assumed, cover temporary maladaptive reactions of normal individuals to unusually stressful life events. Depressed mood is only one of several concomitant symptom patterns of adjustment disorder.

Three new specifiers included in DSM-IV to describe a current mood episode are "With Atypical Features," "With Postpartum Onset," and "With Catatonic Features." A diagnosis of With Atypical Features includes (1) mood reactivity, in which mood brightens in response to actual or potential positive events and (2) two or more of the following features: significant weight gain or increase in appetite, hypersomnia, heaviness in arms or legs, or a long-standing pattern of interpersonal rejection sensitivity that results in significant social or occupational impairment. A diagnosis of atypical features precludes an additional diagnosis of Melancholic or Catatonic features during the same episode.

The Postpartum Onset specifier, which is applied if the onset of the mood disturbance is within 4 weeks after delivery, generally includes the same symptoms in nonpostpartum mood episodes and may include distinct psychotic features. Additional symptoms may involve severe anxiety, panic attacks, disinterest in the infant, and initial insomnia. In early DSMs, postpartum depression was a separate diagnosis. Consensus grew that it was not really distinct from other depressions and could be considered a special case of reactive depression. It was dropped from DSM-III and now reappears in DSM-IV as a specifier.

The specifier "With Catatonic Features" is diagnosed when the clinical situation is characterized by two of the following: motoric immobility such as catalepsy or stupor; excessive, purposeless motor activity that is not influenced by external stimuli; extreme negativism or mutism; peculiarities of voluntary movement such as posturing, stereotyped movements, prominent mannerisms or grimacing, or echolalia or echopraxia.

The Seasonal Pattern Specifier, which was previously established, can be applied to Major Depressive Disorder, Recurrent, or to the depressive episodes in Bipolar I or Bipolar II. The character features are the onset and termination of episodes at particular times of the year. The symptom pattern of seasonal episodes often includes anergy, hypersomnia, overeating, weight gain, and a craving for carbohydrates. The most common seasonal pattern is an onset in fall or winter and a remission in the spring. According to DSM-IV, seasonal depressive episodes must substantially outnumber nonseasonal depressive episodes over the course of one's life.

The symptoms in the depressive disorders are evident within the realms of mood, cognition and perception, and behavior and somatic functioning. Mood is the least varying of these symptoms, and the typical experience of the depressed individual is feeling pervasively sad, blue, or hopeless. Occasionally, individuals do not describe their moods as depressed, yet they are observed by others as appearing so. Depressed mood is often accompanied by excessive tearfulness, although some individuals may experience an inability to cry. Anhedonia, the loss of interest or pleasure in previously pleasant activities, is a common feature of depressed mood and may be experienced as apathy or as a painful inability to experience pleasure. With anhedonia, expression of affect may be blunted. DSM-IV considers that either sadness or anhedonia are essential to the diagnosis of depression. Further, depressed mood is often accompanied by irritable or angry mood, and such moods may be the predominant mood in depressed children and adolescents. The variants of dominant mood associated with depression have been suggested as an important diagnostic dimension with implications for pharmacological treatment selection (Overall & Zisook, 1980).

Cognitive and perceptual symptoms of depression involve the realms of cognitive functioning and of cognitive and perceptual style or content. Impairment of cognitive functioning is indicated by poor concentration, slowed thinking, indecision, and (in cases of depression with psychotic features) hallucinations. Complaints of memory problems are also common, but complaints are often exaggerated and when memory is actually assessed, it is usually not significantly impaired. Such an assessment is sometimes important in differential diagnoses, for example, in differentiating depression from Alzheimer's dementia. Depressive cognitive style or content involves suicidal ideation or preoccupation, ruminative morbid or hypochondriacal thinking, and negatively distorted perceptions and thoughts about oneself, the world, and/or the future, as described later in discussions of cognitive models of depression. Psychotic symptoms of delusions or hallucinations may be evident during depressive episodes. Any psychotic symptoms usually involve content that is clearly consistent with the predominant mood (i.e., mood-congruent), such as delusions of persecution due to some personal inadequacy or transgression. Mood-incongruent psychotic symptoms are relatively rare.

Somatic symptoms, referred to as vegetative signs, include sleep and appetite disturbance, psychomotor agitation or retardation, and decreased energy. Sleep disturbance is among the most pervasive quantifiable and pathognomic symptoms. Insomnia is the most common form of sleep disturbance—sometimes initial insomnia (the inability to fall to sleep), but more commonly among depressed individuals, middle or terminal insomnia, where the individual awakens from sleep and experiences difficulty or inability to return to sleep. Hypersomnia (excessive sleep) is experienced, however, by a smaller but significant portion of depressed individuals. As with sleep disturbance and other somatic symptoms, the direction of appetite disturbance may be that of increase or decrease; more depressed individuals experience appetite and weight loss, but some experience increased appetite and consequent weight gain. Similarly, variance in psychomotor activity is observed across the population of depressed individuals. Psychomotor retardation (a slowing of movement and speech) is most common, although many depressed individuals experience psychomotor agitation in forms such as an inability to sit still or a subjective experience of nervousness or anxiety. Fatigue and decreased energy, as well as decreased libido or sexual interest, are also commonly experienced during a depressive episode.

## Mania and Hypomania Criteria

DSM-IV criteria for a manic episode include (1) a distinct period of abnormally and persistently elevated, expansive, or irritable mood that lasts at least 1 week or less if hospitalization is necessary and (2) three or more associated symptoms such as inflated self-esteem or grandiosity, decreased need for sleep, pressured speech, racing thoughts, distractibility, increased involvement in goal-directed activity, psychomotor agitation, and excessive involvement in pleasurable but potentially harmful activities. Severity of disturbance sufficient to impair occupational, social, interpersonal, or personal functioning, or to necessitate hospitalization to prevent harm to self or others, is a defining criterion. This definition includes psychotic symptoms of delusions, hallucinations, or

catatonia coexisting with the mood disturbance, whether such psychotic symptoms are mood-congruent (i.e., delusions or hallucinations with content consistent with elevated mood) or mood-incongruent.

A hypomanic episode is defined by DSM-IV as a distinct period of abnormally and persistently elevated, expansive, or irritable mood lasting at least 4 days, with the associated manic symptoms but without the presence of delusions, and without disturbance severe enough to cause marked impairment in social or occupational functioning or to require hospitalization. As indicated by DSM-IV, the hypomanic episode must be distinctively different from the individual's typical nondepressed mood, and it must be a clear change in functioning.

The mild-to-moderate degree of symptomatology experienced as hypomania is often experienced by the individual as pleasant and/or productive and may in fact be productive if symptoms do not persist or intensify. The hypomanic mood, ranging from a general sense of well-being to euphoria, is typically enjoyable, and the experiences of increased physical and mental energy and activity and decreased need for sleep may be productive. Further, subjective report is that thought processes often become more fluid, creative, and productive during hypomanic episodes. There is some evidence that bipolar disorder is found at higher than chance levels among particularly creative people (Andreasen & Canter, 1974). These positive experiences of hypomania often prevent the individual from seeking treatment because the symptoms are not subjectively experienced as problematic. However, irritability, anger proneness, and/or affective lability are typically concomitant with such heightened mood states, and the hypomanic episode frequently intensifies into a full manic episode, especially among individuals who have histories of previous manic episodes.

In DSM-III-R, a mixed episode was classified as one subtype of Bipolar Disorder and did not have separate criteria. DSM-IV formalized diagnostic criteria, specifying that a mixed episode consists of criteria for both a Major Depressive Episode and a manic episode lasting almost every day during at least a 1-week period that causes significant functional impairment. Mixed episodes are considered by some the most severe form of bipolar episode.

Manic episodes may cause considerable impairment in functioning and may be quite distressing or dangerous. By definition, mood during a manic episode is elevated, expansive, or irritable, and mania is most frequently described in experiences of elation or grandiosity. In reality, the mood profile across and within individuals who experience mania is more complex and paradoxical, and empirical studies have demonstrated that the mood during a manic episode is depressed and/or labile as often as euphoric, especially in the later stages of the episode. Irritability is the most common mood during a manic episode (Goodwin & Jamison, 1990).

Cognitive symptoms of mania may include both psychotic and nonpsychotic symptoms. The most common content of mania involves grandiosity, occasionally but not usually at a delusional level. This feature can range from unrealistic overconfidence in oneself to acting on unrealistic beliefs that one possesses certain abilities (e.g., creative, political, or medical) to delusional beliefs about identity. In terms of cognitive functioning, one of the most common symptoms during a manic episode is flight of ideas, subjectively experienced as racing thoughts and frequently observed as rapid, pressured speech. Results of empirical studies vary, and the reported proportions of manic patients who experience this symptom ranged from 41 to 100% (Abrams & Taylor, 1976; Braden & Ho, 1981; Carlson & Goodwin, 1973; Clayton, Pitts, & Winokur, 1965; Taylor & Abrams, 1973; Winokur, Clayton, & Reich, 1969). Other common nonpsychotic cognitive symptoms are distractibility, poor concentration, confusion, and (occasionally) disorientation. Psychotic symptoms of delusions and, less commonly, hallucinations have been documented. Delusions (usually of grandiosity or persecution and infrequently of passivity) have been reported across studies in 44 to 75% of manic patients (Black & Narsrallah, 1989; Carlson & Goodwin, 1973; Leff, Fischer, & Bertelsen, 1976; Winokur et al., 1969; Winokur, 1984). Hallucinations, predominantly auditory, have been reported in 14 to 40% of manic patients (Black & Nasrallah, 1989; Carlson & Goodwin, 1973; Winokur, 1984).

The most pervasive somatic and behavioral symptoms demonstrated among manic patients are sleep disturbance, hyperactivity, and speech symptoms. An average of 81% of manic patients experiences insomnia and/or a decreased need for sleep, 87% exhibits hyperactivity, and reports of increased, rapid and/or pressured speech range

from 75 to 100% (Abrams & Taylor, 1976, 1981; Carlson & Goodwin, 1973; Goodwin & Jamison, 1990; Leff et al., 1976; Loudon, Blackburn, & Ashworth, 1977; Winokur et al., 1969). Other behaviors exhibited in significant frequency among manic individuals include hypersexuality, spending sprees, violent or assaultive behavior, and frenzied or aimless activity. The social or occupational impairment and negative social consequences that result from these instances of lapsed judgment in manic episodes are the defining difference between manic and hypomanic episodes. Hypomanic episodes, by definition, do not lead to impairing consequences. This is another instance where the DSM system attempts to make discrete categories from a continuous severity dimension.

## Bipolar Disorder Criteria

In the DSM system, the history of current and past episodes is used to determine the actual mood disorder diagnosis. A bipolar disorder diagnosis is given when both manic and depressive episodes have occurred. The most substantial change in DSM-IV criteria in the mood disorder section is in bipolar disorder. Bipolar disorder is now clearly separated into Types I and II, whereas in DSM-III-R, bipolar II was classified as "not otherwise specified." DSM-IV criteria for bipolar I disorder require one or more manic or mixed episodes, usually accompanied by one or more major depressive episodes. DSM-IV has added three new "most recent episode" categories to the existing mood subtypes. Bipolar I, most recent episode hypomanic, requires at least one manic or mixed episode and a current or most recent hypomanic episode. Bipolar I, most recent episode manic, requires at least one major depressive episode and a current or most recent manic episode. In bipolar I, most recent episode unspecified, there has been at least one manic or mixed episode, and there is a current or most recent manic, mixed, hypomanic, or major depressive episode that has not met the full duration criteria at the time of diagnosis.

Bipolar II, which was previously categorized as bipolar NOS, is now a separate category in DSM-IV. The individual must meet the criteria for at least one hypomanic episode (but not a manic or mixed episode) and one or more major depressive episodes. The presence of a manic or mixed episode changes the diagnosis to bipolar I. Epidemiologic studies suggest that bipolar I is almost equally common in men and women, and bipolar II may be more commonly seen in women. Some authors (Akiskal, Downs, et al., 1985; Cassano et al., 1988; DePue & Monroe, 1978; Giles, Jarrett, Biggs, Guzick, & Rush, 1989; Winokur & Clayton, 1967) have identified and studied a subgroup of mood disorders (alternately referred to as "pseudounipolar," "unipolar II," or "bipolar III") with depressive episodes, no manic episode, and features including a family history of bipolar disorder, hypersomnia, psychomotor retardation, early age of onset, high frequency of depressive episodes, hypomania in response to antidepressant medication, and good prophylactic lithium response. However, this category has not been addressed by DSM-IV, so such individuals are diagnosed under major depression.

Cyclothymia is a chronic mood disturbance of at least two years (one year for children and adolescents), involving numerous hypomanic episodes and numerous periods of depressed mood of insufficient severity or duration to meet the criteria for a major depressive or manic episode. Thus, by definition, this disorder (considered by some a mild form of bipolar disorder) does not involve marked impairment in social or occupational functioning. Cyclothymia is seen in families of bipolar probands, and there is evidence that cyclothymia can be considered a risk factor for late bipolar disorder (DePue et al., 1981).

Overall, the phenomenology of bipolar disorder is varied and multifaceted across individuals and within individuals across time, in both symptom variability and severity previously discussed for depressive and manic episodes and in cyclicity, episode duration, episode sequence, and stability of states. Cyclicity (i.e., the length of time between episodes) can range from less than every 48 hours to many years, and there is considerable intraindividual variability but much greater interindividual variability. Generally, cycle length in bipolar disorder is less than in unipolar major depression. Approximately 13 to 20% of all bipolar patients can be categorized as "rapid-cycling" patients, defined by DSM-IV criteria and others (Goodwin & Jamison, 1990) as experiencing at least four distinct episodes (depressed or manic) per year. Rapid cycling is more common in females; the initial mood disorder episode is usually a depressive episode, and the rapid cycling generally develops later in the course of the disorder, preceded by one or more less frequent episodes. More extreme and rare "ultrarapid cycling" is discussed by Goodwin and Jamison (1990) and, along with rapid cycling, may constitute a separate subgroup of bipolar disorders. Further, distinct from rapid cycling, the cycling may, in some cases, be continuous, in which there is no symptom-free interval between episodes.

Episode duration tends to be independent of cycle length and is also variable across individuals, but with less intraindividual variability. The sequence (or order of manic and depressive episodes within the bipolar spectrum) varies also, so an individual may experience alternate manic and depressive episodes or several episodes of one polarity between consecutive episodes of the other. Frequently, an episode is immediately followed by a short episode of the other kind. Finally, stability and purity of state is a factor related to (but distinct from) cyclicity and is apparently independent of episode severity. This factor is related to the DSM-IV diagnosis of bipolar I disorder, mixed type, in which the full symptoms of both major depressive and manic episodes are present simultaneously or alternating rapidly, often within 1 day's time.

## Other Diagnostic Distinctions

A primary-secondary depression distinction, first proposed by Robins and Guze (1972), differentiates between depression that arises during the course of a serious medical illness or preexisting psychiatric disorder and primary depression that arises in the absence of other disorders. This issue of comorbidity has been insufficiently researched because most depression research excludes subjects who exhibit secondary or even coexisting depression; however, particularly relevant are depression secondary to medical illness, depression secondary to other chronic psychiatric disorders, and substance-induced depression. In DSM-IV, Mood disorder due to a General Medical Condition is diagnosed when the mood disturbance is etiologically related to a specific medical condition, and a substance-induced mood disorder is diagnosed when the disturbance is the result of alcohol or drug usage.

Similarly, secondary mania has been identified in patients shortly after medical, pharmacological, or some somatic dysfunctions. Krauthammer and Klerman (1978) reviewed this literature and concluded that patients with secondary mania are phenomenologically indistinguishable from patients with primary mania, except for a later age of onset for secondary mania. DSM-IV classifies secondary mania as mood disorder due to a general medical condition (if not induced by a substance) or as a substance-induced mood disorder (if manic symptoms are substance-induced).

The primary-secondary distinction causes some confusion as to the nature of hypothesized causes of depressions that might also be considered reactive. For example, as indicated before, depression after the birth of a child is seen as a distinct category. It is unclear whether postpartum depression and mania are most accurately conceptualized as secondary mood disorders or as primary mood disorder episodes precipitated by the psychosocial stress of childbirth. Increased affective episodes have been documented in women during the months following childbirth (Bratfos & Haug, 1968; Kendell, Chalmers, & Platz, 1987; Kendell, Wainwright, Hailey, & Shannon, 1976).

The primary-secondary distinction is further complicated by the fact that depression is often comorbid with a number of other psychiatric disorders. For example, individuals who meet depressive criteria also frequently meet criteria for generalized anxiety disorder. People diagnosed with posttraumatic stress disorder and/or substance abuse often have depression in the clinical picture. Whether one is primary and the other is secondary is generally defined by which came first. This judgment is frequently hard to make and is unreliable.

Bereavement is included in DSM-IV among "other conditions that may be a focus of clinical attention." This condition may resemble a full depressive episode but is considered a normal reaction to the death of a loved one. If impairment is prolonged and severe (still present at 2 months following the loss), the diagnosis of Major Depressive Episode is given. Many losses may produce brief, normal reactions of sadness; it is not clear why DSM-IV considers the death of a loved one a special case.

In DSM-IV, schizoaffective disorder is considered a separate diagnosis in the psychotic disorders section. It is diagnosed when there is a major depressive or a manic syndrome concurrent with psychotic symptoms of the active phase of schizophrenia, there has been an episode in which psychotic symptoms persisted at least 2 weeks in the absence of prominent mood symptoms, and schizophrenia and organic factors have been ruled out.

Another difficult diagnostic distinction is that between mood disorders and certain personality disorders, particularly borderline personality disorder. It has been suggested that borderline personality disorder is best understood as a subsyndromal form of affective illness (Akiskal, Yerevanian, Davis, King, & Lemmi, 1985; Gunderson & Elliott, 1985), whereas others maintain that the personality disorder is independent, although it frequently coexists with mood disorder (McGlashan, 1983; Pope, Jonas, Hudson, Cohen, & Gunderson, 1983). Coexistent unipolar depression has been clearly documented (Charney, Nelson, & Quinlan, 1981). However, the overlapping symptom patterns make it difficult to differentiate bipolar disorder from borderline personality disorder, and data regarding coexistence has been contradictory (Baxter, Edell, Gerner, Fairbanks, & Gwirtsman, 1984; Charney et al., 1981; Friedman, Aronoff, Clarkin, Corn, & Hurt, 1983; Gaviria, Flaherty, & Val, 1982).

## Epidemiology

Affective disorders are among the most prevalent psychiatric disorders in the United States (Weissman et al., 1984). Two of the largest epidemiologic studies that examined the prevalence of mood disorders are the Epidemiologic Catchment Area Study (ECA) (Robins & Regier, 1991) and the National Comorbidity Study (NCS; Kessler et al., 1994). Analyses of data from all five sites of the Epidemiologic Catchment Area (ECA) program of the National Institute of Mental Health, the most comprehensive epidemiologic study of mental illness in the United States to date (Eaton, Regier, Locke, & Taube, 1981), indicates 1-month prevalence rates of 5.1% for all affective disorders, 2.2% for major depressive episodes, 0.4% for manic episodes, and 3.3% for dysthymia (Regier et al., 1988). The 1-year prevalence rate for a major depressive episode in the population is estimated at 10% (Kessler et al., 1994). Lifetime prevalence from the EPA report is estimated at 8.3% for all affective disorders, 5.8% for major depressive episodes, 0.8% for manic episodes, and 3.3% for dysthymia.

A particularly interesting finding of the NIMH study is the increased rate of depression among younger people (Myers et al., 1984; Robins et al.,

1984). The ECA lifetime prevalence rates for major depression in four age groups are 18–29, 5.0%; 30–44, 7.5%; 45–64, 4.0%; 65+, 1.4% (Weissman et al., 1991). Although the finding of increased depression in younger groups might be due, at least in part, to reporting and recollection biases, it has been confirmed in other studies (Klerman et al., 1985), and Seligman (1989) suggested that it may be attributable to historic factors that make individuals more vulnerable to depression now than in earlier eras.

Except for the Amish study (Egeland & Hostetter, 1983), both population studies (Kessler, 1994; Regier et al., 1988; Weissman et al., 1988) and familial investigations (Cadoret, Winokur, & Clayton, 1970; Perris, 1966; Reich, Clayton, & Winokur, 1969) consistently indicate that affective disorders in general are much more common in females than in males. This pattern of differences between males and females is consistent across different cultures (Klerman & Weissman, 1989). Recent reports show that the lifetime prevalence rates of major depression in women range from 7% (Weissman et al., 1991) to 21% (Kessler et al., 1994), and the range for men is reportedly 3% (Weissman et al., 1991) to 13% (Kessler et al., 1994). Conflicting findings have been reported concerning differential sex ratios between unipolar and bipolar disorders. For unipolar depression, estimated female-to-male ratios between 1.5:1 and 3:1 have been reported (Perris, 1973; Radloff, 1975; Regier et al., 1988; Robins et al., 1984; Weissman & Klerman, 1977; Weissman et al., 1988), except for Egeland and Hostetter's (1983) Amish study that revealed equal numbers of male and females with unipolar depression in that population. However, for bipolar disorder, female-to-male ratios of approximately 1:1 were reported by some investigators (Goetzl, Green, Whybrow, & Jackson, 1974; Perris, 1966, 1968, 1973; Weissman et al., 1988), and of as much as 2:1 by others (Cadoret et al., 1970; Robins et al., 1984). Although unipolar depression is clearly more prevalent among women, the sex ratio for bipolar disorder is less clear.

A survey of the empirical literature concerning the clinical course of mood disorders indicates reliable major differences between age at first onset of unipolar and bipolar disorders. Using hospital admissions as a criterion, unipolar subjects typically experience their first hospital admission between ages 40 and 49. ECA data show that in the group of subjects who developed a major depressive episode, 20% had initial symptoms by age 19 and subsequently developed a major depressive episode by age 25; further, 50% showed depressive features by age 26 and developed a depressive episode by age 39 (Mzarek & Haggerty, 1994). Most bipolar first admissions occur between ages 20 and 29 (Angst et al., 1973; Gershon et al., 1971; Perris, 1966). Data from the five sites of the NIMH Epidemiologic Catchment Area (ECA) program reveal a median age at onset of 25 years for unipolar depression and 19 years for bipolar (Burke et al., 1990). Note that these data suggest a rather broad range around these medians and thus many first episodes during adolescence.

Results of urban–rural comparisons of incidence of mood disorders have been inconclusive. Early studies (Jaco, 1960; Malzberg, 1940; Sundby & Nyhus, 1963) reported a higher incidence of mood disorders in urban areas compared with rural areas. More recently, data from three ECA sites have shown nonsignificant increases of the incidence of mood disorders (both manic and major depressive episodes) in urban areas compared to rural (Robins et al., 1984). Initial data from the NCS generally indicated nonsignificant differences between urban and rural samples (Kessler et al., 1994). A closer examination of the ECA data indicated that results from the North Carolina site revealed significantly higher rates of depression in urban than in suburban areas, but no bipolar comparison was made (Blazer et al., 1985). These results suggest the possibility of higher prevalence rates of mood disorders in urban areas, but such differences may involve interactions among region, migration pattern, socioeconomic status, life-style, environment, and other related variables.

Data comparing the incidence of mood disorders among various races has often been inconclusive due to conflicting results, as well as methodological problems such as inconsistent or inadequate diagnostic criteria, confounding variables, and racial biases. A slight majority of studies reports higher rates of bipolar disorder in Whites than Blacks (Jaco, 1960; Marquez, Taintor, & Schwartz, 1985; Prange & Vitols, 1962; Simon, 1965), but many studies (Helzer, 1975; Weissman & Myers, 1978), including the ECA program (Blazer et al., 1985; Robins et al., 1984), report no significant difference between Blacks and Whites. The NCS results contradict those of the ECA by showing that Blacks have significantly lower prevalence rates of affective disorders (along with substance use disorders) than Whites, which cannot be accounted for by education and income. Few comparisons among other races have been reported, but the ECA data from the Los Angeles site revealed nonsignificantly lower rates of manic and major depressive episodes in Mexican-American subjects compared with White subjects. In general, the ECA data found lifetime rates of affective disorders higher among Whites than Hispanics. The NCS, in contrast, reported prevalence rates of current affective disorders significantly higher in Hispanics than in Whites (Kessler et al., 1994). In sum, there is conflicting evidence at present to suggest that a race distinction exists in the prevalence and incidence rates of mood disorders.

As with studies assessing racial differences in mood disorders, studies of socioeconomic status have been hampered by methodological problems. Data from studies that examined social class and prevalence of bipolar disorder suggest a higher incidence of bipolar disorder among upper and possibly middle-class individuals (Coryell et al., 1989; Peterson, 1977; Weissman & Myers, 1978). Data from the NCS are in contrast with these results and show that rates of all psychiatric disorders decline steadily with income and education (Kessler et al., 1994).

Few systematic studies of cross-cultural differences in the prevalence and phenomenology of mood disorders have been reported; most such studies were carried out in industrialized Western nations. Regier et al. (1988) reviewed studies that assessed all major affective disorders and reported 1-month prevalence rates of 7.0% in London, 4.8% in Australia, 7.4% in Athens, 5.9% in Edinburgh, and 18.9% in Uganda. Studies conducted in Denmark, Britain, the United States, and New Zealand reveal remarkably consistent incidence data for bipolar disorder (Fremming, 1951; Helgason, 1979; James & Chapman, 1975; Parsons, 1965; Weissman et al., 1988; Weissman & Myers, 1978). A cross-cultural comparison within the United States is provided by the impressively comprehensive and methodologically sound Amish study (Egeland & Hostetter, 1983), which revealed only a 1% prevalence of mood disorder within the population of this culturally and genetically homogeneous subculture located in Pennsylvania. More surprisingly, the Amish study revealed no gender differences and a slightly higher incidence of bipolar than unipolar disorder.

## Biological Perspectives

### Genetics

Substantial data have been reported from investigations of family history and/or genetic variables for mood disorders. These studies are of four types: family studies, twin concordance, adoption studies, and mode of transmission studies. Case-controlled studies of mood disorder in relatives of patients and normal control subjects consistently show a higher frequency of mood disorders among relatives of bipolar probands compared with those of unipolar probands; reported incidences among first-degree relatives are approximately 12 to 22% versus 7%, respectively (Angst, 1966; Perris, 1966). Family pedigrees of bipolar subjects show a significantly higher incidence (approximately 11%) of bipolar disorder than pedigrees of unipolar subjects (approximately 0.4%; Angst, 1966; Perris, 1966; Winokur et al., 1969). However, these disorders do not necessarily "breed true" because unipolar depression is generally more common in relatives of bipolar subjects (Helzer & Winokur, 1974; James & Chapman, 1975; Loranger, 1975; Reich et al., 1969), although conflicting results have also been reported (Perris, 1966, 1968). Relatives of well-defined unipolar depressives seldom exhibit bipolar disorder (Gershon et al., 1971; Perris, 1966, 1968; Winokur et al., 1969). Based on such findings, Leonhard (1969) estimated the mood disorder morbidity risk for bipolar and unipolar probands' siblings at 10.6% and 4.6%, respectively, and for their parents at 9.5% and 5.3%, respectively, in contrast with the general population morbidity rate of about 2 to 4% (Fieve, 1975). In total, these investigations support the hypothesis of the existence of some genetic factors in mood disorders, particularly bipolar disorder, and more specifically support the unipolar–bipolar distinction within mood disorders. Another interpretation of the data, however, suggests that unipolar and bipolar disorder may be on a continuum. With a polygenetic disorder, the more severe form may be bipolar. With fewer of the genes, unipolar disorder may result. Thus, beginning with a bipolar proband, you may see equally severe bipolars and less severe unipolars. With less severe unipolar probands, more severe bipolar relatives may be rare.

Twin studies consistently show that identical twins are far more concordant for mood disorder than fraternal twins, and this evidence strongly supports a predominantly genetic contribution to vulnerability. Allen's (1976) review of the extant twin literature on mood disorders indicates significant differences between concordance rates for monozygotic unipolar (40%) and bipolar (72%) twins and nonsignificant differences in concordance rates for dizygotic unipolar (11%) and bipolar (14%) twins. These results suggest that genetic factors may be more important in the occurrence of bipolar disorder than in that of unipolar depression.

In attempts to demonstrate that inheritance (or prenatal or perinatal events) is sufficient to determine predisposition to mood disorder, adoption studies have generally yielded inconclusive results. Examining twenty-nine bipolar adoptee probands, Mendlewicz and Rainer (1977) found significantly more biological parents with mood disorders (31%) than adoptive parents (12%), but these results have not been replicated by other methodologically sound studies.

More direct genetic investigations have addressed questions of the exact mode of genetic transmission and what exactly is transmitted. In unipolar depression, parent–child transmission does not follow patterns suggestive of a single dominant or recessive gene, and polygenic transmission seems most probable (Perris, 1968, 1969). Winokur, Cadoret, Dorzab, and Baker (1971) examined families of unipolar depressed patients and identified two subgroups, which they termed "pure depressive disease" and "depressive spectrum disease." The former is typified by late onset and equal numbers of male and female affected relatives; the latter is typified by earlier onset and families with depression among females and alcoholism and antisocial personality among males. In bipolar disorder, the low incidence of father-son pairs has suggested an X-linked genetic transmission (Mendlewicz, Fleiss, & Fieve, 1972; Winokur & Tanna, 1969). Linkage studies have also targeted chromosome 11, where a specific DNA marker was identified by Egeland et al. (1987) in

their study of bipolar disorder among the Amish. This initial report generated considerable excitement, but as additional families entered into the study, the strength of association weakened, and independent replications have not verified the finding (see Merikangas, Spence, & Kupfer, 1989). The current consensus is that bipolar disorder also has a polygenetic pattern.

## Psychopharmacological Treatment

The psychopharmacological research of the past three decades has greatly changed the treatment of depression and has been very influential in the development of biological models of affective disorders. The basic assumption in this particular research area is that differential pharmacological response is associated with differences in biological dysfunctions and thus can be used as a basis for syndrome identification and classification. Although this assumption can be challenged (and indeed has been in many areas of psychopathology), this pharmacological strategy has been powerful in the development of models of mood disorders, particularly bipolar disorder. This is evidenced by the generally accepted view of researchers and clinicians that bipolar disorder is indeed a biological disorder, primarily (if not exclusively) treatable with medication, whereas numerous theories from psychodynamic, behavioral, cognitive, interpersonal, and biological frameworks abound concerning unipolar depression. The result is that psychotherapy for bipolar disorder has largely been ignored in the research literature. In practice, supportive therapy is frequently offered to help patients deal with the consequences of their disorders, and psychoeducational interventions are offered to try to increase medication compliance. This situation is gradually changing and forms of cognitive-behavioral interventions that target stress management, compliance, and manic cognitive distortions are beginning to be described. Comments on these appear later with regard to different approaches to psychotherapy.

Psychopharmacological treatments of mood disorders fall into an increasing number of categories. These include tricyclic antidepressants (TCAs), heterocyclic antidepressants, monoamine re-uptake inhibitors (MAOIs), selective serotonin re-uptake inhibitors (SSRIs), selective serotonin and norepinephrine re-uptake inhibitors (SNRIs), selective norepinephrine re-uptake inhibitors (NRIs), lithium salts, and a variety of additional drug types. A sample of representative generic names, common U.S. brand names, and applications are listed in Table 1 for these categories (*Physician's Desk Reference*, 1998).

Numerous studies with tricyclic antidepressants suggested that these drugs have a significant antidepressant therapeutic effect with some forms of unipolar depression, particularly the more severe episodes of major depression (Bielski & Friedel, 1976; Elkin et al., 1989; Klein & Davis, 1969; Klerman, Mascio, Weissman, Prusoff, & Paykel, 1974). Several studies (Akiskal, Downs, et al., 1985; Cassano et al., 1988; Prein, Klett, & Caffey, 1973) demonstrated the development of manic episodes in response to tricyclic antidepressant treatment of bipolar individuals and of some unipolar depressed individuals ("unipolar II" or "bipolar III" subgroups discussed earlier).

The second-generation heterocyclic antidepressants are modifications of the already well-established tricyclics. Reported advantages of most of these medications in treating depression involve faster onset of therapeutic action and fewer side effects, although some recent reviewers dispute these claims.

Recent reviews of studies of MAOIs suggested their efficacy primarily with "atypical" unipolar depressions (Pare, 1985; White & Simpson, 1985). The MAOIs are often reserved for use only after other antidepressants have failed because they have many side effects, and severe dietary restrictions are required of the patient who takes these medications. Individuals on this medication cannot tolerate tyramine, which is contained in cheese, beans, wine, and various meats.

Selective-serotonin re-uptake inhibitors (SSRI) are a unique class of antidepressants, that act by directly influencing serotonin neurons in the brain. Prozac, which was the first SSRI, is the most widely prescribed antidepressant in the United States. SSRIs are considered suitable first choice antidepressants because they lack lethality in an overdose, have a favorable side-effect profile, and are efficacious with a broad spectrum of symptoms. The limited number of brain chemical systems affected by SSRIs results in fewer side effects than with the tricyclics and MAOIs (Gorman, 1995). SSRIs are considered effective among tricyclic and MAOI nonresponders (Delgado, 1988; Weil-

burg, 1989). Further, SSRIs are efficacious in treating psychiatric disorders that are often comorbid with depression, such as OCD, PTSD, panic disorder, and eating disorders (Charney, Miller, Licinio, & Salomon, 1995; Gorman, 1995).

Selective-serotonin and noradrenaline re-uptake (SNRI) inhibitors are new to the antidepressant medication field. One SNRI, milnacipran, selectively inhibits the re-uptake of serotonin and noradrenaline without directly affecting postsynaptic receptors sites (Lecrubier, 1997). In a controlled trial of milnacipran, this drug was superior in efficacy to SSRIs, particularly in severely depressed patients (Lecrubier, 1997). Like SSRIs, SNRIs work on a limited number of brain chemical systems and therefore produce fewer side effects than the other antidepressants (Gorman, 1995). According to Gorman (1995), the practice of adding a tricyclic antidepressant (which affects the noradrenaline system) to an SSRI nonresponder may be unnecessary with the advent of SNRIs.

New classes of antidepressants continue to come on the market. The NRIs and serotonin receptor agonists act in the neurotransmitter systems traditionally considered most associated with depression. New drugs acting in the dopamine system affect depression as well. One of the newest of these antidepressants, bupropion, may also offer special advantages to depressed bipolar patients due to specific effects on psychomotor retardation and the relatively decreased likelihood of precipitating a manic episode (Benfield, Heel, & Lewis, 1986; Fabre, Brodie, Garver, & Zung, 1983; Gardner, 1983; Shopsin, 1983). Overall, the various classes of drugs used for unipolar depression show about equal effectiveness regardless of the neurotransmitter system impacted. Side effect profiles, however, vary considerably in reliable ways, and the newer classes of drugs are better tolerated by patients. In addition to these regulated pharmaceuticals, an herbal remedy, St. John's Wort (hypericum), has been evaluated for treating depression and is about as effective as the regulated medications (Linde et al., 1996). St. John's Wort, it is thought, is a natural MAOI.

Lithium in the form of various salts such as lithium carbonate was the first and is still the most important of modern antimanic agents. It was discovered to have therapeutic value by physician John Cade (1949) but was not widely used in the United States until the late 1960s. In addition to the

## Table 1. Common Medication for Mood Disorders

| Generic name | Trade name | Indications |
| --- | --- | --- |
| Tricyclic antidepressants | | |
| Amitriptyline | Elavil, Endep, Entrofen | Depression, especially endogenous depression |
| Amoxapine | Ascendin | Reactive, endogenous, and psychotic depression |
| Desipramine | Norpramin, Pertfrane | Depression, especially endogenous depression |
| Doxepin | Adapin, Sinequan | Depression with anxiety; involutional, psychotic, and bipolar depression |
| Imipramine | Tofranil | Depression, especially endogenous depression |
| Nortriptyline | Pamelor | Depression, especially endogenous depression |
| Protriptyline | Vivactil | Depression, especially atypical depression |
| Trinipramine | Surmontil | Depression, especially endogenous depression |
| Second-generation heterocyclics | | |
| Trazadone | Desyrel | Major depression |
| Selective serotonin re-uptake inhibitors | | |
| Fluoxetine | Prozac | Major depression with anxiety symptoms |
| Paroxetine | Paxil | Major depression with anxiety symptoms |
| Sertraline | Zoloft | Major depression with anxiety symptoms |
| Selective serotonin and norepinephrine re-uptake inhibitors | | |
| Venlafaxine | Effexor | Major depression, melancholia, agitated or retarded symptoms, anxiety symptoms |
| Milnacipran | | Major depression, especially severe depression |
| Selective norepinephrine re-uptake inhibitors | | |
| Viloaxzine | Vivalan, Vivarint | Major depression |
| Reboxetine | Edronax | Major depression |
| Dopamine re-uptake inhibitors | | |
| Bupropion | Wellbutrin, Zyban | Major depression, possibly bipolar depression |
| Serotonin receptor agonists | | |
| Nefazodone | Serzone, Dutonin | Major depression |
| Dopamine receptor antagonists | | |
| Amisulpride | Deniban, Solian, Sulamid | Major depression |
| MAO inhibitors | | |
| Phenelzine sulfate | Nardil | Atypical unipolar depression; tricyclic nonresponders |
| Tranylcypronine sulfate | Parnate | Major depression without melancholia; tricyclic nonresponders |
| Antimanic medications | | |
| Lithium carbonate | Eskalith, Lithium, Lithobid | Bipolar disorder treatment and maintenance |
| Carbamazepine | Tegretol | Mania: treatment and maintenance; especially rapid cyclers |
| Divalproex | Depakote | Manic episodes that do not respond to lithium |

widely recognized therapeutic and prophylactic effects of lithium on manic symptoms, numerous controlled empirical studies have demonstrated clear therapeutic and prophylactic effects for lithium in depressed patients; the greatest effect is in depressed bipolar patients (Baron, Gershon, Rudy, Jonas, & Buchsbau, 1975; Goodwin, Murphy, & Bunney, 1969; Goodwin, Murphy, Dunner, & Bunney, 1972; Johnson, 1974; Khan, 1981; Mendels, 1976; Mendels, Secunda, & Dyson, 1972; Noyes, Dempsey, Blum, & Cavanaugh, 1974; Worrall et al., 1979). Despite the significant unipolar-bipolar group differences, it is important to note that a large subgroup of unipolar depressives (up to 40%) exhibits some therapeutic response to lithium and that up to 20% of bipolar depressives do not respond to lithium.

## Other Medical Treatment

Electroconvulsive therapy (ECT) has re-emerged in the last few years due to improvement in the safety of administering it. ECT is typically now administered in six to twelve sessions, unlike in the past, where numerous sessions may have been prescribed unnecessarily. ECT is indicated for various patients, including delusional/psychotic depressives, extremely suicidal patients where it may be dangerous to wait for the effects of an antidepressant, severely malnourished patients who refuse to eat, patients with medical problems where antidepressants are contraindicated, and nonresponders to other antidepressants (Charney et al., 1995; Gorman, 1995). Researchers suggest that ECT is equal or superior in efficacy to tricyclics and monoamine oxidase inhibitors for treating severe depression (Charney et al. 1995).

There are some noted effects of ECT on memory. Abrams (1997) indicates that minimal side effects from bilateral ECT might consist of short-term memory deficits for information immediately before and after treatment that return to normal within a few weeks. More serious effects of bilateral ECT might include deficits for 6 months or more before treatment to 2 months or more afterward. Bilateral ECT does not result in permanent effects on procedural memory or the ability to retain new information. Right unilateral ECT shows considerably fewer side effects than bilateral ECT. Specifically, individuals suffer little or no memory deficits during or immediately after treatment, and any disturbances that occur may be temporary and possibly undetectable (Abrams, 1997).

## Biological Models

The somatic symptom patterns, the genetic findings, and the response to pharmacotherapy of depression have led to the development of biological theories of the disorder. Primarily as an outgrowth of pharmacological studies in humans and animals, much attention has been directed to neurotransmitter deficiencies as core deficits in depression. These monoamine theories have been developed by focusing on deficiencies in the neurochemical systems that involve the catecholamines, norepinephrine and dopamine (Schildkraut, 1965), and the indolamine, serotonin (Glassman, 1969). Mania, conversely, is viewed as due to an excess of neurotransmitters (Schildkraut, 1965).

Many lines of research implicate deficiencies in neurotransmitters. Some examples of the types of evidence include findings that tricyclic antidepressants increase functional levels of norepinephrine and serotonin in the synapse, probably by blocking re-uptake into the cell. The MAO inhibitor antidepressants inhibit the chemicals that break down neurotransmitters. Reserpine, an antihypertensive, depletes storage of monoamines and causes depression in vulnerable individuals (Redmond & Leonard, 1997).

Clinical research with humans has centered around measuring metabolites of the monoamines in blood, urine, and cerebrospinal fluid as possible biological markers of depression. Levels of 3-methoxy-4-hydroxyphenyl glycol (MHPG), a primary metabolic product of norepinephrine, are taken as an indirect index of norepinephrine in the central nervous system. Similarly, homovanillic acid (HVA) is a metabolic index for dopamine, and 5-hydroxy-indoleacetic acid (5-HIAA) is an index of serotonin. Overall, findings have been mixed, and it is clear that many factors influence the levels of these metabolites (Thase, Frank, & Kupfer, 1985). Their utility as diagnostic markers or as symptom or trait measures is questionable; the same neurotransmitters are deficient in other disorders as well (e.g., Nicol & Gottesman, 1983). Recent research has begun to implicate additional neurotransmitters, such as acetylcholine and gamma-aminobutyric acid (GABA), as dysfunctional, suggesting that more generalized processes of neurochemical disregulation may be acting in depression (Thase et al., 1985; Redmond & Leonard, 1997).

Endocrine models of depression have developed because of the observation that diseases of the endocrine glands often present with depressive symptoms and because of the discovery of feedback regulation systems connected to sleep, appetitive, and libido centers and related to the monoamine systems. A finding that has received much attention is that plasma cortisol levels are elevated in a high proportion of depressed persons. Although cortisol elevations occur as a normal response to stress, they are elevated in depression without accompanying stress symptomatology. Clinical research has emphasized the dexamethasone suppression test as a possible biological marker for depression (Carroll, 1982). Dexamethasone, a cortisol-like drug, suppresses cortisol secretion for 24 hours in normals. It is estimated that 30 to 70% of depressed patients fail to suppress; nonsuppression, however, is not specific to depression nor to unipolar versus bipolar type, and it is affected by many conditions such as alcohol and drug use, weight loss, and older age. As such, the test's specificity and sensitivity are not sufficient to make it diagnostically useful. It does not differentially predict drug response, though some argue that its association with indicators of severity suggest it should predict differential response to pharmacological versus psychological intervention. Suppression does return to normal following successful treatment (Redmond & Leonard, 1997).

Studies of thyroid function suggest the possibility that hypothyroidism may be implicated in depression. Low levels of secretion produce symptoms that mimic depression, and thyroid replacement relieves depression in a small percentage of cases. Thyroid-releasing hormone (TRH) has a diminished effect on thyroid-stimulating hormone (TSH) in regulating thyroid hormone production, but this may be due to extraneous factors (Loosen & Prange, 1982).

A number of other endocrine systems have also been studied, including insulin tolerance, growth hormone, somatostatin, prolactin, and endorphins. These are interrelated and involve the monoamine systems (Howland, Thase et al., 1985).

Several of the endocrine systems show abnormalities in their daily or circadian rhythms in depressed individuals, and it has been noted that the symptoms of depression may also show diurnal variation. For these and other reasons, recent attention has been turned to the possibility of disregulating biological clock mechanisms in depression. Neuroendocrine, neurophysiological, and thermal regulation normally cycle on a 24-hour clock. Other biological clocks operate in shorter "ultradian" rhythms, such as 90-minute sleep cycles, and still other clocks operate on a yearly or "cirannual" rhythm. Each has been implicated as dysfunctional in depression. Circadian rhythm research regarding depression has suggested a 4- to 6-hour clock advance in the sleep-wake cycle and in temperature regulation. Basic research, however, suggests that multiple clocks may be implicated in circadian rhythms and that dissociation between systems may be a more likely pattern.

Sleep EEG research has looked at various ultradian factors in sleep. Rapid eye movement (REM) cycles are disrupted in various ways, and measures such as total REM sleep sometimes differentiate depressed samples. The most robust findings is the observation of reduced REM latency in depression. Whereas normals take about 90 minutes to go into their first REM sleep period, this is significantly reduced for many depressed patients (Kupfer & Foster, 1972). Reduced REM latency is currently the most reliable and useful biological marker of depression.

The observation that depression regularly occurs in the fall and winter in some individuals, followed by normal or manic functioning in the spring and summer, has suggested the possibility of circannual disregulation in some persons. The diagnosis of "seasonal affect disorder" (SAD) has been suggested for identifying individuals with this pattern, who have atypical depressions in many ways (Rosenthal et al., 1984). Recent evidence suggests that phototherapy (prolonged exposure to artificial light) may ameliorate SAD, although the hypothetical mechanisms of resetting the annual biological clock may not be valid (Wehr et al., 1986).

Ehlers, Frank, and Kupfer (1988) draw a theoretical connection between the research on biological rhythms and research on stress as precipitants of episodes of depression. They note that biological rhythms are set by the pace of life events, termed zeitgebers ("time givers"). Zeitgebers include persons, social demands, and tasks that we encounter in regular patterns. If social rhythms are disrupted by relationship changes or losses, increases or decreases in demands, or task changes, this social disruption may result in unstable biological rhythms and thus induce depression in vulnerable people.

## Environmental Perspective

The biological contributions to depression are often discussed in terms of a diathesis-stress model. Biological predisposition or risk is a diathesis that is insufficient to produce depression, except in interaction with life stress. Psychological models propose psychological diatheses as well, and these will be discussed later. As with many medical and psychological disorders, there is evidence that periods of stress are likely to precede episodes of depression. It is debatable whether these are a subset of reactive or exogenous depressions, or whether all depressions vary in the degree of contribution of diathesis and stress.

Life events appear to precede depression, and, in some cases, to precipitate episodes (Lloyd, 1980a,b). This appears to be true for bipolar as well as unipolar depressions (Ellicott, Hammen, Gitlin, Brown, & Jamison, 1990). Questions arise as to the specificity of vulnerability and event type. There is evidence that certain types of events may be specific to increased risk for depression. Events linked to depression have included those characterized as long-term or ongoing difficulties and those that involve severe undesirable events, exits by significant others from the person's life, and individual versus shared stresses (see Brown & Harris, 1978; Monroe, 1990).

Brown and Harris (1978; Brown, Bhrolchain, & Harris, 1975) proposed a model in which provoking events interact with psychosocial vulnerability factors. In their study of women in a suburb of London, they found that four vulnerability factors increased the probability that provoking events would produce depression: (1) the lack of a confiding relationship with a male, (2) having three or more children under age 14 in the home, (3) not having a job outside the home, and (4) loss of the subject's mother before the age of eleven. Low socioeconomic status also appears to be a depression vulnerability factor, especially for women (Radloff, 1975). As suggested by Brown and Harris, there is also evidence that social support may have a mitigating effect that decreases the effect of life stress (Barnett & Gotlib, 1988; Monroe, Bromet, Connell, & Steiner, 1986). Hooley, Orley, and Teasdale (1986) presented evidence that the level of expressed emotion in families is a moderator of relapse in depressed persons. In families that are high in conflict and criticism, the probability of relapse is increased.

Overall, the evidence supports the effects of life stress on depression and supports the interaction between life stress and psychosocial vulnerabilities. Some studies also look at interactions with biological vulnerability in the sense of looking at biologically vulnerable individuals based on their own history or their family history.

## Psychological Theory and Research

As with biological models, psychological theories are diathesis-stress theories. Therefore, they assume that reactive depressions are the basic model for the disorder. Psychological diatheses or vulnerability factors interact with environmental stress to precipitate depressions. Each of the theories has led to research that explored implications for assessment, etiology, and psychotherapy for depression. To varying degrees, these approaches have been used to explicate problems of classification, epidemiology, sex differences, and biological interactions.

## Psychodynamic Models

Psychodynamic theory has contributed a number of models to the understanding of depression. Freud's classic psychoanalytic paper "Mourning and Melancholy" (1917/1957) describes depression as the reaction to the loss of an unconscious object. Because of a loss of part of oneself, anger and reproach become self-directed. In mania, Freud speculated that the conflict is the same, but the energy is released outward. A more elaborate early discussion of manic-depressive conditions was offered by Abraham (1911/1949), who speculated that mania represented the failure of repression to contain self-hatred and guilt arising from the need to give up a sexual aim without gratification. The emphasis on internalization of anger seems at odds with the frequency with which anger toward others is expressed in depression, although Abraham suggests that this anger may be a projection of self-hatred.

A number of more recent theorists from this general perspective focused on differentiating two types of depression or depression proneness. Arieti and Bemporad (1980; Bemporad, 1971) emphasized the failure to internalize standards as the basis of dependency depression and internalization of stringent standards as a basis for dominant goal depressions. The individual who has failed to internalize standards depends on the judgments of others for self-esteem. Dominant goal personalities are vulnerable to depression when they fail to meet their own unrealistically high standards.

Other theorists describe similar distinctions. Blatt (1974; Blatt, Wein, Chevron, & Quinlan, 1979) differentiates anaclitic or dependency depressions, which stem from early loss, from introjected or self-criticism depressions that are based on later acceptance of external negative evaluations. The Depressive Experiences Questionnaire (Blatt, D'Affliti, & Quinlan, 1976; Blatt, Quinlan, Chevron, McDonald, & Zuroff, 1982) was devised to differentiate dependency from depressions due to self-criticism. Beck (1983) uses the terms sociotropic versus autonomous depressions. Sociotropic individuals depend on interpersonal relationships for positive self-evaluation, and autonomous individuals depend on achievement and status. The type of loss a person suffers (interpersonal or status) would produce depression only for the person with the corresponding personality type. A Sociotropy–Autonomy Scale (Beck, Epstein, Harrison, & Emery, 1983) was developed to measure the concepts as two independent dimensions. Hammen, Ellicott, Gitlin, and Jamison (1989) reported results supporting the idea that interpersonal life stresses were more likely to precede depression for individuals high on sociotropy, whereas achievement stresses were higher before depression for individuals high on autonomy.

The idea of a depressive personality, defined by various traits, has had a long history in psychodynamic personality theory. Results demonstrating such a personality type have been mixed at best. Recent research seeing personality factors as interacting with life stress are a more fruitful line of inquiry; several reviews cover the area (Barnett & Gotlib, 1988; Chodoff, 1974; Hirschfeld & Cross, 1982; Nietzel & Harris, 1990).

Psychodynamic therapy in a short-term form tailored to depression has been described by Strupp, Sandell, Waterhouse, O'Malley, and Anderson (1982). Relatively little has been published on controlled outcome studies of psychodynamic therapy for depression. Results have not been as strong as for the cognitive and behavioral approaches (Lipman & Covi, 1976; Steuer et al.,

1984; Thompson, Gallagher, & Breckenridge, 1987). However, a recent study by Gallagher-Thompson and Steffen (1994) found that brief dynamic therapy is effective in treating depressed family care givers.

## Reinforcement Model

Behavioral approaches to depression share a basic assumption that depression arises from a disruption of response–reinforcement relationships. Charles Ferster (1973) viewed depression as a generalized reduction of rates of response to external stimuli. His basic analogy in learning terms is to the process of extinction. Major losses in life can be seen as losses of important sources of reinforcement. Generalization of the effects of the loss occur because other behavior was chained to, or organized by, the central source of reinforcement.

Peter M. Lewinsohn's behavioral theory of depression (Lewinsohn, 1974; Lewinsohn, Biglan, & Zeiss, 1976) posits that depression is a response to a loss or lack of response-contingent positive reinforcement. Insufficient reinforcement in major life domains leads to dysphoria and a reduction in behavior, which are the primary phenomena of depression. Other symptoms of depression, such as low self-esteem and hopelessness, follow from the reduced level of functioning.

According to this theory, there are three ways in which insufficient reinforcement may occur. First, the environment may produce a loss of reinforcement or may be inadequate in providing sufficient reinforcement to maintain adequate functioning. For example, the loss of a job would represent a significant loss of a source of reinforcement, and chronic underemployment might represent a continuing lack of sufficient reinforcement. Second, the person may lack the requisite skills to obtain reinforcement in an environment where it is potentially available. For example, poor interpersonal skills might prevent a person from developing satisfactory social relationships. Third, reinforcers might be available to people, but they may be unable to enjoy or receive satisfaction from them. The reason for this condition would ordinarily be interfering anxiety. The socially anxious person does not functionally receive the reinforcers, even if they are emitted by an amiable social environment.

Another feature of the theory is the suggestion

that once depression occurs, depressive behavior functions to elicit reinforcement from others as concern and succor. The person who is experiencing insufficient reinforcement obtains reinforcement for acting in a depressed manner. Depending on the nature of the contingencies, selective reinforcement by others could contribute to a natural resolution of the depression, but importantly, reinforcement of the depressed behavior *per se* can function to maintain the depression. Although depressive behavior elicits positive responses from others in the short run, continued depression is aversive to these others, and eventually they begin to avoid the depressed person, and the ultimate effect is that reinforcement is again lacking. The result is that the depressed behavior is maintained on a thin schedule of reinforcement. Reinforcement continues to be insufficient to overcome the depression and, instead, maintains it in a self-perpetuating cycle.

A primary area of research that stems from Lewinsohn's theory involves the relationship between mood and daily events. On the assumption that positive and negative events can be thought of as rewards and punishments, this research looks at mood as a consequence of reinforcement. Contingency between the event and the person's behavior is assumed, but is usually not demonstrated in these studies. Findings are generally consistent with the theory. Daily mood is positively correlated with pleasant events and negatively correlated with unpleasant events, whereas the two types of events are uncorrelated with each other (Grosscup & Lewinsohn, 1980; Lewinsohn & Graf, 1973; Lewinsohn & Libet, 1972; Rehm, 1978). Depressed persons have lower activity levels, report less pleasure from positive events (i.e., are less able to experience reinforcement), and obtain less total pleasure (i.e., experience a relative lack of reinforcement) compared to normals or psychiatric controls (MacPhillamy & Lewinsohn, 1974, 1982). The corresponding effects occur with unpleasant events, though with somewhat less consistency (Lewinsohn & Talkington, 1979). With treatment, scores improve on event scales in appropriate directions (Lewinsohn, Youngren, & Grosscup, 1979). These studies also support the assumption of continuity between depressed mood and clinical depression. All levels of depression or sadness are seen as responsive to reinforcement conditions.

Lewinsohn's reinforcement theory leads directly to a therapeutic approach based on the three posited causes of a loss or lack of reinforcement (Lewinsohn et al., 1976). Initially, a series of depression therapy "modules" were developed to match the therapy to the primary deficit of the particular depressed person. People with insufficient reinforcement in their environments would be matched to an activity-increase therapy module in which the goal of treatment would be to identify potentially reinforcing activities and to encourage the patient to increase these activities. An interpersonal skill training module was developed to intervene where social skill deficiencies were evident, and a desensitization module was developed for patients who demonstrated interfering anxiety. Later, a cognitive model was also developed. Zeiss, Lewinsohn, and Munoz (1979) found, however, that interpersonal, cognitive, and activity-increase modules were helpful in ameliorating depression, regardless of the pattern of deficits shown by the patients at pretest. Regardless of the therapy module that patients received, they also improved in all three areas. Because matching was not productive, the modules were joined together in a structured therapy program (Lewinsohn, Antonuccio, Breckenridge, & Teri, 1987) that has been effective in various formats (Brown & Lewinsohn, 1984).

Lewinsohn, Hoberman, Teri, and Hautzinger (1985) reviewed research and the theory of depression and developed an expanded version of the behavioral reinforcement approach. They suggested that cognitive factors involving increased self-awareness may mediate between reduced reinforcement and dysphoria/depression. Other modifications of the approach involved considering the ways in which the consequences of depressed behavior may affect depression by influencing evoking events, reinforcement, and self-awareness. The feedback loops created by the consequences of depression amplify and maintain the depression. The elaborated approach attempted to incorporate a wider range of research findings into a more comprehensive theory.

## Social Skill Models

Social skill deficits have been identified as primary causes of depression by a number of theorists. In Lewinsohn's reinforcement model, social skill deficits are one of three causes for a lack of sufficient response-contingent reinforcement.

Wolpe (1979) saw an anxiety-based inability to control interpersonal situations as one route to neurotic or reactive depressions, which he saw as always secondary to anxiety. Gotlib and Colby (1987) make a case for interpersonal deficits as central to depression and review a variety of evidence. Joiner and Coyne (1999) take the argument one step further in a book reviewing interpersonal aspects of depression. They view depression as a phenomenon that should be seen as interpersonal. Other theorists focused on more specific domains of interpersonal behavior as underlying depression. Nezu, Nezu, and Perri (1989) argue that depressed persons are deficient in problem-solving skills, especially interpersonally. The review literature supports the position in terms of comparisons between depressed and nondepressed peoples' performance on multiple components of the problem-solving process.

Several theorists identified marital communication skills as important in depression (Beach & O'Leary, 1986; Jacobson, Holtzworth-Munroe, & Schmaling, 1989; McLean & Hakstian, 1979). The marital relationship is an important basis for interpersonal support, self-esteem, and social satisfaction. A related approach to depression from a different theoretical tradition is the basis for Klerman, Weissman, Rounsaville, and Chevron's (1984) interpersonal therapy for depression. Derived from a Sullivanian or Meyerian psychodynamic paradigm, the underlying rationale is that depression is caused by unresolved disturbances in important interpersonal relationships.

Research evidence from many sources supports the social skill deficit approach to depression. Lewinsohn, Mischel, Chaplin, and Barton (1980) demonstrated that depressed individuals are perceived by themselves and by others as low in social skill. Interestingly, depressed subjects rated their own skills at the same level as they were rated by others. Normals and psychiatric controls rated their own skills higher than they were rated by others. Both self-ratings and the ratings of social skill by others improved with therapy. Several studies demonstrated that depressed persons have a negative impact on those with whom they interact (e.g., Coyne, 1976). What specific behaviors produce this negative reaction has been difficult to determine. Jacobson and Anderson (1982), for example, found that mildly depressed college students who interacted with nondepressed peers

made more negative self-statements and self-disclosed at inappropriate times that switched the focus of the conversation to themselves following a self-disclosure by the other person.

Hammen and Peters (1977) looked at the reactions of male and female college students to written sketches of a depressed fellow student who was given either a male or a female name. Students of both sexes were more sympathetic to the female and more rejecting of the male. These results suggest that depression may be acceptable in our society for women and may actually be reinforced, whereas for males, it is not accepted and might be punished. This is consistent with the idea that males may handle their difficulties through other means, such as alcohol, in circumstances where women might become depressed.

Studies of marital interactions where one spouse is depressed suggest a mutually coercive and aversive pattern of interaction. For example, depressive complaints and nagging may be negatively reinforced by spouses who give in to the complaint (Hautzinger, Linden, & Hoffman, 1982). The nondepressed spouse is reinforced for apology and for giving in and is punished for making requests or demands by further depressive behavior. Bipolar depression has been studied less in terms of social skill issues, but research on the long-term functioning of bipolars indicates poor marital stability (Angst et al., 1973; Brodie & Leff, 1971; Dunner et al., 1976). This could be due to the consequences of the disorder but might also indicate skill deficits.

Another area of research that demonstrates the interpersonal nature of depression consists of studies of the impact of the interaction with depressed parents (primarily mothers) on childhood depression and the psychological development of the child (Gelfand & Teti, 1990). Depressed mothers are less active, less responsive, and less synchronous in their interactions with their infants and young children (e.g., Bettes, 1988; Cole & Rehm, 1986). The children of depressed mothers are less firmly attached and seem less well able to regulate their emotional states (e.g., Cohn & Tronick, 1983; Field, 1984; Zahn-Waxler, Cummings, Iannotti, & Radke-Yarrow, 1984). These effects are lasting and may lead to general or specific vulnerabilities for later psychopathology in the children (Cole & Kaslow, 1988; Zahn-Waxler et al., 1984). The research of Zahn-Waxler et al. is notable for including study of the children of bipolar parents.

For the most part, these theoretical perspectives were developed in developing and evaluating treatment approaches to depression. Each conceptualization of interpersonal skill deficits leads to a corresponding skill training program. A general social skill training approach involving role-playing with coaching and feedback was evaluated by Hersen, Bellack, Himmelhoch, and Thase (1984), who found that this approach compared favorably to treatment with a tricyclic antidepressant. Other studies of social skill training raised the question whether depressed persons have a true skill deficit or whether, when depressed, they merely perform in a less skilled fashion as a symptom of their depression (Rehm, Fuchs, Roth, Kornblith, & Romano, 1979; Rude, 1986).

Interpersonal therapy (Klerman et al., 1984) was evaluated in the large National Institute of Mental Health collaborative research program on the treatment of depression (Elkin et al., 1989). Interpersonal therapy was compared to cognitive therapy, a tricyclic antidepressant plus clinical management, and a drug placebo plus clinical management. Interpersonal therapy did equally as well as the other two active treatments and was superior to the placebo. It is notable that this therapy approach is aimed more at resolving specific current interpersonal disturbances as opposed to teaching more generalizable interpersonal skills.

Problem-solving therapy with a particular orientation to depression was evaluated by Nezu (1986) and found superior to control conditions at posttest and 6-month follow-up. Marital therapy, it has been demonstrated, is effective in treating depression either as the sole focus of treatment (Beach & O'Leary, 1986) or as a component of a larger therapy program (McLean & Hakstian, 1979). Social skill approaches are beginning to be applied to depressed children (e.g., Matson et al., 1980). Parent training of depressed parents is also a viable treatment modality (see Rogers & Forehand, 1983).

Overall, the social skill approaches represent a diverse group of theoretical positions, research strategies, and therapeutic methods. They share the orientation of looking at depression in terms of its interpersonal causes, manifestations, and effects on others. Putting depression and other forms of psychopathology into a more interpersonal perspective is a potentially useful trend that contrasts with the traditional medical model of the disorder.

## Learned Helplessness Theory

Martin E. P. Seligman's (1974, 1975) learned-helplessness theory of depression was derived from an animal model for the disorder. Dogs exposed to unavoidable shock are subsequently deficient in learning an escape or avoidance response in a shuttle-box apparatus (e.g., Seligman & Maier, 1967). These dogs were seen as having acquired a generalized helplessness, that is, a perception of lack of contingency between responses and outcomes. Dogs with equivalent, but response-contingent shock learned later to escape and avoid like dogs with no preconditioned experience. The behavior of these animals is analogous to human depression in several ways. Induction by inescapable shock is a parallel to the traumatic loss that often precipitates depression. The animals' behavior included passivity, weight loss, and lack of appetite. Moreover, the learned helplessness effect dissipated with time, as does normal depression.

In 1978, a more cognitive, attributional revision of the learned-helplessness theory was published (Abramson, Seligman, & Teasdale, 1978). The revision adapted concepts of attribution of responsibility from social psychology (Weiner et al., 1971). The revised model hypothesizes that a particular attributional style is typical of people at risk of depression. Depression-vulnerable individuals habitually attribute negative outcomes to internal, stable, global causes and positive events to external, unstable, specific causes. In other words, following a failure, the depression-prone person accepts blame and assumes that the cause is general and persisting. Following a success, the same person takes no credit and assumes that it has no implication for other behavior or for the future.

A person with this depressive cognitive-diathesis is likely to make a depressive attribution when a major aversive event occurs. To make such an interpretation is to perceive oneself as helpless (e.g., "I am unable to avoid failure and unable to produce success"). The nature of the attribution for a specific aversive experience determines the nature of the depression. An internal attribution determines whether the person's self-esteem is affected, a stable attribution determines the chronicity of the depression, and a global attribution determines the generality of the feelings of depression. The intensity of the depression is determined by the aversiveness of the event and also by the person's consequent attributions.

Later papers concerning the theory have made additional revisions. Alloy, Clements, and Kolden (1985) and Abramson, Alloy, and Metalsky (1988) emphasized the idea that attributional style is neither a necessary nor sufficient cause of depression but only a contributory cause or a risk factor along with many other possible risk factors. A depressive attribution about a particular adverse event is only partly predictable from attributional style. Many other paths to depression may exist, and the model applies to only a subset of depressions. The revisions also add another step in the causal sequence by asserting that helplessness leads to depression when it leads the person to be hopeless about the future. Hopelessness is seen as the proximal antecedent cause of only a subset of depressions. The authors refer to this as a revised "hopelessness model" of depression.

A number of lines of research resulted from the learned-helplessness theoretical position. Studies of helplessness induction in humans have followed the analogy to the animal experiments. Humans who experience noncontingent aversive stimulation show deficits on subsequent task performance that parallel the behavior of depressed persons (e.g., Miller & Seligman, 1975).

The Attributional Style Questionnaire (Peterson et al., 1982) has been employed in many studies to assess the consistent individual difference posited to represent vulnerability to depression. It is clear that a depressive attributional style is a concomitant or symptom of depression, but evidence is less clear that it is a preexisting causal trait (see Barnett & Gotlib, 1988, for a review of the evidence). Evidence is mixed as to whether attributional style remains depressive in remitted patients (Eaves & Rush, 1984); the weight of evidence suggests that it returns to normal levels (e.g., Zeiss & Lewinsohn, 1988). Prospective studies of attributional style as a predictor of depression are few and do not tend to support its predictive value (e.g., Lewinsohn, Steinmetz, Larson, & Franklin, 1981), although positive findings have been found in studies looking at the specific interaction of attributional style and an adverse life event (e.g., Metalsky et al., 1982; O'Hara, Rehm, & Campbell, 1982). An innovative study by Needles and Abramson (1990) demonstrated that a positive attributional style for positive events interacts with the occurrence of positive events to predict recovery from episodes of mild depression.

Seligman's model does not differentiate between unipolar and bipolar depression with regard to attributional style, and most research has excluded bipolars. However, recent studies (Ivens, 1988; Seligman et al., 1988) indicate that attributional styles of unipolar and bipolar depressed patients do not differ significantly.

The learned-helplessness theory has been employed to explicate the problem of differential sex ratio in depression. Dweck suggests that children receive differential feedback as to the causal attributions for their failures (Dweck & Bush, 1976; Dweck, Davidson, Nelson, & Enna, 1978). In effect, boys are told that their failures are due to lack of effort (an unstable cause), whereas girls are more likely to be told that failure is due to lack of ability (a stable cause). The implication is that women are more likely to be socialized to make depressive attributions for failure. Radloff (1975; Radloff & Rae, 1979) employs the helplessness model to explain sex differences in an analysis of epidemiologic data that partition the contributions of marriage, out-of-home employment, and satisfaction with job and marriage to depression in women.

A different tack in dealing with sex differences was proposed by Susan Nolen-Hoeksema (1987). She notes that there are individual differences in cognitive response to aversive experiences. Some people tend to ruminate over the causes and implications of the event and thereby maintain and extend the depressive mood. Others may use strategies to minimize the psychological impact of an aversive event, such as distraction or purposefully focusing on more pleasant topics, which help to terminate a depressive mood. Women are more likely to have a ruminative style, and men are more likely to have a distracting style.

No therapy program has been developed directly from the learned-helplessness perspective. Seligman (1981), however, suggested that four basic therapeutic strategies are consistent with the tenets of the theory. The first is environmental manipulations, which involve putting the person in an environment (such as a psychiatric hospital) that promotes a recovery of a sense of control over daily events. The second is skill training (e.g., in job skills or social skills) to give the person actual increased ability to control the environment. Third, Seligman suggests the possibility of resignation training to help people give up unrealistic goals that they are helpless to achieve and replace them with more realistic and controllable goals. Fourth, attribution retraining would be directed at the depressive attributional style itself to avoid initiating new depressive episodes.

Learned-helplessness theory has been very influential in generating research to test hypotheses that it has generated. It is an evolving approach that has been revised in response to the data generated. It remains to be seen what utility will be added to the theory by the recent hopelessness revision. It may be difficult to operationalize the constructs of attributional style, helplessness, and hopelessness as entities separate from depression itself. Recent extensions of the theory focused on the converse implications of the theory. A pessimistic attribution style as a vulnerability characteristic implies that an optimistic attributional style may be a protective immunity characteristic. Implications of this premise have been elaborated by Seligman (Seligman et al., 1995).

## Self-Control Theory

Models of self-control are concerned with the ways by which people manage their behavior to obtain long-term goals (e.g., quit smoking, or start exercising for long-term health). As applied to depression, the self-control approach focuses on the inability of depressed people to manage their behavior toward long-term goals. Depressed people feel helpless, they are hopeless about the future, and behavior formerly organized by long-term goals is most likely to deteriorate.

Lynn P. Rehm (1977) presented a self-control model of depression that attempted to integrate aspects of the theories of Lewinsohn, Beck, and Seligman in a self-control framework. The framework was an adaptation of Kanfer's (1970) model of self-control; Kanfer described people's efforts at controlling their behavior to obtain long-term goals in terms of a three-stage feedback loop consisting of self-monitoring, self-evaluation, and self-reinforcement. Kanfer assumes that people can control and influence their own behavior using the same reinforcement principles that would ap-

ply to the control of someone else's behavior. Self-reward and self-punishment act as supplements to the external rewards and punishments of the environment and function to maintain behavior when external reinforcement is not immediate.

The self-control model of depression (Rehm, 1977) postulates that the behavior of depressed people could be characterized by one or more of six deficits in self-control behavior. First, depressed persons selectively attend to negative events in their lives, to the relative exclusion of positive events. This self-monitoring deficit describes the phenomenon discussed by Beck (1972) as selective attention in depression. Second, depressed people selectively attend to the immediate (as opposed to the delayed) consequences of their behavior. Depressed persons have difficulty in looking beyond the demands of the present when making behavioral choices.

Third, depressed people set stringent self-evaluative standards for themselves. They are often perfectionistic, and standards for themselves are more stringent than those applied to others. Fourth, depressed people make depressive attributions about their behavior. In the original paper, the internal–external dimension was addressed, and a global–specific dimension was discussed in terms of breadth of standards applied. With the advent of the attributional revision of the learned-helplessness theory (Abramson et al., 1978), later versions of the model incorporated a three-dimensional analysis of helplessness theory.

Fifth, depressed people administer insufficient contingent rewards to themselves to maintain important domains of behavior. Sixth, they administer excessive self-punishment. Self-punishment suppresses constructive behavior in many areas. These deficits in the self-reinforcement phase of self-control are partly the consequence of deficits in the earlier phases of self-control behavior. For example, monitoring negative events and setting high standards minimizes reward and maximizes punishment.

Self-reinforcement is seen as supplementing external reinforcement. The nondepressed person can maintain behavior toward goals, even when the external environment does not reinforce that behavior. The depressed person depends on external sources of reinforcement and becomes depressed when they are insufficient (as suggested by Lewinsohn). When environmental contingencies change, the individual is faced with organizing efforts to readjust and reorient toward distant goals. The self-control model is a vulnerability or diathesis-stress model in the sense that poor self-control skills, as described earlier, place people at risk for depression under adverse conditions of external reinforcement.

Research relevant to the self-control model of depression is diverse (Rehm, 1982, 1988), and only a few examples will be cited here. Roth and Rehm (1980) examined the self-monitoring behavior of depressed and nondepressed psychiatric patients who viewed themselves interacting on videotape, and counted specified positive and negative behaviors. Although there were no objective differences between groups, the depressed patients counted fewer positive and more negative behaviors than the nondepressed patients. Though the study does not distinguish between selective attention and different standards for calling an event positive or negative, it does point to a depressive tendency to self-monitor in a biased fashion.

Rehm and Plakosh (1975) found that mildly depressed college students were more likely to express a preference for a small immediate reward in contrast to a larger delayed reward. In another study, however, when subjects were faced with a real (as opposed to hypothetical) choice, depression scores did not predict the choice of a delayed, but larger payment for research participation (O'Hara & Rehm, 1982).

Studies that show negative self-evaluation in depressed persons are plentiful (e.g., Lewinsohn et al., 1980, discussed earlier). Performance standards of depressed persons appear to be higher because depressed persons often evaluate the same actual performance as less positive than that of nondepressed persons. Shrauger and Terbovic (1976) demonstrated that college students with low self-esteem rated themselves lower on a task than they rated a confederate who was duplicating the subject's performance.

Self-reinforcement studies compared the rate at which depressed and nondepressed subjects administer token rewards and punishments to themselves based on their evaluations of their own performance. For example, on a recognition memory task, Rozensky, Rehm, Pry, and Roth (1977) found that depressed psychiatric patients self-rewarded less and self-punished more than nondepressed patients, even though their actual performance was equivalent. By and large, these studies have not differentiated self-reinforcement from self-evaluation. Gotlib (1981) found that these effects were not specific to depression but characterized psychopathology generally.

Ivens (1988) administered the Self-Control Questionnaire, a scale developed to measure the specific self-control deficits that, it was hypothesized, are related to depression (Rehm et al., 1981), to pharmacologically treated unipolar, bipolar, and schizophrenic outpatients. There were no significant differences between groups, although questionnaire scores within each group correlated with depressive symptoms on the Beck Depression Inventory.

One line of research from this perspective has been the development and evaluation of a therapeutic program based on the self-control model. Self-management therapy is a structured, manual, group-format program that presents the depression concepts of the model to participants and uses weekly homework assignments to modify their self-management behavior. The program was evaluated in outcome studies by Rehm and his colleagues and in a number of independent replications (Flemming & Thorton, 1980; Fuchs & Rehm, 1977; Kornblith, Rehm, O'Hara, & Lamparski, 1983; Rehm et al., 1979; Rehm, Kaslow, & Rabin, 1987; Rehm et al., 1981; Rehm, Lamparski, Romano, & O'Hara, 1985; Rude, 1986). The program was also adapted for children (Stark, Reynolds, & Kaslow, 1987), adolescents (Reynolds & Coats, 1986), and the elderly (Rokke, Tomhave, & Jocic, in press).

Kanfer and Hagerman (1981) presented a revised model of self-control and discussed its applicability to depression. The revision elaborates on the sequences of decisions that are made in the self-control process. For example, attributional processes are incorporated at both the self-monitoring and self-evaluative stages of regulation. The revised model also elaborates on the interaction of short- and long-term goals and standards that may be applied to specific behaviors.

Rehm (1988) used the self-control model to organize current research on depression. He noted the problems of the underlying self-control model, especially regarding the heterogeneity of self-monitoring processes and the concept of self-reinforcement (see Catania, 1975). Alternative models of self-regulation may be desirable to account for the ways in which people solve problems and plan based on biased inferences, negative bias in recall, unrealistic standards, and negative expectancies. Rehm and Naus (1990) present one example of an approach to developing such a model.

## Cognitive Theory

Aaron T. Beck developed a cognitive theory that initially focused on depression and has been expanded to other areas of psychopathology and psychotherapy. Beck's (1972) theory defines depression in cognitive terms. He sees the essential elements of the disorder as the cognitive triad: (1) a negative view of self, (2) a negative view of the world, and (3) a negative view of the future. The depressed person views the world through an organized set of depressive schemata that distort experience about self, world, and future in a negative direction; schemata are complex units of stored information that also serve as templates for interpreting new experience. A number of typical forms of cognitive distortion were identified early in the development of the theory (Beck, 1963). Arbitrary inference involves the arbitrary assumption that some negative event was caused by oneself. Selective abstraction occurs when the person focuses on the negative element in an otherwise positive set of information. Magnification and minimization involve overemphasizing negatives and underemphasizing positives. Inexact labeling involves giving a distorted label to an event and then reacting to the label rather than to the event.

It is a basic tenet of the cognitive approach that a schematic interpretation always mediates between an experience and the emotional response to that experience. The schematic inferences and interpretations that a person makes in a particular situation are termed automatic thoughts. They are automatic in the sense that the person is not aware of the interpretive process and may not even be aware of the thought itself, but only of the emotional consequence of the thought. These specific thoughts can be distinguished from underlying assumptions, which are more basic interpretive rules that form the automatic thoughts. In depression, the theme of the automatic thoughts is the perception of loss. Loss is the cognition that relates to depression. In contrast, perceptions of gain produce euphoria, perceptions of danger produce anxiety, and perceptions of offense produce anger.

Depressive schemata are activated when a major loss is perceived. An organized set of negative schemata is activated that replaces nondistorted schemata when the person becomes depressed. The schemata are formed earlier in life and are reactivated when major losses are experienced. They represent organized and elaborated views of self, world, and future. They may be replaced by more realistic schemata under usual life circumstances, but they remain intact as "latent" schemata with the potential to reactivate under circumstances of loss. With time and the improvement of circumstances, these schemata may again become latent, unless they are modified by some form of intervention.

Beck addresses the problem of mania from the point of view of his model. Systematic positive distortions occur automatically and appear plausible to the patient. In mania, cognitions are less amenable to change by reasoning and contradictory evidence. Manic patients perceive significant gain in life experiences, indiscriminately attribute positive value to experiences, unrealistically expect positive outcomes for endeavors, and have exaggerated estimates of their abilities. These distorted inferences lead to feelings of euphoria and energize high levels of activity. Only a few studies to date have addressed cognitive distortion in mania. The Automatic Thoughts Questionnaire, a measure of negative thinking in a depressed state, discriminates between unipolar and bipolar patients (Hollon & Kendall, 1980). However, the Dysfunctional Attitude Scale, a measure of more trait-like underlying assumptions, has yielded contradictory results in comparisons between unipolars and bipolars (Hollon, Kendall, & Lumrey, 1986; Ivens, 1988; Silverman, Silverman, & Eardley, 1984).

Many areas of research support components of the general cognitive theory, and the theory has been influential in increasing research interest in new areas of cognition and information processing in depression (and in psychopathology generally). The negative biases of the cognitive triad are well established, and the premise that cognition precedes emotion has utility in studying emotion, although it is a debatable assumption (see Zajonc, 1980).

Self-referent encoding research elaborates on the implications of the development of a negative schema regarding self in depression. In an incidental memory task, subjects are asked to recall adjectives that they had seen in another task wherein they had processed the adjectives either by structure (identify as small versus large letters), by semantics (means the same as X), or by self-reference (describes you or not). Self-referent adjectives are recalled best, presumably because the structure of information about oneself serves as a heuristic for organizing the new information. Depressed subjects recall more negative adjectives, suggesting an organized set of negative information (i.e., a negative schema) about oneself (Derry & Kuiper, 1981).

Research on mood-congruent recall (Blaney, 1986) is consistent with the idea that negative schemata influence the processing of information in depression. Current mood affects the recall of personal information. In general, a sad mood leads to enhanced recall of sad memories and poorer ability to recall happy memories (Natole & Hantas, 1982; Teasdale, 1983). The effect is robust in that it occurs with induced mood, naturally occurring mood shifts, and clinical depression, including shifts due to diurnal variation in depression (Clark & Teasdale, 1982).

A related phenomenon has been referred to as mood-state-dependent recall, wherein neutral information learned in a particular mood state is later recalled better in the same than in a different mood state (Bower, 1981). This phenomenon has been difficult to replicate reliably, and Bower believes that mood state dependent learning occurs only when the material is thematically related to the mood state in which it is learned (Bower, 1983). The concept was extended to mania by Weingartner, Miller, and Murphy (1977) in a study of manic-depressives in manic and normal moods. They found that recall of verbal associations was better in the same mood than at contrasting mood points.

The importance of these findings for the cognitive theory of depression is that they provide an empirical base for Beck's concept of a latent schema. Mood activates congruent schemata that facilitate congruent recall and inhibit incongruent recall. Such schemata also organize new information and affect interpretation and inference. Miranda and Persons (1986) demonstrated that scores on the Dysfunctional Attitude Scale (Weissman & Beck, 1978)—thought to assess stable, trait-like underlying assumptions—are influenced by mood for those subjects who have histories of depression. In other words, for those who had developed organized depressive schemata while depressed in the past, current mood activated them to the de-

gree that they affected responses to the questionnaire.

Mood-congruent recall and related phenomena are becoming central data for new developments in cognitive theories of depression and mania (e.g., Ingram, 1984; Rehm & Naus, 1990; Teasdale, 1983). For example, memory models of long-term storage suggest alternative ways of conceptualizing the shift in thinking that occurs in depression. The question has to do with whether alternative "latent" schemata are activated or whether mood simply affects retrieval within one schema system. Other cognitive phenomena have also been the focus of recent theoretical developments in depression, for example, internal focus of attention (Pyszczynski & Greenberg, 1987), control theory (Hyland, 1987), and self-worth contingency (Kuiper & Olinger, 1986).

Beck's cognitive theory was developed in the development of cognitive therapy for depression (Beck, 1976; Beck, Rush, Shaw, & Emery, 1979). Cognitive therapy is a complex collection of behavioral and cognitive techniques that share as their goal identifying and challenging unrealistic automatic thoughts and underlying assumptions. Cognitive therapy is the most thoroughly researched of the cognitive-behavioral approaches to intervention in depression, and several reviews are available (e.g., deRubeis & Beck, 1988; Dobson, 1989; Rehm & Kaslow, 1984; Rehm, 1995; Williams, 1984). Two findings in cognitive therapy research are particularly notable. The first is that cognitive therapy produces effects equal to or superior to tricyclic antidepressants in ameliorating depression (Beck, Hollon, Young, Bedrosian, & Budenz, 1985; Blackburn, Bishop, Glenn, Whalley, & Christie, 1981; Elkin et al., 1989; Murphy, Simons, Wetzel, & Lustman, 1984; Rush, Beck, Kovacs, & Hollon, 1977). Second, evidence suggests that the effects tend to be better maintained, especially in reducing future episodes of depression. The cognitive skills acquired help avoid or diminish future episodes by providing more adaptive ways of coping with stress. Another recent development in cognitive therapy has been extending the therapy to bipolar disorder (Beck, 1997; Scott, 1996). This extension of cognitive therapy has yet to be empirically evaluated.

Beck's theory has been very influential in clinical psychology. It has developed rapidly as a school of psychotherapy with research and application far beyond depression. As a theory, it has borrowed terms and constructs from cognitive psychology and has facilitated the connection between clinical and cognitive psychology.

## Conclusions

The knowledge base for the psychopathology of depression has expanded greatly in recent years. We know much more about its epidemiology, genetics, and biochemistry and about its affective, cognitive, behavioral, and physiological symptomatology. We also know more about the environmental, interpersonal, and psychological antecedents, correlates, and consequences of depression, and we have pharmacological and psychological interventions that are proven effective.

The development of theoretical models has hastened and directed research in depression. In turn, new research findings have led to revisions of existing theory and to the development of new theories and models. As new areas of research develop, theories develop using the new data asa focal points for theory development. For example, the developments in research on memory and emotion have led to models of depression where these phenomena are central (e.g., Ingram, 1984; Rehm & Naus, 1990; Teasdale, 1983). Similarly, new research on biological rhythms has lead to biological models of depression that focus on their disregulation.

Although new developments in theory advance our thinking and point to new research directions, it should also be pointed out that most contemporary theories of depression tend to focus on specific areas and incorporate at most one or two dimensions. Biological models tend to focus narrowly within a single biological system and are largely silent with regard to psychological or social issues. With minor exception, psychological theories do not address the theoretical status of subtypes of depression, nor do they recognize endogenous or bipolar depression. Stress is incorporated as a second dimension in either biological diathesis or psychological diathesis theories, but few theories have addressed the biological–psychological interaction. Although some psychological theorists may acknowledge the contributions of biological factors in etiology, the connection to psychological factors is not articulated, and for the most part, specific mechanisms have not been spelled out.

Research and theory in the future need to take a broader view and to begin to model the interaction between biological, environmental, and psychological factors into a true biopsychosocial model. Some examples of effort in this direction are Akiskal and McKinney's (1973) final common pathway model, the article by Ehlers et al. (1988) on social zeitgebers and biological rhythms, and the integration by Lewinsohn et al. (1985) of a range of factors that influence depression. Integrative theories may be most helpful in directing research into the complex problems of etiology, treatment, and prevention of depression.

## References

Abraham, K. (1949). Notes on the psycho-analytical investigation and treatment of manic-depressive insanity and allied conditions. In K. Abraham (Ed.), *Selected papers of Karl Abraham* (pp. 137–156). London: Hogarth. (Originally published in 1911.)

Abrams, R., & Taylor, M. A. (1976). Mania and schizoaffective disorder, manic type: A comparison. *American Journal of Psychiatry, 133*, 1445–1447.

Abrams, R., & Taylor, M. A. (1981). Importance of schizophrenia symptoms in the diagnosis of mania. *American Journal of Psychiatry, 138*, 658–661.

Abramson, L. Y., Alloy, L. B., & Metalsky, G. I. (1988). The cognitive diathesis-stress theories of depression: Toward an adequate evaluation of the theories' validities. In L. B. Alloy (Ed.), *Cognitive processes in depression* (pp. 3–30). New York: Guilford.

Abramson, L. Y., Seligman, M. E. P., & Teasdale, J. D. (1978). Learned helplessness in humans: Critique and reformulation. *Journal of Abnormal Psychology, 87*, 32–48.

Akiskal, H. S., Downs, J., Jordan, P., Watson, S., Daugherty, D., & Pruitt, D. B. (1985). Affective disorders in referred children and younger siblings of manic-depressives: Mode of onset and prospective course. *Archives of General Psychiatry, 42*, 996–1003.

Akiskal, H. S., & McKinney, W. T., Jr. (1973). Depressive disorder: Toward a unified hypothesis. *Science, 182*, 20–29.

Akiskal, H. S., Yerevanian, B. I., Davis, G. C., King, D., & Lemi, H. (1985). The nosologic status of borderline personality: Clinical and polysomnographic study. *American Journal of Psychiatry, 142*, 192–198.

Allen, M. G. (1976). Twin studies of affective illness. *Archives of General Psychiatry, 33*, 1476–1478.

Alloy, L. B. (Ed.). (1988). *Cognitive processes in depression.* New York: Guilford.

Alloy, L. B., Clements, C., & Kolden, G. (1985). The cognitive diathesis-stress theories of depression: Therapeutic implications. In S. Reiss & R. R. Bootzin (Eds.), *Theoretical issues in behavior therapy* (pp. 379–410). Orlando, FL: Academic Press.

American Psychiatric Association. (1968). *Diagnostic and statistical manual of mental disorders* (2nd ed.). Washington, DC: Author.

American Psychiatric Association. (1980). *Diagnostic and statistical manual of mental disorders* (3rd ed.). Washington, DC: Author.

American Psychiatric Association. (1987). *Diagnostic and statistical manual of mental disorders* (3rd ed., rev.). Washington, DC: Author.

American Psychiatric Association. (1994). *Diagnostic and statistical manual of mental disorders* (4th ed.). Washington, DC: Author.

Andreasen, N. C., & Canter, A. (1974). The creative writer: Psychiatric symptoms and family history. *Comprehensive Psychiatry, 15*, 123–131.

Angst, J. (1966). *Zur atiologie und nosologie endogener depressiveo psychosen.* Berlin: Springer Verlag.

Angst, J., Baastrup, P., Grof, P., Hippius, H., Poldinger, W., & Weis, P. (1973). The course of monopolar depression and bipolar psychoses. *Psychiatrica, Neurologica, et Neurochiarurgia, 76*, 489–500.

Arieti, S., & Bemporad, J. R. (1980). The psychological organization of depression. *American Journal of Psychiatry, 136*, 1369.

Barnett, P. A., & Gotlib, I. H. (1988). Psychosocial functioning and depression: Distinguishing among antecedents, concomitants and consequences. *Psychological Bulletin, 104*, 97–126.

Baron, M., Gershon, E. S., Rudy, V., Jonas, W. Z., & Buchshaum, M. (1975). Lithium carbonate response in depression. *Archives of General Psychiatry, 32*, 1107–1111.

Baxter, L., Edell, W., Gerner, R., Fairbanks, L., & Gwirtsman, H. (1984). Dexamethasone suppression test and Axis I diagnoses of inpatients with DSM-III borderline personality disorder. *Journal of Clinical Psychiatry, 45*, 150–153.

Beach, S. R. H., & O'Leary, K. D. (1986). The treatment of depression occurring in the context of marital discord. *Behavior Therapy, 17*, 43–49.

Beck, A. T. (1963). Thinking and depression: I. Idiosyncratic content and cognitive distortions. *Archives of General Psychiatry, 9*, 324–333.

Beck, A. T., (1972). *Depression: Causes and treatment.* Philadelphia: University of Pennsylvania Press.

Beck, A. T. (1976). *Cognitive therapy and the emotional disorders.* New York: International Universities Press.

Beck, A. T. (1983). *Cognitive therapy of depression: New perspectives—old controversies and new approaches.* New York: Raven Press.

Beck, A. T. (1997). The past and future of cognitive therapy. *Journal of Psychotherapy Practice and Research, 6*, 276–284.

Beck, A. T., Epstein, N., Harrison, R., & Emery, G. (1983). Development of the Sociotropy-Autonomy Scale: A measure of personality factors in psychopathology. Unpublished manuscript, University of Pennsylvania.

Beck, A. T., Hollon, S. D., Young, J. E., Bedrosian, R. C., & Budenz, D. (1985). Treatment of depression with cognitive therapy and amitriptyline. *Archives of General Psychiatry, 42*, 14–152.

Beck, A. T., Rush, A. J., Shaw, B. F., & Emery, G. (1979). *Cognitive therapy for depression.* New York: Guilford.

Beigel, A., & Murphy, D. L. (1971). Unipolar and bipolar affective illness: Differences in clinical characteristics accompanying depression. *Archives of General Psychiatry, 24*, 215–220.

Bemporad, J. R. (1971). New views on the psychodynamics of the depressive character. *World Biennial of Psychiatry and Psychotherapy, 1*, 219–244.

Benfield, P., Heel, R. C., & Lewis, S. P. (1986). Fluoxetine: A review of its pharmacodynamic and pharmacokinetic properties, and therapeutic efficacy in depressive illness. *Drugs, 32*, 481–508.

Bettes, B. A. (1988). Maternal depression and motherese: Temporal and intonational features. *Child Development, 59*, 1089–1096.

Bielski, R. J., & Friedel, R. O. (1976). Prediction of tricyclic antidepressant response: A critical review. *Archives of General Psychiatry, 33*, 1479–1489.

Black, D. W., & Nasrallah, A. (1989). Hallucinations and delusions in 1,715 patients with unipolar and bipolar affective disorders. *Psychopathology, 22*, 28–34.

Blackburn, I. M., Bishop, S., Glenn, A. I. M., Whalley, L. J., & Christie, J. E. (1981). The efficacy of cognitive therapy in depression: A treatment trial using cognitive therapy and pharmacotherapy, each alone and in combination. *British Journal of Psychiatry, 139*, 181–189.

Blaney, P. H. (1986). Affect and memory: A review. *Psychological Bulletin, 49*, 229–246.

Blatt, S. J. (1974). Level of object representation in anaclitic and introjective depression. *Psychoanalytic Study of the Child, 29*, 107–157.

Blatt, S. J., Quinlan, D. M., Chevron, E. S., McDonald, C., & Zuroff, D. (1982). Dependency and self-criticism: Psychological dimensions of depression. *Journal of Consulting and Clinical Psychology, 50*, 113–124.

Blatt, S. J., DiAfflitti, T. P., & Quinlan, D. M. (1976). Experiences of depression in normal young adults. *Journal of Abnormal Psychology, 85*, 383–389.

Blatt, S. J., Wein, S. J., Chevron, E., & Quinlan, D. M. (1979). Parental representations and depression in normal young adults. *Journal of Abnormal Psychology, 88*, 388–397.

Blazer, D., George, L. K., Landerman, R., Pennybacker, M., Melville, W. L., Woodbury, M., Manton, K., Jordan, K., & Locke, B. (1985). Psychiatric disorders: A rural/urban comparison. *Archives of General Psychiatry, 42*, 651–656.

Bower, G. H. (1981). Mood and memory. *American Psychologist, 36*, 129–147.

Bower, G. H. (1983). Affect and cognition. *Philosophic Transaction of the Royal Society of London, B302*, 387–402.

Braden, W., & Ho, C. K. (1981). Racing thoughts in psychiatric inpatients. *Archives of General Psychiatry, 38*, 71–75.

Bratfos, O., & Haug, J. O. (1968). The course of manic-depressive psychosis: A follow-up investigation of 215 patients. *Acta Psychiatrica Scandinavica, 44*, 89–112.

Brodie, H. K. H., & Leff, M. J. (1971). Bipolar depression—a comparative study of patient characteristics. *American Journal of Psychiatry, 127*, 1086–1090.

Brown, G. W., Bhrolchain, M., & Harris, T. (1975). Social class and psychiatric disturbance among women in an urban population. *Sociology, 9*, 225–254.

Brown, G. W., & Harris, T. (1978). *Social origins of depression: A study of psychiatric disorder in women.* New York: Macmillan.

Brown, R. A., & Lewinsohn, P. M. (1984). A psychoeducational approach to the treatment of depression: Comparison of group, individual, and minimal contact procedures. *Journal of Consulting and Clinical Psychology, 52*, 774–783.

Bunney, W. E., Jr., & Murphy, D. L. (1973). The behavioral switch process and psychopathology. In J. Mendel (Ed.),

*Biological psychiatry* (pp. 345–367). New York: Wiley-Interscience.

Burke, K. C., Burke, J. D., Jr., Regier, D. A., & Rae, D. S. (1990). Age at onset of selected mental disorder in five community populations. *Archives of General Psychiatry, 47,* 511–518.

Cade, J. F. J. (1949). Lithium salts in the treatment of psychotic excitement. *Medical Journal of Australia, 36,* 349–352.

Cadoret, R. J., Winokur, G., & Clayton, P. J. (1970). Family history studies: VII. Manic depressive disease versus depressive disease. *British Journal of Psychiatry, 116,* 625–635.

Carlson, G. A., & Goodwin, F. K. (1973). The stages of mania: A longitudinal analysis of the manic episode. *Archives of General Psychiatry, 28,* 221–228.

Carroll, B. J. (1982). The dexamethasone suppression test for melancholia. *British Journal of Psychiatry, 140,* 292–304.

Cassano, G. B., Musetti, L., Perugi, G., Soriani, A., Mignani, V., McNair, D. M., & Akiskal, H. S. (1988). A proposed new approach to the clinical subclassification of depressive illness. *Pharmacopsychiatry, 21,* 19–23.

Catania, A. C. (1975). The myth of self-reinforcement. *Behaviorism, 3,* 192–199.

Charney, D. S., Nelson, J. C., & Quinlan, D. M. (1981). Personality traits and disorder in depression. *American Journal of Psychiatry, 138,* 1601–1604.

Chodoff, P. (1974). The depressive personality: A critical review. In R. J. Friedman and M. M. Katz (Eds.), *The psychology of depression: Contemporary theory and research.* New York: Winston.

Clark, D. M., & Teasdale, J. D. (1982). Diurnal variation in clinical depression and accessibility of memories of positive and negative experiences. *Journal of Abnormal Psychology, 91,* 87–95.

Clayton, P., Pitts, F. N., Jr., & Winokur, G. (1965). Affective disorder: IV. Mania. *Comprehensive Psychiatry, 6,* 313–322.

Cohn, J. F., & Tronick, E. Z. (1983). Three-month-old infants' reaction to simulated maternal depression. *Child Development, 54,* 185–193.

Cole, D. A., & Rehm, L. P. (1986). Family interaction patterns and childhood depression. *Journal of Abnormal Child Psychology, 14,* 297–314.

Cole, P. M., & Kaslow, N. J. (1988). Interactional and cognitive strategies for affect regulation: Developmental perspective on childhood depression. In L. B. Alloy (Ed.), *Cognitive processes in depression* (pp. 310–343). New York: Guilford.

Coryell, W., Endicott, J., Keller, M., Andreasen, N., Grove, W., Hirschfeld, R. M. A., & Scheftner, W. (1989). Bipolar affective disorder and high achievement: A familial association. *American Journal of Psychiatry, 146,* 983–988.

Coyne, J. C. (1976). Depression and the response of others. *Journal of Abnormal Psychology, 85,* 186–193.

DePue, R. A., & Monroe, S. M. (1978). The unipolar-bipolar distinction in the depressive disorders. *Psychological Bulletin, 85,* 1001–1029.

DePue, R. A., Slater, J. F., Wolfstetter-Kausch, H., Klein, D., Goplerud, E., & Farr, D. (1981). A behavioral paradigm for identifying persons at risk for bipolar depressive disorder: A conceptual framework. *Journal of Abnormal Psychology, 90,* 381–438.

Derry, P. A., & Kuiper, N. A. (1981). Schematic processing and self-reference in clinical depression. *Journal of Abnormal Psychology, 90,* 286–297.

deRubeis, R., & Beck, A. T. (1988). Cognitive therapy. In K. S. Dobson (Ed.), *Handbook of cognitive-behavioral therapies* (pp. 273–306). New York: Guilford.

Detre, T., Himmelhoch, J., Swartzburg, M., Anderson, C. M., Byck, R., & Kupfer, D. J. (1972). Hypersomnia and manic-depressive disease. *American Journal of Psychiatry, 128,* 1303–1305.

Dobson, K. S. (1989). A meta-analysis of the efficacy of cognitive therapy for depression. *Journal of Consulting and Clinical Psychology, 57,* 414–419.

Dunner, D. L., Gershon, E. S., & Goodwin, F. K. (1976). Heritable factors in the severity of affective illness. *Biological Psychiatry, 11,* 31–42.

Dweck, C., & Bush, E. (1976). Sex differences in learned helplessness: I. Differential debilitation with peer and adult evaluators. *Developmental Psychology, 12,* 147–156.

Dweck, C., Davidson, W., Nelson, S., & Enna, B. (1978). Sex differences in learned helplessness: II. The contingency of evaluative feedback in the classroom, and III. An experimental analysis. *Developmental Psychology, 14,* 268–276.

Eaton, W. W., Regier, D. A., Locke, B. Z., & Taube, C. A. (1981). The Epidemiologic Catchment Area program of the National Institute of Mental Health. *Public Health Reports, 96,* 319–325.

Eaves, G., & Rush, A. J. (1984). Cognitive patterns in symptomatic and remitted unipolar major depression. *Journal of Abnormal Psychology, 93,* 31–40.

Egeland, J. A., Gerhard, D. S., Pauls, D. L., Sussex, J. N., Kidd, K. K., Allen, C. R., Hostetter, A. M., & Housman, D. (1987). Bipolar affective disorders linked to DNA markers on chromosome II. *Nature, 325,* 783–787.

Egeland, J. A., & Hostetter, A. M. (1983). Amish study: I. Affective disorders among the Amish, 1976–1980. *American Journal of Psychiatry, 140,* 56–61.

Ehlers, C. L., Frank, E., & Kupfer, D. J. (1988). Social zeitgebers and biological rhythms: A unified approach to understanding the etiology of depression. *Archives of General Psychiatry, 45,* 948–952.

Elkin, I., Shea, M. T., Watkins, J. T., Imber, S. D., Sotsky, S. M., Collins, J. F., Glass, D. R., Pilkonis, P. A., Leber, W. R., Docherty, J. P., Fiester, S. J., & Parloff, M. B. (1989). National Institute of Mental Health treatment of depression collaborative research program: General effectiveness of treatments. *Archives of General Psychiatry, 46,* 971–982.

Ellicott, A., Hammen, C., Gitlin, M., Brown, G., & Jamison, K. (1990). Life events and course of bipolar disorder. *American Journal of Psychiatry, 147,* 1194–1198.

Fabre, L. F., Brodie, H. K. H., Garver, D., & Zung, W. W. K. (1983). A multicenter evaluation of bupropion versus placebo in hospitalized depressed patients. *Journal of Clinical Psychiatry, 44,* 88–94.

Ferster, C. B. (1973). A functional analysis of depression. *American Psychologist, 28,* 857–870.

Field, T. M. (1984). Early interactions between infants and their postpartum depressed mothers. *Infant Behavior and Development, 7,* 517–522.

Fieve, R. R. (1975). New developments in manic-depressive illness. In S. Arieti & G. Chuzanowski (Eds.), *New dimensions in psychiatry: A world view* (pp. 3–25). New York: Wiley-Interscience.

Frank, E., Kupfer, D. J., & Perel, J. M. (1989). Early recurrence in unipolar depression. *Archives of General Psychiatry, 46,* 397–400.

Fremming, K. H. (1951). *The expectation of mental infirmity in a sample of the Danish population* (No. 7, Occasional Papers in Eugenics). London: Cassell.

Freud, S. (1957). Mourning and melancholia. In J. Strachey (Ed.), *The standard edition* (Vol. 14). London: Hogarth. (Originally published in 1917.)

Friedman, R. C., Aronoff, M. S., Clarkin, J. F., Corn, R., & Hurt, S. W. (1983). History of suicidal behavior in depressed borderline inpatients. *American Journal of Psychiatry, 140,* 1023–1026.

Fuchs, C. Z., & Rehm, L. P. (1977). A self-control behavior therapy program for depression. *Journal of Consulting and Clinical Psychology, 45,* 206–215.

Gallagher-Thompson, D., & Steffen, A. M. (1994). Comparative effects of cognitive-behavioral and brief dynamic therapy for depressed family caregivers. *Journal of Consulting and Clinical Psychology, 62,* 543–549.

Gardner, E. A. (1983). Long-term preventive care in depression: The use of bupropion in patients intolerant of other antidepressants. *Journal of Clinical Psychiatry, 44,* 157–162.

Gaviria, M., Flaherty, J., & Val, E. (1982). A comparison of bipolar patients with and without a borderline personality disorder. *Psychiatric Journal of University Ottawa, 7,* 190–195.

Gelfand, D. M., & Teti, D. M. (1990). The effects of maternal depression on children. *Clinical Psychology Review, 10,* 329–353.

Gershon, E. S., Dunner, D. L., & Goodwin, F. K. (1971). Toward a biology of affective disorders: Genetic contributions. *Archives of General Psychiatry, 25,* 1–15.

Giles, D. E., Jarrett, R. B., Biggs, M. M., Guzick, D. S., & Rush, A. J. (1989). Clinical predictors of recurrence in depression. *American Journal of Psychiatry, 146,* 764–767.

Glassman, A. H. (1969). Indoleamines and affective disorders. *Psychosomatic Medicine, 31,* 107–114.

Goetzl, U., Green, R., Whybrow, P., & Jackson, R. (1974). X linkage revisited: A further family study of manic-depressive illness. *Archives of General Psychiatry, 31,* 665–672.

Goodwin, K. R., & Jamison, K. R. (1990). *Manic-depressive illness.* New York: Oxford University Press.

Goodwin, F. K., Murphy, D. L., & Bunney, W. E., Jr. (1969). Lithium-carbonate treatment in depression and mania. *Archives of General Psychiatry, 21,* 486–496.

Goodwin, F. K., Murphy, D. L., Dunner, D. L., & Bunney, W. E., Jr. (1972). Lithium response in unipolar versus bipolar depression. *American Journal of Psychiatry, 129,* 44–47.

Gotlib, I. H. (1981). Self-reinforcement and recall: Differential deficits in depressed and nondepressed psychiatric inpatients. *Journal of Abnormal Psychology, 90,* 521–530.

Gotlib, I. H., & Colby, C. A. (1987). *Treatment of depression: An interpersonal systems approach.* New York: Pergamon Press.

Grosscup, S. J., & Lewinsohn, P. M. (1980). Unpleasant and pleasant events, and mood. *Journal of Clinical Psychology, 36,* 252–259.

Gunderson, J. G., & Elliott, G. R. (1985). The interface between borderline personality disorder and affective disorder. *American Journal of Psychiatry, 142,* 277–288.

Hammen, C., Elliott, A., Gitlin, M., & Jamison, K. R. (1989). Sociotrophy/autonomy and vulnerability to specific life events in patients with unipolar depression and bipolar disorders. *Journal of Abnormal Psychology, 98,* 154–160.

Hammen, C. L., & Peters, S. D. (1977). Differential responses to male and female depressive reactions. *Journal of Consulting and Clinical Psychology, 45,* 994–1001.

Hartmann, E. (1968). Longitudinal studies of sleep and dream patterns in manic-depressive patients. *Archives of General Psychiatry, 19,* 312–329.

Hautzinger, M., Linden, M., & Hoffman, N. (1982). Distressed couples with and without a depressed partner: An analysis of their verbal interaction. *Journal of Behavior Therapy and Experimental Psychiatry, 13,* 307–314.

Helgason, T. (1964). Epidemiology of mental disorders in Iceland. *Acta Psychiatrica Scandinavica, 40*(Suppl. No. 173).

Helgason, T. (1979). Epidemiological investigations concerning affective disorders. In M. Schou & E. Stromgren (Eds.), *Origin, prevention and treatment of affective disorders* (pp. 241–255). London: Academic Press.

Helzer, J. E. (1975). Bipolar affective disorder in black and white men: A comparison of symptoms and familial illness. *Archives of General Psychiatry, 32,* 1140–1143.

Helzer, J. E., & Winokur, G. (1974). A family interview study of male manic-depressives. *Archives of General Psychiatry, 31,* 73–77.

Hersen, M., Bellack, A. S., Himmelhoch, J. M., & Thase, M. E. (1984). Effects of social skill training, amitriptyline, and psychotherapy in unipolar depressed women. *Behavior Therapy, 15,* 21–40.

Hirschfeld, R. M. A., & Cross, C. K. (1982). Epidemiology of affective disorders: Psychosocial risk factors. *Archives of General Psychiatry, 39,* 35–46.

Hollon, S. D., & Kendall, P. C. (1980). Cognitive self-statements in depression: Development of an automatic thoughts questionnaire. *Cognitive Therapy and Research, 4,* 383–397.

Hollon, S. D., Kendall, P. C., & Lumey, A. (1986). Specificity of depressotypic cognitions in clinical depression. *Journal of Abnormal Psychology, 95,* 52–59.

Hooley, J. M., Orley, J., & Teasdale, J. D. (1986). Levels of expressed emotion and relapse in depressed patients. *British Journal of Psychiatry, 148,* 642–647.

Hyland, M. E. (1987). Control theory interpretation of psychological mechanisms of depression: Comparison and integration of several theories. *Psychological Bulletin, 102,* 109–121.

Ingram, R. E. (1984). Toward an information-processing analysis of depression. *Cognitive Therapy and Research, 8,* 443–478.

Ivens, C. (1988). Cognitive patterns in unipolar, bipolar, and schizophrenic outpatients. Unpublished doctoral dissertation, University of Houston.

Jaco, E. (1960). *The social epidemiology of mental disorders.* New York: Russell Sage.

Jacobson, N. S., & Anderson, E. A. (1982). Interpersonal skill and depression in college students: An analysis of the timing of self-disclosures. *Behavior Therapy, 13,* 271–282.

Jacobson, N. S., Holtzworth-Munroe, A., & Schmaling, K. B. (1989). Marital therapy and spouse involvement in the treatment of depression, agoraphobia, and alcoholism. *Journal of Consulting and Clinical Psychology, 57,* 5–10.

James, N. M., & Chapman, C. J. (1975). A genetic study of bipolar affective disorder. *British Journal of Psychiatry, 126,* 449–456.

Johnson, G. (1974). Antidepressant effect of lithium. *Comprehensive Psychiatry, 15,* 43–47.

Joiner, T. E., & Coyne, J. C. (1999). *The interactional nature of depression: Advances in interpersonal approaches.* Washington, DC: American Psychological Association.

Kanfer, F. H. (1970). Self-regulation: Research, issues and speculations. In C. Neuringer and J. L. Michael (Eds.), *Behavior modification in clinical psychology* (pp. 178–220). New York: Appleton-Century-Crofts.

Kanfer, F. H., & Hagerman, S. (1981). The role of self-regulation. In L. P. Rehm (Ed.), *Behavior therapy for depression: Present status and future directions* (pp. 143–179). New York: Academic Press.

Kendell, R. E., Chalmers, J. C., & Platz, C. (1987). Epidemiology of puerperal psychoses. *British Journal of Psychiatry, 150*, 662–673.

Kendell, R. E., Wainwright, S., Hailey, A., & Shannon, B. (1976). Influence of childbirth on psychiatric morbidity. *Psychology of Medicine, 6*, 297–302.

Khan, M. C. (1981). Lithium carbonate in the treatment of acute depressive illness. *Biological Psychiatry, 161*, 244–248.

Klein, D. F., & Davis, J. M. (1969). *Diagnosis and drug treatment of psychiatric disorders.* Baltimore: Williams & Wilkins.

Klerman, G., Lavori, P., Rice, J., Reich, T., Endicott, J., Andreasen, N., Keller, M., & Hirschfeld, R. (1985). Birth cohort trends in rates of major depressive disorder among relatives of patients with affective disorder. *Archives of General Psychiatry, 42*, 689–693.

Klerman, G. L., Mascio, A., Weissman, M., Prusoff, B., & Paykel, E. (1974). The treatment of depression by drugs and psychotherapy. *American Journal of Psychiatry, 131*, 186–191.

Klerman, G. L., Weissman, M. M., Rounsaville, B. J., & Chevron, E. S. (1984). *Interpersonal psychotherapy of depression.* New York: Basic Books.

Kornblith, S. J., Rehm, L. P., O'Hara, M. W., & Lamparski, D. M. (1983). The contribution of self-reinforcement training and behavioral assignments to the efficacy of self-control therapy for depression. *Cognitive Therapy and Research, 7*, 499–527.

Kraeplin, E. (1921). *Manic-depressive insanity and paranoia.* Edinburgh, Scotland: Livingstone.

Krauthammer, C., & Klerman, G. L. (1978). Secondary mania: Manic syndromes associated with antecedent physical illness or drugs. *Archives of General Psychiatry, 35*, 1333–1339.

Kuiper, N. A., & Olinger, L. J. (1986). Dysfunctional attitudes and a self-worth contingency model of depression. In P. C. Kendall (Ed.), *Advances in cognitive-behavioral research and therapy*, Vol. 5 (pp. 115–142). New York: Academic Press.

Kupfer, D. J., & Foster, F. G. (1972). Interval between onset of sleep as an indicator of depression. *Lancet, 2*, 684–686.

Kupfer, D. J., Himmelhoch, J. M., Swartzburg, M., Anderson, C., Byck, R., & Detre, T. P. (1972). Hypersomnia in manic-depressive disease: A preliminary report. *Disorders of the Nervous System, 33*, 720–724.

Kupfer, D. J., Weiss, B. L., Foster, G., Detre, T. P., Delgado, J., & McPartland, R. (1974). Psychomotor activity in affective states. *Archives of General Psychiatry, 30*, 765–768.

Leff, J. P., Fischer, M., & Bertelsen, A. C. (1976). A cross-national epidemiological study of mania. *British Journal of Psychiatry, 129*, 428–442.

Leonhard, K. (1969). *Aufteilung der endogenen psychosen* (4th ed.). Berlin, Germany: Akademieverlag.

Lewinsohn, P. M. (1974). A behavioral approach to depression. In R. M. Friedman & M. M. Katz (Eds.), *The psychology of depression: Contemporary theory and research.* New York: Wiley.

Lewinsohn, P. M., Antonuccio, D. O., Breckenridge, J., & Teri, L. (1987). *The coping with depression course: A psychoeducational intervention for unipolar depression.* Eugene, OR: Castalia.

Lewinsohn, P. M., Biglan, A., & Zeiss, A. M. (1976). Behavioral treatment of depression. In P. O. Davidson (Ed.), *The behavioral management of anxiety, depression and pain* (pp. 91–146). New York: Brunner/Mazel.

Lewinsohn, P. M., & Graf, M. (1973). Pleasant activities and depression. *Journal of Consulting and Clinical Psychology, 41*, 261–268.

Lewinsohn, P. M., Hoberman, H., Teri, L., & Hautzinger, M. (1985). An integrative theory of depression. In S. Reiss & R. R. Bootzin (Eds.), *Theoretical issues in behavior therapy.* New York: Academic Press.

Lewinsohn, P. M., & Libet, J. (1972). Pleasant events, activity schedules, and depression. *Journal of Abnormal Psychology, 79*, 291–295.

Lewinsohn, P., Mischel, W., Chaplin, W., & Barton, R. (1980). Social competence and depression: The role of illusory self-perceptions. *Journal of Abnormal Psychology, 89*, 203–213.

Lewinsohn, P. M., Steinmetz, J. L., Larson, D. W., & Franklin, J. (1981). Depression-related cognitions: Antecedent or consequence? *Journal of Abnormal Psychology, 90*, 213–219.

Lewinsohn, P. M., & Talkington, J. (1979). Studies on the measurement of unpleasant events and relations with depression. *Applied Psychological Measurement, 3*, 83–101.

Lewinsohn, P. M., Youngren, M. A., & Grosscup, S. J. (1979). Reinforcement and depression. In R. A. DePue (Ed.), *The psychobiology of the depressive disorders: Implications for the effects of stress* (pp. 291–315). New York: Academic Press.

Linde, K., Ramirez, G., Mulrow, C. D., Pauls, A., Weidenhammer, W., & Melchart, D. (1996). St. John's wort for depression—an overview and meta-analysis of randomised clinical trials. *British Medical Journal, 313*, 253–258.

Lipman, R. S., & Covi, L. (1976). Outpatient treatment of neurotic depression: Medication and group psychotherapy. In R. L. Spitzer & D. F. Klein (Eds.), *Evaluation of psychological therapies.* Baltimore: Johns Hopkins University.

Lloyd, C. (1980a). Life events and depressive disorders reviewed: I. Events as predisposing factors. *Archives of General Psychiatry, 37*, 529–537.

Lloyd, C. (1980b). Life events and depressive disorder reviewed: II. Events as precipitating factors. *Archives of General Psychiatry, 37*, 541–548.

Loosen, P. T., & Prange, A. J. (1982). The serum thyrotropin response to thyrotropic-releasing hormone in psychiatric patients: A review. *American Journal of Psychiatry, 139*, 405–416.

Loranger, A. W. (1975). X-linkage and manic-depressive illness. *British Journal of Psychiatry, 127*, 482–488.

Loudon, J. B., Blackburn, I. M., & Ashworth, C. M. (1977). A study of the symptomatology and course of manic illness using a new scale. *Psychology of Medicine, 7*, 723–729.

MacPhillamy, D. J., & Lewinsohn, P. M. (1974). Depression as a function of levels of desired and obtained pleasure. *Journal of Abnormal Psychology, 83*, 651–657.

MacPhillamy, D. J., & Lewinsohn, P. M. (1982). The Pleasant Events Schedule: Studies on reliability, validity, and scale intercorrelation. *Journal of Consulting and Clinical Psychology, 50,* 363–380.

Malzberg, B. (1940). *Social and biological aspects of mental disease.* Utica, NY: State Hospitals Press.

Marquez, C., Taintor, Z., & Schwartz, M. A. (1985). Diagnosis of manic depressive illness in blacks. *Comprehensive Psychiatry, 26,* 337–341.

Matson, J. L., Esveldt-Dawson, K., Andrasik, F., Ollendick, T. H., Petti, T. A., & Hersen, M. (1980). Observation and generalization effects of social skills training with emotionally disturbed children. *Behavior Therapy, 11,* 522–531.

McGlashan, T. H. (1983). The borderline syndrome: II. Is it a variant of schizophrenia or affective disorder? *Archives of General Psychiatry, 40,* 1319–1323.

McLean, P. D., & Hakstian, A. R. (1979). Clinical depression: Comparative efficacy of outpatient treatments. *Journal of Consulting and Clinical Psychology, 47,* 818–836.

Mendels, J. (1976). Lithium in the treatment of depression. *American Journal of Psychiatry, 133,* 373–378.

Mendels, J., Secunda, S. K., & Dyson, W. C. (1972). A controlled study of the antidepressant effects of lithium carbonate. *Archives of General Psychiatry, 26,* 154–157.

Mendlewicz, J., Fleiss, J., & Fieve, R. (1972). Evidence for X-linkage in the transmission of manic-depressive illness. *Journal of the American Medical Association, 222,* 1624–1627.

Mendlewicz, J., & Rainer, J. D. (1977). Adoption study supporting genetic transmission in manic-depressive illness. *Nature, 268,* 327–329.

Merikangas, K. R., Spence, A., & Kupfer, D. J. (1989). Linkage studies of bipolar disorder—methodologic and analytic issues: Report of MacArthur Foundation workshop on linkage and clinical features in affective disorders. *Archives of General Psychiatry, 46,* 1137–1141.

Metalsky, G. T., Abramson, L. Y., Seligman, M. E. P., Semmel, A., & Peterson, C. (1982). Attributional styles and life events in the classroom: Vulnerability and invulnerability to depressive mood reactions. *Journal of Personality and Social Psychology, 43,* 612–617.

Miller, W. R., & Seligman, M. E. P. (1975). Depression and learned helplessness in man. *Journal of Abnormal Psychology, 84,* 228–238.

Miranda, J., & Persons, J. B. (1986, November). Relationship of dysfunctional attitudes to current mood and history of depression. Paper presented at the *Meeting of the Association for the Advancement of Behavior Therapy,* Chicago.

Monroe, S. M. (1990). Psychological factors in anxiety and depression. In J. D. Maser & C. R. Cloninger (Eds.), *Comorbidity of mood and anxiety disorders* (pp. 463–497). Washington, DC: American Psychiatric Press.

Monroe, S. M., Bromet, E. J., Connell, M. M., & Steiner, S. C. (1986). Social support, life events, and depressive symptoms: A 1-year prospective study. *Journal of Consulting and Clinical Psychology, 54,* 424–431.

Murphy, G. E., Simons, A. D., Wetzel, R. D., & Lustman, P. J. (1984). Cognitive therapy and pharmacotherapy, singly and together, in the treatment of depression. *Archives of General Psychiatry, 41,* 33–41.

Myers, J., Weissman, M., Tischler, G., Holzer, C., Leaf, P., Orvaschel, H., Anthony, J., Boyd, J., Burke, J., Kramer, M., & Stoltzman, R. (1984). Six-month prevalence of psychiatric disorders in three communities. *Archives of General Psychiatry, 41,* 959–967.

Natole, M., & Hantas, M. (1982). Effect of temporary mood states on selective memory about the self. *Journal of Personality and Social Psychology, 42,* 927–934.

Needles, D. J., & Abramson, L. Y. (1990). Positive life events, attributional style, and hopelessness: Testing a model of recovery from depression. *Journal of Abnormal Psychology, 99,* 156–165.

Nezu, A. M. (1986). Efficacy of a social problem-solving therapy approach for unipolar depression. *Journal of Consulting and Clinical Psychology, 54,* 196–202.

Nezu, A. M., Nezu, C. M., & Perri, M. G. (1989). *Problem-solving therapy for depression: Theory research and clinical guidelines.* New York: Wiley.

Nicol, S. E., & Gottesman, I. I. (1983). Clues to the genetics and neurobiology of schizophrenia. *American Scientist, 71,* 398–404.

Nietzel, M. T., & Harris, M. J. (1990). Relationship of dependency and achievement/autonomy to depression. *Clinical Psychology Review, 10,* 279–298.

Nolen-Hoeksema, S. (1987). Sex differences in unipolar depression: Evidence and theory. *Psychological Bulletin, 101*(2), 259–282.

Noyes, R., Dempsey, C. M., Blum, A., & Cavanaugh, G. L. (1974). Lithium treatment of depression. *Comprehensive Psychiatry, 15,* 187–193.

O'Hara, M. W., & Rehm, L. P. (1982). Choice of immediate versus delayed reinforcement and depression. *Psychological Reports, 50,* 925–926.

O'Hara, M. W., Rehm, L. P., & Campbell, S. B. (1982). Predicting depressive symptomatology: Cognitive-behavioral models and postpartum depression. *Journal of Abnormal Psychology, 91,* 457–461.

Overall, J. E., & Zisook, S. (1980). Diagnosis and the phenomenology of depressive disorders. *Journal of Consulting and Clinical Psychology, 48,* 626–635.

Pare, C. M. B. (1985). The present status of monoamine oxidase inhibitors. *British Journal of Psychiatry, 146,* 576–584.

Parsons, P. L. (1965). Mental health of Swansea's old folk. *British Journal of Preventive Social Medicine, 19,* 43–47.

Perris, C. (1966). A study of bipolar (manic-depressive) and unipolar recurrent depressive psychoses. *Acta Psychiatrica Scandinavica, 42*(Suppl. No. 194).

Perris, C. (1968). Genetic transmission of depressive psychoses. *Acta Psychiatrica Scandinavica, 44*(Suppl. No. 203), 45–52.

Perris, C. (1969). The separation of bipolar (manic-depressive) from unipolar recurrent depressive psychoses. *Behavioral Neuropsychiatry, 1,* 17–25.

Perris, C. (1973). The genetics of affective disorders. In J. Mendels (Ed.), *Biological psychiatry* (pp. 385–415). New York: Wiley-Interscience.

Peterson, C., Semmel, A., Von Baeyer, C., Abramson, L. Y., Metalsky, G. I., & Seligman, E. P. (1982). The Attributional Style Questionnaire. *Cognitive Therapy and Research, 6,* 287–299.

Peterson, U. (1977). Manic-depressive illness: A clinical, social and genetic study. *Acta Psychiatrica Scandinavica* (Suppl. No. 269), 1–93.

*Physicians' desk reference* (43rd ed.). (1989). Oradell, NJ: Medical Economics.

Pope, M. G., Jr., Jonas, J. M., Hudson, J. I., Cohen, B. M., & Gunderson, J. G. (1983). The validity of DSM-III borderline personality disorder: A phenomenologic, family history, treatment response, and long-term follow-up study. *Archives of General Psychiatry, 40,* 23–30.

Prange, A. J., Jr., & Vitols, M. M. (1962). Cultural aspects of the relatively low incidence of depression in southern Negroes. *International Journal of Social Psychiatry, 8,* 104–112.

Prein, R. F., Klett, C. J., & Caffey, E. M., Jr. (1973). Lithium carbonate and imipramine in prevention of affective episodes. *Archives of General Psychiatry, 29,* 420–425.

Pyszczynski, T., & Greenberg, J. (1987). Self-regulatory perseveration and the depressive self-focusing style: A self-awareness theory of reactive depression. *Psychological Bulletin, 102,* 122–138.

Radloff, L. (1975). Sex differences in depression: The effects of occupation and marital status. *Sex Roles, 1,* 249–265.

Radloff, L. S., & Rae, D. S. (1979). Susceptibility and precipitating factors in depression: Sex differences and similarities. *Journal of Abnormal Psychology, 88,* 174–180.

Redmond, A. M., & Leonard, B. E. (1997). An evaluation of the role of the noradrenergic system in the neurobiology of depression: A review. *Human Psychopharmacology Clinical and Experimental, 12*(5), 407–430.

Regier, D. A., Boyd, J. H., Burke, J. D., Jr., Rae, D. S., Myers, J. K., Kramer, M., Robins, L. N., George, L. K., Karno, M., & Locke, B. Z. (1988). One-month prevalence of mental disorders in the United States: Based on five Epidemiological Catchment Area sites. *Archives of General Psychiatry, 45,* 977–986.

Rehm, L. P. (1977). A self-control model of depression. *Behavior Therapy, 8,* 787–804.

Rehm, L. P. (1978). Mood, pleasant events and unpleasant events: Two pilot studies. *Journal of Consulting and Clinical Psychology, 46,* 849–853.

Rehm, L. P. (1982). Self-management in depression. In P. Karoly & F. H. Kanfer (Eds.), *Self-management and behavior change: From theory to practice* (pp. 522–570). New York: Pergamon Press.

Rehm, L. P. (1988). Self-management and cognitive processes in depression. In L. B. Alloy (Ed.), *Cognitive processes in depression* (pp. 143–176). New York: Guilford.

Rehm, L. P., & Kaslow, N. T. (1984). Behavioral approaches to depression: Research results and clinical recommendations. In C. M. Franks (Ed.), *New developments in behavior therapy* (pp. 155–229). New York: Haworth Press.

Rehm, L. P., Fuchs, C. Z., Roth, D. M., Kornblith, S. J., & Romano, J. M. (1979). A comparison of self-control and assertion skills treatments of depression. *Behavior Therapy, 10,* 429–442.

Rehm, L. P., Kaslow, N. J., & Rabin, A. S. (1987). Cognitive and behavioral targets in a self-control therapy program for depression. *Journal of Consulting and Clinical Psychology, 55,* 60–67.

Rehm, L. P., Kornblith, S. J., O'Hara, M. W., Lamparski, D. M., Romano, J. M., & Volkin, J. (1981). An evaluation of major components of a self-control behavior therapy program for depression. *Behavior Modification, 5,* 459–490.

Rehm, L. P., Lamparski, D., Romano, J. M., & O'Hara, M. W. (1985). A comparison of behavioral, cognitive and combined target version of a self-control therapy program for depression. Unpublished study, University of Pittsburgh.

Rehm, L. P., & Naus, M. J. (1990). A memory model of emotion. In R. E. Ingram (Ed.), *Contemporary approaches to depression: Treatment, research and therapy* (pp. 23–35). New York: Plenum Press.

Rehm, L. P., & Plakosh, P. (1975). Preference for immediate reinforcement in depression. *Journal of Behavioral Therapy and Experimental Psychiatry, 6,* 101–103.

Reich, T., Clayton, P. J., & Winokur, G. (1969). Family history studies: V. The genetics of mania. *American Journal of Psychiatry, 125,* 1358–1369.

Reynolds, W. M., & Coats, K. I. (1986). A comparison of cognitive-behavioral therapy and relaxation training for the treatment of depression in adolescents. *Journal of Consulting and Clinical Psychology, 54*(5), 653–660.

Robins, E., & Guze, S. B. (1972). Classification of depression. In T. A. Williams, M. M. Katz, & J. A. Shields (Eds.), *Recent advances in the psychobiology of depressive illness* (Publication 70-9053). Washington, DC: Department of Health, Education and Welfare.

Robins, L. N., Helzer, J. E., Weissman, M. M., Orvaschel, H., Gruenberg, E., Burke, J. D., Jr., & Reiger, D. A. (1984). Lifetime prevalence of specific psychiatric disorders in three sites. *Archives of General Psychiatry, 41,* 949–958.

Rogers, T. R., & Forehand, R. (1983). The role of parent depression in interactions between mothers and their clinic referred children. *Cognitive Therapy and Research, 7,* 315–324.

Rokke, P. D., Tomhave, J. A., & Jocic, Z. (in press). Self-management therapy and educational group therapy for depressed elders. *Cognitive Therapy and Research.*

Rosenthal, N. E., Sack, D. A., Gillin, J. C., Lewy, A. J., Goodwin, F. K., Davenport, Y., Mueller, P. S., Newsome, D. A., & Wehr, T. A. (1984). Seasonal affective disorder: A description of a syndrome and preliminary findings with light therapy. *Archives of General Psychiatry, 41,* 72–80.

Roth, D., & Rehm, L. P. (1980). Relationships among self-monitoring processes, memory, and depression. *Cognitive Therapy and Research, 4,* 149–159.

Rozensky, R. A., Rehm, L. P., Pry, G., & Roth, D. (1977). Depression and self-reinforcement behavior in hospital patients. *Journal of Behavior Therapy and Experimental Psychiatry, 8,* 35–38.

Rude, S. S. (1986). Relative benefits of assertion or cognitive self-control treatment for depression as a function of proficiency in each domain. *Journal of Consulting and Clinical Psychology, 54,* 390–394.

Rush, A. J., Beck, A. T., Kovacs, M., & Hollon, S. (1977). Comparative efficacy of cognitive therapy and pharmacotherapy in the treatment of depressed outpatients. *Cognitive Therapy and Research, 1,* 17–38.

Schildkraut, J. J. (1965). The catecholamine hypothesis of affective disorders: A review of supporting evidence. *American Journal of Psychiatry, 112,* 509–522.

Scott, J. (1996). Cognitive therapy of affective disorders: A review. *Journal of Affective Disorders, 37,* 1–11.

Seligman, M. E. P. (1974). Depression and learned helplessness. In R. J. Friedman & M. M. Katz (Eds.), *The psychology of depression: Contemporary theory and research.* New York: Winston-Wiley.

Seligman, M. E. P. (1975). *Helplessness: On depression, development and death.* San Francisco: W. H. Freeman.

Seligman, M. E. P. (1981). A learned helplessness point of view. In L. P. Rehm (Ed.), *Behavior therapy for depression: Present status and future directions.* New York: Academic Press.

Seligman, M. E. P. (1989). Research in clinical psychology: Why is there so much depression today? In I. S. Cohen (Ed.), *The G. Stanley Hall Lecture Series,* Vol. 9 (pp. 75–96). Washington, DC: American Psychological Association.

Seligman, M. E. P., Castellon, C., Cacciola, J., Schulman, P., Luborsky, L., Ollove, M., & Downing, R. (1988). Explanatory style change during cognitive therapy for unipolar depression. *Journal of Abnormal Psychology, 97*, 13–18.

Seligman, M. E. P., & Maier, S. F. (1967). Failure to escape traumatic shock. *Journal of Experimental Psychology, 74*, 1–9.

Seligman, M. E. P., Revich, K., Jaycox, L., & Gillham, J. (1995). *The optimistic child.* Boston: Houghton Mifflin.

Shopsin, B. (1983). Bupropion's prophylactic efficacy in bipolar affective illness. *Journal of Clinical Psychiatry, 44*, 163–169.

Shrauger, J. S., & Terbovic, M. L. (1976). Self-evaluations and assessments of performance by self and others. *Journal of Consulting and Clinical Psychology, 44*, 564–572.

Silverman, J. S., Silverman, J. A., & Eardley, D. A. (1984). Do maladaptive attitudes cause depression? *Archives of General Psychiatry, 41*, 28–30.

Simon, R. I. (1965). Involutional psychosis in Negroes: A report and discussion of low incidence. *Archives of General Psychiatry, 13*, 148–154.

Stark, K. D., Reynolds, W. M., & Kaslow, N. J. (1987). A comparison of the relative efficacy of self-control therapy and a behavioral problem-solving therapy for depression in children. *Journal of Abnormal Child Psychology, 15*, 91–113.

Steuer, J. L., Mintz, J., Hammen, C. L., Hill, M. A., Jarvik, L. F., McCarley, T., Motoike, P., & Rosen, R. (1984). Cognitive-behavioral and psychodynamic group psychotherapy in treatment of geriatric depression. *Journal of Consulting and Clinical Psychology, 52*, 180–189.

Strupp, H. H., Sandell, J. A., Waterhouse, G. J., O'Malley, S. S., & Anderson, J. L. (1982). Psychodynamic therapy: Theory and research. In A. J. Rush (Ed.), *Short-term psychotherapies for depression.* New York: Guilford.

Sundby, P., & Nyhus, P. (1963). Major and minor psychiatric disorders in males in Oslo. *Acta Psychiatrica Scandinavica, 39*, 519–547.

Taylor, M. A., & Abrams, R. (1973). The phenomenology of mania: A new look at some old patients. *Archives of General Psychiatry, 29*, 520–522.

Teasdale, J. D. (1983). Negative thinking in depression: Cause, effect, or reciprocal relationship? *Advances in Behaviour Research and Therapy, 5*, 27–49.

Thase, M. E., Frank, E., & Kupfer, D. J. (1985). Biological processes in major depression. In E. E. Beckham & W. R. Leber (Eds.), *Depression: Basic mechanisms, diagnosis, and treatment* (pp. 816–913). New York: Dow Jones/Irwin.

Thompson, L. W., Gallagher, D., & Breckenridge, J. S. (1987). Comparative effectiveness of psychotherapies for depressed elders. *Journal of Consulting and Clinical Psychology, 55*, 385–390.

Wehr, T. A., Jacobsen, F. M., Sack, D. A., Arendt, J., Tamarkin, L., & Rosenthal, N. E. (1986). Phototherapy of seasonal affective disorder. *Archives of General Psychiatry, 43*, 870–877.

Weiner, B., Frieze, I., Kukla, A., Reed, L., Rest, S., & Rosenbaum, R. M. (1971). *Perceiving the causes of success and failure.* Morristown, NJ: General Learning Press.

Weingartner, H., Miller, H., & Murphy, D. L. (1977). Mood-state-dependent retrieval of verbal associations. *Journal of Abnormal Psychology, 86*, 276–284.

Weissman, A. N. (1979). The Dysfunctional Attitude Scale: A validation study. Dissertation Abstracts International, 40, 1389–1390B. (University Microfilm No. 79-19, 533). Unpublished dissertation, University of Pennsylvania.

Weissman, A. N., & Beck, A. T. (1978, November). Development and validation of the Dysfunctional Attitude Scale. Paper presented at the *Annual Convention of the Association for the Advancement of Behavior Therapy,* Chicago.

Weissman, M. M., & Klerman, G. (1977). Sex differences and the epidemiology of depression. *Archives of General Psychiatry, 34*, 98–111.

Weissman, M. M., Gershon, E. S., Kidd, K. K., Prusoff, B. A., Leckman, J. F., Dibble, E., Hamovit, J., Thompson, W. D., Pauls, D. L., & Guroff, J. J. (1984). Psychiatric disorders in the relatives of probands with affective disorders. *Archives of General Psychiatry, 41*, 13–21.

Weissman, M. M., Leaf, P. J., Tischler, G. L., Blazer, D. G., Karno, M., Bruce, M. L., & Florio, L. P. (1988). Affective disorders in five United States communities. *Psychology of Medicine, 18*, 141–153.

Weissman, M. M., & Myers, J. K. (1978). Affective disorders in a U.S. urban community: The use of Research Diagnostic Criteria in an epidemiological survey. *Archives of General Psychiatry, 35*, 1304–1311.

White, K., & Simpson, G. (1985). Should the use of MAO inhibitors be abandoned? *Integrative Psychiatry, 3*, 34–45.

Williams, J. M. G. (1984). Cognitive-behavioral therapy for depression: Problems and perspectives. *British Journal of Psychiatry, 145*, 254–262.

Winokur, G. (1984). Psychosis in bipolar and unipolar affective illness with special reference to schizo-affective disorder. *British Journal of Psychiatry, 145*, 236–242.

Winokur, G., & Clayton, P. (1967). Family history studies: I. Two types of affective disorders separated according to genetic and clinical factors. In J. Wortis (Ed.), *Recent advances in biological psychiatry,* Vol. 10 (pp. 35–50). New York: Plenum Press.

Winokur, G., Clayton, P. J., & Reich, T. (1969). *Manic depressive disease.* St, Louis, MO: Mosby.

Winokur, G., & Tanna, V. L. (1969). Possible role of X-linked dominant factor in manic depressive disease. *Diseases of the Nervous System, 30*, 89–93.

Winokur, G., Cadoret, R. T., Dorzab, M., & Baker, M. (1971). Depressive disease: A genetic study. *Archives of General Psychiatry, 24*, 135–144.

Wolpe, J. (1979). The experimental model and treatment of neurotic depression. *Behaviour Research and Therapy, 17*, 555–566.

Worrall, E. P., Moody, J. P., Peet, M., Dick, P., Smith, A., Chambers, C., Adams, M., & Naylor, G. J. (1979). Controlled studies of the acute antidepressant effects of lithium. *British Journal of Psychiatry, 135*, 255–262.

Zahn-Waxler, C., Cummings, E. M., Iannotti, R. J., & Radke-Yarrow, M. (1984). Young offspring of depressed parents: A population at risk for affective problems. In D. Cicchetti and K. Schneider-Rosen (Eds.), *Childhood depression* (pp. 81–106). San Francisco: Jossey-Bass.

Zajonc, R. B. (1980). Feeling and thinking: Preferences need no inferences. *American Psychologist, 35*, 151–175.

Zeiss, A. M., Lewinsohn, P. M., & Munoz, R. (1979). Nonspecific improvement effects in depression using interpersonal, cognitive and pleasant events focused treatments. *Journal of Consulting and Clinical Psychology, 47,* 427–439.

Zeiss, A. M., & Lewinsohn, P. M. (1988). Enduring deficits after remissions of depression: A test of the scar hypotheses. *Behaviour Research and Therapy, 26*, 151–159.

CHAPTER 12

# Delusions

## Brendan A. Maher

## Introduction

Delusions are defined in the 4th edition of the *Diagnostic and Statistical Manual of Mental Disorders* (DSM-IV) of the American Psychiatric Association (1994) as follows:

Delusion. A false personal belief based on incorrect inference about external reality and firmly sustained in spite of what almost everyone else believes and in spite of what constitutes incontrovertible and obvious proof or evidence to the contrary. The belief is not one ordinarily accepted by other members of the person's culture or subculture (i.e., it is not an article of religious faith). When a false belief involves an extreme value judgment, it is regarded as a delusion only when the judgment is so extreme as to defy credibility. (DSM-IV, p. 765)

Delusions are reported in connection with a wide range of psychiatric, neurological, and other medical disorders (e.g., Manschreck, 1979). Systematically speaking, a delusion has been regarded as a symptom, a syndrome, or as a component of diseases of the schizophrenic, affective, somatic, or reactive type. Their frequency and importance are such that we might expect that a clear definition of a delusion would have been well established by now. As will be evident in the discussion that follows, the ambiguity of the definition of delusions has plagued the attempt to investigate questions of etiology, pathology, prognosis, course, and treatment.

**Brendan A. Maher** • Department of Psychology, Harvard University, Cambridge, Massachusetts 02138.

*Comprehensive Handbook of Psychopathology* (Third Edition), edited by Patricia B. Sutker and Henry E. Adams. Kluwer Academic/Plenum Publishers, New York, 2001.

## Problems in Defining Delusions

At first sight, the definition given before seems clear enough, but upon close inspection, it becomes clear that there are many problems. The heart of the matter is that it depends upon the following assumptions and that it includes a hypothesis about the underlying pathology:

1. The truth or falsity of a belief statement about external reality can generally be ascertained on the basis of evidence sufficient to confirm or refute it.
2. There are well-established objective principles by which it is possible to draw correct inferences from factual evidence, and normal individuals follow these principles.
3. A belief that is not supported by evidence but that is shared by most people in a culture cannot properly be regarded as arising from a defect of inference similar to that postulated in the case of delusions. This is consistent with the emphasis upon a delusion that it is a *personal* belief.
4. Value judgments may be assessed on a scale of credibility. Extreme cases that "defy credibility" are properly included in the definition of delusion.

The hypothesis is that the core of the pathology that produces delusions lies in a defect in these processes of inference. A corollary of this is the assumption that in the general population, inferences are typically drawn according to the objective principles assumed before.

## Criticisms of the Assumptions

Each of these assumptions has been the subject
of criticism that can be summarized as follows:

1. *The formal criteria for deciding truth and
   falsity.* The definition of truth or falsity has
   long been a matter of debate in the philosophy of knowledge. Space does not permit an
   extended discussion of the issue here. However, we may usefully distinguish between
   the definition of truth as a *correspondence*
   between a statement made and a set of facts
   to which the statement refers. The statement,
   "It is raining outside," may be checked for
   correspondence by looking outside to see if
   rain is falling. The examination will reveal
   that the statement is true or false; it cannot be
   both. A second form of truth is *coherence*.
   The coherence view of truth asserts that a
   statement is true if it is consistent with another set of propositions. In essence, this
   definition is the same as that of the logical
   *validity* of the conclusion of a formal syllogism. It need have no correspondence with
   actual observation.
2. *Physical reality and social reality.* One
   source of criticism comes from the distinction between external facts about physical
   reality and external facts about social reality.
   A patient who states that there is a microchip
   in his frontal lobe is talking about a set of
   allegedly physical facts.* We have clear definitions of the meaning of the term "microchip" and "frontal lobe," and we have
   methods to determine whether the patient's
   statement is literally true or false. When a
   patient states, "I am being deliberately harassed by my neighbors," the definition of
   the relevant "facts" is much more difficult.
   With some difficulty, we might be able to
   establish what the neighbors are doing, but it
   is much harder to establish that their acts are
   deliberate attempts to harass. Consequently
   the clinician is often left with the alternatives
   of making a judgment or abandoning as futile the task of deciding whether the speaker
   has a problem that merits the diagnosis of
   delusion. Psychopathologists who define
   themselves as social constructionists argue

that human clinical judgment that a social
statement is true or false is the major determinant of the diagnosis of delusions (e.g.,
Harper, 1992, 1994). Such fallible judgments
are, they assert, inevitably affected by political, social-power concerns, professional status, and other such scientifically irrelevant
factors. This criticism has not gained much
support in the years since it was first adum-
brated. Critical responses to it may be found
in Garety (1994) and Walkup (1994).

3. *The empirical requirements for demonstrating truth and falsity.* We must also note that
   the task of demonstrating unequivocally that
   some specific factual assertion is true is often difficult, but it is generally even more
   difficult to demonstrate unequivocally that
   something is false. For example, take an
   individual's belief that his mental processes
   are being influenced by emissions from
   high-tension overhead power lines near his
   home. He complains to the power company
   which sends a technician to test the individual's environment for emissions. The technician finds that they are present. We conclude
   that the individual was certainly right about
   the emissions and may possibly be right
   about their effect upon him. If the technician
   fails to find them, we suspect that the individual complainant may be delusional. If we
   challenge his belief, he may respond by
   doubting the reliability of the measuring instruments (measuring instruments do sometimes fail) and persist in the belief. Alternatively, or additionally, he may doubt the
   honesty of the technician (employees of
   large corporations have been known to lie
   about the hazards created by their products).
   Because this argument is extremely difficult
   to rebut, we turn to an alternative criterion
   for identifying a delusion. This is the criterion of *probability*, rather than of unequivocal truth or falsity.

   Because of difficulty in producing definitive evidence of truth or falsity, the diagnosis
   of delusion in actual practice is often based
   on the criterion of probability. As we shall
   see later, this raises many questions about
   calculating the probabilities. Not the least of
   these is the lack of empirical data about the
   actual probabilities of most events.
4. *The rationality of normal inference processes.* Demonstration of the falsity (or im-

---

*Whether or not patients mean such statements literally or
metaphorically is not always clear.

probability) of a delusional belief itself is, of course, insufficient to establish that the belief arises from a process of faulty inference. To escape circularity of reasoning when we seek to establish the cause of a clinically manifest symptom, we must show on the basis of evidence other than the symptom itself, that there is an identifiable pathological process whose existence can be demonstrated in other ways. If we wish to hypothesize that the deluded patient suffers from a basic defect in reasoning, we must demonstrate this defect in other circumstances and in relation to other beliefs. If the alleged defect in reasoning is found only in matters closely related to the core topic of the delusion, we have not discovered a cause. We have merely established the boundaries of the delusional belief.

By and large, it is assumed that rules of inference involve either or both of two sets of rules. One is provided by the logic of syllogistic reasoning; the other by the rules of Bayesian (statistical probability) inference. Correct deduction from the premises created by induction, it is assumed, follows syllogistic rules. Correct induction of empirical probabilities, it is assumed, follows Bayesian rules. From this standpoint, any belief may be judged in terms of the process by which it arose; if that process violates "correct" principles it is, by definition, defective.

According to this perspective, normal human beings form beliefs about their world in about the same way that idealized natural scientists do. At the risk of oversimplifying it, this involves a sequence whereby empirical observations are made and regularities noted, and proper allowance is made for negative instances and for the limitations of sample size. In due course, all of this eventuates in the formulation of a hypothesis about these regularities. This hypothesis is held with a certain degree of confidence—much as an empirical finding is held by a scientist with a degree of probability exemplified by the concept of statistical significance. The individual then conducts empirical tests to see if the hypothesis survives refutation, a step that will, presumably, ultimately lead to retaining or modifying the hypothesis or developing a better hypothesis.

Once the probability value attached to a hypothesis reaches a critical magnitude the hypothesis becomes a basis for action. Most often the scientist's main "action" is acquiring and reporting knowledge. In the general environment, the criterion for action is determined by the individual's assessment of the costs, potential benefits, and potential risks attached to the various options for action.

Before we can employ this paradigm as a guide to the possible loci of impairment in delusional patients, we need to establish that it provides an accurate account of the way in which normal human beings (including scientists) actually form and modify their beliefs. When we examine the data from empirical observation of nondeluded (i.e., "normal") individuals, we find that the alleged rules of correct procedure are quite commonly broken. Hence the crucial objection to the assumption that there are rules of inference (deductive and/or inductive) that guide the belief formation of nondeluded individuals is that this is, in fact, not the case.

Evidence on this point is reviewed later when we consider theories of the etiology of delusions. There is a large and expanding literature about the processes of normal belief formation. In our review, we shall touch only on those aspects of it that are relevant to the definitions of delusion that we presented earlier.

## Other Definitions

### Oltmanns's Definition

Problems in the definition of delusions have led to the development of alternatives. Oltmanns (1988) proposed to use descriptive dimensions as the defining characteristics of or criteria for delusions. He provides a list of seven characteristics that "... draw attention to the fact that specific beliefs may be considered more or less delusional, depending largely upon the number of specific features that are present.... It should be noted that some of these characteristics may not be unique to delusional beliefs" (Oltmanns, 1988, p. 5).

Oltmanns's defining characteristics are as follows:

a. The balance of evidence for and against the belief is such that other people consider it completely incredible.
b. The belief is not shared by others.
c. The belief is held with firm conviction. The

person's statements or behaviors are unresponsive to the presentation of evidence contrary to the belief.

  d. The person is preoccupied with (emotionally committed to) the belief and finds it difficult to avoid thinking or talking about it.
  e. The belief involves personal reference, rather than an unconventional religious, scientific or political conviction.
  f. The belief is a source of subjective distress or interferes with the person's occupational or social functioning.
  g. The person does not report subjective efforts to resist the belief (in contrast to patients with obsessional ideas). (Oltmanns, 1988, p. 5)

Unfortunately, most of the variables listed in these criteria need further definition, ultimately operational. Thus, a reliance on clinical judgment to establish the degree of "preoccupation," "firm conviction," "incredibility," and so on, defers the task of precise definition to a later as yet undefined stage of development.

### Definitional Concepts
### of the Heidelberg School

European psychiatry has been heavily influenced by the work of psychopathologists at the University of Heidelberg. Karl Jaspers—the founder and best-known member of the Heidelberg School—introduced three criteria for the definition of delusions: (1) subjective certainty, (2) incorrigibility, and (3) the realistic impossibility of the content (later attenuated to falsity of content, because many delusions are in principle actually possible). Jaspers took pains to point out that these criteria, especially the third, do not *define* delusions but rather give practical hints for detecting them.

Jaspers drew a distinction between *primary* and *secondary* delusions. He defined the primary delusion (very problematically) as a fully formed belief that appears in consciousness and arises without detectable antecedents. It is incomprehensible, in the sense that neither the patient nor the clinician can understand how it arose. In an attempt to clarify the definition, Jaspers commented,

We find there arises in the patient certain primary sensations, vital feelings, moods, awareness: Something is going on. This general delusional atmosphere with all its vagueness of content

must be unbearable. Patients obviously suffer terribly under it and to reach some definite idea at last is like being relieved of some enormous burden. (Jaspers, 1963, p. 98)

Secondary delusions, on the other hand, arise from identifiable antecedents in the life of the patient. Here the delusion follows from some conscious anomalous perception or experience. The belief, although delusional, is understandable in the context of the patient's experiences.

A somewhat similar dichotomy is that of Kurt Schneider's (1959) concept of *delusional beliefs* and *delusional perceptions*. It rests upon an assumed difference between delusional beliefs that arise autonomously, that is, without any intermediate processing of environmental input, versus those that arise from a mediating process of perceiving some environmental event. The former sound somewhat related to Jasper's primary delusion, whereas the latter correspond to the concept of the secondary delusion.

## The Empirical Approach

Contrasted to the phenomenological position is an approach based upon the search for empirical independent validities for the definitional categories employed. It begins with the observation that reliable descriptive categories may be established based on attributes that have no functionally significant relationship with anything else of clinical importance. For instance, it may be entirely possible to define subsets of delusions based upon the similarity of the specific content of each subset, only to find that the distinction between, let us say, a subset of delusions that refers to control by demonic forces and a subset of those that refer to control by inanimate physical forces is unaccompanied by any correlated difference in their etiologies, related pathologies, natural course, or response to treatment.

Lacking any correlated validities of this kind, the result of purely descriptive definitions is to create a lexicon of technical labels that can be reliably applied by those who have been trained to make the relevant distinctions. Although this is a necessary first step, it is of little scientific value in itself, unless it is followed by further demonstrations that the labeled categories do indeed have predictive relationships to other phenomena. Empirical investigation may, and frequently does, show that phenomena that have been classified into a single category are multifactorial in their relationships to other measures and/or, by the same token, that categories that are differentiated descriptively are unifactorial in their relationships to other measures. Progress in our understanding of pathology accrues by a gradual convergence of a scheme of definitional categories or dimensions with the pattern of construct validities attached to each category. With these reservations in mind, we may turn to historical and current attempts to classify delusions.

## Classification of Delusions

**Early Classification Systems.** Classification of delusions* by content has a long history. In 1806, Thomas Arnold proposed a classification system which included

*Scheming Insanity*: ... the patient thinks himself ... by his superior knowledge or cunning capable of doing great things, which few, or none, but himself, are able to accomplish.

*Vain or Self-Important Insanity*: ... with which they who are possessed, have a very exalted opinion of their own imaginary dignity, opulence ... learning, or some other valuable quality.

*Hypochondriacal Insanity*: in which the patient is forever in distress about his own state of health. (cited in Hunter and Macalpine, 1964, pp. 470–471)

Rejecting content as a basis for classification, Southard (1916a,b) suggested that the grammatical structure of the delusional belief might provide a better framework. At that time, grammarians emphasized the organization of statements into four basic "moods," the indicative, the subjunctive, the imperative, and the optative. He conducted a series of pioneering autopsy studies of deceased deluded patients, from which he was able to demonstrate significant correspondence between the explanations incorporated in the delusions and the conscious concomitants of the diseases from which the patients suffered. Southard's work attracted little attention at the time, no doubt in large part due to the enthusiasm of his later colleagues for psychodynamic explanations of delusional content. Mention of him here is important to acknowledge his early recognition of the function of delusions in explaining anomalous experiences for which no alternative rational explanation has been initially available.

*By classification here, we mean a system for bringing order to various kinds of delusions. It is not intended to imply a system of disease entities.

**Contemporary Classification: DSM-IV.** In the Glossary of the DSM-IV (pp. 765–766), we find a subclassification of delusions divided according to their content. Extracts from descriptions of some of the more common types are listed here.

*Controlled*: A delusion in which feelings, impulses, thoughts, or actions are experienced as being under the control of some external force rather than under one's own control.

*Bizarre*: A false belief that involves a phenomenon that the person's culture would regard as totally implausible.

*Grandiose*: A delusion of inflated worth, power, knowledge, identity, or special relationship to a deity or famous person.

*Jealousy*: The delusion that one's sexual partner is unfaithful.

*Persecutory*: A delusion in which the central theme is that one (or someone to whom one is close) is being attacked, harassed, cheated, persecuted, or conspired against.

*Reference*: A delusion whose theme is that events, objects, or other people in the person's immediate environment have a particular and unusual significance. These delusions are usually negative or pejorative but may also be grandiose in content. This differs from an idea of reference, in which the false belief is not as firmly held nor as fully organized into a true belief.

*Somatic*: A delusion whose main content pertains to the functioning or appearance of one's body.

To this list we may add delusions of poverty, delusions of guilt (the idea that one is responsible for all kind of misery), nihilistic delusions (that one is dead or that the world has come to an end), querulent delusions, and the delusions of misidentification discussed later.

Delusions may be *mood-congruent* or *mood-incongruent*. Mood congruence or incongruence is defined by the relationship between the affective state of the patient and the content of the delusional theme. Depressed patients with delusions of personal worthlessness, guilt, disease, death, etc., have delusions that are congruent with the depressed mood. A patient who is clinically depressed but has delusions of great personal fame or wealth, etc., has mood-incongruent delusions.

Notice that the level of abstraction of the types listed by DSM-IV is not always the same: some types refer to content, others to specific features of delusions, regardless of their content. Thus, delusions of persecution may be systematized or not, and grandiose delusions may be mood-congruent or not. The contents of delusions (guilt, persecution, jealousy), etc., have also been called *themes*; these themes vary from very specific (i.e., a certain person loving oneself, the spouse being involved with a specific person), to quite general (e.g., where "everything" somehow refers to the patient). The list of themes seems to be limited although there is no clear-cut, agreed-upon final total of such themes. Systematization and mood congruency, although related to content, are matters of degree and can be applied to any content. They belong to what we may call the descriptive dimensions of delusions and must be addressed separately.

### Descriptive Dimensions

Some psychopathologists have turned from categorical classifications to dimensional descriptions. The use of continua to describe psychotic phenomena such as hallucinations and delusions was proposed by Strauss (1969). Since then, this proposal has gained some conceptual and empirical support from other authors. A factor analytic study by Heilbrun and Madison (1978), for example, studied a sample of verbatim transcripts of patient interviews from thirty-two schizophrenics. They postulated that four orthogonal factors arise from the content analysis of this material but cautioned that the limited number of patients involved constrains the reliability of their data. Later, in a study involving fifty-two delusional patients, Kendler, Glazer, and Morgenstern (1983) found five dimensions* which turned out to be independent of each other. Garety and Hemsley (1987, 1994) use a scale containing eleven dimensions which, they report, are independent of one another. The eleven characteristics are intensity (strength of conviction), preoccupation (time spent thinking about it), interference (extent to which it affects behavior), resistance (like/dislike of thinking about it), dismissibility (ability to stop thinking about it), absurdity (seems sensible/senseless),

self-evident (seems obvious/implausible), reassurance (seeks reassurance), distress/worry (thinking about it causes worry), distress/mood (thinking about it causes unhappiness), and pervasiveness (cannot think about other things at the same time). In addition to these dimensions, other characteristics are worthy of note. These are the general theme of the delusion (see earlier), other symptoms present (psychic and/or somatic), and time course (rapidity of onset, stability, duration, and remission).

The utility of a system that permits us to identify differences between delusional patients lies in its potential to relate these differences to other clinical and laboratory-based variables.

## Hypotheses about the External World Versus Descriptions of Internal States

Our earlier discussion dealt with the processes by which beliefs about the environment are formed and held, given externally available evidence that is relevant to their validity. Now, we turn to a different aspect of delusional thinking. The question is, are there any judgments about which we are so certain that we would never accept any refutation of them? If the answer is "yes," then these judgments would have something in common with delusions.

There are judgments about which we are perfectly certain so that no counterevidence is possible. These are statements about our primary conscious experience. If I feel pain in my right foot (even if I did not actually have a right foot†) there is no evidence than can refute the fact of the primary experience. The experience that "something in the environment has changed" is a common normal reaction to the existence of a yet undetected actual change. An intense version of this kind of experience, that is, that events, objects, or other people in the immediate environment have changed or acquired a yet unexplained significance, has been reported in about 70% of all schizophrenics (Murray, 1986, p. 342). We cannot refer to the feeling of significance as a "false, idiosyncratic belief," inasmuch as the feeling it-

---

*The five dimensions, assessed by interviewer rating, were (1) conviction, (2) extension (the degree to which the delusional belief involves various areas of the patient's life), (3) bizarreness, (4) disorganization, and (5) pressure (the degree of preoccupation and concern).

†Even if I never had a right foot, I might rightly claim to have pain in it, as findings in patients with phantom limbs from birth on (especially the thalidomide cases) show.

self is primary and undeniable, and the task of providing counterevidence (that things do not have significance) is impossible. Similarly, utterances of depressed patients, that their thoughts have stopped or their feelings of worthlessness should be understood, not as "false beliefs about external reality," but as the patients' best attempts to communicate what they think and how they feel, that is, what their experiences are like. Here, as with schizophrenia, we can make sense about the relatively high frequency of these experiences in depressed patients by interpreting them as direct results of the basic pathological changes brought about by the disorder rather than due to defects of inference about the environment.

## Methods for Investigating Descriptions of Delusions

Idiographic description is surely the oldest method used in studying delusions. Although now rejected as unscientific by many researchers, the descriptive method still has a place among the various attempts to investigate delusions. Single cases do not allow inferences to support a theory; they can disprove theories by providing contradictory ("falsificatory") evidence for general theories. Moreover, single cases can provide the empirical researcher with hypotheses that may be tested later with more rigorous and more quantitative approaches.

### Transcultural Psychiatry

As early as 1904, Kraepelin was the first psychiatrist who tried to determine the extent to which psychiatric symptoms are influenced by culture. Delusions are one of the most difficult symptoms to assess cross-culturally, but we may note that cross-cultural comparisons are addressed to several different kinds of classification: (1) structural (i.e., grandiose, paranoid, etc.), (2) content (i.e., somatic, religious, misidentification, etc.), and (3) frequency (the epidemiology of delusions in terms of both structure and content).

The literature on this general topic is substantial. Studies of frequency are of course also influenced by differential frequency of the psychiatric disorders in which delusions commonly occur. Some authors have reported that the frequency of

paranoid schizophrenia is increasing whereas the catatonic and hebephrenic types of schizophrenia have decreased in this century (Kranz, 1967; Magaro, 1980). For example, Achte (1961), cited in Lenz (1964), investigated 200 schizophrenic patients from 1933–1935 and from 1953–1955 and found an increase of paranoid schizophrenia from 36 to 59%. Others did not find any change in the frequency of subtypes of schizophrenia. Cultural background seems to influence the temporal course of delusions (and influences on prevalence may be explained in those terms). Piedmont (1966) compared German and Polish immigrants with delusions who lived in New York and found that the Germans had more delusions, were more consequential in their elaboration and systematization, and maintained them for a longer time. The authors interpreted this as a reflection of the influence of German culture with its emphasis on "reason" and "consequence." On the other hand, members of cultures, where it is common to be "possessed by a ghost," relinquish their delusions more readily, presumably because one can be abandoned by a ghost as easily as one can be possessed by it. Several authors have interpreted the degree of systematization in delusions to the dominance of rational, materialist thinking in Western cultures (Kiev, 1972; Lambo, 1965).

As the culture changes over time so, it appears, does the specific content of delusions. Kranz examined case reports of 651 schizophrenic and 243 cyclothymic patients (the latter would now most likely be diagnosed as suffering from major affective disorders) from the years 1886, 1916, and 1946 to investigate changes in the themes of delusions. He found that delusions of being controlled occurred in a stable proportion of schizophrenia patients with a frequency of 72% (1886), 75% (1916), and 72% (1946), respectively. Grandiose delusions in schizophrenia patient declined from 24% (1886) to 17% (1916), and to 11% (1946). Similar studies also showed a decline in delusions of grandeur in schizophrenia patients, as well as a decreasing frequency of religious delusions (Lenz, 1964; Streinbrunner & Scharfetter, 1976). The frequency of delusions of grandeur also reportedly decreased in patients with general paralysis (Pauleikhoff, 1962; Vurla, quoted from Lenz, 1964, p. 71).

Kranz reported that the frequencies of the classic delusions of guilt and poverty, as well as hypochondriac delusions in depressed patients, were relatively stable over time, and von Orelli (1954) found a decrease of delusions of guilt and an increase of hypochondriac delusions—a finding which might be related to the decreasing influence of religion.

That the content of delusions varies somewhat with culture is hardly surprising. Studies have shown that delusions mirror culture in broad terms. For example, witches played a role in delusions of the last century in Europe, but this is no longer the case. The frequency of technology as the major theme in delusions of schizophrenia patients has reportedly increased from 12% in 1900 to 31% in 1960 (Achte, 1961). Lenz (1964) gives a vivid account of changes over time in the identity of alleged persecutors in relevant delusions:

In the realm of delusions of persecution before 1880 the content was "the Prussians" as a result of the war between Prussia and Austria in 1866.... In 1921 ... the Social Democrats, who had overthrown the Kaiser, played a major role as the evil enemy who had once been the devil, later the Prussians and, before World War II, the SS and SA, and after World War II the Russians and Communists. (pp. 53–54)

The delusional complaint of having AIDS is now encountered in depressed patients as a substitute for other symbols for the feeling of guilt, being punished for bad life-style, etc. (e.g., Mahorney and Cavenar, 1988; Shetty, 1988).

On the basis of a comprehensive survey of cross-cultural studies, Westermeyer (1988) offered some general conclusions. Chief among them were

1. The structure and content of most delusions are not culture-bound and can readily be identified across cultures. The structure of delusions varies little, if any, across cultures, whereas the content may be influenced by culture.
2. In developing countries, culture-bound delusional content tends to involve religious and traditional world views, especially those that are challenged by modern secular society.
3. Elements of culture-bound content in delusions have been acquired in childhood rather than from later experience or experience in other cultures.
4. Gender differences in delusional content are minimal, except where the socialization of males and females is markedly different.
5. Culture-bound and secular elements in delusions may be found together in the same individual.

6. Where the content of the idea expressed in the delusion is culture-bound, the structure of the delusion becomes more important.

## Hypotheses about the Etiology of Delusions

There is no generally accepted theory of the etiology of delusions. Instead there are some limited models each of which deals with some subset of delusions and invokes an etiological process that may have limited application to the total array of delusions found in clinical practice.

Winters and Neale (1983) organized all of the theories of delusion formation in terms of motivation or defect; this is useful for many instances, but not for all. There is still need for a general strategy of explanation in this field. In this connection, it is crucially important that we take account of the fact that delusions are found in a very wide range of medical disorders, only some of which are regarded as primarily psychopathological. Hence, any attempt to offer a general theory of delusion formation that does not account for their widespread occurrence can hope to gain only limited credence. For our description, it is convenient to place etiological hypotheses about delusion formation into these three broad categories.

1. There is a fundamental cognitive defect by which the patient's capacity to draw valid conclusions from evidence is impaired. A neuropsychological or other biological anomaly is posited to explain the defect.
2. There is a pattern of deviant motivation, such that an otherwise intact cognitive system is distorted in the service of motivation.
3. There is no abnormal cognitive defect. Cognitive processes in the deluded patient are fundamentally the same as those in non-deluded persons. The delusion arises from the operation of normative cognitive activities directed at explaining abnormal experiences. These experiences may be internal; they may be due to improbable but genuine anomalous events in the external environment.

We must note that although these options have been presented as mutually exclusive, this need not be the case. Normal beliefs are acquired by different routes: direct personal experience, indoctrination, observation of the experiences of others, the influence of the popular media, and so forth. Many, perhaps most, of the disorders in which delusions are found are themselves heterogeneous. Schizophrenia is a prime example. It is quite possible—and perhaps probable—that delusional beliefs, like normal beliefs, may arise as the outcome of different etiological sequences.

## Delusions Due to Cognitive Defect

Alternatively, we may decide to compare the belief processes of a psychiatrically defined group with the belief processes of a normal control group. Both groups may violate the rules of correct procedure, but both may do so in similar ways and with similar frequency. If this empirical comparison demonstrates that deluded patients do not differ from controls in their adherence to, or departure from, rules of induction and deduction, we are compelled to conclude that delusional pathology does not lie in the realm of processes of inference, no matter what the DSM-IV definition states to the contrary.

To demonstrate that delusions arise because of a more basic pathology in inferential reasoning or some other cognitive process, certain methodological requirements must be met. First, because our task is to explain why deluded patients have delusions and nondeluded patients do not, it is necessary to compare deluded patients with nondeluded controls, rather than with some formal standard of correct inference. Differences that may be found, however, must be such that the deluded patients' performance departs from the ideal standard more than the performance of controls. In brief, there must be a defect—not an advantage—in inferential processes. Second, we need to show that the putative defect is not confined to the topic of the delusion itself but can be demonstrated independently in other neutral topic areas. Third, but (unfortunately) ideally, we should be able to show that the defect in inferential processes antedated the appearance of the delusion. This latter is a condition met adequately only in high-risk studies, and these are few and far between. A rough approximation to it can be reached in searches for premorbid evidence of reasoning defects, but these are fraught with all of the usual dangers of retrospective investigations. Finally, the experiments that test these hypotheses should have ecological validity for delusional behavior itself, for example, they should demonstrate the

tendency to develop improbable beliefs, incorrigibility of belief in the face of counterevidence, etc.

## Empirical Studies of Normal Belief Formation

Data from several kinds of systematic empirical observation are available. One is the study of the prevalence of irrational beliefs in the general population. Another is the comparison of the performance of deluded and nondeluded samples in formal reasoning tasks. A third is examination of the performance of samples of normal individuals in reasoning tasks evaluated against objective criteria of accuracy.

Broadly speaking, these approaches reflect either a *normative* standard or a *prescriptive* standard of inferential reasoning (Maher, 1992). The prescriptive standard simply assesses the discrepancy between an individual's inferences and some objective standard of what the correct inference should be. By this standard, both deluded and nondeluded persons may make errors.

The basis of the normative standard is the fact that if we are to understand why some people develop delusions and others do not, we must show differences between deluded persons and nondeluded persons. Whether or not deluded persons make errors of inference is irrelevant, unless it is clear that nondeluded persons do not make such errors or make substantially fewer of them. In this latter case, it is also necessary to show that the difference in error-proneness between the two groups is sufficiently large in absolute terms to explain the presumably large difference between delusions and normal beliefs. Some deluded individuals believe that some outside source is transmitting thoughts into their heads, and many normal individuals believe in mental telepathy. If we wish to attribute the first to an inferential process of delusional severity and the second to a normal process, we need to show a comparable difference of severity of impairment in the inferential processes of the two groups.

## The Prevalence of Irrational Beliefs in the General Population

Gallup and Newport (1991) report that 14% of a sample of 1236 adult members of the U.S. population believes that they have seen unidentified flying objects (UFOs); 10% report having seen or been in the presence of ghosts, and 25% believe in telepathy. Ross and Joshi (1992) report that in a sample of 502 adult members of the normal population of Winnipeg, 16% expressed a belief in telepathy, and 5% claimed contact with ghosts. In short, in the normal population, the general prevalence of beliefs that lack adequate support in evidence is quite high. All of these beliefs have the characteristic that evidence sufficient to refute them would require proof of negative propositions, that is, there are no ghosts, there are no witches, no extraterrestrial flying vehicles have ever come within detectable range of earth, etc. As we have already pointed out, many delusional beliefs fit this description, and we are left with the conclusion that the discrimination between delusional beliefs and popular beliefs that lack evidential support is far from clear.

## Studies of Normal Belief Formation

There are two sources of systematic empirical evidence. One is the study of normal samples of the population. The other comes from the behavior of normal control subjects in studies that compare deluded and nondeluded individuals. We turn first to empirical studies limited to normal individuals. This is a large literature, and we shall confine the discussion to those factors that are directly relevant to the definition of delusions.

1. Do people readily change their beliefs in the face of evidence sufficient to refute the beliefs?

   There is a substantial body of evidence to support the conclusion that once a belief has been formed by normal persons, they are reluctant to change it even in the face of clearly contradictory evidence. Studies confirming this have been reported by Wason and Johnson-Laird (1972); Anderson, Lepper, and Ross (1980); Nisbett and Ross (1980); Ross and Lepper (1981); and Ross and Anderson (1981). In this connection, it is interesting to note that Kuhn (1962) and Feyerabend (1970) commented on the incorrigibility of scientists in the face of evidence disconfirming their hypotheses, especially in the early instances of disconfirmation.
2. Do people normally actively check their beliefs by searching for possible counterevidence?

   Mynatt, Doherty, and Tweeny (1977, 1978) investigated the behavior of normal

subjects presented with the choice of either conducting observations that could potentially disconfirm a previously formed hypothesis or of conducting observations that could either confirm or be irrelevant to, but not disconfirm the hypothesis. Their data showed that a significant number of subjects selected the latter option. The investigators termed this effect, "confirmation bias." They found that it was generally unrelated to the capacity of subjects to respond to disconfirming evidence when it turned up. However, when the experimenters made the task of evidence-sifting more complex, the confirmation bias survived, even in the face of contradictory evidence. "The more complex environment," they wrote, "may have made the generation of new hypotheses, and hence, the abandonment of disconfirmed hypotheses, more difficult" (Mynatt et al., 1978, p. 404). Human beings in their natural habitats (in contrast with their situations when serving as experimental subjects) are in very complex environments. Hence Mynatt's comment is particularly pertinent to the question of normative thinking. Wason and Johnson-Laird, summarizing the results of their studies of thought processes in normal individuals who failed to seek appropriate disconfirmation of their hypotheses, commented, "... it is not just particular mechanisms and logical factors which are diagnostic of thought disorder. We have demonstrated that such effects can readily be induced in normal individuals under rather special tasks. Different ways of evading reality are not the prerogative of the mentally ill" (Wason & Johnson-Laird, 1972, p. 239).

What needs to be emphasized here is that patterns of reasoning in normal people in their natural habitats are tested daily, not by their capacity to conform to rules of inference, but by their effectiveness in producing adaptive responses to the actual environments in which individuals live. The notion that behavior ought to be rational in the sense that it ought to and does conform to the rules of deductive and inductive reasoning in a Platonic ideal or academic view of rationality. From the perspective of survival, maladaptive *behavior* is selected against, not illogical deductions or incorrect estimates or objective probabilities (Maher,

1990). Thinking serves purposes, and the purposes that it serves are those of survival and effectiveness in the real world.

This leaves us with the possibility that the kinds of defects of inference involved in delusions differ from the flawed processes of inference found in the nondeluded or that the flaws are similar but that the magnitude of the difference between deluded and nondeluded is very great. We will return to explore this possibility later.

## Comparative Studies of Deluded and Nondeluded Individuals

**Formal Reasoning.** Although it has long been known that intelligence and the capacity for formal reasoning do not protect an individual from developing delusions and although by definition delusions do not involve formal thought disorder, it has often been proposed that a formal thought disorder is their cause. von Domarus (1944) postulated that delusions in schizophrenic patients arise from faulty logical reasoning; the defect consists of the assumption of the identity of two subjects on the grounds of identical predicates ("Napoleon was incarcerated; I am incarcerated; therefore, I am Napoleon"). The hypothesis was quite popular in the 1950s (see Arieti, 1955), but empirical investigations failed to find any evidence in favor of a specific kind of logical error made by paranoid schizophrenic patients (Nims, 1959; Williams, 1964). Spitzer (1989) pointed out that the apparent logical content of delusional statements can be interpreted retroactively as due to any one of several kinds of formal logical error, in addition to the principle of identity proposed by von Domarus, and that the hypothesis implied by the von Domarus principle is not falsifiable and hence not acceptable scientifically.

In Paris, De Bonis, Epelbaum, Féline, Grize, Hardy and Somogyi (1990) investigated the reliability of psychiatric judgments of deficiencies in logical reasoning in a schizophrenic patient. They found nonsignificant levels of agreement between the judgments of thirty-two psychiatrists; furthermore, a logician who performed a detailed analysis of the most contradictory seeming verbal productions of this patient concluded that the internal relationships in his statements were in fact logical.

There have been several studies of what is termed *belief bias*. This refers to a normal bias toward accepting a statement that is believable on the basis of personal experience, even if it is arrived at by an invalid process of reasoning (Garnham & Oakhill, 1994). Kemp, Chua, McKenna, and David (1997) report an investigation of belief bias in delusions. In a task of syllogistic reasoning, deluded and nondeluded subjects were asked to choose between logically fallacious and logically valid conclusions, together with content that was more or less believable. Deluded patients endorsed marginally fewer unbelievable conclusions than the nondelusional subjects. The authors conclude that cognitive deficit is not sufficient to explain delusional thinking. As with other studies, normal controls made many errors of reasoning.

All of the systematic empirical evidence available points strongly to the conclusion that the formation of delusions is not attributable to some defect in formal reasoning that is absent in nondeluded persons but present in the deluded.

**Bayesian Reasoning.** Contemporary models of human reasoning rarely invoke the syllogism as an appropriate paradigm to describe how human beings actually develop beliefs, make decisions, and so forth. Instead, emphasis is placed upon a model of Bayesian processes. According to this model, individuals assign probabilities to propositions about reality. These probabilities range hypothetically from zero to 100% (0.0 to 1.0), although the two extreme values are rarely if ever found in nature. Thus, effective reasoning is based on correctly assessing the probabilities inherent in empirical evidence. This weighing of evidence requires recognizing base rates for the occurrence of classes of events, due allowance for small sample effects and also for the biases that might be inherent in collecting the evidence presented. Contemporary statistical methods provide a clear example of this approach.

Bayesian procedures imply a sequence of steps that go into forming and testing a belief:

1. Identifying and selecting observations and other sources of evidence that are relevant to the validity of the belief.
2. Assessing the significance of the evidence obtained in relation to the belief and to other competing beliefs.
3. Compiling the total data available from all sources (a meta-analysis so to speak) and assessing its impact upon the belief.
4. Selecting an appropriate course of action.

However, the analogy between human decision-making and the scientist/statistician's ascertainment of probabilities to arrive at a decision that a hypothesis ha been rejected or not—the usual standard in the application of tests of statistical significance—has limited validity. Where specific action is contemplated, as in item (4) before, the computation of the probability of Type I and Type II errors is substantially modified by computing the costs and benefits associated with accepting or rejecting the hypothesis. Competent practical application of the Bayesian model requires basing the action decision on an assessment of the *consequences* of the action, not merely on the numerical value assigned to the probability that a belief is valid. Thus the finding that using an experimental drug to treat AIDS has been followed by a slightly better survival rate (with no or minor side effects), than when the drug is not used, may lead to a decision to apply the drug even though the rate of improvement did not reach conventional levels of statistical significance. Low levels of significance are sufficient for action provided that the consequences of inaction are judged sufficiently serious.

Hemsley and Garety (1986) suggested that delusions may result from defects in the ability to weigh evidence along Bayesian lines; the general tenor of the defect is that the deluded patient accepts conclusions at levels of probability too low for acceptance by normal persons. Their hypothesis necessitates, of course, that the kind and quantity of evidence available to, and the costs and benefits of the decision to be made by, the deluded patient are also the same as for the normal individual. One recent test of this hypothesis was reported by Huq, Garety, and Hemsley (1988). Deluded schizophrenic subjects and appropriate controls (psychiatric and nonpsychiatric) were presented with a laboratory task in which the investigator explained that colored beads would be drawn from one of two jars. One jar contained pink and green beads in the ratio 85/15, and the other jar contained beads of the same colors where the ratio was reversed. After this explanation, the jars were concealed, one was selected, and the subject was presented with beads drawn from that jar, one at a time; the bead was returned to the jar after each drawing. Various experimental conditions were employed; the major response element was elicited by asking subjects at each draw to estimate which jar was being used; the degree of probability attached to that estimate and the relative

probabilities that the subject assigned to each of the two possible jars had been chosen. Errors of decision were also recorded. Each subject's first two draws were beads of the same color, thereby creating an objective probability of 0.97 that this was the color of the predominant portion of beads in the jar. Hence the correct application of Bayesian principles should lead a subject to make the decision at that point.

Very few decision errors were made by any group, and there was no significant difference between groups on this measure. In brief, the deluded patients made as many correct decisions as the other subjects. However, the deluded arrived at their correct decisions after significantly fewer draws than the other subjects and did so with greater estimates of confidence in their decision. Their mean total of draws to decision was 2.2, which is the point at which a proper Bayesian decision could be made. The authors state, "Thus it may be argued that the deluded sample reached a decision at an objectively 'rational' point ... the two control groups (being) somewhat overcautious" (p. 809).

This finding clearly fails to support the notion that deluded patients are poorer at Bayesian reasoning than normal subjects. Surprisingly, the authors are uncomfortable with that conclusion, stating that "Although the deluded sample's response ... appears more 'Bayesian,' ... it is not possible to argue that deluded people are better reasoners"* (p. 810). In defense of their own refusal to accept the obvious implication of their findings, the authors suggest that the overcautiousness of the control groups is evidence for a normal "conservatism" bias and that the better performance of the deluded patients can be explained away post hoc by assuming that deluded patients do indeed have a tendency to make hasty judgments on insufficient evidence, but that this is mitigated by the presence of a conservative bias in the deluded patients also; the arithmetical summation of these two tendencies produces a result that is pseudo-reasonable.

---

*The statement that "it is not possible to argue" that people who have performed better than others on a reasoning test are therefore better reasoners is *prima facie* absurd. It can only be impossible to investigators who have already assumed the truth of the proposition that their experiment purported to test, that is, they assume that deluded patients are by definition cognitively impaired. If this is the case, the experiment is a pointless exercise in begging the question.

None of this argument was adduced before the experiment was conducted, nor was any independent evidence provided for the supposed summation. Furthermore, it seems highly likely that had the results come out the other way, where the deluded patients made fewer draws than Bayesian rules prescribe and the controls made the appropriate decision after two draws, the study would have been regarded as good evidence for the original hypothesis of impaired reasoning in the deluded. Post hoc rejection of refutational findings is generally a rather problematic procedure.

In the present writers' opinion, there were important methodological problems in designing the task employed, such that only very limited conclusions can be drawn. The ratios employed made the correct Bayesian decision possible after only two draws had been completed. Hence, the degrees of freedom for being impulsive were extremely limited, whereas the degrees of freedom for being overcautious were considerable. As a result, the test lacked sensitivity to impulsiveness, but not sensitivity to over cautiousness, and was thus psychometrically inadequate to test the hypothesis. Had the ratios been less imbalanced and required more draws before the objectively correct decision could be made, the hypothesis might have been tested more convincingly. At this point, all that we can say is that the control subjects failed to conform to Bayesian rules in this task, whereas the deluded patients, for whatever reason, conformed very closely to them. Hence, a reasoning defect in deluded patients remains to be demonstrated. The failure of the search so far conveys an increment of support for the possibility that there is no defect to be found and that hence the cognitions that produce delusions are fundamentally normal.

## Delusions and Anomalous Experience

A model of delusion formation that emphasized the role of anomalous experience was presented by Maher (Maher, 1970, 1974, 1988a,b,c, 1990, 1999; Maher & Ross, 1984; Maher & Spitzer, 1995). These are the formal propositions of this model:

1. Delusional thinking is not in itself cognitively aberrant. This means that the cognitive processes by which delusions are formed are in no important respect different from those by which normal beliefs are formed. Parenthetically, in neither case are beliefs typically formed by a process of syllogistic deductive reasoning.
2. Delusions are like scientific theories to the extent that they serve the purpose of providing order and meaning for empirical observations.
3. As in the case of normal scientific theorizing, the necessity for a theory arises whenever nature presents us with a puzzle. Puzzles arise when predictable events fail to occur and/or unpredicted events do so in their place, i.e., when observation is discrepant with expectation.

Events appear to be predictable rather than surprising insofar as the individual can process information provided by concurrent or recent prior events in ways that permit effectively anticipating what is normally likely to happen next. If a friend calls to say that he will be coming over to visit in the next ten minutes, and this is followed in order by the sound of a car pulling up outside, a car door opening, and the sound of the doorbell, we are not surprised to find our friend at the door when we open it. We might be mildly surprised but not puzzled to find a stranger at the door, but would assume that the expected visit will follow a little later anyway. We would be very puzzled only if we should find nobody at the door.

On the other hand, if our capacity to process current contexts or sequences so as to generate normal expectancies were impaired, many events would be at least slightly surprising even though they had occurred at the end of a predictable sequence of prior events. Impairment of the capacity to use redundancies to predict events would be likely to make many normal events seem puzzling and thus set the ground for vulnerability to delusional interpretations.

There is substantial evidence that the information processing of many schizophrenic patients exhibits impairment in using contexts and redundancies. Examples are to be found in many studies, including those of Lewinsohn and Elwood (1961); Chapman, Chapman, and Miller (1964); Lawson, McGhie, and Chapman (1964); Salzinger, Portnoy, and Feldman (1964); Gerver (1967); Levy and Maxwell (1968); Truscott (1970); Silverman (1972); Koh, Kayton, and Schwarz (1972);

Hart and Payne (1973); Manschreck, Maher, Rucklos, and White (1979); Maher, Manschreck, and Rucklos (1980); Maher (1983); and Maher, Manschreck, and Molino (1983).

4. When unpredicted and hence discrepant events occur, they attract attention and give rise to an experienced feeling of significance accompanied by some tension.
5. This tension motivates a search for explanation; the search is continued until some explanation is found. The longer the search without an explanation, the greater the tension.
6. Explanations bring relief even if the explanation is not fully adequate to the situation. A partially defective or incomplete explanation is experienced as better than no explanation at all.
7. Once the explanation has been established, dissonant new data are disturbing and will be either ignored or reinterpreted to fit the explanation. Data that are consistent with the explanation give additional relief, and are therefore sought after.

It is important to note that experiences of surprise are not limited to situations in which the individual has been unable to predict events either because the events fail to occur in their predicted pattern or because the individual suffers from an information-processing defect. The same thing can happen when two sequences of events, hitherto believed to be unrelated, turn out to have strikingly similar patterns. In science, of course, similarity of patterns in two seemingly independent phenomena often gives rise to the tentative hypothesis that the processes underlying one may be the same as those underlying the other; scientific theories often gain in generality from evidence sought on the basis of this kind of coincidence.

Noticed coincidences feature with some frequency in the developing stages of delusion formation (Maher, 1988a, pp. 29–30). What seems to characterize the phenomenon in deluded patients is the triviality of the coincidences that are noticed, a circumstance that suggests hyperattentiveness due to either attentional focusing impairment or created by the search process activated by an autonomous sense of significance.

8. Theories will be judged delusional by others if any of the following circumstances exist:

(a) They are based upon observations made by the patient that are unavailable to others. Thus beliefs arising to account for hallucinations, input affected by unrecognized sensory defect or other private sensory anomalies, or from veridical observation of highly improbable events, are likely to be judged delusional. (b) The data are available to others, but they do not appear anomalous to others. Thus where the motor or verbal behavior of the patient is discrepant with the patient's intended behavior, the patient's experience is anomalous ("Somebody else must be speaking through my mouth because the words coming out are not what I want to say"). In like manner, the patient who cannot focus attention but finds that external or internal input disrupts conscious organization has anomalous experiences in an environment that appears normal to others. (c) The feeling of "discrepancy" and "puzzlement" is activated neuropathologically when there is no actual discrepancy in the sequence of external events. Thus there is generated a need to explain, but no clear clue as to what is to be explained.* Activation of this kind has been reported by normal subjects who take psychoactive drugs, are placed in unusual sensory environments, or are hypnotized. As we describe later, many cases of delusions associated with somatic disorders exhibit feelings of puzzlement (often called feelings of significance). The condition is well exemplified by the concept of delusional mood, its vague suspiciousness, and the sense of relief when a delusional resolution of the indefinable "discrepancy" has been created.

Anomalous experience presents a problem to be explained by the person who experiences it. The problem is, How is this experience being induced? Who is doing the inducing? Why are they doing

---

*From time to time, many normal people experience the feeling that "something has changed" in an otherwise familiar environment in which a change has actually taken place; however, it is common to be conscious of the general experience of change some time *before* we manage to identify what specifically has changed. This sequence strongly suggests that the experience of puzzlement may be activated by an automatic detection of a mismatch between an actual observation and expected observation some time before the concrete nature of the discrepancy itself has been identified.

this to me and not to other people? and (sometimes) Why are other people denying the reality of my experience?

Because the anomalous experience, which the delusion is developed to explain, cannot generally be related to visible external causes, answers to the first question frequently have recourse to invisible influences likely to be part of the patient's cultural milieu. Thus, reference to scientific nonvisible forces such as radar, radio, television transmissions, magnetism, cosmic rays, etc., appear quite frequently in delusions; similarly, interpersonal influences such as hypnotism or religious influences such as divine or diabolical power are also common. Because the operation of such influences implies some agency powerful enough to do so, answers to the second question frequently have reference to the FBI, the Communist Party, the government, some specific religious body, God, the Devil and the like. Answers to the third question lead to persecutory and/or grandiose answers: "They are doing this to me because I am evil." "They are doing this to me because I am really a very important person," etc.

Like other explanations, the coherence and quality of the delusion is likely to be influenced by the intelligence and educational level of the patient, the repertoire of culturally common explanations available to the patient, and the degree to which it is couched in nonfalsifiable terms.

What evidence might be adduced in support of this model? Negative evidence that is implicitly supportive comes from (a) the repeated failure of attempts to find a fundamental defect in the cognitive processes of delusional patients and (b) the evidence that the processes of belief formation in normal subjects are indistinguishable in form from those supposed to be characteristic of delusional patients.

Positive evidence comes from (a) the prevalence of delusions in a wide range of disorders in which the deluded individuals have no prior history of cognitive impairment; (b) evidence that delusions can be induced in normal subjects under conditions in which they have anomalous experiences; (c) the presence of delusions in cases of undiagnosed sensory defect; (d) the coexistence (and possibly development) of delusions and (from) psychotic symptoms such as hallucinations, thought insertion, thought withdrawal, passivity phenomena, and the like; (e) the explanatory format of the fully elaborated delusion; and (f) reports that cognitive therapy derived from this model has been effective in some cases (Chadwick & Lowe, 1990).

Empirical studies have reported that anomalies of experience are correlated with the presence of delusions in many different ways.

## Delusions and Time Sense

Melges and Freeman (1975) proposed a cybernetic model of the formation of delusions that is based on the assumption of a temporal disturbance of formal thought as the primary cause of delusions. The disintegration of the temporal sequence of thought is experienced by patients as loss of control that leads in several stages to the formation of delusions. First, the loss of control is experienced as mysterious and "uncanny" and leads to the notion that unidentified others might have taken control of the patient. This is the "premonition stage." This leads to anger and rage and fear that these feelings will be discovered. This is the "pursuit stage," and, later, fear that the others will make reprisals, is the projection stage. This circle of persecution and projection amplifies the fears of loss of control on the patient's part and continued fear of the presumed others. In a final "protest" stage, the patient may take hostile action against the others.

## Delusions and Attention

An attentional defect as the basic disturbance in paranoid patients was proposed in 1903 by Berze. Recent years brought a revival of those ideas, when the concept of attention was refined by experimental psychological methods. However, the concept of attention was used mainly to explain schizophrenic symptoms, which include disordered attention in general rather than single symptoms such as delusions (cf. McGhie & Chapman, 1961; Shakow, 1962). Frith (1979) believed that delusional patients suffer from an abnormal increase in the content of consciousness which is explained—by processes of normal reasoning—in a way that results in developing delusions. Some authors claim that paranoid schizophrenics differ strikingly in their attention deficit from nonparanoid schizophrenics (see Magaro, 1980); the former are extensive scanners of the environment, and the latter are poor scanners.

## Perception

Pavlov (1934) was the first to propose a theory that related delusions of reference and of being controlled to the existence of perceptual disturbances which he conceived to be due to pathological inertness of cells of the sensory cortex. A consequent pathological hyperarousal in other cells causes irrelevant ideas to intrude into consciousness. According to Pavlov, a delusion consists of reflections on such irrelevant ideas. The theory of Pavlov has some resemblance to attributional theories which were formulated much later. However, it had little clinical impact nor did it lead to fruitful hypotheses for empirical research.

It has long been known that delusions may develop in patients with hearing deficits. Kraepelin (1909, pp. 102–103) discusses the "psychosis of the cloth-eared," and empirical studies showed a clear increase in the frequency of delusions in patients with hearing deficits (Houston & Royse, 1954), as well as an increased number of hearing deficits in paranoid patients (Kay & Roth, 1961). Visual disturbances also have been found more frequently in paranoid patients (Herbert & Jacobson, 1967), and Cooper and Curry (1976), Cooper and Porter (1976), as well as Kay (1972), demonstrated that paranoid patients had a much higher incidence of perceptual disturbances in the visual and auditory modality, compared to patients with affective disorders. Further support was provided by the data of Zimbardo, Anderson, and Kabat (1981) who were able to demonstrate that hypnotically induced hearing loss in normal subjects led to higher scores on the paranoia scale of the MMPI.

## Motivational/Affective Models

The idea that delusions may result from some disordered affect dates at least to 1870, when Hagen stated that delusions "grow rapidly in the breast-warmth of affect and passion" (Hagen, 1870, p. 59). He responded to the objection that changes in affect are not frequently seen in delusional patients by emphasizing that delusions may be so striking that the observer simply overlooks

changes in other mental faculties. Kraepelin was another proponent of the affective causation of delusions, "... the roots of which lay in the intellectual processing of intuitions which are influenced for instance by feelings and affects ..." (Kraepelin, 1889, p. 109). About 10 years later, Specht (1908) argued that the incorrigibility of delusions strikingly resembles the way in which strong emotions make human beings resistant to reasoning. By this analogy, delusions and emotions are similar in being resistant to rational argument. In 1906, Eugen Bleuler suggested that emotions weaken "normal" associations between thoughts and lead to the development of delusions in schizophrenic patients, whereas in paranoid patients, emotions lead to pathologically stubborn adherence to the delusional idea.

In contrast, Karl Jaspers and Kurt Schneider proposed that the distinction between primary and secondary delusions (discussed earlier in this chapter) is related to the role of affect. Secondary delusions were "understandable" in terms of some underlying or associated affect, whereas the primary delusion, *by definition*, is not understandable at all in terms of any related factors. The problem of whether emotions play a major role in the genesis of delusions thus was solved by asserting that with respect to primary delusions—those that occur in schizophrenia—this is never the case. This opinion is widely held by clinicians; as stated by Arthur (1964, p. 110), "However many leading psychiatrists deny that delusional persons show any excessive affect, or that it was present before the delusions appeared." Nevertheless, many clinicians, as well as researchers, have been dissatisfied with this approach because it excludes empirical research into the role of affect in the forming of delusions.

Some psychopathologists have emphasized the possible role of specific pathological motivational states in the genesis of delusions. The best known of these and for a long time the most influential single hypothesis in the field was that of Freud.

## The Freudian Hypothesis

Freud's basic hypothesis was that delusions stem from repressed homosexual impulses. He developed his hypothesis from his interpretation of the case of a German judge, Daniel Paul Schreber, who developed what today would have been called schizophrenia, paranoid type. Freud never met Schreber and based his interpretation on an autobiographical account that Schreber published in 1903. It was referred to Freud by C. G. Jung, who also commented on the case in 1908.

Freud's hypothesis was elaborated in his monograph, *Psychoanalytical Remarks on an Autobiographical Case of Paranoia (dementia paranoides)*. It consisted of three parts: the first was the "case report," the second was "interpretational attempts," and the third "on the paranoid mechanism." Freud did not develop his hypothesis through inductive reasoning from the facts of the case. He reported the case quite selectively, ignored certain facts, and emphasized others. Furthermore, he stated directly that he had developed his theory *before* he learned about the Schreber case, having already become convinced of the connection between homosexuality and delusions before he read the Schreber memoirs. In brief, the case was cited not as grounds for the hypothesis, but as a demonstration of a hypothesis that Freud had already developed.

Freud's demonstration of the link between homosexuality and delusions rests on an isolated element in Schreber's book. It went as follows:

... once in the morning lying in bed (I do not know any more whether I was yet half sleeping or already awake) I had a sensation which struck me in a strange way when I later was completely awake and thought about it. It was the idea, that it should be pleasant to be a woman having sexual intercourse. [Schreber comments on this experience in relating it to other experiences of thought control:] This idea was very strange to my whole character. I would have, so to say, consciously rejected it with so much anger that after all I have experienced so far I cannot dismiss the possibility of some external control having given this idea to my mind. (Schreber, 1985, pp. 30–31)

From this comment, Freud proceeded to demonstrate his hypothesis through the systematic examination of the forms of a logical syllogism and its contradictions.

After all it remains curious, Freud remarked, that the most well known main form of paranoia may be conceived entirely as contradictions to the one statement "I (a man) love him (a man)"; furthermore they [the main forms] exhaust all possible formulations of that contradiction. (Freud, 1978/1911, p. 299)

His deductions run as follows: The basic premise or proposition is "I (a man) love him (a man)"; this is unacceptable and cannot come to consciousness. Therefore, it is repressed. However, it finds its way into consciousness after some distortions (i.e., psychodynamics), through delusions each of which takes the form of a contradiction of the basic proposition. Thus,

1. The delusion of *persecution or being followed* contradicts the basic proposition by the statement, "I hate him, and he hates me, and hence he is after me."
2. The delusion of *being loved* provides a contradiction in the form, "I love her and she loves me."
3. The delusion of *jealousy*: a contradiction of the form: "I do not love him, she loves him and he loves her."
4. The delusion of *grandeur*: a contradiction of the form. "I do not love him, I love myself, and others love me."

Despite the tentative formulation in which Freud first put forward his hypothesis, it soon was "accepted as absolute truth" (Klaf & Davis, 1960, p. 1070) and became part of the rock on which further theory was built. In 1915, Freud published a case that seemed to contradict his theory, but having made some additional assumptions post hoc, offered it as further confirmation.

Freud's "theory" may be criticized on different levels with reference to (1) internal consistency, (2) the long accumulated clinically based psychiatric knowledge about delusions, and (3) studies that have been done to test Freud's hypothesis with empirical data. First, from a formal logical viewpoint there is only one negation to a sentence. In this case, the proper and essential contradiction to the statement "I love a man" is simply "I do not love a man." Nothing more is needed. Once this simple principle is overlooked, any delusional statement that does not state "I love a man" can be interpreted as a contradiction of that statement only by virtue of the fact that it does not make the statement.

Second, Freud dealt only with four kinds of delusions, and he provides no basis for defining them as "the main forms." He failed to mention delusions of sin, being poor, of guilt, somatic delusions, delusions of thought insertion or thought control, and so forth. In spite of these fatal weaknesses in the hypothesis, the English translation of Schreber's book as well as Freud's interpretation of it led to a number of empirical studies of the relationship between homosexuality and delusions, mostly in the 1950s and 60s. Although Freud himself showed little interest in the empirical confirmation of his hypotheses, these consequences of this hypothesis can be tested empirically:

1. Delusions should be found more frequently in a homosexual group compared with a nonhomosexual group.
2. Patients with delusions should tend to be homosexual.
3. In the case of a delusion of being followed, the gender of the person who follows and the gender of the patient should be the same.
4. There must not be a homosexual delusion of being loved by a man.

There are few data on the frequency of delusions in homosexuals, and they indicate only a slight correlation at best (Anderson, 1944; Cattel & Morony, 1962). A few studies sought to detect homosexual tendencies in deluded patients (mostly schizophrenics or patients with delusions but without a more specific diagnosis) (Gardner, 1931; Page & Warkentin, 1938; Norman, 1948; Klein & Horowitz, 1948; Klaf & Davis, 1960; Planansky & Johnson, 1962; Moore & Selzer, 1963; Altman, Sletten, Eaton, & Ulett, 1971). There are many problems with these and other studies, quite apart from the inconclusiveness of their results. Many depend on the questionable interpretation of alleged "signs" of homosexuality, interpretations that are made by interpreters who are not blind to either the diagnosis or the hypothesis, and who generally use projective test "signs" of unknown validity (Eriksen, 1951; Aronson, 1952; Grauer, 1954; Daston, 1956; Zamansky, 1958; Watson, 1965).

However, a key problem is the interpretation of results: the finding that patients with delusions show or report more overt homosexuality than normal controls or nondeluded schizophrenics (who would be the only relevant control group) necessarily contradicts the hypothesis because Freud postulated that the homosexual wish had to be repressed and disguised to turn it into a delusion.

The results of studies using test "signs" claim to indicate a tendency toward problems in gender identity related to delusions, but because the validity of the signs themselves is unknown, the findings cannot be accepted with confidence.

Studies of the gender of the "follower" in patients of both sex with delusions of being followed produced inconclusive results (Greenspan, 1963; Klaf, 1961; Modlin, 1963). There are cases of a homosexual delusion of being loved (Doust &

Christie, 1978; Möhr, 1987; Peterson & Davis, 1985).

Finally, it is of interest that there has been a controversy among psychoanalysts about Freudian theory in this matter. Homosexuality in these cases has been seen as a consequence of delusions and termed "pseudohomosexuality" (Ovesey, 1955), and both delusions and homosexuality have been regarded as the consequence of some common underlying pathology (Ehrenwald, 1960). Carr (1963) referred to Hastings (1941), Lagache (1950), and Glick (1959) to explain the finding that homosexuality and delusions were present at the same time by proposing two kinds of homosexuality, one conscious and the other unconscious, a device that renders the hypothesis completely untestable. Lester (1975) tried to explain the co-occurrence of overt homosexuality and delusions by referring to the differential timing with which both occur.

To summarize: There are no studies of purely paranoid patients and homosexuality. The studies and established facts about schizophrenics are inconclusive for the most part. Any existing tendency of some deluded schizophrenics to have problems with gender may easily be understood in terms of the general problems of schizophrenic patients with social identity and need not indicate an underlying homosexual problem.

## Delusions as Expressions of Hatred

Swanson, Bohnert, and Smith (1970) proposed a theory somewhat similar to Freud's but based on hatred rather than homosexuality. Although aggression can frequently be found in schizophrenics, its presence has correlated with the presence of delusions (Overall, Gorham, & Shawver, 1961), and Silverman and Candell (1970) found that the subliminal presentation of aggressive stimuli can aggravate schizophrenic symptoms, these findings are inconclusive (Heilbrun, 1980) and difficult to interpret.

## Delusions as Expressions of Humiliation

Adler (1927) stipulated a loss of self-esteem as the main reason for the development of delusions, and Colby (1975) saw humiliation as the chief cause. Tölle (1987) tries to show how delusions develop in physically disabled patient by using the same concepts. Faught, Colby, and Parkinson (1977, p. 156) refer to the "transfer of blame [that] is reflected in the interpersonal behavior of the paranoid person," thus also referring to some form of projection. This approach to the role of shame in delusions has been extended and applied most recently by Ballerini and Rossi Monti (1990).

## The "Inflammation Model" of Delusions

As we have already seen, the origin of delusions has been linked to disturbances of thought, attention, affect, motivation, perception, and sense of time, as well as homosexuality, humiliation, and hatred. Nevertheless, the formal structure of all of these theories is remarkably similar and may be called the "inflammation model" of delusions. Analogous to the development of an inflammation, delusions have been conceived of as a *normal reaction to some underlying pathology*. The underlying disturbance, it has been thought, refers either to some mental faculty or psychological process; the disturbance of this in most cases is conceived ultimately to be biological.

Hughlings Jackson was among the first to present such a theory of delusions. According to Jackson, the nervous system is such that neurological as well as mental signs and symptoms are to be understood in terms of lesions, on the one hand, and disinhibition (of nonaffected brain structures or functions), on the other hand. "When a general paralytic believes himself to be Emperor of Europe, I submit that this delusion does not arise during activities of any nervous elements touched by any sort of pathological process; but, on the contrary, that it is framed during activities in what remains of his highest centres, that is to say, in what disease has spared ..." (Jackson, 1958, Vol. 2, p. 406). The same approach was proposed by Bickel (1920, p. 132).

## Social Attribution Explanations

Social attribution refers to the processes by which individuals explain their own behavior and that of others by ascribing traits and motives to the persons concerned. Its first consistent formulation is in the seminal works of Heider (1944) and Kel-

ley (1967). Although the underlying model is quite complex, the central concern here is the observation of the seeming universality of the so-called fundamental attribution error, the tendency to ascribe the causes of another person's behavior to characteristics of the person concerned, regardless of the circumstances that exist at the time. Kaney and Bentall (1989) suggested that the development of delusional beliefs might be understood in terms of social attribution processes, specifically that delusions of persecution might be associated with a particular style of social attribution. In their investigations, deluded and nondeluded patients were required to respond to a questionnaire in which they could make attributions to hypothetical situations. By and large, deluded patients did not differ from depressed controls but differed from each other on one or two of the various comparisons made. Given that this rather slight association is reported in patients who had already developed delusions of persecution of sufficient intensity to require psychiatric care, it is quite unclear that any significant causative role can be assigned to attributional style.

In summary, there is no compelling evidence at this time to support the view that processes of deductive or inductive reasoning are impaired in persons with delusional beliefs. When we consider the wide range of conditions in which delusions are found and that in many of these conditions there is no evidence whatever of prior thought disorder in the patients who develop delusions, the most parsimonious and comprehensive conclusion is that delusions arise on the basis of cognitive processes that are indistinguishable from those of nondeluded persons.

## The Neuropsychology of Delusions

Current work on the question of neuropsychological factors in the genesis of delusions centers on the search for identifiable organic lesions or anomalies associated with the presence of delusions in general, and/or with specific types of delusion.

### Hemisphere Differences

One approach has focused on the role of hemisphere specialization, as well as the limbic system, for the formation of delusions. Based on the observation that left temporal brain lesions are correlated with hallucinatory-delusional states and that right parietal damage frequently causes two specific types of abnormal belief, Capgras syndrome and anosognosia, Cutting (1985) stressed the importance of these two brain areas in developing and possibly maintaining delusions. Using hemisphere differences—the left hemisphere is involved in verbal activities, whereas the right hemisphere mediates more perceptual, affective, and visuospatial functions—as his starting point, Cummings (1985) emphasized the role of the limbic system and the basal ganglia in the development of delusions because these structures form an integrated system that mediates mood and motivation.

## The Frontal Lobes

The frontal lobes have been implicated in many kinds of cognitive defects. Stuss and Benson (1986) reviewed much of the relevant data and concluded that the prefrontal areas of the brain were responsible for self-analysis, executive control, sequencing, and drive. They comment, "The ability to self-monitor and to be self-critical must be functional for recognition of the inappropriateness of delusional interpretation or the incorrectness of an imagined sensory perception." Benson and Stuss (1990) report five cases in which delusions were accompanied by direct evidence of frontal damage due to accident or disease.

Malloy and Richardson (1994) reviewed the published literature on monosymptomatic or "content-specific" delusions. These include syndromes such as misidentification syndromes, delusions or jealousy (the "Othello" syndrome), de Clérambault's syndrome, specific hypochondriacal syndromes such as parasitosis, and body dysmorphic syndromes (e.g., Cotard's syndrome, koro). Their conclusions are consistent with the suggestions of Stuss and Benson (1986):

Crucial factors in the persistence of delusions may be the length of time that the perceptual distortion continues and the ability of the patient to correct the misperception on the basis of new information. Frontal lesions may affect the self-corrective function, making it impossible to resolve the conflicting information. (Malloy & Richardson, 1994, p. 463)

In terms of possible neurotransmitter involvement, dopamine is a plausible candidate. Dopaminergic substances that are given to patients with Parkinson's disease frequently cause hallucinatory-delusional syndromes and antidopaminergic substances, that is, neuroleptics, can be used to treat delusions. There is biochemical evidence that cocaine has dopamine-like effects, and recently it was demonstrated that an infusion of cocaine causes suspiciousness and paranoid thinking in normal subjects (Sherer, Kumor, Cone, & Jaffe, 1988). Gawin (1986) had already found that cocaine-induced paranoia can be reduced by neuroleptics. Nevertheless, it is known that delusions may take a while before they gradually disappear when treated with neuroleptics and in many cases—especially when they are highly systematized—may not disappear at all. Because noradrenergic substances like methylphenidate can cause a schizophrenia-like syndrome and because LSD, which acts as serotoninergic receptors, can cause some fleeting delusions, norepinephrine and serotonin are likely to play a role in the genesis of delusions as well.

# Nosology and Classification

As we said in the first section, delusions have been related to schizophrenic, affective, somatic, or reactive disorders. Because these disorders themselves have undergone considerable conceptual changes within the last decades, seemingly simple questions like "What is the frequency of delusions of kind x in disorder y?" are quite difficult to answer. Moreover, mainly for historical reasons, the various concepts that have been developed to account for different delusional syndromes overlap. In this section, we try to give a short summary of the classificatory attempts that have been made.

## Delusional Disorder

Delusional disorder (formerly paranoia) is plagued by the conceptual confusion that surrounds the concept of delusion itself. It has been classified as a subgroup of schizophrenia, an independent third kind (next to mania and depression) of affective disorder, a disorder related to brain damage, and a disorder of personality development, that is, a disorder of a reactive type. In what follows, we will first present the current DSM-IV definition of delusional disorder and then discuss the various approaches that have been taken to evaluate current practice and concepts.

The essential feature of Delusional Disorder is the presence of one or more nonbizarre delusions that persist for at least 1 month (Criterion A). A diagnosis of Delusional Disorder is not given if the individual has ever had a symptom presentation that met Criterion A for Schizophrenia (Criterion B). Auditory or visual hallucinations, if present, are not prominent. Tactile or olfactory delusions may be present (and prominent) if they are related to the delusional theme.... Apart from the direct impact of the delusions, psychosocial functioning is not impaired, and behavior is not markedly odd or bizarre (Criterion C). If mood episodes occur concurrently with the delusions, the total duration of these mood episodes is relatively brief compared to the total duration of the delusional period (Criterion D). The delusions are not due to the direct physiological effects of a substance (e.g., cocaine) or a general medical condition (e.g., Alzheimer's disease, systemic lupus erythematosus (Criterion E). (p. 296)

In Delusional Disorder the following delusional themes are commonly seen: erotomanic, grandiose, jealous, persecutory, and somatic. The type of Delusional Disorder is based on the predominant delusional theme. This way of classifying disorders with delusions as the main symptom has been criticized for being much too narrow (Munro, 1987) and not supported by any empirical facts (Kendler, 1984); there are no specific types of delusions by which a diagnostic distinction may be made without knowing other features of the disorder.

The relationship between delusional disorder and schizophrenia is unclear. The fact that genetic studies show no excess of schizophrenia in first-degree relatives of patients with paranoid disorder (Kendler, Glazer, & Morgenstern, 1983) is usually interpreted as a sign that the two conditions are unrelated. Nevertheless, from a clinical point of view, it is known the cases of paranoia can deteriorate and develop schizophrenic symptoms so that the diagnosis has to be changed to schizophrenia.

Munro (1987) proposes a "paranoid spectrum" with paranoid schizophrenia, on the one hand, and paranoia, on the other hand, and paraphrenia, a condition not included in the DSM-IV but found in the International Classification of Diseases, 9th revision (ICD-9), and characterized by the predominance of delusions and less deterioration and fewer other symptoms than in paranoid schizophrenia, but more than in delusional disorder. Some clinicians such as E. Bleuler, Jaspers, Schneider, and others have argued that all cases of paranoia (delusional disorder) are simply members of a paranoid subgroup of schizophrenia. Clinical experience shows that there certainly are patients who develop a system of delusions without ever having any other sign of psychopathology, but they are comparatively uncommon.

## Delusions in Schizophrenia

Delusions encountered in schizophrenia include the belief or experience that as one's thoughts occur, they are broadcast from one's head to the external world so that others can hear them (thought broadcasting); that thoughts that are not one's own are inserted into one's mind (thought insertion); that thoughts have been removed from one's head (thought withdrawal); or that one's feelings, impulses, thoughts, or actions are not one's own but are imposed by some external force (delusions of being controlled).

Some of these delusions occur with a frequency of up to 70% in all schizophrenic patients across different cultures (Murray, 1986, p. 342). This fact raises interesting questions about the hypothesis that delusions are idiosyncratic and personal. It also suggests that there is a common etiology for these delusions and that they are minimally created by unique personality features or by factors unique to the patient's culture.

The anomalous experience model of delusion formation may contribute to our understanding of this apparent puzzle. There is evidence that several changes happen at the onset of schizophrenia in the way persons experience reality, as well as their own thoughts. These include experiences of passivity ("my thoughts are not thought by me"), of the personal significance of external objects ("this object directly relates to me"), of the significance of the coincidence of one's thoughts and some external event ("this happened because I was thinking about it"), of disordered thought, or of alienation ("there is a wall of glass between me and everything else"). These experiences are likely to arise from internal, endogenous neuropsychological defects that form from the basic pathology of the schizophrenic disorder.

A parallel set of disturbing experiences arises from the discrepancy between the patient's actual action and the intended action. At one level, this appears to arise from a fundamental disjunction in consciousness between the awareness of the action that is performed and the attribution of the action to the self. This explanation has been elaborated by Frith (1987, 1996), Silbersweig, Stern, and Frith (1995), and others with specific reference to the conscious phenomena of hallucinations.

At another level, the experience of discrepancy between intent and action may arise because associative interference in producing language creates utterances that are not congruent with the intended utterance. At the conscious level, the patients' experience is of speaking or (less commonly) writing something that fails to match what they wanted to say (Maher, 1988c; Maher, Manschreck, Seung, & Tsuang, 1995). Similar misattribution about hand movements has been reported in deluded patients by Daprati, Franck, Geogieff, Proust, Pacherie, Dalery, and Jeannerod (1997).

Such experiences are disturbing and they prompt the patient to seek explanations. Thus, the experience of not being able to produce coherent utterances any longer may be interpreted by patients as evidence that somebody else is interfering with their thoughts by some technical device. The experience of not thinking one's own thoughts may become transformed into the idea that someone else is thinking one's thoughts. This, in turn, leads to an attempt to determine who the "someone else" might be. When the patient decides that it must be the FBI, Vatican, or other identifiable agency, the delusional process has begun.

As long as patients focus directly only on changes in their experience—as can be the case for several days or weeks at the beginning of the psychosis—statements that describe these changes should not be defined as delusions but rather understood as veridical descriptions of disordered or anomalous conscious experiences.

## Delusions in Affective Disorders

Estimates of the incidence of delusions in affective disorders are affected by the criteria employed by investigators in defining the cohorts of study. Thus some investigators exclude from their definition of depression those patients who have delusions due to depression. Delusions have been reported by Kantor and Glassman (1977) in 20–30% of depressed inpatients; the most common delusions are of guilt, worthlessness, and hypochondriasis. By definition, delusions in mania and in depression are "mood-congruent," that is, their content can be understood in terms of the prevailing mood or affect of the concomitant disorder. Delusions of grandeur are a common feature of mania, whereas delusions of worthlessness, pov-

erty, or guilt, as well as hypochondriac and nihilistic delusions, are features of depression.

Delusions in affective disorders are meaningfully related to the underlying affect, and they also seem to be causally related to the affective changes brought about by the disorder. Clinically, it is well known that a change in the affect brings about a change in the delusions, although this may take some time. Again, the theory of anomalous experiences—in this case affective—can be used to make those changes plausible. In this framework, delusions in affective disorders can be interpreted as a patients' hypotheses of the reasons and consequences of their affective states.

Research comparing deluded depressed patients with nondeluded depressed patients has been done with inconclusive results. Patients with delusional depression do not differ from nondeluded depressed patients with regard to neurochemical variables (Lykouras, Markianos, Malliaras, & Stefanis, 1988). However, the occurrence of delusions does impact the clinical course of a depressive illness. Kettering, Harrow, Grossman, and Meltzer (1987) reported that delusional depressed patients had more mood-incongruent delusions at a 14-month later follow-up, whereas nondeluded depressed patients suffered from more depressed mood and anxiety, thus suggesting two different underlying disorders. Roose, Glassman, Walsh, Woodring, and Vital-Herne (1983) reported a 25-year retrospective study of the suicidal risk of delusional versus nondelusional depressed patients. They found that the delusional depressed patients had a risk of suicide five times higher than nondeluded patients.

The prevalence of delusions during depressive episodes depends on the diagnostic criteria used to define depression and also schizophrenia and paranoia. As the underlying concepts change over time, the range of prevalences is quite broad, and frequencies range from roughly 5 to 50%. A study with 280 patients reported by Beck (1967, pp. 36–39) reported that there is a correlation between the frequency of delusions and the severity of depression. In this study, the delusions of the main depressive themes, namely, delusions of worthlessness, guilt (sin and punishment), or the patients' body being defective or decaying, occurred with frequencies of about 40 to 50% each. Chambers, Puig-Antich, Tabrizi, and Davies (1982) found that delusions were present in only four out of fifty-eight children with prepubertal major depressive disorder.

Little is known about the exact frequency of delusions of grandeur in mania. Whether other types of delusions are a frequent feature of mania is also not known. As in depression, such figures are highly dependent upon the conceptual boundaries between the affective and schizophrenic disorders.

## Specific Syndromes

There are several syndromes in which delusions are the only or the predominant symptom. In general, these are rare conditions and, perhaps for that reason, the concepts used to describe them are somewhat vague.

### Paranoid Personality Disorder

In the DSM-IV (p. 634), the diagnostic criteria for this disorder are that patients suspect (without adequate basis) that others are exploiting or harming them, are preoccupied with doubts about the loyalty or trustworthiness of friends or associates, are reluctant to confide in others because of unwarranted fear that the information will be used against them, read hidden demeaning or threatening meanings into benign remarks or events, bear grudges, perceive attacks on their character that are not evident to others, and have jealous suspicions of the sexual fidelity of spouse or partner.

Little is known about this disorder with respect to prevalence, family patterns, and predisposing factors. The relationship of this disorder to other paranoid disorders and to paranoid schizophrenia is unclear.

### Delusional Parasitosis

This syndrome is characterized by the delusion that parasites, insects, worms, or foreign bodies are under the skin. The delusion arises on the basis of the patient's sensations of itching under the skin. As a reaction, the patients tend to scratch their skin, sometimes giving rise to severe lesions. At different times, this syndrome has been termed "monosymptomatic hypochondriasis," "epidermozoophobia," "delusion of infestation," "atypi-

cal somatoform disorder," "tactile hallucinosis," and "delusional disorder, somatic type."

Little is known about the prevalence, etiology, predisposing factors, and family patterns of this disorder, perhaps a result of the multiplicity of names under which it has been described. Although the symptomatology is usually circumscribed, delusional parasitosis can lead to considerable impairment. It should be noted that delusions of insects crawling under the skin are a common feature of delusional disorders due to prolonged cocaine abuse. A case of this disorder associated with lesions in frontal white matter was reported by Flynn, Cummings, Scheibel, and Wirshing (1989) and is cited by Benson and Stuss (1990) to support the hypothesis that frontal damage is a critical feature of delusions.

## Delusional Misidentification

### Capgras

In 1923, J. Capgras and J. Reboul-Lachaux first described a syndrome that consisted of the delusional belief that doubles of significant others or oneself or both exist. For instance, patients may claim that their spouses have been replaced by one or more impostors. The syndrome is not a perceptual problem, an illusion, a hallucination, a misrecognition, or an autoscopic phenomenon; it certainly is a very specific circumscribed delusion. The syndrome is also known under the names of "illusion of doubles" and "illusions of false recognition," and is to be distinguished from autoscopy, prosopagnosia, as well as from defects of perception and memory. Berson (1983) summarized 133 cases of this syndrome in the English language literature. The Capgras syndrome appears in both men and women over a wide range of ages and underlying mental disorders. The most common diagnosis was that of schizophrenia (about 60%), especially of paranoid type, whereas 23% of the patients suffered from organic brain disorders.

### Fregoli Syndrome

This syndrome, first described by Courbon and Fail (1927), consists of the delusional belief that familiar persons appear "disguised" in various forms as other people. In one recent case (De

Pauw, Szulecka, & Poltock, 1987), a patient complained that she was being persecuted by a cousin and his friend. She believed that they disguised themselves with false beards, wigs, make-up etc. On this basis, she confronted strangers demanding that they acknowledge their true identity and made complaints to the police. A CT scan revealed a right-sided posterior-temporo-parietal infarct. After recovery from speech slurring, orientation and memory problems, she developed the Frégoli syndrome. It was controllable with trifluoperazine.

## Intermetamorphosis

Courbon and Tusques (1932) described a syndrome wherein the physical appearance of some people, animals, or objects changes radically to match that of someone else. They described the case of a woman who reported that animals or objects that she owned changed to take the form of some other animal or object. Bick (1986) reported four such cases, three of whom had temporal lobe epilepsy.

The frequent appearance of organic disorder in connection with the misidentification syndromes lends support to the model of Ellis and Young (1990), who hypothesized that the critical locus of the pathology lies in a complex neural system of facial recognition units and person identity units. This pathology gives rise to conscious experiences of recognition failure or of false recognition which, in turn, generate delusional explanations. The Ellis-Young model is more specific than other attempts to interpret the misidentification syndromes in broader nonspecific motivational terms (De Pauw, 1994).

## Erotomania
## (de Clérambault's Syndrome)

de Clérambault's syndrome is also called erotomania, or, as in the DSM-IV, delusional disorder, erotomanic type. The central theme of this delusional syndrome is that *one is loved by another.* "The delusion usually concerns idealized romantic love and spiritual union rather than sexual attraction. The person about whom the conviction is held is usually of higher status ..." (DSM-IV, p. 297). The patient's efforts to contact this person by phone calls, letters, etc., are common and can be very distressing for the respective person. Although reportedly more common in females than

males, it does occur in males and may take the form of stalking or other activities that conflict with the law. Signer (1991) argued that at least in some patients, the basic pathology is an affective disorder (rather than a "pure" delusional disorder).

## Folie à Deux
## (Shared Psychotic Disorder)

Folie à deux is the most widely used name for a condition which has been given quite a few names, for example, "shared paranoid disorder" (DSM-III; American Psychiatric Association, 1980)), "induced psychotic disorder" (DSM-III-R; American Psychiatric Association, 1987), "induced insanity," "communicated insanity," "double insanity," and "folie simultanée." The diagnostic criteria listed in the DSM-IV (p. 306) are as follows:

A. A delusion develops (in a second person) in the context of a close relationship with another person, or persons, with an already established delusion.
B. The delusion is similar in content to that of the person who already has the established delusion.
C. The disturbance is not better accounted for by another psychotic disorder ... or by substance abuse ... or a general medical condition.

The disorder develops in a person who is involved with another individual who already has a psychotic disorder with prominent delusions. The disorder is more common among females, and the patients usually are less impaired by it, compared to the patient with the primary person. Cases do not always involve only two patients; cases of three (Dewhurst & Ellenberg, 1961), four (Ropschitz, 1957), five (Kamal, 1965), and twelve (Waltzer, 1963) have been reported.

## Delusions Associated
## with Somatic Disorders

Space does not permit a detailed account of the many reported cases of delusions associated with various bodily disorders. A fairly complete review may be found in Maher and Ross (1984). However, it may be noted summarily here that delusions have been found in the disorders listed following. Although the delusions that are reported cover the range of content that we have already described, many of the cases described in published reports present delusions with persecutory features, and many describe feelings of insignificance or puzzlement. Unsurprisingly much of the delusional content has a somatic theme. Reported cases include patients suffering from temporal lobe epilepsy; narcolepsy; Huntington's chorea; cerebral malaria; hereditary ataxia; multiple sclerosis; hydrocephalus; systemic lupus erythematosus; encephalitis; traumatic brain injury; scleroderma; chronic liver disease; pellagra; manganese intoxication; porphyria; various disorders of the thyroid, as well as many other syndromes. In the majority of cases, the delusions clear up after the basic somatic disorder has been treated successfully.

## Treatment

At the clinical level, a delusion is generally regarded as part of the larger pattern of disturbance that the patient displays. Delusions are generally more likely to respond to appropriate therapeutic action if they are part of a syndrome such as schizophrenia and depression (rather than the only symptoms as in delusional disorder), if they are not systematized (compared to highly systematized delusions that affect almost all realms of a patient's thinking), and if they have not been present for too long. Superior intelligence does not make patients more open to demonstrating the inadequacy of their beliefs. Instead, high IQs may help patients to systematize their delusions, and therefore preserve the disorder against refutation. This is, of course, consistent with our observation that defective reasoning is not a significant causative factor in the genesis of delusions.

### Biological Methods

Our knowledge about the response rate of delusions of various types to drug treatment of the underlying disorder is very limited and can be summarized as follows. Delusions are often harder to cure than other symptoms of mental disorder. In schizophrenia, for example, the anomalous experiences of hallucinations, thought control, thought broadcasting, and the like (i.e., purely subjective experiences), tend to respond quickly to neuroleptic substances, whereas delusional systems that incorporate many aspects of a patient's real life have a tendency to persist, even though the delusion may come to seem more alien to the patient.

Neuroleptic drugs may be taken by the patient either on the basis of the presence of other symptoms such as anxiety or agitation in acutely ill patients or on the basis of an already established therapeutic relationship in nonacutely ill patients.

Glassman, Kantor, and Shostak (1975) found that depressed patients with delusions are markedly unresponsive to tricyclic antidepressants such as imipramine. Good results are reported in treating delusional depression with either a combination of tricyclic antidepressants and neuroleptics or ECT (Minter & Mandel, 1979).

### Psychological Method: Cognitive and Behavioral

Psychotherapists of the various schools agree that establishing a trustful relationship with the patient is a necessary condition of every psychotherapy of a delusional patient. It has long been assumed that it is unwise to confront patients with their delusions because this does not tend to convince the patients that their beliefs are delusional, but rather makes them angry, suspicious, or even hostile. "Initially, the therapist should neither agree with nor challenge the patient's delusions" comment (Kaplan & Sadock, 1985, p. 233). There is no available empirical evidence that would compel us to reject this advice, at least in the initial stages of interaction with the patient. However, whether the therapist should look for psychodynamic reasons and adaptive purposes of delusions, as Kaplan and Sadock propose, is open to question. Although it may be sometimes possible to conclude that a delusional system conveys some "benefit" to the patient, the general hypothesis that delusions serve any purpose other than that of explaining personal experience is highly speculative.

**Behavior Modification.** There are several reports of attempts to modify delusional behavior by manipulating the consequences of the expression of the delusion. Beck (1952) employed direct discussion of delusional ideas that had been held for 7 years by a 28-year-old chronic schizophrenic, a procedure that led to eliminating them. Watts, Powell, and Austin (1973) reported successfully eliminating delusions by presenting counterevidence (without direct confrontation of the delusional belief) and encouraging their clients to develop and voice arguments against their delusional beliefs. Alford (1986, 1994) reported successful outcomes in using a cognitive therapy that centers on helping patients develop the practice of seeking alternative explanations for their experiences. The treatment reportedly reduced the frequency of delusional cognitions and reduced rated levels of confidence in the delusional beliefs of some numbers of patients. Studies using a similar technique were reported by Chadwick and Lowe (1990), Lowe and Chadwick (1990), and Chadwick (1994). In these studies, they were able to obtain substantial reduction in delusional beliefs; the reduction remained in effect at follow-ups carried out for extended periods after the intervention. Mor extensive reports of these interventions and reviews of behavioral interventions may be found in Kingdon and Turkington (1993); Chambon and Marie-Cardine (1994); and Chadwick, Birchwood, and Trower (1996).

Some behavioral aspects of delusions may respond to cognitive explanation training or to adequate contingency management, but the problem remains of determining whether a belief has been modified on the basis of modifying the overt expression of the belief. Supportive counseling and management of the social aspects of the disorder may be the treatment of choice for the chronically ill paranoid patient. If the condition is fluctuating, it is generally agreed that additional drug therapy should not be withheld in stages of acute exacerbation.

## Conclusions

From the material that we have presented, it is clear that our understanding of the etiology, pathology, and therapy of delusions is far from adequate. It is more than likely that the origins of delusional beliefs, as of normal beliefs, are heterogeneous. It is also likely that the factors that give rise to delusions are not the same as those that maintain them over time. With these caveats in mind, we offer the following general conclusions:

1. The criteria by which delusions are to be defined are open to dispute. These disputes center particularly on the ambiguity of concepts of "falsity" and the steps that would serve to establish it. They also include problems with the concept of the "incorrigibility" of a belief and the operational requirements necessary to establish this.

2. There is reason to question the scientific status of the practical distinction whereby culturally accepted, false, and incorrigible beliefs are not defined as delusional, whereas similar beliefs held by one or a few individuals are so defined.

3. After many research studies, there is still no good evidence to support the hypothesis that delusions arise from a cognitive defect in deductive or inductive reasoning or from other processes of inference. Normal individuals employ inferential processes that are indistinguishable from those of deluded patients; the locus of the delusional problem must lie elsewhere.

4. There is no acceptable evidence to support the hypothesis that delusions are reflections of unconscious motives, distorted into delusional form so as to permit entry into consciousness.

5. Given the occurrence of delusions in a very wide range of disorders, it is unlikely that an explanation that is derived from a model of the pathology of a specific disorder will be adequate to explain delusions in general. An adequate model must explain delusions across the spectrum of disorders in which they are found.

6. As an additional comment on the preceding item, it is entirely possible that delusional beliefs have differing etiologies—a possibility that suggests the necessity for fine-grained longitudinal analyses of the origin and development of delusions in clinical populations.

7. The writer has presented a model of delusion formation in which a principal role is played by anomalous conscious experience. As defined in this model, anomalous experience may arise (1) exogenously from the presence of unidentified but genuine atypical and unpredictable features in the external environment or in the somatic functions in the patient's body; (b) from impairment in the sensory and/or information-processing mechanisms involved in attending to, perceiving, and/or processing the redundancies and contexts of an otherwise normal environment; and (c) from endogenous neuropathological states that give rise to conscious experiences such as those of "significance" puzzlement or anomalousness which are in

turn ascribed to undefinable changes in the external environment and/or the patient's bodily functions.

# References

Achte, K. A. (1961). Der Verlauf der schizophrenen und der schizophreniformen Psychosen. *Acta Psychiatrica et Neurologica Scandinavica* (Supplement).

Adler, A. (1927). *Praxis und Theorie der Individualpsychologie*, 3rd ed. Darmstadt, Germany: Bergmann.

Alford, B. A. (1986). Behavioral treatment of schizophrenic delusions: A single-case experimental analysis. *Behavior Therapy, 17*, 637–644.

Alford, B. (1994). Cognitive therapy of delusional beliefs. *Behavior Research and Therapy, 32*, 369–380.

Altman, H., Sletten, I. W., Eaton, M. E., & Ulett, G. A. (1971). Demographic and mental status profiles—patients with homicidal, assaultive, suicidal, persecutory and homosexual ideation. *Psychiatric Quarterly, 45*, 58–64.

American Psychiatric Association. (1980). *Diagnostic and statistical manual of mental disorders* (3rd ed.). Washington, DC: Author.

American Psychiatric Association. (1987). *Diagnostic and statistical manual of mental disorders* (3rd ed., rev.). Washington, DC: Author.

American Psychiatric Association. (1994). *Diagnostic and statistical manual of mental disorders* (4th ed.). Washington, DC: Author.

Anderson, C. A., Lepper, M. A., & Ross, L. (1980). Perseverance of social theories: The role of explanation in the persistence of discredited information. *Journal of Personality and Social Psychology, 39*, 1037–1049.

Arieti, S. (1955). *Interpretation of schizophrenia*. New York: Robert Brunner.

Aronson, M. L. (1952). A study of the Freudian theory of paranoia by means of the Rorschach test. *Journal of Projective Techniques, 16*, 397–411.

Arthur, A. Z. (1964). Theories and explanations of delusions: A review. *American Journal of Psychiatry, 121*, 105–115.

Ballerini, A., & Rossi Monti, M. (1990). *La vergogna e el deliro. Un modello delle sindromi paranoidee*. Turin, Italy: Bollati Boringhieri.

Beck, A. T. (1952). Successful outpatient psychotherapy of a chronic schizophrenia with delusions based on borrowed guilt. *Psychiatry, 15*, 305–312.

Beck, A. T. (1967). *Depression: Causes and treatment*. Philadelphia: University of Pennsylvania Press.

Benson, D. T., & Stuss, D. F. (1990). Frontal lobe influences: A clinical perspective. *Schizophrenia Bulletin, 16*, 403–410.

Berson, R. J. (1983). Capgras' syndrome. *American Journal of Psychiatry, 140*, 969–978.

Bick, P. A. (1986). The syndrome of intermetamorphosis. *Bibliotecha Psychiatrica, 164*, 131–135.

Bickel, H. (1920). Über affektive und intellektuelle Wahnideen. Eine pathopsychologische studie. *Zeitschrift für die gesamte Neurologie und Psychiatrie, 58*, 94–132.

Bleuler, E. (1906). *Affektivität, suggestibilität und paranoia*. Halle, Germany: Marhold.

Carr, A. C. (1963). Observations on paranoia and their relation-ship to the Schreber case. *Medical Journal of Psychoanalysis, 21*, 195–200.

Cattell, R. B., & Moroney, J. H. (1962). The use of the 16PF in distinguishing between homosexuals, normals, and general criminals. *Journal of Consulting Psychology, 26*, 531–540.

Chadwick, P. (1994). A cognitive approach to measuring and modifying delusions. *Behavior Research and Therapy, 32*, 355–367.

Chadwick, P., Birchwood, M., & Trower, P. (1996). *Cognitive therapy for delusions and hallucinations*. New York: Wiley.

Chadwick, P. D. J., & Lowe, C. F. (1990). Measurement and modification of delusional beliefs. *Journal of Consulting and Clinical Psychology, 58*, 225–232.

Chambers, W. J., Puig-Antich, J., Tabrizi, M. A., & Davies, M. (1982). Psychotic symptoms in prepubertal Major Depressive Disorder. *Archives of General Psychiatry, 39*, 921–927.

Chambon, O., & Marie-Cardine, M. (1994). *Psychothérapie cognitive des psychoses chroniques*. Paris: Masson.

Chapman, L. J., Chapman, J. P., & Miller, G. A. (1964). A theory of verbal behavior in schizophrenia. In B. A. Maher (Ed.), *Progress in experimental personality research*, Vol. I. New York: Academic Press.

Colby, K. M. (1975). *Artificial paranoia: A computer simulation of paranoid processes*. New York: Pergamon Press.

Cooper, A. F., & Curry, A. R. (1976). The pathology of deafness in the paranoid and affective psychoses of later life. *Journal of Psychosomatic Research, 20*, 97–105.

Cooper, A. F., & Porter, R. (1976). Visual acuity and ocular pathology in the paranoid and affective psychoses of later life. *Journal of Psychosomatic Research, 20*, 107–114.

Courbon, P., & Fail, G. (1927). Illusion of Frégoli syndrome and schizophrenia. *Bulletin de la Société Clinique de Médicine Mentale, 15*, 121–124.

Courbon, P., & Tusques, J. (1932). Illusions d'intermetamorphose et de charme. *Annales Medico-Psychologiques, 14*, 401–406.

Cummings, J. L. (1985). Organic delusions: Phenomenology, anatomical correlations, and review. *British Journal of Psychiatry, 146*, 184–197.

Cutting, J. (1985). *The psychology of schizophrenia*. Edinburgh, Scotland: Churchill Livingstone.

Deprati, E., Franck, N., Georgieff, N., Proust, J., Pacheria, E., Dalery, J., & Jeannerod, M. (1997). Looking for the agent: An investigation into consciousness of action and self-consciousness in schizophrenic patients. *Cognition, 65*, 71–86.

Daston, P. G. (1956). Perception of homosexual words in paranoid schizophrenia. *Perceptual and Motor Skills, 6*, 45–55.

De Bonis, M., Epelbaum, C., Féline, A., Grize, J.-B., Hardy, P., & Somogyi, M. (1990). Pensée formelle, opérations logico-discursives et schizophrénie: Étude expérimentale d'un cas clinique. *Revue Canadienne de Psychiatrie, 35*, 64–70.

De Pauw, K. W. (1994). Psychodynamic approaches to the Capgras delusion: A critical historical review. *Psychopathology, 27*, 154–160.

De Pauw, K. W., Szulecka, T. K., & Poltock, T. L. (1987). Single case study: Frégoli syndrome after cerebral infarction. *Journal of Nervous and Mental Disease, 175*, 1–6.

Dewhurst, W. G., & Ellenberg, M. D. (1961). Folie a trois. *Journal of Mental Science, 129*, 486–490.

Doust, L., & Christie, H. (1978). The pathology of love: Some clinical variants of de Clérambault's syndrome. *Social Science in Medicine, 12*, 99–106.

Ehrenwald, J. (1960). The symbolic matrix of paranoid delusions and the homosexual alternative. *American Journal of Psychoanalysis, 20,* 49–65.

Ellis, H. D., & Young, A. W. (1990). Accounting for delusional misidentification. *British Journal of Psychiatry, 157,* 239–248.

Eriksen, C. W. (1951). Perceptual defense as a function of unacceptable needs. *Journal of Abnormal Psychology, 60,* 557–564.

Faught, W. S., Colby, K. M., & Parkinson, R. C. (1977). Inferences, affects, and intentions in a model of paranoia. *Cognitive Psychology, 9,* 153–187.

Feyerabend, P. (1970). Against method. In M. Radner & S. Winokur (Eds.), *Studies in the philosophy of science,* Vol. VI. Minneapolis: University of Minnesota Press.

Flynn, F. F., Cummings, J. L., Scheibel, J., & Wirshing, W. (1989). Monosymptomatic delusions of parasitosis associated with ischemic cerebrovascular disease. *Journal of Geriatric Psychiatry and Neurology, 2,* 134–139.

Freud, S. (1978). Psychoanalytische Bemerkungen über einen autobiographisch beschriebenen Fall von Paranoia (Dementia Paranoides). *Gesammelte Werke,* Vol. 8. Frankfurt, Germany: Fischer Verlag. (Originally published in 1911.)

Frith, C. D. (1979). Consciousness, information processing and schizophrenia. *British Journal of Psychiatry, 134,* 225–235.

Frith, C. D. (1987). The positive and negative symptoms of schizophrenia reflect impairments in the perception and initiation of action. *Psychological Medicine, 17,* 631–648.

Frith, C. D. (1996). The role of the prefrontal cortex in self-consciousness: The case of auditory hallucinations. *Philosophical Transactions of the Royal Society, B351,* 1505–1512.

Gallup, G. H., & Newport, F. (1991). Belief in paranormal phenomena among adult Americans. *Skeptical Inquirer, 15,* 137–146.

Gardner, G. E. (1931). Evidences of homosexuality in 120 unanalyzed cases with paranoid content. *Psychoanalytic Review, 18,* 55–72.

Garety, P. A. (1994). Construction of "paranoia": Does Harper enable voices other than his own to be heard? *British Journal of Psychiatry, 67,* 145–146.

Garety, P. A., & Hemsley, D. R. (1987). Characteristics of delusional experience. *European Archives of Psychiatry and Neurological Sciences, 236,* 294–298.

Garety, P. A., & Hemsley, D. R. (1994). *Delusions: Investigation into the psychology of delusional reasoning.* Oxford, England: Oxford University Press.

Garnham, A., & Oakhill, J. (1994). *Thinking and reasoning.* Oxford, England: Basil Blackwell.

Gawin, F. H. (1986). Neuroleptic reduction of cocaine-induced paranoia but not euphoria? *Psychopharmacology, 90,* 142–143.

Gerver, D. (1967). Linguistic rules and the perception and recall of speech by schizophrenic patients. *Journal of Social and Clinical Psychology, 6,* 204–211.

Glassman, A. H., Kantor, S. J., & Shostak, M. (1975). Depression, delusions, and drug response. *American Journal of Psychiatry, 132,* 716–719.

Glick, B. S. (1959). Homosexual panic: Clinical and theoretical considerations. *Journal of Nervous and Mental Diseases, 129,* 20–28.

Grauer, D. (1954). Homosexuality and paranoid schizophrenia as revealed by the Rorschach test. *Journal of Consulting Psychology, 18,* 459–462.

Greenspan, J. (1963). Sex of the persecutor in female paranoid patients. *Archives of General Psychiatry, 9,* 217–223.

Hagen, F. W. (1870). *Studien auf dem gebiet der seelenheilkunde.* Erlangen, Germany: Besold.

Harper, D. J. (1992). Defining delusion and the serving of professional interests: The case of "paranoia." *British Journal of Medical Psychology, 65,* 357–369.

Harper, D. J. (1994). The professional construction of "paranoia" and the discursive use of diagnostic criteria. *British Journal of Medical Psychology, 67,* 131–143.

Hart, D. S., & Payne, R. W. (1973). Language structure and predictability in overinclusive patients. *British Journal of Psychiatry, 123,* 643–662.

Hastings, D. W. (1941). A paranoid reaction with manifest homosexuality. *Archives of Neurology and Psychiatry, 45,* 379–381.

Heider, F. (1944). Social perception and phenomenal causality. *Psychological Review, 51,* 358–374.

Heilbrun, K. S. (1980). Silverman's subliminal psychodynamic activation: A failure to replicate. *Journal of Abnormal Psychology, 89,* 560–566.

Heilbrunn, A. B., & Madison, J. K. (1978). An analysis of structural factors in schizophrenic delusions. *Journal of Clinical Psychology, 34,* 326–329.

Hemsley, D. R., & Garety, P. A. (1986). The formation and maintenance of delusions: A Bayesian analysis. *British Journal of Psychiatry, 149,* 51–56.

Herbert, M. E., & Jacobsen, S. (1967). Late paraphrenia. *British Journal of Psychiatry, 113,* 305–311.

Houston, F., & Royse, A. B. (1954). Relationship between deafness and psychotic illness. *Journal of Mental Science, 100,* 990–993.

Hunter, R., & McAlpine, I. (1963). *Three hundred years of psychiatry.* London: Oxford University Press.

Huq, S. F., Garety, P. A., & Hemsley, D. R. (1988). Probabilistic judgements in deluded and non-deluded subjects. *Quarterly Journal of Experimental Psychology, 40,* 801–812.

Jackson, J. H. (1958). *Selected Writings by J. H. Jackson:* Vols. I and II, J. Taylor (Ed.). New York: Basic Books.

Jaspers, K. (1913/1963). *General Psychopathology* (Allegemeine Psychopathologie, 1913), transl. by M. Hamilton & J. Hoenig. Manchester, England: University of Manchester Press.

Kamal, A. (1965). Folie a cinq: A clinical study. *British Journal of Psychiatry, 111,* 583–586.

Kaney, S., & Bentall, R. P. (1989). Persecutory delusions and attributional style. *British Journal of Medical Psychology, 62,* 191–198.

Kantor, S. J., & Glassman, A. H. (1977). Delusional depressions: Natural history and response to treatment. *British Journal of Psychiatry, 131,* 351–360.

Kaplan, H. I., & Sadock, B. J. (1985). *Modern synopsis of comprehensive textbook of psychiatry* (4th ed.). Baltimore: Williams & Wilkins.

Kay, D. W. K. (1972). Schizophrenia and schizophrenic-like states in the elderly. *British Journal of Hospital Medicine, 8,* 369–376.

Kay, D. W. K., & Roth, M. (1961). Environmental and hereditary factors in the schizophrenias of old age and their bearing on the general problem of causation in schizophrenia. *Journal of Mental Science, 107,* 649–686.

Kelley, H. L. (1967). Attribution theory in social psychology. In D. Levine (Ed.), *Nebraska Symposium on Motivation,* Vol. 15. Lincoln: University of Nebraska Press.

Kemp, R., Chua, S., McKenna, P., & David, A. (1997). Reasoning and delusions. *British Journal of Psychiatry, 170,* 398–405.

Kendler, K. (1984). Paranoia (delusional disorder). *Trends in Neuroscience, 7,* 14–17.

Kendler, K. S., Glazer, W. M., & Morgenstern, H. (1983). Dimensions of delusional experience. *American Journal of Psychiatry, 140,* 466–469.

Kettering, R. L., Harrow, M., Grossman, L., & Meltzer, H. Y. (1987). Prognostic relevance of delusions in depression: Follow-up study. *American Journal of Psychiatry, 144,* 1154–1160.

Kiev, A. (1972). *Transcultural psychiatry.* New York: Free Press.

Kingdon, D., & Turkington, D. (1993). *Cognitive therapy of schizophrenia.* New York: Guilford.

Klaf, F. S. (1961). Female homosexuality and paranoid schizophrenia. *Archives of General Psychiatry, 4,* 84–86.

Klaf, F. S., & Davis, C. A. (1960). Homosexuality and paranoid schizophrenia: A survey of 150 cases and controls. *American Journal of Psychiatry, 116,* 1070–1075.

Klein, H. R., & Horowitz, W. A. (1949). Psychosexual factors in paranoid phenomena. *American Journal of Psychiatry, 105,* 697–701.

Koh, S. D., Kayton, L., & Schwartz, C. (1972). Remembering of connected discourse by young nonpsychotic schizophrenic subjects. (Abstract). Cited in Koh, S. D. (1978). Remembering in schizophrenia. In S. Schwartz (Ed.), *Language and cognition in schizophrenia.* Hillsdale, NJ: Erlbaum.

Kraepelin, E. (1909). *Psychiatrie,* Vol. I. Leipzig, Germany: Barth.

Kraepelin, E. (1889). *Psychiatrie.* Leipzig, Germany: Abel.

Kranz, H. (1967). Wahn und zeitgeist. *Studium Generale, 20,* 606–611.

Kuhn, T. S. (1962). *The structure of scientific revolutions.* Chicago: University of Chicago Press.

Lagache, D. (1950). Homosexuality and jealousy. *International Journal of Psychoanalysis, 31,* 24–31.

Lambo, T. A. (1965). Schizophrenic and borderline states. In A. V. S. De Reuck & R. Porter (Eds.), *Transcultural psychiatry.* London: Churchill.

Lawson, J. S., McGhie, A., & Chapman, J. (1964). Perception of speech in schizophrenia. *British Journal of Psychiatry, 110,* 375–380.

Lenz, H. (1964). *Vergleichende Psychiatrie.* Vienna: Wilhelm Maudrich.

Lester, D. (1975). The relationship between paranoid delusions and homosexuality. *Archives of Sexual Behavior, 4,* 285–293.

Levy, R., & Maxwell, A. E. (1968). The effect of verbal context on the recall of schizophrenics and other psychiatric patients. *British Journal of Psychiatry, 114,* 311–316.

Lewinsohn, P. M., & Elwood, D. L. (1961). The role of contextual constraint on the learning of language samples in schizophrenia. *Journal of Nervous and Mental Diseases, 133,* 79–81.

Lowe, C. F., & Chadwick, P. (1990). Verbal control of delusions. *Behavior Therapy, 21,* 461–479.

Lykouras, E., Markianos, M., Malliaras, D., & Stefanis, C. (1988). Neurochemical variables in delusional depression. *American Journal of Psychiatry, 145,* 214–217.

Magaro, P. A. (1980). *Cognition in schizophrenia and paranoia.* Hillsdale, NJ: Erlbaum.

Maher, B. A. (1970). The psychology of delusions. Paper presented at the *Meeting of the American Psychological Association,* Miami Beach, FL.

Maher, B. A. (1974). Delusional thinking and perceptual disorder. *Journal of Individual Psychology, 30,* 98–113.

Maher, B. A. (1983). A tentative theory of schizophrenic utterance. In B. A. Maher & W. B. Maher (Eds.), *Progress in experimental personality research,* Vol. 12: *Psychopathology.* New York: Academic Press.

Maher, B. A. (1988a). Anomalous experience and delusional thinking: The logic of explanations. In T. F. Oltmanns & B. A. Maher (Eds.), *Delusional beliefs.* New York: Wiley-Interscience.

Maher, B. A. (1988b). Delusions as the product of normal cognitions. In T. F. Oltmanns & B. A. Maher (Eds.), *Delusional beliefs.* New York: Wiley-Interscience.

Maher, B. A. (1988c). Language disorders in psychoses and their impact on delusions. In M. Spitzer, F. A. Uehlein, & G. Oepen (Eds.), *Psychopathology and philosophy.* Berlin: Springer Verlag.

Maher, B. A. (1990). The irrelevance of rationality to adaptive behavior. In M. Spitzer & B. A. Maher (Eds.), *Philosophy and psychopathology.* New York: Springer Verlag.

Maher, B. A. (1992). Models and methods for the study of reasoning in delusions. *Revue Européenne de Psychologie Appliquée, 42,* 97–102.

Maher, B. A. (1999). Anomalous experience in everyday life: Its significance for psychopathology. *The Monist, 82,* 547–570.

Maher, B. A., Manschreck, T. C., & Molino, M. (1983). Redundancy, pause distributions and thought disorder in schizophrenia. *Language and Speech, 26,* 191–199.

Maher, B. A., Manschreck, T. C., & Rucklos, M. E. (1980). Contextual constraint and the recall of verbal material in schizophrenia: The effect of thought disorder. *British Journal of Psychiatry, 137,* 69–73.

Maher, B. A., Manschreck, T. C., Seung, F., & Tsuang, M. (1995). The behavioral correlates of delusions of control in schizophrenia. *Schizophrenia Research, 15,* 16.

Maher, B. A., & Ross, J. S. (1984). Delusions. In H. E. Adams & P. B. Sutker (Eds.), *Comprehensive handbook of psychopathology* (1st ed.). New York: Plenum.

Maher, B. A., & Spitzer, M. (1995). Delusions. In P. B. Sutker & H. E. Adams (Eds.), *Comprehensive handbook of psychopathology* (2nd ed.). New York: Plenum.

Mahorney, S. L., & Cavenar, J. O. (1988). A new and timely delusion: The complaint of having AIDS. *American Journal of Psychiatry, 145,* 1130–1132.

Malloy, P. F., & Richardson, E. D. (1994). The frontal lobes and content-specific delusions. *Journal of Neuropsychiatry, 6,* 455–466.

Manschreck, T. C. (1979). The assessment of paranoid features. *Comprehensive Psychiatry, 20,* 370–377.

Manschreck, T. C., Maher, B. A., Rucklos, M. E., & White, M. T. (1979). The predictability of thought-disordered speech in schizophrenic patients. *British Journal of Psychiatry, 134,* 595–601.

McGhie, A., & Chapman, J. (1961). Disorders of attention and perception in early schizophrenia. *British Journal of Medical Psychology, 34,* 103–116.

Melges, F. T., & Freeman, A. M. (1975). Persecutory delusions: A cybernetic model. *American Journal of Psychiatry, 132,* 1038–1044.

Minter, R. E., & Mandel, M. R. (1979). The treatment of psychotic major depressive disorder with drugs and electroconvulsive therapy. *The Journal of Nervous and Mental Disease, 167,* 726–733.

Modlin, H. C. (1963). Psychodynamics and management of paranoid states in women. *Archives of General Psychiatry, 8,* 263–268.

Moore, R. A., & Selzer, M. L. (1963). Male homosexuality, paranoia, and the schizophrenias. *American Journal of Psychiatry, 119,* 743–747.

Möhr, A. (1987). *Liebeswahn. Phänomenologie und psychodynamik der erotomanie.* Stuttgart: Enke.

Munro, A. (1987). Paranoid (delusional) disorders: DSM-III-R and beyond. *Comprehensive Psychiatry, 28,* 35–39.

Murphy, H. B. M. (1967). Cultural aspects of the delusion. *Studium Generale, 20,* 684–692.

Murray, R. (1986). Schizophrenia. In P. Hill, R. Murray, & A. Thorley (Eds.), *Essentials of postgraduate psychiatry,* 2nd ed. London: Grune and Stratton.

Mynatt, C. R., Doherty, M. E., & Tweeny, R. D. (1977). Confirmation bias in a simulated research environment: An experimental study of scientific interference. *Quarterly Journal of Experimental Psychology, 29,* 85–95.

Mynatt, C. R., Doherty, M. E., & Tweeny, R. D. (1978). Consequences of confirmation and disconfirmation in a simulated research environment. *Quarterly Journal of Experimental Psychology, 30,* 395–406.

Nims, J. P. (1959). Logical reasoning in schizophrenia: The von Domarus principle. Unpublished doctoral dissertation, University of Southern California.

Nisbett, R., & Ross, L. (1980). *Human inference: Strategies and shortcomings of social judgment.* Englewood Cliffs, NJ: Prentice-Hall.

Norman, J. P. (1948). Evidence and clinical significance of homosexuality in 100 unanalyzed cases of dementia praecox. *Journal of Nervous and Mental Disease, 107,* 484–489.

Oltmanns, T. F. (1988). Approaches to the definition and study of delusions. In T. F. Oltmanns & B. A. Maher (Eds.), *Delusional beliefs.* New York: Wiley-Interscience.

Overall, J. E., Gorham, D. R., & Shawver, J. R. (1961). Basic dimensions of change in the symptomatology of chronic schizophrenics. *Journal of Abnormal and Social Psychology, 63,* 597–602.

Ovesey, L. (1955). The pseudohomosexual anxiety. *Psychiatry, 18,* 17–25.

Page, J., & Warkentin, J. (1938). Masculinity and paranoia. *Journal of Abnormal and Social Psychology, 33,* 527–531.

Pauleikhoff, B. (1969). Der liebeswahn. *Fortschritte der Neurologie und Psychiatrie, 37,* 251–279.

Pavlov, I. P. (1934). An attempt at a physiological interpretation of obsessional neurosis and paranoia. *Journal of Mental Science, 80,* 187–197.

Peterson, G. A., & Davis, D. L. (1985). A case of homosexual erotomania. *Journal of Clinical Psychiatry, 46,* 448–449.

Piedmont, E. B. (1966). Ethnicity and schizophrenia: A pilot study. *Mental Hygiene, 50,* 374–379.

Planansky, K., & Johnston, R. (1962). The incidence and relationship of homosexual and paranoid features in schizophrenia. *Journal of Mental Science, 108,* 604.

Rennie, R. A. C. (1942). Prognosis in manic-depressive psychosis. *American Journal of Psychiatry, 98,* 801–814.

Roose, S. P., Glassman, A. H., Walsh, B. T., Woodring, S., & Vital-Herne, J. (1983). Depression, delusions, and suicide. *American Journal of Psychiatry, 140,* 1159–1162.

Ropschitz, D. H. (1957). Folie a deux. A case of folie imposée a

quatre and a trois. *Journal of Mental Science, 103,* 589–596.

Ross, L., & Anderson, C. (1981). Shortcomings in the attribution process: On the origins and maintenance of erroneous social assessments. In D. Kahneman, P. Slovic, & A. Tversky (Eds.), *Judgement under uncertainty: Heuristics and biases.* New York: Cambridge University Press.

Ross, L., & Lepper, M. R. (1981). The perseverance of beliefs: Empirical and normative considerations. In R. A. Shweder & D. Fiske (Eds.), *New directions for methodology of behavioral sciences: Fallible judgment in behavioral research.* San Francisco: Jossey-Bass.

Ross, C. A., & Joshi, S. (1992). Paranormal experiences in the general population. *Journal of Nervous and Mental Disease, 180,* 357–361.

Salzinger, K., Portnoy, S., & Feldman, R. (1964). Verbal behavior in schizophrenics and some comments towards a theory of schizophrenia. Paper presented at *American Psychopathological Association, Annual Meeting.*

Schneider, K. (1959). *Clinical psychopathology* (13th German ed.). (Trans. by M. Hamilton). Philadelphia: Grune and Stratton.

Schreber, D. P. (1988). *Memoirs of my nervous illness* (1903). Translated and edited by I. MacAlpine and R. A. Hunter. Cambridge, MA: Harvard University Press.

Shakow, D. (1962). Segmental set. *Archives of General Psychiatry, 6,* 1–17.

Sherer, M. A., Kumor, K. M., Cone, E. J., & Jaffe, J. H. (1988). Suspiciousness induced by four-hour intravenous transfusions of cocaine. *Archives of General Psychiatry, 45,* 673–677.

Shetty, G. C. (1988). Depressive illness with delusions of AIDS. *American Journal of Psychiatry, 145,* 765.

Silbersweig, D. A., Stern, E., & Frith, C. D. (1995). A functional neuroanatomy of auditory hallucinations. *Nature, 378,* 176–179.

Silverman, G. (1972). Psycholinguistics of schizophrenic language. *Psychological Medicine, 2,* 254–259.

Silverman, L. H., & Candall, P. (1970). On the relationship between aggressive activation, symbolic merging, intactness of body boundaries, and manifest pathology in schizophrenia. *Journal of Nervous and Mental Diseases, 5,* 387–399.

Southard, E. E. (1916a). On descriptive analysis of manifest delusions from the subject's point of view. *Journal of Abnormal Psychology, 11,* 189–202.

Southard, E. E. (1916b). On the application of grammatical categories to the analysis of delusions. *The Philosophical Review, 25,* 424–455.

Specht, G. (1908). Über die klinische kardinalfrage der paranoia. *Zentralblatt für Nervenkrankheiten, 31,* 817–833.

Spitzer, M. (1989). On the logic of thought disorders. In P. Klein (Ed.), *Praktische logik: Traditionen und tendenzen; 350 Jahre Joachimi Jungii "Logica Hamburgensis."* Göttingen, Germany: Vandenhoeck und Ruprecht.

Steinbrunner, E., & Scharfetter, C. (1976). Wahn im wandel der geschicte. *Archiv für Psychiatrie und Nervenkrankheiten, 21,* 581–586.

Strauss, J. S. (1969). Hallucinations and delusions as points on continua functions. *Archives of General Psychiatry, 21,* 581–586.

Stuss, D. T., & Benson, D. F. (1986). *The frontal lobes.* New York: Raven Press.

Swanson, D. W., Bohnert, P. J., & Smith, P. J. (1970). *The paranoid.* Boston: Little, Brown.

Tölle, R. (1987). Wahnentwicklung bei körperlich behinderten. *Nervenartz,* 759–763.

Truscott, I. P. (1970). Contextual constraint and schizophrenic language. *Journal of Consulting and Clinical Psychology, 35,* 189–194.

Tsuang, M. T., Faraone, S. V., & Day, M. (1988). Schizophrenic disorders. In A. M. Nicholi (Ed.), *The new Harvard guide to psychiatry.* Cambridge, MA: Harvard University Press.

von Domarus, E. (1944). The specific laws of logic in schizophrenia. In J. S. Kasanin (Ed.), *Language and thought in schizophrenia.* Berkeley: University of California Press.

von Orelli, A. (1954). Der wandel des inhaltes der depressiven ideen bei der reinen melancholie. *Schweizer Archiev für Neurologie und Psychiatrie, 73,* 217–287.

Walkup, J. (1994). The professional construction of paranoia and the discursive use of diagnostic criteria. *British Journal of Psychiatry, 67,* 147–151.

Waltzer, H. (1963). A psychotic family—folie à douze. *Journal of Nervous and Mental Disease, 137,* 67–75.

Wason, P. C., & Johnson-Laird, P. N. (1972). *Psychology of reasoning: Structure and content.* Cambridge, MA: Harvard University Press.

Watson, C. G. (1965). A test of the relationship between repressed homosexuality and paranoid mechanisms. *Journal of Clinical Psychology, 21,* 380–384.

Watts, F. N., Powell, E. G., & Austin, S. V. (1973). The modification of abnormal beliefs. *British Journal of Medical Psychology, 46,* 359–363.

Westermeyer, J. (1988). Some cross-cultural aspects of delusions. In T. F. Oltmanns & B. A. Maher (Eds.) (1988), *Delusional beliefs.* New York: Wiley-Interscience.

Williams, E. B. (1964). Deductive reasoning in schizophrenia. *Journal of Abnormal and Social Psychology, 69,* 47–61.

Winters, K. C., & Neale, J. M. (1983). Delusions and delusional thinking: A review of the literature. *Clinical Psychology Review, 3,* 227–253.

Zamansky, H. S. (1958). An investigation of the psychoanalytic theory of paranoid delusions. *Journal of Personality, 26,* 410–426.

Zimbardo, P. G., Anderson, S. M., & Kabat, L. G. (1981). Induced hearing deficit generates experimental paranoia. *Science, 212,* 1529–1531.

# CHAPTER 13

# Schizophrenia: Biopsychological Aspects

## Brendan A. Maher and Patricia J. Deldin

## Introduction

The research literature on the biopsychology of schizophrenia is monumental. Any attempt to cover all of it would require that we write a book. Accordingly, we have opted to focus on the literature that relates biological processes to psychological processes in the population of schizophrenia patients and represents lines of investigation that are currently active. This means that we do not include purely biochemical studies, such as those investigating the effect of medications on neurotransmitter activity or other similar associations between the operation of one biological variable on another. It also means, regrettably, that we will have little space for historical references.

Because of the focus that we have chosen, much of the content of this chapter will focus on the general areas of neuropsychology and psychophysiology. In some cases, the inference that a biological variable is involved may itself depend upon a psychological (i.e., nonbiological) measure. Where this is the case, we will point it out.

Brendan A. Maher and Patricia J. Deldin • Department of Psychology, Harvard University, Cambridge, Massachusetts 02138.

*Comprehensive Handbook of Psychopathology* (Third Edition), edited by Patricia B. Sutker and Henry E. Adams. Kluwer Academic/Plenum Publishers, New York, 2001.

## General Methodological Issues in the Investigation of Schizophrenia

### Heterogeneity

Schizophrenia is heterogeneous. That schizophrenia is heterogeneous has been known since the word "schizophrenia" was created. Bleuler's classic *Dementia Praecox or the Group of Schizophrenias*, first published in 1911 (in English in 1950), made it clear that he was talking about a group of diseases with some common symptoms and perhaps some common components in their pathogenesis. This being so, it is ultimately more critical to discover the regularities underlying the differences between subgroups of schizophrenia patients than to demonstrate differences between general unselected samples of schizophrenia patients and patients with some other psychopathological classification or nonpatient controls. The task is rendered difficult because seemingly different manifest aberrant behaviors (i.e., symptoms) may arise from the same prior causes and seemingly similar symptoms may arise from different prior causes. Arguing backward from effect to cause is notoriously unreliable, but it is a constant problem for the research psychopathologist who takes heterogeneity seriously.

The investigation of heterogeneity implies a certain model of a group of illnesses that have been traditionally subsumed under a single diagnostic label. An oversimplified version of this model of this might be stated as follows. A set of independent etiologies creates a set of different basic pathologies. These differences may consist of different biological pathologies and/or differences in the proportional roles played by biology and environment. The differences, however, produce overall clinical presentations that have some striking components in common. These common elements lead to the grouping of the patients under a single diagnostic label. Common elements may arise in part as common, secondary, compensatory responses to the handicaps created by different pathologies and in part because different etiological factors have produced different underlying primary pathologies that have, nonetheless, certain common consequences within the central nervous system itself. Where the common symptom/s are largely in the form of defects, this possibility is particularly likely.

## Etiological Heterogeneity

We have already commented on the complexity of systems that underlie seemingly simple responses. This is especially the case in which we seek to establish the neural basis of a defect. As we have pointed out, a complex system may fail to operate adequately as a result of quite different kinds of damage to the components of the system. Coupled with this is the fact that the brain does not operate on the basis of simple isomorphic linking of behavior with the activity of a specific region of interest; that functional brain regions may develop in response to environmental input, especially in the early years of life; that when regions of the brain are damaged—again, especially early in life—other regions may take over the functions normally mediated by the damaged area; that there are gender differences in normal brain development; and that the brain changes with aging. All of these considerations point to the immense complexity of the task of developing a comprehensive model for understanding the neuropsychological pathologies in a disorder that is as clinically complex as schizophrenia.

## The Concept of Defect

As a general working principle, it may be helpful to consider that human and other organisms rarely do nothing in response to situations in which they find themselves. They may not do,

however, what the observer regards as the correct thing, and what may appear to be normally the most effective thing. When this happens, it is tempting to classify what we observe as an instance of a deficit or lack of capacity to make the normal response. Unfortunately, this is a plausible inference as stated, but this kind of classification tends to distract us from observing what the individual actually does do—an observation that might otherwise have provided a clue to the nature of the active pathological process that determined the "wrong" response. By making this point, we are, of course, simply rephrasing the position of James Hughlings Jackson when he pointed out that much of the disordered behavior seen in cases of CNS damage is produced by the undamaged lower centers (e.g., Jackson, 1887).

A good example of this problem is in the classification of the language utterances of a patient as exhibiting "poverty of content," "derailment," or "incoherence." The very choice of a term such as "incoherent" tells us that we have noticed something that is absent from the utterance, i.e. "coherence," but it does not tell us what was present in the utterance. In one of our own studies, for example, Maher, Manschreck, Hoover, and Weisstein (1987), we found that the counted repetitions of words and phrases in samples of speech in schizophrenic patients significantly correlated with rated levels of Derailment, Understandability, and Poverty of Content as assessed in the Schedule for Affective Disorders and Schizophrenia (SADS; Spitzer & Endicott, 1977) in the same patients at a different time. What the patients were not doing was showing a richness of content; what the patients were doing, at least in part, was repeating and perseverating in speech. This observation leads us to become interested in the positive determinants of repetition and perseveration. The question, "What factors lead to repetitiousness" seems to us a more manageable definition of the research problem than the question "Where did the content go?"

Investigations of heterogeneity have taken certain approaches. One is the attempt to discern independent patterns or clusters within the global spectrum of symptoms, laboratory performance, case histories, and the like. Cluster analysis, the various forms of factor analysis, and other multivariate analyses are the main tools in this search. In themselves, these approaches create models of the possible complexity of the heterogeneity, that is, do the data analyses produce results that are plausibly consistent with the conclusion that there is a specific number of separate entities or subtypes, two, three, or more? If so, can these subtypes be differentiated when we turn to another level of inquiry such as brain structure or patterns of brain functioning?

## The Sequential Emergence of Manifest Phenomena

The timing and the unfolding sequence of the appearance of the various elements of the manifest pathology do not necessarily correspond to the sequential timing of the underlying biopathological processes themselves. We cannot assume that these causes become apparent before their consequences become apparent. This fact creates fundamental problems in retrospective studies of patients who are now manifestly ill. If we turn to relatives for information about the first appearance of the pathology in the premorbid behavior of the future patient, we encounter serious problems. Veridical recall of the past behavior of others is unreliable even when the recall is unaffected by any dramatic later development in the life of the person whose behavior is being described. It may be particularly unreliable when the patient has already been identified as psychiatrically ill.

In the case of biopsychological factors, we can be reasonably confident that structural anomalies in the central nervous system in young patients predate the appearance of pathological behavior. In older patients, our confidence is somewhat reduced because we know that changes in the brain occur with aging. In the case of neurophysiological anomalies unaccompanied by structural anomalies, we must be more cautious in interpreting cause and effect sequences. Once again, caution is more necessary in older patients than in younger ones.

The preferred solution to this problem, namely, the premorbid investigation of populations believed to be at some high risk of later pathology, is complex and difficult. It requires that we have very shrewd ideas about the kinds of variables that should be examined premorbidly and, of course, good epidemiological bases for selecting high-risk subjects. Furthermore, patients in psychopathological research may show deficits in a wide range of tasks for reasons that do not necessarily provide direct clues to their underlying pathology. Problems of diminished motivation, medication, general energy level, and the like can all impair performance. Because of this, hypotheses that predict that patients will fail to equal control groups in performing a specific task are quite likely to receive misleading support from the data.

## Traits and States

Pathological behavior frequently undergoes episodic changes in severity and composition, sufficient at times to warrant discharge from care or to return to care after a previous discharge because some elements of behavior are states that fluctuate over time and others are more permanent traits. The only reliable way to distinguish between these two alternatives is to employ the method of test–retest stability. It is routinely accepted that this be done with formal psychometric tests, such as those of intelligence, but this has been much less often the case with measures developed specifically for psychiatric populations. The method of group comparisons, made cross-sectionally in single time periods, establishes differences between some aspect of the behavior of a group of patients and a group of controls; it cannot establish that the differences obtained are stable and will be found again in the same sample if the comparison is made some time later. Because of this, we can never be sure that a failure to replicate a previous study is due to some methodological flaw in the original or reflects the fact that the behavior under scrutiny is state-like and hence difficult to replicate on demand.

But even more important than the technical questions is the question of functional brain organization itself. Are categories of response that appear similar at the overt behavioral level necessarily mediated by similar topological regions in the brain? What are the conditions under which one part of the brain may take over the functions of a damaged part? What do individual differences in lateralization mean about the brain organization of left-handed and right-handed patients? It is clear that we are making progress in answering these questions, but it is equally clear that a vast territory of information has yet to be acquired.

## Brain-Behavior Isomorphism

Neuropsychological and psychophysiological research in schizophrenia seeks to establish the association between some direct measure of the structure and/or function of the nervous system, on one hand, and either or both of the overt behavior of the patients, measured clinically or in the laboratory, or the patient's conscious experience as described by verbal report. The methods available for assessing brain structure and function are complex. Inferences based on the data produced by these methods rest on assumptions whose validity is sometimes uncertain.

## Methods of Measuring Brain Structure and Activity

The techniques of measurement available for use with the biological side of this link include various methods of imaging and quantifying brain structure and processes: electroencephalography (EEG), pneumoencephalography (PEG), positron emission tomography (PET), magnetoencephalography (MEG), computerized tomography (CT), magnetic resonance imagery (MRI), and MRI images taken while the subject is engaged in a specific activity (fMRI). Brain imaging techniques have their own methodological problems, including, for example, such technical questions as the definition of degrees of level of activity in a specific brain area and how the signal is to be separated from noise. Additionally, the measures vary in their spatial and temporal resolution.

Structural and functional neurophysiological measurements have been used in most psychological paradigms in studying schizophrenia. For example, researchers have attempted to improve differential diagnosis, determine subtypes of schizophrenia, distinguish state versus trait attributes, study abnormal psychological processes, study individual symptoms of the disorder, study populations believed at risk of schizophrenia, examine the environmental factors contributing to the disorder, define the course of the disorder, establish treatment efficacy, understand unique aspects of schizophrenia for special populations (e.g., women and ethnic minorities), and understand associated biological processes. Given the broad nature of neurophysiological research, it would be impossible for us to cover all of their applications in studying schizophrenia. Rather, this chapter will focus on the ability of neurophysiological studies to identify and elucidate possible cortical changes associated with schizo-

phrenia. This chapter will also highlight the psychological constructs associated with the regions of the brain in which abnormalities occur.

## The Search for Markers

At the outset we assume that individuals who later receive a diagnosis of schizophrenia have a preexisting vulnerability to developing the disorder. These individuals are defined as "at risk" for schizophrenia. Psychopathologists generally hypothesize that there will be signs of the presence of this vulnerability for some time before the onset of the illness. These signs are the "markers" for possible future schizophrenia. Implicit in this model is the recognition that biopsychological markers indicate the possibility, not the certainty, of future illness. In principle, a valid marker ought to distinguish reliably between patients and controls, ought to be present in patients even when their clinical condition has remitted, ought be present more frequently in relatives of patients, and ought to present in individuals who show minor subtle features in their perception and thinking that are similar to the more florid symptoms found in patients.

Several methods exist for identifying markers. One is to study the close relatives of patients, especially younger relatives. Because the range of potential biobehavioral features that might be studied is very broad, the usual strategy is to begin by using measures that typically differentiate between schizophrenic patients and the general population. These include measures of language, attention, memory, perception, and so forth.

One example of this approach is the use of the Continuous Performance Test (CPT). This test requires the subject to watch a screen on which stimuli of various kinds appear. Typically these are single digits. All but one of the targets must be ignored. Whenever the designated target appears, the subject must press a button. Stimuli appear briefly (100 milliseconds) at a rapid rate, generally one stimulus per second. Schizophrenic patients have shown defective performance in several studies. The CPT has been interpreted as a measure of sustained attention. Studies of CPT performance have uniformly shown defective performance in schizophrenia patients compared to normal controls. Positron emission tomography (PET) studies suggest that brain activity in normal subjects during the CPT centers in the prefrontal, temporal, and inferior parietal regions of the right hemisphere (Neuchterlein, 1991).

The performance of the parents and siblings of schizophrenia patients has shown deficits compared to controls (e.g., Mirsky et al., 1992; Steinhauer et al., 1991). Examination of the findings from these and other studies (e.g., Cornblatt & Erlenmeyer-Kimling, 1984; Rutschmann, Cornblatt, & Erlenmeyer-Kimling, 1986) indicate that impaired performance on the CPT by the relatives of schizophrenia patients depends on the complexity of the features of the target stimulus that is to be identified. Simple identification of digits is less effective as a test than the identification of complex patterns. Certain components of the deficit in schizophrenia patients' performance on the CPT continue even when the patient's clinical condition is in remission, leading Neuchterlein (1991) to suggest that the CPT is tapping a stable measure of vulnerability to schizophrenia.

Other tasks that have been successful in distinguishing the at-risk relatives of schizophrenia patients from controls are backward masking and span of apprehension. Backward masking involves presenting a rapid sequence of two stimuli located at the same point in the visual field. If the first stimulus has a very brief exposure, such as 20 ms, it can be recognized, unless followed by a second stimulus after an interval of 100 ms or less. In this case, the second stimulus "masks" the first and is not recognized. The interference in recognition is more marked in schizophrenia patients than in normal controls (e.g., Braff, 1981; Knight, 1990). Green, Neuchterlein, and Breitmeyer (1997) demonstrated impairment in backward masking in the siblings of schizophrenia patients, suggesting that this is another possible marker for vulnerability.

The span of apprehension is measured by the capacity of a subject to detect which of two letters, such as T or F, are present in an array of letters briefly flashed on a screen. One or other of the two letters will be present in each array. Schizophrenia patients have been deficient in this task (Asarnow, Granholm, & Sherman, 1991). Remitted patients continue to exhibit the deficit (Asarnow & MacCrimmon, 1978, 1981).

Now, we turn to the investigation of so-called schizotypal individuals. The concept of the schizotypal individual hypothesizes the presence of individuals who are more likely to develop schizophrenia than members of the general population.

Such individuals do not necessarily have family histories of schizophrenia. They are normally functioning individuals in the general population who report experiences and beliefs (minor aberrations that resemble hallucinations, delusions, and other conscious anomalies) that are similar to some of the more evident symptoms in diagnosed schizophrenia patients. These experiences are assessed on questionnaires that can be easily administered to large samples of the population, particularly the population of late adolescents and young adults who are approaching the age at which the onset of schizophrenia is most common. Typical studies have tended to use university students.

Studies of the CPT, backward masking, and the span of apprehension have been conducted on schizotypal individuals with the following results. Lenzenweger, Cornblatt, and Putnick (1991) reported that students who scored high on a schizotypy scale performed significantly less well on the CPT than low scoring students. Keefe et al. (1997) report the presence of anomalous eye tracking and schizotypal features in the nonpsychotic first-degree relatives of patients. Backward masking deficiency has been reported in schizotypal individuals by several investigators (Balogh & Merritt, 1985; Braff, 1981; Saccuzzo & Schubert, 1981; Steronko & Woods, 1978). The latter two studies investigated individuals who had been hospitalized with a diagnosis of schizotypal personality disorder. The span of attention has been examined in schizotypal subjects by Asarnow, Neuchterlein, and Marder (1983). They reported poorer performance in high schizotypes than in low scorers.

The general picture with regard to these stable neuropsychological markers in schizophrenia has been well summarized by Green (1998). In essence, the findings are that CPT deficit has been found in all four relevant groups (patients with schizophrenia, patients in clinical remission, their siblings and/or parents, and schizotypal individuals). A span of apprehension deficit has been found in three of these groups but has not been tested in relatives. Backward masking deficit has been found in all four groups. What we do not know from these studies is (1) Are there subgroups of individuals within these four groups whose performance is not deficient, i.e., do the data reflect heterogeneity? and (2) What are the direct correlates of performance in these tasks with aspects of brain structure or activity?

Research on this question has sometimes taken the form of a search for heterogeneity within schizotypal samples from whom a range of measures has been taken. Recent examples of this approach are in Voglmaier, Seidman, Salisbury, and McCarley (1997) and in Gruzelier and Kaiser (1996).

In the first of these, Voglmaier et al. (1997) compared the neuropsychological profiles of ten individuals who met the *Diagnostic and Statistical Manual of Mental Disorders*, 3rd edition, revised (DSM-III-R; American Psychiatric Association, 1987) criteria for schizotypal personality disorder (SPD) with a group of age-matched normal controls. An array of twenty-four tests covering ten domains (e.g., abstraction, verbal intelligence, semantic memory, visual memory, etc.) was administered. Significant differences were found in two of the ten domains; the SPD group was lower than the controls. The two domains were abstraction, measured by the Wisconsin Card Sorting Test (WCST), and verbal learning, measured with the California Verbal Learning Test (CVLT). In both cases, the difference was at or close to two standard deviations below the mean. The study is suggestive, but the authors point out the limitations of sample size, which includes insufficient power to detect small differences and insufficient size to permit any meaningful assessment of heterogeneity. Additionally, the validity of the study is further limited by the fact that it did not use any biopsychological measure.

Gruzelier and Kaiser (1996) examined the relationship between schizotypy and the onset of puberty. They were guided by the hypothesis that schizophrenia is a disorder related to the termination of the cortical pruning process, whereby synaptic connections are progressively eliminated during adolescence. This process, it is supposed, is terminated by the processes of puberty and maturation into adulthood. Schizophrenia, postulated by Saugstad (1994), is a disorder of late maturity and is characterized, therefore, by low synaptic density, because the pruning process has continued longer than normally. Affective disorders, on the other hand, are attributed to unusually early maturation and its concomitant excessive density of synaptic connections. Sex differences in the major psychoses are consistent with this formulation. Men mature later than women and, according to this model, are therefore more likely to develop schizophrenia. Women on the other hand would be more likely than men to develop affective disorders (Lewine, 1981; De Lisi, Dauphinais, & Hauser, 1989).

Gruzelier and Kaiser offered a modified version of this model. They began with the concept of a three-syndrome classification of the clinical states in schizophrenia. These are the Unreality syndrome, which in schizotypy would be associated with unusual perceptions, magical ideation, and in the psychotic state would include delusions and hallucinations early and late. This syndrome, they suggest, is associated with both extremes of maturation. The Withdrawn syndrome in schizotypy includes social and physical anhedonia that could be associated with early puberty, if depressive in character, or with late puberty if schizophrenic withdrawal was the primary feature. The third syndrome, the Active syndrome, shares some features of hypomania seen in bipolar affective disorder, but are also found in one syndrome of schizophrenia (Hoffman et al., 1986).

With this background, Gruzelier and Kaiser selected three groups, each composed of men and women. These were classified as early, normal, or late maturers. Maturation was defined by the age at growth spurt and menarche in females. In males, it was defined by the age at growth spurt, the age of the first nocturnal emission, and the age at shaving. Composite scores show the expected difference between females and males; the former reached maturity approximately three years earlier than the latter. Schizotypy was measured with the Schizotypy Personality Questionnaire (SPQ) or Raine (1991). The results of this investigation showed that there were significant interactions between gender, age at maturation, and the syndromal features of the schizotypal responses made by the participants. They concluded that the age of onset of puberty is one of the significant components of the determinants of schizophrenia but that the Saugstad model does not fit the data. At this point, it will be helpful to present a summary of the processes that are measured with these methods.

## Electroencephalography

The neurons in the brain are constantly firing and can be recorded as electrical potentials from the scalp or directly from the brain. The recording of such electrical potentials via electrodes is called electroencephalography or EEG. EEG, it is thought reflects the summation of large numbers of neurons whose synchronous firing from cortical and/ or subcortical regions is probably controlled by corticothalamic neurogenerators. The frequency of the electrical activity generally varies according to the degree of psychological arousal. Within this model, it is thought that the more active or aroused a given region of the brain, the faster the frequency of the sinusoidal waveforms; the less active a given region of the brain, the slower the frequency. For example, beta (12–28 Hz) is noted during activation and alpha (8–12 Hz) is noted during relaxation. EEG is generally discussed in terms of the power of a given frequency in a particular region of the brain or in terms of abnormal patterns of response.

Event-related brain potentials are a class of EEG characterized by voltage changes that are time-locked to stimulus presentation or to other relevant events. They are composed of components that, it is thought, reflect specific psychological processes. There are two general types of ERPs, either event-preceding or event-following. Event-preceding ERP components, it is thought, reflect brain activity that is produced in anticipation of an event, and event-following ERP components, it is thought, reflect brain activity that is produced as result of stimulus presentation. Embedded within these temporal categories are psychological categories of ERPs: exogenous and endogenous. Exogenous ERPs, it is thought, reflect changes in the stimulus properties of events. Endogenous ERPs, it is thought, reflect the interaction of the subject with the event. ERPs are generally displayed in a voltage × time function. Positive and negative voltage peaks represented in voltage × time functions are usually characterized by differences in polarity, latency, and voltage. For example, the N200 component of the ERP has a negative shift in polarity and a specific voltage that occurs approximately 200 ms after an eliciting event. Before being statistically analyzed, these voltage changes are subjected to mathematical computation, typically averaging, to enhance the signal-to-noise ratio.

It has been suggested that ERP studies can make a unique contribution to the study of schizophrenia (Roth et al., 1988). Relative to positron emission tomography (PET) and function magnetic resonance imaging (fMRI), scalp recorded ERPs have much better temporal resolution and more thoroughly established substantiation of association with specific psychological processes. However,

ERPs have relatively worse spatial resolution. Except for magnetoencephalography (MEG), EEG and ERPs are the only imaging methods that measure neuronal activity directly as opposed to indirect measures of activity of blood flow via PET and fMRI. Nevertheless, because neuroanotomical generators have been proposed—though in most cases not confirmed—for most ERP components, ERPs can be used to localize and categorize abnormalities associated with schizophrenia. For example, if an ERP component distinguishes patients with schizophrenia from controls, impairment in the region generating that ERP component is implied.

## Magnetic Resonance Imaging

Magnetic resonance imaging of the brain (MRI) refers to a group of procedures that employs common hardware, but has somewhat different emphases. It applies the principles of what is known about nuclear magnetic resonance (NMR) to human physiology. Initially, NMR was used to study various properties of nonorganic objects, providing information about the structural and chemical attributes of these objects. The details of the procedure can be found in De Lisi (1991) and in Coffman and Nasrallah (1986). When employed in the study of brain activity while the patient is engaged in some activity such as speaking, recalling, or identifying stimuli, it is referred to as functional MRI or fMRI.

Examples of the use of MRI to study schizophrenia are found in investigations of patients brain volume and brain volume ratios (e.g., Andreasen, Nasrallah, Dunn, Olsen, Grove, Ehrhardt, Coffman, & Crossett, 1986), and of the use of fMRI to study patient brain activity during verbal production (e.g., Yurgelun-Todd, Waternaux, Cohen, Gruber, Camper, English, & Renshaw, 1996).

## Positron Emission Tomography

Positron emission tomography (PET) measures blood flow by tracing the movement of radioactively labeled substances (oxygen or deoxyglucose) through the body. Brain activity uses oxygen, so that loci of increased activity are reflected by greater rates of oxygen metabolism in the region of the activity. The major limitations of this method are that it is invasive (the labeled substances have to be injected into the patient), it requires the nearby availability of the cyclotron to create the labeled substances, it is expensive, and its capacity to detect rapid activity of brief duration is less than that of either EEG or MRI. A simpler method that embodies the same basic principle as PET is single photon emission cerebral tomography (SPECT) which is less expensive, does not require proximity to a cyclotron and, although it gives a cruder image, is adequate to examine activity in various brain regions.

In the ideal study, direct imaging of the brain and neuropsychological measures are combined. Such studies are costly and complex and are typically confined to limited sample sizes. Because of this, it is common to seek associations between neuropsychological tests believed to reflect a specific regional brain function and other behaviors of interest, from gross diagnostic status to performance in specific behavioral tasks. The obvious advantage of this is that neuropsychological tests are easier and much less expensive to administer and that this may compensate somewhat for the question of their validity as measures of the physical aspect of brain structure and function. However, the disadvantage lies in this invalidity because even large validity coefficients between test performance and brain measurements may translate into a significant potential for error.

Raine et al. (1993) provide an example of the first kind of study. The volume of the prefrontal areas of the brain was assessed with MRI in seventeen schizophrenia patients, eighteen nonschizophrenia psychiatric controls, and nineteen normal controls. These groups were also assessed by three neuropsychological measures, the Wisconsin Card Sorting Test (WCST), the Spatial Delayed Response Matching Test (SDRMT), and the Block Design. The results indicated that schizophrenic patients had smaller frontal areas than either of the two control groups. A comparison of differences in the posterior area of the brain revealed no differences among the three groups. Performance on the three neuropsychological tests were partially parallel to the MRI findings. The main difference was that the WCST discriminated schizophrenics from normal controls, but not from other psychiatric patients. The same was true of the SDRMT. Only the Block Design discriminated between schizophrenic and the other two control groups. No correlation was found between the individual MRI measures and the individual neuropsychological measures.

The investigators point to biasing factors such as the composition of the schizophrenic sample (mainly paranoid schizophrenia), but it is clear that there is a limit to the possible validity of neuropsychological tests as measures of frontal lobe size. Findings of this kind are not uncommon and point to the constraints that exist in trying to establish brain–behavior relationships, using only behavioral measures.

Measurement of brain structure and function may involve many derivative measurements. The absolute size of a brain area may be less predictive of some specific behavior than the ratio of this size to the size of the brain as a whole or to some other brain region with which it is connected. This consideration is complicated further by the hemispheric asymmetry of the human brain, a factor that is discussed extensively later in this chapter in relation to anomalies of cerebral lateralization.

In this general connection we note the problems that exist with a priori assumptions about brain functions that are tapped by a specific test. A simple reaction time task, in which the respondent is instructed to press a key when a light appears, requires maintaining attention in the interval before the light appears, sensory efficiency in detecting the light when it does appear, effectively initiating the central motor program that produces the tapping response, and efficient peripheral motor output of the response itself. This seemingly simple task involves several different brain regions, and it is clear that a defect in any one of them or in the connections between them may lead to a defective response. We now turn to research on particular brain regions in relation to schizophrenia.

## Neuropsychological Profiles in Schizophrenia

Studies of neuropsychological functioning in schizophrenia have identified an array of deficits. These include impairment in abstraction, attention, language, verbal learning, and memory, as well as impairment in motor functioning. The relevant studies are contained in a very large and complex literature. Several strategies have been employed to provide a framework for interpretation that would allow us to hypothesize a smaller number of neurological loci for the complex of impairments.

One approach has been to hypothesize a typology of schizophrenia that could be tested against the correlated clusters of symptoms and quantitative measures that are found in the literature. An example is provided by the work of Liddle (1987) and Liddle and Morris (1991). Liddle proposed that symptom measures in schizophrenia can be subsumed under a three-domain model. The three domains are psychomotor poverty (i.e., poverty of speech, decreased spontaneous movements, and blunting of affect), reality distortion (hallucinations and delusions), and disorganization (thought disorder, inappropriate affect, and poverty of content of speech). To each of these three domains, he assigns a putative dysfunction of brain areas. They are psychomotor poverty—the dorsolateral prefrontal cortex; reality distortion—the medial temporal lobe, and most probably the left medial temporal lobe; and disorganization—the mediobasal prefrontal cortex. Attempts to validate this model have been largely unsuccessful (Liddle, 1987; Liddle & Morris, 1991; Norman et al., 1997). However, the data of Norman et al. did support one component of the model, namely, the relationship between reality distortion and verbal memory. This suggests the possibility of temporal lobe involvement and also of frontal lobe involvement. The other two components of the model received no support.

A second approach begins with the fact that the core neuropsychologies in schizophrenia are difficult to disentangle from the effects of medication, age, length of hospitalization, gender, and other secondary adaptations that the patient makes to the limitations imposed by the illness. In the light of this, there is a promising possibility in the study of individuals at risk for schizophrenia, such as family members, as well as individuals in the general population who meet the criteria for schizotypy. These investigations can be collectively gathered under the rubric of the search for markers of schizophrenia discussed in detail later in this chapter.

### General EEG Dysfunction

It has been established that a significant proportion of patients with schizophrenia have abnormal EEG activity. For example, John et al. (1994) reported that the existing literature demonstrates that 10–80% of schizophrenic patients have nonspecific abnormal brain electrical activity; epileptiform activity, including sharp waves and paroxysmal episodes, is found in as many as 25% of patients studied. In addition, it has been established that patients with schizophrenia have abnormalities in the frequency distribution of their

brain activity. For example, such patients have increased beta, delta, theta, and decreased alpha, whether or not they were first episode or chronic patients, suggesting that it is a stable characteristic of the disorder (Sponheim, Clementz, Iacono, & Beiser, 1993).

It is important to note that these abnormalities have not yet been correlated with overt psychotic symptoms. For example, Stevens et al. (1979) observed behavior while schizophrenic patients' EEGs were collected and transmitted by radio for analysis. In this study, about 40% of the patients demonstrated abnormal activity such as slow waves and spikes. This abnormal activity did not, however, coincide with episodes of abnormal behavior such as hallucinations, stereotypy, catatonia, psychomotor blocking, and other clinical manifestations of schizophrenia. At the most general level, we consider the significance of cerebral lateralization.

## Cerebral Lateralization

### Anomalous Lateralization

There has been a long-standing interest in the role of anomalous cerebral lateralization in at least some schizophrenia patients. This interest is consistent with early reports that there is a greater incidence of left-handedness and mixed-handedness as well as left-footedness in the population of schizophrenia patients than in the general population (Boklage, 1977; Chagule & Mater, 1981; Dvirskii, 1976; Gur, 1977; Piran, Bigler, & Cohen, 1982; Shan-Min, Flor-Henry, Dayi, Tiangi, Shuguang, & Zenxiang, 1985). This is so particularly in male schizophrenia patients (Nasrallah, Keelor, Van Schroeder, & McCalley-Whitters, 1981; Taylor, Brown, & Gunn, 1983; Walker & Birch, 1970). These observations are consistent with the general tenor of those findings, but it should noted that they properly refer to some schizophrenia patients. Most schizophrenia patients do not exhibit manifest anomalies of lateralization. For this reason, we shall consider the subset of patients with left- or mixed-lateralization as a subtype of schizophrenia with possible specific demographic and prognostic neuropsychological features.

### The Measurement of Lateralization

The measurement of lateralization (or the degree of lateral dominance) is a complex matter.

Four different kinds of measures have been employed: preference measures, performance measures, measures of brain structure, and measures of brain activity.

**Preference Measures.** The crudest form of measurement is the simple classification of individuals by the hand preferred for writing. More sophisticated versions of the preference criterion employ self-report questionnaires asking the respondent which hand is used for each of several different tasks. (Which hand do you write with? In which hand do you hold a scissors when cutting? Which hand do you use to throw a ball?) Examples include the Annett Scale (Annett, 1970) and the Edinburgh Scale (Oldfield, 1971), amongst others. Chapman and Chapman (1987) reported a correlation of .83 between a self-report scale of this kind and the actual behavior of subjects when performing the tasks to which the self-report items referred. This is a substantial coefficient but suggests that self-report measures should be interpreted with caution. In this and other studies, participants who describe themselves as left-handed are likely to turn out to be more mixed-handed than participants who describe themselves as right-handed.

**Performance Measures.** Any one preference item necessarily divides respondents dichotomously into left or right; in an occasional case, a respondent reports using either hand for a task. In performance measures, the investigator directly measures the effectiveness with which each hand performs a similar task. The measure of lateral dominance is then computed by subtracting the performance score with one hand from the score with the other, and then dividing the result by the sum of the two scores $(L-R)/(L+R)$. This gives the relative difference in performance in percentage terms, corrected for the absolute magnitude of the scores themselves. Examples of measures of this kind include varieties of pegboard tasks, which assess speed and accuracy in placing wooden pegs in sequence in a row of holes, placing dots in printed squares, finger tapping, and accuracy with which straight lines can be drawn with each hand.

Preference and performance measures give a different picture of the distribution of laterality. Preference measures typically produce a J-curve where very few people are mixed-handed and most are highly right-handed or somewhat left-handed (e.g., Borod, Caron, & Koff, 1984; Maher & Manschreck, 1998). Performance measures, in contrast, give a distribution that is approximately Gaussian, but there is a peak around moderate right laterality. All in all, the data from either type of measure suggests that laterality of manual performance is essentially a continuum stretching from one extreme to the other, and the bulk of cases are somewhere in the middle.

The correlation between dominance measured by the Annett preference scale and the dominance ratio calculated from the line drawing test developed by Maher (Blyler, Maher, Manschreck, & Fenton, 1997) was +.48 (Maher & Manschreck, 1998). Although statistically significant, it is clear that the association between the two kinds of measures reflects only modest common variance and that important relationships between laterality and schizophrenic pathology may not be detected as readily with one as the other.

The intercorrelations between various kinds of manual performance measures are not high, and it is clear that factors specific to the kind of task that is used affect the dominance ratios that are obtained (Borod, Caron, & Koff, 1984). Many questions must be raised about the validity of any of these measures as a valid index of cerebral dominance. The situation has been summed up by Bryden, Bulman-Fleming, and MacDonald (1996), "... handedness is a multidimensional skill. It remains uncertain which dimension is most critical and for what ... if the goal is to predict something about the pattern of cerebral organization, then it is more open to question which aspect of handedness is the most appropriate to measure" (p. 66). However, this question is of lesser concern to psychopathologists who seek to delineate the boundaries of clinically and experimentally measured differences in laterality within the population of schizophrenia patients. Once these are established, their relationship to the putative pathology of cerebral organization becomes the ultimate question.

## Manual Laterality and Schizophrenia

### Handedness and Thought Disorder

Some investigators have turned to the task of identifying what differences of functions, if any, that are relevant to the diagnosis of psychopathology exist between left-handed and right-handed schizophrenia patients when assessed clinically and in the laboratory. Language functions are generally chiefly mediated by areas of the left hemisphere, suggesting that disruption of left-hemisphere function is likely to have consequences in disrupting language as well as impairing right-hand functioning. Because of this, attention has been directed to the possible connection between verbal behavior and left-handedness in schizophrenia. Taylor, Brown, and Gunn (1983), Manoach, Maher, and Manschreck (1988), and Manoach (1994) reported significantly greater disturbances of language and thought in left-handed compared to right-handed schizophrenia patients. Handedness in these studies was defined as the hand used in writing.

## Perseveration (Verbal Repetition)

The production of repetitive perseveration in an array of activities has long been one of the common elements in describing schizophrenia. In summing up the literature on this topic, Crider (1997) concluded that perseveration covaries with positive thought disorder and disturbances of voluntary motor activity. In a study of dominance ratios in the line-drawing task and language production, Maher and Manschreck (1998) reported that there were positive correlations between dominance ratio and repetitions of word types ($-.605$), repeated words ($-.46$), and repeated phrases ($-.43$) in left-handed (by preference) schizophrenia patients. No such correlations were found in the sample of right-handed schizophrenia patients.

## Memory

In an investigation of handedness and verbal memory, Manschreck, Maher, Redmond, Miller, and Beaudette (1996) matched left-handed and right-handed patients for performance on immediate recall in a simple verbal memory task (recall of a list of unrelated words). The two groups showed significant differences in their ability to improve their recall performance for word lists increasingly approximating sentence structure. This difference cannot be readily explained as a general impairment in verbal memory because the groups were matched on this variable, but more plausibly as an impairment in using context as an aid to memory organization. This impairment has been noted in samples of schizophrenia patients not differentiated by handedness (e.g., Gerver,

1967; Truscott, 1970; Williams, 1966). An additional analysis of the same data indicated that the poorer recall performance of left-handed patients was significantly correlated with the presence of thought disorder in the left-handed group, but not in the right-handed group.

## Neuropsychological Aspects of Anomalous Lateralization

Underlying the various reports of anomalous lateralization of performance and preference in schizophrenia patients is the assumption that this arises from some neuropathology that disturbs the normal dominance relationship between the two hemispheres. Two broad possibilities exist. One is that there is a group of schizophrenia patients in whom a biological anomaly (possibly but not necessarily of genetic origin) has led to failed development of normal hemispheric asymmetry. The other is that some early exogenous unilateral damage to the brain has occurred. This possibility envisages perinatal injury, infections or toxic insults, and other such factors that play a role in the genesis of disrupted hemispheric dominance.

## Crow's Hypothesis

One of the most prominent hypotheses of a possible developmental anomaly was presented by Crow and his colleagues (Crow, 1990; Crow, 1995; Crow, Colter, Frith, Johnstone, & Owens, 1989; Crow, Done, & Sacker, 1996; De Lisi, Sakuma, Kushner, Finer, Hoff, & Crow, 1997). Their model proposes that there is a developmental anomaly of genetic origin whereby the normal processes of the development of cerebral asymmetry are impaired. The second decade of life is the period during which the neurodevelopmental processes occur that lead to the emergence of normal hemispheric asymmetry. These processes include the synaptic pruning that has been discussed earlier. The developmental process is usually completed by the end of adolescence (Buchsbaum, Mansour, Teng, Zia, Siegel, & Rice, 1992b; Feinberg, 1982). Benes (1989) reported that this timing for the maturation of the brain is especially the case for the frontal and temporal areas. Normal asymmetry most often consists of left hemisphere dominance but can consist of right hemisphere dominance. Crow's model proposes that the hypothesized genetic anomaly leads to a failure to achieve clear dominance by adulthood. At this point, the effects of this failure become manifest in the behavior of the patient, ultimately leading to the diagnosis of schizophrenia. Therefore, such patients would be most likely to have an early onset. Because the failure to achieve dominance involves the failure of left-hemisphere dominance, language disturbance inevitably becomes a major component in the pathology of schizophrenia. Finally, the model suggests that the genetic disorder is sex-linked and males are more at risk.

Postmortem studies of lack of normal asymmetry have been reported by Falkai et al. (1992), and lack of asymmetry in brain activation was reported by Buchsbaum et al. (1982) and Rossi et al. (1992). Maher, Manschreck, Yurgelun-Todd, and Tsuang (1998) report a volumetric MRI study of the brains of a sample of sixteen schizophrenia patients. Substantial lack of asymmetry in the frontal and temporal areas was found in some patients and was also correlated with age of onset. With a frontal volume dominance ratio, the age-corrected correlation with age of onset was .616 ($p = .01$) and with temporal volume .479 ($p = .05$). This finding is clearly consistent with Crow's hypothesis.

We cannot assume a priori that morphological symmetry will necessarily be reflected in performance symmetry. However, lack of normal asymmetry of manual performance at the age of 11 years was associated with the subsequent onset of schizophrenia in a large scale birth-cohort study of 16,980 persons reported by Crow, Done, and Sacker (1996). In this study, no such lack of manual asymmetry was found in individuals who were later diagnosed with affective disorders or with personality disorders.

All in all, it seems reasonable to conclude that the evidence to date pertinent to Crow's hypothesis is predominantly supportive. In saying so, we remind ourselves that many schizophrenic patients in these studies do not show anomalous asymmetry in either preference, performance, or brain structure. This, in turn, echoes our comments at the beginning of this chapter, namely, that schizophrenias are a heterogeneous group of disorders with some common features. Given this, we should not be overly optimistic about the possibility or usefulness of trying to seek a grand, unifying, reductionist model of the biopsychological aspects of this group of disorders.

## Other Measures of Asymmetry in Schizophrenia

The preceding discussion has centered on brain morphology and manual preference and performance as the core area in which asymmetry might be found. Other studies examined the laterality aspects of such performance as visual recognition of verbal and spatial information. Studies of normal performance in recognition in these tasks has indicated that the left hemisphere is involved in processing verbal information and the right hemisphere in processing spatial information. Studies of left-hemisphere advantage in schizophrenia patients produced inconsistent findings (Gur, 1978; Colbourn, & Lishman, 1979; Pic'l, Magaro, & Wade, 1979; Connolly, Gruzelier, Kleinman, & Hirsch, 1979; Magaro & Chamrad, 1983; George & Neufeld, 1987; Merriam & Gardner, 1987). The general tenor of these findings indicates a deficient left-hemisphere advantage which is consistent with findings of diminished left temporal lobe size. These findings are discussed later under the section dealing with the general topic of temporal lobe anomalies. However, there are inconsistencies in the findings of these studies that are related to variations in the subtype of schizophrenia involved, sample differences in gender, and differences in the kinds of tasks employed. In one recent study, Bruder et al. (1995) reported that a sample of thirty-two schizophrenia patients displayed a smaller right-ear (left-hemisphere) advantage in a dichotic listening task, compared to depressed patients. The smaller advantage was unchanged by the presence or absence of neuroleptic administration and did not depend on gender. This study did look at heterogeneity within the schizophrenic sample and reported significant negative correlations with right-ear advantage and the negative symptom of stereotyped thinking and with the positive symptom of hallucinations. This latter finding is consistent with the findings of Barta et al. (1990) discussed later, in which the same result was obtained when correlating severity of hallucinations with the volume of the left temporal gyrus. Performance measures that offer more consistent findings were reported for right-hemisphere processing of spatial information. Gur (1978), Connolly et al. (1979), George and Neufeld (1987), and Ellis, de Pauw, Christodoulou, Papgeorgiou, Milne, and Joseph (1993) all found that the right hemisphere advantage was preserved in schizophrenia patients in processing spatial visual information.

In a recent study, White, Maher, and Manschreck (1998) reported that the expected right hemisphere advantage in a facial recognition task was not present in schizophrenia patients. However, when the patients were differentiated on the basis of the presence of perceptual aberration, there was a strong negative correlation ($-0.685$) between the perceptual aberration score and a reversal of the normal right-hemisphere advantage. Patients with perceptual aberration showed a left-hemisphere advantage in facial recognition. Patients without perceptual aberration and normal controls showed the expected right-hemisphere advantage. This study underlines once again the importance of seeking the axes of possible heterogeneity in schizophrenic samples.

We turn now to consider general regions of the brain. The division by regions is adopted for convenience in discussion. In dividing our discussion in this way, we remind ourselves that the regions in question are connected reciprocally in many ways. Individual research reports frequently examine multiple regions and report on the interactions between them. Therefore, our decision to cite them under one of the following headings is based on the relative emphasis given to the area by researchers. It is hoped that this organization will have practical usefulness for the reader without distorting the real complexity of the brain structures involved.

# The Investigation of Regions of Interest in the Brain

## The Prefrontal Cortex

The prefrontal cortex is a collection of areas that lies immediately in front of the premotor cortex of the frontal lobe. Its function has been variously described but can be summed up as the one area of the brain that receives information about the external environment and mediates the exchange of this information with neural connections from the internal structures of the brain. It is clear that this makes the question of neuropathology in the prefrontal cortex particularly critical for maintaining organized adaptive behavior in the human being. This crucial role of frontal processes is sometimes summed up by referring to it as the seat of the "executive functions" in the brain.

There is a plethora of evidence that implicates the frontal lobes in the pathology of schizophrenia. Particular attention has been paid to the prefrontal cortex (PFC) and especially to the dorsolateral component of that area (e.g., Berman, Zec, & Weinberger, 1986; Bogerts, 1993; Buchsbaum et al., 1992; Liddle et al., 1992). Adults who suffer lesions in the PFC exhibit some of the characteristics that appear in some schizophrenics, notably the so-called negative symptoms.

Frontal abnormalities in cerebral metabolism were reported by Buchsbaum et al. (1982) and Farkas et al. (1980). Other studies reported abnormalities in regional cerebral blood flow (Berman et al., 1986; Franzen & Ingvar, 1975a,b; Weinberger et al., 1986). Investigators employing neuropsychological tests reported a broad spectrum of findings of anomalous performance. An extensive review is in Goldberg and Seidman (1991).

Many investigators suggested that frontal dysfunction plays a part in memory defect in schizophrenia. A review of these studies was provided by Goldman-Rakic (1991). In a more recent MRI study, Maher, Manschreck, Woods, Yurgelun-Todd, and Tsuang (1995) examined the effect of the ratio of frontal brain volume to that of the brain as a whole in eighteen schizophrenic patients in a memory task that included context-aided and non-context-aided word lists. Absolute frontal volume was not correlated with performance in either kind of task, but relative volume was strongly correlated with context-aided memory ($r = .637, p < .01$). It was not correlated with non-context-aided verbal recall. Correlations with other brain regions produced no significant associations. The significant correlation was attributable mainly to the relative size of the dorsolateral area; the correlations with dorsomedial and orbital areas were negligible. This study points to the importance of examining brain ratios in both structure and function (as is the case in the studies of laterality already described) and the importance of focusing on correlations within samples of schizophrenic patients, rather than focusing exclusively on mean differences between comparison groups.

## Frontal and Prefrontal Dysfunction and ERPs

Three ERP components may be generated in the frontal or prefrontal regions: postimperative negative variation (PINV, e.g., Klein, Rockstroh, Cohen, & Berg, 1996), contingent negative variation (CNV, e.g., Rosahl & Knight, 1995), and P3a (Knight, 1990). CNV, it is thought, is made up of an early (O-wave) component that reflects sensory processing and orienting and a late (E-wave) component that reflects expectancy or motor preparation (Loveless & Sanford, 1974). The psychological interpretation of PINV is less clear, though it is probably related to performance and action uncertainty, as well as control and contingency expectation (Klein, Rockstroh, Cohen, Berg, & Dressel, 1996). P3a, it is thought, is related to novelty stimulus processing (Squires, Squires, & Hillyard, 1975) and has not been studied frequently in schizophrenia. As a guide to the reader, the major ERP components and their functions are presented in Table 1.

CNV and PINV have been studied frequently in patients with schizophrenia and have revealed a relatively consistent pattern of frontal CNV decrements, PINV enhancements, and posterior CNV and PINV normality (for a review, see Pritchard, 1986; for inconsistent results, see Strandburg et al., 1994; van den Bosch, 1983). Patients with schizophrenia have shown unusual CNV and PINV topographical distribution over the frontocentral vertex (Eikmeier & Lodermann, 1994) that suggests inefficient information processing where inadequate frontal functioning commands excessive frontal (relative to central) cortical activation (van den Bosch et al., 1988).

PINV enhancement and CNV decrements are associated with an increase in psychotic symptoms such as emotional withdrawal, incongruous affect, hallucinations, ideas of reference, and a decrease in affective symptoms such as depressed mood, anxious depression, and guilt (for a review, see Pritchard, 1986; Chouinard, Annable, & Dongier, 1977; Eikmeier & Lodermann, 1994; Bachneff & Engelsmann, 1980; Dongier, Dubrovsky, & Englesmann, 1977).

Frontal ERPs are uniquely associated with hallucinations. For example, up to 95% of hallucinating patients with schizophrenia have an enhanced PINV (Dongier, Dubrovsky, & Englesmann, 1977). Additionally, Turetsky, Colbath, and Gur (1998) found that changes in frontal P300 over time were highly inversely related to the severity of auditory hallucinations.

The role of the frontal lobe in negative symptoms is captured by the fact that the difference in amplitude between Fz and Cz for the PINV and CNV is related to anergia, Scale for the Assessment of Negative Symptoms (SANS) total and SANS affective flattening, alogia, and anhedonia, but this difference is negatively related to symptoms of depression, hopelessness, and asociallity (Eikmeier & Lodemann, 1994; van den Bosch et al., 1988). However, it is important to note that some researchers have found no correlation of negative symptoms with PINV (Eikmeier et al., 1992).

There are some hints in the literature that frontal lobes might be modulating ERP attentional decrements typically seen in patients with schizophrenia, even though the components themselves are probably not generated in the frontal lobes. P200 amplitudes, for example, are reduced over frontal brain regions during performance of the SPAN task (Sponheim & Kodalen, 1998). PNs are reduced particularly at the frontal leads (Ward, Catts, Fox, Michie, & McConaghy, 1991), and bilateral N100 amplitudes are reduced at frontocentral sites (Tenke, Bruder, Towey, Leite, Malaspina, Gorman, & Kaufmann, 1992). The amplitude of these components, P200, N100, and Processing Negativity (PN), it is thought, reflect early stimulus processing and selective attention, and they are probably generated, at least in part, by auditory stimuli in the auditory cortex. As discussed in detail later, the frontal lobe probably plays at least a modulatory role in generating PN (Knight, Hillyard, Woods, & Neville, 1981) and P200 (Picton, Hillyard, Krausz, & Galanbos, 1974; Shenton et al., 1989) that may account for group differences found in the frontal lobes.

In summary, frontal dysfunction in schizophrenia is suggested by reduced early CNV amplitude and enhanced PINV amplitude. These differences are evidence of frontal lobe dysfunction in patients with schizophrenia for two reasons: (1) the greatest differences between controls and patients with schizophrenia tend to be in the frontal region and (2) PINV and CNV are likely to be generated over broad frontocentral regions. Additionally, PINV and CNV abnormalities have been related to hallucinations, negative symptoms, and possibly attentional problems. The conclusion that negative symptoms are related to frontal lobe ERP activity agrees with a recent comprehensive study by Gerez and Tello (1995) that concluded that electrocortical variables associated with frontostriatal abnormalities are most related to negative symptoms. Having affective symptoms provides

### Table 1. The Major ERP Components and Their Functions[a]

| Component | Proposed cortical generator | Psychological or mental operation |
|---|---|---|
| Lateralized readiness potential (LRP) Motor potential (MP) Readiness potential | Motor cortex | Motor preparation |
| Contingent negative variation (CNV) Early "O-wave" Late "E-wave" | Cerebral cortex (when excitatory signal from thalamus depolarized neurons over extensive frontal regions) | O wave = orienting, sensory processing E wave = expectancy or readiness or motor prep. |
| Postimperative negative variation (PINV) | Frontocentral cortical structures | Prolongation of CNV State marker for general psychopathology Performance and action uncertainty Sensory perception, attention, time estimation and processing of control and contingency expectation |
| Brain stem (ABR or BAER) | I Distal eighth nerve II Proximal eighth nerve III Cochlear nucleus-trapezoid body IV Superior olivary complex V Lateral lemniscus termination in inferior colliculus VI & VII thalamus (medial geniculate body) to auditory cortex or inferior colliculus | Sensory processing of auditory stimulation |
| P50 | Left and right planum temporale or hippocampus | Sensory gating |
| N100 | Primary auditory cortex in temporal lobe | Selective attention (early selective processing and early stimulus encoding) |
| P200 | Inferior parietal gyrus, auditory temporal cortex, temporoparietal junction | Selective attention, stimulus encoding |
| N200a and MMN | MMN-superior temporal plane— specifically the superior temporal gyrus | MMN-mismatch detector N2a: automatic mismatch detector |
| N2b (auditory) N2b (visual) | Auditory cortex Prestriate cortex of occipital lobe | Deviant stimulus classification (controlled processing) |
| P3a | Frontal lobes, prefrontal cortex, amygdala | Mismatch detector Attention switch Orienting |
| P3b | Hippocampus, temporoparietal junction | Context updating, encoding |
| N400 | Temporal lobes and surrounding areas | Semantic congruity and expectancy |

[a]It is important to note that although these generators have been proposed, most are not universally accepted. Rather, the purpose of this table is to provide a reference for the current state of knowlege, and it should be interpreted with caution.

some protection from these types of frontal abnormalities, presumably due to subtyping differences in patients with affective symptoms. The frontal CNV dysfunction provides convergent evidence of a link between the frontal lobe and orienting deficits. Although the exact psychological significance of PINV is unknown, it may be related to sensory perception, attention, control and contingency expectation, all of which, as has been previously shown, are deficient in patients with schizophrenia and are related to frontal lobe functioning.

At this point, it is clear that the frontal areas of the brain are reliably implicated in the group of disorders that constitute schizophrenia. However, although variations in the Coffman structural features already described (relative frontal volume and lack of frontal hemispheric asymmetry) play a part in the pathology of schizophrenia, we have no clear hypotheses about the heterogeneity that underlies these variations.

## The Temporal Lobe

Disturbances of language and (by inference, from language) thought provide the core of the clinical phenomena that lead to the diagnosis of schizophrenia. The temporal lobe has a central place in organizing language functions in the brain, and it is here that many biopsychologists have turned in their search for the pathology. Changes in the size of temporal lobe structures are closely connected to changes in the size of the ventricles of the brain. Relative ventricular size is computed by the ratio of ventricle size to whole brain size, the ventricle/brain ratio (VBR).

Results of several MRI studies may be summarized by saying that the left temporal lobe of schizophrenia patients, as has often been shown, is smaller than the right temporal lobe (e.g., Coffman et al., 1989; Crow, 1990; Rossi et al., 1990a,b) and that a parallel enlargement of the size of the left ventricle has sometimes been observed. The question to which this gives rise is whether the enlargement of the ventricle is a by-product of the reduction of adjacent cortical structure (or vice versa) or whether both processes have autonomous pathological origins. However, some studies have found the opposite effect, that is, enlargement of the right temporal cortex, and it appears that different effects may be related to differences in the handedness of the patients. An interesting finding by Barta et al. (1990) is that the volume of the left

superior temporal gyrus was inversely related to the severity of hallucinations. This is consistent with the report of Grove and Andreasen (1991) that patients with enlarged VBRs tended to produce negative symptoms, such as catatonia, and patients with small VBRs produced positive symptoms, such as hallucinations and delusions.

With this exception, neuroimaging studies of temporal lobe and ventricular anomalies in schizophrenia have paid little attention to heterogeneity within schizophrenic samples and have been content to measure gross volume or activity levels in comparison with control samples. At this point, it is reasonable to be confident that with more attention to heterogeneity, we will be better able to understand the significance of these biopsychological findings.

## Temporal Dysfunction and ERPs

There has been a flurry of activity examining temporal lobe functioning via event-related brain potential techniques. Components (i.e., P50, N100, P200, N200, and P3b) that are likely to be generated in or near the temporal region have consistently demonstrated reductions in amplitudes of patients with schizophrenia relative to controls. This reduction is not related to general functioning but rather to more specific symptoms of schizophrenia, particularly thought disorder.

**P50.** The ratio of P50 amplitudes in a conditioning testing paradigm is said to be enhanced in patients with schizophrenia (Adler, Pachtman, et al., 1982). This paradigm involves presenting two brief auditory stimuli in pairs (usually 50 ms apart) with long interpair intervals. P50 is reportedly generated in the hippocampus, superior temporal gyrus (STG) (Freedman et al., 1991), or planum temporale (Reite, Teale, Neumann, & Davis, 1987). Although P50 is usually reported in terms of conditioning/testing ratios, both S1 and S2 are reduced in patients with schizophrenia (e.g., Adler, Hoffer Griffith, Waldo, & Freedman, 1992). Recent work (Zouridakus, Boutrous, & Jansen, 1997) has demonstrated that there is a decrease of P50 elicited by S1 in patients with schizophrenia and no further decrease is elicited by S2. The difference in amplitude between the groups is related to the fact that the P50 elicited by S1 is highly synchronized in controls but not in patients. The reduction in P50 elicited by S2 in both patients with schizophrenia and controls results from desynchronization of latency. However, patients with schizophrenia may also have higher S1 P50 trial to trial latency variability, whereas the P50 at S2 shows the same increased variability as controls (Jin, Potkin, Patterson, Sandman, Hetrick, & Bunney, 1997). Consequently, single trial averages eliminated P50 amplitude differences between the groups. Others (Clementz, Geyer, & Braff, 1998), however, disagree with this analysis and believe that the P50 reduction is not due to wave shape or the number of usable trials, rather that the reduction is related to poor suppression.

The P50 reduction in response to the first stimulus is possibly related to stress (Johnson & Adler, 1993; White, Yee, Neuchterlein, & Wirshing, 1997), interference (Jim & Potkin, 1996), and attention deficits (Cullum et al., 1993). This effect is not specific to patients with schizophrenia because approximately 50% of a general psychiatric population has this deficit (Baker et al., 1987). The deficit is not related to global measures of psychopathology (BPRS) or negative symptoms but has been linked to specific symptoms such as anxiety, depression and anergia (Adler et al., 1990; Baker et al., 1990; Yee et al., 1998). The fact that paranoid patients are less likely to show the effect (Boutrous et al., 1992; White, Yee, Neuchterlein, & Wirshing, 1997) suggests that it may be different for subtypes of the disorder.

The P50 ratio is temporarily normalized by nicotine (Adler et al., 1992), clozapine when administered to clozapine responders (Nagamoto, Adler, Waldo, Griffith, & Freedman, 1991), and slow-wave sleep (Griffith & Freedman, 1993), but not REM sleep (Griffith et al., 1995). In contrast, yohimbine causes significant transient decreases in auditory gating in normal controls (Adler, Hoffer, Nagamoto, Waldo, Kisley, & Griffith, 1994). Even though P50 is generated in both the left and right planum temporale (or possibly hippocampus), patients with schizophrenia once again showed an abnormal asymmetric pattern of response. Source localization by MEG suggests that the left-hemisphere source accounts for the difference between the two groups (Reite, Teale, Zimmerman, Davis, Whalen, & Edrich, 1988).

In summary, P50, which may be generated in the temporal lobes, is reduced in schizophrenia. The S1 reduction is likely to be due to the fact that patients with schizophrenia have a more variable P50 response latency. The difference between controls and depressives seems specific to left temporal lobes. The reduction is not related to global measures of psychopathology; rather the reduction is more likely to be related to specific symptoms.

**P300.** P300 is probably the most frequently studied ERP component, and its amplitude, it is almost universally agreed, is reduced in schizophrenia (Souza et al., 1995). P300 is often subdivided into frontal P3a and parietal P3b. Most studies of schizophrenia have studied the classic P3b which is related to expectancy, attention, probability, and stimulus meaning (Duncan-Johnson & Donchin, 1977; Johnson, 1988) and probably reflects encoding or updating of working memory (Fabiani, Gratton, Karis, & Donchin, 1987). There is evidence that P3b (referred to as P300 in the rest of the chapter) may be generated, at least in part, at the temporoparietal junction (Knight, Scabini, Woods, & Clayworth, 1989) or in the inferior parietal lobe (Smith et al., 1990).

The P300 reduction seen in patients with schizophrenia is due to the fact that patients with schizophrenia have fewer, smaller, and more variable latency P300s (Ford, White, Lim, & Pfefferbaum, 1994b; Roschke, Wagner, et al., 1996). And, although P300 amplitude is quite sensitive to schizophrenic psychopathology (e.g., Barrett, McCallum, & Pocock, 1986; Levit, Sutton, & Zubin, 1973), it has failed to be a specific marker for schizophrenia (Ford, Pfefferbaum, & Roth, 1992). For example, no differences have been found between patients with schizophrenia and borderline personality disorder (Kutcher, Blackwood, St. Clair, Gaskell, & Muir, 1987), substance dependence (Brecher, Porjesz, & Begleiter, 1987), major depression (Pfefferbaum, Wenegrat, Ford, Roth, & Kopell, 1984), and bipolar depression (Muir, St. Clair, & Blackwood, 1991; Souza et al., 1995).

Although patients with schizophrenia who have the smallest P300 amplitudes have earlier hospitalizations (Roth & Cannon, 1972), worse social functioning (Strik, Dierks, Kulke, Maurer, & Fallgatter, 1993), poorer premorbid adjustment, pronounced residual symptoms, low relapse, and male predominance (Hergerl, Juckel, Muller-Schubert, Pietzcker, & Gaebel, 1995), P300 amplitude is more likely to be related to specific, rather than general symptoms of schizophrenia. For example, total Brief Psychiatric Rating Scale (BPRS) (Louza & Maurer, 1989; Souza et al., 1995) and the Present State Examination (PSE) (Barrett et al., 1986) and Mini-Mental Status (Louza & Maurer,

1989) fail to be consistently related to P300 amplitude and latency. However, when a relationship is found, P300 amplitude is negatively related to BPRS score (e.g., Strik et al., 1993; Roth et al., 1980).

P300 is related to formal thought disorder that is both active (e.g., Roth, Pfefferbaum, Kelly, Berger, & Kopell, 1981; McConaghy, Catts, Michie, Fox, Ward, & Shelley, 1993; Shenton et al., 1989; O'Donnell et al., 1993—at T3 and Cz), and residual (Juckel, Muller-Schubert, Gaebel, & Hegerl, 1996). However, P300 and Slow Wave (SW) amplitudes are unrelated to delusions and hallucinations (Roth et al., 1980, 1981). Negative symptoms are associated with decreased P300 amplitude (Pfefferbaum, Ford, White, & Roth, 1989; Strik, Deierks, & Maurer, 1993a; Merrin & Floyd, 1994; Eikmeier et al., 1992; Kemali, Galderisi, May, Cesarelli, & DíAmbra, 1988), or unrelated to P300 amplitude (e.g., Ward et al., 1991; Shenton et al., 1989; Blackwood et al., 1991; Brecher & Begleiter, 1983).

The relationship between positive symptoms and P300 is also inconclusive. For example, McCarley's group reported both positive and negative correlations of P300 with positive symptoms in T3 (Shenton et al., 1989; O'Donnell et al., 1993), Brecher and Begleiter (1983) found no relationship, and Egan et al. (1994) found a negative relationship for auditory (but not visual) P300.

Many experimental factors affect whether the P300 amplitude differences appear. Some studies have suggested that P300 is only consistently reduced in the auditory modality and only when low probability stimuli are presented (Duncan, Perlstein, & Morihisa, 1987). Stimulus discriminability plays a role in the P300 amplitude reduction noted in schizophrenia because discriminability is related to enhanced P300 amplitude and decreased latency in controls, but only decreased latency in patients with schizophrenia (Salisbury et al., 1994a). However, even under conditions of enhanced motivation ($1 per correct categorization), P300 is reduced in patients with schizophrenia (Brecher & Begleiter, 1983). Many studies have shown that medication status is not related to P300 amplitudes, whereas others have shown that P300 amplitude to visual stimuli, though not auditory P300, is related ($r = -.88$) to the amount of improvement in neuroleptic medications (Duncan, Morihisa, Fawcett, & Kirch, 1987).

P300 latency, it is thought, reflects stimulus evaluation time (Duncan-Johnson, 1981) and is also probably increased in patients with schizophrenia (e.g., Blackwood et al., 1987; Pfefferbaum et al., 1984), even though it has also failed to distinguish patients with schizophrenia from other groups (Pfefferbaum et al., 1984). P300 latency enhancement in patients with schizophrenia probably reflects slow categorization and decision making (Pfefferbaum et al., 1989). P300 latency has been positively correlated with general functioning, as measured by the BPRS (Blackwood et al., 1987), specific symptoms (e.g., attention; Eikmeier, Loderman, Zerbin, & Gastpar, 1992), and withdrawal (Blackwood et al., 1987).

Some researchers suggested that P300 reduction is particularly sensitive to left temporal lobe dysfunction associated with the illness (e.g., Egan et al., 1994; Morstyn, Duffy, & McCarley, 1982; Salisbury et al., 1994; Heidrich & Strik, 1997; Roemer & Shagass, 1992; Strik, Dierks, Franzek, Sober, & Maurer, 1994). This temporal lobe dysfunction occurs with medicated patients (Ford et al., 1994a; Pfefferbaum et al., 1989) as well as unmedicated patients (Faux et al., 1993). This effect, which appears at the onset of the disorder, is specific to patients with schizophrenia because patients with affective psychosis did not show this reduction (Salisbury et al., 1998).

However, this effect is not universally found (e.g., Pfefferbaum et al., 1989; Kawasaki et al., 1997; Connolly, Manchanda, Gruzlier, & Hirsch, 1985). Proponents of this theory believe that left temporal P300 abnormalities reflect specific left superior temporal gyrus (STG) abnormalities. Indeed, impressive inverse correlations have been found between left temporal lobe structures and left P300 (Egan, Duncan, Suddath, Kirch, Mirsky, & Wyatt (1994) in the auditory but not visual modality (McCarley et al., 1989). The volume of the left STG, in turn, is highly correlated ($r = .81$) with thought disorder (Shenton et al., 1992). T3 is correlated with left sylvian fissure size, both of which are correlated with positive symptoms (CT left sylvian fissure correlates with SAPs .70, delusions, .76, and FTD, .72).

In summary, P300 amplitude, which may have a generator at the temporal-parietal junction, is generally reduced in schizophrenia. This reduction is due to the fact that patients with schizophrenia have fewer, smaller, and more variable P300s. Left temporal P300 is related to specific symptoms such as formal thought disorder but not to hallucinations. The fact that left temporal lobe P300 is particularly sensitive to thought disorder is intuitively appealing, given the proximity of the left temporal lobes to language centers. This effect is particularly robust in response to auditory stimuli and is affected by stimulus discriminability and possibly by medication status (medication enhances P300 under some conditions). P300 amplitude reduction is not related to decreases in motivation. This P300 effect is largest over the left temporal regions perhaps reflecting specific left temporal lobe dysfunction. P300 latency is probably increased in schizophrenia and has occasionally been associated with general functioning, as well as with specific symptoms such as withdrawal.

**N100.** Although not studied as frequently as P300 in clinical samples, N100, generated in the primary auditory cortex in selective attention paradigms (Woldorff, Gallen, Hampson, Hillyard, Pantev, Sobel, & Bloom, 1993), is also reduced in schizophrenia, even though patients with schizophrenia show normal selective attention effects, that is, larger N100 to attended than unattended stimuli at fast but not slow rates of stimulation (Baribeau-Braun, Picton, & Gosselin, 1983). This is the case whether or not subjects are attending to stimuli (O'Donnell et al., 1994; Roth et al., 1981). N100 has not been specifically related to symptoms of psychosis. For example, PSE was unrelated to N1 amplitude except for affective blunting (Barrett et al., 1986).

The selective attention literature about patients with schizophrenia suggests that hemispheric asymmetries may underlie the N100 differences (Hiramatsu, Kameyama, Saitoh, & Niwa, 1984). ERP (and MEG) topographic differences for N100 (and the MEG equivalent, M100) suggest that the dysfunction resides primarily in the left temporal region (Buchsbaum et al., 1982).

**N200.** Auditory N200 is a class of ERP components that are also generally reduced in schizophrenia (e.g., Shelley et al., 1991; Javitt, Doneshka, Zulberman, Ritter, & Vaughn, 1993; Ogura et al., 1991; Salisbury, O'Donnell, McCarley, Shenton, & Benavage, 1994a,b; O'Donnell et al., 1993). This effect occurs using both deviant and non-deviant targets (Pfefferbaum et al., 1984), though this finding is also not universal (Barrett, McCallum, & Pocock, 1986; Roth, Horvath, Pfefferbaum, Berger, & Kopell, 1980).

N200 is a complex component that has been subdivided into three components; each has distinct but related psychological processes associated with it. Specifically, N200 has been related to (1) automatic mismatch detecting, (2) attentionally mediated mismatch detecting, and (3) classification of stimuli that have been associated with the processing of targets (for a review, see Pritchard, Shappell, & Brandt, 1991). The N2 amplitude is correlated with neuroanatomical abnormalities as well, such as reduced neocortical and medial temporal lobe volumes in schizophrenia (O'Donnell et al., 1993; Egan et al., 1994). Symptomatically, subcomponents of N200 over the left and right temporal lobes are correlated with thought disorder and chronicity (O'Donnell et al., 1993) but not affect/volition (Staffansson & Jonsdottir, 1996).

N200 latency differences have been inconsistently found in patients with schizophrenia (Ogura et al., 1991; Salisbury et al., 1994). This difference has been interpreted as suggesting slower classification process or response selection response. The difference between studies may have been due to the fact that there is a large inconsistency in the latency window corresponding to N200 (Anderson et al., 1995). N200 latency, nevertheless, has been associated with negative symptoms (Stefansson & Jonsdottir, 1996).

In general, the N200 literature also suggests greater dysfunction of left than right temporal lobes. The N200 amplitude difference between controls and patients was greater over the left than right temporoparietal sites. This effect was associated with a right ear advantage for perceiving dichotic syllables. Patients with schizophrenia did not show the behavioral or physiological asymmetry suggestive of left temporal lobe dysfunction (Bruder et al., manuscript submitted for publication).

**P200.** Roth and Cannon (1972) were the first to note reduced P200 amplitudes in patients with schizophrenia. Auditory P200 is probably an index of early stimulus processing (Polich, 1993), selective attention, and stimulus encoding (Shenton et al., 1989). The major source of P200 is in the auditory temporal cortex (for a review, see McCarley, Faux, Shenton, Nestor, & Adams, 1991). Some researchers, however, have suggested frontal generation (Picton et al., 1974)—or at least frontal modulation—of the component (Shenton et al., 1989).

P200 amplitude reduction in schizophrenia is probably related to task requirements because

P200 amplitude and latency increased with task requirements in controls but not in patients with schizophrenia (O'Donnell et al., 1994). The P200 deficit is most robust for the left temporal lobe in the presence of nontarget stimuli. Nontarget stimuli presented to the left hemisphere tended to produce a smaller T3 P200 in patients with schizophrenia than in controls, whereas there was no difference in T4 P200 to nontarget stimuli. When nontargets were presented to the right ear, mean amplitudes of T3 and T4 P200s were smaller in patients with schizophrenia than in normals. Patients with schizophrenia had smaller T3 P200 than T4 P200 regardless of the side to which they were attending (Hiramatsu et al., 1984).

The negative symptoms of avolition and anhedonia are significantly related to P200 amplitude at left and right temporal and central sites. Affect was also significantly related to P200 in each of those same regions, except for T4 (Shenton et al., 1989). The relationship of P200 to negative symptoms is unanticipated given the general lack of association between putative temporoparietal regionally generated components. The relationship between ERPs and negative symptoms is more typical of frontally generated ERPs and is consistent with the notion that (1) P200 is generated by broad areas of the frontal lobe (Picton et al., 1974) or (2) the frontal lobe's modulation of P200 is responsible for the relationship between P200 and negative symptoms.

### Right Temporal Dysfunction

Although less frequently found when viewed across studies and components, right-hemisphere differences appear between schizophrenics and controls in both ERPs components and EEG at temporal sites (Shenton et al., 1992) and are related to emotional processes. EEG asymmetry of left/right-hemispheric ratio scores in patients with schizophrenia was associated with BPRS items of anxiety, hypochondriasis, sadness, and depression (Matousek, Capone, & Okawa, 1981). This right-hemisphere association with emotionality has also been supported by imaging studies where right sylvian fissure size correlated with SANS subscales: alogia .67, avolition-apathy .63 (Shenton et al., 1992). Additionally, ERP studies (Shenton et al., 1989) have found that avolition and anhedonia were significantly related to P200 amplitude C4 and T4. Other dysfunctions associated with right-

hemisphere component amplitude includes hallucinations, thought disorder, and chronicity with N200 (O'Donnell et al., 1993). Finally, paranoia has been associated with right-hemisphere Nd amplitude (Oades, Zerbin, & Eggers, 1994) and EEG hypoactivation (Gruzelier, 1984).

**N400.** N400 is an ERP component that is also generated in the temporal lobes and surrounding area (for a review, see Olichney, Iragui, Kutas, Nowacki, & Jeste, 1997). N400 amplitude is related to the processing of semantic incongruity; the more semantically incongruent a sentence ending, the larger the N400 (Kutas & Hillyard, 1980). N400 is an exception to consistent findings of temporal ERP component reductions in schizophrenia. When found, the N400 reduction might be related to asymmetrical dysfunction because greater differences between controls and patients with schizophrenia have been shown over the right lateral leads. For example, Olichney, Iragui, Kutas, Nowacki, and Jeste (1997) found a greater difference between patients with schizophrenia and controls in the right-hemisphere N400. Grillon, Ameli, and Glazer (1991) studied word pairs. Although they found no N400 amplitude differences at left lateral leads, they did report differences at the right lateral leads.

In general, however, N400 results have been inconsistent. Under some conditions, N400 amplitudes are reduced (Adams et al., 1993), equal (Mitchell et al., 1991; Olichney et al., 1997) or enhanced (Andrews et al., 1993; Nestor et al., 1997; Niznikiewicz et al., 1997) relative to controls. These differences emphasize the need to look at clinical symptoms because reduced N400 amplitudes may be related to the severity of negative symptoms, as for example, the correlation of .58 reported by Olichney et al. (1997).

More consistently, N400 latency was reduced in all but one of the studies that reported it (Nestor et al., 1997; Niznikiewicz et al., 1997; Koyama et al., 1991; Grillon et al., 1991; Olichney et al., 1997; Andrews et al., 1993). The exception is Strandburg et al. (1997).

### General Temporal Lobe Summary

The vast majority of studies that examined ERP components generated by a brain system that includes temporal lobe structures show a reduction in amplitude in patients with schizophrenia. Psychologically, the components that are reduced play a role in attention. Left temporal dysfunction may be especially related to thought disorder in schizophrenia. Right temporal lobe dysfunction may be related to the emotional aspects of the disorder. When found, latency reductions in these components are related to negative symptoms of the disorder. It is speculative, but not unreasonable, to assume that schizophrenic temporal lobe ERP reductions recorded at the scalp reflect neuronal pathology such as a general bilateral reduction in temporal volume (for a meta-analytic review of hippocampal volume reductions, see Nelson, Saykin, Flashman, & Riordan, 1998) or less elaborate connections than normal in the hippocampus (for a review, see Weinberger, 1999).

Interestingly, a comprehensive study of ERP components confirmed the specific sensitivity of temporally mediated components in classifying patients according to subtypes and DSM-III-R diagnoses. Boutros et al. (1997) tested five groups of subjects: paranoid schizophrenics (28), disorganized/undifferentiated (22) schizophrenic, schizoaffective (19), bipolar (16) and normal controls (40). Using a standard oddball task, they monitored amplitudes and latencies of P50, N100, P200, and P300. Disorganized subjects could be significantly distinguished from the other groups using N100, P200, and P300 which all may be temporally generated. P200 significantly distinguished all schizophrenic and schizoaffective patients from normal controls. Finally, P300 could differentiate both schizophrenic groups from controls. However, overall, controls had as high a level of misdiagnosis as patients, though the patients with schizophrenia were not often classified as controls.

### Brain Stem and Middle-Latency Components

Brain stem evoked potentials, it is thought, reflect initial sensory processing of auditory stimuli that occur in the brain stem. Brain stem functioning is relatively intact in patients with schizophrenia because there were no reported differences between patients with schizophrenia and controls in brain stem evoked potential amplitudes (Pfefferbaum, Horvath, Roth, Tinklenberg, & Kopell, 1980; Brecher & Begleiter, 1985). They also failed to distinguish between patients with schizophrenia and alcoholics and controls (Sommer, 1985).

However, the latencies of wave III and N3 (not wave V or N15) are different. Harell, Englender, Demer, Kimhi, and Zohar (1986) found N3 latency enhancements but no wave V differences. Kimhi, Englender, Zohar, and Harell (1987) found both wave 3 and wave-V differences. Additionally, they found that the N3–N5 and N1–N5 latency increased in patients with schizophrenia. Grillon, Ameli, and Glazer (1990) also found an increase in wave III-I latency in patients with schizophrenia. N15 latency, which is probably related to hippocampal activity, is normal in patients with schizophrenia (Coger & Serafetinides, 1993). The latency effects are probably modified by clinical status because Szelenberger (1983) found a relationship between the psychoticism score and interpeak conduction time of I–II for patients with schizophrenia and controls, but no group differences.

### Motor Cortex

Reduced readiness and motor potential in schizophrenia were reported (e.g., Chiarenza, Papakostopoulos, Dini, & Cazzullo, 1985; Kornhuber, 1983). For an inconsistent result see Singh et al. (1992). Readiness and motor potentials reflect motor preparation and, it is thought, are generated, at least in part, in the motor cortex. There is a single piece of evidence that there may be differences in motor potential asymmetry between the groups. Terayama, Kumashiro, Kaneko, Suzuki, and Aono (1985, cited by Koyama et al., 1991) found that ERPs recorded from patients with schizophrenia are smaller in the left than the right hemisphere regardless of which hand was used to respond.

## Conclusions

Examination of the research that has been reported in this chapter emphasizes the importance of the heterogeneity of schizophrenia and the complexity of the task of unraveling its components. Some broad themes arise from the neuropsychological evidence. One is the critical role of frontal lobe disturbance in the genesis of many patterns of schizophrenic psychopathology. However, whether the disturbance is due to lack of hemispheric asymmetry, low frontal/whole brain volume, neuronal hypoactivity, neuronal hyperactivity, or any one of a host of other possibilities remains obscure. Nor is it clear that frontal lobe disturbance necessarily brings schizophrenic pathology as an inevitable consequence. Studies of aging, activity balance in the affective disorders, and other disorders implicates frontal functioning in many cases.

It is also clear that the structure and function of the temporal lobes play a critical part in the psychopathology of schizophrenia. The central role of the temporal areas in controlling and mediating language, coupled with the major part that language disturbances play in the diagnosis of schizophrenia, suggests that this link may have more specific significance in schizophrenia than the disturbances of the frontal lobe.

In recent years, particular interest has arisen in the question of anomalous lateralization in schizophrenia. As the present chapter shows, there are now many findings of anomalous laterality in brain volume and in the lateralization of performance. The ramifications of these findings are only now beginning to emerge.

A relatively more coherent story appears when examining schizophrenic symptoms, ERP components, and their neurophysiological generators. Frontally generated ERP components (CNV, PINV, and P3a) are abnormal, and these abnormalities are related to negative symptoms and hallucinations in patients with schizophrenia. Components generated by a brain system that includes temporal lobe structures (i.e., P50, N100, P200, N200, and P300) demonstrate a general reduction in amplitude and are related to decreases in temporal lobe volume. These reductions are most striking in the left temporal lobes. Amplitude reductions in left temporal ERP are not related to global functioning; rather they are related to specific symptoms such as thought disorder. Right temporal reductions are less likely to be observed but might be related to affective symptoms. Early brain stem functioning is relatively intact; later brain stem activity is slowed. Motor cortex functioning has not been studied thoroughly in schizophrenia but has been occasionally reduced.

Hence, ERP and EEG research provides convergent evidence for the frontal and temporal lobe abnormalities in schizophrenia, already mentioned. Additionally, the ERP literature suggests specific relationships between symptoms and these purportedly dysfunctional brain regions.

The picture that is now available gives grounds for optimism about our eventual understanding of the neuropathology of the schizophrenias, but our progress brings with it recognition of the complexity of the problems that lie ahead before that goal can be reached. As is so often the case in the history of science, technological breakthroughs open up new problems more complicated than those that they had solved. With regard to schizophrenia and psychopathology generally, the heart of the matter is the fact that the brain operates as a total system, not as a federation of semiautonomous discrete areas; the activity of each is insulated from that of the others. It is also evident that the relationship of the activity of specific brain areas to categories of behavior is subject to considerable individual variation. For these reasons we will need to develop the concepts necessary to express complex patterns of activity and the mathematical analyses that will permit us to make convincing comparisons between diagnostic groups.

# References

Adams, J., Faux, S. F., Nestor, P. G., Shenton, P. G., Marcy, B., Smith, S., & McCarley, R. W. (1993). ERP abnormalities during semantic processing in schizophrenia. *Schizophrenia Research, 10,* 247–257.

Adler, L. E., Hoffer, L. J., Griffith, J., Waldo, M. C., & Freedman, R. (1992). Normalizations by nicotine of deficient auditory sensory gating in the relatives of schizophrenics. *Biological Psychiatry, 32,* 607–616.

Adler, L. E., Hoffer, L., Nagamoto, H. T., Waldo, M. C., Kisley, M. A., & Griffith, J. M. (1994). Yohimbine impairs P50 auditory sensory gating in normal subjects. *Neuropsychopharmacology, 10,* 249–257.

Adler, L. E., Pachtman, E., Franks, R. D., Pecevich, M., Waldo, M. C., & Freedman, R. (1982). Neurophysiological evidence for a defect in neuronal mechanisms involved in sensory gating in schizophrenia. *Biological Psychiatry, 17,* 639–654.

Adler, L. E., Waldo, M. C., Tatcher, A., Cawthra, E., Baker, N., & Freedman, R. (1990). Lack of relationship of auditory gating defects to negative symptoms in schizophrenia. *Schizophrenia Research, 3,* 131–138.

American Psychiatric Association. (1987). *Diagnostic and statistical manual of mental disorders* (3rd ed., rev.). Washington, DC: Author.

Anderson, J., Gordon, E., Barry, R. J., Rennie, C., Gonsalvez, C., Pettigrew, G., Beumont, P. J. V., & Meares, R. (1995). Event related response variability in schizophrenia: Effect of intratrial target subsets. *Psychiatry Research, 56,* 237–243.

Andreasen, N. C., Nasrallah, H. A., Dunn, V., Olsen, S. C., Grove, W. M., Erhardt, J. C., Coffman, J. A., & Crossett, J. H. (1986). Structural abnormalities in the frontal system in schizophrenia: A magnetic resonance imaging study. *Archives of General Psychiatry, 43,* 136–144.

Andrews, S., Shelley, A. M., Ward, P. B., Fox, A., Catts, S. V., & McConaghy, N. (1993). Event-related potential indices of semantic processing in schizophrenia. *Biological Psychiatry, 34,* 443–458.

Annett, M. (1970). A classification of hand preference by association analysis. *British Journal of Psychology*, *61*, 303–321.

Asarnow, R. F., Granholm, E., & Sherman, T. (1991). Span of apprehension in schizophrenia. In S. R. Steinhauer, J. H. Gruzelier, & J. Zubin (Eds.), *Handbook of schizophrenia. Vol. 5: Neuropsychology, psychopathology and information processing* (pp. 335–370). Amsterdam: Elsevier.

Asarnow, R. F., & MacCrimmon, D. J. (1978). Residual performance deficit in clinically remitted schizophrenics: A marker of schizophrenia? *Journal of Abnormal Psychology*, *87*, 597–608.

Asarnow, R. F., & MacCrimmon, D. J. (1981). Span of apprehension deficits during the post-psychotic stages of schizophrenia. *Archives of General Psychiatry*, *38*, 1006–1011.

Asarnow, R. F., Neuchterlein, K. H., & Marder, S. R. (1983). Span of apprehension performance, neuropsychological functioning, and indices of psychosis proneness. *The Journal of Nervous and Mental Disease*, *171*, 662–669.

Bachneff, S. A., & Engelsmann, F. (1980). Contingent negative variation, postimperative negative variation, and psychopathology. *Biological Psychiatry*, *15*, 323–328.

Baker, N., Adler, L. E., Franks, R. D., Waldo, M., Berry, S., Nagamoto, H., Muckle, A., & Freedman, R. (1987). Neurophysiological assessment of sensory gating in psychiatric inpatients: Comparison between schizophrenia and other diagnoses. *Biological Psychiatry*, *22*, 603–617.

Baker, N. J., Staunton, M., Adler, L. E., Gerhardt, G. A., Drebing, C., Waldo, M., Nagamoto, H., & Freedman, R. (1990). Sensory gating deficits in psychiatric inpatients: Relation to catecholamine metabolites in different diagnostic groups. *Biological Psychiatry*, *27*, 519–528.

Balogh, D. W., & Merritt, R. D. (1985). Susceptibility to Type A backward pattern masking among hypothetically psychosis-prone college students. *Journal of Abnormal Psychology*, *94*, 377–383.

Baribeau-Braun, J., Picton, T. W., & Gosselin, J. Y. (1983). Schizophrenia: A neurophysiological evaluation of abnormal information processing. *Science*, *219*, 874–876.

Barrett, K., McCallum, W. C., & Pocock, P. V. (1986). Brain indicators of altered attention and information processing in schizophrenic patients. *British Journal of Psychiatry*, *148*, 414–420.

Barta, P. E., Pearlson, G. D., Tune, L. E., Powers, R. E., & Richards, S. S. (1990). Superior temporal gyrus volume in schizophrenia. *Schizophrenia Research*, *3*, 22.

Benes, F. (1989). Myelination of cortical-hippocampal relays during late adolescence. *Schizophrenia Bulletin*, *15*, 585–593.

Berman, K. F., Zec, R. F., & Weinberger, D. R. (1986). Physiologic dysfunction of dorsolateral prefrontal cortex in schizophrenia. *Archives of General Psychiatry*, *43*, 126–135.

Blackwood, D. H., Whalley, L. J., Christie, J. E., Blackburn, I. M., St. Clair, D. M., & McInnes, A. (1987). Changes in auditory P3 event-related potential in schizophrenia and depression. *British Journal of Psychiatry*, *150*, 154–160.

Blackwood, D. H., Young, A. H., McQueen, J. K., Martin, M. J., Roxbourough, H. M., Muir, W. J., St. Clair, D. M., & Kean, D. M. (1991). Magnetic resonance imaging in schizophrenia: Altered brain morphology associated with P300 abnormalities and eye tracking dysfunction. *Biological Psychiatry*, *30*, 753–769.

Bleuler, E. (1950). *Dementia praecox or the group of schizo-*

*phrenias* (J. Zinkin, Trans.). New York: International Universities Press. (Original work published in 1911.)

Blyler, C. R., Maher, B. A., Manschreck, T. C., & Fenton, W. S. (1997). Line drawing as a possible measure of lateralized motor performance in schizophrenia. *Schizophrenia Research*, *26*, 15–23.

Bogerts, B. (1993). Recent advances in the neuropathology of schizophrenia. *Schizophrenia Bulletin*, *19*, 431–439.

Boklage, C. C. (1977). Schizophrenia brain asymmetry development and twinning: Cellular relationship with etiologic and possibly prognostic implications. *Biological Psychiatry*, *12*, 19–35.

Borod, J. C., Caron, H. S., & Koff, E. (1984). Left-handers and right-handers compared on performance and preference measures of lateral dominance. *British Journal of Psychology*, *75*, 177–186.

Boutros, N. (1992). A review of indications for routine EEG in clinical psychiatry. *Hospital and Community Psychiatry*, *43*, 716–719.

Boutros, N., Narallah, H., Leighty, R., Torello, M., Tueting, P., & Olson, S. (1997). Auditory evoked potentials, clinical vs. research applications. *Psychiatry Research*, *69*, 183–195.

Braff, D. L. (1981). Impaired speed of information processing in nonmedicated schizotypal patients. *Schizophrenia Bulletin*, *7*, 499–508.

Brecher, M., & Begleiter, H. (1983). Event-related brain potentials to high-incentive stimuli in unmedicated schizophrenic patients. *Biological Psychiatry*, *18*, 661–674.

Brecher, M., & Begleiter, H. (1985). Brain stem auditory evoked potentials in unmedicated schizophrenic patients. *Biological Psychiatry*, *20*, 199–202.

Brecher, M., Porjsez, B., & Begleiter, H. (1987). The N2 component of the event-related potential in schizophrenic patients. *Electroencephalography and Clinical Neurophysiology*, *66*, 369–375.

Bruder, G., Kayser, J., Tenke, C., Amador, X., Friedman, M., Sharif, Z., & Gorman, J. (submitted). Left temporal lobe dysfunction in schizophrenia: Event-related potential and behavioral evidence from phonetic and tonal dichotic listening tasks.

Bruder, G., Rabinowicz, E., Towey, J., Brown, A., Kaufmann, C. A., Amador, X., Malaspina, D., & Gorman, J. M. (1995). Smaller right ear (left hemisphere) advantage with dichotic fused words in patients with schizophrenia. *American Journal of Psychiatry*, *152*, 932–935.

Bryden, M. P., Bulman-Fleming, M. B., & MacDonald, V. (1996). The measurement of handedness and its relation to neuropsychological issues. In D. Elliott & E. A. Roy (Eds.), *Manual asymmetries in motor performance*. Boca Raton, FL: CRC Press.

Buchsbaum, M. S., Ingvar, D. S., Kessler, R., Waters, R. N., Cappalletti, J., van Kammen, D. P., King, A. C., Johnson, J. L., Manning, R. G., Flynn, R. W., Mann, L. S., Bunney, W. E., & Sokoloff, L. (1982). Cerebral glucography with emission tomography: Use in normal subjects and patients with schizophrenia. *Archives of General Psychiatry*, *39*, 251–259.

Buchsbaum, M. S., Haier, R. J., Potkin, S. G., Neuchterlein, K., Bracha, H. S., Katz, M., Lohr, J., Wu, J., Lottenberg, S., Jerabek, P. A., Trenary, M., Tafalla, R., Reynolds, C., & Bunney, W. E., Jr. (1992a). Frontostriatal disorder of cerebral metabolism in never-medicated schizophrenics. *Archives of General Psychiatry*, *49*, 935–942.

Buchsbaum, M. S., King, A. C., Cappelletti, J., Coppola, R., &

van Kammen, D. P. (1982). Visual evoked potential topography in patients with schizophrenia and normal controls. *Advances in Biological Psychiatry*, 9, 50–56.

Buchsbaum, M. S., Mansour, C. S., Teng, D. G., Zia, A. D., Siegel, B. V, & Rice, D. M. (1992b). Adolescent developmental change in topography of EEG amplitude. *Schizophrenia Research*, 7, 101–107.

Chagule, V. B., & Master, R. S. (1981). Impaired cerebral dominance. *British Journal of Psychiatry*, 139, 23–24.

Chapman, L. J., & Chapman, J. P. (1987). The measurement of handedness. *Brain and Cognition*, 6, 175–183.

Chiarenza, G. A, Papakostopoulos, D., Dini, M., & Cazzullo, C. L. (1985). Neuropsychological correlates of psychomotor activity in chronic schizophrenics. *Electroencephalography and Clinical Neurophysiology*, 61, 218–228.

Chouinard, G., Annable, L., & Dongier, M. (1977). Differences in psychopathology of schizophrenic patients with normal and abnormal postimperative negative variation (PINV). *Comprehensive Psychiatry*, 18, 83–87.

Clementz, B. A., Geyer, M. A., & Braff, D. L. (1998). Multiple site evaluation of P50 suppression among schizophrenia and normal comparison subjects. *Schizophrenia Research*, 30, 71–80.

Coffman, J. A., & Nasrallah, H. A. (1986). Magnetic brain imaging in schizophrenia. In H. A. Nasrallah & D. R. Weinberg (Eds.), *Handbook of schizophrenia. Vol. 1: The neurology of schizophrenia* (pp. 251–266). Amsterdam: Elsevier.

Coffman, J. A., Schwartzkopf, S. B., Olson, S. C., Torello, M. W., Bornstein, R. A., & Nasrallah, H. A. (1989). Temporal lobe asymmetry in schizophrenics demonstrated by coronal MRI brain scans. *Schizophrenia Research*, 2, 117.

Coger, R. W., & Serafetinides, E. A. (1993). The N15 component of the brain stem auditory evoked potential: A measure of hippocampal activity in schizophrenics? *International Journal of Neuroscience*, 72, 271–282.

Colbourn, C. J., & Lishman, W. A. (1979). Lateralization of function and psychotic illness: A left hemisphere deficit. In J. Gruzelier & P. Flor-Henry (Eds.), *Hemisphere asymmetries of function in psychopathology* (pp. 539–559). Amsterdam: Elsevier Science.

Connolly, J. F., Gruzelier, J. H., & Hirsch, S. R. (1983). Visual evoked potentials in schizophrenia: Intensity effects and hemispheric asymmetry. *British Journal of Psychiatry*, 142, 152–155.

Connolly, J. F., Gruzelier, J. H., Kleinman, K. M., & Hirsch, S. R. (1979). Lateralized abnormalities in hemisphere-specific tachistoscopic tasks in psychiatric patients and controls. In J. Gruzelier & P. Flor-Henry (Eds.), *Hemisphere asymmetries of function in psychopathology* (pp. 491–509). Amsterdam: Elsevier Science.

Connolly, J. F., Manchanda, R., Gruzelier, J. H., & Hirsch, S. R. (1985). Pathway and hemispheric differences in the event-related potential (ERP) to monaural stimulation: A comparison of schizophrenic patients with normal controls. *Biological Psychiatry*, 20, 293–303.

Crider, A. (1997). Perseveration in schizophrenia. *Schizophrenia Bulletin*, 23, 63–74.

Crow, T. J. (1990). Temporal lobe asymmetries as the key to the etiology of schizophrenia. *Schizophrenia Bulletin*, 16, 433–443.

Crow, T. J. (1995). The relationship between morphological and genetic findings in schizophrenia. In R. Fog, J. Gerlach, & R. Hemmingsen (Eds.), *Schizophrenia: Alfred Benzon symposium* (pp. 15–25). Copenhagen: Munksgaard.

Crow, T. J., Colter, N., Frith, C. D., Johnstone, E. C., & Owens, D. G. C. (1989). Developmental arrest of cerebral asymmetries in early onset schizophrenia. *Psychiatry Research*, 29, 247–253.

Crow, T. J., Done, D. J., & Sacker, A. (1996). Cerebral lateralization is delayed in children who later develop schizophrenia. *Schizophrenia Research*, 22, 181–185.

Cullum, C. M., Harris, J. G., Waldo, M. C., Smernoff, E., Madison, A., Nagamoto, H. T., Griffith, J., Adler, L. E., & Freedman, R. (1993). Neurophysiological and neuropsychological evidence for attentional dysfunction in schizophrenia. *Schizophrenia Research*, 10, 131–141.

De Lisi, L. E. (1991). Brain imaging of cerebral activation. In S. R. Steinhauer, J. H. Gruzelier, & J. Zubin (Eds.), *Handbook of schizophrenia. Vol. 5: Neuropsychology, psychophysiology and information processing* (pp. 147–160). Amsterdam: Elsevier.

De Lisi, L. E., Dauphinais, I. D., & Hauser, P. (1989). Gender differences in the brain. Are they relevant to the pathogenesis of schizophrenia? *Comprehensive Psychiatry*, 30, 197–208.

De Lisi, L. E., Sakuma, M., Kushner, M., Finer, D. L., Hoff, A. L., & Crow, T. J. (1997). Anomalous cerebral asymmetry and language processing in schizophrenia. *Schizophrenia Bulletin*, 23, 255–271.

Dongier, M., Dubrovsky, B., & Englesmann, F. (1977). Event-related slow potentials in psychiatry. In C. Shagass, S. Gershon, & A. J. Friedhoff (Eds.), *Psychopathology and brain dysfunction* (pp. 339–352). New York: Raven Press.

Duncan, C. C., Morishisa, J. M., Fawcett, R. W., & Kirch, D. G. (1987). P300 in schizophrenia: State or trait marker? *Psychopharmacology Bulletin*, 23, 497–501.

Duncan, C. C., Perlstein, W., & Morihisa, J. M. (1987). The P300 metric in schizophrenia: Effects of probability and modality. In R. Johnson, J. Rohrbaugh, & R. Parasuraman (Eds.), *Current trends in event-related potential research* (EEG Suppl. 40), 670–674.

Duncan-Johnson, C. C. (1981). P300 latency: A new metric of information processing. *Psychophysiology*, 18, 207–215.

Duncan-Johnson, C. C., & Donchin, E. (1977). On quantifying surprise: The variation of event-related potentials with subjective probability. *Psychophysiology*, 14, 456–467.

Dvirskii, A. E. (1976). Functional asymmetry of the cerebral hemispheres of clinical types of schizophrenia. *Neuroscience and Behavioral Physiology*, 7, 236–239.

Egan, M. F., Duncan, C. C., Suddath, R. L., Kirch, D. G., Mirsky, A. F., & Wyatt, R. J. (1994). Event-related potential abnormalities correlate with structural brain alterations and clinical features in patients with chronic schizophrenia. *Schizophrenia Research*, 11, 259–271.

Eikmeier, G., & Lodemann, E. (1994). PINV topography and primary negative symptoms in chronic schizophrenia. *Pharmacopsychiatry*, 27, 63–64.

Eikmeier, G., Lodemann, E., Olbrich, H. M., Pach, J., Zerbin, D., & Gastpar, M. (1992). Postimperative negative variation and skin conductance response in chronic DSM-III-R schizophrenia. *Acta Psychiatrica Scandinavica*, 86, 346–350.

Eikmeier, G., Lodemann, E., Zerbin, D., & Gastpar, M. (1992). P300, clinical symptoms, and neuropsychological parameters in acute and remitted schizophrenia: A preliminary report. *Biological Psychiatry*, 31, 1065–1069.

Ellis, H. D., de Pauw, K. W., Christodoulou, G. N., Papageorgiou, L., Milne, A. B., & Joseph, A. B. (1993). Responses to facial and non-facial stimuli presented tachistoscopically in either or both visual fields by patients with Capgras delusion and paranoid schizophrenics. *Journal of Neurology, Neurosurgery, and Psychiatry, 56,* 215–219.

Fabiani, M., Karis, D., & Donchin, E. (1986). P300 and recall in an incidental memory paradigm. *Psychophysiology, 23,* 298–308.

Falkai, P., Bogerts, B., Greve, B., Pfeiffer, U., Machus, B., Folsch-Reetz, B., Majtenyi, C., & Ovary, I. (1992). Loss of sylvian fissure asymmetry in schizophrenia: A quantitative postmortem study. *Schizophrenia Research, 7,* 23–32.

Farkas, T., Reivich, M., & Alavi, A. (1980). The application of [18F] 2-deoxy-fluoro-D-glucose and positron emission tomography in the study of psychiatric conditions. In J. V. Possoneau, R. A. Hawkings, W. E. Lust, & F. A. Welsh (Eds.), *Cerebral metabolism and neural functions.* Baltimore: Williams & Wilkins.

Faux, S. F., McCarley, R. W., Nestor, P. G., Shenton, M. E., Pollak, S. D., Penhune, V., Mondorow, E., Marcy, B., Peterson, A., Horvath, T., & Davis, K. (1993). Auditory P300 abnormalities and left posterior superior temporal gyrus volume reduction in schizophrenia. *Archives of General Psychiatry, 50,* 190–197.

Feinberg, I. (1982). Schizophrenia caused by a fault in programmed synaptic elimination during adolescence? *Journal of Psychiatric Research, 17,* 319–334.

Ford, J. M., Pfefferbaum, A., & Roth, W. (1992). P3 and schizophrenia. In D. Friedman & G. E. Bruder (Eds.), *Psychophysiology and experimental psychopathology: A tribute to Samuel Sutton.* Annals of the New York Academy of Sciences, 658 (pp. 146–162). New York: New York Academy of Sciences.

Ford, J. M., White, P. M., Csernansky, J. G., Faustman, W. O., Roth, W. T., & Pfefferbaum, A. (1994a). ERPs in schizophrenia: Effects of antipsychotic medication. *Biological Psychiatry, 36,* 153–170.

Ford, J. M., White, P., Lim, K. O., & Pfefferbaum, A. (1994b). Schizophrenics have fewer and smaller P300s: A single-trial analysis. *Biological Psychiatry, 35,* 96–103.

Franzen, G., & Ingvar, D. H. (1975a). Abnormal distribution of cerebral activity in chronic schizophrenia. *Journal of Psychiatric Research, 12,* 209–214.

Franzen, G., & Ingvar, D. H. (1975b). Absence of activation in frontal structures during neuropsychological testing in chronic schizophrenics. *Journal of Neurology, Neurosurgery and Psychiatry, 38,* 1027–1032.

Freedman, R., Waldo, M. C., Bickford-Wimer, P., & Nagamoto, H. (1991). Elementary neuronal dysfunctions in schizophrenia. *Schizophrenia Research, 4,* 223–243.

George, L., & Neufeld, R. W. J. (1987). Attentional resources and hemispheric functional asymmetry in schizophrenia. *British Journal of Clinical and Social Psychology, 26,* 35–45.

Gerez, M., & Tello, A. (1995). Selected quantitative EEG (QEEG) and event-related potential (ERP) variables as discriminators for positive and negative schizophrenia. *Biological Psychiatry, 38,* 34–49.

Gerver, D. (1967). Linguistic rules and the perception and recall of speech by schizophrenic patients. *Journal of Social and Clinical Psychology, 6,* 204–211.

Goldberg, E., & Seidman, L. J. (1991). Higher cortical functions in normals and in schizophrenia: A selective review. In S. R. Steinhauer, J. H. Gruzelier, & J. Zubin (Eds.), *Handbook of schizophrenia.* Vol. 5: *Neuropsychology, psychophysiology and information processing* (pp. 397–433). Amsterdam: Elsevier.

Goldman-Rakic, P. (1991). Prefrontal cortical dysfunction in schizophrenia: The relevance of working memory. In B. J. Carroll & J. E. Barrett (Eds.), *Psychopathology and the brain.* New York: Raven Press.

Griffith, J., & Freedman, R. (1993). Normalization of the auditory P50 gating deficit of schizophrenia patients after non-REM but not REM sleep. *Psychiatry Research, 56,* 271–278.

Griffith, J., Hoffer, L. D., Adler, L. E., Zerbe, G. O., & Freedman, R. (1995). Effects of sound intensity on a midlatency evoked response to repeated auditory stimuli in schizophrenic and normal subjects. *Psychophysiology, 32,* 460–466.

Grillon, C., Ameli, R., & Glazer, W. M. (1990). Brain stem auditory-evoked potentials to different rates and intensities of stimulation in schizophrenics. *Biological Psychiatry, 28,* 819–823.

Grillon, C., Ameli, R., & Glazer, W. M. (1991). N400 and semantic categorization in schizophrenia. *Biological Psychiatry, 29,* 467–480.

Grove, W. M., & Andreaasen, N. C. (1991). Thought disorder in relation to brain function. In S. R. Steinhauer, J. H. Gruzelier, & J. Zubin (Eds.), *Handbook of schizophrenia.* Vol. 5: *Neuropsychology, psychophysiology and information processing* (pp. 485–504). Amsterdam: Elsevier.

Gruzelier, J. H. (1984). Hemispheric imbalances in schizophrenia. *International Journal of Psychophysiology, 1,* 227–240.

Gruzelier, J. H., & Kaiser, J. (1996). Syndromes of schizotypy and the timing of puberty. *Schizophrenia Research, 21,* 183–194.

Gur, R. E. (1977). Motoric laterality imbalance in schizophrenia. *Archives of General Psychiatry, 34,* 33–37.

Gur, R. E. (1978). Left hemisphere dysfunction and left hemisphere overactivation in schizophrenia. *Journal of Abnormal Psychology, 87,* 226–238.

Harell, M., Englender, M., Demer, M., Kimhi, R., & Zohar, M. (1986). Auditory brain stem responses in schizophrenic patients. *Laryngoscope, 96,* 908–910.

Heaton, R. K. (1981). *Wisconsin Card Sorting Test manual.* Odessa, FL: Psychological Assessment Resources.

Heidrich, A., & Strik, W. K. (1997). Auditory P300 topography and neuropsychological test performance: Evidence for left hemispheric dysfunction in schizophrenia. *Biological Psychiatry, 41,* 327–335.

Hergerl, U., Juckel, G., Muller-Schubert, A., Pietzcker, A., & Gaebel, W. (1995). Schizophrenics with small P300: A subgroup with a neurodevelopmental disturbance and a high risk for tardive dyskinesia? *Acta Psychiatrica Scandinavica, 91,* 120–125.

Hiramatsu, K., Kameyama, T., Saitoh, O., & Niwa, S. (1984). Correlations of event-related potentials with schizophrenic deficits in information processing and hemispheric dysfunction. *Biological Psychiatry, 19,* 281–294.

Hoffman, R. E., Stopek, S., & Andreasen, N. C. (1986). A comparative study of manic versus schizophrenic speech disorganization. *Archives of General Psychiatry, 43,* 831–838.

Javitt, D. C., Doneshka, P., Zylberman, I., Ritter, W., & Vaughan, H. G., Jr. (1993). Impairment of early cortical processing in schizophrenia: An event-related potential confirmation study. *Biological Psychiatry, 33,* 513–519.

Jin, Y., & Potkin, S. G. (1996). P50 changes with visual interference in normal subjects: A sensory distraction model for schizophrenia. *Clinical Electroencephalography, 27,* 151–154.

Jin, Y., Potkin, S. G., Patterson, J. V., Sandman, C. A., Hetrick, W. P., & Bunney, W. E. (1997). Effect of P50 temporal variability on sensory gating in schizophrenia. *Psychiatry Research, 70,* 71–81.

John, E. R., Prichep, L. S., Alpper, K. R., Mas, F. G., Cancro, R., Easton, P., & Sverdlov, L. (1994). Quantitative electrophysiological characteristics and subtyping of schizophrenia. *Biological Psychiatry, 36,* 801–826.

Johnson, M. R., & Adler, L. E. (1993). Transient impairment in P50 auditory sensory gating induced by a cold-pressor test. *Biological Psychiatry, 33,* 380–387.

Johnson, R. (1988). The amplitude of the P300 component of the event-related potential: Review and synthesis. *Advances in Psychophysiology, 3,* 69–137.

Juckel, G., Muller-Schubert, A., Gaebel, W., & Hergerl, U. (1996). Residual symptoms and P300 in schizophrenic outpatients. *Psychiatry Research, 65,* 23–32.

Kawasaki, Y., Maeda, Y., Higashima, M., Nagasawa, T., Koshino, Y., Suzuki, M., & Ide, Y. (1997). Reduced auditory P300 amplitude, medial temporal volume reduction and psychopathology in schizophrenia. *Schizophrenia Research, 26,* 107–115.

Keefe, R. S. E., Silverman, J. E., Mohs, R. C., Siever, L. J., Harvey, P. D., Friedman, L., Lees Roitman, S. E., DuPre, R. L., Smith, C. J., Schmeidler, J., & Davis, K. (1997). Eye-tracking, attention, and schizotypal symptoms in nonpsychotic relatives of patients with schizophrenia. *Archives of General Psychiatry, 54,* 169–176.

Kemali, D., Galderisi, S., Maj, M., Cesarelli, M., & DíAmbra, L. (1988). Event-related potentials in schizophrenic patients: Clinical and neurophysiological correlates. *Research Communications in Psychology, Psychiatry and Behavior, 13,* 3–16.

Kimhi, R., Englender, M., Zohar, M., & Harell, M. (1987). Brain stem auditory evoked responses in hospitalized unmedicated schizophrenic patients. *Israel Journal of Psychiatry and Related Sciences, 24,* 289–294.

Klein, C., Rockstroh, B., Cohen, R., & Berg, P. (1996). Contingent negative variation (CNV) and determinants of the post-imperative negative variation in schizophrenic patients and healthy controls. *Schizophrenia Research, 21*(2), 97–110.

Klein, C., Rockstroh, B., Cohen, R., Berg, P., & Dressel, M. (1996). The impact of performance uncertainty on the post imperative negative variation. *Psychophysiology, 33,* 426–433.

Knight, R. T., Hillyard, S. A., Woods, D. L., & Neville, H. J. (1981). The effects of frontal cortex lesions on event-related brain potentials during auditory selective attention. *Electroencephalography and Clinical Neurophysiology, 52,* 571–582.

Knight, R. T., Scabini, D., Woods, D. L., & Clayworth, C. C. (1989). Contributions of the temporal-parietal junction to the human auditory P3. *Brain Research, 502,* 109–116.

Knight, R. T. (1990). Neural mechanisms of event-related potentials from human lesions studies. In J. Rohrbaugh, R. Parasuraman, & R. Johnson (Eds.), *Event-related brain potentials: Basic issues and applications* (pp. 3–18). New York: Oxford University Press.

Kornhuber, H. H. (1983). Chemistry, physiology and neuropsychology of schizophrenia: Towards an earlier diagnosis of schizophrenia I. *Archives fur Psychiatrie und Nervenkrankheiten, 233,* 415–422.

Koyami, S., Nageishi, Y., Shimokochi, M., Hokama, H., Miyazato, Y., Miyatani, M., & Ogura, C. (1991). The N400 component of event-related potentials in schizophrenic patients: A preliminary study. *Electroencephalography and Clinical Neurophysiology, 78,* 124–132.

Kutaas, M., & Hillyard, S. (1980). Reading senseless sentences: Brain potentials reflect semantic incongruity. *Science, 207,* 203–205.

Kutcher, S. P., Blackwood, H. R., St. Clair, D., Gaskell, D. F., & Muir, W. J. (1987). Auditory P300 in borderline personality disorder and schizophrenia. *Archives of General Psychiatry, 44,* 645–650.

Lenzenweger, M. F., Cornblatt, B. A., & Putnick, M. (1991). Schizotypy and sustained attention. *Journal of Abnormal Psychology, 100,* 84–89.

Levit, R. A., Sutton, S., & Zubin, J. (1973). Evoked potential correlates of information processing in psychiatric patients. *Psychological Medicine, 3,* 487–494.

Lewine, R. J. (1981). Sex differences in schizophrenia—timing or subtypes? *Psychological Bulletin, 90,* 432–444.

Liddle, P. F. (1987). Schizophrenic syndromes, cognitive performance, and neurological dysfunction. *Psychological Medicine, 17,* 49–57.

Liddle, P. F., & Morris, D. L. (1991). Schizophrenic syndromes and frontal lobe performance. *British Journal of Psychiatry, 158,* 340–345.

Liddle, P. F., Friston, K. J., Frith, C. D., Hirsch, S. R., Jones, T., & Frackowiak, R. S. (1992). Patterns of cerebral blood flow in schizophrenia. *British Journal of Psychiatry, 160,* 179–186.

Louza, M. R., & Maurer, K. (1989). Differences between paranoid and nonparanoid schizophrenic patents on the somatosensory P300 event-related potential. *Neuropsychobiology, 21,* 59–66.

Loveless, N. E., & Sanford, A. J. (1974). Effects of age on the contingent negative variation and preparatory set in a reaction-time task. *Journal of Gerontology, 29,* 52–63.

Magaro, P. A., & Chamrad, D. L. (1983). Information processing and lateralization in schizophrenia. *Biological Psychiatry, 18,* 29–44.

Maher, B. A., & Manschreck, T. C. (1998). Lateralization, memory and language in schizophrenia: Some facts and an artifact. In M. F. Lenzenweger & R. H. Dworkin (Eds.), *Origins and development of schizophrenia* (pp. 211–231). Washington, DC: American Psychological Association.

Maher, B. A., Manschreck, T. C., Woods, B. T., Yurgelun-Todd, D. A., & Tsuang, M. T. (1995). Frontal brain volume and context effects in short-term recall in schizophrenia. *Biological Psychiatry, 37,* 144–150.

Maher, B. A., Manschreck, T. C., Yurgelun-Todd, D. A., & Tsuang, M. T. (1998). Hemispheric asymmetry of frontal and temporal gray matter and age of onset in schizophrenia. *Biological Psychiatry, 44,* 413–417.

Manoach, D. S., Maher, B. A., & Manschreck, T. C. (1988). Left-handedness and thought disorder in the schizophrenias. *Journal of Abnormal Psychology, 97,* 97–99.

Monoach, D. S. (1994). Handedness is related to formal thought disorder and language dysfunction in schizophrenia. *Journal of Clinical and Experimental Neuropsychology, 16,* 2–14.

Manschreck, T. C., Maher, B. A., Redmond, D. A., Miller, C., & Beaudette, S. M. (1996). Laterality, memory and thought disorder in schizophrenia. *Neuropsychiatry, Neuropsychology, and Behavioral Neurology, 8*, 1–7.

Matousek, M., Capone, C., & Okawa, M. (1981). Measurement of the inter-hemispheral differences as a diagnostic tool in psychiatry. *Advances in Biological Psychiatry, 6*, 76–80.

McCarley, R. W., Faux, S. F., Shenton, M. E., LeMay, M., Cane, M., Ballinger, R., & Duffy, F. H. (1989). CT abnormalities in schizophrenia: A preliminary study of their correlations with P300/P200 electrophysiological features and positive/negative symptoms. *Archives of General Psychiatry, 46*, 698–708.

McCarley, R. W., Faux, S. F., Shenton, M. E., Nestor, P. G., & Adams, J. (1991). Event related potentials in schizophrenia: Their biological and clinical correlates and a new model of schizophrenic pathophysiology. *Schizophrenia Research, 4*, 209–231.

McConaghy, N., Catts, S. V., Michie, P. T., Fox, A., Ward, P. B., & Shelley, A. M. (1993). P300 indexes thought disorder in schizophrenics, but allusive thinking in normal subjects. *Journal of Nervous and Mental Disease, 181*, 176–182.

Merriam, A. E., & Gardner, E. B. (1987). Corpus callosum function in schizophrenia: A neuropsychological assessment of inter-hemispheric information processing. *Neuropsychologia, 25*, 185–193.

Merrin, E. L., & Floyd, T. C. (1994). P300 responses to novel auditory stimuli in hospitalized schizophrenic patients. *Biological Psychiatry, 36*, 527–542.

Mirsky, A. F., Lockhead, S. J., Jones, B. P., Kugelmass, S., Walsh, D., & Kendler, K. S. (1992). On familial factors in the attentional deficit in schizophrenia: A review and report of two new subject samples. *Journal of Psychiatric Research, 26*, 383–403.

Mitchell, P. F., Andrews, S., Fox, A. M., Catts, S. V., Ward, P. B., & McConaghy, N. (1991). Active and passive attention in schizophrenia: An ERP study of information processing in a linguistic task. *Biological Psychology, 32*, 101–124.

Morstyn, R., Duffy, F. H., & McCarley, R. W. (1982). Altered P300 topography in schizophrenia. *Archives of General Psychiatry, 40*, 729–734.

Muir, W. J., St. Clair, D. M., & Blackwood, D. H. (1991). Long-latency auditory event-related potentials in schizophrenia and in bipolar and unipolar affective disorder. *Psychological Medicine, 21*, 867–879.

Nagamoto, H. T., Adler, L. E., Waldo, M. C., Griffith, J., & Freedman, R. (1991). Gating of auditory response in schizophrenics and normal controls: Effects of recording site and stimulation interval on the P50 wave. *Schizophrenia Research, 4*, 31–40.

Nasrallah, H. A., Keelor, K., Schroder, C. V., & McCalley-Whitters, M. (1981). Motoric lateralization in schizophrenic males. *American Journal of Psychiatry, 138*, 114–115.

Nelson, A., Saykin, A. J., Flashman, L. A., & Riordan, H. J. (1998). Hippocampal volume reduction in schizophrenia as assessed by magnetic resonance imaging: A meta-analytic study. *Archives of General Psychiatry, 55*, 433–440.

Nestor, P. G., Faux, S. F., McCarley, R. W., Penhune, V., Shenton, M. E., Pollak, S., & Sands, S. F. (1992). Attentional cues in chronic schizophrenia: Abnormal disengagement of attention. *Journal of Abnormal Psychology, 101*, 682–689.

Nestor, P. G., Kimble, M. O., O'Donnell, B. F., Smith, L., Niznikiewicz, M., Shenton, M., & McCarley, R. W. (1997).

Aberrant semantic activation in schizophrenia: A neurophysiological study. *American Journal of Psychiatry, 154*, 640–646.

Neuchterlein, K. (1991). Vigilance in schizophrenia and related disorders. In S. R. Steinhauer, J. H. Gruzelier, & J. Zubin (Eds.), *Handbook of schizophrenia. Vol. 5: Neuropsychology, psychophysiology and information processing* (pp. 397–433). Amsterdam: Elsevier.

Niznikiewicz, M. A., O'Donnell, B. F., Nestor, P. G., Smith, L., Karapelou, M., Shenton, M. E., & McCarley, R. W. (1997). ERP assessment of visual and auditory language processing in schizophrenia. *Journal of Abnormal Psychology, 106*, 85–94.

Norman, R. M. G., Malla, A. K., Morrison-Stewart, S. L., Helmes, E., Williamson, P. C., Thomas, J., & Cortese, L. (1997). Neuropsychological correlates of syndromes in schizophrenia. *British Journal of Psychiatry, 170*, 134–139.

Oades, R. D., Zerbin, D., & Eggers, C. (1994). Negative difference (Nd), and ERP marker of stimulus relevance: Different lateral asymmetries for paranoid and nonparanoid schizophrenics. *Pharmacopsychiatry, 27*, 65–67.

O'Donnell, B. F., Hokama, H., McCarley, R. W., Smith, R. S., Salisbury, D. F., Mondrow, E., Nestor, P. G., & Shenton, M. E. (1994). Auditory ERPs to non-target stimuli in schizophrenia: Relationship to probability, task-demands, and target ERPs. *International Journal of Psychophysiology, 17*, 219–231.

O'Donnell, B. F., Shenton, M. E., McCarley, R. W., Faux, S. F., Smith, R. S., Salisbury, D. F., Nestor, P. G., Pollak, S. D., Kikinis, R., & Jolesz, F. A. (1993). The auditory N2 component in schizophrenia: Relationship to MRI temporal lobe gray matter and to other ERP abnormalities. *Biological Psychiatry, 34*, 26–40.

Ogura, C., Nageishi, Y., Matsubayashi, M., Omura, F., Kishimoto, A., & Shimokochi, M. (1991). Abnormalities in event-related potentials, N100, P200, P300 and slow wave in schizophrenia. *Japanese Journal of Psychiatry and Neurology, 45*, 57–65.

Oldfield, R. C. (1971). The assessment and analysis of handedness: The Edinburgh Inventory. *Neuropsychologia, 9*, 97–113.

Olichney, J. M., Iragui, V. J., Kutas, M., Nowacki, R., & Jeste, D. V. (1997). N400 abnormalities in late life schizophrenia and related psychoses. *Biological Psychiatry, 42*, 13–23.

Pfefferbaum, A., Ford, J. M., White, P. M., & Roth, W. T. (1989). P3 in schizophrenia is affected by stimulus modality, response requirements, medication status, and negative symptoms. *Archives of General Psychiatry, 46*, 1035–1044.

Pfefferbaum, A., Horvath, T. B., Roth, W. T., Tinklenberg, J. R., & Kopell, B. S. (1980). Auditory brain stem and cortical evoked potentials in schizophrenia. *Biological Psychiatry, 15*, 209–223.

Pfefferbaum, A., Wenegrat, B. G., Ford, J. M., Roth, W. T., & Kopell, B. S. (1984). Clinical applications of the P3 component of event-related potentials. II. Dementia, depression and schizophrenia. *Electroencephalography and Clinical Neurophysiology, 59*, 104–124.

Pic'l, A. K., Magaro, P. A., & Wade, E. A. (1979). Hemispheric functioning in paranoid and non-paranoid schizophrenia. *Biological Psychiatry, 14*, 891–903.

Picton, T. W., Hillyard, S. A., Krausz, H. I., & Galambos, R. (1974). Human auditory evoked potentials. I: Evaluation of components. *Electroencephalography and Clinical Neurophysiology, 36*, 179–190.

Piran, N., Bigler, E. D., & Cohen, D. (1982). Motoric laterality and eye dominance suggest a unique pattern of cerebral organization in schizophrenia. *Archives of General Psychiatry, 39,* 1006–1010.

Polich, J. (1993). Hemispheric differences for feature migrations. *Acta Psychologia, 83,* 179–201.

Pritchard, W. S. (1986). Cognitive event-related potential correlates of schizophrenia. *Psychological Bulletin, 100,* 43–66.

Pritchard, W. S., Shappell, S. A., & Brandt, M. E. (1991). Psychophysiology of N200/N400: A review and classification scheme. In J. R. Jennings, P. K. Ackles, et al. (Eds.), *Advances in psychophysiology: A research annual,* Vol. 4 (pp. 43–106). London, England: Jessica Kingsley.

Rainse, A. (1991). The Schizotypal Personality Questionnaire. *Schizophrenia Bulletin, 17,* 554–564.

Raine, A., Lencz, T., Reynolds, G. P., Harrison, G., Sheard, C., Medley, I., Reynolds, L. M., & Cooper, J. E. (1993). An evaluation of structural and functional prefrontal deficits in schizophrenia: MRI and neuropsychological measures. *Psychiatry Research, 45,* 123–127.

Reite, M., Teale, P., Goldstein, L., Whalen, J., & Linnville, S. (1989). Late auditory magnetic sources may differ in the left hemisphere of schizophrenic patients: A preliminary report. *Archives of General Psychiatry, 46,* 565–572.

Reite, M., Teale, P. D., Neumann, R., & Davis, K. (1987). Localization of a 50 msec latency auditory evoked field component. *Current Trends in Event-Related Potential Research* (EEG Suppl. 40), 487–492.

Reite, M., Teale, P., Sheeder, P., Jeanelle, S., Rojas, D. C., et al. (1996). Magnetoencephalographic evidence of abnormal early auditory memory function in schizophrenia. *Biological Psychiatry, 40,* 299–301.

Reite, M., Teale, P., Zimmerman, J., Davis, K., Whalen, J., & Edrich, J. (1988). Source of a 50-msec latency auditory evoked field component in young schizophrenic men. *Biological Psychiatry, 24,* 495–506.

Roemer, R. A., & Shagass, C. (1992). Relationships between receptor occupancy of antipsychotic drugs and human somatosensory evoked potential. *Biological Psychiatry, 31,* 61A.

Rosahl, S. K., & Knight, R. T. (1995). Role of prefrontal cortex in generation of the contingent negative variation. *Cerebral Cortex, 5(2),* 123–125.

Roschke, J., Wagner, P., Mann, K., Fell, J., Grozinger, M., & Frank, C. (1996). Single trial analysis of event related potentials: A comparison between schizophrenics and depressives. *Biological Psychiatry, 40,* 844–852.

Rossi, A., Stratta, P., Matei, P., Cuoillari, M., Bozao, A., Gallucci, M., et al. (1992). Planum temporale in schizophrenia: A magnetic resonance study. *Schizophrenia Research, 7,* 19–22.

Rossi, G. F., Stratta, P., D'Albenzio, L., Tataro, A., Schiazza, G., Di Michele, Bolino, F., & Casacchia, M. (1990a). Reduced temporal lobe area in schizophrenia. *Biological Psychiatry, 27,* 61–68.

Rossi, G. F., Stratta, P., D'Albenzio, L., Tataro, A., Schiazza, G., Di Michele, Bolino, F., & Casacchia, M. (1990b). Reduced temporal lobe areas in schizophrenia: Preliminary evidence from a controlled multiplanar magnetic resonance study. *Schizophrenia Research, 3,* 21.

Roth, W. T., & Cannon, E. H. (1972). Some features of the auditory evoked response in schizophrenics. *Archives of General Psychiatry, 27,* 466–471.

Roth, W., Horvath, T., Pfefferbaum, A., & Kopell, B. (1980). Event-related potentials in schizophrenics. *Electroencephalography and Clinical Neurophysiology, 48,* 127–139.

Roth, W. T., Horvath, T. B., Pfefferbaum, A., Tinklenberg, J. R., Mezzich, J., & Kopell, B. S. (1980). Late event-related potentials and schizophrenia. *Electroencephalography and Clinical Neurophysiology, 49,* 497–505.

Roth, W. T., Pfefferbaum, A., Kelly, A. F., Berger, P. A., & Kopell, B. S. (1981). Auditory event-related potentials in schizophrenia and depression. *Psychiatry Research, 4,* 199–212.

Saccuzzo, D. P., & Schubert, D. L. (1981). Backward masking as a measure of slow processing in schizophrenia disorders. *Journal of Abnormal Psychology, 90,* 305–312.

Salisbury, D. F., O'Donnell, B. F., McCarley, R. W., Nestor, P. G., Faux, S. F., & Smith, R. S. (1994a). Parametric manipulations of auditory stimuli differentially affect P3 amplitude in schizophrenics and controls. *Psychophysiology, 31,* 29–36.

Salisbury, D. F., O'Donnell, B. F., McCarley, R. W., Shenton, M. E., & Benavage, A. (1994b). The N2 event-related potential reflects attention deficit in schizophrenia. *Biological Psychiatry, 39,* 1–13.

Salisbury, D. F., Shenton, M. E., Sherwood, A. R., Fischer, I. A., Yurgelun-Todd, D. A., Tohen, M., & McCarley, R. W. (1998). First-episode schizophrenic psychosis differs from first-episode affective psychosis and controls in P300 amplitude over left temporal lobe. *Archives of General Psychiatry, 55,* 173–180.

Saugstad, L. F. (1994). The maturational theory of brain development and cerebral excitability in the multi-factorially inherited manic-depressive psychosis and schizophrenia. *International Journal of Psychophysiology, 18,* 189–203.

Shan-Min, Y., Flor-Henry, P., Dayi, C., Tiangi, L., Shuguang, Q., & Zenxiang, M. (1985). Imbalance of hemispheric functions in the major psychoses: A study of handedness in the People's Republic of China. *Biological Psychiatry, 20,* 906–917.

Shelley, A. M., Ward, P. B., Catts, S. V., Michie, P. T., Andrews, S., & McConaghy, N. (1991). Mismatch negativity: An index of a preattentive processing deficit in schizophrenia. *Biological Psychiatry, 30,* 1059–1062.

Shenton, M. E., Ballinger, R., Marcy, B., Faux, S. F., Cane, M., Lemay, M., Cassens, G., Coleman, M., Duffy, F. H., & McCarley, R. W. (1989). Two syndromes of schizophrenic psychopathology associated with left vs. right temporal deficits in P300 amplitude. *Journal of Nervous and Mental Disease, 177,* 219–225.

Shenton, M. E., Faux, S. F., McCarley, R. W., Ballinger, R., Coleman, M., Torello, M., & Duffy, F. H. (1989). Correlations between abnormal auditory P300 topography and positive symptoms in schizophrenia: A preliminary report. *Biological Psychiatry, 25,* 710–716.

Shenton, M. E., Kikinis, R., Jolesz, F. A., Pollak, S. D., LeMay, M., Hokama, H., Martin, M. J., Metcalf, D., Coleman, M., & McCarley, R. W. (1992). Abnormalities of the left temporal lobe and thought disorder in schizophrenia: A quantitative magnetic resonance imaging study. *New England Journal of Medicine, 327,* 604–612.

Singh, J., Knight, R. T., Rosenlicht, N., Kotun, J. M., Beckley, D. J., & Woods, D. L. (1992). Abnormal premovement brain potentials in schizophrenia. *Schizophrenia Research, 8,* 31–41.

Smith, M. E., Halgren, E., Sokolik, M., Baudena, P., Musolino,

A., Liegois-Chauvel, C., & Chauvel, P. (1990). The intracranial topography of the P3 event-related potential elicited during auditory oddball. *Electroencephalography and Clinical Neurophysiology, 76,* 235–248.

Sommer, W. (1985). Selective attention differentially affects brain stem auditory evoked potentials of electrodermal responders and nonresponders. *Psychiatry Research, 16,* 227–232.

Souza, V. B. N., Muir, W. J., Walker, M. T., Glabus, M. F., Roxborough, H. M., Sharp, C. W., Dunan, J. R., & Blackwood, D. H. R. (1995). Auditory P300 event-related potentials and neuropsychological performance in schizophrenia and bipolar affective disorder. *Biological Psychiatry, 37,* 300–310.

Spitzer, R., & Endicott, J. (1977). *Schedule for affective disorders and schizophrenia.* New York: Biometrics Research.

Sponheim, S. R., Clementz, B. A., Iacono, W. G., & Beiser, M. (1993). Resting EEG in first-episode and chronic schizophrenia. (unpublished).

Sponheim, S. R., & Kodalen, K. M. (1998, October). Span of apprehension in schizophrenia: An event-related potential study. Paper presented at the *Annual Meeting of the Society for Psychophysiological Research,* Denver, CO.

Squires, N. K., Squires, K., & Hillyard, S. (1975). Two varieties of long latency positive waves evoked by unpredictable auditory stimuli in man. *Electroencephalography and Clinical Neurophysiology, 38,* 387–401.

Stefansson, S. B., & Jonsdottir, T. J. (1996). Auditory event-related potentials, auditory digit span, and clinical schizophrenic men on neuroleptic medication. *Biological Psychiatry, 40,* 19–27.

Stainhauer, S. R., Zubin, J., Condray, R., Shaw, D. B., Peters, J. L., & Van Kammen, D. P. (1991). Electrophysiological and behavioral signs of attentional disturbance in schizophrenics and their siblings. In C. A. Tamminga & S. C. Schulz (Eds.), *Advances in neuropsychiatry and psychopharmacology,* Vol. 1: *Schizophrenia Research* (pp. 169–178). New York: Raven Press.

Steronko, R. J., & Woods, D. J. (1978). Impairment in early stages of visual information processing in nonpsychotic schizotypic individuals. *Journal of Abnormal Psychology, 87,* 481–490.

Stevens, J. R., Bigelow, L., Denney, D., Lipkin, J., Livermore, A. H., Jr., Rauscher, F., & Wyatt, R. J. (1979). Telemetered EEG-EOG during psychotic behaviors of schizophrenia. *Archives of General Psychiatry, 36,* 251–262.

Strandburg, R. J., Marsh, J. T., Brown, W. S., Asarnow, R. F., Guthrie, D., Harper, R., Yee, C. M., & Neuchterlein, K. H. (1997). Event-related potential correlates of linguistic information processing in schizophrenics. *Biological Psychiatry, 42,* 596–608.

Strandburg, R. J., Marsh, J. T., Brown, W. S., Asarnow, R. F., Guthrie, D., Higa, H., Yee-Bradbury, C. M., & Neuchterlein, K. (1994). Reduced attention-related negative potentials in schizophrenic adults. *Psychophysiology, 31,* 272–281.

Strik, W. K., Dierks, T., & Maurer, K. (1993a). Amplitudes of auditory P300 in remitted and residual schizophrenics: Correlations with clinical features. *Neuropsychobiology, 27,* 54–60.

Strik, W. K., Dierks, T., Franzek, E., Sober, G., & Maurer, K. (1993b). P300 asymmetries in schizophrenia revisited with reference-independent methods. *Psychiatry Research and Neuroimaging, 55,* 153–166.

Strik, W. K., Dierks, T., Franzek, E., Sober, G., & Maurer, K. (1994). P300 in schizophrenia: Interactions between amplitudes and topography. *Biological Psychiatry, 35,* 850–856.

Strik, W. K., Dierks, T., Kulke, H., Maurer, K., & Fallgatter, A. (1993). The predictive value of P300-amplitudes in the course of schizophrenic disorders. *Journal of Neural Transmission, 103,* 1351–1359.

Szelenberger, W. (1983). Brain stem auditory evoked potentials and personality. *Biological Psychiatry, 18,* 157–174.

Taylor, P. J., Brown, R., & Gunn, J. (1983). Violence, psychosis, and handedness. In P. Flor-Henry & J. Gruzelier (Eds.), *Laterality and psychopathology* (pp. 181–194). Amsterdam: Elsevier North Holland.

Tenke, C., Bruder, G., Towey, J., Leite, P., Malaspina, D., Gorman, J., & Kaufman, C. (1992). Event-related potentials (ERPs) to complex tones in psychotic patients. Poster presented at the *Society for Research in Psychophysiology,* San Diego, CA.

Terayama, K., Kumashiro, H., Kaneko, Y., Suzuki, A., & Aono, T. (1985). Readiness potential in chronic schizophrenics: Physiological approach for the interhemispheric functional disorder. *Clinical Electroencephalography, 27,* 381–385 (in Japanese). As cited in Koyami, S., Nageishi, Y., Shimokochi, M., Hokama, H., Miyazato, Y., Miyatani, M., & Ogura, C. (1991). The N400 component of event-related potentials in schizophrenic patients: A preliminary study. *Electroencephalography and Clinical Neurophysiology, 78,* 124–132.

Truscott, I. P. (1970). Contextual constraint and schizophrenic language. *Journal of Consulting and Clinical Psychology, 110,* 375–380.

Turetsky, B., Colbath, E. A, & Gur, R. E. (1998). P300 subcomponent abnormalities in schizophrenia. II. Longitudinal stability and relationship to symptom change. *Biological Psychiatry, 43,* 31–39.

van den Bosch, R. J. (1983). Contingent negative variation and psychopathology: Frontal-central distribution, and association with performance measures. *Biological Psychiatry, 18,* 615–633.

van den Bosch, R. J., Rozendaal, N., & Mol, J. M. F. A. (1988). Slow potential correlates of frontal function, psychosis, and negative symptoms. *Psychiatry Research, 23,* 201–208.

Voglmaier, M. M., Seidman, L. J., Salisbury, D., & McCarley, R. (1997). Neuropsychological dysfunction in schizotypal personality disorder. *Biological Psychiatry, 41,* 530–540.

Walker, H. A., & Birch, H. C. (1970). Lateral preference and right-left awareness in schizophrenic children. *Journal of Nervous and Mental Disease, 151,* 341–351.

Ward, P. B., Catts, S. V., Fox, A. M.,. Michie, P. T., & McConaghy, N. (1991). Auditory selective attention and event-related potentials in schizophrenia. *British Journal of Psychiatry, 158,* 534–539.

Ward, P. B., Catts, S. V., & McConaghy, N. (1992). P300 and conceptual loosening in normals: An event-related potential correlate of "thought disorder"? *Biological Psychiatry, 31,* 650–660.

Weinberger, D. R. (1999). Cell biology of the hippocampal formation in schizophrenia. *Biological Psychiatry, 45,* 395–411.

Weinberger, D. R., Berman, K. F., & Zec, R. F. (1986). Physiological dysfunction of dorsolateral prefrontal cortex in schizophrenia: I. Regional cerebral blood flow (rCBF) evidence. *Archives of General Psychiatry, 43,* 114–124.

White, M. S., Maher, B. A., & Manschreck, T. C. (1998). Hemispheric specialization in schizophrenics with perceptual aberration. *Schizophrenia Research, 32*, 161–170.

White, P. M., Yees, C. M., Neuchterlein, K. H., & Wirshing, D. A. (1997, October). P50 gating in schizophrenic patients exposed to a psychological stressor. Presented at the *Meeting of the Society for Research on Psychopathology*, Palm Springs, CA.

Williams, M. (1966). The effect of context on schizophrenic speech. *British Journal of Social and Clinical Psychology, 5*, 161–171.

Woldorff, M., Gallen, S., Hampson, S, Hillyard, S., Pantev, C., Sobel, D., & Bloom, F. E. (1993). Modulation of early sensory processing in human auditory cortex during auditory selective attention. *Proceedings of the National Academy of Science, 90*, 8722–8726.

Yee, C., & Miller, G. A. (1994). A dual-task analysis of resource allocation in dysthymia and anhedonia. *Journal of Abnormal Psychology, 103*, 625–636.

Yee, C., Neuchterlein, K., Morris, S., & White, P. (1998). P50 suppression in recent-onset schizophrenia: Clinical correlates and risperidone effects. *Journal of Abnormal Psychology, 107*, 691–698.

Yurgelun-Todd, D. A., Waternaux, C. M., Cohen, B., Gruber, S. A., English, C. D., & Renshaw, P. F. (1996). Functional magnetic resonance imaging of schizophrenic patients and comparison subjects during word production. *American Journal of Psychiatry, 153*, 200–205.

Zouridakis, G., Boutrous, N. N., & Jansen, B. H. (1997). A fuzzy clustering approach to study the auditory P50 component in schizophrenia. *Psychiatry Research, 69*, 169–181.

# CHAPTER 14

# Genetics and Schizophrenia

Franz Schneider and Patricia J. Deldin

## Introduction

Human beings have had an intuitive understanding of the concept of heredity for centuries. In his 1621 book, *The Anatomy of Melancholy*, Robert Burton wrote, "That ... inbred cause of Melancholy is our [temperament], in whole or part, which we receive from our parents ... it being a hereditary disease;" (Whybrow, 1997, p. 106). A century ago, Gregor Mendel deduced how genes function in heredity through his experiments breeding pea plants, even though he had no knowledge of the physiological mechanisms underlying genetics. The discovery of DNA by Crick and Watson in 1953 provided an understanding of the raw material of genes that has enabled the genetic revolution we have since enjoyed (Watson, 1981).

During this century, perceptions of the significance of genetic etiologies to various illnesses have waxed and waned, as much influenced by social and political trends as by the state of scientific knowledge. Recently, astonishing advances have been achieved in the techniques and understanding of biotechnology, for example, the ability to examine genetic material at the DNA level (Dickerson, 1983). This progress during the last two decades has led to a resurgence of interest in genetic contributions to traits in general and to disease processes in particular.

## Genetics and Mental Illness

During this century, views about the balance between the etiologic components underlying mental illness have been in flux between the poles of the "nature versus nurture" debate. There are many shadings of the perceived etiologic balance, and extreme opinions range from the view of totally genetic etiology, as exemplified by the eugenics movement early in this century, to a totally environmental etiology, for example, Theodore Lidz's concept of schizophrenogenic mothers causing schizophrenia (Lidz, 1973). However, this review of the literature will reveal competing evidence supporting both genetic and environmental etiologies. Thus, the first conclusion is that elements of both etiologies are apparent in schizophrenia.

Two distinct models might account for the fact that both genetic and environmental etiologies are associated with schizophrenia. Some suggest that this reflects the fact that there are actually two or more distinct diseases, which share enough common symptoms that each is called schizophrenia. An alternative possibility is that the presence of both etiologies is a manifestation of a diathesis-stress model. Such a model supposes that genetics provides an individual with a degree of predisposition to a disease but that the onset of the disease is triggered by an environmental stressor(s), depending on the genetic predisposition of the individual. The diathesis-stress model has fit circumstances

**Franz Schneider** • Department of Psychiatry, Harvard Medical School, Boston, Massachusetts 02115. **Patricia J. Deldin** • Department of Psychology, Harvard University, Cambridge, Massachusetts 02138.

*Comprehensive Handbook of Psychopathology* (Third Edition), edited by Patricia B. Sutker and Henry E. Adams. Kluwer Academic / Plenum Publishers, New York, 2001.

well for other mental illnesses with both hereditary and environmental components, such as alcoholism (Vaillant, 1995).

Some dichotomies between possible multiple
diseases will be discussed in the next section, and
in reviewing evidence throughout this review, it
will be important to keep in mind this overall
question of what the appropriate model is. At the
outset, the diathesis-stress model seems better
supported due to the logic of several critical observations; specifically, in the case of families that
are known to be at genetic risk for schizophrenia,
only a minority of the family members actually
develop the disorder. Conversely, to the extent that
whole populations have been exposed to what is
an environmental risk factor, only a small minority
develop the disease.

Because it is likely that schizophrenia at least in
part results from a genetic etiology, the first body
of evidence to be examined will be studies that
may quantify the degree of heritability. These are
observational studies, in particular twin studies.
The existence of both monozygotic and dizygotic
twins is sometimes called an experiment of nature,
and over the years comparison of the concordance
rates for a disease between the two types of twins
has been used to calculate heritability. This review
will examine the limitations of these studies, in
particular, some of their significant methodological problems.

Following a review of evidence for familial
transmission of schizophrenia, a second area of
the literature will examine physiological evidence
that may be relevant to the later review of both
environmental and genetic factors that contribute
to schizophrenia. Such physiological evidence
may be of interest for two reasons. To the extent
physiological traits exist that are associated with
schizophrenia, such features may contribute to
developing and understanding possible mechanisms that might explain how genetic or environmental etiologies, or both, are expressed. Of special interest will be several biological markers that
are associated with schizophrenic patients, and in
some cases, also with the well relatives of patients.

The third area of the schizophrenia literature to
be examined will be that suggesting environmental etiologies. Although an important purpose of
this review is to come to conclusions about the
relative importance of genetic and environmental
etiologies, the base case at the outset is the consensus in the field that schizophrenia has a strong
genetic component. One way to challenge that
predominant view will be to review studies that
have produced evidence suggesting that in some
circumstances the onset of schizophrenia results
from environmental stressors. Examples of reported environmental risk factors that will be
examined below include viral exposure, especially to the fetus; other in utero insults; and season and place of birth, not because these are actual
risk factors, but because they seem to be proxies
for yet unknown stressors.

The fourth and final area to be reviewed will be
evidence that has been reported in the literature to
support genetic etiologies. Given the enormous
interest supporting genetic research, we will focus
primarily on three particular issues: what is the
most likely genetic model for schizophrenia, how
useful have the specific techniques of linkage
analysis been, and what techniques might make
the application of genetic analysis more tractable.
Finally, a review of the results of a number of
studies related to specific chromosomes or specific
candidate genes considered related to schizophrenia will illustrate the current limitations of
genetic analysis techniques.

The conclusions section will summarize the evidence this review has identified that answers the
research questions described before. In addition,
this final section will look beyond the specifics of
the genetic and environmental etiologies to see
how they are related through the diathesis-stress
model and to examine the etiologies that contribute to the incidence of schizophrenia in the general
population. Finally, some comments and suggestions will be offered about the way schizophrenia
research priorities might be altered.

## Taxonomies of Schizophrenia

Several theories related to the etiologies of
schizophrenia have proposed a number of distinctions between the symptoms of schizophrenia and
also between possible subtypes of schizophrenia.
For some studies, these distinctions have provided
a framework for the design of experiments. For
this reason, a number of these distinctions will be
examined now, and the rationale underlying them
will be discussed in the context of the theories they
support.

## Positive and Negative Symptoms

The dichotomy between the positive and negative symptoms of schizophrenia is perhaps the most frequently employed distinction in studying the disorder. This dichotomy is relevant to a review of genetic research because a number of theories and the studies supporting them suggest possibly different etiologies for these two types of symptoms. This dichotomy has also been important in the history of schizophrenia research.

The work of the two pioneers in psychiatric research, Emil Kraepelin, a German psychiatrist, and Eugen Bleuler, a Swiss psychiatrist, took place in the years bracketing the turn of this century. In 1883, Kraepelin first gave the disorder we now know as schizophrenia the name *dementia praecox*, literally precocious dementia; this reflected his belief that this was a progressive neurodegenerative disease (Kendall & Hammen, 1995). Writing in 1911, Bleuler named the disorder schizophrenia, adding the set of symptoms he called *paraphrenia* (hallucinations and delusions) to the dementia described by Kraepelin. Bleuler considered schizophrenia a thought disorder, and its primary symptoms were emotional blunting and an impaired relationship with the outside world; the more dramatic paraphrenia symptoms were secondary (Tsuang & Faraone, 1997).

Reflecting this early insight, the presence or absence of positive or negative symptoms has become a useful classification system. *Positive symptoms* may be considered acute symptoms seen when patients are in their worst states, thus including the hallmark symptoms of delusions and auditory hallucinations, as well as disorganized speech and grossly disorganized or catatonic behavior.

*Negative symptoms*, sometimes called *deficit symptoms*, are usually described as affective flattening or emotional blunting, but often include apathy, lack of motivation, lack of pleasure, and impaired social and personal relationships. The negative symptoms tend to be more chronic than the positive symptoms. Although the bizarre nature of the positive symptoms calls attention to sufferers of schizophrenia, they are usually present only during a minor period of time, and they are often amenable to treatment by pharmaceuticals. The negative symptoms are typically stubbornly persistent and therefore harder to treat.

Some have questioned whether a simple dichotomy between positive and negative symptoms represents an adequate framework for describing schizophrenic patients. Reporting on the results of factor analyses performed in three published studies of schizophrenic patients plus a large pooled sample, one group of researchers concluded that "... more than two distinct dimensions are required to categorise symptoms in schizophrenia" (Arndt, Alliger, & Andreasen, 1991). These investigators' additional dimensionality involved splitting the positive symptom domain into more distinct factors.

More recently, data on 114 sibling pairs afflicted with schizophrenia or schizoaffective disorder were examined to determine what correlations might be detected along three dimensions of symptoms: positive, negative, and disorganized (Loftus, DeLisi, & Crow, 1998). There was a more than chance correlation for the disorganization dimension that led the investigators to conclude that this disorganization subsyndrome might be a suitable phenotypic marker for genetic linkage studies.

## A Neurodevelopmental or Neurodegenerative Disorder?

Although Kraepelin's characterization of schizophrenia as dementia praecox implied that this is a neurodegenerative disease, Bleuler's experience with the disease was such that although he knew complete recovery was rare, he did not necessarily see the irreversible decline of a degenerative disease. His prescience is demonstrated by the fact that debate continues on this point. In a review, Goldberg, Hyde, Kleinman, and Weinberger set out to evaluate evidence to determine whether the nature of cognitive function in schizophrenia was one of progressive dementia or one analogous to a static encephalopathy (1993). Based on their review of longitudinal and cross-sectional studies, they concluded that the latter, nondegenerative, interpretation was strongly supported. Particular data supporting this conclusion was found in a cross-sectional study that administered tests sensitive to progressive dementing diseases to patients in their third through seventh decades of life.

However, a more recent study was designed to address the issue of whether the ventricular neuropathology in schizophrenia is degenerative or is fully expressed at onset and stable thereafter (Nair et al., 1997). MRI volumetric analysis was performed during a two- to three-year period on a group of eighteen patients with symptoms of schizophrenia, as well as on a control group. The measured rate of ventricular expansion (RVE) for the patients was bimodally distributed. The RVE for a group of ten patients was $0.9 \pm 0.5$ cm³/year, a rate similar to that of the controls ($0.7 \pm 0.6$ cm³/year). The other eight patients as a group exhibited a rate of $3.9 \pm 0.7$ cm³/year.

These results support a dichotomy between a more common form of schizophrenia that does not feature neurodegeneration and a less common form that does. Such a finding is consistent with the clinical experience that a minority of schizophrenic patients do suffer progressive cognitive deterioration. A stable neuropathy after onset might be accounted for by a neurodevelopmental model under which the damage is done during the developmental period of the brain, and little further damage occurs once that developmental period has ended, a time that typically coincides with the age of onset of schizophrenia.

As evidence from various studies is reviewed here, it may be useful to keep this possible neurodevelopmental–neurodegeneration dichotomy in mind. In examining the relative merits of claims for genetic and environmental etiologies, it is possible that one etiology may fit one side of this spectrum better than the other.

### Familial and Sporadic Schizophrenia

As research has increasingly focused on possible genetic causes of schizophrenia, some investigators have proposed making a distinction between *familial* and *sporadic* forms of schizophrenia. The defining principle is simple: familial schizophrenia is seen when the family of a patient has a higher prevalence of schizophrenia than the general population. Because those without this familial aspect of the disease lack a readily apparent genetic etiology, their form of the illness is called sporadic schizophrenia. However, this distinction does not necessarily contemplate the existence of two separate disorders. Rather, this is an attempt to define certain characteristics of schizophrenia that may be seen consistently in the familial form and a different constellation of characteristics seen for the sporadic form.

Unfortunately, to develop a consistent familial–sporadic dichotomy requires navigating through a thicket of possibly conflicting evidence. For example, a review of this distinction by two authorities in the field reports that schizophrenia resulting from neurodevelopmental problems early in life is more common among sporadic patients than familial patients (Tsuang & Faraone, 1997). However, they also observe that sporadic schizophrenic patients show evidence of brain atrophy, a characteristic typical of the degenerative form of illness. The most distinctive difference in symptoms that Tsuang and Faraone report are in brain function; familial patients exhibit more problems with attention span and distractibility.

The results of a study of the co-twins and first-degree relatives of thirty-one monozygotic and twenty-eight dizygotic twin probands may shed some light on this issue, although in the process the authors suggest yet another distinction, that between paranoid and nonparanoid schizophrenia (Onstad, Skre, Torgersen, & Kringlen, 1991). These investigators reported that nonparanoid schizophrenia was more commonly observed among the monozygotic probands than the paranoid type, thus implying that the type of disease more likely to be transmitted genetically is the nonparanoid. Considering that the delusions typical of paranoia are hallmark positive symptoms, we might reason that familial schizophrenia is more likely to be characterized by a predominance of negative symptoms. Keeping in mind that positive symptoms can be induced (and reversed) by certain psychoactive drugs, we may conclude that the sporadic type of schizophrenia offers a better long-term prognosis, which in fact has been the clinical experience.

### The Problem of Heterogeneity

In a scientific context, the word heterogeneity usually refers to the problems introduced into an investigation in which the experimental subjects differ in more than one variable. Ideally, in conducting a controlled study of a trait, the clearest results, and thus the most supportable conclusions, are obtained if all of the subjects are exactly alike, except for that one trait. Of course, the real world does not conform to this ideal, and so scientific research usually has to address the potential confounding effects introduced by the heterogeneity of the subjects used in an investigation.

Heterogeneity also emerges as a research problem if the disorder under study may be composed of several different forms with common symptoms as an end point. From this discussion, we can see that schizophrenia is quite likely to be a heterogeneous disorder. Reflecting this, a complicated series of rules have been set out by the authors of DSM-IV to determine a diagnosis of schizophrenia. But beyond problems of diagnosis, substantial heterogeneity is encountered in the symptoms displayed (or not displayed) by patients suffering from schizophrenia. For example, as will be discussed in "Review of Physiological Evidence," about 70% of schizophrenic patients exhibit smooth eye tracking dysfunction, as do 45% of the well relatives of the patients. But the remaining 30% of patients and 55% of relatives show no such eye movement dysfunction. In other mental illnesses, for example, mood disorders, the various defining symptoms are usually observed to a greater or lesser extent but are not likely to be either present or absent.

Finally, heterogeneity should be mentioned in the very technical context of genetic analysis. Here, the problem is the human genome, which contains approximately 100,000 different genes, as specified by approximately 2 billion base pairs of DNA. Given the enormous diversity displayed by the human species, a minefield of potential confounds await those who undertake research in human genetics. As will be seen in "Evidence from Genetic Research," a number of investigative techniques have been developed to minimize the impact of these confounds. Specifically, experience has taught that combining the results of genetic testing from diverse racial, ethnic, and geographical groups must be avoided. Conversely, confining an investigation to a pedigree of related individuals has become the most promising path to obtaining usable data in genetic analysis. These topics will be discussed in more detail in "Evidence from Genetic Research."

# Review of Evidence Indicating Transmission Within Families

In the first section, four general categories of the research literature on schizophrenia were identified for review: evidence of transmission within families, physiological evidence, environmental evidence, and genetic evidence. Evidence of familial transmission of schizophrenia is the logical

place to start because many of the earliest attempts to understand the nature of schizophrenia were prompted by the observation that the disorder runs in families.

Reflecting the wide variety and combinations of symptoms seen in those suffering from schizophrenia, a number of distinctly divergent mechanisms have been proposed as etiologies for the disorder. That there is a genetic component is certainly not in doubt at this time. Over the years, heritability data have been compiled from many observational studies. One consistent result seen in these studies is that the incidence of schizophrenia in first-degree relatives of schizophrenic patients is typically elevated by roughly an order of magnitude over the 1% incidence in the general population.

## Family Association Studies

Family association studies collect data on the incidence of schizophrenia (and sometimes, other mental illnesses) within the families of schizophrenic patients. For example, one study compared the lifetime incidence of schizophrenia in 723 first-degree relatives of schizophrenic patients with the incidence in 1056 first-degree relatives of matched controls (Kendler, Gruenberg, & Tsuang, 1985). A number of analyses were performed using a variety of techniques, and the investigators reported at least an 18-fold greater incidence in the relatives of schizophrenic patients than in the controls. Interestingly, the relatives of schizophrenic patients did not show any elevated incidence for unipolar disorder, anxiety disorder, or alcoholism. This reported elevation in lifetime risk for relatives of schizophrenic patients is somewhat higher than the rates encountered in subsequent studies.

For example, in a study using data from a rural county in Ireland, the relatives of 285 identified schizophrenic patients exhibited a 6.5% lifetime risk for schizophrenia, which can be compared to the generally accepted 1% worldwide lifetime incidence in the general population (Kendler et al., 1993a). In a subsequent report based on additional data from the rural Irish country, the same investigators concluded that a family liability to schizophrenia did not substantially increase the risk to affective disorders, anxiety disorders, or alcoholism (Kendler et al., 1993b). The investigators also concluded that these data did not support a sometimes proposed hypothesis that schizophrenia and

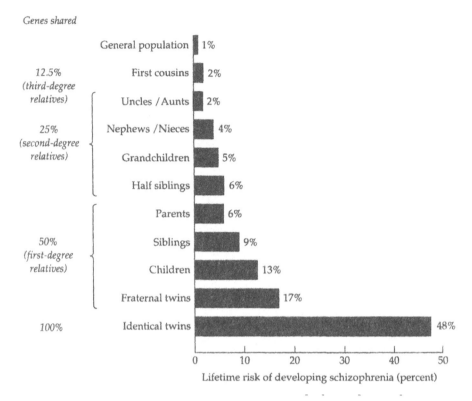

*Genes shared*

**Figure 1.** Lifetime risk of developing schizophrenia based on family relationship. From *Schizophrenia Genesis* by Gottesman. Copyright 1991 by Irving I. Gottesman. Used with permission by W.H. Freeman and Company.

affective illnesses are on a single etiologic continuum from a familial perspective.

Figure 1 depicts data adapted from Gottesman (1991, p. 96) that shows the elevation of lifetime risk of schizophrenia for various family relationships, specifically, for first-degree relatives who share half of their genes, second-degree relatives who share one-quarter of their genes, and third-degree relatives who share one-eighth of their genes. Of particular interest are the differing rates for the four types of first-degree relatives.

The apparently lower lifetime risk for parents (6%) probably reflects the fact that those who suffer from schizophrenia are less likely to reproduce, thus creating an apparent reduction in lifetime risk for the parental generation. Conversely, the higher rate for children of schizophrenic patients (13%) probably reflects the opposite phenomenon. The 9% figure for siblings may indicate a lifetime risk that is not biased by either of these generational effects. Because fraternal twins are

literally just siblings that happened to be born at the same time, the relatively high lifetime incidence of 17% is surprising. Reasons for such an elevation in fraternal twins will be discussed later in the context of twin studies.

One final comment should be made to point out that these observational studies cannot discriminate whether genetic or environmental influences are at work. Thus, elevated lifetime risks are not necessarily derived from a genetic etiology; conceivably, these effects may result from common environmental factors.

## Twin Studies

Twin studies can be designed so that conclusions about heritability can be drawn. They exploit the fact that monozygotic (identical) twins have exactly the same genetic makeup, whereas dizygotic (fraternal) twins, on average, share half of their genes. Specifically, these studies collect data from twin sets in which at least one twin has been diagnosed with schizophrenia. Then concordance rates (the percentage of twin pairs in which both have been diagnosed with schizophrenia) are compared between monozygotic and dizygotic sets of twins. If a disease has a purely genetic etiology, we would expect to see a 100% concordance in monozygotic twins; on the other hand, dizygotic twins should exhibit a significantly lower rate of concordance. Indeed, this is exactly the case with Huntington's disease, which features a purely genetic etiology.

Table 1 provides a summary of the concordance rates observed in eight major twin studies. The pairwise figures are the more useful because the proband method double counts individual twins in some cases, although it is often seen in popular literature.

As seen in the two lines at the bottom of the table, the averaged figures are 26% concordance (identical), compared to 8% (fraternal) if the only three studies considered are those which the authors consider were the best executed. Averaging all of the studies results in a 28% to 6% comparison. Of course, the fact that concordance rates for identical twins, who have exactly the same genes, are less than 30% implies that one or more causative factors other than genetics are also responsible for the disease.

To gain some perspective on the different rates of heritability seen among mental illnesses, Table 2 shows the pairwise concordance rates for twelve disorders. Topping the list is Huntington's disease that is 100% concordant in identical twins, compared to 20% for fraternal twins. This is not surprising because Huntington's disease, it has been shown, results from a single dominant gene. Thus, possession of that gene by one identical twin would make it certain that the other twin would also develop the disease. Schizophrenia is low on the list and has a monozygotic concordance rate about the same as that for multiple sclerosis.

On reflection, there are several issues that imply that results from twin studies may not be entirely applicable to the general population. First, it may be that a twin pregnancy incurs stresses not seen in a normal pregnancy. An additional logical flaw is apparent in the assumption that the concordance rate for identical twins quantifies the genetic component of schizophrenia. This assumes that each identical twin experiences exactly the same environmental effects in utero (Torrey, 1992). But, following this logic, both twins would also be expected to have the same birth weight, which is

### Table 1. Twin Concordance Rates for Schizophrenia[a]

| Study | Identical twins | | Fraternal twins | |
|---|---|---|---|---|
| | Probandwise method (%) | Pairwise method (%) | Probandwise method (%) | Pairwise method (%) |
| Tienari (1975) | 26 (6/23) | 15 (3/20) | 13 (6/45) | 7 (3/42) |
| Kringlen (1967) | 46 (26/57) | 31 (14/45) | 13 (12/96) | 7 (6/90) |
| Fischer (1973) | 39 (9/25) | 24 (5/21) | 18 (8/45) | 10 (4/41) |
| Essen-Moller (1970) | 50 (4/8) | 50 (4/8) | 7 (2/27) | 7 (2/27) |
| Slater & Shields (1953) | 68 (28/41) | 65 (24/37) | 18 (11/61) | 14 (8/58) |
| Gottesman & Shields (1972) | 58 (15/26) | 41 (9/22) | 12 (4/34) | 9 (3/33) |
| Kendler & Robinette (1991) | 31 (60/194) | 18 (30/164) | 7 (18/277) | 3 (9/268) |
| Onstad et al. | 48 (15/31) | 33 (8/24) | 4 (1/28) | 4 (1/28) |
| Total  Tienari, Kringlen, and Fischer only | 39 (41/105) | 26 (22/86) | 14 (26/186) | 8 (13/173) |
| Total  All studies | 40 (163/405) | 28 (97/341) | 15 (62/427) | 6 (36/587) |

[a]Adapted from Are we overestimating the genetic contribution to schizophrenia? by E. F. Torrey, 1992, *Schizophrenia Bulletin, 18*, 159–170; and When assessing twin concordance, use the probandwise not the pairwise rate by M. McGue, 1992, *Schizophrenia Bulletin, 18*, 171–176.

## Table 2. Twin Concordance Rates for Various Nervous System Disorders[a]

| Disorder | Identical twins (%) | Fraternal twins (%) |
|---|---|---|
| Huntington's disease | 100 (14/14) | 20 (1/5) |
| Down's syndrome | 98 (18/19) | 2 (2/127) |
| Epilepsy | 61 (20/46) | 10 (13/126) |
| Mental retardation | 60 (18/30) | 9 (7/77) |
| Bipolar disorder | 56 (44/79) | 14 (16/111) |
| Cerebral palsy | 40 (6/15) | 0 (0/21) |
| Autism | 36 (4/11) | 0 (0/10) |
| Poliomyelitis | 36 (5/14) | 6 (2/31) |
| Congenital anomalies of the CNS | 33 (2/6) | 0 (0/5) |
| Schizophrenia | 28 (97/341) | 6 (36/587) |
| Multiple sclerosis | 27 (17/62) | 2 (2/88) |
| Parkinson's disease | 0 (0/18) | 7 (1/14) |

[a]Adapted from Are we overestimating the genetic contribution to schizophrenia? by E. F. Torrey, 1992, *Schizophrenia Bulletin*, *18*, 159–170.

usually not the case. Thus, although it is clear that identical twins are exactly alike at conception, there are significant ways in which one twin may be subjected to stressors that the other twin escapes. For instance, the way in which twins share the womb and their blood supply can provide an environmental stress on only one twin; however, any changed outcome caused by such a stressor will be counted as a genetic effect. Another potential confound is that whether one or both twins are affected by a stressor such as a virus may be a matter of chance. For example, one study of identical twins born to HIV-infected mothers revealed that of six such twin pairs, three were concordant for the virus, and three discordant (Torrey et al., 1994, p. 19).

Nevertheless, despite these methodological and logical issues, twin studies over the years have provided data that strongly suggests some degree of genetic etiology in schizophrenia. However, the previous discussion has pointed out that the interpretation of the data and certain methodological issues have tended to overstate the likely degree of heritability. Given these limitations, it may be that the use of twin studies has reached a limit in its ability to quantify the genetic etiology of schizophrenia.

## Adoption Studies

Conceptually, adoption studies are designed to control for a potentially significant confound in twin studies; that twins reared together, in addition to sharing genes, are likely to share many environmental influences. Although a number of different designs have been used, the subjects in many adoption studies have been schizophrenic patients who were adopted shortly after birth; typically, matched controls (who were also adopted) are selected as well. An indication of the relative contributions of genetics and family environment can be assessed by comparing the incidence of schizophrenia in the families of both the biological and adoptive parents of the schizophrenic probands.

Unlike twin studies as discussed before, relatively few adoption studies have examined schizophrenia. Although most of these adoption studies have confirmed some likely genetic component, these studies are harder to compare than twin studies because of significant design differences. Nor have their results uniformly produced statistically significant results (for example, see Wender et al., 1986).

One different design produced particularly interesting results from a nationwide Finnish study in which the adopted-away offspring of mothers diagnosed with schizophrenia were compared with matched controls who were adopted away from normal parents (Tienari, 1991: Tienari et al., 1985, 1987). Although the results supported the hypothesized transmission of a genetic predisposition from mothers diagnosed with schizophrenia to schizophrenic probands, a significant effect related to the adoptive family was also detected. Specifically, no cases of schizophrenia were found in forty-three probands raised in relatively normal adoptive families, whereas schizophrenia was present in fifteen of thirty-nine probands (38%) raised in disturbed adoptive families. This led the investigators to conclude that "this combination of findings supports the hypothesis that a possible genetic vulnerability has interacted with the adoptive rearing environment" (Tienari et al., 1985, p. 227).

Although adoption studies in theory should improve the twin study design by separating the genes of subjects from their family environment, adoption studies also suffer from methodological problems; some of them are unique, and some also affect twin studies. In particular, the evidence for environmental effects discussed later makes clear that the in utero period is a likely venue for significant environmental effects. Like twin studies, adoption studies are vulnerable to this potentially substantial confound. If there is an in utero effect, both twin and adoption studies will count it as a genetic effect. Given this uncertainty, it must be concluded that neither twin nor adoption studies can prove genetic etiology, nor can these types of studies rule out other types of etiologies.

## Review of Physiological Evidence

Making the research problem all the more interesting is that unlike many mental illnesses, the study of schizophrenia has revealed a significant number of physiological anomalies that often accompany the disease, and sometimes precede it as well. However, despite these many anomalies, the only physiological evidence relevant to this review is that which may demonstrate a link to the etiology of the disorder. In this regard, the physiological anomalies of most interest are those observed in schizophrenic patients and also in the relatives of patients. For this reason, two specific physiological phenomena will be reviewed: eye movement dysfunction and the inhibition of certain event-related potentials (ERP) that can be recorded by an electroencephalograph, specifically, the P50, a positive wave that occurs 50 ms after an event.

### Eye Movement Dysfunction

It has been known for twenty-five years that eye tracking dysfunction is much more frequently seen in schizophrenic patients than in the general population. In particular, the most consistently seen dysfunction is poor smooth-pursuit eye tracking, that is, in following the track of a moving object, a schizophrenic patient is more likely to exhibit jerky eye movements, rather than the smooth tracking normally seen.

Ten years after such smooth-pursuit eye movement dysfunction had first been noticed, a study was conducted to follow-up on previous studies that found this dysfunction in from 50 to 85% of schizophrenic patients (Holzman, Solomon, Levin, & Waternaux, 1984). Similar smooth-pursuit eye movement dysfunction was found in 34% of the parents (and 55% of the parent pairs) of schizophrenic patients, compared with the 8% rate of the general population. Interestingly, parental eye movement dysfunction was significantly related to the patient's diagnosis and not to the patient's eye tracking performance. This led the investigators to conclude that eye tracking dysfunction represented a familial marker of vulnerability to schizophrenia.

Writing four years later, Holzman et al. (1988) noted that eye movement dysfunctions (EMDs) were found in a majority of schizophrenic patients and in 45% of their first-degree relatives and reported a study in which eye movements of the offspring of monozygotic and dizygotic twins were recorded. Among their conclusions was the statement "the data suggest that EMDs and at least some schizophrenias can be considered expressions of a single underlying trait that is transmitted by an autosomal dominant gene" (p. 641).

In stark contrast to the results obtained in the studies of Holzman et al. were the results of a later study of four normal control pairs of identical twins and eleven pairs discordant for schizophrenia (Torrey et al., 1994). Although the schizophrenic patients showed elevated rates of EMD, the eye tracking scores of their well co-twins were statistically indistinguishable from the scores of the normals. In addition, no correlations for the affected twins were found between EMD and variables associated with the disorder, such as family history for serious mental illnesses, physiological anomalies, and various indices related to medication status.

Because EMD has been discussed as a genetic marker for liability to schizophrenia and because genomic scans have indicated that the short arm of chromosome 6 may be a possible location for a gene related to schizophrenia, an analysis was performed at the 6p21-23 region of the chromosome to test for linkage between chromosomal markers and EMD as well as schizophrenia (Arolt et al., 1996). Testing five models of EMD inheritance, a logarithm of the odds ratio (LOD) score of statistical interest was found. However, after testing with seven models of schizophrenia inheritance, no significant results were obtained; this raised the question whether EMD is a marker for detecting schizophrenia linkage that is more sensitive than the actual disease status.

Finally, a very recent study examined differences in saccadic eye movements (which are reflexive, jerky movements) among twenty-nine schizophrenic patients, fifty of their nonpsychotic first-degree relatives, and thirty-eight unrelated controls (Crawford et al., 1998). They were testing a hypothesis that schizophrenic patients could not reliably inhibit reflexive saccades. Although patients, their relatives, and the controls showed no difference in generating reflexive saccades, the patients showed more saccadic distractibility. Relatives of patients with high distractibility also showed high distractibility. The investigators concluded that the antisaccade anomaly in this distractible subset of patients (and their relatives) might represent a schizophrenia vulnerability marker.

### P50 Inhibition

The connection of ERPs to schizophrenia has been studied since the 1980s. Although much of the earlier research focused on the P300 ERP, more recent research on the P50 may be of more interest because a P50 phenomenon is seen in many schizophrenic patients and also in a significant number of their well relatives (Freedman et al., 1997). The abnormality is related to the inhibition of the second of the two P50 responses to closely paired auditory stimuli. Specifically, when normal people hear pairs of sounds presented close together, they will inhibit their responses to the second sounds, evidence of a rapid habituation reaction to the sound. However, many schizophrenic patients will not inhibit the second wave so that both waves are of the same amplitude, as has been demonstrated in a number of studies (e.g., Clementz, Geyer, & Braff, 1998).

A theory may be proposed that this inability to inhibit specific responses, perhaps symptomatic of a generalized inability to inhibit stimuli, may be the source of various schizophrenic symptoms such as distractibility, confusion, or even some of the more bizarre symptoms, such as hearing multiple voices. A recent study, using forty-seven schizophrenic patients for whom complete neuropsychological and clinical data were available, tested for this P50 abnormality, and then separated the subjects into high- and low-P50 abnormality groups (Erwin, Turetsky, Moberg, Gur, & Gur, 1998). A multivariate analysis of variance for the eleven neuropsychological profile scores showed that the high-abnormality group had relatively greater deficits for attentional profile scores than

for the remaining measures. An analysis of the P50 data and the subjects' Scale for the Assessment of Negative Symptoms (SANS) scores revealed one significant difference: the high-abnormality group was also rated as more severe only on the SANS attention subscale.

This review of physiological evidence has identified two anomalies that may have a bearing on the etiology of schizophrenia. We will revisit these anomalies in the review of genetic analysis contained in "Evidence from Genetic Research," when evidence related to several specific chromosomes and candidate genes is examined. The phenomena of eye tracking dysfunction and P50 inhibition described before may be linked to chromosomes 6 and 15, respectively.

## Review of Environmental Evidence

Decades ago, before a significant genetic etiology had become generally accepted, the common wisdom was that schizophrenia was caused by environmental factors experienced during the patient's youth. In particular, dysfunctional family settings and styles of parenting were believed to cause the disease. Since that time, such ideas have properly receded to the background, and in addition to evidence of heritability, evidence has slowly been uncovered pointing to environmental influences very early in life, specifically, during pregnancy. This section will examine some of that evidence.

However, at the outset it should be kept in mind that because environmental and genetic evidence are being reviewed separately, does not imply that a dichotomy exists such that any specific case of schizophrenia reflects only a genetic etiology or only an environmental etiology. In the first section, the diathesis-stress model was identified as providing a conceptual framework that can incorporate evidence derived from both genetic studies and from studies that identify environmental stressors. In the Conclusions section, the suitability of the diathesis-stress model will be addressed again in the light of the evidence that has been reviewed. However, during the review of evidence, it must be kept in mind that any environmental stressor identified in this section is very likely to interact with some genetic predisposition. Similarly, any genetic mechanism revealed in the evidence considered in the next section is likely to interact with the many and varied stressors that are encountered in life, starting at conception.

## The Dutch Famine

The most dramatic evidence of an in utero effect was provided by a cruel experience of war. During the last winter of World War II, the Nazi forces imposed a severe but relatively short famine on certain parts of the Netherlands. Because of careful Dutch record keeping at the time, accurate assessments of daily food intake are available for this famine period. In a series of studies carried out by Susser and colleagues during eight years, the amount of food deprivation and its timing have been compared with the incidence of schizophrenia several decades later, as derived from a national psychiatric registry.

In the first study published, a hypothesis was tested that first-trimester exposure to acute food deprivation is a risk factor for schizophrenia (Susser & Lin, 1992). The key finding was that in the famine region, birth cohorts exposed to an average daily ration less than 4200 kJ during the first trimester showed a substantial increase in hospitalized schizophrenia for female offspring but not for males. Relative risks (RR) for these women were 2.56 for "restricted" schizophrenia (an International Classifications of Diseases [ICD] diagnosis comparable to current DSM rules for a diagnosis of schizophrenia), and 2.17 for a "broad" variant that included other schizophrenia spectrum disorders. The investigators also concluded that moderate food deprivation, that is, an average daily ration less than 6300 kJ, was not associated with increased risk of schizophrenia.

In their next published study, Susser and colleagues used more precise data on both exposure and outcome (Susser et al., 1996). By comparing the exposed and unexposed cohorts that had been born in western cities of the Netherlands after the famine, they found that the most exposed cohort, those conceived at the peak of the famine, had a twofold and statistically significant increase in the risk of schizophrenia in both men (RR = 1.9) and women (RR = 2.2). The most recently published study (Hoek, Brown, & Susser, 1998) reported on further examination of data related to the famine and concluded that "early prenatal famine was found to be specifically and robustly associated with each of three conditions: (A) congenital anomalies of the central nervous system, (B) schizophrenia, and (C) schizophrenia spectrum personality disorders" (p. 373). They found that the greatest increase in the risk of schizophrenia spectrum disorders occurred among men born in the famine cities in December 1945 (RR = 2.7), who were conceived at the absolute peak of the famine in March and April 1945.

## Viruses

Consistent with this idea of prenatal vulnerability, in utero viral exposure has been investigated as a possible risk factor for later development of schizophrenia. In one study, psychiatric hospital diagnoses were recorded for all individuals in greater Helsinki who had been fetuses during the 1957 type A2 influenza epidemic (Mednick, Machon, Huttunen, & Bonett, 1988). The key finding was that those who were exposed to the viral epidemic during their second trimester in utero had an elevated risk of being admitted to a psychiatric hospital with a diagnosis of schizophrenia. This was true for both males and females and was found independently in several psychiatric hospitals. Among the investigators' conclusions was that the observed viral effects should be considered just one of many possible perturbations in utero. They suggested that the critical factor in triggering future schizophrenia was the timing, rather than the type, of disturbance.

Another study utilized the extensive medical records kept by Denmark to look for any associations between influenza and schizophrenia (Barr, Mednick, & Munk-Jorgensen, 1990). The investigators ascertained the number of live births, births of future schizophrenic patients, and cases of influenza for each month from 1911 to 1950 from health records at the Ministry of Health. The investigators concluded that in periods when influenza rates were higher than seasonally expected, such elevated rates during the sixth month of gestation were correlated, and birth rates of future schizophrenic patients were higher than seasonally expected. They also concluded that this effect was not attributable to other winter-related factors or to climatic variables.

In a 1994 book that described what had been learned to date in their extensive study of mental illness and twins, the authors report finding antibodies to pestiviruses in the plasma of certain subjects (Torrey et al., 1994). Specifically, among the twenty-five identical twin pairs that were discordant for schizophrenia, ten of the patients (40%) had these antibodies, whereas none of the well co-twins did. Also, one of the sixteen normal control twins reacted to the pestivirus antigen. As to the nature of the group of viruses, the authors write, "this group of viruses is well known as animal pathogens but has not previously been found in humans.... Pestiviruses are especially interesting to schizophrenia researchers because the pestivirus that infects cattle is known to be transmitted in utero, but most cows do not develop symptoms for several years" (p. 99).

### Season of Year Effects

If the developing fetus is vulnerable to viruses, then it should not be surprising that a season of birth phenomenon for schizophrenia has been detected; a slight excess of those who will someday suffer from schizophrenia were born during the late winter months, which presumably reflects the lag time after the peak of "flu season." A study examined this phenomenon in detail and collected data as to season of birth and family history for 561 patients with a diagnosis of schizophrenia (O'Callaghan et al., 1991). Patients with no family history of any psychiatric disorder were significantly more likely to be born in winter than patients with a first-degree relative who was affected with schizophrenia. The investigators concluded, "in comparison with normal population controls, only those without a family history exhibited a significant excess of winter births, suggesting an environmental factor of greater aetiological significance in these patients" (p. 764).

A new study reports on data collected from nationwide databases in Denmark (Mortensen et al., 1999). Specifically, the investigators obtained data on every woman born in Denmark during a 43-year period (1935 to 1978), and their offspring born until the end of 1993. Fathers were also identified for 97.7% of these offspring. Of slightly more than 2 million offspring identified, 1.75 million were followed from the later of their fifth birthday or 1970 until the earlier of 1993, their deaths, emigration, or onset of schizophrenia. The diagnosis of interest for this study population was schizophrenia (defined by ICD-8), and using national psychiatric records, 2669 cases were identified among the offspring. Cases were also identified for parents and siblings.

From this data, relative risks were calculated for various categories of family history and for other factors. The calculated relative risks are shown in Table 3. Relative risks for those with affected mothers (9.31), fathers (7.20), and one or more affected siblings (6.99) were consistent with previously published studies. The relative risk for having both an affected mother and father (46.90) was notable not just because of its magnitude, but because it is a novel statistic due to its rarity; even in this population-wide study, both parents were affected in only 4 of the 2669 cases. This small number may support the argument that families heavily loaded for schizophrenia reproduce themselves to a significantly reduced degree.

Risk was also significantly associated with season of birth, was highest for those born in February and March, and lowest for those born in August and September. There was also a relative risk of 2.4 for those born in the capital, compared with those born in rural areas of Denmark; this effect was presumably due to a number of risk factors related to urban life, including a higher likelihood of contracting a virus.

The fact that such a large number of participants was tracked by Mortensen is bound to make conclusions about relative risk factors compelling, but the size of the sample also allowed the investigators to calculate population attributable risks, which the authors define as follows: "the population attributable risk is an estimate of the fraction of the total number of cases of schizophrenia in the population that would not have occurred if the effect of a specific risk factor had been eliminated—that is, if the risk could have been reduced to that of the exposure category with the lowest risk" (p. 604). The population attributable risks calculated by Mortensen and colleagues are given in Table 4.

The most surprising statistic is the very low population attributable risk (5.5%) for schizophrenia in a parent or sibling. The fact that these population attributable risks are not additive is illustrated by the fact that even considering all of the variables used by Mortensen, the population attributable risk was only 46.6%. However, it is striking that a family history accounts for only about 10% of the identified population attributable risks. Thus, although family history for schizophrenia creates much elevated relative risks for the disease, such family histories (or at least family histories that have been identified) account for a small minority of the incidence of schizophrenia in the general population. Accordingly, the two environmental factors chosen by Mortensen ac-

## Table 3. Adjusted Relative Risk of Schizophrenia According to Family History, Place of Birth, and Season of Birth

| Variable | Relative risk (95% CI)[a] |
|---|---|
| Family history | |
| Parent | |
| Father affected, mother affected | 46.90 (17.56–125.26) |
| Father affected, mother not affected | 7.20 (5.10–10.16) |
| Father not affected, mother affected | 9.31 (7.24–11.96) |
| Father not affected, mother not affected[b] | 1.00 |
| Father unknown, mother affected | 14.18 (8.48–23.70) |
| Father unknown, mother not affected | 2.00 (1.72–2.32) |
| Sibling | |
| One or more affected siblings | 6.99 (5.38–9.09) |
| No affected siblings[b] | 1.00 |
| Other factors | |
| Place of birth | |
| Capital | 2.40 (2.13–2.70) |
| Suburb of capital | 1.62 (1.37–1.90) |
| Provincial city (>100,000 population) | 1.57 (1.36–1.81) |
| Provincial town (<10,000 population) | 1.24 (1.10–1.41) |
| Rural area[b] | 1.00 |
| Greenland | 3.71 (2.04–6.76) |
| Other countries | 3.45 (2.69–4.44) |
| Unknown | 1.22 (0.46–3.27) |
| Season of birth (amplitude of sine function)[c] | 1.11 (1.06–1.19) |

[a]The relative risk was adjusted initially for age–sex interaction, calendar year of diagnosis, and ages of the father and mother (first adjustment) and then for family history or, alternatively, other factors as well (second adjustment). The third adjustment (full model) was for all the variables listed. CI denotes confidence interval.
[b]This was the reference category.
[c]For all three adjustments, the estimated peak of the sine function was March 6 (95% confidence interval, February 6 to April 5).
*Note.* From Effects of family history and place and season of birth on the risk of schizophrenia by P. B. Mortensen, C. B. Pedersen, T. Westergaard, J. Wohlfahrt, H. Ewald, O. Mors, P. K. Andersen, and M. Melbye, 1999, *New England Journal of Medicine, 340*(8), 605. Copyright 1999 Massachusetts Medical Society. All rights reserved.

count for the majority of schizophrenia cases. Perhaps retarding the realization that environmental effects are major contributors to the etiology of schizophrenia is the fact that factors like place of birth and season of birth are not the true risk factors, but rather are proxies for environmental agents that are yet unidentified.

## Obstetric Complications

Complications at birth as a risk factor for schizophrenia might seem like a logical extension of the prenatal risks discussed before, but evidence for such a risk factor is less compelling. One Irish study used as a sample population sixty-five patients who had diagnoses of schizophrenia, and their previously born same sex siblings were used as controls (O'Callaghan et al., 1992). Maternity hospital records were evaluated (blindly), and the main outcome measure was the presence of one or more obstetric complications recorded in maternity notes of patients and controls. By using siblings as controls (who share on average 50% of their genes), presumably, any confounding genetic influence would be reduced, thus helping to establish an environmental risk.

The primary finding was that patients with schizophrenia were significantly more likely than

**Table 4. Population Attributable Risk According to Family History, Place of Birth, and Season of Birth[a]**

| Variable | Population attributable risk (%) |
|---|---|
| Schizophrenia in one or both parents | 3.8 |
| Schizophrenia in one or more siblings | 1.9 |
| Schizophrenia in parent or sibling | 5.5 |
| Place of birth | 34.6 |
| Season of birth | 10.5 |
| Place and season of birth | 41.4 |
| All variables listed above | 46.6 |

[a]From Effects of family history and place and season of birth on the risk of schizophrenia by P. B. Mortensen, C. B. Pedersen, T. Westergaard, J. Wohlfahrt, H. Ewald, O. Mors, P. K. Andersen, and M. Melbye, 1999, *New England Journal of Medicine, 340*(8), 606. Copyright 1999 Massachusetts Medical Society. All rights reserved.

the controls to have experienced one or more obstetric complication (odds ratio = 2.44). Patients also showed a greater number, severity of, and total score for obstetric complications, although fetal distress was the only complication that occurred in significant individual excess; it was present in five (8%) patients, and was absent in controls. Obstetric complications in patients were unrelated to family history or season of birth but were associated with a significantly younger age of onset of illness (mean difference = 4.5 years).

However, another study, published several months later, came to the opposite conclusion (Buka, Tsuang, & Lipsett, 1993). To test the hypothesis that pregnancy and delivery complications result in increased risk for developing psychiatric disorders, this study examined the records of 1068 pregnancies classified as chronic fetal hypoxia, other complications, preterm birth, or normal pregnancy/delivery. These pregnancies had initially been followed prospectively from birth to age 7, and the subjects were recontacted at ages ranging from 18 to 27 years. The data did not show that rates of psychiatric disorders were higher for those who had experienced obstetric complications. Two trends were noted that did not achieve statistical significance: subjects born preterm had elevated rates of cognitive impairment, and subjects who experienced chronic fetal hypoxia also had elevated rates of both cognitive impairment and psychotic disorders.

## Signals From Childhood

One of the mysteries of schizophrenia is why the onset of the disorder does not take place until the late teenage years for most men and until the twenties for most women. However, with hindsight, it is possible to find clues that are usually overlooked. For example, in a grand epidemiological undertaking, the British Medical Research Council tracked every child born in the first week of March, 1946, until they reached the age of 43. Within this cohort of 5362, thirty cases of schizophrenia emerged. A group of investigators was able to access the accumulated childhood sociodemographic, neurodevelopmental, cognitive, and behavioral information that had been collected over the years (Jones, Rodgers, Murray, & Marmot, 1994).

Some of the associations they reported included the following: Milestones of motor development were reached later in patients than in controls. For example, whereas about one-third of the general population was two weeks or more late in sitting up, two-thirds were late among the future patients. Also, when patients were compared to the controls, the difference in means for age of walking was 1.2 months, and up to age 15, patients had more speech problems than controls. Predictors of schizophrenia included solitary play preferences at ages 4 and 6 (odds ratio = 2.1); at 15 years, teachers rated cases as more anxious in social situations. Finally, a health visitor's rating of the mother as below average in mothering skills and understanding of her child at age 4 years was a strong predictor of schizophrenia (odds ratio = 5.8).

In an interesting study of developmental precursors of schizophrenia, home movies of adult-onset schizophrenic patients and their healthy siblings were viewed by judges blind to the psychiatric outcome of the subjects (Walker & Lewine, 1990). The films covered the period from infancy until at least age 5. Although none of the children had psychiatric conditions at the time, the trained viewers could correctly identify the children who would go on to become patients. One investigator cited as an example the fact that at 2 years old, some future patients had "slightly odd hand movements," which although not likely to be noticed by a lay person, would be discernible to a trained observer as evidence of troubled motor development. The investigators concluded that "this represents the first demonstration that preschizophrenic subjects can be distinguished from sibling control subjects within the first eight years of life by observing their behavior" (p. 1052).

### Evidence for a Possible Neurodevelopmental Mechanism

Except for obstetric complications at the time of birth, the various environmental influences discussed before are all in utero exposures, particularly during the second trimester of pregnancy. From a neurodevelopmental perspective, this is a very critical time because it is when the individual cells which will become neurons migrate to their eventual positions in the brain. Thus, any insult—whether it be viral infection, malnutrition, and or any other trauma—can upset this migratory progress, thus risking the possibility that the infant brain will grow up lacking some of the intricate interconnections necessary for normal functioning.

A possible mechanism for such an adverse neurodevelopmental course is provided by a study that examined the distribution of various cell types in the prefrontal cortex of twenty deceased schizophrenic patients and twenty matched control subjects (Akbarian, Kim, Potkin, Hetrick, Bunney, & Jones, 1996). They identified three types of cells that represented the remnants of the cortical subplate, a structure that appears in the fourth month of pregnancy and guides migrating nerve cells to their proper locations. As part of programmed cell death, most of these subplate cells die within 30 days of birth, although a few remnants survive that become interstitial cells in the brain. The investigators found that in 35% of the brains of schizophrenic patients (but none of the control brains), there was a maldistribution of these interstitial cells toward the deeper white matter. The investigators concluded that the displacement of these interstitial cells in the frontal lobe of schizophrenic patients suggested alteration in the migration of neurons during brain development or in the pattern of programmed cell death. The investigators concluded that either problem could result in defective circuitry in the cortex.

Such an in utero effect might best explain why a monozygotic twin pair that is identical at conception may become discordant for schizophrenia.

Indeed, this adds to the argument that the heritability of schizophrenia derived from twin studies is overstated. Is it possible that for some monozygotic twin sets concordant for schizophrenia, rather than resulting from a genetic etiology, there was an in utero environmental insult strong enough that it impacted both twins? Keeping in mind schizophrenia's 1% lifetime risk, how much of this relatively low risk derives from genetics and how much from in utero environmental insults?

However, such neurodevelopmental theories do not necessarily exclude a genetic etiology. Given our knowledge of the elevated risk for those with a family history of schizophrenia (roughly an order of magnitude over that of the general public), one avenue of research must be to identify which genes may provide the substrate for increased susceptibility to such developmental influences. We will return to this question of the relationship between genetic and environmental etiologies at the end of "Conclusions."

## Evidence from Genetic Research

In less than two decades, the techniques of molecular biology and genetic analysis have become sophisticated enough that powerful tools are now available to tease out genetic inferences from analysis of the DNA taken from members of a sample population. By using restriction enzymes, it has been possible to map the entire human genome, and in the process, thousands of reference markers spread over all of the chromosomes have been identified. These markers are the guideposts from which a potential disease gene's locus can be triangulated. Thus, to the extent the family members in a pedigree who suffer from schizophrenia may have a common marker in their DNA, it may be inferred that a gene related to schizophrenia may be located someplace physically close to the known position of the marker.

The mathematical model used for the extensive calculations needed for such an analysis gives a result that is expressed as the logarithm of the odds that a finding could have occurred just by chance; this is the LOD score. Thus, if the probability that a result is due to chance is one in ten, the LOD score would be 1.0; the LOD score of a one in a hundred probability would be 2.0, and so on. Because of the vast number of calculations made in a linkage analysis, statistical artifacts are not unusual, and the practical result is that LOD scores less than 3.0 are often not considered noteworthy (Hamer & Copeland, 1994).

Like all mathematical models, the linkage analysis requires making certain assumptions to specify the algorithm used in the calculations. One important input is what the assumed mechanism of inheritance is; for example, is the gene being looked for assumed to be dominant or recessive? For some disorders, definitive empirical evidence on this point is available. For example, Huntington's disease is unusual in that over the years clear evidence accumulated that the disorder is likely to be controlled by a single gene and that the allele that gives rise to the disease is dominant (Barondes, 1998). Although one might expect that a dominant Mendelian disease would lead to the extinction of families carrying that allele, Huntington's has been around for more than 300 years because typically it does not strike until middle age, after the childbearing years.

Given the power of the linkage analysis tools, researchers in this field have become increasing conscious of the problems cause by heterogeneity. Therefore, in finding the Huntington's gene, the research focused on an extended family in Venezuela with a high incidence of the disease. Linkage analysis of data collected in 1982 found a linkage of very high statistical significance on chromosome 4, although it would take another 10 years of effort and the development of new technology to actually identify the exact gene responsible for Huntington's disease (Huntington's Disease Collaborative Research Group, 1993).

Another critical input necessary for linkage analysis is a concise definition of the disorder so that the members of a pedigree whose DNA is being examined are properly classified as affected by the disease or not affected. Therefore, rigorous, clinically derived diagnostic tools, such as DSM-IV, are typically applied to the population studied. Because the quality of a statistical analysis is only as good as the quality of the underlying data, subtle shifts occasioned by varying disease definitions can create widely varying results.

An example of a linkage analysis that produced exciting results followed by disappointment was one undertaken on a number of Amish pedigrees, who exhibited extensive mood disorders, all, it was thought, derived from a small number of founders. Because another study had developed two DNA probes that could be used on chromo-some 11, the Amish linkage analysis was initiated on just this one chromosome. Nevertheless, in 1987, this study produced powerful initial results that linked manic-depressive illness with a gene on that chromosome; the initial statistical analysis indicated that there was only a one in two hundred probability that the results were due to chance (Egeland et al., 1987). However, when two previously healthy members of one extended family exhibited mania and depression, respectively, the recalculation of the statistics to incorporate these new data points reduced the results below the one in twenty odds of chance that are the threshold of statistical significance (Kelsoe et al., 1989).

This ultimate disappointment reflects the fact that LOD statistical analysis is much less effective for more complicated genetic inheritance patterns, even though it is a very effective technique in analyzing Mendelian traits. LOD analysis for disorders resulting from more than one gene may be a high-tech and dangerous version of the old problem of "data dredging," that is, when a large number of variables is examined, some seemingly significant relationships may appear, which turn out to be just chance artifacts.

Another study at about the same time was also affected by these problems (Baron et al., 1987). Several large Israeli families with a high incidence of mood disorders were analyzed; the analysis in this case focused on the X chromosome because no male-to-male inheritance was apparent in the pedigrees in question; evidence suggested an X-linked trait. Here again, the exquisite sensitivity of the LOD technique to small changes in the underlying data was shown. When just two subjects, whose disorder was relatively mild cyclothymia, were reclassified from affected to not affected, the LOD score for linkage dropped from as high as nine (one in twenty million odds that results were due to chance) to scores that indicated a lack of statistical significance.

The point of this discussion is to set out some of the problems presented when attempting to use linkage analysis to locate "schizophrenia genes." An important threshold question is whether a possible genetic liability to schizophrenia is caused by just one gene or by multiple genes. Irving Gottesman first proposed a polygenic theory of schizophrenia in a seminal paper (1967). Almost 20 years later, Gottesman and two coauthors described the results of their goodness-of-fit analysis of pooled data for morbid risks of schizophrenia among the relatives of schizophrenic probands in nine different classes of relatives with five different degrees of genetic relatedness (McGue, Gottesman, & Rao, 1985). They concluded that a pure polygenic threshold model fit the observed risks, although the fit of the model to the data was significantly improved if environmental sources of familial resemblance were also allowed for.

As a result of the extensive genetic analyses performed since, there is a widely accepted consensus that a polygenic model is most likely, with one notable exception, which will be discussed later. One empirical tool argues for such a conclusion as well. In a single gene inheritance model, the gene in question can either be dominant or recessive. If it is dominant, then we would expect that the concordance rate among monozygotic twins would be 100%, which is exactly the case for Huntington's disease, which is determined by one dominant gene. If the single gene is recessive, then we would expect to see that the monozygotic concordance rate would be twice that of the dizygotic concordance rate. However, based on the data reviewed earlier, we have seen that the ratio of monozygotic versus dizygotic concordance rates for schizophrenia is typically between three to five times, depending on the studies considered.

If liability to schizophrenia is likely to be a polygenic phenomenon, one analogy to consider is the existence of another polygenetically determined trait, human height. Common sense tells us that it is not likely that there is a single gene controlling height, but rather that each of us is the result of the influence of many genes that may affect our height. However, even this simple analogy points out possible complications when you consider that in rare cases, one gene may cause pathologies that dramatically affect height, for example, achondroplasia, which includes the symptom of dwarfism.

In addition to the problems occasioned by using linkage analysis to look for genes that are part of a polygenetic process, we must also keep in mind that any input assumptions as to genetic model and penetrance are educated guesses at best. Finally, there is the very legitimate question of how broad a definition of the disorder should be applied to the sample in classifying which pedigree members are affected and which are not. Should the sole criteria be a DSM-IV diagnosis of schizophrenia, or should a schizoaffective diagnosis also merit classification as affected? Or perhaps, family members who exhibit schizotypal personality disorders should also be included as affected. The actual problem created by such choices motivated one author who wrote a review entitled "The maddening hunt for madness genes" to observe that "Some investigators have obtained their most compelling data by using a broad definition of illness, while others prefer to use a narrow one; a narrow definition of schizophrenia resulted in linkage to [chromosome] 5p, a broad definition resulted in linkage to 6p and a still broader one, to 8p in the same pedigree set" (Moldin, 1997, pp. 127–128).

## Genome-Wide Scans

Armed with the caution that the previous discussion should engender, the first step in assessing genetic evidence should be to see what results have been obtained from genome-wide scans. This is the application of the linkage analysis techniques at the macroscale of all of the chromosomes that make up the genome to identify regions that may be worthy of more detailed analysis. A set of markers is chosen (typically numbering in the hundreds), and then the DNA for all members of a pedigree is typed for these markers.

Given the consensus that the heritability of schizophrenia is a polygenetic phenomenon, perhaps not much should be expected from genome-wide scans looking for likely schizophrenia gene sites, and so far, that has proven to be the case. For example, during the past year, several such projects have been reported. The Genetics Initiative of the National Institute of Mental Health reported on genome-wide scans performed on both African-American and European-American pedigrees. The African-American scan comprised thirty nuclear families and ninety-eight subjects, of which seventy-one had received diagnoses of schizophrenia and eight diagnoses of schizoaffective disorder (Kaufmann et al., 1998). There were a total of forty-two independent sib-pairs. The analysis revealed no regions that reached the level of significance that had been previously suggested in the literature (Lander & Kruglyak, 1995), although regions on chromosomes 6, 8, 9, and 15 "showed evidence consistent with linkage" (Kaufmann et al., 1998, p. 282).

The NIMH group reported similar results from their genome scan of forty-three European-American nuclear families with 146 subjects (schizophrenia diagnosis = 82, schizoaffective disorder diagnosis = 14) and fifty independent sib-pairs (Faraone et al., 1998). Once again, no region showed statistically significant evidence for linkage, although evidence that suggested linkage was found at two markers on chromosome 10.

Also in 1998, a California group reported on its genome-wide scan of seventy pedigrees containing three phenotype classifications: schizophrenia only (48 pedigrees, 70 sib-pairs), schizophrenia plus schizoaffective disorder (70 pedigrees, 101 sib-pairs), and a broader category that also included various schizophrenia-related personality disorders plus a number of types of psychoses (70 pedigrees, 111 sib-pairs; Shaw et al., 1998). Using allele-sharing tests, twelve chromosomes had at least one region with a nominal $p$ value less than .05, and of these twelve, two (chromosomes 13 and 16) had nominal $p$ values less than .01. Using two-point LOD score analysis, five chromosomes (1, 2, 4, 11, and 13) had at least one marker whose score was higher than 2.0.

Looking at these three analyses as a group, the African-American scan identified four chromosomes of potential interest (6, 8, 9, and 15), the European-American scan identified just one (on chromosome 10), and the California project pointed to either two chromosomes (13 and 16, if you believed the allele-sharing model) or five chromosome (1, 2, 4, 11, and 13, using LOD score anal-

ysis). No doubt it is more than just a coincidence that these three genome-wide scans identified three mutually exclusive groups of chromosomes that merited further investigation. This certainly suggests that the heritability of schizophrenia is polygenetic, or perhaps even nonexistent!

## Linkage Analysis of Specific Chromosomes

Rather than jumping into a review of the scores of studies of linkage analysis for schizophrenia that have been published, a good place to start is with a table contained in a 1997 review article that assessed the current status of this quest and was written by a skeptic (Crow, 1997). To prove the point implied by the review's subtitle, "Polygenes of vanishingly small effect or multiple false positives?," Table 5 was complied by Crow and lists each of the chromosomes or "candidate genes" for which a successful linkage analysis once reportedly achieved statistical significance (p. 100).

One column in the table gives the author and date for the study that reported such significance, and another column lists at least one, and usually several, studies that failed to replicate a finding of significance. Crow may be a skeptic, but on the question of whether linkage analysis has been successful in locating genes related to schizophrenia, the literature is on his side. Indeed, in

### Table 5. Claims for Linkage and Association in Schizophrenia[a]

| Locus/gene | Claim | Examples of discordant findings (usually the first and/or most salient discrepancy) |
|---|---|---|
| 5q | Sherrington et al. (1988) | St. Clair et al. (1989); McGuffin et al. (1990) |
| 11q | St Clair et al. (1990) | Wang et al. (1993) |
| PSAR | Collinge et al. (1991) | Crow et al. (1994) |
| D3 (homozygosity) | Crocq et al. (1992) | Rietschel et al. (1996) |
| 6p | Straub et al. (1995) | Riley et al. (1996); Garner et al. (1996) |
| 22 | Pulver et al. (1994) | Polymeropoulos et al. (1995); Kalsi et al. (1995) |
| DRD2 | Arinami et al. (1994) | Asherson et al. (1994); Gejman et al. (1994) |
| 8p | Pulver et al. (1995) | Kunugi et al. (1996) |
| 3p | Pulver et al. (1995) | Moises et al. (1995); Kalsi et al. (1996) |
| AR | Crow et al. (1993) | Arranz et al. (1995) |
| 13q | Lin et al. (1995) | |
| 5HT2A | Williams et al. (1996) | Nimgaonkar et al. (1996) |

[a]From Current status of linkage for schizophrenia: Polygenes of vanishingly small effect or multiple false positives, by T. J. Crow, 1997, *American Journal of Medical Genetics*, 74, 100. Copyright 1997 John Wiley & Sons, Inc. Reprinted by permission of John Wiley & Sons, Inc.

commenting on his position as a collaborator for one of these studies, Crow writes "however in contributing to the discussion and writing of the paper I found myself in a small minority in my interpretation of the findings, and in particular in dissent from the widely held assumption that a large number of genes contributing to susceptibility to psychosis are to be found, and that some linkages have already been established" (Crow, 1997, p. 99).

In fact, Crow uses the confusion of so many contrary studies to conclude that just as likely an explanation would be his long-held belief that there is one gene (yet to be discovered) that determines brain asymmetry, and for some individuals, causes schizophrenia. This is the one exception to the polygenic consensus alluded to previously.

The information in Crow's compilation is intended to demonstrate that the mechanisms by which genetics impacts schizophrenia are complex and subtle, and are likely to be the result of more than one gene, and probably many genes, Dr. Crow notwithstanding. There is a large literature reporting on various efforts at genetic linkage analysis for many genes of potential interest located on a number of chromosomes.

However, rather than chronicling the specific results of the many linkage analyses that have been reported, the goal in reviewing this literature will be to look for what this research can tell us about the interaction between genetics and the physiological and environmental evidence discussed earlier.

**Chromosome 5.** Table 5, from Crow's article, listed chronologically the chromosomes for which an association with schizophrenia was claimed at one time. From that table, we see that the earliest linkage claim for schizophrenia, involving chromosome 5, was reported by Sherrington et al. in 1988. Subsequently, a number of failures to replicate this association were reported, and interest waned in chromosome 5 in terms of schizophrenia.

However, several years ago, there were two new reports of possible linkage to chromosome 5; although still on the long arm, the sites were in a different region of the chromosome. In one study using 265 Irish pedigrees (n = 1408), a genome scan highlighted this region as the second most likely for linkage (Straub et al., 1997). More detailed work by the same group identified a locus with a LOD score that exceeded 3. Interestingly, a

significant LOD score was obtained only with a narrow definition of phenotype (schizophrenia only), in contrast with the same group's experience with two other chromosomes, for which broader definitions, applied to the same pedigrees, produced the strongest result. The investigators estimated that the putative vulnerability locus on chromosome 5 was segregated in 10 to 25% of the families. Another study, reported at the same time, found weak indications of an association near the same site, using fifty-four German and Israeli families (Schwab et al., 1997).

**Chromosome 6.** Ironically, the same set of Irish pedigrees was the subject matter of the linkage analysis that produced the strongest indications of linkage to schizophrenia seen to date, but had a locus on the short arm of chromosome 6 (Wang et al., 1995). A LOD score of 3.9 was obtained, although a study published later, which augmented the same pedigrees with more families, found a reduced significance (Straub et al., 1995). Subsequently, a number of published studies was unable to replicate these findings; for example, a 1996 study, which used data from 211 families that had affected sib-pairs, concluded that "the present findings together with the published literature fail to find consistent evidence of a linkage for schizophrenia to a single locus on chromosome 6" (Garner et al., 1996, p. 595).

A more recent study was also unable to confirm these findings, although the investigators obtained LOD scores just over 3 for two markers on the long arm in the region 6q21–q22.3 (Cao et al., 1997). It should be noted that 6q21–6q24 was one of the four regions that demonstrated evidence of significant linkage in a genome-wide scan of African-Americans reported several years later (Kaufmann et al., 1998). This finding will also take on increased relevance later when trinucleotide repeats are discussed.

Among the many studies involving possible linkage with chromosome 6, two stand out because they add dimensions beyond the technicalities of the linkage model and LOD scores. As discussed earlier, eye tracking dysfunction (ETD) has been identified as a trait seen in a significant number of schizophrenic patients and also in their relatives. A German group that has done research into ETD as a marker decided to undertake a linkage analysis focused on the short arm region identified by others (i.e., 6p21–23), using members of the families they had assessed in their ETD research (Arolt et al., 1996). Using schizophrenia as the identified disorder, seven different models failed to detect significant results. However, when the specified disorder was ETD, their work identified two markers with high LOD scores: 3.51 for marker D6S271, and 3.44 for D6S282. Including these markers in a multipoint analysis yielded a LOD score of 4.02. Significantly, these two markers are very close to the three markers (i.e., D6S296, D6S274, and D6S295) that gave the strongest results in the 1995 study of Irish pedigrees that caused the initial excitement about chromosome 6 (Straub et al., 1997).

Another unique approach was taken in a linkage analysis that used twenty-eight markers on chromosome 6 to scan 183 people from ten moderately large Canadian families, for which schizophrenia had been diagnosed in about a quarter of the sample (Brzustowicz et al., 1997). Using various permutations of parametric analysis as well as sibpair analysis based on categorical disease definitions yielded no significant evidence for linkage. However, the investigators then carried out a sibpair analysis using three different quantitative traits as the disease input, specifically scores on a positive symptom scale, a negative symptom scale, and a scale for general psychopathological symptoms. The positive symptom scale found significant evidence of linkage, regardless of the disease diagnosis; nominal $p$ values were $1.2 \times 10^{-5}$ under two-point and $5.4 \times 10^{-6}$ under multipoint analyses. These values corresponded to simulation-calculated empirical $p$ values of .034 and .0085, respectively. For this study, the use of quantitative data rather than categorical disease input greatly increased the detection power of linkage analysis. The field awaits further testing of this approach.

**Chromosome 13.** A study published last year reportedly found evidence from a genome-wide scan for schizophrenia susceptibility loci that suggested associations with chromosomes 8 and 13, although only the chromosome 13 data rose to the level of significance (Blouin et al., 1998). Using a dataset that consisted of fifty-four cases of diagnosed schizophrenia and 309 relatives from European backgrounds and a narrow definition of schizophrenia, LOD scores as high as 4.18 were obtained. When the analysis was performed on another data set consisting of fifty-one cases and 248 relatives, a LOD score of 2.36 was obtained, although a finding of significance was possible only when the definition of the disease was broad-

ened to include categories such as schizophrenia spectrum personality disorders or mood disorder psychoses.

A contemporaneous news report stated that this result was consistent with the findings contained in an unpublished study by S.D. Detera-Wadleigh of the National Institute of Mental health, in which the same chromosome 13 sequence was found often in family members diagnosed with bipolar disorder (Bower, 1998). In the same account, Detera-Wadleigh opined that schizophrenia and bipolar disorder may share some susceptibility genes.

**Chromosome 15.** In the same way that the Arolt study described before focused on a physiological marker (eye tracking dysfunction), a Denver group undertook linkage analysis on members of nine families that exhibited a significant incidence of P50 inhibition. This phenomenon, discussed before with other physiological evidence, is associated with attentional disturbances in schizophrenia (Erwin et al., 1998). The sample population consisted of thirty-six diagnosed cases of schizophrenia; thirty-five of them (97%) exhibited P50 inhibition, and 104 relatives, twenty-two of whom (21%) also displayed this trait (Freedman et al., 1997). The results of a genome-wide scan linked the P50 trait to a dinucleotide polymorphism at chromosome 15q13–14, and yielded a LOD score of 5.3. This site is the same as, or very close to, the site of the gene for the alpha 7-nicotinic receptor, a type of acetylcholine receptor found throughout the brain, which also responds to nicotine. Long-known anecdotal evidence of the extremely high smoking prevalence among schizophrenic patients certainly hints that this may be more than a coincidence.

A later study supported these findings. Using the marker with the highest pairwise LOD score (D15S1360), twenty families, with at least one sibpair concordant for schizophrenia, were tested for linkage (Leonard et al., 1998). Because these families had not been tested for P50 inhibition, the affected phenotype used for the analysis was a DSM-III-R diagnosis of schizophrenia. The sibpair analysis showed a significant proportion of D15S1360 alleles shared identically by descent.

**Chromosome 22.** Findings involving chromosome 22 would probably not merit mention if judged only by the history of claims of significance followed by nonreplication (see commentaries by Crow, 1997, and Moldin, 1997). A 1996 study by the Schizophrenia Collaborative Linkage

Group (Chromosome 22) reported on their combined analysis of genotypic data from eleven independent research groups, which focused on marker D22S278, the marker of most interest in three of these studies (Gill et al., 1996). Using the affected sib-pair method, the combined data set showed 252 alleles shared compared to 188 alleles not shared where parental genotype data was completely known and gave a chi-squared value of 9.31. The chi-squared statistic dropped to 6.12 when the other sib-pairs were added using parental data assigned according to probability.

As will be discussed later under its own heading, chromosome 22 contains a recently discovered gene that specifies a potassium ion channel. This ion channel is of interest because its function could provide a plausible mechanism for a number of the positive symptoms of schizophrenia.

### Candidate Genes

Most of the linkage analyses described before focused on a particular chromosome because it had been identified in a broader, usually genome-wide, scan. However, another logical approach is to focus on certain genes that control structures or functions that might play an important role in the origin or course of the disease in question. By selecting such a candidate gene for investigation, there is the possibility of confirming or rejecting a hypothesized link between the gene and the disease. Of course, the opportunity to discover linkage to sites in the genome unrelated to the candidate gene is foregone, but then again perhaps the chances are also reduced of falling into the type of false positive situation discussed so often before.

**Dopamine.** Until the early 1950s, Western medicine had not found an effective pharmacotherapy for schizophrenia. Then, at about the same time, two drugs were found that were efficacious in treating the positive symptoms of the illness (Veggeberg, 1996). One of these, reserpine, was derived from a plant called *Rauwolfia serpentina*, which had long been used to treat insanity in India; when first administered to schizophrenic patients in 1954, it had a significant calming effect. At about the same time, another drug, chlorpromazine, which had been developed in France as an anesthetic, was similarly effective. These drugs and their successors became the wonder drugs by which a large majority of the mentally ill could be released from mental institutions, which until that time had been considered the only appropriate

forum for treating serious illnesses like schizophrenia.

Until the relatively recent acceptance of *atypical* schizophrenia medications, these first two drugs, and virtually all of the antipsychotic drugs developed subsequently, had their primary effect on dopamine neurotransmission in the brain. Specifically, they reduced dopamine activity in the brain, particularly in the limbic region, the seat of emotions. Not surprisingly, a *dopamine hypothesis* became popular, which considered schizophrenia a disorder characterized by excessive dopamine activity in certain regions of the brain. By reducing dopamine activity, the new antipsychotic agents often dramatically reduced positive symptoms such as hallucinations and delusions. Because these drugs, especially the early ones, were somewhat indiscriminate in terms of which parts of the brain experienced reduced dopamine activity, serious side effects often posed problems. In particular, because dopamine is an important neurotransmitter in the execution of movements, impairment in movement was frequently seen, and symptoms were similar to those seen in Parkinson's disease.

During the last decade or so, improvements in technology at the molecular level have led to the discovery of several subtypes of dopamine receptors. With this new knowledge, it has become harder to support the relatively simple hypothesis that schizophrenia is caused by hyperdopaminergia. It has now been determined that a blockage of the D2 subtype of dopamine receptors is the primary mechanism of action for the older antipsychotic drugs. Presumably the dramatic reduction in positive symptoms which is brought about by these drugs results from decreased activity at D2 receptors. However, the clinical experience was that D2 antagonists had little efficacy in reducing the negative symptoms of schizophrenia, suggesting that negative symptoms may not be related to hyperdopaminergia. Also, a new and more powerful antipsychotic drug, clozapine, has only one-tenth the binding ability to D2 receptors compared to chlorpromazine, even though it has some efficacy in reducing negative symptoms.

Given this history, the likeliest schizophrenia candidate genes are those related to dopamine function. As the number of known types of dopamine receptors has increased, so has the number of dopamine candidate genes. A number of studies during the past decade investigated the D2 receptor with mixed results. One study examined the

DNA of 253 unrelated subjects (106 with schizo-phrenia, 113 with alcoholism, and 34 controls) to determine which alleles of the D2 receptor gene were present (Gejman et al., 1994). Based on their results, the investigators concluded that no abnor-malities in the DRD2 gene were associated with schizophrenia or alcoholism.

However, at about the same time, a study deter-mined the frequency of one variant of the D2 gene (Ser311 → Cys) in 156 Japanese schizophrenic patients and 300 controls (Arinami et al., 1994). They found that the frequency was significantly higher in the patient group (0.054), compared to the control group (0.018). Also within the patient group, the frequency was increased in the before 25 age of onset (0.090), and family history (0.135) subgroups. They also commented that the patients with Cys311 showed significantly less severe thought disorder and negative symptoms. The same group later reported on case control studies with 291 schizophrenic patients, seventy-eight pa-tients with affective disorders, and 579 controls (Arinami et al., 1996). The frequency of the S311C allele was elevated for patients with an absence of negative symptoms (17.1%), compared to both the other patients (5.7%) and the controls (4.1%). The frequency was also significantly higher in familial schizophrenic patients from one local area, but not in those from other areas. Finally, the S311C allele was frequently present in mood-incongruent psy-chotic affective disorders (33.3%), but not in the other affective disorder patients. The investigators concluded that the S311C allele might be a genetic factor for symptomatic dimensions of delusions and hallucinations.

A recently published study tested eight candi-date genes related to dopamine transmission in fifty-nine families from Germany and Israel for association (Schwab et al., 1998). This analysis detected a CA-repeat marker near G-olfalpha on chromosome 18p, which had a corrected $p$ value of .0044. This value decreased to .0007 when nine siblings with recurrent unipolar disorder were in-cluded. A two-point LOD score of 3.1 was also obtained for this marker. The investigators con-cluded that this marker on chromosome 18p repre-sents a potential susceptibility locus for functional psychoses.

**An Ion Channel Gene.** A series of articles by a group from the University of California at Irvine were published last year that created interest in a newly discovered gene for a calcium-activated potassium ion channel (hSKCa3) found in neu-rons. This type of ion channel plays an important role in determining the firing rate of neurons. The new gene was first discovered in a rat model, and when the human version was identified, it was found that it contains CAG repeats (Chandy et al., 1998). CAG repeats have been implicated in other psychiatric disorders, such as Huntington's dis-ease, in which the number of CAG repeats exceeds a certain level for those with a disease condition. This trinucleotide codes for the amino acid glu-tamine so that, as the number of CAG repeats increases, more glutamines are added to the ion channel, perhaps affecting its function in the case of the hSKCa3 gene.

The initial study showed that the number of CAG repeats found in the various alleles ranged from twelve to twenty-eight in samples of both schizophrenic patients and controls (Chandy et al., 1998). However, the overall distribution of alleles was significantly different in the patients com-pared to ethnically matched controls; CAG repeats longer than the modal value were overrepresented in patients. A similar, but nonsignificant, trend was also seen for patients with bipolar disorder. A news account at the time reported that several of the investigators speculated that extra repeats might lead to abnormally active potassium chan-nels, which could suppress NMDA receptors. They also pointed out that when NMDA receptors are inhibited by the drug of abuse PCP, schizo-phrenia-like symptoms can be induced; con-versely, some antipsychotic drugs activate these receptors (Travis, 1997).

Some months later, the same investigators re-ported that when their hypothesis was tested in another case control study, the results provided modest support; schizophrenic probands had a higher frequency of alleles with more than nine-teen repeats than controls (Bowen et al., 1998).

A Chinese group reported on a study in which they tested the hypothesis in ninety-seven family trios with schizophrenia from Southwest China (Li et al., 1998). Based on tests of haplotype rela-tive risk and transmission disequilibrium (TDT), they found no evidence for an excess of longer CAG repeats in patients, although they did find a deficit of transmission of the (CAG)20 repeat al-lele to affected offspring when this allele was considered individually by TDT. A German group also reported on a family-based association study to test the hypothesis in fifty-nine parent/offspring trios (Stober et al., 1998). Contrary to expectations, their findings indicated that short CAG repeats (less than or equal to nineteen repeats) were transmitted at an *increased* frequency to offspring diagnosed with schizophrenia, particularly among familial cases.

### Repeat Trinucleotides

The ion channel gene discussed before is just one example of possible trinucleotide repeat polymorphisms that may have a role in the genetics of schizophrenia. Such a possibility is attractive for several reasons. As mentioned before, such repeat polymorphisms, especially CAG repeats, it has been demonstrated, cause neurodegenerative diseases including Huntington's disease and Alzheimer's disease. From a biological viewpoint, CAG repeats provide a plausible and understandable mechanism, that is, the addition of glutamine amino acids to the ion channel protein affects its functioning.

Finally, repeat polymorphisms also provide a plausible physiological substrate for the phenomenon of genetic anticipation, where the age of onset decreases and/or the severity of a disease increases from generation to generation, presumably because each succeeding generation contains more repeats at one or more critical genes. Such a hypothesis was tested using thirty-three families with at least two affected members in successive generations (Johnson et al., 1997). The disease definition was broad, including schizoaffective disorder, psychoses, and schizotypal personality disorders; various indices measuring age of onset and severity of disease were also used. Anticipation was demonstrated for age of onset regardless of the index used, but anticipation for disease severity was not supported.

Another study used the repeat expansion detection (RED) method to investigate the occurrence of repeat polymorphisms in a group with childhood-onset schizophrenia (COS), as well as in a group with childhood-onset psychosis (Burgess et al., 1998). The difference observed in the CAG/CTG RED product distribution between the normal and the COS samples was only marginally significant. However, the male COS group had a RED product distribution significantly different from the male controls, and longer repeats were detected in the COS group; no significant difference was seen among females. The investigators also reported

that some of the detected trinucleotide repeats in all three populations (COS, childhood-onset psychosis, and control) correlated with expanded alleles found at the CTG18.1 locus on chromosome 18.

A recent study reported on an investigation designed to identify additional candidate genes which might be affected by trinucleotide repeats (Kleiderlein et al., 1998). In this case, complementary DNA (cDNA) libraries (i.e., synthetic DNA without material that may be irrelevant to an analysis; e.g., introns) from the human brain were probed for repeats of a family of six trinucleotides known collectively as the CCG repeats. The cDNA libraries were also compared with the thirty-seven human genes with eight or more consecutive CCG triplets in GenBank. The study reported mapping the repeats to fifteen specific loci, including the following of interest for this review: *6q22*, which was the locus identified by Cao et al., discussed before under the heading Chromosome 6; *18p11*, which may be pertinent to the Burgess et al. study discussed in the previous paragraph; and *22q12*, which is the locus of the gene discussed before in the section Ion Channel Gene. Each of these possible sites for genetic linkage might deserve extra consideration because of the possibility that repeat polymorphisms might also be detected there.

## Conclusions

Like most diseases, both genetics and environmental effects are etiologic factors in schizophrenia. Because of long-standing knowledge that schizophrenia "runs in families," it has been known as a genetic disorder. One of the purposes of this review has been to examine the widely held view that a strong genetic component is a major feature of the disorder. However, when schizophrenia is examined on a societal level, some of the more recent evidence has identified environmental stressors, such as viruses, as significant in the etiology of the disorder.

### Diathesis-Stress Model Favored

At least two models can account for the contribution of both environmental effects and genetics to schizophrenia. One approach might conclude that there are really two separate and distinct disorders that happen to share a number of common symptoms as end points. One disorder would be a familial type that exhibits genetic transmission, and a second disorder would be a sporadic type, caused by environmental stressors. Although these two diseases might share many symptoms, they need not. Indeed, an important aspect of a two-disease model is the research effort to identify symptoms that may be used to distinguish between the disorders. In the review of evidence before, a number of taxonomies were discussed that create dichotomies as an aid to understanding the nature of schizophrenia, for example, positive and negative symptoms and a neurodevelopmental disorder compared to a neurodegenerative disorder. As summarized at the end of "Taxonomies of Schizophrenia," research focused on such distinctions has not produced compelling evidence that multiple disorders exist. Furthermore, results have not been consistent from study to study.

An alternative to a multiple-disease model is a one-disease process that can encompass both genetic and environmental etiologies: the diathesis-stress model. This model explains that the disease results from a genetic predisposition to the disease and environmental stressors that trigger the expression of the disease. A number of common diseases, such as coronary artery disease, fit such a model because it can incorporate the many contributing factors that are observed clinically. Thus, the occurrence of heart disease can be viewed as the confluence of some degree of genetic predisposition with various environmental risk factors, such as obesity, lack of exercise, and improper diet.

Although arguments have been made for both approaches in understanding schizophrenia, the evidence reviewed herein makes a more convincing case for the diathesis-stress model. In particular, in both presumed genetic and environmental situations, the logic of what has been observed strongly supports the diathesis-stress model. For example, when a strong genetic risk factor is likely, such as family loading for schizophrenia, only a minority of the family actually develops the disorder, that is, only a portion of those with the genotype develop the phenotype. Because well relatives may share a number of physiological markers, such as eye tracking dysfunction, we know that some well relatives may also have a genetic risk factor for the disease. Therefore, environmental effects are likely to be the agency by which only some of the family develop the illness. Indeed, if every family member contracted the disease, schizophrenia would quickly become much more rare by reducing reproduction because it strikes in childbearing years.

Conversely, examples of environmental stressors, such as flu epidemics, also provide a logical argument for the diathesis-stress model. The evidence has shown that even if a large population is exposed to an environmental stressor, such as was the case with the 1945 Dutch famine, most of those in utero do not develop schizophrenia later. Rather, the result may be a rate of schizophrenia for those in utero at the time that is elevated from the small 1% lifetime risk to a less small, but still low, several per cent. Unless there is a chance phenomenon at work, it may be argued that the disease occurred in that additional several per cent due to their genetic predisposition.

## The Degree of Heritability

An orthodoxy has developed as to the heritability of schizophrenia. It typically begins with the observation that a number of twin studies demonstrated a concordance for schizophrenia in monozygotic twins of slightly more than 50% (on a probandwise basis), compared to a concordance rate for dizygotic twins of about 15%. This ratio of roughly three to one leads to conclusions that calculate the heritability of schizophrenia as somewhat in excess of 50%.

However, as the evidence reviewed in "Review of Evidence Indicating Transmission within Families" revealed, such logic ignores the fact that behind these average numbers there is great variability in the data collected by different studies. Taking numbers from the eight studies contained in Table 1 (Torrey et al., 1994), we see that monozygotic concordance rates range from 26 to 68%, and the range for dizygotic twins is 4 to 18%.

This lack of consistency reflects important methodological problems that are often encountered in twin studies. Frequently the classification of zygosity has not been determined scientifically, especially where the twins have not actually been examined. Similarly, because many studies predate the development of uniform criteria such as DSM, diagnosis of the subjects is questionable, especially if one or both of the twins have not actually been observed. These are examples of the types of problems that are bound to occur when comparing studies conducted at different times and under different circumstances.

The discussion of Table 1 identified another source of confusion: that concordance rates for schizophrenia have typically been stated on a pro-bandwise basis, rather than the pairwise basis used for many other diseases. However, even allowing for this procedural difference, the higher than 50% rate of concordance for monozygotic twins typ-ically cited is overstated. Using the figures from Table 1, the average probandwise rate for mono-zygotic twins is 40% if all eight studies are in-cluded, or 39% if the only studies counted are the three studies that Torrey considers the least meth-odologically impaired. Average probandwise con-cordance rates for dizygotic twins are 15 or 14%, respectively. Translating these numbers into pair-wise statistics gives a comparison of either 28% (all studies) or 26% (three studies) for mono-zygotic twins, compared to either 6 or 8% for dizygotic twins.

But aside from these methodological concerns, the magnitude of heritability that is calculated prob-ably also suffers from a significant confounding factor. In reviewing the evidence for environmental effects earlier, most studies pointed to the in utero period as the most likely time frame for exposure to environmental stressors that may trigger schizo-phrenia. As discussed in the section "Evidence for a Possible Neurodevelopmental Mechanism," the in utero period also makes sense from a biological perspective, because we can contemplate a plaus-ible mechanism, that is, perturbation during the time when neurons are migrating to their eventual location in the developing brain. However, to the extent that any such environmental stressors occur between the conception and birth of a pair of monozygotic twins, their impact will be counted as a genetic effect in a twin study, further contrib-uting to an overstated heritability.

These types of problems indicate that the use-fulness of twin and other observational studies may have reached a limit as to what they can reveal about the etiology of schizophrenia. If that is the case, then genetic analysis may be the ap-proach that offers the most promising potential for studying heritability.

## Problems with Genetic Analysis

The evidence reviewed before indicates that the genetic etiology of schizophrenia requires a com-plicated model. There are three primary reasons for this: probably more than one gene is involved; there is incomplete penetrance, that is, the disease is not expressed in all those at genetic risk; and there are several definitional problems.

The genetics of schizophrenia almost certainly involves more than one gene. In fact, the more appropriate question is how many genes are in-volved. The evidence we have reviewed points to a model with multiple genes of small effect. One consequence of each gene's small effect is that these effects become difficult to detect. Given this situation, it is not surprising that in the review of genetic studies earlier, many cases were seen of a specific locus on a given chromosome that demon-strated an effect in some studies, but not in other studies.

Even in a family with relatively heavy loading for schizophrenia, only a minority of family mem-bers express the disease, which is evidence of the genetic phenomenon of incomplete penetrance. The conclusion that there is incomplete pene-trance is bolstered by the fact that several physio-logical markers have been identified which are present both in schizophrenic patients and in some of their well relatives. The fact that the degree of penetrance is currently unknown and unpredict-able and that it may vary from pedigree to pedigree makes attempts to fit observed data into mathe-matical models of genetic transmission problem-atical, and perhaps even an impossible task.

An important issue in creating a genetic model is the approach taken in defining the disease. A narrow definition has the virtue of offering a set of quite distinct symptoms (for example, hallucina-tions, delusions), so that the presence of such a constellation reduces the risk that various symp-toms are present by chance or are due to another disorder. However, a broader definition may better reflect the genetic reality. For example, if they are related to the same gene(s), perhaps a related dis-ease, such as schizoaffective disorder, or even usually distinct disorders with a common feature such as psychotic affective disorders, should be included.

The three difficulties in developing a genetic model for schizophrenia described before also have a major impact on linkage analysis. Looking at a converse situation, this technique is most powerful in working with a disorder like Hunt-ington's disease, when it is known that the genetic effect derives from one gene; the genetic model is precisely known, dominant Mendelian in the case of Huntington's; and the outcome measure is bi-nary; either an individual suffers the disease, or does not.

For schizophrenia, to the extent that the number of genes involved in the disease process increases, the mathematics underlying the linkage model is strained in its ability to detect linkage, and the production of false positives that reflect artifacts is increased. Uncertainty about the genetic mechanism forces investigators to test many sets of assumptions, and even then the calculations may not be productive because the penetrance issue is such an unknown in the process. Finally, the issue of the way the disease is defined has a much larger impact on the results produced by linkage models, compared to questions of definition in the real world. In the review of genetic evidence before, investigations were encountered in which the best results were obtained by using narrow, intermediate, or broad definitions. Judgments as to the appropriate broadness of definition for any particular study have to balance the precision gained from a narrow definition against the possible need for a broad definition to reflect genetic realities.

The review of evidence before highlighted several techniques that may increase confidence in using linkage analysis: identification and use of biological markers, the use of quantitative rather than categorical data, and the use of repeat expansion detection techniques.

The use of biological markers may enhance the efficacy of linkage analysis. However, markers that are present only in patients may not help much. For example, according to the most plausible mechanism proposed to explain problems in the neurodevelopmental process (in utero perturbations to migrating neurons), deficits in prefrontal cortex blood flows may be observed only in patients—and not in their well relatives—because such deficits are likely to be markers of an environmental, not genetic, effect. Thus, the utility of markers probably depends on whether they can be found in well relatives, as well as in patients.

Markers in both patients and well relatives may also present an opportunity to overcome the penetrance problem. To the extent that markers such as eye tracking dysfunction (Holzman et al., 1988) can be objectively measured, the issue of how broad a disease definition to choose may be resolved in favor of a narrow definition. The other marker identified in the review of physiological evidence above was an abnormality in P50 inhibition (Freedman et al., 1997).

Another promising technique is that employed by Brzustowicz and her colleagues (1997), in which quantitative data were used as the disease input into the linkage model, rather than categorical judgments. By inputting patients' scores for positive symptoms, a linkage finding of statistical significance was produced, whereas the usual categorical variable could not. This demonstrates the possibility of adding statistical power to the analysis of effects that are so weak that the variables currently being used cannot detect them. There are several other benefits to this approach. By definition, quantitative measures are more objective than an investigator's subjective choice of a disease category. It is possible that significant quantitative data can also be collected from well relatives. For example, relatives with certain personality disorders may exhibit subtle negative symptoms that could be detected by a scale for negative symptoms, even though such relatives would otherwise be categorized only as affected if the broadest possible disease definition had been chosen for the linkage analysis.

Finally, knowledge about mechanisms that involve trinucleotide repeats in genetic transmission, which has been culled from the study of a number of psychiatric illnesses, is accumulating. This is another instance of a phenomenon in which the mechanism is plausible from a biological perspective, that is, including the additional amino acids coded by triplet repeats may impact the structure or function of the protein coded by a particular gene. This developing body of knowledge should spur the use of repeat expansion detection methods. As increasingly refined results are achieved, this may enable identifying more genes that are subject to trinucleotide repeat expansion. Potentially this could powerfully corroborate results obtained by ongoing linkage analyses.

These three relatively new techniques can dramatically increase the productivity of the many scientists wrestling with the genetics of schizophrenia. From the large literature describing linkage analysis efforts that are ongoing worldwide, we know that significant amounts of money and scientists' efforts are being allocated to this question. However, these expenditures may be approaching the point of diminishing returns. Perhaps more research attention should be focused on environmental etiologies.

## Environmental Etiologies in Schizophrenia

Many of the studies reviewed herein have used pedigrees with a history of schizophrenia as the subjects of their research because this increases the ability to detect factors that may contribute to heritability. However, it is important to address the question of the way the phenomenon of family heritability is related to the incidence of schizophrenia in the general population. In other words, can the heritability model that has resulted from the genetic research account for a major portion of the cases of schizophrenia that are seen?

The recently published study of a large Danish cohort, discussed in the section "Season of Year Effects," offers important insights into this question (Mortensen et al., 1999). A major strength of this study is that it considers an entire population by drawing on the thorough health statistics maintained by Denmark. The investigators reported the elevated relative risks that would be expected for those with a family background of schizophrenia; the data in Table 3 display the calculated relative risks. Not surprisingly, relative risks for nonfamily history factors were much lower, for example, 2.40 for birth in the capital city and 1.11 for season of birth. Once again, these relative risks were significant and consistent with several previously published studies.

However, the most interesting statistics calculated by Mortensen and his colleagues were the population attributable risks, which are given in Table 4. The low population attributable risk from a family history of schizophrenia (5.5%) is overshadowed by the two environmental factors chosen by Mortensen, which account for the majority of schizophrenia cases. Thus, although a family history for schizophrenia creates high relative risks for the disease, such family histories (or at least family histories that have been identified) account for a small part of the incidence of schizophrenia in the general population.

The revelation that family background, as defined by Mortensen and colleagues, accounts for a relatively small minority of schizophrenia cases in the general population might argue that genetic factors play a relatively minor role in the etiology of the disorder for the great majority of the population, that is, those without any evidence of family history. However, such an argument unwittingly adopts the assumption that unless the disease is actually exhibited in one or more relatives, a person has zero genetic risk of schizophrenia.

In previously concluding that the diathesis-stress model best fits our understanding of the etiology of schizophrenia, there is an acknowledg-ment that even in the case of an environmental effect that broadly affects a population, such as the Dutch famine, the genetic predisposition of the members of the population will trigger the relatively small number of cases. Thus, although the readily apparent genetic risk of a family loaded for schizophrenia is a small contributor to the population risk, the currently undetectable genetic predisposition of the rest of the population remains important to the etiology of schizophrenia.

# Future Schizophrenia Research Priorities

Because the most significant role of genetics in population attributable risk is in the subtlety of the broad population's genetic predisposition, an interesting question is whether current genetic analysis, which typically focuses on families loaded for schizophrenia, will also provide insights for the much larger population without apparent family loading. The results of linkage analysis among families loaded for schizophrenia may ultimately yield techniques useful for the desirable goals of predictive genetics and/or genetic intervention. But it may be a reasonable question as to whether such techniques will prove useful in evaluating the much less apparent genetic predisposition of the general public.

Genetic research is often viewed as a triumph of high technology and the acquisition of exotic knowledge about the human genome. But, by its nature, it is a very expensive research field and consumes huge resources, measured both in dollars and human effort. Writing in 1992, E. Fuller Torrey, an unabashed advocate for increasing the amount of schizophrenia research focused on environmental effects, made the point that at the time genetics remained the only clearly defined etiological factor for schizophrenia (Torrey, 1992). However, he went on to point out that this might be because genetics is the most important factor in the disorder, but, it might also merely be because other etiological factors are yet to be identified. Certainly, research reported in the six years since Torrey offered these comments demonstrated that there are undeniable environmental effects, even if the mechanisms underlying these effects may still not be known. Studies reviewed earlier that support environmental etiologies include evidence of season of birth effects (O'Callaghan et al., 1991), evidence of delayed childhood motor development (Jones et al., 1994), evidence of in utero effects during periods of famine (Hoek et al., 1998), and flu epidemics (Barr et al., 1990).

Thus, priorities for research funds and efforts should be directed more toward examining the science underlying environmental etiologies of schizophrenia. Specific areas in which such efforts may prove productive include additional epidemiological studies like that of Mortensen et al., especially using data from countries with well-organized health statistics.

Research attention directed at generating new knowledge about in utero risk factors may prove particularly rewarding by adding to our understanding of schizophrenia and also because of its relevance to many other disorders that shatter lives and absorb huge societal resources.

In a comment related to Mortensen's recently published study, it is pointed out that unlike other mental illnesses that affect multiple cognitive systems (e.g., Alzheimer's disease), once the impairments seen at onset stabilize, schizophrenia usually does not exhibit progressive deterioration over time (Andreasen, 1999). This argues for considering the majority of schizophrenia cases as a neurodevelopmental disorder, in which damage to the brain, by definition, occurs during the developmental period between conception and late adolescence. Thus, our revised priorities should include increased research on the processes of brain development and the impact of various stressors on those processes. To the extent that mechanisms can be found that explain such neurodevelopmental problems, our understanding of schizophrenia will be enhanced, and broader gains in medical knowledge can also be achieved.

# References

Akbarian, S., Kim, J. J., Potkin, S. G., Hetrick, W. P., Bunney, W. E. Jr., & Jones, E. G. (1996). Maldistribution of interstitial neurons in prefrontal white matter of the brains of schizophrenic patients. *Archives of General Psychiatry, 53*, 425–436.

American Psychiatric Association. (1987). *Diagnostic and Statistical Manual of Mental Disorders* (3rd ed., rev.). Washington, DC: Author.

American Psychiatric Association. (1994). *Diagnostic and Statistical Manual of Mental Disorders* (4th ed.). Washington, DC: Author.

Andreasen, N. C. (1999). Understanding the causes of schizophrenia. *New England Journal of Medicine, 340*, 645–647.

Arinami, T., Itokawa, M., Aoki, J., Shibuya, H., Ookubo, Y., Iwawaki, A., Ota, K., Shimizu, H., Hamaguchi, H., & Toru, M. (1996). Further association study on dopamine D2 receptor variant S311C in schizophrenia and affective disorders. *American Journal of Medical Genetics, 67*, 133–138.

Arinami, T., Itokawa, M., Enguchi, H., Tagaya, H., Yano, S., Shimizu, H., Hamaguchi, H., & Toru, M. (1994). Association of dopamine D2 receptor molecular variant with schizophrenia. *Lancet, 343*, 703–704.

Arndt, S., Alliger, R. J., & Andreasen, N. C. (1991). The distinction of positive and negative symptoms. The failure of a two-dimensional model. *British Journal of Psychiatry, 158*, 317–322.

Arolt, V., Lencer, R., Nolte, A., Muller-Myhsok, B., Purmann, S., Schurmann, M., Leutelt, J., Pinnow, M., & Schwinger, E. (1996). Eye tracking dysfunction is a putative phenotypic susceptibility marker of schizophrenia and maps to a locus on chromosome 6p in families with multiple occurrence of the disease. *American Journal of Medical Genetics, 67*, 564–579.

Arranz, M., Sharma, T., Sham, P., Kerwin, R., Nanko, S., Owen, M., & Collier, D. (1995). Schizophrenia and the androgen receptor gene: Report of a sibship showing cosegregation with Reifenstein syndrome but no evidence for linkage in 23 multiply affected families. *American Journal of Medical Genetics, 60*, 377–381.

Asherson, P., Williams, N., Roberts, E., McGuffin, P., & Owen, M. (1994). DRD2 Ser311/Cys311 polymorphism in schizophrenia. *Lancet, 343*, 1045.

Baron, M., Risch, N., Hamburger, R., Mandel, B., Kushner, S., Newman, M., Drumer, D., & Belmaker, R. H. (1987). Genetic linkage between X-chromosome markers and bipolar affective illness. *Nature, 326*, 289–292.

Barondes, S. H. (1993). *Molecules and mental illness.* New York: Scientific American Library.

Barondes, S. H. (1998). *Mood genes: Hunting for origins of mania and depression.* New York: W. A. Freeman.

Barr, C. E., Mednick, S. A., & Munk-Jorgensen, P. (1990). Exposure to influenza epidemics during gestation and adult schizophrenia. A 40-year study. *Archives of General Psychiatry, 47*, 869–874.

Blouin, J. L., Dombroski, B. A., Nath, S. K., Lasseter, V. K., Wolyniec, S., Nestadt, G., Thornquist, M., Ullrich, G., McGrath, J., Kasch, L., Lamacz, M., Thomas, M. G., Gehrig, C., Radhakrishna, U., Snyder, S. E., Balk, K. G., Neufeld, K., Swartz, K. L., DeMarchi, N., Papadimitriou, G. N., Dikeos, D. G., Stefanis, C. N., Chakravarti, A., Childs, B., Pulver, A. E., et al. (1998). Schizophrenia susceptibility loci on chromosomes 13q32 and 8p21. *Nature Genetics, 20*, 70–73.

Bowen, T., Guy, C. A., Craddock, N., Cardno, A. G., Williams, N. M., Spurlock, G., Murphy, K. C., Jones, L. A., Gray, M., Sanders, R. D., McCarthy, G., Chandy, K. G., Fantine, E., Kalman, K., Gutman, G. A., Gargus, J. J., Williams, J., McGuffin, P., Owen, M. J., & O'Donovan, M. C. (1998). Further support for an association between a polymorphic CAG repeat in the hKCa3 gene and schizophrenia. *Molecular Psychiatry, 3*, 266–269.

Bower, B. (1998, September 5). DNA links reported for schizophrenia. *Science News*, p. 151.

Brzustowicz, L. M., Honer, W. G., Chow, E. W., Hogan, J., Hodgkinson, K., & Bassett, A. S. (1977). Use of a quantitative trait to map a locus associated with severity of positive symptoms in familial schizophrenia to chromosome 6p. *American Journal of Human Genetics, 61,* 1388–1396.

Buka, S. L., Tsuang, M. T., & Lipsitt, L. (1993). Pregnancy/ delivery complications and psychiatric diagnosis. A prospective study. *Archives of General Psychiatry, 50,* 151–156.

Burgess, C. E., Lindblad, K., Sidransky, E., Yuan, Q., Long, R. T., Breschel, T., Ross, C. A., McInnis, M., Lee, P., Ginns, E. I., Lenane, M., Kumra, S., Jacobsen, L., Rapoport, J. L., & Schalling, M. (1998). Large CAG/CTG repeats are associated with childhood-onset schizophrenia. *Molecular Psychiatry, 3*(4), 321–327.

Cao, Q., Martinez, M., Zhang, J., Sanders, A. R., Badner, J. A., Cravchik, A., Markey, C. J., Beshah, E., Guroff, J. J., Maxwell, M. E., Kazuba, D. M., Whiten, R., Goldin, L. R., Gershon, E. S., & Gejman, P. V. (1997). Suggestive evidence for a schizophrenia susceptibility locus on chromosome 6q and a confirmation in an independent series of pedigrees. *Genomics, 43*(1), 1–8.

Chandy, K. G., Fantino, E., Wittekindt, O., Kalman, K., Tong, L. L., Ho, T. H., Gutman, G. A., Crockq, M. A., Ganguli, R., Nimgaonkar, V., Morris-Rosendahl, D. J., & Gargus, J. J. (1998). Isolation of a novel potassium channel gene hSKCa3 containing a polymorphic CAG repeat: A candidate for schizophrenia and bipolar disorder? *Molecular Psychiatry, 3*(1), 32–37.

Clementz, B. A., Geyer, M. A., & Braff, D. L. (1998). Multiple site evaluation of P50 suppression among schizophrenia and normal comparison subjects. *Schizophrenia Research, 30* (1), 71–80.

Collinge, J., DeLisi, L. E., Boccio, A., Johnstone, E. C., Lane, A., Larkin, C., Leach, M., Lofthouse, R., Owen, F., Poulter, M., Shah, T., Walsh, C., & Crow, T. J. (1991). Evidence for a pseudoautosomal locus for schizophrenia using the method of affected siblings pairs. *British Journal of Psychiatry, 158,* 624–629.

Crawford, T. J., Sharma, T., Puri, B. K., Murray, R. M., Berridge, D. M., & Lewis, S. W. (1998). Saccadic eye movements in families multiply affected with schizophrenia: The Maudsley Family Study. *American Journal of Psychiatry, 155,* 1703–1710.

Crocq, M. A., Mant, R., Asherson, P., Williams, J., Hode, Y., et al. (1992). Association between schizophrenia and homozygosity at the dopamine D3 receptor gene. *Journal of Medical Genetics, 29,* 858–860.

Crow, T. J. (1997). Current status of linkage for schizophrenia: Polygenes of vanishingly small effect or multiple false positives? *American Journal of Medical Genetics, 74,* 99–103.

Crow, T. J., DeLisi, L. E., Lofthouse, R., Poulter, M., Lehner, T., Bass, N., Shah, T., Walsh, C., Boccio-Smith, A., Shields, G., & Ott, J. (1994). An examination of linkage of schizophrenia and schizoaffective disorder to the pseudo-autosomal region (Xp22.3). *British Journal of Psychiatry, 164,* 159–164.

Crow, T. J., Poulter, M., Lofthouse, R., Chin, G., Shah, T., Bass, N., Morganti, C., Vita, A., Smith, C., Boccio-Smith, A., Shields, G., & DeLisi, L. E. (1993). Male siblings with schizophrenia share alleles at the androgen receptor above chance expectation. *American Journal of Medical Genetics, 48,* 159–160.

Dickerson, R. E. (1983, December). The DNA helix and how it is read. *Scientific American, 249*(6), 94.

Egeland, J. A., Gerhard, D. S., Pauls, D. L., Sussex, J. N., Kidd, K. K., Allen, C. R., Hostetter, A. M., & Housman, D. E.

(1987). Bipolar affective disorders linked to DNA markers on chromosome 11. *Nature, 325,* 783–787.

Erwin, R. J., Turetsky, B. I., Moberg, P., Gur, R. C., & Gur, R. E. (1998). P50 abnormalities in schizophrenia: Relationship to clinical and neuropsychological indices of attention. *Schizophrenia Research, 33,* 157–167.

Essen-Moller, E. (1970). Twenty-one psychiatric cases and their MZ cotwins. *Acta Geneticae Medicae et Gemellologiae, 19,* 315–317.

Faraone, S. V., Matise, T., Svrakic, D., Pepple, J., Malaspina, D., Suarez, B., Hampe, C., Zambuto, C. T., Schmitt, K., Meyer, J., Markel, P., Lee, H., Harkavy Friedman, J., Kaufmann, C., Cloninger, C. R., & Tsuang, M. T. (1998). Genome scan of European-American schizophrenia pedigrees: Results of the NIMH Genetics Initiative and Millennium Consortium. *American Journal of Medical Genetics, 81,* 290–295.

Fischer, M. (1973). Genetic and environmental factors in schizophrenia. *Acta Psychiatrica Scandinavica, Supplementum, 238,* 1–153.

Freedman, R., Coon, H., Myles-Worsley, M., Off-Urtreger, A., Olincy, A., Davis, A., Polymeropoulos, M., Holik, J., Hopkins, J., Hoff, M., Rosenthal, J., Waldo, M. C., Reimherr, E., Wender, P., Yaw, J., Young, D. A., Breese, C. R., Adams, C., Patterson, D., Adler, L. E., Kruglyak, L., Leonard, S., & Byerley, W. (1997). Linkage of a neurophysiological deficit in schizophrenia to a chromosome 15 locus. *Proceedings of the National Academy of Sciences, U.S.A., 94,* 587–592.

Garner, C., Kelly, M., Cardon, L., Joslyn, G., Carey, A., LeDuc, C., Lichter, J., Harris, T., Loftus, J., Shields, G., Comazzi, M., Vita, A., Smith, A. M., Dann, J., Crow, T. J., & DeLisi, L. E. (1996). Linkage analyses of schizophrenia to chromosome 6p24-p22: An attempt to replicate. *American Journal of Medical Genetics, 67,* 595–610.

Gejman, P. V., Ram, A., Gelernter, J., Freedman, E., Cao, Q., Picker, D., Blum, K., Noble, E. P., Kranzler, H. R., O'Malley, S., et al. (1994). No structural mutation in the dopamine D2 receptor gene in alcoholism or schizophrenia. Analysis using denaturing gradient gel electrophoresis. *Journal of the American Medical Association, 271,* 204–208.

Gill, M., Vallada, H., Collier, D., Sham, P., Holmans, P., Murray, R., McGuffin, P., Nanko, S., Owen, M., Antonarakis, S., Housman, D., Kazazian, H., Nestadt, G., Pulver, A. E., Straub, R. E., MacLean, C. J., Walsh, D., Kendler, K. S., DeLisi, L., Polymeropoulos, M., Coon, H., Byerley, W., Lofthouse, R., Gerson, E., Read, C. M., et al. (1996). A combined analysis of D22S278 marker alleles in affected sib-pairs: Support for a susceptibility locus for schizophrenia at chromosome 22q12. Schizophrenia Collaborative Linkage Group (Chromosome 22). *American Journal of Medical Genetics, 67,* 40–45.

Goldberg, T. E., Hyde, T. M., Kleinman, J. E., & Weinberger, D. R. (1993). Course of schizophrenia: Neuropsychological evidence for a static encephalopathy. *Schizophrenia Bulletin, 19,* 797–804.

Gottesman, I. I. (1967). A polygenic theory of schizophrenia. *Proceedings of the National Academy of Sciences U.S.A., 58,* 199–205.

Gottesman, I. I. (1991). *Schizophrenia genesis.* New York: W. H. Freeman.

Gottesman, I. I., & Shields, J. (1972). *Schizophrenia and genetics: A twin study vantage point.* New York: Academic Press.

Hamer, D., & Copeland, P. (1994). *The science of desire:*

*The search for the gay gene and the biology of behavior.* New York: Touchstone.

Hoek, H. W., Brown, A. S., & Susser, E. (1998). The Dutch famine and schizophrenia spectrum disorders. *Social Psychiatry and Psychiatric Epidemiology, 33,* 373–379.

Holzman, P. S., Kringlen, E., Matthysse, S., Flanagan, S. D., Lipton, R. B., Cramer, G., Levin, S., Lange, K., & Levy, D. L. (1988). A single dominant gene can account for eye tracking dysfunctions and schizophrenia in offspring of discordant twins. *Archives of General Psychiatry, 45,* 641–647.

Holzman, P. S., Solomon, C. M., Levin, S., & Waternaux, C. S. (1984). Pursuit eye movement dysfunctions in schizophrenia. Family evidence for specificity. *Archives of General Psychiatry, 41,* 136–139.

The Huntington's Disease Collaborative Research Group. (1993). A novel gene containing a trinucleotide repeat that is expanded and unstable on Huntington's disease chromosomes. *Cell, 72,* 971–983.

Johnson, J. E., Cleary, J., Ahsan, H., Harkavy Friedman, J., Malaspina, D., Cloninger, C. R., Faraone, S. V., Tsuang, M. T., & Kaufmann, C. A. (1997). Anticipation in schizophrenia: Biology or bias? *American Journal of Medical Genetics, 74,* 275–280.

Jones, P., Rodgers, B., Murray, R., & Marmot, M. (1994). Child development risk factors for adult schizophrenia in the British 1946 birth cohort. *Lancet, 344,* 1398–1402.

Kaufmann, C. A., Suarez, B., Malaspina, D., Pepple, J., Svrakic, D., Markel, P. D., Meyer, J., Zambuto, C. T., Schmitt, K., Matise, T. C., Harkavy Friedman, J. M., Hampe, C., Lee, H., Shore, D., Wynne, D., Faraone, S. V., Tsuang, M. T., & Cloninger, C. R. (1998). NIMH Genetics Initiative Millennium Schizophrenia Consortium: Linkage analysis of African-American pedigrees. *American Journal of Medical Genetics, 81,* 282–289.

Kalsi, G., Brynjolffson, J., Butler, R., Sherrington, R., Curtis, D., Sigmundsson, D. T., Read, T., Murphy, P., Sharma, T., Petursson, H., & Gurling, H. (1995). Linkage analysis of chromosome 22q12-13 in a United Kingdom/Iceland sample of 23 multiple schizophrenia families. *American Journal of Medical Genetics (Neuropsychiatric Genetics), 60,* 298–301.

Kalsi, G., Curtis, D., Brynjolffson, J., Sigmundsson, T., Butler, R., Read, T., Murphy, P., Petursson, H., & Gurling, H. (1996). Exclusion of linkage between schizophrenia and the putative chromosome 3p24-p26 susceptibility locus. *Psychiatric Genetics, 6,* 148 (Abstract).

Kelsoe, J. R., Ginns, E. I., Egeland, J. A., Gerhard, D. S., Goldstein, A. M., Bale, S. J., Pauls, D. L., Long, R. T., Kidd, K. K., Conte, G., et al. (1989). Re-evaluation of the linkage relationship between chromosome 11p loci and the gene for bipolar affective disorder in the Old Order Amish. *Nature, 342,* 238–243.

Kendall, P. C., & Hammen, C. (1995). *Abnormal psychology.* Boston: Houghton Mifflin.

Kendler, K. S., Gruenberg, A. M., & Tsuang, M. T. (1987). Psychiatric illness in first-degree relatives of schizophrenic and surgical control patients. *Archives of General Psychiatry, 42,* 770–779.

Kendler, K. S., McGuire, M., Gruenberg, A. M., O'Hare, A., Spellman, M., & Walsh, D. (1993a). The Roscommon Family Study. I. Methods, diagnosis of probands, and risk of schizophrenia in relatives. *Archives of General Psychiatry, 50,* 527–540.

Kendler, K. S., McGuire, M., Gruenberg, A. M., O'Hare, A., Spellman, M., & Walsh, D. (1993b). The Roscommon Family Study. IV. Affective illness, anxiety disorders, and alcoholism in relatives. *Archives of General Psychiatry, 50,* 952–960.

Kendler, K. S., & Robinette, C. D. (1983). Schizophrenia in the National Academy of Sciences-National Research Council Twin Registry: A 16-year update. *American Journal of Psychiatry, 140,* 1551–1563.

Kleiderlein, J. J., Nisson, P. E., Jessee, J., Li, W. B., Becker, K. G., Derby, M. L., Ross, C. A., & Margolis, R. L. (1998). CCG repeats in cDNAs from human brain. *Human Genetics, 103,* 666–673.

Kringlen, E. (1967). *Heredity and environment in the functional psychoses.* Vol. 1 (summary of study) and Vol. 2 (case studies). Oslo: Universitetsforlaget.

Kunugi, H., Curtis, D., Vallada, H. P., Nanko, S., Powell, J. F., Murray, R. M., McGuffin, P., Owen, M. J., Gill, M., & Collier, D. A. (1996). A linkage study of schizophrenia with DNA markers from chromosome 8p21-p22 in 25 multiplex families. *Schizophrenia Research, 22,* 61–68.

Lander, E. S., & Kruglyak, L. (1995). Genetic dissection of complex traits: Guidelines for interpreting and reporting linkage results. *Nature Genetics, 11,* 241–247.

Leonard, S., Gault, J., Moore, T., Hopkins, J., Robinson, M., Oliney, A., Adler, L. E., Cloninger, C. R., Kaufmann, C. A., Tsuang, M. T., Faraone, S. V., Malaspina, D., Svrakic, D. M., & Freedman, R. (1998). Further investigation of a chromosome 15 locus in schizophrenia: Analysis of affected sibpairs from the NIMH Genetics Initiative. *American Journal of Medical Genetics, 81,* 308–312.

Li, T., Vallada, H. P., Liu, X., Xie, T., Tang, X., Zhao, J., O'Donovan, M. C., Murray, R. M., Sham, P. C., & Collier, D. A. (1998). Analysis of CAG/CTG repeat size in Chinese subjects with schizophrenia and bipolar affective disorder using the repeat expansion detection method. *Biological Psychiatry, 44,* 1160–1165.

Lidz, T. (1973). *The origin and treatment of schizophrenic disorders.* Madison, CT: International Universities Press.

Lin, M. W., Curtis, D., Williams, N., Arranz, M., Nanko, S., Collier, D., McGuffin, P., Murray, R., Owen, M., Gill, M., & Powell, J. (1995). Suggestive evidence for linkage of schizophrenia to markers on chromosome 13q14.1-q32. *Psychiatric Genetics, 5,* 117–126.

Loftus, J., DeLisi, L. E., & Crow, T. J. (1998). Familial associations of subsyndromes of psychosis in affected sibling pairs with schizophrenia and schizoaffective disorder. *Psychiatry Research, 80*(2), 101–111.

McGue, M., Gottesman, I. I., & Rao, D. C. (1985). Resolving genetic models for the transmission of schizophrenia. *Genetic Epidemiology, 2*(1), 99–110.

McGuffin, P., Sargeant, M., Hetti, S., Tidmarsh, S., Whatley, S., & Marchbanks, R. M. (1990). Exclusion of a schizophrenia susceptibility gene from the chromosome 5q11-q13 region: New data and a reanalysis of previous reports. *American Journal of Human Genetics, 47,* 524–535.

Mednick, S. A., Machon, R. A., Huttunen, M. O., & Bonett, D. (1988). Adult schizophrenia following prenatal exposure to an influenza epidemic. *Archives of General Psychiatry, 45,* 189–192.

Moises, H. W., Yang, L., Kristbjarnarson, H., Wiese, C., Byerley, W., Macciardi, F., Arolt, V., Blackwood, D., Lui, X., Sjogren, B., Aschauer, H. N., Hwu, G., Yang, K., Livesley,

W. J., Kennedy, J. L., Zoega, T., Ivarsson, O., Bui, K., Yu, M., Havsteen, B., Commenges, D., Weissenbach, J., Schwinger, E., Gottesman, I. I., Pakstis, A. J., Wetterberg, L., Kidd, K. K., & Helgason, T. (1995). An international two-stage genome-wide search for schizophrenia susceptibility genes. *Nature Genetics, 6*, 321–324.

Moldin, S. O. (1997). The maddening hunt for madness genes. *Nature Genetics, 17*, 127–129.

Mortensen, P. B., Pedersen, C. B., Westergaard, T., Wohlfahrt, J., Ewald, H., Mors, O., Andersen, P. K., & Melbye, M. (1999). Effects of family history and place and season of birth on the risk of schizophrenia. *New England Journal of Medicine, 340*, 603–608.

Nair, T. R., Christensen, J. D., Kingsbury, S. J., Kumar, N. G., Terry, W. M., & Garver, D. L. (1997). Progression of cerebroventricular enlargement and the subtyping of schizophrenia. *Psychiatry Research, 74*(3), 141–150.

Nimgaonkar, V. L., Zhang, X. R., Brar, J. S., DeLeo, M., & Ganguli, R. (1996). 5-HT2 receptor gene locus: Association with schizophrenia or treatment response not detected. *Psychiatric Genetics, 6*, 23–27.

O'Callaghan, E., Gibson, T., Colohan, H. A., Buckley, P., Walshe, D. G., Larkin, C., & Waddington, J. L. (1992). Risk of schizophrenia in adults born after obstetric complications and their association with early onset of illness: A controlled study. *British Medical Journal, 305*, 1256–1259.

O'Callaghan, E., Gibson, T., Colohan, H. A., Walshe, D., Buckley, P., Larkin, C., & Waddington, J. L. (1991). Season of birth in schizophrenia. Evidence for confinement of an excess of winter births to patients without a family history of mental disorder. *British Journal of Psychiatry, 158*, 764–769.

Onstad, S., Skre, I., Torgersen, S., & Kringlen, E. (1991). Subtypes of schizophrenia—Evidence from a twin-family study. *Acta Psychiatrica Scandinavica, 84*, 203–206.

Onstad, S., Skre, I., Torgersen, S., & Kringlen, E. (1991). Twin concordance for DSM-III-R schizophrenia. *Acta Psychiatrica Scandinavica, 83*, 395–401.

Polymeropoulos, M., Coon, H., DeLisi, L. E., Crow, T. J., Gershon, E. S., Rubenstein, J., Hoff, M., Holis, J., Boccio, M., Shields, G., Bass, N., Poulter, M., Lofthouse, R., Byerley, W., & Merril, C. (1995). Search for a schizophrenia susceptibility locus on chromosome 22. *American Journal of Medical Genetics (Neuropsychiatric Genetics), 54*, 93–99.

Pulver, A. E., Karayiorgou, M., Wolyniec, P. S., Lasseter, V. K., Kasch, L., Nestadt, G., Antonorakis, S. E., Housman, D., Kazazian, H. H., Meyers, D., Ott, J., et al. (1994). Sequential strategy to identify a susceptibility gene for schizophrenia: Report of a potential linkage on chromosome 22q12-q13.1: Part I. *American Journal of Medical Genetics (Neuropsychiatric Genetics), 54*, 36–43.

Pulver, A. E., Lasseter, V. K., Kasch, L., Wolyniec, P., Nestadt, G., Blouin, J., Kimberland, M., Babb, R., Vourlis, S., Chen, H., Lalioti, M., Morris, M. A., Karayiorgou, M., Ott, J., Meyers, D., Antonorakis, S. E., Housman, D., & Kazazian, H. H. (1995). Schizophrenia: A genome scan targets chromosomes 3p and 8p as potential sites of susceptibility genes. *American Journal of Medical Genetics (Neuropsychiatric Genetics), 60*, 252–260.

Rietschel, M. Nothen, M. M., Albus, M., Maier, W., Minges, J., Bondy, B., Koerner, J., Hemmer, S., Fimmers, R., Moeller, H. J., Wildenauer, D., & Propping, P. (1996). Dopamine D-3 receptor Gly-9/Ser-9 polymorphism and schizophrenia: No increased frequency of homozygosity in German familial cases. *Schizophrenia Research, 20*, 181–186.

Riley, B. P., Rajagopalan, S., Mogudi-Carter, M., Jenkins, T., & Williamson, R. (1996). No evidence for linkage of chromosome 6p markers to schizophrenia in Southern African Bantu-speaking families. *Psychiatric Genetics, 6*, 41–49.

Schwab, S. G., Eckstein, G. N., Hallmayer, J., Lere, B., Albus, M., Borrmann, M., Lichtermann, D., Ertl, M. A., Maier, W., & Wildenauer, D. B. (1997). Evidence suggestive of a locus on chromosome 5q31 contributing to susceptibility for schizophrenia in German and Israeli families by multipoint affected sib-pair linkage analysis. *Molecular Psychiatry, 2*(2), 156–160.

Schwab, S. G., Hallmayer, J., Lerer, B., Albus, M., Borrmann, M., Honig, S., Strauss, M., Segman, R., Lichtermann, D., Knapp, M., Trixler, M., Maier, W., & Wildenauer, D. B. (1998). Support for a chromosome 18p locus conferring susceptibility to functional psychoses in families with schizophrenia, by association and linkage analysis. *American Journal of Human Genetics, 63*, 1139–1152.

Shaw, S. H., Kelly, M., Smith, A. B., Shields, G., Hopkins, P. J., Loftus, J., Laval, S. H., Vita, A., De Hert, M., Cardon, L. R., Crow, T. J., Sherrington, R., & DeLisi, L. E. (1998). A genome-wide search for schizophrenia susceptibility genes. *American Journal of Medical Genetics, 81*, 364–376.

Sherrington, R., Brynjolffson, J., Petursson, H., Potter, M., Dudleston, K., Barraclough, B., & Wasmuth, J., et al. (1988). Localization of a susceptibility locus for schizophrenia on chromosome 5. *Nature, 336*, 164–167.

Slater, E., & Shields, J. (1953). *Psychotic and neurotic illnesses in twins*. London: Her Majesty's Stationery Office.

St. Clair, D., Blackwood, D., Muir, W., Baillie, D., Hubbard, A., Wright, A., & Evans, H. J. (1989). No linkage of chromosome 5q11-q13 markers to schizophrenia in Scottish families. *Nature, 339*, 305–309.

St. Clair, D., Blackwood, D. Muir, W., Carothers, A., Maura, W., Spowart, G., Gosden, C., & Evans, H. J. (1990). Association within a family of a balanced autosomal translocation with major mental illness. *Lancet, 336*, 13–16.

Stober, G., Jatzke, S., Meyer, J., Okladnova, O., Knapp, M., Beckmann, H., & Lesch, K. P. (1998). Short CAG repeats within the hSKCa3 gene associated with schizophrenia: Results of a family-based study. *Neuroreport, 9*, 3595–3599.

Straub, R. E., MacLean, C. J., O'Neill, F. A., Burke, J., Murphy, B., Duke, F., Shinkwin, R., Webb, B. T., Zhang, J., Walsh, D., et al. (1995). A potential vulnerability locus for schizophrenia on chromosome 6p24-22: Evidence for genetic heterogeneity. *Nature Genetics, 11*, 287–293.

Straub, R. E., MacLean, C. J., O'Neill, F. A., Walsh, D., & Kendler, K. S. (1997). Support for a possible schizophrenia vulnerability locus in region 5q22-31 in Irish families. *Molecular Psychiatry, 2*, 148–155.

Susser, E. S., & Lin, S. P. (1992). Schizophrenia after prenatal exposure to the Dutch Hunger Winter of 1944–1945. *Archives of General Psychiatry, 49*(12), 983–988.

Susser, E., Neugebauer, R., Hoek, H. W., Borwn, A. S., Lin, S., Labovitz, D., & Gorman, J. M. (1996). Schizophrenia after prenatal famine. Further evidence. *Archives of General Psychiatry, 53*, 25–31.

Tienari, P. (1975). Schizophrenia in Finnish male twins. In *Studies of Schizophrenia: British Journal of Psychiatry Special Publication No. 10*, M. H. Lader, editor. Ashford, Kent: Headley Brothers, 29–35.

Tienari, P. (1991). Interaction between genetic vulnerability and family environment: the Finnish adoptive family study of schizophrenia. *Acta Psychiatrica Scandinavica, 84*, 460–465.

Tienari, P., Sorri, A., Lahti, I., Naarala, M., Wahlberg, K. E., Moring, J., Pohjola, J., & Wynne, L. C. (1987). Genetic and psychosocial factors in schizophrenia: The Finnish adoptive family study. *Schizophrenia Bulletin, 13*, 477–484.

Tiernari, P., Sorri, A., Lahti, I., Naarala, M., Wahlberg, K. E., Ronkko, T., Pohjola, J., & Moring, J. (1985). The Finnish adoptive family study of schizophrenia. *Yale Journal of Biology and Medicine, 58*(3), 227–237.

Torrey, E. F. (1992). Are we overestimating the genetic contribution to schizophrenia? *Schizophrenia Bulletin, 18*, 159–170.

Torrey, E. F., Bowler, A. E., Taylor, E. H., & Gottesman, I. I. (1994). *Schizophrenia and manic-depressive disorder: The biological roots of mental illness as revealed by the landmark study of identical twins.* New York: Basic Books.

Travis, J. (1997, November 8). Repeating DNA linked to schizophrenia. *Science News*, p. 294.

Tsuang, M. T., & Faraone, S. V. (1997). *Schizophrenia: The facts* (2nd ed.). New York: Oxford University Press.

Vaillant, G. E. (1995). *The natural history of alcoholism revisited.* Cambridge, MA: Harvard University Press.

Veggeberg, S. K. (1996). *Medication of the mind.* New York: Henry Holt and Company.

Walker, E., & Lewine, R. J. (1990). Prediction of adult-onset schizophrenia from childhood home movies of the patients. *American Journal of Psychiatry, 147*, 1052–1056.

Wang, S., Sun, C. E., Walczak, C. A., Ziegle, J. S., Kipps, B. R., Goldin, L. R., & Diehl, S. R. (1995). Evidence for a susceptibility locus for schizophrenia on chromosome 6pter-p22. *Nature Genetics, 10*, 41–46.

Wang, Z. W., Black, D., Andreasen, N. C., & Crowe, R. R. (1993). A linkage study of chromosome 11q in schizophrenia. *Archives of General Psychiatry, 50*, 212–216.

Watson, J. D. (1981). *The double helix.* New York: Atheneum.

Wender, P. H., Kety, S. S., Rosenthal, D., Schulsinger, F., Ortmann, J., & Lunde, I. (1986). Psychiatric disorders in the biological and adoptive families of adopted individuals with affective disorders. *Archives of General Psychiatry, 42*, 923–929.

Whybrow, P. C. (1997). *A mood apart: Depression, mania, and other afflictions of the self.* New York: Basic Books.

Williams, J., Spurlock, G., McGuffin, P., Mallet, J., Nothen, M. M., Gill, M., Aschauer, H., Nylander, P., Macclardi, F., & Owen, M. J. (1996). Association between schizophrenia and T102C polymorphism of the 5-hydroxytryptamine type 2a-receptor gene. *Lancet, 347*, 1294.

# CHAPTER 15

# Schizophrenia: A Critical Examination

Charles A. Sanislow and Robert C. Carson

## Introduction

The editors commissioned us to write a chapter that challenges the notion of schizophrenia, thus providing the "other" viewpoint. It seems that the admittedly provocative view taken in the preceding edition of this chapter (Carson & Sanislow, 1993) has earned that request. At once, however, we find ourselves bewildered about what that "other" might be. Are we to represent the antithesis to the prevailing biological zeitgeist of psychopathology? Is this goal to keep alive the epistemological perspectives that have been issued by those of a Szaszian stripe? Or, are we plainly missing the boat? We are, to say the least, uncomfortable with any of these possibilities. However, the mere suggestion that "schizophrenia" may not be a viable construct inspires expectations consistent with at least one of these propositions. We warn against such expectations.

All provocation aside, there is reason for alarm in the light of the lack of progress during the past century. Hegarty and colleagues (1994) conducted an ambitious and rigorous quantitative analysis of worldwide long-term outcomes in schizophrenia over what roughly constitutes the entire span of the construct's existence. The results they found were not good. Overall, the social recovery rate was 40.2% for the period 1895 through 1991. When comparing the contemporary time frame (years 1986–1991) to the period with the most stable plateau (1926–1955), there was no significant difference. Following the introduction of neuroleptics in 1955, the social recovery rates rose to about 50%, but curiously, these rates fell back again around 1975. The authors attributed this drop to the more stringent diagnostic criteria of recent years, a hypothesis related to one of the major impediments of meaningful progress in this area.

On the other hand, the primary focus in this era appeals to the bewildering array of biological correlates in defense of the modern "disease" concept of schizophrenia (because of the lack of progress made during the last century?). In the context of a seemingly endless array of positive results, Crow (1997a) commented as follows on the resultant incoherence of the evidence:

> The problem is that many changes in many different anatomical structures are reported. Which of these is reliably associated with the disease process? If, as seems likely, there is more than one such change, which is primary and which is secondary?... We need to find changes characteristic at least of a subtype of psychopathology.... But there is an embarrassment of riches. (p. 521)

Despite our concerns that the present approaches to biological aspects of the disorder provide resolution that is far less than satisfactory, our position

Charles A. Sanislow • Department of Psychiatry, Yale University School of Medicine, New Haven, Connecticut 06520-8098. Robert C. Carson • Department of Psychology, Duke University, Durham, North Carolina 27708-0085.

*Comprehensive Handbook of Psychopathology* (Third Edition), edited by Patricia B. Sutker and Henry E. Adams. Kluwer Academic / Plenum Publishers, New York, 2001.

should not be mistaken as antibiological. Modern biotechnological methods offer potentially enormous contributions, but there are some serious problems that will be given due consideration later on. Foremost among them, the usual and customary bifurcation of biological and environmental variables lends itself to a dichotomous style of thinking that is at odds with a developmental understanding of psychopathology. We hope that our presentation here will suggest a more productive approach.

Beyond this issue, however, there remains a more fundamental problem: It is still not known exactly what schizophrenia is (this assertion should not be mistaken for deconstruction; we hold the premise that an adequate taxonomy of psychopathology is fundamental to the advancement of knowledge). Noted schizophrenia researcher Nancy Andreasen (1998) pointed out that schizophrenia is a supposed disorder with no visible neuropathology and has warned that, in the light of this fact, the withering dearth of clinical research in this area is a gaping liability. In the absence of a clearly demarcated disorder, advancing research is likely to be accompanied by substantial confusion, thereby undermining the potential knowledge acquired. This, in fact, is the predominant pattern. As will be shown in our review of the multiple changes in the diagnostic approaches, a shifting core without a firm footing is a perennial problem for schizophrenia research.

Having set an appropriately skeptical tone, we remind the reader that the behaviors conventionally associated with the term schizophrenia have been seen for many years and quite properly so, as the most stubbornly opaque, perplexing, frustrating, and in certain eras professionally demoralizing in the entire domain of mental health disciplines and in all probability, of the priestly forebears of the latter. We hope that we have prepared the reader for the idea that much of what can be said for this class of disorder does not cohere in a neat and tidy way, and some of it may be quite disconcerting in its refractoriness to satisfactory conceptualization. Major revisions in the way that the disorder is thought about and studied will be necessary for real progress.

In this chapter, we will address the following areas: The identification of the core, if any, of the disorder(s) (Taxonomic Issues), how genetic and environmental variables are thought about in a developmental context (Etiologic Considerations),

and consideration of the treatment process (Treatment Perspectives). In short, we think that much of what follows will demonstrate that this is not a domain in which simple answers—for example, that schizophrenia is a definite, unitary, but as yet imprecisely localized brain disease—have even a minimal likelihood of achieving convincing confirmation in the foreseeable future.

## Taxonomic Issues

### Background of the Schizophrenia Diagnosis

In 1860, Belgian psychiatrist Benedict Morel described the case of a 13-year-old boy whose functioning severely deteriorated from that of a brilliant pupil to an increasingly withdrawn, lethargic, seclusive, and delusional boy with substantial intellectual decline. Morel hypothesized that the deterioration was the result of irrecoverable brain degeneration of hereditary origin. He used the term *démence précoce* to describe the condition and to distinguish it from the dementing disorders associated with old age. Based on this early belief of intellectual deterioration—a belief that, as will be shown in more detail later, is not well-supported—Kraepelin subsequently adopted the Latin form of this term to refer to a group of conditions that all seemed to have the feature of mental deterioration beginning early in life.

Bleuler (1911/1950) objected to the term in part because he believed that both of its elements were erroneous and misleading. He reportedly observed numerous patients who otherwise met the descriptive criteria for dementia praecox but whose disorders did not progress inexorably into profound cognitive deterioration and did not first appear at a young age. Bleuler felt that he had identified by careful observation a theretofore unrecognized set of "fundamental symptoms" that were invariant and basic properties of the disorder. He believed that these should be its defining features as well as the criterial specifications for rendering the diagnosis. For Bleuler, the central feature of the disorder was that of the "splitting" of different psychic functions, and therefore named the disorder schizophrenia. However, he issued the important caveat (and one that we would submit still holds true today): "For the sake of convenience, I use the word in the singular although it is ... apparent that *the group includes several diseases*" (Bleuler, 1911/1950, p. 8, emphasis added). Indeed, persons who earn the designation "schizophrenic" are an extremely heterogeneous lot both behaviorally and biologically, far more so than "normals" in many dimensions of comparison. The recognition of such heterogeneity has spawned a variety of proposed subtypes of schizophrenia over the years and has led some investigators (e.g., Bellak, 1979) to conclude that "schizophrenia" is merely a final common pathway of varied ego dysfunctions produced by numerous distinct causal patterns. Such a view raises questions about the need for an overarching and potentially misleading construct such as schizophrenia. At the same time, evolving diagnostic systems make zeroing in on the core of a disorder like trying to hit a moving target.

### Developmental History of the DSM-IV Criteria

To fully understand the modern diagnosis of schizophrenia, according to the most prominent system (i.e., DSM), requires a careful look at the history of the ways by which the disorder has been defined. Bleuler was the first to coin the term schizophrenia, but Kraepelin—at least as it appears by the current climate in psychiatric diagnosis—has been credited the status of father of the disorder.

**Early Formulations by Kraepelin.** In outlining the following symptomatology for dementia praecox, Kraepelin noted that the "... disease picture appears so varied that upon superficial observation the fundamental symptoms are not recognized" (Defendorf, 1902, p. 154). He went on to note the moderate effects of what we would now term anxiety (i.e., "clouding of consciousness") and the presence of hallucinations early in the course of the disease, suggesting a source for the distress. It seems that, for Kraepelin, a perplexing aspect of the disorder concerned the fact that those in the throes of it were apparently unaffected in their abilities to perceive the majority of their surroundings and orientation in accurate terms, although delusional states could impose major distortions of specific aspects of the patient's surrounding reality. The other major symptom areas concerned attentional difficulties, primarily the inability to control attentional processes, and disturbance of "emotional field" which referred to a loss of interest or pleasure in routine daily activ-

ities. Finally, in some cases, there was a disturbance of conduct, or a "disappearance of voluntary activity" that also appeared on occasion at the other extreme in the form of impulsive acts (e.g., outbursts of smashing things such as breaking dishes).

Kraepelin noted several areas of progressive deterioration associated with dementia praecox. These, he noted, were primarily in the areas of memory and judgment. For the former, Kraepelin noted that it was the memories formed after the onset of the disorder that were in fact impaired; memories before the onset of the disorder remained intact. The worsening of judgment was largely attributed to behavior that was performed in response to persecutory delusional states. Finally, Kraepelin noted the absence of a definite external cause and the limitation of the methods of the time to establish an anatomical pathological basis for the disease. Indeed, his way of thinking about the disorder has been increasingly embraced in more recent times (i.e., the assumption of a discrete anatomical cause and also, his emphasis on the deterioration feature of the disorder). Kraepelin outlined a clinical description of dementia praecox, but it was somewhat lacking in diagnostic specification, and there was at least some implication of a manic component. For instance, "The whole disturbance can be very gradual ... and the symptoms so ill-defined that relatives see them only as a weakness in character.... He may still show the same or even greater industriousness, apply himself tirelessly to his books, engage in massive, inappropriate and indigestible reading ..." (Kraepelin, 1896/1987, p. 13). It was left to Bleuler to attempt to better isolate the clinical entity in more discrete clinical terms.

**Bleulerian Criteria.** The "splitting" that Bleuler believed characterized the essence of schizophrenic mentation was said to be manifest in three "altered simple functions": association, affectivity, and ambivalence. The other "simple functions"—those of sensation, perception, orientation, and motility—were said to be unaffected in schizophrenia. Certain "compound functions" were also regularly involved in the schizophrenic process, but the only deficit of this type uniformly present was a splitting in the person's relation to reality, termed *autism*. Bleuler's "four A's," as they came to be known, were considered the bedrock characteristics of the disorder for many years, and therefore deserve close attention.

The splitting deficit in *association*—in modern parlance variously termed formal thought disorder, loosening or derailment of association, incoherence, and cognitive slippage—was considered by earlier generations of clinicians the sine qua non of the schizophrenia diagnosis. In severe cases, the phenomenon is very striking and can be utterly baffling to listeners, but its subtler forms are far from obvious and may be detected only post hoc, if then, when clinicians realize on reflection that they have understood hardly anything of prior conversations with patients. The main difficulty is a failure to organize the elements of ideas into linear sequences; the patient's train of thought gets interrupted by intrusions and blockages, and the result is that verbalizations are at best imprecise and at worst mere "word salad."

Bleuler considered that the deficits of affectivity fundamental to schizophrenia are manifold. Often a profound indifference is the most striking feature of the patient's emotional life. Where emotions, even seemingly intense ones, are displayed, they often lack convincing depth and tend to be highly labile. In general, according to Bleuler, there is a discontinuity (splitting) between emotions and the remainder of the patient's mental life, such that thoughts and feelings may seem orthogonal. Unprovoked mood swings are common, as is a certain "blunting" with respect to matters of taste and social propriety. Bleuler gave as an example of the latter a patient's response (conveyed with blissful expression) to being reprimanded for drinking his own urine: "*Herr Direktor*, if you should taste it but once, you would never want to drink anything else" (p. 52). Bleuler (1911/1950) termed as "ambivalence "the tendency of the schizophrenia psyche to endow the most diverse psychisms with both a positive and a negative indicator at one and the same time" (p. 53). Three forms of schizophrenic ambivalence are discernible: (1) affective ambivalence, in which a particular concept or object simultaneously elicits pleasant and unpleasant feelings; (2) ambivalence of will, where the patient experiences co-occurring motives of an opposite or incompatible nature; and (3) intellectual ambivalence, involving the simultaneous maintenance of logically contradictory ideas.

Finally, Bleuler (1911/1950) noted that schizophrenia was always accompanied by a greater or lesser loosening of ties to reality (another type of splitting): "This detachment from reality, together with the relative and absolute predominance of the inner life, we term *autism*" (p. 63, emphasis added). It is interesting that Bleuler, who had been influenced by psychoanalysis, considered that autism was essentially in the service of protecting the patient's "complexes." In other words, the patient's sense of reality tends to fail mostly in matters that have substantial personal import. However, Bleuler doubted that emotional complexes were *etiologically* significant in schizophrenia.

**Schneiderian First-Rank Symptoms.** Notwithstanding Bleuler's extraordinarily detailed and perceptive effort to refine the dementia praecox entity, it had become apparent by the 1950s, at least in the United States, that the distinctions he had proposed were either insufficiently understood (the English translation of Bleuler's major work did not appear until 1950) or too subtle to be adeptly applied by frontline mental health personnel. Interdiagnostician agreement in recognizing the presumed entity, as was shown in repeated studies, was unacceptably, even embarrassingly, low as a general rule, and a tendency had developed to employ idiosyncratic local conventions. The awesomely hopeless prognosis for the unfortunates who acquired the label only complicated matters.

These problems were temporarily alleviated somewhat with the widespread introduction of chlorpromazine, the first of the phenothiazine neuroleptics, in 1955. Now a person could be said to have probably been schizophrenic if he or she responded with notable symptom reduction to a trial on chlorpromazine. But this diagnosis by outcome was still (for various practical and theoretical reasons) a very unsatisfactory gambit. The time was ripe for a new approach to the diagnosis of schizophrenia, one that would permit drawing conclusions upon completion of relatively brief clinical evaluation, but might also yield a reasonable level of interdiagnostician agreement. The work of the German psychiatrist, Kurt Schneider (1959), fit the bill and was seized upon by a number of influential investigators in the United States.

Schneider's approach was organized around eleven pathognomonic signs or "first-rank" symptoms, any one of which, if present, was considered a strong indicator of the presence of a schizophrenic process. In contrast to the subtleties of the Bluelerian criteria, the plainness of Schneider's behaviorally described signs were terms that clinicians have relatively little difficulty in assessing.

1. The patient hears voices speaking his or her thoughts aloud.
2. The patient is the subject of a discussion or argument among hallucinated voices.
3. Hallucinated voices describe the patient's ongoing activity.
4. Delusional percept (a normal perception is interpreted as having special and highly personal significance).
5. Somatic passivity (the patient is a reluctant recipient of bodily sensations imposed by an external agent).
6. Thought insertion (an outside force puts thoughts in the patient's mind).
7. Thought withdrawal (an outside force removes the patient's thoughts).
8. Thought broadcast (the patient experiences his or her thoughts being magically and involuntarily transmitted to others).
9. "Made" feelings (the patient experiences feelings as imposed and controlled by an external agent).
10. "Made" impulses (the patient experiences impulses as similarly imposed from outside).
11. "Made voluntary acts (patients experience their motor activity as similarly imposed from outside).

Schneider's approach to identifying schizophrenia differs fundamentally from that of Bleuler. Whereas Bleuler's criteria focus almost entirely on the formal properties of mentation independent of mental content, Schneider makes distinctive mental content in the form of certain types of delusional and hallucinatory phenomena the central defining property. In fact, Bleuler would have regarded every one of Schneider's signs as having mere "accessory" and inconstant status in instances of true schizophrenia. In any event, Schneider's approach has had a somewhat greater influence in determining the present diagnostic criteria than Bleuler's, as will be seen in what follows.

Whether such prominence is deserved is open to question. Findings from a variety of pertinent studies (e.g., Carpenter, Strauss, & Muleh, 1973; McCabe & Stromgren, 1975; Newmark, Falk, Johns, Boren, & Forehand, 1976; Wing & Nixon, 1975; World Health Organization, 1973) indicate that Schneider's signs show up with distressing frequency in patients for whom a primary diagnosis of schizophrenia would seem on other grounds to be inappropriate. We would also sug-gest that it seems unwise to employ as a cornerstone of diagnosis alleged mental phenomena that have the status of private experience (e.g., the patients' voices) and can never be directly observed by the diagnostician or, for that matter, by anyone else. The standard scientific requirement of interobserver reliability is impossible to satisfy (in fact, meaningless) in such a context, unless it is specified that the focus of inquiry is exclusively on what the patient reports *about* mental happenings of this sort—in which case the observation itself loses much of its intrinsic force.

**Other Diagnostic Systems.** In the early 1970s, several other efforts were made to develop more precise criteria. These efforts were primarily by research investigators. Movements began in some research centers to eschew entirely the often vague, abstract, and theory-driven official criteria in favor of definitions stated in very concrete observational language (i.e., so-called operational criteria). Two proposed sets of such criteria—those of Feighner, Robins, Guze, Woodruff, and Munoz (1972) and a modified version by Spitzer, Endicott, and Robins (1975) that included definitions of schizophrenia—rapidly gained ascendancy among investigators, and it soon became commonplace in the method sections of research reports to read that subjects had been selected according to one or the other of these sets of fairly similar criteria. It was inevitable that the third edition of the *Diagnostic and Statistical Manual of Mental Disorders* (DSM-III; American Psychiatric Association [APA], 1980) would strongly reflect both of these efforts, especially the more current one of Spitzer et al. That is what happened pretty much across the board and particularly in relation to the diagnostic criteria for schizophrenia, which turned out to be largely a reproduction of the Spitzer et al. (1975) Research Diagnostic Criteria rules for making the diagnosis.

Endicott and colleagues (1986) reported in a study in which a given group of patients, after careful clinical study, was diagnosed according to seven different (but considerably overlapping) proposed systems for rendering the schizophrenia diagnosis and obtained results that were not encouraging. They found an eightfold variation among the systems in their rates of applying the diagnosis. *None* of the systems did very well in predicting patient status a mere 6 to 25 months later, although the DSM-III was comparatively among the least inadequate in this respect.

**DSM-IV.** Since the introduction of DSM-III, the changes in subsequent versions have been relatively minor (compared to the changes from DSM-II [APA, 1968] to DSM-III). The primary change concerns the duration of symptoms. From DSM-III to DSM-III-R (APA, 1987), a specification of at least a 1-week duration for the psychotic-delusional (criterion "A") symptoms was added, allegedly to exclude transient psychotic disorders. When DSM-IV (APA, 1994) was introduced, this specification was increased to 1-month, again to "reduce false positive diagnoses" (p. 779). A primary goal of the revisions made in DSM-IV included the provision that "... revisions that would result in substantial reclassification of patients relative to DSM-III-R were to be avoided" (Flaum, Andreasen, & Widiger, 1994, p. 1008). This suggested a recognition of the way changing conceptions of the disorder have stilted progress.

The introduction of the DSM-III began a persistent trend to narrow the schizophrenia diagnosis. There are at least two studies in the literature, those of Winters, Weintraub, and Neale (1981) and Harrow, Carone, and Westermeyer (1985), in which a group of DSM-II-diagnosed schizophrenics was rediagnosed according to DSM-III criteria. The proportions of patients who survived the "cut" (i.e., retained the diagnosis) in the two studies were, respectively, 51 and 41%. Needless to say, such instability renders it uncertain to what extent volumes of pre-1980 research findings apply to the schizophrenias of today. The increase in the duration specification for criterion A, first to 1 week in DSM-III-R, and then to one month in DSM-IV, would be likely to further exclude subjects and perhaps select for a more chronic form of disorder.

To summarize the problems of the main criteria set for DSM-IV schizophrenia, it is neither Bleulerian nor Schneiderian, but a rather complex mixture of both, and considerably favors the latter. Moreover, if there is a clear and unifying concept underlying the various constituent criterial signs, it is not revealed in the accompanying DSM-IV commentary, nor have we been able to discern it on our own. Therefore, the list seems to be something of a hodgepodge of indicators traditionally associated with the concept of schizophrenia, where for the most part each makes an independent contribution to the diagnostic outcome. Certain of the quantitative rules (e.g., "two of the following"; why not one, or three?) are almost

entirely arbitrary. Moreover, for criterion A, only one (not two) of the characteristic symptoms is required if "... delusions are bizarre or hallucinations consist of a voice keeping up a running commentary on a person's behavior or thoughts, or two or more voices conversing with each other" (APA, 1994, p. 285). As can be seen, hallucinatory phenomena are strongly represented and entail the perplexing problems of intersubjective reliability discussed earlier. The naturally occurring overlap with mood disturbance is managed in an artificially exclusionary manner in a cosmetic attempt to enhance diagnostic reliability at the expense of clinical realities. Finally, despite "operational" pretensions, much room remains for subjective judgment in applying the criteria. For example, what is a delusion (see, e.g., Oltmanns & Maher, 1988), and at what intensity level does a phenomenon become "marked"?

No discussion of the schizophrenia diagnosis would be complete without considering the various schizophrenia subtypes that have been proposed, to which we now turn before wrapping up diagnostic issues.

## Schizophrenia Subtypes

Given the pluralistic evidence of schizophrenias, it should be no surprise that the proposed subtypes have existed since the inception of the disorder. We will argue here that given the demonstrated elusiveness of the main category, it would be surprising if any of the subdivisions proved to have extraordinary robustness at the empirical level. Indeed, a major criticism of many of these studies is that too broad a spectrum of psychotic disorders is typically employed, so that it is not necessarily "schizophrenia" that is being subtyped (McGorry, Bell, Dudgeon, & Jackson, 1998). We describe the classical subtypes and also consider the more recent "positive" versus "negative" symptom differentiation.

**The Classical Subtypes.** Kraepelin described hebephrenic, catatonic, and two paranoid subtypes of the disorder (Defendorf, 1902). Later, Bleuler (1911/1950) described simple, hebephrenic, catatonic, and paranoid forms of the basic schizophrenic disorder, but it is clear that he considered that these qualitative distinctions related merely to varying profiles of "accessory" symptoms among different patients who shared the same fundamental deficits. He was not very impressed with them in terms of their prognostic or predictive significance, and a wealth of evidence accumulated over subsequent decades indicates that he was largely right about this. It is, in fact, not uncommon for schizophrenic patients to display mixtures of these symptom clusters and move among them during the course of an episode.

Therefore, it is somewhat puzzling why the practice of applying formal classical subtype diagnoses has persisted, with only minor modification, to the present. From DSM-III on, the "simple" subtype, basically a symptomless personality description, has evidently (and wisely) been relegated to one or another of the Axis II personality disorders, but the other subtypes remain as originally described, and the "hebephrenic" is now called the "disorganized" subtype. The subtype "undifferentiated" was added to the DSMs long ago to apply to the many instances of mixed and/or highly unstable clinical pictures one sees in any psychiatric inpatient setting.

If there is any justification for retaining this seemingly outmoded system of classic subtyping, it resides in a distinction between the paranoid and the remaining subtypes. As a group, paranoids seem different (Magaro, 1980). Schizophrenic patients who remain persistently paranoid often do not show the kind of striking cognitive and/or attentional deficits seen in other forms of the disorder (Rabin, Doneson, & Jentons, 1979). As a group they tend to have a more benign course and outcome (Ritzler, 1981), and they show less evidence of familial concordance (genetic loading?) for schizophrenia (Kendler & Davis, 1981). On the other hand, many patients originally subdiagnosed as paranoid later acquire alternate designations (Kendler & Tsuang, 1981), and it is a venerable item of clinical lore that some paranoid disorders prove extremely intractable and chronic. There is sufficient reason in all of this to maintain a distinction between paranoid and nonparanoid forms of schizophrenia in selecting subjects for research; the groups can always be collapsed if the data prove that the distinction is irrelevant.

**Positive- and Negative-Symptom Schizophrenias.** The changing terminology associated with this distinction has made the long history of these subtypes less obvious than the classical subtypes. This dichotomy can be traced back to the process-reactive distinction forms of schizophrenia. Discrimination between the two was a matter of estimating case characteristics in four bipolar dimensions: (1) slow and insidious versus abrupt onset; (2) absence of identifiable precipitating stress versus severe stress experienced immediately prior to onset; (3) socially shut-in and withdrawn versus socially engaged premorbid functioning; and (4) flat, blunted affect versus volatile, intense affect expression. For each, the first refers more to a *process* pattern, whereas its opposite was said to be associated with the *reactive* one. As these terms suggest, extreme process schizophrenia was considered an endogenously determined pattern of inexorable deterioration, not in concept unlike Kraepelin's dementia praecox, whereas the more reactive variety was seen as induced decompensation in the face of overwhelming life challenge (and therefore had a far more favorable prognosis). Unfortunately, however, the circumstances of many schizophrenic patients were such that they could not definitely be allocated to one or the other of these categories, and some "reactives" showed a distressing tendency over time to drift toward the process end of the continuum.

A later but conceptually similar effort along these lines focused more exclusively on the general competence and adequacy of the person's social functioning before obvious breakdown; the distinction here was "poor premorbid" versus "good premorbid." This strategy yielded a more reliable allocation of patients to the pertinent subtypes, but it too eventually succumbed to a variety of puzzling and contradictory research findings; some of them were undoubtedly attributable to the poorly understood effects of newly introduced phenothiazine drugs. Before its demise, however, this subtyping strategy had modest success in achieving, for the first time, a measure of order in attempts to conceptualize rampant schizophrenic heterogeneity (e.g., Garmezy & Rodnick, 1959).

The newest version of the presumed underlying dichotomy addressed in these efforts is the currently popular distinction between "negative" and "positive" schizophrenia. These terms refer, respectively, to behavioral characteristics that constitute a deficit relative to normal performance and to those that involve some added element not normally present. Thus, flat affect and social withdrawal are negative symptoms, whereas hallucinations and delusions are positive ones (see Andreasen, 1985, 1988; Andreasen et al., 1995, for a more extended discussion on these subtypes). Therefore, negative schizophrenia is roughly equivalent conceptually to the old "process" or "poor premorbid" designations, whereas positive schizophrenia bears the same relationship to the "reactive" or "good premorbid" subtypes. A related differentiation that emphasizes biological variables and speed of onset more refers essentially to these same patterns as Type I (positive) and Type II (negative) schizophrenia (Crow, 1985). Although most patients exhibit both positive and negative signs during the course of their disorders (Breier et al., 1994; Guelfi, Faustman, & Csernansky, 1989), a preponderance of negative symptoms in the clinical picture, it has increasingly been shown, has relatively grave prognostic significance (e.g., Fenton & McGlashan, 1994; McGlashan & Fenton, 1993). Finally, there has been some suggestion that the negative symptoms bear some relationship to medication side effects (Kornhuber et al., 1989; see also Miller and Ereshefsky, 1997).

Disorganized schizophrenia is an independently discerned subtype of schizophrenia that has more recently gained recognition partially independent of the positive and negative subtypes (Ratakonda, Gorman, Yale, & Amador, 1998; Toomey et al., 1997). This subtype is characterized chiefly by chaotic and seemingly directionless speech and behavior, and it has been recognized as the classic hebephrenic subtype of schizophrenia. **Subtypes in the DSM-IV.** The DSM-IV retains subsequent versions of the classic subtypes, including paranoid, disorganized, catatonic, undifferentiated, and residual, despite the criticism that these subtypes evidence poor reliability, poor stability over time, and poor prognostic value (McGlashan and Fenton, 1994). It seems that these subtypes were left in mainly on the basis of "clinical tradition" and the belief that they do possess some prognostic value, despite evidence to the contrary (Flaum, Andreasen, & Widiger, 1994). Interestingly, Appendix B of DSM-IV (APA, 1994) contains a section on "Alternative Dimensional Descriptors for Schizophrenia." These are shown in Table 1.

### Commentary on the Current Diagnostic State of Affairs

In leveling these criticisms, we are in the awkward position of having nothing better to offer (and neither does the field). Debates about ways to

**Table 1. Alternative Dimensional Descriptors for Schizophrenia from the DSM-IV (APA, 1994)[a]**

| Dimension | Description |
|---|---|
| Psychotic | Hallucinations or delusions |
| Disorganized | Disorganized speech or behavior, or inappropriate affect |
| Negative | Affective flattening, alogia, avolition (exclude the effects of medication, depression, and positive symptoms such as hallucinations or delusions) |

[a]The extent to which each dimension is present is rated as absent, mild, moderate, or severe, and ratings can be made for the present episode, and/or the past 6 months, or for the lifetime course of the disorder.

interpret findings from nosological studies of psychosis derived from DSM criteria sets continue along the lines of how many forms of psychosis actually exist. As many as six subclasses have been suggested (e.g., Kendler, Karkowski, & Walsh, 1998; McGorry, Bell, Dudgeon, & Jackson, 1998), and other investigators have provided evidence that suggests four factors (e.g., Dollhus et al., 1996). More parsimonious models have identified criteria sets corresponding to Bleulerian negative symptoms and Schneiderian first-rank systems, results that are not especially surprising in the light of our review of the development of the DSM diagnostic systems.

In any event, the field is presently plagued with debates about where to draw the line on the number of schizophrenic disorders, and the blurry boundary between psychotic and affective disorders has yet to be adequately resolved. We submit that these debates will largely turn out to be fruitless, mainly on the grounds that a multitude of diagnostic approaches drive the interpretation of the data in ways that are not necessarily empirically or theoretically grounded. We further suggest that the current diagnostic system needs a complete overhaul (see Carson, 1997, for careful consideration of this argument). We restrain ourselves from repeating those criticisms here, but it must be mentioned that progress in taxonomy would be better served by a move in the direction of parsimony, with the explicit goal of abandoning the categorical format in favor of a dimensional one (e.g., Bell, Dudgeon, McGorry, & Jackson, 1998; Crow, 1997b). Thus, we view the "alternative" diagnostic scheme presented before as favorable and a step in the right direction.

Where is the field to go from here? An indispensable requirement is that we recognize an urgency to the taxonomic/diagnostic dilemma presented by those diverse aberrations of behavior that are traditionally and somewhat casually allocated to the schizophrenia rubric. In an article often cited in the field of psychiatry, Robins and Guze (1970) suggested minimal requirements for developing validity in psychiatric diagnoses. The basic requirements they put forth have not been adequately followed, and, in particular, a need remains for much neglected basic clinical research (Andreasen, 1998). The haphazard array of diagnostic criteria illustrate the slow progress in this area, and these limitations all but assuredly hamper research efforts aimed at etiology and treatment. In the most basic manner, the DSM system is plainly inadequate for these purposes. Andreasen (1998) made this point in a straightforward manner: "DSM was developed as a clinical manual to serve as a diagnostic 'gatekeeper.' Its descriptions of many disorders are intentionally sparse, simple, and incomplete. (*This is especially true for schizophrenia*)" (p. 1659, emphasis added).

Is the situation hopeless? Perhaps not. The compromise position is simply settling for a definition of the disorder that is more or less acceptable to practitioners and researchers but that is arbitrary in some sense. In fact, this is the strategy adopted by contemporary nosologists such as the authors of the DSMs (i.e., DSM-III and beyond). With such an approach, it is conceivable that systematic and meaningful patterns will be identified over time. And as understanding increases, the defining diagnostic criteria can be sharpened to reflect what might eventually become a valid construct. There is abundant evidence that a program of this sort, "bootstrapping" (Cronbach & Meehl, 1955) our way haltingly toward an understanding of the nature of these disorders, is already in place among mental health researchers. Alas, there is no better alternative, provided that we do not fool ourselves into thinking about "schizophrenia" in unduly reified terms and provided that we continue to seek a much-needed refinement of this *open construct*

in an informed and rigorous manner. This is the sense in which we shall be using the term in the remainder of the chapter.

## Etiologic Considerations

There has been tremendous effort over the years to isolate or otherwise identify a genetic cause of schizophrenia. The process of this research is one that deserves at least parenthetical comment. An answer to "the question" (i.e., What is the cause of schizophrenia?) is never quite obtained, despite intermittent promises that loom on the horizon. The potentially promising results entice researchers, offering hope that the answer to the schizophrenia puzzle will soon be solved. Often, such findings are seized upon by the media, further encouraging simplistic answers to a very complex problem. This is a curious pattern, and one that we speculate is at least partly influenced by the desperation naturally associated with working with such a devastating and disabling disorder in the absence of any truly effective interventions (recall the lack of progress during the last century). Those entering the field should be warned against such potentially seductive claims.

If, as we would anticipate, schizophrenia turns out to be a variety of separate and distinct disorders that happen to share some similar properties at the level of behavioral output (and the class "psychotic," after all, has finite boundaries), it would seem unrealistic to search for some primary etiologic factor that controls a large proportion of morbid outcome variance. Another implication of the multiple-pathway notion is that the search will prove very difficult because such heterogeneity will impede the establishment of reliable commonalities of background across persons who acquire the diagnosis. As will be seen, both of these expectations are amply confirmed in the findings of etiologically relevant research.

It has become customary in discussions of this sort to treat separately purported biological and psychosocial causal influences in schizophrenia, as though it were reasonable to conceive that such influences somehow contribute to the outcome independently of one another; that is, in the merely additive, orthogonal fashion suggested by a simple version of the diathesis-stress model (Zubin & Spring, 1977). It is increasingly clear, however, that some sort of combinatory function that operates between these two broad sources of causation is at least frequent and quite possibly routine in the development of schizophrenia. Accordingly, we will not employ the common but potentially misleading format of biological/psychosocial causation in what follows but will rather try to convey something of what we judge is the enormous complexity of relationships between the two as our discussion of distinct causal factors proceeds.

We have deliberately used the somewhat cumbersome expression *combinatory function* in the preceding paragraph, where in this context the term interaction is doubtless far more commonly employed. But the latter term may suggest a particular kind of joint determination of outcome, whereas we typically do not know the specific form in which the two classes of variables (biological and psychosocial) conjoin in contributing to the schizophrenic outcome. Hardly anyone doubts that some sort of "interaction," loosely defined, occurs among the variables so far identified and that they are probably implicated in producing schizophrenic outcomes. Indeed, the direct and indirect evidence pertaining to the operation of potent modifier variables with respect to essentially every factor suspected of having etiologic significance is so multifaceted and compelling that the task of finding one's way around in the thicket can be stupefying. It is precisely for this reason, we surmise, that investigators generally manifest strong propensities to focus on and treat genetic, other biological, and psychosocial factors as separable entities, even though it makes only limited sense to do so in light of the evidently convoluted etiologic pathways involved. An additional complicating factor is that these pathways will probably turn out to be highly idiosyncratic for individual instances of disorder (Meehl, 1978), thereby seriously compromising the research value of aggregating observations over subjects.

We have little choice but to follow the leads investigators have laid down, but in doing so, we should bear in mind that the strategies employed mask to a great extent the central fact of pervasive and developmentally continuous interplay among the contributory influences. The general problem here is well illustrated in connection with the suspected role of genetic variables in the intergenerational transmission of a propensity to develop schizophrenia. We turn now to a discussion of the evidence supporting this hypothesis.

## Genetic Variables in Schizophrenia

The concept of interaction held by most psychologists derives from the ANOVA statistical model—where, for example, outcomes are allocated to cross-cutting genetic and environmental factors, to their interaction $(G \times E)$, and to "error." This conception of interaction can be quite misleading because the constituent elements are erroneously considered independent and the natural events that unfold in the process of development are removed from the temporal sequences in which they occur. Variance components are extracted and treated as though they were distinct entities unaffected by one another over time. But discrete factors do not occur as such in nature, and the statistical model of necessity ignores the extent to which genes and environment covary over time; in fact, the variable of time, crucial for any developmental process, is discarded. What we are suggesting, then, is the necessity for a decidedly more fine-grained analysis of genetic–environment interaction if there is to be any hope of achieving a true understanding of the contribution of either component to schizophrenic outcomes. With these caveats in mind, we proceed to review the genetic evidence.

Inquiries into the genetics of schizophrenia can be roughly divided into two strategic approaches; each is a function of the progress of knowledge and methods available to scholars and scientists who work in this area. The first approach is based on the traditional Mendelian understanding of genetics, where the occurrence of traits (phenotypes) are identified and observed across generations for trends that will shed light on underlying genetic mechanisms. Working from the other direction, more modern techniques have been developed since the molecular elucidation of DNA and the subsequent development of biochemical techniques to study the encryption and expression of heritable information. The family (including twin and adoption methodologies) belongs to the traditional approaches, though what is in only some ways a less inferential examination of genetic processes is possible in the realm of molecular biology. Either approach faces an extreme limitation: A significant gap remains between what is observed at the behavioral level and that which is observed at the molecular—or inferred at the genetic—level. That gap, partly framed by the nature of the questions asked, will have to be bridged to improve the present rate of progress. More on that later, but first a summary of the currently accepted knowledge.

**Twin Studies.** It is well-established that there is a higher concordance rate among monozygotic twins (MZ) than among dizygotic twins (DZ), a finding that is often cited in defense of the argument that schizophrenia is a "mostly genetic" disease. In a review of the worldwide literature on twin studies, Torrey and colleagues (1994) report an overall pairwise concordance rate of 28% for MZ twins, and 6% for DZ twins. Thus, it seems clear that sharing 100% of the genes with a schizophrenic twin greatly increases the risk (almost fivefold) of developing the disorder. Furthermore, sharing 50% of the genes, as in DZ twins, provides a risk that is substantially greater than in the general population.

Torrey et al. (1994) reported on twenty-seven pairs of MZ twins discordant for schizophrenia, a research strategy that was potentially revealing about nongenetic causal factors. Perinatal factors were important in at least 30% of affected cases, as were widespread early CNS dysfunctions. Evidence from discordant affected twins sheds some light on the complexity of the genetic evidence from twin studies. Of discordant affected twins, 30% were described as having been different during early childhood (e.g., shy and withdrawn, aggressive, or odd), suggesting possible CNS dysfunction. These twins also showed prominent alterations in brain function as assessed by cerebral blood flow, neuropsychological tests, neurological exam, and smooth-pursuit eye movement. Hypofrontality (reduced blood flow to the frontal lobes), it was demonstrated, is associated with reduced size of the anterior hippocampus. Moderate/severe cognitive impairment in neuropsychological tests was observed in fourteen of the twenty-seven affected twins. The nonschizophrenic co-twins of discordant pairs, though less neurologically impaired than their disordered siblings, were more impaired than a set of control MZ twins where both members of the twinship were considered psychiatrically normal. Comparing schizophrenic persons from discordant and concordant pairs, no significant differences in clinical or potential etiologic variables are found.

What can be made of the findings that changes in brain structure were not correlated with clinical aspects of schizophrenia in the affected twins and that there were significant structural deficits in the nonaffected twins? It appears that things are more complicated than can be sorted on the basis of this methodology. Although compelling, several shortcomings must be kept in mind. First, despite the apparent robustness of these findings, it remains impossible to predict schizophrenia outcome for individual cases. Second, there are some inconsistencies in these data. In a few cases, the "well" twin appeared more biologically compromised than the affected co-twin. The authors rightly conclude that these data do not sufficiently resolve the most basic questions of the genetics of schizophrenia. However, it does seem that these neurological abnormalities play a role in the chain of causal events that lead to the disorder. We remind the reader of the problems surrounding the definition of the disorder.

Fischer (1971, 1973) extended the twin methodology by reasoning that the genetic influence would rear itself in the offspring of the nonschizophrenic twin, and bore this out in a search of the official records in Denmark. In a follow-up of these offspring, Gottesman and Bertelson (1989) reported age-corrected incidence rates of 16.8 and 17.4%, respectively, for children of schizophrenic and discordant MZ twins. The age-corrected risk for children of schizophrenic DZ twins was of the same order (also 17.4%), whereas that for the offspring of discordant normal DZs was a mere 2.1%. These data constitute, then, a relatively powerful argument that there is some genetic contribution in some instances of schizophrenia. On the other hand, as Gottesman and Bertelson (1989) note, they also show that this presumed predisposition may remain "unexpressed" unless "released" by unspecified environmental factors.

What can be concluded from the twin studies? It must be remembered that if schizophrenia were an exclusively genetic disorder, the concordance rate would be 100%. As we repeatedly emphasize, however, such typological thinking is erroneous when it comes to conceptualizing unfolding biological or genetic influences or factors. As Torrey and colleagues (1994) pointed out, MZ twins are only genetically identical when the original zygote splits. Phelps, Davis, & Schwartz (1997) report that two-thirds of MZ embryos are monochorionic, meaning that they share blood supply, whereas DZ twins never do. Then, it seems plausible that shared pathogens may account for the increased rate. Chronic hypoxia and other obstetric complications are more likely to be shared by

MZ rather than DZ co-twins (Maier et al., 1995). At the very least, the twin studies have provided an important insight that illustrates the lack of clarity between genetic and environmental boundaries. Environmental-biological events that occur during the pregnancy, as will be discussed in greater detail later on, play a role in the unfolding of genetic material and possibly influence CNS development.

**Adoption Studies.** An additional major approach to examining the genetics of schizophrenia is the adoption strategy. The defining study in this area was carried out by Heston (1966). In a sample obtained from an Oregon state mental hospital, he found a significant difference between the age-corrected incidence of schizophrenia diagnoses among index adoptees (16.6%) compared to controls and a result similar to that for children *not* separated from their schizophrenic mothers. Index adoptees also evidenced an increased range of sociopathic personality disorder, suggesting the possible transmission of a more general sort of psychopathological compromise. Thus, this study provided fairly convincing evidence that enhanced schizophrenia risk was attributable to genetic (or prenatal) causes, and the stage was set to search for genetic causes using the adoption strategy.

The most prominent and extensive of the adoption studies in schizophrenia were initiated by a group of American investigators who were granted access to the exceptionally thorough census and social services database maintained by the government of Denmark. The initial results of this eventually widely reported study became available in 1968 (Kety, Rosenthal, Wender, & Schulsinger, 1968; Rosenthal et al., 1968). The central finding of the original study (Kety et al., 1968) was that a much higher percentage of the biological relatives of the index cases had a schizophrenia spectrum diagnosis than the nonbiological cases (8.7% versus 1.9%, respectively). These results must be tempered because the range of diagnoses included in the schizophrenia spectrum was broad. In fact, subsequent analyses have shown that the finding of heritability specific to schizophrenia does not hold up when more stringent diagnostic criteria for schizophrenia are employed (Rosenthal, Wender, Kety, Welner, & Schulsinger, 1971). Again, the evidence is more supportive for inheritance of some sort of general compromise, a conclusion that is not so surprising in the light of the diagnostic dilemmas reviewed earlier.

Later reports by Kety (Kety, Rosenthal, Wender, Schulsinger, & Jacobsen, 1978; Kety, 1987) have provided results that generally support the original findings. However, one persistent and peculiar finding in which second-degree relatives are persistently more concordant for schizophrenia than those of first degree seemingly disconfirms the genetic transmission hypothesis. Although such an apparent anomaly might be regarded as an important lead to which to devote further effort to unravel the complexities of transmitted—genetic or otherwise—factors, the report by Kety (1987) suggests in narrative format that the balance of first- to second-degree index relatives who show spectrum disorders was "in accord with expectation," presumably implying a preponderance of the effect in parents and full siblings. Unfortunately, that report does not contain the data necessary to fully evaluate the claim.

Kendler and Gruenberg (1984) attempted an independent replication of the Kety et al. (1968, 1978) greater Copenhagen family study. Using the record data already assembled, these investigators rediagnosed all subjects, adoptees, and family members according to the relatively precise criteria of DSM-III. Of the various results of the project, two stand out as especially important: First, schizophrenia spectrum disorders (now systematically defined to include paranoid and schizotypal personality disorders in addition to schizophrenia) are significantly more frequent in index than in control biological families, and the difference is especially pronounced among the *first-degree* relatives. Second, the risk for a schizophrenia spectrum disorder also significantly increased in biological relatives of adoptees who have a predominantly schizophrenic type of schizoaffective disorder or schizotypal personality disorder. These data are relatively convincing and highlight the systematic strengths of the DSM-III-type diagnostic approach in bringing order to a confusing data set with conflicting reports, notwithstanding the limitations of that instrument as a research tool (see Andreasen, 1998).

An important variation on the adoption methodology is the approach of cross-fostering (Wender, Rosenthal, Kety, Schulsinger, & Welner, 1974). This method examines biologically normal adoptees who are placed in foster homes in which one of the adoptive parents subsequently becomes schizophrenic. The schizophrenia incidence rate for these "cross-fostered" adoptees is then compared with (1) adoptees whose adoptive and biological parents are normal and (2) adoptees who have a schizophrenic biological parent and are raised by normal adoptive parents. The "purified" group incidence rates for at least borderline schizophrenia among adoptees in each of the above conditions were, respectively, 4.8, 10.7, and 19.7%, a statistically significant variation. However, it has been independently reported that the schizophrenic adoptive parent of a large majority of the cross-fostered children had not become seriously disturbed until the children's late childhood years (Van Dyke, Rosenthal, & Rasmussen, 1975). Hence, they would not have necessarily presented an unremarkable environmental challenge during the presumably more critical earlier developmental period. In other words, the study basically fails to demonstrate that (adoptive) parental schizophrenia is psychopathologically nonnoxious for children exposed to it (barring the implications of prodromal symptoms).

The adoption method was originally conceived as one that would circumvent the serious problems of other pedigree approaches, such as twin studies, with the hope that the answers provided would be more clear-cut. This was not the outcome, however. Beyond the idea that there is clearly a familial link to the disorder, a proposition that one might reasonably surmise purely by conjecture, evidence that sheds light on the nature of that mechanism is lacking. Evidence does exist, in our view, that whatever is being genetically transferred to the individual lacks specificity to schizophrenia *per se* and more accurately relates to a broader type of compromise, perhaps even beyond the "schizophrenia spectrum." The idea of some sort of general compromise is also consistent with the more recent idea that the most consistent aspect of schizophrenia is poor functioning.

On the other hand, the lack of reports on the environments in which the adoptees were placed is striking. In largely neglecting the environments, a potentially important source of morbidity has been overlooked. This gap has been filled by the work of Tienari and colleagues (1985, 1987, 1994; Tienari, 1991). The design of their study involves a follow-up of the adopted-away children of all women in Finland hospitalized for schizophrenia, beginning around 1960. As these index children grow into adulthood, they are compared with a matched group of control adoptees whose biological mothers were normal. The trend of the results

is already clear and reaches high levels of statistical significance. There is the familiar finding that the index adoptees have developed more, and more serious (including schizophrenia), psychopathology than the controls. Most of this psychopathology, however, is concentrated in the index group reared by poorly functioning adoptive parents—for example, parents who demonstrated high levels of communication deviance. Index adoptees reared by well-functioning adoptive parents had substantially less psychopathology, and control cases reared in disorganized adoptive families experienced more serious psychopathology as adults than their counterparts raised in "healthy" families. We will recall these results when discussing the relationship of schizophrenia to the subculture of the family.

To summarize, the initial promise of the adoption methodology to offer incontrovertible proof of the genetic basis of schizophrenia is now recognized as overstretched. In addition, we would call attention to numerous demonstrations of methodological problems and the erroneously extended conclusions drawn from this evidence (e.g., Benjamin, 1976; Carson & Sanislow, 1993; Lidz & Blatt, 1983; Sarbin & Mancuso, 1980). Aside from methodological concerns, the dichotomization of genetic and environmental components as distinct, assumed to operate in an independent manner *statistically*, overlooks the continual interplay of these factors that actually occurs in reality. It has been established for some time that these methods that treat these components as independent factors are unlikely to elucidate underlying mechanisms of complex traits or disorders (see, for instance, Carson & Sanislow, 1993; Lewontin, 1974; or Wahlsten, 1999). In the light of these limitations, new hope was garnered from the field of molecular biology.

**Molecular Genetics.** Linkage studies, including the physical mapping of genes, presaged the more prominent contemporary research strategies developed in the biological sciences, leading inevitably to the their employment by psychiatric geneticists in attempts to unravel the presumed genetic processes associated with schizophrenia. In the field of genetics, Morgan (1911, 1920) noticed early on that traits could be inherited together, or "linked" on proximal chromosomal locations by the patterns in which combinations of traits were passed on generationally. This idea led to estimating gene distances and locations on particular chromosomes by triangulation from observed trait coinheritances. More recent advances in gene mapping have occurred at the molecular level with the use of restriction enzymes to "cut" DNA at known repetitive DNA sequences (see Botstein, White, Skolnick, & Davis, 1980), thereby providing a sort of anchoring point for determining relative intergene distances and thus to enable a more direct measurement. The resultant construction of more detailed maps has permitted relatively accurate localization of actual "disease" genes and hence isolation and identification of gene products (i.e., enzymes or other proteins) presumably implicated in various medical conditions. Therefore, it is within the realm of possibility that if certain genes are systematically associated with schizophrenic outcomes, we will one day be able to pinpoint their locations and describe in some detail what proximal effects they have. Bear in mind, however, that it is a long way from there to schizophrenia.

The current consensus is that a "large" and very specific gene effect in schizophrenia is unlikely, and many researchers have recognized for some time that the genetic effects involved with schizophrenia are more likely to involve multiple genes in interaction with idiosyncratic environmental experiences (Moldin & Gottesman, 1997). The result of studies in molecular genetics that intend to establish the loci of genes for complex mental disorders such as schizophrenia and bipolar disorder are consistent with this idea; few of the findings implicating single genes have been replicated. Early results, including the announced identification of a gene location for bipolar disorder on chromosome 11 (Egeland et al., 1987), were seized upon by the popular media and are now known to have been premature (DeLisi & Crow, 1989). In schizophrenia, there has been much interest in a specific region of chromosome 5 that was stimulated by the discovery of a Chinese man and his nephew, both schizophrenic, who displayed a particular chromosome 5 aberration (partial trisomy). Sherrington and colleagues (1988) studied five Icelandic and two British families that have multiple occurrences of schizophrenia and presented evidence for a gene locus on chromosome 5 with a dominant schizophrenic-susceptibility allele. This result, however, is inconsistent with data gathered on American (Kaufman, DeLisi, Lehner, & Gilliam, 1989) and Swedish (Kennedy et al., 1988) families that have high concentrations of schizo-

phrenia. DeLisi and Crow (1989) noted that some data indicated that schizophrenia has higher concordance but milder manifestations in females and suggested that the presumably implicated genes have a sex-chromosome locus, but the argument is entirely inferential. Other studies have examined linkage to a marker on chromosome 6 (Lander & Kruglyzk, 1993; Wang et al, 1995), but other studies of this region that used better samples produced equivocal results (Schwab et al., 1995) or failed to replicate (Moises et al., 1995). In the Irish study of high-density schizophrenia families, there has been some suggestion of a locus on chromosome 8p (Kendler et al., 1996). Other results from the Irish sample suggested a locus on chromosome 6 (Wang et al., 1995). However, those are statistically questionable (Straub et al, 1995; Gottesman & Moldin, 1998). In fact, nonreplication for the majority of loci reported is an ongoing problem with linkage studies (Gottesman & Moldin, 1998).

Overall, there has been a general failure to replicate results that identify specific regions in independent samples, and results that implicate a specific chomosomal area are at best suggestive (Moldin, 1997). In the context of these inconsistencies, it has also been pointed out that molecular-linkage strategy simply lacks the necessary statistical power when it comes to testing for anything but large gene effects. We applaud recognition of this limitation, but it seems to us that stacking the deck to detect a small effect size that might be associated with "weak" genetic effects will not ultimately pay off, as in applying alternate strategies such as association analyses (e.g., Risch and Merikangas, 1996). Before leaving this topic, one remaining problem, the fundamental idea of the phenotype, deserves careful consideration.

**The Problem of Phenotype.** It might be reasonably argued that the cardinal factor limiting the acquisition of knowledge of the "genetics of schizophrenia" is a pervasive blurriness of the concept of phenotype. Definitional problems and the diagnostic heterogeneity that surround the schizophrenia diagnosis notwithstanding, the problem of the phenotype is more basic and involves the intricate complexities of the interaction of genes and environment. To illustrate this fact, the "phenotype" (i.e., the resulting expression of the genotype) in schizophrenia can broadly range from the disorder itself, to features associated with the disorder, to some more basic gene product involved with structural development that, it is hypothesized, is related to the disorder. Nowhere in the literature can we find any clarity on this matter, although Scher (1999) succinctly stated the problem when discussing the issue more generally:

Phenotypic psychological mechanisms surely arise through a complicated process. The role of genes is likely to be rather far away and indirect. Certainly, our current understanding of the relationship between mind and body limits our ability to understand how genes—which code for physical structure—contribute to psychological development. (p. 436)

We have stressed that genes and environment continually interplay as the process of development unfolds. In this light, the phenotype is an elusive concept. Is the phenotype the disorder? Or is the phenotype one of the hypothesized components of the disorder such as a manifest neonatal complication? The phenotype might also be related to temperament, to neuronal development of receptor sites, or to the language centers. The "genetics" of schizophrenia will be handicapped until there is consensus on the phenotype. Even with some agreement on a meaningful phenotype, there will still be complications inherent in the level at which the phenotype is implicated in the disorder. Consider, for example, that an abberant gene for a defective receptor site will be limited by our understanding of the way pathological synaptic transmission is implicated in the disorder, something that is, as will become clear shortly, far from settled.

To complicate matters further, exactly what constitutes a gene has varying conceptions that depend on one's approach. In Mendelian (i.e., in pedigree or family) studies, a gene is a hypothesized construct that is related to a particular phenotype and is isolated based on observed patterns of inheritance. In more modern molecular methods, a gene is the smallest sequence of nucleotides in a strand of DNA that codes for the production of a protein. From a molecular point of view, genes are not necessarily unique; they can be overlapping. In other words, genes produce products that undergo programmed biochemical modification to serve their ultimate function, and sometimes these functions include regulating other genes, sometimes the modification of gene products. Such effects are among intricate, interrelated constellations of events that are complex even for the most straightforwardly seeming diseases. For instance, insulin is originally produced as a protein strand that folds back on itself due to the attraction of

branched amino acids within the protein sequence. Related enzymes cleave off the resulting "folds" to produce the final structure. These related enzymes are coded for by other genes, and the final product is produced by a complex system of interdependent regulation and feedback loops. So what causes diabetes? There is no one sole cause, and at least several mechanisms, more or less "genetic," can lead to this disorder. These include problems in the synthesis pathway of insulin either blocking the conversion to the final product or leading to a defective final product, abnormal receptors for insulin, or the intercellular insulin-receptor complex that facilitates insulin binding. These varied mechanisms end with the common final pathway of diabetes that appears isomorphic at the level of clinical pathology. Is diabetes a hereditary disease? Some understanding of the mechanism will undoubtedly aid in determining the best treatment. Unlike schizophrenia, however, there is a clear understanding of the pathophysiology in diabetes, thus enabling meaningful study of genetic aspects at the molecular level to determine various gene influences. In schizophrenia, molecular genetic strategies will not be of full benefit until the pathophysiology of the disorder is clearly understood.

The dearth of knowledge about the pathophysiology of schizophrenia obviates the specification of the layers involved in the regulatory processes and their interactions with environmental insults that result in the disorder. In other words, there is not a clear understanding of what bridges the "nature and nurture." We know that schizophrenia runs in the family and that there is a biological constitution that enhances (creates?) vulnerability to the disorder. It appears that some sort of sequence of traumatic events in the context of development opens the vulnerability, but the role of the timing of such environmental traumas is less clear. It also appears that individuals can undergo traumas similar in magnitude and nature and come out seemingly unscathed, and that not all this can be chalked up to a genetic difference. This has led one of the major thinkers and researcher of the disorder, Paul Meehl (1989), to declare that developing schizophrenia is a matter of "bad luck" in that some idiosyncratic as yet unspecified sequence of traumatizing events opens the vulnerability to the disorder. Finally, evidence also suggests that certain neural pathways function abnormally, but the exact manner of this dysfunction is not entirely clear. Hence, there are many gaps in the knowledge required to understand the "genetics" of the disorder.

The best illustration of this is MZ twins, where one can assume that the genetic material is identical only when the zygote splits. Subsequent to that time, a multitude of levels between the extremes of "nature" and "nurture" exist, and recognition of these levels underscores the artificial aspect of bifurcating developmental events as either genetic or environmental. Seen in this light, adoption and twin methods are obsolete, or as Meehl (1972) had the good foresight to put it, "we have skimmed the cream; we are near the research asymptote" (p. 368). There can be little doubt that now defunct dichotomous positions traditionally taken in the nature/nurture debate which have for many years effectively driven the research on schizophrenia, have reached a point of obsolescence, and it is likely that without a more complete theory of schizophrenia pathology, the same is true for more modern molecular methods.

In the search for the biological, biochemical, or genetic solution, we believe it will someday be accepted that it was simply asking the wrong question. Is schizophrenia genetic? Of course it is—how could the disorder be devoid of genetic influences? We would go so far as to suggest that, for the most part, there are no inherent flaws in the data. Rather, forces driving the conceptualization and interpretation of the science have been obscuring real progress. As it turns out, current views (e.g., Harrison, 1998) clearly recognize the failure of the promise of molecular genetics—the last bastion for a "genetic solution"—to solve the schizophrenia puzzle. Presently, the new emphasis is on its pathophysiology. We will return to review that area shortly.

## Schizophrenia and the Intrafamilial Subculture

Research on the family subculture and interpersonal processes within the family that might contribute to the development of schizophrenia reached its zenith in the late 1950s and, with some exceptions, has been in decline ever since. There appear to be five principal reasons for this decline:

1. Such research is very difficult to carry out in a precise and controlled way, far more so than the high-technology-driven research into biological processes so prevalent today.

2. Relatedly, some early but insufficiently controlled findings of apparent familial aberrancy (e.g., double binding) have proven nonspecific for schizophrenia and indeed somewhat routine in families that have exclusively normal offspring.

3. Dysfunctional behavior in family members, it has been shown, is reactive to the presence of a disturbed family member rather than antecedent to such disturbance; indeed, such circularity in cause–effect sequences in patient–family interaction may be the norm.

4. Research on the possible intrafamilial origins of some schizophrenias has, perhaps understandably, not been popular among parent groups who have (probably accurately) sometimes perceived that they are summarily and unfairly blamed for the disorders of their children.

5. The so-called "decade of the brain" (i.e., the 1980s), for the most part, obviated thinking and research along these lines in mainstream psychiatry.

In the light of the sensitive nature of this topic, we want to be clear about our own position. We find that assigning blame in this area is both counterproductive and based on an oversimplified notion of the way persons become schizophrenic. Parenting is at best an inscrutable task laden with pitfalls throughout the course of child development, and most of the parents we have known, whether they have had the "bad luck" to have raised a son or daughter who became schizophrenic, have done the very best they could to ensure the happiness, health, and success of their children. We have the greatest sympathy for the difficulties faced by the mothers, fathers, and siblings, of schizophrenic persons. Many of these relatives harbor unjustified guilt feelings; we have no wish to induce or augment such feelings—quite the contrary. Nevertheless, we think open inquiry into the developmental process, which necessarily involves attention to the intrafamilial environment, is essential in any comprehensive attempt to discover the sources of schizophrenic outcomes.

Does schizophrenia as a biological disease somehow soften the blow? Admittedly, there seems to have been an impact on destigmatizing the disorder for those afflicted *and* their family members. The downside of the wholesale version of this view is that personal responsibilities are minimized, thereby creating a steadfast system that excludes that examinination of family dynamics, including expressed emotion (EE), and calls into question the contributions of this view to real progress. On the other hand, it is curious that the notion of blame is contingent on the biological–environmental dichotomy. We are skeptical that the biological disease metaphor provides lasting meaningful relief to those exposed to the suffering of schizophrenia. Moreover, it is appalling that the field (either psychiatry or psychology) has yet to find a way to address more kindly the issue of problematic family communication patterns in a direct manner that would foster a posture of curiosity rather than a defensive reaction. We understand that families with a schizophrenic member may well be emotionally volatile, but one only need pay attention to the pejorative nature of many of the family-related concepts about to be discussed for evidence of this shortcoming.

In any event, the heyday of family process research in the 1950s saw the emergence of the double-bind hypothesis of the Palo Alto group (Bateson, Jackson, Haley, & Weakland, 1956), the transmission of irrationality hypothesis of the Yale group (Lidz, Cornelison, Terry, & Fleck, 1958), and the pseudomutuality notion developed by NIMH investigators (Wynne, Ryckoff, Day, & Hirsch, 1958). These and other contributions have been extensively reviewed by numerous scholars (e.g., Goldstein & Rodnick, 1975; Goldstein & Strachan, 1987; Hirsch & Leff, 1975; Jacob, 1975; Mishler & Waxler, 1968; Wynne, Toohey, & Doane, 1979), so we will not repeat the effort here. Suffice it to say that these specific process notions have tended to give way over time to more general ideas that gross intrafamilial communication deviance and a negative affective climate encourages the emergence of schizophrenic behavior. The altered perspective was attributable in no small measure to the success achieved by Singer & Wynne (1965a,b; Singer, Wynne, & Toohey, 1978) in demonstrating that they could postdict the schizophrenia status of offspring from amorphousness and fragmentation in the Rorschach protocols of parents. Subsequent use of a highly similar assessment system in the UCLA high-risk longitudinal sample showed that it could predict schizophrenia spectrum disorders in offspring (Goldstein, 1985). The latter study is particularly significant because the samples of deviant parental communication

were obtained years before the onset of schizophrenia in children, thus ruling out the possibility of parental reactivity to the disordered communication that schizophrenia normally entails.

A nonreactive research design was also employed by Roff and Knight (1981) in a study that related outcomes in diagnosed cases of adult schizophrenia in males to family variables obtained during patients' preschizophrenic childhood years. Data on the latter were obtained from child guidance clinic records that had been prepared at the time these children and their families were seen for various nonpsychotic childhood adjustment difficulties. Particularly interesting was the finding that poor adult outcome was associated with a mothering style remarkably similar to the classic "schizophrenogenic" pattern (Fromm-Reichman, 1948) of rejecting, impervious overconcern, an etiologic concept that had been all but abandoned by researchers by the 1970s. Also in line with the classic notion was some evidence that the effects of such mothering were especially noxious where fathers had been described as critical and noninvolved with their sons. A final instance of this study's rich yield was the confirmation of an association of poor outcome with two particular patterns of parental marital dysfunction that had been described by earlier investigators, in particular, by Lidz, Cornelison, Fleck, and Terry (1957) under the rubrics *marital schism* (extreme distance and hostility between the parents) and *marital skew* (wherein the family subculture is pathologically tilted in the direction of accommodating to serious disturbance in one of the parents).

The notion that familial subcultural aberrancy might promote the development of schizophrenia in offspring must confront at the outset the fact that siblings of the disordered member are usually normal. How have they escaped harm from these presumably relatively constant pathogenic conditions? The answer from proponents of this view is that the subculture of a family is not constant, that it changes appreciably over time, and has its own unique developmental pattern. The early development of the preschizophrenic child just happens to come at a time (Meehl's "bad luck" factor?) of maximum familial pathogenicity. There is some evidence to support this construction.

Taking a direct approach, Stabenau and Pollin (1968; Stabenau, Tupin, Werner, & Pollin, 1965) studied families in which siblings were discordant for schizophrenia and for juvenile delinquency.

They found, in brief, that seventeen of their nineteen "psychopathology siblings" (for schizophrenia alone, nine of ten), compared to only two of twenty-nine controls, encountered periods of maximum family crisis in early childhood identified by the families themselves. The "bad times" included such things as financial disasters, maximum parental strife, and depressive episodes in one or the other parent. A variety of collateral findings confirmed the general picture that these disturbed individuals experienced a world of far less reassuring character in their formative years than their more functional siblings.

Essentially the same type of explanation for normal siblings was offered in the Lidz–Yale family studies (Lidz, Fleck, & Cornelison, 1965). In fact, a criterion for selecting the original families to be studied was that at least one sibling was available who showed no evidence of psychological disturbance. In a series of compelling descriptions, the investigators in this project illustrated how the inherent pathogenicity of a marital dyad can become especially concentrated on a single sibling (owing to gender, concurrent stage of family development, etc), thereby confronting that child with insoluble conflicts and contradictions about the nature of reality that are not necessarily inflicted on other siblings or, if so, at lesser intensity.

As a final entry into this very contracted overview of the extensive literature on family influences in schizophrenia, recall the unique, ongoing project in which independent assessments of child-rearing adequacy were the focus of study by Tienari and colleagues (1985, 1987, 1994; Tienari, 1991) mentioned earlier in the adoption section. There is the familiar finding that the index adoptees have developed more, and more serious (including schizophrenia), psychopathology than the controls. Most of this psychopathology, however, is concentrated in the index group reared by poorly functioning adoptive parents—for example, parents who showed high levels of communication deviance. Index adoptees reared by well-functioning adoptive parents had substantially less psychopathology, and control cases reared in disorganized adoptive families experienced more serious psychopathology as adults than their counterparts raised in "healthy" families. Consistent with their earlier work, these results show a moderate genetic effect—the differential "healthy" and disorder rates of index versus control adoptees, irrespective of adoptive family context. However, parental inadequacy and disturbed communication has a substantial impact on the outcome for both index and control cases. Thus, the findings indicate a strong interaction between genetic vulnerability and an unfavorable family environment in the causal pathway leading to schizophrenia. Unfortunately, we cannot be certain that the emergence of odd or psychotic behavior in adoptees did not precede and cause, in whole or in part, the disorganization of their adoptive families. Analyses to examine this possibility are in progress (e.g., Wahlberg et al., 1997), but so far they provide no definitive support for this alternative interpretation. Some independent work reported by Kinney et al. (1997) also fails to show diminished mental health in adoptive parents raising children who became schizophrenic. Despite additional modest evidence for genetic transmission from these studies, the level of integration of the adoptive family into which the child is placed looms as an extremely critical variable. The most disastrous outcomes occur where children whose mothers have been schizophrenic are placed in chaotic adoptive homes.

Because expressed emotion (EE) has usually been seen as related to the course rather than the causes of schizophrenia, we will postpone discussion of it in families until a later section.

## Soft Neurological Signs, At-Riskness, and Brain Anomalies

Although we find the genetic evidence pertaining to schizophrenia extremely modest in relation to the amount of "play" it gets and, perhaps excepting the case of monozygotic twinship, by itself virtually useless in predicting individual morbidity (as in so-called genetic counseling programs), we do not discount the possibility that other forms of biological compromise may convey a more substantial risk of schizophrenia. Indeed, it is conceivable that much of what appears "genetic" in the etiology of schizophrenia is mediated in some other biological manner. As it turns out, there is no compelling evidence of progressive brain degeneration in the natural course of the disorder (Cannon, 1998a,b; Russell, Munro, Jones, Hemsley, & Murray, 1997). In those instances where progressive degeneration has been observed, it sometimes appears to have resulted from the iatrogenic effects of antipsychotic medications

(Cohen, 1997; Gur et al., 1998). In other instances, it does not seem that reduced volume in at least some brain areas (i.e., hippocampus) is specific to schizophrenia (Velakoulis et al., 1999). In the light of these findings, it is interesting to note that some studies have suggested that deficits associated with the schizophrenias are the most stable element of the disorder (e.g., Amador et al, 1999; Nakaya, Suwa, Komahashi, & Ohmori, 1999).

Among the good candidates is a somewhat ill-defined syndrome consisting of multiple soft neurological signs detectable in early childhood that has possible fetal or perinatal origins (Lyon, Barr, Cannon, Mednick, & Shore, 1989). Obstetrical complications, such as an unduly short gestational period, in the histories of people who later become schizophrenic are well above normative expectations (Cannon et al., 1997; Gureje, Bamidele, & Raji, 1994; Jones, Rantakallio, Hartikainen, Isohanni, & Sipila, 1998; Torrey et al., 1994), although it is possible that resultant early brain injury contributes to schizophrenic outcomes only among genetically predisposed persons (see Marcus, Hans, Auerbach, & Auerbach, 1993; Mednick et al., 1998). The identification of such a syndrome may turn out to be among the most important contribution of longitudinal high-risk research in schizophrenia. First, we examine the more general aspects of neuroanatomical factors.

The advent of modern computer-dependent technologies, such as computerized axial tomography (CAT) and nuclear magnetic resonance imaging (MRI) have made possible research on the structural properties of the brain in living subjects, and the area of schizophrenia research is no exception. The resulting—and rapidly growing—body of research supports the implication of developmental insults and the possible resultant effects on later cognitive development in the pathway to schizophrenia. The nature of this new thinking is by no means completely developed or uniformly expressed, but essentially it involves the idea that the disorder arises from variable aberrations in brain circuitry. Most forms of the idea include the hypothesis of an early, likely prenatal, insult to the brain that may have detectable neurological effects in early childhood but will not necessarily result in the later development of schizophrenia (e.g., Lyon, Barr, Cannon, Mednick, & Shore, 1989). The latter arises where the initial injury somehow interferes with normal brain synapse development during a period of intensive synaptic

reorganization; for most people, it occurs during adolescence or early adulthood. Conceivable candidates here include neuronal cell "pruning," cell migration, and programmed cell death, all processes that occur normally during postnatal phases of brain development (see Harrison, 1999, and Weickert & Weinberger, 1998, for overviews).

Pioneering work in this area was done by Fish (1957, 1977) and by Sobel (1961), both of whom stressed that subtly compromised CNS functioning, possibly attributable to birth complications, predisposed to schizophrenia. Fish (1977) describes the pathogenic pattern as one of "neurointegrative defect" (see Meehl, 1962, 1989, 1990), which leads to "pandevelopmental retardation" in persons who eventually become psychiatric casualties, especially in the schizophrenia range. The notion of premorbid neurological anomalies has been demonstrated by the high-risk studies (e.g., Mednick & Schulsinger, 1968; Mednick, Schulsinger, & Schulsinger, 1975; Mednick et al., 1978), including the suggestion that obstetric complications may factor in as well. Other support has come from the Israeli high-risk study where two neurological assessments carried out 5 years apart showed that index children (offspring of schizophrenic mothers) were markedly more likely than controls to have various neurological anomalies, most of the soft variety (Marcus, Hans, Byhouwer, & Norem, 1985; Silberman & Tassone, 1985).

Ironically, early twin research made a major contribution along the line of compromising neurological events that had pernicious effects later on. Pollin, Stabenau, and Tupin (1965) intensively studied a group of monozygotic twins and their families who were discordant for schizophrenia. Because heredity is a constant in such a sample, it was hoped that thorough investigation of environmental factors that differentiated the members of the discordant pairs would unearth clues as to the causes of schizophrenia in those twins affected. In virtually every instance, the twin who was to become schizophrenic had a relatively unfavorable intrauterine environment, manifested in lower birth weight at the outset and consistent relative retardation in biological developmental milestones. A significant preponderance of soft neurological signs such as praxis difficulties, abnormal reflexes, and abortive clonus, was found in the index twins. In short, the latter were less "competent" than their co-twins over a broad range of behaviors. These indications of compromised functioning were of sufficient magnitude to evoke noticeably differential parenting behavior and to lead to a constellation of personality characteristics best summarized as excessive submissiveness in index co-twins, possibly adding a psychosocial impediment to the biological one.

Fetuses or newborns who sustained the earlier insult, according to the developmental view, are at elevated risk for missing or misconnected circuitry that arises during cell reorganization and thus are more vulnerable to developing schizophrenia (Walker & Diforio, 1997). Such deficiencies in neural circuitry would not be directly observable by currently available methods of brain scanning. Certain research findings of recent years are consistent with this type of etiologic scenario.

The so-called "season-of-birth effect" notion is relevant here. Although there is some controversy on this issue (see Bradbury & Miller, 1985; Lewis, 1989a,b, 1990; Lewis & Griffin, 1981), it has been documented and is largely accepted that people who become schizophrenic are more likely than people in general to have been born in winter and early spring months—about an 8% elevation (DeLisi, Crow, & Hirsch, 1986a). This peculiar observation, although possibly open to dispute on the grounds of statistical artifact (see Lewis, 1990), has given rise to a variety of hypotheses including the question of compromised brain integrity in schizophrenia, an idea suggested early by Bradbury and Miller (1985). Accumulating evidence supports these possibilities. For example, Wright, Takei, Rifkin, and Murray (1995) found that maternal influenza in the second trimester of pregnancy is associated with impaired fetal growth, enhanced obstetrical complications, and later-developing schizophrenia. Several studies have suggested that, historically, influenza epidemics are associated at a higher than chance level with the gestation periods of fetuses who later become schizophrenic. The latest of these studies reported by Takei and colleagues (1996) identifies the supposedly critical peak infectious period as the fifth gestational month. Here, risk of influenza exposure in the critical period was associated with enlarged ventricles and sulci among a group of eighty-three schizophrenic patients, relative to controls. Seemingly important and possibly related findings, reported by Torrey and colleagues (1993), establish a strong correlation between the occurrence of stillbirths and schizophrenia risk, presumably some infectious agent; in one of the cases, according to this hypothesis, it leads to death of the fetus, and in the other to brain changes that enhance vulnerability to schizophrenia.

More recent work using the Finnish registry also demonstrated a relationship between prenatal exposure to polio virus infection during the second trimester and the later development of schizophrenia (Suvisaari, Haukka, Tanskanen, Hovi, & Lonnqvist, 1999). The idea of a virus causing schizophrenia is not new, and simply taken as that, lacks explanatory power in and of itself. However, the relationship between a viral compromise and the subsequent chain of effects in the course of development that might be initiated is something that we find more plausible. On the other hand, work by LaMantia (1999) points to the possible importance of an early insult during the third trimester of pregnancy. This approach focuses on the way the genetic code might be derailed as it unfolds while directing the development of brain areas, including the basal ganglia and hippocampus demonstrated as deficient in schizophrenia.

Despite the promise of findings in this area, it is incumbent on us to conclude this section with a cautionary note. The wealth of findings in this area as an emergent pattern illustrates an impending danger in this promising area of research: Without a clear theory on the way that these neurological insults affect the developmental processes in a manner that relates to identified pathophysiological processes and eventually to the expressed behavior of a taxonomic entity, it is likely that these findings will be merely added to many documented associations with the disorder and will add no real insight to the etiology.

### Traumatizing Events

Clinicians who expend the energy and patience necessary to fully understand the developmental background of schizophrenic persons—and, regrettably, not all are willing to do so—usually come away with a powerful impression of traumatizing life circumstances. Perhaps one of the most stark illustrations of madness and associated horrors concerns the Genain quadruplets, all of whom became schizophrenic (Rosenthal, 1963). All four of these monozygotic sisters acquired the diagnosis before age 25. Though the remarkable concordance might suggest the operation of a genetic pathogen, we choose to mention it here because the sisters were raised in a family context characterized by parental madness of outlandish proportions (e.g., clitoral circumcisions to curb childhood masturbation). Their disorders, moreover, were quite different in respect to course, severity, and relative intractableness, characteristics that in turn were strongly correlated (in the expected direction) with the degree of exposure to pathological parenting. Despite stark clinical examples such as found in the Genain sisters, the yield from studies that compare the backgrounds of schizophrenics and suitable controls has been rather unimpressive in identifying discrete circumstances that differentiate schizophrenics as a group who had particular traumatic experiences while growing up. Perhaps this is another case in which "bad luck" (see Meehl, 1989) such as the occurrence of trauma in particular patterns, sequences, or at key times in development, is more important than the actual events themselves. In any event, we call attention to how little we have to report in this area.

In an early study, Schofield and Balian (1959) compared life history data of 178 schizophrenics with those of a carefully matched normal control group. For even the few significant differences found in the variables that one might assume are critical, the most striking finding was the very considerable overlap of the two groups. Indeed, for the variables of sexual adjustment and "adequacy of sexual outlet," the backgrounds of schizophrenics were significantly superior to those of controls—certainly not the most expected of findings. Some other results, such as excessive maternal overprotection and domination among preschizophrenics, were more consistent with expectations, but again the large majority of schizophrenic persons had normally affectionate relationships with their mothers. The high frequency of supposedly pathogenic circumstances in the backgrounds of their *normal* subjects led these investigators to suggest the need to study the "immunizing" experiences that may have permitted them to overcome their noxious environments. Although we think that the latter is a good idea, the results of the study are equally consistent with the notion that growing up is normatively hard and that preschizophrenic subjects are somehow excessively vulnerable to its vicissitudes.

Schofield and Balian (1959) included assessments of parental loss through separation, divorces, or death in their schedule but failed to find

this a variable that differentiated their groups. In contrast, Roff and Knight (1981), in the retrospective but nonreactive study described before, did find that parental loss before age 7 was associated with poor outcomes among persons diagnosed as schizophrenic. Similarly, in the Mednick et al. (1978) high-risk study, there was some indication that parental loss (here occasioned by maternal hospitalization) is etiologically significant.

Shifting the focus to precipitating as opposed to predisposing environmental life events in schizophrenia, we now have a fair amount of information on the evocations of schizophrenic behavior among persons who had experienced prior schizophrenic episodes. For example, Ventura, Nuechterlein, Lukoff, and Hardesty (1989), in a 1-year prospective study of remitted schizophrenics, presented strong evidence that negative events (independent of symptoms or personal actions) are associated with relapse. By far the largest body of work in this area has been concerned with familial expressed emotion as a precipitant of new episodes of schizophrenic behavior among recovered or near-recovered persons. We turn now to a brief summary of that literature.

Research on expressed emotion (EE), usually defined as a pattern of behavior involving both high intrusiveness and high levels of criticism directed toward the former patient, began in England (Vaughn & Leff, 1976, 1981) and was in due course transported to the United States (Hooley, 1985; Vaughn, Snyder, Jones, Freeman, & Falloon, 1984; Butzlaff & Hooley, 1998; Hooley & Hiller, 1998; Linszen et al., 1997; Miklowitz, Goldstein, & Falloon, 1983). At this point, there can be no doubt that it is associated with rehospitalization of schizophrenia; it occurs in conjunction with familial communication deviance (Doane, Falloon, Goldstein, & Mintz, 1985; Miklowitz, Strachan, Goldstein, Doane, & Snyder, 1986), and its reduction is associated with relapse prevention (Falloon, Boyd, McGill, Williamson, & Razani, 1985; Hogarty, Anderson, Reiss, Kornblith, & Greenwald, 1986). There remains, however, some question of the direction of the effect (i.e., the more disturbed the former patient, the more likely is rehospitalization, *and* the more provocation of EE in family members). Basically, this argument was made by Parker, Johnston, and Hayward (1988), who presented evidence that EE was significantly associated with a poor posthospital course only in one-parent households, where the impact of disturbed behavior would be maximally likely to lead to high EE.

However, this construction is inconsistent with data from the UCLA high-risk study indicating that high family EE (in association with other variables already mentioned) *predicts* schizophrenia spectrum disorders that have their onset much later (Goldstein, 1985), suggesting a causal role in the relapse process (Nuechterlein, Snyder, & Mintz, 1992). Given that attempts to reduce EE and associated behaviors in family members have been very impressive in relapse prevention (e.g., Falloon et al., 1985; Hogarty, Anderson, Reiss, Kornblith, & Greenwald, 1986; Leff, Kuipers, Berkowitz, & Sturgeon, 1982; McFarlane et al., 1995), the time has come to gain a fuller understanding of these processes, as Hooley & Hiller (1998) suggest.

## Aberrations in Pathophysiology

Pathophysiology represents the favored model for an attempted integrative view of the interaction of biochemical, biological, and genetic findings relating to the supposed disease processes of schizophrenia. The history here is characterized by a multitude of hypotheses. The earlier ones involved the idea of autointoxication by substances, sometimes unknown and exotic ones (e.g., "taraxein"; Heath, Martens, Leach, Cohen, & Angel, 1957). The idea of a single, pathognomic agent is now for the most part duly recognized as extremely unlikely, given the complexities of such processes, and so we would assume that the days of searching for a single causative agent are over. The current tack usually entails an "integrative approach" that emphasizes the interplay of different neural systems, which is pretty much the only way to account for the massive and sometimes seemingly contradictory array of findings. Despite these presumably well-accepted cautions, however, a tendency to focus on a specific area as causative of the disorder remains. Along these lines, the dopamine (DA) hypothesis has occupied the attention of researchers for the longest period of time. There has also been some emphasis on neurons that are rich in gamma-aminobutyric acid (GABA) that, it is thought, mediate dopaminergic functioning. With the advent of the "atypical" antipsychotics, there has also been renewed interest in research on the serotonergic mechanisms. It also appears that the latter interacts with at least

some aspects of the dopaminergic system. The often disregarded caveat here is that a therapeutic role does not imply etiology (Harrison & Burnet, 1997).

**Receptor-Site Theories.** Hypotheses related to various receptor sites in the brain have been proposed primarily on the basis that therein lies the site of action for drugs used to treat schizophrenia. Among them is the dopamine hypothesis (e.g., Meltzer & Stahl, 1976) that has sustained the longest period of empirical attention. For interested readers, the lengthy history of this hypothesis is revealed in some detail in an earlier edition of this chapter (Carson, 1984). The basic etiologic hypothesis is that schizophrenia is the product of excess activity in dopaminergic brain pathways, caused by either increased levels of dopamine or by increased sensitivity of the receptor sites. The evidence supporting this hypothesis rests mainly on the observation that the original antipsychotic drugs used to alleviate symptoms of schizophrenia are dopamine antagonists (Creese, Burt, & Snyder, 1976; Seeman, Lee, Chau-Wong, & Wong, 1976). Of the several DA neuronal tracts known to exist in the brain, probably the most attention has been focused on one that originates in the mesencephalon and terminates in the limbic system (hence called the *mesolimbic* tract). In fact, however, the site of action of therapeutic DA blockade— if that is the principal mechanism involved in symptom moderation with neuroleptics—has not yet been precisely determined. It is likely that DA in some way plays a role in schizophrenia, as is the case of other receptor-site theories, but its causal significance is far from clear (Davis, Kahn, Ko, & Davidson, 1991; Joyce & Meador-Woodruff, 1997; Seeman, 1987).

Several basic and well-identified problems with the dopamine hypothesis persist, and it is curious that adherents are reluctant to relinquish the DA hypothesis despite these problems. First, dopamine-blocking drugs are by no means specific for schizophrenia, and their use to treat other psychotic and neuropsychological disorders, affective disorders including mania, and severe personality disorders is relatively commonplace. Second, it has been known for years that the dopamine receptor blocking effect occurs within hours of administering the drug; however, clinical effects do not emerge in some cases for several weeks. Further, the therapeutic effect is obtained not by achieving "normal" levels of dopamine functioning, but at rather abnormally low levels, as evidenced by the correlation of clinical outcome with symptoms of Parkinsonism and more seriously of tardive dyskinesia. Finally, the newer "atypical" neuroleptics exert their symptom-alleviating effects in a wholly different manner, suggesting that the dopamine system plays a complex role in multifaceted sequencing of neurochemical events associated with the expression of schizophrenic psychopathology. Overall, these problems suggest that what is known about the involvement of dopaminergic systems only partially reveals its place in the mechanism of schizophrenia.

Increasing complexities have been discovered regarding DA receptor sites. Snyder, Burt, and Creese (1976) first proposed the idea of two types of dopamine receptors in the brain, now indexed as $D_1$ and $D_2$. $D_1$ receptors stimulate production of the enzyme adenylate cyclase, implicated in the enhancement of cell responsivity, whereas $D_2$ receptors inhibit adenylate cyclase production. The "blocking" effects of neuroleptics, it is now thought, involve binding to the $D_2$ site, thereby in some manner inhibiting DA neurotransmission, possibly by preventing transmitter binding on the $D_1$ site or by a more direct route of inhibiting adenylate cyclase. These DA receptors can exhibit different states of high and low affinity for the reception of neurotransmitters. The dual and bidirectional high–low conversion represents another puzzling variable in the DA regulatory process. The discovery of dopamine receptor subtypes did not stop there. In 1990, a $D_3$ receptor site was identified (Sokoloff, Giros, Martres, Bouthenet, & Schwartz, 1990), and, at this time, no fewer than five dopamine receptor sites have been identified ($D_1$ to $D_5$).

Another source of complexity in the dopamine hypothesis concerns locations of the dopamine neurotransmitter systems. Dopamine is pervasive throughout several different areas of the brain. One study found a decrease—not an increase—in dopamine $D_1$ receptors in the prefrontal cortex of those diagnosed schizophrenic and suggested that this might explain some of the cognitive impairment of the disorder (Okubo et al., 1997). The anterior cingulate cortex, which plays a role in the function of attentional processes, is another area where pathological neuroprocesses associated with dopamine have been investigated. Several studies have implicated the cingulate cortex in schizophrenia psychopathology (e.g., Andreasen,

Paradiso, & O'Leary, 1998; Tamminga et al., 1992).

There is some evidence that the dopamine systems of schizophrenics are fundamentally different. Using challenge methodology, the demonstration of abnormal reactivity of dopaminergic transmission in response to amphetamine in schizophrenic patients appears robust (Abi-Dargham et al., 1998; Breier et al, 1997). However, it has also been suggested that a more accurate model of schizophrenic-like psychosis is gleaned from the more specific action of phenylcyclohexlpiperidine (PCP), a drug that effects the channel that down-modulates glutamatergic processes. It is believed that PCP, which can induce psychotic-like states in normal individuals that last up to three or four hours, can, in schizophrenics, unleash much longer periods of psychosis by virtue of lack of a means to turn the system off (Grace & Moore, 1998).

In one study, subjects were administered a nonselective dopamine agonist, apomorphine, or placebo, and then performed a verbal cognitive task. PET scans were then obtained for two groups— schizophrenic and controls. In schizophrenic patients but not controls, administration of apomorphine enhanced cognitive activation of the cingulate cortex during the verbal task. The results provided *in vivo* evidence that an impaired cognitive-task-induced activation of the anterior cingulate cortex in schizophrenic patients can be modulated by dopaminergic manipulation (Dolan et al., 1995). By studying the interaction of manipulating the dopaminergic system with a verbal task and the effects of the activity of a specific brain area, the authors were able to demonstrate a *systemic* difference in schizophrenic patients. Rather than enabling conclusions in terms of etiology, such an approach begins to recognize the complexity and importantly attempts to bridge mind (i.e., verbal task) with body (i.e., cingulate cortex activation). Still, no doubt, there are many missing pieces to this puzzle.

The "atypical" antipsychotic drugs (e.g., clozapine, olanzapine, risperidone) further complicate the dopamine puzzle. So-called "atypical" because they do not produce the side effects associated with the traditional neuroleptic medications, notably, tardive dyskinesia, these drugs, it is assumed do not impact the same dopamine receptor sites as the traditional ones. However, the demonstration by Nyberg & Farde (1997) estimated that extrapyramidal symptoms (EPS) are not evident until approximately 80% of the $D_2$ receptor sites are occupied. In other words, it may be that the new antipsychotic medications exert a clinical effect before the number of $D_2$ receptor sites required for extrapyramidal symptoms have been affected.

Unfortunately for the dopamine theory, these newer drugs are apparently just as effective as the older neuroleptics, although the more dangerous of these (clozapine) is reserved for those who do not respond to the more traditional drugs. Perhaps due to a desire to preserve the potential for the dopamine hypothesis, it is sometimes concluded that patients who do not respond to the traditional antipsychotics represent a subgroup of schizophrenics who have a variant dopamine pathology. However, Valenstein (1998) has pointed out the inconsistency of this line of reasoning because those patients who do respond to traditional neuroleptics respond to the atypicals as well.

It is clear that the newer antipsychotic medications that exert their effects primarily in systems other than the dopamine system pose particular problems for the dopamine hypothesis. The "atypical" antipsychotics, olanzapine and risperidone, primarily affect serotonergic receptors by decreasing transmission activity, in particular, the subtype receptors that have been labeled "5-HT$_2$." Interestingly, it is believed that these receptors sites are where LSD exerts its hallucinogenic properties (Pierce & Peroutka, 1989; Wing et al., 1990).

Of the atypicals, clozapine is a bit of an anomaly because of its far-reaching and varied effects. Clozapine affects the dopamine system as well as the serotonergic system, and also a wide range of other receptor types (Nyberg & Farde, 1997). There is evidence that clozapine achieves its effects through $D_4$-mediated GABA modulation (Bergson et al., 1995). GABAergic neural systems are another area that, it is thought, plays a role in schizophrenia based on evidence from postmortem and functional imaging studies that demonstrated abnormalities (Akbarian et al., 1995; Benes, Vincent, Alsterberg, Bird, & SanGiovanni, 1992; Busatto et al., 1996; Meltzer, 1994). Further complicating matters, it appears that 5-HT$_2$ receptors have a role in controlling GABAergic neurons (Harrison & Burnet, 1997).

In connecting these systems to behavioral output, there is no more specificity, although some brain areas have been broadly related to either negative (e.g., amygdala) or positive (e.g., the prefrontal cortex) symptoms, mainly on the grounds of speculative reasoning. The serotonergic systems are related to affect, cognition, motor behavior, hormonal, sleep, and body temperature regulation (Cowen, 1991; Stephenson, 1990). Clearly, dopamine and serotonergic systems play critical roles in the schizophrenic process, but where they fall in the cascade of events that undergird the classic psychotic and thought-disordered clinical picture is much less clear (Nyberg and Farde, 1997). It may be that role of neurochemicals will have to include other influences, such as the aberration of neural circuitry, before the role of biochemical abnormalities will more completely elucidate the schizophrenic process. In any event, the limitations of psychopharmacological technology are not unlike those of some forms of cancer treatment, where cellular production of all types, not just cancerous cell growth, is stopped by some chemical interventions and produces well-known iatrogenic effects, an accepted cost given the present limitations of treatment in this area. Similarly, psychotropic drugs used to treat schizophrenia have far-reaching effects such as tardive dyskinesia.

Although perhaps painting too optimistic a picture, Nestler (1997) clearly recognizes this in emphasizing that pinning schizophrenia on a simple increase or decrease of a neurotransmitter is unlikely to pan out and that some sort of integration of brain structures and the various pathways and systems connecting them will be implicated in the emergent etiology of the disorder. Impressive work done by Grace and Moore (1998) makes a comprehensive attempt along these lines. Noting that the nucleus accumbens demonstrates a functional interdependence of the various brain areas that have been implicated in schizophrenia (e.g., the prefrontal cortex, amygdala, and hippocampus), they developed a model of pathophysiology that focuses on the *regulatory* aspects of this brain area on the other areas. Although speculative, they go on to suggest that the development of the various brain systems (including the physiological mechanisms) may be impacted by aberrant processes in the nucleus accumbens. Such an approach takes into account the interrelationships of the various systems, but we suspect that there will be limitations in the knowledge that will be acquired. Specifically, the idea persists that there is a *localized* dysfunctional brain area ostensibly responsible for the dysfunction in other brain areas (i.e., the nucleus accumbens). Simply put, there is no a priori reason to necessarily assume a single causative agent that leads to the malfunction.

**Biology and Disease Commentary.** The idea that "chemical imbalances" in the brain cause serious mental disorder is for some reason an appealing proposition these days. Perhaps the complexity of these physiological processes in some way eludes careful scrutiny by those most involved with the *behavioral* pathology of the disorder. Yet the disease metaphor persists largely based on evidence that has been obtained in a sort of backward fashion. The essential strategy, now commonplace for more than a decade, has been to implicate sites in the brain known to be affected by drugs that are employed to attempt treatment of the disorder. More sophisticated approaches are being attempted with the recognition that multiple brain systems interact *as part of the pathological process*. However, the idea that there is a primary pathological factor or site in the brain persists, even in the most sophisticated of models such as that described before by Grace and Moore (1998). Focusing attention on the nodal areas where the other brain areas connect to each other is a reasonable idea, but it is still driven by the idea that there is a *single, fundamental causative agent* (or area) in the brain that is responsible for the disorder. At the present level of knowledge, such a reductionistic approach is quite possibly an unwarranted step—at least as far as etiology is implied. Observations of brain pathology are merely another level of clinical description. As such, they are important and valid descriptions, but for some reason it seems that they are accorded causal status.

We would not suggest that results from such studies are not worth pursuing, especially in the context of a richly developed theory such as that by Grace and Moore (1998). Indeed, this level of information will be a vital piece of the schizophrenia puzzle. Those models which acknowledge the complexities of interaction in brain systems in the *process* of the disorder will be especially important. For all the pieces to fall into place, however, will require relating these systems to behavioral output, and doing so will require consideration in the developmental context. Importantly, the idea of identifying a primary lesion may be one the field is ready to discard. The unfolding development of these systems, and the accompanying events (molecular and otherwise) will be key to developing an understanding of the etiology of the disorder. Our main contention here is that brain pathology should not be accorded status above clinical description for its explanatory power. Perhaps the results of the varied attempts to treat schizophrenia can serve as a reference point for integrating the molar aspects of the disorder.

## Treatment Perspectives

We cannot attempt here to approach adequately a comprehensive review of research on the treatments and outcomes of schizophrenic disorders. Therefore, we will limit our review here to treatments of historical significance and to those treatments that will hopefully provide some insight into the schizophrenia phenomena. We will be brief with—roughly speaking—the two classes of therapies: the biological approaches because we leave it to the others who present the biological view to provide a comprehensive overview, and the psychosocial therapies because, quite plainly, there is not a lot to report. The essence of our focus is also intended to shed light on the fundamental nature of the psychopathology involved. Before proceeding, we call upon the reader to reflect for a moment that schizophrenia has been a disorder, more so than any other mental disorder, that has consistently *required* multiple levels of intervention.

### Biological Approaches

With the widespread introduction of the phenothiazine drugs, beginning with chlorpromazine, in the mid-1950s, the more drastic forms of biological intervention underwent a rapid decline in use. Psychosurgery, hydrotherapy, and insulin coma, all of them once fairly routinely employed, are for the most part rarely considered today for any form of mental disorder. Electroconcvulsive therapy (ECT), still widely used to treat severe mood disorders and once a mainstay of "therapy" for schizophrenia to the point of abuse (e.g., "regressive" ECT involving multiple administrations per day), is now regarded at best as an improbably useful last resort for schizophrenic patients whose disorders have proven persistently refractory to other therapeutic measures, although there is some evidence to suggest that the threshold for this approach may be relaxing somewhat (e.g., Fink & Sackeim, 1996; Kales, Dequardo, & Tandon, 1999). The fact that these appallingly primitive techniques were still in widespread use only a generation ago speaks to the desperate level to which psychiatry had fallen immediately before the present era of neuroleptics. What sometimes seems to outsiders as an excessive attachment to these drugs among many psychiatric practitioners may be more understandable when viewed in this light.

Nevertheless, that attachment—insofar as it involves a sense of delivery from helplessness by the advent of the neuroleptic era—may be misplaced to some extent. Notwithstanding the seemingly unrestrained advertising claims of pharmaceutical companies about the role of their products in bringing about an alleged mental health revolution, many forces other than the availability of neuroleptics were in operation by the 1950s that were helping to modify views about the hopelessness of severe mental disorders and therefore to transform the previously wretched and iatrogenic environment of the average mental hospital. These positive attitudinal changes were doubtless aided and accelerated by the new drug therapies, but we do not know that they would not have happened anyway.

A look at resident schizophrenic population figures of state and county mental hospitals for the period under consideration is instructive in regard to the general point we are making here. These figures, assembled by Mosher (1989) from data gathered by the National Institute of Mental Health, show that the national peak for resident schizophrenic patients in public hospitals was reached in 1960–1961 at about 269,000. This was 5 years after neuroleptics became readily available and 2 to 3 years after their use had become practically universal, clearly demonstrating that the turnaround from ever-increasing resident schizophrenic hospital populations was not primarily attributable, as is commonly supposed, to the direct clinical effects of these drugs but rather to some other factor or factors. The drop in hospital populations remained modest until 1963, the year when the federal Community Mental Health Centers Act was passed. Thereafter, the rate of decline accelerated dramatically, a trend Mosher attributes primarily to continuing federal legislation (e.g., extension of Social Security benefits to the young mentally disabled) that made community living for the seriously disturbed an increasingly feasible alternative. He points out, interestingly, that in western European countries, with equal access to neuroleptics but with the pertinent social legislation already in place, the sharp decline during the 1960s in hospital residency for schizophrenia did not occur.

There is no denying the relief that can be brought about by neuroleptics—for both the patient and the doctor. Anyone who had seen a mental ward before neuroleptics were introduced can attest to the apparent inhumanity and suffering. But any patient will clearly inform you that the humanity is not fully restored, and the suffering is not fully relieved by drug treatment. Why else would medication compliance be such a preponderant issue in the treatment of schizophrenia? To be clear, drug bashing is not our intent. However, reservations that run counter to the widespread enthusiasm for this type of intervention need to be voiced, especially when some psychologist colleagues want prescription writing privileges. Viewed objectively, the actual record of accomplishment for neuroleptic intervention in schizophrenia is quite modest, especially where unpredictable, serious, and intractable side effects like tardive dyskinesia are factored in.

We have become accustomed in recent years to looking seriously at the results of meta-analytic studies in trying to assess treatment effectiveness. Though it has been largely overlooked in relation to schizophrenia, the original Smith, Glass, and Miller (1980) meta-analysis of the benefits of various therapies for various diagnostic groups included an assessment of drug therapy for schizophrenia. The drugs-alone average effect size (essentially the mean magnitude of the treated group's deviation from the mean of the control group, in control-group standard deviation units) in this assessment was $+0.51$, a figure that is decidedly on the low side for the many effect sizes reported in this remarkable work. Its basic statistical meaning is that the average functionability (as variously assessed) of exclusively drug-treated schizophrenics was at approximately the 70th percentile of that of untreated controls. By comparison, the average effect size for psychosocial interventions with "psychotics" was $+0.68$ (75th percentile of controls), whereas the drug-plus-psychotherapy combination for schizophrenia resulted in a very respectable average effect size of $+0.80$ (79th percentile).

Although these figures on the effectiveness of standard drug treatments in schizophrenia are sobering when viewed against the backdrop that they are often the only treatment offered, they do not convey to a full extent the limitations of an exclusively pharmacological approach. These limitations reside in the virtually complete ineffectiveness of these compounds in enhancing those energies, awarenesses, and skills that form the basis for effective engagement of the social environment, a vital set of personal resources that are strikingly deficient in the behavioral repertoires of the large majority of persons who acquire the schizophrenia designation. Consider in this regard the following remarks of the distinguished Harvard social psychologist Roger Brown, reported on his attendance at a local meeting of Schizophrenics Anonymous:

[The group leader] began with an optimistic testimony about how things were going with him, designed in part to buck up the others. Some of them also spoke hopefully; others were silent and stared at the floor throughout. I gradually felt hope draining out of the group as they began to talk of their inability to hold jobs, of living on welfare, of finding themselves overwhelmed by simple demands. Nothing bizarre was said or done; there was rather a pervasive sense of inadequacy, of lives in which each day was a dreadful trial. Doughnuts and coffee were served, and then each one, still alone, trailed off into the Cambridge night.

What I saw a little of at that meeting of Schizophrenics Anonymous is simply that there is something about schizophrenia that the antipsychotic drugs do not cure or even always remit on a long-term basis. (Brown & Herrnstein, 1977, p. 641)

Brown's observations remind us that perceptive and articulate "laypersons" can often tell simple truths about mental patients in a way that jaded mental health professionals often cannot. We question only his circumspection in suggesting that the antipsychotics "do not ... always remit" the devastating social deficits that normally accompany schizophrenic disorders. We hold that they probably *never* do, and that it is unreasonable to expect that they, or any other currently conceivable drug, might have such an effect. In this sense, we see the pharmacological approach limited indefinitely to a merely palliative role in therapies for schizophrenias. The empirical evidence indicates that long-term rates of *social* recovery in schizophrenia have not improved since the advent of neuroleptic drugs (e.g., Harding, Brooks, Ashikaga, Strauss, & Breier, 1987a,b). The ambitious study by Hegarty and colleagues (1994) mentioned earlier provides compelling evidence. Moreover, a smaller scale but similar study by Warner (1994) confirms the main findings reported by Hegarty and colleagues. It seems obvious to us that our

profession is going to have to look elsewhere for the "cure" to this type of problem.

On a more optimistic note, the disappointing performance of the antipsychotic drugs in the study described relate only to the older "typical" compounds such as chlorpromazine and haloperidol, and may conceivably be overcome with further advances in pharmacological therapy. Sheitman et al. (1998) identify a number of newer "atypical" antipsychotics in various stages of development and use; any of them might produce a better record in terms of social recovery. A primary advantage of the atypical antipsychotic medications is that they are less pernicious in side effects, supporting the hypothesis that the iatrogenic effects of older psychotropic medications may play a role in limiting social recovery. In any event, these newer compounds have yet to be thoroughly evaluated along these lines.

## Psychotherapies of Schizophrenia

Perhaps as a backlash to the days of the "double-bind" and other family approaches that resulted in uncalled for parent bashing and undoubtedly owing some influence to the recent "decade of the brain" that included a heavy emphasis on biologically based research at the National Institutes of Mental Health, there has been a very serious dearth of psychosocial research in schizophrenia. It should not go unnoticed that earlier forms of psychotherapy did not position themselves well in being subjected to empirical evaluation, and this inadequacy likely set the stage for the so-called biological revolution. So dominant became the latter that some extremely promising alternative approaches that appeared in the decades before the 1990s were quite simply ignored by the majority of the professional mental health community. These examples include a therapeutic community-based program of "self-help" for patients moved from the hospital to a commercially failed motel with minimal professional oversight (Fairweather, 1980; Fairweather, Sanders, Maynard, & Cressler, 1969), and a rigorous token economy "social learning" program for chronic state hospital patients (Paul & Lentz, 1977). There was also the report of a well-designed study that demonstrated the superiority of specialized individualized psychotherapy conducted by highly experienced therapists to antipsychotic medication in treating schizophrenia (Karon & Vandenbos, 1981). These studies produced exciting results in patient progress without, for the most part, extensive use of medication. The randomized clinical trial (RCT), ironically borrowed from the medical field concerned with pharmacological efficacy and now a mainstay of psychotherapy research, allowed a more recent examination of the efficacy of some very specific forms of psychotherapeutic intervention for schizophrenia. We now review the various psychotherapies.

**"Moral" and Milieu.** Such "active" (as opposed to prophylactic or maintenance) treatment as occurs in cases of schizophrenia is probably most often conducted in inpatient settings. Even where drugs are the primary mode of intervention, therefore, it is important to ask whether the psychosocial context or milieu of the hospital or ward has any therapeutic significance. A variety of evidence indicates that it does, beginning with the apparently pronounced successes of "moral" (i.e., psychosocial milieu) therapy asylums during the earliest decades of this country's founding.

The era of moral therapy in the United States lasted only roughly through the first half of the nineteenth century, following which it succumbed to paradigmatic social, cultural, and population changes (e.g., a huge influx of non-English speaking immigrants) that, during the subsequent century, produced the disgraceful, overcrowded, "snake-pit" conditions of public mental hospitals of the 1940s and 1950s. The rates of hospital discharge of persons suffering serious mental disorders fell precipitously during that period and resulted in the accumulation of "chronic" cases, most of them doubtless schizophrenic, in the human warehouses that mental hospitals had become. According to the old hospital records unearthed by Brockoven (1972), mental health professionals ironically had done a much better job *before* 1850, lacking as they did access to the subsequent dramatic but evidently largely irrelevant advances in biomedical science that were shortly to begin. In fact, general adoption, for all mental disorders, of the organic model suggested by general paresis, whose connection with syphilis was discovered in 1857, probably contributed significantly to the demise of the moral therapy movement.

The idea that effective treatment of schizophrenic persons should include the planned creation of a benign psychosocial environment surfaced again in the late 1920s with the establishment by Harry Stack Sullivan (1962) of a special ward at the Sheppard and Enoch Pratt Hospital for treating young schizophrenic males. In all probability, Sullivan himself had earlier had some sort of brief personal experience with this type of disorder (see Alexander, 1990, for a detailed examination of this possibility). Whatever the case, he had some insights not widely shared among his professional peers. Revolutionary for its time, this small ward was run with tight control by Sullivan (e.g., he personally selected and trained the nursing attendant staff), and in due course it achieved considerable fame for its innovative philosophy and for the therapeutic results achieved. It was one of the factors that first catapulted Sullivan into a position of prominence in American psychiatry (Chapman, 1976). Unfortunately, few hospital directors were willing to follow his lead in treating schizophrenia, and his influence in this respect seems to have been confined chiefly to the local area around Baltimore, notably including the famed Chestnut Lodge in Rockville.

The notion of milieu therapy (alternatively, therapeutic community) did not really catch on again until approximately the 1950s, undoubtedly aided, as we have seen, by the advent of neuroleptic drugs. Subsequently, the record it compiled (reviewed by Mosher & Gunderson, 1979; Neale & Oltmanns, 1980) may be termed encouraging, although the results achieved are, of course, strongly confounded with drug effects in most settings. In one remarkable study, that of Paul and Lentz (1977), they are not; in these authors' exceptionally well-controlled experiment, chronic patients treated with milieu therapy (in comparison to those who received standard hospital care) fared much better in outcome measures such as release to the community. We shall return to this study shortly in the following section to consider the behavioral aspects employed. In a later report, Mosher and colleagues described the "Soteria Project" and reported the results of milieu treatment, in most cases without neuroleptics that were on a par with treatment as usual for acute psychotic episodes (Mosher, Vallone, & Menn, 1995).

The beneficial effects of a psychologically wholesome milieu for chronically schizophrenic patients can apparently be gained even without hospital confinement. Fairweather and colleagues (1969) with consummate boldness, moved a substantial group of such patients out of the hospital into a commercially defunct motel ("The Lodge") where, after a brief orientation period, the latter were left for the most part on their own with only minimal supervision or medical coverage. The guiding principle was that of self-help. Contrary to the dire predictions many made, after a somewhat rough start, this small society began to organize itself, established a division of labor, and created various other formal arrangements essential to social living. Within a surprisingly short time, it became a truly viable and for the most part sustaining community. In due course, in fact, these "psychotic" citizens established a profitable janitorial and landscaping business! The patient cost per day to the state of California dropped to a fraction of what it had been, although that is perhaps the least of the benefits realized.

The Lodge project was eventually terminated formally, although the expatient community successfully continued on. Despite the evident promise of this approach and the considerable efforts of Fairweather and his associates to promote its consideration on a national scale, the path proved difficult (Fairweather, 1980). Although a few similar projects have been undertaken at scattered locations with comparably impressive results, support in official state or local government budgeting has been rare, as have enthusiastic expressions of interest among members of the traditional mental health disciplines. Why? We can only conjecture that this innovative concept ran so thoroughly counter to institutional bureaucracy and the prevailing professional zeitgeist that it was the victim of a destructive type of cognitive inflexibility or (more sinisterly) of political assassination. Obviously, it still deserves a serious, comprehensive, and extended trial.

**Behavioral.** A similar fate overtook the extraordinarily promising "social learning" program that was part of the large Paul and Lentz (1977) project mentioned before. In this treatment condition, patients were subjected to a closely monitored and continuous token economy, one whose contingencies were unusually rigorous both in behavioral expectations and the range of reinforcements meted out as a consequence of good or substandard patient performance (token acquisition). The outcomes for patients in this program exceeded by a considerable margin the very respectable ones achieved with milieu therapy (which, as noted, were notably superior to standard hospital care), again without significant contribution from drugs. Of a control-matched sample of these chronic patients, 11% achieved wholly independent functioning without readmission during the course of a 4½-

year follow up, whereas 96% of them managed continuous community living for at least 90 days. As we have learned to expect, there was modest postdischarge behavioral deterioration for many of these patients, but nondrug aftercare services were generally effective in reversing this trend. We are baffled by the practically uniform absence of response to these challenging findings—for example, among state mental health authorities— over the years since their original publication.

Although we have yet to see the potential realized in bold and imaginative therapeutic programs, our own conviction is that the real promise of behavioral intervention in schizophrenia resides in the programmed establishment (reestablishment?) of those skills essential to independent adult functioning in an increasingly demanding and complex social environment. As pointed out by Bellack, Morrison, and Mueser (1989), a dearth of significant progress in this area is attributable at least in part to misdirected effort and a related failure to analyze adequately the tasks to be accomplished. The deficits that need to be addressed, for example, are in the main at a more basic level than "problems solving."

**Family.** As in other areas of psychosocial intervention in schizophrenia, research in family therapy has waned substantially in recent years, although its past record is quite respectable (Mosher & Gunderson, 1979). Our reading of the etiologic evidence is that the neglect is a very serious mistake. The primary exception to the pervasive inactivity in family therapy concerns work on the reduction of EE to prevent relapse among persons who have already had one or more hospital admissions. Not surprisingly, such interventions appear quite promising (Faloon et al., 1985; Hogarty et al., 1986). There is some suggestion that intervention to reduce EE may make it feasible to reduce neuroleptic drug dosages, with attendant benefits in instrumental and social role functioning (Hogarty et al., 1988), not to mention reducing the risk of tardive dyskinesia. Family therapy would be an excellent medium for identifying instances of EE and for teaching family members how to avoid it (Tarrier & Barrowclough, 1990).

**Individual.** Though the work of several gifted psychotherapists of schizophrenics, such as Sullivan, Freida Fromm-Reichmann (1950), Green (1964), and John Rosen (1953) is an important part of the history of the field, it must be acknowledged that we lack good data on long-term outcomes for the patients that they treated. The bases for their short-term success are also obscure, although in various writings each of these individuals articulated the principles that supposedly guided their interventions. Because the "principles' are not readily transmitted to others with the assurance of comparable results, our suspicion is that the critical element in each instance was some combination of personality factors that made for facile communication with psychotic persons. Conceivably, they are factors that share some commonality with those identified by Whitehorn and Betz (1954) in isolating a group of psychiatric residents who achieved excellent results in work with schizophrenic patients in the years before neuroleptic drugs washed out the effect.

In the not so distant past, Karon and Vandenbos (1981) published a book on the psychotherapy of schizophrenia which they unabashedly subtitled "The Treatment of Choice." The recommended techniques, ample and fascinatingly illustrated, bear the unmistakable impress of John Rosen. The book ends with a complete report of a research project designed to compare the outcomes of psychotherapy administered by "experienced" and less experienced therapists, neuroleptic drug treatment, and a combination of the two for thirty-three randomly treatment-assigned patients during an effective project period (including follow-up) of 44 months. The multiple-outcome-measure results (which include rehospitalization data) are thoroughly analyzed and discussed. In summary, they showed a strong superiority in the long-term outcomes for the psychotherapy-only treatment group. The drug-plus-psychotherapy group had outcomes only slightly superior to the drug-only group, an effect the authors ascribe chiefly to drug-induced interference with the psychotherapy process.

The report just described also includes a valuable discussion and critique of earlier and probably better known comparative treatment projects of this general type, to which the interested reader is referred (they are omitted here because of space considerations). Overall, the results of these projects are less favorable to the psychotherapeutic approach in schizophrenia than those reported by Karon and Vandenbos (1981), although more encouraging than some secondary reviews have portrayed them. There is a persistent tendency in this literature, by the way, not to recognize the multiple ways in which drug treatment and psycho-

therapy differ that make direct, competitive comparisons of the two more problematic than superficial analysis would suggest. An excellent discussion of some of these considerations was offered by Stiles and Shapiro (1989).

It is striking how relatively little current research on the individual psychotherapy of schizophrenic persons is currently underway, compared to other treatments (i.e., biological) or other disorders. One wonders whether the impact of negative opinions about psychotherapy issued by some has declared the issue moot (e.g., Klerman, 1984). Coursey (1989) expressed this attitude by suggesting that we need a new type of psychotherapy for schizophrenia, one that recognizes the global inefficacy of standard psychotherapy and that accepts schizophrenia as a "biological distortion," the biological revolution in psychiatry, according to Coursey, having "won." As described, this desired form of psychotherapy, which hardly seems new, would be akin to case management for a defective organism. Apart from wondering what research literature Coursey reads and how anything has been won, we are distressed by the unrestrained condescension of his position, as we suspect many intelligent schizophrenic persons would be. Katz (1989) offered a suitable admonishment for this line of thinking.

On the other hand, the tide may be turning. The American Psychiatric Association's (1997) *Practice Guideline for the Treatment of Patients with Schizophrenia* that contains expected comprehensive recommendations on managing medication of patients in various phases and at differing severities of disorder also makes a host of recommendations relating to the desirability of vigorous psychosocial interventions. In making these recommendations, the *Practice Guideline* takes notice of the development in recent years of a number of relatively new psychosocial initiatives demonstrably effective in ameliorating the problems of schizophrenic patients, particularly those problems that seem largely unresponsive to antipsychotic drugs (Kopelowicz & Liberman, 1998). Ironically, it may be that the current scientific standard for demonstrating efficacy in the field, that of the randomized clinical trial or "RCT," is making it possible to gain a foothold in demonstrating the importance of psychotherapy for schizophrenia. In contrast to effectiveness studies (i.e., how treatment interventions hold up in the field under less controlled circumstances), RCTs aimed at efficacy seek to demonstrate how well an intervention works under controlled conditions, thus making it possible to identify a potent treatment. A number of "psychotherapy trials" conducted in this manner reaffirm the role of psychotherapy for schizophrenia.

Hogarty and colleagues (1997a,b) report on a controlled 3-year trial of "Personal Therapy," a form of psychotherapy specifically aimed at schizophrenic individuals. This treatment was very effective in enhancing the social adjustment and social role performance of discharged patients. Personal therapy is described as a staged, nonpsychodynamic approach oriented to learning coping skills for managing emotion and stressful events. In favorably commenting on this program, Fenton and McGlashan (1997) assert the need for a flexible individual psychotherapy component in virtually all treatment packages for schizophrenia.

Training in social skills (see, e.g., Bellack, Mueser, Gingerich, & Agresta, 1997; Dilk & Bond, 1996), as has been demonstrated, has a positive impact on overcoming the embarrassment, ineptitude, awkwardness, and attentional "cluelessness" displayed in social situations by many persons who have undergone episodes of schizophrenia. A broader aspect of social relations concerns integration into a community. Many schizophrenic patients, sometimes abruptly discharged into the community, have great difficulty in marshaling resources and organizing their lives. Included here is some propensity to become involved in substance abuse, often as self-medication for unpleasant antipsychotic drug side effects (Kosten & Ziedonis, 1997). Therefore, there is considerable need for persistent and vigorous community-based follow-up and aid in managing life problems (e.g., Mueser et al., 1998), including coordinating continuing antipsychotic medication (Kopelowicz et al., 1997).

One final, less optimistic point concerns the problem of system inertia. These psychosocially based efforts to compensate for the shortcomings of antipsychotic medication in treating schizophrenia are not at present generally "in place" and functioning up to speed. An intensive effort to assess the degree of conformance of actual practice to a set of previously issued treatment guidelines similar to those described before in the mental health systems of two states found that conformance was generally less than 50%, especially to the psychosocial enhancements recommended (Lehman et al., 1998). We suspect that a national compliance assessment effort covering all fifty states would not produce a more encouraging picture at this time. Actual mental health practice, it seems, fails to keep pace with what is known to be maximally effective in restoring schizophrenic patients to active and productive citizenship. In this sense, we have continued a very long-standing pattern of limited horizons for and neglect of this portion of the population.

## Conclusion

Some behavioral scientists (e.g., Whitaker, 1992) dispute the idea that schizophrenia is caused primarily by biological factors. It is unfortunate and counterproductive that biological and psychosocial research are often conceived as mutually antagonistic and that they rarely make contact with one another. Importantly, although much lip service is paid to the evidence of interaction between biological and psychosocial variables in schizophrenia, studies that actually examine the interaction are rare. Hopefully, interest (and funding) for such endeavors will increase in the near future.

As a good illustration of this type of integration, consider an innovative project that involved rating childhood "home movies" obtained from schizophrenic patients conducted by Walker and colleagues (Grimes & Walker, 1994; Walker, 1994; Walker et al., 1994). The preschizophrenic children showed less—and less positive than negative—emotionality, had poorer motor skills, and showed a higher rate of peculiar movements, such as tic-like muscle contractions, suggestive of neuromotor abnormalities. Bear in mind that the manifest nature of these problems would all but certainly impact the child's social environment negatively. It is extremely likely that the (presumably) neurologically based behavioral deficits observed in the then preschizophrenic children would be noticed and responded to negatively by others who come into contact with them. The child who rarely manifests joy (even on celebratory occasions such as birthdays), whose emotional expressiveness is prevailingly in the bland to negative range, who is motorically clumsy or awkward, and who may evidence peculiar involuntary movements, is likely to have a far less stress-free early life than the child endowed with the opposite characteristics. Minimally, such a scenario suggests that the occurrence of stressful life events may affect social and personality development and is not independent of a potentially pathogenic biological "diathesis." In fact, this idea has been a central element in the important contributions of psychologist Paul Meehl (1962, 1989, 1990) in tracing the developmental course of schizophrenic outcomes. Berenbaum and Fujita (1994) offered a similar conceptualization.

Meehl's (1962, 1989) concepts relating to the genesis of schizophrenia are in broad outline—if not in their details (e.g., we find implausible the notion that a single dominant gene controls vulnerability)—refreshingly closer to what we envisage as a more ideal approach to finding the answers. It seems inescapable in our reading of the evidence that the connections of causal links from the molecular to the molar (behavioral) levels, from the endoenviornment to the ectoenvironment, are both lengthy and intricately interlaced. To unravel the mysteries will require the talents and skills of many different kinds of scientists, from the molecular biologist to the specialist in the social development of children, working in a framework in which some minimal level of collaboration will be essential. Divided research camps devoted primarily to furthering of ideologies are a decided hindrance that we can ill afford in this type of scientific context. Until we can move beyond the clash of genetic/biological *versus* environmental/psychosocial paradigms, we will be limited to a vision holding that the etiology of schizophrenia resides in some imprecisely specified combination of "bad luck."

The simple fact is that in much of the contemporary literature, the psychosocial dimensions of schizophrenia are denied at intensities that approach religious fervor. We fear that the "great and desperate cure" mentality (Valenstein, 1986), the magic-bullet fantasy now embraced by much of psychology as well as our sister discipline of psychiatry, is a step backward in time, one that retards scientific progress and deprives untold numbers of persons designated as schizophrenic of the demonstrable benefits of soundly planned and executed psychosocial intervention. Meanwhile, an egregiously imbalanced allocation of scarce research resources deprives the mental health professions of opportunities to develop vitally needed knowledge that could lead to psychosocially based techniques enhanced in cost-effec-

tiveness, possibly even ones that would enormously potentiate the now rather limited horizons of the growing catalog of antipsychotic drugs.

# References

Abi-Dargham, A., Gil., R., Krystal, J., Baldwin, R. M., Seibyl, J. P., Bowers, M., van Dyck, C. H., Charney, D. S., Innis, R. B., & Laruelle, M. (1998). Increased striatal dopamine transmission of schizophrenia: Confirmation in a second cohort. *American Journal of Psychiatry, 155,* 761–767.

Akbarian, S., Kim, J. J., Potkin, S. G., Hagman, J. O., Tafazzoli, A., & Bunney, W. E. (1995). Gene expression for glutamic acid decarboxylase is reduced without loss of neurons in prefrontal cortex of schizophrenics. *Archives of General Psychiatry, 52,* 258–266.

Alexander, I. E. (1990). *Personology.* Durham, NC: Duke University Press.

Amador, X., Kirkpatrick, B., Buchanan, R. W., Carpenter, W. T., Marcinko, L., & Yale, S. A. (1999). Stability of the Diagnosis of Deficit Syndrome in Schizophrenia. *American Journal of Psychiatry, 156,* 637–639.

American Psychiatric Association (1968). *Diagnostic and statistical manual of mental disorders* (2nd ed.). Washington, DC: Author.

American Psychiatric Association (1980). *Diagnostic and statistical manual of mental disorders* (3rd ed.). Washington, DC: Author.

American Psychiatric Association (1987). *Diagnostic and statistical manual of mental disorders* (3rd ed., rev.). Washington, DC: Author.

American Psychiatric Association (1994). *Diagnostic and statistical manual of mental disorders* (4th ed.). Washington, DC: Author.

American Psychiatric Association (1997). Practice guideline for the treatment of patients with schizophrenia. *American Journal of Psychiatry* (Supplement), *154,* 1–63.

Andreasen, N. C. (1985). Positive vs. negative schizophrenia: A critical evaluation. *Schizophrenia Bulletin, 11,* 380–389.

Andreasen, N. C. (1988). The subtyping of schizophrenia. In F. Flach (Ed.), *The schizoprhenias* (pp. 30–40). New York: W. W. Norton.

Andreasen, N. C. (1994). Changing concepts of schizophrenia and the ahistorical fallacy. *American Journal of Psychiatry, 151,* 1405–1407.

Andreasen, N. C. (1998). Understanding schizophrenia: A silent spring. *American Journal of Psychiatry, 155,* 1657–1659.

Andreasen, N. C., Arndt, S., Alliger, R., Del M. P., & Flaum, M. (1995). Symptoms of schizophrenia: Methods, meanings, and mechanisms. *Archives of General Psychiatry, 52,* 341–351.

Andreasen, N. C., Paradiso, S., & O'Leary, D. S. (1998). "Cognitive dysmetria" as an integrative theory of schizophrenia: A dysfunction in cortical–subcortical–cerebellar circuitry? *Schizophrenia Bulletin, 24,* 203–267.

Bateson, G., Jackson, D. D., Haley, J., & Weakland, J. (1956). Toward a theory of schizophrenia. *Behavioral Science, 1,* 251–264.

Bell, R. C., Dudgeon, P., McGorry, P. D., & Jackson, H. J. (1998). The dimensionality of schizophrenia concepts in first-episode psychosis. *Acta Psychiatrica Scandinavica, 97,* 334–342.

Bellack, A. S., Morrison, R. L., & Mueser, K. T. (1989). Social problem solving in schizophrenia. *Schizophrenia Bulletin, 15,* 101–116.

Bellack, A. S., Mueser, K. T., Gingerich, S., & Agresta, J. (1997). *Social skills training for schizophrenia.* New York: Guilford.

Bellak, L. (1979). Introduction: An idiosyncratic overview. In L. Bellak (Ed.), *Disorders of the schizophrenic syndrome* (pp. 3–24). New York: Basic Books.

Benes, F. M., Vincent, S. L., Alsterberg, G., Bird, E. D., & SanGiovanni, J. P. (1992). Increased GABAA receptor binding in superficial layers of cingulate cortex in schizophrenics. *Journal of Neuroscience, 12,* 924–929.

Benjamin, L. S. (1976). A reconsideration of the Kety and associates study of genetic factors in the transmission of schizophrenia. *American Journal of Psychiatry, 133,* 1129–1133.

Berenbaum, H., & Fujita, F. (1994). Schizophrenia and personality: Exploring the boundaries and connections between vulnerability and outcome. *Journal of Abnormal Psychology, 103,* 148–158.

Bergson, C., Mrzljak, L., Smiley, J. F., Pappy, M., Levenson, R., & Goldman-Rakic, P. S., (1995). Regional, cellular, and subcellular variations in the distribution of D1 and D5 dopamine receptors in the primate brain. *Journal of Neuroscience, 15,* 7821–7836.

Bleuler, E. (1950). *Dementia praecox or the group of schizophrenias* (J. Zinkin, Trans.). New York: International Universities Press. (Original work published in 1911.)

Botstein, D., White, R. L., Skolnick, M., & Davis, R. W. (1980). Construction of a genetic linkage map in a man using restriction fragment length polymorphisms. *American Journal of Human Genetics, 32,* 314–331.

Bradbury, T. N., & Miller, G. A. (1985). Season of birth in schizophrenia: A review of the evidence, methodology, and etiology. *Psychological Bulletin, 98,* 596–594.

Breier, A., Buchanan, R. W., Kirkpatrick, B., Davis, O. R., Irish, D., Summerfelt, A., & Carpenter, W. T. (1994). Effects of clozapine on positive and negative symptoms in outpatients with schizophrenia. *American Journal of Psychiatry, 151,* 20–26.

Breier, A., Malhotra, A. K., Pinals, D. A., Weisenfeld, N. I., & Pickar, E. (1997). Association of ketamine-induced psychosis with focal activation of the prefrontal cortex in healthy volunteers. *American Journal of Psychiatry, 154,* 805–811.

Brockoven, J. S. (1972). *Moral treatment in community mental health.* New York: Springer.

Brown, R., & Hernstein, R. J. (1977). *Psychology.* Boston: Little, Brown.

Busatto, G. F., Pilowsky, L. S., Costa, D. C., Ell, P. J., David, A. S., & Kerwin, R. W. (1996). Reduced benzodiazepine receptor binding correlates with severity of psychotic symptoms in schizophrenia. *American Journal of Psychiatry, 154,* 56–63.

Butzlaff, R. L., & Hooley, J. M. (1998). Expressed emotion and psychiatric relapse: A meta-analysis. *Archives of General Psychiatry, 55,* 547–552.

Cannon, M., Jones, P., Gilvarry, C., Rifkin, L., McKenzie, K., Foerster, A., & Murray, R. M. (1997). Premorbid social functioning in schizophrenia and bipolar disorder: Similarities and differences. *American Journal of Psychiatry, 154,* 1544–1550.

Cannon, T. D. (1998a). Genetic and perinatal influences in the etiology of schizophrenia: A neurodevelopmental model. In M. F. Lenzenweger & R. H. Dworkin (Eds.), *Origins and development of schizophrenia* (pp. 67–92). Washington, DC: American Psychological Association.

Cannon, T. D. (1998b). Neurodevelopmental influences in the genesis and epigenesis of schizophrenia: An overview. *Applied & Preventive Psychology, 7,* 47–62.

Carpenter, W. T., Strauss, J. S., & Muleh, S. (1973). Are there pathognomic symptoms in schizophrenia?: An empiric investigation of Kurt Schneider's first rank symptoms. *Archives of General Psychiatry, 28,* 847–852.

Carson, R. C. (1997). Costly compromises: A critique of the diagnostic and statistical manual of mental disorders. In S. Fisher and R. P. Greenberg (Eds.), *From placebo to panacea: Putting psychiatric drugs to the test* (pp. 98–112). New York: Wiley.

Carson, R. C. (1984). The schizophrenias. In H. E. Adams and P. B. Sutker (Eds.), *Comprehensive handbook of psychopathology* (pp. 411–438). New York: Plenum.

Carson, R. C., & Sanislow, C. A. (1993). The schizophrenias. In H. E. Adams and P. B. Sutker (Eds.), *Comprehensive handbook of psychopathology,* (2nd ed., pp. 295–333). New York: Plenum.

Chapman, A. H. (1976). *Harry Stack Sullivan: His life and his work.* New York: G. P. Putnam's Sons.

Cohen, D. (1997). A critique of the use of neuroleptic drugs in psychiatry. In S. Fisher & R. P. Greenberg (Eds.), *From placebo to panacea: Putting psychiatric drugs to the test* (pp. 173–228). New York: Wiley.

Coursey, R. D. (1989). Psychotherapy with persons suffering from schizophrenia: The need for a new agenda. *Schizophrenia Bulletin, 15,* 349–354.

Cowen, P. J. (1991). Serotonin receptor subtypes: Implications for psychopharmacology. *British Journal of Psychiatry, 159,* 7–14.

Creese, I., Burt, D. R., & Snyder, S. H. (1976). Dopamine receptor binding predicts clinical and pharmacological potencies of antischizophrenic drugs. *Science, 192,* 481–483.

Cronbach, L. J., & Meehl, P. E. (1955). Construct validity in psychological tests. *Psychological Bulletin, 52,* 281–302.

Crow, T. J. (1985). The two syndrome concept: Origins and current status. *Schizophrenia Bulletin, 11,* 471–486.

Crow, T. J. (1997a). Temporolimbic or transcallosal connections: Where is the primary lesion in schizophrenia and what is its nature? *Schizophrenia Bulletin, 23,* 521–524.

Crow, T. J. (1997b). From Kraepelin to Kretschmer leavened by Schneider: The transition from categories of psychosis to dimensions of variation intrinsic to *Homo sapiens. Archives of General Psychiatry, 55,* 502–504.

Davis, K. L., Kahn, R. S., Ko., G., & Davidson, M. (1991). Dopamine in schizophrenia: A review and reconceptualization. *American Journal of Psychiatry, 148,* 1474–1486.

Defendorf, A. R. (1902). *Clinical psychiatry:* Abstracted and adapted from the sixth German edition of Kraepelin's "Lehrbuch Der Psychiatrie." New York: Macmillan.

DeLisi, L. E., & Crow, T. J. (1989). Evidence for sex chromosome locus for schizophrenia. *Schizophrenia Bulletin, 15,* 431–440.

DeLisi, L. E., Crow, T. J., & Hirsch, S. R. (1986). The third biannual winter workshops on schizophrenia. *Archives of General Psychiatry, 43,* 706–711.

Dilk, M. N., & Bond, G. R. (1996). Meta-analytic evaluation of skills training research for individuals with severe mental illness. *Journal of Consulting and Clinical Psychology, 64,* 1337–1346.

Doane, J. A., Falloon, I. R. H., Goldstein, M. J., & Mintz, J. (1985). Parental affective style and the treatment of schizophrenia: Predicting course of illness and social functioning. *Archives of General Psychiatry, 42,* 34–42.

Dolan, R. J., Fletcher, P., Frith, C. D., Friston, K. J., Frackowiak, R. S. J., & Grasby, P. M. (1995). Dopaminergic modulation of impaired cognitive activation in the anterior cingulate cortex in schiozophrenia. *Nature, 378,* 180–182.

Dollhus, S., Everitt, B., Ribeyre, J. M., Assouly-Besse, F., Sharp, C., & Petit, M. (1996). Identifying subtypes of schizophrenia by cluster analysis. *Schizophrenia Bulletin, 22,* 545–555.

Egeland, J. A., Gerhard, D. S., Pauls, D. L., Sussex, J. N., Kidd, K. K., Allen, C. R., Hostetter, A. M., & Housman, D. E. (1987). Bipolar affective disorders linked to DNA markers on chromosome 11. *Nature, 325,* 783–787.

Endicott, J., Nee, J., Cohen, J., Fleiss, J., Williams, J. B. W., & Simon, R. (1986). Diagnostic criteria for schizophrenia: Reliabilities and agreement between systems. *Archives of General Psychiatry, 39,* 884–889.

Fairweather, G. W. (Ed.). (1980). *The Fairweather Lodge: A twenty-five year retrospective.* San Francisco: Jossey-Bass.

Fairweather, G. W., Sanders, D. H., Maynard, H., & Cressler, D. L. (1969). *Community life for the mentally ill: An alternative to institutional care.* Chicago: Aldine.

Falloon, I. R. H., Boyd, J. L., McGill, C. W., Williamson, M., & Razanie, J. (1985). Family management in the prevention of morbidity of schizophrenia: Clinical outcome of a two-year longitudinal study. *Archives of General Psychiatry, 42,* 887–896.

Feighner, J., Robins, E., Guze, S., Woodruff, R., & Munoz, R. (1972). Diagnostic criteria for use in psychiatric research. *Archives of General Psychiatry, 26,* 57–63.

Fenton, W. S., & McGlashan, T. H. (1994). Antecedents, symptom progression, and long-term outcome of the deficit syndrome in schizophrenia. *Archives of General Psychiatry, 151,* 351–356.

Fenton, W. S., & McGlashan, T. H. (1997). We can talk: Individual psychotherapy for schizophrenia. *American Journal of Psychiatry, 154,* 1493–1495.

Fink, M., & Sackeim, H. A. (1996). Convulsive therapy in schizophrenia? *Schizophrenia Bulletin, 22,* 27–39.

Fischer, M. (1971). Psychoses in the offspring of schizophrenic monozygotic twins and their normal co-twins. *British Journal of Psychiatry, 118,* 43–52.

Fischer, M. (1973). Genetic and environmental factors in schizophrenia: A study of schizophrenic twins and their families. *Acta Psychiatrica Scandinavica,* (Suppl. 238), 158.

Fish, B. (1957). The detection of schizophrenia in infancy: A preliminary report. *Journal of Nervous and Mental Disease, 125,* 1–24.

Fish, B. (1977). Neurobiological antecedents of schizophrenia in children: Evidence for an inherited, congenital, neurointegrative defect. *Archives of General Psychiatry, 34,* 1297–1313.

Flaum, M. D., Andreasen, N. C., & Widiger, T. A. (1994). Schizophrenia and other psychotic disorders in DSM-IV: Final overview. In T. A. Widiger, A. J. Frances, H. A. Pincus, R. Ross, M. B. First, W. Davis, & M. Kline (Eds.), *DSM-IV sourcebook* (Vol. 4; pp. 1007–1017). Washington, DC: American Psychiatric Association.

Fromm-Reichman, F. (1948). Notes on the development of treatment of schizophrenics by psychoanalytic psychotherapy. *Psychiatry, 11,* 263–273.

Fromm-Reichman, F. (1950). *Principles of intensive psychotherapy.* Chicago: University of Chicago Press.

Garmezy, N., & Rodnick, E. H. (1959). Premorbid adjustment and performance in schizophrenia. *Journal of Nervous and Mental Disease, 129,* 450–466.

Goldstein, M. J. (1985). Family factors that antedate the onset of schizophrenia and related disorders: The results of a fifteen year prospective longitudinal study. *Acta Psychiatrica Scandinavica, 71* (Suppl. No. 319), 7–18.

Goldstein, M. J., & Rodnick, E. H. (1975). The family's contribution to the etiology of schizophrenia: Current status. *Schizophrenia Bulletin, 1,* 48–63.

Goldstein, M. J., & Strachan, A. M. (1987). The family and schizophrenia. In T. Jacob (Ed.), *Family interaction and psychopathology: Theories, methods, and findings.* New York: Plenum.

Gottesman, I. I., & Bertelson, A. (1989). Confirming unexpressed genotypes for schizophrenia: Risks in the offspring of Fischer's Danish identical and fraternal discordant twins. *Archives of General Psychiatry, 46,* 867–872.

Gottesman, I. I., & Moldin, S. O. (1998). Genotype, genes, genesis, and pathogenesis in schizophrenia. In M. F. Lenzenweger & R. H. Dworkin (Eds.), *Origins and development of schizophrenia* (pp. 5–26). Washington, DC: American Psychological Association.

Grace, A. A., & Moore, H. (1998). Regulation of information flow in the nucleus accumbens: A model for the pathophysiology of schizophrenia. In M. F. Lenzenweger & R. H. Dworkin (Eds.), *Origins and development of schizophrenia* (pp. 123–160). Washington, DC: American Psychological Association.

Green, H. (1964). *I never promised you a rose garden.* New York: Holt, Rinehart & Winston.

Grimes, K., & Walker, E. F. (1994). Childhood emotional expressions, educational attainment, and age at onset of illness in schizophrenia. *Journal of Abnormal Psychology, 103,* 784–790.

Guelfi, G. P., Faustman, W. O., & Csernansky, J. G. (1989). Independence of positive and negative symptoms in a population of schizophrenic patients. *Journal of Nervous and Mental Disease, 177,* 285–290.

Gur, R. E., Manny, V., Mozley, D., Swanson, C., Bilker, W., & Gur, R. C. (1998). Subcortical MRI volumes in neuroleptic-naive and treated patients with schizophrenia. *American Journal of Psychiatry, 155,* 1711–1717.

Gureje, O., Bamidele, R., & Raji, O. (1994). Early brain trauma and schizophrenia in Nigerian patients. *American Journal of Psychiatry, 151,* 368–371.

Harding, C. M., Brooks, G. W., Ashikaga, T., Strauss, J. S., & Breier, A. (1987a). The Vermont longitudinal study of persons with severe mental illness: I. Methodology, study sample, and overall status 32 years later. *American Journal of Psychiatry, 144,* 718–726.

Harding, C. M., Brooks, G. W., Ashikaga, T., Strauss, J. S., & Breier, A. (1987b). The Vermont longitudinal study of persons with severe mental illness: II. Long-term outcome of subjects who retrospectively met DSM-III criteria for schizophrenia. *American Journal of Psychiatry, 144,* 727–735.

Harrison, P. J. (1999). The neuropathology of schizophrenia: A critical review of the data and their interpretation. *Brain, 122,* 593–624.

Harrison, P. J. (1998). Schizophrenia neuropathology: Tortoises and hares. *Journal of Neurology, Neurosurgery, & Psychiatry, 65*, 432.

Harrison, P. J., & Burnet, P. W. J. (1997). The 5-HT2A (serotonin 2A receptor gene in the aetiology, pathophysiology and pharmacotherapy of schizophrenia. *Journal of Psychopharmacology, 11*, 18–20.

Harrow, M., Carone, B. J., & Westermeyer, J. F. (1985). The course of psychosis in early phases of schizophrenia. *American Journal of Psychiatry, 142*, 702–707.

Heath, R. G., Martens, S., Leach, B. E., Cohen, M., & Angel, C. (1957). Effect of behavior in humans with the adminstration of taraxein. *American Journal of Psychiatry, 114*, 14–24.

Hegarty, J. D., Baldessarini, R. J., Tohen, M., Waternaux, C., & Oepen, G. (1994). One hundred years of schizophrenia: A meta-analysis of the outcome literature. *American Journal of Psychiatry, 151*, 1409–1416.

Heston, L. (1966). Psychiatric disorders in foster home reared children of schizophrenic mothers. *British Journal of Psychiatry, 112*, 819–825.

Hirsch, S. R., & Leff, J. P. (1975). *Abnormalities in parents of schizophrenics.* London: Oxford University Press.

Hogarty, G. E., Kornblith, S. J., Greenwald, D., DiBarry, A. L., Cooley, S., Ulrich, R. F., Carter, M., & Flesher, S. (1997a). Three-year trials of personal therapy among schizophrenic patients living with or independent of family, I: Description of study and effects on relapse rate. *American Journal of Psychiatry, 154*, 1504–1513.

Hogarty, G. E., Greenwald, D., Ulrich, R. F., Kornblith, S. J., DiBarry, A. L., Cooley, S., Carter, M., Flesher, S. (1997b). Three-year trials of personal therapy among schizophrenic patients living with or independent of family: II. Effects of adjustment of patients. *American Journal of Psychiatry, 154*, 1514–1524.

Hogarty, G. E., Anderson, C. M., Reiss, D. J., Kornblith, S. J., & Greenwald, D. P. (1986). Family psychoeducation, social skills training, and maintenance chemotherapy in the aftercare treatment of schizophrenia: I. One-year effects of a controlled study. *Archives of General Psychiatry, 43*, 633–642.

Hogarty, G. E., McEvoy, J. P., Munetz, M., DiBarry, A. L., Bartone, P., Cather, R., Cooley, S. J., Ulrich, R. F., Carter, M., & Madonia, M. J. (1988). Dose of fluphenazine, familial expressed emotion, and outcome in schizophrenia: Results of a two-year controlled study. *Archives of General Psychiatry, 45*, 797–805.

Hooley, J. M. (1985). Expressed emotion: A review of the critical literature. *Clinical Psychology Review, 5*, 119–139.

Hooley, J. M., & Hiller, J. B. (1998). Expressed emotion and the pathogenesis of relapse in schizophrenia. In M. F. Lenzenweger & R. H. Dworkin (Eds.), *Origins and development of schizophrenia* (pp. 447–468). Washington, DC: American Psychological Association.

Jacob, T. (1975). Family interaction in disturbed and normal families: A methodological and substantive review. *Psychological Bulletin, 82*, 33–65.

Jones, P. B., Rantakallio, P., Hartikainen, A.-L., Isohanni, M., & Sipila, P. (1998). Schizophrenia as a long-term outcome of pregnancy, delivery, and perinatal complications: A 28-year follow-up of the 1996 North Finland General Population Birth Cohort. *American Journal of Psychiatry, 155*, 355–364.

Joyce, J. N., & Meador-Woodruff, J. H. (1997). Linking the family of D2 receptors to neuronal circuits in human brain: Insights into schizophrenia. *Neuropsychopharmacology, 16*, 375–384.

Kales, H. C., Dequardo, J. R., & Tandon, R. (1999). Combined electroconvulsive therapy and clozapine in treatment-resistant schizophrenia. *Progress in Neuro-Psychopharmacology and Biological Psychiatry, 23*, 547–556.

Karon, B. P., & Vandenbos, G. R. (1981). *Psychotherapy of schizophrenia: Treatment of choice.* New York: Jason Aronson.

Katz, H. M. (1989). A new agenda for psychotherapy of schizophrenia: Response to Coursey. *Schizophrenia Bulletin, 15*, 355–359.

Kaufman, C. A., DeLisi, L. E., Lehner, T., & Gilliam, T. C. (1989). Physical mapping, linkage analysis of a putative schizophrenia locus on chromosome 5q. *Schizophrenia Bulletin, 15*, 441–452.

Kendler, K. S., & Gruenberg, A. M. (1984). An independent analysis of the Danish adoption study of schizophrenia: VI. The relationship between psychiatric disorders as defined by DSM-III in the relatives and adoptees. *Archives of General Psychiatry, 41*, 555–564.

Kendler, K. S., & Davis, K. L. (1981). The genetics and biochemistry of paranoid schizophrenia and other paranoid psychosis. *Schizophrenia Bulletin, 7*, 711–718.

Kendler, K. S., Karkowski, L. M., & Walsh, D. (1998). The structure of psychosis: Latent class analysis of probands from the Roscommon Family Study. *Archives of General Psychiatry, 55*, 494–499.

Kendler, K. S., MacLean, C. J., O'Neill, F. A., Burke, J., Murphy, B., Duke, F., Shinkwin, R., Easter, S. M., Webb, B. T., Walsh, D., & Straub, R. E. (1996). Evidence for a schizophrenia vulnerability locus on chromosome 8p in the Irish Study of High-Density Schizophrenia Families. *American Journal of Psychiatry, 153*, 1534–1540.

Kendler, K. S., Karkowski, L. M., & Walsh, D. (1998). The structure of psychosis. *Archives of General Psychiatry, 55*, 508–509.

Kendler, K. S., & Tsuang, M. T. (1981). Nosology of paranoid schizophrenia and other paranoid psychoses. *Schizophrenia Bulletin, 7*, 594–610.

Kennedy, J. L., Giuffra, L. A., Moises, H. W., Cavallik-Sforza, L. L., Pakstis, A. J., Kidd, J. R., Castiglione, C. M., Sjogren, B., Wetterberg, L., & Kidd, K. K. (1988). Evidence against linkage of schizophrenia to markers on chromosome 5 in a northern Swedish pedigree. *Nature, 336*, 167–170.

Kety, S. S. (1987). The significance of genetic factors in the etiology of schizophrenia. *Journal of Psychiatric Research, 21*, 423–429.

Kety, S. S., Rosenthal, D., Wender, P. H., & Schulsinger, F. (1968). The types and prevalence of mental illness in the biological and adoptive families of adopted schizophrenics. In D. Rosenthal & S. S. Kety (Eds.), *The transmission of schizophrenia* (pp. 345–362). Elmsford, NY: Pergamon Press.

Kety, S. S., Rosenthal, D., Wender, P. H., Schulsinger, F., & Jacobsen, B. (1978). The biologic and adoptive families of adopted individuals who beacme schizophrenic: Prevalence of mental illness and other characteristics. In L. C. Wynne, R. L. Cromwell, & S. Matthysse (Eds.), *The nature of schizophrenia: New approaches to research and treatment* (pp. 25–37). New York: Wiley.

Kinney, D. K., Holzman, P. S., Jacobsen, B., Jansson, L., Faber, B., Hildebrand, W., Kasell, E., & Zimbalist, M. E. (1997). Thought disorder in schizophrenic and control adoptees and their relatives. *Archives of General Psychiatry, 54*, 475–479.

Klerman, G. L. (1984). Ideology and science in the individual psychotherapy of schizophrenia. *Schizophrenia Bulletin, 10,* 608–612.

Kopelowicz, A., & Liberman, R. P. (1998). Psychosocial treatments for schizophrenia. In P. Nathan & J. M. Gorman (Eds), *A guide to treatments that work* (pp. 190–211). New York: Oxford University Press.

Kopelowicz, A., Liberman, R. P., Mintz, J., & Zarate, R. (1997). Comparison of efficacy of social skills training for deficit and nondeficit negative symptoms in schizophrenia. *American Journal of Psychiatry, 154,* 424–425.

Kornhuber, J., Riederer, P., Reynolds, G.P., Beckman, H., Jellinger, K., & Gabriel, E. (1989). 3H-Spiperone binding sites in postmortem brains from schizophrenic patients: Relationship to neuroleptic drug treatment, abnormal movements, and positive symptoms. *Journal of Neural Transmission, 75,* 1–10.

Kosten, T. R., & Ziedonis, D. M. (1997). Substance abuse and schizophrenia: Editors' introduction. *Schizophrenia Bulletin, 23,* 181–186.

Kraepelin, E. (1987). *Dementia praecox* (trans. by J. Cutting & M. Shepherd, 1987). Cambridge, UK: Cambridge University Press. (Original work published in 1896.)

LaMantia, A.-S. (1999). Forebrain induction, retinoic acid, and vulnerability to schizophrenia: Insights from molecular and genetic analysis in developing mice. *Biological Psychiatry, 46,* 19–30.

Lander, E., & Kruglyzk, L. (1993). Genetic dissection of complex traits: Guidelines for interpreting and reporting linkage results. *Nature Genetics, 11,* 241–247.

Leff, J., Kuipers, L., Berkowitz, R., & Sturgeon, D. A. (1982). A controlled trial of social intervention in the families of schizophrenic patients. *British Journal of Psychiatry, 141,* 121–134.

Lehman, A. F., Steinwachs, D. M., Dixon, L. B., Postrado, L., Scott, J. E., Fahey, M. Fischer, P., Hoch, J., Kasper, J. A., Lyles, A., Shore, A., & Skinner, E. A. (1998). Patterns of usual care for schizophrenia: Initial results from the schizophrenia patient outcomes research team (PORT) client survey. *Schizophrenia Bulletin, 24,* 11–19.

Lewis, M. S. (1989a). Age incidence and schizophrenia: Part I. The season of birth controversy. *Schizophrenia Bulletin, 15,* 59–73.

Lewis, M. S. (1989b). Age incidence and schizophrenia: Part II. Beyond age incidence. *Schizophrenia Bulletin, 15,* 75–80.

Lewis, M. S. (1990). Res ipsa loquitur: The author replies. *Schizophrenia Bulletin, 16,* 17–28.

Lewis, M. S., & Griffin, P. A. (1981). An explanation for the season of birth effect in schizophrenia and certain other diseases. *Psychological Bulletin, 89,* 589–596.

Lewontin, R. C. (1974). The analysis of variance and the analysis of genes. *American Journal of Human Genetics, 26,* 400–411.

Lidz, T., & Blatt, S. (1983). Critique of the Danish-American studies of the biological and adoptive relatives of adoptees who became schizophrenic. *American Journal of Psychiatry, 140,* 426–434.

Lidz, T., Cornelison, A., Fleck, S., & Terry, D. (1957). The intrafamilial environment of schizophrenia patients: II. Marital schism and marital skew. *American Journal of Psychiatry, 114,* 241–248.

Lidz, T., Cornelison, A., Terry, D., & Fleck, S. (1958). Intrafamilial environment of the schizophrenic patient: VI. The transmission of irrationality. *Archives of Neurology and Psychiatry, 79,* 305–316.

Lidz, T., Fleck, S., & Cornelison, A. (1965). *Schizophrenia and the family.* New York: International Universities Press.

Linszen, D. H., Dingemans, P. M., Nugter, M. A., & Van der Does, A. J. W. (1997). Patient attributes and expressed emotion as risk factors for psychotic relapse. *Schizophrenia Bulletin, 23,* 119–130.

Lyon, M., Barr, C. E., Cannon, T. D., Mednick, S. A., & Shore, D. (1989). Fetal neural development and schizophrenia. *Schizophrenia Bulletin, 15,* 149–161.

Magaro, P. A. (1980). *Cognition in schizophrenia.* Hillsdale, NJ: Erlbaum.

Maier, R. F., Bialobrzeski, B., Gross, A., Volgel, M., Dudenhausen, J. W., & Obladen, M. (1995). Acute and chronic fetal hypoxia in monochorionic and dichorionic twins. *Obstetrics and Gynecology, 86,* 973–977.

Marcus, J., Hans, S. L., Byhouwer, B., & Norem, J. (1985). Relationships among neurological functioning, intelligence quotients, and physical abnormalities. *Schizophrenia Bulletin, 11,* 85–100.

Marcus, J., Hans, S. L., Auerbach, J. G., & Auerbach, A. G. (1993). Children at risk for schizophrenia: The Jerusalem Infant Development Study: II. Neurobehavioral deficits at school age. *Archives of General Psychiatry, 50,* 797–809.

McCabe, M. S., & Stromgren, E. (1975). Reactive psychoses: A family study. *Archives of General Psychiatry, 32,* 447–454.

McFarlane, W. R., Lukens, E., Link, B., Dushay, R., Deakins, S. A., Newmark, M., Dunne, E. J., Horen, B., & Toran, J. (1995). The multiple family group and psychoeducation in the treatment of schizophrenia. *Archives of General Psychiatry, 52,* 679–687.

McGlashan, T. H., & Fenton, W. S. (1993). Subtype progression and pathophysiologic deterioration in early schizophrenia. *Schizophrenia Bulletin, 19,* 71–84.

McGlashan, T. H., & Fenton, W. S. (1994). Classical subtypes for schizophrenia. In T. A. Widiger, A. J. Frances, & H. A. Pincus (Eds.). *DSM-IV sourcebook* (Vol. 1, pp. 419–440). Washington, DC: American Psychiatric Association.

McGorry, P. D., Bell, R. C., Dudgeon, P. L., & Jackson, H. J. (1998). The dimensional structure of first episode psychosis: An exploratory factor analysis. *Psychological Medicine, 28,* 935–947.

Mednick, S. A., & Schulsinger, F. (1968). Some premorbind characteristics related to breakdown in children with schizophrenic mothers. In D. Rosenthal & S. S. Kety (Eds.), *The transmission of schizophrenia* (pp. 267–292). Elmsford, NY: Pergamon Press.

Mednick, S. A., Schulsinger, H., & Schulsinger, F. (1975). Schizophrenia in children of schizophrenic mothers. In A. Davids (Ed.), *Child personality and psychopathology: Current topics* (Vol. 2, pp. 221–252). New York: Wiley.

Mednick, S. A., Schulsinger, F., Teasdale, T. W., Schulsinger, H., Venables, P., & Rock, D. (1978). Schizophrenia in high risk children: Sex differences in predisposing factors. In G. Serban (Ed.), *Cognitive defects in the development of mental illness* (pp. 169–197). New York: Brunner/Mazel.

Mednick, S. A., Watson, J. B., Huttunen, M., Cannon, T. D., Katila, H., Machon, R., Mednick, B., Hollister, M., Parnas, J., Schulsinger, F., Sajaniemi, N., Voldsgaard, P., Pyhala, R., Gutkind, D., & Wang, X. (1998). A two-hit working model of the etiology of schizophrenia. In M. F. Lenzenweger & R. H. Dworkin (Eds.), *Origins and development of schizophrenia* (pp. 27–66). Washington, DC: American Psychological Association.

Meehl, P. E. (1962). Schizotaxia, schizotypy, schizophrenia. *American Psychologist, 17,* 827–838.

Meehl, P. E. (1972). A critical afterward. In I. I. Gottesman & J. Shields, *Schizophrenia and genetics: A twin study vantage point* (pp. 367–415). New York: Academic Press.

Meehl, P. E. (1978). Theoretical risks and tabular asterisks: Sir Karl, Sir Ronald, and the slow progress of soft psychology. *Journal of Consulting and Clinical Psychology, 46,* 806–834.

Meehl, P. E. (1989). Schizotaxia revisited. *Archives of General Psychiatry, 46,* 935–944.

Meehl, P. E. (1990). Toward an integrated theory of schizotaxia, schizotypy, and schizophrenia. *Journal of Personality Disorders, 4,* 1–99.

Meltzer, H. Y. (1994). An overview of the mechanism of action of clozapine. *Journal of Clinical Psychiatry, 55* (Suppl. B), 47–52.

Meltzer, H. Y., & Stahl, S. M. (1976). The dopamine hypothesis of schizophrenia: A review. *Schizophrenia Bulletin, 2,* 19–76.

Miklowitz, D. J., Goldstein, M. J., & Falloon, I. R. (1983). Premorbid and symptomatic characteristics of schizophrenics from families with high and low levels of expressed emotion. *Journal of Abnormal Psychology, 92,* 359–367.

Miklowitz, D. J., Strachan, A. M., Goldstein, M. J., Doane, J. A., & Snyder, K. S. (1986). Expressed emotion and communication deviance in families of schizophrenics. *Journal of Abnormal Psychology, 95,* 60–66.

Miller, A. L., & Ereshefsky, L. (1997). Schizophrenia: How should we look at it? *Journal of Psychopharmacology, 11,* 21–23.

Mishler, E. G., & Waxler, N. E. (Eds.). (1968). *Family processes and schizophrenia: Theory and selected experimental studies.* New York: Science House.

Moises, H. W., Yang, L., Kristbjarnarson, H., Wiese, C., Byerley, W., Macciardi, F., Arolt, V., Blackwood, D., Liu, X., Sjogren, B., Aschauer, H. N., Hwu, H.-G., Jang, K., Livesley, W. J., Kennedy, J. L., Zoega, T., Ivarsson, O., Bui, M.-T., Yu, M.-H., Havsteen, B., Commenges, D., Weissenbach, J., Schwinger, E., Gottesman, I. I., Pakstis, A. J., Wetterberg, L., Kidd, K. K., & Helgason, T. (1995). An international two-stage genome-wide search for schizophrenia susceptibility genes. *Nature Genetics, 11,* 321–324.

Moldin, S. O. (1997). The maddening hunt for madness genes. *Nature Genetics, 17,* 127–129.

Moldin, S. O., & Gottesman, I. I. (1997). Genes, experience, and chance in schizophrenia—Positioning for the 21st century. *Schizophrenia Bulletin, 23,* 547–561.

Morgan, T. H. (1920). The method of inheritance of two sex-limited characteristics in the same animal. *Proceedings of the Society for Experimental Biology and Medicine, 8,* 17–19.

Morgan, T. H. (1911). The application of the conception of pure lines to sex-limited inheritance and to sexual dimorphism. *American Naturalist, 45,* 65–78.

Mosher, L. R. (1989, August). Schizophrenia: Current myths: The case of neuroleptic drugs. In G. Shean (Chair), Schizophrenia and the current zeitgeist: Antitheses. Symposium conducted at the *Meeting of the American Psychological Association,* New Orleans.

Mosher, L. R., & Gunderson, J. G. (1979). Group, family, milieu and community support systems treatment for schizophrenia. In L. Bellak (Ed.), *Disorders of the schizophrenic syndrome* (pp. 399–452). New York: Basic Books.

Mosher, L. R., Vallone, R., & Menn, A. (1995). The treatment of acute psychosis without neuroleptics: Six-week psycho-pathology outcome data from the Soteria project. *International Journal of Social Psychiatry, 41,* 157–173.

Mueser, K. T., Bond, G. R., Drake, R. E., & Resnick, S. G. (1998). Models of community care for severe mental illness: A review of research on case management. *Schizophrenia Bulletin, 24,* 37–74.

Nakaya, M., Suwa, H., Komahashi, T., & Ohmori, K. (1999). Is schizophrenic symptomatology independent of the phase of illness? *Psychopathology, 32,* 23–29.

Neale, J. M., & Oltmanns, T. F. (1980). *Schizophrenia.* New York: Wiley.

Nestler, E. J. (1997). Schizophrenia: An emerging pathophysiology. *Nature, 385,* 578–579.

Newmark, C. S., Falk, R., Johns, N., Boren, R., & Forehand, R. (1976). Comparing traditional clinical procedures with four systems to diagnose schizophrenia. *Journal of Abnormal Psychology, 85,* 66–72.

Nuechterlein, K. H., Snyder, K. S., & Mintz, J. (1992). Paths to relapse: Possible transactional processes connecting patient illness onset, expressed emotion, and psychotic relapse. *British Journal of Psychiatry, 161* (Suppl. 18), 88–96.

Nyberg, S., & Farde, L. (1997). The relevance of serotonergic mechanisms in the treatment of schizophrenia has not been confirmed. *Journal of Psychopharmacology, 11,* 13–14.

Okubo, Y., Suhara, T., Suzuki, K., Kobayashi, K., Inoue, O., Terasaki, O., Someya, Y., Sassa, T., Sudo, Y., Matsushima, E., Iyo, M., Tateno, Y., & Toru, M. (1997). Decreased prefrontal dopamine D1 in schizophrenia revealed by PET. *Nature, 385,* 634–636.

Oltmanns, T. E., & Maher, B. A. (Eds.). (1988). *Delusional beliefs.* New York: Wiley.

Parker, G., Johnston, P. & Hayward, L. (1988). Parental "expressed emotion" as a predictor of schizophrenic relapse. *Archives of General Psychiatry, 45,* 806–813.

Paul, G. L., & Lentz, R. J. (1977). *Psychosocial treatment of chronic mental patients: Milieu versus social-learning programs.* Cambridge, MA: Harvard University Press.

Phelps, J. A., Davis, J. O., & Schartz, K. M. (1997). Nature, nurture, and twin research strategies. *Current Directions in Psychological Science, 6,* 117–120.

Pierce, P. A., & Peroutka, S. J. (1989). Hallucinogenic drug interactions with neurotransmitter receptor binding sites in human cortex. *Psychopharmacology, 97,* 118–122.

Polin, W., Stabenau, J., & Tupin, J. (1965). Family studies with identical twins discordant for schizophrenia. *Psychiatry, 28,* 60–78.

Rabin, A. I., Doneson, S. L., & Jentons, R. L. (1979). Studies of psychological functions in schizophrenia. In L. Bellak (Ed.), *The schizophrenic syndrome* (pp. 181–231). New York: Basic Books.

Ratakonda, S., Gorman, J., Yale, S., & Amador, X. F. (1998). Characterization of psychotic conditions: Use of the domains of psychopathology model. *Archives of General Psychiatry, 55,* 75–81.

Risch, N., & Merikangas, K. (1996). The future of genetic studies of complex human diseases. *Science, 273,* 1516–1517.

Ritzler, B. A. (1981). Paranoia—prognosis and treatment: A review. *Schizophrenia Bulletin, 7,* 710–728.

Robins, E. & Guze, S. B. (1970). Establishment of diagnostic validity in psychiatric illness: Its application to schizophrenia. *American Journal of Psychiatry, 126,* 983–987.

Roff, J. D., & Knight, R. (1981). Family characteristics, childhood symptoms, and adult outcome in schizophrenia. *Journal of Abnormal Psychology, 90,* 510–520.

Rosen, J. N. (1953). *Direct analysis: Select papers.* New York: Grune & Stratton.

Rosenthal, D. (Ed.). (1963). *The Genain quadruplets.* New York: Basic Books.

Rosenthal, D., Wender, P. H., Kety, S. S., Schulsinger, F., Welner, J., & Ostergaard, L. (1968). Schizophrenics' offspring reared in adoptive homes. In D. Rosenthal & S. S. Kety (Eds.), *The transmission of schizophrenia* (pp. 377–392). Elmsford, NY: Pergamon Press.

Rosenthal, D., Wender, P. H., Kety, S. S., Welner, J., & Schulsinger, F. (1971). The adopted-away offspring of schizophrenics. *American Journal of Psychiatry, 128,* 307–311.

Russell, A. J., Munro, J. C., Jones, P. B., Hemsley, D. R., & Murray, R. M. (1997). Schizophrenia and the myth of intellectual decline. *American Journal of Psychiatry, 154,* 635–639.

Sarbin, T. R., & Mancuso, J. C. (1980). *Schizophrenia: Medical diagnosis or moral verdict?* Elmsford, NY: Pergamon Press.

Scher, S. J. (1999). Are adaptations necessarily genetic? *American Psychologist, 54,* 436–437.

Schneider, K. (1959). *Clinical psychopathology.* New York: Grune & Stratton.

Schofield, W., & Balian, L. (1959). A comparative study of the personal histories of schizophrenic and non-psychiatric patients. *Journal of Abnormal and Social Psychology, 59,* 216–225.

Schwab, S. G., Albus, M., Hallmayer, J., Honig, S., Borrmann, M., Lichtermann, D., Ebstein, R. P., Ackenheil, M., Lerer, B., & Risch, N. (1995). Evaluation of a susceptibility gene for schizophrenia on chromosome 6p by multipoint affected sib-pair linkage analysis. *Nature Genetics, 11,* 325–327.

Seeman, P. (1987). Dopamine receptors and the dopamine hypothesis of schizophrenia. *Synapse, 1,* 133–152.

Seeman, P., Lee, T., Chau-Wong, M., & Wong, K. (1976). Antipsychotic drug doses and neuroleptic/dopamine receptors. *Nature, 261,* 177–179.

Sheitman, B.B., Kinon, B., J., Ridgway, B., A., & Lieberman, J. A., (1998). Pharmacological treatments of schizophrenia. In P. E. Nathan & J. M. Gordon (Eds.), *A guide to treatments that work* (pp. 167–189). New York: Oxford University Press.

Sherrington, R., Brynjolfsson, J., Petursson, H., Potter, M., Dudleston, K., Barraclaugh, B., Wasmuth, J., Dobbs, M., & Gurling, H. (1988). Localization of a susceptibility locus for schizophrenia on chromosome 5. *Nature, 336,* 164–167.

Silberman, E. K., & Tassone, E. P. (1985). The Israeli high-risk study: Statistical overview and discussion. *Schizophrenia Bulletin, 11,* 138–145.

Singer, M. T., & Wynne, L. C. (1965a). Thought disorder and family relations of schizophrenics: III. Methodology using projective techniques. *Archives of General Psychiatry, 12,* 182–200.

Singer, M. T., & Wynne, L. C. (1965b). Thought disorder and family relations of schizophrenics: IV. Results and implications. *Archives of General Psychiatry, 12,* 201–212.

Singer, M. T., Wynne, L. C., & Toohey, M. L. (1978). Communication disorders and the families of schizophrenics. In L. C. Wynne, R. L. Cromwell, & S. Matthysse (Eds.), *The nature of schizophrenia: New approaches to research and treatment* (pp. 499–511). New York: Wiley.

Smith, M. L., Glass, G. V., & Miller, T. I. (1980). *The benefits of psychotherapy.* Baltimore: Johns Hopkins University Press.

Snyder, S. H., Burt, D. R., & Creese, I. (1976). Dopamine receptor of mammalian brain: Direct demonstration of binding to agonist and antagonist states. *Neuroscience Symposia, 1,* 28–49.

Sobel, D. E. (1961). Children of schizophrenic patients: Preliminary observations on early development. *American Journal of Psychiatry, 118,* 512–517.

Sokoloff, P., Giros, B., Martres, M. P., Bouthenet, M. L., & Schwartz, J. C. (1990). Molecular cloning and characterization of a novel dopamine receptor (D3), as a target for neuroleptics. *Nature, 347,* 146–151.

Spitzer, R. L., Endicott, J., & Robins, L. (1975). Research diagnostic criteria. New York: New York State Department of Mental Hygiene, Biometric Research Unit.

Stabenau, J., & Pollin, W. (1968). Comparative life history differences of families of schizophrenics, delinquents, and "normals." *American Journal of Psychiatry, 124,* 1526–1534.

Stabenau, J., Tupin, J., Werner, M., & Pollin, W. (1965). A comparative study of families of schizophrenics, delinquents, and normals. *Psychiatry, 28,* 45–59.

Stephenson, J. D. (1990). Neuropharmacological studies of the serotonergic system. *International Review of Psychiatry, 2,* 157–178.

Stern, E., & Silberszweig, D. A. (1998). Neural mechanisms underlying hallucinations in schizophrenia: The role of abnormal fronto-temporal interactions. In M. F. Lenzenweger & R. H. Dworkin (Eds.), *Origins and development of schizophrenia: Advances in experimental psychopathology* (pp. 235–Washington, DC: American Psychological Association.

Stiles, W. B., & Shapiro, D. A. (1989). Abuse of the drug metaphor in psychotherapy process-outcome research. *Clinical Psychology Review, 9,* 521–543.

Straub, R. E., MacLean, C. J., O'Neill, F. A., Burke, J., Murphy, B., Duke, F., Shinkwin, R., Webb, B. T., Zhang, J., Walsh, D., & Kendler, K. S. (1995). A potential vulnerability locus for schizophrenia on chromosome 6p24-22: Evidence for a genetic heterogeneity. *Nature Genetics, 11,* 287–293.

Sullivan, H. S. (1962). Schizophrenia as a human process. In *The collected works of Harry Stack Sullivan* (Vol. II). New York: W.W. Norton.

Suvisaari, J., Haukka, J., Tanskanen, A., Hovi, T., & Lonnqvist, J. (1999). Association between prenatal exposure to poliovirus infection and adult schizophrenia. *American Journal of Psychiatry, 156,* 1100–1102.

Takei, N., Lewis, S., Jones, P., Harvey, I., & Murray, R. M. (1996). Prenatal exposure to influenza and increased cerebrospinal fluid spaces in schizophrenia. *Schizophrenia Bulletin, 22,* 521–534.

Tamminga, C. A., Thaker, G. K., Buchanan, R., Kirkpatrick, B., Alphs, L. D., Chase, T. N., & Carpenter, W. T. (1992). Limbic system abnormalities identified in schizophrenia using positron emission tomography with fluorodeoxyglucose and neocortical alterations with deficit syndrome. *Archives of General Psychiatry, 49,* 522–530.

Tarrier, N., & Barrowclough, C. (1990). Family interventions for schizophrenia. *Behavior Modification, 14,* 408–440.

Tienari, P. (1991). Interaction between genetic vulnerability and family environment: The Finnish adoptive family study of schizophrenia. *Acta Psychiatrica Scandinavica, 84,* 460–465.

Tienari, P., Lahti, I., Sorri, A., Naarala, M., Moring, J., Wahlberg, K.-E., & Wynne, L. C. (1987). The Finnish adoptive family study of schizophrenia. *Journal of Psychiatric Research, 21,* 437–445.

Tienari, P., Sorri, A., Lahti, I., Naarala, M., Wahlberg, K. E., Pohjola, J., & Moring, J. (1985). Interaction of genetic and psychosocial factors in schizophrenia. *Acta Psychiatrica Scandinavica, 71* (Suppl. No. 319), 19–30.

Tienari, P., Wynne, L. C., Moring, J., Lahti, I., Naaral, M., Sorri, A., Wahlberg, K.-E., Saarento, O., Kaleva, M., & Laksy, K. (1994). The Finnish Adoption Study of schizophrenia: Implications for family research. *British Journal of Psychiatry, 164,* 20–26.

Toomey, R., Kremen, W. S., Simpson, J. C., Samson, J. A., Seidman, L. J., Lyons, M. J., Faraone, S. V., and Tsuang, M. T. (1997). Revisiting the factor structure for positive and negative symptoms: Evidence from a large heterogeneous group of psychiatric patients. *American Journal of Psychiatry, 154,* 371–377.

Torrey, E. F., Bowler, A. E., Rawlings, R., & Terrazas, A. (1993). Seasonality of schizophrenia and stillbirths. *Schizophrenia Bulletin, 19,* 557–562.

Torrey, E. F., Taylor, E. H., Bracha, H. S., Bowler, A. E., McNeil, T. F., Rawlings, R. R., Quinn, P. O., Bigelow, L. B., Rickler, K., Sjostrom, K., Higgins, E. S., & Gottesman, I. I. (1994). Prenatal origin of schizophrenia in a subgroup of discordant monozygotic twins. *Schizophrenia Bulletin, 20,* 423–432.

Umbricht, D., & Kane, J. M. (1997). Medical complications of new antipsychotic drugs. *Schizophrenia Bulletin, 22,* 475–483.

Valenstein, E. S. (1998). *Blaming the brain.* New York: The Free Press.

Valenstein, E. S. (1986). *Great and desperate cures: The rise and decline of psychosurgery and other radical treatments . for mental illness.* New York: Basic Books.

VanDyke, J. L., Rosenthal, D., & Rasmussen, P. V. (1975). Schizophrenia: Effects of inheritance and rearing on reaction time. *Canadian Journal of Behavioral Science, 7,* 223–236.

Vaughn, C. E., & Leff, J. P. (1976). The influences of family and social factors on the course of psychiatry illness: A comparison of schizophrenic and depressed neurotic patients. *British Journal of Psychiatry, 129,* 125–137.

Vaughn, C. E., & Leff, J. P. (1981). Patterns of emotional response in relatives of schizophrenic patients. *Schizophrenia Bulletin, 7,* 43–44.

Vaughn, C. E., Snyder, K. S., Jones, S., Freeman, W. B., & Falloon, I. R. H. (1984). Family factors in schizophrenic relapse: Replication in California of British research on expressed emotion. *Archives of General Psychiatry, 41,* 1169–1177.

Velakoulis, D., Patelis, C., McGorry, P. D., Dudgeon, P., Brewer, W., Cook, M., Desmond, P., Bridle, N., Tierney, P., Murrie, V., Singh, B., & Copolov, D. (1999). Hippocampal volume in first-episode psychoses and chronic schizophrenia: A high-resolution magnetic resonance imaging study. *Archives of General Psychiatry, 56,* 133–141.

Ventura, J., Nuechterlein, K. H., Lukoff, D., & Hardesty, J. P. (1989). A prospective study of stressful life events and schizophrenia relapse. *Journal of Abnormal Pyschology, 98,* 407–411.

Wahlberg, K.-E., Wynne, L. C., Oja, H., Keskitalo, P., Pykalainen, L., Lahti, I., Moring, J., Naarala, M., Sorri, A., Seitamaa, M., Laksy, K., Kolassa, J., Tienari, P. (1997). Gene-environment interaction in vulnerability to schizophrenia:

Findings from the Finnish adoptive family study of schizophrenia. *American Journal of Psychiatry, 154,* 355–362.

Wahlsten, D. (1999). Single-gene influences on brain and behavior. *Annual Review of Psychology, 50,* 599–624.

Walker, E. F. (1994). Developmentally moderated expression of the neuropathology underlying schizophrenia. *Schizophrenia Bulletin, 20,* 453–480.

Walker, E. F., & Diforio, D. (1997). Schizophrenia: A neural diathesis-stress model. *Psychological Review, 104,* 667–685.

Walker, E. F., Grimes, K. E., Davis, D. M., & Smith, A. J. (1993). Childhood precursors of schizophrenia: Facial expressions of emotion. *American Journal of Psychiatry, 150,* 1654–1660.

Walker, E. F., Savoie, T., & Davis, D. (1994). Neuromotor precursors of schizophrenia. *Schizophrenia Bulletin, 20,* 441–451.

Walker, E. F., Baum, K. M., & Diforio, D. (1998). Developmental changes in the behavioral expression of vulnerability for schizophrenia. In M. F. Lenzenweger & R. H. Dworkin (Eds.), *Origins and development of schizophrenia* (pp. 469–492). Washington, DC: American Psychological Association.

Wang, S., Sun, C. E., Walczak, C. A., Ziegle, J. S., Kipps, B. R., Goldin, L. R., & Diehl, S. R. (1995). Evidence for a susceptibility locus for schizophrenia on chromosome 6pter-p22. *Nature Genetics, 10,* 41–46.

Warner, R. (1994). *Recovery from schizophrenia: Psychiatry and political economy* (2nd ed.). New York: Routledge & Kegan Paul.

Weickert, C. S., & Weinberger, D. R. (1998). A candidate molecule approach to defining developmental pathology in schizophrenia. *Schizophrenia Bulletin, 24,* 303–316.

Wender, P. H., Rosenthal, D., Kety, S. S., Schulsinger, F., & Welner, J. (1974). Crossfostering: A research strategy for clarifying the role of genetic and experiential factors in the etiology of schizophrenia. *Archives of General Psychiatry, 30,* 121–138.

Whitaker, L. C. (1992). *Schizophrenic disorders: Sense and nonsense in conceptualization, assessment, and treatment.* New York: Plenum.

Whitehorn, J. C., & Betz, B. J. (1954). A study of psychotherapeutic relationships between physicians and schizophrenic patients. *American Journal of Psychiatry, 111,* 321–331.

Wing, L. L., Tapson, G. S., & Geyer, M. A. (1990). 5HT2 mediation of acute behavioral effects of hallucinogens in rats. *Psychopharmacology, 100,* 417–425.

Wing, J. K., & Nixon, J. (1975). Discriminating symptoms in schizophrenia. *Archives of General Psychiatry, 30,* 853–859.

Winters, K. C., Weintraub, S., & Neale, J. M. (1981). Validity of MMPI code types in identifying DSM-III schizophrenics. *Journal of Consulting and Clinical Psychology, 49,* 486–487.

World Health Organization (1973). *International pilot study of schizophrenia* (Vol. 1). Geneva: World Health Organization Press.

Wright, P., Takei, N., Rifkin, L., & Murray, R. M. (1995). Maternal influenza, obstetric complications, and schizophrenia. *American Journal of Psychiatry, 152,* 1714–1720.

Wynne, L. C., Ryckoff, I. M., Day, J., & Hirsch, S. I. (1958). Pseudomutuality in the family relations of schizophrenics. *Psychiatry, 21,* 205–220.

Wynne, L. C., Toohey, M. L., & Doane, J. (1979). Family studies. In L. Bellak (Ed.), *The nature of schizophrenia: New approaches to research and treatment.* New York: Wiley.

Zubin, J., & Spring, B. J. (1977). Vulnerability: A new view of schizophrenia. *Journal of Abnormal Psychology, 86,* 103–126.

# PART III

# Personality Disorders

# CHAPTER 16

# Antisocial Personality Disorder

## Patricia B. Sutker and Albert N. Allain, Jr.

## Introduction

Behaviors that fly in the face of social convention and legal restraint have provoked interest and argument throughout recorded history. Early clinical accounts described individuals who failed to conform to moral and legal expectations by referring to evil spirits, moral defects, and personal inferiorities. More recent clinical and research work has focused on measuring the antisocial personality and developing a nomenclature for distinguishing antisocial from other categories of character disorder. The literature continues to reflect a deficit model that explains antisocial proclivity, and the search persists for biological and psychological corollaries of blatant nonconformity. This chapter reviews historical and present conceptualizations of antisocial personality from a broad perspective. Competing views concerning classification of the disorder are presented, and etiologic theories that attempt to account for its origins, concomitants, and progression are described. Empirical tests of assumptions derived from these theories are discussed, as are available assessment techniques and current approaches to treatment or behavior change.

Patricia B. Sutker • Departments of Neuropsychiatry and Anesthesiology, Texas Tech University Health Sciences Center, Lubbock, Texas 79430 and Tulane University School of Medicine, New Orleans, Louisiana 70146. **Albert N. Allain, Jr.** • Veterans Affairs Medical Center, New Orleans, Louisiana 70146.

*Comprehensive Handbook of Psychopathology* (Third Edition), edited by Patricia B. Sutker and Henry E. Adams. Kluwer Academic / Plenum Publishers, New York, 2001.

## Labeling of Antisocial Personality

Early nineteenth century accounts described individuals whose behaviors offended normative cultural standards and subgroup ethics yet lacked symptomatology easily classified as psychotically deranged or frankly delusional. Puzzled by persons who seemed to share disregard for conventional mores, observers of behavior disorders sought an explanation in the concept of moral deficiency. In 1801, Phillipe Pinel (1801/1962) identified *"manie sans delire,"* a disorder characterized by aberrant affect, proneness to impulsive rage, but no deficit in reasoning abilities. Also writing in the early nineteenth century, the American psychiatrist Benjamin Rush (1835) described individuals who were constitutionally deficient in moral faculties. These notions were elaborated by the English psychiatrist J. C. Prichard (1835) who popularized the label "moral insanity" and beliefs that antisocial behaviors resulted from organic or constitutional factors with poor prognosis for change. Early German contributions to the classification of behaviorally deviant individuals included references to "psychopathic inferiorities" (Koch, 1891) and typologies of "psychopathic personality" (Kraepelin, 1907/1923; Schneider, 1923).

Contemporary synonyms for the theoretical constructs "psychopathic inferiority" and "psychopathic personality" include "sociopathic personality," "psychopathy," and "antisocial personality disorder." Each label has been a target of criticism and argument, although all refer to a disposition to antisocial behavior and social deviance resulting from personal deficiencies or psychological abnormalities. In the tradition of German nosologists, Cleckley (1982) and Hare (1980) defined psychopaths as individuals who combined deviant personality traits and antisocial behaviors which were often criminal in their severity. Taking a different perspective, Partridge (1930) coined the term "sociopathic personality" to emphasize failure to conform to societal demands and pointed to the role of environmental or cultural factors in the etiology of behavioral deviance. During the 1960s and 1970s, psychosocial theorists and psychiatric clinicians preferred the term sociopathy (Robins, 1966; Vaillant, 1975), and "sociopathic personality" was included in the *Diagnostic and Statistical Manual* of the American Psychiatric Association (APA) in 1952 (DSM-I).

Most widely accepted in recent years has been the label *antisocial personality disorder* (ASPD), which appears in the last three editions of the DSM (APA, 1980, 1987, 1994). DSM-III and DSM-III-R criteria for ASPD differed significantly from those enumerated in DSM-II (APA, 1968). Whereas the 1968 diagnosis was composed largely of attributions regarding personality traits and inferences about underlying processes derived primarily from the Cleckley (1941) conceptualization of psychopathy, the newer criteria constituted a lengthy checklist of antisocial behaviors developed in large measure from criteria proposed by Robins (1966) that must be present in certain frequencies before and after age 15, conveying both the severity and chronicity of the disorder. References to irresponsibility, irritability, aggressiveness, impulsivity, and lack of remorse represented the few psychological characteristics on this list. Critics of the revised nomenclature and diagnostic criteria complained that though reliability was enhanced by criteria operationalization, the clinical meaning of the category had been compromised with definitive criteria both overly inclusive (Wulach, 1983) and exclusive (Hare, 1983; Millon, 1983).

Additionally, critics of the revised diagnostic criteria pointed to a neglect of the trait concepts of psychopathy and the complexity and length of diagnostic criteria (Alterman & Cacciola, 1991; Hare, Hart, & Harpur, 1991; Widiger & Corbitt, 1993; Widiger, Frances, Pincus, Davis, & First, 1991). It was suggested that clinicians often found traits of psychopathy (e.g., disregard for consequences of behavior, disregard for feelings of others) more relevant to ASPD than such DSM-III and DSM-III-R criteria as unemployment for six months and traveling from place to place without a

prearranged job or plans (Tennent, Tennent, Prins, & Bedford, 1990) and that DSM-III and DSM-III-R criteria resulted in overdiagnosis of ASPD in criminal and forensic settings (Hart & Hare, 1989). For example, Hart and Hare (1989) reported that 50% of the men remanded by courts to forensic units met the criteria for ASPD, whereas only 13% met the criteria for psychopathy, as defined by the Psychopathy Checklist (Hare, 1980). In contrast, Robins, Tipp, and Pryzbeck (1991) reviewed Epidemiological Catchment Area (ECA) data and found that only 47% of individuals who met the DSM-III ASPD criteria had significant arrest records and reported that adult symptoms of job troubles (94%), violence (85%), multiple moving traffic offenses (72%), and severe marital difficulties (67%) were more typical of ASPD than criminality. Further, Robins et al. (1991) observed an ASPD prevalence of 50% among prisoners within the ECA database but concluded that a 50% base rate for ASPD in a prison setting is consistent with theoretical and clinical explanations, thus refuting claims that DSM criteria equate ASPD with criminality.

Given this background, two important directions were considered during the development of DSM-IV and in designing and executing the DSM-IV field trial for ASPD: (1) greater emphasis on personality traits of psychopathy and (2) simplification of the criteria set without substantially changing the diagnosis (Widiger et al., 1996). With regard to the first proposal, the DSM-IV ASPD Field Trial considered two alternative criteria sets in addition to that of DSM-III-R: a modified version of the criteria for the Psychopathy Checklist-Revised (PCL-R: Hare, 1991) and research criteria for dissocial personality disorder as derived for the 10th edition of the International Classification of Diseases (ICD-10, World Health Organization, 1990). Thus, the reliability and concurrent validity of the DSM-III-R criteria, a ten-item version of the PCL-R criteria (Hare, Hart, & Harpur, 1991), and ICD-10 criteria were examined as sets and as individual items. The field trial also examined whether the DSM-III-R criteria set could be abbreviated without affecting the diagnosis (Frances, Pincus, Widiger, Davis, & First, 1990).

As a result of this and other field trials, as well as a review of the literature, data reanalyses, and the desire for compatibility with ICD-10 Diagnostic Criteria for Research (APA, 1994), the DSM-IV criteria for ASPD were modified from those of

DSM-III-R in the following manner. Two DSM-III-R items related to behaviors present since age 15 were deleted from ASPD criteria for DSM-IV: parental irresponsibility that included six subitems and failure to sustain a monogamous relationship for more than one year. Items related to failure to meet financial obligations and inconsistent work history were collapsed into a single item reflecting "consistent irresponsibility, as indicated by repeated failures to sustain consistent work behavior or honor financial obligations" (APA, 1994, p. 650). As a result of these deletions and consolidations, the threshold for diagnosis among the items that must be present since age 15 was changed from four of ten items (DSM-III-R) to three of seven items (DSM-IV).

The field trial did not provide conclusive support for the proposal to include traditional traits of psychopathy. Items from the psychopathy criteria set that correlated highest with clinician and interviewer ratings were those that most closely approximated DSM-III-R criteria, that is, early behavior problems and adult antisocial behavior, although in a prison site, items obtaining the highest correlations were those related to traditional conceptualizations of psychopathy, for example, lacks empathy, inflated and arrogant self-appraisal, glib, superficial charm. As a result, in the section on Associated Features and Disorders, DSM-IV specified that traditional conceptions of psychopathy (i.e., lack of empathy, inflated self-appraisal, superficial charm) "may be particularly distinguishing of Antisocial Personality Disorder in prison or forensic settings where criminal, delinquent, or aggressive acts are likely to be nonspecific." (APA, 1994, p. 647).

DSM-IV specified that an individual must exhibit evidence of Conduct Disorder with onset before age 15 years to warrant ASPD diagnosis, whereas DSM-III-R requirements for ASPD included a listing of twelve antisocial behaviors, three of which must have been present before age 15. These behaviors were similar to the thirteen behaviors listed in the DSM-III-R Conduct Disorder standards, but an item describing breaking into someone else's house, building, or car was not included. DSM-IV Conduct Disorder criteria were expanded to include items relating to staying out at night and intimidating others, and the resulting fifteen items were grouped in four categories (aggression against people and animals, destruction of property, deceitfulness or theft, and serious

violations of rules). Consequently, DSM-IV Conduct Disorder diagnosis required the presence of at least three of the fifteen targeted behaviors in the past 12 months and at least one described in the past 6 months. DSM-IV also differentiated Conduct Disorder into Childhood-Onset Type (onset of at least one criterion prior to age 10) and Adolescent-Onset Type (absence of all criteria prior to age 10). Early onset was said to predict a less favorable prognosis and an increased risk in adult life for Antisocial Personality Disorder, as well as Substance-Related Disorders.

Despite the scientific rigor applied to developing DSM-IV ASPD criteria, the current conceptualization is not endorsed universally. Commenting that the traditional conceptualization of psychopathy is not adequately embodied in DSM-IV, Newman and Brinkley (1998) nevertheless concluded that "Cleckley's view of psychopathy as a psychological dysfunction that interferes with self-regulation and precludes the systematic pursuit of long-range personal goals represents an important clinical syndrome" (p. 5) and that continued research into psychopathy in its own right was necessary. This position has been emphasized by Hare (1996b) who referred to psychopathy as a clinical construct whose time has come. However, there is no end to the debate over the nature and meaning of the antisocial personality construct. For example, Blackburn (1988) argued that the DSM-III-R system combined the two universes of personal and social deviance (i.e., those of personality traits and specific acts). Explaining that the contributions of personality characteristics to antisocial behaviors can be unraveled only when the two are identified independently, Blackburn concluded that the diagnostic concept of antisocial personality is "little more than a moral judgment masquerading as a clinical diagnosis." Such arguments recapitulate earlier concerns that the antisocial diagnosis represents a "wastebasket" category limiting assessment of other psychopathology and attenuating treatment efforts (Lewis & Balla, 1975; Rotenberg, 1975), thus creating a "myth" (Karpman, 1948). Nevertheless, the disorder is certainly one of the most researched of the personality disorders (Widiger & Frances, 1985) and accounted for 37% of the personality disorder literature in 1975 and 25% in 1985 (Blashfield & McElroy, 1987). As Robins (1978) pointed out, if the notion of the antisocial personality is a myth, it is one told over and over among different groups of people in different places at varying times—yet with surprising similarity.

## Historical Clinical Perspective

One of the most comprehensive descriptions of the psychopath was offered by Hervey Cleckley in six editions of *The Mask of Sanity* (1941) and related articles (e.g., Cleckley, 1971). Lacking experimental support for his claims, Cleckley nevertheless laid a strong foundation for efforts to define the traits and behavior patterns of antisocial individuals. He outlined sixteen distinguishing characteristics:

Superficial charm and good intelligence; absence of delusions and other signs of irrational thinking; absence of "nervousness" or other psychoneurotic manifestations; unreliability; untruthfulness and insincerity; lack of remorse or shame; inadequately motivated antisocial behavior; poor judgment and failure to learn by experience; pathologic egocentricity and incapacity for love; general poverty in major affective reactions; specific loss of insight; unresponsiveness in general interpersonal relations; fantastic and uninviting behavior, with drink and without; suicide rarely carried out; sex life impersonal, trivial, and poorly integrated; failure to follow any life plan. (Cleckley, 1982, p. 204)

Cleckley (1971) pointed to clear-cut differences between psychopaths and "ordinary lawbreakers" and suggested that psychopaths lack such qualities as purposeful intent, consistency in avoiding consequences, and loyalty to the members of a group. He emphasized that deficits in the experience of emotionality and attachment underlie their callous interpersonal behaviors, coined the term "semantic dementia" to capture their inability to react appropriately to verbal content that typically elicits emotional responses, and characterized their seemingly normal outward appearance as the "mask of sanity." These and other descriptions (McCord & McCord, 1964) were prototypical of the DSM-II (1968) outline of underlying personality traits considered definitive of the antisocial personality.

Vaillant (1975) proposed a more optimistic view of psychopathy and argued that the Cleckley characterization represented a mythical beast. Using the histories of four narcotic addicts, he illustrated the underlying dynamics associated with what he called sociopathy and thus the "humanness" and treatability of individuals so classified. Whereas sociopaths were described as having an apparent absence of anxiety and depression and an inability to learn, Vaillant reasoned that they are more adolescent than ineducable, concealing negative affect by such immature defenses as conversion symptoms, acting out, passive-aggressiveness, and projection. In emphasizing unhealthy defense mechanisms, this view was reminiscent of Thorne's (1959) conceptualization of sociopathy as a lifestyle disorder in which initially normal persons are conditioned to depend upon maladaptive mechanisms for need gratification. Despite this focus on learning or conditioning and affirmation of behavior reversibility, Thorne's view of sociopathy was decidedly negative and included references to an ever-downward spiral of self-hate, alcohol and drug abuse, physical and mental deterioration, and ultimate despair.

During the past four decades, clinical impressions of the psychopathy construct have been subjected to experimental scrutiny. Foremost among these researchers are Robert Hare and his colleagues (Hare, 1978, 1996b; Harpur & Hare, 1994; Hare & Hart, 1993; Harpur, Hare, & Hakstian, 1989; Hart & Hare, 1997; Hemphill, Hare, & Wong, 1998)—who, persuaded by the veracity of Cleckley's clinical description of the entity, attempted to identify the psychological deficits associated with the disorder. Using global ratings of personality traits and behaviors presumed to be characteristic of psychopathy, Hare and his colleagues accumulated a database that describes the Cleckley psychopath primarily among white, male criminal inmates. An array of studies has concentrated in the areas of psychophysiology and autonomic arousal (Hare, 1982; Hare, Frazelle, & Cox, 1978; Williamson, Harpur, & Hare, 1991), information processing and language (Forth & Hare, 1989; Hare & Jutai, 1988; Intrator et al., 1997; Jutai, Hare, & Connolly, 1987; Louth, Williamson, Alpert, Pouget, & Hare, 1998), learning and self-regulatory performances (Hare, 1965, 1984; Hart, Forth, & Hare, 1990), and analysis of criminal behaviors and recidivism (Hart & Hare, 1997; Hart, Kropp, & Hare, 1988; Hemphill et al., 1998). Summarizing much of this work in a series of manuscripts that describe a two-factor conceptualization of psychopathy, Hare and colleagues discussed psychopathy as a unitary clinical syndrome consisting of telltale personality traits, selfish interpersonal style, and shallow affect, as well as a clustering of unstable and antisocial behaviors reflecting social deviance (Harpur et al., 1989; Hart & Hare, 1997).

Although much of the recent research has explored fundamental deficits among psychopaths as defined by personality and behavioral traits, the criteria included in the DSM system since 1980 (DSM-III, 1980; DSM-III-R, 1987; DSM-IV, 1994) draw attention to demonstrably nonconforming, antisocial, and interpersonally disregarding behaviors that are consistent over time. Based in part on the research criteria developed by Spitzer, Endicott, and Robins (1975), diagnostic labeling requires a history of continuous and chronic antisocial behavior in which the rights of others are violated. This conceptualization reflects the well-established association between childhood and adult antisocial behaviors (Bardone, Moffitt, Caspi, & Dickson, 1996; Farrington & West, 1990; Loeber & Dishion, 1983; Robins, 1966; Wells & Forehand, 1985). And as observed earlier, diagnosis of antisocial personality disorder in DSM-III through DSM-IV has required evidence of conduct-disordered behaviors before age 15.

Unlike characterizations of psychopathy that emphasized deficient capacity for genuine human emotion, the DSM system has allowed for significant affective involvement in individuals diagnosed as antisocial by including possibly associated features of dysphoria, such as complaints of tension, inability to tolerate boredom, and depressed mood. Although the disorder has been described as chronic, it has been noted in the DSM-IV that symptom expression may remit with increasing age, particularly by the fourth decade of life, and although such remission tends to be observed primarily with respect to involvement in criminal behaviors, decreases may occur across the full range of antisocial behaviors. Thus, these criteria may be regarded as less pessimistic and significantly more objective than both earlier personality descriptions and the DSM-II (APA, 1968). At the same time, critics have argued that the quest for reliability has resulted in abandoning the personality construct of psychopathy or antisocial personality well known to clinicians and a discrepancy between the disorder and the people it is used to label (Hare, 1996b; Newman & Brinkley, 1998; Widiger & Frances, 1985).

## ASPD Prevalence and Associated Disorders

ASPD diagnosis, defined by a pattern of continuous and chronic antisocial behaviors that are initiated before age 15, persist into adulthood, and disrupt interpersonal and work performances, is often synonymous with criminality. Wulach (1983) estimated that the changes in diagnostic criteria in the 1980s increased ASPD prevalence among criminals by 250%, and Hare (1976) and Hart and Hare (1989) found DSM-III ASPD prevalences of 76% in a male prison sample and 50% in a sample of men remanded to a forensic unit. Similarly, Robins et al. (1991) reported a DSM-III-R prevalence of ASPD among prisoners of 50%, although these investigators considered a base rate of 50% in a prison setting to be consistent with theoretical and clinical explanations. Antisocial psychopathology has traditionally been elevated among samples of opiate addicts (Alterman et al., 1998; Sutker, 1971) and alcoholics (Morgenstern, Langenbucher, Labouvie, & Miller, 1997; Schuckit, 1973), and researchers have reported strong associations between diagnoses of ASPD and substance abuse categories (Gerstley, Alterman, McLellan, & Woody, 1990; Koenigsberg, Kaplan, Gilmore, & Cooper, 1985). For example, Kosten, Rounsaville, and Kleber (1982) found that roughly 55% of opiate addicts met criteria for present and lifetime ASPD, and Hesselbrock, Meyer, and Keener (1985) cited a rate of 49% among hospitalized alcoholics.

More recent estimates of ASPD prevalence among samples of substance abusers have been lower but nevertheless disturbingly high. Kidorf, Brooner, King, and Chutuape (1996) found that 39% of opioid-dependent outpatients met criteria for ASPD, and Alterman et al. (1998) reported a prevalence of ASPD of 33% among a sample of men undergoing methadone maintenance treatment. Ball, Tennen, Poling, Kranzler, and Rounsaville (1997) found an ASPD rate of 32% among a mixed gender sample receiving treatment for various types of substance abuse (e.g., cocaine, opiates, alcohol), and Morgenstern et al. (1997) sampled a group comprised predominantly of women (56%) undergoing treatment primarily for alcohol abuse/dependence, although high rates of concurrent drug use (approximately 50%) were observed, and reported an ASPD prevalence of 23%, including 26% among men and 9% among women. Mueser et al. (1997) assessed ASPD in a community-based sample of dual-diagnosis patients (i.e., those who met DSM-III-R criteria for alcohol or substance use disorder in combination with a DSM-III-R schizophrenia or schizoaffective disorder diagnosis) and found that 22% met criteria for ASPD. Smith and Newman (1990) evaluated the prevalence of DSM-III substance use disorders among a sample of incarcerated psychopaths and reported that 93% met criteria for alcohol dependence or abuse, 74% for dependence or abuse of a drug other than alcohol, and 26% for opioid dependence or abuse.

When prevalence data are collected for ASPD among hospitalized psychiatric patients and in community samples, rates are considerably lower than among those predominantly nonconforming samples in correctional facilities and alcohol and drug rehabilitation programs. Dahl (1986) reported that 14% of 18- to 40-year-old consecutive psychiatric admissions in Oslo, Norway were assigned diagnoses of ASPD, accounting for roughly 18% of personality disorder labels. Studying hospital outpatients, Kass, Skodol, Charles, Spitzer, and Williams (1985) reported that 2% met full and 4% fulfilled partial DSM-III ASPD criteria. Approximately 4% of adult first admissions to public inpatient and outpatient mental health facilities were assigned diagnoses of antisocial personality disorder (Weiss, Davis, Hedlund, & Cho, 1983). Looking at data generated from the community at large, Robins et al. (1984) found that lifetime ASPD prevalences rates varied from 3 to 5% in a community sample using the National Institute of Mental Health (NIMH) Diagnostic Interview Schedule (DIS: Robins, Helzer, Croughan, & Ratcliff, 1981); ASPD was documented in one of forty persons, thereby suggesting a disorder more common than schizophrenia. Similarly, Zimmerman and Coryell (1989) showed that ASPD was the most common disorder among first-degree relatives of normal controls and psychiatric patients (with a rate of 3.3%), and Helzer and Pryzbeck (1988) reported a lifetime prevalence rate of 2.5% in the general population using the five-site ECA data. Newman, Moffitt, Caspi, and Silva (1998) followed a New Zealand birth cohort and reported a DIS-derived DSM-III-R prevalence of ASPD at age 21 of 3.2%, although 74.2% of those assigned an ASPD diagnosis met criteria for a concurrent Axis I disorder. Berman, Fallon, and Coccaro (1998) assessed a community-recruited sample of research volunteers and found a DSM-III-R ASPD prevalence of 5.1%, and Barry, Fleming, Manwell, & Copeland (1997) surveyed 1944 outpatients in the offices of sixty-four primary care physicians and reported that 8% of men and 3% of women met DSM-III-R criteria for ASPD.

Diagnoses of ASPD are more common among men than women across all samples investigated (Blazer et al., 1985; Dahl, 1986; Kass, Spitzer, & Williams, 1983; Robins et al., 1984). Other demographic correlates of ASPD include younger age (Blazer et al., 1985; Robins et al., 1984; Zimmerman & Coryell, 1989), less education (Blazer et al., 1985; Morey & Ochoa, 1989), and lower socioeconomic status (Robins et al., 1984). Few questions have been raised about such characteristics as age and socioeconomic class, but controversy has arisen over explanations for gender differences. The possibilities of stereotyping and sex biases in clinical diagnosis and labeling, sex differences resulting from acculturation experiences, and/or actual sex differences attributed to other factors have been discussed. Kaplan (1983) argued that masculine assumptions about what behaviors are healthy and appropriate influence the behaviors of women and men as well as clinical impressions regarding these behaviors. Kass et al. (1983) described the distribution of DSM-III personality disorder diagnoses in two groups of adult patients and found sex differences in the diagnosis of histrionic and dependent personality disorders (more common among women) and ASPD (more common among men). Nevertheless, they maintained that there were no greater tendencies to label women personality disordered than men and concluded that there was no support for Kaplan's hypothesis of sex bias in DSM-III criteria. Their study, however, neglected Kaplan's charge that sex role stereotyping and societal judgments influence both the behaviors and their perception in the eyes of clinicians.

In a careful and comprehensive test of the hypothesis of sex bias in the diagnosis of personality disorders, Ford and Widiger (1989) assessed bias and base rate explanations, as well as the influence of case presentation ambiguity, clinician gender, and the specificity of individual criteria on diagnostic assignments, using ASPD and Histrionic Personality Disorder (HPD) descriptions. Results indicated that psychologist judges more often failed to diagnose HPD among men than women and ASPD among female compared to male patients and that antisocial female patients were more likely to be diagnosed as HPD than ASPD. Ford and Widiger (1989) minimized the significance of their finding that female psychologists' antisocial ratings for the antisocial case history were not affected by the patient's sex compared to those generated by the male psychologists. They concluded that though the individual criteria may not be intrinsically sex-biased, final diagnoses were influenced by stereotypic expectations elicited by conceptualizations of the disorders themselves.

Clinical meaningfulness or validity, diagnostic reliability, multiple diagnoses, and diagnostic overlap are among the problems highlighted in the literature on personality disorders generally and ASPD specifically (Widiger & Frances, 1985; Jordan, Swartz, George, Woodbury, & Blazer, 1989). The symptoms of one personality disorder, such as disturbed interpersonal relationships, antisocial behaviors, and impulsivity, may represent defining or associated features of other Axis I and II disorders, and strong associations have been observed between certain personality disorders and such Axis I disorders as alcohol and drug abuse and dependence (Grande, Wolf, Schubert, Patterson, & Brocco, 1984). Multiple diagnoses are the likely inevitable consequence of polythetic criteria sets in classification systems where category membership is heterogeneous and boundaries overlap. Therefore, considerable complexity exists in attempts to identify prevalence rates, understand disorder etiologies, and forecast outcomes and treatment responses (Widiger & Frances, 1985). It is important, then, to consider some of the ways in which the diagnosis of ASPD interfaces with the labeling of other psychopathology.

**Overlap within Personality Disorders.** A growing literature reflects considerable overlap among the personality disorders (Morey, 1988; Pope, Jonas, Hudson, Cohen, & Gunderson, 1983; Widiger & Corbitt, 1997; Widiger, Frances, Warner, & Bluhm, 1986) as well as covariation among these diagnoses. Widiger, Frances, Pincus, Davis, and First (1991) reported that diagnostic interviewing yielded an average of four personality disorders per patient, and Widiger and Corbitt (1997) reported that in clinical settings, most individuals who meet criteria for ASPD also meet criteria for at least one other personality disorder. Morgenstern et al. (1997) found that most individuals in a mixed-gender group of substance abusers who met criteria for one personality disorder also satisfied criteria for at least two personality disorders. Berman et al. (1998) reported that 29% of a community-recruited sample of research volunteers met criteria for a personality disorder and that these individuals were assigned an average of 1.55 personality disorder diagnoses. Among a sample of cocaine-dependent outpatients, 48% met criteria for at least one personality disorder diagnosis, and 18% met criteria for two or more. Of those assigned a personality diagnosis, 65%

were diagnosed with a Cluster B personality disorder, and antisocial and borderline personality disorders were the most common (Barber et al., 1996).

The overlap among personality disorders is not surprising in view of the DSM aggregation of personality disorders into clusters, with antisocial, borderline, histrionic, and narcissistic personality disorders forming a constellation that shares such common features as impulsive acting out, unpredictable behaviors, and dramatic presentation. ASPD diagnosis is most often associated with those of borderline, histrionic, narcissistic, and, before DSM-IV, passive-aggressive personality disorders. Pope et al. (1983) found that it was difficult to separate antisocial and borderline personality disorders in men and borderline and histrionic personality disorders in women and suggested that the clustering of borderline, histrionic, and antisocial disorders may reflect a true lack of differentiation. Interviewing psychiatric inpatients for whom personality disorders were the principal treatment issue, Widiger et al. (1986) discovered a particularly strong association between ASPD and borderline, passive-aggressive, histrionic, and schizotypal personality disorders. Widiger and Corbitt (1997) reviewed six studies that assessed Axis II psychopathology in general clinical populations using semistructured interviews and reported high median rates of comorbidity of ASPD and borderline personality disorder (75%), histrionic personality disorder (56%), passive-aggressive personality disorder (36%), paranoid personality disorder (31%), and narcissistic personality disorder (28%).

After reviewing thirteen studies that assessed comorbidity of ASPD and borderline personality disorder, Zanarini and Gunderson (1997) concluded that in samples of individuals with criterion-defined borderline personality disorder, rates of co-occurring ASPD range from 0–60%, with most falling between 10 and 25%, whereas, in samples of nonpsychotic individuals and with study focus solely on rates of Axis II comorbidity, a substantially smaller percentage of patients who met criteria for borderline personality disorder also met criteria for ASPD (i.e., mean = 22.5%, range = 0–68%) than patients who met criteria for ASPD and also met criteria for borderline personality disorder (i.e., mean = 50.25%, range = 0–80%). At the same time, prototypical categorization allows for covariation, and Morey (1988) showed that features of the narcissistic personality disorder combined with nonaggressive antisocial features formed a distinct cluster reminiscent of the Cleckley concept of psychopathy. Similarly, Blashfield, Sprock, Pinkston, and Hodgin (1985), using multidimensional scaling to study relationships among the eleven DSM-III PD diagnoses, suggested a circumplex ordering, with antisocial personality relatively independent from other diagnoses.

The association between antisocial and histrionic personality disorders has sparked recurring speculation that hysteria and antisocial personalities constitute sex-typed versions of the same condition. Cloninger, Reich, and Guze (1975) proposed a multifactorial model in which male sociopathy, female hysteria, and female sociopathy constitute an increasingly severe expression of a shared liability. Reviving the question of whether antisocial personality disorder, somatization disorder or hysteria, and histrionic personality disorder fundamentally constitute the same clinical entity, Lilienfeld, Van Valkenburg, Larntz, and Akiskal (1986) conducted diagnostic interviews among 250 patients sampled from psychiatric care settings. They confirmed reports of a positive relationship between antisocial personality and somatization disorders within individuals of both sexes as well as a strong association of antisocial and histrionic personality, with the latter appearing to moderate the relationship between antisocial personality and somatization disorder. Similarly, Spalt (1980) found close associations between antisocial personality and hysteria in women, but this was not the case for men. It has also been observed that female hysterics and male sociopaths tend to marry each other (Woerner & Guze, 1968) and beget hyperactive children (Morrison & Stewart, 1971) who grow up to be sociopathic (Satterfield, 1978) or hysteric (Cloninger & Guze, 1975).

Whether psychopathy or ASPD and hysteria or histrionic disorder constitute sex-typed expression of the same underlying substrate involves analyzing several complicated hypotheses within the changing climate of psychiatric and psychological assessment. As described before, there are sex-related biases in the conceptualization of antisocial and histrionic personality disorders that may operate differently, depending on the diagnostician's sex (Ford & Widiger, 1989). Moreover, the sociocultural standards for socially appropriate and conforming behaviors may be stronger for women; thus women may depart from societal

constraints less frequently because of cultural pressures. This reasoning is supported by two lines of research. Heilbrun and Gottfried (1988) tested the notion that feminine constraints on physical aggression may decrease with the erosion of traditional sex-role commitments associated with the rise of the feminist movement. They found that although antisociality proved to be a significant predictor of more dangerous criminal behavior from 1965 to 1971 among incarcerated women, this predictiveness was lost for the period 1980–1985, reflecting perhaps lessening of prior role restraints. Second, the literature suggests that for women to display criminality, the congenital predisposition to criminal behavior has to be more severe than for men (Sigvardsson, Cloninger, Bohman, & von Knorring, 1982).

If antisocial behaviors result from stereotyped perceptions and/or less demonstrative display, they may be minimized, overlooked, or mislabeled among women, whereas characteristics defined traditionally as histrionic may be emphasized. Conversely, antisocial behaviors may be more readily recognized among men because such deviance is seen as more male role congruent. Extending this logic, it might be conjectured that women express social nonconformity through different behavioral means, perhaps greater emphasis on sexual promiscuity, neglect of parenting duties, crimes which go undetected, and alcohol and drug abuse. Some years ago, Hammen and Padesky (1977) showed that men and women differed in the behavioral expression of depression. It is conceivable that sociocultural influences lead to sex-typed expression of social deviance as well as difficulties in identifying ASPD among women. Few studies have explored possible differences between male and female patients in measures of personality traits considered antisocial or on behavioral indices of deviance. It has been shown, however, that antisocial women selected more negative adjective self-descriptors than their male antisocial counterparts (Sutker, DeSanto, & Allain, 1985), perhaps reflecting greater internalization of societal prejudice toward deviant or nonconforming behaviors.

## Association with Axis I Disorders

Interrelationships among the major psychiatric illnesses defined on Axis I and those that reflect "inflexible and maladaptive traits" listed on Axis II have constituted a focus for clinical speculation and research activity since the multiaxial classification system was introduced in 1980. Conducting a comprehensive study of the association of personality disorders and Axis I diagnoses among 2462 patients referred for psychiatric evaluation, Koenigsberg et al. (1985) found high overlap between diagnoses of substance abuse and Axis II disorders. Comorbidity was particularly strong for the substance use disorders, categories traditionally identified with neuroses such as the anxiety-based and somatoform disorders, phobic and panic disorders, and dysthymia and atypical depression. Among patients assigned substance use diagnoses, borderline and antisocial were the most common personality disorders, although borderline disorder was distributed across Axis I diagnoses and antisocial disorder clustered strongly with substance abuse. Consistent with these findings, Malow, West, Williams, and Sutker (1989) reported that antisocial and borderline personality disorders were the most prevalent Axis II diagnoses in a drug-abusing sample, and these results were replicated among mixed substance abusers (Ball et al., 1997) and cocaine-dependent outpatients (Barber et al., 1996), as well as in a sample undergoing treatment for alcohol abuse (Morgenstern et al., 1997).

The association between antisocial personality and the substance use disorders has sparked theoretical debate and ongoing research interest. Finding that diagnoses of alcoholism, antisocial personality, and drug dependence form one of two primary psychopathological clusters in a study of DIS-generated diagnoses among psychiatric inpatients, Wolf et al. (1988) concluded that these three disorders constitute a relatively homogeneous triad that is independent of other diagnoses. Strong diagnostic interactions between alcoholism and antisocial personality disorders have been reported in patients referred for psychiatric consultation (Lewis, Rice, & Helzer, 1983), a community sample of black men (Lewis, Robins, & Rice, 1985), and adult male and female adoptees (Cadoret, O'Gorman, Troughton, & Heywood, 1985; Cadoret, Troughton, Bagford, & Woodworth, 1990). Drake and Vaillant (1985, 1988) also pointed to a high degree of association between diagnoses of personality disorders and alcoholism in community samples and called attention to complications of dysphoria among men with personality

disorders; Vaillant and Hiller-Sturmhoefel (1996) summarized longitudinal studies of 268 male college students and 456 inner city 11- to 16-year-old male adolescents selected from 1934 to 1944 and identified co-occurring sociopathy, along with ethnicity and family history of alcoholism, as risk factors for alcoholism.

Koenigsberg et al. (1985) found that borderline, dependent, schizotypal, passive-aggressive, and mixed personality disorders were common among anxiety- and depression-based disorders identified traditionally as neuroses, but antisocial personality disorder was not. However, data derived from studies of comorbidity of ASPD and posttraumatic stress disorder (PTSD), considered an anxiety-based disorder, ranged from 3% in older Vietnam, Korean, and World War II (WWII) veterans (Davidson, Swartz, Storck, Krishnan, & Hammett, 1985), to 10% in an outpatient sample of Vietnam veterans (Uddo-Crane, Thompson, & Sutker, 1991), to 14% among Vietnam veteran outreach clients (Green, Lindy, & Grace, 1985), and to 64% in an outpatient sample of primarily Vietnam veterans (Sierles, Chen, Messing, Besyner, & Taylor, 1986). Although a nonconforming, antisocial flair has often been considered complementary if not integral to diagnosis of PTSD, especially among younger men, rates of ASPD are remarkably low among some samples of patients who suffer anxiety-based PTSD, especially in view of the consistently high rates of substance abuse disorders that often overlap with ASPD. For example, Keane and Wolfe (1990) found that 70% of treatment-seeking PTSD patients met criteria for alcohol abuse or dependence, 42% for drug abuse or dependence, and only 26% for ASPD or mixed personality disorder with antisocial features.

## Typologies and the Psychopathy Construct

Recognition of the heterogeneity among antisocial individuals is not of recent origin or unique to disagreements centered around defining criteria. Kraepelin employed the term psychopathic personality in his textbook *Lehrbuch der Psychiatrie* (1907/1923) and outlined four types of psychopathic personalities that were characterized in varying degrees by antisocial behaviors and traits. Presenting a typology of ten overlapping psychopathic or deviant personalities, Schneider (1923,

1958) described several clinical varieties that might lead to antisocial behavior. In his review of the concept of psychopathic personality, Lykken (1994) characterized the psychopathic personality as a "family of disorders" comprising four subtypes that may then be subdivided. He described dissocial psychopaths whose personality deviations are implied by adherence to the values or code of their predatory, criminal, or other social group, neurotic or impulsive characters in whom antisocial behavior constitutes neurotic acting out or an unconscious need for punishment, antisocial individuals whose behaviors are influenced by organic dysfunction or abnormality in inhibitory control, and primary or idiopathic psychopaths. Lykken (1994) further distinguished two subtypes of primary psychopaths: those whose empathy for others is lessened because of exposure to human suffering and the Cleckley psychopath.

Simple classifications of psychopathic or antisocial personality are based on the presumption of bimodal-like clusterings of individuals using discriminating dimensional constructs such as anxiety (Hare, 1970; Lykken, 1957; Newman & Schmidt, 1998), social withdrawal (Blackburn & Lee-Evans, 1985), and intellectual sophistication (Arieti, 1967). Lykken (1957) distinguished primary and secondary psychopaths on the basis of anxiety, and Weiss et al. (1983) identified a subgroup of "dysphoric psychopaths" who constituted perhaps as many as one-fourth of patients assigned diagnoses of antisocial personality disorder and were characterized by depression, anxiety, difficulties in intellectual functioning, and irritability, in addition to defining antisocial features. Arieti (1967) described simple and complex types differentiated by intelligence level, and the notion that cognitive variables, particularly intelligence, moderate antisocial behaviors, and violence specifically has been a topic for investigation. Heilbrun (1982) reported that psychopathic criminals with low intelligence were impaired in impulse control and empathy compared to psychopathic criminals with greater intelligence and that both empathy and impulse control could contribute to violence. Expanding their model to include Blackburn's social withdrawal variable (Blackburn & Lee-Evans, 1985), Heilbrun and Heilbrun (1985) found that low intelligence predicted dangerousness among psychopathic criminals regardless of situation, whereas social withdrawal enhanced the

prediction of dangerousness within prison, but not in community or parole situations.

A related line of research has attempted to isolate factors that differentiate children at high and low risk for delinquency. Testing the hypothesis that high intelligence may protect individuals at high risk for antisocial outcome, Kandel et al. (1988) showed that high intelligence diminished the risk of criminal behavior in men. Addressing methodological weaknesses in the Kandel et al. (1988) retrospective effort, White, Moffitt, and Silva (1989) replicated findings showing the protective effects of intelligence among male, and to a lesser extent, female youth at risk for delinquency. These investigators reported that average or above average intelligence was associated with less serious and chronic delinquent behaviors among groups of boys and girls at low and high risk. However, high-risk boys may require more sophisticated intellectual functioning than low-risk boys to remain free of delinquent involvement completely. Lynam, Moffitt, and Stouthamer (1993) showed that the protective function of IQ is independent of social status and education, and not due merely to lower intelligence increasing the probability of getting caught (Moffitt & Silva, 1988). Caspi and Moffitt (1995) concluded that perhaps the best focus of study to explain the continuity or stability of antisocial behavior is compromised cognitive ability.

Psychopaths can also be differentiated using such outcome variables as degree of adaptiveness or capacity to avoid negative consequences. In this context, the more positive personal features attributed to psychopaths are relevant. For example, psychopaths have been portrayed as adroit social manipulators (Cleckley, 1982), persistent goal-seekers (Buss, 1966), intellectually capable and observant individuals (Sutker, Moan, & Allain, 1974), survivors in American society (Smith, 1978), and the most adept of human "cheaters" in reproductive strategy (MacMillan & Kofoed, 1984). Clearly, some psychopaths function more adequately in society than others, suggesting a continuum of adaptiveness or gross subdivisions into successful and unsuccessful subtypes. Several research studies have explored the characteristics of these more adaptive psychopaths.

Widom (1977) used newspaper advertisements to identify male psychopaths who were relatively successful in avoiding the negative consequences of antisocial behaviors, and Sutker and Allain (1983) employed MMPI-defined criteria to isolate an even more successful antisocial subgroup among male medical students. In this study, students labeled adaptive sociopaths and normals were compared on measures of cognitive control, planning and organization, interpersonal functioning, and sensation seeking. Adaptive sociopaths produced more qualitative errors on the Porteus Mazes, scored higher on Zuckerman's measure of Experience Seeking (1972) and lower on the California Psychological Inventory (CPI) Scales Socialization (*So*) and Self-Control (*Sc*), reported more arrests, and admitted tendencies to act on impulse. For sociopaths to contemplate an action, deviant or not, suggested greater probability for behavioral execution. This combination of lower self-control, less inhibitory regulation, and greater interest in experience seeking was predictive of greater behavioral deviance among this intellectually sophisticated sample of young adults.

Dichotomous subtypings have been important in conceptualizations of psychopathy, but more complex formulations are required to refine descriptions of prototypical and associated varieties among clinical samples and to characterize disorder expression and severity. Questions of typology have been approached with factor analytic strategies used to define personality traits and behaviors thought to represent psychopathy (Hare et al., 1990; Harpur et al., 1989; Harpur, Hakstian, & Hare, 1988) and to describe the full spectrum of antisocial psychopathology. This latter approach is illustrated by the work of Jordan et al. (1989) who applied grade of membership analysis to identify symptom clusters of antisocial personality and related psychiatric disorders. Results showed seven pure clusters, including two that resembled the DSM-III portrait of ASPD and were strongly associated with DIS-generated diagnoses of ASPD. Two pure types emerged that consisted of alcohol abuse/dependence and recreational illicit drug use symptoms, and two types were identified predominantly among women. Of these, one was characterized by marital instability, other domestic problems, and employment and interpersonal difficulties, and the second was defined by multiple symptoms of depression and selected features of other Axis I disorders. Serving as a comparison group for the other types, the seventh cluster reflected no symptomatology.

These more complex factor and cluster analytic approaches suggest ways to conceptualize predictive and outcome variables relevant to psychopathy, taking into account both person and environment factors. Because a dimensional, prototype model of classification tolerates heterogeneity, there will be variations on the prototypic example, and individuals can be rated on diverse dimensions that transcend simple categorization or bimodal clustering. Psychopathy may best be conceptualized as a cluster of clusters in which the fundamental feature is that of nonconforming or antisocial behaviors persisting over time and usually leading to unfortunate circumstances. Although researchers and clinicians are accustomed to working with the extreme subsets of antisocial individuals or those ranking high or low on various dimensional variables, there appear to be persons whose behaviors approximate the antisocial model but fall short of full expression. There are also factors that operate to protect individuals at genetic or environmental risk for ASPD. An important research task is to guide conceptualizations of cognitive, affective, and behavioral features that are seen as aggregating to create the psychopathy construct and to differentiate subtypes predictive of specific types of antisocial outcomes.

## Etiologic Factors and Antisocial Personality

There has been compelling recognition of the multidetermined nature of antisocial behaviors, including the contributions of biological, psychological, and social variables. Questions of nature versus nurture are less pivotal than those spurring studies that describe the interplay between genetic and environmental variables in predicting antisocial behaviors and gender/sex-related differences in antisocial expression. Cloninger, Reich, and Guze (1978) emphasized that any plausible model of the transmission of antisocial behavior disorders must allow for genetic and environmental factors without making unwarranted assumptions about their relative importance, and the model outlined by Reich, Cloninger, and Guze (1975) assumed that pathogenetic factors relevant to specific disorders are multiple and additive. In search of biological and psychological factors that contribute to antisocial behaviors, investigators have launched twin, family, and adoption studies, the latter being best suited to separating genetic and biological effects from those attributed to social learning and the sociocultural context.

## Genetic and Genetic–Environment Factors

With few exceptions, evidence from twin (Christiansen, 1977; DiLalla, Carey, Gottesman, & Bouchard, 1996; Slutske et al., 1997; van den Oord, Verhulst, & Boomsma, 1996), family (Cloninger et al., 1978), adoption (Mednick, Gabrielli, & Hutchings, 1984), and combined, for example, twin-sibling, (O'Connor, McGuire, Reiss, Hetherington, & Plomin, 1998) research has supported the contributions of genetic and congenital factors in transmitting antisocial behaviors and related personality correlates. Reviewing results of concordant studies, Eysenck and Eysenck (1978) concluded that 55% of monozygous (MZ) twins were concordant for criminal conduct, as opposed to 13% of dizygous (DZ) twins. Cloninger et al. (1978) pointed to concordance rates as high as .70 for MZ twins and .28 for DZ twins. Centerwall and Robinette (1989) searched for a genetic component to antisocial behavior by studying concordance rates for dishonorable discharge among 15,294 pairs of White male twins, both of whom served in the U.S. military. Results indicated greater pairwise concordance for dishonorable discharge in monozygous versus dizygous pairs; the risk of such discharge was fifty-six times more likely among monozygous co-twin dishonorably discharged veterans than among dizygous twins in general. Although these researchers recognized distinctions between dishonorable discharge and antisocial personality, they concluded that results added weight to the presumed importance of genetic contributions to antisocial behavior. More recently, Slutske et al. (1997) examined retrospective reports of conduct disorder in a community-based Australian sample of 2682 twin pairs and reported concordances of .53 for MZ male twins, .37 for DZ male twins, .30 for female MZ twins, and .18 for DZ female twins. Their best-fitting model yielded variance estimates for additive genetic influences of 71%.

Examining prevalences within family units, Cloninger et al. (1978) reported data obtained for 227 first-degree relatives of three types of probands (sociopathic men, sociopathic women, and hysteric women) and 800 subjects in the general population (see Cloninger et al., 1975). Hysteria and sociopathy were more frequently found among the relatives of all three proband types than in the general population, and data were consistent with the notion that hysteria in women is a more prevalent, less deviant manifestation of the same process that causes sociopathy. Cloninger et al. (1978) also concluded that alcoholism and sociopathy may be genetically independent and cited findings that adult sons of Danish alcoholics who were adopted away in infancy showed increased frequency of alcoholism but not antisocial personality, whereas an increased proportion of psychopaths and criminals, but not of alcoholics and drug dependents, was documented among the adopted-away offspring of psychopathic parents.

Carey and Goldman (1997) pointed out that many potential family environment factors, for example, single-parent household, poverty, and housing density, may impact the expression of similar antisocial behaviors among siblings or other relatives and that antisocial behaviors such as aggression can be induced experimentally in the laboratory using social learning techniques (Bandura & Walters, 1959). Hence, they suggested that family studies may not be as appropriate in determining the role of genetics in antisocial behavior as investigating twins, separated relatives, and adoptive relatives. U. S., Danish, and Swedish studies of adopted children of criminals, alcoholics, and otherwise antisocial parents separated at birth suggest significantly increased antisocial behaviors among adoptees with antisocial or criminal backgrounds, but not necessarily parental alcoholism. These investigations revealed increased criminality and personality disorders among the biological, but not adoptive, relatives of psychopathic or criminal probands compared to relatives of controls (Schulsinger, 1972) and pointed to the interaction between genetic factors and the influence of gender and infancy conditions on adult outcomes (Crowe, 1972, 1974). Specificity of inheritance, that is, different heritabilities, of antisocial behaviors such as criminality and alcohol abuse has been reported by Cadoret et al. (1985); Bohman, Cloninger, Sigvardsson, and von Knorring (1982); Crowe (1972, 1974), and Cloninger, Sigvardsson, Bohman, and von Knorring (1982) showed that both genetic and postnatal factors could be sufficient to predispose to criminality, but that specific combinations of gene–environment antecedents may modify the risk factors such as low social status and unstable preadoptive placements may modify the risk factors.

Using data derived from 913 women and 862 men in the Stockholm Adoption Study, Sigvardsson et al. (1982) explored sex differences in criminality and alcoholism, such postnatal antecedents to criminality as prolonged institutional care and urban adoptive placement, and severity of antisocial predisposition. Although the genetic antecedents of petty criminality were qualitatively similar between the sexes, criminal women had more biological parents with petty criminality, and hence a stronger genetic predisposition, than their male counterparts. These researchers concluded that the deviant predisposition must be greater in women than in men to manifest adolescent social maladjustment and adult antisocial personality or petty criminality. Additionally, postnatal antecedents differed according to sex. Results were interpreted as emphasizing the complex pathogenesis of criminality with genetic heterogeneity, sex specificity, heterogeneity in postnatal antecedents, and nonadditive gene–environment interaction.

Cadoret and Cain (1980, 1981) used multiple regression analyses to predict the number of antisocial behaviors in 246 adoptees, a sample that included children and adolescents adopted from psychiatrically disordered parents and matched controls with no evidence of family disorder. Findings pointed to a genetic predisposition to antisocial behavior in offspring who had alcoholic and antisocial biological family members and no apparent sex differences in the biological predictors of antisocial behavior. However, male and female subjects differed in susceptibility to adverse environmental factors such as psychiatric illness in an adoptive parent, adoptive parental divorce, and discontinuous mothering; environmental variables were more predictive of antisocial behavior in male than female participants. Results suggested that men may have a lower threshold for developing antisocial personality in the presence of predisposing environmental factors.

Reporting data derived from a register of 14,427 nonfamilial male adoptions in Denmark, Mednick et al. (1984) described a strong relationship between biological parental criminality and adopted-son criminality, an association that was enhanced if both sets of parents were criminal. These investigators observed, however, that genetic influence was not sufficient to produce criminal convictions

and underscored the finding that 75% of adoptees whose biological parents received three or more convictions were never convicted themselves. Using the same data set, Moffitt (1987) reported that multiple recidivistic nonviolent criminal activity was significantly increased in adopted sons when mental disorder and serious criminal involvement were found in the biological families. Further analyses indicated that the types of mental illness that contributed most strongly to the risk of criminal conviction were personality, drug, and alcohol disorders. Neither parental mental illness nor multiple convictions alone greatly increased the risk of offspring violence, but when both were present in the biological parents, the percentage of adoptees convicted for violence more than doubled.

Results of twin studies of antisocial behavior have been consistent with those of adoption studies in demonstrating a genetic effect for antisocial behavior but not to the exclusion of environmental influences. Grove et al. (1990) studied thirty-two MZ twin pairs raised apart from a very early age and observed the following probandwise concordance rates (i.e., the probability of having an affected co-twin, given that one is an affected twin) for psychiatric diagnoses generated by the Diagnostic Interview Schedule (DIS: Robins, Helzer, Croughan, & Ratcliff, 1981): 29% for antisocial personality disorder, 33% for alcohol abuse and/or dependence, and 36% for drug abuse and/or dependence. These researchers examined frequency counts of DIS symptoms and found greater numbers of symptoms of alcohol problems and childhood and adult antisocial behaviors among men than women and greater numbers of drug problems among younger subjects. Slutske et al. (1997) studied retrospectively genetic and environmental influences in the etiology of conduct disorder among a community-based Australian sample of 2682 MZ and DZ adult twin pairs. The best fitting model demonstrated a substantial genetic influence that accounted for 71% of the variance in DSM-III-R conduct disorder diagnoses. A modest but not significant effect for shared environment was also observed. The magnitude of the genetic and environmental effects for conduct disorder liability did not differ for girls and boys, and the specific genetic and environmental mechanisms important for development of conduct disorder appeared to be similar for both sexes. In the same sample, Slutske et al. (1998) also examined common genetic risk factors for conduct disorder and alcohol dependence and found that genetic factors accounted for most of the association between conduct disorder and alcohol dependence liability in both women and men. These researchers concluded that there are common genetic risk factors for conduct disorder and alcohol dependence, or that conduct disorder itself is an important genetically influenced risk factor for alcohol dependence.

O'Connor, McGuire, Reiss, Hetherington, and Plomin (1998) examined possible genetic and environmental contributions to the co-occurrence of antisocial behavior and depression in adolescents. The sample comprised 720 same-sex adolescent siblings ranging in age from 10 to 18 years and included monozygotic and dizygotic twins, nontwin full siblings, half siblings, and unrelated siblings. The study used a dimensional model of psychopathology based on symptom checklists completed by adolescents and their parents. A composite score for depressive features was derived from self-, mother, and father reports on the Child Depression Inventory (CDI), the depression factors from both the Behavior Problems Inventory (BPI) and Behavior Events Inventory (BEI), and observer reports of depressed mood; an antisocial composite score was derived from self-, mother, and father reports of the antisocial factor of the BPI and BEI and observer reports of antisocial behavior. Approximately 45% of the observed covariation between depressive and antisocial features could be explained by a common genetic liability, although shared (30%) and nonshared (25%) environmental influences were also significant. Results were interpreted to suggest that genetic influences underlie the tendency for developing a specific disorder or dimension (in this case, depressive symptoms and antisocial behavior) and also the co-occurrence of maladjustment and that environmentally mediated risks play an important role in the development of depressive symptoms and antisocial behavior and of the co-occurrence of these dimensions in adolescence. Working with younger children, van den Oord et al. (1996) examined genetic and environmental influences on problem behaviors as determined by mother and father ratings obtained with the Child Behavior Checklist. The sample consisted of 1358 three-year-old twin pairs recruited from the Netherlands Twin Register. On average, genetic, shared environmental, and nonshared environmental influences accounted for 64, 9, and 27% of the variance, respectively, and the strong genetic effect suggests that children with behavior problems are likely to show an innate vulnerability.

The heritability of personality indicators of psychopathology as measured by the Minnesota Multiphasic Personality Inventory (MMPI: Hathaway & McKinley, 1942) was studied in a sample of sixty-five pairs of monozygous twins reared apart (MZA) and fifty-four pairs of dizygous twins reared apart (DZA) (DiLalla, Carey, Gottesman, & Bouchard, 1996). Using the original version of the MMPI, these investigators examined scores on the basic validity and clinical scales and the Wiggins Content Scales (Wiggins, 1966). Consistent with findings of other twin research, MZ twins showed substantial similarity, but there was no significant effect of zygosity, even though the degree of DZA similarity was more variable than the MZA variability. Approximately 44% of the variance in MMPI clinical and content scales was accounted for by genetic variability. Among the clinical scales, there was evidence of strong heritability on the two MMPI scales most typically associated with antisocial personality disorder, the Psychopathic Deviate (Pd) Scale and the Hypomania (Ma) Scale, with heritability estimates of .61 and .55, respectively. Similarly, Miles and Carey (1997) found a substantial heritability estimate of 0.42 for the Socialization Scale (Gough, 1960) of the California Psychological Inventory (Gough 1975).

Carey and Goldman (1997) reviewed and summarized the literature regarding genetic influences on antisocial behavior as follows: (1) identical twins are more similar than fraternal twins, and adoptees correlate more with their biological relatives than with their adoptive relatives—findings that hold for multiple definitions of antisocial behavior, for example, whether defined narrowly such as a felony conviction or more broadly such as symptom counts for antisocial personality disorder or conduct disorder criteria, as self-reported delinquency, or as scores on relevant personality scales; (2) violations of the assumptions of the twin and adoption methods and possible effects of twin imitation cannot account for observed genetic effects; (3) the influences of environmental factors are implicated in all studies; (4) the influences of shared environment are stronger among adolescents than among adults, suggesting that some social factors may contribute to initiating but not maintaining antisocial behavior; (5) genetic effects are implicated in the comorbidity of antisocial behaviors and alcohol abuse/dependence and other substance abuse/dependence; (6) evidence for the heritability of violent behavior is less consistent than evidence for general deviant or antisocial behavior; (7) caution is required in interpreting existing data with regard to a common family environment; and (8) caution is required in extrapolating findings to populations other than those on which they are based.

Review of these studies suggests that we have barely scratched the surface in identifying specific factors, as well as their complex interplay, that constitute risk for criminality and antisocial behavior. In addition to genetic predisposition, environmental variables cited as influencing expression of antisocial personality are unfavorable infancy conditions and delayed home placements (Crowe, 1974); low social status (Cloninger et al., 1982); prolonged institutionalization and urban adoptive placements (Sigvardsson et al., 1982); psychiatric illness in adoptive parents and discontinuous mothering (Cadoret & Cain, 1980, 1981); and single-parent households, poverty, and housing density (Carey & Goldman, 1997). Other studies pointed to the significant impact of assortative mating (Mednick et al., 1984) and adoptive parent criminality (Hutchings & Mednick, 1975).

The study of the heritability of antisocial personality has also included attempts to identify genetic markers (i.e., stable characteristics more readily observable/measurable than the potential pathologic gene) that signal risk for antisocial psychopathology. In the case of schizophrenia, researchers have searched for biochemical abnormalities as well as psychophysiological characteristics (Holzman, 1987; Iacono, 1983); however, this line of investigation is less well developed for antisocial personality disorder. As an example, exploration of the "XYY syndrome" for etiologic significance to antisocial behavior failed to yield useful findings (Witkin et al., 1976). Of greater relevance have been proposed associations between neurological abnormalities and antisocial personality (Fishbein & Thatcher, 1986; Hare, 1970; Henry & Moffitt, 1997), neurotransmitter dysfunction and psychopathy (Berman, Kavoussi, & Caccaro, 1997; Fishbein & Thatcher, 1986; Mawson & Mawson, 1977), EEG and criminality (Raine, 1993), psychopathy and frontal lobe deficiency (Devonshire, Howard, & Sellars, 1988;

Gorenstein, 1982, 1987), anomalous hemisphere lateralization and psychopathy (Day & Wong, 1996), cerebral glucose metabolism and criminality (Goyer et al., 1994; Goyer & Semple, 1996; Raine et al., 1994), and pathological levels of cortical and autonomic arousal and psychopathy (Ellis, 1987; Fowles, 1980; Gorenstein & Newman, 1980; Hare, 1970, 1978; Quay, 1965; Raine, 1997). For example, Raine, Venables, and Williamson reported that electrodermal, cardiovascular, and cortical underarousal (1990a,b) and enhanced attentional processing (1990c) among 15-year-old youths were significantly related to subsequent adult criminality and suggested that underarousal of the autonomic and central nervous systems may represent manifestation of a genetic predisposition to criminality and a possible early predictor of criminal behavior.

## Learning and Behavioral Factors

Speculations regarding family characteristics that influence acquisition of antisocial behaviors originated in psychoanalytic case formulations (Bowlby, 1951). Consensus on specific factors was limited, but most early theorists hypothesized that psychopathy was the result of faulty early childhood processes. For example, insecure attachments during infancy in high-risk families have been associated with increased risk of later disruptive behaviors during toddler, preschool, and school-age periods (Erickson, Sroufe, & Egeland, 1985; Renken, Egeland, Marvinney, Mangelsdorf, & Sroufe, 1989; Shaw & Vondra, 1995). However, economic and social support and quality of alternative care facilities may serve as a buffer to prevent the insecurely attached infant from becoming dysfunctional (Shaw & Vondra, 1995). Research supports the significance of dysfunctional family characteristics and poor parenting techniques in contributing to aggressive, delinquent, and otherwise antisocial behaviors. Olweus (1978) suggested that hostile, rejecting, or power-assertive parental attitudes, combined with minimal demands for responsible, relatively non-aggressive behaviors, were important factors in facilitating aggressive, antisocial childhood involvements. Raine et al. (1994) also pointed to early maternal rejection in combination with birth complications as predictive of violent offending.

Patterson (1982) found that coercive interaction patterns are often found in families with school-age children who exhibit conduct disorder. Similarly, Dumas (1989) and Dumas and Wahler (1985) showed that the parents of antisocial children respond to misbehavior in an aversive, erratic manner, allocate higher levels of positive and negative attention to inappropriate rather than prosocial behaviors, and thereby increase the likelihood of deviant behaviors. Indeed, Shaw and Winslow (1997) suggested that a child who has received less contingent caregiving might act more disruptively to obtain parental attention (Greenberg & Speltz, 1988) and have less to lose by disobeying parental requests (i.e., loss of love, Shaw & Bell, 1993). In a meta-analysis of forty-seven studies, Rothbaum and Weisz (1994) found stronger relationships with child behaviors when multiple parenting characteristics were measured rather than examined individually and that global parenting styles were better predictors than individual dimensions.

Pollock et al. (1990) found that antisocial behavior defined as aggression, criminal acts, and clinician ratings of potential for acting out aggression was associated with a history of physical abuse in a group of young adult Danish men aged 18–21, whereas parental alcoholism and its interaction with childhood physical abuse did not increase the risk of antisocial behaviors. Dodge, Bates, and Pettit (1990) also pointed to the important effect of physical abuse and suggested that physical abuse leads to aggressive behaviors by impacting the development of hostile social information processing patterns, that is, physically abused youths become predisposed to attribute hostile interpretations in social interactions. In a systematic study of the association between childhood physical abuse and neglect and adult antisocial personality disorder, Luntz and Widom (1994) used a prospective cohort design to follow 699 subjects from ages 18 to 35. They found a higher prevalence of DIS-defined ASPD (13.1%) among subjects who had been physically abused or neglected compared to those who had not been abused or neglected (ASPD prevalence = 7.1%). These investigators also reported that a history of childhood abuse and neglect was predictive of the number of ASPD symptoms exhibited in adulthood.

Current thinking about the contributions of learning and behavioral factors to antisocial outcome is heavily influenced by accumulating evidence that antisocial and aggressive behaviors are stable over time (Shaw & Winslow, 1997; Wells & Forehand, 1985). For example, Lahey et al. (1995) found that 88% of clinic-referred conduct-disordered youths still met criteria for the diagnosis in the next three years. Examining childhood predictors of adult antisocial behavior, Robins (1978) found that all childhood antisocial behaviors are strongly predictive of adult antisocial activities, as well as highly intercorrelated. Consistent with her earlier report (1970) that 40% of conduct-disordered children were diagnosed with antisocial personalities in adulthood, she showed that the number of antisocial behaviors or the severity of childhood antisocial involvement was a better predictor of severe adult antisocial behavior than specific childhood behaviors or family variables. The importance of such behavior–behavior relationships has been discussed thoroughly by Hundleby (1978), as has the clustering of various types of antisocial behaviors in adolescents (Sutker, 1982).

Antisocial behaviors tend to cluster and perpetuate, but studies have highlighted particular psychosocial circumstances that increase the probability of antisocial involvement. Recent examples include the work of Farrington (Farrington, 1995, 1997; Farrington & West, 1990) who reported findings from a prospective longitudinal survey of crime and delinquency among 411 male youths drawn from a working-class area of London. Participants were interviewed and tested at ages 8, 10, and 14 and interviewed again at ages 16, 18, and 21 and at ages 25 and 32. Intelligence, academic achievement, school behaviors, personality, psychomotor skills, living circumstances, employment histories, interpersonal relationships, and delinquent acts were assessed, and interviews from teachers and parents yielded additional data. Childhood factors at age 10 that were predictive of future delinquency included teacher ratings as troublesome and dishonest, larger sized families, criminal parents and delinquent older siblings, harsh or erratic parenting techniques, passive or neglectful parental attitudes, and parental conflict. Investigators highlighted the behavioral continuity of this sample and reported that the best independent predictor of offending at any age was troublesome or deviant behaviors at an earlier time. Additional predictors of antisocial offending were economic deprivation, family criminality, poor parenting techniques, and school failure. They also pointed out that the most deviant individuals at one age were the most deviant individuals at later ages, although absolute levels of behavioral deviance could change over time.

These results are consistent with findings that emerged from Loeber and Dishion's (1983) innovative analysis of delinquency data. Attempting to identify variables to improve prediction of the criterion over chance, these researchers reported that parental childrearing techniques, followed by childhood problem behaviors, were most predictive of delinquency. Similarly, Loeber and Stouthamer-Loeber (1987) pointed to such parental factors as supervision, attitude, and involvement as powerful predictors of childhood conduct problems. Reviewing the major epidemiological studies of antisocial behavior in children, Robins (1981) cited a conglomerate of factors that children at risk for antisocial behaviors, including male sex; status as black, urban, and poor; antisocial parents; large sibship size; erratic or excessively lenient parental discipline; and illegitimate or adoptive child status. Robins (1981) underscored the compatibility of these results with explanations that feature social disadvantage, genetic predisposition, family modeling, and psychosocial stress.

## Empirical Tests of Clinical Theory

During the past four decades, researchers have subjected the clinically derived, traditional concept of psychopathy to experimental scrutiny. In addition to efforts to define its inclusionary and exclusionary features, investigators have tested the behavioral excess-deficit hallmarks of psychopathy and attempted to pinpoint shared deficiencies that account for persistently antisocial adjustment. The resulting literature may be summarized by categorizing studies into five subsets, including those that target learning and performance, behavioral extremes and impulsiveness, peculiarities in interpersonal interaction patterns, cognitive or neuropsychological characteristics, and autonomic and cortical arousal phenomena. Although studies have varied in quality, many were executed with sound methodology, and more recent work shows careful regard for multimethod assessment of study participants. Yet, most research has been restricted to prison or drug and alcohol treatment situations, and conclusions based on typically all-male samples are biased by gender effects, as well as by the extreme psychological and physical conditions in which participants are found. Research also suffers from the universal problems of generalizing from the laboratory to the natural environment and inferring individual characteristics from group-derived similarities.

### Learning and Performance Deficits

Theories of psychopathy derived from clinical accounts incorporate the notion that antisocial individuals are inherently deficient in acquiring learned responses. Eysenck (1964) characterized psychopaths as poor learners who extinguish quickly, and Cleckley (1982) described them as incapable of profiting from experience, particularly when the consequences involve punishment. Assumptions of defective learning among psychopaths have captured the interest of researchers since the mid-1950s, and investigators have compared samples of antisocial and control subjects on various tests of learning abilities. The findings generated have not been uniform, but psychopaths have been shown to be inferior in verbal conditioning and verbal learning (Henry & Moffitt, 1997; Johns & Quay, 1962; Quay & Hunt, 1965), semantic processing (Day & Wong, 1996; Hare & Jutai, 1988; Williamson, Harpur, & Hare, 1991), classical conditioning and generalization of autonomic responses (Hare, 1965; Hare & Quinn, 1971), and passive-avoidance learning (Gorenstein & Newman, 1980; Lykken, 1957; Newman, Patterson, & Kosson, 1987; Newman & Schmitt, 1998; Waid & Orne, 1982). At the same time, psychopaths have not necessarily performed more poorly on tasks involving social learning (Kadlub, 1956), learning sets (McCollough & Adams, 1970), verbal conditioning using social reinforcement (Bryan & Kapche, 1967), probability learning where punishment is a near certainty (Siegel, 1978), and paired-associate verbal learning (Gullick, Sutker, & Adams, 1976; Sutker, Gil, & Sutker, 1971). Additionally, psychopaths have not always exhibited deficient avoidance learning (Kosson, Smith, & Newman, 1990; Newman & Kosson, 1986; Newman, Patterson, Howland, & Nichols, 1990; Newman & Schmitt, 1998; Schmauk, 1970; Siegel, 1978).

Given these apparent contradictions, investigators have looked more closely at the parameters of learning, such as the nature of reinforcement, to account for discrepancies. In early studies, Painting (1961) found that primary psychopaths performed as well as controls when incorrect responses resulted in the loss of cigarettes, and

Schmauk (1970) reported that psychopaths behaved comparably to controls when mistakes resulted in monetary losses rather than electric shock or negative social comments. Siegel (1978) found that diminished responsiveness to punishment among psychopathic offenders was greatest when the probability of punishment was most uncertain, whereas Fairweather (1954) showed that psychopaths exhibited maximum performance under conditions of uncertain as opposed to certain or no reward. These studies suggest that both the probability and type of reinforcement can influence learning and performance among psychopaths.

Other aspects of the learning situation may alter performance among psychopaths, such as the timing of reward and response feedback, as well as the sex of the experimenter. In the Painting (1961) study, success rates of primary psychopaths were higher than controls under conditions of reward in which stimuli and responses were delivered in close temporal proximity, but performance decreased as the contiguity between events diminished. Gullick et al. (1976) reported that the acquisition of a paired-associate learning list was slowed by increasing information delay among sociopathic prisoners. Newman, Schmitt, and Voss (1997) demonstrated that low-anxious psychopaths, compared to low-anxious controls, do not exhibit the typical interference due to motivationally neutral contextual cues when the interstimulus interval is short but perform similarly to controls under the long interval–stimulus condition. Newman et al. (1987) compared prison psychopaths and controls on a card-playing task involving monetary rewards and punishments, demands for response set alteration as contingencies changed, and such manipulations as cumulative delay of response feedback and forced postfeedback delays. Psychopaths failed to alter dominant response sets for reward, losing more money than controls, although the combination of postfeedback delays and cumulative feedback reduced their perseverative deficits. Other variables shown to influence learning in psychopaths include the content of the material to be learned (Sutker et al., 1971) and experimenter gender (Bernard & Eisenman, 1967; Stewart & Resnick, 1970).

Several research studies were designed to isolate the factors that contribute to presumed deficiencies in passive-avoidance learning among psychopaths. Linking passive-avoidance deficits

with behavioral disinhibition and pursuit of reward, Newman, Widom, and Nathan (1985) hypothesized that psychopaths falter on passive-avoidance tasks when salient cues for approach responding interfere with processing additional cues that signal the need for response inhibition or behavioral alterations. Testing this notion, Newman et al. (1985) compared psychopathic delinquents and controls using a passive-avoidance paradigm that provided monetary rewards for responding to both positive and negative stimuli. In a second task, rewards were contingent on responding to positive stimuli and withholding responses to negative stimuli. As predicted, psychopathic delinquents committed more passive-avoidance errors than controls on the task that involved both reward and punishment, but not on the reward-only task, that is, delinquent adolescents were deficient in avoiding loss of money when provided competing goals of avoiding punishment while earning rewards.

Newman and Kosson (1986) replicated and extended these findings among White adult prison samples by demonstrating that psychopaths committed more passive-avoidance errors than nonpsychopaths on a computerized task that involved competing reward and punishment contingencies, but performed as well as nonpsychopaths on the same tasks with punishment only. Inconsistent with the authors' reasoning, however, was the absence of performance differences between the two tasks within the psychopathic group. Psychopaths committed no fewer avoidance errors in the punishment-only condition than they did when faced with both reward and punishment. By way of explanation, the researchers suggested that the latter condition may have been more difficult than the former. In a subsequent study involving Black criminal psychopaths and nonpsychopaths, Kosson et al. (1990) found no differences in passive-avoidance performance under competing reward and punishment contingencies, although between-group differences emerged when data from Black subjects were combined with those of White subjects in the earlier study. Newman et al. (1990) also demonstrated a mediating effect of anxiety on passive-avoidance performance among psychopaths such that poor passive-avoidance learning was specific to low-anxiety psychopaths, and Newman and Schmitt (1998) replicated the findings of poor passive-avoidance learning among incarcerated White psychopaths relative to incarcerated White nonpsychopaths. However, consistent with Kosson et al. (1990), Newman and Schmitt (1998) failed to observe the same pattern of results among incarcerated Black psychopaths and nonpsychopaths, and deficits in passive-avoidance learning have not been demonstrated in samples of female psychopaths.

In recent years, Newman and colleagues (Newman, Schmitt, & Voss, 1997; Patterson & Newman, 1993) examined passive-avoidance learning in psychopaths using a response-modulation model, rather than one targeting low fear or insensitivity to punishment cues. Testing this model, Newman, Schmitt, and Voss (1997) studied the effects of peripherally presented motivationally neutral cues on cued recognition in psychopathic and nonpsychopathic (control) prison inmates. Consistent with predictions, low-negative affectivity psychopaths showed significantly less interference when motivationally neutral cues were presented peripherally than low-negative affectivity controls under a short interstimulus interval but not under a long interstimulus interval. These results were not observed in high-negative affectivity psychopaths and controls and were not applicable to Black subjects. Overall, findings were interpreted as supportive of an information-processing response modulation model. On the other hand, Howard, Payamal, and Neo (1997) used a modified version of a cued-reaction task (Howland, Kosson, Patterson, & Newman, 1993) and found no evidence to support response modulation deficits in psychopaths. In fact, subjects showed insensitivity to cues of reward/nonpunishment consistent with an active avoidance deficit, and these investigators interpreted overall performances as congruent with global affective-motivational deficits. Hence, findings remain inconsistent, but the possibility that the passive-avoidance learning deficit among psychopaths may be specific to situations characterized by competing reward and punishment contingencies and to particular subject groups remains an important target for future investigation.

Several studies have shown that psychopaths may not be deficient in acquiring learned responses, learning to avoid punishment, or performing tasks for reward, depending upon the type of comparisons conducted (e.g., Newman & Schmidt, 1998). However, they do behave differently from so-called normal control groups, and the quality of their efforts is more variable and more influenced by salient (and perhaps subtle)

differences in learning context. Type of reward, reinforcement delay, relative probabilities of punishment or reward, timing of discriminative or signaling stimuli, forced response delays, perception of tasks and context, and characteristics of the experimenter have been shown to modify performance. As Lykken (1978) urged, laboratory research must exceed measurement of the obvious situational variables to assess the extent to which the task strikes the fancy of psychopathic subjects. In any case, problem-solving strategies, learning strengths and weaknesses, and characteristic cognitive sets in learning situations remain a fascinating area for research among antisocial individuals.

## Behavior Extremes and Impulsiveness

Clinical observations of behavioral extremes and impulsivity in the face of almost certain untoward consequences led to proposals that psychopaths are characterized by exaggerated needs for sensation-seeking, vulnerability to boredom, and deficits in delay of gratification. Early motivational theories suggest that organisms are driven by needs both to increase and to reduce stimulation. Primate studies show that animals work to glimpse a change of scene (Butler, 1953), manipulate novel stimuli (Harlow, Harlow, & Meyer, 1950), and experience unpatterned light if reared under sensory deprivation (Wendt, Lindsley, Adey, & Fox, 1963), and prolonged sensory deprivation in humans has been associated with severe cognitive and emotional reactions (Zubek, Pushkar, Sansom, & Gowing, 1961). Integrating this knowledge with findings from research with psychopaths (Fairweather, 1954; Fox & Lippert, 1963), Quay (1965) hypothesized that psychopaths require higher, more variable stimulation to maintain positive affect because of their lowered basal reactivity and more rapid adaptation to stimulation. That is, low arousal is seen as representing an aversive physiological state that prompts antisocial individuals to seek out stimulation to increase arousal to optimal or normal levels (Eysenck, 1964; Quay, 1965; Raine, 1993, 1996, 1997). Thus, psychopaths were viewed as fluctuating from baseline stimulus deprivation and affective unpleasantness to states of brief relief associated with sensation-seeking.

Speculations that psychopaths are prompted to exaggerated sensation-seeking and thus to antisocial behaviors were investigated during the

1970s using Zuckerman's Sensation Seeking Scale (SSS: Zuckerman, 1972, 1977). Sensation-seeking reflected by SSS scores has been associated with such antisocial behaviors as gambling among college students (Zuckerman, 1974), prison escapes and disobedience of authority figures among female delinquents (Farley & Farley, 1972), drug use in male veterans and college students (Kilpatrick, Sutker, Roitzsch, & Miller, 1976), arrest chronicity among skid-row alcoholics (Malatesta, Sutker, & Treiber, 1981), college student alcohol and drug use (Zuckerman, Bone, Neary, Mangelsdorff, & Brustman, 1972), and psychopathy in a prison sample (Blackburn, 1978). Additionally, Sutker, Archer, and Allain (1978) found that high sensation seekers among chronic drug using men and women in treatment exhibit Minnesota Multiphasic Personality Inventory (MMPI) responses reflective of greater antisocial inclination, behavioral impulsiveness, and social introversion than their low sensation seeking counterparts. Self-reported behaviors were consistent with SSS and MMPI data, as high sensation seekers reported earlier and more varied drug use as well as pleasure motives for initial alcohol use compared with low sensation seekers who cited peer pressure and conformity as primary motives.

Relationships between sensation-seeking and antisocial behavior have also been implicated in performance studies among children and adults. In two related investigations, DeMyer-Gapin and Scott (1977) and Whitehill, DeMyer-Gapin, and Scott (1976) showed that antisocial children exhibited less time viewing boring material, higher initial levels of attention to novel stimuli, and more extraneous behaviors during experimental tasks than children classified as neurotic. Using a monotonous task called the Prisoner's Dilemma Game, Widom (1976b) found that adult primary psychopaths were as able as nonpsychopaths to tolerate sameness, but that secondary or neurotic psychopaths exhibited greater inability to manage monotony. Widom's (1976b) task required ongoing reciprocal interactions, and results suggested that the conditions under which psychopaths become bored may vary, depending on situational demand characteristics. Her work also highlighted the role of neurotic features in influencing vigilance and other performance behaviors.

Questions concerning capacities for sustained effort and tolerance for sameness among psychopaths have been addressed by evoked potential investigations of attention and information processing. Results from several studies show that psychopaths are capable of proficient selective attention to a video task (Jutai & Hare, 1983) and directing high levels of attention to stimuli of interest (Forth & Hare, 1989; Jutai et al., 1987). Raine and Venables (1987) reported that antisocial 15-year-old boys were more reactive (showed larger P300s) to warning stimuli than their "prosocial" counterparts, and data derived from a subsequent investigation (Raine & Venables, 1988) supported the hypothesis that adult psychopaths are characterized by heightened ability to attend to task-relevant events. Attempting to reconcile these findings with the Cleckley deficit model, Raine and Venables (1988) cautioned that some performance tasks may be too brief to elicit the type of attention deficits described by Cleckley and argued that overly focused short-term attention to events of interest reflects undue emphasis on short-term gratification.

It has been theorized that inability to delay gratification coupled with sensation-seeking contributes to behavioral impulsivity and antisocial outcome (Maher, 1966). Looking at the inability to delay gratification as integrally related to impulsivity, investigators have examined Porteus Maze Test qualitative performance among psychopathic and control groups to assess difficulties in inhibiting impulsive errors. Contrary to expectations, several investigators failed to show performance deficits on this measure. Sutker, Moan, and Swanson (1972) found that prisoner psychopaths showed better qualitative Porteus Maze Test performance than prisoner normals or prisoners labeled antisocial psychotics, differences that could not be attributed to intelligence. Widom (1977) also found relatively fewer Porteus qualitative errors among institutionalized psychopaths than those reported in earlier studies (Fooks & Thomas, 1957; Schalling & Rosen, 1968). Sutker and Allain (1983) reported that male adaptive sociopaths identified among medical students produced significantly more errors on the Porteus qualitative index than their school counterparts who had no detectable psychopathology, whereas overall performance did not differ. In this study, neither group was characterized by significant depression or anxiety, and both showed high levels of intellectual ability. Thus, to some extent, the outcome of psychopath/nonpsychopath comparisons is a function of the subject groups sampled.

Using a different approach, Gullick et al. (1976) investigated the effects of information feedback delay on acquisition rates in paired-associate learning among nonaddict sociopaths, addict sociopaths, and normal controls recruited from male prisoners. Drug use histories were collected by self-report and review of prisoner files, and only primary sociopaths and controls without remarkable psychopathology, defined by a set of MMPI criteria, were recruited. Results showed that reinforcement delay did not interfere with performance among normal subjects, but acquisition rates were significantly slowed under the maximum delay condition in both addicted and nonaddicted sociopathic prisoners. Short delays in information feedback did not impair learning rates, but the maximum delay condition was associated with apparent frustration, annoyance, and self-imposed distractions among primary sociopaths who became restless and bored while waiting for the correct answer. The investigators reasoned that as the structure of the learning task was altered to include frustrating delays, primary sociopaths became impatient for reinforcement and performed less well on task demands than normals who tolerated reinforcement delays without performance changes.

Other factors modified responses to delay conditions when study participants were allowed reward choices. Widom (1977) found that psychopaths recruited from the community chose larger, delayed monetary rewards over smaller, immediate amounts of money and that these decisions were influenced by employment status and MMPI elevations on the Psychopathic Deviate Scale (Pd, or Scale 4). Brown and Gutsch (1985) investigated preferences among primary psychopathic, secondary psychopathic, and nonpsychopathic prisoners for smaller immediate versus larger delayed rewards. Results revealed no significant group differences in reward selection, but neurotic psychopaths were distinguished from primary psychopaths and normal prisoners by what the investigators described as a neurotic cognitive set, including a sense of urgency, indecision, impulsivity, and lack of trust and forethought. By contrast, the other prisoner groups appeared more decisive, agreeable, trusting, and able to delay gratification without accompanying distress. These investigators hypothesized that a relationship exists between deficient ability to delay gratification and neurotic mediating conditions among secondary psycho-

paths. In addition to highlighting the potentially confounding contributions of negative affect, such as depression and anxiety, this study fills an important gap in the psychopathy literature by targeting some of the cognitive underpinnings that prompt behavior in antisocial individuals.

To date, research fails to support the hypothesis that psychopaths cannot postpone gratification or inhibit impulsive errors across situations. Rather, the relationship between impulsivity, at least as related to the delay of gratification, and psychopathy appears to be influenced by such factors as intellectual sophistication, employment status, other types of psychopathology such as anxiety and depression, groups used for comparison, individual learning histories, and other person and situational variables. On the other hand, there is evidence that impulsiveness, eagerness for reward, and antisocial behaviors cluster in association and that the combination may predispose certain individuals to greater impulsivity than might be expected among normal controls. In any case, review of the studies reported here makes it clear that simple generalizing statements about psychopaths are likely to be misleading.

## Peculiarities in Interpersonal Interaction Patterns

Traditional concepts of psychopathy emphasize the blatantly egocentric and unconscionably selfish aspects of associated behaviors. Gough (1948) attributed this deficiency to an inability to view personal actions from another's perspective or to assume another's interpersonal role, and Cleckley (1982) concluded that psychopaths are apathetic to the suffering of others, despite superficial displays of concern. Ullman and Krasner (1975) noted the apparent skillfulness of sociopaths in interpersonal manipulation, and McCord and McCord (1964) pointed to their incapacity to love or form close social attachments. Gorenstein and Newman (1980) wrote that psychopaths disregard totally the sufferings or hardships which may accrue to themselves or others as a result of their behaviors and argued that they adhere to no moral code. These extreme characterizations persist without regard for a growing body of experimental evidence that challenges the assumption of uniform interpersonal deficit and callousness.

Subjecting Cleckley's notion of social insensitivity to experimental scrutiny in a vicarious conditioning paradigm, Sutker (1970) showed that noninstitutionalized sociopathic men were more autonomically responsive than their nonsociopathic counterparts to a stimulus paired with apparently immediate shock to another individual. Sociopaths overresponded to what seemed to be an exciting social stimulus, and it was suggested that sociopaths are sensitive to social cues and emotionally provocative stimuli. In another study, Sutker et al. (1971) reasoned that if this were true, social stimuli might serve as positive reinforcers to modify their behavior more effectively than neutral or nonsocial stimuli. These researchers tested the effects of varied social content ratings of consonant–vowel–consonant (CVC) combinations on speed of acquisition in a serial learning task among imprisoned sociopaths and nonsociopaths. As predicted, sociopaths performed significantly better than nonsociopaths on the list comprised of highly relevant CVCs and acquired this material faster than low social content CVCs, although lists were equated for learning difficulty. Nonsociopaths showed no significant differences in speed of acquisition for the two lists. Complementing these results were those reported by Sutker, Moan, and Allain (1974) who found that noninstitutionalized sociopaths scored significantly better than normals on measures that required observation for detail in the social as well as the tangible environments.

Widom (1976b) investigated interpersonal cooperation during game playing among pairs of primary psychopaths, secondary psychopaths, and controls. Psychopaths did not behave more selfishly or egocentrically, show greater concern with personal gain, or act less responsibly than normal subjects. Widom found that if rewards were sufficient and feedback immediate, psychopaths cooperated with one another, at least for short periods of time. Interestingly, however, psychopaths and normals differed in their perceptions of game partner roles. Nonpsychopathic partners viewed their relationship as a cooperative endeavor, whereas primary and secondary psychopaths regarded their partners as competitors. The strongest support for assumed interpersonal competence deficits among psychopaths was associated with performance among the secondary psychopaths who showed more difficulties in anticipating unpleasant future consequences of their behavior and less accuracy in predicting the behavior of others. Widom reasoned that the discrepancy between primary and

secondary psychopaths represented evidence of the utility of these labels for subtyping antisocial individuals.

Rime, Bouvy, Leborgne, and Rouillon (1978) used videotaped interviews to examine verbal and nonverbal interpersonal behaviors in young male psychopaths aged 12 to 20. Global ratings of their emotional states (e.g., happy, sad, or mad) were also obtained. Compared with controls, psychopathic youths used more hand gestures, leaned toward the interviewer more often, maintained greater eye contact, and tended to smile less frequently. These researchers interpreted their findings as consistent with previous notions about the interpersonal behavior of psychopaths, indicating that the increased levels of nonverbal activity displayed by psychopathic subjects represented intrusive and troublesome behaviors that were likely to be the result of social skill and awareness deficits. Questions can be raised regarding this interpretation, and study findings may be challenged on two counts. Psychopathic subjects in this study received less verbal attention and no tangible reward for participation, and interviews were conducted by an experimenter of the same sex. Both variables have been shown to affect performance among psychopathic participants.

Lee and Prentice (1988) examined empathy, role-taking, cognition, and moral reasoning among incarcerated delinquent boys grouped into psychopathic, neurotic, and subcultural categories and nondelinquent community control subjects. These investigators predicted that psychopathic and neurotic delinquents, compared to subcultural delinquents and nondelinquent controls, would demonstrate relatively deficient performance on such socialization tasks as identifying emotionally with other people, assuming another's perspective, and coping with moral dilemmas. Although delinquents as a group exhibited significantly more immature modes of role-taking, logical cognition, and moral reasoning than nondelinquents, psychopathic and neurotic delinquents did not differ from subcultural delinquents on these measures. Contrary to predictions, no differences in empathy were found among any of the groups. The authors acknowledged that their findings conflict sharply with clinical descriptions of delinquents, particularly psychopaths, as starkly egocentric and deficient in emotional empathy.

Using the repertory grid technique, Widom (1976a) compared the interpersonal and personal construct systems of psychopaths and normals. She found that the construct systems of primary psychopaths were lopsided and idiosyncratic but highly consistent and suggested that they fail to distinguish between their conceptualizations and those of people in general. Secondary psychopaths and controls manifested less lopsidedness, consistency, and social discrepancy. Psychopathic groups showed a significant degree of misperception concerning people in general, but particularly along the dull–exciting construct dimension. Widom concluded that psychopaths failed to entertain adequately the idea that other people construe events differently from them and seem to make little effort to modify their rigid construct systems. These findings underscore the need for continued examination of cognitive inflexibility and idiosyncracies among psychopaths, as well as the extent to which results may be consistent across situations and circumstances.

At least three studies documented bias toward attributions of hostility among aggressive male youths (Dodge & Newman, 1981; Dodge, Pettit, Bates, & Volante, 1995; Nasby, Hayden, & DePaulo, 1980), raising the question whether psychopaths view social situations with overriding negative perceptual sets. Exploring this issue, Blackburn and Lee-Evans (1985) classified sixty offender patients at a psychiatric security hospital into four subgroups using median splits on psychopathy and social withdrawal dimensions. Comparisons of their ratings of reactions to hypothetical situations that represented aspects of frustration, threat, attack, and pain showed more intense responses among psychopaths to anger-provoking situations. Findings were interpreted as evidence of cognitive bias in perceiving interpersonal threat among psychopaths who appeared to be more hypervigilant to violation of their personal domain and more vulnerable to interpersonal than frustrating provocation. Consistent with these data, Sterling and Edelmann (1988) reported that both anxiety and anger situations were perceived as more anger-inducing among psychopaths, compared to nonpsychopathic participants.

Continued study of interpersonal perceptions and behavior among psychopathic or antisocial groups is needed. Research indicates that psychopaths are keen observers of social behavior, are as empathic as nonpsychopaths, find themselves stimulated by socially relevant stimuli, and participate cooperatively in various types of game situations. That psychopaths have been shown to lean toward their interviewers, make longer eye contact, and gesture in conversation is probably as suggestive of facile interpersonal poise as any data yet considered. At the same time, there is evidence that psychopaths share rigid cognitive sets and perceptual biases, particularly with regard to assessing interpersonal threat and the resulting perception of anger. Additionally, psychopaths find difficulty in understanding what others are thinking and feeling because of their own peculiar constructs and assumptions that others perceive circumstances in the same way as themselves. Further investigation of these areas of perceptual and cognitive biases, as well as their implications for communication and interpersonal behavior, may yield results relevant to clinical assessment and management of antisocial individuals.

## Cognitive and Neuropsychological Deficits

Attempts to explain delinquency and antisocial behaviors have included suggestions that there may be relationships between various types of cortical dysfunction and disorders characterized by marked deviations in emotional, motor, and cognitive behaviors. Research speculation in this area has concentrated on frontal lobe dysfunction (e.g., Henry & Moffitt, 1997; Kandel & Freed, 1989), dominant hemisphere dysfunction (Hare, 1979), and weak or unusual lateralization of language function (Day & Wong, 1996; Hare & Jutai, 1988; Raine, O'Brien, Smiley, Scerbo, & Chan, 1990). Probably the most consistently presented of these notions involves positing a relationship between frontal lobe dysfunction and delinquency in youth and antisocial behaviors in adults. As Stuss and Benson (1986) pointed out, however, researchers also attempted to link such major psychiatric disorders as schizophrenia (Benson & Stuss, 1990; Buschbaum, 1990; Robbins, 1990) and depression (Buschbaum, 1986) to frontal lobe pathology.

The special appeal of the frontal lobe hypothesis derives from clinician observations of similarities between problems with cognitive control and uninhibited hedonistic actions thought to characterize psychopaths and the behaviorally restless and apparently gratification-seeking posture often associated with prefrontal pathology. Described as "pseudopsychopathic," the constellation of features often documented following orbital frontal brain damage includes motor disability with the pursuit of immediate gratification, minimal regard for social propriety, and such impulsive, antisocial acts as sexual excesses, crude humor, and unreliability (Stuss & Benson, 1986). Obvious analogies between delinquent and antisocial impulsivity and the disinhibited behaviors of patients with assumed frontal lobe impairment have led to exploration of possible deficits in neuropsychological performance among antisocial subsets which could explain persistent delinquent and antisocial involvements.

Schalling (1978) proposed that some aspects of psychopathy may be attributed to deficiency in frontal lobe processes associated with regulation of attention, emotional responsivity, and behavioral persistence. Integrating evidence that frontal-lobe immaturity may contribute significantly to delinquent behavior, Pontius and her colleagues suggested that delinquency may be tied to frontal lobe system dysfunction (Pontius, 1974; Pontius & Ruttiger, 1976; Pontius & Yudowitz, 1980). A similar line of inquiry offered evidence that anterior neuropsychological dysfunction was associated with criminality, delinquency, and depressive and violent symptoms (Yeudall & Fromm-Auch, 1979; Yeudall, Fromm-Auch, & Davies, 1982). The most clear statement linking frontal lobe dysfunction to neuropsychological deficits among psychopathic subjects, however, was offered by Gorenstein (1982) who classified forty-three male psychiatric patients and eighteen male university students into psychopathic and nonpsychopathic groups. Subjects were administered a battery of cognitive tests, including the Necker Cube, the Wisconsin Card Sorting Test (WCST), a sequential matching memory task (SMMT), the Stroop Color-Word Test, and an anagram task. Group performance did not differ on the latter two measures, but psychopaths exhibited more spontaneous reversals of the Necker Cube, greater numbers of SMMT errors, and more perseverative errors on the WCST. Based upon these data, Gorenstein concluded that psychopaths were deficient in cognitive processes associated with frontal lobe functioning and suffered impaired ability to modulate dominant response sets.

Limitations in the Gorenstein (1982) study conceptualization and methodology, as well as in this researcher's conclusions, have been described in subsequent reports. Hare (1984) criticized Gorenstein (1982) for procedures used to subdivide participants into psychopathic/nonpsychopathic categories and suggested that group differences might be attributed to the influences of age, education, ability, substance abuse, and college student status. Attempting to replicate Gorenstein's (1982) findings, Hare (1984) compared three groups of White prison inmates divided by thirds into high, medium, and low psychopathy categories based on his twenty-two-item psychopathy checklist. Because groups did not differ in intelligence, age, education, or CPI *So* score or in performance on the three cognitive tasks used by Gorenstein (1982), Hare (1984) concluded that the efforts of psychopaths were not at all like those of frontal lobe patients. Subsequently, Hart, Forth, and Hare (1990) found no differences in neuropsychological test performance of two samples of high, moderate, and low psychopathy subjects. Results were consistent with earlier data reported by Sutker, Moan, and Allain (1983) who demonstrated that psychopathic and normal control prisoners showed no differences in tendencies to persist in incorrect responding, to disregard cues suggesting the need to modify behavior, or to proceed impulsively in problem solving as reflected by performances on the WCST and circle drawing and maze tracing tasks.

Sutker and Allain (1987) administered the WCST, Visual Verbal Test, and Porteus Maze Test to nineteen psychopathic and fifteen normal patients undergoing substance abuse treatment, subjects drawn from a population demographically similar to that of Gorenstein's (1982). These investigators assessed the effects of intellectual sophistication by using analyses of covariance and tested the hypothesis that psychopaths are characterized by no greater difficulties in controlling impulsiveness, planning ahead, and exercising cognitive flexibility (such as accommodating shifts and avoiding perseverations) than nonpsychopathic controls. Psychopathic subjects did not differ from controls across the cognitive measures thought to reflect frontal lobe functioning, specifically, planning, flexibility, attention, control, and abstraction. Sutker and Allain (1987) suggested that it may be misleading to conceptualize behavioral or neurophysiological analogies between frontal lobe and psychopathic patients. Hoffman, Hall, and Bartsch (1987) also failed to find evidence that psychopathic individuals performed more poorly than nonpsychopaths on tasks sensitive to frontal lobe functioning.

Devonshire et al. (1988) criticized both Gorenstein (1982) and Hare (1984) for ignoring the distinction drawn by Blackburn (1979b) between primary and secondary psychopaths. Examining performance on a modified version of the Wisconsin Card Sorting Test, these investigators found no differences between subjects classified legally as psychopathically disordered or as mentally ill, and no differences between those classified as high or low in psychopathy using an abbreviated form of Hare's Psychopathy Checklist. A subgroup of primary psychopaths achieved significantly more categories and made fewer errors than a subgroup of secondary psychopaths, leading to the hypothesis that anxious, socially withdrawn individuals, regardless of psychopathy, may be unable to maintain a cognitive set resulting from overappraisal of threat. They proposed that the discrepancy between Gorenstein's (1982) and Hare's (1984) data can be attributed to inconsistent selection criteria and suggested that studies using Hare's Psychopathy Checklist for classification fail to find differences in frontal lobe functioning because of failure to differentiate primary and secondary psychopaths. Supporting this logic in part, Smith, Arnett, and Newman (1992) reported poorer performance among low-anxious psychopaths than high-anxious psychopaths on Trail Making Part B and WAIS-R Block Design tests. However, differences were predicted on six tests of the battery but were found on only two, and the observed significant differences were not apparent when groups were collapsed across anxiety levels.

In a review of the frontal lobe hypothesis and psychopathy, Kandel and Freed (1989) highlighted the complexities in attempting to evaluate frontal lobe dysfunction among antisocial samples. Allowing that such deficits were possible, particularly as regards associations between criminality and dysfunction localized in the anterior regions of the brain, they concluded that existing evidence does not point conclusively to frontal lobe dysfunction in psychopaths. Among the limitations of research studies in the area, they called attention to problems with selecting psychopaths and appropriate control samples, and Henry and Moffitt (1997) concurred and suggested that varied and sometimes unreliable diagnostic procedures

used to define psychopathy may well account for inconsistency of findings. Kandel and Freed (1989) also pointed to contributions of confounding variables such as alcohol and drug abuse, institutionalization, use of questionable frontal lobe measures, lack of dependent measures reflective of other cognitive functions, and absence of corroborative evidence from neuroanatomical indexes. Taking a broader perspective, Stuss and Benson (1986) cautioned that disorders that alter frontal lobe functions exert widespread effects because of frontal anatomical connections with other cortical and subcortical structures; argued against easy localization of mood, behavioral, or cognitive functions to this area; and presented evidence that most measures considered sensitive to frontal lobe impairment can also be affected by impairment in other areas. Clearly then, a hasty diagnosis of frontal lobe malfunction based on the results of several psychological tests may be misleading.

In addition to the complex integrative functions of the frontal lobes and limitations in our expertise to measure such functions with specificity are the problems associated with comparing grossly defined psychopathic and nonpsychopathic groups. Devonshire et al. (1988) criticized Hare (1984) for ignoring differences between primary and neurotic or secondary psychopaths, but more critically limiting factors are failures to employ both exclusionary and inclusionary criteria to define psychopathic and nonpsychopathic groups and to take into account the total range of possible psychopathology that might characterize psychopaths or nonpsychopaths and thereby influence findings. It is insufficient to define psychopaths by reference to psychopathy criteria alone or without regard for the assessment of complicating psychopathology such as depression, anxiety, schizophrenia, and other Axis II disorders. By the same token, selection of control subjects using criteria that solely determine that they are not psychopathic ignores the possibility and perhaps likelihood that other significant psychopathology may exist.

## Arousal Levels and Responsivity

There is a rich tradition of attempts to account for functional disorders and disregulated emotions and behaviors by reference to what has been called arousal theory. Operational definitions of arousal vary widely, depending upon researcher orientation and measurement expertise. Descriptions of arousal may highlight nonspecific baseline or resting levels and changes to such, attentional phenomena and mental control, autonomic responsivity and energization associated with threat, and activation of behaviors in the service of specific appetitive or aversive needs or in response to incentives. Assessment of arousal can incorporate tests of mental alertness and diligence, measures of resting level and reactive electrodermal and heart rate activity, electrophysiological monitoring of event-related potentials and other central nervous system (CNS) phenomena, and, more recently, brain imaging technology such as single photon emission computerized tomography (SPECT). Whether studies target attention and orientation, learning and performance, or autonomic reactivity and conditioning, there is a fundamental interrelatedness to this work, because of commonalities in the neuroanatomical basis for arousal described by Stuss and Benson (1986) as the tripartite neural axis, including the reticular activating system, thalamus, and frontal lobes and their connections.

One of the first investigators to call attention to the relationship between psychopathy and arousal idiosyncracies was Lykken (1957) who showed that psychopaths were slow to condition fear to warning signals, inclined to ignore painful electric shocks that normals learned to avoid, and less influenced by fear reactions. Building on this classic investigation and the arousal literature, Quay (1965) and Eysenck (1964) developed arousal models to account for psychopathy and posited mechanisms of hypoarousal and rapid habituation to stimuli as prompting behaviors which were apparently unfettered by fears of consequences and such psychological deterrents as anxiety and anticipation of shame. There has been no decline in interest in arousal theory related to psychopathy, as evidenced by more than forty years of research by Hare (1970, 1978, 1982; Jutai et al., 1987), work by Raine and colleagues (1987; Raine, Venables, & Williams, 1990a,b,c, 1995, 1996; Brennan et al., 1997), and conceptual papers by Fowles (1980, 1993), Ellis (1987), Gray (1994), Mawson and Mawson (1977), and Quay (1993).

A considerable body of experimental findings has been generated in attempts to elucidate the arousal characteristics of psychopaths. Evidence is reasonably clear-cut that psychopaths do not necessarily differ from nonpsychopaths in cardiovascular activity in resting situations (Blackburn,

1978, 1979a; Hare, 1982; Hare et al., 1978; Steinberg & Schwartz, 1976). Raine (1993, 1997) reviewed this extensive literature and concluded with respect to heart rate that studies of institutionalized criminals and psychopaths have not evidenced lowered resting heart rate levels, whereas research with noninstitutionalized conduct-disordered, delinquent, and antisocial children and adults has consistently shown lowered resting heart rate levels in antisocial youth. Raine (1997) concluded that lowered heart rate is a common predisposition to antisocial behavior in general but not to institutionalized, psychopathic criminal behavior in particular (p. 290).

Studies of electrodermal activity among antisocial individuals have yielded mixed results. Some research has documented significantly lower resting levels of skin conductance among psychopaths (Blankstein, 1969; Dengerink & Bertilson, 1975), whereas other studies showed no differences (Borkovec, 1970; Hare, 1982; Hare & Craigen, 1974; Hare et al. 1978; Schmauk, 1970; Sutker, 1970). In a group of 16-year-old delinquents, Raine et al. (1990b) found lower resting skin conductance levels among those who later became criminals by age 24, compared to those who did not. There are also reports of decreased frequency of nonspecific electrodermal responses in resting situations in psychopaths (Fox & Lippert, 1963; Hare & Quinn, 1971), no differences (Hare et al., 1978; Steinberg & Schwartz, 1976), and higher nonspecific frequency (Blankstein, 1969).

The hyporeactivity hypothesis has led to studies of skin conductance orienting amplitude to unsignaled neutral tone stimuli. Borkovec (1970) found that psychopathic delinquents gave smaller orienting responses to the first in a series of neutral tones than a group of subcultural and neurotic delinquents, results similar to those reported by Siddle, Nicol, and Foggitt (1973). Other investigations of electrodermal responses to unsignaled stimuli have yielded conflicting findings when adult psychopathic and nonpsychopathic groups were compared. In most cases, researchers reported no differences between psychopaths and nonpsychopaths on such measures (Blackburn, 1979a; Hare et al., 1978), whereas other work showed that psychopaths were less responsive (Blankstein, 1969; Hare, 1978). To some extent, the discrepancies in findings may be attributed to inconsistencies in the selection procedures of clinical samples as well as differences in measurement methodology, but results do not necessarily support the hypoarousal hypothesis.

Two additional studies failed to obtain lower than normal skin conductance orienting responses among children with delinquent potential (Mednick, 1977) or antisocial behaviors (Venables, 1987). However, as described earlier in this chapter, Raine et al. (1990b) found lower resting skin conductance levels among 16-year-old youths who later became criminals by age 24, compared to those who did not. With respect to skin conductance levels, reviews were conducted and summarized by Fowles (1993) and Raine (1993, 1997). Fowles (1993) reported that differences in the direction of lowered resting levels of sweat gland activity among psychopaths may occasionally be observed, but the effect sizes are small, and evidence for nonspecific fluctuations is even weaker. Raine (1993, 1997) concluded that there is minimal evidence for lower skin conductance arousal levels in psychopaths. However, when groups are defined on the basis of antisocial behavior in general, there is clear evidence of lower skin conductance levels and fewer nonspecific skin conductance responses during rest.

Contradictory findings weaken the case for the notion that psychopaths share baseline levels of underarousal, although this possibility has not been fully dismissed. Hare (1978) argued that basal skin conductance in psychopaths was lower in absolute magnitude in several studies where significant differences were not necessarily observed. He reported that when data from eight studies were pooled, psychopaths showed significantly lower skin conductance but not differences in nonspecific frequencies. Mawson and Mawson (1977) disagreed with this line of reasoning and proposed a neurochemical model to account for patterns of psychophysiological and behavioral activity manifested by psychopaths. These investigators suggested that rather than higher or lower arousals levels *per se*, psychopaths might best be described as more variable and unpredictable in their arousal tendencies than others. This hypothesis is consistent with accumulating data describing their learning performance, attention characteristics, and interpersonal behaviors. Clearly, psychopaths are more variable in the level to which they apply themselves in structured situations as well as more vulnerable to the influence of factors which do not impact so-called normals.

Some research showed that the amplitude of electrodermal responsivity among normal participants may be proportional to the extent to which the eliciting stimuli evoke emotion or attention (Raskin, 1973). Most data on the psychophysiology of antisocial subjects have been generated in paradigms with low sensory stimulation and relatively uninteresting stimuli, such as tones. However, the extent to which stimuli may be viewed as exciting, either positively or negatively, has relevance to tests of hypoarousal theories of psychopathy, but these parameters have been explored minimally among psychopaths. Studying electrodermal activity as a measure of vicariously instigated autonomic conditioning in a time-delay paradigm and using electric shock to a model as the unconditioned stimulus (UCS), Sutker (1970) found that observing another in discomfort elicited changes in electrodermal activity in sociopathic compared to nonsociopathic men to the stimulus paired with shock. Sociopaths showed less electrodermal anticipation of shock and responded less to the shock stimulus in later conditioning trials. That sociopaths displayed greater initial responsiveness to an exciting stimulus and produced responses out of proportion to the situation suggests a pattern of hyperreactivity and rapid return to the baseline consistent with Quay's (1965) hypoarousal model.

Contrary to diminished anticipatory electrodermal activity in conditioning situations, psychopaths are not deficient in heart-rate (HR) conditioning or anticipatory HR responses preceding noxious stimulation (Hare, 1978). In fact, studies indicate that psychopaths exhibit greater HR increases to signals of impending noxious stimuli than control subjects. For example, Hare and Craigen (1974) requested psychopathic and nonpsychopathic prisoners to administer electric shocks preceded by a 10-second tone to themselves and others. In anticipation of shock to themselves or others, psychopaths showed initial HR acceleration in contrast to nonpsychopaths, whose HR decelerated. In another study, Hare et al. (1978) divided groups of psychopathic prisoners into high and low scorers on the CPI *So* Scale and exposed them to a series of 120-db tones, preceded by 12-second countdown. Subjects defined as high in psychopathy differed from the other groups in showing marked HR acceleration and small increases in electrodermal activity before tone presentation.

Hare (1978) hypothesized that anticipatory HR

acceleration observed among psychopaths in conjunction with small increases in electrodermal arousal may be part of an active process for coping with perceived threat and reducing the salience and arousing functions of premonitory cues. Using a distraction paradigm to determine whether psychopaths exhibit a pattern of HR acceleration and little electrodermal arousal when able to remove themselves physically from the warning signals, Hare (1982) found that small electrodermal responses in psychopaths were associated with decreased HR during trials that included avoidable punishment in conjunction with an opportunity for distraction from premonitory cues, rather than the increase found in previous studies. He speculated that psychopaths may use active coping mechanisms associated with the observed HR increase only when the nature of the situation forces them to attend to premonitory cues (as in countdown and classical conditioning procedures), whereas under other conditions, they may be able to focus on stimuli of immediate interest and effectively ignore warning cues.

In an interesting series of studies of arousal, Raine and colleagues collected psychophysiological data in an unselected school sample of male youths at age 15, followed the youths to determine who exhibited adult criminal behavior, and retrospectively analyzed the data to identify characteristics predictive of subsequent criminality. Raine et al. (1990a,b,c) found that youths who went on to become criminals showed electrodermal, cardiovascular, and cortical underarousal (i.e., fewer nonspecific skin conductance responses, lower resting heart rate levels, excessive theta wave electroencephalograms, and lower amplitudes of skin conductance orienting responses to a tone) and enhanced attentional processing as measured by P300 event-related potentials (ERPs). In later studies (Raine, Venables, & Williams, 1995, 1996), the sample was further subdivided into seventeen antisocial adolescents who desisted from adult crime, seventeen antisocial adolescents who became criminals by age 29, and seventeen nonantisocial, noncriminal controls. The groups were matched in demographic and, where appropriate, adolescent antisocial behavior variables. Compared to those who became criminals, subjects who desisted from adult crime exhibited significantly higher heart rate levels at age 15, more nonspecific skin conductance responses, higher amplitudes of skin conductance orienting responses, better skin conductance conditioning, and faster half-recovery time of the skin conductance response. Findings were specific to autonomic arousal because the groups did not differ in resting EEG levels, and were interpreted as suggesting that higher levels of autonomic activity during adolescence may act as a protective factor against the development of adult antisocial behavior defined by criminal conviction.

Raine and colleagues further investigated the possible protective effects of elevated autonomic arousal in different samples. Brennan et al. (1997) collected skin conductance and heart rate data in an orienting paradigm in four groups of Danish men: criminal sons with criminal fathers, noncriminal sons with criminal fathers, criminal sons with noncriminal fathers, and noncriminal sons with noncriminal fathers. Skin conductance, heart rate orienting activity, and the percentage of subjects who evidenced a skin conductance orienting response were greater among the noncriminal sons with criminal fathers than in the other groups. These results were consistent with earlier work by Raine et al. (1995, 1996) who identified elevated autonomic nervous system reactivity as an apparent protective factor for male subjects at high risk of criminal behavior, i.e., elevated skin conductance and heart rate orienting reactivity was associated with a lower likelihood of a criminal outcome. Additionally, Scarpa, Raine, Venables, and Mednick (1997) measured heart rate and skin conductance arousal in a large sample of 3-year-old Mauritian children classified on the basis of social behavior as inhibited, uninhibited, or neither inhibited nor uninhibited. They found that at this young age, inhibited children could be differentiated from uninhibited children by faster heart rate and higher skin conductance in response to a tone stimulus and, given that reduced behavioral inhibition may underlie psychopathic behavior, suggested that early detection of inhibited and uninhibited individuals may have implications for prevention of antisocial behaviors.

Two attempts to create order from the complex array of data extracted from the studies that targeted arousal characteristics among psychopaths are papers by Fowles (1980, 1984, 2001) and Ellis (1987). Both are important for their integrative perspective and suggestions of promising research directions. Drawing from a broadly-based literature on learning and motivation, Fowles (1980, 1984, 2001) called attention to Gray's (1975, 1976,

1985) hypothesized antagonistic appetitive and aversive motivational systems. The proposed aversive system is labeled the behavioral inhibition system (BIS) and is conceptualized as responsible for inhibiting behavior in punishment and extinction situations and, hence, as the substrate for anxiety. In this model, the BIS has input into the nonspecific arousal system associated with the reticular activating system. Arousal effects are thereby inferred when there is increased behavioral vigor without an increase in incentive. The BIS acts in opposition to the approach system, the Behavioral Approach System (BAS), that activates behavior in response to conditioned stimuli for rewards. Thus, two mutually antagonistic systems determine whether behavior will be activated or inhibited, and both are assumed to have positive input into the arousal system that increases behavioral vigor or intensity.

Given this background, Fowles (1980, 2001) hypothesized that the clinical aspects of psychopathy are interpretable as direct manifestations of a weak or deficient BIS in combination with a normal or strong BAS that predicts reduced sensitivity to threatening stimuli and attenuated anxiety in normally stressful situations. This assumption also predicts that reward-seeking behavior will be disinhibited by virtue of the inability of punishing conditioned stimuli and rewarding conditioned stimuli to inhibit approach responses. Fowles noted that this notion has appeal because it complements the psychophysiological evidence reviewed by Hare (1978) as well as data collected in animal experiments, where septal lesions produced similar behavioral deviance. He observed that psychopaths are not deficient in their behavioral activation system and that, therefore, reward-seeking and active-avoidance behaviors are not implicated or deficient. In a variant on this theme, Gorenstein and Newman (1980) and Newman and Wallace (1993) presented psychopaths as characterized by the most extreme form of human disinhibition and posited a functional analogy between animals with septal lesions or septohippocampal system dysfunction and psychopathy. Deriving from this "septal model" is the hypothesis that the psychopath's apparent insensitivity to punishment reflects a deficiency in response modulation, that is, difficulty in suspending a dominant set to accommodate feedback from the environment.

Taking a somewhat different approach, Ellis (1987) proposed that if psychopathy and criminality were integrally associated with suboptimal arousal, they should correlate positively with other hypothesized behavioral systems of arousal deficiency. After reviewing of the literature on arousal theory applied to criminality and psychopathy, he suggested that eight behavior patterns besides criminality and psychopathy should be enhanced by suboptimal arousal: resistance to punishment, impulsivity, childhood hyperactivity, sensation-seeking and risk-taking, neurologically active recreational drug use including heavy alcohol use, extraversion, sexual promiscuity, and poor academic performance. He concluded that the data reviewed supported the proposed relationship between criminality and psychopathy and the hypothesized behavioral manifestations of suboptimal arousal. Attempting to account for variations in these arousal tendencies, Ellis (1987) cast arousal theory in an evolutionary context and argued that hormonal and genetic factors combined to contribute to variations in criminal behavior and psychopathy.

An exciting and promising advance in the study of arousal and antisocial behavior involves recent applications of brain imaging technology. Intrator et al. (1997) used single photon emission computerized tomography (SPECT) to investigate relative cerebral blood flow (rCBF) during a semantic and affective processing task in two patient groups, PCL-R-defined psychopaths (n = 8) and nonpsychopaths (n = 9), and a normal control group (n = 9). Patient groups were recruited from an inpatient substance abuse program at a Veterans Affairs Medical Center. Subjects were administered a lexical decision task that required rapid identification of strings of letters as real words or nonwords. Words and nonwords were presented in separate blocks counterbalanced across subjects. One block consisted of neutral words, whereas the other block comprised emotional words. Psychopaths showed greater activation (i.e., perfusion) in the emotional condition relative to the neutral condition in four areas—the left and right frontal temporal regions and the left and right subcortical regions contiguous to them. In contrast, nonpsychopaths and controls exhibited the opposite pattern—greater activation in the neutral condition relative to the emotional condition in these areas. Groups did not differ in decision times or accuracy levels on the lexical decision task. Thus, it was unlikely that SPECT findings reflected group differences in levels of alertness or motivation.

Other studies applying brain imaging technology to the study of social deviance focused on specific antisocial behaviors such as violence. For example, Raine and colleagues used positron emission tomography (PET) to study glucose metabolism in murderers (or attempted murderers) who pleaded not guilty by reason of insanity (Raine, Buschbaum, & LaCasse, 1997). Compared to age- and sex-matched normal controls, murderers showed lowered glucose metabolism in the prefrontal cortex, superior parietal gyrus, left angular gyrus, and the corpus callosum, as well as abnormal asymmetries of activity (i.e., left hemisphere lower than right hemisphere) in the amygdala, thalamus, and medial temporal lobe (Raine et al., 1997). Subsequently, Raine et al. (1998) reanalyzed these data after subdividing the murderer group into affective murderers who acted impulsively and predatory murderers who planned their crimes. Of the forty-one murderers, fifteen were categorized as strongly predatory and constituted the predatory group, and nine murderers classified as strongly affective comprised the affective group. Murderers who were rated as neither strongly predatory nor strongly affective (n = 17) were eliminated from data analyses. Relative to control subjects, affective murderers showed lower left and right prefrontal functioning, higher right-hemisphere subcortical functioning, and lower right-hemisphere prefrontal/subcortical ratios. Predatory murderers exhibited prefrontal functioning similar to that of controls but significantly higher right subcortical activity. Raine et al. (1998) suggested that although excessive subcortical activity may predispose to aggressive behaviors, murderers who act emotionally, impulsively, and without planning are less able to control aggressive impulses generated from subcortical structures because of deficits in prefrontal regulatory functioning. In contrast, predatory murderers who act purposefully to achieve a goal have sufficient prefrontal functioning to regulate aggressive impulses deriving from excessive subcortical activity.

Regardless of the differences in subject selection procedures and measurement methodology, the conglomerate of attention, learning, conditioning, and arousal studies suggests certain commonalities in responding by psychopaths that set them apart from so-called normal individuals and in some instances from other clinical groups. Comparisons with psychotic and other clinical groups

have been conspicuous for their absence, although attention has been focused on clinical samples that share antisocial and schizoid or schizophrenic-like symptomatology (Crider, 1993; Goodwin & Guze, 1989; Raine, 1987; Sutker et al., 1972). The most uniform and salient findings to be extracted from the literature on arousal and psychopathy are those suggesting that psychopaths are slow to condition fear to warning signals, are less influenced by threats of punishment, are capable of anticipating negative consequences at least on some level, and are inclined to overrespond to unusual or exciting stimuli. Implications for arousal theory in accounting for sensation-seeking behaviors, problems with delay of gratification, peculiarities in attention to cues that are relevant and irrelevant, and performance in a variety of learning situations have yet to be explored fully. That such neurotic features as anxiety and depression may influence responses on many dependent variables employed in research with psychopaths suggests the need for more careful definition of subject groups, and comparisons of psychopaths with other clinical groups might shed light on both their relative areas of deficiency and their strengths.

## Assessment of Antisocial Personality

Beginning with publication of the DSM-III (1980) and continuing through the publication of DSM-III-R (1987) and DSM-IV (1994), clinicians and researchers have refined their conceptualizations of psychological assessment and methodologies for identifying and describing psychopathology. Renewed interest in the area of clinical diagnosis has increased recognition of the need for multimethod, multivariate measurement and widespread attention to the problems of assuring diagnostic validity and reliability. Disorders or symptom clusters are less likely to be viewed in isolation, and requirements for uncovering comorbidities and areas of symptom overlap and differentiation are better understood. Hence, the appropriateness of simple distinctions between pathological and nonpathological groups has been called into question. Topics in clinical assessment are now scrutinized in the light of the literature on behavioral consistency over time and situations, the relationships of traits and symptoms to biological substrates, and the perspectives on continuity in behavioral normality and disorder. Assessment researchers have also become more interested in the results of studies describing relationships between specific disorders and models of personality superstructures (Cloninger, 1987; Eysenck & Eysenck, 1985; Tellegen, 1985), including the DSM-III-R and DSM-IV defined personality disorder clusters (Axelrod, Widiger, Trull, & Corbitt, 1997; O'Connor & Dyce, 1998).

Issues in classifying and labeling psychopathology are presented by Adams, Luscher, and Bernat in Chapter 1 of this volume. This discussion calls attention to the changing nature of clinical and research assessment and the proliferation of instruments developed to measure personality disorders and antisocial personality in particular. A series of reviews describes these changes in standardized measurement (Lilienfeld, Purcell, & Jones-Alexander, 1997; Reich, 1987, 1989; Widiger & Frances, 1987), and a discussion of the instruments developed for this purpose and their relative strengths and weaknesses is presented by Widiger and Trull (1993). It is worth noting, however, that unstructured approaches to clinical diagnosis have declined in popularity and usefulness, and behavior rating and symptom checklists are being superseded by more sophisticated techniques that accomplish many of the same purposes and considerably more. Complementing similar approaches to Axis I disorders, a variety of structured interview and self-report inventory methodologies is available for personality disorder diagnosis, facilitating multimethod, multivariate assessment and offer options to enhance reliability and validity.

## Structured and Semistructured Interviews

Widiger and Frances (1987) described nine structured interviews for personality disorder diagnosis, and Reich (1989) added three to the list. With ongoing data collection and instrument revisions, it becomes difficult to select measures appropriate to clinical or research tasks and likely to yield data comparable to those collected by others, especially in the future. Among the more widely used instruments is the Structured Clinical Interview for DSM-IV Personality Disorders (SCID-II: First, Spitzer, Williams, Gibbon, & Benjamin, 1994), companion to the SCID-I for Axis I disorders and said to be relatively efficient in time

demands. The eighty-one-item Personality Interview Questions (PIQ-II) developed by Widiger (1987) yields nine-point ratings based on reported behaviors and patient self-evaluations, and interviewers solicit behavioral examples or supporting incidents for each symptom. Other useful interviews are the Structured Interview for DSM-III-R Personality Disorders (SIDP: Pfohl, Coryell, Zimmerman, & Stangl, 1986) and the Personality Disorder Examination (PDE) developed by Loranger and colleagues (Loranger, 1988; Loranger, Susman, Oldham, and Russakoff, 1987).

## Self-Report Inventories

Multiscale inventories have been published for personality disorder diagnosis, including the Personality Diagnostic Questionnaire (PDQ: Hyler et al., 1989), Personality Adjective Checklist (Strack, 1987), and Wisconsin Personality Inventory (WISPI: Klein, Benjamin, Greist, Rosenfeld, & Treece, 1989). The most popular and widely applied instruments are the Millon Clinical Multiaxial Inventory (MCMI: Millon, 1983) and its successors, the MCMI-II (Millon, 1987) and MCMI-III (Millon, 1994), which are probably more reflective of Millon's (1981) comprehensive explication of personality disorder psychopathology than that offered by the DSM-III, -III-R, and -IV. Cloninger's (1987) Tridimensional Personality Questionnaire (TPQ) reflects an ambitious theoretical integration of relationships among neurochemical substrates and the behavioral traits of novelty seeking (dopamine system), harm avoidance (serotonergic system), and reward dependence (norepinephrine system). Presented in a 100-item forced-choice format, the TPQ may stimulate brain–behavior investigations innovatively.

Morey, Waugh, and Blashfield (1985) introduced a set of eleven scales for diagnosing personality disorder using a combined rational/empirical strategy for selecting 164 items from the MMPI pool. Although correlations among the scales in a sample of 475 patients were consistent with theoretical expectations regarding personality disorder relationships, questions have been raised about the diagnostic efficiency and validity of the MMPI personality disorder scales (Widiger & Frances, 1987). Dubro, Wetzler, and Kahn (1988) found that the scales are sensitive and specific for diagnosing any DSM-III personality disorder and for diagnosing Cluster 2 and 3 disorders; however, the instrument tended to underdiagnose borderline, histrionic, and dependent psychopathology. The personality disorder scales appear to discriminate patients with specific personality disorders from normal and other personality-disordered patients (Morey, Blashfield, Webb, & Jewell, 1988), and robust correlations between MMPI PD and MCMI scale scores have been reported (Dubro & Wetzler, 1989). Preliminary studies suggest that although the PD scales warrant further testing and validation, they hold promise for clinical and research applications (Wiggins & Pincus, 1989).

Several unidimensional self-report scales have been widely accepted for identifying antisocial features. These include the MMPI and MMPI-2 Psychopathic Deviate ($Pd$) Scale, often used in combination with the MMPI Hypomania ($Ma$) Scale, and the Socialization Scale ($So$) derived from the CPI. The $Pd$ Scale (Scale 4), particularly when combined with $Ma$ (Scale 9), has become synonymous with the hallmark features of psychopathy or antisocial personality. Developed to identify nonconforming and antisocial individuals, or psychopathic personalities (McKinley & Hathaway, 1944), the $Pd$ Scales derived from the MMPI and now the MMPI-2 have been associated with textbook definitions of the characteristics traditionally assigned to psychopaths (Gilberstadt & Duker, 1965; Graham, 1993; Marks, Seeman, & Haller, 1974). Clinical descriptions of the 4–9/9–4 and spike 4 code types emphasize irresponsible, egocentric, demanding, impulsive, poor socialization, and acting-out features. Additionally, research showed associations between $Pd$ elevations and criminality (Sutker & Moan, 1973), antisocial personality in offender populations (Walters, 1985), illicit drug dependence in men and women (Sutker, 1971; Sutker, Patsiokas, & Allain, 1981), alcoholism (Kammeier, Hoffman, & Loper, 1973; Overall, 1973), and more general antisocial features (Graham, 1987, 1993). Scores on $Pd$ have been used effectively in combination with $So$ and indexes of psychopathology such as anxiety and depression to derive antisocial or psychopathic groups (Brown & Gutsch, 1985; Gullick et al., 1976; Heilbrun, 1979, 1982; Newman et al., 1985; Sutker & Allain, 1987), although Hare and his colleagues (Harpur et al., 1989) cautioned against usng them for these purposes.

Predicated on Gough's (1948, 1960) view of sociopathy as a defect in role-taking and socialization, Gough and Peterson (1952) developed a De-

linquency ($De$) Scale which was cross-validated and revised to form the $So$. Lower scores on the fifty-four-item $So$ have been related to rule breaking and norm violations (Megargee, 1972) and to performance and physiological correlates of psychopathy (Rosen & Schalling, 1971; Waid & Orne, 1982). Widom (1976a) found that lower $So$ scores were associated with lopsided and idiosyncratic personal construct systems among psychopaths, and Rosen (1977) concluded that subjects can be ordered along a latent dimension of differences in role-taking ability that relate to varying degrees of general socialized behavior. Gough (1975) contended that scale scores were not significantly influenced by socioeconomic status or intelligence and could be expected to predict, as a broad dispositional variable, a range of interpersonal behaviors and social activities that in themselves might not be highly correlated. Among other scales developed to measure the psychopathy construct is Hare's (1985) Self-Report Psychopathy Scale (SRP) and the revised Self-Report Psychopathy Scale-II (SRP-II: 1996a), designed to complement his behavioral checklist. Although Hart and Hare (1997) pointed out that the SRP-II constituted part of the DSM-IV field trial for antisocial personality disorder (Widiger et al., 1996), they cautioned that scores on self-report scales should not be confused with clinical or behavioral assessments based on reliable and valid criteria for the disorder (p. 26).

Attempting to isolate the emotional and interpersonal features fundamental to a working concept of psychopathy, Blackburn (1974, 1979b) constructed the Special Hospitals Assessment of Personality and Socialization (SHAPS), a 213-item, ten-scale self-report inventory composed of MMPI items, including some from the MMPI $Pd$ Scale and items from the Buss–Durkee Hostility Inventory (Bendig, 1962) and Psychopathic Delinquency Scale of Peterson, Quay, and Cameron (1959). Cluster analysis of the SHAPS indicated four broad offender classes (primary psychopathic, secondary psychopathic, controlled, and inhibited) and two factors (one defined by psychopathy and antisocial aggression; the other by shyness, introversion, anxiety, and depression). Emerging from this research, Blackburn (1987) developed forty-item Belligerence ($B$) and twenty-seven-item Withdrawal ($W$) Scales which were highly correlated with factor scores among psychiatric offender samples. Blackburn (1987) argued that the $B$ Scale offered advantages over $Pd$

as a unitary measure of psychopathy, because it tapped an interpersonal dimension reflecting mistrust and lack of regard that is expressed in punitive and coercive behaviors and correlates highly with *Pd*, observer ratings of antisocial aggression, and Cleckley's criteria of psychopathy.

## Behavior and Symptom Checklists

Several behavior checklists have been designed for assessing psychopathy and antisocial personality. One of their primary advantages has been to collect objective, performance-based ratings of specific symptoms and their severity applicable to individuals at certain times. Judgments are rendered by clinicians or by significant others (e.g., by parents or teachers in the case of children and adolescents), and descriptions may be generated from behavioral observations and/or reviews of medical and institutional records. Robins' (1966, 1978) research contributions have been significant in pinpointing the behavioral symptoms associated with the natural course of ASPD, as has the work of Quay and his colleagues (Peterson, Quay, & Cameron, 1959; Peterson, Quay, & Tiffany, 1961; Quay, 1964; Quay & Parsons, 1970). This latter group of investigators developed two scales, the Behavior Problem Checklist and the Checklist for the Analysis of Life History Data, to distinguish among delinquent groups, particularly for comparisons of neurotic and psychopathic delinquents (Ellis, 1982; Johns & Quay, 1962; Lee & Prentice, 1988; Orris, 1969).

The Psychopathy Checklist (PCL) and its successor, the Psychopathy Checklist-Revised (PCL-R) were developed by Hare (1980, 1991) to assess psychopathy in adult, male criminal populations. Based on Cleckley's view of the necessary and sufficient features for definiting psychopathy, the PCL consisted originally of twenty-two items (twenty items in the revised 1991 version) rated on three-point scales from both interview and file information. It included items that assess personality traits such as lack of remorse or guilt and lack of empathy as well as overt behaviors such as pathological lying, irresponsible parenting, and juvenile delinquency. Interrater reliabilities have been reported in the range of .84 to .90 (Hare, 1985; Harpur et al., 1988; Hart, Forth, & Hare, 1990; Schroeder, Schroeder, & Hare, 1983), and convergent and construct validity data have been similarly supportive (Hare, 1985; Hart et al., 1988).

The PCL obtained high correlations with subjective, global ratings of psychopathy (.80) and antisocial diagnoses based on DSM-III criteria (.67), and research has suggested that the correlation of PCL-R scores with DSM-IV ASPD diagnoses may be enhanced compared to that observed with ASPD diagnoses based on DSM-III-R criteria (Stalenheim & von Knorring, 1996, 1998). As discussed earlier, much of the research with the PCL and PCL-R has focused on factors underlying the items, in addition to total scores (Harpur et al., 1988, 1989). Kosson et al. (1990) administered the PCL to a multiracial sample and noted similarities in interrater reliabilities and indexes of internal consistency for PCL ratings of Blacks and Whites; however, they reported racial differences in the distributions of PCL scores and the underlying factor structure. Other investigators found sex differences in the PCL-R factor structure (Salekin, Rogers, & Sewell, 1997).

In addition to possible racial and sex differences, concerns may be raised regarding the intended use and appropriate target populations for the PCL and PCL-R, given the nature of samples on which much of the research has been based. The instruments have been used primarily with White institutionalized men, although there are examples of application in other populations (e.g., Alterman et al., 1998). Lack of clarity concerning instrument purpose and target populations is evidenced in marketing materials for the PCL-R from the publisher, Multi-Health Systems. Catalog descriptions specify that the PCL-R is intended for use with forensic populations; however, the Hare Psychopathy Checklist: Screening Version (PCL: SV; Hart, Cox, & Hare, 1995) is listed for use with individuals in the general population as well as forensic or psychiatric populations (Multi-Health Systems, 1999). In any event, there have been increasing efforts to apply the PCL and PCL-R to diverse samples (see Hart & Hare, 1997), and recently, researchers have attempted to extend the concept of psychopathy to adolescents by using assessment instruments modeled on the PCL-R. These include the Childhood Psychopathy Scale (Lynam, 1997, 1998) and the Psychopathy Screening Device (Frick, O'Brien, Wootton, & McBurnett, 1994).

In summary, investigators and clinicians can now select from structured interview, self-report inventory, and behavioral rating technologies and can employ the more traditional types of clinical assessment to identify personality disorders, antisocial personality in particular, and the potentially complicating psychiatric disorders listed on Axis I. Decisions are required regarding the comprehensiveness of assessment goals versus specificity of symptom definition as well as the appropriateness of measurement content. Questions of whether to sample from both normal and disordered behaviors are pivotal, and resolution of this dilemma may not be accomplished without carefully considering the samples to be selected for measurement and criterion validation, for example, community, psychiatric, and forensic samples. Hare (1985) documented the fact that convergence among self-report and interview measures for assessment of psychopathy is disappointing, but more fundamental to assessment is the absence of a universally agreed upon conceptualization of the nature of psychopathy. Thus, there is the problem of establishing validity for both assessment instruments and the construct they are purported to measure.

## Summary and Conclusions

Despite arguments regarding their validity or usefulness, constructs describing persistent antisocial behaviors without demonstrable loss of reality contact have found their place in the literature on general psychopathology. The fascination of psychosocial and biological scientists with habitual rule breaking and chronic disregard for sociolegal restraints in the face of predictably negative consequences is documented by an ever-increasing bibliography of books and articles. Confusion in this literature derives from using several different labels to describe similar behavioral phenomena, from arguments centered on the significance of these definitions and their unique meanings, and from lack of clarity in defining terms. The term sociopathy and the more prevalent label psychopathy have been popularized in the psychological literature, whereas the construct of antisocial personality disorder has assumed importance for psychiatric diagnosis. This divergence between psychological research with its emphasis on psychopathy and psychiatric nomenclature positing an antisocial personality disorder has widened in the past two decades. The confusion resulting from either equating or differentiating these terms has yet to be resolved.

Dating to conceptualizations of the psychopath as morally deranged and pathologically inferior, the notion of a psychopathic personality is founded on a behavioral deficit-excess model that is defined, on the one hand, by deficiencies in interpersonal warmth, capacity to empathize, autonomic conditioning and fear arousal, learning and other cognitive performances, and control of impulsiveness and, on the other hand, by behavioral excesses in the service of aggressive, sexual, and sensation-seeking needs. Gough (1948) proposed that psychopaths are pathologically deficient in role-playing ability, but Cleckley's (1971, 1982) clinical observations and the research of Hare and his colleagues (Hare, 1978, 1980; Harpur et al., 1989; Hart & Hare, 1997) have pointed to the psychopathic personality as prototypical of individuals who are deficient across multiple domains. Evidence is disregarded that, at least in some aspects of behavior, individuals labeled psychopathic may be similar to those considered to be functioning normally. More complex psychopathy constructs were proposed by Blackburn (1988) and Heilbrun (1982; Heilbrun & Heilbrun, 1985) who posited that fundamental deficits in socialization define the core of the psychopathy construct but tied predictions regarding severity and specificity to individual variations in such moderator variables as social withdrawal, impulsivity, and intelligence.

If psychopaths are seen as incapable of profiting from experience, are rarely distressed by their behaviors or interpersonal suffering, are unable to form emotional attachments, and are concerned primarily with the circumstances of immediate gratification, it is not surprising that predictions for response to treatment, regardless of type of intervention, have been pessimistic (Suedfeld & Landon, 1978). As greater attention has been focused on personality disorders, several papers have been published which offer hope for behavior change among antisocial individuals (Davidson & Tyrer, 1996; Kellner, 1986; Sutker & King, 1985). Treatment successes have been documented among antisocial patients enrolled in a therapeutic community (Copas, O'Brien, Roberts, & Whiteley, 1984) and methadone maintenance patients diagnosed with antisocial personality (Alterman, 2001; Brooner, Kidorf, King, & Stoller, 1998; Gerstley et al., 1989). Studies with antisocial children have shown even more promising results (Kazdin, Bass, Siegel, & Thomas, 1989; Kazdin, Siegel, & Bass, 1992; Kazdin & Weisz, 1998;

Wells & Forehand, 1985). These findings, combined with results derived from empirical tests of the psychopathy construct, suggest that antisocial behaviors, ranging from idiosyncratic to maladaptive, are subject to prescribed principles of acquisition and modification, as are any sets of behaviors that might be described in categorical terms. The contingencies for altering antisocial expression may be less apparent than for normals but need not be assumed to be nonexistent.

The research and clinical data reviewed in this chapter call into question the viability of a unitary conceptualization of psychopathy defined by pervasive personal deficits. At the same time, the construct of psychopathy has been important from the standpoint of stimulating research that describes the evolution of behavioral deviance from childhood; the contributions of genetic, familial, environmental, and learning factors to the etiology of antisocial behaviors; and the complexities involved in attempting to account for persistent behavioral deviance and specific types of nonconformity. The construct has been also useful when it has been understood that it represents a set of personality traits, cognitive styles, and emotional dispositions that may be combined in certain clusters and with varying degrees of intensity to predict severity and type of antisocial behaviors. If we assume that these characteristics are dimensional and can be identified among all population subgroups, it is possible to extend the knowledge of behavioral maladjustment and the circumstances under which it becomes exacerbated by studying personality deviation in pathological and normal samples of both sexes.

After more than five decades of clinical observations and research, it is timely to turn greater empirical scrutiny to understanding the full range of personal and situational characteristics associated with antisocial behaviors. Rather than focusing exclusively on the behavioral deficit-excess model, especially among the more disadvantaged and antisocial of our population, greater attention can be directed toward studying the strengths and weaknesses of individuals who are considered fundamentally psychopathic, particularly within the community context. This line of work might well yield findings that will enhance efforts to encourage prosocial behaviors generally and foster more effective behavioral change strategies for severely antisocial persons. It may also lead to better understanding of the mechanisms by which psychopaths cope with fears and insecurities under trying circumstances and thus find application to stress management approaches among persons who are rendered ineffective by anxieties and fearfulness.

# References

Alterman, A. (2001). Opioid and cocaine abuse disorders. In H. E. Adams & P. B. Sutker (Eds.), *Comprehensive handbook of psychopathology* (3rd ed., pp. 623–640) New York: Plenum.

Alterman, A., & Cacciola, J. S. (1991). The antisocial personality disorder diagnosis in substance abusers: Problems and issues. *Journal of Nervous and Mental Disease, 179,* 401–409.

Alterman, A. I., McDermott, P. A., Cacciola, J. S., Rutherford, M. J., Boardman, C. R., McKay, J. R., & Cook, T. G. (1998). A typology of antisociality in methadone patients. *Journal of Abnormal Psychology, 107,* 412–422.

American Psychiatric Association. (1952). *Diagnostic and statistical manual of mental disorders.* Washington, DC: Author.

American Psychiatric Association. (1968). *Diagnostic and statistical manual of mental disorders* (2nd ed.). Washington, DC: Author.

American Psychiatric Association. (1980). *Diagnostic and statistical manual of mental disorders* (3rd ed.). Washington, DC: Author.

American Psychiatric Association. (1987). *Diagnostic and statistical manual of mental disorders* (3rd ed., rev.). Washington, DC: Author.

American Psychiatric Association. (1994). *Diagnostic and statistical manual of mental disorders* (4th ed.). Washington, DC: Author.

Arieti, S. (1967). *The intrapsychic self.* New York: Basic Books.

Axelrod, S. R., Widiger, T. A., Trull, T. J., & Corbitt, E. M. (1997). Relation of five-factor model antagonism facets with personality disorder symptomatology. *Journal of Personality Assessment, 69,* 297–313.

Ball, S. A., Tennen, H., Poling, J. C., Kranzler, H. R. A., & Rounsaville, B. J. (1997). Personality, temperament, and character dimensions and the DSM-IV personality disorders in substance abusers. *Journal of Abnormal Psychology, 106,* 545–553.

Bandura, A., & Walters, R. H. (1959). *Adolescent aggression.* New York: Ronald Press.

Barber, J. P., Frank, A., Weiss, R. D., Blaine, J., Siqueland, L., Moras, K., Calvo, N., Chittams, J., Mercer, D., & Salloum, I. M. (1996). Prevalence and correlates of personality disorder diagnoses among cocaine dependent outpatients. *Journal of Personality Disorders, 10,* 297–311.

Bardone, A. M., Moffitt, T., Caspi, A., & Dickson, N. (1996). Adult mental health and social outcomes of adolescent girls with depression and conduct disorder. *Development and Psychopathology, 8,* 811–829.

Barry, K. L., Fleming, M. F., Manwell, L. B., & Copeland, L. A. (1997). Conduct disorder and antisocial personality (ASP) disorder in adult primary care patients. *Journal of Family Practice, 45,* 151–158.

Bendig, A. W. (1962). Factor analytic scales of covert and overt hostility. *Journal of Consulting Psychology, 26,* 200.

Benson, D. F., & Stuss, D. T. (1990). Frontal lobe influences on delusions. *Schizophrenia Bulletin, 16,* 403–411.

Berman, M. E., Fallon, A. E., & Coccaro, E. F. (1998). The relationship between personality psychopathology and aggressive behavior in research volunteers. *Journal of Abnormal Psychology, 107,* 651–658.

Berman, M. E., Kavoussi, R. J., & Coccaro, E. F. (1997). Neurotransmitter correlates of human aggression. In D. M. Stoff, J. Breiling, & J. D. Maser (Eds.), *Handbook of antisocial behavior* (pp. 305–313). New York: Wiley.

Bernard, J. L., & Eisenman, R. (1967). Verbal conditioning in sociopaths with social and monetary reinforcement. *Journal of Personality and Social Psychology, 6,* 203–206.

Blackburn, R. (1974). *Development and validation of scales to measure hostility and aggression* (Rep. No. 12). London: Special Hospitals Research Unit.

Blackburn, R. (1978). Psychopathy, arousal, and the need for stimulation. In R. D. Hare & D. Schalling (Eds.), *Psychopathic behaviour: Approaches to research* (pp. 157–164). New York: Wiley.

Blackburn, R. (1979a). Cortical and autonomic arousal in primary and secondary psychopaths. *Psychophysiology, 16,* 143–150.

Blackburn, R. (1979b). Psychopathy and personality: The dimensionality of self-report and behaviour rating data in abnormal offenders. *British Journal of Social and Clinical Psychology, 18,* 111–119.

Blackburn, R. (1987). Two scales for the assessment of personality disorder in antisocial populations. *Personality and Individual Differences, 8,* 81–93.

Blackburn, R. (1988). On moral judgments and personality disorders: The myth of psychopathic personality revisited. *British Journal of Psychiatry, 153,* 505–512.

Blackburn, R., & Lee-Evans, M. J. (1985). Reactions of primary and secondary psychopaths to anger-evoking situations. *British Journal of Clinical Psychology, 24,* 93–100.

Blankstein, K. R. (1969). Patterns of autonomic functioning in primary and secondary psychopaths. Unpublished master's thesis, University of Waterloo, Waterloo, Ontario, Canada.

Blashfield, R. K., & McElroy, R. A. (1987). The 1985 journal literature on the personality disorders. *Comprehensive Psychiatry, 28,* 536–546.

Blashfield, R. K., Sprock, J., Pinkston, K., & Hodgin, J. (1985). Exemplar prototypes of personality disorder diagnoses. *Comprehensive Psychiatry, 26,* 11–21.

Blazer, D., George, L. K., Landerman, R., Pennybacker, M., Melville, M. L., Woodbury, M., Manton, K. G., Jordan, K., & Locke, B. (1985). Psychiatric disorders: A rural/urban comparison. *Archives of General Psychiatry, 42,* 651–656.

Bohman, M., Cloninger, C. R., Sigvardsson, S., & von Knorring, A. (1982). Predisposition to petty criminality in Swedish adoptees: I. Genetic and environmental heterogeneity. *Archives of General Psychiatry, 39,* 1233–1241.

Borkovec, T. (1970). Autonomic reactivity to stimulation in psychopathic, neurotic, and normal juvenile delinquents. *Journal of Consulting and Clinical Psychology, 35,* 217–222.

Bowlby, J. (1951). Maternal care and mental health. *Bulletin of the World Health Organization, 3,* 355–533.

Brennan, P. A., Raine, A., Schulsinger, F., Kirkegaard-Sorensen, L., Knop, J., Hutchings, B., Rosenberg, R., & Mednick, S. A. (1997). Psychophysiological protective factors for male subjects at high risk for criminal behaviors. *American Journal of Psychiatry, 154,* 853–855.

Brooner, R. K., Kidorf, M., King, V. L., & Stoller, K. (1998). Preliminary evidence of good treatment response in antisocial drug abusers. *Drug and Alcohol Dependence, 49,* 249–260.

Brown, H. J. D., & Gutsch, K. U. (1985). Cognitions associated with a delay of gratification task. *Criminal Justice and Behavior, 12,* 453–462.

Bryan, J. H., & Kapche, R. (1967). Psychopathy and verbal conditioning. *Journal of Abnormal Psychology, 72,* 71–73.

Buschbaum, M. S. (1986). Brain imaging in the search for biological markers in affective disorder. *Journal of Clinical Psychiatry, 47,* 7–10.

Buschbaum, M. S. (1990). The frontal lobes, basal ganglia, and temporal lobes as sites for schizophrenia. *Schizophrenia Bulletin, 16,* 379–389.

Buss, A. H. (1966). *Psychopathology.* New York: Wiley.

Butler, R. A. (1953). Discrimination learning by rhesus monkeys to visual-exploration motivation. *Journal of Comparative and Physiological Psychology, 46,* 95–98.

Cadoret, R. J., & Cain, C. (1980). Sex differences in predictions of antisocial behavior. *Archives of General Psychiatry, 37,* 1171–1175.

Cadoret, R. J., & Cain, C. A. (1981). Environmental and genetic factors in predicting adolescent antisocial behaviors in adoptees. *Psychiatric Journal of the University of Ottawa, 6,* 220–225.

Cadoret, R. J., O'Gorman, T. W., Troughton, E., & Heywood, E. (1985). Alcoholism and antisocial personality: Interrelationships, genetic and environmental factors. *Archives of General Psychiatry, 42,* 161–167.

Cadoret, R., Troughton, E., Bagford, J., & Woodworth, G. (1990). Genetic and environmental factors in adoptee antisocial personality. *European Archives of Psychiatry and Neurological Sciences, 239,* 231–240.

Carey, G., & Goldman, D. (1997). The genetics of antisocial behavior. In D. M. Stoff, J. Breiling, & J. D. Maser (Eds.), *Handbook of antisocial behavior* (pp. 243–254). New York: Wiley.

Caspi, A., & Moffitt, T. E. (1995). The continuity of maladaptive behavior. In D. Chichetti & D. J. Cohen (Eds.), *Developmental psychopathology.* Vol. 2: *Risk, disorder and adaptation* (pp. 472–511). New York: Wiley.

Centerwall, B. S., & Robinette, C. D. (1989). Twin concordance for dishonorable discharge from the military: With a review of the genetics of antisocial behavior. *Comprehensive Psychiatry, 30,* 442–446.

Christiansen, K. O. (1977). A review of studies of criminality among twins. In S. A. Mednick & K. O. Christiansen (Eds.), *Biosocial bases of criminal behavior* (pp. 45–88). New York: Gardner.

Christianson, S.-A., Forth, A. E., Hare, R. D., Strachan, C., Lidberg, L., & Thorell, L.-H. (1996). Remembering details of emotional events: A comparison between psychopathic and nonpsychopathic offenders. *Personality and Individual Differences, 20,* 437–443.

Cleckley, H. (1941). *The mask of sanity.* St. Louis: Mosby.

Cleckley, H. (1982). *The mask of sanity* (Rev. ed.). New York: Plume.

Cleckley, H. M. (1971). Psychopathic states. In S. Arieti (Ed.), *American handbook of psychotherapy and behavior change* (pp. 566–588). New York: Wiley.

Cloninger, C. R. (1987). A systematic method for clinical description and classification of personality variants. *Archives of General Psychiatry, 44*, 573–588.

Cloninger, C. R., & Guze, S. B. (1975). Hysteria and parental psychiatric illness. *Psychological Medicine, 5*, 27–31.

Cloninger, C. R., Reich, T., & Guze, S. B. (1975). The multifactorial model of disease transmission: III. Familial relationships between sociopathy and hysteria (Briquet's syndrome). *British Journal of Psychiatry, 127*, 23–32.

Cloninger, C. R., Reich, T., & Guze, S. B. (1978). Genetic-environmental interactions and antisocial behaviour. In R. D. Hare & D. Schalling (Eds.), *Psychopathic behaviour: Approaches to research* (pp. 225–237). New York: Wiley.

Cloninger, C. R., Sigvardsson, S., Bohman, M., & von Knorring, A-L. (1982). Predisposition to petty criminality in Swedish adoptees: II. Cross-fostering analysis of gene-environment interaction. *Archives of General Psychiatry, 39*, 1242–1247.

Copas, J. B., O'Brien, M., Roberts, J., & Whiteley, J. S. (1984). Treatment outcome in personality disorder: The effect of social psychological and behavioural variables. *Personality and Individual Differences, 5*, 565–573.

Crider, A. (1993). Electrodermal response lability-stability: Individual difference correlates. In J.-C. Roy, W. Boucsein, D. C. Fowles, & J. Gruzelier (Eds.), *Electrodermal activity: From physiology to psychology* (pp. 173–186). New York: Plenum.

Crowe, R. R. (1972). The adopted offspring of women criminal offenders: A study of their arrest records. *Archives of General Psychiatry, 27*, 600–603.

Crowe, R. R. (1974). An adoption study of antisocial personality. *Archives of General Psychiatry, 31*, 785–791.

Dahl, A. (1986). Some aspects of DSM-III personality disorders illustrated by a consecutive sample of hospitalized patients. *Acta Psychiatrica Scandinavica, 73*(Suppl. 328), 61–67.

Davidson, J., Swartz, M., Storck, M., Krishnan, R. R., & Hammett, E. (1985). A diagnostic and family study of posttraumatic stress disorder. *American Journal of Psychiatry, 142*, 90–93.

Davidson, K. M., & Tyrer, P. (1996). Cognitive therapy for antisocial and borderline personality disorders: Single case study series. *British Journal of Psychiatry, 35*, 413–429.

Day, R., & Wong, S. (1996). Anomalous perceptual asymmetries for negative emotional stimuli in the psychopath. *Journal of Abnormal Psychology, 105*, 648–652.

DeMyer-Gapin, S., & Scott, T. J. (1977). Effect of stimulus novelty on stimulation seeking in antisocial and neurotic children. *Journal of Abnormal Psychology, 86*, 96–98.

Dengerink, H. A., & Bertilson, H. S. (1975). Psychopathy and physiological arousal in an aggressive task. *Psychophysiology, 12*, 682–684.

Devonshire, P. A., Howard, R. C., & Sellars, C. (1988). Frontal lobe dysfunction and personality in mentally abnormal offenders. *Personality and Individual Differences, 9*, 339–344.

DiLalla, D. L., Carey, G., Gottesman, I. I., & Bouchard, T. J. (1996). Heritability of MMPI personality indicators of psychopathology in twins reared apart. *Journal of Abnormal Psychology, 105*, 491–499.

Dodge, K. A., Bates, J. E., & Pettit, G. S. (1990). Mechanisms in the cycle of violence. *Science, 250*, 1678–1683.

Dodge, K. A., & Newman, J. P. (1981). Biased decision making processes in aggressive boys. *Journal of Abnormal Psychology, 90*, 375–379.

Dodge, K. A., Pettit, G. S., Bates, J. E., & Valente, E. (1995). Social-information-processing patterns partially mediate the effect of early physical abuse on later conduct problems. *Journal of Abnormal Psychology, 104*, 632–643.

Drake, R. E., & Vaillant, G. E. (1985). A validity study of axis II of DSM-III. *American Journal of Psychiatry, 142*, 553–558.

Drake, R. E., & Vaillant, G. E. (1988). Predicting alcoholism and personality disorder in a 33-year longitudinal study of children of alcoholics. *British Journal of Addiction, 83*, 799–807.

Dubro, A. F., & Wetzler, S. (1989). An external validity study of the MMPI personality disorder scales. *Journal of Clinical Psychology, 45*, 570–575.

Dubro, A. F., Wetzler, S., & Kahn, M. W. (1988). A comparison of three self-report questionnaires for the diagnosis of DSM-III personality disorders. *Journal of Personality Disorders, 2*, 256–266.

Dumas, J. E. (1989). Treating antisocial behavior in children: Child and family approaches. *Clinical Psychology Review, 9*, 197–222.

Dumas, J. E., & Wahler, R. G. (1985). Indiscriminate mothering as a contextual factor in aggressive-oppositional child behavior: "Damned if you do, damned if you don't." *Journal of Abnormal Child Psychology, 13*, 1–17.

Ellis, P. L. (1982). Empathy: A factor in antisocial behaviors. *Journal of Abnormal Child Psychology, 10*, 123–134.

Ellis, L. (1987). Relationships of criminality and psychopathy with eight other apparent behavioral manifestations of suboptimal arousal. *Personality and Individual Differences, 8*, 905–925.

Erickson, M. F., Sroufe, L. A., & Egeland, B. (1985). The relationship between quality of attachment and behavior problems in preschool in a high-risk sample. In I. Bretherton & E. Waters (Eds.), *Growing points of attachment theory and research. Monographs of the Society for Research in Child Development, 50*(12), 147–167.

Eysenck, H. J. (1964). *Crime and personality.* London: Methuen.

Eysenck, H. J., & Eysenck, M. W. (1985). *Personality and individual differences: A natural science approach.* New York: Plenum.

Eysenck, H. J., & Eysenck, S. B. G. (1978). Psychopathy, personality, and genetics. In R. D. Hare & D. Schalling (Eds.), *Psychopathic behaviour: Approaches to research* (pp. 197–223). New York: Wiley.

Fairweather, G. W. (1954). The effect of selective incentive conditions on the performance of psychopathic, neurotic, and normal criminals in a serial rote learning situation. *Dissertation Abstracts International, 14*, 394–395. (University Microfilms No. 6940)

Farley, F. H., & Farley, S. V. (1972). Stimulus-seeking motivation and delinquent behavior among institutionalized delinquent girls. *Journal of Consulting and Clinical Psychology, 39*, 94–97.

Farrington, D. P. (1995). The development of offending and antisocial behavior from childhood: Key findings from the Cambridge study in delinquent development. *Journal of Child Psychology and Psychiatry, 36*, 929–964.

Farrington, D. P. (1997). A critical analysis of research on the development of antisocial behavior from birth to adulthood. In D. M. Stoff, J. Breiling, & J. D. Maser (Eds.), *Handbook of antisocial behavior* (pp. 234–240). New York: Wiley.

Farrington, D. P., & West, D. J. (1990). The Cambridge study in delinquent development: A long-term follow-up of 411 London males. In H. J. Kerner & G. Kaiser (Eds.), *Criminality: Personality, behaviour, life history*. Heidelberg: Springer Verlag.

First, M. B., Spitzer, R. L, Williams, J. B. W., Gibbon, M., & Benjamin, L. (1994). *Structured Clinical Interview for DSM-IV Axis II Personality Disorders (Version 2.0)*. New York: Biometrics Research Department, New York State Psychiatric Institute.

Fishbein, D. H., & Thatcher, R. W. (1986). New diagnostic methods in criminology: Assessing organic sources of behavioral disorders. *Journal of Research in Crime and Delinquency, 23*, 240–267.

Fooks, G., & Thomas, R. R. (1957). Differential qualitative performance of delinquents on the Porteus Maze. *Journal of Consulting Psychology, 21*, 351–353.

Ford, M. R., & Widiger, T. A. (1989). Sex bias in the diagnosis of histrionic and antisocial personality disorders. *Journal of Consulting and Clinical Psychology, 57*, 301–305.

Forth, A. E., & Hare, R. D. (1989). The contingent negative variation in psychopaths. *Psychophysiology, 26*, 676–682.

Fowles, D. C. (1980). The three arousal model: Implications of Gray's two-factor learning theory for heart rate, electrodermal activity, and psychopathy. *Psychophysiology, 17*, 87–104.

Fowles, D. C. (1984). Biological variables in psychopathology. In H. E. Adams & P. B. Sutker (Eds.), *Comprehensive handbook of psychopathology* (pp. 77–110). New York: Plenum.

Fowles, D. C. (1993). Electrodermal activity and antisocial behavior: Empirical findings and theoretical issues. In J.-C. Roy, W. Boucsein, D. Fowles, & J. Gruzelier (Eds.), *Progress in electrodermal research* (pp. 223–237). London: Plenum.

Fowles, D. C. (2001). Biological variables in psychopathology: A psychobiological perspective. In H. E. Adams & P. B. Sutker (Eds.), *Comprehensive handbook of psychopathology* (3rd ed., pp. 85–104). New York: Plenum.

Fox, R., & Lippert, W. (1963). Spontaneous GSR and anxiety level in sociopathic delinquents. *Journal of Consulting Psychology, 27*, 368.

Frances, A. J., Pincus, H. A., Widiger, T. A., Davis, W. W., & First, M. B. (1990). DSM-IV: Work in progress. *American Journal of Psychiatry, 147*, 1439–1448.

Frick, P. J., O'Brien, B. S., Wootton, J. M., & McBurnett, K. (1994). Psychopathy and conduct disorder in children. *Journal of Abnormal Psychology, 103*, 700–707.

Gerstley, L. J., Alterman, A. I., McLellan, A. T., & Woody, G. E. (1990). Antisocial personality disorder with substance abuse disorders: A problematic diagnosis. *American Journal of Psychiatry, 147*, 173–178.

Gerstley, L., McLellan, A. T., Alterman, A. I., Woody, G. E., Luborsky, L., & Prout, M. (1989). Ability to form an alliance with the therapist: A possible marker of prognosis for patients with antisocial personality disorder. *American Journal of Psychiatry, 146*, 508–512.

Gilberstadt, H., & Duker, J. (1965). *A handbook for clinical and actuarial MMPI interpretation*. Philadelphia: Saunders.

Goodwin, D. W., & Guze, S. B. (1989). *Psychiatric diagnosis* (4th ed.). New York: Oxford University Press.

Gorenstein, E. E. (1982). Frontal lobe functions in psychopaths. *Journal of Abnormal Psychology, 91*, 368–379.

Gorenstein, E. E. (1987). Cognitive-perceptual deficit in an alcoholism spectrum disorder. *Journal of Studies on Alcohol, 48*, 310–318.

Gorenstein, E. E., & Newman, J. P. (1980). Disinhibitory psychopathology: A new perspective and a model for research. *Psychological Review, 87*, 301–315.

Gough, H. G. (1948). A sociological theory of psychopathology. *American Journal of Sociology, 53*, 359–366.

Gough, H. G. (1960). Theory and measurement of socialization. *Journal of Consulting Psychology, 24*, 23–30.

Gough, H. G. (1975). *Manual for the California Psychological Inventory*. Palo Alto, CA: Consulting Psychologists Press.

Gough, H. G., & Peterson, D. R. (1952). The identification and measurement of predispositional factors in crime and delinquency. *Journal of Consulting Psychology, 16*, 207–212.

Goyer, P., Andreason, P., Semple, W., Clayton, A., King, A., Compton-Toth, B., Schulz, S. C., & Cohen, R. (1994). Positron-emission tomography and personality disorders. *Neuropsychopharmacology, 10*, 21–28.

Goyer, P. F., & Semple, W. E. (1996). PET studies of aggression in personality disorder and other nonpsychotic patients. In D. M. Stoff & R. F. Cairns (Eds.), *The neurobiology of clinical aggression* (pp. 219–236). Hillsdale, NJ: Erlbaum.

Graham, J. R. (1987). *The MMPI: A practical guide* (2nd ed.). New York: Oxford University Press.

Graham, J. R. (1993). *MMPI-2: Assessing personality and psychopathology* (2nd ed.). New York: Oxford University Press.

Grande, T. P., Wolf, A. W., Schubert, D. S. P., Patterson, M. B., & Brocco, K. (1984). Associations among alcoholism, drug abuse, and antisocial personality: A review of the literature. *Psychological Reports, 55*, 455–474.

Gray, J. A. (1975). *Elements of a two-process theory of learning*. New York: Academic Press.

Gray, J. A. (1976). The behavioural inhibition system: A possible substrate for anxiety. In M. P. Feldman & A. Broadhurst (Eds.), *Theoretical and experimental bases of the behaviour therapies* (pp. 3–41). London: Wiley.

Gray, J. A. (1985). A whole and its parts: Behavior, the brain, cognition and emotion. *Bulletin of the British Psychological Society, 3*, 99–112.

Gray, J. A. (1994). Framework for a taxonomy of psychiatric disorder. In S. H. M. van Goozen, N. E. Van de Poll, & J. A. Sergeant (Eds.), *Emotions: Essays on emotion theory* (pp. 29–60). Hillsdale, NJ: Erlbaum.

Green, B. L., Lindy, J. D., & Grace, M. C. (1985). Posttraumatic stress disorder: Toward DSM-IV. *Journal of Nervous and Mental Disease, 173*, 406–411.

Greenberg, M. T., & Speltz, M. (1988). Attachment and the ontogeny of conduct problems. In J. Belsky & T. Nezworski (Eds.), *Clinical implications of attachment* (pp. 177–218). Hillsdale, NJ: Erlbaum.

Grove, W. M., Eckert, E. D., Heston, L., Bouchard, T. J., Segal, N., & Lykken, D. T. (1990). Heritability of substance abuse and antisocial behavior: A study of monozygotic twins raised apart. *Biological Psychiatry, 27*, 1293–1304.

Gullick, E. L., Sutker, P. B., & Adams, H. E. (1976). Delay of information in paired-associate learning among incarcerated groups of sociopaths and heroin addicts. *Psychological Reports, 38*, 143–151.

Hammen, C. L., & Padesky, C. A. (1977). Sex differences in the expression of depressive responses on the Beck Depression Inventory. *Journal of Abnormal Psychology, 86*, 609–614.

Hare, R. D. (1965). Acquisition and generalization of a conditioned-fear response in psychopathic and nonpsychopathic criminals. *Journal of Psychology, 59,* 367–370.

Hare, R. D. (1970). *Psychopathy: Theory and research.* New York: Wiley.

Hare, R. D. (1978). Electrodermal and cardiovascular correlates of psychopathy. In R. D. Hare & D. Schalling (Eds.), *Psychopathic behaviour: Approaches to research* (pp. 107–143). New York: Wiley.

Hare, R. D. (1979). Psychopathy and laterality of cerebral function. *Journal of Abnormal Psychology, 88,* 605–610.

Hare, R. D. (1980). The assessment of psychopathy in criminal populations. *Personality and Individual Differences, 1,* 111–119.

Hare, R. D. (1982). Psychopathy and physiological activity during anticipation of an aversive stimulus in a distraction paradigm. *Psychophysiology, 19,* 266–271.

Hare, R. D. (1983). Diagnosis of antisocial personality disorder in two prison populations. *American Journal of Psychiatry, 140,* 887–890.

Hare, R. D. (1984). Performance of psychopaths on cognitive tasks related to frontal lobe function. *Journal of Abnormal Psychology, 93,* 133–140.

Hare, R. D. (1985). Comparison of procedures for the assessment of psychopathy. *Journal of Consulting and Clinical Psychology, 53,* 7–16.

Hare, R. D. (1991). *The Hare Psychopathy Checklist-Revised.* Toronto, Ontario, Canada: Multi-Health Systems.

Hare, R. D. (1996a). *The Hare Self-Report Psychopathy Scale-II.* Toronto, Ontario, Canada: Multi-Health Systems.

Hare, R. D. (1996b). Psychopathy: A clinical construct whose time has come. *Criminal Justice and Behavior, 23,* 25–54.

Hare, R. D., & Connolly, J. F. (1987). Perceptual asymmetries and information processing in psychopaths. In S. A. Mednick, T. E. Moffitt, & S. A. Stack (Eds.), *The causes of crime: New biological approaches* (pp. 218–238). Cambridge, England: Cambridge University Press.

Hare, R. D., & Craigen, D. (1974). Psychopathy and physiological activity in a mixed-motive game situation. *Psychophysiology, 11,* 197–206.

Hare, R. D., Frazelle, J., & Cox, D. N. (1978). Psychopathy and physiological responses to threat of aversive stimulus. *Psychophysiology, 15,* 165–172.

Hare, R. D., Harpur, T. J., Hakstian, A. R., Forth, A. D., & Hart, S. D. (1990). The Revised Psychopathy Checklist: Reliability and factor structure. *Psychological Assessment: A Journal of Consulting and Clinical Psychology, 2,* 338–341.

Hare, R. D., & Hart, S. D. (1993). Psychopathy, mental disorder, and crime. In S. Hodgins (Ed.), *Mental disorder and crime* (pp. 104–115). Newbury Park, CA: Sage.

Hare, R. D., Hart, S. D., & Harpur, T. J. (1991). Psychopathy and DSM-IV criteria for antisocial personality disorder. *Journal of Abnormal Psychology, 100,* 391–398.

Hare, R. D., & Jutai, J. W. (1988). Psychopathy and cerebral asymmetry in semantic processing. *Personality and Individual Differences, 9,* 329–337.

Hare, R. D., & Quinn, M. J. (1971). Psychopathy and autonomic conditioning. *Journal of Abnormal Psychology, 79,* 223–226.

Harlow, H. F., Harlow, M. K., & Meyer, D. F. (1950). Learning motivated by a manipulation drive. *Journal of Experimental Psychology, 40,* 228–234.

Harpur, T. J., Hakstian, A. R., & Hare, R. D. (1988). Factor structure of the Psychopathy Checklist. *Journal of Consulting and Clinical Psychology, 56,* 741–747.

Harpur, T. J., & Hare, R. D. (1994). The assessment of psychopathy as a function of age. *Journal of Abnormal Psychology, 103,* 604–609.

Harpur, T. J., Hare, R. D., & Hakstian, A. R. (1989). Two-factor conceptualization of psychopathy: Construct validity and assessment implications. *Psychological Assessment: A Journal of Consulting and Clinical Psychology, 1,* 6–17.

Hart, S. D., & Hare, R. D. (1989). Discriminant validity of the Psychopathy Checklist in a forensic psychiatric population. *Psychological Assessment: A Journal of Consulting and Clinical Psychology, 1,* 211–218.

Hart, S. D., & Hare, R. D. (1997). Psychopathy: Assessment and association with criminal conduct. In D. M. Stoff, J. Breiling, & J. D. Maser (Eds.), *Handbook of antisocial behavior* (pp. 22–35). New York: Wiley.

Hart, S. D., Kropp, P. R., & Hare, R. D. (1988). Performance of psychopaths following conditional release from prison. *Journal of Consulting and Clinical Psychology, 56,* 227–232.

Hart, S. D., Forth, A. E., & Hare, R. D. (1990). Performance of criminal psychopaths on selected neuropsychological tests. *Journal of Abnormal Psychology, 99,* 374–379.

Hart, S. D., Cox, D. N., & Hare, R. D. (1995). *Manual for the Hare Psychopathy Checklist-Revised: Screening Version (PCL:SV).* Toronto. Ontario, Canada: Multi-Health Systems.

Hathaway, S. R., & McKinley, J. C. (1983). *Minnesota Multiphasic Personality Inventory: Manual for administration and scoring.* Minneapolis: University of Minnesota Press. Distributed by NCS Interpretive Systems, a division of National Computers Systems, Inc.

Heilbrun, A. B. (1979). Psychopathy and violent crime. *Journal of Consulting and Clinical Psychology, 47,* 509–516.

Heilbrun, A. B. (1982). Cognitive models of criminal violence based upon intelligence and psychopathy levels. *Journal of Consulting and Clinical Psychology, 50,* 546–557.

Heilbrun, A. B., & Gottfried, D. M. (1988). Antisociality and dangerousness in women before and after the women's movement. *Psychological Reports, 62,* 37–38.

Heilbrun, A. B., & Heilbrun, M. R. (1985). Psychopathy and dangerousness: Comparison, integration, and extension of two psychopathic typologies. *British Journal of Clinical Psychology, 24,* 181–195.

Helzer, J. E., & Pryzbeck, T. R. (1988). The co-occurrence of alcoholism with other psychiatric disorders in the general population and its impact on treatment. *Journal of Studies on Alcohol, 49,* 219–224.

Hemphill, J. F., Hare, R. D., & Wong, S. (1998). Psychopathy and recidivism: A review. *Legal and Criminological Psychology, 3,* 139–170.

Hemphill, J. F., Hart, S. D., & Hare, R. D. (1995). Psychopathy and substance use. *Journal of Personality Disorders, 8,* 169–180.

Henry, B., & Moffitt, T. E. (1997). Neuropsychological and neuroimaging studies of juvenile delinquency and adult criminal behavior. In D. M. Stoff, J. Breiling, & J. D. Maser (Eds.), *Handbook of antisocial behavior* (pp. 280–288). New York: Wiley.

Hesselbrock, M. N., Meyer, R. E., & Keener, J. J. (1985). Psychopathology in hospitalized alcoholics. *Archives of General Psychiatry, 42,* 1050–1055.

Hoffman, J. J., Hall, R. W., & Bartsch, T. W. (1987). On the relative importance of "psychopathic" personality and alcoholism on neuropsychological measures of frontal lobe dysfunction. *Journal of Abnormal Psychology, 96,* 158–160.

Holzman, P. S. (1987). Recent studies of psychophysiology in schizophrenia. *Schizophrenia Bulletin, 13,* 49–75.

Howard, R., Payamal, L. T., & Neo, L. H. (1997). Response modulation deficits in psychopaths: A failure to replicate and a reconsideration of the Patterson-Newman model. *Personality and Individual Differences, 22,* 707–717.

Howland, E. W., Kosson, D. S., Patterson, C. M., & Newman, J. P. (1993). Altering a dominant response: Performance of psychopaths and low-socialization college students on a cued reaction time task. *Journal of Abnormal Psychology, 102,* 379–387.

Hundleby, J. D. (1978). Using other behaviors in the study of adolescent drug usage. In R. P. Schlegel (Chair), Social psychological aspects of nonmedical drug use. Symposium conducted at the *Meeting of the American Psychological Association,* Toronto, Ontario, Canada.

Hutchings, B., & Mednick, S. A. (1975). Registered criminality in the adoptive and biological parents of registered male criminal adoptees. In R. Fieve, D. Rosenthal, & H. Brill (Eds.), *Genetic research in psychiatry* (pp. 105–116). Baltimore: Johns Hopkins University Press.

Hyler, S. E., Reider, R. O., Williams, J. B. W., Spitzer, R. L., Lyons, M., & Hendler, J. (1989). A comparison of clinical and self-report diagnoses of DSM-III personality disorders in 552 patients. *Comprehensive Psychiatry, 30,* 170–178.

Iacono, W. G. (1983). Psychophysiology and genetics: A key to psychopathology research. *Psychophysiology, 20,* 371–383.

Intrator, J., Hare, R., Stritzke, P., Brichtswein, K., Dorfman, D., Harpur, T., Bernstein, D., Handelsman, L., Schaefer, C., Keilp, J., Rosen, J., & Machac, J. (1997). A brain imaging (single photon emission computerized tomography) study of semantic and affective processing in psychopaths. *Biological Psychiatry, 42,* 96–103.

Johns, J. H., & Quay, H. C. (1962). The effect of social reward on verbal conditioning in psychopathic and neurotic military offenders. *Journal of Consulting Psychology, 26,* 217–220.

Jordan, B. K., Swartz, M. S., George, L. K., Woodbury, M. A., & Blazer, D. G. (1989). Antisocial and related disorders in a Southern community: An application of grade of membership analysis. *Journal of Nervous and Mental Disease, 177,* 529–541.

Jutai, J. W., & Hare, R. D. (1983). Psychopathy and selective attention during performance of a complex perceptual-motor task. *Psychophysiology, 20,* 146–151.

Jutai, J. W., Hare, R. D., & Connolly, J. F. (1987). Psychopathy and event-related potentials (ERPs) associated with attention to speech stimuli. *Personality and Individual Differences, 8,* 175–184.

Kadlub, K. J. (1956). The effects of two types of reinforcements on the performance of psychopathic and normal criminals. Unpublished doctoral dissertation, University of Illinois, Champaign.

Kammeier, M. L., Hoffman, H., & Loper, R. G. (1973). Personality characteristics of alcoholics as college freshmen and at time of treatment. *Quarterly Journal of Studies on Alcohol, 34,* 390–399.

Kandel, E., & Freed, D. (1989). Frontal-lobe dysfunction and antisocial behavior: A review. *Journal of Clinical Psychology, 45,* 404–413.

Kandel, E., Mednick, S. A., Kirkegaard-Sorensen, L., Hutchings, B., Knop, J., Rosenberg, R., & Schulsinger, F. (1988). IQ as a protective factor for subjects at high risk for antisocial behavior. *Journal of Consulting and Clinical Psychology, 56,* 224–226.

Kaplan, M. (1983). A woman's view of DSM-III. *American Psychologist, 38,* 786–792.

Karpman, B. (1948). Myth of psychopathic personality. *American Journal of Psychiatry, 104,* 523–534.

Kass, F., Skodol, A. E., Charles, E., Spitzer, R. L., & Williams, J. B. W. (1985). Scaled ratings of DSM-III personality disorders. *American Journal of Psychiatry, 142,* 627–630.

Kass, F., Spitzer, R. L., & Williams, J. B. W. (1983). An empirical study of the issue of sex bias in the diagnostic criteria of DSM-III Axis II personality disorders. *American Psychologist, 38,* 799–801.

Kazdin, A. E., Bass, D., Siegel, T., & Thomas, C. (1989). Cognitive-behavioral therapy and relationship therapy in the treatment of children referred for antisocial behavior. *Journal of Consulting and Clinical Psychology, 57,* 522–535.

Kazdin, A. E., Siegel, T. C., & Bass, D. (1992). Cognitive problem solving skills training and parent management training in the treatment of antisocial child behavior. *Journal of Consulting and Clinical Psychology, 60,* 733–740.

Kazdin, A. E., & Weisz, J. R. (1998). Identifying and developing empirically supported child and adolescent treatments. *Journal of Consulting and Clinical Psychology, 66,* 19–36.

Keane, T. M., & Wolfe, J. (1990). Comorbidity in posttraumatic stress disorder: An analysis of community and clinical studies. *Journal of Applied Social Psychology, 20,* 1776–1788.

Kellner, R. (1986). Personality disorders. *Psychotherapy and Psychosomatics, 46,* 58–66.

Kidorf, M., Brooner, R. K., King, V. L., & Chutuape, M. A. (1996). Concurrent validity of cocaine and sedative dependence diagnoses in opioid-dependent outpatients. *Drug and Alcohol Dependence, 42,* 117–123.

Kilpatrick, D. G., Sutker, P. B., Roitzsch, J. C., & Miller, W. C. (1976). Personality correlates of polydrug use. *Psychological Reports, 38,* 311–317.

Klein, M. H., Benjamin, L. S., Greist, J. H., Rosenfeld, R., & Treece, C. (1989). The Wisconsin Personality Inventory (WISPI): Validation studies. Unpublished manuscript, University of Wisconsin, Madison.

Koch, J. A. L. (1891). *Die psychopathischen Minderwertigkeiten.* Ravensburg, Germany: Maier.

Koenigsberg, H. W., Kaplan, R. D., Gilmore, M. M., & Cooper, A. M. (1985). The relationship between syndrome and personality disorder in DSM-III: Experience with 2,462 patients. *American Journal of Psychiatry, 142,* 207–212.

Kosson, D. S., Smith, S. S., & Newman, J. P. (1990). Evaluating the construct validity of psychopathy in black and white male inmates: Three preliminary studies. *Journal of Abnormal Psychology, 99,* 250–259.

Kosten, T. R., Rounsaville, B. J., & Kleber, H. D. (1982). DSM-III personality disorders in opiate addicts. *Comprehensive Psychiatry, 23,* 572–581.

Kraepelin, E. (1923). *Clinical psychiatry: A textbook for students and physicians.* Abstracted and adapted from the 7th German edition of Kraepelin's *Lehrbuch der Psychiatrie* by A. R. Diefendorf. New York: Macmillan. (Original work published in 1907.)

Lahey, B. B., Loeber, R., Hart, E. L., Frick, P. J., Applegate, B.,

Zhang, Q., Green, S. M., & Russo, M. F. (1995). Four-year longitudinal study of conduct disorder in boys: Patterns and predictors of persistence. *Journal of Abnormal Psychology, 104,* 83–93.

Lee, M., & Prentice, N. M. (1988). Interrelations of empathy, cognition, and moral reasoning with dimensions of juvenile delinquency. *Journal of Abnormal Child Psychology, 16,* 127–139.

Lewis, C. E., Rice, J., & Helzer, J. E. (1983). Diagnostic interactions: Alcoholism and antisocial personality. *Journal of Nervous and Mental Disease, 171,* 105–113.

Lewis, C. E., Robins, L. N., & Rice, J. (1985). Association of alcoholism with antisocial personality in urban men. *Journal of Nervous and Mental Disease, 173,* 166–174.

Lewis, D. O., & Balla, D. (1975). "Sociopathy" and its synonyms: Inappropriate diagnoses in child psychiatry. *American Journal of Psychiatry, 132,* 720–722.

Lilienfeld, S. O., Purcell, C., & Jones-Alexander, J. (1997). Assessment of antisocial behavior in adults. In D. M. Stoff, J. Breiling, & J. D. Maser (Eds.), *Handbook of antisocial behavior* (pp. 234–240). New York: Wiley.

Lilienfeld, S., Van Valkenburg, C., Larntz, K., & Akiskal, H. (1986). The relationship of histrionic personality disorder to antisocial personality and somatization disorders. *American Journal of Psychiatry, 143,* 718–722.

Loeber, R., & Dishion, T. (1983). Early predictors of male delinquency. *Psychological Bulletin, 94,* 68–99.

Loeber, R., & Stouthamer-Loeber, M. (1987). Prediction. In H. C. Quay (Ed.), *Handbook of juvenile delinquency* (pp. 325–382). New York: Wiley.

Loranger, A. W. (1988). *Personality Disorders Examination (PDE) manual.* Yonkers, NY: DV Communications.

Loranger, A. W., Susman, V. L., Oldham, J. M., & Russakoff, L. M. (1987). The Personality Disorder Examination: A preliminary report. *Journal of Personality Disorders, 1,* 1–13.

Louth, S. M., Williamson, S., Alpert, M., Pouget, E. R., & Hare, R. D. (1998). Acoustic distinctions in the speech of male psychopaths. *Journal of Psycholinguistic Research, 27,* 375–384.

Luntz, B. K., & Widom, C. S. (1994). Antisocial personality disorder in abused and neglected children grown up. *American Journal of Psychiatry, 151,* 670–674.

Lykken, D. T. (1957). A study of anxiety in the sociopathic personality. *Journal of Abnormal and Social Psychology, 55,* 6–10.

Lykken, D. T. (1978). The psychopath and the lie detector. *Psychophysiology, 15,* 137–142.

Lykken, D. T. (1994). Psychoneurology. In R. J. Corsini (Ed.), *Encyclopedia of psychology* (2nd ed., Vol. 3, pp. 231–234). New York: Wiley-Interscience.

Lynam, D. R. (1997). Pursuing the psychopath: Capturing the fledgling psychopath in a nomological net. *Journal of Abnormal Psychology, 106,* 425–438.

Lynam, D. R. (1998). Early identification of the fledgling psychopath: Locating the psychopathic child in the current nomenclature. *Journal of Abnormal Psychology, 107,* 566–575.

Lynam, D., Moffitt, T. E., & Stouthamer-Loeber, J. (1993). Explaining the relation between IQ and delinquency: Race, class, test motivation, school failure, or self-control. *Journal of Abnormal Psychology, 102,* 187–196.

McCollough, J. P., & Adams, H. E. (1970). Anxiety, learning sets, and sociopathy. *Psychological Reports, 27,* 47–52.

McCord, W. M., & McCord, J. (1964). *The psychopath.* Princeton, NJ: Van Nostrand.

McKinley, J. C., & Hathaway, S. R. (1944). The MMPI: V. Hysteria, hypomania, and psychopathic deviate. *Journal of Applied Psychology, 28,* 153–174.

MacMillan, J., & Kofoed, L. (1984). Sociobiology and antisocial personality: An alternative perspective. *Journal of Nervous and Mental Disease, 172,* 701–706.

Maher, B. (1966). *Principles of psychopathology.* New York: McGraw-Hill.

Malatesta, V. J., Sutker, P. B., & Treiber, F. A. (1981). Sensation seeking and chronic public drunkenness. *Journal of Consulting and Clinical Psychology, 49,* 292–294.

Malow, R. M., West, J. A., Williams, J. L., & Sutker, P. B. (1989). Personality disorders classification and symptoms in cocaine and opioid addicts. *Journal of Consulting and Clinical Psychology, 57,* 765–767.

Mawson, A. R., & Mawson, D. C. (1977). Personality and arousal: New interpretation of the psychophysiological literature. *Biological Psychiatry, 12,* 49–74.

Mednick, S. A. (1977). A biosocial theory of the learning of law-abiding behavior. In S. A. Mednick & K. O. Christiansen (Eds.), *Biosocial bases of criminal behavior* (pp. 1–8). New York: Gardner.

Mednick, S. A., Gabrielli, W. I., & Hutchings, B. (1984). Genetic factors in criminal behavior: Evidence from an adoption cohort. *Science, 224,* 891–893.

Megargee, E. I. (1972). *The California Psychological Inventory handbook.* San Francisco: Jossey-Bass.

Miles, D. R., & Carey, G. (1997). The genetic and environmental architecture of human aggression. *Journal of Personality and Social Psychology, 72,* 207–217.

Millon, T. (1981). *Disorders of personality: DSM-III: Axis II.* New York: Wiley.

Millon, T. (1983). *Millon Clinical Multiaxial Inventory manual* (3rd ed.). Minneapolis: National Computer Systems.

Millon, T. (1987). *Millon Clinical Multiaxial Inventory-II.* Minneapolis: National Computer Systems.

Millon, T. (1994). *Millon Clinical Multiaxial Inventory-III.* Minneapolis: National Computer Systems.

Moffitt, T. E. (1987). Parental mental disorder and offspring criminal behavior: An adoption study. *Psychiatry, 50,* 346–360.

Moffitt, T. E., & Silva, P. A. (1988). Self-reported delinquency, neuropsychological deficit, and history of attention deficit disorder. *Journal of Abnormal Child Psychology, 16,* 553–569.

Morey, L. C. (1988). The categorical representation of personality disorders: A cluster analysis of DSM-III-R personality features. *Journal of Abnormal Psychology, 97,* 314–321.

Morey, L., Blashfield, R., Webb, W., & Jewell, J. (1988). MMPI scales for DSM-III personality disorders: A preliminary validation. *Journal of Clinical Psychology, 44,* 47–50.

Morey, L., & Ochoa, E. (1989). An investigation of adherence to diagnostic criteria: Clinical diagnosis of the DSM-III personality disorders. *Journal of Personality Disorders, 3,* 180–192.

Morey, L. C., Waugh, M. H., & Blashfield, R. K. (1985). MMPI scales for DSM-III personality disorders: Their derivation and correlates. *Journal of Personality Assessment, 49,* 245–251.

Morgenstern, J., Langenbucher, J., Labouvie, E., & Miller, K. J. (1997). The comorbidity of alcoholism and personality disorders in a clinical population: Prevalence rates and relation to alcohol typology variables. *Journal of Abnormal Psychology, 106*, 74–84.

Morrison, J. R., & Stewart, M. A. (1971). A family study of the hyperactive child syndrome. *Biological Psychiatry, 3*, 189–195.

Mueser. K. T., Drake, R. E., Ackerson, T. H., Alterman, A. I., Miles, K. M., & Noordsy, D. L. (1997). Antisocial personality disorder, conduct disorder, and substance abuse in schizophrenia. *Journal of Abnormal Psychology, 106*, 473–477.

Nasby, W., Hayden, B., & DePaulo, B. M. (1980). Attributional bias among boys to interpret unambiguous social stimuli as displays of hostility. *Journal of Abnormal Psychology, 89*, 459–468.

Newman, D. L., Moffitt, T. E., Caspi, A., & Silva, P. A. (1998). Comorbid mental disorders: Implications for treatment and sample selection. *Journal of Abnormal Psychology, 107*, 305–311.

Newman, J. P., & Brinkley, C. A. (1998). Psychopathy: Rediscovering Cleckley's construct. *Psychopathology Research: The Newsletter of the Society for Research in Psychopathology, 9*(1), 1–5, 7–8.

Newman, J. P., & Kosson, D. S. (1986). Passive avoidance learning in psychopathic and nonpsychopathic offenders. *Journal of Abnormal Psychology, 95*, 252–256.

Newman, J. P., Patterson, C. M., Howland, E. W., & Nichols, S. L. (1990). Passive avoidance in psychopaths: The effects of reward. *Personality and Individual Differences, 11*, 1101–1114.

Newman, J. P., Patterson, C. M., & Kosson, D. S. (1987). Response perseveration in psychopaths. *Journal of Abnormal Psychology, 96*, 145–148.

Newman, J. P., & Schmidt, W. A. (1998). Passive avoidance in psychopathic offenders: A replication and extension. *Journal of Abnormal Psychology, 107*, 527–532.

Newman, J. P., Schmidt, W. A., & Voss, W. D. (1997). The impact of motivationally neutral cues on psychopathic individuals: Assessing the generality of the response modulation hypothesis. *Journal of Abnormal Psychology, 106*, 563–575.

Newman, J. P., & Wallace, J. F. (1993). Psychopathy and cognition. In P. C. Kendall & K. S. Dobson (Eds.), *Psychopathology and cognition* (pp. 293–349). New York: Academic Press.

Newman, J. P., Widom, C. S., & Nathan, S. (1985). Passive avoidance in syndromes of disinhibition: Psychopathy and extraversion. *Journal of Personality and Social Psychology, 48*, 1316–1327.

O'Connor, B. P., & Dyce, J. A. (1998). A test of models of personality disorder configuration. *Journal of Abnormal Psychology, 107*, 3–16.

O'Connor, T. G., McGuire, S., Reiss, D., Hetherington, E. M., & Plomin, R. (1998). Co-occurrence of depressive symptoms and antisocial behavior in adolescence: A common genetic liability. *Journal of Abnormal Psychology, 107*, 27–37.

Olweus, D. (1978). Antisocial behaviour in the school setting. In R.D. Hare & D. Schalling (Eds.), *Psychopathic behaviour: Approaches to research* (pp. 319–327). New York: Wiley.

Orris, J. B. (1969). Visual monitoring performance in three subgroups of male delinquents. *Journal of Abnormal Psychology, 74*, 227–229.

Overall, J. E. (1973). MMPI personality patterns of alcoholics and narcotic addicts. *Quarterly Journal of Studies on Alcohol, 34*, 104–111.

Painting, D. H. (1961). The performance of psychopathic individuals under conditions of positive and negative partial reinforcement. *Journal of Abnormal Psychology, 62*, 352–355.

Partridge, G. E. (1930). Current conceptions of psychopathic personality: I. The concept of "psychopathic personality." *American Journal of Psychiatry, 10*, 53–99.

Patterson, C. M., & Newman, J. P. (1993). Reflectivity and learning from aversive events: Toward a psychological mechanism for the syndromes of disinhibition. *Psychological Review, 100*, 699–720.

Patterson, G. R. (1982). *Coercive family processes* (Vol. 3). Eugene, OR: Castalia.

Peterson, D. R., Quay, H. C., & Cameron, G. E. (1959). Personality and background factors in juvenile delinquency as inferred from questionnaire responses. *Journal of Consulting Psychology, 23*, 395–399.

Peterson, D. R., Quay, H. C., & Tiffany, T. L. (1961). Personality factors related to juvenile delinquency. *Child Development, 32*, 355–372.

Pfohl, B., Coryell, W., Zimmerman, M., & Stangl, D. (1986). DSM-III personality disorders: Diagnostic overlap and internal consistency of individual DSM-III criteria. *Comprehensive Psychiatry, 27*, 21–34.

Pinel, P. (1962). *A treatise on insanity.* (D. D. Davis, Trans.). New York: Published under the auspices of the Library of the New York Academy of Medicine by Hafner Publishing Company. (Original work published in 1801.)

Pollock, V. E., Briere, J., Schneider, L., Knop, J., Mednick, S. A., & Goodwin, D. W. (1990). Childhood antecedents of antisocial behavior: Parental alcoholism and physical abusiveness. *American Journal of Psychiatry, 147*, 1290–1293.

Pontius, A. A. (1974). Basis for a neurological test of frontal lobe function in adolescents. *Adolescence, 9*, 221–232.

Pontius, A. A., & Ruttiger, K. F. (1976). Frontal lobe system maturational lag in juvenile delinquents shown in the Narratives Test. *Adolescence, 11*, 509–518.

Pontius, A. A., & Yudowitz, B. S. (1980). Frontal lobe system dysfunction in some criminal actions as shown in the Narratives Test. *Journal of Nervous and Mental Disease, 168*, 111–117.

Pope, H. G., Jonas, J. M., Hudson, J. I., Cohen, B. M., & Gunderson, J. G. (1983). The validity of DSM-III borderline personality disorder: A phenomenologic, family history, treatment response, and long-term follow-up study. *Archives of General Psychiatry, 40*, 23–30.

Prichard, J. C. (1835). *A treatise on insanity.* London: Sherwood, Gilbert, & Piper.

Quay, H. C. (1964). Personality dimensions in delinquent males as inferred from the factor analysis of behavior ratings. *Journal of Research in Crime and Delinquency, 1*, 33–37.

Quay, H. C. (1965). Psychopathic personality as pathological stimulation-seeking. *American Journal of Psychiatry, 122*, 180–183.

Quay, H. C. (1993). The psychobiology of undersocialized aggressive conduct disorder: A theoretical perspective. *Development and Psychopathology, 5*, 165–180.

Quay, H. C., & Hunt, W. A. (1965). Psychopathy, neuroticism, and verbal conditioning: A replication and extension. *Journal of Consulting Psychology, 29*, 283.

Quay, H. C., & Parsons, L. (1970). The differential behavioral classification of the juvenile offender. Washington, DC: Bureau of Prisons, U.S. Department of Justice.

Raine, A. (1987). Effect of early environment on electrodermal and cognitive correlates of schizotypy and psychopathy in criminals. *International Journal of Psychophysiology, 4,* 277–287.

Raine, A. (1993). *The psychopathology of crime: Criminal behavior as a clinical disorder.* San Diego, CA: Academic Press.

Raine, A. (1996). Autonomic nervous system activity and violence. In D. M. Stoff & R. F. Cairns (Eds.), *The neurobiology of clinical aggression* (pp. 145–168). Hillsdale, NJ: Erlbaum.

Raine, A. (1997). Antisocial behavior and psychophysiology: A biosocial perspective and a prefrontal dysfunction hypothesis. In D. M. Stoff, J. Breiling, & J. D. Maser (Eds.), *Handbook of antisocial behavior* (pp. 289–304). New York: Wiley.

Raine, A., & Venables, P. H. (1987). Contingent negative variation, P3 evoked potentials, and antisocial behaviour. *Psychophysiology, 24,* 191–199.

Raine, A., & Venables, P. H. (1988). Enhanced P3 evoked potentials and longer P3 recovery time in psychopaths. *Psychophysiology, 25,* 30–38.

Raine, A., O'Brien, M., Smiley, N., Scerbo, A., & Chan, C-J. (1990). Reduced lateralization in verbal dichotic listening in adolescent psychopaths. *Journal of Abnormal Psychology, 99,* 272–277.

Raine, A., Venables, P. H., & Williams, M. (1990a). Autonomic orienting responses in 15-year-old male subjects and criminal behavior at age 24. *American Journal of Psychiatry, 147,* 933–937.

Raine, A., Venables, P. H., & Williams, M. (1990b). Relationships between central and autonomic measures of arousal at age 15 and criminality at age 24 years. *Archives of General Psychiatry, 47,* 1003–1007.

Raine, A., Venables, P. H., & Williams, M. (1990c). Relationships between N1, P300, and contingent negative variation recorded at age 15 and criminal behavior at age 24. *Psychophysiology, 27,* 567–574.

Raine, A., Buschbaum, M., Stanley, J., Lottenbreg, S., Abel, L., & Stoddard, J. (1994). Selective reductions in prefrontal glucose metabolism in murderers. *Biological Psychiatry, 36,* 365–373.

Raine, A., Venables, P. H., & Williams, M. (1995). High autonomic arousal and electrodermal orienting at age 15 years as protective factors against criminal behavior at age 29 years. *American Journal of Psychiatry, 152,* 1595–1600.

Raine, A., Venables, P. H., & Williams, M. (1996). Better autonomic conditioning and faster electrodermal half-recovery time at age 15 years as protective factors against crime at age 29 years. *Developmental Psychology, 32,* 624–630.

Raine, A., Buschbaum, M., & LaCasse, L. (1997). Brain abnormalities in murderers indicated by positron emission tomography. *Biological Psychiatry, 42,* 495–508.

Raine, A., Meloy, J. R., Bihrle, S., Stoddard, J., LaCasse, L., & Buschbaum, M. S. (1998). Reduced prefrontal and increased subcortical functioning assessed using positron emission tomography in predatory and affective murderers. *Behavioral Sciences and the Law, 16,* 319–332.

Raskin, D. C. (1973). Anxiety and arousal. In W. F. Prokasy &

D. C. Raskin (Eds.), *Electrodermal activity in psychological research* (pp. 125–155). New York: Academic.

Reich, J. (1987). Sex distribution of DSM-III personality disorders in psychiatric outpatients. *American Journal of Psychiatry, 144,* 485–488.

Reich, J. H. (1989). Update on instruments to measure DSM-III and DSM-III-R personality disorders. *Journal of Nervous and Mental Disease, 177,* 366–370.

Reich, T., Cloninger, C. R., & Guze, S. B. (1975). The multifactorial model of disease transmission: I. Description of the model and its use in psychiatry. *British Journal of Psychiatry, 127,* 1–10.

Renken, B., Egeland, B., Marvinney, D., Mangelsdorf, S., & Sroufe, A. (1989). Early childhood antecedents of aggression and passive-withdrawal in early elementary school. *Journal of Personality, 57,* 257–281.

Rime, B., Bouvy, H., Leborgne, B., & Rouillon, F. (1978). Psychopathy and nonverbal behavior in an interpersonal situation. *Journal of Consulting and Clinical Psychology, 42,* 833–841.

Robbins, T. W. (1990). The case for frontostriatal dysfunction in schizophrenia. *Schizophrenia Bulletin, 16,* 391–402.

Robins, L. N. (1966). *Deviant children grown up.* Baltimore: Williams & Wilkins.

Robins, L. N. (1970). The adult development of the antisocial child. *Seminars in Psychiatry, 2,* 420–434.

Robins, L. N. (1978). Sturdy childhood predictors of adult antisocial behaviour: Replications from longitudinal studies. *Psychological Medicine, 8,* 611–622.

Robins, L. N. (1981). Epidemiological approaches to natural history research. *Journal of the American Academy of Child Psychiatry, 20,* 566–580.

Robins, L. N., Helzer, J. E., Croughan, J., & Ratcliff, K. S. (1981). National Institute of Mental Health Diagnostic Interview Schedule: Its history, characteristics, and validity. *Archives of General Psychiatry, 38,* 381–389.

Robins, L. N., Helzer, J. E., Weissman, M. M., Orvaschel, H., Gruenberg, E., Burke, J. D., & Regier, D. A. (1984). Lifetime prevalence of specific psychiatric disorders in three sites. *Archives of General Psychiatry, 41,* 949–958.

Robins, L. N., Tipp, J., & Przybeck, T. (1991). Antisocial personality. In L. N. Robins & D. A. Regier (Eds.), *Psychiatric disorders in America* (pp. 258–290). New York: Free Press.

Rosen, A.-S. (1977). On the dimensionality of the California Psychological Inventory Socialization Scale. *Journal of Consulting and Clinical Psychology, 45,* 583–591.

Rosen, A.-S., & Schalling, D. (1971). Probability learning in psychopathic and nonpsychopathic criminals. *Journal of Experimental Research in Personality, 5,* 191–198.

Rotenberg, M. (1975). Psychopathy, insensitivity, and sensitization. *Professional Psychology, 6,* 382–392.

Rothbaum, F., & Weisz, J. (1994). Parental caregiving and child externalizing behavior in nonclinical samples: A meta-analysis. *Psychological Bulletin, 116,* 994–1003.

Rush, B. (1835). *Medical inquiries and observations upon the diseases of the mind* (5th ed.). Philadelphia: Grigg & Elliott.

Salekin, R. T., Rogers, R., & Sewell, K. W. (1997). Construct validity of psychopathy in a female offender sample: A multitrait-multimethod evaluation. *Journal of Abnormal Psychology, 106,* 576–585.

Satterfield, J. H. (1978). The hyperactive child syndrome: A precursor of adult psychopathy? In R. D. Hare & D. Schalling (Eds.), *Psychopathic behaviour: Approaches to research* (pp. 329–346). New York: Wiley.

Scarpa, A., Raine, A., Venables, P. H., & Mednick, S. A. (1997). Heart rate and skin conductance in behaviorally inhibited Mauritian children. *Journal of Abnormal Psychology, 106,* 182–190.

Schalling, D. (1978). Psychopathy-related personality variables and the psychophysiology of socialization. In R. D. Hare & D. Schalling (Eds.), *Psychopathic behaviour: Approaches to research* (pp. 85–106). New York: Wiley.

Schalling, D., & Rosen, A.-S. (1968). Porteus Maze differences between psychopathic and nonpsychopathic criminals. *British Journal of Social and Clinical Psychology, 7,* 224–228.

Schmauk, F. J. (1970). Punishment, arousal, and avoidance learning in sociopaths. *Journal of Abnormal Psychology, 76,* 325–335.

Schneider, K. (1923). *Psychopathic personalities.* London: Cassell.

Schneider, K. (1958). *Psychopathic personalities* (M. W. Hamilton, Trans.). Springfield, IL: Charles C. Thomas. (Translated from *Die psychopathischen Personlichkeiten,* 9th ed., 1950.)

Schroeder, M., Schroeder, K., & Hare, R. D. (1983). Generalizability of a checklist for assessment of psychopathy. *Journal of Consulting and Clinical Psychology, 51,* 511–516.

Schuckit, M. A. (1973). Alcoholism and sociopathy: Diagnostic confusion. *Quarterly Journal of Studies on Alcohol, 34,* 157–164.

Schulsinger, F. (1972). Psychopathy: Heredity and environment. *International Journal of Mental Health, 1,* 190–206.

Shaw, D. S., & Bell, R. Q. (1993). Developmental theories of parental contributors to antisocial behavior. *Journal of Abnormal Child Psychology, 21,* 493–518.

Shaw, D. S., & Vondra, J. I. (1995). Attachment security and maternal predictors of early behavior problems: A longitudinal study of low-income families. *Journal of Abnormal Child Psychology, 23,* 335–357.

Shaw, D. S., & Winslow, E. B. (1997). Precursors and correlates of antisocial behavior from infancy to preschool. In D. M. Stoff, J. Breiling, & J. D. Maser (Eds.), *Handbook of antisocial behavior* (pp. 148–158). New York: Wiley.

Siddle, D. A. T., Nicol, A. R., & Foggitt, R. H. (1973). Habituation and over-extinction of the GSR component of the orienting response in anti-social adolescents. *British Journal of Social and Clinical Psychology, 12,* 303–308.

Siegel, R. A. (1978). Probability of punishment and suppression of behavior in psychopathic and nonpsychopathic offenders. *Journal of Abnormal Psychology, 87,* 514–522.

Sierles, F. S., Chen, J.-J., Messing, M. L., Besyner, J. K., & Taylor, M. A. (1986). Concurrent psychiatric illness in non-Hispanic outpatients diagnosed as having posttraumatic stress disorder. *Journal of Nervous and Mental Disease, 174,* 171–173.

Sigvardsson, S., Cloninger, C. R., Bohman, M., & von Knorring, A.-L. (1982). Predisposition to petty criminality in Swedish adoptees: III. Sex differences and validation of the male typology. *Archives of General Psychiatry, 39,* 1248–1253.

Slutske, W. S., Heath, A. C., Dinwiddie, S. H., Madden, P. A. F., Buckholz, K. K., Dunne, M. P., Statham, D. J., & Martin, N. G. (1997). Modeling genetic and environmental influences in the etiology of conduct disorder: A study of 2,682 adult twin pairs. *Journal of Abnormal Psychology, 106,* 266–279.

Slutske, W. S., Heath, A. C., Dinwiddie, S. H., Madden, P. A. F., Buckholz, K. K., Dunne, M. P., Statham, D. J., & Martin, N. G. (1998). Common genetic risk factors for conduct disorder and alcohol dependence. *Journal of Abnormal Psychology, 107,* 363–374.

Smith, R. J. (1978). The psychopath in society. In D. T. Lykken (Ed.), *Personality and psychopathology* (Vol. 19). New York: Academic Press.

Smith, S. S., Arnett, P. A., & Newman, J. P. (1992). Neuropsychological differentiation of psychopathic and nonpsychopathic criminal offenders. *Personality and Individual Differences, 13,* 1233–1245.

Smith, S. S., & Newman, J. P. (1990). Alcohol and drug abuse-dependence disorders in psychopathic and nonpsychopathic criminal offenders. *Journal of Abnormal Psychology, 99,* 430–439.

Spalt, L. (1980). Hysteria and antisocial personality: A single disorder? *Journal of Nervous and Mental Disease, 168,* 456–464.

Spitzer, R. L., Endicott, J., & Robins, E. (1975). Research diagnostic criteria. New York: Biometrics Research, New York State Department of Mental Health.

Stalenheim, E. G., & von Knorring, L. (1996) Psychopathy and Axis I and Axis II psychiatric disorders in a forensic psychiatric population in Sweden. *Acta Psychiatrica Scandinavica, 94,* 217–223.

Stalenheim, E. G., & von Knorring, L. (1998). Personality traits and psychopathy in a forensic psychiatric population. *European Journal of Psychiatry, 12,* 83–94.

Steinberg, E. P., & Schwartz, G. E. (1976). Biofeedback and electrodermal self-regulation in psychopathy. *Journal of Abnormal Psychology, 85,* 408–415.

Sterling, S., & Edelmann, R. J. (1988). Reactions to anger and anxiety-provoking events: Psychopathic and nonpsychopathic groups compared. *Journal of Clinical Psychology, 44,* 96–100.

Stewart, D. J., & Resnick, H. J. (1970). Verbal conditioning of psychopaths as a function of experimenter-subject sex differences. *Journal of Abnormal Psychology, 75,* 90–92.

Strack, S. (1987). Development and validation of an adjective check list to assess the Millon personality types in a normal population. *Journal of Personality Assessment, 51,* 572–587.

Stuss, D. T., & Benson, D. F. (1986). *The frontal lobes.* New York: Raven Press.

Suedfeld, P., & Landon, P. B. (1978). Approaches to treatment. In R. D. Hare & D. Schalling (Eds.), *Psychopathic behaviour: Approaches to research* (pp. 347–376). New York: Wiley.

Sutker, P. B. (1970). Vicarious conditioning and sociopathy. *Journal of Abnormal Psychology, 76,* 380–386.

Sutker, P. B. (1971). Personality differences and sociopathy in heroin addicts and nonaddict prisoners. *Journal of Abnormal Psychology, 78,* 247–251.

Sutker, P. B. (1982). Adolescent drug and alcohol behaviors. In T. M. Field, A. Huston, H. C. Quay, L. Troll, & G. E. Finley (Eds.), *Review of human development* (pp. 356–380). New York: Wiley-Interscience.

Sutker, P. B., & Allain, A. N. (1983). Behavior and personality assessment in men labeled adaptive sociopaths. *Journal of Behavioral Assessment, 5,* 65–79.

Sutker, P. B., & Allain, A. N. (1987). Cognitive abstraction, shifting, and control: Clinical sample comparisons of psychopaths and nonpsychopaths. *Journal of Abnormal Psychology, 96,* 73–75.

Sutker, P. B., Archer, R. P., & Allain, A. N. (1978). Drug abuse patterns, personality characteristics, and relationships with sex, race, and sensation seeking. *Journal of Consulting and Clinical Psychology, 46,* 1374–1378.

Sutker, P. B., DeSanto, N. A., & Allain, A. N. (1985). Adjective self-descriptions in antisocial men and women. *Journal of Psychopathology and Behavioral Assessment, 7,* 175–181.

Sutker, P. B., Gil, S. H., & Sutker, L. W. (1971). Sociopathy and serial learning of CVC combinations with high and low social-content ratings. *Journal of Personality and Social Psychology, 17,* 158–162.

Sutker, P. B., & King, A. R. (1985). Antisocial personality disorder: Assessment and case formulation. In I. D. Turkat (Ed.), *Behavioral case formulation* (pp. 115–153). New York: Plenum.

Sutker, P. B., & Moan, C. E. (1973). A psychosocial description of penitentiary inmates. *Archives of General Psychiatry, 29,* 663–667.

Sutker, P. B., Moan, C. E., & Allain, A. N. (1974). WAIS performance in unincarcerated groups of MMPI-defined sociopaths and normal controls. *Journal of Consulting and Clinical Psychology, 42,* 307–308.

Sutker, P. B., Moan, C. E., & Allain, A. N. (1983). Assessment of cognitive control in psychopathic and normal prisoners. *Journal of Behavioral Assessment, 5,* 275–287.

Sutker, P. B., Moan, C. E., & Swanson, W. C. (1972). Porteus Maze Test qualitative performance in pure sociopaths, prison normals, and antisocial psychotics. *Journal of Clinical Psychology, 28,* 349–353.

Sutker, P. B., Patsiokas, A. T., & Allain, A. N. (1981). Chronic illicit drug abusers: Gender comparisons. *Psychological Reports, 49,* 383–390.

Tellegen, A. (1985). Structures of mood and personality and their relevance to assessing anxiety with an emphasis on self-report. In A. H. Tuma & J. D. Maser (Eds.), *Anxiety and the anxiety disorders* (pp. 681–706). Hillsdale, NJ: Erlbaum.

Tennent, G., Tennent, D., Prins, H., & Bedford, A. (1990). Psychopathic disorder—A useful clinical concept? *Medicine, Science, and Law, 30,* 39–44.

Thorne, F. C. (1959). The etiology of sociopathic reactions. *American Journal of Psychotherapy, 13,* 319–330.

Uddo-Crane, M., Thompson, K. E., & Sutker, P. B. (1991, October). Post-traumatic stress disorder and antisocial personality disorder in combat veterans. Paper presented at the *Meeting of the International Society for Traumatic Stress Studies,* Washington, DC.

Ullman, L. P., & Krasner, L. (1975). *A psychological approach to abnormal behavior* (2nd ed.). Englewood Cliffs, NJ: Prentice-Hall.

Vaillant, G. E. (1975). Sociopathy as a human process: A viewpoint. *Archives of General Psychiatry, 32,* 178–183.

Vaillant, G. E., & Hiller-Sturmhoefel, S. (1996). The natural history of alcoholism. *Alcohol Health and Research World, 20,* 152–161.

Van den Oord, E. J. C. G., Verhulst, F. C., & Boomsma, D. I. (1996). A genetic study of maternal and paternal ratings of problem behaviors in 3-year-old twins. *Journal of Abnormal Psychology, 105,* 349–357.

Venables, P. H. (1987). Autonomic nervous system factors in criminal behavior. In S. A. Mednick, T. E. Moffitt, & S. A. Stack (Eds.), *The causes of crime: New biological approaches* (pp. 110–136). New York: Cambridge University Press.

Waid, W. M., & Orne, M. T. (1982). Reduced electrodermal

response to conflict, failure to inhibit dominant behaviors, and delinquency proneness. *Journal of Personality and Social Psychology, 43,* 769–774.

Walters, G. D. (1985). Scale 4 *(Pd)* of the MMPI and the diagnosis of antisocial personality. *Journal of Personality Assessment, 49,* 474–476.

Weiss, J. M. A., Davis, D., Hedlund, J. L., & Cho, D. W. (1983). The dysphoric psychopath: A comparison of 524 cases of antisocial personality disorder with matched controls. *Comprehensive Psychiatry, 24,* 355–369.

Wells, K. C., & Forehand, R. (1985). Conduct and oppositional disorders. In P. H. Bornstein & A. E. Kazdin (Eds.), *Handbook of clinical behavior therapy with children* (pp. 219–265). Homewood, IL: Dorsey Press.

Wendt, R. H., Lindsley, D. F., Adey, W. R., & Fox, S. S. (1963). Self-maintained visual stimulation in monkeys after long-term visual deprivation. *Science, 139,* 336–338.

White, J. L., Moffitt, T. E., & Silva, P. A. (1989). A prospective replication of the protective effects of IQ in subjects at high risk for juvenile delinquency. *Journal of Consulting and Clinical Psychology, 57,* 719–724.

Whitehill, M., DeMyer-Gapin, S., & Scott, T. J. (1976). Stimulation seeking in antisocial preadolescent children. *Journal of Abnormal Psychology, 85,* 101–104.

Widiger, T. A. (1985). *Personality interview questions.* Unpublished manuscript, University of Kentucky, Lexington.

Widiger, T. A. (1987). *Personality Interview Questions-II.* Unpublished manuscript, University of Kentucky, Lexington.

Widiger, T. A., Cadoret, R., Hare, R., Robins, L., Rutherford, M., Zanarini, M., Alterman, A., Apple, M., Corbitt, E., Forth, A., Hart, S., Kulterman, J., Woody, G., & Frances, A. (1996). DSM-IV antisocial personality disorder field trial. *Journal of Abnormal Psychology, 105,* 3–16.

Widiger, T. A., & Corbitt, E. M. (1993). Antisocial personality disorder: Proposals for DSM-IV. *Journal of Personality Disorders, 7,* 63–77.

Widiger, T. A., & Corbitt, E. M. (1997). Comorbidity of antisocial personality disorder with other personality disorders. In D. M. Stoff, J. Breiling, & J. D. Maser (Eds.), *Handbook of antisocial behavior* (pp. 75–82). New York: Wiley.

Widiger, T. A., & Frances, A. (1985). The DSM-III personality disorders: Perspectives from psychology. *Archives of General Psychiatry, 42,* 615–623.

Widiger, T. A., & Frances, A. (1987). Interviews and inventories for the measurement of personality disorders. *Clinical Psychology Review, 7,* 49–75.

Widiger, T. A., Frances, A. J., Pincus, H. A., Davis, W. W., & First, M. B. (1991). Toward an empirical classification for the DSM-IV. *Journal of Abnormal Psychology, 100,* 280–288.

Widiger, T. A., Frances, A., Warner, L., & Bluhm, C. (1986). Diagnostic criteria for the borderline and schizotypal personality disorders. *Journal of Abnormal Psychology, 95,* 43–51.

Widiger, T. A., & Trull, T. J. (1993). Borderline and narcissistic personality disorders. In P. B. Sutker & H. E. Adams (Eds.), *Comprehensive handbook of psychopathology* (pp. 371–394). New York: Plenum.

Widom, C. S. (1976a). Interpersonal and construct systems in psychopaths. *Journal of Consulting and Clinical Psychology, 44,* 614–623.

Widom, C. S. (1976b). Interpersonal conflict and cooperation in psychopaths. *Journal of Abnormal Psychology, 85,* 330–334.

Widom, C. S. (1977). A methodology for studying noninstitutionalized psychopaths. *Journal of Consulting and Clinical Psychology, 45,* 674–683.

Wiggins, J. S. (1966). Substantive dimensions of self-report in the MMPI item pool. *Psychological Monographs, 80* (Whole No. 630), 1–42.

Wiggins, J. S., & Pincus, A. L. (1989). Conceptions of personality disorders and dimensions of personality. *Psychological Assessment: A Journal of Consulting and Clinical Psychology, 1,* 305–316.

Williamson, S., Harpur, T. J., & Hare, R. D. (1991). Abnormal processing of affective words by psychopaths. *Psychophysiology, 28,* 260–273

Witkin, H. A., Mednick, S. A., Schulsinger, F., Bakkestrom, E., Christiansen, K. O., Goodenough, D. R., Hirschhorn, K., Lundesteen, C., Owen, D. R., Philip, J., Rubin, D. B., & Stocking, M. (1976). Criminality in XYY and XXY men. *Science, 193,* 547–555.

Woerner, P. I., & Guze, S. B. (1968). A family and marital study of hysteria. *British Journal of Psychiatry, 114,* 161–168.

Wolf, A. W., Schubert, D. S. P., Patterson, M. B., Grande, T. P., Brocco, K., & Pendleton, L. (1988). Association among major psychiatric diagnoses. *Journal of Consulting and Clinical Psychology, 56,* 292–294.

World Health Organization. (1990). ICD-10 Chapter V. Mental and behavioral disorders. Diagnostic criteria for research. Geneva: Author.

Wulach, J. S. (1983). Diagnosis of the DSM-III antisocial personality disorder. *Professional Psychology: Research and Practice, 14,* 330–340.

Yeudall, L. T., & Fromm-Auch, D. (1979). Neuropsychological impairments in various psychopathological populations. In J. Gruzelier & P. Flor-Henry (Eds), *Hemisphere asymmetries of function in psychopathology* (pp. 401–428). Amsterdam: Elsevier.

Yeudall, L. T., Fromm-Auch, D., & Davies, P. (1982). Neuropsychological impairment of persistent delinquency. *Journal of Nervous and Mental Disease, 170,* 257–265.

Zanarini, M. C., & Gunderson, J. G. (1997). Differential diagnosis of antisocial and borderline personality disorders. In D. M. Stoff, J. Breiling, & J. D. Maser (Eds.), *Handbook of antisocial behavior* (pp. 83–91). New York: Wiley.

Zimmerman, M., & Coryell, W. (1989). DSM-III personality disorder diagnoses in a nonpatient sample. *Archives of General Psychiatry, 46,* 682–689.

Zubek, J. P., Pushkar, D., Sansom, W., & Gowing, J. (1961). Perceptual changes after prolonged sensory isolation. *Canadian Journal of Psychology, 15,* 83–100.

Zuckerman, M. (1972). *Manual and research report for the Sensation Seeking Scale (SSS).* Newark: University of Delaware.

Zuckerman, M. (1974). The sensation seeking motive. In B. A. Maher (Ed.), *Progress in experimental personality research* (Vol. 7) (pp. 79–148). New York: Academic Press.

Zuckerman, M. (1977). *Preliminary manual with scoring keys and norms for Form V of the Sensation Seeking Scale.* Newark: University of Delaware.

Zuckerman, M., Bone, R. N., Neary, R., Mangelsdorff, D., & Brustman, B. (1972). Personality trait and experience correlates of the Sensation Seeking Scale. *Journal of Consulting and Clinical Psychology, 43,* 308–321.

# CHAPTER 17

# Borderline Personality Disorder: An Overview

Henry E. Adams, Jeffrey A. Bernat, and Kristen A. Luscher

## Introduction

The diagnosis of Borderline Personality Disorder (BPD) is new. It first appeared as a diagnostic entity in the *Diagnostic and Statistical Manual of Mental Disorders*, third edition (DSM-III; American Psychiatric Association, 1980), but the concept has a long history first delineated by Stern (1938) to describe a group of patients who did not profit from psychoanalysis and did not seem to fit into the categories of neurotic or psychotic. Patients with affective lability, unstable interpersonal relationships, transient psychotic disturbances, impulsivity, and chronic suicide attempts seemed to defy categorization, and the term "borderline" denoted this diagnostic ambiguity. These confusing cases were often labeled pervert personality, psychotic personality, inadequate personality (Green, 1977), schizophrenia, latent type, pseudoneurotic schizophrenia (Hoch & Polatin, 1949), and patients with borderline states (Knight, 1953). These early conceptualizations emphasized the belief that borderline patients were suffering from a milder form or an atypical presentation of schizophrenia.

For the next 35 years, the concept of borderline was largely confined to the psychoanalytic literature and did not appear in either the DSM-I or DSM-II (Paris, 1999). Kernberg (1975, 1984) was largely responsible for the resurgence in interest in borderline personality, particularly among psychoanalysts. Although Kernberg popularized the concept of "borderline," he used the term to describe a level of personality organization that reflected the most serious forms of character pathology rather than a discrete personality disorder. In fact, borderline personality organization (BPO) is not specific to those patients who meet the current DSM-IV (American Psychiatric Association, 1994) diagnosis of BPD.

A turning point came in the 1970s when Gunderson and Singer (1975) developed the first operational definition of BPD, based on integrating findings in the existing empirical literature. Gunderson and colleagues were the first to demonstrate that BPD could be reliably observed, scored, and differentiated from other psychiatric disorders (Gunderson & Kolb, 1978). This empirical work, coupled with the research of others (Perry & Klerman, 1978, 1980), led to a formalized and accepted diagnosis of BPD. BPD became an "official" disorder with the publication of the DSM-III. In DSM-III, the diagnosis of BPD was reserved for the more interpersonally unstable and affectively labile patients. Schizotypal personality disorder,

Henry E. Adams, Jeffrey A. Bernat, and Kristen A. Luscher • Department of Psychology, University of Georgia, Athens, Georgia 30602-3013.

*Comprehensive Handbook of Psychopathology* (Third Edition), edited by Patricia B. Sutker and Henry E. Adams. Kluwer Academic/Plenum Publishers, New York, 2001.

on the other hand, was used to describe patients who were more closely connected to schizophrenia and more closely related to earlier descriptors of borderline patients (e.g., "pseudoneurotic schizophrenia" and "schizophrenia latent-type") (Spitzer et al., 1979). Although BPD has undergone considerable revision since 1980, many of the essential features remain the same in DSM-IV (for a comprehensive review of criterion changes, see Gunderson, Zanarini, & Kigiel, 1995).

## DSM-IV Diagnostic Criteria

BPD is characterized by a pattern of instability and disregulation across emotional, interpersonal, behavioral, and cognitive domains. In the DSM-IV, a new criterion was added to capture cognitive aspects of the disorder (i.e., transient stress-related paranoid ideation or severe dissociative symptoms). Table 1 provides the DSM-IV criteria for BPD, in which five of nine specified criteria are required. Both Linehan (1993), who reorganized and summarized the DSM-IV criteria, and Paris (1999) described the essential features of BPD. First, individuals with BPD experience *emotional disregulation* or *affective instability*. The moods of borderline individuals are highly reactive, labile, and depend on environmental stimuli. Radical shifts in mood may occur during the course of a day. For example, Freeman and colleagues (1990) described the case of a woman who was performing competently in an advanced work setting. However, at the end of the day, she would experience extreme depression and struggled with impulses to cut herself with broken glass. These mood shifts were so transient that her supervisor was unaware of the extent or seriousness of her problems. Because of episodic mood changes, individuals with BPD are often misdiagnosed as bipolar disordered. However, the key difference is that the time frame for mood changes in BPD is hours rather than weeks or months, as in bipolar disorder (Paris, 1999). Moreover, episodes of anxiety, depression, irritability, and dysphoria usually occur in response to environmental stressors that the borderline individual feels helpless to influence (Gunderson & Phillips, 1991; Linehan, 1993; Paris, 1999). Emotion disregulation is also exemplified by difficulty controlling and expressing anger.

Second, individuals with BPD experience *inter-

## Table 1. DSM-IV Criteria for Borderline Personality Disorder[a]

A pervasive pattern of instability of interpersonal relationships, self-image, and affects, and marked impulsivity beginning by early adulthood and present in a variety of contexts, as indicated by five (or more) of the following:

1. Frantic efforts to avoid real or imagined abandonment (do not include suicidal or self-mutilating behavior covered in criterion 5)
2. A pattern of unstable and intense interpersonal relationships characterized by alternating between extremes of idealization and devaluation.
3. Identity disturbance: markedly and persistently unstable self-image or sense of self.
4. Impulsivity in at least two areas that are potentially self-damaging (e.g., spending, sex, substance abuse, reckless driving, binge eating) (do not include suicidal or self-mutilating behavior covered in criterion 5)
5. Recurrent suicidal behavior, gestures, or threats, or self-mutilating behavior
6. Affective instability due to a marked reactivity of mood (e.g., intense episodic dysphoria, irritability, or anxiety usually lasting a few hours and only rarely more than a few days)
7. Chronic feelings of emptiness
8. Inappropriate, intense anger or difficulty controlling anger (e.g., frequent displays of temper, constant anger, recurrent physical fights)
9. Transient, stress-related paranoid ideation or severe dissociative symptoms

[a]APA (1994, pp. 650–654).

*personal difficulties*. Although they become easily involved with people, their relationships tend to be chaotic, intense, and marked with difficulty (Linehan, 1993). They may alternate from feeling completely consumed by other people to feeling totally abandoned (Megles & Swartz, 1989; Paris, 1999). Individuals with BPD are exquisitely sensitive to perceived threats of abandonment or rejection. These fears make it very difficult for them to maintain stable, close relationships. Consequently, long-standing difficulties with relationships are common. Many engage in frantic efforts to prevent significant others from leaving them. For example, it is not uncommon for individuals with BPD to take pills or self-mutilate (e.g., cut themselves) following an argument. Paris (1999) described this *impulsive behavior* (i.e., *behavioral disregulation*) as the sine qua non of BPD. Self-destructive, impulsive behavior, which may take the form of substance abuse, sexual promiscuity, overdosing, binge eating, and reckless behavior, is viewed as a maladaptive strategy for coping with dysphoric affect (Linehan, 1993). Indeed, the impulsive behavior pattern that is most important in identifying BPD patients is a pattern of self-injurious behaviors and suicide attempts (Gunderson, 1984; Linehan, 1993; Morey, 1988).

Another central feature of BPD is *cognitive disregulation*. In response to stressful situations, many borderline patients experience transient, quasi-psychotic forms of thought disturbance, including auditory and visual hallucinations, dissociation, depersonalization, and paranoid ideation. Because many borderline individuals hear voices, they may be misdiagnosed as schizophrenic (Paris, 1999). However, unlike schizophrenics, individuals with BPD recognize that voices are produced from their own minds; moreover, they do not respond to them with delusional thinking (Paris, 1999). Paranoid thinking can also occur in response to stress. However, symptoms are rarely of delusional intensity and usually abate by removing or ameliorating the stressor (Linehan, 1993; Paris, 1999). Finally, borderline individuals experience *self-disregulation*. They are often confused about their own identities and may look to the environment for clues on how to behave, what to think, and how to feel (Linehan, 1993). They may experience a profound and intolerable sense of emptiness and loneliness (Gunderson & Phillips, 1991; Linehan, 1993; Paris, 1999), and some patients report no sense of self at all.

## Assessment

There are several methods for assessing personality disorders, including BPD. The most common method of assessment in clinical practice is the unstructured clinical interview (Western, 1997), but the preferred method is the semistructured or structured interview. The main advantage of the structured interview is that it provides a comprehensive, reliable, and objective assessment of personality disorder diagnosis (Segal, 1997). Zimmerman and Mattin (1999), for example, demonstrated that clinicians who used a semistructured clinical interview (i.e., the Structured Interview for DSM-

IV Personality Disorders) were significantly more likely to diagnose patients with BPD than clinicians who relied on routine unstructured clinical interviews. Moreover, without the benefit of detailed information from the semistructured clinical interview, clinicians rarely diagnosed BPD during a routine intake evaluation.

There are a number of semistructured and structured clinical interviews for categorically diagnosing DSM-IV personality disorders, including the Structured Interview for DSM-IV Personality Disorders (SIDP-IV; Pfohl, Blum, & Zimmerman, 1995), Structured Clinical Interview for DSM Personality Disorders (SCID-II; First, Spitzer, Biggon, Spitzer, Williams, & Benjamin, 1997), International Personality Disorder Examination (IPDE; Loranger et al., 1994), Personality Disorder Interview-IV (Widiger, Mangine, Corbitt, Ellis, & Thomas, 1995), and Diagnostic Interview for Personality Disorders (DIPD; Zanarini, Frankenburg, Sickel, & Yong, 1996). For a review of the reliability and validity of these instruments, the interested reader is referred to Segal (1997). Unfortunately some of these instruments may diagnose different individuals as borderline (Perry, 1992). Thus, some researchers and clinicians prefer the Diagnostic Interview for Borderlines-Revised (DIB-R; Zanarini, Gunderson, Frankenburg, & Chauncey, 1989), which is a semistructured clinical interview designed specifically to measure BPD criteria. The DIB-R has 136 questions, which correspond to four scales: affect, cognition, impulsivity, and interpersonal relationships. In scoring the DIB-R, the latter two criteria (impulsivity and interpersonal relationships) are assigned heavier weighting; BPD is assigned if the individual scores at least eight on a ten-point total score (Paris, 1999; Reich, 1992).

Because administration of structured interviews can be extremely time-consuming, especially in clinical settings, one strategy is first to administer a screening instrument to determine whether a patient may meet criteria for BPD and then to assess further using a structured interview format (Lezenweger, Loranger, Korfine, & Neff, 1997; Widiger & Bornstein, this book). There are several screening and self-report instruments to assess personality disorder criteria, including the Minnesota Multiphasic Personality Inventory-2 (MMPI-2) personality disorders scales developed by Morey, Waugh, and Blashfield (1985), Millon Clinical Multiaxal Inventory-III (Millon, Davis, & Millon,

1997), Personality Diagnostic Questionnaire-IV (PDQ-IV; Hyler, 1994), Wisconsin Personality Inventory (WISPI; Klein et al., 1993), Personality Assessment Inventory (PAI; Morey, 1991), and Schedule for Normal and Abnormal Personality (SNAP; Clark, 1993). The MMPI-2 and MCMI-III enjoy the most empirical support. The PAI has a Borderline Features Scale that taps four empirically derived dimensions that underlie borderline phenomenology: affective instability, identity problems, negative relationships, and self-harm. Studies have demonstrated that this scale has good internal consistency, high test–retest stability, and good convergent and discriminant validity (Morey, 1991; Trull, 1995).

## Prevalence

Interest in BPD increased greatly in the last 20 years, primarily due to the growing number of individuals presenting to mental health centers and practitioner's offices. Although the prevalence of BPD was not determined in the Epidemiological Catchment Area (ECA) study or in the recent National Comorbidity Survey, several studies (e.g., Ross, 1991; Swartz, Blazer, George, & Winfield, 1990) indicate that approximately 2% of the general population meet criteria for BPD (Paris, 1999). As would be expected, this figure is elevated in clinical samples. For example, approximately 11% of individuals seen in outpatient mental health settings meet criteria for BPD (Widiger & Frances, 1989). The prevalence of BPD again increases in psychiatric inpatient settings, where approximately 19% of individuals receive a diagnosis of BPD (Widiger & Frances, 1989). Additionally, among patients diagnosed exclusively with personality disorders, the prevalence rate of BPD ranges from 30 to 60% (Widiger & Trull, 1993), which is consistent with data showing that BPD is the most common personality disorder in clinical settings around the world (Loranger et al., 1994).

Social factors, it has been hypothesized, play a role in the development of BPD (Millon, 1993), although there are no existing cross-cultural studies examining the prevalence of BPD (Paris, 1999). In the United States, approximately 75% of individuals diagnosed with BPD are women (Swartz et al., 1990; Widiger & Trull, 1993), although many have argued that this gender difference is an arti-

fact of a diagnostic sex bias (e.g., Brown, 1992; Caplan, 1991, 1995). Widiger (1998) asserts that clinicians tend to apply a sex-biased style of diagnosing personality disorders, particularly when one considers that certain personality disorders are more common in women than in men. For example, many features of BPD (emotional displays, dependence in relationships) are associated with stereotypical feminine rather than masculine characteristics. Overgeneralizations such as these ultimately can lead to an overrepresentation of women diagnosed with BPD and an underrepresentation of men diagnosed with BPD (even if they meet criteria).

The influence of sex bias was revealed in one study. Becker and Lamb (1994) mailed surveys to a variety of mental health providers, who were asked to assign diagnoses to hypothetical scenarios in which a patient met criteria either for BPD or posttraumatic stress disorder. Half of those surveyed received a "male" case, whereas half received a "female" case. "Female" cases were more frequently diagnosed with BPD than "male" cases, even when the scenarios for both men and women met criteria for BPD. An article by Zanarini and Gunderson (1997) discusses the overlap of symptoms in antisocial personality disorder (APD) and BPD. As a result of this overlap, a man presenting with behaviors that meet criteria for BPD is more likely to be diagnosed with APD, which may be a function of assigning diagnoses that are consistent with sex biases related to these disorders. Again, remaining cognizant of the natural inclination to attribute particular behaviors to one gender rather than the other is extremely important when assigning personality diagnoses, such as BPD.

## Comorbidity

### Axis I Disorders

Substantial evidence exists to support the fact that BPD is comorbid with many Axis I disorders, specifically, mood, panic, substance abuse, impulse discontrol, eating, gender identity, attention-deficit, and posttraumatic stress disorders (Gunderson & Zanarini, 1987; Herman, Perry, & van der Kolk, 1989; van der Kolk, 1987; Widiger & Frances, 1989). Zanarini et al. (1998), for example, compared patients with criteria-defined BPD and participants with personality disorders to investigate DSM-III-R Axis I disorders. In a sample of 504 participants, it was found that anxiety, mood, and posttraumatic stress disorders were highly comorbid with BPD compared with participants with other personality disorders.

BPD occurs regularly with mood disorders, which is highlighted in the DSM-IV. The DSM-IV points to the fact that many of the symptoms of BPD can mimic an episode of Mood Disorder, and it becomes necessary to differentiate between common symptoms. Despite diagnostic overlap, there has been a considerable amount of research to support the notion that these two disorders are frequently comorbid. Widiger and Trull (1993) compiled all studies (though May 1989) that reported the diagnosis of a mood disorder in individuals diagnosed with BPD. Among 2015 BPD patients, it was found that 32% were diagnosed with major depression, 17% were diagnosed with dysthymic disorder, and 4% were diagnosed with bipolar disorder. As evidenced by this review, it becomes increasingly clear that a significant number of BPD patients also present with a mood disorder during the diagnostic phase.

Some concern has been raised about the comorbidity of BPD and affective disorders. As a matter of fact, some researchers have suggested that BPD is best understood as a subsyndrome or form of depression (Akiskal, Yerevanian, Davis, King, & Lemmi, 1985). Although a detailed review of the relevant literature on the overlap between BPD and affective disorders is beyond the scope of this chapter, Gunderson and Phillips (1991) provided a comprehensive review of the disorders that examined data on phenomenology, family history, comorbidity, psychopharmacology, biological markers, and pathogenesis. Briefly, the data failed to confirm a close or specific relationship between affective disorder and BPD (Gunderson, 1994). Moreover, as noted by Widiger and Trull (1993, p. 383), "what makes BPD a personality disorder is the course and phenomenology of the symptomatology, not whether there is an underlying biogenetic etiology shared by another disorder."

In addition to the comorbidity between BPD and mood disorders, evidence regarding the co-occurrence of BPD and posttraumatic stress disorder (PTSD) has surfaced in recent years. Research has indicated that a vast number of psychiatric patients with histories of childhood trauma often meet criteria for BPD (Herman, Perry, & van der Kolk, 1989). In a study by Bryer, Nelson, Miller, and Kroll (1987), it was found that child sexual abuse was reported by 86% of inpatients diagnosed with BPD. It has been found that a history of trauma is usually common among inpatients populations, but the severity of trauma tends to be more pronounced in BPD patients (Herman & van der Kolk, 1987). Given the commonality of childhood sexual abuse in both PTSD and BPD, it becomes apparent why these disorders might be comorbid.

Dissociation is a common feature that is often associated with both BPD and PTSD. Dissociation is correlated with both the intensity of BPD symptomatology and the severity of childhood trauma (Kluft, 1990; Putnam, 1989). Given this commonality, the issue of overlapping symptomatology again becomes important in considering the comorbidity between BPD and PTSD. Considering this issue, appropriate use of criteria for both disorders is essential for determining if an individual clearly meets diagnostic standards, because the possibility for misdiagnosis can be great.

## Axis II Disorders

BPD coexists with other Axis II disorders, specifically, Cluster B disorders (Zittel & Westen, 1998). Intuitively, this makes sense considering that a common element underlying Cluster B disorders (antisocial, histrionic, and narcissistic personality disorder) is impulsive and dramatic or erratic behavior. Widiger and Trull (1993) reviewed a number of studies and found that many individuals who received a diagnosis of BPD also received a diagnosis for another personality disorder. Although clinicians routinely differentiate between Axis II disorders, researchers have continually struggled with issues of diagnostic validity (e.g., high rates of comorbidity and diagnostic overlap between Axis II categories) (Zanarini & Gunderson, 1997; Zittel & Westen, 1998). Some have argued that validity problems might be resolved by replacing categories with a dimensional classification system (Widiger, 1993). In a categorical system, prototypical cases of personality disorders are relatively easy to differentiate overlapping symptomatology (Gunderson, 1984; Gunderson & Zanarini, 1987; Widiger & Frances, 1989). However, difficulty increases considerably in cases that do not present with clearly defined behavioral patterns consistent with a particular disorder. In an attempt to remedy this situation, a great deal of time was spent clarifying diagnostic criteria for Axis II disorders during the revision of the DSM-III-R to the DSM-IV. The available evidence indicates an improvement in reliability and divergence among the DSM-IV Cluster B categories, although issues of diagnostic efficiency and convergence of criteria sets remain a problem (Blais, Hilsenroth, & Castlebury, 1997; Blais, Hilsenroth, & Fowler, 1999; Fossati et al., 1999).

Zanarini and Gunderson (1997) highlighted the overlap between BPD and other Axis II disorders and devoted specific attention to the comorbidity between BPD and antisocial personality disorder (ASPD). In an analysis of all studies that investigated the relationship between BPD and ASPD, they found that "in studies focusing on criteria-defined BPD samples, rates of ASPD comorbidity ranged from 0% to 60%, with most studies reporting rates of co-occurrence between about 10% to 25%" (p. 85). Impulsivity and instability in interpersonal relationships, common features of both disorders, may account, in part, for the high degree of comorbidity between the disorders. As Zanarini (1993) demonstrated, converging lines of evidence (reviewed later) link BPD with other psychiatric disorders that have impulsivity as a predominant feature (e.g., ASPD, substance abuse).

In addition to Cluster B disorders, BPD co-occurs with other Axis II disorders, and specific attention is given to its co-occurrence with schizotypal personality disorder (STP) (Zittel & Westen, 1998; Widiger & Trull, 1993). Research has indicated that diagnostic criteria for both STP and BPD can often be applied to the same individual (Rosenberger & Miller, 1989; Widiger, Frances, & Trull, 1987). However, with careful consideration and specific attention to subtle differences (e.g., cognitive functioning and affect), the ability to differentiate the two disorders becomes less troublesome. For example, Widiger and Trull (1993) noted that the correlation between DSM-III-R BPD and STP criterion sets was often minimal, suggesting that the two disorders represent distinct dimensions or categories. Moreover, although the inclusion of stress-induced, quasi-psychotic symptoms in the DSM-IV definition of BPD was vociferously debated mainly because of the possibility of increasing diagnostic overlap with STP, the weight of the available empirical evidence suggests that the two disorders remain readily distinguishable (Blais et al., 1997). In general, STP belongs along a spectrum of schizophrenia pathology (Meehl, 1989), whereas BPD occurs along a spectrum of impulsivity and affective pathology (Siever & Davis, 1991; Zanarini, 1993).

This issue of comorbidity obviously presents itself when considering the diagnosis of Axis II disorders, given the commonality of personality characteristics within this subset of disorders. With this in mind, the importance of accurate assignment of personality characteristics in diagnosis becomes germane. Thorough assessment of personality characteristics is an essential component in accurately distinguishing Axis II disorders. Assessment will allow adequately diagnosing comorbid personality disorders when required. Given the evidence of high comorbidity between BPD and other Axis II disorders, appropriate consideration should be given during diagnosis to avoid incorrectly assigning diagnostic labels.

## Course and Outcome of BPD

When reviewing the data on the outcome and course of the disorder, it is important to remember that the majority of studies has followed borderline patients in treatment, and thus little is known about the natural history or course of the disorder (Stone, 1989; Widiger & Trull, 1993). BPD usually begins in adolescence and peaks in young adulthood (Paris, 1999). If borderline individuals survive their 20s and early 30s, the symptoms tend to "burn out" by age 40 or 50 (Zittel & Westen, 1998).

Short-term follow-up studies (e.g., Barasch et al., 1985; Stevenson & Meares, 1992) indicate that 60–70% of individuals who are diagnosed with BPD continue to meet diagnostic criteria 2 to 3 years after the initial assessment. Intermediate outcome studies (e.g., Pope, Jonas, Hudson, Cohen, & Gunderson, 1983) indicate that 57–67% of BPD patients continue to meet diagnostic criteria 4 to 7 years after the index assessment (Linehan & Heard, 1999). At 5-year follow-up, most patients show little to no improvement in functioning (e.g., Paris, 1988; Stone, 1989; Zanarini, Chauncey, Grady, & Gunderson, 1991). However, more recent studies (e.g., Linehan, Armstrong, Suarez, Allmon, & Heard, 1991; Najavits & Gunderson, 1995) indicate that borderline patients can show functional improvement in 1 to 3 years, which may reflect advancements in treatment.

Long-term outcome studies (e.g., McGlashan, 1986; Paris, Brown, & Nowlins, 1987; Plakun, Burkhardt & Muller, 1985; Stone, 1990) indicate that diagnosable BPD usually remits by middle age. Both Stone (1990) and Paris et al. (1987) found that 75% of patients diagnosed as borderline during early adulthood no longer met criteria at 15-year follow-up. Nonetheless, considerable variability exists in functional outcome, and long-term recovery was rarely complete (Paris, 1999; Widiger & Trull, 1993). For example, 10 to 30 years after initial diagnosis, about one in five patients in Stone's (1990) sample were living normal symptom-free lives, whereas about one in three still showed major symptoms. Prognosis was better for patients who were intelligent, attractive, had artistic talents, or who were described as more likable, whereas prognosis was poorer for patients who had alcohol or substance abuse problems, histories of physical or sexual abuse, severe problems with impulsive behavior, and comorbid antisocial or schizotypal personality features. McGlashan (1992), who conducted a review of the literature on the course of BPD, concluded that better long-term outcome was associated with higher intelligence; lower-affective lability; less chronicity; and an ability to experience pleasure, contain aggression in relationships, and tolerate psychological pain.

Suicide is one of the major risks for borderline patients observed in these and other studies (Zittel & Westen, 1998). In general, BPD patients have a high rate of suicide completion. Although McGlashan (1986) found a suicide rate of 3%, both Paris (1993) and Stone (1990) found completed suicide rates of 8 to 9%. Based on a review of eight outcome studies, Linehan and Heard (1999) estimated the average suicide rates at 7.8%. Breaking this down over time periods, the average suicide rate among patients followed in short-term studies (i.e., 3 years after the index point) was 4.22%, whereas for studies that estimated suicide rates from 4 to 7 years and 13 to 20 years, the average rates were 7.53 and 7.65%, respectively. A consistent finding among all of these studies is that most suicides occur within the first 5 years of the index assessment (Linehan & Heard, 1999; Paris, 1999; Zittel & Westen, 1998).

## Etiology

When examining etiologic factors associated with BPD, it is important to note that biological and psychological factors interact in multiple ways to shape the course of the disorder. Paris

(1999) distinguished between necessary and sufficient conditions for BPD. He applied a diathesis-stress model (Monroe & Simmons, 1991) to explain the etiology of the disorder. In his biopsychosocial model (Paris, 1994, 1999), biological factors are considered necessary for borderline psychopathology to take particular form, but genetic vulnerabilities by themselves are not sufficient causes of the disorder. Psychological and social factors, although insufficient causal factors, probably best determine which vulnerable individuals develop BPD. Therefore, psychological conditions may be necessary but not sufficient causes for developing BPD (Paris, 1999). With this biopsychosocial model in mind, we review the empirical literature on biological and psychological factors implicated in BPD.

### Biological Factors

There has been limited genetic research on BPD. To date, there are no adoption studies of BPD. The only twin study was conducted by Torgersen (1984), who did not find any concordance for BPD among seven monozygotic pairs, although his original sample was too small to make definitive conclusions. In subsequent work, Torgersen (1986) examined a larger sample of twins and established that BPD has a particularly low index of heritability, compared with most of the other personality disorders. Paris (1999) noted that studies of normal twin populations (e.g., Jang, Livesley, Vernon, & Jackson, 1996; Livesley, Jang, Schroeder, & Jackson, 1993) provide support for the heritability of certain personality traits seen in BPD (e.g., impulsivity, affective instability, and cognitive symptoms) (see also Plomin, Defries, McClearn, & Rutter, 1997). However, evidence for the genetic heritability of the specific disorder is essentially nonexistent, which makes BPD no different from other Axis II disorders (McGuffin & Thapar, 1992; Nigg & Goldsmith, 1994; Paris, 1994).

Family history studies (e.g., Akiskal et al., 1985; Andrulonis & Vogel, 1984; Links, Steiner, & Huxley, 1988; Zanarini et al., 1988) examined the prevalence of psychiatric disorders among the first-degree relatives of individuals with BPD. One of the most consistent findings is that BPD tends to "breed true" (Links et al., 1988; Zanarini & Frankenberg, 1997) because borderline individuals are five times more likely to have first-degree relatives with BPD than by chance alone (Gunderson, 1994; Zittel & Westen, 1998). Some have suggested that this represents genetic transmission of the disorder (e.g., Baron, Risch, Levitt & Gruen, 1985), although only twin and adoption studies can separate genetic from environmental influences. In addition, family history studies have documented a higher frequency of relatives with other impulse spectrum disorders, namely, alcoholism, substance abuse, and antisocial behavior (Paris, 1999; Zanarini et al., 1993). There is also a greater frequency of unipolar major depression, but only in the relatives of BPD patients with concurrent major depression (Pope et al., 1983; Gunderson & Phillips, 1991; Paris, 1999).

Research has yet to reveal any biological markers that are specific to BPD (Gunderson & Phillips, 1991; Paris, 1999). For example, biological markers for depression, such as abnormal dexamethasone suppression (DST) or decreased REM latency, occur only in BPD patients who are also depressed (Gunderson & Phillips, 1991; Gunderson, 1994). Zanarini and Frankenburg (1997), who summarized the results of EEG studies, arrived at a similar conclusion. At least two studies reported a significantly higher rate of abnormal EEG findings among BPD patients relative to depressed controls (Cowdry, Pickar, & Davies, 1985–1986; Snyder & Pitts, 1984). However, two other studies found that the rates of abnormal EEG findings in BPD patients and Axis II control patients were roughly comparable (Cornelius, Brenner, Soloff, Schulz, & Tumuluru, 1986; Zanarini, Kimble, & Williams, 1994). Paris (1999) noted that a more sophisticated EEG study, which examined "P-300" event related potentials (Kutcher, Blackwood, Clair, Gaskell, & Muir, 1987), revealed that BPD patients had abnormal EEG findings resembling those seen in schizophrenia. However, it should be underscored that biological markers, even when found, do not necessarily demonstrate a biological etiological factor (Paris, 1994, 1999). Moreover, research strategies that attempt to localize specific brain deficits may be far too simplistic because the causes of BPD, it is thought, are multidimensional, complex, and interactive.

Thus, it is not surprising that studies that have used neuroimaging techniques with BPD patients have also produced mixed findings. Two studies found that BPD patients had normal CT scans (Schulz et al., 1983; Snyder, Pitts, & Gustin, 1983). By contrast, two other studies found that a small percentage of borderline patients had abnormal CT scans, although the rates of abnormal scans were not significantly different from those seen in normal participants or patients with other personality disorders (Lucas, Gardner, Cowdry, & Pickar, 1989; Zanarini, Kimble, & Williams, 1994). To date, only two studies examined PET scans in BPD patients (Goyer, Konicki, & Schulz, 1994; Leyton et al., 1997), although the sample sizes were rather small. Goyer et al. (1994) found reduced brain activity in the frontal and parietal lobes of BPD patients. The strongest findings link brain metabolism with aggressive and impulsive traits, suggesting that biological markers are more specific to borderline traits than the disorder *per se* (Paris, 1994, 1999).

Similar conclusions were reached from biochemical studies that examined markers associated with impulsivity (Coccaro et al., 1989; Hollander et al., 1994; Martial et al., 1997). In these studies, that typically assess serotonergic activity by the flenfluramine challenge test, BPD patients show decreased serotonergic activity relative to control subjects. However, this deficit is more specific to those patients who score high on traits of impulsivity and aggression than BPD *per se*. Moreover, levels of the serotonin metabolite 5-HIAA in the cerebrospinal fluid are not significantly lower in BPD than in control patients unless the BPD patients also have histories of suicide attempts (Gardner, Lucas, & Cowdry, 1990; Paris, 1999).

Additionally, some evidence supports the notion of a biological relationship between affective instability and increased sensitivity of the cholinergic and noradrenergic systems, although there are no clear biological markers related specifically to BPD or other personality disorders (Figueroa & Silk, 1997; Steinberg, Trestman, & Siever, 1994). Finally, several researchers (Andrulonis, Blueck, Stroebel, & Vogel, 1982; Gardner, Lucas, & Cowdry, 1987; van Reekum, Links, & Boiago, 1993) found that individuals with BPD have a significantly greater number of soft neurological signs, compared to normal controls. However, these markers are rather nonspecific (e.g., they occur in other patient populations as well) (Zanarini et al., 1994).

In summary, existing evidence implicates a number of biological systems that may play a role in BPD, although no biological markers are specific to BPD. Some BPD patients, particularly those with comorbid depression, may share some of the hypothylamic-pituitary-adrenal (HPA) abnormalities of depressed patients, as revealed by the DST and REM-latency onset studies (Figueroa & Silk, 1997). Other BPD patients, mainly those with impulsive traits, may have abnormalities in the serotonergic system. There are also nonspecific abnormalities in the cholinergic and adrenergic systems, which may be related to symptoms of dysphoria, emotional lability, and hyperreactivity to environmental stimuli (Figueroa & Silk, 1997).

## Psychological Factors

There is a substantial amount of evidence that psychological factors play a role in the development of BPD (Paris, 1994, 1999). The risk factors tend to be related to a variety of childhood experiences and fall into three broad categories: childhood trauma, early parental separation and loss, and disturbed family environment and abnormal parental bonding (Paris, 1994, 1999; Zanarini & Frankenburg, 1997).

## Childhood Trauma

Research findings suggest that borderline individuals report a high rate of childhood trauma. A number of studies showed that childhood physical abuse is more commonly reported by BPD patients than by controls (Herman et al., 1989), but some researchers have not found such associations (Ogata, Silk, Goodrich, et al., 1990). The most consistent finding is the association between childhood sexual abuse (CSA) and BPD. Approximately 50 to 70% of BPD patients report CSA (Paris, 1994; Zanarini et al., 1993; Zittel & Westen, 1998). Additionally, CSA has a strong association with BPD independent of other factors such as neglect or loss (Ogata et al., 1990; Paris et al., 1994a). In the light of these findings, childhood trauma has been proposed by some (Herman & van der Kolk, 1987) as an explanation for the etiology of BPD. However, Paris (1999) identified several problems in interpreting findings on CSA.

First, CSA lacks specificity as an etiologic risk factor for BPD. For example, childhood trauma is frequently reported in both BPD patients and patients with other personality disorders (Paris et al.,

1994a,b). More fundamentally, many individuals who experience childhood trauma, including sexual abuse, do not go on to develop BPD. In fact, there is a wide range of clinical outcomes in individuals with CSA (e.g., depression, PTSD, substance abuse, normal presentation). Thus, childhood trauma, it is thought, represents a general risk factor for psychopathology rather than a cause of any one specific disorder (Browne & Finkelhor, 1986; Paris, 1999).

Another problem is that most studies have not systematically examined that parameters or characteristics of sexual abuse (e.g., the identity of the perpetrator and the severity, frequency and duration of the abuse), which are better predictors of clinical outcome than sexual abuse alone (Browne & Finkelhor, 1986; Paris, 1999). In a series of studies, Paris et al. (1994a,b) measured parameters of CSA severity in a sample of BPD patients. Severity of sexual abuse was much more strongly related to BPD than abuse alone. Thus, it appears that the long-term outcome of sexual abuse partially depends on these parameters.

Additionally, Paris (1999) noted that most research has not systematically teased apart the relationship between CSA and concomitant risk factors. For example, CSA frequently occurs in a chaotic and pathological family environment (Finkelhor, Hotaling, Lewis, & Smith, 1990). In community studies, the long-term effects of CSA were explained by their intercorrelations with abnormalities in family functioning (Nash et al., 1993). Additionally, research has not considered how CSA might interact with biological risk factors, such as childhood temperament and personality features (Paris, 1999). Finally, the effect size of the association between CSA and BPD is not very large. Fossati et al. (1999) conducted a meta-analysis of twenty-one published studies and found only a moderate pooled correlation (.279) between CSA and BPD.

In summary, childhood trauma, and sexual abuse in particular, represent psychological risk factors in the development of BPD. However, the magnitude of their effects are not specific and probably depend on multiple interacting factors, such as the parameters or characteristics of the abuse, the presence or absence of a supportive family environment, the temperament of the child, and the existence of additional biological and psychological risk factors. Future research needs to sort out these interactions by examining the impact of childhood trauma using a multidimensional framework (Paris, 1997). Additionally, longitudinal studies need to be carried out to examine changes in functioning over time.

## Parental Separation and Loss

Several studies examined the prevalence of early separations and losses in the childhood histories of BPD patients (e.g., Akiskal et al., 1985; Links, Steiner, Offord, & Eppel, 1988; Soloff & Millward, 1983; Zanarini, Gunderson, Marino, Schwartz & Frankenburg, 1988). Zanarini and Frankenburg (1997) summarized the major findings of these studies. First, early separations and losses are common among patients with BPD (approximately 37–64% of BPD patients report early parental separation or loss, depending on the study). Second, prolonged separations and early losses tend to discriminate BPD patients from other psychiatric patients, including those with psychotic, affective, or other personality disorder diagnoses.

However, Paris (1999), who also reviewed studies on parental separation and loss, reached a somewhat different conclusion. He noted that most studies that supported a relationship between BPD and parental separation/loss compared borderline patients with depressed patients. Moreover, some studies failed to confirm these differences (Ogata et al., 1990). For example, Paris et al. (1994a,b) compared BPD patients with patients who had other personality disorders. Although early separation and losses were frequent in BPD patients, they occurred just as frequently in individuals with other Axis II disorders. Indeed, Paris (1999) noted that a history of early separation and loss is quite frequent in normal populations (Tennant, 1988) and is not specific to any type of psychopathology. Most likely, if early separation and loss does play an etiological role in BPD, it does not lead to the disorder by itself (Paris, 1999; Rutter, 1989).

## Disturbed Family Environment and Parental Bonding

Although the data on family environment and parental bonding are largely based on retrospective accounts of childhood experiences, if we are to believe the reports of BPD patients, then malig-

nant family experiences cannot be overlooked. The early clinical literature suggested that BPD arose out of overinvolved, hostile-dependent, and separation-resistant families (Gunderson, 1994). However, empirically studies indicated that rather than overinvolvement, there was significant emotional neglect of children who later developed BPD (Gunderson, Kerr, & Englund, 1980). Family history studies consistently documented the fact that many borderline individuals grew up in severely dysfunctional family environments characterized by neglect, conflict, hostility, and chaotic unpredictability (Links, 1990; Gunderson & Zanarini, 1989). In addition to living in chaotic and unpredictable home environments, many BPD patients perceive having had abnormal bonding with their parents that involve both neglectful and overprotective responses (Frank & Paris, 1981; Soloff & Millward, 1983; Zanarini et al., 1993). These findings are consistent with environmental and biosocial theories of BPD (Adler, 1985; Linehan, 1993) that emphasize the etiological significance of chaotic and unpredictable environments in the development of BPD.

Adler (1985), for example, postulated that parents who fail to provide a supportive and protective environment do not allow their children to develop the skills necessary to regulate emotions and buffer emotional distress. One consequence of emotional neglect is that children learn to regulate negative emotions through impulsive behavior (Paris, 1999). According to Linehan (1993), an "invalidating environment" consistently communicates to the individual that his or her behaviors and reactions are not appropriate or valid responses to events. Children who are raised in an "invalidating environment" never receive adequate training or parental modeling to learn necessary skills to regulate arousal and tolerate emotional distress. Children instead learn that drug abuse, promiscuity, and self-injurious behavior produce temporary relief from stress. Additionally, children do not learn to trust their own reactions as valid, and consequently may have to rely on the environment to provide information about how to feel, think, and act (Linehan, 1993). BPD, it is thought, arises from a combination of these malignant environmental influences (e.g., chaotic and unpredictable family environments, sexual abuse, neglect, etc.) interacting with biologically based deficits in emotional processing and their transaction over time (Linehan, 1993). For a comprehensive review of the theories of BPD, the interested reader is referred to Millon (1992) and Paris (1999).

## Treatment

Few clinicians would disagree that individuals with BPD represent one of the most challenging and difficult to treat populations. Although various psychosocial treatments have been developed (e.g., psychodynamic, interpersonal, behavioral, and cognitive treatments), few enjoy strong empirical support. Pharmacotherapy has proven useful as an adjunctive treatment of BPD. These treatments are briefly described and evidence supporting their efficacy is reviewed.

### Dialectical Behavior Therapy

Dialectical Behavior Therapy (DBT) is a form of cognitive behavioral therapy that was originally developed as a treatment for chronically suicidal individuals who meet criteria for BPD (Linehan, 1993). DBT uses a combination of directive, problem-solving, and behavioral change strategies, coupled with nondirective techniques that promote acceptance and empathy. DBT includes individual and group therapy. The group component involves psychoeducation and teaching patients behavioral coping skills, including distress tolerance, interpersonal effectiveness, emotion regulation, and mindfulness (Linehan, 1993). Individual therapy focuses on six goals addressed in hierarchical priority: suicidal behavior, therapy-interfering behavior, behaviors that interfere with quality of life, behavioral skill acquisition, post-traumatic stress symptoms, and self-respect behaviors.

DBT is one of the only treatments for BPD that has been subjected to careful empirical scrutiny. Linehan et al. (1991) conducted the first randomized controlled clinical trial with BPD patients. Forty-four women diagnosed with BPD and histories of parasuicidal behavior were randomly assigned to either 1-year DBT or treatment as usual (TAU) in the community. At the end of 1 year of outpatient treatment, women who received DBT were significantly less likely to attempt suicide or drop out of therapy than women in the TAU group. Women who received DBT also spent significantly less time in psychiatric inpatient hospi-

tals, had fewer and less medically severe episodes of parasuicidal behavior, were better adjusted interpersonally, and reported less anger (Linehan et al., 1991, 1994). However, the groups did not differ on measures of depression, hopelessness, or suicidal ideation at the completion of the trial.

DBT has also proven effective for treating more severely dysfunctional BPD patients. For example, Barley et al. (1993) found that BPD inpatients who received DBT in conjunction with standard inpatient treatment (SIT) had significantly fewer incidents of parasuicidal behavior than inpatients who received only SIT. Moreover, Linehan et al. (1999) demonstrated that DBT is more effective than treatment as usual in reducing drug use among women with BPD and comorbid substance abuse problems. Future empirical studies are needed to determine the long-term effectiveness of DBT.

### Psychodynamic Treatment

Psychodynamic approaches enjoy a long-standing history in treating BPD. Many studies reported significant improvements in patient functioning following psychodynamic treatment (e.g., Adler, 1985, 1989; Buie & Adler, 1982; Kernberg, 1984, 1987; Masterson, 1976, 1981; Stevenson & Meares, 1992). Unfortunately, most psychodynamic clinicians have supported claims of effectiveness on the basis of data from case studies and uncontrolled outcome or longitudinal studies (Linehan & Heard, 1999).

The exceptions are two independent groups of investigators who evaluated psychodynamic treatment approaches using controlled outcome designs. The first studies were conducted by Marziali and colleagues (Clarkin, Marziali & Munroe-Blum, 1991; Munroe-Blum & Marziali, 1988, 1995) who compared psychodynamic group therapy with individual psychodynamic therapy (control condition). The psychodynamic group treatment, called relationship management therapy (RMT), is a time-limited approach that uses a cotherapist model and focuses on interpersonal transactions and their outcomes. Within the group setting, individuals are encouraged to express internalized conflicts around self-attributes, and feedback is provided by cotherapists and other group members. At 12- and 24-month follow-up, the investigators found no significant differences between the treatment groups on major outcome measures.

However, both groups demonstrated significant improvements on all major outcomes at follow-up, which suggests that psychodynamic group therapy may be a more cost-effective method of delivering services than individual psychodynamic therapy (Linehan & Heard, 1999).

In a more recent randomized clinical trial, Bateman and Fonagy (1999) compared the efficacy of a psychodynamically oriented partial hospitalization treatment (PHT) with standard psychiatric care for patients with BPD. PHT included both individual and group psychodynamic treatment and occurred for a maximum of 18 months. At the end of 18 months, patients who were partially hospitalized were significantly less likely to attempt suicide, engage in self-mutilatory acts, or to be admitted inpatient for psychiatric hospitalization, compared to patients who received standard psychiatric care. Additionally, patients who were partially hospitalized reported significant reductions in anxiety, depression, and general distress, and improvements in interpersonal functioning and social adjustment, whereas patients who received standard psychiatric care demonstrated either limited changes or deterioration during the 18-month period. For most outcomes, improvements in the partial hospitalization group began at 6 months and were maintained at 18 months. Although replication is needed with larger groups, these findings suggest that partial hospitalization may represent an effective alternative to standard inpatient treatment, especially for severely dysfunctional BPD patients.

### Pharmacotherapy

A number of pharmacotherapeutic studies were conducted using randomized controlled procedures (for reviews, see Brinkley, 1993; Dimeff, McDavid, & Linehan, 1999; and Soloff, 1994). The four major BPD symptoms at which pharmacotherapy has been targeted are affective instability, impulsive behavior, transient psychotic symptoms, and anxiety (Soloff, 1994). The effects of a number of drugs have been tested, including neuroleptics (Cowdry & Gardner, 1988; Goldberg et al., 1986), antidepressants (Cornelius, Soloff, Perel, & Ulrich, 1990; Parsons et al., 1989), anticonvulsants (Cowdry & Gardner, 1988), and lithium carbonate (Links, Steiner, Boiago, & Irwin, 1990). In general, pharmacotherapeutic agents have proven effective in decreasing depression,

anger, impulsive behavior, psychosis, and other forms of cognitive disturbance (Linehan & Heard, 1999); however, treatment effects are generally considered modest, and most agents have been tested only during short periods of time (Soloff, 1994). Additionally, medications should be monitored carefully in this population because of the potential for misuse, drug abuse, or use for suicide attempts (Linehan, 1993). Pharmacotherapy should be considered a useful adjunct to psychotherapy in treating BPD (Linehan & Heard, 1999; Soloff, 1994).

### Summary

The overview of the borderline personality disorder literature reveals that this category continues to evolve, despite its relative recent history in the DSM. Perhaps the most significant improvements will come from systematic research that attempts to resolve the controversy whether the disorder is best conceptualized as a category or personality dimension. Nonetheless, the DSM-IV diagnosis describes a reliable and valid construct. Additional research is also needed to gain a better understanding of the etiology of the disorder, including systematic investigations of the interplay among biological factors, genetic vulnerabilities, and psychological and social risk factors. The use of prospective, longitudinal designs studying large cohorts of children will provide a better understanding of the development, etiology, course, and prevention of the disorder. It is expected that advances in basic research will also translate into breakthroughs in treatment, which ultimately may improve the quality of life for BPD patients.

### References

Adler, G. (1985). *Borderline psychopathology and its treatment*. New York: Jason Aronson.

Adler, G. (1989). Psychodynamic therapies in borderline personality disorder. In A. Tasman, R. E. Hales, & A. J. Frances (Eds.), *American Psychiatric Press Review of Psychiatry* Vol. 8 (pp. 48–64).

Akiskal, H., Yerevanian, B., Davis, G., King, D., & Lemmi, H (1985). The nosologic status of borderline personality: Clinical and polysomnographic study. *American Journal of Psychiatry, 142*, 192–198.

American Psychiatric Association. (1980). *Diagnostic and statistical manual of mental disorders* (3rd ed.). Washington DC: Author.

American Psychiatric Association. (1987). *Diagnostic and statistical manual of mental disorders* (3rd ed., rev.). Washington, DC: Author.

American Psychiatric Association. (1994). *Diagnostic and statistical manual of mental disorders* (4th ed.). Washington, DC: Author.

Andrulonis, P. A., & Vogel, N. G. (1984). Comparison of borderline personality subcategories to schizophrenic and affective disorders. *British Journal of Psychiatry, 144,* 358–363.

Andrulonis, P. A., Bluek, B. C., Stroebel, O. F., & Vogel, N. G. (1982). Borderline personality subcategories. *Journal of Nervous and Mental Diseases, 174,* 727–734.

Barasch, A., Frances, A., Hurt, S., Clarkin, J., & Cohen, S. (1985). Stability and distinctness of borderline personality disorder. *American Journal of Psychiatry, 142,* 1484–1486.

Barley, W. D., Buie, S. E., Peterson, E. W., Hollingsworth, A. S., Oriva, M., Hickerson, S. C., Lawson, J. E., & Bailey, B. J. (1993). Development of an inpatient cognitive-behavioral treatment program for borderline personality disorder. *Journal of Personality Disorders, 7,* 232–240.

Baron, M., Risch, N., Levitt, M., & Gruen, R. (1985). Familial transmission of schizotypal and borderline personality disorders. *American Journal of Psychiatry, 142,* 927–934.

Bateman, A., & Fonagy, P. (1999). Effectiveness of partial hospitalization in the treatment of borderline personality disorder: A randomized control trial. *American Journal of Psychiatry, 156,* 1563–1569.

Becker, D., & Lamb, S. (1994). Sex bias in the diagnosis of borderline personality disorder and posttraumatic stress disorder. *Professional Psychology: Research and Practice, 25,* 55–61.

Blais, M. A., & Norman, D. K. (1997). A psychometric evaluation of the DSM-IV personality disorder criteria. *Journal of Personality Disorders, 11,* 168–176.

Blais, M. A., Hilsenroth, M. J., & Catlebury, F. D. (1997). Psychometric characteristics of the cluster B Personality Disorders under DSM-III-R and DSM-IV. *Journal of Personality Disorders, 11,* 270–278.

Blais, M. A., Hilsenroth, M. J., & Fowler, C. (1999). Diagnostic efficiency and hierarchical functioning of the DSM-IV borderline personality disorder criteria. *Journal of Nervous and Mental Disease, 187,* 167–173.

Brinkley, J. R. (1993). Pharmacotherapy of borderline states. *Psychiatric Clinics of North America, 16,* 853–884.

Brown, L. S. (1992). A feminist critique of the personality disorders. In L. S. Brown & M. Ballou (Eds.), *Personality and psychopathology: Feminist reappraisals* (pp. 206–228). New York: Guilford.

Browne, A., & Finkelhor, D. (1986). Impact of child sexual abuse: A review of the literature. *Psychological Bulletin, 99,* 66–77.

Bryer, J. B., Nelson, B. A., Miller, J. B., & Krol, P. A. (1987). Childhood sexual abuse and physical abuse as factors in adult psychiatric illness. *American Journal of Psychiatry, 144,* 1426–1430.

Buie, D. H., & Adler, G. (1982). The definitive treatment of borderline personality. *International Journal of Psychoanalytic Psychotherapy, 9,* 51–87.

Caplan, P. J. (1991). How do they decide who is normal? The bizarre, but true, tale of the DSM process. *Canadian Psychology, 32,* 162–170.

Caplan, P. J. (1995). *They say you're crazy: How the world's most powerful psychiatrists decide who is normal.* Reading, MA: Addison-Wesley.

Clark, L. A. (1993). *Manual for the schedule for nonadaptive and adaptive personality.* Minneapolis, MN: University of Minnesota Press.

Clark, L. A., Livesley, J., & Morey, L. (1997). Special feature: Personality disorder assessment: The challenge of construct validity. *Journal of Personality Disorders, 11,* 205–231.

Clarkin, J. E., Marziali, E., & Munroe-Blum, H. (1991). Group and family treatments for borderline personality disorder. *Hospital and Community Psychiatry, 42,* 1038–1043.

Coccaro, E. F., Siever, L. J., Klar, H. M., Maurer, G., Cochrane, K., Cooper, T. B., Mohs, R. C., & Davis, K. L. (1989). Serotonergic studies in patients with affective and personality disorders. *Archives of General Psychiatry, 46,* 587–599.

Cornelius, J. R., Brenner, R. P., Soloff, P. H., Schulz, S. C., & Tumuluru, R. V. (1986). EEG abnormalities in borderline personality disorder: Specific or nonspecific. *Biological Psychiatry, 21,* 977–980.

Cornelius, J. R., Soloff, P. H., Perel, J. M., & Urlich, R. F. (1990). Fluoxetine trial in borderline personality disorder. *Psychopharmacological Bulletin, 26,* 149–152.

Cowdry, R. W., Pickar, D., & Davies, R. (1985–1986). Symptoms and EEG findings in borderline syndrome. *International Journal of Psychiatric Medicine, 15,* 201–211.

Cowdry, R. W., & Gardner, D. L. (1988). Pharmacotherapy of borderline personality disorder: Alprazolam, carbamazepine, trifluoperazine and tranylcypromine. *Archives of General Psychiatry, 45,* 111–119.

Dimeff, L. A., McDavid, J., & Linehan, M. M. (1999). Pharmacotherapy for borderline personality disorder: A review of the literature and recommendations for treatment. *Journal of Clinical Psychology in Medical Settings, 6,* 113–138.

Figueroa, E., & Silk, K. R. (1997). Biological implications of childhood sexual abuse in borderline personality disorder. *Journal of Personality Disorders, 11,* 71–92.

Finkelhor, D., Hotaling, G., Lewis, I. A., & Smith, C. (1990). Sexual abuse in a national survey of adult men and women: Prevalence characteristics and risk factors. *Child Abuse and Neglect, 14,* 19–28.

First, M., Gibbon, M., Spitzer, R. L., Williams, J. B. W., & Benjamin, L. S. (1997). *User's guide for the Structured Clinical Interview for the DSM-IV Axis II Personality Disorders.* Washington, DC: American Psychiatric Press.

Fossati, A., Maffei, C., Bagnato, M., Donati, D., Namia, C., & Novella, L. (1999). Latent structure analysis of DSM-IV borderline personality disorder criteria. *Comprehensive Psychiatry, 40,* 72–79.

Fossati, A., Madeddu, F., & Maffei, C. (1999). Borderline personality disorder and childhood sexual abuse: A meta-analytic study. *Journal of Personality Disorders, 13,* 268–280.

Frank, H., & Paris, J. (1981). Recollections of family experience in borderline patients. *Archives of General Psychiatry, 38,* 1031–1034.

Freeman, A. M., Pretzer, J. L., Fleming, B., & Simon, K. M. (1990). *Clinical applications of cognitive therapy.* New York: Plenum.

Gardner, D. L., Lucas, P. B., & Cowdry, R. W. (1990). CSF metabolites in borderline personality disorder compared with normal controls. *Biological Psychiatry, 28,* 247–254.

Goldberg, S. C., Schulz, S. C., Schulz, P. M., Resnick, R. J.,

Hamer, R. M., & Friedel, R. O. (1986). Borderline and schizotypal personality disorders treated with low-dose thiothixene vs. placebo. *Archives of General Psychiatry, 45,* 111–119.

Goyer, P. F., Konicki, P. E., & Schulz, S. C. (1994). Brain imaging in personality disorders. In K. R. Silk (Ed.), *Biological and neurobehavioral studies of borderline personality disorder* (pp. 109–127). Washington, DC: American Psychiatric Press.

Green, A. (1977). The borderline concept. In P. Hartocollis (Ed.), *Borderline personality disorders.* New York: International Universities Press.

Gunderson, J. (1984). *Borderline personality disorder.* Washington, DC: American Psychiatric Press.

Gunderson, J. (1994). Building structure for the borderline construct. *Acta Psychiatrica Scandinavica, 89*(Suppl. 379), 12–18.

Gunderson, J., & Singer, M. (1975). Defining borderline patients: An overview. *American Journal of Psychiatry, 132,* 1–9.

Gunderson, J., & Kolb, J. (1978). Discriminating features of borderline patients. *American Journal of Psychiatry, 135,* 792–796.

Gunderson, J., Zanarini, M., & Kigiel, C. (1995). Borderline personality disorder. In W. J. Livesley (Ed.), *The DSM-IV personality disorders* (pp. 141–157). New York: Guilford.

Gunderson, J., & Phillips, K. A. (1991). A current view of the interface between borderline personality disorder and depression. *American Journal of Psychiatry, 148,* 967–975.

Gunderson, J., & Zanarini, M. (1987). Current overview of the borderline personality diagnosis. *Journal of Clinical Psychiatry, 48*(Suppl. 8), 5–11.

Gunderson, J., Kerr, J., & Eklund, D. (1980). The families of borderlines: A comparative study. *Archives of General Psychiatry, 37,* 27–33.

Gunderson, J., & Zanarini, M. (1989). Pathogenesis of borderline personality disorder. In A. Tasman, R. E. Hales, & A. J. Frances (Eds.), *American Psychiatric Press review of psychiatry,* Vol. 8. Washington, DC: American Psychiatric Press.

Herman, J. L., Perry, J. C., & van der Kolk, B. A. (1989). Childhood trauma in borderline personality disorder. *American Journal of Psychiatry, 146,* 490–495.

Herman, J. L., & van der Kolb, B. A. (1987). Traumatic origins of borderline personality disorder. In B. A. van der Kolb (Ed.), *Psychological trauma.* Washington, DC: American Psychiatric Press.

Hoch, J., & Palatin, J. (1949). Pseudoneurotic forms of schizophrenia. *Psychiatric Quarterly, 23,* 248–276.

Hollander, E., Stein, D. J., DeCaria, C. M., Cohen, L., Saoud, J. B., Skodol, A. E., Kellman, D., Rosnick, L., Oldham, J. M. (1994). Serotonergic sensitivity in borderline personality disorder: Preliminary findings. *American Journal of Psychiatry, 151,* 277–280.

Hyler, S. E. (1994). *Personality Diagnostic Questionnaire-4.* New York: New York State Psychiatric Institute.

Jang, K. L., Livesley, W. J., Vernon, P. A., & Jackson, D. N. (1996). Heritability of personality traits: A twin study. *Acta Psychiatrica Scandinavica, 94,* 438–444.

Kaplan, M. (1983). A woman's view of the DSM-III. *American Psychologist, 38,* 786–792.

Kernberg, O. (1975). *Borderline conditions and pathological narcissism.* New York: Jason Aronson.

Kernberg, O. (1984). *Severe personality disorders.* New Haven, CT: Yale University Press.

Kernberg, O. (1987). A psychodynamic approach. *Journal of Personality Disorders, 1,* 344–346.

Klein, M. H., Benjamin, L. S., Rosenfeld, R., Treece, C., Husted, J., & Griest, J. H. (1993). The Wisconsin Personality Disorders Interview: Development, reliability, and validity. *Journal of Personality Disorders, 7,* 285–303.

Kluft, R. P. (Ed.). (1990). *Incest-related syndromes of adult psychopathology.* Washington, DC: American Psychiatric Press.

Knight, R. (1953). Borderline states. *Bulletin of the Menninger Clinic, 17,* 1–12.

Kroll, J. (1988). *The challenge of the borderline patient.* New York: W.W. Norton.

Kutcher, S. P., Blackwood, D. H. R., Clair, D., Gaskell, D. F., & Muir, W. J. (1987). Auditory P300 in borderline personality disorder and schizophrenia. *Archives of General Psychiatry, 44,* 645–650.

Langbehn, D. R., Pfohl, B. M., Reynolds, S., Clark, L. A., Battaglia, M., Bellodi, L., Cadoret, R., Grove, W., Pilkonis, P., & Links, P. (1999). The Iowa Personality Disorder Screen: Development and preliminary validation of a brief screening interview. *Journal of Personality Disorders, 13,* 75–89.

Lenzenweger, M. F., Loranger, A. W., Korfine, L., & Neff, C. (1997). Detecting personality disorders in a nonclinical population. Application of a 2-stage procedure for case identification. *Archives of General Psychiatry, 54,* 345–351.

Leyton, M., Diksic, M., Young, S. N., Okazawa, H., Nishizawa, S., Paris, J., Mzaengeza, S., & Benkelfat, C. (1997). Brain regional rate of 5HT synthesis in borderline personality patients: PET study using $^{11}C$-α-methyl-l-tryptophan. Presented to *Society for Biological Psychiatry.*

Linehan, M. M. (1993). *Cognitive behavioral therapy for borderline personality disorder.* New York: Guilford.

Linehan, M. M., & Heard, H. L. (1999). Borderline personality disorder: Costs, course, and treatment outcomes. In N. E. Miller & K. M. Magruder (Eds.), *Cost-effectiveness of psychotherapy: A guide for practitioners, researchers, and policymakers* (pp. 291–305). New York: Oxford University Press.

Linehan, M. M., Armstrong, H. E., Suarez, A., Allmon, D., & Heard, H. L. (1991). Cognitive-behavioral treatment of chronically parasuicidal borderline patients. *Archives of General Psychiatry, 48,* 1060–1064.

Linehan, M. M., Tutek, D. A., Heard, H. L., & Armstrong, H. E. (1994). Cognitive behavioral treatment for chronically suicidal borderline patients: Interpersonal outcomes. *American Journal of Psychiatry, 151,* 1771–1776.

Linehan, M. M., Schmidt, H., Dimeff, L. A., Craft, J. C., Kanter, J., & Comtois, K. A. (1999). Dialectical behavior therapy for patients with borderline personality disorder and drug-dependence. *American Journal on Addictions, 8,* 279–292.

Links, P. S. (1990). *Family environment and borderline personality disorder.* Washington, DC: American Psychiatry Press.

Links, P. S., Steiner, M., & Huxley, G. (1988). The occurrence of borderline personality disorder in the families of borderline patients. *Journal of Personality Disorders, 2,* 14–20.

Links, P. S., Steiner, M., Offord, D. R., & Eppel, A. (1988). Characteristics of borderline personality disorder: A Canadian study. *Canadian Journal of Psychiatry, 33,* 336–340.

Links, P. S., Steiner, M., Boiago, I., & Irwin, D. (1990). Lithium therapy for borderline patients: Preliminary findings. *Journal of Personality Disorders, 4,* 173–181.

Livesley, W. J., Jang, K., Schroeder, M. L., & Jackson, D. N. (1993). Genetic and environmental factors in personality dimensions. *American Journal of Psychiatry, 150,* 1826–1831.

Loranger, A. W., Sartorius, N., Andreoli, A., Berger, P., Buchheim, P., Channabasavanna, S. M., Coid, B., Dahl, A., Diekstra, R. F. W., Ferguson, B., Jacobsberg, L. B., Mombour, W., Pull, C., Ono, J., & Regier, D. A. (1994). The International Personality Disorder Examination. The World Health Organization/Alcohol, Drug Abuse, and Mental Health Administration International pilot study of personality disorders. *Archives of General Psychiatry, 51,* 215–224.

Lucas, P. B., Gardner, D. L., Cowdry, R. W., & Pickar, D. (1989). Cerebral structure in borderline personality disorder. *Psychiatry Research, 27,* 111–115.

Martial, J., Paris, J., Leyton, M., Zweig-Frank, H., Schwartz, G., Teboul, E., Thavuyandil, J., Larue, S., Ng, Y. J., & Nair, N. P. V. (1997). Neuroendocrine study of serotonergic sensitivity in female borderline personality disorder patients. *Biological Psychiatry, 42,* 737–739.

Masterson, J. F. (1976). *Psychotherapy of the borderline adult: A developmental approach.* New York: Brunner/Mazel.

Masterson, J. F. (1981). *The narcissistic and borderline disorders.* New York: Brunner/Mazel.

McGlashan, T. (1986). The Chestnut Lodge follow-up study: III. Long-term outcome of borderline personalities. *Archives of General Psychiatry, 43,* 2–30.

McGlashan, T. (1992). The longitudinal profile of borderline personality disorder: Contributions from the Chestnut Lodge follow-up study. In P. Silver & M. Rosenbluth (Eds.), *Handbook of borderline disorders* (pp. 53–86). Madison, CT: International Universities Press.

McGuffin, P., & Thapar, A. (1992). The genetics of personality disorder. *British Journal of Psychiatry, 160,* 12–23.

Meehl, P. (1989). Schizotaxia revisited. *Archives of General Psychiatry, 46,* 935–944.

Megles, F. T., & Schwartz, M. S. (1989). Oscillations of attachment in borderline personality disorder. *American Journal of Psychiatry, 146,* 1115–1120.

Millon, T. (1993). Borderline personality disorder: A psychosocial epidemic. In J. Paris (Ed.), *Borderline personality disorder: Etiology and treatment* (pp. 197–210). Washington, DC: American Psychiatric Press.

Millon, T. (1992). The borderline construct: Introductory notes on its history, theory, and empirical grounding. In J. F. Clarkin, E. Marziali, & H. Munroe-Blum (Eds.), *Borderline personality disorder: Clinical and empirical perspectives* (pp. 116–148). New York: Guilford.

Millon, T., Davis, R. D., & Millon, C. M. (1997). *MCMI-III manual* (2nd ed.). Minneapolis, MN: National Computer Systems.

Monroe, S. M., & Simmons, A. D. (1991). Diathesis-stress theories in the context of life stress research. *Psychological Bulletin, 110,* 406–425.

Morey, L. C. (1988). A psychometric analysis of the DSM-III-R personality disorder criteria. *Journal of Personality Disorders, 2,* 109–124.

Morey, L. C. (1991). *Personality Assessment Inventory: Professional manual.* Odessa, FL: Psychological Assessment Resources.

Morey, L. C., Waugh, M. H., & Blashfield, R. K. (1985). MMPI scales for DSM-III personality disorders: Their derivation and correlates. *Journal of Personality Disorders, 3,* 180–192.

Munroe-Blum, H., & Marziali, E. (1988). Time limited, group psychotherapy for borderline patients. *Canadian Journal of Psychiatry, 33,* 364–269.

Munroe-Blum, H., & Marziali, E. (1995). A controlled trial of short-term group treatment for borderline personality disorder. *Journal of Personality Disorders, 9,* 190–198.

Najavitz, L. M., & Gunderson, J. G. (1995). Better than expected: Improvements in borderline personality disorder in a 3-year prospective outcome study. *Comprehensive Psychiatry, 36,* 296–302.

Nash, M. R., Hulsely, T. L., Sexton, M. C., Haralson, T. L., & Lambert, W. (1993). Long-term effects of childhood sexual abuse: Perceived family environment, psychopathology, and dissociation. *Journal of Consulting and Clinical Psychology, 61,* 276–283.

Nigg, J. T., & Goldsmith, H. H. (1994) Genetics of personality disorders: Perspectives from personality and psychopathology research. *Psychological Bulletin, 115,* 346–380.

Ogata, S. N., Silk, K. R., Goodrich, S., Lohr, N. E., Westen, D., & Hill, E. M. (1990). Childhood sexual and physical abuse in adult patients with borderline personality disorder. *American Journal of Psychiatry, 147,* 1008–1013.

Paris, J. (1988). Follow-up studies of borderline personality: A critical review. *Journal of Personality Disorders, 2,* 189–197.

Paris, J. (1994a). The etiology of borderline personality disorder: A biopsychosocial model. *Psychiatry, 57,* 300–307.

Paris, J. (1994b). *Borderline personality disorder: A multidimensional approach.* Washington, DC: American Psychiatric Press.

Paris, J. (1997). Childhood trauma as an etiological factor in the personality disorders. *Journal of Personality Disorders, 11,* 34–49.

Paris, J. (1999). Borderline personality disorder. In T. Millon, P. H. Blaney, & R. D. Davis (Eds.), *Oxford textbook of psychopathology* (pp. 625–652). New York: Oxford University Press.

Paris, J., Brown, R., & Nowlins, D. (1987). Long-term follow-up of borderline patients in a general hospital. *Comprehensive Psychiatry, 28,* 530–535.

Paris, J., Zweig-Frank, H., & Gudzer, J. (1994a). Psychological risk factors for borderline personality disorder in female patients. *Comprehensive Psychiatry, 35,* 301–305.

Paris, J., Zweig-Frank, H., & Gudzer, J. (1994b). Risk factors for borderline personality disorder in male outpatients. *Journal of Nervous and Mental Disease, 182,* 375–380.

Parsons, B., Quitkin, F. M., McGrath, P. J., et al. (1989). Phenelzine, imipramine, and placebo in borderline patients meeting criteria for atypical depression. *Psychopharmacological Bulletin, 25,* 524–534.

Perry, J. C. (1992). Problems and considerations in the valid assessment of personality disorders. *American Journal of Psychiatry, 149,* 1645–1653.

Perry, C. J., & Klerman, G. L. (1976). Clinical features of borderline personality disorder. *American Journal of Psychiatry, 137,* 165–173.

Perry, C. J., & Klerman, G. L. (1980). The borderline patient: A comparative analysis of four sets of diagnostic criteria. *Archives of General Psychiatry, 35,* 141–150.

Pfohl, B., Blum, N., & Zimmerman, M. (1995). *Structured Clinical Interview for DSM-IV Personality SIDP-IV*. Iowa City: University of Iowa.

Plakun, E. M., Burkhardt, P. E., & Muller, J. P. (1985). 14 year follow-up of borderline and schizotypal personality disorder. *Comparative Psychiatry, 26*, 448–455.

Plomin, R., DeFries, J. C., McClearn, G. E., & Rutter, M. M. (1997). *Behavioral genetics: A primer*. New York: W.H. Freeman.

Pope, H., Jonas, J., Hudson, J., Cohen, B., & Gunderson, J. (1983). The validity of the DSM-III borderline personality disorder. *Archives of General Psychiatry, 40*, 23–30.

Putnam, F. W. (1989). *Diagnosis and treatment of multiple personality disorder*. New York: Guilford.

Reich, J. (1992). Measurement of DSM-III and DSM-III-R borderline personality disorder. In J. F. Clarkin, E. Marziali, & H. Munroe-Blum (Eds.), *Borderline personality disorder: Clinical and empirical perspectives* (pp. 116–148). New York: Guilford.

Rosenberger, P., & Miller, G. (1989). Comparing borderline definitions: DSM-III borderline and schizotypal personality disorders. *Journal of Abnormal Psychology, 98*, 161–169.

Ross, C. (1991). Epidemiology of multiple personality and dissociation. *Psychiatric Clinics of North America, 14*, 503–518.

Ross, R., Frances, A. J., & Widiger, T. A. (1995). Gender issues in the DSM-IV. In J. M. Oldham & M. B. Riba (Eds.), *Review of psychiatry*, Vol. 14 (pp. 205–226). Washington, DC: American Psychiatric Press.

Rutter, M. (1989). Pathways from childhood to adult life. *Journal of Child Psychology and Psychiatry, 30*, 23–51.

Schulz, S. C., Koller, M. M., Kishoore, P. R., Hamer, R. M., Gehl, J. J., & Friedel, R. O. (1983). Ventricular enlargement in teenage patients with schizophrenia spectrum disorder. *American Journal of Psychiatry, 140*, 1592–1595.

Segal, D. L. (1997). Structured interviewing and DSM classification. In S. M. Turner & M. Hersen (Eds.), *Adult psychopathology and diagnosis* (pp. 24–57). New York: Wiley.

Siever, L. J., & Davis, K. L. (1991). A psychobiological perspective on the personality disorders. *American Journal of Psychiatry, 148*, 1647–1658.

Snyder, S., & Pitts, W. M. (1984). Electroencephalography of DSM-III borderline personality disorder. *Acta Psychiatrica Scandinavica, 69*, 129–134.

Snyder, S., Pitts, W. M., & Gustin, Q. (1983). CT scans in patients with borderline personality disorder. *American Journal of Psychiatry, 140*, 272.

Soloff, P. H. (1994). Is there any drug treatment of choice for the borderline patient? *Acta Psychiatrica Scandinavica, 379*, 50–55.

Soloff, P. H., & Millward, J. W. (1983). Developmental histories of borderline patients. *Comprehensive Psychiatry, 24*, 574–588.

Spitzer, R. L., Endicott, J., & Gibbon, M. (1979). Crossing the border into borderline personality and borderline schizophrenia. *Archives of General Psychiatry, 36*, 17–24.

Steinberg, B. J., Trestman, R. L., & Siever, L. J. (1994). The cholinergic and noradrenergic neurotransmitter systems and affective instability in borderline personality disorder. In K. R. Silk (Ed.), *Biological and neurobiological studies of borderline personality disorder* (pp. 41–62). Washington, DC: American Psychiatric Press.

Stern, A. (1938). Psychoanalytic investigations of and therapy in the borderline group of neuroses. *Psychoanalytic Quarterly, 7*, 467–489.

Stevenson, J., & Meares, R. (1992). An outcome study of psychotherapy for patients with borderline personality disorder. *American Journal of Psychiatry, 149*, 358–362.

Stone, M. H. (1989). The course of borderline personality disorder. In A. Tasman, R. Hales, & A. Frances (Eds.), *Review of psychiatry* (pp. 103–122). Washington, DC: American Psychiatric Press.

Stone, M. H. (1990). *The fate of borderline patients*. New York: Guilford.

Swartz, M., Blazer, D., George, L.,& Winfield, L. (1990). Estimating the prevalence of borderline personality disorder in the community. *Journal of Personality Disorders, 4*, 257–272.

Tennant, C. (1988). Parental loss in childhood to adult life. *Archives of General Psychiatry, 45*, 1045–1050.

Torgersen, S. (1984). Genetic and nosological aspects of schizotypal and borderline disorders: A twin study. *Archives of General Psychiatry, 41*, 546–554.

Togersen, S. (1986). Genetics in borderline conditions, *Acta Psychiatrica Scandinavica, 89*(Suppl. 379), 19–25.

Trull, T. (1995). Borderline personality disorder features in nonclinical young adults: I. Identification and validation. *Psychological Assessment, 7*, 33–41.

van der Kolk, B. (1987). *Psychological trauma*. Washington, DC: American Psychiatric Press.

van Reekum, R., Links, P. S., & Boiago, I. (1993). Constitutional factors in borderline personality disorder. In J. Paris (Ed.), *Borderline personality disorder: Etiology and treatment* (pp. 13–38). Washington, DC: American Psychiatric Press.

Westen, D. (1997). Divergences between clinical and research methods for assessing personality disorders: Implications for research and the evolution of axis II. *American Journal of Psychiatry, 154*, 895–903.

Widiger, T. A. (1998). Invited essay: Sex biases in the diagnosis of personality disorders. *Journal of Personality Disorders, 12*, 95–118.

Widiger, T. A. (1993). The DSM-III-R categorical personality disorder diagnoses: A critique and an alternative. *Psychological Inquiry, 4*, 75–90.

Widiger, T. A., Mangine, S., Corbitt, E. M., Ellis, C. G., & Thomas, G. V. (1995). *Personality Disorder Interview-IV: A semistructured interview for the assessment of personality disorders*. Odessa, FL: Psychological Assessment Resources.

Widiger, T. A., & Frances, A. J. (1989). Epidemiology, diagnosis, and comorbidity of borderline personality disorders. In A. Tasman, R. E. Hale, & A. J. Frances (Eds.), *Review of psychiatry*, Vol. 8 (pp. 8–24). Washington, DC: American Psychiatric Press.

Widiger, T. A., & Trull, T. J. (1993). Borderline and narcissistic personality disorders. In P. B. Sutker & H. E. Adams (Eds.), *Comprehensive handbook of psychopathology* (pp. 371–394). New York: Plenum.

Widiger, T. A., Frances, A. J., & Trull, T. J. (1987). A psychometric analysis of the social-interpersonal and cognitive-perceptual items for the schizotypal personality disorder. *Archives of General Psychiatry, 44*, 741–745.

Zanarini, M. C. (1993). BPD is an impulse spectrum disorder. In J. Paris (Ed.), *Borderline personality disorder: Etiology and treatment* (p. 67–85). Washington, DC: American Psychiatric Press.

Zanarini, M., Frankenburg, F. R., Sickel, A. E., & Yong, L. (1996). *Diagnostic Interview for DSM-IV Personality Disorders*. Laboratory for the Study of Adult Development, MacLean Hospital, and the Department of Psychiatry, Harvard University.

Zanarini, M., Gunderson, J., Frankenburg, F. R., & Chauncey, D. L. (1989). The revised diagnostic interview for borderlines: Discriminating BPD from other Axis II disorders. *Journal of Personality Disorders, 3,* 10–18.

Zanarini, M. C., & Gunderson, J. (1997). Differential diagnosis of antisocial and borderline personality disorders. In D. M. Stoff, J. Breiling et al. (Eds.), *Handbook of antisocial behavior* (pp. 83–91). New York: Wiley.

Zanarini, M. C., Frankenburg, F. R., Dubo, E. D., Sickel, A. E., Trikha, A., Levin, A., & Reynolds, V. (1998). Axis I comorbidity of borderline personality disorder. *American Journal of Psychiatry, 155,* 1733–1739.

Zanarini, M. C., Chauncey, D. L., Grady, R. A., & Gunderson, J. G. (1991). Outcome studies of borderline personality disorder. In S. M. Mirin, J. T. Gossett, & M. C. Grob (Eds.), *Psychiatric treatment: Advances in outcome research.* Washington, DC: American Psychiatric Press.

Zanarini, M. C., Gunderson, J. G., Marino, M. F., Schwartz, E. O., & Frankenburg, F. R. (1988). DSM-III disorders in the families of borderline outpatients. *Journal of Personality Disorders, 2,* 292–302.

Zanarini, M. C., & Frankenburg, F. R. (1997). Pathways to the development of borderline personality disorder. *Journal of Personality Disorders, 11,* 93–104.

Zanarini, M. C., Kimble, C. R., & Williams, A. A. (1994). Neurological dysfunction in borderline patients and Axis II control subjects. In K. R. Silk (Ed.), *Biological and neurobiological studies of borderline personality disorder* (pp. 159–175). Washington, DC: American Psychiatric Press.

Zimmerman, M., & Mattin, J. I. (1999). Differences between clinical and research practices in diagnosing borderline personality disorder. *American Journal of Psychiatry, 159,* 1570–1574.

Zittel, C., & Westen, D. (1998). Conceptual issues and research findings on borderline personality disorder: What every clinician should know. *Psychotherapy in Practice, 4,* 5–20.

# CHAPTER 18

# Histrionic, Narcissistic, and Dependent Personality Disorders

## Thomas A. Widiger and Robert F. Bornstein

## Introduction

All of the DSM-IV personality disorders share at least some features in common (e.g., impaired interpersonal relationships, distortions in self-concept). Numerous classification systems have been proposed to organize personality disorder pathology into categories, dimensions, or clusters that would share certain underlying commonalities and would be distinguished with respect to others. Only a few of these systems have been widely accepted, and most have been widely criticized. Perhaps any grouping of personality disorders, and particularly any categorical distinctions, will create certain difficulties, even as it resolves others.

This chapter is concerned with histrionic, narcissistic, and dependent personality disorders. The inclusion of these disorders within the same chapter does not necessarily suggest a common issue or unifying theme that naturally joins them or distinguishes them from other disorders of personality. All three have their roots within psychodynamic

theory, but this can also be said for other personality disorders (e.g., obsessive-compulsive and borderline). All three disorders may also be characterized by high levels of dependency needs (including the histrionic and the narcissistic, if one includes implicit needs), but the same may again be equally true for other personality disorders (e.g., borderline). Histrionic, narcissistic, and dependent personality disorders also share some common issues and controversies (e.g., gender and cultural biases), but whatever issues they share will apply as well to the other personality disorders. Historically, they have been among the less frequently researched personality disorders, but now there is a substantial amount of research supporting their validity, particularly for the dependent and narcissistic personality disorders. Each will be discussed in turn, and each presentation is organized with respect to its diagnosis, assessment, epidemiolology, etiology, and pathology.

## Histrionic Personality Disorder

Histrionic personality disorder is defined in the 4th edition of the American Psychiatric Association's (APA) *Diagnostic and Statistical Manual of Mental Disorders* (DSM-IV) as "a pervasive pattern of excessive emotionality and attention seeking, beginning by early adulthood and present in a variety of contexts" (APA, 1994, p. 657). The

**Thomas A. Widiger** • Department of Psychology, University of Kentucky, Lexington, Kentucky 40506-0044.    **Robert F. Bornstein** • Department of Psychology, Gettysburg College, Gettysburg, Pennsylvania 17325-1486.

*Comprehensive Handbook of Psychopathology* (Third Edition), edited by Patricia B. Sutker and Henry E. Adams. Kluwer Academic / Plenum Publishers, New York, 2001.

diagnosis was not included in the first edition of the DSM (APA, 1952), although some of the persons who were given the DSM-I diagnosis of emotionally unstable personality were probably given the DSM-II diagnosis of hysterical personality (APA, 1968). The narrative description of the disorder provided in DSM-II is still applicable today:

These behavior patterns are characterized by excitability, emotional instability, over-reactivity, and self-dramatization. This self-dramatization is always attention-seeking and often seductive, whether or not the patient is aware of its purpose. These personalities are also immature, self-centered, often vain, and usually dependent on others. (APA, 1968, p. 43)

The DSM-III-R diagnostic criteria referred to such traits as constantly seeking reassurance, approval, or praise; inappropriately sexually seductive; overly concerned with physical attractiveness; exaggerated emotional expression; uncomfortable when not the center of attention; rapidly shifting and shallow expression of emotions; self-centeredness; and impressionistic speech (APA, 1987). These diagnostic indicators were consistent with the descriptions provided within the recent and past clinical literature (Pfohl, 1991), but significant concerns have also been raised regarding their validity, consistency with clinical theory, and consistency with clinical practice (Blashfield & Davis, 1993; Bornstein, 1999).

Blashfield and Breen (1989) presented the 142 DSM-III-R personality disorder diagnostic criteria to sixty-one clinicians and asked them to indicate the personality disorder "with which [they] believe this criterion is associated" (p. 1576). The histrionic criteria were assigned to the histrionic personality disorder only 41% of the time, consistent with an earlier study by Blashfield and Haymaker (1988). Five of the eight criteria were misassigned more than half of the time. The worst criterion from this perspective was self-centeredness. This criterion was assigned to the histrionic diagnosis by only 8% of the clinicians; assigned instead to the narcissistic by 66%. Blashfield and Breen (1989) concluded that "these results strongly suggest that the DSM-III-R definition of histrionic does not match the definition for this category that is used by contemporary American clinicians [and] this category needs a major change in definition in DSM-IV" (p. 1578).

Blashfield and Herkov (1996) asked 320 clinicians to select one of their patients whom they knew well and was considered to have a person-

ality disorder. They were asked to indicate the personality disorder diagnosis they had assigned to the patient and to indicate on a scrambled list which of the DSM-III-R personality disorder diagnostic criteria were present. Thirty-nine of the patients had been given a clinical diagnosis of histrionic personality disorder, but sixty-five were assigned a sufficient number of histrionic diagnostic criteria to be given the diagnosis. Kappa for the agreement between their clinical diagnoses and the diagnoses that would be provided on the basis of their own assessments of the diagnostic criteria was only .30, consistent with the kappa of .27 in a comparable study by Morey and Ochoa (1989) with the DSM-III criteria sets. "Our study supports the Morey and Ochoa finding that there is a poor correspondence between the clinicians' diagnoses of patients and what DSM-III-R disorders these patients would meet if the clinicians strictly adhered to the DSM-III-R rules" (Blashfield & Herkov, 1996, p. 223).

When diagnosticians do adhere to the rules, the histrionic criteria set does not identify a qualitatively distinct personality disorder. Widiger and Rogers (1989) summarized the results across prior published studies and indicated that at least 80% of the persons who met the DSM-III-R criteria for histrionic personality disorder were likely to meet the criteria set for another personality disorder. Widiger and Trull (1998) reported the percentage of co-occurrence for the diagnosis of DSM-III-R histrionic personality disorder averaged across unpublished data sets involving more than 1000 patients obtained from six independent research teams. A singular diagnosis was rare, and "at least a third of those with histrionic personality disorder met the criteria for borderline and narcissistic" (Widiger & Trull, 1998, p. 362). Stuart et al. (1998) reported the co-occurrence rates obtained from data for 1116 patients pooled from several research sites that had administered the same semistructured interview. Ninety-three of the patients (8.3%) met the DSM-III-R criteria for histrionic personality disorder, and more than 40% met the criteria for the paranoid, narcissistic, borderline, dependent, and passive-aggressive personality disorders. Consistent with Widiger and Trull, the greatest overlap was with the borderline and narcissistic personality disorders (51% met the criteria for borderline, and 73% met the criteria for narcissistic).

Table 1 provides the DSM-IV diagnostic criteria

## Table 1. DSM-IV Criteria
### for Histrionic Personality Disorder[a]

A pervasive pattern of excessive emotionality and attention seeking, beginning by early adulthood and present in a variety of contexts, as indicated by five (or more) of the following:

(1) is uncomfortable in situations in which he or she is not the center of attention

(2) interaction with others is often characterized by inappropriate sexually seductive or provocative behavior

(3) displays rapidly shifting and shallow expression of emotions

(4) consistently uses physical appearance to draw attention to self

(5) has a style of speech that is excessively impressionistic and lacking in detail

(6) shows self-dramatization, theatricality, and exaggerated expression of emotion

(7) is suggestible, i.e., easily influenced by others or circumstances

(8) considers relationships to be more intimate than they actually are

[a]APA (1994, pp. 657–658).

for histrionic personality disorder. A major intention of the revision was to increase the criteria set's specificity and its consistency with clinical theory (Pfohl, 1991). The two most problematic DSM-III-R criteria, as suggested by the psychometric data, were (1) constantly seeks or demands reassurance, approval, and praise; and (2) self-centeredness (Pfohl, 1991). Both were deleted. Constantly seeking or demanding reassurance, approval, and praise was replaced by the DSM-IV seventh criterion of suggestibility; self-centeredness was replaced by the DSM-IV eighth criterion of considering relationships more intimate than they really are. The latter criterion was obtained from the clinical literature and from suggestions by consultants to DSM-IV who were experts in the diagnosis of histrionic personality disorder (Pfohl, 1991, 1995). Pfohl (1995) has suggested that DSM-IV suggestibility was simply a rewording of DSM-III-R constantly seeking or demanding reassurance, approval, or praise. However, it is perhaps better understood as a new criterion because it was obtained from the World Health Organization's (1992) research criteria set and was included in

large part to increase the congruence of DSM-IV with the international nomenclature (Widiger et al., 1995). Being suggestible or easily influenced by others is consistent with clinical descriptions of the disorder (Pfohl, 1991), but these traits are unlikely to correlate highly with constantly seeking or demanding approval or praise (Schooler & Loftus, 1986).

The order in which the personality disorder diagnostic criteria are provided in DSM-IV is consistent with their validity in the diagnosis of the disorder, based largely on psychometric research using the DSM-III-R criteria sets (Widiger et al., 1995). The exceptions to this rank ordering are the new diagnostic criteria. They are typically placed at the end of the list not because they might be less diagnostic of the disorder, but simply because there was inadequate data to justify placing them above any of the other diagnostic criteria. Suggestibility and misperceiving the intimacy of relationships are placed at the end of the list in DSM-IV because they are new diagnostic criteria. Being uncomfortable in situations in which they are not the center of attention and inappropriately sexually seductive behavior are placed at the beginning of the list because they are considered the most highly diagnostic indicators. DSM-IV also provides substantially more discussion and explication of the meaning and application of each diagnostic criterion within the text than was provided in DSM-III-R (Frances, First, & Pincus, 1995). Further discussions of each diagnostic criterion are provided by Widiger et al. (1995), and additional experimental criteria for histrionic personality disorder are provided by Pfohl (1995) and Shedler and Westen (1998).

It is unclear whether the revisions to the histrionic criteria set will appreciably affect those who now receive the diagnosis. Morey (1988) indicated that the DSM-III-R and DSM-III criteria sets for histrionic personality diagnosed the same percentage of persons (22%) in their sample of 291 patients, but not necessarily the same persons. Kappa for the agreement between the two criteria sets was .66, which was significant and was the third highest of the criteria sets. Blashfield, Blum, and Pfohl (1992) obtained a comparable rate of agreement (kappa = .55) but they indicated that they had expected much more disagreement, given the substantial revisions to the DSM-III criteria set provided by DSM-III-R (Widiger, Frances, Spitzer, & Williams, 1988). Blais, Hilsenroth, and Castlebury

(1997) reported a substantial decrease in the number of persons likely to receive the histrionic diagnosis using DSM-IV in comparison to DSM-III-R, from 14% in their sample of ninety-four patients with DSM-III-R to only 4% with DSM-IV (kappa = .34).

Linde and Clark (1998) replicated the methodology of Blashfield and Breen (1989), using the DSM-IV criteria set and providing a comparison to criteria sets for various Axis I mental disorders. Linde and Clark indicated that 71% of the DSM-IV histrionic criteria set were correctly assigned (compared to only 41% for DSM-III-R). They also indicated that misassignment occurred significantly less often for the personality disorder criteria sets, compared to the criteria sets for childhood, mood, and anxiety disorders. If one of the goals of DSM-IV was to generate a more clinically meaningful criteria set, "our results suggest that the goals of the most recent Task Force have been met to a large degree" (Linde & Clark, 1998, p. 132). The improvement in face validity might be due in part to the increasing familiarity with and acceptance of the APA diagnostic nomenclature, but the weak findings obtained earlier by Blashfield and Breen (1989) might also be attributed to a lack of understanding or adequate appreciation of the APA diagnostic nomenclature.

Blais, Benedict, and Norman (1996) administered the DSM-III-R and initial drafts of the DSM-IV criteria sets for histrionic personality disorder to a sample of thirty-three clinicians at their medical center and to thirty college students, along with the DSM-III-R criteria set for major depressive disorder. They asked each participant to rate the clarity and understandability of each criterion on a 1- to 5-point scale. The professional clinicians rated the major depressive criteria as more understandable than the histrionic criteria (3.88 vs. 3.16, respectively), but the nonprofessionals rated the histrionic criteria more understandable than the professionals (4.36 vs. 3.16, respectively) and more understandable than the major depressive criteria (4.36 vs. 3.81, respectively). A mean rating of 3.16 indicated that the professional clinicians considered the criteria set at least "fairly clear" and "this finding can be interpreted as indicating that the personality disorder criteria sets are adequately clear" (Blais et al., 1996, p. 20). However, the rating of 3.16 was the lowest for any personality disorder. The fact that the histrionic criteria are less clear than the criteria set for major depres-

sive disorder is an inevitable requirement when describing personality compared simply to an episode of major depression. The lower rating of clarity by the professionals compared to the college students may suggest that the professional clinicians have a better appreciation of this complexity, that they might be reading too much complexity into the criteria, or that they might have higher standards than college students for clarity within diagnostic criteria (Westen, 1997).

Blais, Hilsenroth, and Castlebury (1997) and Blais and Norman (1997) reported initial psychometric studies on the DSM-IV criteria set for histrionic personality disorder. Blais and Norman indicated that the DSM-IV histrionic criteria set obtained relatively weak internal consistency, with Cronbach's alpha = .66, and many of the items continued to correlate with the narcissistic and borderline criteria sets. They also noted that the impressionistic speech and suggestibility criteria failed to correlate appreciably with the other histrionic criteria. "Our findings indicate that DSM-IV personality disorders will continue to demonstrate high comorbidity rates" (Blais & Norman, 1997, p. 175). Blais et al. (1997) were more complimentary. "For example, in the present study the DSM-III-R histrionic personality disorder was significantly correlated with both the narcissistic and borderline personality disorders ... while the DSM-IV version ... showed no significant correlations with [these] other [personality disorders]" (Blais et al., 1997, pp. 275–276). They also indicated that there had been an improvement in the internal consistency of the histrionic criteria set (from .61 to .67) that was well above a coefficient of .35 that would be obtained by nine randomly selected diagnostic criteria of personality disorder. Blais et al. (197) did indicate relatively weak correlations for the criteria concerned with discomfort when not the center of attention, rapidly shifting emotions, and suggestibility. The poor results for discomfort when not the center of attention is particularly surprising because it was the most diagnostic in prior research (Pfohl, 1991). The criterion that had the highest correlation with the other diagnostic criteria was the new criterion of considering relationships more intimate than they really are.

It is stated in DSM-IV that "in the common situation in which an individual has more than one Axis II [personality disorder] diagnosis, all should be reported" (APA, 1994, p. 26). If a histrionic person meets the DSM-IV diagnostic criteria for a borderline, dependent, or antisocial personality disorder, then these additional diagnoses should be provided. These personality disorders do overlap, but a histrionic person with only a few borderline or antisocial traits will be much different from a histrionic person with many borderline and antisocial traits. Nevertheless, most practicing clinicians provide only one diagnosis of personality disorder per patient, perhaps finding the presence of multiple diagnoses theoretically and clinically problematic (Gunderson, 1992; Widiger & Sanderson, 1995b). An implicit hierarchical structure occurs in general clinical practice, and the presence of one personality disorder trumps the presence of others (Herkov & Blashfield, 1995). DSM-IV provides suggestions within the text for differentiating among the individual personality disorders. This additional information will be useful at times to clinicians who are attempting to determine which personality disorder would provide the most valid diagnosis. For example, it is stated that "individuals with antisocial personality disorder and histrionic personality disorder share a tendency to be impulsive, superficial, excitement seeking, reckless, seductive, and manipulative, but persons with histrionic personality disorder ... are manipulative to gain nurturance, whereas those with antisocial personality disorder are manipulative to gain profit, power, or some other material gratification" (APA, 1994, p. 657). This additional information goes significantly beyond the individual diagnostic criteria because an assessment of the underlying motivation for a manipulation is not required within the diagnostic criteria for antisocial or histrionic personality disorder. Further discussion of the individual diagnostic criteria and differential diagnosis is also provided in many of the manuals that accompany semistructured interviews (e.g., Widiger et al., 1995).

Problematic differential diagnosis and excessive co-occurrence, however, might be an inevitable result of the attempt to construct qualitatively distinct diagnostic categories from constellations of maladaptive personality traits (Bornstein, 1998b; Tyrer & Johnson, 1996; Widiger, 1993). The empirical fact is that many histrionic patients will have other clinically significant personality traits (e.g., Oldham et al., 1992; Stuart et al., 1998). Providing only one diagnosis to these patients might eliminate this complexity only by ignoring

its existence. "Although clinicians and researchers can describe prototypic personality disorder symptom patterns that reflect different diagnostic ideals, in real-life clinical settings most personality disorder patients show an array of symptoms from several (or even many) different categories" (Bornstein, 1998b, p. 336).

## Assessment

There are four primary methods for assessing a personality disorder: an unstructured clinical interview, a semistructured clinical interview, a self-report inventory, and/or a projective test (Widiger & Saylor, 1998). There are advantages and disadvantages to each approach that will apply to each of the personality disorders considered in this chapter (Perry, 1992; Westen, 1997; Widiger & Sanderson, 1995a; Zimmerman, 1994).

The single most popular method for assessing personality disorders within general clinical practice is an unstructured interview (Watkins, Campbell, Nieberding, & Hallmark, 1995; Westen, 1997), whereas the preferred method for clinical research is the semistructured interview (Rogers, 1995; Segal, 1997; Widiger & Saylor, 1998; Zimmerman, 1994). The reluctance to use semistructured interviews in general clinical practice is understandable because they are constraining, may at times be impractical, and can appear superficial. However, they are advisable when questions regarding the reliability or validity of an assessment are likely to be raised (Widiger & Saylor, 1998). Semistructured interviews are helpful in ensuring that the interview will be systematic, comprehensive, replicable, and objective. Unstructured clinical interviews are problematic because they tend to be unreliable, idiosyncratic, and more susceptible to attributional errors and false assumptions (Garb, 1997; Rogers, 1995; Segal, 1997). Minimally, semistructured interviews will provide the clinician with a set of useful suggestions regarding alternative inquiries to assess each diagnostic criterion.

A recommended approach in clinical practice would be to administer first a self-report inventory to identify a subset of personality disorders whose diagnoses are then confirmed by administering a semistructured interview. There are currently five semistructured interviews for assessing the DSM-IV personality disorders: (1) Diagnostic Interview for DSM-IV Personality Disorders (DIPD; Zanarini, Frankenburg, Sickel, & Yong, 1996), (2) International Personality Disorder Examination (IPDE; Loranger, Sartorius, & Janca, 1997), (3) Personality Disorder Interview-IV (PDI-IV; Widiger et al., 1995), (4) Structured Clinical Interview for DSM-IV Axis II Personality Disorders (SCID-II; First, Gibbon, Spitzer, Williams, & Benjamin, 1997), and (5) Structured Interview for DSM-IV Personality Disorders (SIDP-IV: Pfohl, Blum, & Zimmerman, 1997). The SIDP-IV, SCID-II, and IPDE have the most empirical support (Segal, 1997; Zimmerman, 1994), but the PDI-IV has the most extensive manual (Rogers, 1995), including a detailed discussion of the history, rationale, and assessment issues for each of the 94 DSM-IV personality disorder diagnostic criteria.

The single most popular method for assessing personality by researchers of normal personality functioning is a self-report inventory (Butcher & Rouse, 1996). The advantages of a self-report inventory are self-evident. It is relatively less expensive and time-consuming to administer, it is systematic, comprehensive, and reliable in its assessment, and it will often be supported by a substantial amount of normative and clinical research that will facilitate interpreting it (Widiger & Saylor, 1998). There are six self-report inventories that can be and have often been used for assessing the DSM-IV personality disorders: (1) Minnesota Multiphasic Personality Inventory-2 (MMPI-2) personality disorder scales developed originally by Morey, Waugh, and Blashfield (1985); (2) Millon Clinical Multiaxial Inventory-III (Millon, Davis, & Millon, 1997); (3) Personality Diagnostic Questionnaire-IV (PDQ-IV; Hyler, 1994); (4) Personality Assessment Inventory (PAI; Morey, 1991); (5) Wisconsin Personality Inventory (WISPI; Klein et al., 1993); and (6) Coolidge Axis II Inventory (CATI; Coolidge & Merwin, 1992). The MMPI-2 and the MCMI-III have the most empirical support; the CATI and WISPI might be comparably valid but are more recent instruments that need further research; the PAI assessment of personality disorders is confined largely to the borderline, antisocial, and paranoid personality disorders; and the PDQ-IV is the least valid but most commonly used due to its brevity and close coordination with the DSM-IV diagnostic criteria (Widiger & Saylor, 1998; Zimmerman, 1994).

A potential disadvantage of self-report inventories and semistructured interviews is their relative emphasis on self-report (Bornstein, 1995; Perry, 1992; Westen, 1997). Personality disorders are characterized in part by characteristic distortions in self-image and self-presentation, which may not be assessed adequately simply by asking respondents if they have each diagnostic criterion. However, many of these instruments can also be administered to persons who know the patient well and have observed firsthand the maladaptive personality traits. In addition, self-report inventories and semistructured interviews do not necessarily rely on accurate self-description. Many of the inquiries within these instruments are subtle and indirect. Most projective tests depend less on the ability or willingness of the person to provide an accurate self-description, although there is currently only limited empirical support for using projective techniques to assess histrionic personality traits (Blais, Hilsenroth, & Fowler, 1998).

## Epidemiology

Approximately 1 to 3% of the general population would be diagnosed with histrionic personality disorder (Maier et al., 1992; Nestadt et al., 1990; Zimmerman & Coryell, 1989), and approximately 10 to 15% of patients within clinical settings (Pfohl, 1991). This disorder is typically diagnosed more frequently in females, but this gender ratio has been highly controversial (Bornstein, 1999; Kaplan, 1983; Widiger, 1998). The diagnostic criteria for histrionic personality disorder include behaviors or traits that are significantly correlated with stereotypically feminine behavior (Sprock, Blashfield, & Smith, 1990), clinicians will at times overdiagnose histrionic personality disorder in female patients (Ford & Widiger, 1989; Hamilton, Rothbart, & Dawes, 1986), and some studies that used semistructured interviews failed to obtain a differential sex prevalence rate (Corbitt & Widiger, 1995; Nestadt et al., 1990; Pfohl, 1991). It is even suggested in DSM-IV that the differential sex prevalence rate might be an illusory artifact of a higher base rate of females within clinical settings, biased clinical assessments, or perhaps even biased diagnostic criteria. "Histrionic personality disorder as defined in DSM-IV may continue to represent an exaggerated version of stereotypical feminine traits and may place too little emphasis on items and examples that would tap the parallel 'macho' male version expressing exaggerated masculine traits" (Frances et al., 1995, p. 373). The text discussion of the disorder in

DSM-IV emphasizes the consideration of masculine variants of the diagnostic criteria. "For example, a man with this disorder may dress and behave in a manner often identified as 'macho' and may seek to be the center of attention by bragging about athletic skills" (APA, 1994, p. 656).

If "a healthy woman automatically earns the diagnosis of histrionic personality disorder" (Kaplan, 1983, p. 789), the diagnosis would indeed be invalid and sex-biased. Funtowicz and Widiger (1995, 1999), however, indicated that the diagnostic criteria for histrionic personality disorder (with perhaps one exception) do not diagnose women who are actually lacking in clinically significant impairments in social or occupational dysfunction or personal distress. Some of the women might be only mildly impaired, but they will be at least as impaired as men who meet the criteria for personality disorders that are diagnosed more frequently in males (e.g., antisocial, obsessive-compulsive, and narcissistic). To the extent that personality disorders are extreme maladaptive variants of commonly occurring personality traits (Livesley, Schroeder, Jackson, & Jang, 1994; Widiger & Costa, 1994), differential sex prevalence rates consistent with the normative differences between men and women (Feingold, 1994) would be expected (Corbitt & Widiger, 1995). Some personality disorders may indeed involve maladaptive variants of gender-related traits; some personality disorders occur more often in males (e.g., antisocial and narcissistic), and others occur more often in females (e.g., histrionic and dependent). It has even been suggested that histrionic and antisocial personality disorders are complementary gender-related variants; the antisocial male tends to manipulate others through antagonistic intimidation, and the histrionic female manipulates others through extraverted, seductive flirtation (Hamburger, Lilienfeld, & Hogben, 1996). However, the presence of these gender-related traits substantially complicates the development of gender-neutral, or at least unbiased, diagnostic criteria (Widiger, 1998). A more valid diagnosis of histrionic personality disorder might not be achieved by revising the criteria to be more masculine or to diagnose an equal number of males and females with the disorder. A more valid diagnosis might be obtained by revising "the criteria to decrease the likelihood that there will be false positive errors in their application to women, perhaps by increasing (for example) their behavioral specificity to reduce their ambiguity, misinterpretation, and misapplication" (Widiger, 1998, pp. 114–115).

Concerns may also be raised with respect to other demographic variables. For example, histrionic personality disorder is likely to be diagnosed in some cultural groups more than others. For example, the disorder might be seen less frequently in Asian cultures, where overt sexual seductiveness is less frequent (Johnson, 1993), and more frequently within Hispanic and Latin American cultures, where more overt and uninhibited sexuality is evident (Padilla, 1995). However, it will be unclear at times whether adjustments to the diagnostic criteria should be made within these different cultural contexts because the DSM-IV criteria may also reflect biases or assumptions regarding seductiveness that are not shared within other societies (Alarcon, 1996; Rogler, 1996).

Histrionic personality disorder and the validity of the diagnostic criteria may also change across the life span. As the disorder is currently described in the DSM-IV, it is most appropriate for a young adult (Bornstein, 1999). Sexual seductiveness will become less apparent as a person ages or at least may become a less effective means of capturing the attention of or manipulating others. On the other hand, histrionic psychopathology might become more evident as a person ages because the histrionic person continues to rely on an increasingly ineffective means of obtaining attention. In the only study to assess the relationship of age to diagnosis, Nestadt et al. (1990) reported no differential sex prevalence rate for the disorder within younger adults. A differential sex prevalence rate did not emerge until the persons were older than 45. It is possible that many of the behaviors were considered more normative within the younger females (Sprock, 1996) and contributed to an underdiagnosis of the disorder at this time.

## Etiology and Pathology

There is some limited support for the heritability of histrionic personality traits, although there has not yet been a familial aggregation, twin, or adoption study of this disorder (McGuffin & Thapar, 1992; Nigg & Goldsmith, 1994). Substantial data suggest that the disorder is a constellation of maladaptive variants of common personality traits within the broad domains of neuroticism and extraversion (e.g., Trull, 1992; Trull et al., 1998). For example, extraversion includes the dispositions to be outgoing, talkative, and affectionate; to be convivial, to have many friends, and to seek social contact; to be energetic, fast-paced, and vigorous; to be flashy, seek stimulation, and take risks; and to be high-spirited. Costa and McCrae (1992) organized these traits of extraversion into facets of warmth, gregariousness, activity, excitement-seeking, and positive emotionality (respectively). Traits of extraversion are, for the most part, desirable and adaptive. However, persons who are at the most extreme variants of these traits of extraversion are likely to experience a number of maladaptive consequences and would be characterized as being histrionic. "Histrionic individuals express emotions with an inappropriate exaggeration (excessively high positive emotions); they crave excitement and stimulation (high excitement seeking); they are quick to form numerous, generally superficial relationships (high gregariousness); and they display inappropriate affection, intimacy, and seductiveness (high warmth)" (Widiger et al., 1994, p. 47). To the extent that histrionic personality disorder does indeed include maladaptively extreme variants of traits of extraversion, there would be support for its heritability (Jang et al., 1998; Nigg & Goldsmith, 1994).

The pathology of the disorder is to some extent evident by the diagnostic criteria provided in DSM-IV (APA, 1994). Persons with this disorder are said to have a pathological need to be loved, desired, and intensely involved with others intimately, and they will use a variety of means to get this involvement (Horowitz, 1991). They will use their physical appearance to draw attention to themselves, they will be melodramatically emotional, and they will be inappropriately seductive. They may even perceive that a relationship is more intimate than is really the case, in part because of their need for and fantasies of close intimacies. They will be highly suggestible or easily influenced by others because they want to be closely involved and engaged within an intense personal relationship. An extreme example of this suggestibility would be the development of symptoms or memories suggested by a clinician to develop a special, significant relationship.

This description of the disorder is largely consistent with psychodynamic descriptions of oral-dependent pathology (Bornstein, 1999), and a variety of parent–child relationships may contribute to its development. The excessive needs may develop in part through an overly eroticized parent–child relationship. For example, a father might repeatedly indicate through a variety of verbal and nonverbal communications that his love and attention for a daughter are largely contingent upon her being attractive, desirable, and provocative to him. Her sense of self-worth and meaning might depend in large part on the way he relates to her, and she might then value herself primarily in terms of the way she is valued by men (Stone, 1993). She may learn that to get what she needs from others, she must be highly provocative, intrusive, and manipulative (Millon et al., 1996).

Neurochemical models of the disorder have emphasized a hyperresponsiveness of the noradrenergic system. This disregulation in catecholamine functioning may contribute to a pronounced emotional reactivity to signs of rejection (Klein, 1999). There may be a naturally occurring neurochemical mechanism for regulating mood in response to signs of social applause and rejection. This regulatory mechanism would be helpful sociobiologically in making a person appropriately responsive to cues of social interest. "Perhaps in hysteroid dysphoric patients this mechanism had become overresponsive and ... monoamine oxidase inhibitors [are] reparative for this dysfunction" (Klein, 1999, p. 425).

Cognitive theorists have emphasized irrational schemata associated with these interpersonal dynamics. Horowitz (1991), for example, describes how histrionic persons view themselves as a "sexy star, wounded hero [or] worthy invalid" (p. 6), and the rest of the world plays the supporting roles of "interested suitor [or] devoted rescuer" (p. 6). Beck and Freeman (1990) address what they consider are irrational core beliefs, such as "Unless I captivate people I am nothing" or "If I can't entertain people they will abandon me." Complicating the treatment of persons with this disorder is their impressionistic and diffuse cognitive style, described well by Shapiro (1965): "hysterical cognition in general is global, relatively diffuse, and lacking in sharpness.... The hysterical person tends to respond quickly and is highly susceptible to what is immediately impressive, striking, or merely obvious" (pp. 111–112). This diffuse, impressionistic cognitive style will contribute to their suggestibility, and also in part results from their excessive emotionality. The histrionic person relies primarily on feelings rather than rationality to make decisions. This might be in part biogenetic in origin, but it may also be encouraged through social learning because impressionistic suggestibility can be appealing to and can be reinforced by others.

## Narcissistic Personality Disorder

Narcissistic personality disorder is described in DSM-IV as "a pervasive pattern of grandiosity (in fantasy or behavior), need for admiration, and lack of empathy, beginning by early adulthood and present in a variety of contexts" (APA, 1994, p. 661). This disorder was not included in the first or second editions of the APA DSM, nor is it included in the current, 10th edition of the World Health Organization's (1992) international nomenclature. Its inclusion in DSM-III (APA, 1980) "was suggested by an increasing psychoanalytic literature and by the isolation of narcissism as a personality factor in a variety of psychological studies" (Frances, 1980, p. 1053).

The criteria set for DSM-III consisted of a grandiose sense of self-importance or uniqueness; preoccupation with fantasies of success, power, brilliance, beauty, or ideal love; exhibitionism; indifference, rage, shame, humiliation, or emptiness in response to criticism or defeat; feelings of entitlement; interpersonal exploitativeness; overidealization and devaluation of others; and lack of empathy (APA, 1980). The revisions for DSM-III-R added feelings of envy and the belief that one's problems are unique; the alternation between feelings of idealization and devaluation was deleted due to its overlap with borderline personality disorder (Widiger et al., 1988). The revisions for DSM-III-R were not intended to be substantial, but Morey (1988) suggested that the revisions did change the recipients of the diagnosis. Only 6% of the 291 patients in his study met the DSM-III criteria, compared to 22% with the DSM-III-R criteria that contributed to a kappa of only .38 across the two editions (the third lowest rate of agreement). Blashfield et al. (1992), however, reported a better agreement rate of .57 across the two editions. They concluded that "the concordance of the DSM-III and DSM-III-R was relatively high" (Blashfield et al., 1992, p. 250).

The face validity studies of the DSM-III-R criteria set by Blashfield and Breen (1989) and Blashfield and Haymaker (1988) suggested that there were only a few problematic criteria. In the study by Blashfield and Breen, the diagnostic criteria were correctly assigned 69% of the time, and there was no consistent misassignment to an alternative diagnostic category. Interpersonal exploitativeness and preoccupation with feelings of envy, however, were misassigned by a majority of the clinicians. Blashfield and Haymaker (1988) indicated that interpersonal exploitativeness was consistently misassigned to the antisocial personality disorder. Morey and Ochoa (1989) reported a kappa of only .31 between the narcissistic personality disorder diagnoses provided by clinicians and the diagnoses that would be provided by their own assessments of the DSM-III criteria. Blashfield and Herkov (1996), however, reported a substantial improvement to .54 for the DSM-III-R criteria set, the third highest among the personality disorders.

A narcissistic personality disorder diagnosis tends to co-occur with other personality disorder diagnoses, particularly the paranoid, borderline, and histrionic (Stuart et al., 1998; Widiger & Rogers, 1989; Widiger & Trull, 1998). There has been surprisingly little co-occurrence with the antisocial personality disorder, despite the presence of the criterion concerned with interpersonal exploitativeness (Blashfield & Breen, 1989; Blashfield & Haymaker, 1988) and the presence of features included within Hare's (1991) checklist for psychopathy (i.e., lack of empathy, glib charm, and arrogance).

Gunderson, Ronningstam, and Smith (1991) summarized the results of a number of psychometric studies of the DSM-III-R criteria set. They concluded that the most problematic criteria were (1) reactions to criticism with feelings of rage, shame, or humiliation, even if not expressed; (2) lack of empathy; and (3) preoccupation with feelings of envy. Gunderson et al. (1991) did not suggest that these items should be deleted but argued that they needed substantial revision. The first criterion occurred frequently in persons with borderline and paranoid personality disorders. Gunderson et al. suggested that feelings of disdain might be more specific to narcissism than feelings of rage. Subsequent recommendations included the deletion of unexpressed feelings because unexpressed feelings can be quite difficult to assess reliably (Widiger et al., 1995). Lack of empathy is often described in narcissism, but it is also difficult to assess reliably (Ronningstam & Gunderson, 1990) and often occurs in persons with antisocial personality disorder. Gunderson et al. (1991) concluded that feelings of envy were "not found that often and ... [are] not necessarily found in [narcissistic] subjects" (p. 173). Ronningstam and Gunderson (1990) suggested that a belief that others envy them would be more diagnostic than feeling envious of others. Advisors to the DSM-IV Personality Disorders Work Group also suggested including feelings of resentment for the privileges or achievements of others (Gunderson et al., 1991).

Table 2 provides the DSM-IV diagnostic criteria. The reaction to criticism with feelings of rage, shame, or humiliation, even if not expressed, was deleted. DSM-III-R preoccupation with feelings of envy was also revised to include a belief that others envy them. A new criterion was added that generally described arrogant, haughty behaviors or attitudes (Ronningstam & Gunderson, 1990). Significant revisions were also made to five of

the other diagnostic criteria (Widiger et al., 1995). For example, the DSM-III-R need for constant attention and admiration was confined only to a need for admiration to facilitate the differentiation from the histrionic personality disorder, and lack of empathy was revised to indicate that narcissistic persons may be able to recognize cognitively how others feel but may not be at all concerned with these feelings (Gunderson et al., 1991; Widiger et al., 1995).

Linde and Clark (1998) indicated in their face validity study that the DSM-IV narcissistic criteria were correctly assigned 74% of the time. However, they did indicate that, once again, interpersonal exploitation was misassigned frequently to antisocial personality disorder. "Indeed, [interpersonal exploitation] appears closer to this antisocial core concept [disregard for the rights of others] than to the narcissistic personality disorder core concept of 'grandiosity and lack of empathy,' which was appropriately assigned to narcissistic personality disorder by 97% of clinicians" (Linde & Clark, 1998, p. 134).

Blais and Norman (1997) reported a Cronbach's alpha of .82 for the DSM-IV narcissistic personality disorder criteria set, the highest obtained by any personality disorder. Many of the narcissistic criteria, however, obtained significant correlations with the antisocial and histrionic criteria sets (e.g., interpersonal exploitation correlated .48 with the antisocial). The lowest internal consistency coefficient was obtained by envy (.35) and the highest by a grandiose sense of self-importance (.64). These findings are consistent with the rank order of the diagnostic criteria because the prior research indicated that grandiosity was the most diagnostic criterion and feelings of envy was the least diagnostic (Gunderson et al., 1991). Blais et al. (1997) found weak agreement between the DSM-III-R and DSM-IV criteria sets with respect to who received the diagnosis (kappa = .44), but they also concluded that "the changes to the narcissitic personality disorder criteria set appear beneficial, as the alpha coefficient for the DSM-IV versions was substantially improved over that obtained by the DSM-III-R version" (p. 276). Further discussions of each diagnostic criterion and additional experimental criteria are provided in Cooper (1998), Ronningstam and Gunderson (1990), Shedler and Westen (1998), and Widiger et al. (1995).

### Table 2. DSM-IV Criteria for Narcissistic Personality Disorder[a]

A pervasive pattern of grandiosity (in fantasy or behavior), need for admiration, and lack of empathy, beginning by early adulthood and present in a variety of contexts, as indicated by five (or more) of the following:

(1) has a grandiose sense of self-importance (e.g., exaggerates achievements and talents, expects to be recognized as superior without commensurate achievements)

(2) is preoccupied with fantasies or unlimited success, power, brilliance, beauty, or ideal love

(3) believes that he or she is "special" and unique and can only by understood by, or should associate with, other special or high-status people (or institutions)

(4) requires excessive admiration

(5) has a sense of entitlement, i.e., unreasonable expectations of especially favorable treatment or automatic compliance with his or her expectations

(6) is interpersonally exploitative, i.e., takes advantage of others to achieve his or her own ends

(7) lacks empathy: is unwilling to recognize or identify with the feelings and needs of others

(8) is often envious of others or believes that others are envious of him or her

(9) shows arrogant, haughty behaviors or attitudes

[a]APA (1994, pp. 661).

## Assessment

All of the semistructured interviews and self-report inventories cited earlier (except the PAI; Morey, 1991) include scales for assessing the narcissistic personality disorder (Morey & Jones, 1998, however, review how the PAI can be used for assessing narcissism). There is also a semi-structured interview devoted to assessing narcissism (Diagnostic Interview for Narcissism; Gunderson, Ronningstam, & Bodkin, 1990); the research with it was highly influential in developing the DSM-IV diagnostic criteria (Gunderson et al., 1991). There are also a number of self-report inventories devoted to assessing narcissistic personality traits, including the Narcissistic Personality Inventory (NPI; Raskin & Terry, 1988), that has been used in a number of personality and social-psychological studies of narcissism (Rhodewalt & Morf, 1995) and has the particularly useful feature of subscales for assessing various components of narcissism (i.e., superiority, vanity, leadership, authority, entitlement, exploitativeness, and exhibitionism).

Hilsenroth, Handler, and Blais (1996) provide an informative overview of the assessment of narcissistic personality disorder, and considerable discussion is devoted to projective instruments. Narcissism is one of the more heavily researched domains of Rorschach assessment, and also one of the more controversial. Nezworski and Wood (1995) provided a thorough critique of the empirical support for Rorschach indicators such as pair responses, reflections, and the egocentricity index. They indicated that the diagnostic criteria for narcissism were unspecified in most studies, and, more importantly, the "diagnosticians were aware of Rorschach scores and incorporated them into their diagnoses" (Nezworski & Wood, 1995, p. 192). Nezworski and Wood also indicated that none of these Rorschach indicators correlated significantly with such well-researched self-report measures of narcissism as the NPI (Raskin & Terry, 1988). "In summary, research has not yet demonstrated that Rorschach measures of narcissism are related to diagnoses or self-report measures of narcissism" (Nezworski & Wood, 1995, p. 193).

Exner (1995) responded in part by indicating that his scoring system "does not and never has contained a formal index of narcissism" (p. 200) and therefore should not be faulted for the failure to correlate with measures of narcissism. Persons with high scores on the egocentricity index will tend to be self-involved, but self-involvement does not necessarily suggest an inflated sense of self-worth. "It may simply indicate an unusual preoccupation with the self, generated by a sense of dissatisfaction" (Exner, 1995, p. 203). Exner (1995) did suggest that the reflection response "does seem to have a relationship to narcissism" (p. 200), but it would still be considered only a "narcissistic-like feature" (p. 202) rather than a direct indication of narcissism, narcissistic pathology, or a narcissistic personality disorder.

Hilsenroth et al. (1996) cited six studies that "have used the Rorschach in differential diagnostic research for narcissistic personality disorder" (p. 673); only one was cited by Nezworski and Wood (1995), and they concluded "that the Rorschach may be helpful to identify narcissistic personality disorder patients from different clinical groups" (p. 675). Hilsenroth et al. did not address the methodological criticisms raised by Nezworski and Wood (1995), but Hilsenroth, Fowler, Padawer, and Handler (1997) did address them in their own Rorschach study. Hilsenroth et al. (1997) compared the frequency of Rorschach reflection, personalization, idealization, and egocentricity scores in a university clinic and student sample. The personality disorder diagnoses were obtained from systematic reviews of material available in the patients' charts (excluding the original Rorschach data and clinicians' diagnoses). The results were particularly strong for idealization and reflection responses. "Narcissistic personality disorder patients had significantly more idealization responses than did the antisocial personality disorder group and more reflection responses than did both the antisocial and the borderline personality disorder groups" (Hilsenroth et al., 1997, p. 116). The number of reflection responses correlated significantly ($r = .33$) with the total number of DSM-IV narcissistic personality disorder diagnostic criteria and correlated significantly with the frequency of the individual narcissistic diagnostic criteria that, it would be predicted, is most closely associated with the disorder, including grandiose sense of self-importance, fantasies of unlimited success, and sense of entitlement. Hilsenroth et al. also correlated the Rorschach scores with the Morey et al. (1985) MMPI-2 narcissistic self-report measure (which could not have been affected by a knowledge of the Rorschach scores). Both the reflection and idealization scores correlated significantly with the MMPI-2 scale. Hilsenroth et al. (1997) concluded that their "findings reflect converging lines of evidence and support the use of the Rorschach as a valuable instrument in the diagnosis of narcissistic personality disorder as well as contributing to a conceptual understanding of narcissism and narcissistic pathology" (pp. 119–120).

## Epidemiology

Narcissistic is among the least frequently diagnosed personality disorders within clinical settings (Gunderson et al., 1991); estimates of prevalence are as low as 2%, but at times as high as 16% (APA, 1994). A curious finding is that none of the published community studies that have used a semistructured interview have identified any cases. In fact, three community studies that used semistructured interviews failed to identify a single case of narcissistic personality disorder, despite interviews of more than 2000 persons (Maier et al., 1992; Nestadt et al., 1990; Zimmerman & Coryell, 1989) and despite the substantial amount of research on maladaptive narcissistic personality traits within normal community and college samples (Rhodewalt & Morf, 1995). Modesty versus conceit is one of the facets of one of the fundamental domains of personality functioning (i.e., agreeableness versus antagonism), and approximately 18% of men and 6% of women might be characterized as excessively immodest, arrogant, or conceited (Costa & McCrae, 1992). DSM-IV narcissistic personality disorder is diagnosed more frequently in males (APA, 1994).

Cross-cultural studies of narcissism and narcissistic personality disorder would be of interest. Narcissistic is the only DSM-IV personality disorder that is not officially recognized within the World Health Organization's (1992) international nomenclature. Loranger et al. (1994) demonstrated that the DSM-IV can be applied within a wide variety of cultures and suggested that there were few difficulties with the application. With only a few minor exceptions, "the clinicians viewed the [DSM-IV] as applicable to their particular cultures" (Loranger et al., 1994, p. 223). However, being able to apply a diagnostic criteria set within another culture does not necessarily mean that the disorder diagnosed is valid or even

meaningful within that culture (Alarcon, 1996; Rogler, 1996). Theorists have suggested that narcissistic personality disorder is distinctly cultural and that pathological narcissism is the manifestation of a modern, Western society that has become overly self-centered and materialistic, coupled with a decreasing importance of familial (interpersonal) bonds (Cooper & Ronningstam, 1992; Lasch, 1978).

A life-span developmental model for the disorder would also be of interest for future research. Persons with this disorder might be seemingly well adjusted and even successful as young adults, based on substantial achievements in education, career, and perhaps even within relationships (Ronningstam & Gunderson, 1990). However, their relationships with their colleagues, peers, and intimates might become strained as their lack of consideration for and even exploitative use of others becomes more evident across time. Successes might also become more infrequent as their inability to accurately perceive or address criticism and setback contributes to a mounting number of failures. Persons with this disorder may at times not recognize their pathology until they have had a substantial number of setbacks or have finally recognized that the excessive importance they have given to achievement, success, and status has led to an emptiness and loneliness in their older age (Stone, 1993). As a result, mid-life and late-life transitions may be particularly difficult for persons with this disorder.

## Etiology and Pathology

There has not yet been a familial aggregation, twin, or adoption study of the narcissistic personality disorder (McGuffin & Thapar, 1992). The central construct of arrogance (versus modesty) is one of the facets of the broad domain of antagonism (versus agreeableness) that, it has been shown, are closely related to narcissistic personality disorder (Trull, 1992; Trull et al., 1998), and there has been consistent empirical support for the heritability of this broad domain of personality functioning (Nigg & Goldsmith, 1992). Jang et al. (1998), for example, estimated its heritability at .48 in a German and Canadian study. Jang et al. also explored the heritability for each facet of each broad domain after the common heritable component had been removed. Whereas the antagonism facets of mistrust, manipulativeness, oppositionalism, and tough-mindedness demonstrated unique heritability (.25 to .31), arrogance versus modesty did not. Much of its unique variance was attributed to shared and nonshared environmental influences.

The predominant psychosocial models for the etiology of narcissism have been largely social learning or psychodynamic (Auberbach, 1993; Cooper & Ronningstam, 1992). One model proposes that narcissism develops through an excessive idealization by parental figures, which is then incorporated by the child into his or her self-image (Benjamin, 1993; Millon et al., 1996). Narcissism may also develop through unempathic, neglectful, inconsistent, or even devaluing parental figures who have failed to adequately mirror a child's natural need for idealization (Kernberg, 1998). The child may find that the attention, interest, and perceived love of a parent are contingent largely on achievements or successes. The child may fail to perceive that the parents value or love them for their own sake, but may instead recognize that the love and attention are largely conditional on successful accomplishments. The child might then develop the belief that its own feelings of self-worth depend on continued recognition by others of such achievements, status, or success.

Conflicts and deficits with respect to self-esteem are central to the pathology of the disorder (Gabbard, 1994; Kernberg, 1998; Stone, 1993). Narcissistic persons must continually seek and obtain signs and symbols of recognition to compensate for conscious or perhaps even unconscious feelings of inadequacy (Auerbach, 1993). Empirical support for the validity of hypotheses concerning narcissistic pathology are being provided by social-psychological and personality, as well as clinical, research. Rhodewalt, Madrian, and Cheney (1998), for example, indicated how narcissism is more highly correlated with instability in self-esteem, rather than simply a consistently high self-confidence. Narcissistic persons may not consider themselves persons who are valued for their own sake because their own worthiness depends on a success, accomplishment, or status, and the value of others is measured as well in terms of the contributions they can make to a success or status. Their feelings of insecurity may at times be masked by disdainful indifference to criticism or by overt expressions of arrogance and conceit. Narcissism is perhaps a maladaptive process of regulating or protecting fragile self-esteem (Morf & Rhodewalt, 1993; Raskin, Novacek, & Hogan, 1991) in part through gaining the approval and admiration of others. Narcissistic persons may at times claim that it is not narcissism if they are in fact brilliant, talented, and successful. However, the pathology would still be evidenced by an excessive need for and reliance on recognition of their achievements. They are not persons who are comfortable when they are not adequately appreciated for their accomplishments, brilliance, or talent and may feel grossly insulted or enraged when they feel unjustly slighted (Stone, 1993).

In this context, in a series of studies Baumeister and his colleagues have been exploring the contribution of narcissistic conflicts to the occurrence of aggressive, violent behavior (Baumeister, Smart, & Boden, 1996). Bushman and Baumeister, for example demonstrated empirically that neither low nor high self-esteem was predictive of reacting aggressively to threat. It was "the combination of narcissism and insult [that] led to exceptionally high levels of aggression toward the source of the insult" (Bushman & Baumeister, 1998, p. 219). "It is not so much the people who regard themselves as superior beings who are the most dangerous but, rather, those who have a strong desire to regard themselves as superior beings" (Bushman & Baumesiter, 1998, p. 228). Some narcissistic persons may (perhaps appropriately) envy persons who are truly indifferent to success and who can enjoy a simple, modest, and unassuming life.

## Dependent Personality Disorder

The dependent personality disorder is described in DSM-IV as "a pervasive and excessive need to be taken care of that leads to submissive and clinging behavior and fears of separation, beginning by early adulthood and present in a variety of contexts" (APA, 1994, p. 668). A diagnosis of dependent personality disorder was included in the 1st edition of the DSM, but as a subtype to the passive-aggressive personality disorder, "characterized by helplessness, indecisiveness, and a tendency to cling to others as a dependent child to a supporting parent" (APA, 1952, p. 37). It was not included in DSM-II (APA, 1968; Hirschfeld, Shea, & Weise, 1991).

The DSM-III criteria for dependent personality disorder were grossly inadequate and were confined to the requirement of the three criteria of passively allowing others to assume responsibility for major areas of life because of an inability to function independently, subordinating own needs to avoid any possibility of having to rely on themselves, and lacking in self-confidence (APA, 1980). Morey and Ochoa (1989) reported a kappa agreement of only .23 between diagnoses of dependent personality disorder provided by clinicians and the presence of the three diagnostic criteria assessed by the same clinicians.

The criteria set was expanded substantially in DSM-III-R to include feelings of submissiveness and fears of separation (Widiger et al., 1988), and it is not surprising that the revisions for DSM-III-R did substantially change those who received the diagnosis. Whereas only 14% of the 291 patients studied by Morey (1988) met the DSM-III criteria, 22% met the criteria set for DSM-III-R (kappa = .54). Blashfield et al. (1992) reported a comparably low kappa of agreement between the two editions (k = .47), but they indicated that the DSM-III-R criteria resulted, in a reduction in the prevalence of the diagnosis (from 22 to 17%). "Given the substantial change in definitions, the low diagnostic concordance (k = .471) and the relatively low correlation (r = .622) were expected" (Blashfield et al., 1992, p. 250).

The face validity study of Blashfield and Breen (1989) indicated that 73% of the criteria were correctly assigned; this was the third highest rate obtained (after the paranoid and obsessive-compulsive criteria sets). Only one of the diagnostic criteria was not assigned to the dependent personality disorder by a majority of the clinicians: easily hurt by criticism or disapproval. This criterion also obtained the weakest results in the earlier face validity study by Blashfield and Haymaker (1988). Blais et al. (1996) indicated that the DSM-III-R criteria set for dependent personality disorder obtained the highest rating of clarity by their college students, 4.48 on a scale of 1 to 5 (where 5 = very clear). The ratings by the clinicians were significantly lower (3.35) but still well within the "fairly clear" range.

However, despite their apparent face validity, Blashfield and Herkov (1996) reported no improvement in the agreement between the diagnoses of dependent personality disorder provided by clinicians and their own assessment of the presence of the nine diagnostic criteria. The clinicians and the criteria set diagnosed approximately the same percentage of patients (61% and 57%, respectively), but the kappa value for agreement with respect to those who received the diagnosis was only .29, the second lowest for any personality disorder in this study. Blashfield and Herkov indicated that an allowance of others to assume responsibility for major areas of life was given particular weight in the clinicians' diagnoses.

Most of the patients who meet the criteria for dependent personality disorder will meet the diagnostic criteria for other personality disorders, particularly the borderline, histrionic, and avoidant (Stuart et al., 1998; Widiger & Rogers, 1989). Widiger and Trull (1998) indicated (in their summary of the findings for more than 1000 patients obtained from six unpublished data sets that were analyzed for DSM-IV) that 48% of the dependent patients met the DSM-III-R criteria for borderline personality disorder and 57% met the DSM-III-R criteria for avoidant. The most problematic item with respect to differentiating among these personality disorders was being easily hurt by criticism or disapproval. This diagnostic criterion occurred in more than 85% of the avoidant patients and in more than 70% of the borderline at four of the six research sites (Widiger & Trull, 1998). Feeling devastated or helpless when a close relationship ended was the second most problematic criterion because it was the next most frequent dependent criterion among borderline patients at four of the six sites and was the third most frequent symptom at the remaining two sites.

Hirschfeld, Shea, and Weise (1991) based their recommendations for DSM-IV on this prior research and on clinical and theoretical literature concerning attachment and dependency. Table 3 provides the DSM-IV diagnostic criteria. Being easily hurt by criticism or disapproval was deleted because it "is not specific to dependent personality disorder" (Hirschfeld et al., 1991, p. 147). No item was added to the criteria set to replace this deletion, but all of them were revised significantly (Hirschfeld et al., 1991; Widiger et al., 1995). Feeling devastated or helpless when a close relationship ends was revised to "urgently seeks another relationship as a source of care and support when a close relationship ends" (APA, 1994, p. 669). "Avoidant and dependent persons may act quite similarly when they have someone, but not when they are alone" (Widiger et al., 1995, p. 116). Avoidant and dependent persons are often clinging, insecure, and dependent when they are involved with someone, but when the relationship

### Table 3. DSM-IV Dependent Personality Disorder Criteria[a]

A pervasive and excessive need to be taken care of that leads to submissive and clinging behavior and fears of separation, beginning by early adulthood and present in a variety of contexts, as indicated by five (or more) of the following:

1. Has difficulty making everyday decision without an excessive amount of advice and reassurance from others.
2. Needs others to assume responsibility for most major areas of his or her life.
3. Has difficulty expressing disagreement with others because of fear of loss of support or approval (Note: Do not include realistic fears of retribution).
4. Has difficulty initiating projects or doing things on his or her own (because of a lack of self-confidence in judgment or abilities rather than to a lack of motivation or energy).
5. Goes to excessive lengths to obtain nurturance and support from others, to the point of volunteering to do things that are unpleasant.
6. Feels uncomfortable or helpless when alone, because of exaggerated fears of being unable to care for himself or herself.
7. Urgently seeks another relationship as a source of care and support when a close relationship ends.
8. Is unrealistically preoccupied with fears of being left to take care of himself or herself.

[a]APA (1994, pp. 668–669).

ends, avoidant persons are slow to find replacements, whereas in "dependent persons, the history of negligent, abusive, unreliable, or exploitative partners is due, in large part, to their failure to be careful, selective, or discriminating" (Widiger et al., 1995, p. 116) in selecting new partners. Many of the other revisions were made to emphasize attachment issues and an emotional reliance on others, rather than simply feelings of low self-confidence (Benjamin, 1993; Hirschfeld et al., 1991; Livesley, Schroeder, & Jackson, 1990). This is evident in the references to need for or a seeking of nurturance and, most significantly, in the revision to the definition of the disorder from simply a "pervasive pattern of dependent and submissive behavior" (APA, 1987, p. 354) to "a pervasive and excessive need to be taken care of that leads to

submissive and clinging behavior and fears of separation" (APA, 1994, p. 665).

Linde and Clark (1998) reported that the DSM-IV criteria for dependent personality disorder were correctly assigned by their participants 78% of the time; this was the fourth highest rate obtained among the personality disorders and was higher than the average rate of 69% obtained for the Axis I disorders. Blais and Norman (1997), however, suggested that some of the diagnostic criteria are still problematic. They reported an internal consistency (Cronbach's alpha) coefficient of .67; this was among the second lowest but still well above the coefficient of .35 obtained by nine randomly selected diagnostic criteria. The two weakest criteria were going to excessive lengths to obtain nurturance and support and urgently seeking another relationship as a source of care and support when a close relationship ends. The latter item, however, was only one of three dependent criteria that was uncorrelated with the avoidant criteria.

## Assessment

All of the semistructured interviews and self-report inventories cited before (except the PAI; Morey, 1991) include scales for assessing the DSM-IV dependent personality disorder. There are also a number of self-report inventories devoted to assessing dependent personality traits, including the Interpersonal Dependency Inventory (Hirschfeld et al., 1977), the dependency scale from the Blatt Depressive Experience Questionnaire (Blatt & Zuroff, 1992; Santor, Zuroff, & Fielding, 1997), and the sociotropy scale from the Beck Sociotropy-Autonomy Scale (Robins, Hayes, Block, Kramer, & Villena, 1995).

Bornstein (1993, 1995) provides a thorough overview of the assessment of dependent personality traits, including the use of projective techniques. The Rorschach Oral Dependency (ROD) scale developed by Masling, Rabie, and Blondheim (1967) "is far and away the most widely used projective dependency measure" (Bornstein, 1993, p. 25). The ROD is a content scoring system for the Rorschach, including explicitly dependent or dependency-related imagery or oral imagery. Interrater reliability is typically quite high; agreement ranges from 85 to 95%, correlation in total score is typically greater than .90, and kappa coefficients for cutoff point classifications often exceed

.80 (Bornstein, 1996a). Significant correlations have been obtained with thematic apperception measures of dependency ($r =. 58$; Masling et al., 1967) and with the Hirschfeld et al. (1977) self-report IDI, ranging from .32 to .67 in women and .37 to .48 in men. Behavioral correlates of ROD dependency have included increased yielding in Asch-type conformity experiments, completing introductory psychology research requirements earlier in the semester, and difficulty terminating psychotherapy. "Laboratory, clinical, and field studies confirm that the ROD scale does, in fact, predict dependency-related behavior in a variety of participant groups" (Bornstein, 1996a, p. 203). There has not yet been a published study on the correlation of the ROD scale with any measure of dependent personality disorder. "The relationship between ROD scores and Axis II psychopathology remains unexamined" (Bornstein, 1996a, p. 204), and Bornstein (1995) does suggest that self-report inventory and semistructured interview assessments of dependency are probably better predictors of a DSM-IV dependent personality disorder diagnosis than projective measures. However, clinicians who prefer to assess implicit, perhaps even unconscious, dependency needs might prefer a projective assessment rather than a self-report inventory or a semistructured interview (Bornstein, 1998a; Westen, 1997).

## Epidemiology

Dependent personality disorder is among the most frequently diagnosed personality disorders (APA, 1994); it occurs in 5 to 30% of patients (Hirschfeld et al., 1991) and 2 to 4% of the general population (Maier et al., 1992; Nestadt et al., 1990; Zimmerman & Coryell, 1989). It is diagnosed more frequently in females than in males, although this differential sex prevalence rate is controversial in a manner comparable to histrionic personality disorder (see earlier discussion), and it is again suggested in DSM-IV that the differential sex prevalence rate might be an illusory artifact of biased clinical assessments and the base rate of females within clinical settings (APA, 1994).

A few studies that used semistructured interviews have failed to identify a differential sex prevalence rate for dependent personality disorder (e.g., Glolomb, Fava, Abraham, & Rosenbaum, 1995; Grilo et al., 1996). However, most studies that used semistructured interviews indicated that more women than men are likely to have dependent personality disorders (Corbitt & Widiger, 1995). Bornstein (1996b) conducted a meta-analysis of studies that assessed for dependent personality traits. "All dependent personality disorder prevalence rate studies published before 1993 that (a) used structured interviews to derive dependent personality disorder diagnoses and (b) involved random samples of psychiatric inpatients, outpatients, or community subjects were included in this analysis (n of studies = 18)" (Bornstein, 1996b, p. 4). He found "a highly significant difference that indicates that a woman is nearly 40% more likely than a man to receive a dependent personality disorder diagnosis" (Bornstein, 1996a, p. 4).

It should be noted, however, that Bornstein (1996b) did not suggest that the differential sex prevalence rate obtained with semistructured interviews is necessarily correct. On the contrary, he suggested that instruments of assessment with high face validity (e.g., semistructured interviews or self-report inventories whose questions obviously assess for dependent personality traits) will tend to underestimate the prevalence of the disorder in males given the higher likelihood that they unconsciously or consciously deny the extent of their dependency needs. Bornstein (1995) also conducted a meta-analysis of all studies published since 1950 that provided data on sex differences in dependency. A total of ninety-seven studies was identified, and the findings "revealed that (a) women of all ages consistently obtain higher dependency scores than do men on objective dependency tests; and (b) adult men obtain slightly higher scores than do adult women on projective dependency tests" (Bornstein, 1995, p. 319). These results suggest that although women almost invariably obtain higher scores than men on measures of self-attributed (i.e., overt or conscious) dependency needs, women and men might not differ with respect to their levels of implicit (underlying or unconscious) dependency needs.

The prevalence and diagnosis of dependent personality disorder may also vary across cultures (Foulks, 1996) because there are profound differences in the extent to which societies encourage and value dependency-related behaviors. Many Western societies place more emphasis and value on expressions of autonomy and self-reliance and might then be prone to overdiagnose the disorder (Bornstein, 1992, 1993). In some cultures, such as the Japanese (Johnson, 1993) or Indian (Singh & Ojha, 19878), interpersonal connectedness and interdependency are more highly valued, and what is considered dependency within the American culture might not be considered pathological within another culture.

The controversies concerning gender may also interact with issues concerning culture. Within many societies, females are encouraged to be more dependent than males and are diagnosed as disordered for having conformed to this sex role (Kaplan, 1983). It is not always clear whether this diagnosis represents an accurate assessment of a pathology created by maladaptive socialization of women (Widiger & Spitzer, 1991) or a masculine bias with respect to these judgments (Kaplan, 1983). Some researchers have even suggested that there might not be many dependent females if there were more dependable males (Coyne & Whiffen, 1995). Dependent behavior in females is often in reaction to irresponsible, indifferent, or negligent behavior of the persons with whom they are involved. If males, including fathers, were more consistently dependable, there might indeed be less dependency in females.

There is also substantial need for research on the relationship of aging to the presence and the diagnosis of this disorder (Abrams & Horowitz, 1996; Segal, Hersen, Van Hasselt, Silberman, & Roth, 1996). Dependent personality disorder is one of the more commonly discussed and researched personality disorders among the aged (Baltes, 1996; Loranger, 1996). However, it is not always clear if this dependency results from the aging process (e.g., secondary to a deterioration in capacity to care for oneself and loss of supportive relationships) or if it represents the characteristic manner in which the person functioned throughout life. Studies have suggested that the increased dependency levels in older adults are due primarily to increases in instrumental dependency (i.e., reliance on others for assistance in daily living), rather than to increases in an emotional dependency (as suggested by a clinging insecurity). Emotional dependency is more closely linked with the diagnosis of a dependent personality disorder (Baltes, 1996; Bornstein, 1993). In any event, one cannot currently diagnose a personality disorder with DSM-IV unless the disorder was evident since late childhood or early adulthood. DSM-IV does recognize adult-onset personality change if it is the direct result of a neurochemical change

secondary to a medical disorder (i.e., personality change due to a general medical condition), but not if the change is the direct result of social-environmental experiences or is an indirect result of a medical incapacitation.

## Etiology and Pathology

There has been a study of the heritability of dependent personality disorder, but the methodology was too weak to be adequately conclusive (Nigg & Goldsmith, 1994). O'Neill and Kendler (1998) reported the results of a longitudinal study of 2230 twins to whom an interpersonal dependency subscale of the IDI had been administered (Hirschfeld et al., 1977). The results suggested a modest genetic influence and a large specific environmental contribution. Dependent personality disorder may also involve maladaptive variants of common personality traits within the broad domains of neuroticism and agreeableness (Mongrain, 1993; Widiger et al., 1995; Zuroff, 1994). Facets of agreeableness that are closely involved with dependency are excessive trust (gullibility), altruism (self-sacrificing), compliance (submissiveness), modesty (self-effacing), and tender-mindedness (Widiger et al., 1995). These traits appear to be heritable (Nigg & Goldsmith, 1992). A closely related dimensional model of personality pathology is provided by Livesley and his colleagues; included within it is a dimension of insecure attachment that may represent a fundamental pathology of dependent personality disorder (Bornstein, 1992, 1993) that, it has been shown, is heritable within both clinical and nonclinical populations (Livesley, Jang, & Vernon, 1998).

Dependent personality disorder may represent an interaction of an anxious, fearful temperament with an insecure attachment to an inconsistent or unreliable parental figure (McGuffin & Thapar, 1992). Dependent persons may turn to parental figures to provide reassurance and a sense of security that they are unable to generate for themselves. This empirically supported etiologic model (Rothbart & Ahadi, 1994) is consistent with current object relations theory in which dependent personality traits are considered an internalization of the mental representation of the self as weak and ineffectual and contribute to a disposition to look to others to provide protection and support, to become preoccupied with fears of abandonment, and to develop feelings of helplessness and insecurity

(Blatt, Cornell, & Eshkol, 1993; Bornstein, 1992, 1993).

Parental figures might exacerbate genetically based dispositions toward feelings of anxiousness and insecurity by not encouraging the development of interpersonal skills and coping strategies and by validating an inadequate, powerless, or ineffectual self-image through authoritarian or overprotective behavior (Bornstein, 1993, 1999). Efforts toward autonomy and individuation might be discouraged, whereas continued infantilization and dependency are encouraged. In an intriguing cross-generational laboratory study, Thompson and Zuroff (1998) demonstrated how dependent mothers tended to reward mediocre rather than excellent performance by their daughters. Positive regard by parental figures might not be unconditional, but conditional instead the continued (and perhaps inconsistent) communication of their value or worth to them. Persons with this disorder might then develop the belief that their worth is contingent on their worth or importance to another person.

Cognitive theorists describe an irrational schema that conveys this pathological sense of self-worth. Beck and Freeman (1990) suggest that the core belief is that "I am completely helpless," coupled with the sense that "I can function only if I have access to somebody competent" (p. 290). "They conclude that the solution to the dilemma of being inadequate in a frightening world is to try to find someone who seems able to handle life and who will protect and take care of them" (Beck & Freeman, 1990, p. 290). However, their neediness and desperation will often prevent them from carefully selecting people who will indeed be protective and nurturant. They often choose indiscriminately and become quickly attached to persons who are unreliable, unempathic, and even exploitative and abusive. They might feel that either they deserve inadequate partners or may even select inadequate partners to try to work through or resolve their long-standing interpersonal conflicts and feelings of inadequacy (Stone, 1993).

A substantial number of studies has now confirmed that the dependent person's self-image as weak and ineffectual and the excessive need to please others contributes to a variety of interpersonal problems and maladaptive consequences (Bornstein, 1999; Overholser, 1996). Bornstein, Riggs, Hill, and Calabrese (1996), for example, demonstrated in a series of experiments how de-

pendent persons might do whatever is necessary when competing with peers to please an authority figure, even if it means acting aggressively. Santor and Zuroff (1997) demonstrated how dependent persons were excessively concerned with maintaining interpersonal relatedness, adopting the responses of friends who outperformed, minimizing disagreement with disagreeing friends, and praising friends even when they disagreed with them. A number of studies have also indicated that dependent personality traits provide vulnerability to the development of clinically significant episodes of depression, particularly in response to interpersonal rejection or loss (Blatt & Zuroff, 1992). Valid methodological concerns are often raised with respect to this research (e.g., Coyne & Whiffen, 1995; Widiger, Verheul, and van den Brink, 1999), but a sufficient number of replicated, well-designed prospective studies support the hypothesis that dependency does indeed provide vulnerability to episodes of depression (Robins et al., 1995). For example, Hammen et al. (1995) obtained 6-month and 12-month follow-up assessments of 129 high school senior women. They conducted multiple regression analyses to predict depression on the basis of dependency cognitions, prior interpersonal stress, and the interaction between them, controlling for initial levels of depression. All of the young women experienced stressful life events during this period of their lives, including moving away from home, separating from an important relationship, and losing a romantic partner, but most of them did not become depressed. "It was the women with cognitions about relationships representing concerns about rejection or untrustworthiness of others who were especially challenged by normative changes" (p. 441). Hammen et al. (1995) concluded that "overall, the results suggest that dysfunctional attachment cognitions contribute to both onset and severity of symptomatology" (p. 441).

## Conclusions

A substantial amount of clinical, personality, and social-psychological research has been conducted on histrionic, narcissistic, and dependent personality disorders since the last edition of this text (Blashfield & Davis, 1993). It is no longer the case that these are weakly validated diagnostic constructs. Much is now known regarding their diagnosis, assessment, epidemiology, etiology, and pathology.

Many issues, of course, remain to be resolved. For example, additional studies are needed to understand more completely the myriad ways in which gender, ethnicity, and age influence the likelihood of actually having or simply receiving a diagnosis of histrionic, narcissistic, or dependent personality disorder. For each disorder, the interaction of hypothesized genetic and neurochemical diatheses with early environmental influences that may exacerbate or minimize these predispositions needs to be more carefully examined. Many issues of excessive diagnostic co-occurrence and inadequate differentiation must also be addressed, and future revisions of the diagnostic system will have a substantial amount of clinical, theoretical, and empirical literature that will be of substantial help in these deliberations. Finally, it would also be useful to consider adaptive consequences of histrionic, narcissistic, and dependent personality traits. These personality traits are present in part because they have adaptive consequences and useful benefits. Individuals who select (or perhaps modify) environments that accommodate their vulnerabilities and value their strengths may experience substantially fewer consequences of the maladaptive nature of the personality disorder symptomatology. This chapter has hopefully been helpful in highlighting some of the more significant findings that have occurred since the prior edition of this text and also in stimulating the development of useful research for future editions of this text.

# References

Abrams, R. C., & Horowitz, S. V. (1996). Personality disorders after age 50: a meta-analysis. *Journal of Personality Disorders, 10,* 271–282.

Alarcon, R. D. (1996). Personality disorders and culture in DSM-IV: A critique. *Journal of Personality Disorders, 10,* 260–270.

American Psychiatric Association. (1952). *Diagnostic and statistical manual of mental disorders.* Washington, DC: Author.

American Psychiatric Association. (1968). *Diagnostic and statistical manual of mental disorders* (2nd ed.). Washington, DC: Author.

American Psychiatric Association. (1980). *Diagnostic and statistical manual of mental disorders* (3rd ed.). Washington, DC: Author.

American Psychiatric Association. (1987). *Diagnostic and statistical manual of mental disorders* (3rd ed., rev.). Washington, DC: Author.

American Psychiatric Association. (1994). *Diagnostic and statistical manual of mental disorders* (4th ed.). Washington, DC: Author.

Auerbach, J. S. (1993). The origins of narcissism and narcissistic personality disorder: A theoretical and empirical reformulation. In J. M. Masling & R. F. Bornstein (Eds.), *Psychoanalytic perspectives on psychopathology* (pp. 43–110). Washington, DC: American Psychological Association.

Baltes, M. M. (1996). *The many faces of dependency in old age.* New York: Cambridge University Press.

Baumeister, R. F., Smart, L., & Boden, J. M. (1996). Relation of threatened egoism to violence and aggression: The dark side of high self-esteem. *Psychological Review, 103,* 5–33.

Beck, A. T., & Freeman, A. (1990). *Cognitive therapy of personality disorders.* New York: Guilford.

Benjamin, L. S. (1993). *Interpersonal diagnosis and treatment of personality disorders.* New York: Guilford.

Blais, M. A., Benedict, K. B., & Norman, D. K. (1996). The perceived clarity of the Axis II criteria. *Journal of Personality Disorders, 10,* 16–22.

Blais, M. A., Hilsenroth, M. J., & Castlebury, F. D. (1997). Psychometric characteristics of the Cluster B personality disorders under DSM-III-R and DSM-IV. *Journal of Personality Disorders, 11,* 270–278.

Blais, M. A., Hilsenroth, M. J., & Fowler, J. C. (1998). Rorschach correlates of the DSM-IV histrionic personality. *Journal of Personality Assessment, 70,* 355–364.

Blais, M. A., & Norman, D. K. (1997). A psychometric evaluation of the DSM-IV personality disorder criteria. *Journal of Personality Disorders, 11,* 168–176.

Blashfield, R. K., Blum, N., & Pfohl, B. (1992). The effects of changing Axis II diagnostic criteria. *Comprehensive Psychiatry, 33,* 245–252.

Blashfield, R. K., & Breen, M. J. (1989). Face validity of the DSM-III-R personality disorders. *American Journal of Psychiatry, 146,* 1575–1579.

Blashfield, R. K., & Davis, R. T. (1993). Dependent and histrionic personality disorders. In P. B. Sutker & H. E. Adams (Eds.), *Comprehensive handbook of psychopathology* (pp. 395–409). New York: Plenum.

Blashfield, R. K., & Haymaker, D. (1988). A prototype analysis of the diagnostic criteria for DSM-III-R personality disorders. *Journal of Personality Disorders, 2,* 272–280.

Blashfield, R. K., & Herkov, M. J. (1996). Investigating clinician adherence to diagnosis by criteria: A replication of Morey and Ochoa (1989). *Journal of Personality Disorders, 10,* 219–228.

Blatt, S. J., Cornell, C. E., & Eshkol, E. (1993). Personality style, differential vulnerability, and clinical course in immunological and cardiovascular disease. *Clinical Psychology Review, 13,* 421–450.

Blatt, S. J., & Zuroff, D. (1992). Interpersonal relatedness and self-definition: Two prototypes for depression. *Clinical Psychology Review, 12,* 527–562.

Bornstein, R. F. (1992). The dependent personality: Developmental, social, and clinical perspectives. *Psychological Bulletin, 112,* 3–23.

Bornstein, R. F. (1993). *The dependent personality.* New York: Guilford.

Bornstein, R. F. (1995). Sex differences in objective and projective dependency tests: A meta-analytic review. *Assessment, 2,* 319–331.

Bornstein, R. F. (1996a). Construct validity of the Rorschach oral dependency scale: 1967–1995. *Psychological Assessment, 8,* 200–205.

Bornstein, R. F. (1996b). Sex differences in dependent personality disorder prevalence rates. *Clinical Psychology: Science and Practice, 3,* 1–12.

Bornstein, R. F. (1997). Dependent personality disorder in the DSM-IV and beyond. *Clinical Psychology: Science and Practice, 4,* 175–187.

Bornstein, R. F. (1998a). Implicit and self-attributed dependency strivings: Differential relationships to laboratory and field measures of help-seeking. *Journal of Personality and Social Psychology, 75,* 778–787.

Bornstein, R. F. (1998b). Reconceptualizing personality disorder diagnosis in the DSM-V: The discriminant validity challenge. *Clinical Psychology: Science and Practice, 5,* 333–343.

Bornstein, R. F. (1999). Dependent and histrionic personality disorders. In T. Millon, P. Blaney, & R. Davis (Eds.), *Oxford textbook of psychopathology* (pp. 535–554). Oxford, England: Oxford University Press.

Bornstein, R. F., Riggs, J. M., Hill, E. L., & Calebrese, C. (1996). Rorschach measures of oral dependence and the internalized self-representation in normal college students. *Journal of Personality Assessment, 52,* 648–657.

Bushman, B. J., & Baumeister, R. F. (1998). Threatened egotism, narcissism, self-esteem, and direct and displaced aggression: Does self-love or self-hate lead to violence? *Journal of Personality and Social Psychology, 75,* 219–229.

Butcher, J. N., & Rouse, S. V. (1996). Personality: Individual differences and clinical assessment. *Annual Review of Psychology, 47,* 87–111.

Coolidge, F. L., & Merwin, M. M. (1992). Reliability and validity of the Coolidge Axis II inventory: A new inventory for the assessment of personality disorders. *Journal of Personality Assessment, 59,* 223–228.

Cooper, A. M. (1998). Further developments in the clinical diagnosis of narcissistic personality disorder. In E. F. Ronningstam (Ed.), *Disorders of narcissism. Diagnostic, clinical, and empirical implications* (pp. 53–74). Washington, DC: American Psychiatric Press.

Cooper, A. M., & Ronningstam, E. (992). Narcissistic personality disorder. In A. Tasman & M. B. Riba (Eds.), *Review of psychiatry,* Vol. 11 (pp. 80–97). Washington, DC: American Psychiatric Press.

Corbitt, E. M., & Widiger, T. A. (1995). Sex differences among the personality disorders: An exploration of the data. *Clinical Psychology: Science and Practice, 2,* 225–238.

Costa, P. T., & McCrae, R. R. (1992). *Revised NEO Personality Inventory (NEO-PI-R) and NEO Five-Factor Inventory (NEO-FFI) professional manual.* Odessa, FL: Psychological Assessment Resources.

Coyne, J. C., & Whiffen, V. E. (1995). Issues in personality as diathesis for depression: The case of sociotropy-dependency and autonomy-self-criticism. *Psychological Bulletin, 118,* 358–378.

Exner, J. (1995). Comment on "Narcissistic in the Comprehensive System for the Rorschach." *Clinical Psychology: Science and Practice, 2,* 200–206.

Feingold, A. (1994). Gender differences in personality: A meta-analysis. *Psychological Bulletin, 116,* 429–456.

First, M., Gibbon, M., Spitzer, R. L., Williams, J. B. W., & Benjamin, L. S. (1997). *User's guide for the Structured Clinical Interview for DSM-IV Axis II Personality Disorders.* Washington, DC: American Psychiatric Press.

Ford, M., & Widiger, T. A. (1989). Sex bias in the diagnosis of histrionic and antisocial personality disorders. *Journal of Consulting and Clinical Psychology, 57,* 301–305.

Foulks, E. F. (1996). Culture and personality disorders. In J. E. Mezzich, A. Kleinman, H. Fabrega, & D. L. Parron (Eds.), *Culture and psychiatric diagnosis. A DSM-IV perspective* (pp. 243–252). Washington, DC: American Psychiatric Press.

Frances, A. J. (1980). The DSM-III personality disorders section: A commentary. *American Journal of Psychiatry, 137,* 1050–1054.

Frances, A. J., First, M. B., & Pincus, H. A. (1995). *DSM-IV guidebook.* Washington, DC: American Psychiatric Press.

Funtowicz, M. N., & Widiger, T. A. (1995). Sex bias in the diagnosis of personality disorders: A different approach. *Journal of Psychopathology and Behavioral Assessment, 17,* 145–165.

Funtowicz, M. N., & Widiger, T. A. (1999). Sex bias in the diagnosis of personality disorders: An evaluation of the DSM-IV criteria. *Journal of Abnormal Psychology, 108,* 195–202.

Gabbard, G. O. (1994). *Psychodynamic psychiatry in clinical practice. The DSM-IV Edition.* Washington, DC: American Psychiatric Press.

Garb, H. N. (1997). Race bias, social class bias, and gender bias in clinical judgment. *Clinical Psychology: Science and Practice, 4,* 99–120.

Golomb, M., Fava, M., Abraham, M., & Rosenbaum, J. F. (1995). Gender differences in personality disorders. *American Journal of Psychiatry, 152,* 579–582.

Grilo, C. M., Becker, D. F., Fehon, D. C., Walker, M. L., Edell, W. S., & McGlashan, T. H. (1996). Gender differences in personality disorders in psychiatrically hospitalized adolescents. *American Journal of Psychiatry, 153,* 1089–1091.

Gunderson, J. G. (1992). Diagnostic controversies. In A. Tasman & M. B. Riba (Eds.), *Review of psychiatry,* Vol. 11 (pp. 9–24). Washington, DC: American Psychiatric Press.

Gunderson, J. G., Ronningstam, E., & Bodkin, A. (1990). The diagnostic interview for narcissistic patients. *Archives of General Psychiatry, 47,* 676–680.

Gunderson, J. G., Ronningstam, E., & Smith, L. E. (1991). Narcissistic personality disorder: A review of data on DSM-III-R descriptions. *Journal of Personality Disorder, 5,* 167–177.

Hamburger, M. E., Lilienfield, S. O., & Hogben, M. (1996). Psychopathy, gender, and gender roles: Implications for antisocial and histrionic personality disorder. *Journal of Personality Disorders, 10,* 41–55.

Hamilton, S., Rothbart, M., & Dawes, R. (1986). Sex bias, diagnosis, and DSM-III. *Sex Roles, 15,* 269–274.

Hammen, C. L., Burge, D., Daley, S. E., Davila, J., Paley, B., & Rudolph, K. D. (1995). Interpersonal attachment cognitions and predictions of symptomatic responses to interpersonal stress. *Journal of Abnormal Psychology, 104,* 436–443.

Hare, R. D. (1991). *The Revised Psychopathy Checklist.* Toronto, Ontario, Canada: Multi-Health Systems, Inc.

Herkov, M. J., & Blashfield, R. K. (1995). Clinical diagnoses of personality disorders: evidence of a hierarchical structure. *Journal of Personality Assessment, 65,* 313–321.

Hilsenroth, M. J., Fowler, J. C., Padawer, J. R., & Handler, L. (1997). Narcissism in the Rorschach revisited: Some reflections on empirical data. *Psychological Assessment, 9,* 113–121.

Hilsenroth, M. J., Handler, L., & Blais, M. A. (1996). Assessment of narcissistic personality disorder: A multi-method review. *Clinical Psychology Review, 16,* 655–683.

Hirschfeld, R. M. A., Klerman, G. L., Gough, H. G., Barrett, J., Korchin, S. J., & Chodoff, P. (1977). A measure of interpersonal dependency. *Journal of Personality Assessment, 41,* 610–618.

Hirschfeld, R. M. A., Shea, M. T., & Weise, R. (1991). Dependent personality disorder: perspectives for DSM-IV. *Journal of Personality Disorders, 5,* 135–149.

Horowitz, M. J. (1991). *Hysterical personality style and the histrionic personality disorder.* Northvale, NJ: Jason Aronson.

Hyler, S. E. (1994). *Personality Diagnostic Questionnaire-4.* New York: New York State Psychiatric Institute.

Jang, K. L., McCrae, R. R., Angleitner, A., Reimann, R., & Livesley, W. J. (1998). Heritability of facet-level traits in a cross-cultural twin sample: Support for a hierarchical model of personality. *Journal of Personality and Social Psychology, 74,* 1556–1565.

Johnson, F. F. (1993). *Dependency and Japanese socialization.* New York: New York University Press.

Kaplan, M. (1983). A woman's view of DSM-III. *American Psychologist, 38,* 786–792.

Kernberg, O. F. (1998). Pathological narcissism and narcissistic personality disorder: Theoretical background and diagnostic classification. In E. F. Ronningstam (Ed.), *Disorders of narcissism. Diagnostic, clinical, and empirical implications* (pp. 29–51). Washington, DC: American Psychiatric Press.

Klein, D. F. (1999). Harmful dysfunction, disorder, disease, illness, and evolution. *Journal of Abnormal Psychology, 108,* 421–429.

Klein, M. H., Benjamin, L. S., Rosenfeld, R., Treece, C., Husted, J., & Greist, J. H. (1993). The Wisconsin Personality Disorders Interview: Development, reliability, and validity. *Journal of Personality Disorders, 7,* 285–303.

Lasch, C. (1978). *The culture of narcissism.* New York: W.W. Norton.

Linde, J. A., & Clark, L. E. A. (1998). Diagnostic assignment of criteria: clinicians and DSM-IV. *Journal of Personality Disorders, 12,* 126–137.

Livesley, W. J., Jang, K. L., & Vernon, P. A. (1998). Phenotypic and genetic structure of traits delineating personality disorder. *Archives of General Psychiatry, 55,* 941–948.

Livesley, W. J., Schroeder, M. L., & Jackson, D. N. (1990). Dependent personality disorder and attachment problems. *Journal of Personality Disorders, 4,* 232–240.

Livesley, W. J., Schroeder, M. L., Jackson, D. N., & Jang, K. L. (1994). Categorical distinctions in the study of personality disorder: Implications for classification. *Journal of Abnormal Psychology, 103,* 6–17.

Loranger, A. W. (1996). Dependent personality disorder. Age, sex, and axis I comorbidity. *Journal of Nervous and Mental Disease, 184,* 17–21.

Loranger, A. W., Sartorius, N., Andreoli, A., Berger, P., Buchheim, P., Channabasavanna, S. M., Coid, B., Dahl, A., Diekstra, R. F. W., Ferguson, B., Jacobsberg, L. B., Mombour, W., Pull, C., Ono, J., & Regier, D. A. (1994). The International Personality Disorder Examination. The World Health Organization/Alcohol, Drug Abuse, and Mental Health Administration international pilot study of personality disorders. *Archives of General Psychiatry, 51,* 215–224.

Loranger, A. W., Sartorius, N., Janca, A. (Eds.). (1997). *Assess-ment and diagnosis of personality disorders: The ICD-10 International Personality Disorder Examination (IPDE).* Cambridge, England: Cambridge University Press.

Maier, W., Lichtermann, D., Klingler, T., Heun, R., & Hallmayer, J. (1992). Prevalences of personality disorders (DSM-III-R) in the community. *Journal of Personality Disorders, 6,* 187–196.

Masling, J. M., Rabie, I., & Blondheim, S. H. (1967). Obesity, level of aspiration, and Rorschach and TAT measures of oral dependence. *Journal of Counseling Psychology, 31,* 233–239.

McGuffin, P., & Thapar, A. (1992). The genetics of personality disorder. *British Journal of Psychiatry, 160,* 12–23.

Millon, T., Davis, R. D., & Millon, C. M. (1997). *MCMI-III manual* (2nd ed.). Minneapolis, MN: National Computer Systems.

Millon, T., Davis, R. D., Millon, C. M., Wenger, A., Van Zullen, M. H., Fuchs, M., & Millon, R. B. (1996). *Disorders of personality. DSM-IV and beyond* (2nd ed.). New York: Wiley.

Mongrain, M. (1993). Dependency and self-criticism located within the five-factor model of personality. *Personality and Individual Differences, 15,* 455–462.

Morey, L. C. (1988). Personality disorders in DSM-III and DSM-III-R: convergence, coverage, and internal consistency. *American Journal of Psychiatry, 145,* 573–577.

Morey, L. C. (1991). *Personality Assessment Inventory: Professional manual.* Odessa, FL: Psychological Assessment Resources.

Morey, L. C., & Jones, J. K. (1998). Empirical studies of the construct validity of narcissistic personality disorder. In E. F. Ronningstam (Ed.), *Disorders of narcissism. Diagnostic, clinical, and empirical implications* (pp. 351–373). Washington, DC: American Psychiatric Press.

Morey, L. C., & Ochoa, E. S. (1989). An investigation of clinical adherence to diagnostic criteria: clinical diagnosis of DSM-III personality disorders. *Journal of Personality Disorders, 3,* 180–192.

Morey, L. C., Waugh, M. H., & Blashfield, R. K. (1985). MMPI scales for DSM-III personality disorders: Their derivation and correlates. *Journal of Personality Assessment, 49,* 245–251.

Morf, C. C., & Rhodewalt, F. (1993). Narcissism and self-evaluation maintenance: Explorations in object relations. *Personality and Social Psychology Bulletin, 19,* 666–676.

Nestadt, G., Romanoski, A., Chahal, R., Merchant, A., Folstein, M., Gruenberg, E., & McHugh, P. (1990). An epidemiological study of histrionic personality disorder. *Psychological Medicine, 20,* 413–422.

Nezworski, M. T., & Wood, J. M. (1995). Narcissism in the Comprehensive System for the Rorschach. *Clinical Psychology: Science and Practice, 2,* 179–206.

Nigg, J. T., & Goldsmith, H. H. (1994). Genetics of personality disorders: Perspectives from personality and psychopathology research. *Psychological Bulletin, 115,* 346–380.

Oldham, J. M., Skodol, A. E., Kellman, H. D., Hyler, S. E., Rosnick, L., & Davies, M. (1992). Diagnosis of DSM-III-R personality disorders by two semistructured interviews: Patterns of comorbidity. *American Journal of Psychiatry, 149,* 213–220.

O'Neill, F. A., & Kendler, K. S. (1998). Longitudinal study of interpersonal dependency in female twins. *British Journal of Psychiatry, 172,* 154–158.

Overholser, J. C. (1996). The dependent personality and interpersonal problems. *Journal of Nervous and Mental Disease,* *184,* 8–16.

Padilla, A. M. (1995). *Hispanic psychology: Critierial issues in theory and research.* Newbury Park, CA: Sage.

Perry, J. C. (1992). Problems and considerations in the valid assessment of personality disorders. *American Journal of Psychiatry, 149,* 1645–1653.

Pfohl, B. (1991). Histrionic personality disorder: A review of available data and recommendations for DSM-IV. *Journal of Personality Disorders, 5,* 150–166.

Pfohl, B. (1995). Histrionic personality disorder. In W. J. Livesley (Ed.), *The DSM-IV personality disorders* (pp. 173–192). New York: Guilford.

Pfohl, B., Blum, N., & Zimmerman, M. (1997). *Structured Interview for DSM-IV Personality.* Washington, DC: American Psychiatric Press.

Raskin, R., & Novacek, J., & Hogan, R. (1991). Narcissistic self-esteem management. *Journal of Personality and Social Psychology, 60,* 911–918.

Raskin, R., & Terry, H. (1988). A principal-components analysis of the Narcissistic Personality Inventory and further evidence of its construct validity. *Journal of Personality and Social Psychology, 54,* 890–902.

Rhodewalt, F., Madrian, J. C., & Cheney, S. (1998). Narcissism, self-knowledge, organization, and emotional reactivity: The effect of daily experience on self-esteem and affect. *Personality and Social Psychology Bulletin, 24,* 75–87.

Rhodewalt, F., & Morf, C. C. (1995). Self and interpersonal correlates of the Narcissistic Personality Inventory: A review and new findings. *Journal of Research in Personality, 29,* 1–23.

Robins, C. J., Hayes, A. H., Block, P., Kramer, R. J., & Villena, M. (1995). Interpersonal and achievement concerns and the depressive vulnerability and symptom specificity hypothesis: A prospective study. *Cognitive Therapy and Research, 19,* 1–20.

Rogers, R. (1995). *Diagnostic and structured interviewing. A handbook for psychologists.* Odessa, FL: Psychological Assessment Resources.

Rogler, L. H. (1996). Framing research on culture in psychiatric diagnosis: The case of the DSM-IV. *Psychiatry, 59,* 145–155.

Ronningstam, E., & Gunderson, J. G. (1990). Identifying criteria for narcissistic personality disorder. *American Journal of Psychiatry, 147,* 585–601.

Rothbart, M. K., & Ahadi, S. A. (1994). Temperament and the development of personality. *Journal of Abnormal Psychology, 103,* 55–66.

Santor, D. A., & Zuroff, D. C. (1997). Interpersonal responses to threats of status and interpersonal relatedness: Effects of dependency and self-criticism. *British Journal of Clinical Psychology, 36,* 521–541.

Santor, D. A., Zuroff, D. C., & Fielding, A. (1997). Analysis and revision of the Depressive Experiences Questionnaire: Examining scale performance as a function of scale length. *Journal of Personality Assessment, 69,* 145–163.

Schooler, J. W., & Loftus, E. F. (1986). Individual differences and experimentation: Complementary approaches to interrogative suggestibility. *Social Behavior, 1,* 105–112.

Segal, D. L. (1997). Structured interviewing and DSM classification. In S. M. Turner & M. Hersen (Eds.), *Adult psychopathology and diagnosis* (pp. 24–57). New York: Wiley.

Segal, D. L., Hersen, M., Van Hasselt, V. B., Silberman, C. S., & Roth, L. (1996). Diagnosis and assessment of personality disorders in older adults: A critical review. *Journal of Personality Disorders, 10,* 384–399.

Shapiro, D. (1965). *Neurotic styles.* New York: Basic Books.

Shedler, J., & Westen, D. (1998). Refining the measurement of Axis II: A Q-sort procedure for assessing personality pathology. *Assessment, 5,* 333–354.

Singh, R. R., & Ojha, S. K. (1987). Sex difference in dependence proneness, insecurity, and self-concept. *Manas, 34,* 61–66.

Sprock, J. (1996). Abnormality ratings of the DSM-III-R personality disorder criteria for males vs. females. *Journal of Nervous and Mental Disease, 184,* 314–316.

Sprock, J., Blashfield, R. K., & Smith, B. (1990). Gender weighting of DSM-III-R personality disorder criteria. *American Journal of Psychiatry, 147,* 586–590.

Stone, M. H. (1993). *Abnormalities of personality. Within the beyond the realm of treatment.* New York: W.W. Norton.

Stuart, S., Pfohl, B., Battaglia, M., Bellodi, L., Grove, W., & Cadoret, R. (1998). The cooccurrence of DSM-III-R personality disorders. *Journal of Personality Disorders, 12,* 302–315.

Thompson, S., & Zuroff, D. C. (1998). Dependent and self-critical mothers' responses to adolescent autonomy and competence. *Personality and Individual Differences, 24,* 311–324.

Trull, T. J. (1992). DSM-III-R personality disorders and the five factor model of personality: An empirical comparison. *Journal of Abnormal Psychology, 101,* 553–560.

Trull, T. J., Widiger, T. A., Useda, J. D., Holcomb, J., Doan, B.-T., Axelrod, S. R., Stern, B. L., & Gershuny, B. S. (1998). A structured interview for the assessment of the five-factor model of personality. *Psychological Assessment, 10,* 229–240.

Tyrer, P., & Johnson, T. (1996). Establishing the severity of personality disorder. *American Journal of Psychiatry, 153,* 1593–1597.

Watkins, C. E., Campbell, V. L., Nieberding, R., & Hallmark, R. (1995). Contemporary practice of psychological assessment by clinical psychologists. *Professional Psychology: Research and Practice, 26,* 54–60.

Westen, D. (1997). Divergences between clinical and research methods for assessing personality disorders: Implications for research and the evolution of Axis II. *American Journal of Psychiatry, 154,* 895–903.

Widiger, T. A. (1993). The DSM-III-R categorical personality disorder diagnoses: A critique and an alternative. *Psychological Inquiry, 4,* 75–90.

Widiger, T. A. (1998). Sex biases in the diagnosis of personality disorders. *Journal of Personality Disorders, 12,* 95–118.

Widiger, T. A., & Costa, P. T. (1994). Personality and personality disorders. *Journal of Abnormal Psychology, 103,* 78–91.

Widiger, T. A., Frances, A. J., Spitzer, R. L., & Williams, J. B. W. (1988). The DSM-III-R personality disorders: An overview. *American Journal of Psychiatry, 145,* 786–795.

Widiger, T. A., Mangine, S., Corbitt, E. M., Ellis, C. G., & Thomas, G. V. (1995). *Personality Disorder Interview-IV. A semistructured interview for the assessment of personality disorders.* Odessa, FL: Psychological Assessment Resources.

Widiger, T., & Rogers, J. H. (1989). Prevalence and comorbidity of personality disorders. *Psychiatric Annals, 19,* 132–136.

Widiger, T. A., & Sanderson, C. J. (1995a). Assessing personality disorders. In J. N. Butcher (Ed.), *Clinical personality assessment. Practical approaches* (pp. 380–394). New York: Oxford University Press.

Widiger, T. A., & Sanderson, C. J. (1995b). Towards a dimensional model of personality disorders in DSM-IV and DSM-V. In W. J. Livesley (Ed.), *The DSM-IV personality disorders* (pp. 433–458). New York: Guilford.

Widiger, T. A., & Saylor, K. I. (1998). Personality assessment. In A. S. Bellack & M. Hersen (Eds.), *Comprehensive clinical psychology* (pp. 145–167). New York: Pergamon Press.

Widiger, T. A., & Spitzer, R. L. (1991). Sex bias in the diagnosis of personality disorders: Conceptual and methodological issues. *Clinical Psychology Review, 11,* 1–22.

Widiger, T. A., & Trull, T. J. (1998). Performance characteristics of the DSM-III-R personality disorder criteria sets. In T. A. Widiger et al. (Eds.), *DSM-IV sourcebook,* Vol. 4 (pp. 357–363). Washington, DC: American Psychiatric Association.

Widiger, T. A. Trull, T. J., Clarkin, J. F., Sanderson, C., & Costa, P. T. (1994). A desription of the DSM-III-R and DSM-IV personality disorders with the five-factor model of personality. In P. T. Costa & T. A. Widiger (Eds.), *Personality disorders and the five-factor model of personality* (pp. 41–

56). Washington, DC: American Psychological Association.

Widiger, T. A., Verheul, R., & van den Brink, W. (1999). Personality and psychopathology. In L. Pervin & O. John (Eds.), *Handbook of personality* (2nd ed., pp. 347–366). New York: Guilford.

World Health Organization. (1992). The ICD-10 classification of mental and behavioural disorders. Clinical descriptions and diagnostic guidelines. Geneva, Switzerland: Author.

Zanarini, M. C., Frankenburg, F. R., Sickel, A. E., & Yong, L. (1996). *Diagnostic Interview for DSM-IV Personality Disorders (DIPD-IV).* Boston, MA: McLean Hospital.

Zimmerman, M. (1994). Diagnosing personality disorders. A review of issues and research methods. *Archives of General Psychiatry, 51,* 225–245.

Zimmerman, M., & Coryell, W. (1989). DSM-III personality disorder diagnosis in a nonpatient sample. *Archives of General Psychiatry, 46,* 682–689.

Zuroff, D. C. (1994). Depressive personality styles and the five-factor model of personality. *Journal of Personality Assessment, 63,* 453–472.

# PART IV

# Disorders Associated with Social and Situational Problems

# CHAPTER 19

# Paranoid, Schizoid, and Schizotypal Personality Disorders

## Michael B. Miller, J. David Useda, Timothy J. Trull, Rachel M. Burr, and Christa Minks-Brown

## Introduction

Our personalities are collections of behavioral, mental, and social characteristics that define us as individuals. Characteristics that are not temporally stable cannot establish replicable individual differences and therefore are not considered aspects of personality. For some of us, our personalities interfere with our abilities to form relationships, to control our impulses or emotions, to perceive ourselves and others accurately, and to enjoy life or to function at work. When such problems reach a sufficiently pathological extreme, personality is said to be disordered.

According to the *Diagnostic and Statistical Manual of Mental Disorders*, 4th ed. (DSM-IV; American Psychiatric Association [APA], 1994), Personality Disorders (PDs) are characterized by inflexible, pervasive, stable, and enduring patterns of inner experience and behavior that deviate markedly from the expectations of the individual's culture and lead to clinically significant distress or impairment in important areas of functioning. The maladaptive patterns of thought or behavior must be present at least by early adulthood, they must not be manifestations or consequences of other mental disorders, and they must not be caused by drug use or by medical conditions (see DSM-IV, p. 633, for general diagnostic criteria for a Personality Disorder).

In the DSM system of psychiatric diagnosis, PDs are grouped into three clusters (called A, B, and C) based on phenotypic similarity. Cluster A disorders include Paranoid, Schizoid, and Schizotypal PDs. The major commonality for these disorders is that affected individuals generally have very weak or nonexistent social attachments and odd or eccentric behavior. A second source of similarity for these disorders is that all three of them are found at higher rates in the families of schizophrenia patients, so that all three disorders may be alternative expressions of a similar genetic predisposition.

In this chapter, we focus on three Cluster A disorders. Seven major topics are presented: (1) a historical overview of both the schizophrenia spectrum concept and of the Cluster A personality disorders; (2) detailed descriptions of the disorders based on their modern (DSM-IV) diagnostic criteria; (3) epidemiology, including preva-

Michael B. Miller, J. David Useda, Timothy J. Trull, Rachel M. Burr, and Christa Minks-Brown • University of Missouri-Columbia, Columbia, Missouri 65211.

*Comprehensive Handbook of Psychopathology* (Third Edition), edited by Patricia B. Sutker and Henry E. Adams. Kluwer Academic / Plenum Publishers, New York, 2001.

lence rates and intercorrelations (comorbidity rates) of the disorders; (4) methods of assessment; (5) dimensional (continuous) alternatives to diagnostic classification; (6) major theories of etiology; and (7) leading treatments for Cluster A disorders.

## Historical Overviews

### History of the Schizophrenia Spectrum of Disorders

It has been observed for many years that the family members of psychotic patients often exhibit symptoms similar to those of their psychotic relatives, but of lesser severity. Nineteenth-century American psychiatrist Isaac Ray was one of the first to write on this topic. According to Ray (1863), "the current philosophy ... supposes that the hereditary affection must appear in the offspring in precisely the same degree of intensity which it had in the parent.... Such views are not warranted by the present state of our knowledge respecting the hereditary transmission of disease" (p. 30). Ray believed that subtler aspects of mental disorder deserved more attention than they were receiving. He believed that mentally sound and unsound elements could coexist in one individual and he wrote of persons who "may get on very well in their allotted part, and even achieve distinction, while the insane element is often cropping out in the shape of extravagancies or irregularities of thought or action, which, according to the standpoint they are viewed from, are regarded as gross eccentricity, or undisciplined powers, or downright insanity" (Ray, 1863, p. 31). Psychiatrists of the early part of the twentieth century, such as Eugen Bleuler, Emil Kraepelin, and Ernst Kretschmer, also described individuals who were not frankly psychotic but had features of psychotic illness. Bleuler and Kretschmer described the family members of those with schizophrenia by using terms such as schizoid, shut in, or suspicious (Kendler, 1985). Bleuler coined the term *schizophrenia* for what he believed was a *group* of psychotic disorders, and he also coined the term *latent schizophrenia* to describe cases where features of schizophrenic illness were present but in attenuated form. Gregory Zilboorg's (1941) *ambulatory schizophrenia* was merely schizophrenia that was not striking enough to be easily recognizable. Paul Hoch and colleagues

developed the diagnostic category of *pseudoneurotic schizophrenia* (Hoch & Cattell, 1959; Hoch & Polatin, 1949; Hoch et al., 1962), whose primary clinical symptoms were similar to the symptoms of today's Schizotypal PD. Rado (1953) coined the term *schizotypal*, and Meehl (1962) introduced the concept of *schizotypy* to define a condition with an underlying inherited neural integrative defect that could be manifested as anything from mild distortions of thought and perception to full-blown schizophrenia.

Even though these different writers seemed to be describing very similar individuals, no single term became clearly favored. During the middle of the twentieth century, up to the 1970s, the adjective *schizoid* (noun *schizoidia*) was often used to describe schizophrenic-like individuals (e.g., Heston, 1970; Kallmann, 1938). This often confuses today's readers because the term *schizotypal* has taken on the meaning once held by *schizoid*, and the diagnostic criteria for Schizotypal PD criteria are much more schizophrenia-like that those for Schizoid PD.

In the late 1960s, Paul Wender, Seymour Kety, and David Rosenthal used Danish adoption and psychiatric records to undertake a series of studies of the genetics of schizophrenia. Their research methods were impeccable, and the published results of their "Danish adoption studies" were extremely influential—truly a watershed in the history of psychiatric research. Like the clinicians and researchers who preceded them, these researchers observed that biological relatives of schizophrenic patients, even those who were not schizophrenic themselves, sometimes exhibited schizophrenic behaviors. The researchers interpreted the range of psychopathology in the family members as evidence of a continuum or spectrum of schizophrenic-like disorders with a similar genetic basis:

We had recognized certain qualitative similarities in the features that characterized the diagnoses of schizophrenia, uncertain schizophrenia, and inadequate personality, which suggested that these syndromes formed a continuum; this we called the schizophrenia spectrum of disorders. If schizophrenia were to some extent genetically transmitted, there should be a higher prevalence of disorders in the schizophrenia spectrum among the biological relatives of the index cases than in those of their controls. (Kety, Rosenthal, Wender, & Schulsinger, 1968, p. 353)

In later papers, the same authors used the term "borderline schizophrenia" for individuals who did not meet their criteria for schizophrenia but had some schizophrenic personality features. The term "schizophrenia spectrum" is still widely used, but which disorders should be included in the spectrum is still not fully resolved.

The DSM-II was published in 1968, but it did not include reference to personality types with schizophrenic features. It contained terse descriptions (three sentences each) of Paranoid and Schizoid PDs, but no formal diagnostic criteria, and Schizotypal and Borderline PDs were not listed. Psychiatrists of the day used the term "borderline" inconsistently to refer to either an unstable "borderline personality" or to "borderline schizophrenia." Some psychiatric researchers of the 1970s wisely sought to clarify the meanings of the diagnostic labels by refining the DSM diagnostic approach to include explicit criteria and more complete descriptions. The DSM-III, which appeared in 1980, marked a dramatic change in diagnostic rigor. The addition of Schizotypal PD and Borderline PD in DSM-III was influenced greatly by the work of Spitzer, Endicott, and Gibbon (1979). Spitzer et al. sought to clarify the meaning of the term "borderline" as it was being used by psychiatrists at that time. Spitzer mailed letters to a randomly selected sample of 4000 APA members asking for their help in developing the criteria for DSM-III borderline personality disorder and requesting that they use items developed by Spitzer et al. to rate two of their patients, one "who warrants a diagnosis of borderline personality, borderline personality organization or borderline schizophrenia" (p. 20) and one who is "moderately to severely ill but [does] not have a diagnosis of psychosis or any of the borderline categories" (p. 20). Exactly 808 psychiatrists responded, and statistical analysis of their data showed that the two types of borderline patients could be partially distinguished from each other (but with a 54% overlap!) and readily distinguished from the non-borderline controls. The items used to rate patients in the Spitzer et al. (1979) study were later developed into the DSM-III criteria for Borderline PD (corresponding to the unstable personality) and Schizotypal PD (corresponding to borderline schizophrenia).

## History of Schizotypal PD

Schizotypal PD is the major schizophrenia-spectrum personality disorder, so much of the history of Schizotypal PD was covered in the preceding section, but we will add a discussion of the historical development of the terms *schizotype* and *schizotypal*. The term *schizotype* was used by Kretschmer early in the twentieth century (Brueel, 1936), but most of today's scholars attribute the term to Rado (1953). Rado created *schizotype* by combining *schizo*phrenia and pheno*type*. Paul Meehl (1962, 1964, 1990) elaborated extensively on Rado's concepts and developed a complex theory of a trait he called *schizotypy*. In Meehl's theory, a single dominant gene carried by 10% of the population causes, in every carrier, a "neural integrative defect" which he called *schizotaxia* (combining schizo- with ataxia). He did not specify the exact nature of the defect. In addition, Meehl (1962) stated that "All schizotaxics become, *on all actually existing social learning regimes*, schizotypic in personality organization" (p. 231, italics in original). Meehl's schizotype (an individual with a schizotypic personality organization) is characterized by cognitive slippage (mild thought disorder), anhedonia or hypohedonia (lack of pleasure), ambivalence, and interpersonal aversiveness (social fear). It follows that, in our world, every carrier of the dominant gene will have a schizotypic personality organization; also, according to Meehl (1990), 10% of such individuals will develop frank schizophrenia, and the remaining 90% will have varying degrees of personality psychopathology. Individuals who do not carry the gene are protected from developing schizophrenia, but they might very rarely develop a psychotic disorder that mimics schizophrenia. Meehl's (1964) descriptions of schizotypic personality traits were very clear and detailed, and they have played an important role in research (viz., the psychometric scales developed by the Chapmans and described in the section of this chapter on dimensional approaches).

Meehl's concepts and terminology were not adopted by the DSM when the category of Schizotypal PD was added in 1980. In fact, Spitzer et al. (1979) cited neither Meehl nor Rado and simply claimed to adopt the term schizotypal because "the term means 'like schizophrenia'" (p. 18). Meehl's theory of schizotaxia, schizotypy, and schizophrenia has inspired a tremendous amount of research in the decades since it was published. Some of the findings of that research will be discussed later in this chapter. We should add that the single-gene aspect of Meehl's theory, while perhaps not refuted outright, seems unlikely to be correct in the face of a large number of genetic linkage analysis studies of schizophrenia that have failed to find evidence of a strong single-gene effect.

## History of Paranoid PD

The study of paranoid phenomena has a long and rich history within philosophy, psychiatry, and psychology. The literature has focused on the existence and description of distinct subtypes of paranoia, the relation of paranoid states to other diagnostic entities, as well as the etiology and course of the various paranoid diagnoses. The definitions and terms used to described paranoid disorders have varied and evolved over time. The evolution of the Paranoid PD construct will be described briefly (see Millon & Davis [1996] for a more in-depth discussion).

Early descriptions of paranoia do not resemble contemporary conceptualizations of this phenomenon. In Greek literature, paranoia was often used to describe madness in general or thinking amiss (Akhtar, 1990; Lewis, 1970; Manschreck, 1979). Various formulations through the 1700s attempted to define conditions which had exhibited some aspects of paranoia, but none received the attention that was accorded to Heinroth's (1818) conceptualization (Akhtar, 1990; Lewis, 1970; Tanna, 1974). Heinroth's description included four types of paranoia: a gross distortion of an individual's reality due to a single misconception; delusions of the supernatural; megalomania; and a mixture of cognitive, emotional, and volitional problems (Lewis, 1970). Heinroth believed that paranoia predominantly affected understanding and rarely occurred in a pure form, a nineteenth-century observation that still rings true today. He asserted that paranoia usually co-occurs with disorders of the will or affect or both (i.e., delusions and bizarre behavior, mood disturbance).

Kahlbaum's 1863 definition of paranoia is widely regarded as resembling a modern-day conceptualization of this phenomenon (Tanna, 1974). Yet, the classification of paranoid syndromes posed a challenge for diagnosticians of the nineteenth-century. Turn-of-the-century German diagnosticians, particularly Emil Kraepelin and Eugene Bleuler, continued to examine paranoia and its subtypes, and delusions of persecution figured prominently in

their conceptions of the various paranoid disorders. The greatest challenge in classifying paranoia lay in the nineteenth-century observation that paranoid states were seen in many different psychiatric conditions, an observation that is still valid today (Manschreck & Petri, 1978). Central to the diagnostic dilemma of the time was whether to classify paranoia as a separate disorder that could co-occur with schizophrenia (or dementia praecox, as it was then called) or to classify paranoia as a subtype of schizophrenia (Lewis, 1970; Manschreck, 1979), a controversy that continues to this day (Coryell & Zimmerman, 1989; Kendler & Gruenberg, 1982; Kendler, Masterson, & Davis, 1985; Maier, Lichtermann, Minges, & Heun, 1994).

By the end of the nineteenth century, Emil Kraepelin's classification of psychiatric disorders recognized three forms of paranoia; (1) a subtype of dementia praecox (like modern Schizophrenia, Paranoid Type); (2) a form associated with a milder type of dementia praecox which did not display the deterioration of personality Kraepelin expected to see in dementia praecox (like modern Delusional Disorder, Persecutory Type); and (3) most importantly for this discussion, another form of paranoid disorder described was an insidious, chronic illness characterized by a fixed delusional system, without hallucinations or deterioration of personality (see Manschreck, 1979). This third form most closely resembles the present-day Paranoid PD.

Paranoid PD has been recognized formally in the U.S. psychiatric nomenclature since 1942 and has been included in every edition of the DSM since its inception in 1952. In this century, the defining features of Paranoid PD, as described in the clinical literature, have included a pervasive and unwarranted mistrust of others (Kraepelin, 1921), hypersensitivity to criticism (Cameron, 1943, 1963; Kretschmer, 1925), antagonism and aggressiveness (Sheldon, 1940; Sheldon & Stevens, 1942), an excessive need for autonomy (Millon, 1969, 1981), hypervigilance (Cameron, 1963; Millon, 1981; Shapiro, 1965), and rigidity (Shapiro, 1965). Although Paranoid PD had already been a part of the DSM system, this body of literature was the basis for the formulation of explicit diagnostic criteria for Paranoid PD in the DSM-III (APA, 1980). The DSM-III criteria were meant to be representative of the clinical literature; yet not all have agreed to the comprehensiveness of the construct as defined by the DSM and have described additional criteria for assessing Paranoid PD (Akhtar, 1990; Millon, 1983, 1987; WHO, 1992).

## History of Schizoid PD

The term *schizoid* was coined by Bleuler (1922), but descriptions of individuals who would meet today's criteria for Schizoid PD preceded Bleuler by many years. Millon and Davis (2000) note that Ribot (1890) coined the term *anhedonia* for the lack of physical and social pleasure that is central to the schizoid experience. August Hoch (1910) described a "shut-in" personality that he saw as highly vulnerable to dementia praecox (schizophrenia). Hock's shut-ins were seclusive and quiet, stubborn, rigid, and prone to fantasy. Bleuler's concept of the schizoid was similar to Hoch's, but Bleuler focused more on the indifference of schizoid individuals and on their self-absorption—their autistic focus on an inner world. Kretschmer (1925) interpreted the inner focus of schizoid persons as a necessary consequence of their detachment from other human beings.

The Schizoid personality has been included in the DSM diagnostic system since its inception in 1952. The earliest description noted that "Inherent traits in such personalities are (1) avoidance of close relations with others, (2) inability to express directly hostile or even ordinary aggressive feelings, and (3) autistic thinking" (APA, 1952), DSM-II (APA, 1968) retained a similar description, but DSM-III (APA, 1980) introduced diagnostic criteria in place of mere descriptions and added an emphasis on the emotion in the Schizoid PD. Rather than simply avoiding interpersonal relationships, the schizoid is said to show "(A) Emotional coldness and aloofness, absence of warm, tender feelings for others; (B) indifference to praise or criticism or to the feelings of others" (APA, 1980, p. 311). A new diagnostic category called Avoidant PD was added in the DSM-III. The Avoidant PD was said to be socially withdrawn, like the schizoid, but the avoidant was hypersensitive to rejection and derogation instead of being indifferent like the schizoid. So the fundamental distinction among these disorders was that the *cause* of social isolation differed among them: The avoidant was isolated because of social anxiety, whereas the schizoid was isolated because of social aloofness and indifference. DSM-III-R enhanced this difference in emotionality by adding "rarely, if ever, claims to experience strong emotions, such as anger and joy" (APA, 1987, p. 340) to the list of symptoms of Schizoid PD and simultaneously more strongly emphasized the neurotic emotionality of the Avoidant PD. The DSM-IV (1994) has deemphasized the emotionality issue for both PDs, and the DSM-III-R schizoid symptom shown in the previous sentence was removed in DSM-IV.

The vacillation in DSM criteria for Schizoid and Avoidant PDs reflects a controversy that dates to Kretschmer's (1925) writings on schizoid personality. Kretschmer distinguished between two schizoid types: the anesthetic and the hyperaesthetic. This dichotomy was revised and elaborated by Millon (1969) in his theory of personality, and it became the basis for the schizoid (anesthetic) and avoidant (hyperaesthetic) PDs. According to Kretschmer (1925), hyperaesthetic individuals tend to feel their isolation strongly and "they seek as far as possible to deaden all stimulation from the outside" (p. 161). Anesthetic individuals were considered indifferent and withdrawn because they were so lacking capacity for affective responsiveness: "He draws back into himself ... because all that is about him can offer him nothing" (p. 162). This dichotomization of socially withdrawn individuals into schizoid and avoidant PDs has always been controversial and remains so. Several writers (e.g., Akhtar, 1987) have doubted that individuals with schizoid personalities are truly unemotional, even though they appear so to observers. Gunderson (1983) questioned the need for the Avoidant PD category in DSM-III on the grounds that empirical support for the schizoid/avoidant distinction was weak and the theoretical rationale for the distinction was not widely accepted.

Today, we are left in the awkward position of having two DSM personality disorders—schizoid and avoidant—that are similar enough that some experts feel that they are not distinct disorders, but these same two disorders are grouped in different DSM personality disorder clusters because of their theoretical dissimilarity. Bleuler originally conceived of schizoid individuals as schizophrenic-like and, despite relatively weak empirical affirmation for the relationship of Schizoid PD to schizophrenia, Schizoid PD is grouped with Schizo-

### Table 1. DSM-IV Diagnostic Criteria for Schizotypal Personality Disorder

A. A pervasive pattern of social and interpersonal deficits marked by acute discomfort with, and reduced capacity for, close relationships as well as by cognitive or perceptual distortions and eccentricities of behavior, beginning by early adulthood and present in a variety of contexts, as indicated by five (or more) of the following:

(1) ideas of reference (excluding delusions of reference)

(2) odd beliefs or magical thinking that influences behavior and is inconsistent with subcultural norms (e.g., superstitiousness, belief in clairvoyance, telepathy, or "sixth sense"; in children and adolescents, bizarre fantasies or preoccupations)

(3) unusual perceptual experiences, including bodily illusions

(4) odd thinking and speech (e.g., vague, circumstantial, metaphorical, overelaborate, or stereotyped)

(5) suspiciousness or paranoid ideation

(6) inappropriate or constricted affect

(7) behavior or appearance that is odd, eccentric, or peculiar

(8) lack of close friends or confidants other than first-degree relatives

(9) excessive social anxiety that does not diminish with familiarity and tends to be associated with paranoid fears rather than negative judgments about self

B. Does not occur exclusively during the course of Schizophrenia, a Mood Disorder With Psychotic Features, another Psychotic Disorder, or a Pervasive Developmental Disorder.

---

tricities of behavior which begins by early adulthood and is present in a variety of situations. At least five of nine criteria listed in Table 1 must be evident for this diagnosis to be given (American Psychiatric Association, 1994). These criteria include ideas of reference (Criterion A1) that are incorrect interpretations of events as having a particular and unusual meaning specifically meant for the individual. Ideas of reference must be distinguished from delusions of reference, which may be similar in content but are held with greater conviction. For example, a person who exhibits ideas of reference may have the *feeling* that strangers are talking about him/her, but if challenged, acknowledges that the people may be talking about something else. In contrast, individuals with delusions of reference would consistently *believe* that people are talking about them and could probably give specific examples of what those people are saying. Individuals with Schizotypal PD may have odd beliefs or magical thinking that influence their behavior and are inconsistent with subcultural norms (Criterion A2). For example, they may be superstitious and/or believe in clairvoyance, telepathy, or a "sixth sense." Unusual perceptual experiences, such as feeling the presence of another person or hearing someone call their name when no one is there, may be present as well (Criterion A3).

In addition, individuals with Schizotypal PD may exhibit odd thinking and speech (Criterion A4). Speech patterns may be vague, circumstantial, metaphorical, over elaborate, or stereotyped. Suspiciousness or paranoid ideation (Criterion A5) may also be characteristic of these individuals. For example, they may believe that their coworkers are trying to undermine their reputations with their boss. They frequently lack close friends or confidants other than first-degree relatives (Criterion A8). This may be due, in part, to their interactional style. They often experience excessive social anxiety that does not diminish with familiarity and tends to be associated with paranoid fears (Criterion A9). At social events, schizotypal people tend to become more uncomfortable rather than relaxed as time passes. In addition, they often are unable to express the full range of affects and thus may seem to interact with others in an inappropriate, stiff, or constricted manner (Criterion A6). These individuals' behavior or appearance may seem odd, eccentric, or peculiar (Criterion A7) which, again makes maintaining relationships difficult.

typal and Paranoid PDs in DSM-IVs Cluster A. Following Kretschmer (1925) and Millon (1969), the DSM-IV Avoidant PD is marked by feelings of inadequacy, hypersensitivity, and fear of rejection. So it is grouped with the anxious/inhibited Dependent and Obsessive-Compulsive PDs in Cluster C.

## Descriptions of Cluster A PDs

### Description of Schizotypal PD

Schizotypal PD is characterized by a pervasive pattern of acute discomfort in close relationships, cognitive or perceptual distortions, and eccen-

It is important to note that Schizotypal PD should not be diagnosed if these behaviors occur only during the course of Schizophrenia, other psychotic conditions (e.g., mood disorder with psychotic features), or a pervasive developmental disorder (APA, 1994). The following is a vignette of a person with schizotypal PD.

Although Jim was viewed by his high school teachers as "bright" and "creative," he never seemed to live up to his potential. Further, at times his "creativity" seemed to border on the bizarre. For example, he made it clear to several people that he believed in "fairies" who were invisible but did good deeds. According to Jim, you can sometimes "feel" their presence, and these fairies may in fact be responsible for day-to-day events that transpire. Fairly mundane or routine happenings seem to take on personal significance to Jim. For example, thunderstorms might be interpreted by Jim as a message not to shower for one day. Discussions with Jim about fairies or otherwise tend to be hard to follow. Jim often is quite vague, and he frequently uses metaphors that are difficult to connect to the topic at hand. Another "odd" feature of Jim's behavior is that he frequently breaks out into a silly grin and laughs for no apparent reason. This makes those around him feel very uncomfortable. For the last ten years, Jim has had no real friends, lives by himself, and prefers to be alone. He "lives off the land" and is much more comfortable being "out in nature" rather than around people.

## Description of Paranoid PD

Nearly anyone can describe an individual who would be called "paranoid" or who has acted "paranoid" to some degree at some time. Nearly everyone has experienced fleeting feelings of suspicion, felt unduly criticized, or felt the need to be alone. We all know what is means to "read between the lines" of what someone is saying for other meanings, such as implied criticisms. Perhaps, we have sometimes have been unwilling to be flexible about what we think, or we have reacted angrily to a mild insult. These experiences are at the core of the way a person with Paranoid PD experiences the world, and they carry these feelings, thoughts, and actions to such an extreme, and so consistently, across a wide variety of circumstances that their lives are full of threat, anger, and interpersonal problems.

### Table 2. DSM-IV Diagnostic Criteria for Paranoid Personality Disorder

A. A pervasive distrust and suspiciousness of others such that their motives are interpreted as malevolent, beginning by early adulthood and present in a variety of contexts, as indicated by four (or more) of the following:

(10) suspects, without sufficient basis, that others are exploiting, harming, or deceiving him or her

(11) is preoccupied with unjustified doubts about the loyalty or trustworthiness of friends or associates

(12) is reluctant to confide in others because of unwarranted fear that the information will be used maliciously against him or her

(13) reads hidden demeaning or threatening meanings into benign remarks or events

(14) persistently bears grudges, i.e., is unforgiving of insults, injuries, or slights

(15) perceives attacks on his or her character or reputation that are not apparent to others and is quick to react angrily or to counterattack

(16) has recurrent suspicions, without justification, regarding fidelity of spouse or sexual partner

B. Does not occur exclusively during the course of Schizophrenia, a Mood Disorder With Psychotic Features, another Psychotic Disorder and is not due to the direct physiological effects of a general medical condition.

Note: If criteria are met prior to the onset of Schizophrenia, add "Premorbid," e.g., "Paranoid Personality Disorder (Premorbid)."

According to the DSM-IV (see Table 2), "The essential feature of Paranoid Personality Disorder is a pattern of pervasive distrust and suspiciousness of others such that their motives are interpreted as malevolent. This pattern begins by early adulthood and is present in a variety of contexts" (p. 634). Paranoid PD is comprised of maladaptive variants of six personality traits: mistrust/suspicion, antagonism, autonomy, hypersensitivity, hypervigilance, and rigidity. It is differentiated from transitory suspicious states that we all may experience, as well as from systematized paranoid delusional states associated with certain Axis I disorders (e.g., schizophrenia, delusional disorder). Paranoid PD individuals experience transitory psychotic symptoms during periods of extreme stress. Paranoid PD is considered among the more severe PD in terms of the defensive style employed (e.g., projection, acting out) and the level of dysfunction (Millon & Davis, 1996; Shapiro, 1994; Vaillant, 1994). Paranoid PD is rarely diagnosed alone (Morey, 1988; Weissman, 1993; Widiger & Rogers, 1989; Widiger & Trull, 1998). The comorbidity with other Axis II disorders observed in these individuals may, in part, also explain the severity associated with this diagnosis (Weissman, 1993). A "pure" Paranoid PD case is rarely, if ever, seen (Millon & Davis, 1996). Thus, what is described herein is a prototype of the disorder. As this list of traits indicates, the term "paranoid" as applied to Paranoid PD is not just feelings or thoughts of persecution. The diagnosis describes individuals who lack trust, are hypersensitive to criticism, are prepared to act in a hostile manner to defend their sense of autonomy, incessantly seek out examples to confirm their maladaptive beliefs, are intensely preoccupied with suspicions about others' intent to harm or threaten them, and are rigid in their beliefs about others. In addition, Paranoid PD individuals tend to be tense and affectively inhibited.

## Interpersonal Style

The DSM-IV's General Diagnostic Criteria for a Personality Disorder indicate that interpersonal dysfunction is a defining characteristic of PDs. It is stated that the interpersonal dysfunction must be observed in a variety of personal and social situations. This is particularly true of Paranoid PD. Paranoid PD individuals suffer from problematic interpersonal relationships primarily due to their propensity for suspiciousness, mistrust of others, and hostile reactions to perceived threat. A vicious cycle occurs in the interpersonal lives of Paranoid PD individuals. Their lack of trust and expressed hostility tend to push people out of their lives. Expressions of hostility may provoke hostile reactions, which in turn only confirm the Paranoid PD individual's maladaptive belief that the world is generally threatening and hostile. They do not tend to check with others whether their beliefs are sensible.

Individuals with Paranoid PD are impaired in their ability to examine their own beliefs. Their rigid style of thinking often restricts their ability to take another perspective. They will often act on their suspicious ideas regarding others' intentions, reasoning that others are "out to get them." They

often look for examples of their suspicious ideas in the actions of others and are reluctant to interpret events differently. This interpersonal style typically leads to problems in initiating or maintaining romantic relationships and is associated with lack of trust and pathological jealousy, divorce, intolerance of indifference, difficulties keeping a job, and recurrent litigation for perceived injustices (Auchincloss & Weiss, 1994; DSM-IV, APA, 1994; Meissner, 1995; Millon, 1981; Sullivan, 1932/1965; Turkat, 1985). Paranoid PD individuals have an excessive need for autonomy and lack trust in others, which disrupts the formation of stable interpersonal relationships. The following is a vignette of a person with Paranoid PD.

George is a 30-year-old single man with a long history of problems with co-workers at the small high-tech company where he works. He keeps to himself at work, does not confide in others about his work or personal life, and is viewed by most as very difficult to get along with. It is not unusual for George to lash out verbally at others, accusing them of lying or trying to make him look bad. This has led to an extremely tense work environment. Co-workers frequently complain to work supervisors about George's hostility and uncooperativeness. George's immediate supervisor has tried to talk to him about these issues, but George maintains that the problem lies with his co-workers, not himself. Most recently, George has begun to accuse his supervisor of trying to make him look bad as well. George has threatened to sue his supervisor and the company because of "harassment." Although very little is known about George outside of the workplace, it does not appear that he has any long-standing friendships. Previous acquaintances have complained that George soon became hostile and accusatory, leading to the end of the relationship.

**Cognitive Style.** According to Shapiro (1965), the paranoid type is hyperalert and possesses a rigid attentional style to environmental stimuli. This cognitive style is representative of a cognitive mode that "is not merely occasionally or sporadically characteristic of paranoid people, but is continuous," (p. 59) and confirms a paranoid's anticipations. Magaro (1980, 1981) also discussed cognitive distortions displayed by paranoid individuals such as intolerance for ambiguous stimuli; rigid response styles; and distortions of perceptions, attention, and encoding. Although Magaro (1981) argues for a distinct paranoid cognitive style that differentiates the paranoid from the schizophrenic (as mentioned before, a focus of historical controversy), this work relied on the study of paranoid psychotics (i.e., delusional and/or hallucinating). Unfortunately, Magaro's (1981) information-processing perspective has not received empirical attention in relation to the cognitive style of those with Paranoid PD. It is unclear to what extent paranoid thought processes in the more severe paranoid disorders (i.e., the paranoid subtype of Schizophrenia and Delusional Disorder) can be generalized to the less severe but chronic form of paranoia in Paranoid PD. Munro (1982, 1992) has also argued for a distinct paranoid dimension as well, but Paranoid PD is not firmly established as part of this dimension within this perspective. The study of Paranoid PD from an information-processing perspective warrants further research.

Beck and Freeman (1990) offer the most extensive theory on the cognitive style of individuals with Paranoid PD. They postulate that the paranoid behaviors themselves are not at the center of the disorder. According to Beck and colleagues, beliefs and feelings of inadequacy and the inability to cope effectively in interpersonal situations are essential features of Paranoid PD. The resulting anxiety associated with these negative self-perceptions is reduced when one searches for an explanation external to oneself and blames others. From this perspective, the terms schemas and misattributions replace the theoretically cumbersome term "projection" (to be discussed later), often described in a variety of other theoretical perspectives. Paranoid individuals will search incessantly for reasons in their environment to confirm their maladaptive beliefs; this self-perpetuating cycle reinforces their maladaptive ideas even further. Any sign of criticism or mistreatment confirms their cognitions and feelings regarding the disloyalty and threatening stance of others (Beck et al., 1990). Unfortunately, there is little empirical data for a cognitive profile representative of Paranoid PD (Schmidt, Joiner, Young, & Telch, 1995).

The defense mechanism of projection must be discussed in any discussion of the cognitive nature of paranoia or Paranoid PD. The clinical utility of using projection as a diagnostic indicator of Paranoid PD has been demonstrated empirically (Drake & Vaillant, 1985). Defense mechanisms refer to innate involuntary regulatory processes that allow individuals to reduce cognitive dissonance and to minimize sudden changes in internal and external environments by altering the way these events are perceived. Defense mechanisms can alter our perception of any or all of the following: subject (self), object (other), idea, or feeling (Vaillant, 1994, p. 44).

The terms projection, introjection, and projective identification have long been widely accepted to describe the paranoid's intrapsychic processes, and the use of projection as a defense mechanism is a defining characteristic of Paranoid PD (Vaillant, 1994). The psychoanalytic writings on the defense mechanism of projection are vast and often complicated theoretically (Freud, 1911/1963; Klein, 1946/1986; Meissner, 1978). Summarizing these psychoanalytic viewpoints on projection is beyond the scope of this chapter. Briefly, the construct entails recognizing characteristics in another individual that are in conflict within the Paranoid PD individual's own self-esteem, but out of conscious awareness. This is experienced by Paranoid PD individuals as something wrong with the other, not with themselves. From the Paranoid PD individual's perspective, the other is faulty, threatening, or critical. The Paranoid PD individual often acts on this perception.

Projection in the clinical literature is often synonymous with paranoid conditions. This view of projection may be a limited interpretation of this defense mechanism (see Shapiro, 1994). More recent psychodynamic and interpersonal perspectives offer assistance in clarifying the description of projection (O'Leary & Watson, 1995; Shapiro, 1994). Briefly, similar to the description by Beck et al. (1990) and broader than more traditional views, the process of projection in Paranoid PD can be simply stated as the attribution of self-blame and anxiety associated with negative self-concepts (I feel shame) to external sources (I am being humiliated). The rigidity of Paranoid PD individuals' cognitive processes inclines them to perceive threat from external sources (as opposed to from within) and direct anger outward to alleviate internal anxieties. Projection or substitution of blame is central to understanding the cognitive style of Paranoid PD. Unfortunately, empirical investigation of defense mechanisms has only recently become systematic (Morey, 1993).

Note that social psychologists have systematically studied the constructs known as self-serving biases, attribution, and schemas as well as their moderation by motivation. The process of projection could easily be encompassed within this literature. These constructs may provide a more parsimonious theoretical foundation, as well as established empirical evidence for the cognitive processes involved in the individuals' tendencies to blame others for their problems (for a review of these classic social psychology constructs, see Fiske & Taylor, 1991). The applicability of these constructs to a clinical sample of Paranoid PD individuals may be fruitful in the empirical investigation of projection. In summary, although the clinical literature has consistently regarded projection as a hallmark of Paranoid PD and there is indication as to this construct's clinical utility, the empirical study of projection in Paranoid PD remains to be conducted systematically.

**Affective Style.** The DSM-IV does not include Paranoid PD criteria that refer specifically to affect or mood. However, the Associated Features section of the manual describes correlates of the disorder such as being cold to others or having restricted affect with little sense of humor. Paranoid PD individuals have also been described as tense and nervous (DSM-II-R; APA, 1987, p. 337). This criterion refers to the Paranoid PD individual's proclivity to appear to others as guarded, generally cold, emotionally reserved, and as noted before, uses the ability to blame others to defend against anxieties. Evidence presented by Trull (1992) found significant positive correlations between the NEO-Personality Inventory-Revised (NEO-PI-R; Costa & McCrae, 1992), the Neuroticism domain (regarded as an index for the proclivity to experience negative affect-depression/anxiety), and Paranoid PD symptom counts. Thus, despite appearing emotionally reserved to others generally, the Paranoid PD individual experiences anxiety and is prone to angry outbursts in response to perceived slights. This apparent contradiction between the external presentation of those with Paranoid PD and their internal emotional state has been a characteristic common to Paranoid PD within the clinical literature (Akhtar, 1990).

### Description of Schizoid PD

According to the Diagnostic and statistical manual of mental disorders, 4th ed. (DSM-IV; APA, 1994), Schizoid PD is characterized by a "pervasive pattern of detachment from social relationships and a restricted range of expression of emotions in interpersonal settings" (p. 638; see Table 3). Individuals with Schizoid PD do not seem to enjoy interpersonal contact and derive little or no pleasure from close personal relationships. They demonstrate little interest in sexual experiences with another person and rarely marry. Individuals with Schizoid PD tend to lack emotional attachments and do not seek out close friendships, except pos-

**Table 3. DSM-IV Diagnostic Criteria for Schizoid Personality Disorder**

A. A pervasive pattern of detachment from social relationships and a restricted range of expression of emotions in interpersonal settings, beginning by early adulthood and present in a variety of contexts, as indicated by four (or more) of the following:

(1) neither desires nor enjoys close relationships, including being part of a family
(2) almost always chooses solitary activities
(3) has little, of any, interest in having sexual experiences with another person
(4) takes pleasures in few, if any, activities
(5) lacks close friends or confidants other than first-degree relatives
(6) appears indifferent to the praise or criticism of others
(7) shows emotional coldness, detachment, or flattened affectivity

B. Does not occur exclusively during the course of Schizophrenia, a Mood Disorder with Psychotic Features, another Psychotic Disorder, or a Pervasive Developmental Disorder and is not due to the direct physiological effects of a general medical condition.

sibly with a first-degree relative. Persons with Schizoid PD typically prefer to spend time in solitary pastimes rather than engaging in social activities. Therefore, these individuals tend to perform better in those occupations that require minimum interpersonal contact.

Those interactions in which persons with Schizoid PD do engage do not seem to provide these individuals with much pleasure or satisfaction. They appear indifferent and unaffected by typically pleasurable or emotional experiences (e.g., "walking on a beach at sunset or having sex;" APA, 1994, p. 638). In fact, Schizoid PD individuals usually have a difficult time expressing emotion, especially anger, and may report never having experienced a strong emotional response. Their lack of subjective emotional experience and paucity of expression may cause individuals with Schizoid PD to appear cold and detached. They seem to be affected by neither criticism nor commendation, and they appear generally unaware of social nuances, such as body language and facial expressions. Due to their lack of social acuity, Schizoid PD individuals tend to be socially inept and are perceived by others as impassive and self-absorbed.

Finally, individuals with Schizoid PD may also experience brief psychotic episodes, especially under stress. In fact, according to DSM-IV, Schizoid PD may be present premorbidly in individuals with Delusional Disorder or Schizophrenia. Table 3 presents the DSM-IV criteria for Schizoid PD.

In summary, Schizoid PD is a pattern of emotional detachment and social isolation. Individuals with Schizoid PD do not appear to need, nor do they seem to desire close interpersonal relationships with other people, including sexual experiences. It is necessary to differentiate individuals with Schizoid PD from those who are considered "loners." Although behaviorally these individuals may appear quite similar, it is "only when these traits are inflexible and maladaptive and cause significant functional impairment or subjective distress do they constitute Schizoid Personality Disorder" (APA, 1994, p. 640). The following vignette is typical of Schizoid PD.

Sandy is a 28-year-old single woman who has always been viewed as a "loner." Even as a child and as a teenager, she had little interest in being around or interacting with others, including her own family members. Her school record was unremarkable, and she moved away from home as soon as she finished high school. Her parents have been concerned about her for some time. She rarely leaves her small apartment, does not have any hobbies or interests, and only occasionally works at "odd jobs." Her financial situation is bleak, and her parents pay her rent, so that she is not evicted. This all goes on without Sandy's knowledge; if left up to her, it is likely she would lose her apartment. Although the threat of loss of one's apartment would concern most people, Sandy does not seem to care one way or another. This is typical of her. She shows very little emotion regardless of the situation. Those who come into contact with her see her as "cold" and "detached."

## Epidemiology of Cluster A PDs

### Epidemiology of Schizotypal PD

According to DSM-IV, Schizotypal PD has a prevalence of approximately 3% of the general population (APA, 1994), but DSM cites no empirical support for that claim. Prevalence rates for Schizotypal PD in clinical samples range widely from 2 to 31%, and higher rates are found in inpatient samples (Widiger & Trull, 1998). The 3% prevalence for the general population presented by DSM-IV seems high, given that systematic studies of psychiatric patients and their relatives have found lower values (Loranger, 1990; Zimmerman & Coryell, 1990). Some evidence suggests a higher rate for Schizotypal PD in men than in women (Essen-Möller, et al., 1956), and the same may be true of schizophrenia (Iacono & Beiser, 1992).

### Epidemiology of Paranoid PD

Despite the general paucity of empirical research on Paranoid PD, estimates of the prevalence rates of Paranoid PD across a variety of settings have been offered. The prevalence rates of Paranoid PD in clinical samples, it has been noted, have increased since the revisions of DSM-III to DSM-III-R (Bernstein et al., 1993b; Morey, 1988). Prevalence estimates available from nonpsychiatric control subjects of the New York High-Risk Project range from 0–1.1% for DSM-III-R Paranoid PD (Erlenmyer-Kimling et al., 1995; Squires-Wheeler et al., 1993). An epidemiological study estimated the prevalence of Paranoid PD at 3.3% in young adults aged 18–21 (Bernstein, Cohen, Velez, Schwab-Stone, Siever, & Shinsato, 1993a). The DSM-IV (1994) reports Paranoid PD prevalence rates of 0.5–2.5% in the general population, 10–30% in psychiatric inpatient settings, and 2–10% in outpatient mental health clinics (p. 636). Unfortunately, there are no recent studies that provide prevalence rates of Paranoid PD according to the DSM-IV criteria set. It has been commonly believed that Paranoid PD is more prevalent in males, and empirical evidence has suggested this as well (Alnaes & Torgersen, 1988a; Reich, 1987).

### Comorbidity with Other Personality Disorders

Another challenging area of research that has implications for assessing Paranoid PD involves the high degree of overlap among the PDs defined by the DSM classification system. Zimmerman (1994) reviews the many studies that report the high rate of overlap among the PDs defined by the DSM categorical classification system. It is clear that the DSM system has improved the interrater reliability (i.e., the concurrence of assessment between two different raters) of the PDs, yet, the diagnostic scheme itself may have some problems of its own. As noted before, the emphasis on behavioral criteria in the DSM-III-R and DSM-IV (an effort that has increased the interrater reliability of the PD diagnoses by reducing the need for inferences when diagnosing these disorders) may cause artifactual overlap among the disorders. Simply put, the same *behaviors* may occur across PDs but for different reasons.

High comorbidity rates among PDs raise the issue of whether present diagnostic categories are clinically discrete or useful (Millon, 1981). Nearly all studies of inpatient samples indicate that those diagnosed with Paranoid PD receive additional PD diagnoses (Widiger & Rogers, 1989; Zimmerman, 1994). The defining characteristics (i.e., "odd and eccentric") of Cluster A PDs (DSM-IV; APA, 1994, p. 629) it has been shown, are poor predictors for inclusion into this cluster (Schopp & Trull, 1993). Morey (1988) refers to the boundary problem in PD diagnosis and reported that 22% of 291 outpatients who were receiving treatment for PDs met the criteria for a Paranoid PD diagnosis. Yet, those diagnosed with Paranoid PD frequently received additional diagnoses of Borderline PD (48%), Narcissistic PD (35.9%), and Avoidant PD (48.4%). Widiger and Trull (1998) in their review of DSM-III-R criteria set's performance across a variety of published and unpublished data sets report problematic co-occurrence (> 41%) among Paranoid PD, Borderline PD, and Avoidant PD. In addition, problematic co-occurrence (> 38%) among Schizoid PD, Schizotypal PD, Narcissistic PD, and Paranoid PD was found as well. Borderline PD, Narcissistic PD, and Avoidant PD are not included in the Cluster A grouping. This indicates that PD overlap is not restricted to cluster membership.

Parnoid PD is viewed as a syndrome of covarying traits that together define the boundaries of this disorder. It is becoming more accepted that Paranoid PD may be viewed as a dimensional construct that spans a continuum of severity and impairment (Auchincloss & Weiss, 1994; Sperry, 1995). Empirical and theoretical support for assessing Paranoid PD from a dimensional perspective is growing (Clark, Livesley, Schroeder, & Irish, 1996; Tien et al., 1992; Trull, 1992; Widiger, Trull, Clarkin, Sanderson, & Costa, 1994). It would serve both clinicians and researchers to assess the *degree* of significant maladaptive paranoid traits one possesses, as defined by the DSM-IV, as opposed to simply rating the presence or absence of symptoms associated with Paranoid PD, called for by the DSM-IV categorical diagnostic system. A dimensional approach that takes maladaptive variants of normal personality into account offers more diagnostic information than merely assessing the presence or absence of a PD and its behavioral expressions. An increase in diagnostic information may in turn facilitate the differentiation of PDs. The differentiation of Paranoid PD from other PDs in empirical research could also have the effect of (1) refining both the construct of Paranoid PD, as well as the criteria that assess Paranoid PD; and (2) increasing the reliability of conclusions based on empirical studies of Paranoid PD samples.

## Epidemiology of Schizoid PD

Few studies have assessed the prevalence of Schizoid PD, but it is one of the rarest PDs. Bernstein, Cohen, and Velez (1993) assessed PDs in a large, community-based sample of adolescents and diagnosed 1.8% with Schizoid PD. Of course, the diagnostic criteria have changed over the years, and the DSM-IV criteria might yield a different prevalence than observed when DSM-III-R was used. Schizoid PD is somewhat more common in men than in women (Kass, Spitzer, & Williams, 1983). Unfortunately, very few epidemiological studies of personality disorders have been undertaken.

## Dimensional Approaches

Psychiatry and the DSM take a medical approach to understanding personality psychopathology. Symptoms are assessed and counted, and individuals are classified either as "disordered" if they have sufficient symptoms for a particular PD, or as not disordered if they do not have sufficiently many symptoms. Unfortunately, nearly any symptom can be assessed on a continuum of severity, and the implicit threshold for determining the presence of the symptom is usually arbitrary and vaguely defined. For example, DSM-IV criteria often use phrases such as "has little, if any, interest" and "almost always…" which leave room for interpretation.

Personality psychologists have developed systems for measuring personality along sets of correlated dimensions. Many attempts have been made to use factor analytic techniques to reduce the system to a small number of interpretable dimensions, but no one approach has been satisfactory to all researchers. We will focus on one popular system called the five-factor model (FFM). Using a dimensional system, like the FFM, researchers and clinicians can understand personality pathology as an extreme deviation from normality along some dimension or along some combination of dimensions. In this approach, a set of scores replaces diagnosis as an approach to assessing personality. It should be very appealing to both clinicians and researchers to have an informative collection of numbers that rates a patient or subject instead of a simple yes/no diagnosis.

We distinguish from the preceding general approach to personality measurement by a second dimensional approach that does not attempt to measure every aspect of personality. This second approach, which we will call the *specific-traits approach*, focuses the measurement problem on a single trait dimension, usually one that has an important relationship to psychopathology. For example, one might develop a scale for measuring social anxiety. Perhaps most of the variance of such a scale can be accounted for by dimensions of the FFM (e.g., neuroticism and extroversion), but researchers and clinicians who want to assess social anxiety might prefer a more focused tool. The specific-traits approach has been used extensively in psychopathology research.

## Trait Dimensions and
## the Five-Factor Model

An alternative way to conceptualize and understand PDs is to examine the major personality traits that underlie each disorder. Currently, one of the more popular personality models is the five-factor model of personality (FFM) or Big Five. There are a number of measures of the FFM or Big Five available; most use a self-report format (Widiger & Trull, 1997). As operationalized by Costa and McCrae (1992) in the NEO-Personality Inventory-Revised (NEO-PI-R), the FFM consists of the personality domains of neuroticism (vs. emotional stability), extraversion (vs. introversion), openness to experience (vs. closed to experience), agreeableness (vs. antagonism), and con-

scientiousness (vs. carelessness). Further, each domain of personality consists of six personality trait facets. For example, Costa and McCrae (1992) propose that the facets of neuroticism are anxiety, depression, self-consciousness, vulnerability, impulsiveness, and angry hostility.

On the surface, the scores on FFM measures should demonstrate at least moderate correlations with PD pathology. After all, by definition, PDs are comprised of maladaptive personality traits and represent some of the more commonly encountered variants of personality pathology. In general, studies have demonstrated that the FFM is relevant to the official PD categories. This has held true regardless of the clinical status of the samples examined or the specific FFM instrument employed.

To provide personality trait information on the Paranoid, Schizoid, and Schizotypal PDs, we present FFM trait correlation predictions based on understanding the criteria for these three disorders, as well as some examples of studies that presented data relevant to these predictions.

In their five-factor "translation" of the PDs, Widiger, Trull, Clarkin, Sanderson, and Costa (1994) predicted that Paranoid PD would be characterized primarily by low levels of Agreeableness (low scores of facets of Trust, Straightforwardness, and Compliance), high scores on the Neuroticism facet of Hostility, and low scores on the facet Openness to Actions. Widiger et al. proposed that Schizoid PD is characterized primarily by low levels of Extraversion (low scores on Warmth, Gregariousness, Excitement Seeking, and Positive Emotions), low levels of the Neuroticism facets of Hostility and Self-Consciousness, and low levels of the facet Openness to Feelings. Finally, the authors predicted that Schizotypal PD is characterized primarily by high levels of Neuroticism (especially the facet of Self-Consciousness), high levels of Openness to Experience (especially the facets of Openness to Fantasy and Openness to Ideas), low scores on the Extraversion facets of Warmth and Gregariousness, and low scores on the Agreeableness facet of Trust.

In general, empirical studies have supported these predicted associations in both clinical (Soldz, Budman, Demby, & Merry, 1993; Trull, 1992) and nonclinical samples (Costa & McCrae, 1990; Wiggins & Pincus, 1989). For example, Paranoid PD scores were negatively related to Agreeableness scores (Costa & McCrae, 1990; Trull, 1992; Wiggins & Pincus, 1989) and positively related to Neuroticism scores (Costa & McCrae, 1990; Trull, 1992). Further, Schizoid PD scores were negatively related to Extraversion scores (Costa & McCrae, 1990; Soldz et al., 1993; Trull, 1992; Wiggins & Pincus, 1989), negatively related to Warmth and Gregariousness facet scores (Wiggins & Pincus, 1989), and negatively related to Openness scores (Trull, 1992; Wiggins & Pincus, 1989). Finally, Schizotypal PD scores were positively related to Neuroticism scores (Costa & McCrae, 1990; Soldz et al., 1993; Trull, 1992), positively related to Openness scores (Wiggins & Pincus, 1989), negatively related to Extraversion scores (Costa & McCrae, 1990; Soldz et al., 1993; Trull, 1992), and negatively related to Agreeableness scores (Costa & McCrae, 1990; Soldz et al., 1993; Trull, 1992).

One limitation of these early studies is that they all used questionnaire measures of the FFM, and in addition, few facet level relationships were reported. Recently, an interview-based measure of the FFM has been developed, the Structured Interview for the Five-Factor Model of Personality (SIFFM; Trull & Widiger, 1997). The SIFFM provides both domain and facet-level personality trait scores and contains items that tap more maladaptive variants of these personality traits (Trull et al., 1998). Similar to the findings of previous investigators who used questionnaire measures of the FFM, Trull & Widiger (1997) found that Paranoid PD scores correlated positively with Neuroticism scores and negatively with Agreeableness scores, that Schizoid PD scores correlated negatively with Extraversion scores, and that Schizotypal PD scores correlated positively with Neuroticism and Openness scores and negatively with Extraversion scores. Further, Trull & Widiger's (1997) results supported several of the facet-level predictions noted before. For example, Schizotypal PD scores were positively correlated with Self-Consciousness, Openness to Fantasy, and Openness to Ideas scores, and negatively correlated with Warmth and Trust scores. Finally, in a more recent study, Trull, Widiger, and Burr (in press) found that once comorbid personality disorder symptoms were controlled for, Paranoid PD was characterized primarily by low levels of Trust; Schizoid PD was characterized primarily by low Warmth, low Gregariousness, and low Positive Emotions; and Schizotypal PD was characterized by low levels of Openness to Feelings and Trust and high levels of Anxiety, Self-Consciousness, Openness to Fantasy, and Openness to Ideas. Thus, more fine-grained differentiation among these schizophrenia

spectrum personality disorders was possible by considering first-order/facet-level personality traits.

In summary, the FFM is a promising scheme for assessing and conceptualizing the PDs, including Paranoid, Schizoid, and Schizotypal PDs.

## Specific-Traits Approach

In the factor analytic approach of the FFM, a relatively small number of dimensions is used to describe all other personality traits and disorders. As an alternative to the actor analytic approach, one might prefer to design scales that focus on specific symptom dimensions. The advantage of this approach, which we are calling the *specific-traits approach*, is that highly refined measurements of the targeted trait dimension can be produced for use in research. The reliability and validity of scale scores can be determined, and individuals at the extremes of trait dimensions can be selected for study. Use of linear combinations of FFM factor scores would probably never produce measures of the desired traits that are as valid as those produced by scales designed specifically for that purpose.

Loren and Jean Chapman and their students at the University of Wisconsin developed several paper and pencil self-report scales for specific dimensions of schizotypal personality described by Meehl in his manual of schizotypic signs (Meehl, 1964). These scales (sometimes called the "Wisconsin scales") include the thirty-item Magical Ideation (MagId) Scale (Eckblad & Chapman, 1983), which measures beliefs in forms of causation that are conventionally regarded as invalid and magical; the thirty-five item Perceptual Aberration (PerAb) Scale (Chapman et al., 1978), which measures schizophrenic-like distortions in the perception of one's own body (twenty-eight items) and other perceptual distortions (seven items); the forty-item Social Anhedonia (SocAnh) Scale, first developed by Chapman et al. (1976) and revised by Eckblad et al. (1982), which measures schizoid indifference to other people; and the fifty-one item Impulsive Nonconformity (NonCon) Scale (Chapman et al., 1984), which measures impulsive antisocial behavior like that observed in some premorbid schizophrenics. All of the Wisconsin scales are highly reliable measures of individual differences and have internal consistency reliability coefficients of .80 to .90 (Chapman et al., 1982). College students identified by high scores on these scales are schizophrenic-like in many aspects of cognitive and social behavior

(Edell, 1993) and psychophysiology (Miller & Yee, 1993). Chapman, Chapman, Kwapil, Eckblad, and Zinser (1994) conducted 10-year follow-up interviews of a sample of several hundred college students selected for high scores on one or more of the scales or for moderately low scores on all of the scales (a control group). They found that former students selected for high scores on MagId or PerAb were significantly more likely than control participants to have experienced a psychotic episode during the follow-up period and to have heightened schizotypal and psychotic-like symptoms. In addition, participants in the MagId/PerAb group with elevated scores on SocAnh were at especially high risk for schizotypal symptomatology, and this was replicated by Kwapil et al. (1997). Furthermore, Kwapil (1998) has shown that high SocAnh scores are specifically related to schizophrenia-spectrum disorders and not to mood disorders.

The Chapman approach has been influential, and the Wisconsin scales have been used widely by psychopathology researchers. Much of the research has used individuals (usually college students) with high scores on the PerAb and/or MagId scales (usually placing them in the upper 3–5% on those scales). Few of these selected individuals meet criteria for PD diagnoses, but they often have multiple PD symptoms, psychotic-like symptoms, or mood disorders. The approach is popular partly because it is inexpensive to screen and select college students for research. The studies of selected college students are not studies of PDs per se, but they certainly tell us something about the nature of the schizophrenia-spectrum PDs.

# Etiological Theories of Cluster A Personality Disorders

### Etiological Theories of Schizotypal PD

Genetic influences are important in the etiology of Cluster A PDs. Adoption studies have shown that biological relatives of schizophrenic probands are at higher risk of Schizotypal PD than control subjects, even when they have had no contact with the schizophrenic relative (see Kety et al., 1994). This is a strong indication that Schizotypal PD and schizophrenia share some common genetic risk factors.

Less is known about environmental etiological factors. Mednick, Parnas, & Schulsinger (1987)

suggested that schizophrenia would emerge in high-risk individuals (e.g., children of mothers with schizophrenia) who were exposed to a "deleterious environment." They found that high-risk children who later developed schizophrenia had more often endured traumatic births than those who developed Schizotypical PD and that those who developed Schizotypal PD experienced even fewer birth complications than children of normal mothers who never developed a mental disorder. These findings suggest that schizotypal PD might be caused by a schizophrenia-prone genotype in an especially salutary environment.

### Etiological Theories of Paranoid PD

As with other pertinent nosological issues that surround Paranoid PD, etiological factors such as associated risk factors or developmental processes have been based on case studies, clinical consensus, and speculation. Many theorists from different perspectives (e.g., psychoanalytic, interpersonal, behavioral-cognitive) provide etiological conjectures of Paranoid PD. Yet, most do not explicate the connection between a risk factor and the development of maladaptive personality traits or provide empirical support for their assertions. There is a consensus in clinical literature as to what the antecedents of Paranoid PD should be. In the psychosocial realm, parental neglect or domination, abuse, isolation, exposure to violent adults, and infliction of pain have been cited as risk factors.

Limited empirical support has been found for a relationship between DSM-III-R Paranoid PD and retrospective self-reported ratings of a negative paternal relationship during childhood (e.g., criticism, rejection, lack of confiding, rarely feeling loved) as well as childhood traumatic experiences (e.g., physical/sexual abuse) (Modestin, Oberson, & Erni, 1998; Norden, Klein, Donaldson, Pepper, & Klein, 1995). There is evidence suggesting a relationship between parental aggressiveness and later development of aggression and hypervigilance (two core traits of Paranoid PD) in offspring (Lewis, 1992). Yet, these relationships were found for other PDs as well. Overall, these findings point to the nonspecificity of trauma and problems with parental bonding as possible antecedents of PD pathology in general. There is no empirical evidence suggesting that early home environmental factors are associated *specifically* with the development of Paranoid PD (Modestin et al., 1998; Norden et al., 1995). Furthermore, the studies that have been conducted on early home environments or abuse in childhood and the development of PDs are plagued by methodological issues (e.g., small sample sizes, use of retrospective report, differing treatment settings, lack of normal controls, not accounting for the effects of comorbidity between Axis-I and Axis-II disorders, or selection and response biases) and limit the conclusions that can be drawn (Crowell, Waters, Kring, & Riso, 1993; Ruegg & Frances, 1995). There are presently no prospective empirical studies that have examined familial factors in the development of Paranoid PD.

**Genetic Relationship to Schizophrenia.** Paranoid PD (along with Schizotypal and possibly Schizoid PD) is believed to be genetically related to schizophrenia and therefore is considered a schizophrenia-spectrum disorder. The hypothesis of a common genetic mechanism(s) underlying schizophrenia-spectrum disorders has been tested extensively. A major diagnostic question pervading this research is the relationship of Paranoid PD to schizophrenia disorders and to Axis I Delusional Disorder (Kendler et al., 1985b; Kendler & Gruenberg, 1982; Siever & Davis, 1991; Winokur, 1985, 1986). The schizophrenic-delusional disorder dichotomy has become increasingly controversial. Researchers have attempted to study the familial rates of Paranoid PD, Schizotypal PD, and Schizoid PD in those identified with a schizophrenic or delusional disorder (Baron et al., 1985; Coryell & Zimmerman, 1989; Dorfman, Shields, & DiLisi, 1993; Frangos, Athanassenas, Tsitourides, Katsanou, & Alexandrakou, 1985; Kendler & Gruenberg, 1982; Kendler et al., 1985a,b, 1993; Lowing, Mirsky, & Pereira, 1983; Parnas et al., 1993; Yeung, Lyons, Waternaux, Farone, & Tsuang, 1993) or alternatively and to a lesser degree, the familial rates of Paranoid PD, Schizotypal PD, and Schizoid PD in those identified with the same Cluster A disorders (Fulton & Winokur, 1993; Kendler et al., 1993; Siever et al., 1990; Thaker, Adami, Moran, Lahti, & Cassady, 1993). These studies have demonstrated an inconsistent, weak relationship of Paranoid PD to schizophrenia as well as a weak relationship to delusional disorder (for reviews of these studies see Nigg & Goldsmith, 1994; Ruegg & Frances, 1995; Webb & Levinson, 1993). Some empirical data have supported the contention that Paranoid PD may lie on a continuum of paranoia and Axis I delusional disorder (paranoid psychosis) in its most severe form (Kendler et al., 1985b; Winokur, 1985) and is distinct from schizophrenia (Kendler et al., 1985b).

Methodological issues in this literature limit the strength of inferences that can be drawn from the body of data gathered to date.

Paranoid PD has also been found at increased rates in families identified through a depressed proband (Alnaes & Torgersen, 1988b), and it may have an etiological relationship to anxiety disorders (Reich & Braginsky, 1994). The reported relationship of Paranoid PD to depressive or anxiety disorders presents evidence contrary to including Paranoid PD as strictly a schizophrenia-spectrum disorder. However, more research is needed to address these hypotheses before conclusions can be drawn.

Siever and Davis (1991) provide the most relevant description of an inherited psychobiological dimension as a risk factor in developing Cluster A disorders. From this perspective, it is hypothesized that attention/selection deficits in Cluster A disorders negatively impact cognitive/perceptual apparatus that results in misunderstandings, social isolation, mistrust, and poor reality testing. Siever and Davis assert that persistent mild disturbances in this dimension could contribute to the development of specific defense mechanisms and adaptive strategies. If these susceptibilities crystallize to define the pervasive characteristic ways in which an individual reacts to others or stress, then a Cluster A PD is possible. Although Siever and Davis bridge the gap between a risk factor and the development of a PD (and the available data suggest that there may be a substantial genetic component to the development of PD), the specific mode of inheritance or what is inherited remains unclear (Weissman, 1993). Furthermore, although the effects of punitive or abusive traumatic experiences are believed to interact with a genetic predisposition toward a paranoid style or core features of Paranoid PD (Siever & Davis, 1991), specific environmental or genetic influences that may moderate or mediate the development of Paranoid PD traits have not been identified (Nigg & Goldsmith, 1994).

## Etiology of Schizoid PD

Very little is known about the etiology of Schizoid PD. It has long been believed that Schizoid PD is genetically related to schizophrenia, but the empirical support for that hypothesis is very weak. For example, Kety et al. (1994) found a similar rate of Schizoid PD among the biological relatives of adoptees with chronic schizophrenia (5.7%) as among the biological relatives of control adoptees (8.1%).

Schizoid PD may be genetically related to autism. Wolff, Narayan, and Moyes (1988) selected twenty-one children with autism and twenty-one control children with other handicaps and compared the parents of the two types of children on schizoid symptomatology. They rated sixteen of thirty-five parents of autistic children (eight of fourteen fathers and eight of twenty-one mothers) as having schizoid traits compared with none of the thirty-nine parents of the control children. Wolff et al. suggested that this effect might be attributable to a genetic influence shared by parent and offspring that is sometimes expressed as schizoid traits and sometimes as autism. An adoption study would help to clarify if the effect is genetic or from other causes.

Millon (1981) noted that schizoid individuals often report that their parents were cold and unaffectionate toward them. This observation has not been confirmed in systematic research, but even if it were, it would not prove a cause–effect relationship between parental warmth and the development of schizoid personality traits. It is possible that parents of schizoid people are schizoid themselves (perhaps due to a genetic effect) and therefore are unaffectionate. Another possibility is that schizoid adults were aloof schizoid children who were so unresponsive to parental affection that their parents learned to be less affectionate. The causal picture is potentially very complex, but we have some suggestive leads.

# Treatment of Cluster A Personality Disorders

## Treatment of Schizotypal PD

Clinicians should consider patients individually and tailor treatments to match patients' symptom profiles. Patients with extensive thought disorder problems or with transient psychotic experiences might be more responsive to antipsychotic medication. Medication might enhance the patient's responsiveness to other forms of psychotherapy. Few controlled treatment studies of Schizotypal PD exist, but Hymnowitz et al. (1986) treated seventeen schizotypal outpatients with haloperidol in a single-blind trial and noted improvement on overall schizotypal symptoms, particularly on the scales that measure ideas of reference, odd com-

munication, and social isolation. Unfortunately, half of their patients dropped out of the study complaining of side effects, particularly sedation. The newer "novel" antipsychotic medications have superior side-effect profiles, are successful in treating schizophrenia, and might also be effective with schizotypal patients.

Cognitive therapy is another appealing approach for treating Schizotypal PD. Cognitive therapies for treating depression and anxiety disorders have empirical support for effectiveness, and similar therapies designed to treat Schizotypal PD might be effective, but we were not able to identify any empirical studies to support that claim. Odd beliefs and magical thinking are common symptoms of the disorder and seem well suited for a cognitive-behavioral approach. Beck et al. (1990) listed four types of cognitive distortions in Schizotypal PD: (1) suspicious or paranoid ideation, (2) ideas of reference, (3) odd beliefs and magical thinking, and (4) illusions. If therapists can develop enough of a relationship with schizotypal patients to gain their compliance with the treatment program, it might be possible to start dialogue about automatic thoughts and cognitive distortions. The difficulty of establishing a productive relationship should not be understated. Schizotypal individuals are often suspicious and socially awkward. They probably do not seek treatment often and may terminate treatment before it is complete.

Psychodynamic therapies generally lack empirical support, and this is certainly true of psychodynamic therapies for treating Schizotypal PD. Stone (1985) reviewed the literature on psychodynamic treatment in Schizotypal PD. Even if the psychodynamic approaches are not effective, reading the literature on such treatments can be helpful to clinicians who are trying to develop working relationships with schizotypal clients.

## Treatment of Paranoid PD

The pervasiveness of suspicion and lack of trust in others that is associated with Paranoid PD presents difficulty in assessment and treating it. The therapeutic environment itself, with its emphasis on trust and disclosure, may be overwhelming to the Paranoid PD client (Meissner, 1995; Millon & Davis, 1996; Stone, 1993). In general, very little is known about treating PDs (Shea, 1993). A small number of empirical studies is relevant to treating Paranoid PD, but what is known about this topic comes primarily from clinical observation. Parnas et al. (1993) noted that 51% of those with a DSM-III-R Cluster A disorder in their sample reported that they had never sought treatment. In a study of 339 Australian psychiatrists given a vignette of a DSM-III-R Paranoid PD case, two-thirds responded that they saw patients like this at a rate of two per year, 62% said that this treatment was beyond their expertise or untreatable, and only 11% thought the case would continue treatment. Almost all thought that supportive therapy that reduced suspicion and hostility was the method of treatment to use, and difficulty in establishing therapeutic relationships with these individuals, as well as noncompliance, were areas of concern (Quality Assurance Project, 1990).

Accurate and efficient assessment of Paranoid PD is essential in treatment. Without an initial understanding of the client's paranoid perception of the world, clinicians who approach Paranoid PD clients in a manner that may threaten their excessive need for autonomy and privacy may never see those clients again after the first session. Clinicians and researchers alike are faced with the often difficult task of attempting to differentiate between relatively transitory mistrustful beliefs, an overly valued belief, and delusions, as well as of ascertaining the level of impairment and dysfunction associated with a suspicious and antagonistic interpersonal style. For this reason, there is often difficulty in initially assessing Paranoid PD features in individuals who suffer from the disorder.

Paranoid PD clients' suspicious and antagonistic interpersonal style often challenges assessment and therapeutic skills. A clinician should not be too warm or friendly or question the validity of claims prematurely without becoming included in the Paranoid PD individual's suspicions. Furthermore, the client may not be capable of distinguishing presenting problems (such as stress, depression, and anxiety) from a paranoid perspective of the world. A lack of insight into the nature of their problems and difficulties with self-disclosure delay the gathering of pertinent information relevant to verifying a Paranoid PD diagnosis. Often, Paranoid PD individuals do not view their perspective of the world as related to their problems; rather, they view it as the way they need to be to survive. It would not be typical of a Paranoid PD client to present with complaints of paranoia. Turkat et al. (1990) report that, "clinically the Paranoid PD [client] may present with symptoms that initially appear unrelated to DSM-III-R criteria, which leads to misdiagnosis" (p. 264). An assessment of motivation for change and ability to tolerate the therapeutic process is indicated, given the Paranoid PD individual's rigidity and the problems cited before. Those who are coming to therapy to alleviate the symptoms (e.g., depression, anxiety) often associated with stress related to interpersonal problems are believed to be poor candidates for successful therapy, but those who are willing to confront their paranoid styles may fare better (Meissner, 1995). Furthermore, informants could be interviewed and prior psychological and medical history should be reviewed, given the Paranoid PD individual's tendency toward secretiveness, deception, or defensiveness. Ironically, Paranoid PD may be overdiagnosed by inexperienced clinicians who may underappreciate the severity of this disorder and view "normal" suspicious tendencies as meeting criteria for severe maladaptive paranoid traits (The Quality Assurance Project, 1990). Paranoid individuals will often drop out of therapy, will be resistant to self-disclosure, or will resist following treatment regimens (Turkat, 1985; Williams, 1988). Furthermore, they have been characterized as difficult patients who exhibit more dysfunctional behavior relative to other clinical populations and have poorer prognoses (Auchincloss & Weiss, 1994; Meissner, 1995; Millon, 1981). Interpersonalists may not share this negative prognostic view (O'Leary & Watson, 1995).

The psychodynamic and interpersonal literature offers may theoretical perspectives of both the etiology and treatment of paranoid states (e.g., Blum, 1980; Meissner, 1978; O'Leary & Watson, 1995). Only recently, there have been efforts by psychodynamically oriented clinicians to establish time-limited treatment approaches to PDs. It should be noted that these treatments of PDs focus on gaining insight into features of personality (e.g., introversion, misattributions of others' intent, anger control, excessive fear of social evaluation, interpersonal problems) that are relevant to Paranoid PD and thus offer techniques that are applicable (see Luborsky, 1984; Strupp & Binder, 1984). The cognitive-behavioral, interpersonal, and behavioral approaches offer more specific treatment guidelines (e.g., Beck & Freeman, 1990; Benjamin, 1993; Linehan, 1987; Turkat & Maisto, 1985; Turkat, 1990; Williams, 1988). Briefly, these prescriptions include increasing the Paranoid PD individual's sense of self-efficacy, reducing anxiety in response to perceived negative evaluation by others, increasing interpersonal skills (e.g., trust, communication, perspective-taking), and increasing more realistic attributions to the motives of others. It should be noted, however, that there are presently no treatment studies that assess the relative effectiveness of any of the cognitive-behavioral (or of the interpersonal and psychodynamic) interventions for Paranoid PD. It has also been suggested that during periods of extreme stress, anxiolitic medication may be indicated as is the use of antipsychotic medication (Coccaro, 1993; Manschreck, 1992; Quality Assurance Project, 1990), but Paranoid PD individuals may be resistant to taking medications, and the effects of this request on the therapeutic relationship could be negative (Meissner, 1995). The efficacy of medications in alleviating Paranoid PD symptoms is unknown.

### Treatment of Schizoid PD

As noted by Millon and Davis (1996, 2000), the prognosis is poor for those with Schizoid PD to make significant changes in their interpersonal styles. Individuals with Schizoid PD typically come to the attention of mental health professionals because of Axis I conditions (e.g., Major Depression). Once these Axis I symptoms have abated, the Schizoid PD patient may not have much motivation to stay in treatment. Further, and most importantly, those with Schizoid PD are unlikely to see their characteristic pattern of passive avoidance and indifference to others as problematic. Schizoid PD patients see little value in increasing social contact or in learning to identify emotional states in themselves and others. However, there may be situations in which the social isolation is so maladaptive or dysfunctional as to suggest to the therapist and hopefully to the Schizoid PD patient that treatment is warranted.

Several general strategies and techniques are recommended in these cases (Beck & Freeman, 1990; Millon & Davis, 2000). The two major overarching treatment goals are to increase social contact and improve social skills and to help the patient begin to identify and differentiate emotional states in self and others. Increased social contact and improved interpersonal skills may be accomplished through homework assignments, role-playing, and ultimately through group therapy (Beck & Freeman, 1990). Group therapy may

be especially useful for Schizoid PD because group members model appropriate self-disclosure, provide a "safe" interpersonal environment, and give feedback regarding interpersonal style. Beck and Freeman (1990) also recommend the use of Dysfunctional Thought Records (DTRs) with Schizoid PD patients. DTRs document patients' thoughts, emotional reactions, and behaviors in specified situations that are tailored to the individual patient. In the case of Schizoid PD, the DTR can be used to challenge maladaptive thoughts and reactions concerning social interactions and to help the patient identify and differentiate emotions and gradations of emotions in self and others (Beck & Freeman, 1990).

Despite their appeal, it is worth remembering that no well-controlled studies of the efficacy or effectiveness of these techniques in treating Schizoid PD exist. Further, the majority of Schizoid PD patients, by virtue of the nature of the disorder, are unlikely to be interested in treatment aimed at increasing social interaction or improving interpersonal skills. Therefore, the treating mental health professional should not expect quick and significant changes and should guard against feeling overly frustrated or discouraged (Millon & Davis, 2000).

## General Conclusion

Schizotypal, Paranoid, and Schizoid personality disorders are all marked by serious problems in interpersonal relationships. Because of this, such individuals have been hard to study. They avoid psychotherapy and participation in research. As a result, data on epidemiology, etiology, and treatment for these disorders are sparse. It is not even clear that these three disorders truly belong in the same personality disorder cluster. Future research focused on the causes of variation in the general population in the individual symptoms of these PDs might lead to greater understanding of their natures and causes.

## References

Akhtar, S. (1987). Schizoid personality disorder: A synthesis of developmental, dynamic, and descriptive features. *American Journal of Psychotherapy, 41*, 499–518.

Akhtar, S. (1990). Paranoid personality disorder: A synthesis of developmental, dynamic, and descriptive features. *American Journal of Psychotherapy, 44,* 5–25.

Alnaes, R., & Torgersen, S. (1988a). DSM-III symptom disorders (Axis I) and personality disorders (Axis II) in an outpatient population. *Acta Psychiatrica Scandinavica, 78,* 348–355.

Alnaes, R., & Torgersen, S. (1988b). The relationship between DSM-III symptom disorders (Axis I) and personality disorders (Axis II) in an outpatient population. *Acta Psychiatrica Scandinavica, 78,* 485–492.

American Psychiatric Association. (1952). *Diagnostic and statistical manual of mental disorders.* Washington, DC: Author.

American Psychiatric Association. (1968). *Diagnostic and statistical manual of mental disorders* (2nd ed.). Washington, DC: Author.

American Psychiatric Association. (1980). *Diagnostic and statistical manual of mental disorders* (3rd ed.). Washington, DC: Author.

American Psychiatric Association. (1987). *Diagnostic and statistical manual of mental disorders* (3rd ed., rev.). Washington, DC: Author.

American Psychiatric Association. (1994). *Diagnostic and statistical manual of mental disorders* (4th ed.). Washington, DC: Author.

Auchincloss, E. L., & Weiss, R. W. (1994). Paranoid character and the intolerance of indifference. In J. Oldham & S. Bone (Eds.), *Paranoia: New psychoanalytic perspectives* (pp. 27–48). Madison, CT: International Universities Press.

Baron, M., Gruen, R., Rainer, J. D., Kane, J., Asnis, L., & Lord, S. (1985). A family study of schizophrenic and normal control probands: Implications for the spectrum concept of schizophrenia. *American Journal of Psychiatry, 142,* 447–455.

Beck, A. T., Freeman, A. T., et al. (1990). *Cognitive therapy of personality disorders.* New York: Guilford.

Benjamin, L. S. (1993). *Interpersonal diagnosis and treatment of personality disorders.* New York: Guilford.

Bernstein, D. P., Cohen, P., Velez, C. N., Schwab-Stone, M., Siever, L., & Shinsato, L. (1993). Prevalence and stability of the DSM-III-R personality disorders in a community-based survey of adolescents. *American Journal of Psychiatry, 150,* 1237–1243.

Bernstein, D. P., Useda, D., & Siever, L. J. (1993b). Paranoid personality disorder: Review of the literature and recommendations for DSM-IV. *Journal of Personality Disorders, 7,* 53–62.

Bleuler, E. (1922). Die probleme der schizoidie und der syntonie. Zeitschrift fuer die gesamte. *Nurologie und Psychiatrie, 78,* 373–388.

Blum, H. P. (1980). Paranoia and beating fantasy: An inquiry into the psychoanalytic theory of paranoia. *Journal of the American Psychoanalytic Association, 28,* 331–361.

Brueel, O. (1936). On the psychopathogenesis of schizophrenia. *Acta Psychiatrica et Neurologica (Kjobenhavn), 11,* 575–584.

Cameron, N. (1943). The paranoid pseudo-community. *American Journal of Sociology, 49,* 32–38.

Cameron, N. (1963). *Personality development and psychopathology.* Boston: Houghton Mifflin.

Chapman, L. J., et al. (1984). Impulsive nonconformity as a trait contributing to the prediction of psychotic-like and schizotypal symptoms. *Journal of Nervous and Mental Disease, 172,* 681–691.

Chapman, L. J., Chapman, J. P., & Raulin, M. L. (1976). Scales for physical and social anhedonia. *Journal of Abnormal Psychology, 85,* 374–382.

Chapman, L. J., Chapman, J. P., & Raulin, M. L. (1978). Body image aberration in schizophrenia. *Journal of Abnormal Psychology, 87,* 399–407.

Chapman, L. J., Chapman, J. P., Kwapil, T. R., Eckblad, M., & Zinser, M. C. (1994). Putatively psychosis-prone subjects 10 years later. *Journal of Abnormal Psychology, 103,* 171–183.

Chapman, L. J., Chapman, J. P., & Miller, E. N. (1982). Reliabilities and intercorrelations of eight measures of proneness to psychosis. *Journal of Consulting & Clinical Psychology, 50,* 187–195.

Clark, L. A., Livesley, W. J., Schroeder, M. L., & Irish, S. L. (1996). Convergence of two systems for assessing specific traits of personality. *Journal of Personality Disorders, 8,* 294–303.

Coccaro, E. F. (1993). Psychopharmacological studies in patients with personality disorders: Review and perspective. *Journal of Personality Disorders,* Supplement 1, 181–192.

Coryell, W. H., & Zimmerman, M. (1989). Personality disorder in the families of depressed, schizophrenic, and never-ill probands. *American Journal of Psychiatry, 146,* 496–502.

Costa, P. T., Jr., & McCrae, R. R. (1990). Personality disorders and the five-factor model of personality. *Journal of Personality Disorders, 4,* 362–371.

Costa, P. T., & McCrae, R. (1992). *The NEO Personality Inventory-Revised: Manual.* Odessa, FL: Psychological Assessment Resources.

Crowell, J. A., Waters, E., Kring, A., & Riso, L. P. (1993). The psychosocial etiologies of personality disorders: What is the answer like? *Journal of Personality Disorders,* Supplement 1, 118–128.

Dorfman, A., Shields, G., & DeLisi, L. E. (1993). DSM-II-R personality disorders in parents of schizophrenic patients. *American Journal of Medical Genetics, 48,* 60–62.

Drake, R. E., & Vaillant, G. E. (1985). A validity study of Axis II of DSM-III. *American Journal of Psychiatry, 142,* 553–558.

Eckblad, M., & Chapman, L. J. (1983). Magical ideation as an indicator of schizotypy. *Journal of Consulting and Clinical Psychology, 51,* 215–225.

Eckblad, M. Chapman, L. J., Chapman, J. P., & Mishlove, M. (1982). [The Revised Social Anhedonia Scale]. Unpublished test (copies available from L. J. Chapman), University of Wisconsin, Madison, WI.

Edell, W. S. (1993). The psychometric measurement of schizotypy using the Wisconsin scales of psychosis proneness. In G. A. Miller (Ed.), *The behavioral high-risk paradigm in psychopathology.* New York: Springer Verlag.

Erlenmyer-Kimling, L., Squires-Wheeler, E., Adamo, U. H., Basset, A. S., Cornblatt, B. A., Kestenbaum, C. J., Rock, D., Roberts, S. A., & Gottesman, I. I. (1995). The New York High Risk Project: Psychoses and cluster A personality disorders in offspring of schizophrenic parents at 23 years follow-up. *Archives of General Psychiatry, 52,* 857–865.

Essen-Möller, E., Larson, H., Uddenberg, C. E., & White, G. (1956). Individual traits and morbidity in a Swedish rural population. *Acta Psychiatrica et Neurologica Scandinavica* (Supplement 100).

Fiske, S. T., & Taylor, S. E. (1991). *Social cognition* (2nd Edition). New York: McGraw-Hill.

Frangos, E., Athanassenas, G., Tsitourides, G., Katsanou, N., & Alexandrakou, P. (1985). Prevalence of DSM-III schizophrenia among the first-degree relatives of schizophrenic probands. *Acta Psychiatrica Scandinavica, 72,* 382–386.

Freud, S. (1911/1963). Psychoanalytic notes upon an autobiographical account of a case of paranoia. In P. Rieff (Ed.), *Three case histories.* New York: Collier Books.

Fulton, M., & Winokur, G. (1993). A comparative study of paranoid and schizoid personality disorders. *American Journal of Psychiatry, 150,* 1363–1367.

Gunderson, J. G. (1983). DSM-III diagnoses of personality disorders. In J. P. Forsch (Ed.), *Current perspectives on personality disorders.* Washington, DC: American Psychiatric Press.

Herbert, M. E., & Jacobson, S. (1967). Late paraphrenia. *British Journal of Psychiatry, 113,* 461–469.

Heston, L. L. (1970). The genetics of schizophrenia and schizoid disease. *Science, 167,* 249–256.

Hoch, A. (1910). Constitutional factors in the dementia praecox group. *Review of Neurology and Psychiatry, 8,* 463–475.

Hoch, P. H., Cattell, J. P., Strahl, M. O., & Pennes, H. H. (1962). The course and outcome of pseudoneurotic schizophrenia. *American Journal of Psychiatry, 119,* 106–115.

Hoch, P. H., & Cattell, J. P. (1959). The diagnosis of pseudoneurotic schizophrenia. *Psychiatric Quarterly, 33,* 17–43.

Hoch, P. H., & Polatin, P. (1949). Pseudoneurotic forms of schizophrenia. *Psychiatric Quarterly, 23,* 248–276.

Howard, R., & Levy, R. (1993). Personality structure in the paranoid psychoses of later life. *European Psychiatry, 8,* 59–66.

Hymnowitz, P., Frances, A., Jacobsberg, L. B., Sickles, M., & Hoyt, R. (1986). Neuroleptic treatment of schizotypal personality disorders. *Comprehensive Psychiatry, 27,* 267–271.

Iacono, W. G., & Beiser, M. (1992). Where are the women in first-episode studies of schizophrenia? *Schizophrenia Bulletin, 18,* 471–480.

Kallmann, F. J. (1938). *The genetics of schizophrenia.* New York: J.J. Augustin.

Kass, F., Spitzer, R. L., & Williams, J. B. (1983). An empirical study of the issue of sex bias in the diagnostic criteria of DSM-III axis II personality disorders. *American Psychologist, 38,* 799–803.

Kendler, K. S. (1988). Familial aggregation of schizophrenia spectrum disorders: Evaluation of conflicting results. *Archives of General Psychiatry, 45,* 377–383.

Kendler, K. S. (1985). Diagnostic approaches to schizotypal personality disorder: A historical perspective. *Schizophrenia Bulletin, 11,* 538–553.

Kendler, K. S., & Gruenberg, A. M. (1982). Genetic relationship between paranoid personality disorder and the "schizophrenic spectrum" disorders. *American Journal of Psychiatry, 139,* 1185–1186.

Kendler, K. S., Gruenberg, A. M., & Tsuang, M. T. (1985a). Psychiatric illness in first-degree relatives of schizophrenic and surgical control patients: A family study using DSM-III criteria. *Archives of General Psychiatry, 42,* 770–779.

Kendler, K. S., Heath, A., & Martin, N. G. (1987). A genetic epidemiological study of self-report suspiciousness. *Comprehensive Psychiatry, 28,* 187–195.

Kendler, K. S., Masterson, C. C., & Davis, K. (1985b). Psychiatric illness in first-degree relatives of patients with paranoid psychosis, schizophrenia and medical illness. *British Journal of Psychiatry, 147,* 524–531.

Kendler, K. S., McGuire, M., Gruenberg, A. M., O'Hare, A., Spellman, M., & Walsh, D. (1993). The Roscommon Family Study III: Schizophrenia-related personality disorders in relatives. *Archives General Psychiatry, 50,* 781–788.

Kendler, K. S., Neal, M. C., & Walsh, D. (1995). Evaluating the spectrum concept of schizophrenia in the Roscommon Family Study. *American Journal of Psychiatry, 152* 749–754.

Kety, S. S., Rosenthal, D., Wender, P. H., & Schulsinger, F. (1968). The types and prevalence of mental illness in the biological and adoptive families of adopted schizophrenics. In D. Rosenthal & S. S. Kety (Eds.), *The transmission of schizophrenia* (pp. 345–362). Oxford: Pergamon Press.

Kety, S. S., Wender, P. H., et al. (1994). Mental illness in the biological and adoptive relatives of schizophrenic adoptees. Replication of the Copenhagen Study in the rest of Denmark. *Archives of General Psychiatry, 51,* 442–455.

Klein, M. (1946/1986). Notes on some schizoid mechanisms. In Juliet Mitchell (Ed.), *The selected Melanie Klein.* New York: The Free Press.

Kraepelin, E. (1921). *Manic-depressive insanity and paranoia.* Edinburgh, Scotland: Livingstone.

Kretschmer, E. (1925). *Physique and character.* London: Kegan Paul.

Kwapil, T. R., Miller, M. B., Zinser, M. C., Chapman, J., & Chapman, L. J. (1997). Magical ideation and social anhedonia as predictors of psychosis proneness: A partial replication. *Journal of Abnormal Psychology, 106,* 491–495.

Kwapil, T. R. (1998). Social anhedonia as a predictor of the development of schizophrenia-spectrum disorders. *Journal of Abnormal Psychology, 107,* 558–565.

Lewis, A. (1970). Paranoia and paranoid: A historical perspective. *Psychological Medicine, 1,* 2–12.

Lewis, D. O. (1992). From abuse to violence: Psychophysiological consequences of maltreatment. *Journal of the American Academy of Child and Adolescent Psychiatry, 31,* 383–391.

Lineham, M. M. (1987). Dialectical behavior therapy for borderline personality disorder. *Bulletin of the Menninger Clinic, 51,* 261–276.

Loranger, A. (1990). The impact of DSM-III on diagnostic practice in a university hospital: A comparison of DSM-II and DSM-III in 10,914 patients. *Archives of General Psychiatry, 47,* 672–675.

Lowing, P., Mirsky, A. F., & Pereira, R. (1983). The inheritance of schizophrenia spectrum disorders: A reanalysis of the Danish Adoption Study. *American Journal of Psychiatry, 140,* 1167–1171.

Luborsky, L. (1984). *Principles of psychoanalytic psychotherapy—a manual for supportive-expressive treatment.* New York: Basic Books.

Magaro, P. A. (1980). *Cognition in schizophrenia and paranoia: Integration of cognitive processes.* Hillsdale, NJ: Erlbaum.

Magaro, P. A. (1981). The paranoid and the schizophrenic: The case for distinct cognitive style. *Schizophrenia Bulletin, 7,* 632–660.

Maier, W., Lichterman, D., Minges, J., & Heun, R. (1994). Personality disorders among the relatives of schizophrenic patients. *Schizophrenia Bulletin, 20,* 481–493.

Manschreck, T. C. (1979). The assessment of paranoid features. *Comprehensive Psychiatry, 20,* 370–377.

Manschreck, T. C. (1992). Delusional disorders: Clinical concepts and diagnostic strategies. *Psychiatric Annals, 22,* 241–251.

Manschreck, T. C., & Petri, M. (1978). The paranoid syndrome. *Lancet, 2,* 251–259.

Mednick, S. A., Parnas, J., & Schulsinger, F. (1987). The Copenhagen high-risk project, 1962–86. *Schizophrenia Bulletin, 13*(3), 485–495.

Meehl, P. E. (1962). Schizotaxia, schizotypy, schizophrenia. *American Psychologist, 17,* 827–838.

Meehl, P. E. (1964). *Manual for use with the checklist of schizotypic signs.* Unpublished manuscript, University of Minnesota, Minneapolis, MN, copies available from author.

Meehl, P. E. (1990). Toward an integrated theory of schizophrenia. *Journal of Personality Disorders, 4,* 1–99.

Meissner, W. W. (1978). *The paranoid process.* New York: Jason Aronson.

Meissner, W. W. (1995). Paranoid personality disorder. In G. O. Gabbard (Ed.), *Treatments of psychiatric disorders* (Vol. 2, 2nd ed., pp. 2250–2259). Washington, DC: APA Press.

Miller, G. A., & Yee, C. M. (1993). Risk for severe psychopathology: Psychometric screening and psychophysiological assessment. In P. K. Ackles, J. R. Jennings, & M. G. H. Coles (Eds.), *Advances in psychophysiology,* Vol. 5. London: Jessica Kingsley.

psychophysiology, Vol. 5. London: Jessica Kingsley.

Millon, T. (1969). *Modern psychopathology: A biosocial approach to maladaptive learning and functioning.* Philadelphia: W.B. Saunders.

Millon, T. (1981). *Disorders of personality: DSM-III Axis II.* New York: Wiley.

Millon, T. (1983). *Millon clinical multiaxial inventory* [Professional Manual]. Minneapolis: Interpretive Scoring Systems.

Millon, T. (1987). *Millon clinical multiaxial inventory MCMI-II* (2nd ed.) [Professional Manual]. Minneapolis, MN: National Computer Systems.

Millon, T., & Davis, R. (1996). *Disorders of personality: DSM-IV and beyond.* New York: Wiley.

Millon, T., & Davis, R. D. (2000). *Personality disorders in modern life.* New York: Wiley.

Modestin, J., Oberson, B., & Erni, T. (1998). Possible antecedents of DSM-III-R personality disorders. *Acta Psychiatrica Scandinavica, 97,* 260–266.

Morey, L. C. (1988). Personality disorders in DSM-III and DSM-III-R: Convergence, coverage, and internal consistency. *American Journal of Psychiatry, 145,* 573–577.

Morey, L. C. (1993). Psychological correlates of personality disorders. *Journal of Personality Disorders,* Supplement 1, 149–166.

Munro, A. (1982). Paranoia revisited. *British Journal of Psychiatry, 141,* 344–349.

Munro, A. (1992). Psychiatric disorders characterized by delusions: Treatment in relation to specific types. *Psychiatric Annals, 22,* 232–240.

Nigg, J. T., & Goldsmith, H. H. (1994). Genetics of personality disorders: Perspectives from personality and psychopathology research. *Psychological Bulletin, 115,* 346–380.

Norden, K. A., Klein, D. N., Donaldson, S. K., Pepper, C. M., & Klein, L. M. (1995). Reports of the early home environment in DSM-III-R personality disorders. *Journal of Personality Disorders, 9,* 213–223.

O'Leary, J., & Watson, R. I. (1995). Paranoia. In M. Lionells, J. Fiscalini, C. H. Mann, & D. B. Stern (Eds.), *Handbook of interpersonal psychoanalysis* (pp. 397–417). Hillsdale, NJ: Analytic Press.

Parnas, J., Cannon, T. D., Jacobsen, B., Schulsinger, H., Schulsinger, F., & Mednick, S. A. (1993). Lifetime DSM-III-R diagnostic outcomes in the offspring of schizophrenic mothers: Results from the Copenhagen High Risk Study. *Archives of General Psychiatry, 50,* 707–714.

The Quality Assurance Project. (1990). Treatment outlines for paranoid, schizotypal, and schizoid personality disorders. *Australian & New Zealand Journal of Psychiatry, 24,* 339–350.

Rado, S. (1953). Dynamics and classification of disordered behavior. *American Journal of Psychiatry, 110,* 406–416.

Ray, I. (1863/1968). *Mental hygiene.* New York: Hafner.

Reich, J. (1987). Sex distribution of DSM-III personality disorders in psychiatric outpatients. *American Journal of Psychiatry, 144,* 485–488.

Reich, J., & Braginsky, Y. (1994). Paranoid personality traits in a panic disorder population. *Comprehensive Psychiatry, 35,* 260–264.

Ribot, T. (1890). *Psychologie des sentiments.* Paris: Delahaye and Lecrosnier.

Ruegg, R., & Frances, A. (1995). New research in personality disorders. *Journal of Personality Disorders, 9,* 1–48.

Schmidt, N. B., Joiner, T. E., Young, J. E., & Telch, M. (1995). The Schema Questionnaire: Investigation of psychometric properties and the hierarchical structure of a measure of maladaptive schemas. *Cognitive Therapy and Research, 19,* 295–321.

Schopp, L., & Trull, T. J. (1993). Validity of the DSM-III-R personality disorder clusters. *Journal of Psychopathology and Behavioral Assessment, 15,* 219–237.

Shapiro, D. (1965). *Neurotic styles.* New York: Basic Books.

Shapiro, D. (1994). Paranoia from a characterological standpoint. In J. Oldham & S. Bone (Eds.), *Paranoia: New psychoanalytic perspectives* (pp. 49–57). Madison, CT: International Universities Press.

Shea, M. T. (1993). Psychosocial treatment of personality disorders. *Journal of Personality Disorders,* Supplement 1, 167–180.

Sheldon, W. H. (1940). *The varieties of human physique: An introduction to constitutional psychology.* New York: Harper.

Sheldon, W. H., & Stevens, S. S. (1942). *The varieties of temperament: A psychology of individual differences.* New York: Harper.

Siever, L. J., & Davis, K. (1991). A psychobiologic perspective on the personality disorders. *American Journal of Psychiatry, 148,* 1647–1658.

Siever, L. J., Silverman, J. M., Horvath, T. B., Klar, H., Coccaro, E., Keefe, R. S., Pinkham, L., Rinaldi, P., Mohs, R. C., & Davis, K. L. (1990). Increased morbid risk for schizophrenia related disorders in relatives of schizotypal personality disordered patients. *Archives General Psychiatry, 47,* 634–640.

Soldz, S., Budman, S., Demby, A., & Merry, J. (1993). Representation of personality disorders in circumplex and five-factor space: Explorations with a clinical sample. *Psychological Assessment, 5,* 41–52.

Sperry, L. (1995). *Handbook of diagnosis and treatment of the DSM-IV personality disorders.* New York: Brunner/Mazel.

Spitzer, R. L., Endicott, J., & Gibbon, M. (1979). Crossing the border into borderline personality and borderline schizophrenia: The development of criteria. *Archives of General Psychiatry, 36,* 17–24.

Spitzer, R. L., Endicott, J., & Robins, E. (1978). Research diagnostic criteria: Rationale and reliability. *Archives of General Psychiatry, 35,* 773–782.

Squires-Wheeler, E., Skodol, A. E., Adamo, U. H., Basset, A. S., Gewirtz, G. R., Honer, W. G., Cornblatt, B. A., Roberts, S. A., & Erlenmyer-Kimling, L. (1993). Personality features and disorder in the subjects in the New York High-Risk Project. *Journal of Psychiatric Research, 27,* 379–393.

Stone, M. H. (1993). Long-term outcome in personality disorders. *British Journal of Psychiatry, 162,* 299–313.

Stone, M. (1985). Schizotypal personality: Psychotherapeutic aspects. *Schizophrenia Bulletin, 11,* 576–589.

Strupp, H., & Binder, J. L. (1984). *Psychotyperapy in a new key: A guide to time-limited dynamic psychotherapy.* New York: Basic Books.

Sullivan, H. S. (1932/1965). *Presonal psychopathology.* New York: W.W. Norton.

Tanna, V. L. (1974). Paranoid states: A selected review. *Comprehensive Psychiatry, 15,* 453–470.

Thaker, G., Adami, H., Moran, M., Lahti, A., & Cassady, S. (1993). Psychiatric illnesses in families of subjects with schizophrenia-spectrum personality disorders: High morbidity risks for unspecified functional psychoses and schizophrenia. *American Journal of Psychiatry, 150,* 66–71.

Tien, A. Y., Costa, P. T., & Eaton, W. W. (1992). Covariance of personality, neurocognition, and schizophrenia spectrum traits in the community. *Schizophrenia Research, 7,* 149–158.

Torgersen, S. (1995). Commentary on paranoid, schizoid, and schizotypal personality disorders. In W. J. Livesley (Ed.), *The DSM-IV personality disorders* (pp. 91–102). New York: Guilford.

Trull, T. J. (1992). DSM-II-R personality disorders and the five factor model of personality: An empirical comparison. *Journal of Abnormal Psychology, 101,* 553–560.

Trull, T. J., & Widiger, T. A. (1997). *Structured Interview for the Five-Factor Model of Personality (SIFFM): Professional manual.* Odessa, FL: Psychological Assessment Resources.

Trull, T. J., Widiger, T. A., & Burr, R. (in press). A structured interview for the assessment of the five-factor model of personality: Facet-level relations to the Axis II personality disorders. *Journal of Personality.*

Trull, T. J., Widiger, T. A., Useda, J. D., Holcomb, J., Doan, B., Axelrod, S. R., Stern, B. L., & Gershuny, B. S. (1998): A structured interview for the assessment of the five-factor model of personality. *Psychological Assessment, 10,* 229–240.

Tsuang, M. T., Bucher, K. D., & Flemin, J. (1983). A search for 'schizophrenia spectrum disorders': An application of a multiple threshold model to blind family study data. *British Journal of Psychiatry, 143,* 572–577.

Turkat, I. D. (1985). Paranoid personality disorder. In I. D. Turkat (Ed.), *Behavioral case formulation* (pp. 155–198). New York: Plenum.

Turkat, I. D. (1990). *The personality disorders: A psychological approach to clinical management.* New York: Pergamon Press.

Turkat, I. D., & Banks, D. (1987). Paranoid and its disorder. *Journal of Psychopathology and Behavioral Assessment, 9,* 295–304.

Turkat, I. D., Keane, S. P., & Thompson-Pope, S. K. (1990). Social processing errors among paranoid personalities. *Journal of Psychopathology and Behavioral Assessment, 12,* 263–269.

Turkat, I. D., & Maisto, S. A. (1985). Application of the experimental method to the formation and modification of personality disorders. In D. H. Barlow (Ed.), *Clinical hand-* book of psychological disorders: A step-by-step treatment manual (pp. 502–570). New York: Guilford.

Vaillant, G. E. (1994). Ego mechanisms of defense and personality psychopathology. *Journal of Abnormal Psychology, 103,* 44–50.

Webb, C. T., & Levinson, D. F. (1993). Schizotypal and paranoid personality disorder in the relatives of patients with schizophrenia and affective disorders: A review. *Schizophrenia Research, 11,* 81–92.

Weissman, M. M. (1993). The epidemiology of personality disorders: A 1990 update. *Journal of Personality Disorders,* Supplement 1, 44–62.

Widiger, T. A., & Rogers, J. H. (1989). Prevalence and comorbidity of personality disorders. *Psychiatric Annals, 19,* 132–136.

Widiger, T. A., & Trull, T. J. (1990). Assessment of the five-factor model of personality. *Journal of Personality Assessment, 68,* 228–250.

Widiger, T. A., & Trull, T. J. (1997). Assessment of the five-factor model of personality. *Journal of Personality Assessment, 68,* 228–250.

Widiger, T. A., & Trull, T. J. (1998). Performance characteristics of the DSM-III-R personality disorder criteria sets. In T. Widiger, A. Frances, H. Pincus, R. Ross, M. First, W. Davis, & M. Kline (Eds.), *DSM-IV sourcebook,* Vol. 4 (pp. 357–373). Washington, DC: American Psychological Association.

Widiger, T. A., Trull, T. J., Clarkin, J. F., Sanderson, C., & Costa, P. T., Jr. (1994). A description of the DSM-III-R and DSM-IV personality disorders with the five factor model of personality. In P. T. Costa, Jr. & T. A. Widiger (Eds.), *Personality disorders and the five factor model of personality* (pp. 41–56). Washington, DC: American Psychological Association.

Wiggins, J. S., & Pincus, A. L. (1989). Conceptions of personality disorders and dimensions of personality. *Psychological Assessment, 1,* 305–316.

Williams, J. G. (1988). Cognitive intervention for a paranoid personality disorder. *Psychotherapy, 25,* 570–575.

Winokur, G. (1985). Familial psychopathology in delusional disorder. *Comprehensive Psychiatry, 26,* 241–248.

Winokur, G. (1986). Classification of chronic psychoses including delusional disorders and schizophrenias. *Psychopathology, 19,* 30–34.

Wolff, S., Narayan, S., & Moyes, B. (1988). Personality characteristics of parents of autistic children: A controlled study. *Journal of Child Psychology & Psychiatry & Allied Disciplines, 29,* 143–153.

World Health Organization (1992). *Tenth Revision of the International Classification of Diseases (ICD-10).* Geneva: WHO.

Yeung, A. S., Lyons, M. J., Waternaux, C. M., Farone, S. V., & Tsuang, M. T. (1993). A family study of self-reported personality traits and DSM-III-R personality disorders. *Psychiatry Research, 48,* 243–255.

Zilboorg, G. (1941). Ambulatory schizophrenia. *Psychiatry, 4,* 149–155.

Zimmerman, M. (1994). Diagnosing personality disorders: A review of issues and research methods. *Archives of General Psychiatry, 51,* 225–245.

Zimmerman, M., & Coryell, W. (1990). Diagnosing personality disorders in the community: A comparison of self-report and interview measures. *Archives of General Psychiatry, 47,* 526–531.

# CHAPTER 20

# Substance Abuse: An Overview

Susan F. Tapert, Susan R. Tate,
and Sandra A. Brown

## Introduction

Substance abuse and other addictive behavior disorders are among the most prevalent mental health disorders in our society. Significant health and societal costs are attributed to excessive involvement with alcohol, nicotine, illicit drugs, prescription drugs, industrial solvents, and impulse control problems (e.g., gambling, binge eating, risky sexual behaviors). This chapter will discuss conceptual models, assessment, and treatment of substance abuse, covering alcohol, illicit drugs, misused prescription drugs, and nicotine problems. Gambling disorders will be briefly reviewed. Although eating disorders and compulsive sexual disorders share features of addictive behaviors, these issues will be addressed in other chapters of this volume.

### Prevalence

Current substance abuse or dependence is present in 11% of the U.S. population, and nearly 27% percent have met criteria during their lifetime, based on the results of a national survey (Kessler et al., 1994). Alcohol is the most widely used intoxicating substance. National household surveys report that 82% of Americans ages 12 and above have used alcohol and half drank alcohol in the past month (Substance Abuse and Mental Health Services Administration [SAMHSA], 1998), as shown in Table 1. Binge drinking, consuming five or more drinks on a single occasion, is most common among young adults ages 18 to 25, although evident among adolescents (Johnston, O'Malley, & Bachman, 1999). Frequent bingeing (5 times in the past month) indicates unhealthy drinking and was reported by 11% of young adults. Over 13% of the population has met diagnostic criteria for alcohol dependence at some point in their lifetimes, and more than 4% currently meet criteria (Grant, 1997). Alcohol-related economic losses due to decreased productivity, health care costs, and motor vehicle crashes are estimated at $148 billion annually (Harwood, Fountain, Livermore, & The Lewin Group, 1998). Alcohol is the third most prominent contributor to mortality in the United States (McGinnis & Foege, 1993).

Illicit drug use has increased in recent decades, and prevalence rates of individual substances fluctuate over time. Nearly 36% of the population over age 12, it is estimated, has used an illicit drug in their lifetimes (see Table 1). Marijuana is the most commonly used illicit drug, used by an estimated 9% of the population during 1997. Almost 12% of males aged 18 to 25 years have used marijuana more than fifty times in the past year. In 1997, 1.9% of the U.S. adult population used cocaine, 1.9% used hallucinogens, 1.1% used inhalants (the rate is 4.4% for 12–17-year-olds), 0.3% used heroin, and 2.8% reported nonmedical use of prescription

Susan F. Tapert, Susan R. Tate, and Sandra A. Brown • University of California, San Diego and VA San Diego Healthcare System, San Diego, California 92161-0002.

*Comprehensive Handbook of Psychopathology* (Third Edition), edited by Patricia B. Sutker and Henry E. Adams. Kluwer Academic / Plenum Publishers, New York, 2001.

**Table 1. Percent of U.S. Adolescents, Young Adults, and Adults
who Used Alcohol, Binge Drank, Used Illicit Drugs,
and Used Nicotine in the Past Month[a]**

| Age group | Any alcohol use | Binge drinking[b] | Illicit drug use | Nicotine use |
|---|---|---|---|---|
| 12–17 | 21% | 8% | 11% | 20% |
| 18–25 | 58% | 28% | 15% | 41% |
| 26–34 | 60% | 23% | 7% | 34% |
| 35 and older | 53% | 12% | 4% | 28% |

[a]SAMHSA, 1998.
[b]Indicates consumption of five or more drinks on a single occasion.

medications (SAMHSA, 1998). Nearly 8% of the national population, it is estimated, met criteria for drug dependence at some point in their lifetimes, and almost 3% met criteria in the past year (Kessler et al., 1994). Illicit drugs present particular medical risks because the content of any drug obtained on the street is difficult to specify. Drug injectors are at risk for HIV, hepatitis, infections, vein deterioration, and endocarditis (Peterson, Dimeff, Tapert, & Stern, 1998). Drug use alone costs the United States an estimated $89 billion annually due to loss in productivity, crime, medical consequences, and treatment services (Harwood et al., 1998).

Nicotine is the most abused addictive substance in our society. More than 70% of the U.S. population over age 12 has smoked at some point, and 30% currently smoke (see Table 1). Approximately three million people start smoking each year at the average age of 15.6 years. Current smokers are more likely to drink heavily and use illicit drugs than nonsmokers (SAMHSA, 1998). Although not considered an intoxicant, nicotine is associated with significant health problems across the lifespan (e.g., Myers & Brown, 1997), and tobacco is the leading preventable cause of mortality in the United States (McGinnis & Foege, 1993).

Gambling is an increasing problem in the United States. The expanding presence of casinos on U.S. Indian reservations and Internet gambling provide easily accessible means of risking monetary loss for a chance at quick winnings. Pathological gambling refers to a diagnosable disorder (American Psychiatric Association [APA], 1994) involving recurrent gambling, preoccupation, gambling with increasing amounts of money, loss of control, unsuccessful attempts to cut back, and jeopardizing

jobs and relationships. A recent epidemiological survey reported that 46% of the population has gambled recreationally, 9% reported at least one gambling-related problem, and 1% met criteria for pathological gambling. Problem gamblers are commonly tobacco- and alcohol-dependent (Cunningham-Williams, Cottler, Compton, & Spitznagel, 1998).

**Definitions.** Before we discuss theories of substance abuse, we will define key terms in this field of study. *Addictive behaviors* refer to "any compulsive habit pattern in which the individual seeks a state of immediate gratification" (Marlatt, 1985, p. 4). The gratification may be in the form of relief from discomforts such as tension, negative mood, or withdrawal states, or it may be the introduction of pleasure or euphoria. Addiction involves continued involvement with the behavior despite adverse consequences and attempts to stop (Roberts & Koob, 1997). Addictive behaviors include excessive use of psychoactive substances, such as alcohol, nicotine, and other drugs, or excessive, unhealthy levels of other behaviors with compulsive characteristics, such as gambling, eating, or sexual acts.

Substance dependence and substance abuse are clinical disorder diagnoses of the *Diagnostic and Statistical Manual of Mental Disorders*, 4th ed. (DSM-IV; APA, 1994) that require fulfilling specific criteria. The diagnostic criteria have changed with each revision of the DSM-IV (see Nathan, Skinstad, & Dolan, Chapter 21, this volume). *Substance dependence* implies an addiction to the drug, whereas *substance abuse* refers to a less severe condition involving continued use of a mind-altering substance despite problems caused by such use (American Psychiatric Association, 1994; Schuckit, 1995). Substance dependence is diagnosed in individuals who demonstrate at least three of seven criteria within the same year: (1) tolerance to the substance, (2) withdrawal from the substance upon cessation of use, (3) taking more of the substance or over longer periods of time, (4) loss of control over the substance use, (5) loss of time related to use, (6) activities forsaken, and (7) continued use despite knowledge of consequences. A diagnosis of substance abuse applies to maladaptive patterns of substance use that do not meet the more severe criteria for substance dependence. Specifically, a person is diagnosed with substance abuse if one of the four following criterion are met as a result of the substance use: (1) failure to meet role obligations, (2) recurrent use in dangerous situations, (3) recurrent legal problems, or (4) continued use despite persistent social problems, and criteria for substance dependence are not met.

Substance dependence implies a psychological and/or a physical need for the drug. *Psychological* dependence can occur following repeated use of any drug of abuse and refers to users' perceptions that they need the substance to feel or function optimally. For example, regular marijuana smokers who feel they cannot relax at the end of the day without an evening joint have developed psychological dependence on marijuana. *Physical dependence* indicates the physiological adaptation of the body to prolonged exposure to the substance. Two aspects of this adaptation are tolerance and withdrawal. *Tolerance* refers to cellular and metabolic adaptations in response to continued presence of the substance (Koob & Bloom, 1988). As tolerance develops, more of the drug is necessary to obtain the desired effects, and use becomes more frequent. *Cross-tolerance* occurs when tolerance to one drug has developed and more of any drugs in that class is necessary to produce comparable effects, based on the similar organic structure of active ingredients and nervous system response. If a user simultaneously administers multiple drugs of the same class, *potentiation* occurs, and the additive or synergistic effects can result in an overdose.

*Withdrawal* is experienced when administering a substance to a physically dependent organism is halted. Characteristic withdrawal syndromes ensue, depending on the drug class used, and the withdrawal syndromes tend to involve opposite symptoms as intoxication effects of the substance (Koob & Bloom, 1988). For example, opiate intox-

ication reduces pain sensations, but opiate withdrawal involves increased sensitivity to pain. This neuroadaptation is illustrated by the opponent process model. Positive hedonic effects (e.g., a cocaine rush) are followed by compensatory negative hedonic experiences (e.g., negative mood and withdrawal symptoms after cessation of use; Koob, Caine, Parsons, Markou, & Weiss, 1997).

From a public health perspective, substance use and abuse can be conceptualized along a continuum, in which excessive use of a variety of substances is associated with increasing levels of the risk of negative consequences (Newcomb & Bentler, 1988a). The risk of adverse consequences decreases at moderate use levels and declines further with abstinence (Marlatt & Tapert, 1993).

## Models of Addiction

As the substance abuse field has developed during the past several decades, controversies have arisen over the way to conceptualize addiction problems. The first controversy relates to the cause of substance abuse. Is it the fault of the addicted individuals, or is it due to circumstances beyond their control? The second controversy concerns treating substance abuse problems. Is recovery the responsibility of the addicted person, or are external entities responsible for recovery (Marlatt, 1992)? Opposing perspectives on these issues are summarized by four competing models of addiction (Brickman et al., 1982), highlighted here.

### Moral Model

The moral model of addictive behaviors refers to movements such as the temperance movement that preceded the prohibition on alcohol and law enforcement approaches in the recent "War on Drugs" (Trebach & Zeese, 1990). In this model, responsibility for developing and resolving the addiction is attributed to the individual with the substance use disorder. Drinking, for example, is viewed as a "sign of weak character" (Brickman et al., 1982), and the only way out is to exert willpower. Genetic and environmental etiological factors do not modify this responsibility. The moral stance can foster guilt for developing the addiction problem and failing to change. From this perspective, relapse is ascribed to moral weakness (Marlatt, 1992).

## Medical Model

The medical or disease model, which is the most common theoretical view employed in the United States, places responsibility for developing the addictive disorder on physiological factors, such as a family history of addiction or pathological metabolism (Jellinek, 1960). Treatment relies on external sources for specialized medical intervention into the pathological process. The addictive process, it is thought, has a deteriorating course, and, if left untreated, may result in death (Miller & Hester, 1995). Total abstinence from all intoxicating substances is the only acceptable treatment outcome and must be maintained lifelong to arrest disease progression (McCrady, 1994). Relapses are viewed as triggered by factors beyond the individual's control, often with a physiological basis. Taking a biological perspective, drug properties appear to interact with genetics to determine the reinforcement of drug taking, thereby influencing repeated use (Koob et al., 1998). The advantage of the medical model over the moral model is that addicted individuals are not blamed for the problem and they are encouraged to seek help from specialists, rather than attempt to treat the problem alone. In addition, research on the biological substrates of addictive processes has greatly advanced our understanding of genetic risk and protective factors and enhanced treatment of these disorders.

## Spiritual Model

The spiritual or enlightenment model is espoused by twelve-step programs such as Alcoholics Anonymous and Narcotics Anonymous (Alcoholics Anonymous, 1980; Miller, 1998b). The development of addiction is seen as related to a spiritual weakness. The concept of a "higher power" is emphasized for overcoming the addiction problem, and the individual must admit helplessness over the substance of abuse. Attending group meetings is considered imperative to prevent recurrence of the spiritual disease. A major advantage of this model is the social support and supplementary resources that members receive from meetings. Criticisms of the spiritual model include difficulty incorporating nonspiritual individuals into group processes that rely on religious beliefs and that peers or paraprofessionals with past histories of addiction deliver the intervention in lieu of addiction-trained professionals (Miller & Brown, 1997).

## Biobehavioral and Interactionist Models

Several integrative models have been proposed to incorporate the accumulating knowledge base of addictive behaviors from both biological and psychological sciences. The compensatory model (Brickman et al., 1982) posits that people with addiction problems need not be held at fault for developing the problem but are responsible for changing the behaviors, either independently or by seeking assistance. Substance abuse acquisition is conceptualized as a maladaptive response that occurs when stressors overpower appropriate coping strategies (e.g., Windle & Windle, 1996). Physiological, conditioning, social learning, and cultural factors exacerbate this process (Roberts & Koob, 1997; Vogel-Sprott, 1995). A relapse is viewed as a mistake in a new learning process (Marlatt, 1992). Recent refinements of interactionist theories of addictions include behavioral-genetic perspectives on the development of substance use disorders (McGue, 1997; Rose, Kaprio, Winter, Koskenvuo, & Viken, 1999) and behavioral economics views on addictive behavior problem resolution (Tucker, Vuchinich, & Pukish, 1995; Vuchinich & Tucker, 1998). In summary, the accumulating knowledge base of factors involved in developing addiction problems strongly suggests a multifaceted process, involving biological, psychological, and cultural components.

# Initiation, Maintenance, and Remission of Addiction

Substances of abuse have unique pharmacological properties and somewhat distinct use consequences, but they also share a great deal in common. A number of risk factors and developmental pathways in and out of addictive behaviors are shared across substances. The initial experimentation with substances of abuse is primarily determined by social and environmental risks. Biological and environmental factors combine to influence decisions to use again, the development of adverse consequences, and ultimately, efforts to reduce or stop substance involvement.

## Genetic Risk

Genetically influenced factors, it has been shown, affect the risk of developing substance use disorders (e.g., Pickens et al., 1991; Schuckit, 1985; Wall & Ehlers, 1995), although the heritability of dependence on drugs other than alcohol is less clear. Sons of male alcoholics are two to four times more likely to develop alcohol problems than sons of nonalcoholics (Cloninger, Bohman, & Sigvardsson, 1981). Approximately a quarter to half of the variability in drug abuse or dependence is attributable to heredity (Grove et al., 1990; Pickens, Svikis, McGue, & LaBuda, 1995), and the genetic risk is greater for male offspring. High rates of comorbidity with antisocial personality disorder complicate determining the genetic risk of drug dependence (Kessler et al., 1997). The risk of behavior control problems are also elevated for offspring of alcoholics (Sher, 1997), whereas risk of depression and anxiety problems has not been demonstrated (Schuckit & Smith, 1996).

## Learning Influences

**Classical Conditioning.** Self-administration of a variety of substances of abuse has been conditioned across several species. Drug-induced euphoria (unconditioned stimulus) over time becomes associated with environmental stimuli present during the euphoric state (conditioned stimuli), such as drug-taking paraphernalia, locations, behavior, and people (Vogel-Sprott, 1995). After continued pairing with the drug-induced euphoria, these associated stimuli may produce intense urges or cravings to take the substance again (Roberts & Koob, 1997). However, not all individuals with substance dependence use drugs in response to cravings (Vogel-Sprott, 1995). Similarly, stimuli associated with unpleasant periods of abstinence may elicit withdrawal-like symptoms. This conditioning principle can be observed in individuals who attempt to quit substance use and are constantly reminded of the addictive substance by a wide range of cues in the environment (Ludwig, Wickler, & Stark, 1974; Vogel-Sprott, 1995).

**Instrumental Learning.** Any reward following a behavior will increase the chance that the behavior will occur again. With substance use, both the acute pharmacological impact and social/environmental factors may produce rewards following drug self-administration, which increase the chance that drug taking will recur. For example, if individuals smoked marijuana, then experienced pleasurable pharmacological effects or experienced social approval, they would be likely to smoke marijuana again. Additionally, relief from aversive states, such as withdrawal or distress following drug self-administration also increases the likelihood of repeated drug-taking behaviors (Alexander & Hadaway, 1982). Euphoric sensations associated with drug taking are mediated by specific groups of connected neurons in the brain. Extant research indicates that the brain's reward circuitry involves connections between the ventral tegmental area and the basal forebrain, encompassing the dopaminergic neurotransmitter system, as well as opioid, serotonergic, and gamma-aminobutyric acid (GABA) neurotransmitter systems. These brain regions and systems, it has been demonstrated, subserve reinforcement of using a variety of addictive substances, including repeated alcohol, cocaine, and opiate self-administration, as well as other addiction cycles such as pathological gambling, binge eating, and compulsive sexual behaviors (Koob & Le Moal, 1997).

## Environmental factors

**Family.** Aspects of an individual's environment may act independently or in concert with biological factors to protect or imperil the chance of developing an addiction (Sher, Gershuny, Peterson, & Raskin, 1997). Positive, loving parent–child bonds reduce the risk of substance abuse (Kandel, 1978). Conversely, high levels of parent–adolescent conflict (Needle, Glynn, & Needle, 1983) and lack of familial cohesion (Hundleby & Mercer, 1987) increase this risk. Offspring of substance abusing parents have a significantly increased risk of using substances above and beyond genetic risks because substance use is often a common coping response modeled to offspring (Chassin, Pillow, Curran, Molina, & Barrera, 1993; Holden, Brown, & Mott, 1988). Parental monitoring and attitudes influence teen substance use directly by limiting opportunities to engage in deviant behavior (Forehand, Miller, Dutra, & Chance, 1997) and indirectly by influencing peer selection (Brown, Mott, & Stewart, 1992; Dishion, Patterson, & Reid, 1988). In general, three family characteristics elevate the risk of subsequent substance abuse: (1) parental dysfunction (e.g., substance dependence), including antisocial behaviors, alcoholism, and drug abuse; (2) minimal parental involvement with their children; and (3) dearth of affectionate, supportive parent–child interactions (Sadava, 1987). These family climate factors may interact with shared genes to contribute to the development of substance problems (McGue, Sharma, & Benson, 1996). Some studies of adoptees have indicated that siblings may be a greater source of environmental influence than parents for risk of substance use disorder (McGue, 1997; Rose et al., 1999).

**Life Stress.** Researchers have associated a variety of stressful life circumstances with the onset and progression of substance involvement. Life adversity, such as relationship problems, familial difficulties, legal troubles, and academic failure, increases the risk factors of substance abuse during adolescence (Duncan, 1977; Pandina & Schuele, 1983). Life stress is higher in families with substance abusers, suggesting an interactive mechanism by which positive family histories may increase the risk of substance abuse (Brown et al., 1995; Sher, 1991). Among adults treated for substance use disorders, those experiencing taxing psychosocial stressors appear more vulnerable to rapid posttreatment relapses (Brown, Vik, Patterson, Grant, & Schuckit, 1995).

## Cognitions

**Expectancies.** Expectations regarding the effects of substances are related to consumption patterns in youth and adults. These expectancies mediate initiation of use and progression to problematic use (Brown, 1993; Goldman, Brown, Christiansen, & Smith, 1991; Smith, Goldman, Greenbaum, & Christiansen, 1995). Expectancies develop from both direct and vicarious experiences with substances and reflect culturally held beliefs, as well as personal learning about substances in school, in the media, and from peers and family (Goldman et al., 1991). Research has also linked family histories of substance use disorders, particularly when exposed to abusing models during youth, with increased positive expectancies of certain substance effects (Brown, Tate, Vik, Haas, & Aarons, 1999; Sher, 1993). Although very young

children of substance abusers may hold more negative expectancies for substance effects, these expectancies are more likely to become quite positive as offspring acquire personal substance use experiences (Lundahl, Davis, Adesso, & Lukas, 1997; Wiers, Gunning, & Sergeant, 1998). Expectancies are generally substance-specific, but some (e.g., tension-reduction effects) are common to several classes of substances. Overall, individuals who anticipate that substances will produce positive effects have a greater chance of developing substance-related problems than those who do not hold this belief. In contrast, expectancies of negative substance effects may deter the initiation of involvement with certain substances (Brown, 1993). Expectancies may also result in anticipatory psychological responses of a compensatory nature (Ross & Pihl, 1988) that are linked to behavioral tolerance.

**Perceptions of Normative Use.** Users of alcohol and other drugs tend to perceive that others use amounts similar to those they use (Baer, Stacy, & Larimer, 1991). Erroneous perceptions of normative use are particularly notable among substance abusing adolescents and college students. These biases preserve cognitions of personal use patterns as nonproblematic and accelerate consumption to conform to perceived normative use levels (Marks & Miller, 1987; Perkins & Berkowitz, 1986).

## Personality

Individuals with substance abuse or dependence are quite heterogeneous with regard to lifestyle, social background, and personality characteristics (Babor, Hesselbrock, Meyer, & Shoemaker, 1994). Several personality traits are more common among people with addiction problems. These include rebelliousness, autonomy striving, liberalism, willingness to try new experiences, and independence (Segal, Huba, & Singer, 1980). Similarly, research has linked sensation seeking (Kohn & Annis, 1977; Zuckerman et al., 1994), impulsivity (Vistor, Crossman, & Eiserman, 1973), low self-esteem (Kaplan, 1977), reduced self-efficacy (Schinke, Botvin, & Orlandi, 1991), nonconventionality (Brook, Whiteman, & Gordon, 1983), behavioral undercontrol (Jessor & Jessor, 1977), and aggressive tendencies (Krueger, Caspi, Moffitt, Silva, & McGee, 1996) to high rates of substance involvement. Children with personalities characterized by deviance, emotional lability, inattention, lack of involvement in activities, and stubbornness are at greater risk of using substances frequently in late adolescence (Shedler & Block, 1990). Although evidence for a unitary "addictive personality" has not received empirical support (Sutker & Allain, 1988), more individuals with substance use disorders meet criteria for antisocial personality disorder and other mental health problems (e.g., anxiety and depressive disorders), even after substance-related pathology is excluded (Verheul, Hartgers, van den Brink, & Koeter, 1998). These personality characteristics that are relatively common among substance abusers appear to be inherited traits which may exacerbate or mediate familial substance abuse or dependence (McGue, 1997; Sher, 1997).

### Developmental Issues

In the past decade, increased awareness of the prevalence of youthful substance use and the risks involved has brought about growth in research focused on developmental issues. Experimentation with a variety of socially unapproved behaviors during adolescence is fairly common. Approximately 54% of eighth-grade students in the United States have used alcohol, and 38% have used an illicit drug (Johnston, O'Malley, & Bachman, 1998). This experimentation, especially with alcohol, cigarettes, and marijuana, can be part of the developmental process of individuation (Hawkins, 1982; Schinke et al., 1991). However, age of onset of substance use has recently been linked to lifetime risk of both alcohol abuse and dependence (Grant, 1997).

The relevance of various risk and protective factors for substance abuse fluctuates across developmental stages (Newcomb & Bentler, 1989). For example, the influence of peer behaviors and attitudes is greatest during adolescence (Hawkins, 1982), and spousal support among adults is a significant predictor of successful recovery without treatment (Sobell & Sobell, 1998). Personality traits and substance expectancies stabilize with maturity and play a powerful role in perpetuating substance involvement in young adulthood (Tapert, Stewart, & Brown, 1999). The consequences of adolescent substance use may develop slowly and include physical problems, psychological mal-

adjustment, unstable employment patterns, higher divorce rates (Brown, Myers, Mott, & Vik, 1994; Kandel, Davies, Karus, & Yamaguchi, 1986; Newcomb & Bentler, 1988a), and impaired social development (Baumrind & Moselle, 1985). Troubled life trajectories are particularly associated with multiple drug problems during adolescence (Brown et al., 1994; Newcomb & Bentler, 1988b, 1989).

The natural course of substance abuse involves fluctuating levels of use across time (Schuckit, Tipp, Smith, & Bucholz, 1997), including reductions and cessation without formal treatment. For example, only 12% of opiate-dependent Vietnam veterans continued their addiction after returning to the United States (Robins, Davis, & Nurco, 1974), likely due to major reductions in both stress and drug-related cues (Alexander & Hadaway, 1982; Robins, 1993). Individuals who remedy addictions without professional assistance have become a recent focus of attention, because the majority of adults who develop alcohol problems and resolve them do not seek treatment (Sobell & Sobell, 1998). Several studies of adolescents also demonstrate that many high school students deescalate their alcohol and drug involvement over the course of a school year (Stice, Myers, & Brown, 1998) and that youth routinely make serious attempts to reduce or stop their tobacco, alcohol, and other drug use (Wagner, Brown, Monti, Myers, & Waldron, 1999). The availability of desirable activities other than substance use greatly enhances the chance of natural recovery for adults (Tucker, 1995; Vuchinich, 1998), and youth use multiple strategies simultaneously (e.g., social supports, alternative activities) to sustain their behavior change efforts (Wagner, Brown, Monti, Myers, & Waldron, 1999). Investigations of the natural change process suggest that many individuals initiate behavior change before entering formal treatment and that interventions may assist primarily in maintaining change efforts (Tucker et al., 1995).

### Substances of Abuse

The principles underlying development of substance abuse problems are quite similar across different substances of abuse, but substances differ in intoxication effects, withdrawal syndromes, resulting consequences, and the sequence in which experimentation tends to occur.

## Sequence of Substance Experimentation

Substance involvement tends to follow a predictable sequence, from the use of "gateway" substances that are legal for adults (i.e., alcohol or cigarettes) to the use of marijuana, hard drugs, and prescribed psychoactives in adulthood (Ellickson, Hays, & Bell, 1992). This common sequence was investigated in more than 1000 high school students followed through young adulthood (Kandel, Yamaguchi, & Chen, 1992). Alcohol use has a stronger link to progression in this sequence for males than for females, whereas cigarette use has a stronger link for females than for males. The use of a substance at a particular stage in the sequence does not necessarily dictate progression to the next stage; rather, entry into a use stage is a prerequisite for the next stage.

The following section details the properties and consequences of specific substances of abuse. It should be remembered that polysubstance use involving multiple substances used concurrently is relatively common (Earleywine & Newcomb, 1997), particularly among adolescents and young adults (Stein, Newcomb, & Bentler, 1987; Stewart & Brown, 1995), complicating acute effects, withdrawal, and clinical course.

## CNS Depressants

Central nervous system depressants include alcohol, sedatives, and anxiolytic drugs. These drugs depress excitable tissues at all brain levels, produce a subjective sensation of intoxication, and are physically addictive (Schuckit, 1995).

**Alcohol.** Properties specific to alcohol are discussed in detail by Nathan and colleagues (this volume). Briefly, intoxication generally involves subjective sensations of relaxation, tension reduction, sociability, disinhibition, and euphoria. Toxic reactions occur at higher doses or with potentiation from other CNS depressants and involve confusion, irritability, slowed pulse, reduced body temperature, low blood pressure, and possible respiratory failure. Some degree of alcohol withdrawal is generally observed in daily drinkers who quit drinking and involves sweating, increased heart rate and respiratory rate, increased body temperature, tremor, nausea, vomiting, depressed mood, and muscle aches. More severe symptoms of seizure and delirium tremens, a condition marked by increased tremor, profound confusion, and hallucinations, appear in 5% of those who experience alcohol withdrawal (for a review, see Schuckit, 1995).

Approximately half of adults with alcohol dependence evidence cognitive impairments in visuospatial functioning, verbal learning and memory, visual memory, psychomotor functioning, or nonverbal abstract reasoning (Beatty, Hames, Blanco, Nixon, & Tivis, 1996; Brandt, Butters, Ryan, & Bayog, 1983) and tend to be more pronounced in older drinkers (Adams et al., 1993). The majority of these cognitive deficits improve with extended abstinence (Reed, Grant, & Rourke, 1992). Neuroimaging studies also demonstrate adverse brain changes associated with alcohol dependence (Jernigan, Pfefferbaum, & Zatz, 1986) that tend to resolve with abstinence (Carlen et al., 1986) and worsen following alcohol relapse (Pfefferbaum et al., 1995).

**Depressant drugs.** This class of drugs includes hypnotics (e.g., barbiturates, methaqualone, chloral hydrate), anxiolytics, and benzodiazepines (e.g., Xanax®, Valium®, Librium®, Ativan®). These drugs are prescribed at high rates (approximately 15% of the U.S. population), and although used effectively for most, misuse is observed in 5–10% of patients for whom these medications are prescribed. Effects experienced after ingestion include euphoria, disinhibition, cognitive impairment, loss of motor coordination, and slurred speech. High doses can produce hallucinations or paranoia, ataxia, sedation, and increased risk of accidents (e.g., vehicular). Very high doses can produce depressed heart rate, respiratory failure, coma, or death. These substances show crosstolerance and present a high risk of lethal overdose if used simultaneously with alcohol or other CNS depressants. Abrupt cessation can be fatal and is especially dangerous from agents with short halflives (e.g., Xanax®—10 hours). The typical withdrawal syndrome is characterized by anxiety, insomnia, headaches, tremors, muscle aches, increased heart and respiratory rates, fatigue, and, sometimes, disorientation, hallucinations, depression, and convulsions. This withdrawal syndrome can persist for days to weeks. Individuals who withdraw from depressant drugs should receive medical monitoring (Schuckit, 1995). The chronic use of barbiturates is associated with persisting deficits in abstraction, psychomotor processing, and nonverbal learning (Bergman, Borg, Engelbrektson, & Vikander, 1989).

## Stimulants

CNS stimulants include caffeine and nicotine, but the major intoxicating stimulants of abuse are cocaine and amphetamines. Drugs of this class typically produce physiological arousal, euphoria, insomnia, and diminished appetite.

**Cocaine.** Users can insufflate (snort) or smoke cocaine powder, sprinkle the powder in rolled cigarettes, smoke it in cooked form ("crack" or "rock"), or inject it in a dissolved form. Crack is more potent than powdered cocaine and causes intense effects that diminish rapidly. Cocaine use produces euphoria, expansive mood, loquaciousness, restlessness, mood swings, irritability, aggression, and insomnia. In higher doses, loss of control, paranoia, panic attacks, and hallucinations may occur. Common physical effects include elevated heart rate, dry mouth, sweating, numbness of the mucous membranes, and hand tremors. Tolerance develops rapidly, usually within days of continued use. Withdrawal symptoms include fatigue, depressed mood, craving, agitation, and, in some cases, physical aggression. The half-life of cocaine is 1 hour, and withdrawal lasts for days to months (Kuhn, Swartzwelder, & Wilson, 1998). Chronic cocaine use adversely influences short-term memory (Ardila, Rosselli, & Strumwasser, 1991; Manschreck et al., 1990), verbal recall (Mittenberg & Motta, 1993), speed of information processing, attention (Ardila, 1991; O'Malley & Gawin, 1990), and abstraction (O'Malley, Adamse, Heaton, & Gawin, 1992).

**Amphetamines.** Amphetamines include pharmaceutically prepared substances (e.g., Benzedrine®, Dexedrine®, Ritalin®, and other drugs prescribed for obesity, attention deficit/hyperactivity disorder, and narcolepsy) as well as substances produced illegally, such as methamphetamine ("crystal meth," "speed," or "ice"). Users can snort powder forms of these drugs, dissolve and inject the substances, smoke them, or ingest the drugs orally. Amphetamines produce subjective experiences of euphoria, sociability, hypervigilance, anxiety, stereotyped behaviors, and impaired judgment. As with cocaine, smoked and injected forms are more concentrated, and behaviors are more dramatically altered than with use of other forms. The primary difference between cocaine and amphetamines is the longer half-life of the latter (6 to 12 hours). Physical effects include increased heart rate, pupil dilation, and psychomotor agitation. Withdrawal symptoms involve 1 week to 6 months of depression, irritability, fatigue, and hypersomnia and can involve aggression and hallucinations (Maxmen & Ward, 1995).

**Tobacco.** Nicotine, the addictive substance in tobacco, is delivered through cigarettes, cigars, and smokeless tobacco products such as chew and snuff. Long-term use of tobacco has been associated with a wide range of health problems, particularly cancers (of the lung, mouth, and esophagus), coronary artery disease, atherosclerosis, cerebrovascular disease, emphysema, compromised immune function, decreased fertility, and low birth-weight offspring (see review by Baer & Brady Murch, 1998). Although a third of smokers attempt to quit each year, less than 5% remain smoke-free longer than 12 months (see review by Haaga & Kirk, 1998). Cigarette smoking is the leading preventable cause of mortality in the United States (McGinnis & Foege, 1993), and elevated rates of respiratory problems have been noted in youth with as little as 2- to 4-year histories of smoking (Myers & Brown, 1997).

The acute effects of nicotine are less dramatic than those of other substances of abuse; intoxication is mild and generally nonimpairing. Nicotine delivery products tend to be used throughout the day: the half-life of nicotine is only 30 to 120 minutes and increases the environmental associations that may cue the user to smoke. Significant withdrawal symptoms of depressed mood, fatigue, irritability, and craving that last 2–3 weeks are reported in youth and adults who stop or cut down nicotine intake and make the quitting process particularly arduous.

## Opiates

This drug class includes derivatives of the opium poppy (e.g., opium, morphine), semi-synthetics (heroin), medication preparations synthesized to have morphine-like properties (e.g., codeine, hydromorphone, methadone, oxycodone, meperidine, and fentanyl), and medications with both opiate agonist and antagonist properties (buprenorphine, pentazocine). Opiates are prescribed for pain relief, cough suppression, or to alleviate opiate withdrawal symptoms. Opiate users inject, snort, smoke, and swallow the drug.

Opiate users report the intoxicating effects of euphoria, especially during the "rush" immediately following administration, as well as apathy, dysphoria, impaired judgment, and relaxation. Physical effects of intoxication include suppressed respiratory functioning, slurred speech, psychomotor retardation, reduced pain sensations, impairment of attention and memory, constricted pupils, and constipation. Tolerance develops rapidly. Due to the comparatively short half-life of heroin (30 minutes versus 2 to 3.5 hours for morphine), administration four times per day is common in addicts. Thus, daily activities revolve around obtaining and administering opiates. Withdrawal is generally very unpleasant and involves nausea, vomiting, diarrhea, muscle aches, tremor, fatigue, insomnia, fever, dysphoric mood, and cravings and can last up to 8 days (Tapert et al., 1998). Administration of street opiates poses a particular risk for overdose because purity levels remain unknown to the user. Because many opiate users inject, additional risks of HIV infection, hepatitis, cellulitis, endocarditis, and tuberculosis are imminent. Death from opiate overdose most commonly results from respiratory depression. No consistent neuropsychological deficits have been identified among tolerant users or detoxified former users (Zacny, 1995).

## Cannabinols

Marijuana is the most commonly used illicit drug in the United States. Users ingest THC by smoking marijuana leaves ("pot," "weed"), smoking resin ("hashish"), or eating cannabinoids mixed with food. Intoxicating effects include relaxation, euphoria, altered perception, impaired motor coordination, the sensation of slowed time, impaired judgment, and social withdrawal (APA, 1994). THC has a relatively long half-life of 2 to 7 days. Anxiety, paranoia, attention and memory impairment, panic, and hallucinations may occur acutely. Physical symptoms include increased appetite, dry mouth, bloodshot eyes, and tachycardia (Tapert et al., 1999). Although its use involves fewer physiological changes than most other drugs of abuse, the consequences of chronic use may include amotivational syndrome as well as lung diseases similar to those experienced by tobacco smokers. Males may suffer impaired sperm production, decreased testosterone secretion, and decreased size of prostate and testes. Females can experience blocked ovulation (Cohen, 1981; McGlothlin & West, 1968, Tapert et al., 1998).

Studies of marijuana's influence on cognition have yielded mixed results (Culver & King, 1974;

Wert & Raulin, 1986). Recent studies have demonstrated some mild impairments in attention, problem solving, and verbal learning following at least 1 day of abstinence among chronic, heavy users (Pope & Yurgelun-Todd, 1996), visuospatial memory problems in chronic female users (Pope, Jacobs, Mialet, Yurgelun-Todd, & Gruber, 1997), and complex problem solving (Block, Farinpour, & Braverman, 1992).

## Hallucinogens

These drugs produce dramatic alterations in sensation and perception and include lysergic acid diethylamide (LSD), psilocybin (from certain mushrooms), dimethyltryptamine (DMT), mescaline (from the peyote cactus), 2,5-dimethoxy-4-methylamphetamine (DOM or STP), methylene dioxyamphetamine (MDA), methylene dioxymethamphetamine (MDMA, "ecstasy," "E," or "X"), 2C-B ("Nexus"), ibotenic acid, and muscimol. Hallucinogens are usually taken orally. Users experience intensification of perceptions, visual hallucinations, derealization, euphoria, alertness, and emotional lability. Confusion, paranoia, panic, loss of control, and depression may result. The most imminent risk during intoxication is acting on delusional beliefs (e.g., ability to fly). Physical effects include pupillary dilation, tachycardia, tremors, nausea, and sweating (Tapert et al., 1998). Heavy, long-term LSD use has been inconsistently associated with mild deficits in speeded visuomotor scanning abilities (Culver & King, 1974), and MDMA ("ecstasy") may produce verbal learning and memory impairments (Krystal & Price, 1992). Incorrect chemical synthesis of MDMA and MDA can produce substances that cause severe Parkinsonian symptoms (e.g., MTPT). Hallucinogenic effects tend to be more intense for younger users than for older users. Tolerance can develop with frequent use (Tapert et al., 1999).

## Dissociatives

Phencyclidine (PCP, Sernylan®, "Angel Dust") and related compounds (Ketamine®, Ketaject®) were developed as anesthetics and became street drugs in the 1960s. Users can smoke, snort, orally ingest, or inject them. Because PCP is relatively inexpensive, drug dealers often mix it with other drugs (particularly marijuana) to intensify effects. Intoxicating effects include marked behavioral change, assaultiveness, belligerence, unpredictability, impaired judgment, euphoria, hallucinations, intensified perceptions, and heightened emotions. Some users experience hyperactivity, panic, paranoia, and confusion. Physical effects include numbness and diminished response to pain, psychomotor agitation and discoordination, tachycardia, slurred speech, and sometimes, catatonia, convulsions, respiratory depression, coma, and death (see review by Tapert et al., 1999). PCP has a half-life of approximately 18 hours, and, due to profoundly impaired judgment and reduced fear of pain, users may engage in very violent or destructive behaviors while high. PCP use is associated with long-term impairments in abstraction and motor skills (Carlin, Grant, Adams, & Reed, 1979).

### Inhalants

Inhalants of abuse include industrial and household compounds, such as glues, aerosol sprays, gasoline, paints, paint thinners, nail polish remover, correction fluid, certain cleaning solvents, and nitrous oxide ("poppers," "rush"). Due to availability and low cost, children, adolescents, and youth from economically disadvantaged regions comprise the majority of inhalant users. Euphoria, floating sensations, temporal distortion, and visual hallucinations occur acutely, followed by apathy, confusion, irritability, assaultiveness, and panic. Physical effects include loss of coordination, dizziness, headache, slurred speech, lethargy, psychomotor retardation, tremor, and blurred vision. Inhalant abuse can lead to serious physiological problems, including respiratory damage, eye, nose, and throat damage, as well as kidney, liver, heart, gastrointestinal, and nervous system damage (Morton, 1990). Death can occur from heart arrhythmias or suffocation from breathing out of plastic bags containing the solvent. Inhalant abuse is robustly associated with impaired attention, memory, fine motor, and visuospatial functioning (Allison & Jerrom, 1984).

### Assessment

Treatment planning and evaluation of treatment response are accomplished by assessment procedures developed specifically for the field of substance use disorders. Methods for assessing substance use may involve screening for alcohol or drug problems, assessing substance use behaviors,

determining diagnosis, or evaluating outcomes. Measures of substance involvement described in this chapter are exemplars of instruments available to assist treatment providers and researchers in tailoring interventions and evaluating substance use behaviors. Although substances differ in consumption patterns and physiological properties, broad similarities across psychoactive substances guide diagnostic procedures, as evidenced by the adoption of uniform dependence criteria across substances in the DSM-IV (APA, 1994). Thorough assessments should include evaluating alcohol and illicit drug use, given the prevalence and poorer treatment outcomes associated with polysubstance disorders (Kolar, Brown, Weddington, & Ball, 1990; Rounsaville, Dolinsky, Babor, & Meyer, 1987).

### Self-Report Assessment Issues and Strategies

The accuracy of self-reported substance use has been questioned due to acute and chronic memory problems associated with substance use, motivation to avoid the negative consequences of use, stigmatization, and minimization of personal problems (Carroll, 1995). However, empirical investigations have found that self-reports of substance use are relatively reliable and valid. Studies have substantiated the reliability and validity of alcohol use self-reports across populations (e.g., adolescents, college students, inpatients, outpatient, and normal drinkers; Babor, Brown, & Del Boca, 1990; Babor, Stephens, & Marlatt, 1987; Brown, Myers, et al., 1998; Maisto, Sobell, Cooper, & Sobell, 1979), as well as the accuracy of self-reported tobacco and other substance use (Brown, Myers, et al., 1998; Ehrman & Robbins, 1994).

Specific strategies enhance the accuracy of substance-related assessments (Babor et al., 1987). A critical first step is to verify that the client is not intoxicated or experiencing withdrawal states that may compromise memory or attention at the time of assessment. Unlike many other clinical symptoms, substance use and associated problems are observable or detectable. Methods of increasing self-report accuracy capitalize on these features by obtaining corroborating information from spouses, relatives, friends, records (e.g., medical and legal), and biological tests (Babor et al., 1987; Maisto, McKay, & Connors, 1990). Informing a client that these resources will be used improves reliability. Assuring both the client and collateral contacts of confidentiality encourages disclosure without concern for repercussions. In the event of discrepancies among informants, the source indicating that substance use has occurred usually is more accurate (Carroll, 1995). Calendar prompts are helpful (i.e., linking dates to holidays, anniversaries, and important life events).

Computer versions are available for many diagnostic and screening assessment instruments. Individuals may be more comfortable and provide more accurate information on sensitive topics when reporting to a computer, as opposed to a live interviewer. Comparisons of interview, self-report, and computer assessments have typically revealed few differences in the information provided (Davis, Hoffman, Morse, & Luehr, 1992; Skinner & Allen, 1983), and clients may prefer computer assessments to interviews or paper-and-pencil self-reports (Millstein, 1987; Skinner & Allen, 1983) and respond to computer measures more completely (Erdman, Klein, & Greist, 1983).

## Screening

Because substance use disorders are highly prevalent but treatment is sought at disproportionately low frequencies, identifying the need for intervention among non-treatment-seeking individuals may be beneficial. For example, alcohol and drug use problems are prevalent in medical patients (Rydon, Redman, Sanson-Fisher, & Reid, 1992), military personnel (Bray, Guess, Marsden, & Herbold, 1989), and college students (Gfroerer, Greenblatt, & Wright, 1997). Screening measures are designed to identify individuals who need intervention or who are at risk of developing substance-related problems in a time-efficient manner (Connors, 1995), and include brief self-report measures, short interviews, and biological markers of substance use.

Widely used self-report instruments developed to screen for alcohol problems include the ten-item Alcohol Use Disorders Identification Test (AUDIT), developed and tested cross-culturally by the World Health Organization (Saunders, Aasland, Babor, De La Fuente, & Grant, 1993), the Michigan Alcoholism Screening Test (MAST; Selzer, 1971), that consists of twenty-five questions, and the four-item Cut down, Annoyed, Guilty, Eye opener (CAGE; Adams, Barry, & Fleming 1996; Mayfield, McLeod, & Hall, 1974), which is widely used in medical facilities. A comparison of the AUDIT and CAGE showed that the AUDIT performed significantly better in detecting drinking problems among general medical patients (Bradley, Bush, McDonell, Malone, & Finn, 1998). Even briefer versions of the AUDIT, using only the three questions related to alcohol consumption (frequency, typical quantity, frequency of six or more drinks in a single sitting), performed comparably to the full AUDIT for identifying individuals with current alcohol abuse or dependence. The single item on frequency of binge drinking detected 81% of patients with alcohol abuse or dependence, and only 17% of patients were falsely identified as positive (Bush, Kivlahan, McDonnell, Finn, & Bradley, 1998). Thus, the AUDIT is a preferable alcohol problem screening measure.

The Personal Experience Screening Questionnaire (PESQ; Winters, 1991) is a brief self-report instrument designed to screen for alcohol and drug use problems in adolescents. This forty-item measure takes approximately 10 minutes to complete. Sound psychometric properties have been demonstrated (Winters, 1991, 1992). The PESQ does not provide diagnoses but efficiently assists clinicians and schools in identifying teens who may need substance abuse assessment.

## Biological Markers of Substance Use

In addition to self-report screening instruments, biological markers are available for a range of substances including nicotine, alcohol, and both licit and illicit drugs. Biological tests vary in cost, biological specimen (e.g., saliva, breath, urine, and blood), sensitivity, and specificity. Sensitivity refers to the likelihood that a substance will be identified by the test if the substance is present. Specificity refers to the proportion of biological samples that is accurately identified. Generally, tests that are very accurate (both highly sensitive and highly specific) are more costly. Thus, it is advisable to begin biological screening with a very sensitive method and follow positive results using a more expensive test with high specificity (Schuckit, 1995).

The majority of alcohol and other drug testing occurs through urine toxicology due to its relatively low cost. A limitation is that results indicate only the recent presence of the substance, not the quantity or timing of use. Alcohol use is detectable for approximately 24 hours postconsumption, amphetamines for 48 hours, opiates for 48 hours, cocaine for 3–5 days, barbiturates for for 1–7 days, and cannabinols approximately for 5–7 days. Positive tests may result from regular cannabinol use for up to 3–4 weeks (Schuckit, 1995).

Expired carbon monoxide (CO) and cotinine improve the accuracy of self-reported nicotine use (Hughes, 1993). CO breath samples are less expensive, easily collected, and provide immediate results and reasonable sensitivity to past 24-hour nicotine use (Velicer, Prochaska, Rossi, & Snow, 1992). Cotinine can be tested using saliva, blood, or urine samples and has superior sensitivity and specificity for detecting nicotine use in the past 3–7 days.

Biological markers are also available for detecting prolonged heavy alcohol consumption and corroborating a suspicion of relapse. These include relatively inexpensive liver function tests such as gamma-glutamyltransferase (GGT), aspartate aminotransferase (SGOT), alanine aminotransferase (SGPT), and a red blood cell test for mean corpuscular volume (MCV). Medical problems can cause false positive results. These tests are most useful in combination (Irwin, Baird, Smith, & Schuckit, 1988). A newer test, carbohydrate-deficient transferrin (CDT), is more expensive but is more accurate than GGT or MCV in men under age 40, smokers (Yersin, Nicolet, Decrey, Burnier, van Mele, & Pecoud, 1995), patients with liver disease, and early relapsers (Schmidt et al., 1997).

A less studied biological screening method analyzes hair follicles. Most drugs are carried by the bloodstream to the scalp, where the substance is incorporated into the hair follicles. Because hair grows predictably over time, separate sections of hair samples can provide estimates of the months in which various drugs were used (Strang, Black, March, & Smith, 1993).

## Diagnosis

Diagnostic assessment involves following a set of diagnostic criteria to determine if an individual has a clinical disorder. The DSM-IV (APA, 1994) is the most widely used diagnostic system in the United States and has criteria for substance disorders similar to the *International Classification of Diseases and Related Health Problems* (ICD-10;

World Health Organization, 1992) which is used worldwide. In selecting diagnostic measures, considerations include available resources, administrative time, training required, cost of the measure, scoring methods, and client characteristics (e.g., age and culture). Many instruments were originally developed with predominantly Caucasian adult male samples and should be reviewed for reliability and validity for use with adolescents, older adults, women, and non-Caucasians.

Methods for diagnosis include structured and semistructured interviews distinguished by the level of interviewer judgment and flexibility incorporated in the assessment process. The NIMH Diagnostic Interview Schedule (DIS; Spitzer, 1983) and the WHO Composite International Diagnostic Interview—Substance Abuse Module (CIDI-SAM; Cottler et al., 1995) are reliable structured interviews that do not require professional training, but some clinicians report a mechanical quality to this type of interview. Semistructured measures allow more discretion on the part of interviewers to determine when more detailed questioning is needed, but require more professional training. The Psychiatric Research Interview for Substance and Mental Disorders (PRISM; formerly known as the Structured Clinical Interview for DSM-III-R, Alcohol/Drug Version; SCID-A/D) is a widely used semistructured measure with more flexibility, that provides diagnoses for other Axis I and II disorders as well.

Specifiers that indicate severity and other characteristics (e.g., physiological dependence) can be useful in both clinical and research settings. For example, the Alcohol Dependence Scale (Horn, Skinner, Wanberg, & Foster, 1984) provides a reliable quantitative measure of the severity of alcohol dependence based on twenty-five questions covering withdrawal symptoms, impaired control over drinking, compulsion to drink, tolerance, and alcohol-seeking behaviors.

The Addiction Severity Index (ASI; McLellan et al., 1992) is a structured interview that queries personal/family characteristics and provides severity estimates for problems in six life areas frequently impacted by substance abuse (medical, employment/financial support, drug/alcohol use, legal/criminal justice involvement, family/social, and psychological/psychiatric). Separate categories of substances assessed include alcohol, heroin, methadone, other opiates/analgesics, barbiturates, other sedatives/hypnotics/tranquilizers, cocaine, amphetamines, cannabis, hallucinogens, inhalants, and polysubstance use. The ASI requires 45–60 minutes to administer and 10–15 minutes to score and has been normed on multiple samples that consistently demonstrate strong psychometric characteristics (Friedman & Granick, 1994). The composite score for drugs is a weighted sum of the frequencies of several different types of drug use, and consequently heavy users of a single substance are likely to receive lower scores than less frequent users of multiple drugs (Carroll et al., 1994). Therefore, evaluation of clinical progress may be influenced by the pattern of drug use for a particular client, and this measure may be less sensitive to change for some substance users (Carroll, 1995).

The Customary Drinking and Drug Use Record (CDDR; Brown, Myers, et al., 1998) is a structured interview that assesses recent (prior 3 months) and lifetime characteristics of adolescent alcohol and other drug involvement; it queries separately for marijuana, amphetamines, barbiturates, hallucinogens, cocaine, inhalants, opiates, prescription medications, and other substance not previously identified. Additionally, age of initiation and progression to regular use, negative consequences, withdrawal, and dependence are assessed. Reliability and validity have been demonstrated for community and clinical samples of adolescents and young adults (Brown, Myers et al., 1998).

## Detailed Substance Assessments

Detailed assessments provide valuable information on patterns of substance use, including quantity and frequency of use, binge use, high-risk situations, and progress in treatment. Methods for assessing substance use have been classified into two categories: summary (also called aggregate or quantity-frequency) measures and detailed daily assessments (Room, 1990). Clients report the quantity of alcohol that they typically consume, the maximum number of drinks consumed in one sitting, how frequently they drink, and how frequently they use a variety of drugs. The three major types of alcoholic beverages (beer, wine, and hard liquor) are often queried for separately. Drug use is more difficult to quantify due to differences in quantity descriptions and quality of "street" drugs; thus, frequency of drug use is more reliable,

although money spent on heroin or cocaine may estimate the quantity (Ehrman & Robbins, 1994).

Daily instruments such as the Timeline Followback (TLFB; Sobell, Kwan, & Sobell, 1995; Sobell, Toneatto, Sobell, 1994) use a calendar to prompt detailed assessment of a client's substance use over a period of time up to 1 year. Individuals retrospectively estimate daily substance use. Salient event anchors (e.g., incarcerations, hospitalizations, pay days, birthdates, and holidays) aid recall. The TLFB was initially developed for assessing alcohol use, and has been adapted to assess other drug and tobacco use (Brown, Burgess, et al., 1998; Ehrman & Robbins, 1994). Daily techniques permit examining substance use patterns over time. Clients can record substance use on an ongoing basis with self-monitoring diaries and cards.

Other facets of drug involvement are useful in treatment planning, evaluation, and research. For example, self-efficacy (confidence in one's ability to execute a given behavior) is related to alcohol and drug treatment outcomes (Marlatt, Baer, & Quigley, 1995). The Situational Confidence Questionnaire (Annis & Graham, 1988), Drug-Taking Confidence Questionnaire (Sklar et al., 1997), and Smoking Self-Efficacy Questionnaire (Colletti, Supnick, & Payne, 1985) assess self-efficacy related to alcohol, other drugs, and cigarette use. The Inventory of Drinking Situations (Annis, 1982) and Inventory of Drug-Taking Situations (Annis & Martin, 1985) identify situations in which the client drank or used drugs during the past year, based on eight relapse precipitant categories developed by Marlatt and Gordon (1985). Personal expectancies about the effects of alcohol or drugs have also been associated with use patterns (e.g., Brown et al., 1985; Schafer & Brown, 1991). The Alcohol Expectancy Questionnaire (Brown, Christiansen, & Goldman, 1987) assesses the anticipated effects of alcohol use and has been adapted for adolescent populations (Christiansen, Goldman, & Brown, 1996) and for other substances (e.g., stimulants, marijuana, and nicotine; Schafer & Brown, 1991). Profiles on these scales help identify relapse risks and can focus interventions on situations that require strategies and skills for avoiding future substance use. Summaries of a variety of substance use measures are described in a manual published by the National Institute on Alcohol Abuse and Alcoholism (Allen & Columbus, 1995).

# Treatment

In any given month, an estimated 2.3 million adults meet clinical criteria for drug dependence or abuse based on household interviews (Regier et al., 1990). Including criminal justice populations (inmates, probationers, or parolees), homeless people, and pregnant women (bearing a lower threshold for treatment need), an estimated 5.5 million individuals need treatment at any given time (Institute of Medicine, 1990). People transition in and out of these diagnostic labels as a function of biology, conditioning, and social factors. Due to the heterogeneity among individuals with substance use disorders, different forms of treatment are needed (Institute of Medicine, 1990).

In response to this need for treatment, therapeutic strategies developed to treat addictive disorders have evolved over time. Because initial alcohol and drug cessation attempts were most commonly followed by resuming substance use (Hunt, Barnett, & Branch, 1971), the need for a more extensive framework for addressing addictive behaviors became evident. Addiction theory and therapies began to incorporate behavioral principles. Limitations of early behavioral theories that focused on immediate environmental contingencies led to consideration of cognitive and affective factors associated with substance use patterns (e.g., Blane & Leonard, 1987). Behavioral principles, cognitive and affective factors, and behavioral choice theory have been combined to form sophisticated models of addiction. Behavioral choice theory extended the scope of earlier behavior theories, recognizing that behaviors (such as substance use) depend on immediate environmental contingencies and also on the availability of valued alternate activities and environmental constraints (Vuchinich & Tucker, 1996). Contemporary interventions may encompass components of these theoretical contributions.

Thus, the clinician and client have a wide variety of treatment options. Alcohol and drug abuse treatments vary in multiple ways: the format of treatment services (individual, family, group), type of treatment provider (peers, paraprofessionals, professionals), length of treatment (brief interventions to lifelong participation), treatment intensity (inpatient hospitalization, outpatient treatment, or community meetings on an as needed basis), and treatment modality (pharmacological therapy, psychotherapy, therapeutic communities). These multiple facets coexist in various combinations, often with little empirical information to guide optimal treatment choices. In initial therapeutic sessions, interventions specifically developed to enhance motivation and engage the client in the treatment process have proven useful.

## Motivational Enhancement Therapy (MET)

Because client motivation is a central concern in addressing addictive behaviors clients are often ambivalent about initiating or continuing treatment. A treatment approach specifically aimed at enhancing motivation was developed by Miller and Rollnick (1991) based on therapeutic elements found effective across interventions. Therapists work in an empathic manner with clients to develop cognitive dissonance between current substance use behaviors and personal goals or values, such as health, self-esteem, or role responsibilities. Therapists avoid confrontation with client statements and instead, "roll with resistance" to explore and resolve ambivalence. Therapists support client self-efficacy to change by examining alternative avenues for achieving desired goals, problem solving to remove barriers to behavior change, and encouraging clients to mobilize personal resources. These MET interview techniques have been empirically supported for treating less severe alcohol and nicotine problems. Although initially considered effective mostly for mildly dependent individuals, recent studies have shown efficacy with a variety of patients, including those who express high levels of anger (Miller & Hester, 1995; Project MATCH Research Group, 1998).

Changing substance abuse behaviors is challenging and complex. The transtheoretical model is a useful heuristic that illustrates the five steps of the change process (DiClemente & Prochaska, 1998): (1) precontemplation (unaware of the problem or unwilling to change), (2) contemplation (considering change), (3) preparation (deciding to change), (4) action (implementing change), and (5) maintenance (behavior change sustained several months and integrated into lifestyle; DiClemente & Prochaska, 1998). Individuals may progress or revert to previous stages. This model is helpful in depicting the complexities and motivational levels involved in behavior change (Miller, 1998a).

For some clients, brief motivational interventions may be adequate to inspire behavior change. Short-term approaches include a variety of low-intensity interventions, collectively known as brief interventions, that have proven beneficial in a range of settings.

## Brief Interventions (BI)

BIs are a collection of techniques that generally involve one to three sessions of counseling, psychoeducation, professional advice, and/or bibliotherapy (Miller et al., 1995). Commonly, reducing use or preventing problem use, not necessarily abstinence, is the therapeutic goal. Research findings demonstrate that not all substance users require protracted, intensive therapy for healthy behavior change. Four types of clients have been the primary focus of this type of intervention: (1) hazardous drivers, (2) smokers, (3) mildly to moderately alcohol-dependent individuals, and (4) highly dependent drinkers not reached by other services (Heather, 1995). BI is frequently administered in emergency departments or primary care settings. Providers include primary care physicians, nurses, and social workers. An extension of this cost-effective approach is Guided Self-Change (Sobell & Sobell, 1998), which provides readings, exercises, assessment, and personalized feedback regarding substance use patterns, high-risk situations, and relapse prevention techniques. Positive treatment outcomes have been reported following just two–four sessions for alcohol and tobacco problems (Sobell & Sobell, 1998).

Motivational Enhancement, Brief Interventions, and Guided Self-Change are typically delivered individually in outpatient contexts by professionals or paraprofessionals during brief time frames with flexible treatment goals. These approaches all strive to engage clients in initiating changes in substance use behaviors; at times they use personal and community resources.

## Self-Help Groups

Self-help groups, one of the most widely recognized and readily available addiction resources, are composed of peers who face similar difficulties and shared goals for change. The most widely known contemporary self-help group, Alcoholics Anonymous (AA; Alcoholics Anonymous World Services, 1976), has 96,000 weekly group meetings throughout the United States and 150 countries. Similar groups have been developed for other substance use disorders (e.g., Narcotics Anonymous, Cocaine Anonymous, and Nicotine Anonymous) and other addictive behaviors (e.g., Gamblers Anonymous, Overeaters Anonymous). Twelve-step participants share experiences at meetings, obtain sponsorships by successful members, read literature on the principles and steps, and use a spiritual focus to achieve abstinence and seek life meaning. Recovery is considered a lifelong process, and complete abstinence is the only means of managing addiction. Groups are also available to support friends and families of those with addictions (e.g., Al-anon, Adult Children of Alcoholics).

Although twelve-step groups are dominant in the United States, the majority of individuals referred to them do not follow through with long-term attendance (National Academy of Sciences, 1990). Alternative support groups (e.g., Women for Sobriety, Men for Sobriety, Rational Recovery, Moderation Management, and Self-Management and Recovery Training) have emerged that differ from twelve-step groups by emphasizing self-reliance and secular methods of recovery. The primary drawback of these alternatives is limited availability outside of major metropolitan areas. Detailed descriptions of self-help and alternative support groups are provided by McCrady and Delaney (1995) and Horvath (1997), respectively.

In the event that low-intensity approaches prove ineffective for a particular client, short-term inpatient or outpatient treatment formats may be indicated. Treatment providers are professionals or paraprofessionals, and often combinations of individual and group formats are included. Group modalities offer unique therapeutic features, including observational learning and social support (Yalom, 1985). In addition, group counseling may be cost-efficient (Schuckit, 1995). Short-term inpatient treatment programs typically encourage continuing participation in more extended intervention programs following discharge, including outpatient aftercare, self-help groups, residential treatment facilities, or therapeutic communities.

A range of therapeutic approaches that have proven useful in outpatient and inpatient treatment settings is described next. It should be remembered that the features of these interventions overlap at times and multiple techniques are often provided in combination within a single treatment setting. Treatments developed by psychologists based on theoretical and empirical foundations will be presented first, followed by a brief presentation of effective pharmacotherapies available in these settings.

## Relapse Prevention

Relapse Prevention (RP), developed by Marlatt and Gordon (1985), was based on empirical observations that substance use disordered individuals could cease addictive behaviors briefly but had difficulty maintaining the change over time. RP provides behavioral and cognitive skills training to avoid or minimize relapse. Clients are taught to identify and anticipate situations that increase the risk for relapse and to prepare coping strategies to avoid or manage these high-risk situations. If a relapse occurs, it is viewed as a learning experience for fine-tuning strategies and efforts for the future. Balanced lifestyles are encouraged to reduce the reliance on psychoactive substances for pleasurable experiences.

## Coping and Social Skills Training

Coping and Social Skills Training (CSST; Monti et al., 1990; Monti, Gulliver, & Myers, 1994) developed from social cognitive learning theory based on the premise that substance abusing individuals exhibit deficits in coping and social skills necessary for adaptive daily living. CSST interventions develop interpersonal skills, affect regulation, stress management, and coping with substance availability cues (Monti, Rohsenow, Colby, & Abrams, 1995). Treatment begins with assessing client strengths and weaknesses in these domains and specifying risky situations for relapse. Because alcohol and drug use cues are not always avoidable in natural environments, exposure to substance-use cues in the safety of the treatment setting seeks to extinguish craving responses (Niaura, Rohsenow, Binkoff, & Monti, 1988).

## Contingency Contracting

Contingency contracting, based on operant behavior principles, involves creating a contract between the patient and treatment provider for reinforcers (or punishers) to eliminate substance use and shape goal-directed behaviors (e.g., attending therapy sessions, working). For example, cocaine abusers have been paid with vouchers for not using cocaine, and increases in voucher amounts escalate for successive weeks of abstinence (Silverman et al., 1996, 1998). Alternatively, clients may agree to an aversive consequence for relapse, such as having employers notified of their drug use (Anker & Crowley, 1982). Another study used small fines ($5) to patients for not attending therapy appointments without appropriate prior notification (Boudin et al., 1977). Contingency contracting has proven effective in reducing substance use (Dolan, Black, Penk, Robinowitz, & DeFord, 1985; Silverman et al., 1996, 1998) although effects have been transient in some studies (Magura, Casriel, Goldsmith, Strug, & Lipton, 1988). The success of contingency contracting relies on behavioral principles, and careful design and implementation are required. For example, voucher-reinforcement for smoking cessation demonstrated differing outcomes for fixed versus progressive rate reinforcement schedules (Roll, Higgins, & Badger, 1996).

## Interpersonal Psychotherapy (IPT)

Long-term substance abuse is associated with multiple social and interpersonal problems, and relationships often become severely strained. Based on the principle that disturbances in interpersonal functioning are related to depressive disorders, IPT techniques were initially developed to focus on clients' difficulties, improve interpersonal skills, expand social support, and decrease depressive symptoms (Klerman, Weissman, Rounsaville, & Chevron, 1984; Rounsaville, Glazer, Wilber, Weissman, & Kleber, 1983; Rounsaville, Gawin, & Kleber, 1985). IPT is adapted to substance use disorders, and the therapist helps clients identify and change maladaptive interpersonal patterns in relationships and recognize the influence of substance use on interactions. IPT is designed as a time-limited, supportive intervention, and has been applied to eating disorders as well (Fairburn, Jones, Peveler, Connor, & Hope, 1991; Wilfley et al., 1993).

Extending this approach focused on interpersonal relationships, approaches that include couples, family members, and multiple systems (e.g., home, school, and work in multisystemic therapy) have also demonstrated efficacy in addressing addictive behaviors (Henggeler & Borduin, 1995; Stanton & Shadish, 1997; Waldron, 1997).

## Couple and Family Therapies

Positive couple and family environments are associated with better treatment outcomes (Moos, Finney, & Cronkite, 1990). Because interpersonal conflict is associated with relapse after treatment (Marlatt & Gordon, 1985), interventions to enhance couple and family functioning hold promise for improving treatment outcomes of substance use disorder. Couple and family treatment interventions motivate the substance abusing family member to enter treatment, support change efforts once initiated, and alter family interactions to provide a more conducive environment for maintaining abstinence. Strategies for reestablishing trust, increasing positive interactions, enhancing communication skills, and increasing problem solving and conflict resolution are established components of empirically validated couple and family therapies (O'Farrell, 1995). An important preliminary step involves evaluating the potential for domestic violence and appropriate provisions for the safety of all involved.

Multidimensional family therapy (MDFT) is a promising family-based therapy for adolescent substance abusers, with intervention strategies for teen, parent, and extrafamilial relationships (Liddle, 1995). Work with parents may include supportive therapy, education about adolescence, training in parental monitoring, family-management skills, and appropriate negotiating skills. The clinician provides support and empathy, problem solving, and assistance to the teen in making changes. Parents and teens are seen together to work on communication facilitation. MDFT interventions have been effective in treating adolescent drug abuse and improving conflictual teen–parent interactions (Diamond & Liddle, 1996; Liddle, 1995).

Multisystemic therapy (MST) has shown favorable results with adolescents who are involved in a variety of antisocial behaviors, including substance abuse (Henggeler, Melton, & Smith, 1992; Henggeler, Schoenwald, & Pickrel, 1995). Interventions are developed in collaboration with family members and delivered in the natural setting (e.g., home and school) to enhance generalization. Emphasis is placed on preserving the family system. Family, school, community, and peer influences on adolescent development and behaviors are addressed. Therapy intensity is adjusted based on client need (Henggeler et al., 1997). Positive outcomes have included improvements in family cohesion, peer relations, and reductions in future arrests, criminal behaviors, and substance use.

## Community Reinforcement

The Community reinforcement approach (CRA) recognizes the powerful influence of environmental contingencies and was developed to incorporate social, recreational, family, and job-related reinforcers into treatment (Smith & Meyers, 1995). Individually tailored skills training to improve these areas, as well as substance-related skills, are important elements of this behavioral treatment approach (e.g., communication skills, problem solving, drink refusal training, job counseling, recreational counseling, marital therapy). A key component of CRA is functional analysis of both substance-related and non-substance-related behaviors. Thoughts, feelings, events, and behaviors preceding and following substance use are assessed, and the function of substance use is explored with the client. This analysis helps to identify "high-risk" situations and develop coping strategies to manage or avoid these situations without resuming substance use. Additionally, a similar analysis is conducted for non-substance-related activities to assist the client in identifying pleasurable experiences other than alcohol or drug use. Strong support has been demonstrated for CRA with alcohol, cocaine, marijuana, and heroin abusers (Azrin, Sisson, Meyers, & Godley, 1982; Higgins et al., 1993; Smith, Meyers, & Delaney, 1998).

Couples, family, multisystemic, and community reinforcement approaches extend the influence of interventions beyond the specialized substance treatment setting to incorporate the client's environment. Generalization of skills learned in therapy settings is likely to be enhanced by including natural environmental contexts, and environmental contingencies can be enlisted to aid in the recovery process. In addition to these psychotherapeutic and environmental interventions, pharmacological interventions to address physiological aspects of substance dependence, it has been shown are effective for some substances of abuse.

## Pharmacotherapies

Pharmacotherapies for substance-related addictions work through various mechanisms: relieving withdrawal, reducing craving (replacement), blocking the reinforcing effects of drug consumption, or counterconditioning aversive responses. No medication can cure substance use disorders, but some pharmacotherapies reduce substance-related problems, as well as symptoms, associated with concomitant psychiatric disorders.

Short-term interventions for alcohol detoxification and short-term withdrawal include administration of benzodiazepines, slowly tapering the dose during a 5–7 day period (Schuckit, 1996). Long term pharmacotherapies include disulfiram (Antabuse®), which causes a severe adverse reaction to alcohol shortly after consumption and reduces the likelihood of relapses. Naltrexone, an opiate antagonist, has shown promising results in reducing relapse and severity of relapse to alcohol (O'Malley, Jaffe, et al., 1992; Volpicelli, Alterman, Hayashida, & O'Brien, 1992). Variable compliance with disulfiram and naltrexone therapy compromises the efficacy of these treatments. Acamprosate is a medication that increases GABA activity and decreases glutamate action with few side effects. Although not yet available in the United States, acamprosate has shown modest clinical benefits in extending initial abstinence, reducing drinking days, and increasing the proportion of patients who remained abstinent in initial human trials in Europe (Sass, Soyka, Mann, & Zieglgansberger, 1996; Whitworth et al., 1996).

Two opiate replacement therapies have significantly improved outcomes for opiate disorders. Methadone is a long-acting (~24 hours), orally administered opiate that shares many pharmacological features with heroin. Due to cross-tolerance and the long half-life of methadone, the risks of illicit injection opiate use (e.g., impurity of "street" drugs, crime, HIV risk) are significantly reduced (Ball & Ross, 1991). L-alpha-Acetylmethadol (LAAM) is even longer acting (48–72 hours) and has also shown evidence that it reduces illicit opiate use, increases the duration of treatment participation, and reduces criminal behaviors (Hubbard, Craddock, Flynn, Anderson, & Etheridge, 1997; Ling, Charuvastra, Kaim, & Klett, 1976). Although improved outcomes have clearly been demonstrated, opiate replacement therapies continue to be stigmatized by some, based on the premise that one addiction is just being replaced by another. Although technically correct, a properly dosed methadone treatment coupled with ancillary services (e.g., self-help groups, psychotherapy, and access to condoms; Calsyn, Meinecke, Saxon, & Stanton, 1992; Calsyn et al., 1994) facili-

tates stable functioning. The long-acting properties of replacement therapies reduce the rapid cycling of euphoria, withdrawal, and drug seeking associated with short-acting, illegally obtained opiates such as heroin (Zweben & Sorensen, 1988). Naltrexone, an opiate antagonist, demonstrated modest reduction in heroin use in clinical trials. However, heroin addicts are more difficult to retain in this type of pharmacotherapy than in opiate replacement therapies (O'Brien, 1996; Tapert et al., 1998).

Nicotine replacement therapies (e.g., nicotine transdermal patch, gum, and nasal sprays) reduce the symptoms of nicotine withdrawal and have been helpful in achieving initial abstinence among smokers (Hughes, 1993). Modest but long-term (6–12 months) improved rates of abstinence have been achieved using these products as adjuncts to cognitive-behavioral relapse prevention approaches (O'Brien, 1996). One study examined the effect of the dose of nicotine patches and found that abstinence rates improved with increased doses (0, 7, 14, 21 mg; Transdermal Nicotine Study Group, 1991). Replacement therapies are the most developed pharmacotherapies for smoking cessation, but antidepressant medications such as buproprion (Wellbutrin®, Zyban®) may reduce nicotine craving (O'Brien & McKay, 1998). Clonidine, an antihypertensive agent that reduces alcohol and opiate withdrawal, also reduces tobacco withdrawal and craving, although beneficial effects are short-lived (Covey & Glassman, 1991; Niaura, Brown, Goldstein, Murphy, & Abrams, 1996). The mechanism of action for clonidine is not clear, and some studies suggest that effects may be limited to women (Covey & Glassman, 1991; Hughes, 1993). Mecamylamine, a nicotinic blocking agent that prevents the subjective reinforcing effects of tobacco use, is under investigation but has significant side effects that reduce treatment compliance (Hughes, 1993).

For patients with concomitant mental health disorders, treating persisting psychiatric symptoms improves substance abuse outcome. Negative affective states, frequently experienced by those with comorbid disorders, have been identified as relapse precursors (Marlatt, 1985). Thus, pharmacological interventions to reduce negative mood would also be likely to improve substance use outcomes. As an example, the selective serotonergic re-uptake inhibitor, fluoxetine, is effective in treating major depression, and decreases in both depressive symptoms and alcohol consumption have been demonstrated among depressed individuals with alcohol dependence (Cornelius et al., 1997).

In summary, medications have demonstrated robust effectiveness in ameliorating withdrawal symptoms, modest efficacy in reducing alcohol and nicotine cravings, and significant benefits in replacing illicit opiates. Pharmacotherapies are most useful in a comprehensive treatment program that involves psychological interventions described previously (O'Brien, 1996; Schuckit, 1996). To date, medications have not been identified that are effective in treating other substances of abuse (O'Brien, 1996).

Research has repeatedly demonstrated that initial addictive behavior changes, like other behavioral changes, are difficult to maintain over time. Often, a complete lifestyle change is beneficial. Various residential arrangements designed to promote substance-free living help extend gains achieved through psychosocial interventions and pharmacotherapy. Extended living arrangements following addictions treatment are also needed due to the prevalence of substance use disorders among homeless individuals (e.g., Bassuk, Rubin, & Lauriat, 1984).

## Therapeutic Communities and Residential Treatment Facilities

Abstinence-focused residential facilities are known by a variety of names: sober living environments, halfway houses, recovery homes, residential treatment programs, and therapeutic communities, to name a few. They all share a common emphasis on providing substance-free living environments but vary in the methods and services offered. Many short-term inpatient and outpatient substance abuse treatment programs advise clients to reside in this type of environment for at least several months after initial abstinence, based on empirical findings of improved outcomes (Hubbard et al., 1997; Moos, King, & Patterson, 1996).

Community residential facilities provide substance-free environments to assist substance abusers between hospital discharge and subsequent independent living. Typically, continuous staffing is provided and is available for emergencies (Moos et al., 1994). Individual and group counseling, vocational and discharge planning, and connection with community resources such as self-help programs are common components of

these facilities. Contracts for this type of residential program have been provided for 60 days of care and 30-day extensions, if needed, by the Department of Veterans Affairs since 1980 in response to the need for a transitional environment. Research on outcomes has evidenced reduced readmission rates for patients who participated in these residential programs (Moos et al., 1994).

Therapeutic communities (TCs) are based on "family" models; members of the program act as a surrogate family, helping each other to change substance-related behaviors (De Leon, 1989; Sorensen, Acampora, & Iscoff, 1984). TCs emphasize increasing residents' self-esteem, self-reliance, and use of social supports, and provide education, vocational services, and, after several months of abstinence, independent living arrangements. Any substance use usually results in immediate expulsion to preserve the drug-free environment. Length of stay varies, but a year or longer is common to accomplish the complete transition to drug-free living.

Alternatively, if an individual is not considering treatment or is resistant to abstinence-focused interventions, alternative intervention strategies that target reducing the negative or harmful consequences of alcohol and drug use may be beneficial.

## Harm Reduction

Harm reduction techniques, which emerged from a public health approach to substance abuse, focus on strategies for reducing the negative consequences of substance use (Marlatt, 1998). Harm reduction interventions operate at both the individual and public policy levels. The approach is pragmatic and nonjudgmental and is designed to engage individuals on their own terms while reducing personal and societal harm due to substance use. An advantage of harm reduction approaches is the potential to engage non-treatment-seeking individuals. Abstinence is viewed as an ideal (no risk for harm), but behavior changes that move the individual along a continuum away from harm are viewed as steps in the right direction. These approaches address risky behaviors that co-occur with substance use, such as unsafe sexual practices, violence, and driving while intoxicated. Harm reduction strategies for illicit drug users include drug replacement interventions (e.g., methadone) and programs to reduce the risks of drug administration (e.g., clean needle exchange programs and education to reduce the risks of needle use; Tapert et al., 1998). Reviews of studies on needle exchange programs (NEPs) report decreased rates of HIV risk behaviors (e.g., reductions in needle sharing and giving away used needles) and some evidence of reductions in subcutaneous abscesses and hepatitis B and C (Lurie et al., 1993). As another example of harm reduction strategies, a harm reduction intervention with college students was associated with significant reductions in both drinking and harmful consequences, compared to students assigned to a nonintervention group (Marlatt et al., 1998). An excellent, comprehensive presentation on harm reduction principles and strategies is provided by Marlatt (1998).

Project MATCH (Project MATCH Research Group, 1997) compared three different treatments and tested the hypothesis that matching substance abusers to treatments based on personal attributes would result in superior treatment outcomes. Clients were randomly assigned to 12-Step Facilitation (TSF), Cognitive Behavioral Coping Skills Therapy (CBT), or Motivational Enhancement Therapy (MET), and received the manual-driven, individually administered treatment. Extensive baseline assessments of client attributes facilitated evaluation of outcomes as a function of the type of treatment received (see Nathan et al., this volume for details). At 12 months posttreatment, clients had substantially reduced drinking from pretreatment levels in all three treatments. However, few client-treatment matching hypotheses were supported. Generalizations of results are limited by the sample studied, which excluded drug-dependent, homeless, psychiatrically diagnosed, and cognitively impaired individuals, and by delivery of treatment in a format not typical of standard practice. Thus, efficacy, but not effectiveness, of treatments was addressed by Project MATCH. Finally, the absence of a control group prohibits investigating the natural course in this specialized population.

The Drug Abuse Treatment Outcome Study (DATOS; Hubbard et al., 1997) examined substance use and life functioning outcomes of 3000 patients in eleven metropolitan areas during the 12 months following treatment. Four types of treatments were evaluated: long-term residential, outpatient drug-free programs, short-term inpatient, and methadone maintenance. Major reductions in most types of drug use were observed in the year following treatment relative to pretreatment use in all four treatment formats. In long-term residential programs, weekly heroin and cocaine use dropped by 66%, and marijuana and heavy alcohol use were reduced by more than 50% from the pretreatment to the posttreatment year. The weekly use of alcohol and all drugs was reduced by 50% in outpatient drug-free programs, and weekly use was 33% of pretreatment levels for those treated in short-term inpatient programs. In methadone maintenance programs, weekly heroin use declined by 33%, and weekly cocaine use was reduced by 50% from pretreatment levels, although marijuana and heavy alcohol use did not change after treatment. Rates of suicidal thoughts and attempts declined in all groups except the methadone clients. Predatory criminal activities and risky sexual behaviors were significantly reduced, but physical health limitations and less than full-time employment remained high in all treatment types.

DATOS evaluated the effect of treatment length on outcome. Clients who received 3 months or more of treatment in long-term residential programs and outpatient drug-free programs reported lower rates of drug use at 12-month follow-up than clients who were treated for less than 3 months. Methadone maintenance clients who remained in the programs used significantly less heroin than clients who dropped out. Reduced illegal activity, risky sexual behaviors, and unemployment were also associated with longer treatment duration, but cocaine, marijuana, and alcohol use were not. These findings were generally consistent with previous major drug treatment studies (Drug Abuse Reporting Program [Simpson & Sells, 1982] and Treatment Outcome Prospective Study [Hubbard et al., 1989]). In summary, the DATOS results confirmed that participation in drug treatment is associated with positive changes in substance use and life functioning in the year after treatment and that clients who remain in treatment longer than 3 months receive more benefits. DATOS findings must be considered in the context of two study limitations: data relied solely on self-reports without corroboration from biological tests or collateral interviews, and only 70% of follow-up interviews were completed.

## Special Populations

No understanding of substance use is complete without acknowledging the special circumstances and variations in use, assessment, treatment, and outcome for different populations. Sensitivity to the unique characteristics and issues potentially relevant to individual clients is important in all phases of therapeutic contact. Following are some factors associated with commonly encountered special populations.

### Women

Men and women experience many aspects of substance abuse similarly, but some important gender differences affect consequences and treatment for females. The most widely recognized issue for women is the teratogenic effect of substances on fetal development. Fetal alcohol syndrome (FAS) seen in the infants of women who consume large amounts of alcohol during pregnancy involves a cluster of physical (e.g., facial dysmorphology and small stature) and neuropsychological (e.g., mental retardation and attentional impairment) effects that persist throughout the life-span. Less severe fetal alcohol effects (FAE) have been documented at lower levels of alcohol consumption. Alcohol is not uniformly teratogenic, suggesting complex relationships with factors such as drinking patterns, gestational period, nutrition, and genetics.

Cigarette smoking is related to retarded fetal growth, premature birth, and low birth weight, and effects appear related to smoking levels (Collins, 1993). Cocaine use during pregnancy increases the likelihood of slow fetal growth, low birth weight, early labor, spontaneous abortion, and sudden infant death syndrome (Fox, 1994; Miller & Hyatt, 1992; Zuckerman et al., 1989), although other studies demonstrate modest effects of cocaine when drinking, smoking, and nutrition are considered (Lester, LaGasse, Freier, & Brunner, 1996). Infants born to mothers addicted to cocaine are irritable, respond excessively to stimulation, and show impaired motor coordination, and these effects are detectable months later (Cole & Cole, 1993). Mothers addicted to heroin or methadone give birth to babies who are also addicted; treatment is often necessary shortly after birth to avoid potentially life-threatening withdrawal. These infants are more likely to be premature, underweight, and at risk for respiratory illnesses. Mortality is twice as high for neonates of opiate-addicted mothers (Bolton, 1983; Ostrea & Chavez, 1979). Detoxification causes irritability, tremors,

disturbed sleep, and diminished motor control in these infants. Impaired attention and motor control have been documented up to a year later (Jones & Lopez, 1990). Other gynecologic and obstetric problems are more common for women who smoke cigarettes, or abuse alcohol or drugs (Collins, 1993).

A relationship between victimization and trauma (e.g., childhood sexual abuse, domestic violence) and substance abuse has been documented in female populations (Downs, Miller, & Gondoli, 1987; Miller, Downs, & Gondoli, 1989), increasing the need for comprehensive assessment in these domains and treatment to address concomitant posttraumatic stress disorder, if indicated. Although women may face more consequences for substance abuse than men, services may be less available and less utilized by women (Dawson, 1996). Child-care responsibilities, limited financial resources, and societal stigmatization can be greater barriers to treatment for substance-abusing women than for men (Collins, 1993).

### Adolescents

Substance use and related disorders are relatively common during adolescence (typically defined as ages 13 to 20) and have implications for adult functioning. Unique risk factors, consequences, diagnostic criteria, assessment approaches, and treatment methods are pertinent to understanding substance abuse and dependence during the teenage years. For youth, substance abuse may be considered a cluster of problem behaviors, rather than an independent diagnosis (Donovan & Jessor, 1985). Problem behavior theory describes adolescent deviance as a single factor of unconventionality in which a variety of problematic behaviors co-occur, such as drug taking, smoking, precocious sexual involvement, gambling, and involvement in other criminal and health-threatening behaviors (Donovan & Jessor, 1985; Newcomb & Bentler, 1989).

Families and peers influence problem behavior and initiation of substance involvement. The influence of peers and the desire to "fit in" with group norms increases throughout child and adolescent development and is the most robust risk factor for early substance use (Bentler, 1992; Costanzo & Shaw, 1966). Peers influence exposure and access to drugs, model use or abstinence, and act as powerful reinforcers regarding substance use decisions. Youths select their peer groups and are selected by peers largely on the basis of shared values and interests (Dishion, Patterson, & Reid, 1988). Youths with social networks composed of substance users are likely to assume beliefs and values consistent with a substance-using lifestyle (Tapert et al., 1999). Youths without role models who reinforce healthy coping strategies are more likely to use (Holden et al., 1988; Tucker, 1982) or continue to abuse substances (Myers & Brown, 1990; Richter, Brown, & Mott, 1991). By contrast, positive social supports offset potential substance-related problems that may emerge in youth (Newcomb & Bentler, 1988b).

Negative health consequences for youth have been linked to abuse or dependence on the most commonly used substances. Teen smokers have increased rates of respiratory problems, and teen drinkers and drug users are more likely to experience motor vehicle crashes and other traumatic injuries (Aarons et al., 1999). Modest cognitive deficits have been associated with substance abuse in adolescence (Moss, Kirisci, Gordon, & Tarter, 1994), and withdrawal symptoms have been related to decreased retention of information and poor visuospatial functioning (Tapert & Brown, 1999).

Diagnostic criteria for substance abuse and dependence are based on adult symptom patterns. However, adolescents have characteristic substance use profiles and life consequences. Substance-involved adolescents typically use multiple intoxicating substances (Brown et al., 1994; Stewart & Brown, 1995). Adolescents can experience preoccupation with substances, loss of control over substance use, and reckless behavior while using, but are less likely than adults to report continued use despite medical problems (Martin, Arria, Mezzich, & Bukstein, 1993; Stewart & Brown, 1995). Current diagnostic criteria may not accurately capture all adolescent problematic substance use patterns. For example, abuse criteria lack applicability to adolescent life demands and form a less useful diagnostic construct (Martin, Kaczynski, Maisto, Bukstein, & Moss, 1995; Martin, Langenbucher, Kaczynski, & Chung, 1996).

Optimal assessment tools used with adolescents tailor wording to an appropriate reading level, acknowledge that polysubstance use is the norm for adolescent substance abusers, use computer administration formats when possible (Wright, Aquilino, & Supple, 1998), and consider the previously mentioned diagnostic challenges. The Personal Experience Inventory (Winters & Henly, 1989) is a self-report measure that assesses the severity of substance use and psychosocial functioning in adolescents. The Problem Severity scales in this well-validated self-report instrument discriminate between clinical and nonclinical adolescent samples (Henly & Winters, 1988). The Adolescent Diagnostic Interview (Winters & Henly, 1993) is a structured interview developed to assess substance use disorders, global functioning, psychosocial stressors, and cognitive functioning. Extensive information beneficial in treatment planning for adolescents is attained with this instrument which has demonstrated sound psychometric characteristics. Similarly, the Teen Addiction Severity Index (Kaminer, Bukstein, & Tarter, 1991), modeled after the adult Addiction Severity Index, collects substance-related information across domains of adolescent life functioning. Adequate psychometric properties have been reported (Kaminer, Wagner, Plummer, & Seifer, 1993).

Avenues to success for youths with substance use disorders, include (1) engaging in treatment programs that incorporate family involvement or (2) participating in activities that are incompatible with substance use (e.g., sports, jobs, active participation in academics, and volunteer activities; Brown et al., 1994). Multidimensional family therapy (Liddle, 1995) is a family-based therapy that focuses on engaging the youth in the treatment process. Multisystemic therapy (Henggeler et al., 1992, 1995) works with teens, parents, school systems, community resources, and peers to decrease problem behaviors (see previous section on Treatments for more detail on these therapies). Incorporating families to the extent possible helps many recovering teens. However, involvement in healthy activities is critical for success for teens whose parents have substance use disorders or other major problems.

## Elderly

Substance use and substance-related disorders are less prevalent among the elderly (over age 65) than in younger populations (Graham, 1986). However, characterization of substance use problems in older adults is hampered by assessment challenges. Older drinkers often underreport consumption and problems (Atkinson & Kofoed, 1982; Graham, 1986), and many assessment instruments have not been validated with older adults. Diagnostic criteria for role obligations and social functioning are insensitive for seniors with limited responsibilities and social networks and cause substance problems to go unnoticed. Additionally, symptoms of substance use disorders may resemble other age-related illnesses (e.g., dementia, malnutrition, or bone damage) and may complicate the diagnostic picture (Schuckit, 1990). Identifying substance abuse in this population is important, however, because more than 75% of adults over the age of 65 take prescription medications; many of them interact adversely with alcohol, tobacco, and illicit drugs (e.g., Adams, 1995). Due to physiological changes and medical problems associated with aging, the elderly are more sensitive to alcohol and drug effects and the synergistic effects of substances; Morgan et al., 1996; Smith, 1995). The MAST has been adapted specifically to assess problem drinking in older adults (Michigan Alcohol Screening Test—Geriatric Version; Blow et al., 1992).

Suggestions for treating older problem substance users include (1) avoiding confrontation and increasing the supportive nature of therapy; (2) focusing on coping skills related to loneliness, depression, and social isolation rather than occupational or relationship issues; (3) slowing the pace of group-based skills training; (4) addressing medical and transportation needs (Schonfeld & Dupree, 1995); and (5) specifically tailoring printed materials to an older audience (including seniors in photos and graphics, content specific to older age groups, especially the benefits of quitting at any age (Morgan et al., 1996). Older adults have treatment outcomes similar to those of adults in general (Kashner, Rodell, Ogden, Guggenheim, & Karson, 1992; Kofoed, Tolson, Atkinson, Toth, & Turner, 1987).

## Psychiatric Comorbidity

Individuals with other mental health disorders have a twofold increase in lifetime risk of alcohol abuse or dependence and a fourfold increase in lifetime risk of drug abuse or dependence. Among individuals with alcohol use disorders, 37% had another psychiatric disorder. Over half of those with drug use disorders have also had histories of psychiatric disorders (Regier et al., 1990). Substance use disorders and concomitant psychiatric comorbidity are often associated with a poor prog-

nosis (e.g., Dickey & Azeni, 1996; Ouimette, Finney, & Moos, 1997; Rounsaville, Kosten, Weissman, & Kleber, 1986). Many clients with severe mental health disorders have difficulty connecting with substance-related self-help organizations for a variety of reasons (Noordsy, Schwab, Fox, & Drake, 1996). Youths with comorbid mood disorders and who start abusing substances at younger ages evidence greater difficulty maintaining problem-free status after treatment (Brown et al., 1994; Tapert et al., 1999).

Substance intoxication, chronic use effects, and withdrawal states can mimic symptoms of other psychiatric disorders, including depression, anxiety, paranoia, delusions, and hallucinations (Boutros & Bowers, 1996; Brown & Schuckit, 1988; Brown, Irwin, & Schuckit, 1991). Many alcohol-dependent individuals report clinical levels of depression when admitted for treatment, but only a small minority remains clinically depressed 4 weeks later (Brown & Schuckit, 1988). Similar findings have been reported for cocaine abusers (Brown, Monti et al., 1998). Correspondingly, many in treatment for alcohol problems report elevated levels of state anxiety at admission, which typically reduce to normal levels following several weeks of abstinence (Brown et al., 1991). Psychotic symptoms induced by substance intoxication or withdrawal (e.g., alcohol, stimulants, and cannabinols) also tend to remit within days of abstinence. Exceptions include amphetamine-induced psychotic symptoms experienced by some abusers for up to a year or more of abstinence and PCP-induced psychotic symptoms that last for up to 30 days following the most recent use (Bacon, Granholm, & Withers, 1998). Accurate assessment determines whether psychiatric symptoms are substance-induced and likely to remit with abstinence or are indicative of an independent psychiatric disorder that requires specific treatments. Making this evaluation can be difficult, and the following guidelines are suggested:

1. The Timeline Technique (Bacon et al., 1998; Schuckit & Hesselbrock, 1994) involves constructing a lifetime calendar delineating the timing of specific substance dependence symptoms, psychiatric symptoms, and periods of abstinence. The clinician can evaluate whether psychiatric symptoms occurred before or after the onset of substance dependence, as well as whether psychiatric symp-

toms were experienced during periods of abstinence.

2. Familiarity with the quality and severity of substance-specific intoxication and withdrawal symptoms (Bacon et al., 1998) and the duration of abstinence required for substance-induced symptom remission (e.g., Brown et al., 1991, 1994) will aid clinical evaluation.

3. A family history of psychiatric disorders with evidence of genetic influence (e.g., schizophrenia, bipolar disorders) may be indicative of independent psychiatric disorders.

4. Patients with concomitant psychiatric disorders are more likely to require repeated treatment for substance dependence (Rounsaville, Dolinsky, Babor, & Meyer, 1987).

### Ethnicity and Culture

Substance use and problem development is influenced by genetic, social, and environmental factors, all of which may interact with culture. The Epidemiological Catchment Area (ECA) Study found prevalence rates of lifetime substance abuse or dependence comparable between African-American and Caucasian adults (Helzer, Burnam, & McEvoy, 1991), but African-Americans experience more social and medical consequences than Caucasians (Caetano & Schafer, 1996). Hispanic men have relatively high rates of alcohol use and abuse, whereas Hispanic women have low rates (Lex, 1987), and drug use rates are lower for Hispanics than Caucasians (Robins & Regier, 1991). Acculturation and U.S. nativity have been reported as risk factors for illicit drug use among Mexican-Americans (Vega, Alderete, Kolody, & Anguila-Gaxiola, 1998). Alcohol abuse and dependence are high among American Indians and Alaskan natives. The age-adjusted death rate due to alcohol dependence is nearly seven times higher than the overall U. S. rate (U. S. Department of Health and Human Services, 1997). Substantial variations are found in substance use patterns in relation to tribal affiliation, and some tribes now report high rates of abstinence.

Asian-Americans have lower rates of alcohol consumption, abuse, and dependence (Klatsky, Siegelaub, Landy, & Friedman, 1983), partially due to genetic influences that reduce their ability to metabolize alcohol, resulting in aversive physi-ological reactions to drinking among some Asian individuals. Jewish samples evidence particularly low rates of alcohol abuse and dependence (Weissman, Myers, & Harding, 1980).

### HIV

Substance use continues to be significantly associated with HIV transmission. Methadone maintenance, LAAM, needle exchange programs, and community information programs demonstrate favorable HIV risk reduction for injection drug users (Ling et al., 1976; Magura, Rosenblum, & Rodriguez, 1998). Needle exchange and community outreach programs reach injection drug users who are not in treatment programs (Peterson, Dimeff, Tapert, & Stern, 1998). Risky sexual behaviors are more resistant to change (Haverkos, 1998). Alcohol reduces inhibitions and increases the likelihood of risky sexual activity (Steele & Josephs, 1990). Stimulant intoxication is associated with participation in highly risky sexual behaviors, but substance abuse treatment can result in reduced numbers of sexual partners (Shoptaw, Reback, Frosch, & Rawson, 1998). In summary, interventions decrease HIV risk by reducing the frequency of injection, decreasing needle sharing, and reducing risky sexual behaviors (Iguchi, 1998; Shoptaw et al., 1998).

## General Recommendations

Substance use disorders are common mental health problems in our society and bear significant personal and societal consequences. The severity of problems may range from brief experimentation to protracted, life-threatening alcohol or drug involvement. Several models were presented that have been employed to conceptualize why people repeatedly engage in these harmful behaviors. Current models incorporate evidence from studies of genetics, conditioning, social learning, behavioral economics, and cognitive psychology. These theories guide our understanding of the way addiction processes are developed, maintained, and best treated.

Given the documented prevalence of substance use disorders, particularly in mental health settings, it is recommended that brief screening assessments for substance involvement and substance-related problems be conducted routinely. Positive results on screening assessments indicate the need for more extensive assessment. Detailed substance assessments should incorporate evaluation of comorbid mental health disorders that may influence clinical course and treatment planning decisions. In the event that assessments indicate problem substance use, the client's current motivation to change should be discussed, and motivational enhancement strategies should be initiated based on the motivational level or stage.

Diverse treatment options are available for substance use disorders. Enlisting client participation in the treatment planning process and willingness to "meet the client" toward goal establishment have been empirically supported. Consideration of nonabstinence goals can be discussed openly and nonjudgmentally, weighing the advisability of this alternative goal in view of the client's unique characteristics. Clear professional advice should be provided in support of abstinence when indicated, but research findings indicate that confrontation should be avoided. Situations in which abstinence should clearly be advised include the presence of liver disease, pregnancy, severe dependence, and the use of prescription medications. Studies support the involvement of family members in substance disorder treatments. Increasing availability and access to valued alternative nondrug activities will support the long-term process of behavior change. Pharmacotherapies in conjunction with psychotherapy interventions often enhance substance use outcomes for some substances, including tobacco, alcohol, and opiates.

Although significant progress has been made in understanding and treating substance use disorders in recent decades, significant limitations in our knowledge remain. Findings have not yet provided many clear guidelines to clinicians in attempting to optimally match clients to types of treatments. Some researchers have advised that clinicians maintain a stance of "informed eclecticism, an openness to a variety of approaches that is guided by scientific evidence" (Miller & Hester, 1995). Additionally, little is known regarding the efficacy and effectiveness of group versus individual interventions for substance use disorders.

A third limitation in the substance abuse treatment field is the lack of information on whether comorbid psychiatric disorders are best treated simultaneously or independently and whether treatments should be integrated. Researchers are working to address these questions, and client prefer-

ences may be the best guide for treatment selection at this time. For example, preliminary studies of tobacco cessation interventions conducted concurrently with other substance abuse treatment have suggested some success in outcomes. Researchers have proposed dual-diagnosis treatments for substance abusers with severe mental health disorders such as schizophrenia and bipolar disorders (Drake, 1996; Osher & Kofoed, 1989), and research findings are beginning to support such integrated treatments (e.g., Drake, McHugo, & Noordsy, 1993; Drake, Mueser, Clark, & Wallach, 1996).

# References

Aarons, G. A., Brown, S. A., Coe, M. T., Myers, M. G., Garland, A. F., Ezzet-Lofstram, R., Hazen, A. L., & Hough, R. L. (1999). Adolescent alcohol and drug abuse and health. *Journal of Adolescent Health, 6,* 412–421.

Adams, K. M., Gilman, S., Koeppe, R. A., Kluin, K. J., Brunberg, J. A., Dede, D., Berent, S., & Kroll, P. D. (1993). Neuropsychological deficits are correlated with frontal hypometabolism in positron emission tomography studies of older alcoholic patients. *Alcoholism: Clinical and Experimental Research, 17,* 205–210.

Adams, W. L. (1995). Interactions between alcohol and other drugs. *International Journal of the Addictions, 30,* 1903–1923.

Adams, W. L., Barry, K. L., & Fleming, M. F. (1996). Screening for problem drinking in older primary care patient. *Journal of the American Medical Association, 276,* 1964–1967.

Alcoholics Anonymous. (1980). *Alcoholics Anonymous.* New York: Author.

Alcoholics Anonymous World Services. (1976). *Alcoholics Anonymous: The story of how many thousands of men and women have recovered from alcoholism* (3rd ed.). New York: Author.

Alexander, B. K., & Hadaway, P. F. (1982). Opiate addiction: The case for an adaptive orientation. *Psychological Bulletin, 92,* 367–381.

Allen, J. P., & Columbus, M. (Eds.). (1995). *Assessing alcohol problems: A guide for clinicians and researchers.* Bethesda, MD: National Institute on Alcohol Abuse and Alcoholism.

Allison, W. M., & Jerrom, D. W. (1984). Glue sniffing: A pilot study of the cognitive effects of long-term use. *International Journal of the Addictions, 19,* 453–458.

American Psychiatric Association. (1994). *Diagnostic and statistical manual of mental disorders* (4th ed.). Washington, DC: Author.

Anker, A. L., & Crowley, T. J. (1982). Use of contingency contracts in specialty clinics for cocaine abuse. In L. S. Harris (Ed.), *Problems on drug dependence* (pp. 452–459). Rockville, MD: National Institute on Drug Abuse.

Annis, H. M. (1982). *Inventory of drinking situations.* Toronto, Ontario, Canada: Addiction Research Foundation.

Annis, H. M., & Martin, G. (1985). *Inventory of drug-taking situations*. Toronto, Ontario, Canada: Addiction Research Foundation of Ontario.

Annis, H. M., & Graham, J. M. (1988). *Situational Confidence questionnaire (SCQ-39): User's guide*. Toronto, Ontario, Canada: Addiction Research Foundation of Ontario.

Ardila, A., Rosselli, M., & Strumwasser, S. (1991). Neuropsychological deficits in chronic cocaine abusers. *International Journal of Neuroscience, 57*, 73–79.

Atkinson, R. M., & Kofoed, L. L. (1982). Alcohol and drug abuse in old age: A clinical perspective. *Substance & Alcohol Actions/Misuse, 3*, 353–368.

Azrin, N. H., Sisson, W., Meyers, R., & Godley, M. (1982). Alcoholism treatment by disulfiram and community reinforcement therapy. *Journal of Behavior Therapy & Experimental Psychiatry, 13*, 105–112.

Babor, T. F., Stephens, R. S., & Marlatt, G. A. (1987). Verbal report methods in clinical research on alcoholism: Response bias and its minimization. *Journal of Studies on Alcohol, 48*, 410–424.

Babor, T. F., Brown, J., & Del Boca, F. K. (1990). Validity of self-reports in applied research on addictive behaviors: Fact or fiction? *Addictive Behaviors, 12*, 5–32.

Babor, T. F., Hesselbrock. V., Meyer, R. E., & Shoemaker, W. (1994). *Types of alcoholics: Evidence from clinical, experimental, and genetic research* (Vol. 708). New York: New York Academy of Sciences.

Bacon, A., Granholm, E., & Withers, N. (1998). Substance-induced psychosis. *Seminars in Clinical Neuropsychiatry, 3*, 70–79.

Baer, J. S., Stacy, A., & Larimer, M. (1991). Biases in the perception of drinking norms among college students. *Journal of Studies on Alcohol, 52*, 580–586.

Baer, J. S., & Brady Murch, H. (1998). Harm reduction, nicotine, and smoking. In G. A. Marlatt (Ed.), *Harm reduction: Pragmatic strategies for managing high-risk behaviors* (pp. 122–144). New York: Guilford.

Ball, J. C., & Ross, A. (1991). *The effectiveness of methadone maintenance treatment*. New York: Springer Verlag.

Bassuk, E. L., Rubin, L., & Lauriat, A. (1984). Is homelessness a mental health problem? *American Journal of Psychiatry, 141*, 1546–1550.

Baumrind, D., & Moselle, K. A. (1985). A developmental perspective on adolescent drug use. *Advances in Alcohol and Substance Use, 5*, 41–67.

Beatty, W. W., Hames, K. A., Blanco, C. R., Nixon, S. J., & Tivis, L. J. (1996). Visuospatial perception, construction and memory in alcoholism. *Journal of Studies on Alcohol, 57*, 136–143.

Bentler, P. M. (1992). Etiologies and consequences of adolescent drug use: Implications for prevention. *Journal of Addictive Diseases, 11*, 47–61.

Bergman, H., Borg, S., Engelbrektson, K., & Vikander, B. (1989). Dependence on sedative-hypnotics: Neuropsychological impairment, field dependence and clinical course in a 5-year follow-up study. *British Journal of Addiction, 84*, 547–553.

Blane, H. T., & Leonard, K. E. (1987). *Psychological theories of drinking and alcoholism*. New York: Guilford.

Block, R. I., Farinpour, R., & Braverman, K. (1992). Acute effects of marijuana on cognition: Relationship to chronic effects and smoking techniques. *Pharmacology, Biochemistry and Behavior, 43*, 907–917.

Blow, F. C., Brower, K. J., Schulenberg, J. E., Demo-Dananberg, L. M., Young, K. J., & Beresford, T. P. (1992). The Michigan Alcoholism Screening Test: Geriatric version (MAST-G): A new elderly-specific screening instrument. *Alcoholism: Clinical and Experimental Research, 16*, 172.

Bolton, P. J. (1983). Drugs of abuse. In D. F. Hawkins (Ed.) *Drugs and pregnancy: Human teratogenesis and related problems*. Edinburgh, Scotland: Churchill Livingstone.

Boudin, H. M., Valentine, V. E., III, Inghram, R. D., Jr., Brantley, J. M., Ruiz, M. R., Smith, G. G., Catlin, R. P., III, & Regan, E. J., Jr. (1977). Contingency contracting with drug abusers in the natural environment. *The International Journal of the Addictions, 12*(1), 1–16.

Boutros, N. N., & Bowers, M. D. (1996). Chronic substance-induced psychotic disorders: State of the literature. *Journal of Neuropsychiatry and Clinical Neuroscience, 8*, 262–269.

Bradley, K. A., Bush, K., McDonell, M. B., Malone, T., & Fihn, S. D. (1998). Screening or problem drinking: Comparison of CAGE and AUDIT. *Journal of General Internal Medicine, 13*, 379–388.

Brandt, J., Butters, N., Ryan, C., & Bayog, R. (1983). Cognitive loss and recovery in long-term alcohol abusers. *Archives of General Psychiatry, 40*, 435–442.

Bray, R. M., Guess, L. L., Marsden, M. E., & Herbold, J. R. (1989). Prevalence, trends, and correlates of alcohol use, nonmedical drug use, and tobacco use among U.S. military personnel. *Military Medicine, 154*, 1–11.

Brickman, P., Robinowitz, V. C., Karuza, J., Jr., Coates, D., Cohn, E., & Kidder, L. (1982). Models of helping and coping. *American Psychologist, 37*, 368–384.

Brook, J. S., Whiteman, M., & Gordon, A. S. (1983). Stages of drug use in adolescence: Personality, peer, and family correlates. *Developmental Psychology, 19*, 269–277.

Brown, R. A., Burgess, E. S., Sales, S. D., Evans, D. M., & Miller, I. W. (1998). Reliability and validity of a smoking timeline follow-back interview. *Psychology of Addictive Behaviors, 12*, 101–112.

Brown, R. A., Monti, P. M., Myers, M. G., Martin, R. A., Rivinus, T., Dubreuil, M. E., & Rohsenow, D. J. (1998). Depression among cocaine abusers in treatment: Relation to cocaine and alcohol use and treatment outcome. *American Journal of Psychiatry, 155*, 220–225.

Brown, S. A. (1985). Reinforcement expectancies and alcoholism treatment outcome after a one-year follow-up. *Journal of Studies on Alcohol, 46*, 304–308.

Brown, S. A., Christiansen, B. A., & Goldman, M. A. (1987). The Alcohol Expectancy Questionnaire: An instrument for the assessment of adolescent and adult alcohol expectancies. *Journal of Studies on Alcohol, 48*, 483–491.

Brown, S. A., & Schuckit, M. A. (1988). Changes in depression among abstinent alcoholics. *Journal of Studies on Alcohol, 49*, 412–417.

Brown, S. A., Irwin, M., & Schuckit, M. A. (1991). Changes in anxiety among abstinent male alcoholics. *Journal of Studies on Alcohol, 52*, 55–61.

Brown, S. A., Mott, M. A., & Stewart, M. A. (1992). Adolescent alcohol and drug abuse. In C. E. Walker & M. C. Roberts (Eds.), *Handbook of clinical child psychology* (2nd ed., pp. 677–693). New York: Wiley.

Brown, S. A. (1993). Drug effect expectancies and addictive behavior change. *Experimental and Clinical Psychopharmacology, 1*, 55–67.

Brown, S. A., Myers, M. G., Mott, M. A., & Vik, P. W. (1994). Correlates of success following treatment for adolescent substance abuse. *Applied & Preventive Psychology, 3*, 61–73.

Brown, S. A., Vik, P. W., Patterson, T. L., Grant, I., & Schuckit, M. A. (1995). Stress, vulnerability and adult alcohol relapse. *Journal of Studies on Alcohol, 56*, 538–545.

Brown, S. A., Myers, M. G., Lippke, L., Tapert, S. F., Stewart, D. G., & Vik, P. W. (1998). Psychometric evaluation of the Customary Drinking and Drug Use Record (CDDR): A measure of adolescent alcohol and drug involvement. *Journal of Studies on Alcohol, 59*, 427–438.

Brown, S. A., Tate, S.R., Vik, P.W., Haas, A. L., & Aarons, G. A. (1999). Modeling of alcohol use mediates the effect of family history of alcoholism on adolescent alcohol expectancies. *Experimental and Clinical Psychopharmacology, 7*, 20–27.

Bush, K., Kivlahan, D. R., McDonell, M. B., Fihn, S. D., & Bradley, K. A. (1998). The AUDIT alcohol consumption questions (AUDIT-C): An effective brief screening test for problem drinking. *Archives of Internal Medicine, 158*, 1789–1795.

Caetano, R., & Schafer, J. (1996). DSM-IV alcohol dependence and drug abuse/dependence in a treatment sample of whites, blacks, and Mexican Americans. *Drug and Alcohol Dependence, 43*, 93–101.

Calsyn, D. A., Meinecke, C., Saxon, A. J., & Stanton, V. (1992). Risk reduction in sexual behavior: A condom giveaway program in a drug abuse treatment clinic. *American Journal of Public Health, 82*, 1536–1658.

Calsyn, D. A., Wells, E. A., Saxon, A. J., Jackson, T. R., Wrede, A. F., Stanton, V., & Fleming, C. (1994). Contingency management of urinalysis results and intensity of counseling services have an interactive impact on methadone maintenance treatment outcome. *Journal of Addictive Diseases, 13*, 47–63.

Carlen, P. L., Penn, R. D., Fornazzari, L., Bennett, J., Wilkinson, A., & Wortzman, G. (1986). Computerized tomographic scan assessment of alcoholic brain damage and its potential reversibility. *Alcoholism: Clinical & Experimental, 10*, 226–232.

Carlin, A. S., Grant, I., Adams, K. M., & Reed, R. (1979). Is phencyclidine (PCP) abuse associated with organic mental impairment? *American Journal of Drug and Alcohol Abuse, 6*, 273–281.

Carroll, K. M., Rounsaville, B. J., Nick, C., Gordon, L. T., Wirtz, P. W., & Gawin, F. H. (1994). One year follow-up of psychotherapy and pharmacotherapy for cocaine dependence: Delayed emergence of psychotherapy effects. *Archives of General Psychiatry, 51*, 989–997.

Carroll, K. M. (1995). Methodological issues and problems in the assessment of substance use. *Psychological Assessment, 7*, 349–358.

Chassin, L., Pillow, D. R., Curran, P. J., Molina, B. S. G., & Barrera, M. (1993). Relation of parental alcoholism to early adolescent substance use: A test of three mediating mechanisms. *Journal of Abnormal Psychology, 102*, 3–19.

Christiansen, B. A., Goldman, M. S., & Brown, S. A. (1996). Alcohol Expectancy Questionnaire Adolescent Form. *NIAAA Treatment Assessment Instrument Handbook*. Rockville, MD: National Institute of Alcohol Abuse and Alcoholism.

Cloninger, C. R., Bohman, M., & Sigvardsson, S. (1981). Inheritance of alcohol abuse: Cross-fostering analysis of adopted men. *Archives of General Psychiatry, 38*, 861–868.

Cohen, S. (1981). Adolescence and drug abuse: Biomedical consequences. *NIDA Research Monograph, 38*, 104–112.

Cole, M. C., & Cole, S. R. (1993). *The development of children* (2nd ed.). New York: Scientific American Books.

Colletti, G., Supnick, J. A., & Payne, T. J. (1985). The Smoking Self-Efficacy Questionnaire (SSEQ): Preliminary scale development and validation. *Behavioral Assessment, 7*, 249–260.

Collins, R. L. (1993). Women's issues in alcohol use and cigarette smoking. In J. S. Baer, G. A. Marlatt, & R. J. McMahon (Eds.), *Addictive behaviors across the life span* (pp. 274–306). Newbury Park, CA: Sage.

Connors, G. J. (1995). Screening for alcohol problems. In J. P. Allen & M. Columbus (Eds.), *Assessing alcohol problems: A guide for clinicians and researchers*. Bethesda, MD: National Institute on Alcohol Abuse & Alcoholism.

Cornelius, J. R., Salloum, I. M., Ehler, J. G., Jarrett, P. J., Cornelius, M. D., Perel, J. M., Thase, M. E., & Black, A. (1997). Fluoxetine in depressed alcoholics. A double-blind, placebo-controlled trial. *Archives of General Psychiatry, 54*, 700–705.

Costanzo, P., & Shaw, M. (1966). Conformity as a function of age level. *Child Development, 37*, 967–975.

Cottler, L. B., Schuckit, M. A., Helzer, J. E., Crowley, T., Woody, G., Nathan, P., & Hughes, J. (1995). The DSM-IV field trial for substance use disorders: Major results. *Drug & Alcohol Dependence, 38*, 59–69.

Covey, L. S., & Glassman, A. H. (1991). A meta-analysis of double-blind placebo-controlled trials of clonidine for smoking cessation. *British Journal of Addiction, 86*, 991–998.

Culver, C. M., & King, F. W. (1974). Neuropsychological assessment of undergraduate marijuana and LSD users. *Archives of General Psychiatry, 31*, 707–711.

Cunningham-Williams, R. M., Cottler, L. B., Compton, W. M., III, & Spitznagel, E. L. (1998). Taking chances: Problem gamblers and mental health disorders: Results from the St. Louis Epidemiologic Catchment Area study. *American Journal of Public Health, 88*, 1093–1096.

Davis, L. J., Hoffman, N. G., Morse, R. M., & Luehr, J. G. (1992). Substance Use Disorder Schedule (SUDDS): The equivalence and validity of a computer administered and an interviewer administered format. *Alcoholism: Clinical & Experimental Research, 16*, 250–254.

Dawson, D. A. (1996). Gender differences in the probability of alcohol treatment. *Journal of Substance Abuse, 8*, 211–225.

De Leon, G. (1989). Psychopathology and substance abuse: What we are learning from research in therapeutic communities. *Journal of Psychoactive Drugs, 21*, 177–188.

Diamond, G., & Liddle, H. A. (1996). Resolving a therapeutic impasse between parents and adolescents in multidimensional family therapy. *Journal of Consulting and Clinical Psychology, 64*, 481–488.

Dickey, B., & Azeni, H. (1996). Persons with dual diagnoses of substance abuse and major mental illness: Their excess costs of psychiatric care. *American Journal of Public Health, 86*, 973–977.

DiClemente, C. C., & Prochaska, J. O. (1998). Toward a comprehensive, transtheoretical model of change: Stages of change and addictive behaviors. In W. R. Miller & N. Heather (Eds.), *Treating addictive behaviors* (2nd ed., pp. 3–24). New York: Plenum.

Dishion, T. J., Patterson, G. R., & Reid, J. R. (1988). Parent and peer factors associated with drug sampling in early adolescence: Implications for treatment. *NIDA Research Monograph, 77*, 69–93.

Dolan, M. P., Black, J. L., Penk, W. E., Robinowitz, R., & DeFord, H. A. (1985). Contracting for treatment termination to reduce illicit drug use among methadone maintenance treatment failures. *Journal of Consulting and Clinical Psychology, 53*, 549–551.

Donovan, J. E., & Jessor, R. (1985). Structure of problem behavior in adolescence and young adulthood. *Journal of Consulting and Clinical Psychology, 53*, 890–904.

Downs, W. R., Miller, B. A., & Gondoli, D. M. (1987). Childhood experiences of parental physical violence for alcoholic women as compared with a randomly selected household sample of women. *Violence & Victims, 2*, 225–240.

Drake, R. E. (1996). Substance use reduction among patients with severe mental illness. *Community Mental Health Journal, 32*, 311–314.

Drake, R. E., McHugo, G. J., & Noordsy, D. L. (1993). Treatment of alcoholism among schizophrenic outpatients: 4-year outcomes. *American Journal of Psychiatry, 150*, 328–329.

Drake, R. E., Mueser, K. T., Clark, R. E., & Wallach, M. E. (1996). The course, treatment, and outcome of substance disorder in persons with severe mental illness. *American Journal of Orthopsychiatry, 66*, 42–51.

Duncan, D. F. (1977). Life stress as a precursor to adolescent drug dependence. *International Journal of the Addictions, 12*, 1047–1056.

Earleywine, M., & Newcomb, M. D. (1997). Concurrent versus simultaneous polydrug use: Prevalence, correlates, discriminant validity, and prospective effects on health outcomes. *Experimental & Clinical Pharmacology, 5*, 353–364.

Ehrman, R. N., & Robbins, S. J. (1994). Reliability and validity of 6-month timeline reports of cocaine and heroin use in a methadone population. *Journal of Consulting and Clinical Psychology, 62*, 843–850.

Ellickson, P. L., Hays, R. D., & Bell, R. M. (1992). Stepping through the drug use sequence: Longitudinal scalogram analysis of initiation and regular use. *Journal of Abnormal Psychology, 101*, 441–451.

Erdman, H., Klein, M. H., & Greist, J. H. (1983). The reliability of a computer interview for drug use/abuse information. *Behavior Research Methods and Instrumentation, 15*, 66–68.

Escobedo, L. G., Chorba, T. L., & Waxweiler, R. (1995). Patterns of alcohol use and the risk of drinking and driving among US high school students. *American Journal of Public Health, 85*, 976–978.

Fairburn, C. G., Jones, R., Peveler, R. C. O., Connor, M. E., & Hope, R. A. (1991). Three psychological treatments for bulimia nervosa: A comparative trial. *Archives of General Psychiatry, 48*, 463–469.

Forehand, R., Miller, K. S., Dutra, R., & Chance, M. W. (1997). Role of parenting in adolescent deviant behavior: Replication across and within two ethnic groups. *Journal of Consulting and Clinical Psychology, 65*, 1036–1041.

Fox, C. H. (1994). Cocaine use in pregnancy. *Journal of the American Board of Family Practices, 7*, 225–228.

Friedman, A. S., & Granick, S. (1994). Assessing drug abuse among adolescents and adults: Standardized instruments. Clinical Report Series. Rockville, MD: National Institute on Drug Abuse, NIH Publication No. 94-3757.

Gfroerer, J. C., Greenblatt, J. C., & Wright, D. A. (1997). Substance use in the US college-age population: Differences according to educational status and living arrangement. *American Journal of Public Health, 87*, 62–65.

Goldman, M. S., Brown, S. A., Christiansen, B. A., & Smith, G. T. (1991). Alcoholism and memory: Broadening the scope of alcohol-expectancy research. *Psychological Bulletin, 110*, 137–146.

Graham, K. (1986). Identifying and measuring alcohol abuse among the elderly: Serious problems with existing instrumentation. *Journal of Studies on Alcohol, 47*, 322–326.

Grant, B. (1997). Prevalence and correlates of alcohol use and DSM-IV alcohol dependence in the United States: Results of the National Longitudinal Alcohol Epidemiologic Survey. *Journal of Studies on Alcohol, 58*, 464–473.

Grove, W. M., Eckert, E. D., Heston, L., Bouchard, T. J., Jr., Segal, N., & Lykken, D. T. (1990). Heritability of substance abuse and antisocial behavior: A study of monozygotic twins raised apart. *Biological Psychiatry, 27*, 1293–1304.

Grunbaum, J. A., Basern-Engquist, K., & El Souki, R. (1996). Tobacco, alcohol, and illicit drug use among Mexican-American and non-Hispanic white high school students. *Substance Use & Misuse, 31*, 1279–1310.

Haaga, D. A. F., & Kirk, L. (1998). Strategies for tobacco cessation. In W. R. Miller & N. Heather (Eds.), *Treating addictive behaviors* (2nd ed., pp. 245–258). New York: Plenum.

Harwood, H., Fountain, D., Livermore, G., & The Lewin Group. (1998). The economic costs of alcohol and drug abuse in the United States, 1992. Rockville, MD: National Institute on Drug Abuse and National Institute on Alcohol Abuse and Alcoholism.

Haverkos, H. W. (1998). HIV/AIDS and drug abuse: Epidemiology and prevention. *Journal of Addictive Diseases, 17*, 91–103.

Hawkins, R. O. (1982). Adolescent alcohol abuse: A review. *Developmental and Behavioral Pediatrics, 3*, 83–87.

Heather, N. (1995). Brief intervention strategies. In R. K. Hester & W. R. Miller (Eds.), *Handbook of alcoholism treatment approaches: Effective alternatives* (2nd ed.). Boston: Allyn & Bacon.

Helzer, J. E., Burnam, A., & McEvoy, L. (1991). Alcohol abuse and dependence. In L. N. Robins & D. A. Regier (Eds.), *Psychiatric disorders in America: The Epidemiologic Catchment Area Study* (pp. 81–115). New York: The Free Press.

Henggeler, S. W., Borduin, C. M., Melton, G. B., Mann, B. J., et al. (1991). Effects of multisystemic therapy on drug use and abuse in serious juvenile offenders: A progress report from two outcome studies. *Family Dynamics of Addiction Quarterly, 1*, 40–51.

Henggeler, S. W., Melton, G. V., & Smith, L. A. (1992). Family preservation using multisystemic therapy: An effective alternative to incarcerating serious juvenile offenders. *Journal of Consulting and Clinical Psychology, 60*, 953–961.

Henggeler, S. W., & Borduin, C. M. (1995). Multisystemic treatment of serious juvenile offenders and their families. In I. M. Schwartz & P. AuClaire (Eds.), *Home-based services for troubled children.* (pp. 113–130). Lincoln: University of Nebraska Press.

Henggeler, S. W., Schoenwald, S. K., & Pickrel, S. G. (1995). Multisystemic therapy: Bridging the gap between university- and community-based treatment. *Journal of Consulting and Clinical Psychology, 63*, 709–717.

Henggeler, S. W., Rowland, M. D., Pickrel, S. G., Miller, S. L., Cunningham, P. B., Santos, A. B., Schoenwald, S. K., Randall, J., & Edwards, J. E. (1997). Investigating family-based alternatives to institution-based mental health services for youth:

Lessons learned from the pilot study of a randomized field trial. *Journal of Clinical Child Psychology, 26,* 226–233.

Henly, G. A., & Winters, K. C. (1988). Development of problems severity scales for the assessment of adolescent alcohol and drug abuse. *International Journal of the Addictions, 23,* 65–85.

Higgins, S. T., Budney, A. J., Bickel, W. K., Hughes, J. R., Foerg, F., & Badger, G. (1993). Achieving cocaine abstinence with a behavioral approach. *American Journal of Psychiatry, 150,* 763–769.

Holden, M. G., Brown, S. A., & Mott, M. A. (1988). Social support network of adolescents: Relation to family alcohol abuse. *American Journal of Drug and Alcohol Abuse, 14,* 487–498.

Horn, J. I., Skinner, H. A., Wanberg, K., & Foster, F. M. (1984). *Alcohol Dependence Scale (ADS).* Toronto, Ontario, Canada: Addiction Research Foundation.

Horvath, A. T. (1997). Alternative support groups. In J. H. Lowinson, P. Ruiz, R. B. Millman, & J. G. Langrod (Eds.), *Substance abuse: A comprehensive textbook* (3rd ed.). Baltimore: Williams & Wilkins.

Hubbard, R. L., Marsden, M. E., Rachal, J. V., Harwood, H. J., Cavanaugh, E. R., & Ginsburg, H. M. (1989). *Drug abuse treatment: A national study of effectiveness.* Chapel Hill: University of North Carolina Press.

Hubbard, R. L., Craddock, S. G., Flynn, P. M., Anderson, J., & Etheridge, R. M. (1997). Overview of 1-year follow-up outcomes in the Drug Abuse Treatment Outcome Study (DATOS). *Psychology of Addictive Behaviors, 11,* 261–278.

Hughes, J. R. (1993). Pharmacotherapy for smoking cessation: Unvalidated assumptions, anomalies, and suggestions for future research. *Journal of Consulting and Clinical Psychology, 61,* 751–760.

Hundleby, J. D., & Mercer, G. W. (1987). Family and friends as social environments and their relationship to young adolescents' use of alcohol, tobacco, and marijuana. *Journal of Marriage and the Family, 49,* 151–164.

Hunt, W. A., Barnett, L. W., & Branch, L. G. (1971). Relapse rates in addiction programs. *Journal of Consulting and Clinical Psychology, 27,* 455–456.

Iguchi, M. R. (1998). Drug abuse treatment as HIV prevention: Changes in social drug use patterns might also reduce risk. *Journal of Addictive Diseases, 17,* 9–18.

Institute of Medicine. (1990). *Treating drug problems,* Vol. 1. Washington, DC: National Academy Press.

Irwin, M., Baird, S., Smith, T. L., & Schuckit, M. (1988). Use of laboratory tests to monitor heavy drinking by alcoholic men discharged from a treatment program. *American Journal of Psychiatry, 145,* 595–599.

Jellinek, E. M. (1960). *The disease model of alcoholism.* Highland Park, NJ: Hillhouse Press.

Jernigan, T. L., Pfefferbaum, A., & Zatz, L. M. (1986). CT correlates in alcoholism. In I. Grant (Ed.), *Neuropsychiatric correlates in alcoholism* (pp. 21–36). Washington, DC: American Psychiatric Association.

Jessor, R., & Jessor S. L. (1977). *Problem behavior and psychosocial development: A longitudinal study of youth:* New York: Academic Press.

Johnston, L. D., O'Malley, P. M., & Bachman, J. G. (1998). National survey results on drug use from the Monitoring the Future study, 1975–1997. Volume I: Secondary school students. Rockville, MD: National Institute on Drug Abuse.

Johnston, L. D., O'Malley, P. M., & Bachman, J. G. (1999).

National survey results on drug use from the Monitoring the Future study, 1975–1998. Volume I: Secondary school students. Rockville, MD: National Institute on Drug Abuse.

Jones, C. L., & Lopez, R. E. (1990). Drug abuse and pregnancy. In I. R. Merkatz & J. E. Thompson (Eds.), *New perspectives on prenatal care.* New York: Elsevier.

Kaminer, Y., Bukstein, O., & Tarter, R. E. (1991). The Teen-Addiction Severity Index: Rationale and reliability. *International Journal of the Addictions, 26,* 219–226.

Kaminer, Y., Wagner, E., Plummer, B., & Seifer, R. (1993). Validation of the Teen Severity Index (T-ASI): Preliminary findings. *American Journal of Addictions, 2,* 250–254.

Kandel, D. (1978). Convergences in prospective longitudinal surveys of drug use in normal populations. In D. Kandel (Ed.), *Longitudinal research in drug use: Empirical findings and methodological issues.* Washington, DC: Hemisphere-Wiley.

Kandel, D. B., Davies, M., Karus, D., & Yamaguchi, K. (1986). The consequences in young adulthood of adolescent drug involvement. *Archives of General Psychiatry, 43,* 746–754.

Kandel, D. B., Yamaguchi, K., & Chen, K. (1992). Stages of progression in drug involvement from adolescence to adulthood: Further evidence for the gateway theory. *Journal of Studies on Alcohol, 53,* 447–457.

Kaplan, H. B. (1977). Antecedents of deviant responses: Predicting from a general theory of deviant behavior. *Journal of Youth and Adolescence, 7,* 253–277.

Kashner, T. M., Rodell, D. E., Ogden, S. R., Guggenheim, F. G., & Karson, C. N. (1992). Outcomes and costs of two VA inpatient programs for older alcoholics. *Hospital Community Psychiatry, 43,* 985–989.

Kessler, R. C., McGonagle, K. A., Zhao, S., Nelson, C. B., Hughes, M., Eshlemen, S., Wittchen, H., & Kendler, K. S. (1994). Lifetime and 12-month prevalence of DSM-III-R psychiatric disorders in the United States: Results from the National Comorbidity Survey. *Archives of General Psychiatry, 51,* 8–19.

Kessler, R. C., Crum, R. M., Warner, L. A., Nelson, C. B., Schulenberg, J., & Anthony, J. C. (1997). Lifetime of-occurrence of DSM-III-R alcohol abuse and dependence with other psychiatric disorders in the national Comorbidity Survey. *Archives of General Psychiatry, 54,* 313–321.

Klatsky, A. L., Siegelaub, A. B., Landy, C., & Friedman, G. D. (1983). Racial patterns of alcoholic beverage use. *Alcoholism: Clinical & Experimental Research, 7,* 372–377.

Klerman, G. L., Weissman, M. M., Rounsaville, B. J., & Chevron, E. S. (1984). *Interpersonal Psychotherapy of Depression.* New York: Basic Books.

Kofoed, L., Tolson, R., Atkinson, R. M., Toth, R., & Turner, J. (1987). Treatment compliance of older alcoholics: An elder-specific approach is superior to "mainstreaming". *Journal of Studies on Alcohol, 48,* 47–51.

Kohn, P. M., & Annis, H. M. (1977). Drug use and four kinds of novelty-seeking. *British Journal of Addiction, 72,* 135–141.

Kolar, A. F., Brown, B. S., Weddington, W. W., & Ball, J. C. (1990). A treatment crisis: Cocaine use by clients in methadone maintenance programs. *Journal of Substance Abuse Treatment, 7,* 101–107.

Koob, G. F., & Bloom, F. E. (1988). Cellular and molecular mechanisms of drug dependence. *Science, 242,* 715–723.

Koob, G. F., Caine, S. B., Parsons, L., Markou, A., & Weiss, F. (1997). Opponent process model and psychostimulant addiction. *Pharmacology, Biochemistry & Behavior, 57,* 513–521.

Koob, G. F., & Le Moal, M. (1997). Drug abuse: Hedonic homeostatic dysregulation. *Science, 278,* 52–58.

Koob, G. F., Rocio, M., Carrera, A., Gold, L. H., Heyser, C. J., Maldonado-Irizarry, C., Markou, A., Parsons, L. H., Roberts, A. J., Schulteis, G., Stinus, L., Walker, J. R., Weissenborn, R., & Weiss, F. (1998). Substance dependence as a compulsive behavior. *Journal of Psychopharmacology, 12,* 39–48.

Krueger, R. F., Caspi, A., Moffitt, T. E., Silva, P. A., & McGee, R. (1996). Personality traits are differentially linked to mental disorders: A multitrait-multidiagnosis study of an adolescent birth cohort. *Journal of Abnormal Psychology, 105,* 299–312.

Krystal, J. H., & Price, L. H. (1992). Chronic 3,4-methylenedioxymethamphetamine (MDMA) use: Effects on mood and neuropsychological function. *American Journal of Drug and Alcohol Abuse, 18,* 331–341.

Kuhn, C., Swartzwelder, S., & Wilson, W. (1998). *Buzzed.* New York–London: W.W. Norton.

Lester, B. M., LaGasse, L., Freier, K., & Brunner, S. (1996). Studies of cocaine-exposed human infants. In *Behavioral studies of drug-exposed offspring: Methodological issues in human and animal* (pp. 175–210). Rockville, MD: U.S. Department of Health and Human Services.

Lex, B. W. (1987). Review of alcohol problems in ethnic minority groups. *Journal of Consulting and Clinical Psychology, 55,* 293–300.

Liddle, H. A. (1995). Conceptual and clinical dimensions of a multidimensional, multisystems engagement strategy in family-based adolescent treatment. *Psychotherapy, 32*(1), 39–58.

Liddle, H. L., & Dakof, G. (1995). Family-based treatment for adolescent drug use: State of the science. In E. Rahdert & D. Czechowicz (Eds.), Adolescent drug abuse: Clinical assessment and therapeutic interventions (pp. 218–254). Rockville, MD: National Institute on Drug Abuse.

Ling, W., Charuvastra, V. C., Kaim, S. C., & Klett, J. (1976). Methadryl acetate and methadone as maintenance treatments for heroin addicts. *Archives of General Psychiatry, 33,* 709–720.

Ludwig, A. M., Wickler, A., & Stark, L. H. (1974). The first drink: Psychobiological aspects of craving. *Archives of General Psychiatry, 30,* 539–547.

Lundahl, L. H., Davis, T. M., Adesso, V. J., & Lukas, S. E. (1997). Alcohol expectancies: Effects of gender, age, and family history of alcoholism. *Addictive Behaviors, 22*(1), 115–125.

Lurie, P., Reingold, A. L., Lee, P. R., Bowser, B., Chen, D., Foley, J., Guydish, J., Kahn, J. G., Lane, S., & Sorenson, J. (1993). The public health impact of needle exchange programs in the United States and abroad, Vols. 1 and 2. Atlanta, GA: Centers for Disease Control.

Magura, S., Casriel, C., Goldsmith, D. S., Strug, D. L., & Lipton, D. S. (1988). Contingency contracting with polydrug-abusing methadone patients. *Addictive Behaviors, 13*(1), 113–118.

Magura, S., Rosenblum, A., & Rodriguez, E. M. (1998). Changes in HIV risk behaviors among cocaine-using methadone patients. *Journal of Addictive Diseases, 17,* 71–90.

Maisto, S. A., Sobell, M. B., Cooper, A. M., & Sobell, L. C. (1979). Test-retest reliability of retrospective self-reports in three populations of alcohol abusers. *Journal of Behavioral Assessment, 1,* 315–326.

Maisto, S. A., McKay, J. R., & Connors, G. J. (1990). Self-report issues in substance abuse: State of the art and future directions. *Behavioral Assessment, 12,* 117–134.

Manschreck, T. C., Schneyer, M. L., Weisstein, C., Laughery, J., Rosenthal, J., Celada, T., & Bemer, J. (1990). Freebase cocaine and memory. *Comprehensive Psychiatry, 4,* 369–375.

Marks, G., & Miller, N. (1987). Ten years of research on the false-consensus effect: An empirical and theoretical review. *Psychological Bulletin, 102,* 72–90.

Marlatt, G. A. (1985). Relapse prevention: Theoretical rationale and overview of the model. In G. A. Marlatt & J. R. Gordon (Eds.), *Relapse prevention: Maintenance strategies in the treatment of addictive behaviors* (pp. 3–70). New York: Guilford.

Marlatt, G. A., & Gordon, J. R. (Eds.). (1985). *Relapse prevention: Maintenance strategies in the treatment of addictive behaviors.* New York: Guilford.

Marlatt, G. A. (1992). Substance abuse: Implications of a biopsychosocial model for prevention, treatment, and relapse prevention. In J. Grabowski & G. R. VandenBos (Eds.), *Psychopharmacology: Basic mechanisms and applied interventions* (pp. 131-162). Washington, DC: American Psychological Association.

Marlatt, G. A., & Tapert, S. F. (1993). Harm reduction: Reducing the risks of addictive behaviors. In J. S. Baer, G. A. Marlatt, & R. J. McMahon (Eds.), *Addictive behaviors across the life span: Prevention, treatment, and policy issues* (pp. 243–273). Newbury Park, CA: Sage.

Marlatt, G. A., Baer, J. S., & Quigley, L. A. (1995). Self-efficacy and addictive behavior. In A. Bandura (Ed.), *Self-efficacy in changing societies* (pp. 289–315). New York: Cambridge University Press.

Marlatt, G. A. (Ed.). (1998). *Harm reduction: Pragmatic strategies for managing high-risk behaviors.* New York: Guilford.

Marlatt, G. A. (1998). Harm reduction around the world: A brief history. In G. A. Marlatt (Ed.), *Harm reduction: Pragmatic strategies for managing high-risk behaviors* (pp. 30–48). New York: Guilford.

Marlatt, G. A., Baer, J. S., Kivlahan, D. R., Dimeff, L. A., Larimer, M. E., Quigley, L. A., Somers, J. M., & Williams, E. (1998). Screening and brief intervention for high-risk college student drinkers: Results from a 2-year follow-up assessment. *Journal of Consulting & Clinical Psychology, 66,* 604–615.

Martin, C. S., Arria, A. M., Mezzich, A. C., & Bukstein, O. G. (1993). Patterns of polydrug use in adolescent alcohol abusers. *American Journal of Drug and Alcohol Abuse, 19,* 511–521.

Martin, C. S., Kaczynski, N. A., Maisto, S. A., Bukstein, O. M., & Moss, H. B. (1995). Patterns of DSM-IV alcohol abuse and dependence symptoms in adolescent drinkers. *Journal of Studies on Alcohol, 56,* 672–680.

Martin, C. S., Langenbucher, J. W., Kaczynski, N. A., & Chung, T. (1996). Staging in the onset of DSM-IV alcohol symptoms in adolescents: Survival/hazard analyses. *Journal of Studies on Alcohol, 57,* 549–558.

Maxmen, J. S., & Ward, N. G. (1995). *Psychotropic drugs fast facts.* New York–London: W.W. Norton.

Mayfield, D., McLeod, G., & Hall, P. (1974). The CAGE Questionnaire: Validation of a new alcoholism screening instrument. *American Journal of Psychiatry, 131,* 1121–1123.

McCrady, B. S. (1994). Alcoholics Anonymous and behavior therapy: Can habits be treated as diseases? Can diseases be treated as habits? *Journal of Consulting and Clinical Psychology, 62,* 1159–1166.

McCrady, B. S., & Delaney, S. I. (1995). Self-help groups. In R. K. Hester & W. R. Miller (Eds.), *Handbook of alcoholism treatment approaches: Effective alternatives* (2nd ed., pp. 160–175). Boston: Allyn & Bacon

McGinnis, J. M., & Foege, W. H. (1993). Actual causes of death in the United States. *Journal of the American Medical Association, 270,* 2207–2212.

McGlothlin, W. H., & West, L. J. (1968). The marijuana problem: An overview. *American Journal of Psychiatry, 125,* 1126–1134.

McGue, M. (1993). From proteins to cognitions: The behavioral genetics of alcoholism. In E. R. Plomin & G. E. McClearn (Eds.), *Nature, nurture & psychology* (pp. 245–268). Washington, DC: American Psychological Association.

McGue, M., Sharma, A., & Benson, P. (1996). Parent and sibling influences on adolescent alcohol use and misuse: Evidence from a U.S. adoption cohort. *Journal of Studies on Alcohol, 57,* 8–18.

McGue, M. (1997). A behavioral-genetic perspective on children of alcoholics. *Alcohol Health & Research World, 21,* 210–217.

McLellan, A. T., Kusher, H., Metzger, D., Peters, R., Smith, I., Grissom, G., Pettinati H., & Argerious, M. (1992). The fifth edition of the Addiction Severity Index. *Journal of Substance Abuse Treatment, 9,* 199–213.

Miller, B. A., Downs, W. R., & Gondoli, D. M. (1989). Spousal violence among alcoholic women as compared to a random household sample of women. *Journal of Studies on Alcohol, 50,* 533–540.

Miller, W. R., & Rollnick, S. (1991). *Motivational interviewing: Preparing people to change addictive behavior.* New York: Guilford.

Miller, W. H., & Hyatt, M. C. (1992). Perinatal substance abuse. *American Journal of Drug and Alcohol Abuse, 18,* 247–261.

Miller, W. R. (1995). Increasing motivation for change. In R. K. Hester & W. R. Miller (Eds.), *Handbook of alcoholism treatment approaches: Effective alternatives* (2nd ed., pp. 89–104). Boston: Allyn & Bacon.

Miller, W. R., Brown, J. M., Simpson, R. L., Handmaker, N. S., Bien, T. H., Luckie, L. F., Montgomery, H. A., Hester, R. K., & Tonigan, J. S. (1995). What works? A methodological analysis of the alcohol treatment outcome literature. In R. K. Hester & W. R. Miller (Eds.), *Handbook of alcoholism treatment approaches: Effective alternatives* (2nd ed., pp. 12–44). Boston: Allyn & Bacon.

Miller, W. R., & Hester, R. K. (1995). Treatment for alcohol problems: Toward an informed eclecticism. In R. K. Hester & W. R. Miller (Eds.), *Handbook of alcoholism treatment approaches: Effective alternatives* (2nd ed., pp. 1–11). Boston: Allyn & Bacon.

Miller, W. R., & Brown, S. A. (1997). Why psychologists should treat alcohol and drug problems. *American Psychologist, 52,* 1269–1279.

Miller, W. R. (1998a). Enhancing motivation for change. In W. R. Miller & N. Heather (Eds.), *Treating addictive behaviors* (2nd ed., pp. 121–132). New York: Plenum.

Miller, W. R. (1998b). Researching the spiritual dimensions of alcohol and other drug problems. *Addiction, 93,* 979–990.

Millstein, S. G. (1987). Acceptability and reliability of sensitive information collected via computer interview. *Educational & Psychological Measurement, 47,* 523–533.

Mittenberg, W., & Motta, S. (1993). Effects of chronic cocaine abuse on memory and learning. *Archives of Clinical Neuropsychology, 8,* 477–483.

Monti, P. M., Abrams, D. B., Binkoff, J. A., & Zwick, W. R. (1990). Communication skills training, communication skills training with family and cognitive behavioral mood management training for alcoholics. *Journal of Studies on Alcohol, 51,* 263–270.

Monti, P. M., Rohsenow, D. J., Colby, S. M., & Abrams, D. B. (1995). Coping and social skills training. In R. K. Hester & W. R. Miller (Eds.), *Handbook of alcoholism treatment approaches: Effective alternatives* (2nd ed., pp. 221–241). Boston: Allyn & Bacon.

Monti, P. M., Gulliver, S. B., & Myers, M. G. (1994). Social skills training for alcoholics: Assessment and treatment. *Alcohol & Alcoholism, 29,* 627–637.

Moos, R. H., Finney, J. W., & Cronkite, R. C. (1990). *Alcoholism treatment: Context, process, and outcome.* New York: Oxford University Press.

Moos, R. H., Mertens, J. R., & Brennan, P. L. (1994). Rates and predictors of four-year readmission among late-middle-aged and older substance abuse patients. *Journal of Studies on Alcohol, 55,* 561–570.

Moos, R. H., King, M. J., & Patterson, M. A. (1996). Outcomes of residential treatment of substance abuse in hospital- and community-based programs. *Psychiatric Services, 47*(1), 68–74.

Morgan, G. D., Noll, E. L., Orleans, C. T., Rimer, B. K., Amfoh, P. H. K., & Bonney, G. (1996). Reaching midlife and older smokers: Tailored interventions for routine medical care. *Preventive Medicine, 25,* 346–354.

Morton, H. G. (1990). Occurrence and treatment of solvent abuse in children and adolescents. In D. J. K. Balfour (Ed.), *Psychotropic drugs of abuse* (pp. 431–451). New York: Pergamon Press.

Moss, H. B., Kirisci, L., Gordon, H. W., & Tarter, R. E. (1994). A neuropsychologic profile of adolescent alcoholics. *Alcoholism: Clinical & Experimental Research, 18,* 159–163.

Myers, M. G., & Brown, S. A. (1990). Coping responses and relapse among adolescent substance abusers. *Journal of Substance Abuse, 2,* 177–189.

Myers, M. G., & Brown, S. A. (1997). Cigarette smoking four years following treatment for adolescent substance abuse. *Journal of Child & Adolescent Substance Abuse, 7,* 1–15.

National Academy of Sciences. (1990). *Broadening the base of treatment for alcohol problems.* Washington, DC: National Academy Press.

Needle, R., Glynn, T., & Needle, M. (1983). Drug abuse: Adolescent addictions and the family. In R. Figley & H. McCubbin (Eds.), *Stress and the family* (pp. 37–52). New York: Brunner/Mazel.

Newcomb, M. D., & Bentler, P. M. (1988a). *Consequences of adolescent drug use: Impact on the lives of young adults.* Newbury Park, CA: Sage.

Newcomb, M. D., & Bentler, P. M. (1988b). Impact of adolescent drug use and social support on problems of young adults: A longitudinal study. *Journal of Abnormal Psychology, 97,* 64–75.

Newcomb, M. D., & Bentler, P. M. (1989). Substance use and abuse among children and teenagers. *American Psychologist, 44,* 242–248.

Niaura, R. S., Rohsenow, D. J., Binkoff, J. A., & Monti, P. M. (1988). Relevance of cue reactivity to understanding alcohol and smoking relapse. *Journal of Abnormal Psychology, 97,* 133–152.

Niaura, R., Brown, R. A., Goldstein, M. G., Murphy, J. K., & Abrams, D. B. (1996). Transdermal clonidine for smoking cessation: A double-blind randomized dose-response study. *Experimental and Clinical Psychopharmacology, 4,* 285–291.

Noordsy, D. L., Schwab, B., Fox, L., & Drake, R. E. (1996). The role of self-help programs in the rehabilitation of persons with severe mental illness and substance use disorders. *Community Mental Health Journal, 32*(1), 71–81; discussion 83–86.

O'Brien, C. P. (1996). Recent developments in the pharmacotherapy of substance abuse. *Journal of Consulting and Clinical Psychology, 64,* 677–686.

O'Brien, C. P., & McKay, J. R. (1998). Psychopharmacological treatments of substance use disorders. In P. E. Nathan & J. M. Gorman (Eds.), *A guide to treatments that work* (pp. 127–155). New York: Oxford University Press.

O'Farrell, T. J. (1995). Marital and family therapy. In R. K. Hester & W. R. Miller (Eds.), *Handbook of alcoholism treatment approaches: Effective alternatives* (2nd ed., pp. 195–220). Needham Heights, MA: Allyn & Bacon.

O'Malley, S., & Gawin, F. H. (1990). Abstinence symptomatology and neuropsychological impairment in chronic cocaine abusers. *NIDA Research Monograph, 101,* 179–190.

O'Malley, S., Adamse, M., Heaton, R. K., & Gawin, F. H. (1992). Neuropsychological impairment in chronic cocaine abusers. *American Journal of Drug and Alcohol Abuse, 18,* 131–144.

O'Malley, S. S., Jaffe, A., Change, G., Schottenfeld, R. S., Meyer, R. E., & Rounsaville, B. (1992). Naltrexone and coping skills therapy for alcohol dependence: A controlled study. *Archives of General Psychiatry, 49,* 881–887.

Osher, F. C., & Kofoed, L. L. (1989). Treatment of patients with psychiatric and psychoactive substance abuse disorders. *Hospital & Community Psychiatry, 40,* 1025–1030.

Ostrea, E. M., & Chavez, C. J. (1979). Perinatal problems (excluding neonatal withdrawal) in maternal drug addiction: A study of 830 cases. *Journal of Pediatrics, 94,* 292–295.

Ouimette, P. C., Finney, J. W., & Moos, R. H. (1997). Twelve-step and cognitive-behavioral treatment for substance abuse: A comparison of treatment effectiveness. *Journal of Consulting and Clinical Psychology, 65,* 230–240.

Pandina, R., & Schuele, J. (1983). Psychosocial correlates of alcohol and drug use of adolescent students and adolescents in treatment. *Journal of Studies on Alcohol, 44,* 950–973.

Perkins, H. W., & Berkowitz, A. D. (1986). Perceiving the community norms of alcohol use among students: Some research implications for campus alcohol education programming. *International Journal of the Addictions, 21,* 961–976.

Peterson, P. G., Dimeff, L. A., Tapert, S. F., & Stern, M. S. (1998). Harm reduction and HIV/AIDS prevention. In G. A. Marlatt (Ed.), *Harm reduction: Pragmatic strategies for managing high-risk behaviors* (pp. 218–297). New York: Guilford.

Pfefferbaum, A., Sullivan, E. V., Mathalon, D. H., Shear, P. K., Rosenbloom, M. J., & Lim, K. O. (1995). Longitudinal changes in magnetic resonance imaging brain volumes in abstinent and relapsed alcoholics. *Alcoholism: Clinical & Experimental Research, 19,* 1177–1191.

Pickens, R. W., Svikis, D. S., McGue, M., Lykken, D. T., Heston, L. L., & Clayton, P. J. (1991). Heterogeneity in the inheritance of alcoholism: A study of male and female twins. *Archives of General Psychiatry, 48,* 19–28.

Pickens, R. W., Svikis, D. S., McGue, M., & LaBuda, M. C. (1995). Common genetic mechanisms in alcohol, drug, and mental disorder comorbidity. *Drug & Alcohol Dependence, 39,* 129–138.

Pope, H. G., Jr., & Yurgelun-Todd, D. (1996). The residual cognitive effects of heavy marijuana use in college students. *Journal of the American Medical Association, 275,* 521–527.

Pope, H. G., Jr., Jacobs, A., Mialet, J.-P., Yurgelun-Todd, D., & Gruber, S. (1997). Evidence for a sex-specific residual effect of cannabis on visuospatial memory. *Psychotherapy & Psychosomatics, 66*(4), 179–184.

Project MATCH Research Group. (1997). Matching alcoholism treatments to client heterogeneity: Project MATCH posttreatment drinking outcomes. *Journal of Studies on Alcohol, 58,* 7–29.

Project MATCH Research Group. (1998). Matching alcoholism treatments to client heterogeneity: Project MATCH three-year drinking outcomes. *Alcoholism: Clinical & Experimental Research, 22,* 1300–1311.

Reed, R. J., Grant, I., & Rourke, S. B. (1992). Long-term abstinent alcoholics have normal memory. *Alcoholism: Clinical & Experimental Research, 16,* 677–683.

Regier, D. A., Farmer, M. E., Rae, D. S., Locke, B. Z., Keith, S. J., Judd, L. L., & Goodwin, F. K. (1990). Comorbidity of mental disorders with alcohol and other drug abuse: Results from the Epidemiological Catchment Area (ECA) study. *Journal of the American Medical Association, 264,* 2511–2518.

Richter, S. S., Brown, S. A., & Mott, M. A. (1991). The impact of social support and self-esteem on adolescent substance abuse treatment outcome. *Journal of Substance Abuse, 3,* 371–385.

Roberts, A. J., & Koob, G. F. (1997). The neurobiology of addiction: An overview. *Alcohol Health & Research World, 21,* 101–106.

Robins, L. N., Davis, D. H., & Nurco, D. N. (1974). How permanent was Vietnam drug addiction? In M. H. Greene & R. L. DuPont (Eds.), The epidemiology of drug abuse (NIDA Journal Supplement, Part 2, Vol. 64) . Washington, DC: U.S. Government Printing Office.

Robins, L. N., & Regier, D. A. (1991). *Psychiatric disorders in America: The Epidemiologic Catchment Area Study.* New York: The Free Press.

Robins, L. N. (1993). Vietnam veterans' rapid recovery from heroin addiction: A fluke or normal expectation? *Addiction, 88,* 1041–1054.

Roll, J. M., Higgins, S. T., & Badger, G. J. (1996). An experimental comparison of three different schedules of reinforcement of drug abstinence using cigarette smoking as an exemplar. *Journal of Applied Behavior Analysis, 29,* 495–505.

Room, R. (1990). Measuring alcohol consumption in the United States: Methods and rationales. In L. T. Kozlowski, H. M. Annis, H. D. Cappell, F. B. Glaser, M. S. Goodstadt, Y. Israel, H. Kalant, E. M. Sellers, & E. R. Vingilis (Eds.), *Research advances in alcohol and drug problems* (Vol. 10). New York: Plenum.

Rose, R. J., Kaprio, J., Winter, T., Koskenvuo, M., & Viken, R. J. (1999). Familial and socioregional environmental effects on abstinence from alcohol at age sixteen. *Journal of Studies on Alcohol, 13,* 63–74.

Ross, D. F., & Pihl, R. O. (1988). Alcohol, self-focus, and complex reaction-time performance. *Journal of Studies on Alcohol, 49,* 115–125.

Rounsaville, B. J., Glazer, W., Wilber, C. H., Weissman, M. M., & Kleber, H. D. (1983). Short-term interpersonal psychotherapy in methadone-maintained opiate addicts. *Archives of General Psychiatry, 40,* 629–636.

Rounsaville, B. J., Gawin, F., & Kleber, H. (1985). Interpersonal psychotherapy adapted for ambulatory cocaine abusers. *American Journal of Drug and Alcohol Abuse, 11,* 171–191.

Rounsaville, B. J., Kosten, T. R., Weissman, M. M., & Kleber, H. D. (1986). Prognostic significance of psychopathology in treated opiate addicts. A 2.5-year follow-up study. *Archives of General Psychiatry, 43,* 739–745.

Rounsaville, B. J., Dolinsky, Z. A., Babor, T. F., & Meyer, R. E. (1987). Psychopathology as a predictor of treatment outcome in alcoholics. *Archives of General Psychiatry, 44,* 505–513.

Rydon, P., Redman, S., Sanson-Fisher, R. W., & Reid, A. L. A. (1992). Detection of alcohol-related problems in general practice. *Journal of Studies on Alcohol, 53,* 197–202.

Sadava, S. W. (1987). Interactionist theories. In H. T. Blane & K. E. Leonard (Eds.), *Psychological theories of drinking and alcoholism* (pp. 90–130). New York: Guilford.

Sass, H., Soyka, M., Mann, K., & Zieglgansberger, W. (1996). Relapse prevention by acamprosate: Results from a placebo-controlled study on alcohol dependence. *Archives of General Psychiatry, 53,* 673–680.

Saunders, J. B., Aasland, O. G., Babor, T. F., De La Fuente, J. R., & Grant, M. (1993). Development of the Alcohol Use Disorders Identification Test (AUDIT): WHO Collaborative Project on Early Detection of Persons with Harmful Alcohol Consumption II. *Addiction, 88,* 791–804.

Schafer, J., & Brown, S. A. (1991). Marijuana and cocaine effect expectancies and drug use patterns. *Journal of Consulting & Clinical Psychology, 59,* 558–565.

Schinke, S. P., Botvin, G. J., & Orlandi, M. A. (1991). *Substance abuse in children and adolescents: Evaluation and intervention.* Newbury Park, CA: Sage.

Schmidt, L. G., Schmidt, K., Dufeu, P., Ohse, A., Rommelspacher, H., & Muller, C. (1997). Superiority of carbohydrate-deficient transferrin to g-glutamyltransferase in detecting relapse in alcoholism. *American Journal of Psychiatry, 154,* 75–80.

Schonfeld, L., & Dupree, L. W. (1995). Treatment approaches for older problem drinkers. *International Journal of the Addictions, 30,* 1819–1842.

Schuckit, M. A. (1985). Genetics and the risk for alcoholism. *Journal of the American Medical Association, 254,* 2614–2617.

Schuckit, M. A. (1989). *Drug and alcohol abuse: A clinical guide to diagnosis and treatment* (3rd ed.). New York: Plenum.

Schuckit, M. A. (1990). Introduction: Assessment and treatment strategies with the late life alcoholic. *Journal of Geriatric Psychiatry, 23,* 83–89.

Schuckit, M. A., & Hesselbrock, V. (1994). Alcohol dependence and anxiety disorders: What is the relationship? *American Journal of Psychiatry, 151,* 1723–1734.

Schuckit, M. A. (1995). *Drug and alcohol abuse: A clinical guide to diagnosis and treatment* (4th ed.). New York: Plenum.

Schuckit, M. A. (1996). Recent developments in the pharmacotherapy of alcohol dependence. *Journal of Consulting & Clinical Psychology, 64,* 669–676.

Schuckit, M. A., & Smith, T. L. (1996). An 8-year follow-up of 450 sons of alcoholic and control subjects. *Archives of General Psychiatry, 53,* 202–210.

Schuckit, M. A., Tipp, J. E., Smith, T. L., & Bucholz, K. K. (1997). Periods of abstinence following the onset of alcohol dependence in 1,853 men and women. *Journal of Studies on Alcohol, 58,* 581–589.

Segal, B., Huba, G. J., & Singer, J. L. (1980). *Drugs, daydreaming, and personality: A study of college youth.* City?, NJ: Erlbaum.

Selzer, M. L. (1971). The Michigan Alcoholism Screening Test: The quest for a new diagnostic instrument. *American Journal of Psychiatry, 127,* 1653–1658.

Shedler, J., & Block, J. (1990). Adolescent drug use and psychological health. *American Psychologist, 45,* 612–630.

Sher, K. J. (1991). *Children of alcoholics: A critical appraisal of theory and research.* Chicago: University of Chicago Press.

Sher, K. J. (1993). Children of alcoholics and the intergenerational transmission of alcoholism: A biopsychosocial perspective. In J. S. Baer, G. A. Marlatt, & R. J. McMahon (Eds.), *Addictive behaviors across the life span* (pp. 3–33). Newbury Park, CA: Sage.

Sher, K. J. (1997). Psychological characteristics of children of alcoholics. *Alcohol Health & Research World, 21,* 247–254.

Sher, K. J., Gershuny, B. S., Peterson, L., & Raskin, G. (1997). The role of childhood stressors in the intergenerational transmission of alcohol use disorders. *Journal of Studies on Alcohol, 58,* 414–427.

Shoptaw, S., Reback, C. J., Frosch, D. L., & Rawson, R. A. (1998). Stimulant abuse treatment as HIV prevention. *Journal of Addictive Diseases, 17,* 19–32.

Silverman, K., Higgins, S. T., Brooner, R. K., Montoya, I. D., Cone, E. J., Schuster, C. R., & Preston, K. L. (1996). Sustained cocaine abstinence in methadone maintenance patients through voucher-based reinforcement therapy. *Archives of General Psychiatry, 53,* 409–415.

Silverman, K., Wong, C. J., Umbrickt-Schneiter, A., Montoya, I. D., Schuster, C. R., & Preston, K. L. (1998). Broad beneficial effects of cocaine abstinence reinforcement among methadone patients. *Journal of Consulting and Clinical Psychology, 66,* 811–824.

Simpson, D. D., & Sells, S. B. (1982). Effectiveness of treatment for drug abuse: An overview of the DARP research program. *Advances in Alcohol and Substance Abuse, 2,* 7–29.

Skinner, H. A., & Allen, B. A. (1983). Does the computer make a difference? Computerized versus face-to-face self-report assessments of alcohol, drug and tobacco use. *Journal of Consulting and Clinical Psychology, 51,* 267–275.

Sklar, S. M., Annis, H. M., & Turner, N. E. (1997). Development and validation of the Drug-Taking Confidence Questionnaire: A measure of coping self-efficacy. *Addictive Behaviors, 22,* 655–670.

Smith, G. T., Goldman, M. S., Greenbaum, P. E., & Christiansen, B. A. (1995). Expectancy for social facilitation from drinking: The divergent paths of high-expectancy and low-expectancy adolescents. *Journal of Abnormal Psychology, 104,* 32–40.

Smith, J. E., & Meyers, R. J. (1995). The community reinforcement approach. In R. K. Hester & W. R. Miller (Eds.), *Handbook of alcoholism treatment approaches: Effective alternatives* (pp. 251–266). New York: Allyn & Bacon.

Smith, J. E., Meyers, R. J. & Delaney, H. D. (1998). The community reinforcement approach with homeless alcohol-dependent individuals. *Journal of Consulting and Clinical Psychology, 66,* 541–548.

Smith, J. W. (1995). Medical manifestations of alcoholism in the elderly. *The International Journal of the Addictions, 30,* 1749–1798.

Sobell, L. C., Toneatto, T., & Sobell, M. B. (1994). Behavioral assessment and treatment planning for alcohol, tobacco, and other drug problems: Current status with an emphasis on clinical applications. *Behavior Therapy, 25,* 533–580.

Sobell, L. C., Kwan, E., & Sobell, M. B. (1995). Reliability of a drug history questionnaire (DHQ). *Addictive Behaviors, 20,* 233–241.

Sobell, M. B., & Sobell, L. C. (1998). Guiding self-change. In W. R. Miller & N. Heather (Eds.), *Treating addictive behaviors* (2nd ed., pp. 189–202). New York: Plenum.

Sorensen, J. L., Acampora, A. P., & Iscoff, D. (1984). From maintenance to abstinence in a therapeutic community: Clinical treatment methods. *Journal of Psychoactive Drugs, 16,* 229–239.

Spitzer, R. L. (1983). Psychiatric diagnosis: Are clinicians still necessary? *Comprehensive Psychiatry, 24,* 399–411.

Stanton, M. D., & Shadish, W. R. (1997). Outcome attrition and family/couples treatment for drug abuse: A meta-analysis and review of the controlled, comparative studies. *Psychological Bulletin, 122,* 170–191.

Steele, C. M., & Josephs, R. A. (1990). Alcohol myopia: Its prized and dangerous effects. *American Psychologist, 45,* 921–933.

Stein, J., Newcomb, M., & Bentler, P. (1987). An 8-year study of multiple influences on drug use and drug use consequences. *Journal of Personality and Social Psychology, 53,* 1094–1105.

Stewart, D. G., & Brown, S. A. (1995). Withdrawal and dependency symptoms among adolescent alcohol and drug abusers. *Addictions, 90,* 627–635.

Stice, E., Myers, M. G., & Brown, S. A. (1998). A longitudinal grouping analysis of adolescent substance use escalation and de-escalation. *Psychology of Addictive Behaviors, 12,* 14–27.

Strang, J., Black, J., March, A., & Smith, B. (1993). Hair analysis for drugs: Technological break-through or ethical quagmire? *Addiction, 88,* 163–166.

Substance Abuse and Mental Health Services Administration. (1998). *1997 National Household Survey on Drug Abuse.* Rockville, MD: Office of Applied Studies.

Sutker, P. B., & Allain, A. N., Jr. (1988). Issues in personality conceptualizations of addictive behaviors. *Journal of Consulting and Clinical Psychology, 56,* 172–182.

Tapert, S. F., Kilmer, J. R., Quigley, L. A., Larimer, M. E., Roberts, L. J., & Miller, E. T. (1998). Harm reduction strategies for illicit substance use and abuse. In G. A. Marlatt (Ed.), *Harm reduction: Pragmatic strategies for managing high-risk behaviors* (pp. 145–217). New York: Guilford.

Tapert, S. F., Stewart, D. G., & Brown, S. A. (1999). Drug abuse in adolescence. In A. J. Goreczny & M. Hersen (Eds.), *Handbook of pediatric and adolescent health psychology* (pp. 161–178). Boston, MA: Allyn & Bacon.

Tapert, S. F., & Brown, S. A. (1999). Neuropsychological correlates of adolescent substance abuse: Four year outcomes. *Journal of the International Neuropsychological Society, 5,* 481–493.

Transdermal Nicotine Study Group. (1991). Transdermal nicotine for smoking cessation: Results of two multicenter controlled trials. *Journal of the American Medical Association, 266,* 3133–3138.

Trebach, A. S., & Zeese, K. B. (1990). *Drug prohibition and the conscience of nations.* Washington, DC: Drug Policy Foundation.

Tucker, J. A., Vuchinich, R. E., & Pukish, M. M. (1995). Molar environmental contexts surrounding recovery from alcohol problems by treated and untreated problems drinkers. *Experimental and Clinical Psychopharmacology, 3,* 195–204.

Tucker, M. B. (1982). Social support and coping: Applications for the study of female drug abuse. *Journal of Social Issues, 38,* 117–137.

U.S. Department of Health and Human Services. (1997). Highlights of 1997 trends in Indian health. Rockville, MD: Indian Health Service Office of Public Health, Division of Community and Environmental Health Program Statistics Team.

Vaillant, G. E., & Hiller-Sturmhofel, S. (1996). The natural history of alcoholism. *Alcohol Health & Research World, 20,* 152–161.

Vega, W. A., Alderete, E., Kolody, B., & Aguilar-Gaxiola, S. (1998). Illicit drug use among Mexicans and Mexican Americans in California: The effects of gender and acculturation. *Addiction, 93,* 1839–1850.

Velicer, W. F., Prochaska, J. O., Rossi, J. S., & Snow, M. G. (1992). Assessing outcome in smoking cessation studies. *Psychological Bulletin, 111,* 23–41.

Verheul, R., Hartgers, C., van den Brink, W., & Koeter, M. W. J. (1998). The effect of sampling, diagnostic criteria and assessment procedures on the observed prevalence of DSM-III-R personality disorders among treated alcoholics. *Journal of Studies on Alcohol, 59,* 227–236.

Vistor, H. R., Crossman, J. C., & Eiserman, R. (1973). Openness to experience and marijuana use in high school students. *Journal of Consulting and Clinical Psychology, 41,* 78–85.

Vogel-Sprott, M. (1995). The psychobiology of conditioning, reinforcement and craving. In B. Tabakoff & P. L. Hoffman (Eds.), *Biological aspects of alcoholism* (pp. 225–244). Seattle, WA: Hogrefe & Huber.

Volpicelli, J. R., Alterman, A. I., Hayashida, M., & O'Brien, C. P. (1992). Naltrexone in the treatment of alcohol dependence. *Archives of General Psychiatry, 49,* 876–880.

Vuchinich, R. E., & Tucker, J. A. (1996). The molar context of alcohol abuse. In L. Green & J. Kagel (Eds.), *Advances in behavioral economics:* Vol. 3. *Substance use and abuse* (pp. 133–162). Norwood, NJ: Ablex.

Vuchinich, R. E., & Tucker, J. A. (1998). Choice, behavioral economics, and addictive behavior patterns. In W. R. Miller & N. Heather (Eds.), *Treating addictive behaviors* (2nd ed., pp. 93–104). New York: Plenum.

Wagner, E. F., Brown, S. A., Monti, P. M., Myers, M. G., & Waldron, H. B. (1999). Innovations in adolescent substance abuse intervention. *Alcoholism: Clinical and Experimental Research, 23,* 236–249.

Waldron, H. B. (1997). Adolescent substance abuse and family therapy outcome: A review of randomized trials. In T. H. Ollendick & R. J. Rinz (Eds.), *Advances in clinical child psychology.* New York: Plenum.

Wall, T. L., & Ehlers, C. L. (1995). Genetic influences affecting alcohol use among Asians. *Alcohol Health & Research World, 19,* 184–189.

Weissman, M. M., Myers, J. K., & Harding, P. (1980). Prevalence and psychiatric heterogeneity of alcoholism in a United States urban community. *Journal of Studies on Alcohol, 41,* 672–681.

Wert, R. C., & Raulin, M. L. (1986). The chronic cerebral

effects of cannabis use. I. Methodological issues and neurological findings. *International Journal of the Addictions, 21*, 605–628.

Whitworth, A. B., Fischer, F., Lesch, O. M., Nimmerrichter, A., Oberbauer, H., Platz, T., Potgieter, A., Walter, H., & Fleischhacker, W. W. (1996). Comparison of acamprosate and placebo in long-term treatment of alcohol dependence. *Lancet, 347*, 1438–1442.

Wiers, R. W., Gunning, W. B., & Sergeant, J. A. (1998). Do young children of alcoholics hold more positive or negative alcohol-related expectancies than controls? *Alcoholism: Clinical & Experimental Research, 22*, 1855–1863.

Wilfley, D. E., Agras, W. S., Telch, C. T. F., Rossiter, E. M., Schneider, J. A., Cole, A. G., Sifford, L., & Raeburn, S. D. (1993). Group cognitive-behavioral therapy and group interpersonal psychotherapy for the nonpurging bulimic: A controlled comparison. *Journal of Consulting and Clinical Psychology, 61*, 296–305.

Windle, M., & Windle, R. C. (1996). Coping strategies, drinking motives, and stressful life events among middle adolescents: Associations with emotional and behavioral problems and with academic functioning. *Journal of Abnormal Psychology, 105*, 551–560.

Winters, K. C. (1991). *Manual for the Personal Experience Screening Questionnaire (PESQ)*. Los Angeles: Western Psychological Services.

Winters, K. C. (1992). Development of an adolescent alcohol and other drug abuse screening scale: Personal Experience Screening Questionnaire. *Addictive Behaviors, 17*, 479–490.

Winters, K. C., & Henly, G. A. (1989). *Personal Experience Inventory Test and Manual*. Los Angeles: Western Psychological Services.

Winters, K. C., & Henly, G. A. (1993). *Adolescent Diagnostic Interview (ADI) Manual*. Los Angeles: Western Psychological Services.

World Health Organization. (1992). ICD-10. Geneva, Switzerland: World Health Organization Press Office.

Wright, D. L., Aquilino, W. S., & Supple, A. J. (1998). A comparison of computer-assisted paper-and-pencil self-administered questionnaires in a survey on smoking, alcohol, and drug use. *Public Opinion Quarterly, 62*, 331–353.

Yalom, I. D. (1985). *The theory and practice of group psychotherapy* (3rd ed.). New York: Basic Books.

Yersin, B., Nicolet, J., Decrey, H., Burnier, M., van Mele, G., & Pecoud, A. (1995). Screening for excessive alcohol drinking. *Archives of Internal Medicine, 155*, 1907–1911.

Zacny, J. P. (1995). A review of the effects of opioids on psychomotor and cognitive functioning in humans. *Experimental and Clinical Psychopharmacology, 3*, 432–466.

Zuckerman, B., Frank, D. A., Hingson, R., Amaro, H., Levenson, S. M., Kayne, H., Parker, S., Vinci, R., Aboagye, K., Fried, L. E., Cabral, H., Timperi, R., & Bauchner, H. (1989). Effects of maternal marijuana and cocaine use on fetal growth. *New England Journal of Medicine, 320*, 762–768.

Zuckerman, M. (1994). *Behavioral expressions and biosocial bases of sensation seeking*. New York: Cambridge University Press.

Zweben, J. E., & Sorensen, J. L. (1988). Misunderstandings about methadone. *Journal of Psychoactive Drugs, 20*, 275–281.

# CHAPTER 21

# Alcohol-Related Disorders: Psychopathology, Diagnosis, Etiology, and Treatment

## Peter E. Nathan, Anne Helene Skinstad, and Sara Dolan

## Introduction

Alcohol-related disorders in DSM-IV (APA, 1994) include the alcohol use disorders and the alcohol-induced disorders. Alcohol abuse and alcohol dependence comprise the alcohol use disorders. These conditions exact substantial costs from both society and individual abusers; they are the principal focus of this chapter. Alcohol-induced disorders, which include alcohol intoxication delirium, alcohol withdrawal delirium, alcohol-induced persisting dementia, and alcohol-induced persisting amnestic disorder, are serious sequelae of alcohol abuse and dependence; they are a secondary focus of the chapter.

## Alcohol Use Disorders

*Alcohol abuse* comprises "a maladaptive pattern of alcohol use leading to clinically significant impairment or distress" (American Psychiatric Association [APA], 1994, p. 182) that involves

recurrent, significant, social or occupational problems caused by alcohol. These problems include failure to meet major role obligations at home, school, or work; the use of alcohol in physically hazardous situations; recurrent alcohol-related legal problems; and continued use of alcohol despite the substantial problems it has already caused.

*Alcohol dependence* encompasses "a cluster of cognitive, behavioral, and physiological symptoms indicating that the individual continues use of alcohol despite significant alcohol-related problems" (APA, 1994, p. 176). Physiological symptoms typically include tolerance and withdrawal symptoms. Other behaviors attest to the loss of control over alcohol consumption, including ingesting more alcohol over a longer period of time than intended; experiencing a persistent desire or having a history of unsuccessful efforts to reduce or control the alcohol use; spending a great deal of time obtaining, ingesting, or recovering from the effects of alcohol; giving up or reducing important activities because of alcohol; and continuing to ingest alcohol despite a physical or psychological problem caused or made worse by the drug.

The latest figures on alcohol use in the United States (Grant, 1997), derived from a large and representative sample of the U.S. population, indicate that 66.0% of Americans over the age of 18 years has consumed alcohol at some time in their lives and that 44.4% of them are currently doing it.

Peter E. Nathan, Anne Helene Skinstad, and Sara Dolan • University of Iowa, Iowa City, Iowa 52242-1316.

*Comprehensive Handbook of Psychopathology* (Third Edition), edited by Patricia B. Sutker and Henry E. Adams. Kluwer Academic / Plenum Publishers, New York, 2001.

Grant (1997) also estimated lifetime and current prevalences of DSM-IV alcohol dependence: 13.3% of the population (about 34.5 million Americans) met the criteria for alcohol dependence at some time in their lives and 4.4% (about 11.4 citizens) currently meet those criteria. Given these figures, it is not surprising that alcohol dependence is one of the nation's leading public health problems.

## Alcohol-Induced Disorders

*Alcohol intoxication delirium* is characterized by a disturbance of consciousness (that is, reduced clarity of awareness of the environment) that results in diminished ability to focus, sustain, or shift attention and deterioration in cognition (typically involving memory deficit, disorientation, and/or language disturbance) or the development of perceptual disturbances. All of these symptoms may develop during alcohol intoxication.

*Alcohol withdrawal delirium* develops during alcohol withdrawal; it is known more commonly as *delirium tremens*. This syndrome, which affects fewer than 5% of alcoholics hospitalized for severe withdrawal, develops within the week following a reduction in or the cessation of heavy drinking. It is characterized by confusion, disorientation, and severe tremulousness ("the shakes"). Alternating periods of agitation and calm may be punctuated by vivid visual and tactile hallucinations, illusions, and autonomic hyperactivity. The disorder is generally of short duration (15% of those who experience it recover within 24 hours), but it has a mortality rate of 10–15%, if it is not recognized and treated.

*Alcohol-induced persisting dementia* is signaled by the irreversible development of multiple cognitive deficits (including aphasia, apraxia, agnosia, and/or disturbance in executive functioning), as well as impaired memory (impaired ability to learn new information or to recall previously learned information). These symptoms reflect the persisting effects of alcohol on the brain, sometimes long after the patient has stopped abusive drinking.

*Alcohol-induced persisting amnestic disorder* involves a profound impairment in the ability to learn new information or to recall previously learned information or past events; these symptoms are etiologically related to the persisting effects of alcohol and are marked enough to impair social or occupational functioning. Otherwise known as *Korsakoff's syndrome*, this irreversible condition results from a long-term deficiency in vitamin $B_1$ (thiamin) that sometimes accompanies chronic alcohol abuse.

## Diagnosis

### A Brief Historical Perspective

The first *Diagnostic and Statistical Manual of Mental Disorders* (APA, 1952) clustered alcoholism and drug addiction, sexual deviations (later renamed the paraphilias), and antisocial and dissocial reactions (now termed antisocial personality disorder) as a single diagnostic entity called sociopathic personality disturbances. This phrase was meant to imply that persons who behave in one or more of these ways have chosen to flaunt society's rules. Alcoholism and drug addiction were similarly grouped with personality disorders and sexual deviations in DSM-II (APA, 1968) for the same reason. Both of these initial diagnostic arrangements reflected the distaste that the drafters of the first two *Diagnostic and Statistical Manuals* felt for behaviors that seriously transgressed contemporary social norms.

When a rapidly growing research literature began to point to the roles of genetic and environmental factors in the etiology of many psychopathological disorders, the developers of DSM-III (APA, 1980) and DSM-III-R (APA, 1987) moved away from the psychoanalytic underpinnings of their 1952 and 1968 predecessors toward empirically supported diagnostic and etiologic information. For the same reason, alcohol and drug abuse and dependence were separated in 1980 from the renamed paraphilias and personality disorders when voluminous research began to suggest profound differences in the signs, symptoms, etiology, and courses of these conditions.

The 1980 and 1987 diagnostic manuals, unlike their predecessors, distinguished the behavioral consequences of alcohol and drug abuse and dependence from their central nervous system consequences. They also differentiated the signs and symptoms of alcohol and drug abuse much more clearly from those of dependence. However, whereas DSM-III required the presence of signs of tolerance or withdrawal to confirm the diagnosis of substance dependence, DSM-III-R deemphasized tolerance and withdrawal symptoms in favor of the complex of behaviors associated with loss of control over drinking, which Edwards and Gross

(1976) termed the substance dependence syndrome.

The DSM-IV Substance Use Disorders Work Group attempted to resolve the long-standing diagnostic question how to conceptualize alcohol dependence best, as well as several other important unresolved issues, by undertaking an extensive, multisite field trial (Cottler et al., 1995). Data from the field trial were used to address the following four questions:

*Should the new diagnostic criteria reemphasize or deemphasize tolerance and physical withdrawal symptoms for the diagnosis of dependence?* Substantial proportions of dependent users of amphetamines, hallucinogens, inhalants, PCP, and sedatives in the field trial failed to experience tolerance or withdrawal symptoms, even though from 86 to 99% of persons dependent on alcohol, cannabis, cocaine, opiates, sedatives, and nicotine did so. Because these conflicting data prevented it from generalizing across substances on this key diagnostic issue, the Work Group decided to request clinicians to specify one of two criteria set qualifiers, "with physiological dependence" or "without physiological dependence," to highlight this issue in anticipation of DSM-V.

*Should the new diagnostic criteria deemphasize social consequences and occupational impairment as criteria for dependence?* Substantial numbers of all substance users, except those using cocaine, failed to report either social consequences or occupational impairment. As a consequence, the Work Group decided that the social and occupational consequences of alcohol and drug use better described abuse than dependence, so these criteria became the principal cues to substance abuse.

*Could DSM-IV offer a shorter list of criteria for dependence, thereby easing the diagnostic task of clinicians and researchers?* As just noted, the Work Group moved the diagnostic criteria relating to social and occupational consequences from dependence to abuse. As a result, abuse came to represent substance misuse with adverse social or occupational consequences but without evidence of compulsive use, tolerance, or withdrawal, whereas dependence signaled compulsive use with or without physiological accompaniments. In making these changes, the Work Group substantially clarified the separate conceptual bases for substance abuse and dependence.

*Should abuse be made more distinct from dependence (as it was in DSM-III), not just a resid-*ual category (as it became in DSM-III-R)? As noted before, in reconceptualizing substance abuse and dependence, the DSM-IV Work Group provided specific contexts and distinct sets of criteria for the abuse and dependence diagnoses, thereby making both more distinct and more meaningful.

The alcohol dependence syndrome (Edwards & Gross, 1976), which substantially influenced the diagnostic conception of dependence in DSM-III-R (APA, 1987) and, to a lesser extent, DSM-IV, posits that a combination of behavioral conditioning and physiological processes best define the dependence syndrome. The syndrome's most important symptom is impaired control over drinking: "loss of control" drinking. A recent examination of the validity of DSM-IV alcohol dependence and abuse diagnoses in a randomly selected community sample of 936 household residents strongly supported the validity of the alcohol dependence diagnosis but not the validity of the alcohol abuse diagnosis (Hasin et al., 1997). These findings suggest that although clinicians and researchers can have substantial confidence in the validity of DSM-IV diagnoses of alcohol dependence, the validity of the alcohol abuse diagnosis is a good deal more problematic.

### The Research Diagnostic Project

The Research Diagnostic Project (RDP) of the Center of Alcohol Studies, Rutgers University, recently explored a range of issues in substance abuse diagnosis by gathering clinical data from patients treated in four public and four private treatment settings, balanced across inpatient and outpatient facilities, that are located in five Northeastern states.

The reliability of lifetime DSM-IV diagnoses of alcohol, cannabis, cocaine, and opiate abuse and dependence was explored in an early RDP study (Langenbucher, Morgenstern, Labouvie, & Nathan, 1994a). The reliability of the new DSM-IV decision rules, it was found, is excellent, and an especially strong relationship was observed between the reliability of a symptom and its centrality to the individual abuse pattern.

Agreement among diagnostic systems was a particular concern of the DSM-IV Task Force, which worked hard to bring DSM-IV and ICD-10 (World Health Organization, 1992) into greater diagnostic concordance so that mental health workers across the world could better communicate diagnostically. Langenbucher, Morgenstern,

Labouvie, and Nathan (1994b) examined diagnostic agreement among DSM-III, DSM-IV and ICD-10 for alcohol, amphetamines, cannabis, cocaine, hallucinogens, opiates, PCP, and sedative/hypnotics. They concluded that ICD-10 is the most sensitive diagnostic system, because it diagnoses a larger number of cases than either of the two versions of the DSM. Generally satisfactory statistical agreement was found between ICD-10 "harmful use" and DSM "abuse." The three diagnostic systems diverged strongly, however, in cases whose symptoms barely reached the diagnostic threshold.

As we noted earlier, the predictive validity of tolerance and withdrawal symptoms remains an important unanswered question (e.g., Blaine, Horton & Towle, 1995; Schuckit, 1996). Although it has been assumed that both signal increased risk of dependence-related medical problems and relapse, two recent studies (Carroll, Rounsaville & Bryant, 1994; Rounsaville & Bryant, 1992) reported that tolerance and withdrawal symptoms did not predict deterioration in physical status or a return to substance misuse. With like aims in mind, Langenbucher and his colleagues (in press) compared the predictive validity of four sets of dependence criteria: the DSM-IV criteria for alcohol dependence with and without physiological dependence, an alternative dichotomous criterion for physiological dependence, and a dimensional measure of physiological dependence specifically designed to predict multiple indexes of medical problems and relapse behavior. As Rounsaville and his colleagues previously reported, DSM-IV physiological alcohol dependence failed to predict either medical problems or relapse. Langenbucher, however, blamed this failure on operational problems in DSM-IV, rather than on a specific lack of predictive validity for physiological dependence: he concluded as a consequence that physiological dependence can serve as a course specifier for alcohol problems. However, to serve this purpose, it must be more sensitively scaled than it is in DSM-IV, either by using alternative criteria for coding physiological dependence or by developing a dimensional measure.

Diagnosticians must differentiate among cases varying within as well as those varying between diagnostic categories. Severity is one of the most important within-category descriptive dimensions that influences patient/treatment matching (McCrady & Langenbucher, 1996), reimbursement for various levels of care (Jencks & Goldman, 1987), and determination of the length-of-stay (Mezzich & Sharfstein, 1985). Langenbucher, Sulesund, Chung and Morgenstern (1996) compared the relapse prediction efficiency of illness severity (reflected by the DSM-IV symptom count and scores on the Alcohol Dependence Scale and the Addiction Severity Index) and self-efficacy (reflecting patients' estimates of the likelihood of remaining sober). The Alcohol Dependence Scale predicted four of five relapse indicators; self-efficacy did not contribute to this prediction. These findings favor illness severity, particularly, severity of physiological dependence, over self-efficacy as the best predictor of treatment outcome, thereby suggesting that physiological aspects of dependence may be more important than cognitive mechanisms in influencing the likelihood of relapse.

The order of appearance of the symptoms of a given disorder is often predictable, in which case it contributes to valid diagnoses; when the sequencing of symptoms is not predictable, the validity of the diagnosis is lower. A study of the onset and staging of symptoms of alcohol abuse and dependence (Langenbucher & Chung, 1995) identified three successive stages: alcohol abuse, alcohol dependence, and accommodation to the illness. The model survived a rigorous series of tests for goodness-of-fit that support the construct validity of alcohol abuse as a discrete first illness phase and of alcohol dependence as distinct from and succeeding abuse. These findings support the common perception that alcohol abuse is a distinct stop along the road to alcohol dependence for many individuals (Helzer, 1994).

## Etiology

### Genetic/Biological Factors

Alcoholism runs in families. Does it do so because alcoholic parents transmit a genetic predisposition to alcohol abuse or dependence to their children, because the environment alcoholic parents create produces psychological or behavioral consequences for their children that lead to abuse or dependence, or both, or neither? We review here the data, increasingly substantial over the past 25 years, that point to the heightened risk of alcohol abuse and dependence transmitted genetically from alcoholic parent to child. However, the review does not extend to research on the molecular genetics of alcoholism, which is still growing and still conflicted. That research now focuses on the function of the DRD2 gene, located on chromosome 11q22-q23. The DRD2 gene encodes the dopamine D2 receptor, which many neuroscientists believe is involved in the genetic transmission of alcoholism (Edenberg et al., 1998).

**Concordance Rates for Alcoholism in Twins.** If there is a genetic component in the risk of alcoholism, then identical twins, who possess identical genes, should exhibit similar consumption and abuse histories, and fraternal twins, who share an average of 50% of their genetic material, should differ more in consumption and abuse histories. In fact, researchers using the twin method to study the genetics of alcoholism confirmed these expectations.

In one of the earliest twin studies of the genetics of alcoholism, Kaij (1960) reported concordance rates of 54% for alcohol abuse among Swedish monozygotic twins; it was 28% among dizygotic twins. A number of subsequent twin studies confirmed these initial findings on the genetics of abuse. In a study of 850 pairs of American like-sex twins who were high school juniors at the time, Leohlin (1977) reported that identical twins were also significantly more concordant for heavy drinking than fraternal twins. And, in a recent study of 1030 female-female twin pairs in Virginia, Kendler and his colleagues (1992) found that concordance for alcohol dependence was significantly higher among monozygotic than dizygotic twin pairs; overall, 58% of identical twin pairs and only 29% of fraternal twin pairs were concordant for alcoholism.

**Adoption Studies of Children of Alcoholics.** Adoption studies hold environmental influences constant, which twin studies may not, and they permit systematic variation in genetic factors. Many behavioral scientists believe that adoption studies provide the clearest perspective to date on the role of genetic factors in mental disorders.

The first adoption studies of children of alcoholics compared four groups of young adult children of Danish alcoholics (Goodwin, 1976, 1979, 1985). Sons of alcoholics raised by nonalcoholic foster parents, sons of alcoholics raised by their biological parents, and daughters of alcoholics raised, respectively, by nonalcoholic foster parents and by their biological parents were included. Paired with each of these four groups was a control group matched for age, gender, and adoption sta-

tus. All adoptees had been separated from their biological parents during the first few weeks of life and then adopted by nonrelatives. The studies yielded two principal findings: (1) sons of alcoholics were about four times more likely than sons of nonalcoholics to become alcoholics as adults, regardless of whether they were raised by their biological parents or by nonalcoholic adoptive parents; (2) the influence of genetics on the daughters of alcoholics was not as strong as on the sons of alcoholics.

Subsequent adoption research in Sweden (Bohman, Cloninger, von Knorring, & Sigvardsson, 1984) confirmed Goodwin's conclusions about the impact of genetic factors on the sons of alcoholics and showed, as well, that genetic factors also significantly affect daughters of alcoholics. The Swedish research also suggested the existence of two forms of inherited alcoholism. Analyzing data from 2000 Swedish adoptees, Bohman, Sigvardsson, and Cloninger (1981) and Cloninger, Bohman, and Sigvardsson (1981) identified two groups of alcoholics that differed in alcoholism heritability. The more numerous, lower heritability, Type I alcoholics began drinking in their mid-twenties to thirties, although typically they did not develop alcohol problems until middle age; they had a high risk of liver disease and showed little antisocial behavior and relatively few social and occupational problems. Children of Type I alcoholics were twice as likely to develop alcoholism as persons without a family history of alcoholism; sons of Type I alcoholics raised in troubled adoptive homes were at even greater risk of developing alcoholism. In contrast, the higher heritability Type II alcoholics, whose alcoholism began very early, experienced profound social and occupational problems but relatively few medical difficulties. Their biological sons—but not their biological daughters—were nine times more likely to develop alcoholism, regardless of environmental influences.

Although a number of investigators have been unable to validate Cloninger's typology, it has generated a great deal of fruitful research (e.g., Fils-Aime et al., 1996; Hallman, von Knorring, & Oreland, 1996; Howard, Kivlahan, & Walker, 1997).

**A Biological/Genetic Basis for Alcohol Abuse and Dependence?** Do these data prove that the children of alcoholics are destined to follow in their parents' footsteps? No, they do not. Despite the enhanced risk of alcoholism that adult children of alcoholics carry, most children of alcoholics do not become substance abusers, and most alcoholics are not the children of alcoholics, affirming the importance of sociocultural, learning-based, and other factors in the development of substance abuse (Prescott et al., 1994; Schuckit, 1994a).

To this end, Sher and his colleagues (1997) recently explored possible relationships among childhood stressors (including disrupted family rituals, embarrassment, abuse and neglect), paternal alcoholism, and alcohol abuse and dependence in the adolescent and early adult children of alcoholic fathers. Sher and his colleagues asked whether exposure to stressors during childhood further increases the substantial risk of developing alcoholism that children of alcoholic fathers already have. Not unexpectedly, the answer was qualified. Paternal alcoholism was associated with every childhood stressor studied, and a number of these stressors (specifically, verbal, emotional, physical, and sexual abuse) were related to alcohol use disorder in adolescence or early adulthood, but self-reported childhood stressors overall were only moderately and inconsistently related to the development of alcohol problems. In other words, environmental stressors like parental abuse in childhood do affect the genetic burden of familial alcoholism, but how and why they do so is not yet well understood.

## Sociocultural Influences

**Demographic Factors.** The racial, religious, national, and ethnic groups to which our parents and we belong, as well as our gender, profession, education, and age, influence who we are, including the likelihood that we will abuse alcohol and drugs (Johnson et al., 1990). This is hardly surprising. Our parents' sociocultural group memberships shaped their child-rearing practices, just as our own membership in these groups influenced our behavior during childhood and impacts it now.

Hispanics and African-Americans are at greater risk than Caucasians of developing alcohol-related problems. This was the conclusion from a recent U.S. adult household survey of alcohol-related problems and social consequences among representative groups of Caucasians, African-Americans, and Hispanics between 1984 and 1992 (Caetano, 1997). Caetano hypothesized that these ethnic differences in risk status reflect inequalities in in-

come distribution, employment, education, and access to adequate health care among these groups.

Age also strongly affects rates of alcohol and drug consumption and risk of abuse. Both men and women drink most heavily between the ages of 18 and 25. Substantially lower rates characterize persons over 45 years of age, especially those over 65 (Grant, 1997; NIAAA, 1997). Wechsler and his colleagues (1994) recently reported some startling data on drinking by college students, who represent a highly visible subgroup of this heavy drinking, young adult cohort. Surveying the drinking practices of 17,592 undergraduates at 140 U.S. colleges and universities, these researchers found that almost half (44%) of their sample met criteria as binge drinkers and almost one-fifth (19%) were frequent binge drinkers. Binge drinking was defined as consumption of five or more drinks (for men) and four or more drinks (for women) on a single occasion during the 2 weeks before the survey; frequent binge drinkers reported three or more binges during the same period. A strong, positive relationship linked frequency of binge drinking and significant alcohol-related health and other problems. Frequent binge drinkers were seven to ten times more likely than nonbinge drinkers to fail to use protection when having sex, to engage in unplanned sexual activity, to get into trouble with campus police, to damage property, or to get hurt or injured. Binge drinking was strongly age-related: students between 17 and 23 years of age had much higher bingeing rates than older students.

Grant's 1997 survey of more than 40,000 Americans, referred to previously, confirmed that gender powerfully affects the risk of alcoholism in this country: Males were much more likely than females to abuse alcohol at every age. An earlier population survey of alcohol abuse and addiction in five sites across the globe in the late 1980s—in St. Louis, Missouri; Edmonton, Canada; San Juan, Puerto Rico; Seoul, South Korea; and Taipei City, Taiwan—came to the same conclusion (Helzer et al., 1990). Marked disparities between men and women in lifetime prevalence of alcohol dependence were observed in all five geographically diverse sites, confirming in every instance that men were at markedly higher risk of alcoholism than women. As an example, the survey found that lifetime prevalence rates for alcoholism in St. Louis were 29% for men and only 4% for women.

Two factors have been weighed most heavily in

efforts to explain these marked differences between men and women in alcohol abuse and dependence. First, because of women's traditional child-care role, our society tolerates alcohol abuse by women much less readily than it does alcohol abuse by men. Second, recent empirical data on differential rates of metabolism of alcohol by men and women (Frezza et al., 1990) suggest that women possess smaller amounts than men of a crucial enzyme that detoxifies alcohol in the stomach and small intestine. This gender-based metabolic difference explains why alcohol consumed in equivalent doses by men and women has greater behavioral and physiological effects on women (Gallant, 1987). Simply put, fewer women than men drink to excess because alcohol produces more aversive behavioral, bodily, and interpersonal consequences for women than for men.

**Peer Influences.** Heavy drinking and drug use and rebellious and delinquent behavior by peers are significant risk factors in adolescent substance abuse (Newcomb & Bentler, 1986). Conversely, having peers who do not drink abusively, use drugs, or commit rebellious or delinquent acts protects adolescents against substance use and abuse (Jessor & Jessor, 1977).

Gottfredson and Koper (1996) found that adolescent peer drinking, drug use, rebelliousness, and delinquency were more closely linked to initiating substance use in Caucasians than in African-Americans and more in African-American males than in African-American females, a finding which Reifman et al. (1998) subsequently confirmed. Reifman and his colleagues (1998) also reported that peer drinking alone did not predict progression to heavier drinking in Caucasian and African-American adolescents. The degree of parental monitoring of drinking and the extent of parental efforts to control other troubling aspects of the behavior of their adolescents interacted with peer influences to influence the likelihood that heavier drinking by the adolescents would progress.

In a study of 25,411 male and female undergraduates from sixty-one U.S. colleges and universities that replicated and extended the 1994 study by Wechsler and his colleagues reviewed earlier, Cashin, Presley, and Meilman (1998) related alcohol consumption, binge drinking, the consequences of use, and beliefs about drinking to membership in fraternities and sororities. It has long been assumed that fraternities and sororities represent a powerful source of peer influence on their members. As predicted, students in the Greek system averaged significantly more drinks per week, engaged in heavy drinking significantly more often, and suffered significantly more negative consequences of their drinking than non-Greeks. The officers of fraternities and sororities consumed alcohol, engaged in heavy drinking, and experienced negative consequences at levels at least as high and, in some cases, higher than that of other Greek members. Whether these heavy drinking officers were leading or following their fellow Greeks could not be determined from the design of this study.

### Learning-Based Factors

**Classical Conditioning.** Such common symptoms of alcohol dependence as craving and tolerance have been interpreted as classical conditioning mechanisms. For example, a series of experiments with alcohol (Crowell, Hinson, & Siegel, 1981) and morphine (Siegel, 1978) showed that substance-dependent rats that developed drug tolerance maintained it only when they were tested under the environmental conditions originally associated with the drug or alcohol administration. Tolerance was not observed when the drug was given in a novel environment. These experiments led Siegel and his colleagues to propose the *conditioned compensatory response model*, a classical conditioning model of drug tolerance. According to Siegel (1978), environmental stimuli linked with drug intake become associated with the drug's effects on the body to elicit a conditioned response opposite to the drug's effect, thus creating a compensating response designed to maintain bodily homeostasis. As this conditioned response increases in magnitude with continued drug intake, the drug's effects decrease and tolerance increases.

The *conditioned appetitive motivational model* is a classical conditioning model of craving (Stewart, deWit, & Eikelboom, 1984). It explains the common observation that the conditioned stimuli associated with the positive reinforcing effects of drugs (for example, the smell, sounds, and lighting of the place where alcohol is most often ingested) sometimes become capable themselves of eliciting a positive motivational state similar to that elicited by a preferred alcoholic beverage itself. This state, in turn, creates strong, continuing urges to seek and use alcohol. This model helps explain the great difficulty that recovering alcoholics have in maintaining abstinence when they must return to the environments in which they originally developed their dependence.

**Operant Conditioning.** Nathan and O'Brien (1971) described a series of studies of operant conditioning mechanisms in alcohol self-administration by humans. They explored the behavior of alcoholic subjects who lived for up to 33 days in a self-contained experimental environment at Boston City Hospital. The social behavior, mood, and drinking behavior of matched groups of alcoholics and nonalcoholics were compared during this prolonged period. Operant procedures assessed the differential reinforcement value of alcohol and social interaction, both of which are extremely powerful reinforcers for these subjects. All subjects had to press an operant panel's push-button repeatedly, on a high fixed-ratio schedule, to earn points to "purchase" alcohol, time out of their rooms in a social area, or both.

Comparisons of the operant behavior of the alcoholic and nonalcoholic groups revealed the following:

- Alcoholics worked much longer and harder to earn points to purchase alcohol. As a result, though both alcoholics and nonalcoholics reached the same high blood-alcohol levels early in drinking, alcoholics remained at these levels longer and returned to them more frequently. They drank almost twice as much as the nonalcoholics.
- Nonalcoholics worked much longer and harder to earn points that permitted them to leave their rooms and spend time with each other in a social area. By contrast, alcoholics remained social isolates before, during, and after drinking.
- Once drinking began, alcoholics became significantly more depressed and less active and demonstrated significantly more psychopathology (including anxiety, manic behavior, depression, paranoia, and phobic and compulsive behavior) than nonalcoholics.

This research program ultimately led a number of other clinical researchers to explore operant programs designed to reinforce alcoholics to reduce or stop their drinking. Bigelow, Cohen, Liebson, and Faillace (1972) and Bigelow, Liebson, and Griffiths (1974), for example, reported marked reductions in drinking by alcoholics when they were reinforced with money and other rewards for

maintaining limited periods of abstinence in a laboratory setting.

## A Biopsychosocial View of Alcoholism Etiology

The past two decades have witnessed great progress in establishing empirically the key factors associated with the etiology of alcohol abuse and dependence. Much more remains to be understood, but we certainly know enough now to advocate a biopsychosocial view of the etiology of alcoholism. We make this claim convinced that genetic/biological, sociocultural, and learning-based factors exert their own distinct influences on the etiology of these conditions. It is also clear that emphasizing one or another of these factors over the others provides a limiting view of etiology, whereas stressing their coordinate power to impact the development of alcohol abuse and dependence most accurately describes our current knowledge about the etiology of these conditions.

## Markers of Risk for Alcohol-Related Disorders

### Family History

A family history of alcoholism is the strongest single predictor of heightened risk of alcoholism (Cadoret, 1980; Cotton, 1979). Three different research programs conducted during three different recent decades (Cloninger et al., 1981; Goodwin et al., 1974; Kendler et al., 1992) demonstrated that a family history of alcoholism substantially increases the risk of alcoholism in the children of alcoholics. The risk of alcoholism is increased, presumably, because still-unidentified mediators of risk are genetically transmitted.

Schuckit (1997) describes an ongoing prospective study, now in its fifteenth year, of 453 sons of alcoholics and controls originally chosen at random from lists of university students and nonacademic staff at the University of California, San Diego. We refer here to data from this study on the level of reaction to an alcohol challenge as a marker of heightened risk of alcoholism. Here, we call readers' attention to a recent article by Schuckit and Smith (1996), which compared the men in their sample who were family history positive (FH+) for paternal alcoholism with a matched family history negative (FH−) comparison group;

in all other relevant respects, the two groups were indistinguishable from one another. At the 8.2 year follow-up mark, when the men were in their early 30s, the prevalence of DSM-III-R alcohol abuse and dependence among the FH+ men was 14.1 and 28.6%, respectively, compared to 6 and 10.8% for the FH− men, thereby affirming the impact of a family history of alcoholism on the rates of alcoholism in the FH+ men in this sample.

## Neurophysiological Index

**ERP: Auditory and Visual P300.** The event-related potential (ERP) is an electroencephalographic (EEG) technique that reflects the electrical events that arise during the processing of information by the brain following an external auditory or visual stimulus. Testing the hypothesis that the visual P300 wave deficit, a distinct ERP waveform, was a genetically determined marker of enhanced risk for alcoholism, Begleiter and his colleagues (1984) compared the ERPs of a group of 12-year-old boys who had alcoholic fathers with those of a matched group without a history of paternal alcoholism. Significant differences in the P300 voltage distinguished the two groups. Moreover, the boys with a paternal history of alcoholism showed a P300 pattern similar to that previously seen in abstinent chronic alcoholics (Porjesz & Begleiter, 1983). Subsequent reports of diminished P300 voltage in groups of boys and girls with family histories of alcoholism (Hill & Steinhauer, 1993; O'Connor, Hesselbrock, & Tasman, 1986; Steinhauer & Hill, 1993) supported the validity of the Begleiter group's initial findings, although other researchers—most recently, Holguin, Corral, and Cadaveira (1998)—failed to do so.

Auditory stimuli have not been associated with P300 amplitude reductions as consistently as visual stimuli. For example, Hill, Steinhauer, and Locke (1995) observed no differences in the amplitude of the P300 component of the ERP to two auditory stimuli among alcoholics from "high-density, multigenerational families," first-degree nonalcoholic relatives from the same families, and nonalcoholic controls from low-density families. This finding contrasts with the same authors' report of reliable visual P300 amplitude differences in high- and low-risk children from the same high- and low-density families (Hill & Steinhauer, 1993; Steinhauer & Hill, 1993).

Ramachandran and his colleagues (1996) hypothesized that reduced P300 amplitudes are signs of cortical inhibition that interferes with the ability to respond to novel stimuli and reflects a developmental lag in high-risk youth. Ramsey and Finn (1997) propose, instead, that diminished P300 amplitudes may reflect deficits in the motivational-cognitive system of children of alcoholics. They drew this conclusion after comparing visual P300 amplitudes of family-history positive (FH+) and family-history negative (FH−) men under both monetary incentive and no-incentive conditions and found that only the FH− men increased the amplitude of their P300 in the incentive condition.

**Level of Reaction to Alcohol.** Twenty years ago, Nathan and Lipscomb (1979) and Lipscomb, Carpenter, and Nathan (1979) reported that some nonalcoholic individuals given a challenge dose of alcohol showed little body sway in response to the challenge, whereas others swayed substantially. The degree of body sway in response to the challenge dose of alcohol turned out to be associated with subsequent development of tolerance to alcohol: Subjects who were relatively unresponsive to the challenge dose were more likely to demonstrate substantial tolerance following a period of sustained drinking than those who showed significant body sway following ingestion of the challenge dose. Nathan and his colleagues hypothesized that body sway following an alcohol challenge in nondependent drinkers might be a marker for heightened risk of alcoholism.

Subsequently, Schuckit and his colleagues (Schuckit, 1985; Schuckit, 1994b; Schuckit & Gold, 1988) compared the level of response to alcohol challenge (LR) in the family history positive (FH+) and family history negative (FH−) subjects of their longitudinal study of multiple markers of risk of developing alcoholism. In two of the most recent reports of this research, Schuckit and Smith (1996, 1997) reported that LR at the age of 20 years had turned out to be a marker for increased risk of later alcoholism: FH+ males with low LR scores were significantly more likely than FH− males with low LR scores to develop alcoholism, and FH+ males with low LR scores were significantly more likely than FH+ males with high LR scores to develop later alcoholism. These authors concluded, as had Nathan and his colleagues (1979), that "these data are consistent with the conclusion that LR might be a mediator of the alcoholism risk" (Schuckit & Smith, 1996, p. 202). They posit that young drinkers in whom alcohol consumption induces little effect, especially those with family histories of alcoholism, might well drink more over time to achieve a stronger effect than those on whom alcohol has a stronger initial effect.

## Personality Traits

Despite repeated attempts, efforts to identify a predominant personality style in alcohol- or drug-dependent individuals—the "addictive personality"—have failed to yield a single trait dimension or pattern of dimensions characteristic of many, most, or all such persons (e.g., Nathan, 1988; Sutker & Allain, 1988). However, substantial data have been gathered in recent years which suggest that personality traits are markers of the risk of alcoholism and probably contribute to the development and/or persistence of an addiction.

To this end, Allen, Fertig, and Mattson (1994) identified five discrete personality trait patterns in a group of 400 primary alcoholics; each trait pattern was associated with a different set of motivations to use alcohol and drugs. For example, alcohol-dependent individuals who were dependent on others and hostile toward peers most often used alcohol to dampen dysphoric mood and respond to peer pressure, and alcoholics who admitted to feeling socially isolated used alcohol to alleviate the emotional distress that accompanies social alienation.

Reviewing data on the personality topography of individuals diagnosed with alcohol dependence or antisocial personality disorder (the two are often comorbid), Sher and Trull (1994) identified three broad dimensions of personality common to both disorders. Neuroticism/negative emotionality, impulsivity/disinhibition and, to a lesser extent, extroversion/sociability all contribute to the development and persistence of these conditions. These three personality dimensions have emerged repeatedly in efforts to characterize the personality traits of alcohol and drug abusers. What remains, above all, is to determine whether and how these dimensions of personality differ between substance abusers and persons with antisocial personality disorder.

## Alcohol Expectancies

Alcohol expectancies are the attitudes and beliefs that we hold about the effects that alcohol will have on our thoughts, feelings, and behavior. In 1980, Brown and her colleagues (Brown et al.,

1980) developed the first questionnaire to assess alcohol expectancies. Since then, a number of other expectancy questionnaires have been developed to address methodological problems in Brown's Alcohol Expectancy Questionnaire (AEQ; Brown et al., 1980). These instruments include the Effects of Drinking Alcohol (EDA; Leigh, 1987; Leigh & Stacy, 1993), the Comprehensive Effects of Alcohol (CEOA; Fromme, Stroot, & Kaplan, 1993), and the Drinking Expectancy Questionnaire (DEQ; Young & Oei, 1990).

These instruments, along with the AEQ, have successfully predicted a number of variables related to alcohol consumption in both adults (e.g., Brown, Goldman, & Christiansen, 1985) and children (Smith et al., 1995). Alcohol expectancies also differentiate between heavy and light drinkers (see review by Goldman et al., 1991) and, interacting with personality variables (Earlywine, Finn, & Martin, 1990; Leonard & Blane, 1988), moderate relationships between drinking and stress (Cooper et al., 1992) and drinking and anxiety (Kushner et al., 1994).

Alcohol expectancies also influence the risk of alcoholism. In a one-year longitudinal study, Christiansen et al. (1989) found that alcohol expectancies in adolescents who had not yet begun regular drinking, predicted eventual alcohol consumption levels by differentiating between those who ultimately became problem drinkers and those who did not. The same research group (Smith et al., 1995) also examined the divergent paths of adolescents with high and low expectations for alcohol's positive effects. Following their subjects for 2 years, they reported a direct relationship between expectancy endorsement and subsequent drinking: The greater their expectations of alcohol's positive effects on social functioning, the greater their alcohol use. Smith and his colleagues also found that expectancies and drinking influenced each other reciprocally: Greater expectancy endorsements led to higher subsequent drinking which led, in turn, to even greater expectancy levels.

Expectancies have also recently been linked to anterior brain functioning in young men at risk of alcoholism (Deckel, Hesselbrock, & Bauer, 1995). Ninety-one young men without significant drug or alcohol histories completed EEGs, batteries of neuropsychological tests, and AEQs. Regression analysis revealed that four of the neuropsychological tests of anterior brain functioning predicted a number of AEQ scales; moreover, frontal, but not parietal, EEG scores were also associated with AEQ scales. These findings suggest that alcohol-related expectancies may be biologically determined in part by frontal/prefrontal systems and that inherited dysfunctions in these systems might function as risk factors for alcohol abuse or dependence.

The relationship between alcohol expectancies and memory has been another recent focus of expectancy research. Goldman and his colleagues (e.g., Dunn & Goldman, 1996; Rather & Goldman, 1994; Rather, Goldman, Roehrich, & Brannick, 1992; Roehrich & Goldman, 1995) attempted to model alcohol expectancy memory networks, using theories from cognitive psychology. They posit that expectancies are stored as memories and that these memories may implicitly affect future drinking decisions. In the study by Roehrich and Goldman (1995), the effect of implicit priming of drinking on actual consumption was studied. In a 2 × 2 factorial design, participants were exposed to clips from TV sitcoms (*Cheers* or *Newhart*) in the videotape prime condition and a Stroop task with either alcohol expectancy or neutral words in the semantic prime condition. Subjects were then asked to participate in an alcohol "taste test" in which they rated three different nonalcoholic beers. The dependent measure was how much alcohol each participant consumed. Participants who viewed a clip from *Cheers*, a program set in a Boston bar, consumed significantly more than those who viewed *Newhart* (a program set in a Vermont inn); those in the expectancy word conditions consumed significantly more than those in the control word conditions. Roehrich and Goldman concluded from these findings that memory processes do influence drinking decisions and that alcohol expectancies, as well as other contents of memory, play roles in these processes.

## Psychopathology

### Interpersonal Aggression

Alcohol intoxication reliably induces aggression in some individuals (Nathan, 1993). Extensive data also implicate alcohol intoxication, alcohol abuse, and alcohol dependence in criminal behavior and family and sexual abuse (NIAAA, 1997). Summarizing two decades of research, Nathan (1993) concluded that

the relationship linking alcohol and aggression remains firmly established in our culture. This relationship appears to depend on a balance of expectancies and drug effects ... [However], when beverage alcohol consumed in moderate quantities exerts an aggression-inducing effect, it most likely does so because the drinker believes that to be its effect rather than because of any drug-induced effect. (p. 463)

Successful efforts to trace the link of alcohol and aggression have taken place in both laboratory settings and the real world.

Using a laboratory-based aggression analogue, Giancola and Zeichner (1995) examined the impact of aggressive personality traits, the degree of subjective intoxication, and the blood alcohol concentration (BAC) on aggression in young adult males and females. Subjects competed against a nonexistent "opponent" by giving electric shocks to, and receiving them from, the opponent under both provocative and nonprovocative conditions. Provocation was defined by the strength of shocks subjects received. Aggression was defined by the intensity of shocks that subjects gave. For males in the high provocation condition, aggressive personality traits, subjective intoxication, and BAC all predicted physical aggression. However, none of these variables was an effective predictor of aggression in women; this finding replicates prior failures to observe heightened aggressivity following intoxication among females in experimental settings (e.g., Gustafson, 1991). Perhaps heightened aggression could be observed in intoxicated women if a different laboratory analogue, one in which the aggression were not as blatantly physical, were employed.

Chermack and Taylor (1995) used the same experimental paradigm to contrast the two principal competing explanations for alcohol's effects on aggression: its pharmacological actions and its effects on expectancy/disinhibition. Male college students were divided into a group already convinced that alcohol increases aggression and a group convinced that it decreases aggression,. Subjects were then randomly assigned to active-placebo or high alcohol dose conditions. Subjects who consumed the high alcohol dose delivered significantly higher levels of shock than those who consumed the active-placebo, regardless of preexisting alcohol expectancies. Intoxicated subjects who believed that alcohol increases aggressive behavior delivered more intense shocks in high but not low provocation conditions. Chermack and Taylor's conclusion: The pharmacological effects of alcohol on aggression play the primary role in the alcohol–aggression nexus. This represents one of the first times that disinhibitory effects of alcohol on aggression were not emphasized following a laboratory demonstration of the alcohol–aggression connection. Chermack and Taylor's use of an analogue aggression measure, however, tempers our acceptance of this explanation. Real-world aggression is typically expressed in a more complex manner.

A number of authors recently examined linkages between real-world aggressivity and alcohol intoxication and dependence. Moss and Kirisci (1995), for example, undertook a correlational study of alcohol- and drug-misusing dependent adolescents; they found that aggressivity in the real world and symptoms of conduct disorder, which include overt aggressivity, correlated significantly and positively with alcohol consumption. Mezzich and her colleagues (1997) compared a group of alcohol- and drug-abusing adolescent females with a group of nonabusing controls and confirmed that the severity of alcohol/drug use has significant impact on relationships between personality disorder, mood disorder and family impairment, on the one hand, and suicide and violence on the other. Reviewing the extensive literature on the connection between alcohol and violent crime, Zhang, Wieczorek, and Welte (1997) identified four different roles that alcohol plays in crime and violence; these correspond to four major causes of crime at the individual level.

## Cognitive Dysfunction

Chronic alcohol abuse causes cognitive impairment, which may involve visual, spatial, or verbal memory; problem-solving; cognitive efficiency; or visuospatial perception (Beatty et al., 1996; Nixon, Tivis, & Parsons, 1995). From one-third to one-half of all chronic alcohol abusers suffer from demonstrable cognitive deficits (e.g., Fals-Stewart, 1996; Fals-Stewart & Lucente, 1994). Speculations on the etiology of these deficits range from alcoholic neurotoxicity (Freund, 1982), heredity (Hegadus et al., 1984), avitaminosis (Victor, Adams, & Collins, 1971), and physical trauma (Wetzig & Hardin, 1990). Cognitive dysfunctions diminish with continued abstinence; after a few months of sobriety, they may largely or completely disappear, depending on the length and severity of the

alcohol abuse, the length of abstinence, and the age of the abuser (Eckardt et al., 1995). Surprisingly, a family history of alcoholism does not affect the prognosis for recovery from alcohol-induced cognitive impairment (Adams et al., 1998). In older abusers, especially those whose abuse histories have been severe, the cognitive impairments may never completely disappear (Goldman et al., 1983).

Research on the long-term cognitive impact of alcohol use and abuse has recently shifted from an exclusive focus on the severe deficits of older alcohol abusers to the more modest impairments of younger social drinkers that may be premonitory to more severe dysfunction. For example, Nichols and Martin (1996) recorded visual ERPs from young, male, heavy and light social drinkers under an alcohol condition designed to induce mild disorientation or an alcohol placebo. The amplitude of the P300 ERP component was significantly more diminished in heavy than in light social drinkers, suggesting that the heavy social drinkers may already have begun to develop an alcohol-induced deficit in information processing. Given prior findings, reviewed before, that alcoholics typically demonstrate a diminished visual P300, these results suggest that this marker of impairment in information processing may constitute an early sign in heavy social drinkers of the serious impairments in cognitive functioning that afflict many chronic alcoholics.

Scheier and Botvin (1995) found that early adolescent alcohol and drug use are associated with small but significant declines in cognitive and self-management strategies that increase in magnitude in middle adolescence if substance use continues. These substance-induced effects may be more than epiphenomena. Scheier and Botvin hypothesize that "early drug use may impede acquisition of critical thinking skills and hinder the learning of important cognitive strategies required for successful transition to adulthood" (1995, p. 379).

Reviewing the nineteen pertinent studies on cognitive functioning in sober social drinkers published since 1986, Parsons and Nixon (1998) propose "an alcohol-causal-threshold hypothesis" that led them to propose that "persons drinking five or six U.S. standard drinks per day over extended time periods manifest some cognitive inefficiencies; at seven to nine drinks per day, mild cognitive deficits are present; and at 10 or more drinks per day, moderate cognitive deficits equivalent to those found in diagnosed alcoholics are present" (p. 180).

## Impaired Sexual Functioning and Increased Sexual Risk-Taking

Prolonged alcohol abuse, it has long been thought, impairs sexual functioning (Fahrner, 1987; Schiavi, 1990), probably by affecting hormonal mechanisms and testicular function in males (Bannister & Lowosky, 1987; Van Thiel et al., 1980). The impact of a history of alcoholism on sexual functioning, marital adjustment, sleep-related erections, sleep disorders, and hormone levels was recently studied in a small sample of abstinent male alcoholics by Schiavi and his colleagues (1995), with unexpected results. Two months to three years after achieving stable sobriety, the recovering alcoholics were compared to a group of nonalcoholic males; both groups of subjects were from 28–50 years of age. Subjects and their sexual partners all received thorough psychosexual evaluations, as well as a polygraphic assessment of sleep pattern, assessment of nocturnal penile tumescence, and nocturnal sequential blood sampling. Surprisingly, the alcoholic men did not differ from the comparison group along any dimension of sexuality or in the number of sexual problems, even though their sexual partners reported significant marital dissatisfaction. Despite a history of severe alcohol dependence, these men had been able to maintain normal sexual function, even in disturbed marriages. Schiavi and his coauthors observed, however, that their alcoholic subjects were not suffering from hepatic or gonadal disease or taking medication; in prior studies, these factors have been associated with impaired sexual function.

Alcohol use and abuse also increases sexual risk-taking (Kim, Celentano, & Crum, 1998). For example, Gordon and Carey (1996) studied the consequences of alcohol intoxication on condom use in a laboratory-based inquiry. Moderate to heavy drinking, young male nonalcoholic subjects were randomly assigned to either alcohol or alcohol placebo conditions. Those in the alcohol condition drank sufficient vodka and tonic to achieve blood alcohol levels of 0.08%; controls drank only tonic. All subjects then completed a battery of self-report measures of condom and AIDS-related knowledge, motivation to use condoms, and be-havioral self-efficacy for condom use. Subjects who had consumed alcohol reported more negative attitudes toward condom use and lower self-efficacy about the ability to use condoms than subjects who had consumed only tonic.

Parker, Harford, and Rosenstock (1994) explored real-world relationships between sexual risk-taking and alcohol and drug use in a large group of nonabusing young adults. After controlling for age, education, and family income, they found that the quantity and frequency of alcohol use (and that of marijuana and cocaine) were related significantly to sexual risk-taking, which they defined as the degree to which these men and women failed to take reasonable precautions against unintended pregnancy and sexually transmitted disease. Koopman and her colleagues (1994) observed the same phenomenon when they examined relationships between both lifetime and current alcohol and drug use and sexual risk-taking in several hundred male and female adolescent runaways, predominantly African-American and Hispanic, who lived in four residential centers in New York City. Greater frequency of substance use, which included marijuana and cocaine as well as alcohol, was related significantly to more sexual partners and less frequent condom use.

## Comorbidity

Alcohol abusers demonstrate more comorbid psychopathology than persons with any other psychiatric syndrome (Ross, Glaser, & Germanson, 1988; Wilson et al., 1996). According to Schuckit (1994c), however, the frequent co-occurrence of alcohol abuse and common forms of psychopathology like depression and anxiety partly reflects base rates, that is, because the prevalence rates of substance abuse, depression, and anxiety are all very high (Helzer et al., 1988), chance alone helps explain their frequent co-occurrence. It is also the case, Schuckit (1994c) continues, that persons with symptoms of two or more disorders—alcoholism and a mood or anxiety disorder, for example—are more likely to seek treatment than those with only one and, for that reason, to be represented in studies of comorbidity based on treatment populations.

A recent general population survey of the comorbidity of major depression and several substance use disorders revealed pervasive comorbidity among these conditions (Grant, 1995). The association between alcohol and other drug dependence and major depression was greater among older than younger subjects, consistent with the use of alcohol and other sedatives by older people to self-medicate for depression. This association was also greater for women than for men; Grant explained that this relationship derived at least in part from interaction between women's greater vulnerability to stigmatization for alcohol and drug abuse and the DSM-IV abuse criteria, which emphasize strongly the adverse consequences arising from abuse.

Many of the drugs of abuse, including alcohol, produce symptoms that mimic major psychiatric disorders (Schuckit, 1994c). These behaviors have been studied most extensively as a consequence of central nervous system depressant (alcohol, barbiturates, and benzodiazepines) and stimulant (the amphetamines and cocaine) use:

... intoxication with *brain stimulants* can cause many symptoms of *anxiety*, with intake of larger doses even producing syndromes that can look similar to obsessive-compulsive disorder, panic disorder, and generalized anxiety disorder. Withdrawal from brain stimulants as well as repeated and prolonged intoxication with *brain depressants* can cause sadness that might even produce severe and incapacitating *depression* that resembles a major depressive episode. Withdrawal from brain depressant drugs is likely to produce intense and acute anxiety, with the probability of prolonged, but less severe, anxiety during what might be considered a protracted abstinence syndrome. Repeated stimulant intoxication, especially with amphetamines and cocaine, is likely to produce a syndrome of auditory hallucinations along with paranoid delusions that can temporarily resemble *schizophrenia*. (Schuckit, 1994c, p. 46)

Because alcohol sometimes functions briefly as a CNS stimulant, even though its major effect is as a CNS depressant, it can induce symptoms of both anxiety and depression.

## Schizophrenia and Other Psychoses

The Epidemiological Catchment Area (ECA) study (Regier et al., 1990) surveyed the mental health status of a large representative sample of the U.S. population in five cities around the country and found that persons diagnosed with schizophrenia experience an elevated lifetime prevalence of alcohol-related disorder, that more than a quarter of persons with schizophrenia simultaneously experience comorbid alcohol-related disorder, and that persons diagnosed with schizophrenia are much more likely to have histories of

alcohol-related disorder than those without the disorder. All three findings confirm the common co-occurrence of alcohol-related disorder and psychosis, prominently including schizophrenia. These conditions co-occur for several reasons: schizophrenic persons, as well as those suffering from other psychotic disorders, tend to be intemperate (e.g., Barbee et al., 1989; Drake, Osher, & Wallach, 1989); alcohol is commonly self-administered by schizophrenic persons in an effort to dampen psychotic symptoms; and persons with the dual diagnoses of schizophrenia and substance abuse are substantially more likely to come to the attention of mental health professionals than those with only one or the other of these disorders (Schuckit, 1994c).

## Attention-Deficit/Hyperactivity Disorder (ADHD)

Symptoms of ADHD in persons with alcohol-related disorders are quite common (e.g., Biederman et al., 1995; Wilens et al., 1994). Because ADHD is often a feature of the childhood of individuals who develop alcohol-related disorders as adults, ADHD has been portrayed, most notably, by Tarter and his colleagues (1977) as a precursor of alcohol abuse and possibly shares a common genotype in some individuals. However, questions remain whether ADHD itself or the mood, anxiety, and conduct disorders that often accompany it is primarily responsible for the co-occurrence of alcohol-related disorders and ADHD.

## Personality Disorders

Personality disorders and substance-related disorders very often co-occur (Verheul et al., 1998; Zimmerman & Coryell, 1990). The most prevalent of personality disorders comorbid with substance-related disorders is antisocial personality disorder (ASPD). ASPD is most common among persons who abuse illegal drugs, but it also accompanies high rates of alcohol abuse and dependence (Verheul, van den Brink, & Hartgers, 1995), with which it shares personality trait dimensions.

The co-occurrence of ASPD and depression in alcohol-dependent persons is particularly familiar. Holdcraft, Iacono, and McGue (1998) explored these comorbid conditions in more than 200 alcoholic men recruited from a community-based sample (the Minnesota Twin-Family Study); subjects were further divided into four groups: alcoholics with ASPD, alcoholics with depression, alcoholics with neither ASPD nor depression, and alcoholics with no other psychiatric comorbidity. Depression was associated with a less severe course of alcoholism, but ASPD and alcoholism co-occurred in persons who reported an earlier age of first alcohol intoxication, a more chronic and severe form of alcoholism, more social consequences of drinking, and higher levels of drug use. These findings, which support Cloninger's two-fold alcoholism typology (Bohman, Sigvardsson, & Cloninger, 1981; Cloninger, Bohman, & Sigvardsson, 1981), emphasize the importance of carefully diagnosing comorbid conditions in alcohol abusers for better treatment planning and more accurate prognoses.

## Mood Disorders

The mood disorders that include major depressive disorder, dysthymic disorder, and bipolar disorder are among the conditions most commonly comorbid with alcohol-related disorder.

In a longitudinal study designed to examine the impact of alcohol use on the course of depressive disorder (Mueller et al., 1994), patients with dual diagnoses of major depression and alcoholism, as well as those diagnosed only with major depressive disorder, were followed over a 10-year time span. To determine more precisely the impact of alcohol abuse on the course of depression, three patient subtypes based on alcohol usage were constituted; they included patients who were never alcoholic, those who did not meet criteria for current alcoholism, and those who were currently alcoholic. Patients who had never been alcoholic or were not actively alcoholic were twice as likely to recover from major depressive disorder as actively alcoholic patients; this strongly suggests that active alcoholism has a decidedly malignant effect on recovery from major depressive disorder.

In a study with similar goals, Brown and her colleagues (1995) compared changes in the severity of depressive symptoms among men with alcohol dependence, affective disorder, or both during 4 weeks of inpatient treatment for either alcohol dependence or affective disorder. Symptoms of depression remitted more rapidly in men with primary alcoholism than in those with primary depression. Alcohol dependence in persons suffering from primary affective disorder neither intensified symptoms of depression nor interfered with their treatment. These findings, in apparent conflict

with those from the study by Mueller and his colleagues (1994), may reflect the fact that Mueller and his colleagues, unlike Brown and her coworkers, did not distinguish between primary and secondary depression—which appears to be an important distinction to make. Moreover, the severity of the depressive conditions treated in the two studies may also have differed.

Pettinati et al. (1997) explored gender differences in ninety-three alcohol-dependent outpatients divided into approximately equal groups of males with current or lifetime depressive disorders, females with current or lifetime depressive disorders, females without a history of depressive disorder, and males without a history of depressive disorder. Substantial differences between males and females were found. Depressed males had more serious alcoholism—more drinking, more drinking-related problems, and greater alcoholism severity—than depressed females and never-depressed males, whereas depressed female alcoholics were more severely depressed—reported more intense symptoms of depression—than depressed male alcoholics. The significant interaction between gender and comorbid depression observed in this study reinforces the accepted view that gender has important implications for predicting success in treating comorbid alcoholism and depression.

We conclude that depression, for some individuals, is an antecedent to, and for others, it is a consequence of alcohol use and alcohol abuse. Severe depression exacerbates alcohol problems and makes treating them effectively more difficult. Depression, the comorbid behavioral disorder most intimately linked to alcohol abuse and dependence, is also its most troubling accompaniment. The differing expressions of both depression and alcohol dependence in men and women require considering gender when planning treatment for these frequently comorbid conditions.

## Social Anxiety, Tension Reduction, and Anxiety Disorders

The first viable alternative to the psychodynamic theory of alcoholism etiology, which held sway during the decades immediately preceding World War II, was the tension-reduction hypothesis (TRH). Buttressed by anecdotal reports from both social drinkers and alcoholics that alcohol reduces anxiety, the TRH gained additional support from empirical research (e.g., Conger, 1951; Masserman &

Yum, 1946) that documented alcohol's capacity to reduce experimentally induced conflict ("anxiety") in rats and cats. The TRH did not fare so well, however, when it was tested in alcoholics. This research (see reviews by Cappell, 1974, and Langenbucher & Nathan, 1993) revealed that alcoholics do not respond consistently to alcohol. Some experience tension relief, others an increase in tension, and still others show no effect at all.

The importance of attitudes toward the tension-reducing effects of alcohol were underlined in research completed a number of years ago (e.g., Abrams & Wilson, 1979; Polivy, Schueneman, & Carlson, 1976; Wilson & Abrams, 1977). This research suggested that the sedative effects of alcohol at low to moderate doses do tend to reduce tension and anxiety in the short run—unless the drinkers' attitudes toward drinking are so conflicted (as are those of many alcoholics) that they experience anxiety rather than tension-relief when beginning to drink again.

A review of contemporary research on alcohol and anxiety by Schuckit and Hesselbrock (1994) was motivated by the observation that although many alcoholics report symptoms of severe anxiety during periods of abstinence, it is unclear whether the anxiety is primarily associated with independent psychiatric syndromes, with the abstinence syndrome, or with the two in combination. Schuckit and Hesselbrock (1994) conclude that

the available data, while imperfect, do not prove a close relationship between lifelong anxiety disorders and alcohol dependence. Further, prospective studies of children of alcoholics and individuals from the general population do not indicate a high rate of anxiety disorders preceding alcohol dependence. The high rates of comorbidity (of alcohol dependence and anxiety disorder) in some studies likely reflect a mixture of true anxiety disorders among alcoholics at a rate equal to or slightly higher than that for the general population, along with temporary, but at times severe, substance-induced anxiety syndromes. (p. 1723)

These conclusions point to a fairly remote relationship between anxiety and alcohol abuse and contrast with the much closer relationship between alcohol abuse and depression reviewed earlier.

## Treatment

The search for effective treatments for alcohol use disorders continues. Despite intense efforts over many years, available treatments still help only some alcoholic patients some of the time. Many persons who abuse alcohol are motivated to moderate or stop their drinking on their own or in treatment, but substantial numbers eventually return to abusive drinking. That is the nature of the disorder: Alcohol dependence is a chronic recurrent disorder, characterized by periods of drinking that are out of control, periods of more moderate drinking, and periods of abstinence (Schuckit, 1995; Vaillant, 1995). Nonetheless, as this section of the chapter demonstrates, the search for effective treatments for alcoholism continues to attract substantial resources and numerous highly motivated research workers.

Nathan summarized the status of alcoholism treatment in the early part of the 90s in the second edition of this volume (1993). The material that follows surveys subsequent developments.

### Reviews of Psychosocial Treatment Outcomes

Most reviews have concluded that outcomes of psychosocial treatments for alcoholism depend primarily on two factors, the treatment provided and the characteristics patients bring to it (especially the length and severity of their substance abuse, but also marital, educational, and employment history; physical health status; and comorbid psychopathology). However, recent reviews suggest that other factors, including therapist characteristics, the duration and amount of treatment, and the setting of treatment, also impact treatment outcomes substantially.

**Treatments.** In their recent review of the treatment outcome research literature, Finney and Moos (1998) ranked fifteen psychosocial treatments on the basis of results from three or more empirical studies of each, as evaluated by Holder et al. (1991), Miller et al. (1995), and Finney and Monahan (1996). Treatments with the highest effectiveness ratings in these reviews all fell into the cognitive-behavioral domain. All aimed to help patients develop skills to cope more effectively with the environmental stressors often implicated in relapse from abstinence. The top four treatments, all cognitive-behavioral, included social skills training, community reinforcement, brief motivational counseling, and behavioral marital therapy.

*Social skills training* (e.g., Smith & McCrady,

1991) aims to develop more effective assertive and communicative skills, on the assumption that persons who lack these skills may abuse alcohol because it dampens their feelings of social inadequacy or gives them the illusion that they are socially skilled. *Community reinforcement* (Azrin et al., 1982) initially involved interventions that assisted patients with job-related, legal, and family problems and provided them access to an alcohol-free club. Later, the club was dropped and a buddy-support system, group counseling, and behavioral contracting to encourage maintenance of Antabuse treatment were added. Throughout, the focus was on behavioral efforts to modify patients' drinking and enhance their relationships with their families and employers. *Brief motivation counseling* (Miller & Sanchez, 1993) is intended to enhance patients' motivation to modify their abusive drinking, partly by emphasizing the serious consequences of continued abuse, including the negative effects of alcohol abuse on lifespan. *Behavioral marital therapy* (O'Farrell et al., 1993) simultaneously uses behavioral and Antabuse contracts to address the abusive drinking of the alcoholic spouse; it also includes a variety of behavioral approaches designed to improve the marital relationship.

In sharp contrast to these four underused but empirically supported treatments are the three most widely used alcoholism treatment methods, which turn out to have the least documented effectiveness of all of the fifteen treatments cited by Finney and Moos (1998). Even though they lack proven efficacy, *educational films, confrontational interventions*, and *general alcoholism counseling* are at the core of many alcoholism programs nationwide.

**Therapist Characteristics.** What do we know about therapist characteristics that contribute to successful treatment for alcoholism? A great deal of research on the therapist characteristics that affect therapy outcomes more generally has been reported (Beutler, Machado, & Neufeldt, 1994, review this extensive literature), but only Najavits and Weiss (1994) addressed this issue specifically for outcomes of alcoholism treatment. After reviewing seven studies that found marked differences among different therapists in treatment retention or outcome, these authors conclude that therapist characteristics play a more important role in therapy outcome than techniques. Predictably, therapists who were more skilled interper-

sonally, less confrontational, and more empathic produced better outcomes for their alcoholic patients.

**Duration and Amount of Treatment.** There is considerable support for the effectiveness of brief interventions for alcohol problems (Miller et al., 1995). Most efforts to compare brief with more extended treatments for alcoholism concluded that briefer treatments are generally as efficacious as more extended ones; some observers even concluded that brief treatments have better outcomes (Bien, Miller, & Tonigan, 1993). Miller and Sanchez (1993) proposed the acronym FRAMES as a reminder of the six ingredients of brief therapy for alcoholism that they believe predict favorable outcomes: *F*eedback of personal risk or impairment, emphasis on personal *R*esponsibility for change, clear *A*dvice to change, a *M*enu of alternative change options, therapeutic *E*mpathy, and enhancement of patients' *S*elf-efficacy or optimism about successful change efforts.

Because most studies of brief interventions for alcohol problems have recruited persons with only mild to moderate problems, it is not clear how effective brief interventions are for more severe alcohol dependence. Finney and Moos (1998) and Monahan and Finney (1996) suggest that more serious substance abuse probably benefits from more intensive, longer lasting treatments.

**Length of Stay in Treatment.** The data on the impact of length of stay in residential treatment facilities on outcomes of treatment for alcoholism are equivocal. Reviews by Miller and Hester (1986) and Mattick and Jarvis (1994) persuaded their authors that the length of inpatient treatment is unrelated to outcome differences, but Monahan and Finney (1996) reached a different conclusion. Their "quantitative synthesis of patient, research design, and treatment effects" convinced them that amount of treatment across 150 treatment groups in 100 studies bore a significant relationship to abstinence rates. In an attempt to explain their divergent findings, they emphasized the 10:1 difference in the amount of treatment received by high- (148 hours of treatment) versus low-intensity (14 hours) treatment groups; a ratio of this magnitude had not been represented in previous randomized trials of treatment duration.

Finney and Moos (1998) submit that "beneficial effects of longer stays in inpatient/residential treatment apply only to more impaired patients with fewer social resources" (p. 161), a conclusion supported by Welte, Hynes, and Sokolow (1981), who found a clear relationship between length of stay and outcome for patients who had lower but not higher social stability.

## Project MATCH (Matching Alcoholism Treatments to Client Heterogeneity)

Only recently, large-scale randomized clinical trials of alcoholism treatments, the "gold standard" for treatment outcomes, have been undertaken. In 1997, results from two such studies, the National Institute on Alcohol Abuse and Alcoholism's Project MATCH (Project MATCH Research Group, 1993, 1997a,b) and the Veterans Administration's cooperative study (Ouimette, Finney, & Moos, 1997), were reported.

Project MATCH was a large national multisite clinical trial designed to evaluate a set of patient–treatment matching hypotheses. A priori hypotheses that linked eleven client attributes to three treatments proposed that certain attributes would be associated with better outcomes (in terms of the percentage of days abstinent and drinks per drinking day) when patients received one of the treatments rather than either of the other two. The basic assumption underlying Project MATCH and its series of matching hypotheses was that substance abusers appropriately matched to treatments will experience better outcomes than those who are unmatched or mismatched. An extensive history of research successfully matching patients to treatments supported the validity of these hypotheses (e.g., Longabaugh et al., 1994; Mattson & Allen, 1991; Mattson et al., 1994; Moos, Finney, & Cronkite, 1990).

Project MATCH's secondary purpose was to compare outcomes of three different, manual-guided, individually delivered 12-week treatments: *Cognitive-Behavioral Coping Skills Treatment* (CBT), *Motivational Enhancement Therapy* (MET), and *Twelve-Step Facilitation* (TSF). The treatments were described as follows:

CBT was based on social learning theory and viewed drinking behavior as functionally related to major problems in an individual's life, with emphasis placed on overcoming skills deficits and increasing the ability to cope with situations that commonly precipitate relapse. TST was grounded in the concept of alcoholism as a spiritual and medical disease with stated objectives of fostering acceptance of the disease of alcoholism, developing a commitment to participate in AA and beginning to work through the 12 steps ... MET was based on principles of

motivational psychology and focused on producing internally-motivated change. This treatment was not designed to guide the client, step by step, through recovery, but instead employed motivational strategies to mobilize the individual's own resources. (Project MATCH Research Group, 1997a, p. 13)

Detailed treatment manuals were provided to each therapist who participated in the study (Kadden et al., 1992; Miller et al., 1992; Nowinski, Baker, & Carroll, 1992) to ensure to the extent possible that different therapists at different sites would deliver the same treatment in the same way.

Two independent, parallel matching studies were conducted, one with 952 patients (72% male) recruited from outpatient settings, the other with 774 patients (80% male) in aftercare treatment after a period of inpatient treatment. Patients were contacted for follow-up every 3 months for a year after the 12-week treatment period; as noted before, primary outcome measures were the percentage of days abstinent and drinks per drinking day. At the 12-month mark, 92 and 93%, respectively, of patients originally treated were successfully contacted.

Contrary to expectation, only two a priori contrasts produced significant posttreatment attribute by treatment interactions (Project MATCH Research Group, 1997b): (1) Outpatients high in anger treated in MET drank less on follow-up than in CBT; (2) Aftercare patients high in alcohol dependence drank less on follow-up in TSF; aftercare patients low in alcohol dependence drank less in CBT. Commenting on this paucity of anticipated matching effects, the Project MATCH Research Group (1997a) frankly observed that "the power of the present study to detect matching effects, and its careful, rigorous implementation, make the lack of substantial findings particularly notable." The logical inference: "... little evidence to support widely held views regarding the potential value of matching clients, at least on the basis of nine of the client attributes tested, to any of the treatments offered as individual therapy in this study" (Project MATCH Research Group, 1997a, p. 23).

Of primary importance to us, although a secondary focus of Project MATCH, was that "significant and sustained improvements in drinking outcomes were achieved from baseline to 1-year posttreatment by the clients assigned to each of these well-defined and individually delivered psychosocial treatments. There was little difference in outcomes by type of treatment" (Project MATCH Research Group, 1997a, p. 7).

What were the "significant and sustained improvements in drinking outcomes" to which the Project MATCH Research Group refers? The aftercare group was abstinent only about 1 in 5 days, and the outpatient group was abstinent only about 1 in 4 days before treatment began, but the aftercare group was abstinent about 95% of the days following treatment, and the outpatient group maintained abstinence a bit more than 80% of posttreatment days. Drinks per drinking day for the aftercare group dropped from fifteen to twenty during the pretreatment period to two to three drinks per drinking day posttreatment; the comparable figures for the outpatient group were eleven to thirteen and three to four drinks. Approximately 35% of the aftercare subjects and 19% of the outpatient subjects reported continued complete abstinence throughout the 12 follow-up months.

When these data are weighed in the light of the study's design, they permit either a positive or a negative evaluation of the effectiveness of the three Project MATCH treatments, depending on which findings are emphasized. The positive view sees that the findings documented marked reductions in the percentage of days abstinent and drinks per drinking day that reflected the effects of three equally robust treatments, all capable of inducing marked changes in drinking that lasted through a full year of follow-up.

The negative view laments the absence of a control group, which makes it impossible to know whether the changes in drinking were related specifically to the treatments or to other factors. The absence of data beyond the 1-year follow-up mark prevents us from knowing to what extent these gains were sustained. Exclusion criteria which ruled out potential clients who lacked residential stability; showed signs of organic impairment; or met diagnostic criteria for cocaine, sedative/hypnotic, stimulant, or opiate-dependence may have yielded a sample population unrepresentative of clients typically seen at public alcoholism treatment facilities nowadays.

Of concern, as well, is the MATCH authors' decision not to provide detailed data on the numbers of clients who established and maintained abstinence during the follow-up period. The relatively incomplete data that are provided on abstinence make it difficult to compare Project MATCH

outcomes with those from most other alcoholism treatment outcome studies, including the VA cooperative study. In the absence of detailed data on abstinence, we know only that a substantial majority of Project MATCH clients (65% of the aftercare group and 81% of the outpatient group) consumed alcohol during the follow-up period. These data, although scanty, are telling. Most studies and reviews of recovering alcoholics have concluded that those who continue to drink after treatment, however minimally, are at substantial risk of resuming abusive drinking at some point (Nathan & McCrady, 1987; Nathan & Skinstad, 1987; Schuckit, 1995; Vaillant, 1995).

## Veterans Administration Medical Centers Cooperative Study

Ouimette, Finney, and Moos (1997) compared the effectiveness of twelve-step, cognitive-behavioral (C-B), and combined twelve-step-C-B models of substance abuse treatment in a nonrandom clinical trial of 3018 detoxified inpatients in the substance abuse treatment programs of fifteen Department of Veterans Affairs Medical Centers (VAMC). Unlike Project MATCH, the major focus of the VAMC study was a direct comparison of two widely used models for substance abuse treatment. The fifteen sites were selected because they offered twelve-step, cognitive-behavioral, and combined cognitive-behavioral inpatient treatment programs that met the investigators' criteria for quality and theoretical integrity. The desired length of stay in the programs ranged from 21 to 28 days; all provided both individual and group therapy, and all had multidisciplinary staffing.

Follow-up of treatment extended for a year. Eleven outcome measures were used; five reflected alcohol and drug use, two tapped symptoms of anxiety and depression, and three measured social variables, including arrests, employment, and living situation.

The treatments were described as follows:

Twelve-step programs emphasized treatment activities such as 12-step meetings in the community and hospital, and psychotherapy groups covering topics such as working the steps, the *Big Book*, and writing an autobiography. Treatment targeted the patient's acceptance of an alcoholic-addict identity, acknowledgment of a loss of control-powerlessness over the abused substance, and adherence to abstinence as a treatment goal.... C-B programs required participation in relapse prevention groups, cognitive skills training, behavioral skills training, abstinence skills training, and small C-B therapy groups. The goals of C-B treatment were to teach more adaptive ways of coping, to enhance the patient's sense of self-efficacy to cope with high-risk relapse-inducing situations, and to modify the patient's expectations of the abused substances' effects such that they were more realistic and appropriate. (Ouimette, Finney, & Moos, 1997, p. 232)

Unlike Project MATCH, which randomized assignment of patients to treatments, the VAMC study used a quasi-experimental design that resulted in significant differences among patients in the three treatment conditions. To this end, C-B programs enrolled significantly higher percentages of non-African Americans; mixed twelve-step-C-B programs inducted patients whose alcohol consumption and heroin use were significantly higher at intake and who were most likely to have had prior outpatient substance abuse treatment; and twelve-step programs treated the highest percentage of African-Americans, the lowest percentage of clients ever to inject heroin, and the lowest percentage of clients with prior detoxification-inpatient substance abuse treatment experience or outpatient treatment experience.

Although twelve-step patients were somewhat more likely to be abstinent and to be employed at the 1-year follow-up mark, patients in all three treatments reduced substance use and improved most other areas of functioning equally at both the end of inpatient treatment and the 1-year follow-up. The finding of equal effectiveness was consistent over several treatment subgroups, including patients who attended the "purest" twelve-step and C-B treatment programs and patients who had received the "full dose" of treatment. Moreover, patients with substance abuse diagnoses alone, those with comorbid psychiatric diagnoses, and those who had not entered treatment of their own volition all showed similar improvement at 1-year follow-up, regardless of the type of treatment received.

At the 1-year mark, however, only 25–30% of the patients were judged to be without a substance abuse problem, only 23–29% were considered to be in remission from their substance use disorder, and only 18–25% had been able to maintain abstinence. These figures represent marked improvements over pretreatment rates, but they are nonetheless disturbing in their prognostic significance. As we noted earlier, a great deal of research suggests that many or most recovering alcoholics who continue to drink even in a controlled fashion

following treatment will ultimately return to abusive drinking.

### Pharmacological Interventions

**Alcohol-Sensitizing Agents.** Antabuse (disulfiram) blocks the chemical breakdown of alcohol; individuals who have ingested Antabuse cannot metabolize alcohol beyond the point at which it has been metabolized in the bloodstream to acetaldehyde. Because acetaldehyde is toxic to the body in very small quantities, when even the smallest amount of alcohol has been consumed by someone who has disulfiram in the bloodstream, an acetaldehyde reaction takes place (Christensen et al., 1991). The alcoholic quickly experiences nausea, vomiting, profuse sweating, and markedly increased respiration and heart rate. Alcoholics who have had an Antabuse reaction say it is an experience that they would do almost anything to avoid.

Alcoholics who take an Antabuse tablet every day are "protected" from the impulse to drink even if they are tempted to do so by alcohol-related cues. Because of the dangers of the acetaldehyde reaction, however, physicians in the United States prescribe disulfiram only to patients who are physically fit, motivated to stop drinking, and fully able to appreciate the consequences if they drink while they are taking the drug.

Some experienced clinicians swear by Antabuse; others find it ineffective. The data on its effectiveness are equivocal (Wright & Moore, 1989), largely because it works well for some patients and not at all for others. Patient differences in sensitivity to the effects of the drug may explain its inconsistent effectiveness. In general, clinicians prescribe Antabuse to give alcoholics a recovery "window" that reduces their risk of succumbing to craving. This grace period permits psychological and behavioral gains that will allow discontinuing Antabuse at some point.

**Agents for Managing Withdrawal and Maintaining Sobriety.** Two decades ago, clinicians in this country routinely gave alcoholics a benzodiazepine, generally, Librium or Valium, during withdrawal. It was widely assumed that these drugs eased the physical and psychological pains of detoxification and prevented the development of more serious withdrawal phenomena like delirium tremens. Nowadays, however, many clinicians have concluded that relatively few alcoholics experience serious enough withdrawal symptoms to warrant pharmacological intervention (Wartenburg et al., 1990); as a result, many more patients are routinely detoxified nonpharmacologically.

In years past, antianxiety agents were also given to alcoholics in hopes that the drugs would dampen the anxiety for which many alcoholics self-medicate. Instead, however, many alcohol abusers simply added the abuse of these highly addictive drugs to their abuse of alcohol and other substances. As a result, these drugs are now rarely given to persons dependent on alcohol or other drugs (O'Brien & McKay, 1998).

**Anticraving Agents.** During the past decade, investigations of several drug classes that act on neurotransmitters in the brain, including serotonin re-uptake inhibitors, dopamine agonists, and opioid antagonists, have led to the development of drugs that have the exciting potential to decrease craving and the reinforcing effects of alcohol. These drugs are promising because they have the potential to prevent, rather than simply treat the effects of, alcohol abuse and dependence.

Serotonin re-uptake inhibitors increase quantities of serotonin in the brain. They have produced modest decreases in alcohol consumption in male heavy drinkers with mild to moderate alcohol dependence (Naranjo et al., 1990); serotonin exerts an anticraving effect. Dopamine agonists also decrease alcohol consumption and self-reported craving because of their effect on concentrations of dopamine in the brain (Dongier et al., 1991); dopamine increases craving. Finally, the opioid antagonist, naltrexone, originally developed to treat opioid dependence by inducing withdrawal and blocking subsequent dependence in opioid addicts, has a substantial impact on alcohol consumption by alcoholics. O'Malley and her colleagues (1992), for example, reported that naltrexone led to a marked decrease in alcohol consumption by outpatient alcoholics because the drug reduces the pleasurable feelings that alcohol induces.

## Resolution of Alcohol Problems without Treatment

Although we all know people who have recovered from serious alcohol problems on their own, resolution of alcohol problems without treatment has only recently become a focus of research attention. Watson and Sher (1998) reviewed this literature. Perhaps the most surprising of their conclusions is that natural recovery may be the major path to recovery from alcohol use disorders; estimates range up to three-quarters of all recovering alcoholics who do so without treatment (Sobell, Cunningham, & Sobell, 1996; Vaillant, 1995).

Unfortunately, methodological problems prevent abundant generalization across empirical studies about self-changers, defined as alcoholics who have recovered without treatment. Watson and Sher (1998) noted that differences across studies in the criteria for judging drinking status pre- and postrecovery, in the time that must pass before a person is considered recovered, and in definitions of what constitutes treatment all make it difficult to generalize across these studies. Lack of sample heterogeneity, a problem of a very different nature, also afflicts this literature. Most reports of alcoholics who recover without treatment are of White, middle-aged males, so there is a paucity of data about self-changers who are non-White, older or younger, and/or female. An additional problem stems from the diverse strategies employed to study natural recovery. Some studies have relied on retrospective assessments either systematically from community samples or unsystematically from volunteers, and others have used prospective designs that assess groups of treatment seekers or nonclinical samples. Although each of these strategies can be justified, they differ sufficiently to further impede efforts to generalize their findings.

Despite these formidable methodological problems, some findings have emerged from this literature with enough consistency to consider them valid generalizations. One of the most intriguing concerns *the processes of self-directed change*, which are the strategies self-changers use to recover and the environmental events that precipitate their recovery. Of the ten processes associated with the well-known change model proposed by Prochaska and his colleagues (Prochaska, DiClemente, & Norcross, 1992), eight frequently mentioned in the self-change literature include consciousness raising, self-reevaluation, environmental evaluation, self-liberation, counterconditioning, stimulus control, reinforcement management, and helping relationships.

The *circumstances that surround the decision to stop drinking on one's own* are also a focus of interest. They include the events that lead to self-recognition of the existence of a drinking problem, concerns about alcohol-related health problems, and role transitions (e.g., marrying, taking a new job). Researchers have also attempted to study the impact of *individual difference variables on success in self-changing*, including the severity of the alcohol problem, a family history of alcoholism, comorbid psychopathology, antisocial personality disorder, other substance use disorders, and a range of personality traits.

These generalizations are tentative because of the methodological shortcomings in the research to date on self-changers. Nonetheless, they might help clinicians identify persons most likely to self-change, to whom less intensive interventions might be offered to encourage their propensity for self-change. What we learn about self-changers also might help us design more effective treatments for alcoholics who require formal treatment because they are unlikely to change on their own.

### Conclusions about Treatment

Despite the results of two large-scale, multisite clinical trials of alcoholism treatments, and several recent comprehensive reviews, we cannot yet point to psychosocial or pharmacological treatments for alcohol abuse and dependence whose efficacy has been proven. Regretfully, significant methodological problems make unequivocal interpretation of the findings from Project MATCH and the VAMC Cooperative Study impossible. Both found that cognitive-behavioral and twelve-step treatments are associated with significant reductions in consumption, and Project MATCH provided additional data attesting to the efficacy of motivational enhancement counseling as well, but the absence of control groups and, in the case of Project MATCH, the form in which the follow-up data were reported make us uncertain whether it was the treatments themselves that brought about the positive changes and what the actual dimensions of those changes were. The fact that substantial numbers of treated patients in both studies were drinking at the conclusion of the follow-up periods convinces us they were at substantial risk of returning to abusive drinking at some point.

At the same time, there is reason for optimism. A start has been made. Project MATCH and the VAMC Cooperative Study have identified three treatments that impact drinking by alcoholics markedly, at least for a time. Nonetheless, controlled research on these treatments that documents their centrality in the change process is necessary, as is research designed to explore effec-

tive treatment variations, including combining promising new medications designed to reduce craving with psychosocial interventions designed to heighten motivation to change, to develop alternatives to the alcoholic lifestyle, and to provide clients with a supportive, alcohol-free social environment.

## References

Abrams, D. B., & Wilson, G. T. (1979). Effects of alcohol on social anxiety in women: Cognitive versus physiological processes. *Journal of Abnormal Psychology, 88*, 161–173.

Adams, K. M., Gilman, S., Johnson-Greene, D., Koeppe, R. A., Junck, L., Kluin, K. J., Martello, S., Johnson, M. J., Heumann, M., & Hill, E. (1998). The significance of family history status in relation to neuropsychological test performance and cerebral glucose metabolism studied with positron emission tomography in older alcoholic patients. *Alcoholism: Clinical and Experimental Research, 22*, 105–110.

Allen, J. P., Fertig, J. B., & Mattson, M. E. (1994). Personality-based subtypes of chemically dependent patients. *Annals of the New York Academy of Sciences, 708*, 7–22.

American Psychiatric Association. (1952). *Diagnostic and statistical manual of mental disorders* (1st ed.). Washington, DC: Author.

American Psychiatric Association. (1968). *Diagnostic and statistical manual of mental disorders* (2nd ed.). Washington, DC: Author.

American Psychiatric Association. (1980). *Diagnostic and statistical manual of mental disorders* (3rd ed.). Washington, DC: Author.

American Psychiatric Association. (1987). *Diagnostic and statistical manual of mental disorders* (3rd ed., rev.). Washington, DC: Author.

American Psychiatric Association. (1994). *Diagnostic and statistical manual of mental disorders* (4th ed.). Washington, DC: Author.

Azrin, N. H., Sisson, R. W., Meyers, R., & Godley, M. (1982). Alcoholism treatment by disulfiram and community reinforcement therapy. *Journal of Behavior Therapy and Experimental Psychiatry, 13*, 105–112.

Bannister, P., & Lowosky, M. S. (1987). Ethanol and hypogonadism. *Alcohol, 22*, 213–217.

Barbee, J. G., Clark, P. D., Crapanzo, B. S., et al. (1989). Alcohol and substance abuse among schizophrenic patients presenting to an emergency psychiatric service. *Journal of Nervous and Mental Disease, 177*, 400–407.

Beatty, W. W., Hames, K. A., Blanco, C. R., Nixon, S. J., & Tivis, L. J. (1996). Visuospatial perception, construction and memory in alcoholism. *Journal of Studies on Alcohol, 57*, 136–143.

Begleiter, H., Porjesz, B., Bihari, B., & Kissin, B. (1984). Event-related potentials in boys at risk for alcoholism. *Science, 225*, 1493–1496.

Beutler, L. E., Machado, P. P. P., & Neufeldt, S. A. (1994). Therapist variables. In A. E. Bergin & S. L. Garfield (Eds.), *Handbook of psychotherapy and behavior change* (pp. 229–269). New York: Wiley.

Biederman, J., Wilens, T., Mick, E., Milberger, S., Spencer, T. J., & Faraone, S. V. (1995). Psychoactive substance use disorders in adults with attention deficit hyperactivity disorder (ADHD): Effects of ADHD and psychiatry comorbidity. *American Journal of Psychiatry, 152,* 1652–1658.

Bien, T. H., Miller, W. R., & Tonigan, J. S. (1993). Brief interventions for alcohol problems: A review. *Addiction, 88,* 315–336.

Bigelow, G., Cohen, M., Liebson, I., & Faillace, L. (1972). Abstinence or moderation? Choice by alcoholics. *Behaviour Research and Therapy, 10,* 209–214.

Bigelow, G., Liebson, I., & Griffiths, R. R. (1974). Alcohol drinking: Suppression by a behavioral time-out procedure. *Behaviour Research and Therapy, 12,* 107–115.

Blaine, J. D., Horton, A. H., & Towle, L. H. (Eds.). (1995). *Diagnosis and severity of drug abuse and drug dependence.* NIH Pub. No. 95-3884. Rockville, MD: National Institute on Drug Abuse.

Bohman, M., Cloninger, C. R., von Knorring, A. L., & Sigvardsson, S. (1984). An adoption study of somatoform disorders. III. Cross fostering analysis and genetic relationship to alcoholism and criminality. *Archives of General Psychiatry, 41,* 872–878.

Bohman, M., Sigvardsson, S., & Cloninger, C. R. (1981). Maternal inheritance of alcohol abuse. *Archives of General Psychiatry, 38,* 965–969.

Brown, S. A., Goldman, M. S., & Christiansen B. A. (1985). Do alcohol expectancies mediate drinking patterns of adults? *Journal of Consulting and Clinical Psychology, 53,* 512–519.

Brown, S. A., Goldman, M. S., Inn, A., & Anderson, L. (1980). Expectations of reinforcement from alcohol: Their domain and relation to drinking patterns. *Journal of Consulting and Clinical Psychology, 48,* 419–426.

Brown, S. A., Inaba, R. K., Gillin, J. C., Schuckit, M. A., Stewart, M. A., & Irwin, M. R. (1995). Alcoholism and affective disorder: Clinical course and depressive symptoms. *American Journal of Psychiatry, 152,* 45–52.

Cadoret, R. J. (1980). Development of alcoholism in adoptees raised apart from alcoholic biologic relatives. *Archives of General Psychiatry, 37,* 561–563.

Caetano, R. (1997). Prevalence, incidence, and stability of drinking problems among whites, blacks, and Hispanics: 1984–1992. *Journal of Studies on Alcohol, 58,* 565–572.

Cappell, H. (1974). An evaluation of tension models of alcohol consumption. In Y. Israel (Ed.), *Research advances in alcohol and drug problems.* New York: Wiley.

Carroll, K. M., Rounsaville, B. J., & Bryant, K. J. (1994). Should tolerance and withdrawal be required for substance dependence disorders? *Drug and Alcohol Dependence, 36,* 15–22.

Cashin, J. R., Presley, C. A., & Meilman, P. W. (1998). Alcohol use in the Greek system: Follow the leader? *Journal of Studies on Alcohol, 59,* 63–70.

Chermack, S. T., & Taylor, S. W. P. (1995). Alcohol and human physical aggression: Pharmacological versus expectancy effects. *Journal of Studies on Alcohol, 56,* 449–456.

Christensen, J. K., Moller, I. W., Ronsted, P., Angelo, H. R., & Johansson, B. (1991). Dose-effect relationship of disulfiram in human volunteers: I. Clinical studies. *Pharmacology and Toxicology, 68,* 163–165.

Christiansen, B. A., Smith, G. T., Roehling, P. V., & Goldman, M. S. (1989). Using alcohol expectancies to predict adolescent drinking behavior after one year. *Journal of Consulting and Clinical Psychology, 57,* 93–99.

Cloninger, C. R., Bohman, M., & Sigvardsson, S. (1981). Inheritance of alcohol abuse: Cross-fostering analysis of adopted men. *Archives of General Psychiatry, 38,* 861–868.

Conger, J. J. (1951). The effects of alcohol on conflict behavior in the albino rat. *Quarterly Journal of Studies on Alcohol, 12,* 1–29.

Cooper, M. L., Russell, M., Skinner, J. B., Frone, M. R., & Mudar, P. (1992). Stress and alcohol use: Moderating effects of gender, coping, and alcohol expectancies. *Journal of Abnormal Psychology, 101,* 139–152.

Cottler, L. B., Schuckit, M. A., Helzer, J. E., Crowley, T., Woody, G., Nathan, P. E., & Hughes, J. (1995). The DSM-IV field trial for substance use disorders: Major results. *Drug and Alcohol Dependence, 38,* 59–69.

Cotton, N. S. (1979). The familial incidence of alcoholism. *Journal of Studies on Alcohol, 40,* 89–116.

Crowell, C. R., Hinson, R. E., & Siegel, S. (1981). The role of conditional drug responses in tolerance to the hypothermic effects of alcohol. *Psychopharmacology, 73,* 51–54.

Deckel, A. W., Hesselbrock, V., & Bauer, L. (1995). Relationship between alcohol-related expectancies and anterior brain functioning in young men at risk for developing alcoholism. *Alcoholism: Clinical and Experimental Research, 19,* 476–481.

Dongier, M., Vachon, L., & Schwartz, G. (1991). Bromocriptine in the treatment of alcohol dependence. *Alcoholism: Clinical and Experimental Research, 15,* 970–977.

Drake, R. E., Osher, F. C., & Wallach, M. A. (1989). Alcohol use and abuse in schizophrenia: A prospective community study. *Journal of Nervous and Mental Disease, 177,* 408–414.

Dunn M. E., & Goldman, M. S. (1996). Empirical modeling of an alcohol expectancy memory network in elementary school children as a function of grade. *Experimental and Clinical Psychopharmacology, 4,* 209–217.

Earlywine, M., Finn, P. R., & Martin, C. S. (1990). Personality risk and alcohol consumption: A latent variable analysis. *Addictive Behaviors, 15,* 183–187.

Eckardt, M. J., Stapleton, J. M., Rawlings, R. R., Davis, E. Z., & Grodin, D. M. (1995). Neuropsychological functioning in detoxified alcoholics between 18 and 35 years of age. *American Journal of Psychiatry, 152,* 53–59.

Edenberg, H. J., Foroud, T., Koller, D. L., Goate, A., et al. (1998). A family-based analysis of the association of the dopamine D2 receptor (DRD2) with alcoholism. *Alcoholism: Clinical and Experimental Research, 22,* 505–512.

Edwards, G. & Gross, M. M. (1976). Alcohol dependence: Provisional description of a clinical syndrome. *British Journal of Psychiatry, 1,* 1058–1061.

Fahrner, E. M. (1987). Sexual dysfunction in male alcohol addicts: Prevalence and treatment. *Archives of Sexual Behavior, 16,* 247–257.

Fals-Stewart, W. (1996). Intermediate length neuropsychological screening of impairment among psychoactive substance-abusing patients: A comparison of two batteries. *Journal of Substance Abuse, 8,* 1–17.

Fals-Stewart, W., & Lucente, S. (1994). The effect of neurocognitive status and personality functioning on length of stay on residential substance abuse treatment. *Psychology of Addictive Behaviors, 8,* 1–12.

Fils-Aime, M.-L., Eckardt, M. J., George, D. T., Brown, G. L., Mefford, I., & Linnoila, M. (1996). Early-onset alcoholics have lower cerebrospinal fluid 5-hydroxyindoleacetic acid levels than late-onset alcoholics. *Archives of General Psychiatry, 53,* 211–216.

Finney, J. W., & Monahan, S. C. (1996). The cost-effectiveness of treatment for alcoholism: A second approximation. *Journal of Studies on Alcohol, 57,* 229–243.

Finney, J. W., & Moos, R. H. (1998). Psychosocial treatments for alcohol use disorders. In P. E. Nathan & J. M. Gorman (Eds.), *A guide to treatments that work* (pp. 156–166). New York & Oxford: Oxford University Press.

Freund, G. (1982). The interaction of chronic alcohol consumption and aging on brain structures and function. *Alcoholism: Clinical and Experimental Research, 6,* 13–21.

Frezza, M., DiPadova, C., Pozzato, G., Terpin, M., Baraona, E., & Lieber, C. S. (1990). High blood alcohol levels in women: Role of decreased gastric alcohol dehydrogenase activity and first pass metabolism. *New England Journal of Medicine, 322,* 95–99.

Fromme, K., Stroot, E., & Kaplan, D. (1993). Comprehensive effects of alcohol: Development and psychometric assessment of a new expectancy questionnaire. *Psychological Assessment, 5,* 19–26.

Gallant, D. M. (1987). The female alcoholic: Early onset of brain damage. *Alcoholism, 11,* 190–191.

Giancola, P. R., & Zeichner, A. (1995). Alcohol-related aggression in males and females: Effects of blood alcohol concentration, subjective intoxication, personality, and provocation. *Alcoholism: Clinical and Experimental Research, 19,* 130–134.

Goldman, M. S., Brown, S. A., Christiansen, B. A., & Smith, G. T. (1991). Alcoholism and memory: Broadening the scope of alcohol-expectancy research. *Psychological Bulletin, 110,* 137–146.

Goldman, M. S., Williams, D. L., & Klisz, D. K. (1983). Recoverability of psychological functioning following alcohol abuse: Prolonged visual-spatial dysfunction in older alcoholics. *Journal of Consulting and Clinical Psychology, 51,* 370–378.

Goodwin, D. W. (1976). *Is alcoholism hereditary?* New York: Oxford University Press.

Goodwin, D. W. (1979). Alcoholism and heredity. *Archives of General Psychiatry, 36,* 57–61.

Goodwin, D. W. (1985). Genetic determinants of alcoholism. In J. H. Mendelson & N. K. Mello (Eds.), *The diagnosis and treatment of alcoholism* (pp. 65–87). New York: McGraw-Hill.

Goodwin, D. W., Schulsinger, F., Mollen, N., Hermansen, L., Winokur, G., & Guze, S. B. (1974). Drinking problems in adopted and nonadopted sons of alcoholics. *Archives of General Psychiatry, 31,* 164–169.

Gordon, C. M., & Carey, M. P. (1996). Alcohol's effects on requisites for sexual risk reduction in men: An initial experimental investigation. *Health Psychology, 15,* 56–60.

Gottfredson, D. C., & Koper, C. S. (1996). Race and sex differences in the prediction of drug use. *Journal of Consulting and Clinical Psychology, 64,* 305–313.

Grant, B. F. (1995). Comorbidity between DSM-IV drug use disorders and major depression: Results of a national survey of adults. *Journal of Substance Abuse, 7,* 481–497.

Grant, B. F. (1997). Prevalence and correlates of alcohol use and DSM-IV alcohol dependence in the United States: Results of the National Longitudinal Alcohol Epidemiologic Survey. *Journal of Studies on Alcohol, 58,* 464–473.

Gustafson, R. (1991). Aggressive and nonaggressive behavior as a function of alcohol intoxication and frustration in women. *Alcoholism: Clinical and Experimental Research, 15,* 886–892.

Hallman, J., von Knorring, L., & Oreland, L. (1996). Personality disorders according to DSM-III-R and thrombocyte monoamine oxidase activity in Type 1 and Type 2 alcoholics. *Journal of Studies on Alcohol, 57,* 155–161.

Hasin, D., Van Rossem, R., McCloud, S., & Endicott, J. (1997). Alcohol dependence and abuse diagnoses: Validity in community sample heavy drinkers. *Alcoholism: Clinical and Experimental Research, 21,* 213–219.

Hegadus, A., Tarter, R., Hill, S., Jacob, T., & Winsten, N. (1984). Static ataxia: A possible marker for alcoholism. *Alcoholism: Clinical and Experimental Research, 8,* 580–582.

Helzer, J. E. (1994). Psychoactive substance abuse and its relation to dependence. In T. A. Widiger, A. J. Frances, H. A. Pincus, M. B. First, R. Ross, & W. Davis (Eds.), *DSM-IV sourcebook,* Vol. 1 (pp. 21–32). Washington, DC: American Psychiatric Association.

Helzer, J. E., Canino, G. J., Hwu, H. G., et al. (1988). Alcoholism: A cross-national comparison of population surveys with the Diagnostic Interview Schedule. In R. M. Rose & J. Barrett (Eds.), *Alcoholism: Origins and outcome.* New York: Raven Press.

Helzer, J. E., Canino, G. J., Yeh, E.-K., Bland, R. C., Lee, C. K., Hwu, H.-G., & Newman, S. (1990). Alcoholism—North America and Asia. *Archives of General Psychiatry, 47,* 313–319.

Hill, S. Y., & Steinhauer, S. R. (1993). Assessment of prepubertal and postpubertal boys and girls at risk for developing alcohol with P300 from a visual discrimination task. *Journal of Studies on Alcohol, 54,* 350–358.

Hill, S. Y., Steinhauer, S. R., & Locke, J. (1995). Event-related potentials in alcoholic men, their high-risk male relatives, and low-risk male controls. *Alcoholism: Clinical and Experimental Research, 19,* 567–576.

Holdcraft, L. C., Iacono, W. G., & McGue, M. K. (1998). Antisocial personality disorder and depression in relation to alcoholism: A community-based sample. *Journal of Studies on Alcohol, 59,* 222–226.

Holder, H., Longabaugh, R., Miller, W. R., & Rubonis, A. V. (1991). The cost effectiveness of treatment for alcoholism: A first approximation. *Journal of Studies on Alcohol, 52,* 517–540.

Holguin, S. R., Corral, M., & Cadaveira, F. (1998). Visual and auditory event-related potentials in young children of alcoholics from high- and low-density families. *Alcoholism: Clinical and Experimental Research, 22,* 87–96.

Howard, M. O., Kivlahan, D., & Walker, R. D. (1997). Cloninger's Tridimensional Theory of personality and psychopathology: Applications to substance use disorders. *Journal of Studies on Alcohol, 58,* 48–66.

Jencks, S. F., & Goldman, H. H. (1987). Implications of research for psychiatric prospective payment. *Medical Care, 25,* 542–551.

Jessor, R., & Jessor, S. (1977). *Problem behavior and psychosocial development: A longitudinal study of youth.* New York: Academic Press.

Johnson, R. C., Nagoshi, C. T., Danko, G. P., Honbo, K. A. M. & Chau, L. L. (1990). Familial transmission of alcohol use norms and expectancies and reported alcohol use. *Alcoholism: Clinical and Experimental Research, 14,* 216–220.

Kadden, R., Carroll, K. M., Donovan, D., Cooney, N., Monti, P., Abrams, D., Litt, M., & Hester, R. (1992). Cognitive-behavioral coping skills therapy manual: A clinical research guide for therapists treating individuals with alcohol abuse and dependence. NIAAA Project MATCH Monograph, Vol. 3, DHHS Publication No. (ADM) 92-1895. Washington, DC: U.S. Government Printing Office.

Kaij, J. (1960). *Studies in the etiology and sequels of abuse of alcohol.* Lund, Sweden: University of Lund.

Kendler, K. S., Heath, A. C., Neale, M. C., Kessler, R. C., & Eaves, L. J. (1992). A population-based twin study of alcoholism in women. *Journal of the American Medical Association, 268,* 1877–1882.

Kim, J., Celentano, D. D., & Crum, R. M. (1998). Alcohol consumption and sexually transmitted disease risk behavior: Partner mix among male Korean University students. *Alcoholism: Clinical and Experimental Research, 22,* 126–131.

Koopman, C., Rosario, M., & Rotheram-Borus, M. J. (1994). Alcohol and drug use and sexual behaviors placing runaways at risk for HIV infection. *Addictive Behaviors, 19,* 95–103.

Kushner, M. G., Sher, K. J., Wood, M. D., & Wood, P. K. (1994). Anxiety and drinking behavior: Moderating effects of tension-reduction alcohol outcome expectancies. *Alcoholism: Clinical and Experimental Research, 18,* 852–860.

Langenbucher, J. W., & Chung, T. (1995). Onset and staging of DSM-IV alcohol dependence using mean age and survival/hazard methods. *Journal of Abnormal Psychology, 104,* 346–354.

Langenbucher, J. W., Chung, T., Morgenstern, J., Labouvie, E., Nathan, P. E., & Bavly, L. (in press). Physiological alcohol dependence as a "specifier" of risk for medical problems and relapse liability in DSM-IV. *Journal of Studies on Alcohol.*

Langenbucher, J. W., Morgenstern, J., Labouvie, E., & Nathan, P. E. (1994a). Lifetime DSM-IV diagnosis of alcohol, cannabis, cocaine and opiate dependence: Six-month reliability in a multi-site clinical sample. *Addiction, 89,* 1115–1127.

Langenbucher, J. W., Morgenstern, J., Labouvie, E., & Nathan, P. E. (1994b). Diagnostic concordance of substance use disorders in DSM-III, DSM-IV and ICD-10. *Drug and Alcohol Dependence, 36,* 193–203.

Langenbucher, J. W., & Nathan, P. E. (1993). Alcohol, affect, and the tension-reduction hypothesis: The reanalysis of some crucial early data. In W. M. Cox (Ed.), *Why people drink: Parameters of alcohol as a reinforcer.* New York: Gardner Press.

Langenbucher, J. W., Sulesund, D., Chung, T., & Morgenstern, J. (1996). Illness severity and self-efficacy as course predictors of DSM-IV alcohol dependence in a multisite clinical sample. *Addictive Behaviors, 21,* 543–553.

Leigh, B. C. (1987). Beliefs about the effects of alcohol on self and others. *Journal of Studies on Alcohol, 48,* 467–475.

Leigh, B. C., & Stacy, A. W. (1993). Alcohol outcome expectancies: Construction and predictive utility in higher order confirmatory models. *Psychological Assessment, 5,* 216–229.

Leohlin, J. C. (1977). An analysis of alcohol-related questionnaire items from the National Merit twin study. In F. A. Seixas, G. S. Omenn, E. D. Burk, & S. Eggleston (Eds.), *Annals of the New York Academy of Sciences, 197,* 117–120.

Leonard, K. E., & Blane, H. T. (1988). Alcohol expectancies and personality characteristics in young men. *Addictive Behaviors, 13,* 353–357.

Lipscomb, T. R., Carpenter, J. A., & Nathan, P. E. (1979). Static ataxia: A predictor of alcoholism? *British Journal of Addiction, 74,* 289–294.

Longabaugh, R., Wirtz, P. W., DiClemente, C. C., & Litt, M. (1994). Issues in the development of client-treatment matching hypotheses. In D. M. Donovan & M. E. Mattson (Eds.), *Alcoholism treatment matching research: Methodological and clinical approaches, Journal of Studies on Alcohol, 12*(Suppl.), 46–59.

Masserman, J. H., & Yum, K. S. (1946). An analysis of the influence of alcohol and experimental neurosis in cats. *Psychological Medicine, 8,* 36–52.

Mattick, R. P., & Jarvis, T. (1994). Inpatient setting and long duration for the treatment of alcohol dependence? Outpatient care is as good. *Drug and Alcohol Review, 13,* 127–135.

Mattson, M. E., & Allen, J. P. (1991). Research on matching alcoholic patients to treatments: Findings, issues, and implications. *Journal of Addictive Diseases, 11,* 33–49.

Mattson, M. E., Allen, J. P., Longabaugh, R. L., et al. (1994). A chronological review of empirical studies matching alcoholic clients to treatments. In D. M. Donovan & M. E. Mattson (Eds.), Alcoholism treatment matching research: Methodological and clinical approaches. *Journal of Studies on Alcohol, 12*(Suppl.), 16–29.

McCrady, B. S., & Langenbucher, J. W. (1996). Alcoholism treatment and health care system reform. *Archives of General Psychiatry, 53,* 737–746.

Mezzich, A. C., Giancola, P. R., Tarter, R. E., Lu, S., Parks, S. M., & Barrett, C. M. (1997). Violence, suicidality, and alcohol/drug use involvement in adolescent females with a psychoactive substance use disorder and controls. *Alcoholism: Clinical and Experimental Research, 21,* 1300–1307.

Mezzich, J. E., & Sharfstein, S. S. (1985). Severity of illness and diagnostic formulation: Classifying patients for prospective payment systems. *Hospital and Community Psychiatry, 36,* 770–772.

Miller, W. R., Brown, J. M., Simpson, T. L., Handmaker, N. S., Bien, T. H., Luckie, L. F., Montgomery, H. A., Hester, R. K., & Tonigan, J. S. (1995). What works? A methodological analysis of the alcohol treatment literature. In R. K. Hester & W. R. Miller (Eds.), *Handbook of alcoholism treatment approaches: Effective alternatives* (pp. 12–44). Boston, MA: Allyn & Bacon.

Miller, W. R., & Hester, R. K. (1986). Inpatient alcoholism treatment: Who benefits? *American Psychologist, 41,* 794–805.

Miller, W. R., & Sanchez, V. C. (1993). Motivating young adults for treatment and lifestyle change. In G. Howard & P. E. Nathan (Eds.), *Issues in alcohol use and misuse by young adults.* Notre Dame, IN: University of Notre Dame Press.

Miller, W. R., Zweben, A., DiClemente, C. C., & Rychtarik, R. G. (1992). Motivational enhancement therapy manual: A clinical research guide for therapists treating individuals with alcohol abuse and dependence. NIAAA Project MATCH Monograph, Vol. 2, DHHS Publication No. (ADM) 92-1894. Washington, DC: U.S. Government Printing Office.

Monahan, S. C., & Finney, J. W. (1996). Explaining abstinence rates following treatment for alcohol abuse: A quantitative synthesis of patient, research design, and treatment effects. *Addiction, 91,* 787–805.

Moos, R. H., Finney, J. W., & Cronkite, R. C. (1990). *Alcoholism treatment: Context, process, and outcome.* New York: Oxford University Press.

Moss, H. B., & Kirisci, L. (1995). Aggressivity in adolescent alcohol abusers: Relationship with conduct disorder. *Alcoholism: Clinical and Experimental Research, 19,* 642–646.

Mueller, T. I., Lavori, P. W., Keller, M. B., Swartz, A., Warshaw, M., Hasin, D., Coryell, W., Endicott, J., Rice, J., & Akiskal, H. (1994). Prognostic effect of the variable course of alcoholism on the 10-year course of depression. *American Journal of Psychiatry, 151,* 701–706.

Najavits, L. M., & Weiss, R. D. (1994). Variations in therapist effectiveness in the treatment of patients with substance abuse disorders: An empirical review. *Addiction, 89,* 679–688.

Naranjo, C. A., Kadlec, K. E., Sanhueza, P., Woodley-Remus, D., & Sellers, E. M. (1990). Fluoxetine differentially alters alcohol intake and other consummatory behaviors in problem drinkers. *Clinical Pharmacological Therapy, 47,* 490–498.

Nathan, P. E. (1988). The addictive personality is the behavior of the addict. *Journal of Consulting and Clinical Psychology, 56,* 183–188.

Nathan, P. E. (1993). Alcoholism: Psychopathology, etiology, and treatment. In P. B. Sutker & H. E. Adams (Eds.), *Comprehensive handbook of psychopathology* (2nd ed, pp. 451–476). New York: Plenum.

Nathan, P. E., & Lipscomb, T. R. (1979). Studies in blood alcohol level discrimination: Etiologic cues to alcoholism. In N. A. Krasnegor (Ed.), Behavioral analysis and treatment of substance abuse (pp. 178–190). Washington, DC: National Institute on Drug Abuse.

Nathan, P. E., & McCrady, B. S. (1987). Bases for the use of abstinence as a goal in the behavioral treatment of alcohol abusers. *Drugs and Society, 2,* 109–131.

Nathan, P. E., & O'Brien, J. S. (1971). An experimental analysis of the behavior of alcoholics and nonalcoholics during prolonged experimental drinking. *Behavior Therapy, 2,* 455–476.

Nathan, P. E., & Skinstad, A. H. (1987). Outcomes of treatment for alcohol problems: Current methods, problems, and results. *Journal of Consulting and Clinical Psychology, 55,* 332–340.

National Institute on Alcohol Abuse and Alcoholism (NIAAA). (1997). Ninth Special Report to Congress on Alcohol and Health. Washington, DC: U.S. Department of Health and Human Services.

Newcomb, M. D., & Bentler, P. M. (1986). Substance use and ethnicity: Differential impact of peer and adult models. *Journal of Psychology, 120,* 83–95.

Nichols, J. M., & Martin, F. (1996). The effect of heavy social drinking on recall and event-related potential. *Journal of Studies on Alcohol, 57,* 125–135.

Nixon, S. J., Tivis, R., & Parsons, O. A. (1995). Behavioral dysfunction and cognitive efficiency in male and female alcoholics. *Alcoholism: Clinical and Experimental Research, 19,* 577–581.

Nowinski, J., Baker, S., & Carroll, K. (1992). Twelve step facilitation therapy manual: A clinical research guide for therapists treating individuals with alcohol abuse and dependence. NIAAA Project MATCH Monograph, Vol. 1, DHHS Publication No. (ADM) 92-1893. Washington, D.C.: U.S. Government Printing Office.

O'Brien, C. P., & McKay, J. (1998). Psychopharmacological treatments of substance use disorders. In P. E. Nathan & J. M. Gorman (Eds.), *A guide to treatments that work* (pp. 127–155). New York & Oxford: Oxford University Press.

O'Connor, S. J., Hesselbrock, V., & Tasman, A. (1986). Corre-

lates of increased risk for alcoholism in young men. *Progress in Neuropsychopharmacology and Biological Psychiatry, 10,* 211–218.

O'Farrell, T. J., Choquette, K. A., Cutter, H. S. G., Brown, E. D., & McCourt, W. F. (1993). Behavioral marital therapy with and without additional couples relapse prevention sessions for alcoholics and their wives. *Journal of Studies on Alcohol, 54,* 652–666.

O'Malley, S. S., Jaffe, A., Chang, G., Witte, G., Schottenfeld, R. S., & Rounsaville, B. J. (1992). Naltrexone in the treatment of alcohol dependence: Preliminary findings. In C. A. Naranjo & E. M. Sellars (Eds.), *Novel pharmacological interventions for alcoholism* (pp. 148–157). New York: Springer Verlag.

Ouimette, P. C., Finney, J. W., & Moos, R. H. (1997). Twelve-step and cognitive-behavioral treatment for substance abuse: A comparison of treatment effectiveness. *Journal of Consulting and Clinical Psychology, 65,* 230–240.

Parker, D. A., Harford, T. C., & Rosenstock, I. M. (1994). Alcohol, other drugs, and sexual risk-taking among young adults. *Journal of Substance Abuse, 6,* 87–93.

Parsons, O. A., & Nixon, S. J. (1998). Cognitive functioning in sober social drinkers: A review of the research since 1986. *Journal of Studies on Alcohol, 59,* 180–190.

Pettinati, H. M., Pierce, J. D., Jr., Wolf, A. L., Rukstalis, M. R., & O'Brien, C. P. (1997). Gender differences in comorbidly depressed alcohol-dependent outpatients. *Alcoholism: Clinical and Experimental Research, 21,* 1742–1746.

Polivy, J., Schueneman, A. L., & Carlson, K. (1976). Alcohol and tension reduction: Cognitive and physiological effects. *Journal of Abnormal Psychology, 85,* 595–600.

Porjesz, B., & Begleiter, H. (1983). Brain dysfunction and alcohol. In B. Kissin & H. Begleiter (Eds.), *The pathogenesis of alcoholism* (pp. 415–483). New York: Plenum.

Prescott, C. A., Hewitt, J. K., Truett, K. R., Heath, A. C., Neale, M. C., & Eaves, L. J. (1994). Genetic and environmental influences on lifetime alcohol-related problems in a volunteer sample of older twins. *Journal of Studies on Alcohol, 55,* 184–202.

Prochaska, J. O., DiClemente, C. C., & Norcross, J. C. (1992). In search of how people change. *American Psychologist, 47,* 1102–1114.

Project MATCH Research Group. (1993). Project MATCH: Rationale and methods for a multisite clinical trial matching patients to alcoholism treatment. *Alcoholism: Clinical and Experimental Research, 17,* 1130–1145.

Project MATCH Research Group. (1997a). Matching alcoholism treatment to client heterogeneity: Project MATCH posttreatment drinking outcomes. *Journal of Studies on Alcohol, 58,* 7–29.

Project MATCH Research Group. (1997b). Project MATCH secondary *a priori* hypotheses. *Addiction, 92,* 1671–1698.

Ramachandran, G., Porjesz, B., Begleiter, H., & Litke, A. (1996). A simple auditory oddball task in young adult males at high risk for alcoholism. *Alcoholism: Clinical and Experimental Research, 20,* 9–15.

Ramsey, S. E., & Finn, P. R. (1997). P300 from men with a family history of alcoholism under different incentive conditions. *Journal of Studies on Alcohol, 58,* 606–616.

Rather, B. C., & Goldman, M. S. (1994). Drinking-related differences in the memory organization of alcohol expectancies. *Experimental and Clinical Psychopharmacology, 2,* 167–183.

Rather, B. C., Goldman, M. S., Roehrich, L., & Brannick, M.

(1992). Empirical modeling of an alcohol expectancy memory network using multidimensional scaling. *Journal of Abnormal Psychology, 101*, 174–183.

Regier, D. A., Farmer, M. E., Rae, D. S., Locke, B. Z., Keith, S. J., Judd, L. L., & Goodwin, F. K. (1990). Comorbidity of mental disorders with alcohol and other drug abuse: Results from the Epidemiological Catchment Area (ECA) study. *Journal of the American Medical Association, 264*, 2511–2518.

Reifman, A., Barnes, G. M., Dintcheff, B. A., Farrell, M. P., & Uhteg, L. (1998). Parental and peer influences on the onset of heavier drinking among adolescents. *Journal of Studies on Alcohol, 59*, 311–317.

Roehrich, L., & Goldman, M. S. (1995). Implicit priming of alcohol expectancy memory processes and subsequent drinking behavior. *Experimental and Clinical Psychopharmacology, 3*, 402–410.

Ross, H. E., Glaser, F. B., & Germanson, T. (1988). The prevalence of psychiatric disorders in patients with alcohol and other drug problems. *Archives of General Psychiatry, 45*, 1023–1031.

Rounsaville, B. J., & Bryant, K. J. (1992). Tolerance and withdrawal in the DSM-III-R diagnosis of substance dependence: Utility in a cocaine-using population. *American Journal of the Addictions, 1*, 50–60.

Scheier, L. M., & Botvin, G. J. (1995). Effects of early adolescent drug use on cognitive efficiency in early-late adolescence: A developmental structural model. *Journal of Substance Abuse, 7*, 379–404.

Schiavi, R. C. (1990). Chronic alcoholism and male sexual dysfunction. *Journal of Sex and Marital Therapy, 16*, 23–33.

Schiavi, R. C., Stimmel, B. B., Mandeli, J., & White, D. (1995). Chronic alcoholism and male sexual function. *American Journal of Psychiatry, 152*, 1045–1051.

Schuckit, M. A. (1985). Ethanol-induced changes in body sway in men at high alcoholism risk. *Archives of General Psychiatry, 42*, 375–379.

Schuckit, M. A. (1994a). A clinical model of genetic influence in alcohol dependence. *Journal of Studies on Alcohol, 55*, 5–17.

Schuckit, M. A. (1994b). Low level of response to alcohol as a predictor of future alcoholism. *American Journal of Psychiatry, 151*, 184–189.

Schuckit, M. A. (1994c). The relationship between alcohol problems, substance abuse, and psychiatric syndromes. In T. A. Widiger, A. J. Frances, H. A. Pincus, M. B. First, R. Ross, & W. Davis (Eds.), *DSM-IV sourcebook*, Vol. 1 (pp. 45–66). Washington, DC: American Psychiatric Association.

Schuckit, M. A. (1995). *Drug and alcohol abuse: A critical guide to diagnosis and treatment*, 4th edition. New York: Plenum Medical.

Schuckit, M. A. (1996). DSM-V: There's work to be done. *Journal of Studies on Alcohol, 57*, 469–470.

Schuckit, M. A. (1997). *The 1997 Mark Keller Memorial Lecture: An evaluation of the alcoholism risk in three generations of 453 men.* New Brunswick, NJ: Rutgers Center of Alcohol Studies.

Schuckit, M. A., & Gold, E. O. (1988). A simultaneous evaluation of multiple markers of ethanol/placebo challenges in sons of alcoholics and controls. *Archives of General Psychiatry, 45*, 211–216.

Schuckit, M. A., & Hesselbrock, V. (1994). Alcohol dependence and anxiety disorders: What is the relationship? *American Journal of Psychiatry, 151*, 1723–1734.

Schuckit, M. A., & Smith, T. L. (1996). An 8-year follow-up of 450 sons of alcoholic and control subjects. *Archives of General Psychiatry, 53*, 202–210.

Schuckit, M. A., & Smith, T. L. (1997). Assessing the risk for alcoholism among sons of alcoholics. *Journal of Studies on Alcohol, 58*, 141–145.

Sher, K. J., Gershuny, B. S., Peterson, L., & Raskin, G. (1997). The role of childhood stressors in the intergenerational transmission of alcohol use disorders. *Journal of Studies on Alcohol, 58*, 414–427.

Sher, K. J., & Trull, T. J. (1994). Personality and disinhibitory psychopathology: Alcoholism and antisocial personality disorder. *Journal of Abnormal Psychology, 103*, 92–102.

Siegel, S. (1978), A Pavlovian conditioning analysis of morphine tolerance. In N. A. Krasnegor (Ed.), *Behavioral tolerance*. Washington, DC: National Institute on Drug Abuse.

Smith, D. E., & McCrady, B. S. (1991). Cognitive impairment among alcoholics: Impact on drink refusal skill acquisition and treatment outcome. *Addictive Behaviors, 16*, 265–274.

Smith, G. T., Goldman, M. S., Greenbaum, P. E., & Christiansen, B. A. (1995). Expectancy for social facilitation from drinking: The divergent paths of high-expectancy and low-expectancy adolescents. *Journal of Abnormal Psychology, 104*, 32–40.

Sobell, L. C., Cunningham, J. A., & Sobell, M. B. (1996). Recovery from alcohol problems with and without treatment: Prevalence in two population surveys. *Journal of Public Health, 86*, 966–972.

Steinhauer, S. R., & Hill, S. Y. (1993). Auditory event-related potentials in children at high risk for alcoholism. *Journal of Studies on Alcohol, 54*, 408–421.

Stewart, J., deWit, H., & Eikelboom, R. (1984). The role of unconditioned and conditioned drug effects in the self-administration of opiates and stimulants. *Psychological Review, 91*, 251–268.

Sutker, P. B., & Allain, A. N. (1988). Issues in personality conceptualizations of addictive behaviors. *Journal of Consulting and Clinical Psychology, 56*, 172–183.

Tarter, R. E., McBride, H., Buonpane, N., & Schneider, D. U. (1977). Differentiation of alcoholics. *Archives of General Psychiatry, 34*, 761–768.

Vaillant, G. E. (1995). *The natural history of alcoholism revisited*. Cambridge, MA: Harvard University Press.

Van Thiel, D. H., Gavaler, J. S., Eagan, P. K., Chiao, Y. B., Cobb, C. F., & Lester, R. (1980). Alcohol and sexual function. *Pharmacology and Biochemistry of Behavior, 13*(Suppl. 1), 125–129.

Verheul, R., van den Brink, W., & Hartgers, C. (1995). Prevalence of personality disorders among alcoholics and drug addicts: An overview. *European Addiction Research, 1*, 166–177.

Verheul, R., Hartgers, C., van den Brink, W., & Koeter, M. W. J. (1998). The effect of sampling, diagnostic criteria and assessment procedures on the observed prevalence of DSM-III-R personality disorders among treated alcoholics. *Journal of Studies on Alcohol, 59*, 227–236.

Victor, M., Adams, R. D., & Collins, G. H. (1971). *The Wernicke-Korsakoff syndrome*. Philadelphia: Davis.

Wartenburg, A. A., Nirenberg, T. D., Liepman, M. R., Silvia, L. Y., Begin, A. M., & Monti, P. M. (1990). Detoxification of alcoholics: Improving care by symptom-triggered sedation. *Alcoholism: Clinical and Experimental Research, 14*, 71–75.

Watson, A. L., & Sher, K. J. (1998). Resolution of alcohol problems without treatment: Methodological issues and future directions of natural recovery research. *Clinical Psychology: Science and Practice, 5,* 1–18.

Wechsler, H., Davenport, A., Dowdall, G., Moeykens, B., & Castillo, S. (1994). Health and behavioral consequences of binge drinking in college: A national survey of students at 140 campuses. *Journal of the American Medical Association, 272,* 1672–1677.

Welte, J., Hynes, G., & Sokolow, L. (1981). Effect of length of stay in inpatient alcoholism treatment on outcome. *Journal of Studies on Alcohol, 42,* 483–499.

Wetzig, D., & Hardin, S. I. (1990). Neurocognitive deficits of alcoholism. *Journal of Clinical Psychology, 46,* 219–221.

Wilens, T. E., Biederman, J., Spencer, T. J., & Frances, R. J. (1994). Comorbidity of attention deficit hyperactivity disorder and the psychoactive substance use disorders. *Hospital and Community Psychiatry, 45,* 421–435.

Wilson, G. T. & Abrams, D. B. (1977). Effects of alcohol on social anxiety and physiological arousal: Cognitive versus pharmacological processes. *Cognitive Therapy and Research, 1,* 195–210.

Wilson, G. T., Nathan, P. E., O'Leary, K. D., & Clark, L. A. (1996). *Abnormal psychology: Integrating perspectives.* Needham Heights, MA: Allyn & Bacon.

World Health Organization. (1992). *International classification of diseases* (10th ed.). Geneva: World Health Organization.

Wright, C. & Moore, R. D. (1989). Disulfiram treatment of alcoholism: Position paper of the *American College of Physicians.*

Young, R., & Oei, T. P. S. (1990). Drinking Expectancy Profile: A manual. Brisbane, Australia: University of Queensland.

Zhang, L., Wieczorek, W. F., & Weite, J. W. (1997). The nexus between alcohol and violent crime. *Alcoholism: Clinical and Experimental Research, 21,* 1264–1271.

Zimmerman, M., & Coryell, W. H. (1990). Diagnosing personality disorders in the community: A comparison of self-reports and interviews. *Archives of General Psychiatry, 47,* 527–531.

# CHAPTER 22

# Cocaine and Opioid Abuse/ Dependence Disorders

Arthur I. Alterman, Charles P. O'Brien, A. Thomas McLellan, and James R. McKay

## Introduction

This chapter is concerned primarily with the consequences of cocaine and opioid use, with the psychopathology associated with cocaine and opioid dependence, and with the available treatments to address these disorders. These two disorders are associated, directly or indirectly, with very serious biomedical and psychosocial consequences, particularly because both often involve intravenous drug administration and intercourse with multiple sex partners, the two primary modalities for transmitting the AIDS virus. Significant involvement in criminal behavior may also be associated with drug procurement. These patients generally are very difficult to treat because by the time they are seen for treatment, many of them have multiple biomedical problems, directly or indirectly traceable to their substance dependence, as well as psychosocial problems and psychiatric disorders including polysubstance abuse. Thus, a treatment model that considers that substance dependence disorders are chronic over the lifetime in the same sense as diabetes or hypertension is in-

creasingly being adopted (Majewska, 1996; O'Brien & McLellan, 1996). Although we will consider each of the disorders separately in this chapter, it is important at the outset to appreciate that polydrug abuse/dependence is likely to be more common than abuse/dependence of only one drug in many, perhaps the majority, of patients seen (Bartzokis, Beckson, & Ling, 1996). For example, cocaine, benzodiazepine, and alcohol abuse/dependence are clearly problems in many patients who are opioid-dependent, and concurrent alcohol abuse/ dependence is present in the majority of cocaine-dependent patients. Marijuana dependence is also highly prevalent in both opioid and cocaine dependence. The existence of these multiple substance dependence disorders clearly complicates treatment, and the adverse interactive effects between two drugs can be far more serious than the combination of their individual effects. For example, in cocaine use, even limited exposure to amphetamines can have severe neurotoxic consequences (Bartzokis et al., 1996). Finally, the geometric growth of managed care treatment systems that have and are taking place in the United States makes it clear that the nature of treatments for substance abuse/dependence are and will be changing markedly. Although there is yet only limited research knowledge about the effects of managed care practices on substance abuse treatment, it has become increasingly clear that cost considerations are greatly influencing the nature and quantity of the treatment services dispensed.

Arthur I. Alterman, Charles P. O'Brien, A. Thomas McLellan, and James R. McKay • University of Pennsylvania School of Medicine and Veterans Affairs Medical Center, Philadelphia, Pennsylvania 19104.

*Comprehensive Handbook of Psychopathology* (Third Edition), edited by Patricia B. Sutker and Henry E. Adams. Kluwer Academic / Plenum Publishers, New York, 2001.

## Cocaine Abuse/Dependence

### Medical Consequences of Use

Coca leaves have been chewed by South American Indians for several centuries, and cocaine hydrochloride (HCl) has been used since it was isolated in the middle of the nineteenth century by Niemann (Daras, 1996; O'Brien, 1995). Untoward effects related to chewing the leaves or intranasal insufflation of cocaine HCl had been rare. The introduction in 1983 of the alkaloidal form of cocaine, known as crack (Jekel, Allen, Pollewski, Clarke, Dean-Paterson, & Cartwright, 1986), led to the cocaine epidemic in the United States followed by a corresponding rise in the incidence of medical, neurological, and psychiatric complications. Cocaine toxicity manifests itself at the level of nearly every organ system; the most dramatic changes occur in the cardiovascular system, liver, and the brain (Majewska, 1996). "In the cardiovascular system, tachycardia, hypertension, ruptures of blood vessels, arrhythmias, and arteriosclerotic lesions are typical complications that often precede myocardial ischemia and infarction" (Majewska, 1996, p. 2; also see Karch, 1993). Cocaine is directly toxic to the myocardium (Volkow, Fowler, & Ding, 1996). Cocaine is hepatotoxic in humans (Marks & Chapple, 1967) and in animals (Mehanny & Abdel-Rahman, 1991). This hepatoxicity is enhanced by other drugs such as barbiturates, alcohol, and cocaine adulterants such as amphetamine (Majewska, 1996). Cocaine also induces pulmonary disorders that are particularly severe in cocaine smokers. These disorders include inflammation of and lung infections, pulmonary congestion, edema, hypertrophy of pulmonary arteries, and pulmonary necrosis (Karch, 1993). Cocaine abuse in humans can lead to seizures (Holand, Marx, Earnest, & Ranninger, 1992), optic neuropathy, cerebral infarction (Sloan & Mattioni, 1992), subarachnoid and intracerebral hemorrhage, multifocal cerebral ischemia, cerebral atrophy, and myocardial infarction that leads to global brain ischemia and edema (Daras, Tuchman, & Marks, 1991; Fredericks, Lefkowitz, Challa, & Troost, 1991). Of note, cocaine abuse is a significant risk factor for cerebrovascular complications in young adults (Kaku & Lowenstein, 1990) in whom traditional risk factors are frequently missing (Levine, Brust, Futrell, et al., 1990). Ethanol intoxication has also been associated with strokes (Gorelick, 1987). Combining both drugs induces more adverse cardiovascular effects in healthy volunteers than cocaine alone (Perez-Reyes & Jeffcoat, 1992). Seizures are not confined to those who abuse cocaine but have also been observed in recreational users of cocaine (Daras, 1996). Headaches are frequently experienced following cocaine use (Dhopesh, Maany, & Herring, 1990; Washton & Gold, 1984). These are not always benign and may herald the onset of an acute cerebrovascular accident (CVA; Daras, 1996). There have also been reports of CVAs in neonates whose mothers were addicted to cocaine (Daras, 1996). Thus, cocaine is truly a medically dangerous drug. Importantly, more than 23 million people in the United States have used cocaine at some time in their lives (O'Brien 1996).

### Psychopathology Associated with Cocaine Abuse

Morphological, physiological, and neurochemical neurological abnormalities in chronic drug abusers have been demonstrated by using modern diagnostic techniques such as positron emission tomography (PET), computed axial tomography (CAT), magnetic resonance imaging (MRI), and single photon emission computed tomography (SPECT; Bartzokis et al., 1996; Cascella, Perrlson, Wong, Broussole, et al., 1991; Langendorf, Anderson, Tupper, Rottenberg, & Weisman, 1996; Pascual-Leone, Dhuna, & Anderson, 1991). Various degrees of cerebral atrophy and brain lesions, particularly in the frontal cortex and basal ganglia, have been found in cocaine abusers (Bartzokis et al., 1996; Langendorf et al., 1996; Pascual-Leone et al., 1991). Cerebral circulatory deficits have also been noted by other investigators (Kosten, Malison, & Wallace, 1996). Typically, frontal lobe degeneration is accompanied by dementia, neuropsychological deficits, apathy, depression, and social disinhibition. Such brain changes in conjunction with abnormalities in catecholamine receptors and re-uptake carriers induced by chronic cocaine usage may underlie the apathy and depression that are common in cocaine abusers (Kosten et al., 1996). Cognitive impairments in cocaine users were described as long ago as 1908 (Daras, 1996). Buck and colleagues (Buck, Sasaki, Hewitt, & Macrae, 1968) described psychological impairment and poor work performance in South American coca leaf chewers. Subsequent studies demonstrated subtle deficits in auditory recall, concentration, and reaction time (O'Malley, Adamse, Heaton, & Gawin, 1992b; Weinrieb & O'Brien, 1993) that suggest an underlying problem in information processing (Herning & King, 1996). Theoretically, such deficits should adversely influence the ability to benefit from psychosocial treatment, although there is still surprisingly little evidence that superior cognitive abilities are associated with better treatment response by substance abusers (Alterman, Kushner, & Holahan, 1990).

Just as for other substance abuse/dependent patients, the majority of cocaine-dependent patients have considerable Axis I pathology, including additional substance abuse disorders (Halikas, Crosby, Pearson, Nugent, & Carlson, 1994; Rounsaville, Anton, Carroll, Budde, Prusoff, & Gawin, 1991; Ziedonis, Rayford, Bryant, & Rounsaville, 1994). The more common diagnoses include alcohol dependence, major depression, bipolar disorder, phobias, posttraumatic stress disorder (Cottler, Compton, Mager, Spitznagel, & Janca, 1992), antisocial personality disorder (APD), and a history of childhood attention deficit disorder (ADD). APD is as common a diagnosis in cocaine abuser/dependent patients as in opioid abuser/dependent patients (see later), contrasted with the relatively lower rates found in alcohol abuser/dependent patients. The presence of ADD may reflect the efforts of these patients at self-medication. Phobias, ADD, and APD precede the onset of cocaine addiction, whereas depression and alcoholism frequently follow it. In this regard, a residual mood disorder may be seen after cocaine withdrawal and may in some cases require antidepressant medication (O'Brien, 1996). Paranoia and anhedonia are also often observed in chronic cocaine abusers (Kosten et al., 1996; O'Brien, 1996). Thus, the majority of cocaine patients present with comorbid psychopathology. Unemployment, absence of housing arrangements, and legal and family problems are also barriers to effective treatment that often need to be addressed in the treatment process.

## Treatment of Cocaine Abuse/Dependence

Lacking a drug substitution method analogous to methadone maintenance or a specific antagonist similar to naltrexone, the initial response of the treatment community to cocaine dependence was to adopt the abstinence-oriented, staged model of alcoholism treatment. The data on the effectiveness of psychosocial treatments for cocaine dependence as well as recent intensive efforts to facilitate the initiation of abstinence by pharmacological means will be described.

**Withdrawal.** Although there is no definitive evidence that cocaine produces a withdrawal syndrome such as seen with alcohol, opiates, or sedatives, there is definitely a period of physical and mental instability following continuous use of cocaine, and this has been termed the "withdrawal" period (Schuckit, 1997). The withdrawal effects of cocaine are irritability, weakness, a marked reduction in energy, hypersomnia, depression, loss of concentration, increased appetite, and paranoid ideation (hallucinations and delusions). If paranoid effects occur, they usually last from 2 to 14 days, but can last longer. Kleber (1995) indicates that the symptomatology following the initial barrage of unpleasant symptoms, commonly called the "crash," differs for outpatients and inpatients. In cocaine inpatients, the crash appears "to be followed by gradual improvement in the cocaine-induced impairment with normalization of sleep, energy, and hedonic response" (p. S97). By contrast, "In outpatients, where cocaine availability and craving remain high, the crash is followed by a few days of apparent normalcy. The next phase is a prolonged period of chronic dysphoria and diminished pleasurable responses to the environment" (Kleber, 1995, p. S97). Because cocaine is typically used intermittently, even heavy users experience periods of withdrawal or "crash" (O'Brien, 1996). As indicated, a residual mood disorder may be seen after cocaine withdrawal in some patients (O'Brien, 1996). Because of limited bed capacities, inpatient detoxification is generally limited to cases in need of immediate psychiatric (drug-induced psychosis) or medical (pregnancy, myocardial damage) attention, as there is no effective existing treatment for the abstinence symptomatology during the withdrawal period.

Whether or not the withdrawal symptomatology following cocaine abstinence qualifies for the formal designation of a withdrawal syndrome, the dysphoric psychological state and the physiological instability associated with cocaine abstinence contribute to the considerable difficulties in retaining cocaine-dependent patients in outpatient treatment (Hoffman, Caudill, Koman, Luckey, Flynn, & Hubbard, 1994). Consequently, there has been an intensive effort to evaluate effective psychosocial and pharmacological treatments for cocaine abstinence symptomatology. A recent study at our University of Pennsylvania Center indicated that a measure of cocaine withdrawal/ abstinence symptomatology, the Cocaine Selective Severity Assessment (CSSA), modeled after measures of the alcohol withdrawal syndrome (AWS), was successful in predicting early dropouts from treatment (Kampman et al., 1998). More effective ways of dealing with this abstinence symptomatology are an important starting point in increasing the effectiveness of treating cocaine dependence.

## Psychosocial Treatments

**High Attrition Rates.** As indicated, one of the more difficult problems for the outpatient treatment of cocaine dependence is the high attrition rates. In this regard, Kang and colleagues (Kang, Kleinman, Woody, et al., 1991) found that a treatment program that provided once weekly psychotherapy, nearly half of the treatment candidates (47%) dropped out before the treatment began and 31% completed fewer than six sessions. In a 12-week study of once weekly psychotherapy and/or pharmacotherapy, Carroll et al. (Carroll, Rounsaville, Gordon, Nich, Jatlow, Bisighini, & Gawin, 1994a) reported that 21% of the patients failed to complete 2 weeks of treatment and that only 49/139 (35.2%) completed the full 12 weeks of treatment. In an earlier comparison of two forms of psychosocial treatment for cocaine dependence, Carroll and colleagues (Carroll, Rounsaville, & Gawin, 1991) reported that 24% of the patients dropped out after 1 week of the projected 12-week, once per week course of treatment. Similarly, Higgins et al. (Higgins, Budney, Bickel, Hughes, Foerg, & Badger, 1993) reported that eight (42%) of the patients attending a 3.5-hour per week twelve-step treatment program failed to attend more than one treatment session. Hoffman et al. (1994) also found drop-out rates of 56% within the first week of treatment that provided 90 minutes of group therapy twice weekly.

**Effective Psychosocial Treatments.** Notwithstanding the evidence for high attrition rates, there is accumulating evidence that treatment for cocaine dependence can be relatively effective, even for patients with relatively limited social resources.

Higgins and colleagues (Higgins, Delaney, Budney, Bickel, Hughes, Foerg, & Fenwick, 1991;

Higgins, et al., 1993) presented evidence that a behavioral treatment that combined contingency reinforcement for those whose urines are negative for cocaine (not for other drugs) and aspects of Azrin's community reinforcement (CRF) treatment approach—marital, job, and recreational counseling (Azrin & Besalel, 1980; Azrin, Naster, & Jones, 1973)—was effective in bringing about abstinence from cocaine during a 12-week study/treatment period. Subjects were thirteen consecutively admitted outpatients who received the behavioral treatment and fifteen consecutively admitted outpatients offered twelve-step counseling. Thus, the study participants were not randomly assigned. Urines were taken four times weekly for all subjects, and no contingencies were attached for the twelve-step patients. Patients who participated in the behavioral program could earn approximately $1000 worth of points for abstinence during the course of the twelve treatment weeks which could be exchanged for merchandise or services, and twelve-step patients could earn $240 for giving forty-eight urines during this period. The CRF component of treatment was implemented in twice weekly 1-hour sessions, and the twelve-step counseling consisted of 2 hours of treatment weekly and encouragement to attend at least one self-help group weekly.

Eleven of thirteen behavioral patients completed treatment, as contrasted with five of fifteen 12-step patients. This treatment completion rate for the behavioral program, in itself, is relatively remarkable. Ten of thirteen behavioral patients achieved 4 weeks of abstinence compared with only 3/15 for the twelve-step treatment, and 3/13 were abstinent for all 12 weeks. None of the twelve-step patients achieved even 8 weeks of abstinence. Ninety percent of 552 urines obtained in the behavioral treatment program and 78% of the 312 from the patients who received twelve-step counseling were free of cocaine.

In a second study (Higgins et al., 1993), thirty-eight patients were randomly assigned to either the behavioral or drug abuse counseling treatment. The behavioral treatment was much like that in the earlier study, and the drug counseling program was similar to the twelve-step program implemented in the earlier program. The counseling consisted of one 2.5-hour group and one 1-hour individual therapy session per week for 12 weeks. Both treatment programs were extended an additional 12 weeks through 24 weeks. During weeks

13–24, counseling was reduced to once weekly for both treatment groups, and three times weekly urine monitoring was reduced to twice weekly. Behavioral subjects could earn approximately $1000 exchangeable for merchandise/services during the first 12 treatment weeks and they were given a $1 state lottery ticket for each clean urine during the weeks 13–24 treatment "fading" period. Drug counseling patients continued to receive $5 for each urine, independent of its status.

The results for this latter study were similar to those obtained for the earlier study. A 58% treatment completion rate was obtained for the behavioral patients for the 24 weeks of treatment versus only 11% for drug counseling patients. Although 68 and 42% of the behavioral patients achieved at least 8 and 16 weeks of continuous cocaine abstinence, respectively, these rates were 11 and 5% for drug abuse counseling patients. There was little evidence of a precipitous decline in functioning for the behavioral patients following the removal of the higher intensity treatment/contingency. A subsequent study has now extended the outcome findings to 1-year posttreatment entry and shows that the gains can be sustained through this period (Higgins, Budney, Bickel, Badger, Foerg, & Ogden, 1995).

A study of cocaine dependence treatment by Alterman and colleagues (1994) compared the effectiveness of 4 weeks of intensive, highly structured day hospital (DH—27 hours weekly) treatment with that of inpatient treatment (INP—48 hours of weekly scheduled treatment) with the same treatment elements. The subjects were primarily inner city, male African-Americans treated at a Veterans Administration Medical Center. Fifty-six patients were randomly assigned to the DH and fifty-five to the INP. Group therapy was the primary treatment, and emphasis was on initiating abstinence, a drug-free lifestyle, and education about substance abuse. Both programs endorsed the self-help philosophy and expected participation in self-help groups. Both cocaine- and alcohol-dependent patients were concurrently treated in both programs. Additional treatments available were individual counseling and case management, pharmacotherapy, medical treatment, and recreational and family therapies.

The INP treatment completion rate of 89% was significantly higher than that of the DH treatment (54%). However, at 7 months posttreatment entry, self-reported outcomes indicated considerable improvements in both groups for drug and alcohol use, family/social, legal, employment, and psychiatric problems in a variety of Addiction Severity Index measures. The finding of reduced cocaine use was supported by urine data. Both self-report and urine data indicated 50–60% abstinence for both groups at the follow-up assessment. The costs of the DH were about 40% lower than those of the INP treatment.

Several studies by Carroll and colleagues provide further indication of the effectiveness of outpatient treatment for cocaine dependence. An initial study (Carroll et al., 1991) compared the effectiveness of a once per week, 12-week treatment course of individual relapse prevention therapy (RPT) with that of individual interpersonal therapy (IPT) for forty-two randomly assigned patients. Overall, 31% of the subjects were classified as recovered when treatment ended, and 52% completed treatment.

In a subsequent study, Carroll and her colleagues compared the effectiveness of RPT with that of clinical management (CM—standardized form of basic administrative management and minimal clinical support) in an evaluation of the effectiveness of the medication, desipramine (DMI). In that study of 139 cocaine-dependent patients (Carroll, Power, Bryant, & Rounsaville, 1993; Carroll, et al., 1994a), the investigators found evidence of reduced cocaine use and psychosocial and medical problems over the course of treatment, and these reductions were maintained during a 1-year posttreatment follow-up period. As in their earlier work, there was an indication that RPT was the more effective psychosocial treatment. One interesting aspect of that study was a delayed effect of the RPT treatment. At 6 months posttreatment, there were modest differences between the RPT and CM groups; but at the 12-month point, the differences (favoring RPT) were much greater (Carroll, Rounsaville, Nich, Gordon, Wirtz, & Gawin, 1994b). These findings are similar to those of two studies by Woody and colleagues who compared professional psychotherapy with standard drug counseling for methadone maintained patients (Woody, Luborsky, McLellan, O'Brien, Beck, Blaine, et al., 1983; Woody, McLellan, Luborsky, & O'Brien 1995).

Finally, research by Hoffman et al. (1994) shows the contribution of more intensive treatment to increased treatment retention during a 4-month treatment period. This study compared two levels of intensity of group treatment: either 90 minutes, twice weekly or 120 minutes, five times weekly. Each group therapy condition was also supplemented by one of three individual therapy conditions varying in intensity: (1) no additional treatment, (2) individual psychotherapy (twice weekly in the first month and weekly thereafter), and (3) individual psychotherapy plus weekly family therapy beginning in the second month. The findings revealed that the highest drop-out rates were for the low-intensity group treatment without supplemental individual treatment. Fifty-six percent of the patients in this group dropped out of treatment within the first week. This contrasts with an average drop-out rate of about 35% for five other groups. Similar findings obtained for predicting retention in treatment for 3 months or more. This was only 14% for the low-intensity treatment and about 30% for the five other treatment conditions. Thus, any increase in intensity of treatment above that provided by the twice weekly group therapy, whether it took the form of additional individual therapy or more intensive group therapy, resulted in notable increases in retention. Adding individual treatments to the intensive group therapy condition failed to increase treatment retention.

**Summary of Psychosocial Treatment.** It is likely that the inability to treat the symptomatology associated with initial abstinence from cocaine in an outpatient setting is a significant contributor to the high early patient drop-out rates that are found in most outpatient treatment programs for cocaine dependence. As indicated previously, higher scores on the CSSA, a measure of withdrawal/abstinence symptomatology, predicts treatment dropout. In addition, we have found in two separate studies (Alterman, McKay, Mulvaney, & McLellan, 1996a; Alterman, Kampman, Boardman, Rutherford, Cacciola, McKay, & Maany, 1997) that a positive initial cocaine urine toxicology, an indication of the patient's inability to achieve abstinence, as well of the severity of cocaine dependence, is highly predictive of treatment dropout. Thus, a beginning is being made in identifying individuals at "high risk" of dropping out of outpatient treatment. Providing incentives to patients or more intensive treatment can help to mitigate the adverse influences which bring about early treatment dropout. Other forms of psychosocial treatment such as motivational enhancement treatment (MET; Miller, Zweben, DiClemente, & Rychtarik, 1992), derived from the alcoholism

field, are being examined for their effectiveness. Additionally, the stage of change measures (Prochaska & DiClemente, 1984) that have recently been used in the alcoholism treatment field (Project Match Research Group, 1997) are being introduced to the field in another effort to enhance the effectiveness of treatment for cocaine dependence. Pharmacotherapy is an alternative/complementary approach to treating cocaine dependence.

## Pharmacotherapy

**Primary Medications Studied.** The reinforcing effects of cocaine and cocaine analogues correlate best with their effectiveness in blocking the dopamine (DA) transporter. This re-uptake blockage results in excess synaptic DA and thus increased DA stimulation at critical brain sites. Cocaine also blocks both norepinephrine (NE) and serotonin (5HT) re-uptake, and chronic use produces changes in these systems, as measured by reductions in the neurotransmitter metabolites MHPG (3-methoxy-4 hydroxphenetyleneglycol) and 5-HIAA (5-hydroxyindoleacetic acid). Thus, neurotransmitters other than DA may be involved after a period of heavy cocaine use (O'Brien, 1996). Most efforts to identify medications that would be effective in treating patients with cocaine use disorders have been directed toward finding agents that either correct alterations in neurochemical substrates brought on by chronic cocaine use or block the reinforcing effects of cocaine (Kleber, 1995). Although there have been a number of promising leads, no pharmacological agent has yet generated consistent evidence of effectiveness in reducing cocaine use (Kleber, 1995; O'Brien, 1996; O'Brien & McKay, 1997). Several studies evaluated the effects of tricyclic antidepressants, selective serotonin re-uptake inhibitors (SSRIs), and MAO-Is (monoamine oxidase inhibitors). The findings of Nunes and colleagues (Nunes, McGrath, Quitkin, Ocepek-Welikson, Stewart, Koenig, et al., 1995), for a 12-week placebo-controlled trial of imipramine (150–300 mg/daily) in 113 cocaine abusers, are noteworthy. In this study, there was some indication of higher abstinence rates, defined as three consecutive confirmed urine-negative weeks, in the group on imipramine (IMI; 19 vs. 7%). There was also suggestive evidence that these effects were stronger for depressed users of IMI (26% IMI versus 13% PL). Other drugs that influence the DA system have also been tried. Amantadine, a drug that stimulates dopaminergic transmission may have short-term efficacy as an aid in detoxification because cocaine urines for twenty-one subjects on amantadine during a 10-day trial were significantly more negative during a 1-month period than those of twenty-one placebo subjects (Alterman, Droba, Cornish, Antello, Sweeney, Parikh, & O'Brien, 1992). This study was conducted in the context of the 27-hour per week DH psychosocial treatment. A second study (Kampman, Volpicelli, Alterman, Cornish, Weinrieb, Epperson, et al., 1996) by investigators at the same Center did not replicate these findings, although unpublished findings from this latter study indicate that patients with high CSSA scores at treatment outset did benefit from amantadine (Kampman, 1999). It should be noted that the psychosocial treatment was much less intensive in this latter study.

**Other Medications.** The kindling phenomenon has been the target of studies using carbamazepine, an anticonvulsant, but several controlled studies failed to demonstrate any benefit (Cornish, Maany, Fudala, Neal, Poole, Volpicelli, & O'Brien, 1995; O'Brien, 1996). Selective serotonin re-uptake inhibitors were also studied. Fluoxetine reportedly produces a significant reduction of cocaine use in methadone maintenance patients, as measured by lower average urinary levels of the cocaine metabolite benzoylecgonine. It is not clear that the reduced levels of benzoylecognine represent a clinically significant hange in patient outcome (Batki, Manfredi, Jacob, & Jones, 1993). These findings have thus far not been replicated in primary cocaine abuse patients (Grabowski, Rhoades, Elk, Schmitz, Davis, Creson, & Kirby, 1995). An interesting line of research recently described by (Kosten, 1996) involves the use of an N-methyl-D-aspartate (NMDA) regulated neurotransmitter, lamotragine, to combat neurotoxicity resulting from chronic cocaine use. Initial findings demonstrated the drug's safety during acute cocaine administration, a reduction in cocaine use by the outpatient subjects, and selective improvement in cognitive functioning. Finally, open-label pilot research conducted at our Center showed that the medication propranolol had higher retention rates (80%) during the 7-week drug trial than nefazodone, a combination of phentermine and fenfluramine, or a multivitamin control condition (Kampman, McGinnis, Volpicelli, Ehrman, Robbins, & O'Brien, 1996). A trend for reduced cocaine use, as measured by urine toxicologies, was also revealed for propranolol. A number of potential mechanisms may underlie the effect of propranolol, including a reduction in noradrenergic activity that may ameliorate cocaine craving and in the anxiety associated with abstinence from the drug. A double-blind study is underway to further evaluate effectiveness.

## Summary of Treatment for Cocaine Dependence

Our review of psychosocial treatments for cocaine dependence indicated that intensive outpatient treatments in various forms can be relatively effective. The major problem in outpatient treatment is treatment dropout. However, given the current environment in which treatments are becoming increasingly less, rather than more, intensive, it is quite possible that the effectiveness of treatment will decline in the coming years. With regard to pharmacological treatment, several promising drugs are being evaluated that take advantage of distinctive mechanisms. Further, the National Institute of Drug Abuse is currently funding a number of Centers nationally that are dedicated to evaluating the efficacy of promising medications. Thus, there is the possibility that evidence for one or more effective drugs will be established within the coming 5 to 10 years. However, in the same sense that most opiate-dependent persons choose not to use naltrexone (see later), the question remains whether the majority of patients will be inclined to use this medication(s). Finally, an important consideration in regard to the effectiveness of medications is the psychosocial treatment context within which the medication is administered. Research by Carroll and her colleagues with cocaine-dependent patients (Carroll et al., 1994a,b), by Volpicelli and O'Malley and their colleagues (O'Malley, Jaffe, Chang, Schottenfeld, Meyer, & Rounsaville, 1992a; Volpicelli, Alterman, Hayashida, O'Brien, & Muentz, 1992) with alcohol-dependent patients, by Rounsaville and colleagues (Rounsaville, Glazer, Wilber, Weissman, & Kleber, 1983) and Woody and colleagues (Woody et al., 1983) with opiate-dependent patients, and by Glassman and Covey (1995) and Hall and colleagues (Hall, Munoz, Reus, & Sees, 1996) working with nicotine-dependent patients uniformly suggests that psychosocial interventions can be combined with pharmacological interventions in treating dependence disorders and also that the addition of psychosocial support and services may be necessary to achieve the full potential from even clearly effective medications. Ultimately, there is a need for studies that will specify the optimal mix of medication and psychosocial interventions for these disorders. In addition, there is a need for research designed to identify methods for increasing medication compliance so that the full potential from efficacious medications can be realized in real-world settings.

## Opioid Abuse/Dependence

### Overview

There is some evidence that opioid dependence is increasing in the United States (Kosten & Stine, 1997), and there is the possibility that opioid dependence will replace cocaine dependence as the latest major epidemic in this country. An influx of new users of heroin is being seen, which is one indicator of an epidemic. This epidemic is attributable to a change in the supply side of heroin; new sources are available from Mexico and South America with a much greater purity and lower cost than was available 5 years ago (Kosten & Stine, 1997; O'Brien & McKay, 1997). Because of higher purity, snorting and smoking of heroin is now possible and is being seen. Thus, recent estimates were that there are currently 2 million heroin abusers in the United States (Woody & McNicholas, 1996), but the prevalence may become substantially higher in the near future.

It is important to point out that opioid dependence has been a serious problem in this country for a considerably longer time than cocaine dependence and also that the nature of the two forms of illicit drugs also differ markedly. Accordingly, research and treatment for opioid dependence do not always follow a course parallel to that for cocaine dependence.

A large body of studies conducted in the 1970s revealed that opioid-dependent patients, just as the cocaine-dependent patients previously described, suffer from other forms of psychopathology (Brooner, King, Kidorf, Schmidt, & Bigelow, 1997). Later in this chapter, we describe the findings of a series of studies that systematically examined psychopathology and the relationship between psychopathology and treatment response in

opioid-dependent patients. Investigations of the relationship between psychopathology and treatment response was not described for cocaine-dependent patients because the investigation of this question for these patients has not been nearly as systematic or thorough.

The medical consequences of opioid dependence are also not discussed in this section, because unlike cocaine use, there are virtually no toxic effects from normal doses of opiates or opioids (Kreek, 1992). The significant medical problems associated with opioid dependence result primarily from drug overdose (Kosten & Stine, 1997) or the use of contaminated injection equipment (HIV/AIDS, hepatitis; Woody & McNicholas, 1996).

Just as for other addicting drugs, opiate addiction is seen as a chronic, relapsing disorder (Cooper, 1989; O'Brien & McLellan, 1996; Woody & McNicholas, 1996). There are four major forms of treatment for this disorder: maintenance drug treatment, antagonist drug treatment, residential/ therapeutic community treatment, and outpatient drug-free treatment. Managed care restrictions on funding during the past several years have restricted the availability of therapeutic community treatment (National Academy of Sciences, 1996), but residential treatments still exist for selected patients.

Many addicts who relapse need detoxification. Opioids produce marked physiological dependence and withdrawal symptomatology, in contrast to cocaine (Kleber, 1994; Woody & McNicholas, 1996) which requires medical detoxification. Detoxification is often presented as a treatment (and reimbursed by insurance), but research continues to suggest that it should be considered only a first step in a comprehensive rehabilitation program. The distinctions between rehabilitation and "continuing care" are not clear in the treatment of opiate addiction—at least not as it pertains to agonist or antagonist (e.g., methadone, naltrexone, or other medication) maintenance models of treatment. The term aftercare has been applied to the treatment of opioid dependence, but its meaning differs from that connoted for alcohol/cocaine dependence, that is, aftercare has been used to describe a much reduced schedule of treatment for highly stabilized, methadone maintained addicts which could be of value in opening up resources for a greater number of new patients (Cooper, 1989), rather than an emphasis on a qualitatively different form of treatment. This stage of treatment is often also called the supportive phase (Woody & McNicholas, 1996). The following section of this chapter will discuss the detoxification process for opioid dependence. This section will be followed by a discussion of pharmacological and psychosocial treatments for opiate dependence.

## Detoxification

Opiate detoxification is generally implemented in one of two situations. If a patient has been stabilized on methadone for a number of years, appears to have the ability to be drug-free, and communicates this interest, detoxification can be accomplished by using a tapered methadone schedule for several months, which in limited cases can extend over an even longer period (Woody & McNicholas, 1996). This process can be implemented on an outpatient basis, although hospitalization is sometimes helpful at the end of detoxification when the dose is less than 20 to 25 mg. Clonidine or lofexidine are often helpful in blocking signs and symptoms of withdrawal related to autonomic hyperactivity. However, Cushman (1974) showed more than two decades ago, that only a small proportion of detoxification candidates can remain free of opiates for an extended period of time. As with detoxification alone for alcohol/cocaine dependence, detoxification without additional treatment is not recommended. Detoxification is also properly used as an initial stage of treatment for opiate dependence, usually for heroin addicts who prefer not to participate in methadone maintenance and wish to enter into a drug-free outpatient treatment or narcotic antagonist (naltrexone) treatment or into drug-free therapeutic communities.

Numerous detoxification techniques have been proposed. The most commonly used method involves transferring a patient from a short-acting opiate such as heroin to a long-acting opioid such as methadone which blocks symptoms of withdrawal by cross-tolerance. The dose of methadone can then be gradually reduced according to a predetermined schedule, adjusted as needed if the patient reports discomfort or shows signs of a withdrawal syndrome. Clonidine and lofexidine are two nonopioid medications that can block many of the signs and symptoms of opiate withdrawal. The effectiveness of lofexidine in this regard is currently undergoing evaluation. These drugs can be quite useful when opioids for detoxification are not available. In all detoxification methods, prompt relapse is likely unless the patient becomes engaged in a long-term aftercare program (O'Brien, 1996; O'Brien & McKay, 1997). A relatively new form of detoxification has received considerable attention during the past several years. Twenty-four hour detoxifications from opiates have been accomplished in offices using a combination of a nonopiate sedative to put patients to sleep, followed by administration of increasing doses of a short-acting opiate antagonist, such as naloxone, to displace all opiates from receptor sites. This process can be accomplished while the patient is asleep and, it has been claimed, produces a drug-free state that is unaccompanied by withdrawal symptoms (benzodiazepines and clonidine are sometimes used to medicate low-level residual withdrawal). This rapid detoxification procedure (Loimer, Lenz, Schmid, Presslich, 1991) has been attractive to many clients because of its speed and the claims that it avoids withdrawal symptoms. However, at this time, this process has not been carefully evaluated for efficacy or safety, and it remains controversial because it requires anesthetization. Research is needed to determine the effectiveness of this technique.

## Rehabilitation

Maintenance substitution treatment with methadone, levo-alpha-acetylmethadol (LAAM), or buprenorphine are first discussed followed by consideration of antagonist treatment. This is then followed by consideration of psychosocial treatments for opioid dependence.

**Maintenance Treatment.** *Methadone.* Some opioid addicts can detoxify and remain drug-free, but the majority relapses, even after intensive psychotherapy (Cushman, 1974; State of Oregon, 1996; Gerstein, Johnson, Harwood, Fountain, Suter, & Malloy, 1994). More important, many heroin addicts will not even consider drug-free treatment. In this regard, it is noteworthy that although the sustained stimulation from cocaine cannot be maintained over long periods, the sedation from heroin leads to sustainable long-term dependence (Kosten & Stine, 1997). Thus, the majority of opioid-dependent patients are treated by a form of substitution therapy. Approximately 120,000 individuals currently receive methadone maintenance

(MM) treatment in the United States. MM, developed in the 1960s, consists of transferring the patient from heroin, a short-acting opiate that must be taken by injection two to four times daily, to methadone, a long-acting opioid that need be taken only once daily by mouth. Methadone substitutes for heroin, reduces drug-seeking behavior, and blocks opiate withdrawal symptoms (O'Brien, 1996). It stabilizes physiological systems because of its long duration of action in contrast to the short action of heroin which produces ups and downs (Kreek, 1992). Typically, patients continue to use some heroin during the first few weeks or months on methadone, but usually in reduced amounts and frequency. Methadone does not block the effects of heroin, but it produces cross-tolerance to heroin and all similar drugs. Thus, the effects of usual doses of heroin are diminished; over time the typical patient decreases heroin use further and may stop using heroin entirely (O'Brien & McKay, 1997; Woody & McNicholas, 1996).

The changes produced by transfer to a long-acting opioid are significant. Several reviews of the opioid dependence literature have concluded that in-treatment performance, measured by decreased use of narcotics and other illicit drugs, decreased criminal activity, and increased social productivity, improves in a direct linear relationship to the length of time spent in treatment (Cooper, 1989; Ball & Ross, 1991; O'Brien, 1996). With respect to length of time in treatment, on average, 40 to 50% of newly admitted patients leave outpatient or residential drug-free treatment within the first 3 months of treatment, compared with an average 14% dropout rate in well-run methadone maintenance programs (Cooper, 1989). Importantly, a large number of studies based on a variety of nonexperimental strategies have produced consistent evidence that MM is associated with lower HIV positive rates (Caplehorn & Ross, 1995; Metzger et al., 1993; Metzger, Navaline, & Woody, 1998; Moss, Vranizan, Gorter, Bachetti, Watters, & Osmond, 1994; Novick, Joseph, Croxon, et al., 1994; Serpelloni, Carriere, Rezza, Morganti, Gomma, & Binkin, 1994). The primary mechanism for this reduction is lower needle injection rates associated with treatment participation (Caplehorn & Ross, 1995; Metzger et al., 1998). Indeed, as Metzger and his colleagues (1998, p. 98) point out, "Given the hidden nature of drug use and its social stigmatization, substance abuse treatment provides a location for the delivery and evaluation of HIV prevention interventions." In this light, research such as that reported by Zanis and colleagues (Zanis, McLellan, Alterman, & Cnaan, 1996), in which outreach efforts may be successfully employed to return discharged MM patients to treatment, takes on increased importance. Thus, there are reasons related to public health to retain patients in methadone maintenance.

As indicated, considerable evidence has been reported that well-run methadone maintenance (MM) programs, which include structured counseling and other problem-oriented treatment, are effective (Cooper, 1989; Dole, 1989). One of the primary requirements is prescribing a sufficient daily dose of methadone. Dole (1989) described unpublished data by Ball (also see Ball & Ross, 1991) that revealed an inverse relationship between the percentage who used heroin during the past month and the dose of methadone hydrochloride prescribed. Daily doses of 60 mg/day and above were associated with no heroin use. That is, a blood level of methadone at concentrations greater than 150 ng/mL is necessary to stop illicit opiate use. However, it is not as clear that the dose levels described by Dole (1989) are as effective now as they once were. Recently, high purity heroin in the United States has become cheaper (Kosten & Stine, 1997). Thus, the average street heroin addict is likely to have a higher level of physiological dependence. This has necessitated higher doses of methadone to prevent withdrawal and to produce sufficient cross-tolerance to counter the effects of very potent heroin. Although very few treatment outcome studies have been done under these new circumstances, there is anecdotal evidence that methadone treatment may be less effective or at least more difficult in the era of cheap and potent heroin (Bickel & Amass, 1995; O'Brien & McKay, 1997). Thus, a survey by the U.S. General Accounting Office (1995) found that rates of recent illicit drug use ranged from 13 to 63% in a sample of methadone maintenance programs. Data from our Center indicate that approximately 50% of the urine toxicologies for heroin and cocaine are positive for patients in the first 6 months of treatment (Alterman, Rutherford, Cacciola, McKay, & Woody, 1996b). Research by Morral and colleagues (Morral, Iguchi, Belding, & Lamb, 1997) revealed that only about 30% of new patients have relatively few drug-free urines by the end of 4 months of treatment. The increased cocaine abuse that has been seen in the past decade in opioid-dependent patients is associated with poorer outcomes (Woody & McNicholas, 1996). Additionally, the knowledge that HIV positivity can be substantially reduced by retaining users in treatment weakens the contingency-based treatment contract that has been used in MM programs, whereby continued use of other nonprescribed drugs resulted in gradual detoxification and program discharge and is thereby likely to be associated with higher use rates by patients in treatment.

*LAAM.* Levo-alpha-acetyl methadol (LAAM) is a slower acting substance whose pharmacological effects are similar to that of methadone. It was studied extensively in clinical trials before its approval by the Food and Drug Administration (FDA) in 1993 (O'Brien & McKay, 1997). Its long half-life and even longer acting metabolites produce opiate effects for about 72 hours after a single daily ingestion. This makes LAAM very convenient because it requires dosing only three times per week and still provides physiological stability (O'Brien, 1996). Studies done to date show that treatment results for those who remain on LAAM compare favorably with those obtained with methadone, although LAAM's slower onset probably contributes to the higher initial dropout rate seen when LAAM is compared with methadone (Woody & O'Brien, 1986).

*Buprenorphine.* Buprenorphine belongs to another class of medications called partial agonists. It is currently approved for treating pain, and it has shown good efficacy as a maintenance medication in addiction treatment in several clinical trials among heroin addicts (Bickel & Amass, 1995). As a partial opiate agonist, operating primarily at the mu receptor, buprenorphine activates opiate receptors and produces effects similar to heroin and methadone, but there is a "ceiling" above which higher doses produce no greater effect. In studies so far, overdose from buprenorphine has not been seen, and if heroin or other opioids are taken, their effects are attenuated or blocked by the presence of buprenorphine (O'Brien, 1996). At the same time, buprenorphine (like all other opiate agonist medications) will produce euphoria, and there are reports that buprenorphine is diverted and sold on the street. A new preparation for this medication is likely to reduce buprenorphine diversion and illicit use. By combining buprenorphine with naloxone (an opiate antagonist), injection can be prevented, thus reducing one important side effect of the medication. An additional potential benefit

from this medication is that, even after protracted periods of maintenance with this drug, it can be terminated at the will of the patient with no need for dose reduction schedules and very few withdrawal effects—due in large part to its very long half-life (Jasinski, Pevnick, & Griffith, 1978). This medication is expected to receive FDA approval and to join methadone and LAAM as a third option for maintenance in treating heroin addicts. Based on experience from clinical trials, there are some heroin addicts who prefer methadone, others who prefer LAAM, and still others who feel that they are most stable and alert on buprenorphine. As with other classes of medications, it is helpful for the clinician to have a choice of medications.

**Antagonist Treatment.** The discovery of specific opiate receptor antagonists in the early 1970s gave rise to hopes for the "perfect" medication for treating heroin addiction. Naltrexone seemed to be the answer because it specifically blocks mu opiate receptors and kappa receptors to a lesser extent (Raynor, Kong, Chen, Yasuda, Yu, Bell, & Reisine, 1994), but it has little or no direct or agonistic effects of its own. Naltrexone and its short-acting analogue naloxone have high affinity for opiate receptors and will displace drugs like morphine or methadone, resulting in the sudden onset of withdrawal symptoms when given to people who are opioid-dependent. If the heroin addict is first detoxified so that opiate receptors are gradually evacuated, naltrexone will bind to the receptors and prevent subsequent injections of heroin from having an effect. Numerous clinical trials have shown that naltrexone is effective in blocking opiate receptors and safe; thus, it was approved by the FDA in 1983. Unfortunately, naltrexone is a very underused medication for treating heroin addiction. Unlike methadone, it has no positive psychoactive effects. Few street heroin addicts show any interest in this type of treatment, and few programs encourage patients to try it. Opioid antagonists are more complicated to prescribe than methadone, and most physicians have not been trained in their use. Opioid-dependent health care workers such as physicians, pharmacists and nurses often do well on naltrexone because it enables them to return to work with no risk of relapse, even though they work in areas of high drug availability (Washton, Pottash, & Gold, 1984). It should be noted that naltrexone has been found most effective when additional psychosocial treatment services are also provided (Farren, O'Malley, & Rounsaville, 1997). There is also preliminary evidence that naltrexone is helpful in preventing relapse in probationers who have conditional releases from prison after drug-related crimes (Cornish et al., 1997). Naltrexone is a viable treatment for highly motivated patients whose continued careers depend on completing successful treatment (Farren et al., 1997).

**Psychosocial Treatment.** A large body of research, thus far, has shown that methadone maintenance is most successful when coupled with a variety of services, including regular client contact and urine drug monitoring (Cooper, 1989). Particularly, because many opiate-dependent patients need assistance with vocational and legal problems and many come to treatment with additional psychiatric symptomatology (Rounsaville, Weissman, Kleber & Wilbur, 1982; McLellan, 1986), there is a need for drug counseling by a certified drug counselor and sometimes a need for psychotherapy or psychotropic medication to combat coexisting psychopathology (Woody & O'Brien, 1986). Yet, the amount of psychosocial treatment provided in MM programs is typically quite modest compared to that which has been provided to alcohol and other substance-dependent patients in the past. At our own Center, for example, patients are usually seen weekly for several months and then are tapered to less frequent meetings (biweekly to monthly), once the patient shows evidence of stabilization. Even this amount of treatment exceeds that provided in most community methadone programs. Assessment of treatment services received even by patients who participated in a research-enhanced program of treatment revealed relatively few treatment services in many problem areas—employment, legal, family/social—despite the stated policies of MM programs to provide such services (McLellan, Arndt, Metzger, Woody, & O'Brien, 1993). Not surprisingly, then, little improvement in functioning is seen for many patients beyond the first 2 months of treatment (Cacciola, Alterman, Rutherford, McKay, & McLellan, 1998; also see Morral et al., 1997).

There is clear evidence that methadone patients respond positively to supplemental psychosocial services, particularly professional services. For example, a study conducted at our Center 15 years ago showed that psychotherapy is highly beneficial to Veterans' Administration MM patients (Woody et al., 1983). A second study extended

these findings to community-based MM programs (Woody et al., 1995). Nonetheless, there is a continuing effort to further reduce the amount of psychosocial treatment provided to MM patients on the justification that more patients could be pharmacologically treated with methadone alone and that there is a public health benefit to having more patients improve somewhat than fewer patients improving more (Cooper, 1989). A recent study by McLellan and colleagues (McLellan et al., 1993) showed that increasing the amount and range of psychosocial treatments produced superior outcomes in methadone patients. An equally important finding is that the majority of methadone patients who received minimal counseling, a level of treatment below that usually provided under standard counseling conditions, did very poorly. Thus, though opioid-dependent patients need a markedly greater amount of treatment, current cost considerations are leading to even greater reductions in the amount of treatment provided. It should be noted, however, that a small subgroup of patients in the McLellan et al. (1993) study was able to function reasonably well under the minimal counseling condition. This finding is supported by data that show that about 20% of treatment candidates can achieve relatively stable functioning when put on a waiting list for methadone treatment (Yancovitz et al., 1991). Thus, the majority of, but possibly not all, patients need and can benefit from psychosocial treatment services within the context of methadone or other treatment.

There is a limited amount of research using behavioral contingency contracting procedures with methadone patients. Several approaches have been employed. One of these specifies that the patient must accomplish certain behaviors within a specified period of time or face suspension from the program (Bigelow, Spitzer, & Liebson, 1984). This approach may extend to reducing the methadone dose in response to problematic behaviors. When this is the case, it is in direct conflict with the medical approach to methadone treatment which strongly opposes a reduction in the medications prescribed for a patient based on the patient's poor compliance with treatment requirements (Kreek, 1986). Accordingly, this is an approach rarely seen in practice. Several recent studies by Iguchi and colleagues (Iguchi, Lamb, Belding, Platt, Husband, & Morral, 1996; Iguchi, Belding, Morral, Lamb, & Husband, 1997), provide another example of the use of behavioral approaches to enhance MM treatment outcomes. In the first study (Iguchi et al., 1996), take-home medications were used to reinforce either the provision of drug-free urines (UA) or attendance in groups that provide training in interpersonal problem solving (TIPS). During the 24-week intervention period, UA participants showed greater improvement than TIPS participants in rates of abstinence from unauthorized drugs. In the second study (Iguchi et al., 1997), vouchers were used to reinforce either provision of urine samples testing negative for illicit drugs (UA group) or the completion of objective, individually defined, treatment-plan-related tasks (TP group). A third group was assigned to the clinic's standard treatment (STD group). Results of urinalysis indicated that the TP condition was significantly more effective than the other two conditions during the 12-week contingency period and tended to retain this superiority for 12-weeks following termination of the specialized treatments.

# Psychopathology and the Relationship of Treatment Response to Psychopathology

Opioids are known to produce changes in mood and feeling. It is likely that repeated opioid use is motivated by a desire to reexperience this sense of euphoria. The complex of euphoria and decreased concern with anticipated problems produced by opioids is often referred to as a "high" (Jaffe, 1992; Woody & McNicholas, 1996). "For some individuals, opioids appear to have the capacity to ameliorate certain varieties of depression, to control anxiety, to reduce anger, and to blunt paranoid feelings and ideation" (Jaffe, 1992, p. 187). In this regard, it has been recognized for some time that substance-dependent patients as a group suffer from considerably more psychiatric pathology (other than substance dependence) than the general population (Rounsaville, Weissman, Kleber, & Wilber, 1982; Rounsaville et al., 1986; Rounsaville, Dolinsky, Babor, et al., 1987), particularly major depression and APD. A recent methodologically rigorous diagnostic study by Brooner and colleagues (Brooner et al., 1997) with 716 MM patients interviewed 1 month after admission confirmed these earlier findings and revealed that 25% of the patients qualified for APD (significantly

more men than women—34 vs. 15%) and nearly 16% for lifetime major depression disorder (significantly more women than men—24 vs. 9%). Overall, nearly half of the patients (47.5%) qualified for a lifetime nonsubstance dependence Axis I or Axis II diagnosis.

A number of studies showed that patients with additional psychopathology such as major depression, another substance dependence disorder, or APD, have a poorer response to treatment than patients without additional psychopathology (Gerstley, McLellan, Alterman & Woody, 1990; Rounsaville et al., 1986, 1987; Woody, McLellan, Luborsky, & O'Brien 1985). A seminal investigation by McLellan and colleagues (McLellan et al., 1983; McLellan, 1986) that has been upheld over the years (Kosten, Rounsaville, & Kleber, 1985; Rounsaville et al., 1986) showed that patients with more psychiatric pathology at baseline, as reflected in the psychiatric interviewer severity rating of the Addiction Severity Index (ASI), strongly predicted negative outcomes in several life areas. Indeed, a study by Rounsaville et al. (1986) showed that this index was a better predictor of negative outcomes than various psychiatric disorders.

As noted, APD is a particularly common disorder in opiate-dependent patients and occurs in as many as 50% of male patients (Gerstley et al., 1990; Brooner et al., 1997). In a study extending their initial study on the effectiveness of psychotherapy, Woody and colleagues (Woody et al., 1985) found that patients with an APD diagnosis plus a lifetime diagnosis of major depression were functioning as well at 6 months posttreatment intake as patients with no additional psychiatric diagnoses (other than substance dependence) or those with lifetime major depression. However, patients with the APD diagnosis without major depression generally responded more poorly than the other patients. The insight of this study was the distinction between APD patients with and without major depression that pointed to a possible subtyping of APD patients. It is noteworthy that no further effort has been made to replicate these findings. In a recent effort to extend the findings to MM patients who receive counseling rather than psychotherapy, Alterman and colleagues (Alterman, Rutherford, Cacciola, McKay, & Woody, 1996b) found no differences in outcomes between APD patients with and without lifetime major depression and little indication that APD is a negative prognostic indicator in MM patients. Because counseling is an overwhelmingly more common treatment than psychotherapy in the current treatment environment, the findings take on increased import.

As previously indicated, the cocaine epidemic added a dimension to MM treatment that has reduced its effectiveness in treating illicit substance use. Many of the particularly recalcitrant patients who continue to use throughout treatment are those implicated in a cycle of opiate and cocaine use (Woody & McNicholas, 1996). In an effort to address this problem, several investigations were conducted to determine whether treatment with a tricyclic antidepressant such as desipramine was effective in reducing cocaine use (Arndt, Dorozynsky, Woody, McLellan, & O'Brien, 1992; Kosten, Morgan, Falcione, & Schottenfield, 1992). The findings of these investigations have not been very encouraging. For example, although there was modest evidence in one study that desipramine was associated with reduced cocaine use in those who did not drop out of the drug trial, the drop-out rate was markedly higher for desipramine than for placebo (Arndt et al., 1992). Thus, provision of specialized treatments for cocaine abuse within the context of MM treatment is still quite limited, and thus far there is little evidence for an effective treatment. Alcohol abuse, although generally not as common as cocaine abuse in MM patients, still constitutes a considerable problem (Bickel, Marion, & Lowinson, 1987). There is little indication of specialized treatment for this problem, although a recent investigation revealed that an increase in problems related to alcohol in the first 6 months of treatment were highly predictive of violent crime and also significantly predicted nonviolent crime (Alterman, McDermott, Cook, et al., 1998). The typical approach to this problem in MM programs is to make methadone dosing contingent on a clean breath alcohol reading. The extent to which this procedure is effective or even actually implemented in practice is unclear.

## Summary of Treatment for Opioid Dependence

MM is the dominant treatment for opioid dependence in the United States. It is believed to be associated with reduced HIV risk, reductions in crime, and some modest improvements in other areas of life functioning. In the past decade, however, several developments have limited the effectiveness of this treatment for reducing illicit drug use. These include the cocaine epidemic and higher purity of heroin on the street. Additionally, the existence of the AIDS epidemic has resulted in a loosening of the behavioral contract that was originally at the foundation of MM treatment. Thus, although MM is still a useful treatment in many ways, particularly from a public health standpoint, it is not achieving the same levels of improvement in patients that were shown earlier.

ACKNOWLEDGMENTS. This work was supported by grants from NIDA, NIAAA, and the Department of Veterans Affairs.

## References

Alterman, A. I., Kushner, H., & Holahan, J. M. (1990). Cognitive functioning and treatment outcome in alcoholics. *Journal of Nervous and Mental Disease, 178*, 494–499.

Alterman, A. I., Droba, M., Cornish, J., Antello, R., Sweeney, K., Parikh, G., & O'Brien, C. P. (1992). Amantadine may facilitate detoxification of cocaine addicts. *Drug and Alcohol Dependence, 31*, 19–29.

Alterman, A. I., McLellan, A. T., O'Brien, C. P., August, D. S., Snider, E . C., Droba, M., Cornish, J. W., Hall, C. P., Raphaelson, A. H., & Schrade, F. (1994). Effectiveness and costs of inpatient vs. day hospital treatment for cocaine dependence. *Journal of Nervous and Mental Disease, 182*, 157–163.

Alterman, A. I., McKay, J. R., Mulvaney, F., & McLellan, A. T. (1996a). Prediction of attrition from day hospital treatment in lower socioeconomic cocaine dependent men. *Drug and Alcohol Dependence, 40*, 227–233.

Alterman, A. I., Rutherford, M. J., Cacciola, J. S., McKay, J. R., & Woody, G. E. (1996b). Response to methadone maintenance and counseling among antisocial patients with and without major depression. *Journal of Nervous and Mental Disease, 184*, 695–702.

Alterman, A. I., Kampman, K., Boardman, C., Rutherford, M. J., Cacciola, J. S., McKay, J. R., & Maany, I. (1997). An initial clean cocaine urine predicts favorable outpatient treatment response. *Drug and Alcohol Dependence, 46*, 79–85.

Alterman, A. I., McDermott, P. A., Cook, T. G., Metzger, D., Rutherford, M. J., Cacciola J. S., & Brown, L. S. (1998). New scales to assess change in the Addiction Severity Index for the opioid, cocaine, and alcohol dependent. *Psychology of Addictive Behavior, 12*(4), 233–246.

Arndt, I. O., Dorozynsky, L., Woody, G. E., McLellan, A. T., & O'Brien, C. P. (1992). Desipramine treatment of cocaine dependence in methadone patients. *Archives of General Psychiatry, 49*, 904–908.

Azrin, N. H., & Besalel, V. A. (1980). *Job club counselor's manual*. Baltimore: University Park Press.

Azrin, N. H., Naster, B. J., & Jones, R. (1973). Reciprocity counseling: A rapid learning based procedure for marital counseling. *Behaviour and Therapy, 11*, 364–382.

Ball, J., & Ross, A. (1991). *The effectiveness of methadone maintenance treatment.* New York: Springer Verlag.

Bartzokis, G., Beckson, M., & Ling, W. (1996). Clinical and MRI evaluation of psychostimulant neurotoxicity. In M. D. Majewska (Ed.), *Neurotoxicity and neuropathology associated with cocaine abuse.* NIDA Research Monograph 163 (pp. 300–317), Rockville, MD: United States Department of Health and Human Services.

Batki, S. L., Manfredi, L., Jacob, P., III, & Jones, R. T. (1993). Fluoxetine for cocaine dependence in methadone maintenance: Quantitative plasma and urine cocaine/benzoylecgonine concentrations. *Journal of Clinical Psychopharmacology, 13,* 243–250.

Bickel, W. K., & Amass, L. (1995). Buprenorphine treatment of opioid dependence. *Experimental and Clinical Psychopharmacology, 3,* 477–489.

Bickel, W. K., Marion, I., & Lowinson, J. H. (1987). The treatment of alcoholic methadone patients: A review. *Journal of Substance Abuse Treatment, 4,* 15–19.

Bigelow, G. E., Stitzer, M. L., & Liebson, I. (1984). The role of behavioral contingency management in drug abuse treatment. In J. Grabowski, M. L. Stitzer, & J. C. Henningfield (Eds.), *Behavioral intervention techniques in drug abuse treatment.* NIDA Research Monographs No. 46 (pp. 36–52). Rockville, MD: United States Department of Health and Human Services.

Brooner, R. K., King, V. L., Kidorf, M., Schmidt, C. W., & Bigelow, G. E. (1997). Psychiatric and substance use comorbidity among treatment-seeking opioid abusers. *Archives of General Psychiatry, 54,* 71–80.

Buck, A. A., Sasaki, T. T., Hewitt, J. J., & Macrae, A. A. (1968). Coca chewing and health. An epidemiologic study among residents of a Peruvian village. *American Journal of Epidemiology, 88,* 159–177.

Cacciola, J. S., Alterman, A. I., Rutherford, M. J., McKay, J. R., & McLellan, A. T. (1998). The course of change in methadone maintenance. *Addictions, 93,* 41–49.

Caplehorn, J. R. M., & Ross, M. W. (1995). Methadone maintenance and the likelihood of risky needle sharing. *International Journal of the Addictions, 30,* 685–698.

Carroll, K. M., Power, M. D., Bryant, K., & Rounsaville, B. J. (1993). One year followup status of treatment-seeking cocaine abusers: Psychopathology and dependent severity as predictors of outcome. *Journal of Nervous and Mental Disease, 181,* 71–79.

Carroll, K. M., Rounsaville, B. J., & Gawin, F. H. (1991). A comparative trial of psychotherapies for ambulatory cocaine abusers: Relapse prevention and interpersonal psychotherapy. *American Journal of Drug and Alcohol Abuse, 17,* 229–247.

Carroll, K. M., Rounsaville, B. J., Gordon, L. T., Nich, C., Jatlow, P., Bisighini, R. M., & Gawin, F. H. (1994a). Psychotherapy and pharmacotherapy for ambulatory cocaine abusers. *Archives of General Psychiatry, 51,* 177–187.

Carroll, K. M., Rounsaville, B. J., Nich, C., Gordon, L. T., Wirtz, P. W., & Gawin, F. H. (1994b). One year follow-up of psychotherapy and pharmacotherapy for cocaine dependence: Delayed emergence of psychotherapy effects. *Archives of General Psychiatry, 51,* 989–997.

Cascella, N. G., Perrlson, G., Wong, D. F., Broussole, E., Nagoshi, C., Margolin, R. A., & London, E. D. (1991). Effects of substance abuse on ventricular and sulcal measures assessed by computerized tomography. *British Journal of Psychiatry, 159,* 217–221.

Cooper, J. R. (1989). Methadone treatment and acquired immuno-deficiency syndrome. *Journal of the American Medical Association, 262,* 1664–1668.

Cornish, J. W., Maany, I., Fudala, P. J., Neal, S., Poole, S. A., Volpicelli, P. & O'Brien, C. P. (1995). Carbamazepine treatment for cocaine dependence. *Drug and Alcohol Dependence, 38,* 221–227.

Cornish, J. W., Metzger, D., Woody, G. E., Wilson, D., McLellan, A. T., Vandergrift, B., & O'Brien, C. P. (1997). Naltrexone pharmacotherapy for opioid dependent federal probationers. *Journal of Substance Abuse Treatment, 14,* 529–534.

Cottler, L. B., Compton, W. M., Mager, D., Spitznagel, E. L., & Janca, A. (1992). Posttraumatic stress disorder among substance users from the general population. *American Journal of Psychiatry, 149,* 664–670.

Cushman, P. (1974). Detoxification of rehabilitated methadone patients: Frequency and predictors of long-term success. *American Journal of Drug and Alcohol Abuse, 1,* 393–408.

Daras, M. (1996). Neurologic complications of cocaine. In M. D. Majewska (Ed.), *Neurotoxicity and neuropathology associated with cocaine abuse.* NIDA Research Monograph 163 (pp. 43–65). Rockville, MD: United States Department of Health and Human Services.

Daras, M., Tuchman, A. J., & Marks, S. (1991). Central nervous system infarction related to cocaine abuse. *Stroke, 22,* 1320–1326.

Dhopesh, V., Maany, I., & Herring, C. (1990). The relationship of cocaine to headache in polydrug abusers. *Headache, 31,* 17–19.

Dole, V.P. (1989). Methadone treatment and the acquired immunodeficiency syndrome epidemic. *Journal of the American Medical Association, 262,* 1681–1682.

Farren, C. K., O'Malley, S., & Rounsaville, B. (1997). Naltrexone and opiate. In S. M. Stine & T. R. Kosten (Eds.), *New treatments for opiate dependence.* New York: Guilford.

Fredericks, R. K., Lefkowitz, D. S., Challa, V. R., & Troost, B. T. (1991). Cerebral vasculitis associated with cocaine abuse. *Stroke, 22,* 1437–1439.

Gerstein, D. R., Johnson, R. A., Harwood, H. J., Fountain, D., Suter, N., & Malloy, K. (1994). Evaluating recovery services: The California Drug and Alcohol Assessment (CALDATA). Sacramento: California Department of Alcohol and Drug Programs.

Gerstley, L. J., Alterman, A. I., McLellan, A. T., & Woody, G. E. (1990). Antisocial personality disorders in patients with substance abuse disorders: A problematic diagnosis? *American Journal of Psychiatry, 147,* 173–178.

Glassman, A. H., & Covey, L.S. (1995). Nicotine dependence and treatment (1995). In R. Michels (Ed.), *Psychiatry.* Bethesda, MD: National Institute on Drug Abuse.

Gorelick, P. B. (1987). Alcohol and stroke: Current concepts of cerebrovascular disease. *Stroke, 18,* 268–270.

Grabowski, J., Rhoades, H., Elk, R., Schmitz, J., Davis, C., Creson, D., & Kirby, K. (1995). Fluoxetine is ineffective for treatment of cocaine dependence or concurrent opiate and cocaine dependence: Two placebo-controlled, double blind trials. *Journal of Clinical Psychopharmacology, 15,* 163–174.

Halikas, J. A., Crosby, R. D., Pearson, V. L., Nugent, S. M., & Carlson, G. A. (1994). Psychiatric comorbidity in treatment-seeking cocaine abusers. *American Journal of Addiction, 3,* 25–35.

Hall, S. M., Munoz, R. F., Resu, V. I., & Sees, K. L. (1996).

Mood management and nicotine gum in smoking treatment: A therapeutic contact and placebo-controlled study. *Journal of Consulting and Clinical Psychology, 64,* 1003–1009.

Herning, R. I., & King, D. I. (1996). EEG and evoked potentials alterations in cocaine-dependent individuals. In M. D. Majewska (Ed.), *Neurotoxicity and neuropathology associated with cocaine abuse.* NIDA Research Monograph No. 163 (pp. 203–223). Rockville, MD: United States Department of Health and Human Services.

Higgins, S. T., Delaney, D. D., Budney, A. J., Bickel, W. K., Hughes, J. R., Foerg, F., & Fenwick, J. W. (1991). A behavioral approach to achieving initial cocaine abstinence. *American Journal of Psychiatry, 148,* 1218–1224.

Higgins, S. T., Budney, A. J., Bickel, W. K., Hughes, J. R., Foerg, F., & Badger, G. (1993). Achieving cocaine abstinence with a behavioral approach. *American Journal of Psychiatry, 150,* 763–769.

Higgins, S. T., Budney, A. J., Bickel, W. K., Badger, G., Foerg, F., & Ogden, D. (1995). Outpatient behavioral treatment for cocaine dependence: One-year outcome. *Experimental and Clinical Psychopharmacology, 3,* 205–212.

Hoffman, J. A., Caudill, B. D., Koman, J. J., Luckey, J. W., Flynn, P. M., & Hubbard, R. L. (1994). Comparative cocaine abuse treatment strategies: Enhancing client retention and treatment exposure. *Journal of Addictive Diseases, 13,* 115–128.

Holand, R. W., Marx, J. A., Earnest, M. P., & Ranninger, S. (1992). Grand mal seizures temporally related to cocaine use: Clinical and diagnostic features. *Annals Emergency Medicine, 21,* 772–776.

Iguchi, M. Y., Lamb, R. J., Belding, M. A., Platt, J. J., Husband, S. D., & Morral, A. R. (1996). Contingent reinforcement of group participation versus abstinence in a methadone maintenance program. *Experimental and Clinical Psychopharmacology, 4,* 315–321.

Iguchi, M. Y., Belding, M. A., Morral, A. R., Lamb, R. J., & Husband, S. D. (1997). Reinforcing operants other than abstinence in drug abuse treatment: An effective alternative for reducing drug use. *Journal of Consulting and Clinical Psychology, 65,* 421–428.

Jaffe, J. H. (1992). Opiates: Clinical aspects. In J. H. Lowinson, P. Ruiz, R. B. Millman, & J. G. Langrod (Eds.), *Substance abuse: A comprehensive textbook.* Baltimore, MD: Williams & Wilkins.

Jasinski, D. R., Pevnick, J. S., & Griffith, J. D. (1978). Human pharmacology and abuse potential of the analgesic buprenorphine. *Archives of General Psychiatry, 35,* 501–516.

Jekel, J. F., Allen, D. F., Pollewski, H., Clarke, N., Dean-Paterson, S., & Cartwright, P. (1986). Epidemic free-base cocaine abuse. *Lancet, 1,* 459–462.

Kaku, D. A., & Lowenstein, D. H. (1990). Emergence of recreational drug abuse as a major risk factor for stroke in young adults. *Annals of International Medicine, 113,* 821–827.

Kampman, K. M. (1999). Unpublished data. Philadelphia: University of Pennsylvania School of Medicine.

Kampman, K. M., McGinnis, D., Volpicelli, J., Ehrman, R., Robbins, S., & O'Brien, C. P. (1996). A case series of newly abstinent cocaine dependent outpatients treated with propranolol. Presented at *The College on Problems of Drug Dependence Annual Meeting,* San Juan, PR.

Kampman, K., Volpicelli, J. R., Alterman, A. I., Cornish, J., Weinrieb, R., Epperson, L., Sparkman, T., & O'Brien, C. P. (1996). Amantadine in the early treatment of cocaine depen-

dence: A double-blind, placebo-controlled trial. *Drug and Alcohol Dependence, 41,* 25–33.

Kampman, K., Volpicelli, J. R., McGinnis, D., Alterman, A. I., Weinrieb, R., D'Angelo, L., & Epperson L. ( 1998). Reliability and validity of the Cocaine Selective Severity Assessment. *Addictive Behaviors, 23,* 449–461.

Kang, S., Kleinman, P. H., Woody, G. E., Millman, R. B., Todd, T. C., Kemp, J., & Lipton, D. S. (1991). Outcomes for cocaine abusers after once-a-week psychosocial therapy. *American Journal of Psychiatry, 148,* 630–635.

Karch, S. B. (1993). *The pathology of drug abuse.* Boca Raton, FL: CRC Press.

Kleber, H. (1994). Opioids: Detoxification. In M. Galanter & H. D. Kleber (Eds.), *Textbook of substance abuse treatment.* Washington, DC: American Psychiatric Press.

Kleber, H. (1995). Pharmacotherapy, current and potential, for the treatment of cocaine dependence. *Clinical Neuropharmacology, 18,* S96–S109.

Kosten, T. R. (1996). NMDA regulated calcium channels as targets to prevent cocaine neurotoxicity. Presented at *35th Annual Meeting of the American College of Neuropharmacology,* San Juan, PR.

Kosten, T. R., Rounsaville, B. J., & Kleber, H. D. (1985). Concurrent validity of the Addiction Severity Index. *Journal of Nervous and Mental Disease, 171,* 606–610.

Kosten, T. R., Morgan, C. M., Falcione, J., & Schottenfeld, R. S. (1992). Pharmacotherapy for cocaine abusing methadone maintained patients using amantadine or desipramine. *Archives of General Psychiatry, 49,* 904–908.

Kosten, T. R., & Stine, S. M. (1997). Introduction and overview. In S. M. Stine & T. R. Kosten (Eds.), *New treatments for opiate dependence.* New York: Guilford.

Kosten, T. R., Malison, R., & Wallace, E. (1996). In M. D. Majewska (Ed.), *Neurotoxicity and neuropathology associated with cocaine abuse.* NIDA Research Monograph No. 163 (pp. 175–192). Rockville, MD: United States Department of Health and Human Services.

Kreek, M. J. (1986). Factors modifying the pharmacological effectiveness of methadone. NIDA Monograph, DHHS Publication No. ADM 87-1281. Rockville, MD: National Institute on Drug Abuse.

Kreek, M. J. (1992). Rationale for maintenance pharmacotherapy of opiate dependence. In C. P. O'Brien & J. H. Jaffe (Eds.), *Addictive states* (pp. 205–330). New York: Raven Press.

Langendorf, F. G., Anderson, D. C., Tupper, D. E., Rottenberg, D. A., & Weisman, I. D. (1996). In M. D. Majewska (Ed.), *Neurotoxicity and neuropathology associated with cocaine abuse.* NIDA Research Monograph No. 163 (pp. 43–65). Rockville, MD: United States Department of Health and Human Services.

Levine, S. R., Brust, J. C. M., Futrell, N., Ho, K. L., Blake, D., Millikan, C. H., Brass, L. M., et al. (1990). Cerebrovascular complications of the use of the "crack" form of alkaloidal cocaine. *New England Journal of Medicine, 323,* 699–704.

Loimer, N., Lenz, K., Schmid, R., & Presslich, O. (1991). Technique for greatly shortening the transition from methadone to naltrexone maintenance of patients addicted to opiates. *American Journal of Psychiatry, 148,* 933–935.

Majewska, M. D. (1996). Cocaine addiction as a neurological disorder: Implications for treatment. In M. D. Majewska (Ed.), *Neurotoxicity and neuropathology associated with cocaine abuse.* NIDA Research Monograph No. 163 (pp. 1–26). Rockville, MD: United States Department of Health and Human Services.

Marks, V., & Chapple, P. (1967). Hepatic dysfunction in heroin and cocaine users. *British Journal of Addiction, 62,* 189–195.

McLellan, A. T. (1986). "Psychiatric severity" as a predictor of outcome from substance abuse treatments. In R. Meyer (Ed.), *Psychopathology and addictive disorders.* New York: Guilford.

McLellan, A. T., Arndt, I. O., Metzger, D., Woody, G., & O'Brien, C. P. (1993). The effects of psychosocial services in substance abuse treatment. *Journal of the American Medical Association, 269,* 1953–1959.

McLellan, A. T., Luborsky, L., Woody, G. E., Druley, K. A., & O'Brien, C. P. (1983). Predicting response to drug and alcohol treatments: Role of psychiatric severity. *Archives of General Psychiatry, 140,* 620–625.

Mehanny, S. Z., & Abdel-Rahman, M. (1991). Cocaine hepatoxicity in mice. Histologic and enzymatic studies. *Toxicological Pathology, 19,* 24–29.

Metzger D. S., Woody, G. E., McLellan, A. T., O'Brien, C. P., Druley, P., Navaline, H., DePhilippis, D., Stolley, P., & Abrutyn, E. (1993). Human immunodeficiency virus seroconversion among in- and out-of-treatment intravenous drug users: An 18-month prospective follow-up. *Journal of Acquired Immune Deficiency Syndromes, 6,* 1049–1056.

Metzger D. S., Navaline, H., & Woody, G. E. (1998). Drug abuse treatment as AIDS prevention. *Public Health Reports, 113,* 97–106.

Miller, W. R., Zweben, A., DiClemente, C. C., & Rychtarik, R. G. (1992). Motivational enhancement therapy manual: A clinical research guide for therapists treating individuals with alcohol abuse and dependence. NIAAA Project MATCH Monograph Series, Vol. 2, DHHHS Publication No. (ADM) 92-1894, Washington, DC: U.S. Government Printing Office.

Morral, A. R., Iguchi, M. Y., Belding, M. A., & Lamb, R. J. (1997). Natural classes of treatment response. *Journal of Consulting and Clinical Psychology, 65*(4), 673–685.

Moss, A. R., Vranizan, K., Gorter, R., Bachetti, P., Watters, J., & Osmond, D. (1994). HIV seroconversion in intravenous drug users in San Francisco 1985–1990. *AIDS, 8,* 223–231.

National Academy of Sciences, Institute of Medicine (1996). Managing managed care: Quality improvement in behavioral health. M. Edmunds, R. Frank, M. Hogan, D. McCarty, R. Robinson-Beale & C. Weisner (Eds.). Washington, DC: National Academy Press.

Novick, D. M., Joseph, H., Croxon, T. S., Salsitz, E. A., Wang, G., Richman, B. L., Poretsky, L., Keefe, J. B., & Whimbey, E. (1990). Absence of antibody to human immunodeficiency virus in long term, socially rehabilitated methadone maintenance patients. *Archives of Internal Medicine, 150,* 97–99.

Nunes, E. V., McGrath, P. J., Quitkin, F. M., Ocepek-Welikson, K., Stewart, J. W., Koenig, T., Wager, S., & Klein, D. F. (1995). Imipramine treatment of cocaine abuse: Possible boundaries of efficacy. *Drug and Alcohol Dependence, 39,* 185–195.

O'Brien, C. P. (1995). Drug addiction and drug abuse. In J. G. Hardman & L. E. Limbird (Eds.), *Goodman & Gilman's The Pharmacological Basis of Therapeutics* (9th ed.) (pp. 557–577). New York: McGraw-Hill.

O'Brien, C. P. (1996). Recent developments in the pharmacotherapy of substance abuse. *Journal of Consulting and Clinical Psychology, 64,* 677–686.

O'Brien, C. P., & McKay, J. R. (1997). Psychopharmacological treatments of substance use disorders. In P. E. Nathan, & J. M. Gorman (Eds.), *Effective treatments for DSM-IV disorders* (pp. 127–155). New York: Oxford University Press.

O'Brien, C. P., & McLellan, A. T. (1996). Myths about the treatment of addiction. *Lancet, 347,* 237–240.

O'Malley, S. S., Jaffe, A., Chang, G., Schottenfeld, R. S., Meyer, R. E., & Rounsaville, B. (1992a). Naltrexone and coping skills therapy for alcohol dependence: A controlled study. *Archives of General Psychiatry, 49,* 881–887.

O'Malley, S. S., Adamse, M., Heaton, R.J., & Gawin, F.H. (1992b). Neuropsychological impairment in chronic cocaine abusers. *American Journal of Drug and Alcohol Abuse, 18,* 131–144.

Pascual-Leone, A., Dhuna, A., & Anderson, D. C. (1991). Long-term neurological complications of chronic, habitual cocaine abuse. *Neurotoxicology, 12,* 393–400.

Perez-Reyes, M., & Jeffcoat, A. R. (1992). Ethanol/cocaine interaction: Cocaine and cocaethylene plasma concentrations and their relations to subjective and cardiovascular effects. *Life Science, 51,* 553–563.

Prochaska, J. O., & DiClemente, C. C. (1984). *The transtheoretical approach: Crossing traditional boundaries of therapy.* Homewood, IL: Dow Jones, Irwin.

Project Match Research Group. (1997). Matching alcoholism treatments to client heterogeneity: Project MATCH posttreatment drinking outcomes. *Journal of Studies on Alcohol, 58,* 7–29.

Raynor, K., Kong, H., Chen, Y., Yasuda, K., Yu, L., Bell, G. I., & Reisine, T. (1994). Pharmacological characterization of the cloned k-, d-, and m-opioid receptors. *Molecular Pharmacology, 45,* 330–334.

Rounsaville, B., Weissman, M., Kleber, H., & Wilber, C. (1982). Heterogeneity of psychiatric diagnosis in treated opiate addicts. *Archives of General Psychiatry, 39,* 161–166.

Rounsaville, B., Glazer, W., Wilber, C. H., Weissman, M. M., & Kleber, H. D. (1983). Short-term interpersonal psychotherapy in methadone-maintained opiate addicts. *Archives of General Psychiatry, 40,* 630–636.

Rounsaville, B. J., Anton, S. F., Carroll, K., Budde, D., Prusoff, B. A., & Gawin, F. (1991). Psychiatric diagnoses of treatment-seeking cocaine abusers. *Archives of General Psychiatry, 48,* 43–51.

Rounsaville, B., Dolinsky, Z., Babor, T., et al. (1987). Psychopathology as a predictor of treatment outcome in alcoholics. *Archives of General Psychiatry, 44,* 505–513.

Rounsaville, B., Kosten, T., Weissman, M. M., Kleber, H. D. (1986). Prognostic significance of psychopathology in treated opiate addicts. *Archives of General Psychiatry, 43,* 739–745.

Schuckit, M. A. (1997). Outpatient detoxification from alcohol, opiates, and stimulants. *Drug Abuse and Alcoholism Newsletter, 26*(4), San Diego, CA: Vista Hill Foundation.

Serpelloni, G., Carriere, M. P., Rezza, G., Morganti, S., Gomma, M., & Binkin, N. (1994) Methadone treatment as a determinant of HIV risk reduction among injecting drug users: A nested case-controlled study. *AIDS Care, 6,* 215–220.

Sloan, M. A., & Mattioni, T. A. (1992). Concurrent myocardial and cerebral infarctions after intranasal use. *Stroke, 23,* 427–430.

State of Oregon, Department of Substance Abuse Services (1996). Evaluation of alcohol and drug abuse treatments in the State of Oregon. Oregon Office of Publications.

United States General Accounting Office Report on Methadone Treatment (1995). Washington, DC: United States Government Printing Office.

Volkow, N. D., Fowler, J. S., & Ding, Y. S. (1996). Cardiotoxic properties of cocaine. In M. D. Majewska (Ed.), *Neurotoxicity and neuropathology associated with cocaine abuse.* NIDA Research Monograph No. 163 (pp. 159–174). Rockville, MD: United States Department of Health and Human Services.

Volpicelli, J. R., Alterman, A. I., Hayashida, M., O'Brien, C. P., & Muentz, L. (1992). Naltrexone in the treatment of alcohol dependence: Initial findings. *Archives of General Psychiatry, 49*, 876–880.

Washton, A. M., & Gold, M. S. (1984). Chronic cocaine abuse: Evidence for adverse effects on health and functioning. *Psychiatric Annals, 14*, 733–743.

Washton, A. M., Pottash, A. C., & Gold, M. S. (1984). Naltrexone in addicted business executives and physicians. *Journal of Clinical Psychiatry, 45*, 39–41.

Weinrieb, R. M., & O'Brien, C. P. (1993). Persistent cognitive deficits attributed to substance abuse. In: J. C. M. Brust (Ed.), *Neurologic clinics. Neurologic complications of drug and alcohol abuse*, Vol. 11 (pp. 663–691). Philadelphia: W.B. Saunders.

Woody, G. E., & O'Brien, C. P. (1986). Update on methadone maintenance. In D. Cappell, F. Glaser, Y. Israel, et al. (Eds.), *Research advances in alcohol and drug dependence.* New York: Plenum.

Woody, G. E., Luborsky, L., McLellan, A. T., O'Brien, C. P., Beck, A. T., Blaine, J., Herman, I., & Hole, A. (1983). Psychotherapy for opiate addicts: Does it help? *Archives of General Psychiatry, 40*, 639–645.

Woody, G., McLellan, A. T., Luborsky, L., & O'Brien, C. P. (1985). Sociopathy and psychotherapy outcome. *Archives of General Psychiatry, 42*, 1081–1086.

Woody, G. E., McLellan, A. T., Luborsky, L., & O'Brien, C. P. (1995). Psychotherapy in community methadone programs: A validation study. *American Journal of Psychiatry, 152*, 1302–1308.

Woody, G. E., & McNicholas, L. (1996). Opioid use disorders. In A. Tasman, J. Kay, & J. Lieberman (Eds.), *Psychiatry*, Vol. 1 (pp. 867–880). W.B. Saunders.

Yancovitz, S. R., Des Jarlais, D. C., Peskoe Peyser, N., Drew, E., Friedmann, P., Trigg, H., & Robinson, J. W. (1991). A randomized trial of an interim methadone maintenance clinic. *American Journal of Public Health, 81*, 1185–1191.

Zanis, D. A., McLellan, A. T., Alterman, A. I., & Cnaan, R. A. (1996). Efficacy of enhanced outreach counseling to reenroll high-risk drug users 1 year after discharge from treatment. *American Journal of Psychiatry, 156*, 1095–1096.

Ziedonis, D. M., Rayford, B. S., Bryant, K. J., & Rounsaville, B. J. (1994). Psychiatric comorbidity in White and Black cocaine addicts seeking substance abuse treatment. *Hospital and Community Psychiatry, 45*, 43–49.

# CHAPTER 23

# Etiology and Management of Eating Disorders

## Donald A. Williamson, Nancy L. Zucker, Corby K. Martin, and Monique A. M. Smeets

## Introduction

The American Psychiatric Association specifies three eating disorders in the current *Diagnostic and Statistical Manual of Mental Disorders* (DSM-IV) (American Psychiatric Association, 1994): anorexia nervosa, bulimia nervosa, and eating disorder not otherwise specified (NOS). The public has become increasingly aware of eating disorders such as anorexia nervosa and bulimia nervosa in the past two decades largely from descriptions of these disorders in the mass media. However, anorexia nervosa has been known to the medical community since the 1870s, and the symptom of intentional self-starvation has been reported since medieval Europe (Brumberg, 1989). There is some debate as to whether the early reported episodes of anorexia nervosa in the medical literature (e.g., Gull, 1874; Laségue, 1873; Marcé, 1860; Morton, 1694) are equivalent to the modern manifestation of the disease (Parry-Jones & Parry-Jones, 1994). However, several perspectives hold that, although the function of anorexic symptoms may have changed over time, depending on cultural and environmental contexts, fear of weight gain has been the underlying motivational factor for most cases of anorexia nervosa since the early 1800s (Habermas, 1996).

Bulimia nervosa has a more recent history; the syndrome was first formally delineated by Russell in 1979. However, the Greek term boulimis, literally "ox hunger," or ravenous hunger, can be traced back for 2000 years. Symptoms of binge eating may have appeared in reaction to scarce food supplies when individuals would overeat in times of prosperity to prepare for periods when supplies were more scarce (Atkinson & Stern, 1997). Later reports of hyperphagia in the sixteenth through nineteenth centuries described a few extreme cases of gluttony associated with morbid obesity (Parry-Jones & Parry-Jones, 1995). These case descriptions probably reflect the earliest identification of a syndrome now called binge-eating disorder (APA, 1994).

To understand the etiology of eating disorders, one must also understand the etiology of obesity. Obesity is generally defined in terms of excess body fat content (Mayer, 1973). One's percentage of body fat is determined by the relative amount of adipose tissue to muscle and other tissue. Adiposity is conceptualized in terms of adipose (or fat) cellularity. When one gains weight, adipose cells increase in size; when weight is lost, they decrease in size. Of significance is the fact that dieting shrinks only the size of fat cells. Thus, people with excess adipose cellularity will be

Donald A. Williamson, Nancy L. Zucker, Corby K. Martin, and Monique A. M. Smeets • Pennington Biomedical Research Center, Louisiana State University, Baton Rouge, Louisiana 70803.

*Comprehensive Handbook of Psychopathology* (Third Edition), edited by Patricia B. Sutker and Henry E. Adams. Kluwer Academic / Plenum Publishers, New York, 2001.

likely to gain weight if their body weights are below a "set-point" weight, a hypothetical biologically determined body weight or body energy level that is maintained by the mechanisms of homeostasis (Keesey, 1995). In many ways, eating disorders are motivated by the individual's desire to override the biological mechanisms that determine body size and shape. Longitudinal studies have reported that having a high body weight as an adolescent may increase the likelihood of developing later eating disorder symptoms (Attie & Brooks-Gunn, 1989; Killen, Hayward, et al., 1994). Persons diagnosed with anorexia nervosa are almost certainly maintaining a body weight below the biological "set point." It is probable that many cases of bulimia nervosa are also at a weight level below the person's "set point." Thus, regulating body weight is an important consideration when trying to understand the etiology of eating disorders.

Obesity is influenced by genetic (Bouchard, 1995), physiological, and behavioral factors (Blundell, 1995; Blundell & Hill, 1993). Despite the complex factors that interact to determine body weight, a gain in body mass is predicted by a simple formula: energy input is greater than energy output (Garrow, 1995). Obesity is not considered a psychiatric disorder, however, and it is not regarded as an eating disorder. Most persons diagnosed with binge-eating disorder and some who have bulimia nervosa are obese. For the purposes of this chapter, we have elected to review the psychopathology of anorexia nervosa, bulimia nervosa, and Eating Disorder-NOS, which includes binge-eating disorder. We will not review the research literature pertaining to obesity.

## Anorexia Nervosa

### Diagnosis and Clinical Description

The DSM-IV lists four criteria necessary for a diagnosis of anorexia nervosa. New to this fourth edition of the DSM is the delineation of two subtypes of anorexic patients: the restricting subtype and the binge-eating/purging subtype. The diagnostic criteria are summarized in Table 1. The first diagnostic criterion requires that individuals intentionally maintain a body weight below weight levels recommended for health. The low weight level suggested as a guideline is less than 85% of one's expected weight level or a failure to make expected gains if the individual has not yet reached

**Table 1. Summary of DSM-IV Diagnostic Criteria for Anorexia Nervosa**

A. Refusal to maintain normal body weight (e.g., less than 85% of that expected).

B. Fear of gaining weight, even though below normal weight.

C. The presence of body weight or shape disturbance, self-evaluation being overly influenced by body weight or shape, or refusal of the significance of low body weight.

D. The presence of amenorrhea in postmenarcheal females (i.e., the absence of at least three consecutive menstrual cycles).

**Restricting Type**: The person has not regularly engaged in binge-eating or purgative behaviors. Purgative behaviors include self-induced vomiting and the misuse of laxatives, diuretics, and enemas.

**Binge-Eating/Purging Type**: The person has regularly engaged in binge-eating or purging behavior.

biological maturity. Walsh and Garner (1997) recommend a flexible interpretation of this guideline. For example, if individuals meet all of the diagnostic criteria for anorexia nervosa but their current weight levels are 90% below that expected, the diagnosis of anorexia nervosa is still warranted (Walsh & Garner, 1997). Factors such as the length of time during which weight loss has occurred (less time is more diagnostic) and the degree of weight loss (more weight loss is more diagnostic) can aid in this decision. In addition, this criterion requires that individuals "refuse" to keep their weight levels in a healthy range. Thus, this criterion excludes those individuals whose biological set-point weight is naturally low and who are continually trying to gain weight or do not experience distress if possible weight gain should occur.

The second diagnostic criterion specifies that the individuals exhibit intense fear of becoming fat or of gaining weight despite their current low weight status. This fear of fatness can be distinguished from the "normative" fear of weight gain present among a majority of adult females in Western society by its intensity, by its irrationality, and by its degree of interference in daily activities and social relationships (Striegel-Moore, Silberstein, & Rodin, 1986). The fear of gaining weight associated with anorexia nervosa is notably inconsistent with their current emaciated weight status (Walsh & Garner, 1997). These individuals will often eat the same foods and conduct their daily routines in exactly the same way for fear that any minor deviation will cause weight gain. In addition, such individuals will often avoid social activities if such activities will bring them into possible contact with food or will interfere with their ability to engage in restrictive eating or excessive exercise habits.

The third criterion specifies that the individuals experience a disturbance in body image. For example, the individuals may overvalue weight as a determinant of personal worth, may deny the seriousness of their current weight level, or may have an impression of their physical appearance that does not correspond to objective evidence. This criterion describes a disturbance in the way in which one's body size and shape is experienced. This disturbance can be manifested in several ways. There has been much debate as to whether the body-image disturbance seen among patients with anorexia nervosa is perceptual, affective, or a combination of both of these components (Heinberg, 1996). Recent conceptualizations have hypothesized that individuals with anorexia nervosa perceive themselves accurately but are mistaken in the selective interpretation of their bodily experiences (Williamson, 1996). In addition, weight level may have multiple meanings for the anorexic patient. Rather than being an indicator of body mass, the ability to control one's weight represents extreme self-control and feelings of accomplishment for the anorexic patient, whereas weight gain is associated with feelings of self-hatred, personal failure, and intense anxiety (Garner, Vitousek, & Pike, 1997).

The final criterion specifies that normal menstrual functioning is disrupted, such that the individual fails to menstruate for three consecutive menstrual cycles. The clinical significance of the presence of amenorrhea is debated because this symptom is considered an effect of the physical consequences of starvation and not a diagnostic indicator of specific psychological symptoms (Beaumont, Garner, & Touyz, 1994). Historically, this criterion has been used as an indicator of the severity of the individual's current physical status. This criterion specifies that the onset of the symptoms of anorexia nervosa among girls who have attained biological maturity interferes with healthy physiological functioning that results in losing the menstrual cycle. Adolescents may experience primary amenorrhea, the failure to have ever experienced a healthy menstrual cycle. Individuals who can menstruate only when ovarian steroids are prescribed are also considered to have amenorrhea.

Once a diagnosis of anorexia nervosa has been established, the clinician must classify the individual into one of two subtypes: *the restricting type* (the lack of binge-eating or purgative behavior) or the *binge-eating/purging type* (the person has regularly engaged in binge-eating or purging behavior: self-induced vomiting or the misuse of laxatives, diuretics, or enemas). This distinction is based on recent research evidence that documents a difference in clinical presentation between these two subtypes (e.g., Vitousek & Manke, 1994). Research has demonstrated that anorexics with the binge-eating/purging subtype are more similar to bulimia nervosa patients in their clinical presentation and often demonstrate impulsive behavior patterns and affective instability, whereas restrictor anorexic patients are more likely to exhibit rigid and obsessional personality styles (Vitousek & Manke, 1994; Wonderlich, 1995).

### Prevalence

In a recent study, Lucas, Beard, O'Fallon, and Kurland (1988) estimated the incidence of anorexia nervosa during a 45-year period (1935–1979) in the population of Rochester, Minnesota at 7.3 per 100,000 person-years, and the point-prevalence rate was 113.1 per 100,000 person-years in January of 1980. Screened data from the General Practice Research Database in Britain from 1988–1994 for newly diagnosed cases of anorexia nervosa revealed incidence rates of 4.2 per 100,000 (Turnbull et al., 1996). In a population-based sample of 2163 female Caucasian twins, the prevalence of anorexia nervosa was 0.51% (Walters & Kendler, 1995). A recent review that aggregated the data from twelve retrospective cohort incidence studies across cultures that spanned the period from 1950–1992. The study reported that the incidence of anorexia in the female cohort aged 13–19 years was five times greater than the incidence among other age groups and that a nearly threefold increase reported in the past 40 years among women in their 20s and 30s resulted in an incidence rate of 17.7 per 100,000 person-years (Pawluck & Gorey, 1998). Thus, the accumulation of evidence from these studies and other studies that examined prevalence rates for anorexia nervosa indicate that the point prevalence ranges from 0.1–1% of the population and may be higher among certain subgroups of the population, particularly among adolescent girls in later early adulthood.

## Etiology

**Cognitive-Behavioral Perspectives.** Cognitive-behavioral perspectives of anorexia nervosa emphasize the interaction between environmental pressures for thinness, social modeling of dieting, cognitive bias for body-related information, and principles of reinforcement. Current Western cultural values unduly emphasize that attaining a thin physique is vital to attain rewards such as social acceptance, financial prosperity, and happiness (Rothblum, 1994). Researchers have documented that the ideal body type depicted in the media has become progressively thinner (Garner, Garfinkel, Schwartz, & Thompson, 1980) and within the last two decades, progressively more toned (Brownell, 1991). The effect of this cultural emphasis has been more pronounced in women, and various political, social, and developmental perspectives have been offered to explain this trend (Fallon, Katzman, & Wooley, 1994). However, the sociocultural idealization of a lean and toned physique may also be promoting extreme levels of body dissatisfaction among growing segments of the male population who subsequently "feel too small" and engage in extreme weight gain behaviors such as the abuse of steroids to achieve weight gain. This phenomenon has been referred to as "reverse anorexia" or "muscle dysmorphia" (Pope, Katz, & Hudson, 1983).

Individuals who are vulnerable to such sociocultural influences due to the combination of personality variables, affective instability, and/or biological precursors, it is thought, adopt these cultural messages and subsequently develop a fear of fatness and/or a drive for thinness. According to cognitive-behavioral theories, fear of gaining weight, it is thought, is the primary motivational factor driving extreme food restriction, excessive exercise, and/or purgative behavior. These behaviors are negatively reinforced in that engaging in restrictive eating, excessive exercise, and/or purgative behavior reduces the anxiety associated with a fear of gaining weight. Principles of negative reinforcement may also be operative in helping the individual avoid stressful situations that involve expectations of high performance and family conflicts (Garner, Vitousek, & Pike, 1997).

Among the subset of individuals with anorexia nervosa who engage in binge eating , it is believed that the extreme biological deprivation caused by fasting leads to episodes of binge eating. The anxiety associated with the consumption of a large amount of food promotes purgative behaviors such as self-induced vomiting, the abuse of laxatives, or the abuse of diuretics to decrease anxiety. Thus, the use of purgative methods is negatively reinforced because it decreases the anxiety associated with excessive food consumption. Fasting can be viewed as the avoidance of eating, which is also motivated by the fear of weight gain (Garner, Vitousek, & Pike, 1997). Thus, cognitive-behavioral theory conceives that dietary restriction, purgative habits, and binge eating are motivated either directly or indirectly by fear of weight gain.

Cognitive schemata are viewed as knowledge structures that direct attention, perception, and the processing of information. In individuals with eating disorders, schemata are related to the "self" and, it is hypothesized, contain stereotyped, affectively-loaded, and overvalued information concerning weight and shape (Williamson, Muller, Reas, & Thaw, in press). Because of the anxiety associated with possible weight gain, the person with an eating disorder becomes vigilant to stimuli that may be interpreted as weight-related. Due to the salience of such stimuli, the individual's attention may be biased to attend to weight-related stimuli and to block other information from awareness (Fairburn, Cooper, Cooper, McKenna, & Anastasiades, 1991). Such processing occurs beyond the level of conscious awareness; thus, this biased interpretation may be given an air of reality (Williamson et al., in press).

There are also significant positive consequences associated with anorexic behaviors. Behaviors resulting in weight loss are positively reinforced by feelings of achievement and self-control. Individuals with anorexia may derive satisfaction from their ability to deny strong biological urges and may engage in behaviors that emphasize these "abilities" such as preparing rich foods for others while refusing to eat.

**Biological Perspectives.** Recent investigations of biological theories of eating disorders have examined the association between premorbid temperament, patterns of comorbid diagnoses, and persistent personality characteristics following weight restoration. Such investigations have raised the possibility that these traits may contribute to the pathogenesis of the disorder. For example, the rigidity, obsessionality, and behavioral inhibition consistently seen in patients with anorexia nervosa, it has been found, exist retrospectively before eating disorder symptom onset and persist following weight maintenance (Kaye, 1995, 1997). Bulik, Sullivan, Fear, and Joyce (1997) investigated the differential age of onset for anorexia nervosa, bulimia nervosa, and comorbid anxiety disorders and compared incidence rates with women with major depression or no diagnosis. Results indicated that in 90% of anorexic subjects, 94% of bulimic subjects, and 71% of depressed subjects, anxiety disorders preceded the onset of these other disorders. Subjects diagnosed with anorexia were most likely to have received a prior diagnosis of obsessive compulsive disorder or overanxious disorders, and patients diagnosed with bulimia nervosa were most likely to have received a prior diagnosis of social phobia or overanxious disorder (Bulik et al., 1997). The authors concluded that certain anxiety disorders may serve as nonspecific risk factors for the later development of affective and eating disorders.

Serotonergic systems have often been investigated as a cause of anorexia nervosa due to their influence in modulating appetite, mood, and personality variables such as impulsiveness and aggressiveness (Kaye, 1997). Elevated cerebral spinal fluid (CSF) 5-HIAA levels, the major metabolite of brain serotonin, were found in long-term weight-restored anorexic patients (Kaye, Gwirtsman, George, & Ebert, 1991). Such findings are of interest because low levels of CSF 5-HIAA are associated with impulsive, suicidal, and aggressive behavior—behaviors not traditionally associated with restrictor anorexics.

Further support of potential serotonergic influences on symptom development has been provided by the examination of familial symptom prevalence and inheritance patterns (Kaye, 1997). Family and twin studies, and more recently, behavioral genetic studies have found a high incidence of eating disorders among relatives of anorexics (e.g. Allison & Faith, 1997; Strober, Lampert, Morrell, & Burroughs, 1990). Twin studies have documented a possible genetic basis for anorexia nervosa. A population-based examination of 2163 Caucasian female twin pairs reported that the twin of a person with anorexia nervosa was at risk for anorexia nervosa relative to control subjects (Walters & Kendler, 1995). However, due to the low prevalence of anorexia nervosa in the general pop-

ulation, the number of concordant twins in this study was small. In this study, the dizygotic probandwise concordance rates were larger than the monozygotic rates. The authors concluded that the variance of this sample could not be effectively partitioned into genetic and environmental influences (Walters & Kendler, 1995). Previous reviews of concordance for anorexia among twin pairs relied on treatment samples, but this study may reflect a more accurate estimate of genetic influence on the development of anorexia nervosa. Future research using adoptive and half-sibling studies will be necessary to establish the contribution of genetics to this disorder. It is possible that other characteristics (e.g., obsessiveness) may be transmitted that predispose individuals reared in a certain sociocultural environment to develop anorexia (Strober et al., 1990). However, the difficulty of separating environmental and genetic influences complicates the conclusions drawn from such studies (Hayes, 1998).

**Psychodynamic Perspectives.** Psychodynamic perspectives encompass a variety of conceptualizations regarding the etiology of anorexia nervosa. For example, Bruch (1973) described antecedent feelings of ineffectiveness and helplessness and deficits in interoceptive awareness that are etiologically related to the development of anorexia nervosa. Persons with anorexia nervosa, it is hypothesized, use extreme discipline over biological urges to compensate for their perceived lack of identity and concomitant sense of loss of control (Bruch, 1973).

Proponents of self-psychology suggest that undeveloped psychic structures result in feelings of dysphoria, tension, numbness, and emptiness (Goodsitt, 1997). Symptoms are viewed as a way to restore a sense of wholeness and often serve to "drown out" the aversive self-states of devitalization (Goodsitt, 1997). For example, principles of self-psychology espouse that the constant activity of an individual with anorexia is an attempt to escape from painful internal conditions of boredom, emptiness, and aimlessness (Goodsitt, 1997).

In other psychodynamic perspectives, anorexia nervosa is conceptualized as a phobic avoidance disorder in which the feared object is adult weight and body shape and concomitantly, adult sexuality (Crisp, 1997). The anorexic is able to avoid these fears by maintaining body weight at a subpubertal level and thus prevents the onset of the menstrual cycle and sexual maturity. Strong drives to ingest food and grow cause the individual to lose more weight as "insurance" against possible weight gain. Avoidance of eating enables the individual to manage fears of maturation. Over time, the initial motivational drives to achieve an emaciated state may be forgotten while only the drive to lose weight remains.

The initial fears that promoted this deprivation can take many forms, including fears of aging and death, denial of sexuality, or fear of succeeding as an adult (Crisp, 1997). Thus, the individual successfully regresses to a prior state of functioning through physiological and biological deprivation and avoids the challenges of adulthood.

Family-systems theories emphasize that the successful negotiation of developmental stages is essential for healthy adult maturation. Anorexic symptomatology is viewed as a symbolic representation of the individual's failure to negotiate the separation/individuation stage. Anorexic symptoms serve as an attempt to achieve power, autonomy, and independence while at the same time retreating from the developmental challenge of adolescence (Casper, 1982). Family characteristics such as parental overcontrol, discouragement of self-sufficiency, and enmeshment have been described in families of anorexic patients (Johnson & Conners, 1987) and may contribute to this conflict. The development of anorexia, it is thought, provides an individual with a secure self-identity that was not achieved as a result of negotiating development stages.

## Comorbidity

Investigators have examined patterns of comorbidity among persons diagnosed with anorexia nervosa to inform treatment planning and to determine possible etiological mechanisms. Affective disorders, anxiety disorders, and personality disorders have received the greatest amount of attention from researchers.

**Affective Disorders.** The most widely reported comorbid feature of anorexia nervosa is depression; prevalence rates range from 21–91% of individuals who exhibit symptoms of depression during the acute phase of anorexia nervosa (Hudson, Pope, Jonas, & Yergelun-Todd, 1983; Rothenberg, 1990; Wonderlich, 1995). Such high prevalence rates have raised speculation about a common diathesis between the two disorders. However, the physical and behavioral concomitants of the star-

vation process (Keys, Brozek, Henschel, Mickelsen, & Taylor, 1950) often resemble depressive symptoms and may inflate reported prevalence levels. In addition, critical reviews of the research, including patterns of family transmission, response to anti-depressant medication, and time of disorder onset, fail to support a common diathesis for these disorders (Rothenberg, 1990). Rather, Rothenberg (1990) hypothesized that the depression seen in anorexia nervosa may be secondary to a more intrinsic relationship with obsessive-compulsive symptoms.

**Anxiety Disorders.** Given the obsessive concern with body size and shape among anorexics, much research has been devoted to investigating obsessive symptoms in this population. In a review of the comorbidity literature, Rothenberg (1990) reported that between 11 and 83% of patients displayed obsessive symptoms during the acute phase of anorexia nervosa or after weight restoration. In addition, Rothenberg (1990) concluded that if strict diagnostic criteria for depression were used, then obsessive-compulsive disorders are more prevalent among anorexic patients in the majority of studies. Lifetime prevalence rates of any anxiety disorder in anorectic individuals has ranged from 20–65%, and the most prevalent anxiety diagnoses found among anorexic patients are obsessive-compulsive disorder and social phobia (Herzog, Keller, Sacks, Yeh, & Lavori, 1992; Wonderlich & Mitchell, 1997).

**Personality Disorders.** The personality characteristics of anorexia nervosa have generated a great deal of interest among researchers and clinicians (Vitousek & Manke, 1994). However, delineation of the personality features of anorexic patients is seriously confounded by the effects of the starvation process on personality features and the lack of reliability in diagnosing personality disorders (Keys et al., 1950; Vitousek & Manke, 1994). Given these limitations, research has suggested that restrictor anorexics are most likely to exhibit personality diagnoses from the anxious-fearful cluster and bulimic anorexics are most likely to exhibit personality diagnoses from the dramatic-erratic cluster (Dennis & Sansone, 1997; Herzog et al., 1992; Wonderlich, 1995).

## Long-Term Course of Anorexia Nervosa

Strober, Freeman, and Morrell (1997) assessed the long-term course of recovery and relapse in eighty-five female and ten male anorexic patients annually for a period of 10–15 years following the index admission. Results indicated that approximately 30% of patients experienced a relapse in anorexic symptoms before recovery and nearly 76% of the sample met criteria for full recovery. However, the length of time to recovery was protracted and ranged from 57 to 79 months (Strober, Freeman, & Morrell, 1997). Steinhausen (1995) reviewed the treatment outcome literature for anorexia nervosa from the 1950s to the 1980s, but methodological shortcomings precluded definitive conclusions regarding treatment outcome. Despite these reservations, means across studies indicate that approximately 40% of anorexic patients recover, one-third improve, and 20% exhibit a chronic course (Steinhausen, 1995).

## Bulimia Nervosa

### Diagnosis and Clinical Description

Bulimia nervosa is an eating disorder characterized by episodes of binge eating followed by the use of inappropriate compensatory behaviors to prevent weight gain. The most common methods for controlling weight are self-induced vomiting, laxative and diuretic abuse, excessive exercise, and restrictive eating. These behaviors, it is thought, are motivated by an intense fear of weight gain and body-image disturbances, similar to those described for anorexia nervosa. Unlike persons diagnosed with anorexia nervosa, persons diagnosed with bulimia nervosa are usually within the normal weight range, as a result of binge eating and less restrictive eating.

The diagnostic criteria for bulimia nervosa have changed considerably over the years. Russell (1979) first described a variant of anorexia nervosa he called *bulimia nervosa*, and in 1980 the term *bulimia* was included in the DSM-III (APA, 1980). The DSM-III described a syndrome marked by binge eating, followed by negative mood. Purging was not required for the diagnosis; therefore, persons who binge ate, but did not purge, could be diagnosed with bulimia (Williamson, Kelley, Cavell, & Prather, 1987). In the revision of the DSM-III, the DSM-III-R (APA, 1987), the name of the disorder was changed to *bulimia nervosa* and required the presence of purgative behavior and lack of control over eating during binge-eating episodes.

**Table 2. Summary of DSM-IV Diagnostic Criteria for Bulimia Nervosa**

A. Recurrent episodes of binge eating. Binge eating episodes are marked by both:
1) eating an amount of food that is larger than others would eat in a similar time period and under similar circumstances;
2) a sense of lack of control over eating during the episode.

B. Recurrent use of inappropriate compensatory behaviors including fasting, excessive exercise, self-induced vomiting, and the misuse of laxatives, diuretics, or enemas.

C. Binge eating and inappropriate compensative behaviors must occur at least twice a week for 3 months, on average.

D. Body weight and shape must influence self-evaluation.

E. The disturbance does not occur during Anorexia Nervosa.

**Purging Type**: The person has regularly engaged in self-induced vomiting or the misuse of laxatives, diuretics, or enemas in order to prevent weight gain.

**Nonpurging Type**: The person has used fasting or excessive exercise, but not self-induced vomiting or the misuse of laxatives, diuretics, or enemas in order to prevent weight gain.

With the publication of the DSM-IV (APA, 1994), the diagnostic criteria for bulimia nervosa, summarized in Table 2, underwent additional changes. The diagnosis of bulimia nervosa requires recurrent episodes of binge eating that are marked by (1) eating an amount of food that is larger than others would eat in a similar time period under similar circumstances and (2) a sense of loss of control over eating during the episode. Some binge-eating episodes involve consuming measurably large amounts of food (e.g., one gallon of ice cream). However, other binges are subjective and may include a piece of candy or eating small amounts of a "forbidden food." Because of these variations, there is considerable controversy about the most appropriate definition of "binge eating." For example, Schlundt and Johnson (1990) suggested defining binge eating as eating any food or quantity of food that violates one's idea of dieting and creates anxiety about gaining weight. However, Garfinkel (1995) recommends that the most appropriate way to define a binge-eating episode is by comparing the amount of food consumed to what others might eat, taking into consideration the time and social circumstances of the individual's last meal.

The second criterion required for diagnosing bulimia nervosa is recurrent use of inappropriate compensatory behaviors to prevent weight gain such as self-induced vomiting, excessive exercise, or misusing laxatives, diuretics, enemas, and other medications (APA, 1994). The DSM-IV also indicates that both binge eating and inappropriate compensatory behaviors must occur, on average, at least twice per week for three months. This criterion has been often criticized. It may be desirable to set a minimum frequency for binge eating and purging to eliminate those who occasionally engage in bulimic behavior but who do not meet the full syndrome, setting the frequency at two episodes per week, on average, is arbitrary and lacks empirical support (Garfinkel, 1995).

A diagnosis of bulimia nervosa requires that body shape and weight unduly influence the individual's self-evaluation. Concerns about weight and shape appear to be an important factor in developing and maintaining bulimia nervosa (Walsh & Kahn, 1997). Many women who do not have eating disorders also express considerable concern about body size and shape (Hadigan & Walsh, 1991). Therefore, as noted in the discussion of anorexia nervosa, it is important to assess the intensity of concerns about weight and shape before concluding that this criterion has been met.

Finally, the disturbance of bulimia nervosa may not occur exclusively during episodes of anorexia nervosa. This criterion allows the diagnosis of anorexia nervosa to "override," so to speak, the diagnosis of bulimia nervosa. Thus, only one eating disorder may be diagnosed, and priority is given to the diagnosis of anorexia nervosa and the seriousness of the low body weight associated with its diagnosis (Walsh & Garner, 1997).

Following the diagnosis of bulimia nervosa, one of two subtypes, *purging* or *nonpurging*, is required by the DSM-IV. The purging type is diagnosed when the person uses self-induced vomiting or misuses laxatives, diuretics, or enemas to control body weight. The nonpurging type indicates that the person has used fasting, excessive exercise, or other inappropriate compensatory behaviors but has not regularly engaged in self-induced vomiting or misused laxatives, diuretics, or enemas. This system of subtyping has been sup-

ported empirically (Hay, Fairburn, & Doll, 1996) and accommodates findings which demonstrate that persons who have the purging subtype demonstrate greater levels of body-image disturbance and increased levels of anxiety about eating, compared to those who have the nonpurging subtype (Garfinkel, 1995). However, other authors have failed to find differences in measures of eating disturbance and psychopathology between those who purge or do not purge (Hay & Fairburn, 1998).

## Prevalence

The prevalence rate of bulimia nervosa varies widely from study to study, depending on the definition of bulimia nervosa and the method of diagnosis. Findings based solely on questionnaires produce higher prevalence rates compared to studies that have used interviews to diagnose bulimia nervosa. Using strict diagnostic criteria, the point-prevalence rate of bulimia nervosa among young females is about 1.0% (Hoek, 1995). This finding is in keeping with the DSM-IV (APA, 1994) reported prevalence rate of approximately 1–3% among adolescent females. The prevalence rate of bulimia nervosa in males is roughly one-tenth that of females (APA, 1994). However, recent findings suggest that male homosexuality may be a specific risk factor for the development of eating disorders (Heffernan, 1994).

Minority populations reportedly have lower prevalence rates of bulimia nervosa than Caucasian populations; however, the estimates of bulimia nervosa in minority populations are likely to be misleading (Smith, 1995). Studies using strict methodology may provide prevalence-rate estimates in minority samples that are higher than once believed, yet are still below those of Caucasian samples (Smith, 1995). This hypothesis is supported by evidence indicating that Caucasian and ethnic minority participants scored similarly on measures of both eating disorder and general psychopathology (le Grange, Telch, & Agras, 1997). Additional evidence suggests that an ethnic subculture does not protect adolescent females from sociocultural factors that influence body dissatisfaction (French et al., 1996).

## Etiology

**Cognitive-Behavioral Theories.** Cognitive-behavioral theories of bulimia nervosa take into consideration the concept of dietary restraint and anxiety about weight gain. From this perspective, sociocultural pressure for thinness contributes to dissatisfaction with body size among young females (Williamson, Davis, Duchmann, McKenzie, & Watkins, 1990). Young women develop rigid rules about dieting and attempt to restrict caloric intake to avoid the negative connotations of weight gain. If restrictive eating cannot be maintained, dietary restriction may be broken and may lead to binge eating (Polivy & Herman, 1985). Following binge eating, there is an increase in anxiety and feelings of fullness (Rosen & Leitenberg, 1982) that is alleviated following compensatory behavior (Johnson, Jarrell, Chupurdia, & Williamson, 1994). Compensatory behavior subsequently depletes energy stores, increasing the likelihood of future binge-eating episodes (Jarrell, Johnson, & Williamson, 1986). Therefore, dietary restraint is important in initiating binge eating, and fear of weight gain motivates compensatory behavior that reduces anxiety caused by binge eating.

It is clear that dietary restraint is associated with initiating binge eating in bulimia nervosa; however, recent evidence suggests that the role of restraint may be complex. Findings indicate that restraint is a risk factor for bulimia nervosa rather than a necessary precursor (Mussell, Mitchell, Fenna, et al., 1997). From this perspective, predisposing factors such as depression qualitatively alter the experience of restraint or dieting (Lowe, Gleaves, & Murphy-Eberenz, 1998). Therefore, restraint may combine with other factors to contribute to the development of bulimia nervosa (Wilson, 1993). For instance, stressful major life events may combine with restraint to develop bulimia nervosa (Troop & Treasure, 1997). Bulimia nervosa patients, it has been found, experience significantly more stressful life events compared to controls in the year before the onset of their eating disorder (Troop & Treasure, 1997). Evidence also suggests that restraint may combine with excessive exercise or physical activity to contribute to the development of bulimia nervosa (Davis et al., 1997).

Other research has questioned the association of dietary restraint and binge eating. Stice (1998) found that dietary restraint did not predict future bulimic behavior, as the restraint model of bulimia nervosa would predict, but that bulimic behavior predicted future restraint. From this perspective, dietary restraint may be conceptualized as a conse-quence of binge eating. Ongoing research is needed to explicate the role of restraint in the etiology of bulimia nervosa and to examine other potential factors.

Heatherton and Baumeister (1991) proposed an alternative model of binge eating. They hypothesized that binge eating is motivated by an "escape from self-awareness." Heatherton and Baumeister (1991) hypothesized that binge eaters subject themselves to high standards and when these standards are not met, an aversive emotional state ensues. To escape from this aversive state, cognitive narrowing takes place, and greater attention is given to the environment, contributing to disinhibition of eating.

**Biological Theories.** Biological evidence suggests that bulimia nervosa may be related to substance use disorders and that both are mediated by endogenous opioids (Hardy & Waller, 1988). Support for this theory comes from findings that altered endogenous opioid activity is related to food cravings and intake (Mercer & Holder, 1997). Patients with bulimia and anorexia nervosa have significantly higher levels of endogenous opioid alkaloids (codeine and morphine) than noneating disorder controls (Marrazzi, Luby, Kinzie, Munjal, & Specker, 1997). Thus, an "auto-addiction opioid model" has been proposed which hypothesizes that endogenous opioids are released when dieting is initiated and this reinforces a state of starvation (Marrazzi et al., 1997). Additionally, the opiate antagonist, naltrexone, it has been found, significantly reduces binge-eating frequency (Marrazzi, Markham, Kinzie, & Luby, 1995), and naloxone, it has been found, reduces the consumption of sweet and high fat foods in persons who binge eat (Drewnowski, Krahn, Demitrack, Nairn, & Gosnell, 1995).

Other biological theories have examined the role of neurotransmitters, particularly serotonin. Serotonin has been linked to the regulation of hunger and satiety, and decreased serotonin in the central nervous system, it is hypothesized, is a predisposing factor in the development of bulimia nervosa (Pike, 1995). Diminished serotonin activity may contribute to, or even precipitate, binge eating. Thus, binge eating may be viewed as a form of self-medication used to alter the negative consequences of decreased serotonin in the brain.

Behavioral genetics can be defined as the study of the way genetics and the environment determine behavioral characteristics (Hewitt, 1997).

Behavioral genetics relies on twin, family, or adoption designs to determine the genetic and environmental contributions to behaviors and disorders. Behavioral genetics has investigated bulimia nervosa and found that there may be a substantial heritable component to bulimia nervosa (Hewitt, 1997). For example, Kendler et al. (1991) found that DSM-III-R bulimia nervosa is more common in monozygotic than in dizygotic twins and that the development of bulimia nervosa is substantially influenced by genetic factors.

**Psychoanalytic Theories.** Early psychoanalytic theories explained eating disorders as a fear of oral impregnation and a rejection of femininity (Bruch, 1973). Later theories emphasized early mother–child interactions (Lerner, 1983). Lerner (1983) conceptualized a bulimic patient as overreliant on external structure as a consequence of the failure to develop an adequate "self." This failure of ego development leaves the person with a false sense of self. Food becomes a symbol of the failed mother–daughter relationship, and binge eating and purging represent the conflict between a desperate need for the mother and the desire to reject her. Support for psychoanalytic theory is limited; tests of the theory relied on measures of autonomy and found that developing autonomy was not problematic for bulimic patients (Teusch, 1988).

## Comorbidity

**Affective Disorders.** Depressive disorders are consistently associated with bulimia nervosa (Cooper, 1995). Comorbidity studies have found that a majority of cases can be diagnosed with a comorbid affective disorder (Hinz & Williamson, 1987).

**Anxiety Disorders.** Generalized anxiety and obsessional worry frequently coexist with bulimia nervosa. Pope, Hudson, and Yurgelun-Todd (1984) reported that 50% of the bulimic patients in their sample received an anxiety disorder diagnosis. Obsessive-compulsive disorder commonly accompanies bulimia nervosa. For example, 65% of bulimia nervosa patients in Hudson, Pope, Yurgelun-Todd, Jonas, and Frankenberg's (1987) sample could have been diagnosed with obsessive-compulsive disorder at some point in their lives. Obsessive-compulsive disorder, it is hypothesized, is premorbid to the development of the eating disorder (Thornton & Russell, 1997), and Cooper (1995) reports that OCD may be secondary

to depressed mood in bulimia nervosa patients, as depression and obsessionality appear to be associated. Additionally, OCD may be a consequence of energy deprivation, or it may be related to the eating disorder itself.

**Personality Disorders.** Estimates of the prevalence rates of comorbid personality disorders associated with bulimia nervosa patients vary widely. Wonderlich (1995) reports that 21–77% of bulimia nervosa patients suffer from comorbid personality disorders, particularly Cluster B personality disorders. Estimates of borderline personality disorder range from 2–47% in bulimia nervosa samples (Wonderlich, 1995). Dennis and Sansone (1997) report that the average prevalence rate is about 34%. Investigators have hypothesized that bulimia nervosa may mimic borderline personality disorder and may contribute to diagnostic confusion and misdiagnosis (Wonderlich, 1995); however, this hypothesis has not been investigated thoroughly. The presence of comorbid personality disorders in bulimia nervosa patients has been known to interfere with eating disorder treatment and to contribute to poor outcome.

**Substance Use Disorders.** Substance use disorders are common among bulimia nervosa patients; approximately 23% suffer from alcohol abuse or dependence (Holderness, Brookes-Gunn, & Warren, 1994). Bulimia nervosa patients with comorbid substance use disorders may demonstrate greater levels of impulsivity compared to those without such secondary psychopathology (Wonderlich & Mitchell, 1997).

# Eating Disorder Not Otherwise Specified

### Diagnosis and Clinical Description

Recently, there has been an increased emphasis in the eating disorder literature on the prevalence and subsequent severity of eating disorder symptoms in the general population. There has been increased attention and recognition that the segment of the population that exhibits eating disorder symptoms at a "subclinical level" constitutes a significant proportion of clinic patients (Beaumont et al., 1994; Shisslak, Crago, & Estes, 1995; Walsh & Garner, 1997; Williamson, Gleaves, & Savin, 1992). These disorders have been called by various names, including atypical eating disorders, subclinical eating disorders, and Eating Disorder-NOS.

## Epidemiology

The DSM-IV (APA, 1994) provided greater specificity in the designation of Eating Disorder-NOS diagnoses (Williamson et al., 1992). According to Walsh and Garner (1997), the Eating Disorder-NOS diagnosis represents the presence of clinically significant eating disorder symptoms that do not meet the DSM-IV diagnostic criteria for anorexia nervosa or bulimia nervosa. For example, subclinical bulimia nervosa is defined by a constellation of symptoms, including binge-eating or purgative behavior that occur at a lower frequency or for a shorter duration than that required for the formal diagnosis of bulimia nervosa (Walsh & Garner, 1997). Of additional significance is that a long-term follow-up study reported that 40% of partial eating disorder syndrome patients met the full criteria for a "typical" eating disorder at follow-up (Herzog, Hopkins, & Burns, 1993).

## Prevalence

Studies of the prevalence rates of partial syndrome eating disorders indicate that they may occur at a prevalence rate equal to or greater than the diagnoses of bulimia nervosa (1–3%) or anorexia nervosa (0.5%) (Fairburn & Beglin, 1990; Kendler et al., 1991; Patton, 1992). For example, Kendler et al. (1991) documented a prevalence rate of 3% for partial syndrome eating disorders in an epidemiological investigation of eating disorder prevalence among 2163 twins from a population-based register. In a community-based investigation of 8116 subjects, the prevalence of bulimia nervosa was 1.1% and the presence of partial syndrome eating disorder was 1.4% for female participants (Garfinkel et al., 1995). Button and Whitehouse (1995) reported a prevalence rate of 5% for partial syndrome eating disorders among a population of London schoolgirls, and Patton, Johnson-Sabine, Wood, Mann, and Wakeling (1990) reported that 10% of the population had a partial syndrome eating disorder. These disorders also constitute a substantial proportion (40–46%) of adult clients who sought treatment for eating disorder symptoms in the United States (Herzog et al., 1993; Williamson et al., 1992). Prevalence rates for adolescent females referred for eating disorder treat-

ment are similar and range from 35–50% (Bunnell, Cooper, Hertz, & Shenker, 1992).

## Comorbidity

Two community studies examined the prevalence rates of comorbid psychiatric diagnoses with subclinical bulimia nervosa (Garfinkel et al., 1995; Kendler et al., 1991). Community-based studies, it is thought, provide more reliable prevalence estimates than clinical samples due to sampling biases of clinical samples (Pedhazer & Schmelkin, 1991; Wonderlich & Mitchell, 1997). These studies found no significant differences between prevalence rates of comorbid diagnoses of persons with bulimia nervosa or subclinical bulimia nervosa (Garfinkel et al., 1995; Kendler et al., 1991). Reported lifetime prevalence rates of comorbid diagnoses that occur with subclinical bulimia nervosa in these studies are as follows: alcohol dependence: 15.5–30.9%, generalized anxiety disorder: 9.1–11.4%, and major depressive disorder: 36.4–51%.

## Etiology

Given the similarity of these disorders to the formal diagnosis of anorexia or bulimia nervosa, the etiologies of the subclinical forms of these disorders are presumed to be the same as those for the full syndromes of anorexia nervosa and bulimia nervosa.

# Binge-Eating Disorder

### Diagnosis and Clinical Description

Research on eating disorders has occasionally described cases of "nonpurging bulimia" or "obese binge eaters" throughout the years, following Stunkard's (1959) initial case description of an obese binge-eater in 1959. However, it was not until the early 1990s that a formal definition was developed to classify individuals who engage in binge eating, but who do not regularly engage in the compensatory behaviors indicative of bulimia nervosa (Marcus, 1993). This syndrome became known as "binge-eating disorder" (BED) and was included in the DSM-IV (APA, 1994) as a diagnostic category in need of further study. The development of a definition for BED stimulated research in the area and contributed to an accumulating database on the subject. Much of the earlier research relied on samples that met the binge-eating disorder criteria proposed by Spitzer et al. (1992, 1993); however, recent studies relied on the DSM-IV definition of BED. This chapter will not differentiate between the two because the two sets of criteria varied only minimally.

Persons diagnosed with binge-eating disorder exhibit chaotic eating patterns and consume more calories at normal meals and during binge-eating episodes, compared to weight matched non-binge-eating persons (Yanovski et al., 1992). Most of these individuals are obese and seek weight loss treatment primarily, not eating disorder treatment (Marcus, 1997). The finding that binge-eating disorder most often occurs in obese individuals helps differentiate it from bulimia nervosa, which occurs mostly in individuals of normal weight (Marcus, 1997). However, the key distinction between bulimia nervosa and BED is the absence of inappropriate compensatory behavior in BED.

The research criteria for binge-eating disorder, summarized in Table 3, require recurrent episodes of binge eating, as defined in the diagnostic crite-

### Table 3. Summary of DSM-IV Research Criteria for Binge-Eating Disorder

A. Recurrent episodes of binge eating. Binge eating episodes are marked by both:
1) eating an amount of food that is larger than others would eat in a similar time period and under similar circumstances;
2) a sense of lack of control over eating during the episode.
B. The binge-eating episodes are associated with at least three of the following:
1) eating faster than normal
2) eating until feeling uncomfortably full
3) eating when not feeling hungry
4) eating alone due to embarrassment of the amount of food one is eating
5) feeling disgusted, depressed, or guilty after overeating
C. The presence of distress concerning binge eating.
D. Binge eating occurs at least 2 days a week for 6 months, on average.
E. The binge eating is not associated with the regular use of inappropriate compensatory behaviors and Anorexia Nervosa or Bulimia Nervosa are not present.

ria for bulimia nervosa. Specifically, the amount of food eaten must be greater than others would eat in a similar circumstance, and a sense of loss of control over eating must be present. The problems discussed earlier in defining a binge-eating episode in bulimia nervosa are also present in BED's criteria. Similarly, it is concluded that the most appropriate way to define a binge-eating episode is by comparing the amount of food consumed to that which others might eat, taking into consideration the time and social circumstances of the individual's last meal (Garfinkel, 1995).

The second criterion for binge-eating disorder requires the presence of three or more of the following characteristics associated with binge-eating episodes: (1) eating more rapidly than normal; (2) eating until feeling uncomfortably full; (3) eating large amounts of food when not feeling hungry; (4) eating alone due to embarrassment over the amount one is eating; or (5) feeling disgusted, depressed, or guilty after overeating.

The diagnostic criteria for bulimia nervosa require that binge eating (and inappropriate compensatory behaviors) occurs, on average, at least twice a week for 3 months. However, the diagnostic criteria for binge-eating disorder require that the binge eating occurs at least 2 days a week for 6 months. Therefore, in binge-eating disorder, the focus is not on the *number of binge-eating episodes*, but rather the *number of days on which binge eating occurred*. This definition is advantageous because obese binge eaters frequently report binge-eating episodes that last throughout the day, making it difficult to determine the "number" of episodes (Marcus, Smith, Santelli, & Kaye, 1992). Nonetheless, the diagnostic validity of the frequency criterion has been questioned by findings that individuals who meet all of the BED criteria except the frequency criterion are indistinguishable in a number of psychological and behavioral variables from individuals diagnosed with binge-eating disorder (Striegel-Moore, Wilson, Wilfley, Elder, & Brownell, 1998).

The diagnosis of binge-eating disorder requires distress concerning binge eating, and the binge eating may not be associated with the regular use of inappropriate compensatory behaviors. This criterion is problematic due to the difficulty in defining "regular use" of inappropriate compensatory behaviors which dictates the differential diagnosis between binge-eating disorder and non-purging bulimia nervosa. Finally, the binge eating may not occur exclusively during the course of anorexia or bulimia nervosa.

Examination of the diagnostic criteria for binge-eating disorder illustrates the importance of refining the criteria. This may entail eliminating, modifying, or adding criteria. For example, Eldredge and Agras (1996) found that overconcern with weight and shape should be investigated as a diagnostic feature of binge-eating disorder and that emotional eating is associated with binge-eating disorder, not obesity *per se*.

## Prevalence

Studies that examined the prevalence of binge-eating disorder have yielded inconsistent findings. Earlier studies reported prevalence rates of 30% in persons who sought weight loss treatment and 2% in community samples (Spitzer, et al., 1992, 1993). These studies relied on self-report instruments; however, other studies relied on interviews to assess binge-eating disorder. For example, Varnado et al. (1997) used the Interview for the Diagnosis of Eating Disorders, Fourth Revision (IDED-IV; Kutlesic, Williamson, Gleaves, Barbin, & Murphey-Eberenz, 1998) to define binge-eating disorder and found prevalence rates of 1.3% in adults who sought weight loss treatment. Studies investigating the efficacy of interviews and questionnaires in defining BED indicate that questionnaires are less reliable than interviews (Greeno, Marcus, & Wing, 1995).

Binge-eating disorder is more common in females than in males (Spitzer, et al., 1992). A recent study that relied on two obese samples found that 77% of those diagnosed with BED were female (Varnado et al., 1997). However, other authors argue that more males are afflicted with BED than have been reported (Fairburn & Walsh, 1995).

Ethnic differences associated with binge-eating disorder are not pronounced (Smith, 1995). In obese samples, Caucasians and African-Americans demonstrated similar prevalence rates of binge-eating disorder (Spitzer et al., 1993).

## Etiology

**Cognitive-Behavioral Theories.** The dietary restraint model of binge eating has been the primary behavioral theory of BED. The dietary restraint model suggests that individuals restrict caloric intake which leads to energy deprivation and increased internal cues to consume food. Thus, the individual is more susceptible to disinhibition of eating and subsequently binge eats (Polivy & Herman, 1985). Although this theory provides a parsimonious explanation of binge eating in binge-eating disorder, recent research indicates otherwise.

First, evidence suggests that persons diagnosed with BED often do not report restrictive eating (Castonguay, Eldredge, & Agras, 1995). Second, binge eating reportedly occurs before dieting or attempts to restrict caloric consumption (Mussell et al., 1995). These findings argue against the dietary restraint model. Instead, disinhibition appears to be important in mediating binge eating in BED (Mussell, Mitchell, de Zwaan, et al., 1996); however, research is needed to clarify its role.

An alternative theory to the restraint model involves depression and negative mood. Depression, it is hypothesized, is a risk factor for the development of binge-eating disorder (Marcus, 1995), and negative mood is an immediate trigger to initiate binge eating (Castonguay, Eldredge, & Agras, 1995). The manner in which negative mood triggers binge eating may be explained by the "trade-off" hypothesis (Kenardy, Arnow, & Agras, 1996). This hypothesis states that in persons diagnosed with BED, the prebinge emotions (e.g., anger) are experienced as more aversive than the postbinge emotions (e.g., guilt). Therefore, binge eating is perpetuated by the "trade-off" of the less aversive postbinge emotions for the more aversive prebinge emotions.

A final alternative theory to the dietary restraint model is Heatherton and Baumeister's (1991) theory involving an "escape from self-awareness" which was discussed earlier in this chapter. Heatherton and Baumeister (1991) hypothesized that binge eaters subject themselves to high standards, and when these standards are not met, an aversive emotional state ensues. Cognitive narrowing takes place to escape from this aversive state, and greater attention is given to the environment, which leads to disinhibition of eating. This was a broad theory of binge eating proposed before the development of the criteria for binge-eating disorder, but it holds promise in enhancing our understanding of the disinhibition process and the relationship of negative emotional states and binge eating.

**Biological Theories.** Undoubtedly, the physiological mechanisms involved in regulating food intake are associated with binge-eating disorder. Evidence suggests that a psychobiological mechanism is involved in binge-eating disorder where a physiological event triggers binge eating (Drewnowski, 1995). Therefore, binge eating is seen as an expression of obesity and is more likely to occur in those individuals susceptible to genetically influenced obesity (Drewnowski, 1995). This model can accommodate the findings that binge eating increases with increasing adiposity (Telch, Agras, & Rossiter, 1988) and that binge-eating disorder is overrepresented in the obese population (Spitzer et al., 1992, 1993).

Binge-eating disorder, it has been hypothesized, shares a common biological determinant with affective disorders. However, evidence indicates that binge eating precedes the first major depressive episode (Mussell et al., 1995) and that binge-eating disorder is not a variant of an affective disorder (Cooper, 1995).

## Comorbidity

Binge-eating disorder is associated with depression, anxiety, substance abuse, personality disorders, and eating- and weight-related disturbances. Psychopathology is associated with binge eating and is not an expression of obesity alone (Telch & Agras, 1994).

**Affective Disorders.** Major depression is one of the most common forms of psychopathology associated with binge-eating disorder. In samples of persons diagnosed with binge-eating disorder, 37–51% of individuals also have major depression compared to 14–26% for non-binge-eating persons (Mussell, Peterson, et al., 1996; Specker, de Zwaan, Raymond, & Mitchell, 1994; Yanovski, Nelson, Dubbert, & Spitzer, 1993).

**Anxiety Disorders.** Evidence suggests that binge-eating disorder is associated with elevated trait anxiety (Antony, Johnson, Carr-Nangle, & Abel, 1994) and with high rates of anxiety disorders (Marcus, 1995).

**Personality Disorders.** Personality disorders are more common in persons diagnosed with BED, compared to non-binge-eating controls or the general population. A study that used questionnaires to assess personality disorders obtained prevalence rates of 56% in persons diagnosed with BED and 23% in non-binge-eating controls (Specker et al., 1994). However, interviews obtained personality disorder prevalence rates of 35% in persons with binge-eating disorder compared to 16% in controls (Yanovski, Nelson, Dubbert, & Spitzer, 1993). The types of personality disorders that are more common in persons diagnosed with binge-eating disorder include histrionic, borderline, and avoidant personality disorders (Specker et al., 1994).

**Eating- and Weight-Related Psychopathology.** Binge-eating disorder is associated with significant eating- and weight-related psychopathology. Persons with binge-eating disorder score significantly higher than non-binge-eating persons on measures of disinhibited eating, drive for thinness (de Zwaan et al., 1994), and body dissatisfaction (Mussell, Peterson et al., 1996), and they have difficulty interpreting hunger and satiety signals (Kuehnel & Wadden, 1994). Additionally, these individuals exhibit greater concern for weight and shape and are more likely to eat in response to negative emotions, compared to non-binge-eating persons (Eldredge & Agras, 1996). Weight cycling may be associated with binge eating (Yanovski & Sebring, 1994), although others have failed to find that association (Kuehnel & Wadden, 1994).

**Substance Abuse.** Substance abuse or dependence is significantly more common in persons with BED, compared to non-binge-eating persons (Eldredge & Agras, 1996; Mussell, Mitchell, et al., 1996). Researchers have found that 31% of persons diagnosed with BED have histories of alcohol abuse, compared to 9% of non-binge-eating controls (Eldredge & Agras, 1996).

## Dimensional Models of Eating Disorders

The existence of these subclinical eating disorders, the ambiguity with which some eating disorder diagnostic criteria are defined, and the prevalence of subclinical eating disorders have led to criticism of the diagnostic nomenclature of eating disorders, namely, whether eating disorders would be better encapsulated by a dimensional as opposed to a categorical approach (Shisslak et al., 1995). Proponents of the latter viewpoint argue that many eating disorder patients are not consistent in their symptomatology but rather alternate between various eating disorder diagnoses, depending on their current weight levels, the presence of binge eating, and the presence of purgative behavior (Beaumont et al., 1994). Other researchers cite that the lack of a clear distinction between clinical versus subclinical levels of pathology precludes a categorical approach (Kendler et al.,

1991). These researchers endorse defining patients on relevant symptom continua rather than applying a blanket categorical label. Critics of these criteria describe the frequency criteria for binge eating, purging, and the absence of menstrual cycles as arbitrary and the criterion of body-image disturbance as ambiguous. The end result is that a substantial segment of the population that seeks treatment does not "fit" the definitions of anorexia nervosa or bulimia nervosa and, therefore, must be classified as Eating Disorder-NOS.

## Assessment

Psychological assessment of anorexia nervosa, bulimia nervosa, and Eating Disorder-NOS can be very useful when establishing a case formulation and planning treatment. However, assessing the eating disorder patient is often complicated by the ego-syntonic nature of the symptoms (Garner et al., 1997). Because the eating disorder patients value their thinness and may desire to maintain their current body weights and eating habits, establishing rapport is essential to obtain accurate information and to initiate effective treatment processes (Vitousek, Daly, & Heiser, 1991). In contrast, the bulimic patient may not disclose information about current symptomatology due to shame or embarrassment (Vitousek et al., 1991). The assessment process will proceed most effectively if the interviewer empathizes with the patient's current ambivalence about engaging in the treatment process.

Assessment is best conceptualized as an ongoing process of information gathering in which hypotheses of etiology and symptom maintenance are formulated and revised as new information is gathered during the course of treatment. There are several important domains that require thorough investigation. First, a detailed weight history should be obtained that includes the individuals highest and lowest weights, the relationship between interpersonal stressors and weight fluctuations, early childhood weight and incidents of teasing, and the client's ideal weight. Additional areas of assessment include the presence of body-image disturbance, dysfunctional eating behaviors, and comorbid psychopathology. Finally, a thorough assessment involves using multiple methods of data collection, including structured interviews, self-report measures, behavioral observations, and collateral interviews.

## Structured Interviews

Structured interviews offer the benefit of a systematized collection of information that may minimize investigator bias. However, such interviews can interfere with the establishment of rapport due to their structured format. Despite this limitation, the structured interview is a useful tool for collecting assessment data.

The patient and family members are often interviewed separately to help establish the validity of the patient's reports and to begin formulating hypotheses about the relationships among family variables and eating disorder symptom development. A functional analysis of disordered eating behavior is important for effective treatment planning because it can elicit variables that may have contributed to the initiation of disordered eating. Additionally, foods that are avoided because of a belief that they will lead to rapid weight gain (i.e., "forbidden" foods) should be identified for use in exposure therapy to reduce irrational fears associated with such foods.

Several structured interview formats for diagnosing eating disorders have been developed. The Eating Disorder Examination, 12th ed. is the most extensively researched of the structured interviews (Fairburn & Cooper, 1993). The EDE has four subscales that assess different dimensions of pathology associated with disordered eating (restraint, eating concern, shape concern, and weight concern) as well as a global measure of overall severity. The EDE provides operationally defined eating disorder diagnoses and is sensitive to the effects of treatment (Fairburn, Jones, Peveler, Hope, & O'Connor, 1993). Acceptable psychometric properties have been reported (Fairburn & Cooper, 1993).

The Interview for Diagnosis of Eating Disorders, 4th ed. (IDED-IV) was designed specifically for the differential diagnosis of anorexia nervosa, bulimia nervosa, and eating disorder, not otherwise specified, based on the DSM-IV criteria (Kutlesic, Williamson, Gleaves, Barbin, & Murphy-Eberenz, 1998). Satisfactory reliability and validity have been reported (Kutlesic et al., 1998).

## Self-Report Inventories

The Eating Attitudes Test (EAT) is a forty-item self-report measure developed to assess anorexic attitudes, beliefs, and behaviors (Garner & Garfinkel, 1979). A factor analysis of the original measure produced a twenty-six-item measure that is widely utilized in research as a screening tool (Garner, 1997). The EAT discriminates eating disorder patients from nonclinical controls and differentiates binge eaters from individuals diagnosed with bulimia nervosa (Williamson, Prather, McKenzie, & Blouin, 1990). However, the EAT does not discriminate patients diagnosed with anorexia nervosa from patients diagnosed with bulimia nervosa (Williamson, 1990). Psychometric properties of the EAT are reportedly satisfactory (Gross, Rosen, Leitenberg, & Willmuth, 1986).

The Eating Disorder Inventory Revised (EDI-2) was developed to assess the cognitive and behavioral characteristics of anorexia and bulimia nervosa (Garner, 1991). The EDI-2 has eleven subscales: (1) drive for thinness, (2) bulimia, (3) body dissatisfaction, (4) ineffectiveness, (5) perfectionism, (6) interpersonal distrust, (7) interoceptive awareness, (8) maturity fears, (9) asceticism, (10) impulse regulation, and (11) social insecurity. Internal consistency for each of the eleven subscales except asceticism was above .65, and the criterion validity for each subscale is satisfactory. Extensive norms have been established for this measure.

The Bulimia Test-Revised (BULIT-R; Thelen, Farmer, Wonderlich, & Smith, 1991) was developed to assess the symptoms of bulimia nervosa according to the DSM-III-R (APA, 1987). Satisfactory psychometric data have been reported, and the BULIT-R, it was found, discriminates subjects with bulimia nervosa, binge-eating disorder, obesity, and nonclinical subjects (Williamson et al., 1990).

The Binge Eating Scale (BES; Gormally, Black, Daston, & Rardin, 1982) and the Questionnaire on Eating and Weight Patterns (QEWP; Spitzer et al., 1992) have been used to assess BED. However, research has found that the BES and QEWP agree poorly in classifying binge eaters (Gladis, Wadden, Foster, Vogt, & Wingate, 1998). Both scales overestimate the presence of BED, compared to the results of structured interviews for diagnosing BED (Varnado et al., 1997).

## Test Meals

Direct observation of eating can be used to assess behavioral avoidance of anxiety-producing foods. This procedure usually consists of informing the patient that purging will be prohibited, measuring the amounts and types of food con-sumed, and obtaining ratings of fear, anxiety, and the urge to engage in self-induced vomiting or other purgative behavior (Williamson, 1990).

## Self-Monitoring

Self-monitoring data can assist behavioral analysis, diagnosis, and evaluation of treatment outcome. This procedure requires that the individual record the amounts and types of food eaten, as well as the behavioral, cognitive, and emotional antecedents and consequences of eating (Schlundt & Johnson, 1990; Williamson et al., 1990). Analysis of these data allows an evaluation of the variations in eating behavior as a function of environmental events. Fairburn and colleagues have used this methodology as an important component of their efficacious and specific treatment protocol for treating bulimia nervosa and more recently, for binge eating disorder (Chambliss & Hollon, 1998; Fairburn et al., 1991; Wilfrey et al., 1993). Williamson (1990) developed a self-monitoring procedure that has been validated for eating disorders (Williamson et al., 1990). Using this method, the person records the type and amount of food intake, the mood before and after eating, hunger before and after eating, and the environmental circumstances before and during eating. For bulimic and purging anorexics, a section allowing reports of the occurrence of purging and associated moods and hunger is included. Self-monitoring for two weeks before entering therapy is recommended to aid in diagnosis and case formulation (Williamson, Prather, Goreczny, Davis, & McKenzie, 1989) and to provide baseline data.

## Body Composition

A central diagnostic feature of anorexia nervosa is low body weight. Estimates of body fat percentage are useful for determining the extent of emaciation. Methods employed to determine body fat percentage include neuron activation analysis, underwater weighing, electrical resistance techniques, radioactive potassium studies, and sum of skinfolds. Except for skinfold measurements, however, these techniques are costly and impractical for most clinicians. Quetelet's Body Mass Index (BMI) is a valid and economical means of estimating body mass. BMI is obtained by dividing weight in kilograms by the square of height in meters. It has been suggested that a BMI of 17.5 to

18 or lower is generally used as the criterion for low weight level in anorexia nervosa (WHO, 1992). This measure is highly correlated with body density, total body water, and total potassium estimates of body fat (Webster, Hesp, & Garrow, 1984). Skinfold measurement is another economical and convenient method for determining body fat. Body fat estimates derived from BMI and skinfold measurement may be compared using the norms compiled by Durnin and Womersley (1974).

## Body Image

One of the core features of anorexia nervosa and bulimia nervosa is a disturbance of body image. Researchers have often conceptualized that body image consists of two components: perceptual components, which focus on size perception accuracy of body image; and subjective indexes, which assess the attitudinal or cognitive aspect of body-image disturbance (Thompson, 1990).

Numerous questionnaires have been developed to assess attitudes toward the degree of satisfaction with body size. These measures include the EDI-2 subscale that assesses body dissatisfaction (Garner, 1991); the Body Shape Questionnaire (Cooper, Taylor, Cooper, & Fairburn, 1987), which assesses the frequency of thoughts or feelings that express body dissatisfaction; and the Body-Self Relations Questionnaire (Butters & Cash, 1987), which measures attitudes toward appearance, physical fitness, and health.

Perceptual methods for assessing body-image distortion require the person to estimate body size, and the degree of error made in this estimation is determined. A body-distortion index can be computed by dividing the estimated size by actual size, yielding a ratio of over- or underestimation of body size. Numerous methods for estimating body size have been developed during the past 20 years, including (1) manipulation of light beams (Thompson, 1990; Thompson & Spana, 1988); (2) image marking procedures (Bowden, Touyz, Rodriguez, Henley, & Beaumont, 1989); and (3) distorting mirrors, photographs, lenses, or video (Touyz, Beaumont, Collins, McCabe, & Jupp, 1984).

A simple procedure to assess body-image disturbances has been developed by Williamson, Davis, Goreczny, Bennett, and Gleaves (1989). This procedure requires that the individual compare perception of body size to ideal body size. Female figures that vary from extremely thin to obese are represented on nine cards, from which the subject is instructed to choose the card closest to actual body size and then ideal body size. Body size distortion, body size dissatisfaction, and preference for thinness may be ascertained from this procedure by using normative data. The procedure was found to be reliable and valid in a series of studies (Williamson et al., 1989).

## Treatment Planning for Anorexia Nervosa and Bulimia Nervosa

Due to the serious medical consequences and potential mortality of eating disorder symptoms, the initial stage of treatment planning must determine the appropriate level of care for the patient's current medical status. Potential levels of care include inpatient hospitalization, partial day hospitalization, intensive outpatient treatment, and outpatient treatment. Factors to be taken into account when determining the level of care are given in Table 4.

### Inpatient Treatment

Before initiating an inpatient hospital stay, a treatment contract is usually formulated with the patient to delineate the goals to be achieved during the inpatient stay and the progress that must be achieved before a less intense level of care can be considered. These goals usually focus on medical stabilization, establishing regular patterns of eating, identifying issues that contribute to current disturbances with eating, identifying and beginning to resolve major cognitive distortions regarding body weight and body image, and relapse prevention plans and readmission criteria (Anderson, Bowers, & Evans, 1997).

Alterations in eating habits, improvement in nutritional status, and a decrease of purgative behavior are usually accomplished by using behavioral approaches (Williamson, Duchmann, Barker, & Bruno, 1998). A primary goal of inpatient hospitalization for anorexic patients is to create a positive energy balance through increased caloric intake and decreased energy expenditure (Anderson et al., 1997). A primary goal of inpatient hospitalization for bulimia nervosa patients is establishing regular eating patterns and eliminating purgative behavior. Behavior is altered by meal planning,

**Table 4. Criteria to Determine Level of Care**

Inpatient
1. Extreme emaciation (e.g., body weight is 15% or more below normal).
2. Severe medical complications (e.g., end stage renal disease, diabetes mellitus, extreme dehydration or malnutrition).
3. Repeated failure of less intense levels of treatment.
4. Psychiatric crises (e.g., suicidal attempt or intent).
5. Extreme exacerbation in frequency of purgative behavior.

Partial day hospital
1. Moderate level of emaciation (e.g., body weight is 5% to 15% below normal).
2. Rapid weight loss (e.g., patient is losing 2 lbs. per week over the past 4 weeks).
3. Repeated failure of outpatient treatment.

Intensive outpatient treatment
1. Moderate level of emaciation (e.g., body weight is 5% to 15% below normal).
2. Failure to fully comply with meal plan on an outpatient basis.
3. Repeated failure of outpatient treatment alone.

Outpatient
1. Normal body weight status.
2. Good family/social support system.

behavioral contracting, and education regarding myths about nutrition that patients may have endorsed. Meal planning is initially conducted by a registered dietician who is the "expert" on questions of nutrition and prescribes a plan of eating in the format of a medication regimen emphasizing that for the eating disorder patient, food is medicine.

Reinforcement of behavior change is accomplished by increasing patient privileges and by increasing staff social reinforcement (Williamson et al., 1998; Touyz & Beaumont, 1997). Because one of the primary motivating constructs of anorexic behavior is a fear of weight gain, food is viewed as a feared object. Thus, according to the principles of exposure with response prevention, each meal consumed in the hospital involves exposing the patient to a feared stimulus (food) and preventing the patient from engaging in behaviors that may have previously reduced anxiety (i.e., exercise, purgative behavior). Through the process of extinction, anxiety is reduced during the hospital stay. Repeated exposure to feared situations in which the feared negative consequences do not ensue is intended to help to modify dysfunctional beliefs about eating and weight gain.

## Partial Day Hospitalization

Once the individual is medically stabilized, the patient may be transitioned to a reduced level of care, referred to as partial day hospitalization. This treatment program usually requires the patient to attend hospital treatment groups during the day, to be supervised for the majority of meals, and to spend evenings at home. In this manner, the patient is gradually reintroduced to the stressors of the family and social environment while still receiving an intensive level of care and medical supervision.

## Intensive Outpatient Therapy

Intensive outpatient requires the individual to attend a prescribed number of treatment groups per week, along with a limited number of meals. This level of care is a further transition to outpatient treatment because the patient usually has contact with the eating disorder treatment program for several afternoons during the week. Targets for this level of treatment include maintaining a healthy weight level and increasing patient responsibility for meal planning outside of the hospital.

## Outpatient Therapy

Given the limitations imposed on the length of inpatient hospital stays due to current health care policies, the preponderance of treatment for eating disorders occurs on an outpatient basis. Outpatient therapy focuses on the issues identified during the inpatient hospital stay; helps the patient to identify and modify dysfunctional thoughts, schemas, and thinking patterns associated with body image and interpersonal difficulties; and continues to address dysfunctional eating behaviors. Cognitive restructuring is often an important component of outpatient treatment as patients are taught to reevaluate their previous overvaluation of body size and shape as a determination of self-worth. Relapse prevention planning is often a component of outpatient treatment; patients are often provided with behavioral expectations that must be maintained to avoid readmission to the hospital.

## Components of Treatment

**Body-Image Therapy.** As weight gain occurs, body size distortion and dissatisfaction are likely to worsen. Cognitive behavioral techniques, such as challenging pertinent irrational beliefs and body-image desensitization, can be incorporated into treatment to address these body-image disturbances (Rosen, 1997). Once these beliefs are identified and monitored, patients are taught to challenge irrational thoughts and to generate more rational thinking. Recently published self-help manuals for treating body-image disturbance can be useful adjuncts to an intensive body-image program (Cash, 1997).

**Family Therapy.** Family therapy has been increasingly recognized as an important component in the effective treatment of anorexia nervosa and is strongly recommended for young anorexic patients. Evidence of the effectiveness of family therapy for treating bulimia nervosa has been less conclusive. However, recent successful interventions have demonstrated the potential utility of this mode of therapy for bulimia nervosa (Russell, Szmukler, Dare, & Eisler, 1987). Family therapy encompasses a variety of theoretical orientations that may focus on the nature of alliances between family members, the function of the eating disorder within the family system, and the communication styles of the family members (Dare & Eisler, 1997). Often the eating disorder has come to serve specific functions within the interacting family system that need to be identified and replaced with more adaptive behaviors, if treatment is to be effective. Family therapy often begins with education about eating disorders and gradually progresses to investigating the family's communication styles and skill deficits through the examples of family interactions that occur during the therapeutic session (Williamson et al., 1998). Recently, Robin and colleagues empirically validated their behavioral family systems treatment protocol for treating adolescent anorexic patients (Robin, Bedway, Siegel, & Gilroy, 1996). In addition, Dare, Eisler, Russell, and Smucker (1990) reported robust findings that adolescents with symptoms of short duration respond well to family therapy.

**Treatment of Secondary Psychopathology.** As noted in earlier sections, a substantial propor-

tion of patients with eating disorders may have been diagnosed with comorbid psychiatric disorders. The presence of comorbid diagnoses often complicates the treatment of an eating disorder, and the potential interference of secondary psychopathology on treatment adherence must be considered in treatment planning. For example, it may be more difficult to treat the food rituals often seen among anorexic patients when a patient has also been diagnosed with obsessive-compulsive disorder. Effective treatment planning must take into account how these individual diagnostic variables can affect such factors as the therapeutic alliance, the client's motivation for treatment, and the treatment outcome.

**Pharmacological Treatment.** Advances in using pharmacological agents for treating mental disorders has stimulated research into using such agents for treating eating disorders. The use of antidepressant medications, it has been shown, is efficacious in treating bulimia nervosa (Agras, 1997). In a review of the treatment of bulimia nervosa with antidepressants, the overall effectiveness of these pharmacological agents in reducing the frequency of binge eating and purging was 70% (Agras, 1997). Agras (1997) reported that approximately one-third of patients have full-recovery. However, several factors have been found that affect treatment effectiveness. For example, treatment of short duration with antidepressants, that is, 12–16 weeks, leads to relapse when the medication is withdrawn (Agras et al., 1992). Agras (1997) recommends a treatment trial of antidepressant medication of at least 6 months. In addition, in a study in which sequential antidepressant medication was given, medication was as effective as cognitive-behavior therapy plus placebo (Agras, 1997). Thus, more sophisticated drug regimens may have increased effectiveness. Other classes of drugs such as anxiolytics, opiate antagonists, and mood stabilizers had limited effectiveness in treating bulimia nervosa (Garfinkel & Walsh, 1997).

Despite significant advances in the pharmacological treatment of bulimia nervosa, the core psychopathology of anorexia nervosa remains relatively refractory to pharmacological treatment (Garfinkel & Walsh, 1997). Several types of psychotropic medications have been used to treat anorexia nervosa without significant success. These included antipsychotic medications (Dally & Sargant, 1966), antidepressants (Kaye, Weltzin, Hsu,

& Bulik, 1991), anxiolytics (Garfinkel et al., 1997), appetite-enhancing agents (Vaccarino, Kennedy, Ralevski, & Black, 1994), and prokinetic agents (Szmukler, Young, Miller, Lichtenstein, & Binns, 1995). Further, the significant side effects often associated with using these medications in a patient population with substantial medical complications further precludes their use.

A recent investigation examined the effectiveness of administering fluoxetine, a selective serotonergic re-uptake inhibitor, to the standard outpatient treatment protocol for a group of anorexic patients that had previously received intensive inpatient treatment (Strober, Freeman, DeAntonio, Lampert, & Diamond, 1997). Patients were followed for 24 months postinpatient hospitalization. Results indicated that fluoxetine failed to have a significant effect on maintaining target weight during the follow-up period, on risk of sustained weight loss, or on other clinical measures of outcome (Strober et al., 1997). Anxiolytics have been used by some clinicians to reduce the significant anxiety experienced by patients before a meal, when the patient fails to respond to supportive measures (Anderson, 1987). However, it is recommended that the use of minor tranquilizers be time-limited (Garfinkel & Walsh, 1997). Finally, prokinetic agents, medications that promote gastric emptying, have been investigated (Szmukler et al., 1995). Although such agents do not significantly improve the rate of weight gain, prokinetic agents may improve patient compliance for those individuals who experience significant distress from food consumption (Szmukler et al., 1995).

## Treatment Planning for Binge-Eating Disorder

Treatment planning for persons diagnosed with binge-eating disorder is unique because most individuals present for weight loss treatment, not treatment for an eating disorder (Marcus, 1997). Therefore, treatment planning must incorporate problems related to obesity, as well as to comorbid psychopathology. The most popular treatment modality for binge-eating disorder is outpatient cognitive-behavioral therapy (CBT) which was adapted from Fairburn's (1985) treatment for bulimia nervosa (Fairburn, Marcus, & Wilson, 1993). In CBT for binge-eating disorder, overall moderation of food intake and decreasing binge-eating

episodes are targeted as primary treatment goals, and special attention is given to obesity education (Marcus, 1997). The normalization of eating uses the same techniques as CBT for bulimia nervosa, and cognitive restructuring is used to change maladaptive thoughts, beliefs, and values related to eating (Marcus, 1997). Exercise is important in the treatment due to its effects in stress management and increasing energy expenditure, and calorie counting may be used to help define "normal eating" and promote a healthy, balanced diet (Marcus, 1997).

Research has supported the efficacy of CBT for treating binge-eating disorder (Smith, Marcus, & Kaye, 1992). CBT, it has been found, significantly reduces binge-eating frequency and maladaptive attitudes about shape, weight, and eating (Smith, Marcus, & Kaye, 1992). Follow-up studies indicate that CBT maintained significant reductions in binge eating at 1 year follow-up (Wilfrey et al., 1993).

Interpersonal psychotherapy (IPT) asserts that binge eating results from negative affect induced by interpersonal difficulties such as social isolation. Therefore, IPT is not focused on the symptoms of binge eating but on alleviating interpersonal distress and problems. Evidence suggests that IPT is effective in significantly reducing binge eating, and these reductions remain at 1 year follow-up (Wilfrey et al., 1993).

### Pharmacotherapy

Medications that have been effective for bulimia nervosa and for depression have been examined in obese persons who binge. Tricyclic antidepressants reduce binge eating compared to placebo in persons diagnosed with nonpurging bulimia (McCann & Agras, 1990). The selective serotonin re-uptake inhibiting antidepressants fluoxetine and fluvoxamine (SSRI) also reduce binge-eating frequency in persons diagnosed with binge-eating disorder (Greeno & Wing, 1996; Hudson, Carter, & Pope, 1996). Opiate antagonists reduce binge-eating frequency in persons diagnosed with binge-eating disorder (Marrazzi, Markham, Kinzie, & Luby, 1995); however, others have failed to replicate these findings (Alger et al., 1991).

Despite the effectiveness of pharmacological interventions, binge-eating frequency and weight often return to baseline levels when the use of medication stops. The use of behavioral interventions, relapse prevention, longer medication trials, and combinations of pharmacotherapy and psychotherapy are advocated to increase the effectiveness of BED treatment (Agras, 1997).

# Future Research Directions

## Cognitive Bias

When this volume was last published, research into cognitive biases associated with eating disorders was just beginning (Williamson, Barker, & Norris, 1993). During the intervening years, considerable progress has been made. Two recent reviews have summarized these research findings (Williamson, 1996; Williamson, Muller, Reas, & Thaw, in press). Three types of information-processing biases have been reported: (1) selective attentional bias, (2) selective recall (from memory) bias, and (3) selective interpretation bias. For each type of cognitive bias, research has found that information-processing errors are specific to information related to body size/shape and/or eating "fattening" foods. Cognitive biases have also been observed in women of normal weight who are preoccupied with body size/shape (Baker, Williamson, & Sylve, 1995; Jackmann, Williamson, Netemeyer, & Anderson, 1995). These findings suggest that cognitive bias may be a central feature of the eating disorders and may play an important role in maintaining eating disorders (Williamson, Muller, Reas, & Thaw, in press). Williamson (1996) hypothesized that body-image disturbances associated with eating disorders may be conceptualized as a type of cognitive bias. Several longitudinal investigations have identified body concerns and body-image disturbances (Killen, Taylor, et al., 1994, 1996; Thompson, Coovert, Richards, Johnson, & Cattarin, 1995) as an important precursor to the development of a clinical eating disorder syndrome. Given these findings, it would be of considerable interest to assess the relationships among body concerns, cognitive biases related to body and eating, and eating disorder symptoms in developmental studies of girls that span the age ranges before and after puberty, the developmental period of greatest risk for developing eating disorders. Developmental psychopathology studies of cognitive bias could answer questions about the role of body concerns and cognitive bias related to body size/shape as causative versus maintenance

factors for eating disorders. For example, if body concerns consistently precede cognitive biases and the development of eating disorder symptoms, this pattern of findings would argue that the obsession with body size/shape is the earliest indicator of an eating disorder. However, if the presence of cognitive bias for body size/shape is the strongest predictor of eating disorder symptoms, this pattern of findings would argue that information-processing errors may be causative. On the other hand, if cognitive biases covary only with eating disorder symptoms, this pattern of results would argue that cognitive biases are likely to play a maintenance role in eating disorders.

Another approach to answering this question would be to evaluate changes in cognitive bias as a function of treatment. If cognitive biases for body size/shape improve with a reduction of eating disorder symptoms and worsen before relapse, this pattern of findings would suggest a causative role for cognitive bias. Whereas, if cognitive biases covary only with eating disorder symptoms, this pattern of results would argue for a maintenance role for cognitive bias. For persons who respond positively to treatment, it would be of interest to assess the effect of activating weight concerns on the presence of cognitive biases. It is possible that cognitive biases are present only when weight concerns are very active. Research on body image (Baker et al., 1995; McKenzie, Williamson, & Cubic, 1993) has found that body-image disturbances are most pronounced when weight concerns and/or negative affect are elicited. If body-image disturbances are a type of cognitive bias (Williamson, 1996), these findings can be regarded as preliminary evidence to support this hypothesis. This line of research would help clarify whether body concerns and/or cognitive biases for body size/shape are central features of eating disorders. If these body shape concerns are central, then they must be primary targets for treatment and prevention programs for eating disorders or secondary factors that improve with behavioral symptoms, for example, restrictive eating, binge eating, and purging.

## Cost-Effective Treatment

Treatment of eating disorders, and especially treatment of anorexia nervosa, is often lengthy and costly (Williamson, Duchmann, et al., 1998). During the past 5 years, managed care (in the United

States) has provided a strong challenge to traditional inpatient treatment programs for eating disorders, because they are very expensive. Because of the limitations of health care insurance benefits for managed care, there is a need to evaluate treatment options that are less intensive and less expensive than inpatient treatment. It will be important to evaluate the treatment outcome of these programs, so that both cost and effectiveness can be determined. As noted earlier, modern treatment programs for eating disorders (e.g., Williamson, Duchmann, et al., 1998) have introduced multiple levels of care: inpatient; day hospital, intensive outpatient, and outpatient levels. This approach to treatment allows reserving the most expensive treatment, inpatient, for patients who are very ill, and it allows limiting intensive treatment to the most critical stages of treatment. This approach also makes it possible to treat less severely ill patients at a less expensive level of care, day hospital or intensive outpatient therapy. At this time, very few reports have described the relative costs and outcomes of different levels of treatment. Williamson, Bruno, Thaw, and Muller (1998) reported that cases of severe eating disorder that were treated in a partial hospital program had outcomes equivalent to those of patients initially treated in an inpatient program. The costs of treatment for patients treated in a partial day hospital program were approximately two-thirds of the costs of inpatient treatment. This type of clinical research is needed if health professionals are to discover effective but less costly approaches to treatment.

## Prevention of Eating Disorders

Given the cost and difficulty of effectively treating eating disorders in tertiary care settings, there has been considerable interest in developing prevention programs for eating disorders. Most prevention programs have targeted preadolescent or adolescent girls in school-based prevention programs (e.g., Killen, Hayward et al., 1994; Shisslak et al., 1990). These programs can be conceptualized as primary prevention. When these programs have been evaluated for efficacy, they have generally reported some changes in knowledge about eating disorders, nutrition, and/or dieting, but very limited changes in attitudes about body or eating or in actual behaviors, such as dieting, binge eating, or the use of extreme weight control

behaviors. There has been some discussion of targeting persons who are "at risk" of developing eating disorders (Taylor & Altman, 1997), but very few studies have actually evaluated the impact of the prevention program on "at-risk" cases (Varnado, Zucker, Williamson, Reas, & Thaw, 1998). There is also very little research on the merits of early intervention for eating disorders that can be viewed as secondary prevention for eating disorders. Research on early intervention for anorexia nervosa has yielded mixed results (Schoemaker, 1997), and only a few studies provide evidence that early treatment is more effective, compared to treatment after the eating disorder has become chronic. A recent study on long-term outcome for bulimia nervosa (Reas, Williamson, Martin & Zucker, in press) found that outpatient treatment during the first few years of the onset of bulimia resulted in an 80% recovery rate. Further research on secondary prevention and prevention interventions for "at-risk" children and adolescents is needed.

## Risk Factors for Eating Disorders

As noted in the previous sections, there has been much discussion of identifying persons who are "at risk" for eating disorders and there has been considerable interest in identifying *risk factors* for eating disorders. Risk factors have traditionally been viewed as psychosocial or biological variables that are highly correlated with eating disorder symptoms. In recent years, the concept of risk has been the source of considerable debate, and much of the research which was initially described as risk factor studies is now viewed as having identified *correlates* of eating disorder symptoms (Kraemer, Kazdin, Offord, Kessler, Jensen, & Kupfer, 1997). As we discuss following, these correlational studies offer very little insight into risk factors for eating disorders.

To understand this modern literature, it is necessary to define the terms "risk" and "risk factors." In general, the term "risk" refers to the probability of an outcome, for example, development of eating disorder symptoms, within a sample of subjects. The term "risk factor" indicates a measurable characterization of each subject that precedes the outcome of interest and can be used to divide the population into two groups: the high-risk and low-risk population that comprise the whole population (Mrazek & Haggerty, 1994). The term characteristic may refer to a feature of the individual as well as to its context. To demonstrate that a characterization is a risk factor, first, it must be measured in a sample of subjects who are free of the outcome of interest. Second, those who do have the outcome, for example, development of eating disorder symptoms, must be distinguished from those who do not subsequently have the outcome of interest. A statistically significant association between the risk factor and the outcome must be established, which can be used to define a risk factor's *potency*. Kraemer, Kazdin et al. (1997) conceptualize potency as the maximal discrepancy achievable by using a risk factor to dichotomize the population into high- and low-risk groups (e.g., odds ratio).

In view of these considerations, there are two primary problems with most of the earlier risk factor studies. The first problem is that most studies of risk factors for eating disorders have used cross-sectional research designs that simply compared one or more characteristics of an eating disorder group to those of a control group. Other studies simply reported the correlation between a purported risk factor and some measure of eating disorder symptoms. In all of these cross-sectional studies, the precedence of the risk factor to the onset of eating disorder symptoms was not established. Thus, these studies cannot determine whether the purported risk factor is an antecedent or consequence of the eating disorder. For a variable to be a risk factor, it must precede the onset of eating disorder symptoms. The second problem with most of this literature is that few studies indicated the potency of the risk factor. The implication of these considerations is that only longitudinal studies can be viewed as true risk factor research. Unfortunately, there have been only a few longitudinal studies of eating disorders, and they have yielded quite varied results. Of the variables that have been studied in these longitudinal studies, concerns about body weight and shape have been most significantly predictive of the onset of eating disorder symptoms several years later. For example, several studies of girls in the seventh through tenth grades have reported that concern with body size was the strongest predictor of eating disorder symptoms 2 to 4 years later (Attie & Brooks-Gunn, 1989; Killen, Taylor, et al., 1994, 1996; Thompson, Coovert, et al., 1995). Other studies reported that self-esteem (Button, Sonuga-Barke, Davies, & Thompson, 1996) and body mass index

and early pubertal development (Keel, Fulkerson, & Leon, 1997) were significant predictors of eating disorder symptoms in young girls followed for several years.

A few recommendations can be made for future studies on risk factors. In many studies, the best predictor of disordered eating at Time 2 was disordered eating at Time 1 (Leon, Keel, Klump, & Fulkerson, 1997) . In these studies, a subset of subjects already experienced some eating-related problems at the first period of assessment. The implication of this observation is that it is important for risk factor studies of eating disorders to begin the studies with children at ages before puberty, the most common period for developing concerns about body size (Lask & Bryant-Waugh, 1997). Self-report questionnaires such as the EAT are frequently used to measure problematic eating behavior. It is most convenient to use questionnaires for this purpose, but most researchers believe that structured interviews such as the EDE (Fairburn & Cooper, 1993) or the IDED-IV (Kutlesic et al., 1998) are the most valid method for assessing symptoms of an eating disorder. The field of risk factor research could benefit from greater use of structured interviews. We also found a general absence of reports of potency in most risk factor studies, though two recent reports (Killen, Taylor, et al., 1994, 1996) reported on the potency of weight concerns as a risk factor for eating disorders.

## Summary

Research into the psychopathology of eating disorders has expanded rapidly during the past 10 years. Most authorities on this topic agree that overconcern with body size, fear of fatness, drive for thinness, and disturbances of body image are central cognitive and emotional features of anorexia and bulimia nervosa. The behavioral features of anorexia and bulimia nervosa, for example, restrictive eating, binge eating, and purging, are generally viewed as being motivated by these cognitive and emotional factors. Binge-eating disorder is a new and controversial syndrome. The authors of the DSM-IV (APA, 1994) concluded that more research is needed before BED is sanctioned as a new form of eating disorder. There are important questions about the psychopathology of BED: What are the essential characteristics of this disorder? What is the prevalence of BED? How does it differ from simple obesity and bulimia nervosa, nonpurging type? Treatment methods for anorexia and bulimia nervosa are advancing, and efforts to improve effectiveness and control the costs of treatment are being made. Treatment for BED is still in its infancy. Prevention programs for eating disorders have been developed, but true tests of the effectiveness of these programs for preventing the onset of an eating disorder have not been conducted. It is now clear that primary and secondary prevention of eating disorders is the direction that is needed for this field of research, and we anticipate that research in this area will become increasingly more sophisticated in the next 10 years.

# References

Agras, W. S. (1987). *Eating disorders: Management of obesity, bulimia, and anorexia nervosa.* New York: Pergamon Press.

Agras, W. S. (1997). Pharmacotherapy of bulimia nervosa and binge eating disorder: Longer-term outcomes. *Psychopharmacology Bulletin, 33*(3), 433–436.

Agras, W. S., Rossiter, E. M., Arnow, B., Schneider, J. A., Telch, C. F., Raeburn, S. D., Bruce, B., Perl, M., & Koran, L. M. (1992). Pharmacologic and cognitive-behavioral treatment for bulimia nervosa: A controlled comparison. *American Journal of Psychiatry, 149*, 82–87.

Alger, S. A., Schwalberg, M. D., Bigaouette, J. M., Michalek, A. V., & Howard, L. J. (1991). Effect of a tricyclic antidepressant and opiate antagonist on binge-eating behavior in normoweight bulimic and obese, binge eating-subjects. *American Journal of Clinical Nutrition, 53*, 865–871.

Allison, D. B., & Faith, M. S. (1997). Issues in mapping genes for eating disorders. *Psychopharmacology Bulletin, 33*, 359–368.

American Psychiatric Association. (1980). *Diagnostic and statistical manual of mental disorders* (3rd ed.). Washington, DC: Author.

American Psychiatric Association. (1987). *Diagnostic and statistical manual of mental disorders* (3rd ed., rev.). Washington, DC: Author.

American Psychiatric Association. (1994). *Diagnostic and statistical manual of mental disorders* (4th ed.). Washington, DC: Author.

Anderson, A. E. (1987). Uses and potential misuses of antianxiety agents in the treatment of anorexia nervosa and bulimia nervosa. In P. E. Garfinkel & D. M. Garner (Eds.), *The role of drug treatments for eating disorders* (pp. 59–72). New York: Brunner/Mazel.

Anderson, A. E., Bowers, W., & Evans, K. (1997). Inpatient treatment of anorexia nervosa. In D. M. Garner & P. E. Garfinkel (Eds.), *Handbook of treatment for eating disorders*, 2nd ed. (pp. 327–353). New York: Guilford.

Antony, M. M., Johnson, W. G., Carr-Nangle, R. E., Abel, J. L. (1994). Psychopathology correlates of binge eating and

binge eating disorder. *Comprehensive Psychiatry, 35*(5), 386–392.

Atkinson, R. L., & Stern, J. S. (1997). Weight cycling: Definitions, mechanisms, and problems with interpretation. In G. A. Bray, C. Bouchard, & W. P. T. James (Eds.), *Handbook of obesity* (pp. 791–804). New York: Marcel Dekker.

Attie, I., & Brooks-Gunn, J. (1989). Development of eating problems in adolescent girls: A longitudinal study. *Developmental Psychology, 25*, 70–79.

Baker, J. D., Williamson, D. A., & Sylve, C. (1995). Body image disturbance, memory bias, and body dysphoria: Effects of negative mood induction. *Behavior Therapy, 26*, 747–759.

Beaumont, J. V., Garner, D. M., & Touyz, S. W. (1994). Diagnoses of eating or dieting disorders: What may we learn from past mistakes? *International Journal of Eating Disorders, 16*, 349–362.

Blundell, J. E., & Hill, A. J. (1993). Binge eating: Psychobiological mechanisms. In C. G. Fairburn & G. T. Wilson (Eds.), *Binge eating: Nature, assessment, and treatment* (pp. 206–226). New York: Guilford.

Blundell, J. E. (1995). The psychobiological approach to appetite and weight control. In K. D. Brownell & C. G. Fairburn (Eds.), *Eating disorders and obesity: A comprehensive handbook* (pp. 13–20). New York: Guilford.

Bouchard, C. (1995). Genetic influences on body weight and shape. In K. D. Brownell & C. G. Fairburn (Eds.), *Eating disorders and obesity: A comprehensive handbook* (pp. 21–26). New York: Guilford.

Bowden, P. K., Touyz, S. W., Rodriguez, P. J., Hensley, R., & Beaumont, P. J. V. (1989). Distorting patient or distorting instrument? Body shape disturbance in patients with anorexia nervosa and bulimia. *British Journal of Psychiatry, 155*, 196–201.

Brownell, K. D. (1991). Dieting and the search for the perfect body: Where physiology and culture collide. *Behavior Therapy, 22*, 1–12.

Bruch, H. (1973). *Eating disorders: Obesity, anorexia nervosa, and the person within.* New York: Harper Collins.

Brumberg, J. J. (1989). *Fasting girls.* New York: Penguin Group.

Bulik, C. M., Sullivan, P. F., Fear, J. L., & Joyce, P. R. (1997). Eating disorders and antecedent anxiety disorders: A controlled study. *Acta Psychiatrica Scandinavica, 96*, 101–107.

Bunnell, D. W., Cooper, P. J., Hertz, S., & Shenker, I. R. (1992). Body shape concerns among adolescents. *International Journal of Eating Disorders, 11*, 79–83.

Bunnell, D. W., Shenker, I. R., Nussbaum, M. P., Jacobson, M. S., & Cooper, P. J. (1990). Subclinical versus formal eating disorders: Differentiating psychological features. *International Journal of Eating Disorders, 9*, 357–362.

Butters, J. W., & Cash, T. F. (1987). Cognitive behavioral treatment of women's body-image dissatisfaction. *Journal of Consulting and Clinical Psychology, 55*, 889–897.

Button, E. J., Sonuga-Barke, E. J. S., Davies, J., & Thompson, M. (1996). A prospective study of self-esteem in the prediction of eating problems in adolescent schoolgirls: Questionnaire findings. *British Journal of Clinical Psychology, 35*, 193–203.

Button, E. J., & Whitehouse, A. (1995). A prospective study of self-esteem in the prediction of eating problems in adolescent schoolgirls: Questionnaire findings. *British Journal of Clinical Psychology, 35*, 193–203.

Cash, T. F. (1997). *The body image workbook: An 8-step program for learning to like your looks*. Oakland, CA: New Harbinger.

Casper, R. C. (1982). Treatment principles in anorexia nervosa. *Adolescent Psychiatry, 10,* 86–100.

Castonguay, L. G., Eldredge, K. L., & Agras, W. S. (1995). Binge eating disorder: Current state and future directions. *Clinical Psychology Review, 15*(8), 865–890.

Chambless, D. L., & Hollon, S. D. (1998). Defining empirically supported therapies. *Journal of Consulting and Clinical Psychology, 66,* 7–18.

Cooper, P. J. (1995). Eating disorders and their relationship to mood and anxiety disorders. In K. D. Brownell & C. G. Fairburn (Eds.), *Eating disorder and obesity: A comprehensive handbook* (pp. 159–164). New York: Guilford.

Cooper, P. J., Taylor, J. J., Cooper, Z., & Fairburn, C. G. (1987). The development and validation of the Body Shape Questionnaire. *International Journal of Eating Disorders, 6,* 485–494.

Crisp, A. H. (1970). Anorexia nervosa: "Feeding disorder," "nervous malnutrition," or "weight phobia?" *World Review of Nutrition and Diet, 12,* 452–504.

Crisp, A. H. (1997). Anorexia nervosa as flight from growth: Assessment and treatment based on the model. In D. M. Garner & P. E. Garfinkel (Eds.), *Handbook of treatment for eating disorders,* 2nd ed. (pp. 248–277). New York: Guilford.

Dally, P., & Sargant, W. (1966). Treatment and outcome of anorexia nervosa. *British Medical Journal, ii,* 793–795.

Dare, C., & Eisler, I. (1997). Family therapy for anorexia nervosa. In D. M. Garner & P. E. Garfinkel (Eds.), *Handbook of treatment for eating disorders,* 2nd ed. (pp. 307–326). New York: Guilford.

Dare, C., Eisler, I., Russell, G. S. F., & Smuckler, G. I. (1990). Family therapy for anorexia nervosa: Implications from the results of a controlled trial of family and individual therapy. *Journal of Marital and Family Therapy, 16,* 39–57.

Davis, C., Katzman, D. K., Kaptein, S., Kirsh, C., Brewer, H., Kalmbach, K., Olmsted, M. P., Woodside, D. B., & Kaplan, A. S. (1997). The prevalence of high-level exercise in the eating disorders: Etiological implications. *Comprehensive Psychiatry, 38*(6), 321–326.

de Zwaan, M., Mitchell, J. E., Seim, H. C., Specker, S. M., Pyle, R. L., Raymond, N. C., & Crosby, R. B. (1994). Eating related and general psychopathology in obese females with binge eating disorder. *International Journal of Eating Disorders, 15,* 43–52.

Dennis, A. B., & Sansone, R. A. (1997). Treatment of patients' personality disorders. In D. M. Garner & P. E. Garfinkel (Eds.), *Handbook of treatment for eating disorders,* 2nd ed. (pp. 437–449). New York: Guilford.

Doerr, P., Fichter, M., Pirke, K. M., & Lund, R. (1980). Relationship between weight gain and hypothalamic-pituitary-adrenal function in patients with anorexia nervosa. *Journal of Steroid Biochemistry, 13,* 529–537.

Drewnowski, A. (1995). Metabolic determinants of binge eating. *Addictive Behaviors, 20*(6), 733–745.

Drewnowski, A., Krahn, D. D., Demitrack, M. A., Nairn, K., & Gosnell, B. A. (1995). Naloxone, an opiate blocker, reduces the consumption of sweet high-fat foods in obese and lean female binge eaters. *American Journal of Clinical Nutrition, 61,* 1206–1212.

Durnin, J. V. G. A., & Womersley, J. (1974). Body fat assessed from total body density and its estimation from skinfold thickness: Measurement on 481 men and women aged from 16 to 72 years. *British Journal of Psychiatry, 32,* 32–37.

Eldredge, K. L., & Agras, W. S. (1996). Weight and shape overconcern and emotional eating in binge eating disorder. *International Journal of Eating Disorders, 19,* 73–82.

Fairburn, C. G. (1985). Cognitive-behavioral treatment for bulimia. In D. M. Garner & P. E. Garfinkel (Eds.), *Handbook of psychotherapy for anorexia nervosa and bulimia* (pp. 160–192). New York: Guilford.

Fairburn, C. G. (1996). *Overcoming binge eating*. New York: Guilford.

Fairburn, C. G., & Beglin, S. J. (1990). Studies of the epidemiology of bulimia nervosa. *American Journal of Psychiatry, 147,* 401–408.

Fairburn, C. G., & Cooper, Z. (1993). The Eating Disorder Examination, 12th ed. In C. G. Fairburn & G. T. Wilson (Eds.), *Binge eating: Nature, assessment, and treatment* (pp. 317–360). New York: Guilford.

Fairburn, C. G., Cooper, P. J., Cooper, M. J., McKenna, F. P., & Anastasiades, P. (1991). Selective information processing in bulimia nervosa. *International Journal of Eating Disorders, 10,* 415–422.

Fairburn, C. G., Jones, R., Peveler, R. C., Carr, S. J., Solomon, R. A., O'Connor, M. E., Burton, J., & Hope, R. A. (1991). Three psychological treatments for bulimia nervosa. *Archives of General Psychiatry, 48,* 463–469.

Fairburn, C. G., Jones, R., Peveler, R. C., Hope, R. A., & O'Connor, M. E. (1993). Psychotherapy and bulimia nervosa: The longer-term effects of interpersonal therapy, behaviour therapy, and cognitive-behaviour therapy. *Archives of General Psychiatry, 50,* 419–428.

Fairburn, C. G., Marcus, M. D., & Wilson, G. T. (1993). Cognitive-behavioral treatment for binge eating and bulimia nervosa: A comprehensive treatment manual. In C. G. Fairburn & G. T. Wilson (Eds.), *Binge eating: Nature, assessment and treatment* (pp. 361–404). New York: Guilford.

Fairburn, C. G., & Walsh, B. T. (1995). Atypical eating disorders. In K. D. Brownell & C. G. Fairburn (Eds.), *Eating disorder and obesity: A comprehensive handbook* (pp. 135–140). New York: Guilford.

Fallon, P., Katzman, M. A., & Wooley, S. C. (1994). *Feminist perspectives on eating disorders*. New York: Guilford.

French, S. A., Story, M., Remafedi, G., Resnick, M. D., & Blum, R. W. (1996). Sexual orientation and prevalence of body dissatisfaction and eating disordered behaviors: A population-based study of adolescents. *International Journal of Eating Disorders, 19*(2), 119–126.

Garfinkel, P. E. (1995). Classification and diagnosis of eating disorders. In K. D. Brownell & C. G. Fairburn (Eds.), *Eating disorder and obesity: A comprehensive handbook* (pp. 125–134). New York: Guilford.

Garfinkel, P. E., & Walsh, B. T. (1997). Drug therapies. In D. M. Garner & P. E. Garfinkel (Eds.), *Handbook of treatment for eating disorders* 2nd ed., (pp. 372–380). New York: Guilford.

Garfinkel, P. E., Lin, E., Goering, P., Spegg, C., Goldbloom, D. S., Kennedy, S., Kaplan, A. S., & Woodside, D. B. (1995). Bulimia nervosa in a Canadian community sample: Prevalence and comparison of subgroups. *American Journal of Psychiatry, 152,* 1052–1058.

Garner, D. M. (1991). *Eating Disorders Inventory-2*. Odessa, FL: Psychological Assessment Resources.

Garner, D. M. (1997). Psychoeducational principles in treatment. In D.M. Garner & P.E. Garfinkel (Eds.), *Handbook of treatment for eating disorders*, 2nd ed. (pp. 145-177). New York: Guilford.

Garner, D. M., & Garfinkel, P. E. (1979). The Eating Attitudes Test: An index of the symptoms of anorexia nervosa. *Psychological Medicine*, *9*, 273-279.

Garner, D. M., Garfinkel, P. E., Schwartz, D., & Thompson, M. (1980). Cultural expectations of thinness in women. *Psychological Reports*, *47*, 483-491.

Garner, D. M., Vitousek, K. M., & Pike, K. M. (1997). Cognitive-behavioral therapy for anorexia nervosa. In D. M. Garner & P. E. Garfinkel (Eds.), *Handbook of treatment for eating disorders*, 2nd ed. (pp. 94-144). New York: Guilford.

Garrow, J. S. (1995). Effect of energy imbalance on energy stores and body weight. In K. D. Brownell & C. G. Fairburn (Eds.), *Eating disorders and obesity: A comprehensive handbook* (pp. 38-41). New York: Guilford.

Gladis, M. M., Wadden, T. A., Foster, G. D., Vogt, R. A., & Wingate, B. J. (1998). A comparison of two approaches to the assessment of binge eating in obesity. *International Journal of Eating Disorders*, *23*, 17-26.

Goodsitt, A. (1997). Eating disorders: A self-psychological perspective. In D. M. Garner & P. E. Garfinkel (Eds.), *Handbook of treatment for eating disorders*, 2nd ed. (pp. 94-144). New York: Guilford.

Gormally, J., Black, S., Daston, S., & Rardin, D. (1982). The assessment of binge eating severity among obese persons. *Addictive Behaviors*, *7*, 47-55.

Greeno, C. G., Marcus, M. D., & Wing, R. R. (1995). Diagnosis of binge eating disorder: Discrepancies between a questionnaire and clinical interview. *International Journal of Eating Disorders*, *17*, 563-160.

Greeno, C. G., & Wing, R. R. (1996). A double-blind, placebo-controlled trial of the effect of fluoxetine on dietary intake in overweight women with and without binge-eating disorder. *American Journal of Clinical Nutrition*, *64*, 267-273.

Gross, J., Rosen, J. C., Leitenberg, H., & Willmuth, M. (1986). Validity of Eating Attitudes Test and the Eating Disorders Inventory in bulimia nervosa. *Journal of Consulting and Clinical Psychology*, *54*, 875-876.

Gull, W. W. (1874). Anorexia nervosa. *Transactions of the Clinical Society of London*, *7*, 22-28.

Habermas, T. (1996). In defense of weight phobia as the central organizing motive in anorexia nervosa: Historical and cultural arguments for a culture-sensitive psychological conception. *International Journal of Eating Disorders*, *19*, 317-334.

Hadigan, C. M., & Walsh, B. T. (1991). Body shape concerns in bulimia nervosa. *International Journal of Eating Disorders*, *10*, 323-331.

Halmi, K. A., Eckert, E., LaDu, T. J., & Cohen, J. (1986). Anorexia nervosa: Treatment efficacy of cyproheptadine and amitriptyline. *Archives of General Psychiatry*, *43*, 177-181.

Hardy, B. W., & Waller, D. A. (1988). Bulimia as substance abuse. In W. G. Johnson (Ed.), *Advances in eating disorders*, Vol. 2. New York: JAI.

Hay, P., & Fairburn, C. (1998). The validity of the DSM-IV scheme for classifying bulimic eating disorders. *International Journal of Eating Disorders*, *23*, 7-15.

Hay, P. J., Fairburn, C. G., & Doll, H. A. (1996). The classification of bulimic eating disorders: A community based cluster analysis study. *Psychological Medicine*, *26*, 801-812.

Hayes, S. C. (1998). Resisting biologism. *Behavior Therapist*, *21*, 95-97.

Heatherton, T. F., & Baumeister, R. F. (1991). Binge eating as escape from self-awareness. *Psychological Bulletin*, *110*, 86-108.

Heffernan, K. (1994). Sexual orientation as a factor in risk for binge eating and bulimia nervosa: A review. *International Journal of Eating Disorders*, *16*(4), 335-347.

Heinberg, L. (1996). Theories of body image disturbance: Perceptual, developmental, and sociocultural factors. In J. K. Thompson (Ed.), *Body image, eating disorders, and obesity: An integrative guide for assessment and treatment* (pp. 27-48). Washington, DC: American Psychological Association.

Herzog, D. B., Hopkins, J. D., & Burns, C. D. (1993). A follow-up study of 33 subdiagnostic eating disordered women. *International Journal of Eating Disorders*, *14*, 261-267.

Herzog, T. A., Keller, M., Sacks, N., Yeh, C., & Lavori, P. (1992). Psychiatric comorbidity in treatment seeking anorexics and bulimics. *Journal of the American Academy of Child and Adolescent Psychiatry*, *31*, 810-818.

Hewitt, J. K. (1997). Behavior genetics and eating disorders. *Psychopharmacology Bulletin*, *33*(3), 355-358.

Hinz, L. D., & Williamson, D. A. (1987). Bulimia and depression: A review of the affective variant hypothesis. *Psychological Bulletin*, *102*, 150-158.

Hoek, H. W. (1995). The distribution of eating disorders. In K. D. Brownell & C. G. Fairburn (Eds.), *Eating disorder and obesity: A comprehensive handbook* (pp. 207-211). New York: Guilford.

Holderness, C., Brooks-Gunn, J., & Warren, M. (1994). Comorbidity of eating disorders and substance abuse. Review of the literature. *International Journal of Eating Disorders*, *16*, 1-35.

Hudson, J. I., Carter, W. P., & Pope, H. G. (1996). Antidepressant treatment of binge-eating disorder: Research findings and clinical guidelines. *Journal of Clinical Psychiatry*, *57*(Suppl. 8), 73-79.

Hudson, J. I. Pope, H. G., Jonas, J. M., & Yurgelun-Todd, D. (1983). Phenomenologic relationship of eating disorders to major affective disorder. *Psychiatry Research*, *9*, 345-354.

Hudson, J. I., Pope, H. G., Jr., Yurgelun-Todd, D., Jonas, J. M., & Frankenberg, F. R. (1987). A controlled study of lifetime prevalence of affective and other psychiatric disorders in bulimic outpatients. *American Journal of Psychiatry*, *144*, 1283-1287.

Jackman, L. P., Williamson, D. A., Netemeyer, R. G., & Anderson, D. A. (1995). Do weight preoccupied women misinterpret ambiguous stimuli related to body size? *Cognitive Therapy and Research*, *19*(3), 341-355.

Jarrell, M. P., Johnson, W. G., & Williamson, D. A. (1986). Insulin and glucose responses in the binge/purge episode of bulimic women. Presented at the *Annual Meeting of the Association for Advancement of Behavior Therapy*, Chicago.

Johnson, W. G., Jarrell, M. P., Chupurdia, K. M., & Williamson, D. A. (1994). Repeated binge/purge cycles in bulimia nervosa: The role of glucose and insulin. *International Journal of Eating Disorders*, *15*, 331-341.

Johnson, C. L., & Connors, M. E. (1987). *The etiology and treatment of bulimia nervosa*. New York: Basic Books.

Kapen, S., Sternthal, E., & Braverman, L. (1981). A "pubertal" 24-hour luteinizing (LH) secretory pattern following weight loss in the absence of anorexia nervosa. *Psychosomatic Medicine*, *4*, 177-182.

Katz, J. L., Boyar, R. M., Roffwarg, H., Hellmans, L., & Weiner, H. (1978). Weight and circadian luteinizing hormone secretory pattern in anorexia nervosa. *Psychosomatic Medicine, 40*, 549–567.

Kaye, W. H. (1995). Neurotransmitters in anorexia nervosa. In K. D. Brownell & C. G. Fairburn (Eds.), *Eating disorders and obesity: A comprehensive handbook* (pp. 255–260). New York: Guilford.

Kaye, W. H. (1997). Anorexia nervosa, obsessional behavior, and serotonin. *Psychopharmacology Bulletin, 33*, 335–344.

Kaye, W. H., Gwirtsman, H. E., George, D. T., & Ebert, M. H. (1991). Altered serotonin activity in anorexia nervosa after long-term weight restoration: Does elevated CSF 5-HIAA correlate with rigid and obsessive behavior? *Archives of General Psychiatry, 48*, 556–562.

Kaye, W. H., Weltzin, T. C., Hsu, L. K. G., & Bulik, C. M. (1991). An open trial of fluoxetine in patients with anorexia nervosa. *Journal of Clinical Psychiatry, 52*, 464–471.

Keel, P. K., Fulkerson, J. A., & Leon, G. R. (1997). Disordered eating precursors in pre- and early adolescent girls and boys. *Journal of Youth and Adolescence, 26*, 203–216.

Keesey, R. E. (1995). A set-point model of body weight composition. In K. D. Brownell & C. G. Fairburn (Eds.), *Eating disorders and obesity: A comprehensive handbook* (pp. 46–50). New York: Guilford.

Keesey, R. E., & Corbett, S. W. (1984). Metabolic defense of the body weight set-point. In A. J. Stunkard & E. Stellar (Eds.), *Eating and its disorders*. New York: Raven Press.

Kenardy, J., Arnow, B., & Agras, W. S. (1996). The aversiveness of specific emotional states associated with binge-eating in obese subjects. *Australian and New Zealand Journal of Psychiatry, 30*, 839–844.

Kendler, K. S., MacLean, C., Neale, M., Kessler, R., Heath, A., & Eaves, L. (1991). The genetic epidemiology of bulimia nervosa. *American Journal of Psychiatry, 148*(12), 1627–1636.

Keys, A., Brozek, J., Henschel, A., Mickelsen, O., & Taylor, H. L. (1950). *The biology of human starvation*. Minneapolis: University of Minnesota Press.

Killen, J. D., Hayward, C., Wilson, D. M., Taylor, C. B., Hammer, L. D., Litt, I., Simmonds, B., & Haydel, F. (1994). Factors associated with eating disorder symptoms in a community sample of 6th and 7th grade girls. *International Journal of Eating Disorders, 15*, 357–367.

Killen, J. D., Taylor, C. B., Hayward, C., Haydel, K. F., Wilson, D. M., Hammer, L. D., Kraemer, H., Blair-Greiner, A., & Strachowski, D. (1996). Weight concerns influence the development of eating disorders: A 4-year prospective study. *Journal of Consulting and Clinical Psychology, 64*, 936–940.

Killen, J. D., Taylor, C. B., Hayward, C., Wilson, D. M., Haydel, K. F., Hammer, L. D., Simmonds, B., Robinson, T. N., Litt, I., Varady, A., & Kraemer, H. (1994). Pursuit of thinness and onset of eating disorder symptoms in a community sample of adolescent girls: A three-year prospective analysis. *International Journal of Eating Disorders, 16*, 227–238.

Kraemer, H. C., Kazdin, A. E., Offord, D. R., Kessler, R. C., Jensen, P. S., & Kupfer, D. J. (1997). Coming to terms with the terms of risk. *Archives of General Psychiatry, 54*, 337–343.

Kuehnel, R. H., & Wadden, T. A. (1994). Binge eating disorder, weight cycling, and psychopathology. *International Journal of Eating Disorders, 15*(4), 321–329.

Kutlesic, V., Williamson, D. A., Gleaves, D. H., Barbin, J. M., & Murphy-Eberenz, K. P. (1998). The Interview for the Diagnosis of Eating Disorders IV: Application to DSM-IV diagnostic criteria. *Psychological Assessment, 10*, 41–48.

Laségue, C. (1873). On hysterical anorexia. *Medical Times and Gazette, 2*, 367–369.

Lask, B., & Bryant-Waugh, R. (1997). Prepubertal eating disorders. In D. M. Garner & P. E. Garfinkel (Eds.), *Handbook of treatment of eating disorders*, 2nd ed. (pp. 476–483). New York: Guilford.

le Grange, D., Telch, C. F., & Agras, S. W. (1997). Eating and general psychopathology in a sample of Caucasian and ethnic minority subjects. *International Journal of Eating Disorders, 21*(3), 285–293.

Leon, G. R., Keel, P. K., Klump, K. L., & Fulkerson, J. A. (1997). The future of risk factor research in understanding the etiology of eating disorders. *Psychological Bulletin, 33*(3), 405–411.

Lerner, H. D. (1983). Contemporary psychoanalytic perspectives on gorge-vomiting: A case illustration. *International Journal of Eating Disorders, 3*, 47–63.

Lilenfeld, L. R., Kaye, W. H., Greeno, C. G., Merikangas, K. R., Plotnicov, K., Pollice, C., Rao, R., Strober, M., Bulik, C. M., & Nagy, L. (1997). Psychiatric disorders in women with bulimia nervosa and their first-degree relatives: Effects of comorbid substance dependence. *International Journal of Eating Disorders, 22*(3), 253–264.

Lowe, M. R., Gleaves, D. H., & Murphy-Eberenz, K. (1998). On the relation of dieting and bingeing in bulimia nervosa. *Journal of Abnormal Psychology, 107*(2), 263–271.

Lucas, A. R., Beard, C. M., O'Fallon, W. M., & Kurland, L. T. (1988). Anorexia nervosa in Rochester, Minnesota: A 45-year study. *Mayo Clinic Proceedings, 63*, 433–442.

Marcé, L. V. (1860). On a form of hypochondriacal delirium occurring consecutive to dyspepsia, and characterized by refusal of food. *Journal of Psychological Medicine and Mental Pathology, 13*, 264–266.

Marcus, M. (1993). Binge eating in obesity. In C. G. Fairburn & G. T. Wilson (Eds.), *Binge eating: Nature assessment and treatment*. New York: Guilford.

Marcus, M. D. (1995). Binge eating and obesity. In K. D. Brownell & C. G. Fairburn (Eds.), *Eating disorder and obesity: A comprehensive handbook* (pp. 441–444). New York: Guilford.

Marcus, M. D. (1997). Adapting treatment for patients with binge-eating disorder. In D. M. Garner & P. E. Garfinkel (Eds.), *Handbook of treatment for eating disorders*, 2nd ed. (pp. 484–493). New York: Guilford.

Marcus, M. D., Smith, D. E., Santelli, R., & Kaye, W. (1992). Characterization of eating disordered behavior in obese binge eaters. *International Journal of Eating Disorders, 12*, 249–255.

Marrazzi, M. A., Luby, E. D., Kinzie, J., Munjal, I. D., & Specker, S. (1997). Endogenous codeine and morphine in anorexia and bulimia nervosa. *Life Sciences, 60*(20), 1741–1747.

Marrazzi, M. A., Markham, K. M., Kinzie, J., & Luby, E. D. (1995). Binge eating disorder: Response to naltrexone. *International Journal of Obesity, 19*, 143–145.

Mayer, J. (1973). Fat babies grow into fat people. *Family Health, 5*, 24–38.

McCann, U. D., & Agras, W. S. (1990). Successful treatment of nonpurging bulimia nervosa with desipramine: A double-blind, placebo-controlled study. *American Journal of Psychiatry, 147,* 1509–1513.

McKenzie, S. J., Williamson, D. A., & Cubic, B. A. (1993). Stable and reactive body image disturbances in bulimia nervosa. *Behavior Therapy, 24,* 195–207.

Mercer, M. E., & Holder, M. D. (1997). Food cravings, endogenous opioid peptides, and food intake: A review. *Appetite, 29*(3), 325–352.

Morton, R. (1694). *Phthisiologia, or a treatise of consumptions.* London: Smith & Walford.

Moshang, T., Jr., & Utiger, R. D. (1977). Low triiodothyronine euthyroidism in anorexia nervosa. In R. Vigersky (Ed.), *Anorexia nervosa* (pp. 265–270). New York: Raven Press.

Mrazek, P. J., & Haggerty, R. J. (1994). Reducing risks for mental disorders: Frontiers for prevention intervention research. Washington, DC: National Academy Press. In H. C. Kraemer, A. E. Kazdin, D. R. Offord, R. C. Kessler, P. S. Jensen, & D. J. Kupfer (Eds.). Coming to terms with the terms of risk. *Archives of General Psychiatry, 54,* 337–343.

Mussell, M. P., Mitchell, J. E., de Zwaan, M., Crosby, R. D., Seim, H. C., & Crow, S. J. (1996). Clinical characteristics associated with binge eating in obese females: A descriptive study. *International Journal of Obesity, 20,* 324–331.

Mussell, M. P., Mitchell, J. E., Fenna, C. J., Crosby, R. D., Miller, J. P., & Hoberman, H. M. (1997). A comparison of onset of binge eating versus dieting in the development of bulimia nervosa. *International Journal of Eating Disorders, 21*(4), 353–360.

Mussell, M. P., Mitchell, J. E., Weller, C. L., Raymond, N. C., Crow, S. J., & Crosby, R. D. (1995). Onset of binge eating, dieting, obesity, and mood disorder among subjects seeking treatment for binge eating disorder. *International Journal of Eating Disorders, 17*(4), 395–401.

Mussell, M. D., Peterson, C. B., Weller, C. L., Crosby, R. D., de Zwaan, M., & Mitchell, J. E. (1996). Differences in body image and depression among obese women with and without binge eating disorder. *Obesity Research, 4*(5), 431–439.

Parry-Jones, W. L., & Parry-Jones, B. (1994). Implications and historical evidence for the classification of eating disorders: A dimension overlooked in DSM-III-R and ICD-10. *British Journal of Psychiatry, 65,* 287–292.

Parry-Jones, B., & Parry-Jones, W. L. (1995). History of bulimia and bulimia nervosa. In K. D. Brownell & C. G. Fairburn (Eds.), *Eating disorders and obesity: A comprehensive handbook* (pp. 145–150). New York: Guilford.

Patton, G. C. (1992). Eating disorders: Antecedents, evolution, and course. *Annals of Medicine, 24,* 281–285.

Patton, G. C., Johnson-Sabine, E., Wood, K., Mann, A. H., & Wakeling, A. (1990). Abnormal eating attitudes in London schoolgirls: A prospective epidemiological study, outcome at 12 months. *Psychological Medicine, 20,* 383–394.

Pawluck, D. E., & Gorey, K. M. (1998). Secular trends in the incidence of anorexia nervosa: Integrative review of population-based studies. *International Journal of Eating Disorders, 23,* 347–352.

Pedhazur, E. J., & Schmelkin, L. P. (1991). *Measurement, design, and analysis.* Hillsdale, NJ: Erlbaum.

Pike, K. M. (1995). Physiology of bulimia nervosa. In K. D. Brownell & C. G. Fairburn (Eds.), *Eating disorder and obesity: A comprehensive handbook* (pp. 261–265). New York: Guilford.

Polivy, J., & Herman, C. P. (1985). Dieting and binging: A causal analysis. *American Psychologist, 40,* 193–201.

Pope, H. G., Hudson, J. L., & Yurgelun-Todd, D. (1984). Anorexia nervosa and bulimia among 300 suburban women shoppers. *American Journal of Psychiatry, 141,* 292–294.

Pope, H. G., Katz, D. L., & Hudson, J. I. (1983). Anorexia nervosa and "reverse anorexia" among 108 male body builders. *Comprehensive Psychiatry, 34,* 406–409.

Prather, R. C., & Williamson, D. A. (1988). Psychopathology associated with bulimia, binge eating, and obesity. *International Journal of Eating Disorders, 7,* 177–184.

Reas, D. L., Williamson, D. A., Martin, C. K., & Zucker, N. (in press). Duration of illness predicts outcome for bulimia nervosa: A long term follow-up study. *International Journal of Eating Disorders.*

Robin, A. R., Bedway, M., Siegel, P. T., & Gilroy, M. (1996). Therapy for adolescent anorexia nervosa: Addressing cognitions, feelings, and the family's role. In E. D. Hibbs & P. S. Jensen (Eds.), *Psychosocial treatments for child and adolescent disorders: Empirically based strategies for clinical practice* (pp. 239–262). Washington, DC: American Psychiatric Association.

Rosen, J. C. (1997). Cognitive-behavioral body image therapy. In D. M. Garner & P. E. Garfinkel (Eds.), *Handbook of treatment for eating disorders,* 2nd ed. (pp. 188–204). New York: Guilford.

Rosen, J. C., & Leitenberg, H. (1982). Bulimia nervosa: Treatment with exposure and response prevention. *Behavior Therapy, 13,* 117–124.

Rothblum, E. D. (1994). "I'll die for the revolution but don't ask me not to diet": Feminism and the continuing stigmatization of obesity. In P. Fallon, M. A. Katzman, & S. C. Wooley (Eds.), *Feminist perspectives on eating disorders* (pp. 53–76). New York: Guilford.

Rothenberg, A. (1990). Adolescence and eating disorder: The obsessive-compulsive syndrome. *Psychiatric Clinics of North America, 13,* 469–486.

Russell, G. F. M. (1979). Bulimia nervosa: An ominous variant of anorexia nervosa. *Psychological Medicine, 9,* 429–448.

Russell, G. F. M., Szmukler, G. I., Dare, C., & Eisler, I. (1987). An evaluation of family therapy in anorexia nervosa and bulimia nervosa. *Archives of General Psychiatry, 44,* 1047–1056.

Schlundt, D. G., & Johnson, W. G. (1990). *Eating disorders: Assessment and treatment.* Boston, MA: Allyn & Bacon.

Schoemaker, C. (1997). Does early intervention improve the prognosis in anorexia nervosa? A systematic review of the treatment-outcome literature. *International Journal of Eating Disorders, 21*(1), 1–15

Shisslak, C. M., Crago, M., & Estes, L. S. (1995). The spectrum of eating disorders. *International Journal of Eating Disorders, 18,* 209–219.

Smith, D. E. (1995). Binge eating in ethnic minority groups. *Addictive Behaviors, 20*(6), 695–703.

Smith, D. E., Marcus, M. D., & Kaye, W. (1992). Cognitive-behavioral treatment of obese binge eaters. *International Journal of Eating Disorders, 12*(3), 257–262.

Specker, S., de Zwaan, M., Raymond, N., & Mitchell, J. (1994). Psychopathology in subgroups of obese women with and without binge eating disorder. *Comprehensive Psychiatry, 35*(3), 185–190.

Spitzer, R. L., Devlin, M, Walsh, B. T., Hasin, D., Wing, R., Marcus, M., Stunkard, A., Wadden, T., Yanovski, S., Agras, S., Mitchell, J., & Nonas, C. (1992). Binge eating disorder: A multisite field trial of the diagnostic criteria. *International Journal of Eating Disorders, 11*(3), 191–203.

Spitzer, R. L., Yanovski, S., Wadden, T., Wing, R., Marcus, M. D., Stunkard, A., Devlin, M., Mitchell, J., Hasin, D., & Horne, R. L. (1993). Binge eating disorder: Its further validation in a multisite study. *International Journal of Eating Disorders, 13*(2), 137–153.

Steinhausen, H. C. (1995). The course and outcome of anorexia nervosa. In K. D. Brownell & C. G. Fairburn (Eds.), *Eating disorders and obesity: A comprehensive handbook* (pp. 234–237). New York: Guilford.

Stice, E. (1998). Relations of restraint and negative affect to bulimic pathology: A longitudinal test of three competing models. *International Journal of Eating Disorders, 23*, 243–260.

Striegel-Moore, R. H., Silberstein, L. R., & Rodin, J. (1986). Toward an understanding of risk factors for bulimia. *American Psychologist, 41*, 246–263.

Striegel-Moore, R. H., Silberstein, L. R., Frensch, P., & Rodin, J. (1989). A prospective study of disordered eating among college students. *International Journal of Eating Disorders, 8*, 499–509.

Striegel-Moore, R. H., Wilson, G. T., Wilfley, D. E., Elder, K. A., & Brownell, K. D. (1998). Binge eating in an obese community sample. *International Journal of Eating Disorders, 23*, 27–37.

Strober, M., Freeman, R., DeAntonio, M., Lampert, C., & Diamond, J. (1997). Does adjunctive fluoxetine influence the post-hospital course of restrictor-type anorexia nervosa? A 24-month prospective longitudinal follow-up and comparison with historical controls. *Psychopharmacology Bulletin, 33*, 425–431.

Strober, M., Freeman, R., & Morrell, W. (1997). The long-term course of severe anorexia nervosa in adolescent: Survival analysis of recovery, relapse, and outcome predictors over 10–15 years in a prospective study. *International Journal of Eating Disorders, 22*, 339–360.

Strober, M., Lampert, C., Morrell, W., & Burroughs, J. (1990). A controlled family study of anorexia nervosa: Evidence of familial aggregation and lack of shared transmission with affective disorders. *International Journal of Eating Disorders, 9*, 239–253.

Stunkard, A. J. (1959). Eating patterns and obesity. *Psychiatry Quarterly, 33*, 284–295.

Szmukler, G. I., Young, G. P., Miller, G., Lichtenstein, M., & Binns, D. S. (1995). A controlled trial of cisapride in anorexia nervosa. *International Journal of Eating Disorders, 17*, 345–357.

Taylor, C. B., & Altman, T. (1997). Priorities in prevention research for eating disorders. *Psychopharmacology Bulletin, 33*, 413–417.

Telch, C. F., & Agras, W. S. (1994). Obesity, binge eating and psychopathology: Are they related? *International Journal of Eating Disorders, 15*, 53–61.

Telch, C. F., Agras, W. S., & Rossiter, E. M. (1988). Binge eating increases with increasing adiposity. *International Journal of Eating Disorders, 7*, 115–119.

Teusch, R. (1988). Level of ego development and bulimics' conceptualization of their disorder. *International Journal of Eating Disorders, 7*, 607–615.

Thelen, M. H., Farmer, J., Wonderlich, S., & Smith, M. (1991). A revision of the Bulimia Test: The BULIT-R. *Psychological Assessment: A Journal of Consulting and Clinical Psychology, 3*, 119–124.

Thompson, J. K. (1990). *Body image disturbance: Assessment and treatment*. Elmsford, NY: Pergamon Press.

Thompson, J. K., & Spana, R. E. (1988). The adjustable light beam method for the assessment of size estimation accuracy description, psychometrics, and normative data. *International Journal of Eating Disorders, 7*, 521–526.

Thompson, J. K., Coovert, M. D., Richards, K. J., Johnson, S., & Cattarin, J. (1995). Development of body image, eating disturbance, and general psychological functioning in female adolescents: Covariance structure modeling and longitudinal investigations. *International Journal of Eating Disorders, 18*, 221–236.

Thornton, C., & Russell, J. (1997). Obsessive compulsive comorbidity in the dieting disorders. *International Journal of Eating Disorders, 21*, 83–87.

Touyz, S. W., & Beaumont, P. J. V. (1997). Behavioral treatment to promote weight gain in anorexia nervosa. In D. M. Garner & P. E. Garfinkel (Eds.), *Handbook of treatment for eating disorders*, 2nd ed. (pp. 361–371). New York: Guilford.

Touyz, S. W., Beaumont, P. J. V., Collins, J. K., McCabe, M. P., & Jupp, J. J. (1984). Body shape perception and its disturbance in anorexia nervosa. *British Journal of Psychiatry, 144*, 167–171.

Troop, N. A., & Treasure, J. L. (1997). Psychosocial factors in the onset of eating disorders: Response to life-events and difficulties. *British Journal of Medical Psychology, 70*(4), 373–385.

Turnbull, S., Ward, A., Treasure, J., Jick, H., & Derby, L. (1996). The demand for eating disorder care: An epidemiological study using the General Practice Research Database. *British Journal of Psychiatry, 169*, 705–712.

Vaccarino, F. J., Kennedy, S. H., Ralevski, E., & Black, R. (1994). The effects of growth-hormone releasing-factor on food consumption in anorexia nervosa patients and normals. *Biological Psychiatry, 35*, 445–451.

Varnado, P. J., Williamson, D. A., Bentz, B. G., Ryan, D. H., Rhodes, S. K., O'Neil, P. M., Sebastian, S. B., & Barker, S. E. (1997). Prevalence of binge eating disorder in obese adults seeking weight loss treatment. *Eating and Weight Related Disorders, 2*, 117–124.

Varnado, P. J., Zucker, N., Williamson, D. A., Reas, D. L., & Thaw, J. M. (1998). Development and implementation of the body logic program for adolescents: A primary prevention program for eating disorders. Paper presented at the *8th New York International Conference on Eating Disorders*, New York.

Vitousek, K. B., Daly, J., & Heiser, C. (1991). Reconstructing the internal world of the eating-disordered individual: Overcoming self-denial and distortion in self-report. *International Journal of Eating Disorders, 10*, 647–666.

Vitousek, K., & Manke, F. (1994). Personality variables and disorders in anorexia nervosa and bulimia nervosa. *Journal of Abnormal Psychology, 103*, 137–147.

Wakeling, A. (1985). Neurobiological aspects of feeding disorders. *Journal of Psychiatric Research, 19*, 191–201.

Walsh, B. T., & Garner, D. M. (1997). Diagnostic issues. In D. M. Garner & P. E. Garfinkel (Eds.), *Handbook of treatment for eating disorders* 2nd ed., (pp. 25–33). New York: Guilford.

Walsh, B. T., & Kahn, C. B. (1997). Diagnostic criteria for eating disorders: Current concerns and future directions. *Psychopharmacology Bulletin, 33*(3), 369–372.

Walters, E. E., & Kendler, K. S. (1995). Anorexia nervosa and anorexic-like syndromes in a population-based female twin sample. *American Journal of Psychiatry, 152*, 64–71.

Webster, J. D., Hesp, R., & Garrow, J. S. (1984). The composition of excess weight in obese women estimated by body density, total body water, and total body potassium. *Human Nutrition; Clinical Nutrition, 38,* 299–306.

Wilfrey, D. E., Agras, W. S., Telch, C. F., Rossiter, E. M., Schneider, J. A., Cole, A. G., Sifford, L., & Raeburn, S. D. (1993). Group cognitive-behavioral therapy and group interpersonal psychotherapy for the nonpurging bulimic individual: A controlled comparison. *Journal of Consulting and Clinical Psychology, 61*(2), 296–305.

Williamson, D. A. (1990). *The assessment eating disorders: Obesity, anorexia, and bulimia nervosa.* Elmsford, NY: Pergamon Press.

Williamson, D. A. (1996). Body image disturbances in eating disorders: A form of cognitive bias? *Eating Disorders: Journal of Treatment and Prevention, 5,* 15–27.

Williamson, D. A., Barker, S. E., & Norris, L. E. (1993). Etiology and management of eating disorders. In P. B. Sutker & H. E. Adams (Eds.), *Comprehensive handbook of psychopathology,* 2nd ed. (pp. 505–530). New York: Plenum.

Williamson, D. A., Bruno, R., Thaw, J. M., & Muller, S. L. (1998). Inpatient, day hospital, and outpatient treatment: A continuum of care. Paper presented at the *8th New York International Conference on Eating Disorders,* New York.

Williamson, D. A., Davis, C. J., Duchmann, E. G., McKenzie, S. J., & Watkins, P. C. (1990). *Assessment of eating disorders: Obesity, anorexia and bulimia nervosa.* New York: Pergamon Press.

Williamson, D. A., Davis, C. J., Goreczny, A. J., Bennett, S. M., & Gleaves, D.H. (1989). Development of a simple procedure for assessing body image disturbances. *Behavioral Assessment, 11,* 433–446.

Williamson, D. A., Duchmann, E. G., Barker, S. E., & Bruno, R. M. (1998). Anorexia nervosa. In V. B. Van Hasselt & M. Hersen (Eds.), *Handbook of psychological treatment protocols for children and adolescents* (pp. 413–434). Hillsdale, NJ: Erlbaum.

Williamson, D. A., Gleaves, D. H., & Savin, S. S. (1992). Empirical classification of eating disorder not otherwise specified: Support for DSM-IV changes. *Journal of Psychopathology and Behavioral Assessment, 14,* 201–216.

Williamson, D. A., Kelley, M. L., Cavell, T. A., & Prather, R. C. (1987). Eating and eliminating disorders. In C. L. Frame & J. L. Matson (Eds.), *Handbook of assessment in childhood psychology: Applied issues in differential diagnosis and treatment evaluation* (pp. 461–487). New York: Plenum.

Williamson, D. A., Muller, S. L., Reas, D. L., & Thaw, J. M. (in press). Cognitive bias in eating disorders: Implications for theory and treatment. *Behavior Modification.*

Williamson, D. A., Prather, R. C., Goreczny, A. J., Davis, C. J., & McKenzie, S. J. (1989). A comprehensive model of bulimia nervosa: Empirical evaluation. In W. G. Johnson (Ed.), *Advances in eating disorders* (pp. 137–156). Greenwich, CT: JAI.

Williamson, D. A., Prather, R. C., McKenzie, S. J., & Blouin, D. C. (1990). Behavioral assessment procedures can differentiate bulimia nervosa, compulsive overeater, obese, and normal subjects. *Behavioral Assessment, 12,* 239–252.

Wilmore, J. H., & Costill, D. L. (1994). *Physiology of sport and exercise.* Champaign, IL: Human Kinetics.

Wilson, G. T. (1993). Relation of dieting and voluntary weight loss to psychological functioning and binge eating. *Annals of Internal Medicine, 199*(7 pt 2), 727–730.

Wonderlich, S. A. (1995). Personality and eating disorders. In K. D. Brownell & C. G. Fairburn (Eds.), *Eating disorder and obesity: A comprehensive handbook* (pp. 171–176). New York: Guilford.

Wonderlich, S. A., & Mitchell, J. E. (1997). Eating disorders and comorbidity: Empirical, conceptual, and clinical implications. *Psychopharmacology Bulletin, 33*(3), 381–390.

World Health Organization (WHO). (1992). *The ICD-10 classification of mental and behavioral disorders: Clinical descriptions and diagnostic guidelines.* Geneva: Author.

Yanovski, S. Z., Leet, M., Yanovski, J. A., Flood, M., Gold, P. W., Kissileff, H. R., & Walsh, B. T. (1992). Food selection and intake of obese women with binge-eating disorder. *American Journal of Clinical Nutrition, 56,* 975–980.

Yanovski, S. Z., Nelson, J. E., Dubbert, B. K., & Spitzer, R. L. (1993). Association of binge eating disorder and psychiatric comorbidity in the obese. *American Journal of Psychiatry, 150,* 1472–1479.

Yanovski, S. Z., & Sebring, N. G. (1994). Recorded food intake of obese women with binge eating disorder before and after weight loss. *International Journal of Eating Disorders, 2,* 135–150.

CHAPTER 24

# Sleep Disorders

## Richard R. Bootzin, Rachel Manber, Derek H. Loewy, Tracy F. Kuo, and Peter L. Franzen

## Introduction

During the past 15 years there has been an explosion of research on sleep and sleep disorders. Much has been learned about the causes and treatment of sleep disorders, including insomnia, sleep apnea, and narcolepsy. In addition, alterations in sleep patterns are so commonly associated with some disorders, such as affective disorders, post-traumatic stress disorder, and fibromyalgia, that they are used as diagnostic criteria for those disorders. More generally, we are all affected by the amount and quality of the sleep we obtain. Sleep has broad, systemic effects on mood, performance, and physical functioning. Thus, understanding sleep is essential to complete understanding of normal and abnormal behavior.

The current chapter is a revision of the chapter by Bootzin, Manber, Perlis, Salvio, and Wyatt (1993). References to research that appeared since the last chapter was written have been added; some sections have been substantially rewritten, new sections have been added, and some sections have been deleted. This chapter must, by necessity, be selective. Sources for additional information are the *International Classification of Sleep Disorders, Revised: Diagnostic and Coding Manual* (American Sleep Disorders Association, ASDA, 1997) and *Principles and Practice of Sleep Medicine*, 3rd ed. (Kryger, Roth, & Dement, 2000).

## Basic Sleep Information

Sleep must be understood within the context of the 24-hour day. Now, there is substantial evidence that sleep-wake behavior has an endogenous rhythm, that is, a rhythm that persists in the absence of environmental cues. Core body temperature is used to measure the underlying sleep-wake circadian rhythm. Within the normal range, higher core body temperatures are associated with alertness, and lower temperatures are associated with sleep and sleepiness.

The presence of an endogenous sleep-wake rhythm of 24.2 to 25.1, rather than 24, hours has been observed under free-running conditions in which participants were kept in isolation from cues of the time of day (Czeisler et al., 1999). Under normal circumstances, environmental influences, such as sunlight, meals, and social activity, entrain the endogenous rhythm to a 24-hour cycle. The combination of bright light during wake and total darkness during sleep is a particularly strong entraining influence and can facilitate adjustment to changes in sleep schedules (Czeisler et al., 1989).

The fact that the endogenous sleep circadian rhythm is longer than 24 hours may help explain some findings regarding jet lag. It has been ob-

**Richard R. Bootzin and Peter L. Franzen** • Department of Psychology, University of Arizona, Tucson, Arizona 85712. **Rachel Manber, Derek H. Loewy, and Tracy F. Kuo** •Stanford University, Stanford, California 94305.

*Comprehensive Handbook of Psychopathology* (Third Edition), edited by Patricia B. Sutker and Henry E. Adams. Kluwer Academic / Plenum Publishers, New York, 2001.

served that it takes twice as long to adjust to time changes produced by eastward than westward travel (Moore-Ede, Sulzman, & Fuller, 1982). When traveling east, one is shortening the day, thereby increasing the difference between the endogenous sleep-wake rhythm and the new time zone.

## Electrophysiology of Sleep

It is possible to distinguish sleep from wakefulness based solely on behavioral criteria. Stereotypical postures are associated with sleep periods, reductions in responsiveness to the environment, and reductions in activity. These distinctions between sleep and wake can be seen throughout the phylogenetic scale from insects through mammals (Amlaner & Ball, 1994; Hartse, 1994; Zepelin, 1994). In birds and mammals, there are also detectable changes in brain activity associated with sleep.

Sleep recording in humans, called polysomnography, is scored using information from the electroencephalogram (EEG), eye movements (EOG), and muscle activity from the chin (EMG) following the Rechtshaffen and Kales (1968) scoring manual. When an individual is awake, the EEG is characterized by a low-voltage, fast-frequency signal. This signal is dominated by beta (14–20 Hz) and alpha (8–12 Hz) EEG frequencies. As one becomes drowsy, the EEG pattern slows down to a slightly higher amplitude theta rhythm (3–7.5 Hz). If more than 50% of an EEG epoch of 20 or 30 seconds consists of theta, the individual is considered to be in stage 1 sleep. Stage 1, a transitional stage, may also contain slow, rolling, eye movements. Although the first epoch of stage 1 sleep is often used to define sleep onset operationally, individuals aroused from stage 1 usually report that they were about to fall asleep. A more conservative criterion for sleep onset is the appearance of stage 2 sleep.

Stage 2 sleep occurs when certain phasic events, sleep spindles and K-complexes, appear in the EEG. Sleep spindles, named for their sewing-spindle appearance, are short bursts of 12–14 Hz activity and, it is thought, are due to inhibitory neuronal activity during sleep. K-complexes are slow, high-amplitude voltage bursts that consist of a large negative deflection followed by a large positive deflection and, it is thought, are brain responses to external or internal stimuli. The appearance of high-amplitude, slow delta waves

(0.5–2.5 Hz) marks the presence of stages 3 and 4, also called slow-wave sleep. Stage 3 contains 20 to 50% delta waves in an epoch, and stage 4 has more than 50%. The progression from stage 1 to stage 4 sleep is characterized by decreases in frequency and increases in amplitude of the EEG. Arousal thresholds to external stimuli increase with increases in sleep stage.

Rapid-eye-movement (REM) sleep is an activated stage of sleep that occurs cyclically, about every 90 minutes throughout the night and is associated with dreaming. Reports of cognition obtained from REM sleep are longer, more visual, more story-like, and more bizarre than reports from stages 1 through 4 (NREM sleep) that are similar to reports of waking cognition. REM sleep is also quite different physiologically from NREM sleep. In addition to rapid eye movements, postural muscle atonia, irregular respiration, increased heartrate, disrupted temperature regulation, and penile erections occur during REM sleep.

As seen in Figure 1, most slow-wave sleep occurs during the first half of the night. As night progresses, REM sleep periods are longer. Thus, more REM sleep occurs during the last half, than the first half, of the sleep period.

## Sleep Deprivation

The short-term effects of one or two days of sleep deprivation are increased irritability, deficits in sustained attention, and sleepiness, particularly at night. With longer periods of sleep deprivation, there is an increase in sleepiness, a loss in fine motor control, and the appearance of mild flu-like symptoms. Extended periods of partial sleep deprivation can also lead to decrements in vigilance and objective, as well as subjective, measures of sleepiness (Dinges et al., 1997). Recovery sleep following three or four nights of sleep deprivation consists mostly of slow-wave and REM sleep. Most of the lost slow-wave sleep and about half of the lost REM sleep are made-up during recovery nights (Horne, 1988).

Circadian sleep-wake and temperature cycles persist even during sleep deprivation. Thus, sleep-deprived individuals are more alert during the hours they would normally be awake and more sleepy when they would normally be asleep. Many industrial accidents such as Three-Mile-Island and Chernobyl occurred during the night shift when individuals would be sleepiest.

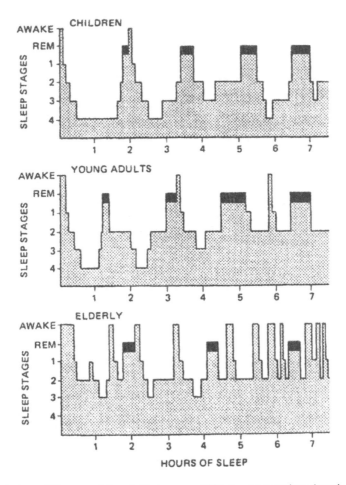

**Figure 1.** A typical night for a child, young adult, and elderly person. REM sleep reoccurs throughout the night; the differences that are most noticeable as individuals age are the decrease in stage 4 sleep and the increase in the frequency of awakenings. Reprinted by permission of the *New England Journal of Medicine* from Kales, A., & Kales, J. D. (1974), "Sleep disorders: Recent findings in the diagnosis and treatment of disturbed sleep," *New England Journal of Medicine, 290,* P. 487.

### Developmental Changes in Sleep

Sleep, its duration, architecture, and diurnal distribution, changes across the human life-span. These developmental changes in sleep parameters are accompanied by corresponding changes in the types and prevalence rates of sleep disorders. Childhood sleep problems are usually transient, but when they persist, they may influence the child's daytime functioning and impact other family members.

A neonate's sleep is comprised of active and quiet phases, similar but not identical to REM and NREM sleep seen in older children and adults. During the first 6 months of life, slow waves become more continuous, sleep spindles and K-complexes emerge, and the four stages that characterize adult NREM sleep become distinguishable (Williams et al., 1974). During the same period, there are changes in the distribution and duration of sleep stages. The percentage of time spent in REM sleep decreases from 50 to 30%, and the latency to REM sleep, which is zero minutes at birth, gradually increases and starts to exhibit circadian rhythmicity (Schulz et al., 1983). The percentage of REM sleep gradually decreases during childhood and reaches the adult level of 20 to 25% at adolescence. The number of sleep cycles decreases from a childhood level of seven cycles to four or five cycles during adolescence (Karacan et al., 1975); this reflects a lengthening of the sleep cycle and a shortening of total sleep duration.

The amount of slow-wave sleep increases in the first 3 years of life, stays constant until the teens, and then gradually declines. Beginning in the teens, the amplitude of slow waves declines with age (Smith et al., 1977). These changes in slow-wave sleep, as individuals age, are associated with lightening in the depth of sleep, as measured by arousal thresholds and the frequency of brief arousals from sleep.

**Infants and Toddlers.** The total duration of sleep declines sharply during the first year of life from about 17 hours at birth to about 13 hours by the end of the first year and continues to decline gradually to about 11 hours at age 2. By the fourth month of life, the circadian sleep-wake cycle becomes more prominent and more synchronized with the light-dark cycle (Harper et al., 1981). The changes in sleep duration are accompanied by changes in the distribution of sleep throughout the day. By 6 months, most infants have one extended period of sleep at night and two naps.

The most common parental concerns about their children's sleep during infancy and toddlerhood are difficulties in settling to sleep and waking up at night. Treatments are commonly based on stimulus control principles. Parents are informed about the importance of a consistent and relaxing bedtime routine and on the importance of teaching their children to fall asleep on their own, so that the parent's presence will not become a distinguishing stimulus for sleep onset. Often, treatment involves extinguishing old habits and establishing a new and consistent bedtime routine. Extinction of parental presence in the room at bedtime can be accomplished abruptly or by successive approximations in which parents gradually decrease the interval of contact time with their children at bedtime (Ferber, 1985). Estimates of the efficacy of this approach are very high (Adair et al, 1992; Durand & Mindell, 1990; Richman et al., 1985; Sadeh, 1994), and its benefits often generalize beyond the sleep problem (Minde, Faucon, & Faulkner, 1994). When an infant's or toddler's sleep difficulties are a manifestation of separation anxiety, an alternative and effective approach is for a parent to sleep in the child's bedroom for about a week and avoid interactions with the child during the night (Sadeh, 1994). Some form of co-sleeping with infants (sharing the same room or sharing the same bed) is customary in the majority of the world's cultures. The impact on the mother's sleep indicates a small reduction in slow-wave sleep and an increase in arousal frequency (Mosko, Richard, & McKenna, 1997) that allows increased monitoring of the infant.

**Preschool and Early Childhood.** Sleep problems common in this age group are those of initiating and maintaining sleep and parasomnias. The results of prospective investigations suggest that childhood complaints about sleep onset and sleep maintenance difficulties are transient (Strauch & Meier, 1988). However, Hauri and Olmstead (1980) found that childhood insomnia persists into adulthood in some cases. They coined the term childhood onset insomnia to describe adult insomniacs whose problems started before age ten.

Sleep onset difficulties during early childhood may be manifested as bedtime struggle stemming from oppositional struggle with parents, fear of going to sleep, or difficulty in settling down. Distress at bedtime may be related to developmental changes that affect the prevalence of fears in children (Ollendick et al., 1985). One treatment approach for cases in which fear and anxiety are central to the child's difficulty in initiating sleep consists of cognitive rehearsal of appropriate bedtime behaviors during the day and positive reinforcement in the morning (Cashman & McCann, 1988). Children's anxiety at bedtime may also benefit from a relaxation routine designed to match their cognitive and attention levels. Relaxation routines designed for use with children typically include imagery such as a melting snowmen as well as tense-release instructions (Oaklander, 1988; Ollendick & Cerny, 1981; Schumann, 1981). Older children may be helped by a comprehensive intervention based on self-management strategies that include relaxation, self-statements, self-assessment, and self-reinforcement (Graziano & Mooney, 1982). Sleep onset problems that, it is judged, stem primarily from oppositional factors are commonly treated by positive reinforcement or by paradoxical intention. When oppositional struggles mark daytime behavior, treatment focuses on the most urgent oppositional problem which often results in improvement at bedtime as well (Cashman & McCann, 1988). Stimulus control instructions (see later) can be tailored to school aged children when poor association between the bed and sleep are apparent.

The prevalence rate of sleep maintenance problems decreases sharply from 30 to 35% at ages four–five to about 15% at age six and continues to decline to 8% at age ten (Klackenberg, 1982). Sleep maintenance problems during the preschool years are often found in conjunction with sleep onset problems and tend to disappear as the latter problems are solved (Mindell, 1990).

Parasomnias, including sleep walking, sleep talking, night terrors, and enuresis, are most prevalent in children aged five–twelve. The presence of parasomnias beyond the teens is commonly associated with psychopathology. Parasomnias are discussed in detail later in the chapter.

**The Second Decade of Life.** Physical and endocrinological maturation associated with puberty may result in an increase in sleep need (Carskadon & Dement, 1987). Nevertheless, there is a decline in total sleep time from 10 to 7 hours per night from pre- to late puberty. The reduction of total sleep time reflects the increasing demands on adolescents' time from school, work, and social interactions.

Epidemiological studies examining sleep-wake problems in adolescence found that the most common complaint is daytime sleepiness (Carskadon & Dement, 1987; Strauch & Meier, 1988). More than half of the adolescents surveyed complained of daytime sleepiness. The prevalence rate of daytime sleepiness, which is very low at preadolescence (Palm et al., 1989), increases with the onset of puberty and peaks at midpuberty.

Another common, though less prevalent, complaint is frequent or severe insomnia reported by about 12 to 14% of adolescents (Price et al., 1978; White et al., 1980). Henschel and Lack (1987) suggested the possibility that adolescent sleep onset difficulties may reflect a mild form of circadian rhythm disturbance. Life-style patterns typical in adolescence are likely to contribute to irregular sleep-wake schedules and to sleep deprivation on school nights. Teenagers who work after school and who have a heavy load of extracurricular activities are particularly sleepy during the day (Carskadon, Mancuso, & Rosekind, 1989). Nevertheless, in addition to psychosocial factors, the tendency to delay sleep in some cases is related to the biological pubertal process itself (Carskadon, Viera, & Acebo, 1993).

Sleep deprivation during adolescence may result in irritability, vulnerability to minor illness, inability to sustain attention, sleepiness, and fewer personal resources for dealing with emotional stresses. In addition, emotional stresses and alcohol and drug abuse are likely to amplify the effects of sleep deprivation.

To help meet the demands of adolescence and reduce sleepiness, teenagers should be encouraged to get more regular and longer durations of sleep (Ferber, 1990). The treatment of severe daytime sleepiness due to intrinsic sleep disorders such as narcolepsy and sleep apnea are discussed later. The treatment of disturbed sleep during adolescence is similar to its treatment during adulthood and is outlined later in this chapter.

**Adults and the Elderly.** From early adulthood to old age, sleep continues to change due to normal aging, psychosocial/life-style factors, and concomitant medical and/or psychiatric conditions (Vitiello, 1997). Although the sleep need of most individuals remains constant throughout adulthood, the ability to maintain uninterrupted sleep, unfortunately, diminishes with age (Ancoli-Isreal, 1997). Increased sleep disturbance at night often leads to increased daytime sleepiness and fatigue. People differ in the amount of sleep changes that are associated with aging; some show little change in their sleep patterns, whereas others experience dramatic deterioration (Webb, 1992).

The nightly amounts of total sleep, stage 4 sleep, and REM sleep level off at puberty, remain stable throughout adulthood, and decrease with advancing age (Smallwood, Vitiello, Giblin, & Prinz, 1983). Gross sleep architecture also remains relatively stable and is comprised of approximately 70–75% of NREM sleep and 20–25% of REM sleep relative to total sleep throughout adulthood (Carskadon & Dement, 1994). There are some differences in monthly sleep patterns between men and women that are likely to relate to hormonal changes associated with the menstrual cycle. As many as 15% of women experience a significant increase in sleep disturbance in the late luteal or premenstrual part of their cycles (Manber & Armitage, 1999).

During the middle-age years, most people first notice a shallowing of sleep along with a growing sense of fatiguing more easily in the daytime. Sleep becomes less continuous beginning in middle age and becomes progressively more fragmented with advancing age and declining health. Of all of the age-related changes in sleep, the reduction of slow wave sleep (SWS) is the most prominent. With the reduction in SWS, there is a corresponding increase in the lighter stages of non-REM sleep, especially stage 1, and increased time is spent awake during the nocturnal sleep period. A pattern of lighter, more fragmented sleep with frequent and prolonged awakenings is common in the elderly (Webb & Campbell, 1980; Bliwise, 2000a). Thus, the elderly get less total sleep at night than their younger counterparts, although they may spend more time in bed (Dement, Miles, & Carskadon, 1982). When sleep across the entire 24-hour day is accounted for (including naps), the elderly get about the same amount of total sleep as middle-aged adults.

The effect of aging differs in men and women. This gender difference emerges between ages thirty and forty. Men and women in their twenties have similar percentages of SWS, a significant reduction in the percentage of SWS occurs in men during their thirties, but not in women (Ehlers & Kupfer, 1997). Objective measures of sleep reveal that the sleep of women tends to be better preserved with aging than that of men. In contrast, the subjective rating of sleep is worse in elderly women than in elderly men; the former report more sleep complaints than the latter (Rediehs, Reis, & Creason, 1990).

There are many biological and psychological consequences of aging that may affect sleep, either directly or indirectly. Biological processes include decreased bladder control, degenerative diseases, dementing disorders, poor health, and sleep disorders such as sleep apnea and periodic leg movements. Psychological processes include bereavement, anxiety about health and financial security, and enforced changes from daily routine (Morgan, 1987). It has been commonly assumed that depression, anxiety, and poor health account for many instances of poor sleep in the elderly, but research on the healthy elderly has found that frequent awakenings and decreased amounts of stage 4 and REM sleep occur, even in the absence of depression, anxiety, or overt disease processes (Feinberg, Koresko, & Heller, 1967; Prinz et al., 1984).

The deterioration of sleep that parallels aging can also result directly from sleep disorders such as sleep apnea (see later section) and periodic limb movement disorder (PLMs; see later section. Sleep apnea and PLMs, which can be primary or secondary to other medical conditions, are increasingly prevalent with age and affect a high percentage of the geriatric population (Carskadon, van den Hoed, & Dement, 1980), and PLMs occur in up to 44% of residents of nursing homes (Ancoli-Israel, Kripke, Mason, & Massin, 1981). The rate of PLMs in the aged population is due in part to the high prevalence of renal disease, arthritis, diabetic neuropathy, iron deficiency anemia, and venous insufficiency in this population; PLMs are often associated with theses disorders (Bliwise, 2000a).

Some researchers believe that age-dependent changes in circadian rhythm also contribute to the gradual deterioration of sleep at night and the increased propensity to nap during the day seen in the elderly (Bliwise, 2000a). The sleep-wake pattern of many elderly, especially those in nursing homes, resembles the polyphasic sleep-wake cycle of infancy and may be secondary to the weak entrainment of the sleep-wake cycle into the circadian rhythm that occurs in these institutions (Dement, Miles, & Carskadon, 1982; Schnelle, Cruise, Alessi, et al. 1998). The most commonly described circadian rhythm disturbance in the elderly is a gradual phase advance of the sleep period relative to the desired sleep time (see section on advanced sleep phase syndrome). This phase-advanced rhythm results in early evening drowsiness and sleep and concurrent early morning awakening and difficulty returning back to sleep (Czeisler et al., 1986; Miles & Dement, 1980; Weitzman et al., 1982). Although the elderly show a clear phase advance in their circadian rhythms, this may not be due to differences between elderly and younger adults in the length of the endogenous daily rhythm. A recent study found no differences in age in the length of the endogenous rhythm, when no light cues were available (Czeisler et al., 1999). Age differences in sleep are more likely to be due to changes in sleep-wake schedules and changes in sleep architecture such as increased frequency of awakenings.

Naps are seldom reported in the 20-year-old working population, but nearly all 60-year-olds report some napping that averages approximately two naps per week (Webb, 1992). Two factors that may lead to daytime napping in the elderly are (1) attempts to compensate for lost sleep and (2) understimulation and weakening of social constraints (Morgan, 1987). In addition, napping may not interfere with nighttime sleep in the elderly to the same extent that it does in young adults (Feinberg et al., 1985; Morin & Gramling, 1989; see section on sleep-wake schedules). Although napping can be adaptive because it can supplement nocturnal sleep, excessive napping can disrupt the circadian entrainment of the sleep-wake cycle and exacerbate nocturnal sleep disturbance.

Changes in sleep patterns in the elderly do not necessarily lead to the subjective experience of insomnia. Some complain about sleep problems, others notice but do not complain, and still others do not notice. Morin and Gramling (1989) compared self-identified poor and good older sleepers on measures of sleep, mood, life-style, health, and expectations of sleep requirements and found that the poor sleepers showed greater discrepancies between their current sleep patterns and expectations and acknowledged more depression and anxiety than the good sleepers.

Many biological and psychological consequences of aging may affect sleep, either directly or indirectly. Practice of good sleep hygiene, such as keeping a regular sleep-wake schedule, avoiding alcohol, tobacco, and caffeine, reducing excessive time awake in bed, and treating underlying sleep disorders will facilitate the preservation of good sleep.

# Assessment of Sleep and Sleepiness

To identify sleep disorders, it is necessary to have reliable and valid measures of sleep and sleepiness. Although substantial information about sleep can be obtained from a detailed history, more direct assessment is usually desirable. There are many methods from which to choose, and each method has advantages and disadvantages.

## Assessment of Sleep Variables

**Polysomnography.** As mentioned earlier, the progression of sleep stages throughout the night, as well as transitions from wakefulness to sleep, are typically assessed by all-night recording of brain wave activities at one or more sites (EEG) and by monitoring eye movements (EOG) and muscle activity from the chin (EMG). Additional physiological measures may be used for special purposes such as evaluating sleep apnea and periodic leg movements. Evaluating sleep apnea requires measuring respiratory effort, air flow, and blood oxygen saturation. Periodic leg movements are measured by recording EMG from the anterior tibialis muscles of the legs.

Several factors indicate the need for more than one night of recording in insomnia. Among these factors are night-to-night variability in sleep parameters and the fact that an unfamiliar sleep environment, such as a sleep laboratory, may result in disrupted sleep. This is often called a "first-night effect." In addition, rare events, such as sleep terrors, may not be observed in a single night of recording.

Polysomnographic recording can be done in the sleep laboratory or at home. The effects of a unfamiliar setting on sleep can be reduced by using home recording (Palm et al., 1989). Recording at home can be by telephone transmission of the recording signals to the laboratory or by recording the signals on tape or computer for later analysis.

**Auditory Event-Related Potentials.** Neurophysiological assessment of sleep and waking states may also be conducted by using auditory event-related potential (ERP) measurements. ERPs are microelectrical EEG events that are elicited by and time-locked to the presentation of a stimulus. The ERP is comprised of a series of positive- and negative-going waves (components) labeled either sequentially or according to their peak amplitude latency (i.e., a positive wave at 300 ms is labeled the "P300"). The waking auditory ERP is comprised of a series of components which, labeled sequentially, are the P1, N1, P2, N2, and P3. The onset of stage 1 sleep is associated with increased amplitudes of the P1, P2, and N2 components, whereas the N1 and P3 amplitudes are diminished (Campbell, Bastien, & Bell, 1992). During sleep stages 2, 3, and 4, the amplitude and latency of the N2 increase dramatically and a large amplitude, non-REM-sleep-specific wave complex emerges, called the "evoked" K-Complex (N550–P900). ERP component structure in REM sleep resembles waking, however, amplitudes are reduced.

Auditory ERPs show reliable variations with states of consciousness and levels of cognitive processing. ERPs have shown enhanced cognitive processing in insomniacs, relative to good sleepers, during evening wakefulness and initial stage 2 sleep (Loewy & Bootzin, 1998). Cognitive impairment in healthy adults, due to prolonged sleep deprivation, is positively related to reductions in P300 amplitude (Morris, So, Lee, Lash, & Becker, 1992).

**Activity Monitoring.** When the focus of the evaluation is the distribution of sleep and wakefulness across the night, including sleep parameters such as sleep latency, time awake after sleep onset, and total sleep time, it is possible to use activity monitoring devices that are typically worn on the wrist. A wrist actigraph is a small, solid-state, computerized movement detector that continuously records wrist movement throughout the night. Several studies support the reliability and validity of the assessment of different sleep parameters based on actigraphs and its validity as an assessment tool of sleep disorders (ASDA, 1995b; Sadeh et al., 1989, 1991). A wrist actigraph provides a relatively unobtrusive, objective, all-night measure of several sleep parameters that allows monitoring the patient's sleep for extended periods of time in the patient's own environment. To evaluate circadian rhythm disturbances, some versions of wrist actigraphs can be equipped with light meters that allow continuously measuring light exposure. When worn continuously, day and night, actigraphs can be used to evaluate rest-activity behaviors, and versions that are equipped with a behavioral response capacity can assess reaction time upon a prompt and assist in evaluating alertness.

**Sleep Questionnaires.** Sleep questionnaires provide valuable information about the perceived severity of a presenting sleep complaint, as well as the perceived efficacy of treatment. In addition, they allow collecting data on a wide variety of behavioral variables. However, the retrospective nature of the questionnaires may introduce intentional or unintentional biases (Bootzin & Engle-Friedman, 1981). Therefore, though sleep questionnaires are of value in providing adjunctive data, they should not be used alone in assessing sleep. The use of multiple measures (e.g., collateral reports, mechanical devices, or PSG) will improve reliability and validity.

**Daily Sleep Diaries.** Daily sleep-wake diaries are a valuable assessment tool that can provide continuous daily information on sleep parameters, as well as on daytime functioning. Unlike polysomnography that usually records only one or two nights of sleep, sleep diaries can provide information about sleep behavior for weeks and even months. Although insomniacs often overestimate sleep onset latency and underestimate total sleep, compared to polysomnography, the correlation between diaries and polysomnography is substantial (e.g., Carskadon et al., 1976). The validity of diaries with other measures increases over time. Individuals become more exact at assessing their sleep as they continue to monitor it (Franklin, 1981).

To be maximally useful, care must be taken to ensure that daily sleep diaries are completed each morning. If diaries are collected infrequently, patients may not fill them out until immediately before they are collected. Under these circumstances, the diaries would be no more useful than retrospective questionnaires (Bootzin & Engle-Friedman, 1981). One way to eliminate this problem is to have patients call in their data each morning to a telephone answering machine (Spielman, Saskin, & Thorpy, 1987). In this way, problems with compliance can be detected immediately, and corrective actions can be taken.

**Observers.** Observers such as nurses, spouses, or parents can be used to assess sleep onset, movement, respiration, and reaction to noise. In addition to general problems common to observational data, some specific problems arise in using observers to assess sleep-related variables. For example, spouses may fall asleep before their to-be-observed partners and may be unaware of their sleep later at night. Sleep reports by parents and children are similarly often in poor agreement (Clarkson et al., 1986). The relatively low validity of observer data suggests using observers primarily as supplemental, rather than primary sources of information.

### Assessment of Daytime Sleepiness

The measurement of sleepiness is complex because it is an inferred construct that has multiple indicators. There are cognitive, physiological, and behavioral indicators of sleepiness that are reflected in self-report, physiological, and performance measures. Further, there are a number of related constructs such as fatigue and lowered arousal that, although they overlap with sleepiness, are not identical. In addition, daytime sleepiness is not solely a function of the length and quality of the previous night's sleep. Sleepiness and alertness are strongly influenced by the sleep-wake circadian rhythm and by factors such as threat, motivation, and interest in the activities being undertaken.

**Stanford Sleepiness Scale (SSS).** The subjective evaluation of an individual's current level of sleepiness is most commonly measured by the SSS, which consists of seven descriptively anchored points (Hoddes et al., 1973). The statements reflect the severity of sleepiness from "Feeling active and vital; alert and wide awake" to "Almost in reverie; sleep onset soon; lost struggle to remain awake." Hoddes et al. (1973) found that the scale was sensitive to sleep loss and validated it with performance measures when mental tasks were long (at least an hour), monotonous, and boring. Polysomnographically measured sleep latency, it has also been shown, correlates highly with the subjective feeling of sleepiness, as measured by the SSS.

**Epworth Sleepiness Scale (ESS).** In a clinical setting, it is often useful to have a measure of the extent to which individuals exhibit excessive sleepiness in different situations. The ESS (Johns, 1991) asks respondents how likely they are to doze off or fall asleep in different situations such as while a passenger in a car for an hour or while sitting or talking to someone. The test-retest reliability during five months is .81, and the correlation between spouses and respondents is .74 (Johns, 1994). Self-report measures, such as the ESS, are useful as quick screens for sleepiness and as a supplement to objective measures.

**Multiple Sleep Latency Test (MSLT).** The MSLT is arguably the most important assessment device for quantifying daytime sleepiness in human subjects. Since its development at Stanford University in the mid 1970s, it has been used to measure sleepiness in a wide range of experiments that examined normal and abnormal functioning (Carskadon, 1994).

The MSLT measures how long it takes to fall asleep on multiple opportunities throughout the day. It is intended to be a standardized set of procedures for obtaining an objective measurement of an individual's "physiological sleepiness" at different times of the day. Physiological sleepiness should be distinguished from "manifest sleepiness," an individual's behavioral or subjective level of arousal. Manifest sleepiness is influenced by other physiological needs, motivation, and demands from the immediate environment.

The MSLT consists of a series of four to seven polysomnographically monitored naps, administered every 2 hours (see Carskadon et al., 1986, for detailed procedures). Subjects should not be given caffeine or alcohol during the day of MSLTs to avoid confounding effects on sleep latency. Similarly, investigators should be aware of any medications being taken by the subject that might influence the latency to sleep onset.

The nap is considered to have begun as soon as the lights are turned off and is terminated after 20 minutes, three consecutive 30-second periods of stage 1 NREM sleep, or one 30-second period of any other sleep stage. The latency to sleep is defined as the amount of time between "lights out" and the first 30-second period of any sleep stage.

Different average MSLT scores indicate different levels of sleepiness, and shorter scores indicate a higher degree of physiological sleepiness. MSLT averages less than 5 minutes are considered "pathological" and indicate a severe degree of sleepiness. Scores in this range are often seen in individuals with narcolepsy, sleep apnea, and those with either acute or chronic sleep deprivation (Carskadon & Dement, 1981; Dement, Carskadon, & Richardson, 1978; Richardson et al., 1978). Pathological levels of sleepiness, it has been found, correlate with performance deficits (Carskadon, Littell, & Dement, 1985). Nocturnal values such as sleep duration on the previous night, respiratory disturbance index, and lowest oxygen desaturation do not correlate well with MSLT measures and account for less than 25% of the variance in MSLT scores (Pollak, 1997). A greater percentage of the variance can be explained (over 40%) if multivariate (rather than bivariate correlations) analyses are used. In a community sample, six variables (chronic daytime tiredness, body-mass index, psychological distress, nocturnal motor activity, serum thyrotropin level, and age) independently and significantly predicted MSLT scores (Kronholm, Hyyppä, Alanen, Halonen, & Partinen, 1995).

Although the MSLT has been helpful in identifying excessive sleepiness due to narcolepsy and sleep apnea, it is not a pure measure of physiological sleepiness in all individuals. There are determinants, in addition to sleepiness, that affect the capacity to fall asleep. Insomniacs tend to take a long time to fall asleep on the MSLT, even following a poor night's sleep. The same variables that produce insomnia at night result in elevated MSLT scores. On the other hand, many individuals who fall asleep quickly at night can fall asleep quickly on the MSLT, even when they are not sleep deprived (Dorsey & Bootzin, 1987). Thus, the MSLT measures both sleepiness and individual differences in sleep tendency.

**Maintenance of Wakefulness Test (MWT).** The MWT, a variant of the MSLT, measures the ability to remain awake, rather than the ability to fall asleep (Mitler, Gujavarty, & Browman, 1982). This test has been used clinically to assess daytime sleepiness and treatment efficacy. The procedure involves sitting in a comfortable chair or sitting up in bed in a darkened room for either a 20- or 40-minute period or until the beginning of sleep onset. The criteria used for sleep onset includes either the first consecutive 10 seconds of sleep or the same criteria as in the MSLT: three consecutive 30-second epochs of NREM stage 1 or a single epoch of any other stage of sleep. The first trial occurs 2 hours following the final morning awakening and is repeated three more times every 2 hours.

A normative study found that healthy sleepers had an average sleep latency of 18.1 minutes for a 20-minute MWT and 32.6 minutes for a 40-minute MWT (Doghramji et al., 1997). Sleep latency values in clinical populations (e.g., narcolepsy and obstructive sleep apnea syndrome) are significantly lower. Using a statistical criterion of two standard deviations below the mean, the lower limit of the normal range is 10.9 and 12.9 minutes for a 20- and 40-minute MWT, respectively, using the first 30-second epoch of stage 1 as the criterion for sleep onset. Using the more stringent criterion, the lower limit of the normal range is 13.5 and 19.4 minutes, respectively. Based on their normative data, Doghramji and colleagues (1997) recommend the 20-minute over the 40-minute protocol because it is not as susceptible to age effects (older people can maintain wakefulness longer than younger people) and is more cost effective.

The MWT is more sensitive than the MSLT to the effects of treatment. Many patients' MSLT scores remain pathological after treatment. In people with disordered sleep (i.e., obstructive sleep apnea, narcolepsy, idiopathic hypersomnia, depression, periodic limb movement, and head trauma), MSLT scores showed a slight, nonsignificant increase after treatment, whereas the MWT scores showed large increases 1–6 months after treatment (Sangal, Thomas, & Mitler, 1992).

**Pupillometry.** The pupil is fully dilated in a darkened room but constricts as the individual begins to fall asleep. This has led to measures of sleepiness based on the degree of constriction and the degree of stability of pupil size. Untreated patients with excessive sleepiness have pupils of smaller diameter than normals, and their pupils show frequent constrictions and dilation, whereas normals show only minor changes in pupil diameter (Lin et al., 1990; Yoss, 1969). Research on the pupillary light reflex, which measures the time taken for a pupil's diameter to dilate to baseline levels after light flashes, indicates that sleep apnea patients show increased latencies to recovery with increased sleepiness, as measured by the MSLT (Pressman & Fry, 1989). Although there have been encouraging results with pupillometry for those who are severely sleepy during the day, such as those with narcolepsy and severe sleep apnea, it has been less consistently useful for use with other sleep disorders.

**Performance Measures.** Performance measures provide objective data in assessing the effect of sleepiness and can be use to evaluate the efficacy of treatment. The most commonly used performance measures are reaction time, attention and vigilance, mental arithmetic, tracking and memory tasks (see Bootzin & Engle-Friedman, 1981). Slow reaction time, lack of response, or errors are indicators of sleepiness. A common finding in sleep deprivation studies is that sleep loss impairs performance in most cognitive and sustained attention tasks. Such impaired performance is most consistently documented when the task is long (30–60 min), repetitive, and boring. In general, when severely sleep deprived subjects are motivated, they can sustain attention for short periods of time and perform no differently than nonsleep deprived subjects. Even on simple tasks of short duration (3–10 min), however, researchers have found performance decrements in sleepy subjects (Dinges, 1992). Lapsing, which refers to a period of marked response delay or response omission, is the foremost effect of sleep loss. Characteristic performance patterns in sleep deprived individuals include a slowing in self-paced cognitive tasks and the speed of the fastest response time, progressive and accelerated performance degradation, increased variability in response time, and erratic or unevenness in performance across trails (Kribb & Dinges, 1994; Dinges, 1992).

# Sleep Disorders

In providing a review of sleep disorders, we will use the diagnostic categories of the recently published, *International Classification of Sleep Disorders, Revised: Diagnostic and Coding Manual* (ASDA, 1997). The major categories are dyssomnias, parasomnias, and sleep disorders associated with medical or psychiatric disorders.

## Dyssomnias

Dyssomnias include disorders of initiating and maintaining sleep and disorders of excessive sleepiness. There are three major categories: circadian rhythm disorders, intrinsic sleep disorders, and extrinsic sleep disorders.

### Circadian Rhythm Disorders

Circadian rhythm disorders occur when individuals attempt to sleep at times that are inconsistent with their underlying biological clocks. Intrinsic circadian rhythm disorders refer to desynchronies between attempts to sleep and the sleep-wake circadian rhythm that are due presumably to internal rather than external causes. These disorders might result from a weak circadian rhythm or from an inability to entrain the rhythm to the environment. Extrinsic circadian rhythm sleep disorders occur when environmental conditions, such as working night shifts or traveling across time zones, result in disrupted sleep-wake circadian rhythms.

**Intrinsic Circadian Rhythm Disorders.** *Delayed Sleep Phase Syndrome (DSPS).* In DSPS, the sleep-wake circadian rhythm is delayed compared to the time the individual attempts to sleep. DSPS was first identified by Weitzman et al. (1981) as a "chronobiological disorder with sleep-onset insomnia." Individuals report difficulty falling asleep at a desired bedtime but have normal sleep if they attempt to sleep a few hours later. Daily sleep-wake diaries of individuals with DSPS show late sleep onset, few awakenings, early wake-up times when work or social demands are present, and late (midafternoon) wake-up times when there are no such demands on their time. The disorder is associated with daytime sleepiness that is most pronounced in the morning (Thorpy et al., 1988). Polysomnography shows that, compared to age matched norms, patients with DSPS have longer latencies to stages 2 and 3 and decreased sleep efficiency (Allen et al., 1989). In addition, DSPS patients have more awakenings and less slow-wave sleep in the first part of the night. These findings indicate a reduced depth and quality of sleep in the first part of the night which is consistent with the phase delay.

Delayed sleep phase individuals commonly identify themselves as "night people" and report being most alert during the late evening and night hours. Many case study reports on the disorder come from adolescent and young adult populations (Ferber, 1985). Adults who suffer from DSPS often report childhood onset of the symptoms Weitzman et al., 1981). The prevalence of the diagnosis among patients in sleep disorders cen-

ters is estimated at 7%. The prevalence of the disorder in the general population is unknown, but some researchers estimate that the prevalence is higher, particularly with adolescents and young adults (Henschel & Lack, 1987; Thorpy et al., 1988).

Although patients with delayed sleep phase experience an inability to phase advance their rhythm, they usually have no such difficulty with phase delay. This is the basis for chronotherapy (Czeisler et al., 1981). In chronotherapy, bedtime is successively delayed by daily increments of 3 hours until a desired bedtime is reached. This strategy is often augmented with appropriately timed light exposure (see later). Although chronotherapy with or without light exposure is effective (Czeisler et al., 1981), it requires high motivation and, in the case of adolescents, clear behavioral contracts and monitoring (Dahl, 1992). The efficacy of chronotherapy with adolescents who manifest school refusal or when other motivational factors are present is not very high (Ferber, 1985). In these cases, treatment needs to explicitly address intrinsic and environmental factors that reinforce the delayed bedtime behavior. Even when treatment successfully shifts the sleep-wake rhythm to a desired time, the risk of relapse is high, and maintaining a regular sleep-wake schedule is important to prevent relapse.

*Advanced Sleep Phase Syndrome (ASPS).* Patients with ASPS present with a set of complaints converse from those with DSPS, namely, inability to stay awake until the desired bedtime and inability to remain asleep until the desired wake-up time. Other than a shift in the major sleep episode toward earlier sleep-onset time with respect to a 24-hour day, the sleep of individuals with ASPS is normal in quality and duration. Typical sleep-onset times are between 6 P.M. and 8 P.M., and no later than 9 P.M., and wake times are between 1 A.M. and 3 A.M., and no later than 5 A.M. Unlike other sleep maintenance disorders, early morning awakening occurs after a normal amount of otherwise undisturbed sleep (ASDA, 1997).

As with DSPS, individuals afflicted with ASPS come to clinical attention only when the inherent sleep-wake schedule interferes with social activities and/or a work schedule. Problems may also occur as a result of attempting to adhere to a conventional sleep schedule. For example, when a patient attempts to remain awake until the desired bedtime, the early awakening aspect of the syndrome can lead to chronic insufficient sleep and excessive daytime sleepiness (Richardson & Malin, 1996).

ASPS is much more common in older individuals than in the young, and the complaint of waking up too early in the morning may be confused with depression. It is thought that the higher prevalence of ASPS in elderly individuals is due to shortening of the endogenous circadian timing system that accompanies normal aging. However, sleep maintenance insomnia in the elderly may be due to an intrinsic sleep disorder or secondary to a mental, neurological, or other medical disorder (see the sections on intrinsic sleep disorders and sleep disorders associated with neurological disorders). Some types of depression, for example, also exhibit phase-advance features. The early morning awakening of patients with depression is usually accompanied by other sleep and somatic symptoms and altered mood (see the section on depression).

The current approach to treating ASPS is bright light exposure in the evening and avoidance of light exposure (e.g. wearing dark, wraparound sunglasses) in the morning. Bright light exposure in the evening and the avoidance of bright light in the morning, it is thought, help to reentrain the sleep-wake cycle into the circadian rhythm (Allen, 1991; Wagner, 1996; see the section on light treatment).

*Irregular Sleep-Wake Pattern.* This rare disorder is characterized by a variable and disorganized sleep-wake pattern that suggests the absence of circadian rhythmicity. Sleep is broken into several short sleep episodes, but the cumulative sleep for a 24-hour period is at normal levels. Polysomnographic studies show no abnormalities in sleep parameters except for the short duration of each episode (Roehrs, Zorick, & Roth, 1994). The absence of a sleep-wake rhythm is confirmed by the absence of a temperature rhythm. This pattern, it has been found, is common in elderly people with dementia compared to age matched controls (Okawa, Mishima, Hishikawa, Hozumi, Hori, & Takahashi, 1991). Treatment consists of a gradual decrease in the number and duration of daily naps. Increase in activity levels and social interaction is recommended to facilitate the process (Hauri, 1982; Okawa et al., 1991).

*Non-24-Hour Sleep-Wake Syndrome.* This is a disorder in which individuals are unable to entrain to a 24-hour day and instead maintain 25- to 27-hour sleep-wake cycles. Some individuals with this syndrome tend to progressively phase delay. The disorder is rare in the general population and is assumed to have higher prevalence among blind people (Miles et al., 1977). Treatment focuses on entraining the circadian rhythm to a 24-hour day through social interaction, exposure to light, and melatonin. Melatonin has been successful in treating this disorder in blind individuals (Palm, Blennow, & Wetterberg, 1997).

**Extrinsic Circadian Rhythm Disorders.**
*Shift Work.* Because of family and social demands, night shift workers usually attempt to live their days off on a schedule different from that of their workdays. A disrupted sleep-wake schedule often results in disturbed and shortened sleep, sleepiness on the job, reduced performance levels, and psychological distress due to disruptions in family and social life. Workers on rotating shift schedules have greater difficulty than those on permanent night shifts. The severity of the problem increases with age. Ascoff (1978) and Reinberg et al. (1978) found that individuals whose temperature rhythm had low amplitude could better adapt to shift work.

Polysomnographic studies of the sleep and sleepiness of night shift workers show short durations of sleep following work nights (5 to 6 hours) and reduced sleep efficiency (Walsh et al., 1984), reduced amounts of stage 2 and REM sleep (Akerstedt, 1985), and increased sleepiness on the MSLT during waking hours (Akerstedt et al., 1982).

Many researchers recommend that rotating shift schedules should be designed to be consistent with the natural tendency to phase delay, that is, the direction of rotation should be progressively later, and the duration of the shift should be long enough to allow adaptation (Roehrs, Zorick, & Roth 1994). European researchers, on the other hand prefer a very rapidly rotating system of two days on each shift because that allows the circadian rhythm to remain constant (Akerstedt, 1985). A variety of methods for enhancing alertness and performance among shift workers have been suggested (Penn & Bootzin, 1990). The optimal timing of work breaks, social activity during breaks bright light and other sensory stimulation have the most potential for short-term alerting effects Stress coping techniques, sleep hygiene informa tion, and family counseling have the most poten tial for addressing the long-term effects of shift work.

*Time-Zone Change Disorders.* Dyssomnia associated with rapid time-zone change ("jet lag") is due to desynchrony between the endogenous sleep-wake rhythm and the light/dark cycle. Symptoms include an inability to sustain sleep and excessive sleepiness. For most people, these symptoms subside after a few days, depending on the number of time zones crossed. Frequent travelers, such as transatlantic airline crews, may experience more persistent difficulties. Westward travel is associated with disturbed sleep at the end of the sleep period, which coincides with habitual wake-up time, and eastward travel is associated with sleep onset insomnia (Roehrs, Zorick, & Roth, 1994). Due to the natural tendency to phase delay, travel westbound is easier to adjust to than travel eastbound.

*Light Treatment.* Results show that properly timed exposures to bright light (7,000–12,000 lux) for 2 to 3 days can shift the phase of the sleep rhythm (Czeisler et al., 1989). For comparison, typical indoor room light is less than 500 lux; sunlight produces about 2500 lux a few minutes after dawn; and at noon, sunlight is in the 100,000 lux range (Terman, 1994). The direction of the shift depends on the timing of the exposure to light. A phase advance is achieved by light exposure in the morning, and a phase delay is achieved by light exposure in the evening. In addition to the proper timing of bright light, it is also important to have periods of darkness during which no bright light is allowed (Czeisler et al., 1989; Rosenthal et al., 1990).

Preliminary results indicate that bright light treatment may be effective for a number of circadian rhythm sleep disorders. Bright light treatment during night shift work resulted in increased duration of daytime sleep and improved alertness on the job (Czeisler et al., 1990). Bright light treatment, it has also been shown, benefits jet lag sufferers (Daan & Lewy, 1984; Sasaki et al., 1989), insomnia during the "dark period" in northern Norway (Lingjaerde et al., 1985), early morning awakening (Lack & Wright, 1993), and delayed sleep phase syndrome (Rosenthal et al., 1990).

The disruptive effects of time-zone travel on circadian rhythms can also be alleviated through melatonin administration about an hour before bedtime in the new time zone. Melatonin is a circadian-setting hormone released by the pineal gland and, it has been shown, induces drowsiness and shortens sleep latency. Thus, timely adminis-

tration may advance or delay the circadian phase. However, research concerning the optimal dose and the effects of long-term use are lacking (Chase & Gidal, 1997; Sack, Hughes, Edgar, & Lewy, 1997).

## Intrinsic Sleep Disorders

Intrinsic sleep disorders are those due primarily to internal mechanisms. They include insomnia, narcolepsy, sleep apnea, periodic limb movements, and restless legs.

**Insomnia.** Insomnia includes difficulty falling asleep, frequent or prolonged awakenings during the night, early morning awakenings, and the experience of poor quality sleep. Epidemiological surveys indicate that about 15% of adults report severe or frequent insomnia and another 15% report mild or occasional insomnia (Bixler et al., 1979; Mellinger, Balter, & Uhlenhuth, 1985). The prevalence of insomnia increases with age. More than 25% of those over 65 years of age report having had considerable difficulty in falling or staying asleep during the preceding 12 months (Mellinger et al., 1985). The two most common types of intrinsic insomnia are psychophysiological insomnia and sleep state misperception.

*Psychophysiological Insomnia.* Psychophysiological insomnia refers to sleep disturbances that can be verified by objective measures (such as polysomnography) and are not associated with either extrinsic determinants such as noise or drugs or with other disorders such as major depression. About 15% of patients seen at sleep disorder centers with complaints of insomnia receive this diagnosis (ASDA, 1997).

The major determinants of psychophysiological insomnia are stress, expectations of disturbed sleep, and poor sleep habits. Other determinants such as circadian rhythm disturbances, changes associated with aging, drug abuse, and misinformation about sleep may contribute to the problem. Learned sleep-preventing associations are often central in psychophysiological insomnia and may also contribute to exacerbating and maintaining other sleep disturbances.

Insomniacs frequently engage in activities at bedtime that are incompatible with falling asleep. Many insomniacs organize their activities around their bedrooms with television, telephone, books, and food within easy reach. For others, bedtime is the first time during the day that is available to think about the day's events and to plan and worry about the next day. Under these conditions, bed and bedtime become cues for arousal rather than cues for sleep (Bootzin & Nicassio, 1978).

Another source of arousal for the insomniac is that the bedroom can become a cue for the anxiety and frustration associated with trying to fall asleep. Insomniacs can often sleep any place other than their own beds. They may fall asleep in chairs or on couches and often have less difficulty sleeping away from home. In contrast, good sleepers often have difficulty in strange surroundings. For them, there are strong cues for sleep associated with their beds and they have difficulty sleeping only when these cues are not available (Bootzin & Nicassio, 1978).

*Sleep State Misperception.* Sleep state misperception is the most recent label for instances in which the complaint of insomnia is not verified by objective measures. In the past, this disorder has been called pseudoinsomnia, subjective insomnia, and disorder of initiating or maintaining sleep without objective findings. Fewer than 5% of patients seen at sleep disorder centers for complaints of insomnia receive this diagnosis (ASDA, 1997).

A number of investigations have indicated that insomniacs of all types overestimate sleep latency and underestimate total sleep and the number of nocturnal awakenings, compared to polysomnography (e.g., Borkovec & Weerts, 1976; Carskadon et al., 1976). Those with sleep state misperception are the most extreme on this dimension. It should be emphasized that this diagnosis is not the sleep equivalent of hypochondria. Sleep state misperception often involves perceptual and cognitive dysfunctions that are not detected by polysomnography.

Some patients who have this diagnosis have difficulty distinguishing sleep states from wake-sleep transition states (Perlis et al., 1997) due perhaps to increased access to cognitive rumination during sleep. Other patients are hypervigilant to environmental stimuli during sleep and can remember and report on their occurrence (Anch, Saskin, & Moldofsky, 1989; Loewy & Bootzin, 1998).

*CAPS and Alpha Sleep.* Two arousal-related electrophysiological patterns have been found in the sleep of insomniacs: cyclic alternating pattern sequences (CAPS) and alpha sleep. CAPS, a biphasic electrical pattern that is found in the microstructure of NREM sleep stages (Terzano, Mancia, Salati, Costani, Decembrino, & Parrino, 1985),

consists of an arousal phase (composed of arousal-related phasic events distinct to each particular NREM sleep stage) that lasts between 2 and 60 seconds and is followed by a return to tonic or baseline activity. CAPS are a normal pattern of NREM sleep. Such arousal and de-arousal patterns occupy about 25% of NREM sleep in young, healthy, adult sleepers. CAPS are significantly more elevated (68%) in the sleep of insomniacs and suggest a hyperaroused state during sleep. The exact relationship of CAPS to the pathophysiology of insomnia is currently unknown, however, treatment of insomnia with hypnotics, it has been shown, reduces CAPS to a normal level (Terzano & Parrino, 1992).

Alpha rhythm, 8–12 Hz, is the dominant electrical pattern found in people who are awake, but relaxed. Many hypervigilant patients with insomnia have simultaneous alpha and sleep EEG waves. This has been called alpha-delta sleep (Hauri & Hawkins, 1973) or, more recently, alpha sleep. During wake, alpha is seen primarily from occipital leads, whereas during sleep, the alpha rhythm is more frontal and central. Alpha sleep is often experienced as nonrestorative sleep (i.e., not feeling rested after sleeping). Alpha sleep has been found in insomnia-affected patients who have fibromyalgia, rheumatoid arthritis, posttraumatic stress disorder, chronic pain disorders, depression, chronic fatigue syndrome, AIDS, and alcoholism (Fredrickson & Krueger, 1994; Moldofsky, Scarisbrick, England, & Smythe, 1975; Norman et al., 1992; Ware, Russell & Campos, 1986; Whelton, Saskin, Salit, & Moldofsky, 1988; for additional information, see the section on fibromyalgia).

**Treatment of Insomnia.** The prescription of sedative/hypnotics is the most frequently used treatment for insomnia. About 4.3% of adults in the United States use medically prescribed psychoactive medication to promote sleep (i.e., hypnotics, anxiolytics, and antidepressants; Mellinger, Balter, & Uhlenhuth, 1985). Of the sedative/hypnotics, benzodiazepines are the most frequently prescribed and have almost completely replaced barbiturates (Morin & Kwentus, 1988). Five principles of pharmacotherapy for persistent insomnia have been summarized by Kupfer and Reynolds (1997): use the lowest effective dose, use intermittent dosing to delay tolerance (two to four times weekly), prescribe medication for short-term use, discontinue medication gradually, and be alert for rebound insomnia following discontinuation. The use of sedative/hypnotics to induce sleep is effective for short-term use; effects last 2–4 weeks. However, there have been no published randomized clinical trials of hypnotics for periods longer than 35 days (Kupfer & Reynolds, 1997). Thus, long-term effectiveness is unknown, and long-term use of hypnotics has generally been discouraged because of problems of tolerance, side effects, and dependence (see the section on hypnotic-dependent sleep disorder).

A number of nonpharmacological treatments, it has been found, are effective for insomnia, In a recent review by the American Academy of Sleep Medicine, the task force report concluded that nonpharmacological therapies produce reliable and durable changes in sleep and that between 70 and 80% of patients improve (Morin, Hauri, Espie, et al., 1999). The most frequently used nonpharmacological treatments include stimulus control instructions, sleep restriction, relaxation training, paradoxical intention, and cognitive therapy.

Stimulus control instructions consist of a set of instructions designed to help the insomniac establish a consistent sleep-wake rhythm, strengthen the bed and bedroom as cues for sleep, and weaken them as cues for activities that might interfere with sleep. The following rules constitute the stimulus control instructions (Bootzin, 1972, 1977; Bootzin, Epstein, & Wood, 1991).

1. Lie down intending to go to sleep only when you are sleepy.
2. Do not use your bed for anything except sleep, that is, do not read, watch television, eat, or worry in bed. Sexual activity is the only exception to this rule. On such occasions, the instructions are to be followed afterward when you intend to go to sleep.
3. If you find yourself unable to fall asleep, get up and go into another room. Stay up as long as you wish, and then return to the bedroom to sleep. Although we do not want you to watch the clock, we want you to get out of bed if you do not fall asleep immediately. Remember the goal is to associate your bed with falling asleep *quickly*! If you are in bed more than about 10 minutes without falling asleep and have not gotten up, you are not following this instruction.
4. If you still cannot fall asleep, repeat Step 3. Do this as often as is necessary throughout the night.
5. Set your alarm, and get up at the same time every morning irrespective of how much

sleep you got during the night. This will help your body acquire a consistent sleep rhythm.
6. Do not nap during the day.

Stimulus control therapy, it has been found, is effective for both sleep onset and sleep maintenance insomnia. Meta-analyses of the treatment outcome literature for insomnia have found that stimulus control is one of the most effective of the nonpharmacological treatments (Morin, Culbert, & Schwartz, 1994; Murtagh & Greenwood, 1995).

Sleep restriction (Spielman, Saskin, & Thorpy, 1987) is based on the observation that many insomniacs have low sleep efficiency, that is, the proportion of time during which they are in bed and are actually asleep is less than 85%. To help consolidate sleep, insomniacs are instructed to limit the time during which they are in bed to the number of hours of sleep that they normally obtain. At first, patients experience partial sleep deprivation because they usually underestimate how much sleep they normally get. Sleep deprivation, however, helps to consolidate sleep. Patients are then instructed to follow a gradual schedule of increasing the amount of time spent in bed while maintaining the improved sleep efficiency. Sleep restriction has been effectively used in combination with sleep education and stimulus control instructions for treating sleep maintenance insomnia in older adults (Hoelscher & Edinger, 1988).

A commonly recommended treatment for insomnia is some type of relaxation training. This includes a variety of procedures such as progressive relaxation, autogenic training, transcendental meditation, yoga, hypnosis, and EMG biofeedback. As treatments for insomnia, all of these procedures are based on the same premise: if people can learn to be relaxed at bedtime, they will fall asleep faster. Because many insomniacs are aroused and anxious during the day, relaxation training may provide a double benefit—first, to help induce sleep, and second, as a general coping skill for dealing more effectively with the stresses of the day (Bootzin & Nicassio, 1978). The different types of relaxation procedures have all been found about equally effective in controlled studies (Bootzin & Rider, 1997).

Progressive relaxation training has been found effective in producing sleep onset latency improvement in both sleep state misperception and psychophysiological insomniacs (Borkovec et al., 1979). Improvement of the sleep state misperception patients was found for daily sleep diaries and subjective estimates while in the sleep laboratory. Because these patients did not exhibit a problem on polysomnographic measures, no improvement was observed on those measures. Improvement of psychophysiological insomniacs, on the other hand, was found on both sleep diaries and polysomnography.

Cognitive treatments have focused on patients' beliefs and expectations. Insomniacs often subscribe to a number of irrational beliefs about sleep. Examples of these beliefs are that the individual must get at least 8 hours of sleep to feel refreshed and function well the next day; the worry that if individuals go for one or two nights without sleep, they will have nervous breakdowns; or the belief that individuals should avoid or cancel social, family, and work obligations after a poor night's sleep (Morin, 1993). Treatment involves providing accurate information and having the insomniac identify and rehearse alternative belief statements. These techniques have been effective as part of multicomponent treatments (Morin et al., 1999; Morin, Stone, McDonald, & Jones, 1994).

Paradoxical intention (PI) is a cognitive intervention that has been frequently evaluated. Many insomniacs exacerbate their problem by worrying whether they will be able to fall asleep. To reduce the anticipatory anxiety associated with "trying" to fall asleep, insomniacs are instructed to stay awake as long as possible. Controlled evaluations of PI for sleep onset insomnia have been mixed. The rationale provided by the therapist for the paradoxical instruction may be a crucial component of its effectiveness. In a meta-analysis of the application of PI to a number of different problems, Shoham-Salomon and Rosenthal (1987) found that rationales that emphasize a positive benefit or the positive qualities of the person who has the problem are more effective than rationales that are neutral or that emphasize negative aspects of the problem.

Many controlled studies have examined the efficacy and durability of psychological treatments for chronic insomnia. Two separate meta-analyses have been published (Morin, Culbert, & Schwartz, 1994; Murtagh & Greenwood, 1995). Both meta-analyses concluded that psychological treatments improve the sleep of insomniacs over control conditions, and improvements were maintained at 6-month follow-ups. Murtagh and Greenwood (1995) concluded that there are few differences between different active treatments, although stim-

ulus control instructions had the strongest effects. Morin, Culbert, & Schwartz (1994) concluded that both stimulus control instructions and sleep restriction, as single-component treatments, had the strongest effects.

In recent years, the focus has shifted from efficacy studies of single-component treatments to effectiveness studies of multicomponent treatments. In one study, primary care nurses within a community general medical clinic were trained to deliver a multicomponent treatment consisting of stimulus control instructions, sleep restriction, and cognitive therapy (Espie, Inglis, Tessier, & Harvey, 2001). The treatment was more effective than a control condition in improving sleep, and 84% of patients who were initially using hypnotics remained drug-free during the follow-up period. Another innovative intervention presented a course of eight television programs broadcast in the Netherlands. About 200,000 people viewed the course of whom 23,000 ordered course materials. An evaluation of a sample of those who participated found that the course produced improvements in sleep latency and total sleep and decreases in hypnotic drug use (Oosterhuis & Klip, 1997).

## Narcolepsy

Narcolepsy is characterized by excessive daytime sleepiness and abnormal manifestations of REM sleep (ASDA, 1997). The REM abnormalities associated with narcolepsy include sleep onset REM periods and dissociated REM processes such as cataplexy, sleep paralysis, and hypnagogic hallucinations.

Narcolepsy has a prevalence of between 5 and 10 per 10,000 individuals (Guilleminault, 1994a). Age at onset can range from childhood to the fifth decade, but it peaks in the second decade. Researchers have documented a strong association between narcolepsy and the human leukocyte antigen HLA-DR2 phenotype that lends support to genetic theories of narcolepsy (Honda, Asaka, Tanimura, & Furusho, 1983). However, it has not been a useful diagnostic measure because as many as 25% of nonnarcoleptics also have the HLA-DR2 phenotype. The gene for canine narcolepsy, which is characterized primarily by symptoms of cataplexy (see later), is due to a recessive gene that affects the hypocretin (orexin) receptor 2 gene (Lin et al., 1999). Although genetics is definitely involved in the development of narcolepsy, there is also a strong environmental component because only 30% of identical twins are concordant for narcolepsy (Mignot, 1998).

Narcolepsy is classified as a disorder of excessive somnolence. However, narcoleptics do not sleep abnormally long within a 24-hour period. Narcoleptics may sleep 8 hours a night and be awake 16 hours during the day, but they will have repeated naps or lapse into sleep of short duration that lasts about 10 to 20 minutes. They awaken feeling refreshed but begin to feel sleepy again within 2 to 3 hours, at which point the pattern repeats itself (ASDA, 1997). These sudden and irresistible sleep attacks, also called excessive daytime sleepiness (EDS), are most common in, but not limited to, sleep-inducing circumstances such as sedentary activities. They may occur when the individual is actively involved in a task such as taking an examination, eating, walking, driving, or talking.

An accurate diagnosis of narcolepsy depends on differentiating it from two other medical conditions associated with the symptoms of excessive somnolence, breathing disorders during sleep, and central nervous system hypersomnia (Guilleminault, 1994a). The four classic symptoms of narcolepsy include (1) sleep attacks—characterized by an irresistible urge to sleep; (2) cataplexy—an abrupt and reversible decrease or loss of muscle tone that ranges in severity from mild weakness to complete postural collapse, with no loss of consciousness, elicited by emotion (usually pleasant or exciting emotions, e.g., laughter, pride, anger, and surprise) and ranging from a few seconds to several minutes; (3) hypnagogic hallucinations—frightening and vivid visual or auditory hallucinations that occur at the onset of sleep; and (4) sleep paralysis—muscle paralysis upon falling asleep or awakening, characterized by the inability to move limbs, speak, or breathe deeply, that lasts from one to several minutes, and is often a frightening experience. Only 20–25% of narcoleptics have all four of the core symptoms, and the latter three typically decrease over time. Sleep disruption and frequent nocturnal awakenings are common, as are reports of memory problems and automatic behavior (ASDA, 1997).

A positive diagnosis of narcolepsy requires either irresistible sleepiness or cataplexy plus sleep onset REM episodes documented by polysomnogram (ASDA, 1997). On the basis of polysomnographic recording, confirmatory diagnosis can

be made if the mean MSLT score is less than 5, two or more sleep onset REM periods occur during a MSLT, and REM sleep occurs within 20 minutes of sleep onset during a nighttime recording (Association of Professional Sleep Societies, 1986). Caution must be exercised, however, because individuals without complaints of daytime sleepiness occasionally have two or more sleep onset REM periods (Aldrich, Chervin, & Malow, 1997; Bishop, Rosenthal, Helmus, Roehrs, & Roth, 1996) and some individuals with narcolepsy do not have multiple sleep onset REM periods on the first day of a MSLT (Choo & Guilleminault, 1998).

Conventional treatment of narcolepsy focuses on the separate symptoms. Stimulants (methylphenidate and dextroamphetamine) are often used to treat EDS, and antidepressants (protriptyline and viloxazine) are used for the REM-related symptoms of cataplexy, sleep paralysis, and hypnagogic hallucinations (Guilleminault et al., 1986; Mitler et al., 1986). A routine of medication and naps (Roehrs et al., 1986) can reduce sleep attacks from three per day to one or two per month (Mitler, Nelson, & Hajdukovich, 1987). Support groups (Guilleminault, 1994a) and counseling for the families of narcoleptics (Karacan & Howell, 1988) are useful in helping patients and their families deal with the psychological and social effects of narcolepsy, including loss of self-esteem, depressive reactions, and family discord.

## Sleep Apnea

Sleep apnea is a respiratory disorder characterized by repetitive episodes of cessation of airflow that last at least 10 seconds. Sleep apnea is one of the most common causes of sleep disturbance. The prevalence is higher in men than in women and increases with age. An occasional pause in breathing is normal, but sleep apnea becomes a health problem when apneas occur frequently and are associated with significant reduction in blood oxygen saturation, cardiac arrhythmia, or impaired daytime functioning secondary to frequent arousals and fragmented sleep. In general, more than five apneas per hour of sleep in adults is considered abnormal (Guilleminault & Dement, 1988). Three types of sleep apnea have been defined: (1) *obstructive*—cessation of airflow secondary to upper airway obstruction; (2) *central*—cessation of airflow secondary to lack of ventilatory effort; (3) *mixed*—cessation of airflow in a pattern that suggests lack of ventilation effort initially and subsequent upper airway obstruction. As mentioned, the term *apnea* refers to a complete cessation of airflow; *hypopnea* refers to a partial reduction in airflow, again usually accompanied by an arousal. Hypopnea and apnea have similar clinical features (e.g., unrefreshed sleep, excessive daytime sleepiness). Patients with obstructive sleep apnea can demonstrate obstructive, central, or mixed apneas, in addition to hypopneas throughout the night. Thus, the severity of the disorder is measured by combining all of these events in a total score, referred to as the respiratory disturbance index (RDI). Many individuals with sleep apnea have obstructive, central, and mixed events in one night and as many as 300 such events per night.

**Obstructive Sleep Apnea (OSA).** OSA is the most common of the three types of sleep apnea. The term *sleep disordered breathing* (SDB) is sometimes used synonymously for OSA. A recent epidemiological study reported that the prevalence of OSA is higher than previously estimated, approximately 4 and 2% in middle-aged men and women, respectively (Young et al. 1993). On the basis of a group of community dwelling adults ages 40–60 years, Kripke et al. (1997) estimated that the prevalence of OSA is even higher at 9.3% for men and 5.2% for women. Patients with OSA are often overweight. Although OSA is a common disorder in middle-aged adults and increases the risk of or exacerbates already existing cardiovascular diseases, it remains underrecognized and underdiagnosed (Young et al., 1997; Chan et al., 1998; Partinen & Guilleminault, 1990). The onset of OSA is usually insidious, and if untreated, complications including mortality can ensue (Redline & Strohl, 1998).

During sleep, the upper airway musculature relaxes, reducing the caliber of the airway and leading to increased respiratory effort. Snoring, which has been reported in up to 50% of males over age 40, is an indication of partial airway obstruction and is produced by the vibration of pharyngeal tissues on inspiration, as the airflow becomes increasingly turbulent in the narrowed oropharyngeal space. Further narrowing produces hypopnea or with complete obstruction, apnea. Factors that reduce the diameter of the upper airway and predispose patients to snoring and OSA include obesity (via fat deposition), enlarged tonsillar tissue mass, and craniofacial abnormalities. In addition, excessive upper airway muscle relaxation and narrow-

ing occur from using alcohol, or other respiratory depressants (Bootzin, Quan, Bamford, & Wyatt, 1995; Redline & Stroh, 1998).

Patients with obstructive sleep apnea usually snore loudly, as reported by their bed partners, and their snoring is irregular and interrupted by pauses. These pauses end with a loud snort as the patient's progressively stronger ventilatory efforts finally produce arousals, contraction of the upper airway muscles, and normal breathing. Arousals can be brief and not recalled by the patient or prolonged with complete awakening. As the patient returns to sleep, the cycle of progressive upper airway narrowing begins again.

In addition to the hallmark symptom, loud snoring, nighttime symptoms of OSA may include restlessness, frequent awakenings, choking, tachycardia, heartburn, enuresis, nocturia, and profuse sweating. Daytime symptoms include waking up feeling unrefreshed with feelings of disorientation or grogginess, sometimes accompanied by a headache. Additionally, some patients may also experience decreased libido and changes in personality (e.g., increased irritability, depression, and aggressiveness) (Guilleminault, 1994b; ASDA, 1997). Daytime sleepiness is common and can range from fatigue to involuntary sleep attacks, which can occur while the patient is driving or conversing. Definitive diagnosis and determination of appropriate treatment require that the patient undergo a polysomnographic study.

The treatment of OSA depends on the severity of the condition, as expressed by disturbance in nocturnal sleep, cardiac or neurological complications, and daytime symptoms. The goals of treatment are to eliminate snoring and upper airway obstruction, maintain nocturnal oxygenation and ventilation, and normalize sleep architecture (Chan et al., 1998). Several treatment modalities are available for OSA, including behavioral, medical, and surgical interventions. Behavioral interventions to modify risk factors generally are considered first or are sometimes recommended as adjuncts to more aggressive therapies. In patients with mild to moderate OSA weight loss (Brownman et al., 1984), avoidance of alcohol and other CNS depressants (Issa & Sullivan, 1982; Robinson & Zwillich, 1985) and position therapy (measures designed to keep the patient in the lateral rather than the supine position when asleep) (Cartwright, Lloyd, Lilie, & Kravitz, 1985) can be effective interventions.

Because the pathophysiology of OSA is due

primarily to the intermittent collapse of a narrowed airway, mechanical or surgical techniques to enlarge the airway are the most logical treatment approach. Nasal continuous positive airway pressure (CPAP) is by far the treatment of choice for moderate to severe OSA. CPAP is applied by an airtight nasal mask connected to a flow generator and acts as a pneumatic internal splint of the upper airway to prevent it from collapsing. Nasal CPAP is highly effective in abolishing apneic events and produces immediate improvement in symptoms, quality of life, and cognitive function (Engleman, Martin, Deary & Douglas, 1997; Sullivan, Issa, Berthon-Jones, & Eves, 1981). Many patients, however, do not tolerate the CPAP appliance, which leads to poor compliance. Kribbs and colleagues (1993) have reported that although the majority of patients claim to use CPAP nightly, only sixteen of thirty-five (46%) in their study met criteria for regular use. And when used, the mean duration of CPAP use was less than 5 hours per night.

Surgical procedures for OSA include tonsillectomy, nasal surgery (e.g., correcting deviated septum, removing nasal polyps), and uvulopalatopharyngoplasty (UPPP). The long-term efficacy of UPPP is highest in patients with mild to moderate disease, but even in this population, satisfactory results occur in less than 50% of patients (Conway, Fujita, Zorick, et al., 1985). Mandibular advancement devices (MRD) that reposition the mandible, the tongue, and other structures to increase the upper airway dimensions are effective in treating snoring and mild OSA. The long-term efficacy of MRD, however, is still unclear (Chan et al., 1998; Chervin & Guilleminault, 1996).

**Central Sleep Apnea (CSA).** CSA represents a loss of ventilatory drive or rhythmicity. Most CSA episodes occur at sleep onset and are benign. CSA is considered pathological only when the events are sufficiently frequent to disturb sleep, result in hypoxemia or cardiac arrhythmias, or disturb daytime functioning. The severity of CSA and the extent of sleep disturbance depend partially on the underlying pathophysiology. Clinical presentation of patients with CSA differs from patients with OSA in a number of ways, however, there is also considerable overlap. Pure CSA is rare; patients with this condition constitute fewer than 10% of patients evaluated in sleep laboratories. Compared to patients with OSA, CSA patients less commonly complain of daytime hypersomnolence; although obesity and snoring are sometimes present,

they are not prominent features. The primary complaints of CSA patients are usually insomnia and frequent awakenings during the night, sometimes accompanied by a gasp for air and shortness of breath. Daytime symptoms may include morning headache, tiredness, fatigue, sleepiness, difficulty in memory and other cognitive functions, sexual dysfunction, and depression (ASDA, 1997).

CSA occurs secondary to lesions that affect the neural systems involved in ventilation (White, 1994). For example, CSA is a known complication of several neuromuscular diseases (e.g., amyotrophic lateral sclerosis (ALS), motor-sensory neuropathy, and myotonic dystrophy). These patients usually demonstrate daytime hypoventilation manifested by an elevated blood carbon dioxide level. At night, at the onset of sleep, loss of the behavioral control of ventilation, the so-called "wakefulness" stimulus, leads to further hypoventilation and oxygen desaturation. Typically, CSA worsens during REM sleep because these patients lose the use of accessory muscles of respiration that compensate for diaphragmatic weakness due to the muscle atonia that occurs in REM sleep. Profound hypoxemia can result (Guilleminault & Robinson, 1996).

Because CSA remains a disorder that is not well understood, currently available treatments are not entirely satisfactory. Central respiratory stimulants such as medroxyprogesterone are effective in central sleep apnea for a short time, but result have been variable in long-term use (Bootzin et al., 1995). Tricyclic antidepressant agents that suppress REM sleep and increase respiratory musculature tone have been used with little success to treat both CSA and OSA (Guilleminault & Robinson, 1996). Oxygen therapy helps some patients by decreasing the wide swings in blood oxygen content that characterize some forms of CSA and affect central nervous system rhythmicity. Nighttime ventilatory support, usually administered through appliances similar to CPAP devices, can be effective treatment for patients with CSA secondary to neuromuscular disorders. The boost in ventilation provided compensates for muscle weakness, corrects oxygen and carbon dioxide abnormalities, leading to none consolidated sleep.

### Periodic Limb Movements and Restless Legs Syndrome

Periodic limb movement (PLM) disorder is characterized by periodic episodes of repetitive and stereotypic limb movements during sleep. Also known as nocturnal myoclonus, periodic movements during sleep, and periodic leg movements, PLMs are described as episodes of rhythmic extensions of the big toe and dorsiflexions of the ankle, sometimes with flexions of the knee and hip.

The most common sleep characteristics associated with PLMs are frequent arousals and complaints of nonrestorative sleep. Patients are often unaware of PLMs and present with complaints of insomnia or excessive daytime sleepiness or seek help as a result of a bed partner's complaints of excessive nighttime movement.

Accurate diagnosis of PLMs is complex. The incidence of PLMs increases with age. It is known to exist concurrently with other disorders of excessive somnolence such as narcolepsy, sleep apnea, or restless legs syndrome (Moore & Gurakar, 1988) and may be associated with medical conditions such as chronic uremia, anemia, chronic lung disease, and fibromyalgia (Montplaisir et al., 1994). PLMs may be induced or aggravated by using tricyclic antidepressants and monoamine oxidase inhibitors, as well as by withdrawal from drugs such as anticonvulsants, benzodiazepines, barbiturates, and other hypnotic agents (ASDA, 1997). A polysomnogram with leg EMG is necessary to establish a final diagnosis of PLMs.

Polysomnographic recording of PLMs reveals repetitive episodes of muscle contraction measured by EMG that occur every 20 to 40 seconds (ASDA, 1997). These episodes usually occur in stages 1 and 2 sleep, decrease in stages 3 and 4, and are usually absent during REM sleep (Montplaisir et al., 1985). A PLM index (number of PLMs per hour of sleep) greater than 5 is considered pathological.

Restless legs syndrome (RLS) is a disorder characterized by irresistible leg movements usually before sleep onset (ASDA, 1997) and often described as an "aching" sensation. The most prominent characteristic of this disorder is the partial or complete relief of the sensation with leg motion and return of the symptom with cessation of movement. Symptoms are often exacerbated soon after getting into bed and tend to cease long enough for the patient to fall asleep, only to reappear later in the night. However, RLS may occur at times during the day after prolonged periods of sitting. The severity of symptoms with RLS may wax and wane throughout a patient's lifetime. Remissions may last for years, and symptoms

reappear suddenly without warning. Most patients with RLS also show PLMs during sleep. Symptoms are associated with a number of conditions such as the last trimester of pregnancy, caffeine intake, fatigue, exceptionally warm environment, prolonged exposure to cold (Montplaisir et al., 1994), anemia, and rheumatoid arthritis (ASDA, 1997).

Treatment for PLMs and RLS is pharmacological. The most effective drugs to date are carbidopa/ levodopa, benzodiazepines (clonazepam, temazepam, lorazepam, and nitrazepam), and opioids. Carbidopa/levodopa are considered the drugs of choice and, it has been shown, reduce the quantity of movements and increase the quality of sleep (Bootzin, Quan, Bamford, & Wyatt, 1995). Benzodiazepines may be considered in milder cases (Mitler, Brownman, Gujavarty, Timms, & Menn, 1984; Moldofsky, Tullis, Quance, & Lue, 1985), however, their use should be considered carefully, especially in the elderly, because they may induce or exacerbate sleep apnea and prevent arousal from apneic episodes (Montplaisir et al., 1994).

### Extrinsic Sleep Disorders

External factors such as sleep schedules, light, noise, drugs, nicotine, alcohol, and activity levels may cause disrupted sleep. In some instances, even chronic insomnia may be due to these factors.

**Inadequate Sleep Hygiene.** Inadequate sleep hygiene is defined as "a sleep disorder due to the performance of daily living activities that are inconsistent with the maintenance of good quality sleep and full daytime alertness" (p. 73, ASDA, 1997).

The likelihood that sleep disorders will be produced by inadequate sleep hygiene depends on predisposing factors, on the persistence of the behavior, and on the degree to which it deviates from normal practices. For example, some individuals who maintain highly irregular sleep-wake schedules never experience sleep disturbances, but others will report great difficulties in initiating or maintaining sleep even when their schedules are less irregular. The probability that an individual will engage in behavior that is inconsistent with maintaining good sleep is increased for individuals with low tolerance for daytime sleepiness. Such individuals may take naps, increase caffeine consumption, or go to bed too early. Although these behaviors may increase alertness in the short run, they may weaken the underlying biological clock and lead to insomnia when practiced for a long time.

Three aspects of sleep hygiene will be discussed: (1) the regularity of sleep-wake schedules, (2) regular exercise, and (3) the use of caffeine and nicotine.

*Sleep–Wake Schedules.* The relationship between biological rhythms and the sleep-wake cycle is the basis for the common recommendation to maintain a regular sleep schedule. Those who keep irregular schedules for long periods of time are at risk of developing sleep disturbances. Conversely, those with sleep disturbances frequently benefit from regularizing their sleep schedules. Indeed, when irregular sleepers regularize their nocturnal sleep and at the same time make sure their sleep is adequately long, their sleep and daytime alertness improve, and these improvements are greater than those observed when an intervention includes only the provision of adequate sleep duration without attempts to regularize the sleep schedule (Manber, Bootzin, Acebo, & Carskadon, 1996).

The role of naps within the sleep-wake schedule is complex. In polysomnographic terms, afternoon and evening naps begin the night's sleep, and morning naps are a continuation of the previous night's sleep. Thus, afternoon and evening naps have more slow-wave sleep, and morning naps have more REM sleep. The sleep on a night that follows an afternoon nap resembles sleep in the latter part of a normal night, which is lighter and has more awakenings. Thus, afternoon and evening naps should be avoided to preserve the quality of sleep at night. If they are taken, they should be short and should be made a regular part of the daily schedule at about the same time each day.

*Regular Exercise.* For exercise to be effective in improving sleep, individuals have to engage in programs of regular exercise. Recommendations to exercise are not always effective because of variability in compliance. A meta-analysis concluded that exercise must last for at least an hour to have reliable effects on sleep (Youngstedt, O'Connor, & Dishman, 1997). Regular exercise programs in older men produce increased continuous sleep, increased slow-wave sleep, and decreased nighttime awakenings (Edinger et al., 1993; Vitiello et al., 1992).

*Use of Caffeine and Nicotine.* Caffeine and nicotine are central nervous system stimulants that lighten sleep and produce arousals (ASDA, 1997).

Caffeine is present in chocolate and in coffee (100–200 mg, depending on the strength of the brew), tea (50–75 mg), and many carbonated beverages (50–75 mg). There are individual differences in the degree of sensitivity to caffeine. Some individuals may experience sleep disturbances from consuming chocolate and soft drinks alone. Other medications, including analgesics (those that contain caffeine), bronchodilators, decongestants, and appetite suppressants, are or contain stimulants that increase sleep latency, decrease total sleep time, and increase spontaneous awakenings (ASDA, 1997; Brown et al., 1995). Cessation of caffeine or nicotine intake may cause withdrawal symptoms such as sleepiness, irritability, lassitude, and severe depression (ASDA, 1997).

Complaints of insomnia and/or anxiety may be due to excessive ingestion of caffeine, nicotine, or other stimulants. Because caffeine has a plasma half-life of approximately 6 hours, individuals continue to experience its effects long after it has been ingested. Reducing or eliminating the intake of caffeine, particularly in the afternoon and evening, and quitting smoking can lead to substantial improvement in sleep. However, an increase in disturbed sleep can be expected during the initial period of smoking withdrawal (Wetter, Fiore, Baker, & Young, 1995).

**Environmental Sleep Disorders.** Among the many environmental factors that affect sleep are noise, temperature, room or bed sharing, institutionalization, and the need for vigilance during sleep. The presenting complaints consist of insomnia symptoms or marked impairment of daytime functioning. This diagnosis is given only when the environmental causes are judged the primary cause for the complaints. Its prevalence rate in patients seen in sleep disorder centers is estimated at less than 5% (ASDA, 1997). Sensitivity to environmental factors increases with age and is subject to great individual variability.

Noise decreases the amount of deep sleep and the continuity of sleep. There is an increase in body movements and sleep stage shifts. Studies show that a presentation of an auditory stimulus is often followed by very brief arousal (3–15 seconds). The fragmentation of sleep often leads to increased daytime sleepiness (Stepansky et al., 1984). Unpredictable noise is particularly disturbing (Sanchez & Bootzin, 1985). Thus, continuous white noise, such as that from a fan, is often useful for noisy environments.

People can adjust to a wide range of room temperatures but have more difficulty adjusting to cold than to heat. Uncomfortable room temperatures, particularly cold rooms, affect the quality of sleep more than the capacity to fall asleep (Haskell et al., 1981).

Recommendations for reducing environmental disturbances and strengthening good sleep hygiene have become an integral part of many treatments for insomnia. Frequent recommendations include maintaining regular sleep-wake schedules, establishing an environment conducive to sleep (quiet, dark, and secure), increasing exposure to light and other sensory stimuli upon awakening, and carefully timing and limiting the use of caffeine and alcohol. The importance of a comprehensive treatment approach, based on a thorough analysis of the problem, should be emphasized.

**Drug-Dependent Sleep Disorders.** Chronic use of drugs to induce or to suppress sleepiness may cause adverse effects. Although alcohol and sedative/hypnotics, it is thought, induce a state of unconsciousness that resembles sleep, in fact the resemblance to natural sleep is weak. Hypnotics produce disruptions in sleep architecture and increases in arousal threshold (Kay & Samiuddin, 1988). Using stimulants to suppress sleep can produce persistent insomnia.

*Hypnotic-Dependent Sleep Disorder.* Hypnotic-dependent sleep disorder is characterized by insomnia or excessive sleepiness associated with the tolerance to or withdrawal from hypnotic medications (ASDA, 1997).

Sedative/hypnotics are the most frequently used method for treating insomnia. With continued use, tolerance rapidly develops, and larger doses are required to achieve a soporific effect. As dosage is increased to offset tolerance, daytime carryover effects also increase and may include symptoms such as excessive sleepiness, poor motor coordination, visual–motor problems, and late afternoon restlessness (ASDA, 1997). These symptoms promote psychological dependency as the individual becomes convinced that the daytime effects are symptoms related to poor sleep the night before. This leads to a continued search for pharmacological relief from the insomnia, possibly by consulting several physicians or trying a variety of sleep-inducing medications. Polysomnographic monitoring of chronic sedative/hypnotic users shows decreases in stages 1, 3, 4, and REM sleep, an increase in stage 2 sleep, and fragmented

NREM and REM sleep with frequent stage changes (ASDA, 1997).

Once benzodiazepine hypnotics or anxiolytics are begun, it is often difficult for individuals to withdraw. In a study of abrupt discontinuation by individuals who had been taking benzodiazepines for 1 year or longer, 56% who took long half-life and 62% who took short half-life benzodiazepines failed to remain free of drugs during a 5-week follow-up (Rickels et al., 1990). In a companion study of gradual taper, 32% of long half-life and 42% of short half-life benzodiazepine-treated patients failed to achieve a drug-free state (Schweizer et al., 1990).

Cessation of sedative/hypnotics results in withdrawal symptoms that may also promote psychological dependence. Insomnia, it has been shown, is among the most frequent withdrawal symptoms from the long-term use of benzodiazepines (Busto et al., 1986; Schneider-Helmert, 1988). Other withdrawal symptoms include a dramatic increase in REM and stage 2 sleep percentages and daytime sleepiness (Schneider-Helmert, 1988). Total sleep time does not decrease with the withdrawal of medication, but the subjective perception of rebound insomnia is judged much worse than before drug therapy and often leads the patient to resume sedative/hypnotic use.

*Alcohol-Dependent Sleep Disorder.* About 10–15% of patients with chronic insomnia have problems with substance abuse, particularly alcohol and other sedatives (Gillin & Byerley, 1990). Alcohol, like other depressants, is a REM suppressant. Withdrawal from heavy drinking produces a REM rebound effect that is accompanied by restless sleep and nightmares. Alcohol also exacerbates sleep apnea because it affects ventilation during sleep by increasing upper airway resistance (Issa & Sullivan, 1982; Taasan et al., 1981). The effects of alcohol on sleep can persist as long as 2–3 hours after plasma alcohol levels return to zero (Zarcone, 1994).

Alcohol-dependent sleep disorder is characterized by the use of alcohol for initiating sleep onset (ASDA, 1997). Usually, the ingestion of alcohol begins about 3–4 hours before bedtime, and consumption is equivalent to about 6–8 ounces of liquor. This condition is not associated with other alcoholic patterns of drinking (drinking during the day and related socioeconomic problems) and is usually considered clinically relevant if the alcohol has been used daily for a minimum of 30 days. Continued use results in tolerance to alcohol as a sleep-inducing agent, and sleep fragmentation becomes more prominent. Often, patients will become desperate and increase the amount of alcohol or add other sedatives to sleep. Patients will often report that they have no sleep disturbance, as long as they continue to take the alcohol nightly.

Polysomnographic monitoring of this type of alcohol user shows an increase in stages 3 and 4, fragmentation of REM sleep, and frequent awakenings and sleep stage transitions (ASDA, 1997). Frequent sleep transitions are usually seen later in the sleep period, as the alcohol blood level begins to decline. In addition to polysomnogram recordings, diagnosis is confirmed if the patient complains of insomnia, has unsuccessfully attempted to withdraw from bedtime alcohol ingestion, and there is no evidence of medical or psychiatric disorder responsible for the insomnia (ASDA, 1997).

*Stimulant-Dependent Sleep Disorder.* Stimulant-dependent sleep disorder is characterized by the reduction of sleepiness or the suppression of sleep through the use of central stimulants that result in alterations in wakefulness following drug abstinence (ASDA, 1997). Many stimulants are used to combat daytime sleepiness. Cocaine, amphetamines, and inhalants have sleep suppressing effects. They increase the time to fall asleep and REM sleep latency and decrease total sleep time and REM time (Gillin, 1994). Tolerance may develop with chronic use and results in increased dosages. During episodes of stimulant abuse, individuals may go for days without sleep followed by periods of hypersomnia and accompanied psychological and mood problems of paranoia, psychosis, social withdrawal, and sleep disturbances. Individuals may use sedatives or alcohol to counteract the sleep suppressing effects of stimulants and reduce anxiety.

Withdrawal from stimulants is associated with hypersomnia and depression that can last 2 weeks (Gillin, 1994). At the end of the 2-week period, the individual may experience a few days of insomnia and poor quality sleep. Both sleep disturbances and hypersomnia may be risk factors for the reuse of stimulants or the use of other drugs.

## Parasomnias

Parasomnias are phenomena that intrude into sleep, although they are not primarily part of sleep *per se.* The more common examples include sleep talking, sleepwalking, sleep terrors, enuresis, and bruxism. These disorders reflect central nervous system activation and are divided into the following categories: (1) arousal disorders, (2) sleep-wake transition disorders, (3) parasomnias usually associated with REM sleep, and (4) other parasomnias.

### Arousal Disorders

Arousal disorders, such as sleep terrors and sleepwalking occur during arousal from slow-wave sleep.

**Sleep Terrors.** Sleep, or night, terrors, also called "pavor nocturnus" in children and "incubus" in adults, arise out of slow-wave sleep. They are characterized by the subjective experience of panic, rapid autonomic arousal, and behavioral activation. The individual will appear to be in great distress, emit a piercing scream, frequently will sit up, and may flee from the bedroom.

Despite behavioral activation and the experience of intense emotion, the individual may have either partial or total amnesia for the details of the event. If awakened during the sleep terror, the individual is likely to be confused, may report a sense of terror or dread, but reported sleep mentation will be vague, unlike the detail that occurs during nightmares. Because sleep terrors arise out of slow-wave sleep, they tend to occur during the first few hours of sleep. Nightmares, in contrast, are REM phenomena and are more likely to occur during the latter half of the night. Sleep terrors need also to be distinguished from nocturnal panic episodes, though the latter are usually not associated with screaming and do not produce vivid fearful imagery. Another differential diagnosis for sleep terrors is nocturnal seizures. Like sleep terrors, they are associated with difficulty to arouse during the event and with confusion upon arousal. However, whereas nocturnal seizures are often associated with daytime sleepiness, sleep terrors usually are not. Sleep terrors are not associated with daytime EEG abnormalities. Unless the clinical presentation suggests the possibility of a seizure disorder or other sleep disorders, an all night sleep study is not necessary to diagnose sleep terrors.

Recurring episodes of sleep terrors occur in from 1–6% of prepubertal children, and the typical age range for the disorder is from 5–7 years (Thorpy

& Glovinsky, 1987). Sleep terrors occur in about 1% of the adult population (Thorpy & Glovinsky, 1987). Although sleep terrors tend to abate after the onset of puberty, sleepwalking sometimes occurs or persists in those who had sleep terrors during childhood.

Pharmacological treatment of sleep terrors is based upon attempts to reduce the amount of slow-wave sleep experienced and usually involves using benzodiazepines or tricyclic antidepressants (Thorpy & Glovinsky, 1987). More recently, non-pharmacological treatments have also shown promise. Self-hypnosis (Hurwitz, 1986; Hurwitz & Mahowald, 1988) and scheduled awakenings with children (Lask, 1988) have been reportedly effective. In the scheduled awakening treatment, parents note how long after the child goes to sleep that a sleep terror is typically experienced. On subsequent nights, the parents are instructed to awaken the child 10–15 minutes before the sleep terror would have occurred. This procedure has been reportedly highly successful and may disrupt and lighten slow-wave sleep. It is also easier to comfort a child after a planned awakening than from one in which the child is frightened. Because both insufficient sleep and increased stress often exacerbate disorders of partial arousal (Guilleminault et al., 1995; Moldofsky et al., 1995), including sleep terrors, treatment should include education about the contribution of these factors and specific suggestions for managing stress and ensuring sufficient sleep.

**Sleepwalking.** Sleepwalking, or somnambulism, occurs during the first few hours of sleep, out of slow-wave sleep, not REM. Thus, sleepwalkers are not acting out their dreams. Their movements are coordinated with their environments, they typically avoid objects, may go to the bathroom, and even return to bed, if left alone. If awakened, sleepwalkers are confused and have little memory of dream mentation. Sleepwalking episodes may last from 15 seconds to 30 minutes (Aldrich, 2000a). Sleepwalking should be differentiated from REM behavior disorder (see parasomnias associated with REM) in which individuals lack the muscle atonia that accompanies REM, so that they do act out their dreams.

Sleepwalking is more common among children than adults. It is estimated that 15–30% of healthy children have at least one episode and 2–3% have more frequent episodes (Thorpy & Glovinsky, 1987). Generally, sleepwalking first occurs during prepubescence, reaches a peak prevalence at 12 years of age, and only infrequently occurs in children older than 15 years old. The prevalence in adults is less than 1%. There do not appear to be sex-related differences, but there is evidence for a familial tendency. Sleepwalking occurs ten times more frequently among first-degree relatives than in the general population (Karacan, 1988).

There is no known pathophysiology that corresponds to sleepwalking. Fatigue, stress, sleep deprivation, and drug use (especially sedative/hypnotics) may precipitate episodes. Psychopathology is not usually associated with sleepwalking in children, but it is in adults. Kales, Soldatos, Cadwell, et al. (1980) reported that adult sleepwalkers had elevated MMPI profiles (Pd, Sc, and Ma) and 72% of his sample had psychiatric diagnoses.

Parents of sleepwalking children should be cautioned to take safety precautions such as locking doors and windows. It is usually better to direct sleepwalkers back to bed rather than to awaken them. The very process of awakening may frighten and confuse them. When sleepwalking occurs frequently and is associated with potentially injurious or harmful behaviors, the intervention and preventive measures that are used for sleep terrors are also effective with the sleepwalker. These include preventing sleep deprivation, introducing stress coping strategies, and using scheduled awakening (Stores, 1990; Thorpy & Glovinsky, 1987).

Although there is a higher incidence of psychopathology among adults who sleepwalk than among those who do not, a complaint of sleepwalking does not necessarily indicate psychopathology. Sometimes sleepwalking persists well into the second decade of life, particularly among individuals with a history of parasomnias who report being sound sleepers and difficult to arouse. These individuals are likely to need more sleep, to have higher than average slow-wave sleep, and to suffer from sleep deprivation. Nevertheless, a complete psychological evaluation is often recommended for adults who sleepwalk. For sleepwalking adults, a motion-detection alarm is often useful. In addition to the other nonpharmacological interventions described earlier, pharmacological therapy is indicated when the sleepwalker is in particular danger. It includes medications such as benzodiazipines and antidepressants that suppress slow-wave sleep and reduce nocturnal arousals (Karacan, 1988).

### Sleep–Wake Transition Disorders

This category includes sleep talking and sleep starts. These disorders usually occur in the transitions between wakefulness and sleep and, more rarely, in the transitions between sleep stages. They occur in otherwise healthy subjects (ASDA, 1997).

**Sleep Talking.** Sleep talking, also called somniloquy, occurs during all stages of sleep. About 80% of sleep talking takes place during NREM sleep (Arkin, 1978). Dream mentation is recalled in association with 79% of the episodes that occur in REM sleep, 46% of the episodes that occur in stage 2, and 21% of the episodes that occur during slow-wave sleep (ASDA, 1997). Usually, sleep utterances occur spontaneously, are brief, and are devoid of signs of emotional distress. Occasionally, sleep talking may be induced or prolonged by conversation with the sleeper. Laughing, singing, and crying occasionally occur during sleep, as well (Anch et al., 1988).

Almost everyone has experienced an episode of sleep talking. In a survey of 1508 college undergraduates, 83% reported having had at least one episode of sleep talking (Perlis, 1989). Sleep talking may be precipitated by emotional distress or physical illness and may also accompany other parasomnias. Sleep talking is considered benign, so there is no recommended treatment.

**Sleep Starts.** Sleep starts, also called hypnic jerks, are sudden brief contraction of the legs, sometimes also involving the arms and head, that occur during the transitions from wakefulness to sleep. They occur mainly at the beginning of the sleep episode. Sleep starts are sometimes associated with sensory experiences, including the subjective impression of falling, a visual hypnagogic dream, and fragmentary auditory (e.g., loud bangs, snapping noises) or somesthetic (e.g., pain, floating) hallucination. Sleep starts are considered a normal phenomenon of the sleep onset process and should not be confused with seizures or movement disorders that occur at sleep onset or during sleep. Prevalence of 60–70% in the population has been reported (ASDA, 1997; Mahowald & Schenck, 1998).

Sleep starts may be exacerbated by excessive caffeine, the use of stimulants, strenuous exercise prior to sleep, and stress. Although sleep starts are generally considered of little consequence, if they occur frequently and cause repeated awakenings of the sleeper or bed partner, they may lead to sleep onset insomnia.

### Parasomnias Usually Associated with REM

This category includes nightmares, sleep paralysis, and REM sleep behavior disorder. These disorders are associated with or occur during REM sleep.

**Nightmares.** Nightmares are frightening dreams. They are often long and complicated, become increasingly frightening, and wake up the dreamer. Fear or anxiety are always associated with nightmares but sometimes seem out of proportion to the content being reported.

Nightmares occur during REM sleep, whereas sleep terrors and sleep panic attacks occur during NREM sleep. Two important features that differentiate nightmares are the time of the night when they occur and the detail of dream content that is reported. Nightmares, as REM sleep phenomena, are more likely to occur during the latter half of the night, and the dream content can be recalled in detail. Sleep terrors, associated with slow-wave sleep, and sleep panic attacks, associated with transitions between stages 2 and 3, are more likely to occur during the first half of the night. In both sleep terrors and sleep panic attacks, the sleeper awakens very frightened but is able to recall only fragmentary images, if any, and general feelings of fear and anxiety or of being attacked or suffocated.

Nightmares are a common feature of sleep. From 10–50% of children aged three to five have frequent enough nightmares to concern their parents (ASDA, 1997), and 5–8% of adults report having problems with nightmares (Bixler et al., 1979; Klink & Quan, 1987). The frequency of nightmares decreases with age. About 10% of adolescents (Muller & Wood, 1991) and college students (Wood & Bootzin, 1990) have at least one nightmare a week, compared to about 1% of healthy elderly (Salvio, Wood, & Schwartz, 1991).

The occurrence of frequent nightmares in adults has been considered a primary diagnostic criterion for anxiety and stress disorders. However, no relationship was found between frequent nightmares and trait anxiety in a study of college students (Wood & Bootzin, 1990). This suggests that other criteria, in addition to nightmares, are necessary to diagnose anxiety disorders.

**Sleep Paralysis.** Sleep paralysis, also called familial sleep paralysis or hypnagogic or hypnapompic paralysis, is a phenomenon during which individuals cannot perform voluntary movements at either sleep onset (hypnagogic paralysis) or upon awakening from sleep (hypnapompic paralysis). Although temporary, the paralysis immobilizes the head, trunk, limb and, sometimes, speech-related musculature. Episodes usually last less than 5 minutes and can sometimes be terminated by intense efforts to move (Anch et al., 1988). Sleep paralysis, it is hypothesized, is due to a dysfunction in REM sleep mechanisms in which the muscle atonia associated with REM sleep occurs during wake-sleep transitions. Sleep paralysis resembles cataplexy seen in narcolepsy. The two states differ in that sleep paralysis occurs during sleep-wake transitions, whereas cataplexy occurs during the day and is often triggered by an intense emotional stimulus. Both cataplexy and sleep paralysis may be symptoms of narcolepsy.

As an isolated symptom, sleep paralysis occurs in 40–50% of normal individuals sometime during their lifetimes (ASDA, 1997). Recurrent episodes of sleep paralysis, in the absence of a primary diagnosis of narcolepsy, are rare. From 17–40% of narcoleptics experience frequent episodes of sleep paralysis. Irregular sleep habits, sleep deprivation, stress, and sleep position have all been reported as predisposing factors for sleep paralysis.

**REM Sleep Behavior Disorder (RBD).** RBD is characterized by the intermittent loss of muscle atonia during REM sleep. Individuals with RBD may engage in elaborate behavioral sequences during REM sleep. If awakened during an episode, individuals are likely to report dreams that correspond to their behavior. Episodes typically occur once a week but may occur several times per night on consecutive nights. Polysomnographically, REM behavior disordered individuals exhibit normal, more rapid eye movements than usual, and substantial muscle tonus.

Little is known about the overall prevalence of RBD; the largest series of cases consists of sixty-eight patients (Schenck & Mahowald, 1990). The disorder occurs primarily in elderly men, and there is some evidence of a familial pattern (ASDA, 1997).

RBD has been considered a human analog of experimental work in animals that found that REM without atonia could be produced by ablating regions in the pons and medulla (Morrison, 1988). Extensive neurological and neuropsychological evaluation of twenty-one RBD patients revealed that 38% evidenced discernible brain damage and the remaining were classified as "idiopathic" (Mahowald & Schenck, 1994).

## Other Parasomnias

Other parasomnias that are not easily classified include sleep enuresis, sleep bruxism, and sudden infant death syndrome.

**Sleep Enuresis.** Sleep, or nocturnal, enuresis is involuntary urination during the night that occurs primarily in children. Enuretic children are commonly described by their parents as very deep sleepers, a report consistent with laboratory findings of increased duration of slow-wave sleep relative to nonenuretic children (Andres & Weinstein, 1972). Enuresis should not be considered an indication of psychopathology in children under age five, particularly boys, because its prevalence among 4-year-old boys is 14–38% (Feldman, 1983).

There are two types of sleep enuresis, primary and secondary. A child with primary enuresis has always had bed-wetting problems and has never had any extended dry periods. Typically, children with primary bed-wetting problems are less than 8 years old. A child with secondary enuresis is one who develops enuresis after having had extended dry periods. The onset of secondary enuresis is often at times of emotional distress. Primary enuresis is more likely to be genetic than secondary enuresis (Kales, Soldatos, & Kales, 1980) and is more likely to be influenced by biological factors such as a smaller bladder (Troup & Hodgson, 1971). Enuresis can occur in any stage of sleep, including nocturnal awakenings, and is most common during the first third of the night (ASDA, 1997).

Treatment for sleep enuresis includes bladder training aimed at increasing bladder capacity and control, use of the "bell and pad" system based on classical conditioning, and a combination of information, support, and reinforcement strategies. The efficacy of bladder training is about 30%, but the bell-and-pad treatment has success rates as high as 70%; with the best results have been in children older than 7 years (McClain, 1979). A common pharmacological treatment involves desmopressin, an antidiuretic hormone, which, it has been shown, reduces the number of wet nights in primary enuresis (Hansen & Jorgessen, 1997). The efficacy of desmopressin treatment may be greater for children who exhibit decreased levels of psychosocial distress (Dittmann & Wolter, 1996). Tricyclic antidepressants have relatively low success rates and high relapse rates upon withdrawal (Kales, Soldatos, & Kales, 1980).

**Sleep Bruxism.** Bruxism involves grinding or clenching teeth during sleep. Bruxism can occur during all stages of sleep but most commonly occurs during stage 2. As much as 90% of the population reports that they have ground their teeth some time during their lifetimes. In about 5% of them, the problem may be severe enough to require treatment (ASDA, 1997) and can lead to dental damage and temporomandibular joint (TMJ) disorders. Severe bruxism is often associated with daytime anxiety.

A common treatment is a rubber mouth guard worn over the teeth (Lavigne & Manzini, 2000). In some cases, relaxation training or biofeedback has been effective. In a double-blind clinical trial, the administration of L-dopa, it was shown, significantly decreased the number of bruxism episodes (Lobbezzo et al., 1997).

**Sudden Infant Death Syndrome (SIDS).** SIDS is characterized by sudden death during nocturnal sleep in the absence of definable pathology. Epidemiological studies have indicated that the following groups are at increased risk (ASDA, 1997): premature infants, twin or triple births, subsequent siblings of SIDS infants, infants born to substance-abusing mothers, infants who previously experienced apparent life-threatening events (ALTEs) that required mouth-to-mouth resuscitation or vigorous stimulation, infants of low socioeconomic parents, and African-American or Eskimo infants. SIDS, it is estimated, occurs in 1 to 2 per 1000 live births and is most likely to occur between the tenth and twelfth weeks of life. SIDS occurs slightly more frequently in males then females.

Polysomnographic evaluation in one group of infants who subsequently died of SIDS found three variables that differentiated SIDS victims from matched controls (Blum et al., 1988). All of the variables were related to respiratory function. More specifically, the authors found that the maximal duration of central apneas, the number of sighs followed by a central apnea, and the presence of obstructive or mixed apneas "significantly characterized the future SIDS victims." However, only 7% of those infants who had ALTEs show evidence of apnea (Ariagno, 1987). Thus, infant sleep apnea may not be the primary cause of SIDS.

# Sleep Disorders Associated with Other Disorders

## Sleep Disorders Associated with Mental Disorders

**Schizophrenia.** The majority of schizophrenics who undergo acute psychotic phases experience some sleep disturbance. It has been proposed that different sleep architectures might be useful diagnosing whether an acute psychotic episode is approaching or dissolving (Kupfer et al., 1970). Schizophrenics in the waxing phase of an acute psychotic period have low total sleep times and very disrupted sleep. These patients took an average of 152 minutes to fall asleep. Their quantities of slow-wave sleep and REM sleep were also significantly less than those of the controls. In contrast to these findings, schizophrenics in the waning phase displayed a slight return of their sleep parameters toward those of the controls. During remission, the schizophrenics' sleep resembled the controls' sleep values.

A number of studies have found shortened REM latencies in schizophrenics (Hiatt et al., 1985; Zarcone et al., 1987) and decreases in slow-wave sleep (Feinberg et al., 1969; Hiatt et al., 1985). An exception to these findings come from studies of young schizophrenics who had never been medicated. They exhibited normal REM latencies (Ganguli et al., 1987). In contrast to the findings for REM latency, a recent study of medicated and neuroleptic-naive, first-episode, schizophrenic patients found decreased amounts of slow-wave sleep in both groups (Keshavan et al., 1998), which may indicate that slow-wave sleep is more related to the pathophysiology of schizophrenia than REM sleep.

One puzzling observation about the sleep of schizophrenics concerns their response to experimental REM deprivation. It has been a consistent finding that acutely psychotic schizophrenics fail to exhibit REM rebound after REM deprivation (Gillin et al., 1974; Zarcone et al., 1969). One possible explanation is that hallucinations and other positive symptoms may be an expression of a REM process (Cartwright, 1978). Because acutely psychotic schizophrenics have hallucinations, they may not need as much REM during the night as nonpsychotic individuals. Another REM phenomena, dreaming, seems to be deficient in schizophrenics. Schizophrenics awakened during REM sleep often report sparse dream content. Patients have reported dreams that consisted of single objects alone without contextual cues (Dement, 1955).

The effect of antipsychotic medications on the sleep of schizophrenics remains somewhat unclear. There have been contradictory reports whether there are increases in slow-wave sleep, total sleep, and REM sleep in schizophrenics due to clorpromazine, flenfluradol, and haloperidol (Zarcone, 1988). In a longitudinal study, schizophrenic patients, free from medication for at least two weeks, were studied at baseline, 4 weeks, and 1 year after beginning treatment (Keshavan, Reynolds, Miewald, & Montrose, 1996). At 4 weeks, sleep continuity significantly improved, and REM latency showed a modest, nonsignificant increase; at the 1-year assessment, REM latency, time, and density significantly increased. It is unclear, however, whether these changes resulted from medication or a change in the illness state, or both. Slow-wave sleep did not change from baseline to the 1 year follow-up. The effects of clozapine were recently assessed in a population of long-term medication-free schizophrenics (Hinze-Selch, Mullington, Orth, Lauer, & Pollmächer, 1997). Clozapine significantly increased sleep continuity, REM density (but not REM time), and NREM sleep, particularly, stage 2 sleep, whereas stage 4 sleep significantly decreased.

## Mood Disorders

**Depression.** Sleep problems are one of the primary symptoms of a major depressive episode (DSM-IV, 1994). It is estimated that approximately 90% of all individuals with depression will have at least a mild degree of abnormality in sleep architecture (Reynolds, 1989). Conversely, about 21% of persons who reported serious insomnia have major depression (Mellinger et al., 1985).

An extensive body of research identifies sleep EEG abnormalities of patients with major depression (see Benca et al., 1992, for a meta-analytic review of these results). These abnormalities can be grouped into three general categories. The first category, sleep continuity disturbances, includes prolonged sleep latency, increased wakefulness after sleep onset, and, most notably, early morning awakenings; all contribute to decreased sleep efficiency (see Benca, 1994). Sleep continuity disturbances lead depressed patients to complain about poor sleep and such complaints often precede the relapse of remitted depression (Perlis et al., 1997). The second category, slow-wave sleep (SWS) deficits, includes a reduction of amount and percent SWS primarily during the first non-REM period (Kupfer et al., 1986; Reynolds et al., 1985). Depressed men show a greater reduction in slow-wave sleep than depressed women (Reynolds et al., 1990). The third category, REM sleep abnormalities, includes reduced latency to the first REM episode, prolonged duration of the first REM episode, and an increased rate of rapid eye movement, also referred to as increased REM density (Vogel, 1981). This category includes the most robust findings regarding the sleep of depressed

patients. Approximately 60% of depressed outpatients (Rush et al., 1982a) have reduced REM latencies, compared with only about 9% of matched controls. Note, however, that shortened REM latency is not specific to major depression. Short REM latencies have been found in patients with narcolepsy, schizophrenia, alcoholism, and post-traumatic stress disorder (Benca, 1994).

The relationship between sleep abnormalities, particularly REM sleep abnormalities and depression, is also evidenced by the fact that REM sleep deprivation in the laboratory, as well as total sleep deprivation, often improves depressive symptoms with a time course that parallels the effects of antidepressants (King, 1977; Mendelson, 1987; Vogel, 1975). Some EEG sleep disturbances such as high REM density and low sleep efficiency are often normalized after successful treatment, whereas others, such as SWS abnormalities, remain unaffected. Normalization of sleep occurs following successful treatment regardless of modality. This includes electroconvulsive therapy (Lahmeyer et al., 1989), pharmacotherapy, and psychotherapy. Antidepressants have a suppressant effect on REM sleep (Vogel et al., 1990) and often lengthen the REM latency significantly (Roth et al., 1982). Successful psychotherapy reduces REM density but does not alter REM latencies. It has been suggested that individuals with short latency to REM sleep and with increased eye movements during REM sleep (REM density) have a better response to pharmacotherapy. In contrast, EEG sleep abnormalities do not predict response to psychotherapy regardless of the type therapy, be it individual (Buysse et al., 1992; Jarret et al., 1990) or group therapy (Corbishley et al., 1990) or interpersonal (Buysse et al., 1992) or cognitive behavioral therapy (Jarret et al., 1990) in a sample of outpatients (Thase et al., 1994) or inpatients (Thase, Simons, & Reynolds, 1993). However, a recent study that used a composite of EEG sleep parameters in a large sample of outpatients with a definite or probable endogenous subtype of depression to predict response to individual CBT (Thase, Simons, & Reynolds, 1993) found that abnormal sleep profiles and higher severity of pretreatment depression were independently associated with poorer outcome, including lower recovery rates and higher risks of recurrence.

The extensive body of research on sleep and depression has led to formulation of several theories on the etiology of depression, including malfunction of either a REM sleep activation mechanism, a slow-wave activating and REM sleep inhibition system, some component of a circadian timing circuit, or some combination of the three. The fact that some sleep abnormalities persist beyond the active phase of the depression and may be present even before the first episode of depression indicates that sleep abnormalities may reflect a vulnerability for depression (Giles et al., 1990; Hauri et al., 1974).

**Mania.** In comparison to unipolar depression, there is a dearth of research on mania and sleep. Manic patients have extended periods of wakefulness, short total sleep times, long sleep latencies, and deficits in slow-wave sleep (ASDA, 1997). Manic patients also have the same shortened REM latencies and more dense REM episodes as depressed patients (Hudson et al., 1990).

**Seasonal Affective Disorder (SAD).** SAD is a disorder involving an annual fluctuation in mood which has been correlatively linked to seasonal fluctuations of melatonin levels and variations in the period of sunlight. SAD patients present with problems in sleep quantity, sleep quality, and circadian phase position or the timing of sleep and wake. SAD has become one of the most rapidly expanding areas in sleep research as well as in affective disorder research. Strengthening the circadian oscillation in these individuals through light therapy alleviates the sleep problems and improves mood (Rosenthal et al., 1984). Light therapy clears up both the nocturnal sleep problems and the daytime sleepiness (Terman, 1994).

### Anxiety Disorders

This category includes generalized anxiety disorder, obsessive-compulsive disorder, simple and social phobias, and posttraumatic stress disorder. Sleep disturbances involve sleep onset or sleep maintenance insomnia (ASDA, 1997).

**Generalized Anxiety Disorder (GAD).** Patients with GAD have increased sleep latencies, diminished REM and slow-wave sleep, a higher number of transitions to light NREM sleep, increased waking during the sleep period, and decreased efficiency of sleep (Fuller, Waters, Binks, & Anderson, 1997; Reynolds, Shaw, Newton, Coble, & Kupfer, 1983). GAD patients are distinguishable from depressed patients by longer REM latencies and from psychophysiological insomniacs by persistently poor sleep efficiency.

**Obsessive-Compulsive Disorder (OCD).** OCD patients have lower total sleep times, more awakenings, less NREM stage 4, and significantly shorter REM latencies than controls (Insel et al., 1982). Short REM latencies for OCD patients, similar to those seen in depressives, have been reported by some (Insel et al., 1982) but not by others (Hohagen et al., 1994).

**Posttraumatic Stress Disorder (PTSD).** The sleep of PTSD patients often includes terrifying nightmares. Estimates of the percentage of Vietnam veterans who suffer from nightmares have ranged from about 59–68% (DeFazio et al., 1975; van der Kolk et al., 1980). In PTSD patients, nightmares reportedly involve the same near-real-life scenes that occur over and over again, as opposed to the changing nightmare content of the chronic, non-PTSD nightmare sufferers (Hartmann, 1987). As mentioned earlier, nightmares occur frequently in normal populations (Wood & Bootzin, 1990). Thus, nightmares alone are insufficient for a diagnosis of PTSD.

Polysomnographic evaluations of the sleep of PTSD patients have revealed inconsistent and inconclusive abnormal sleep parameters. Some PTSD patients exhibit short REM latencies and high REM densities (Greenberg et al., 1972; Kauffman et al., 1987). Others exhibit increased REM latencies and less total REM time (Lavie, et al., 1979).

### Panic Disorder

Panic attacks during sleep are sudden awakenings associated with intense fear. Although very similar to sleep terrors, panic attacks do not begin with a piercing scream, and they occur in stage 2 or 3, rather than stage 4 sleep. Sleep panic attacks usually occur in individuals who have daytime panic attacks. Out of a group of forty-five patients who had panic attacks, thirty-one (69%) reportedly had at least one nocturnal panic attack in their lives. Occasional or frequent sleep panic attacks were reported by fifteen (33%) of the group (Mellman & Uhde, 1989b).

Several findings emerge consistently in the literature on sleep panic attacks. Panic attack patients have increased sleep latencies, decreased sleep efficiency, and increased duration and number of body movements (Hauri et al., 1989; Mellman & Uhde, 1989a,b; Uhde et al., 1985). There is no consistent evidence of any abnormality of REM in panic attack patients.

Roy-Byrne et al. (1986) examined the effects of a night of total sleep deprivation on patients with panic disorder, along with depressed patients and normal controls. Unlike the improvement in mood and anxiety ratings evidenced in the depressed patients, the panic attack patients and controls showed no significant effects. However, when analyzing the data from the patients with panic disorder, two subgroups emerged. One group showed no change, whereas the other actually displayed an increase in next-day panic attacks and anxiety ratings. Although panic disorder and depression, it has been hypothesized, are related because both respond to antidepressants, the sleep findings indicate that they are independent disorders. Patients with nocturnal panic respond to cognitive-behavioral treatments for panic disorder (Craske & Rowe, 1997), indicating that the same principles are likely to operate in both types of panic disorder patients.

## Alcoholism

Insomnia or excessive sleepiness is a common feature of alcoholism (ASDA, 1997). Alcohol often enhances early slow-wave sleep in alcoholics and decreases early REM. There is increased REM and wakefulness during the second half of the night. The acute effects of withdrawal are somewhat inconsistent. Sleep may be more fragmented soon after drinking stops, and associated increases occur in REM sleep (Johnson, 1972). In two samples of nondepressed alcoholics, shortened REM latency and increased REM percentage upon admission to an alcohol treatment program predicted relapse within a 3-month abstinence period (Gillin et al., 1994). Fragmented and reduced slow-wave sleep has been recorded in recovering alcoholics as long as 2 years after drinking ceased (Adamson & Burdick, 1973). Acute alcohol use may also precipitate or exacerbate snoring and sleep apnea (ASDA, 1997).

## Sleep Disorders Associated with Neurological Disorders

A variety of neurological disorders affect sleep. For more detail, see Aldrich (2000b), Bliwise (2000b), and Lugaresi et al. (1988).

**Cerebral Degenerative Disorders.** Cerebral degenerative disorders encompass a group of heterogeneous diseases (e.g., Huntington's disease, torsion dystonia, supranuclear palsy, and multiple system atrophy) that affect one or more systems and are progressive conditions characterized by abnormal behaviors or involuntary movements, often with evidence of motor system dysfunction. Complaints of insomnia and hypersomnia are common. Sleep disturbance manifestations of these disorders include sleep fragmentation, abnormal motor activities, and disorganization of the circadian sleep-wake cycle. Polysomnography may reveal sleep fragmentation, decreased slow-wave sleep or REM sleep, disordered breathing, fragmentary myoclonus, periodic arm or leg movements, dystonic postures, and prolonged tonic contractions of one or more limb (ASDA, 1997; Chokroverty, 1996).

**Dementia and Parkinsonism.** Dementia refers to a loss of higher cortical functions due to a chronic, progressive degenerative disease process of the brain. Dementing illnesses include a wide variety of nonreversible conditions, including Alzheimer's disease (AD), Pick's disease, and certain forms of hydrocephalus. AD, the most common cause of dementia, accounts for as much as 70% of all cases (Bliwise, 2000b). Sleep disturbances in demented patients are very common. Their severity parallels the progression of the underlying illness, and their pathophysiology is probably related to the dementia process itself. In addition, demented patients are often treated with psychotropic medicines, and these drugs may worsen sleep disturbances and daytime symptoms. Nighttime behavior of demented patients is characterized by delirium, agitation, and sundown syndrome (ASDA, 1997). *Sundowning* is to the phenomenon of agitation strongly associated with darkness and is characterized by nocturnal wandering and confusion. Polysomnographic studies of AD patients have documented altered sleep architecture, including decreased sleep efficiency, slow-wave, and REM sleep, increased Stage 1 sleep, and an increase in the number of and duration of nocturnal awakenings (Prinz, 1995). Some patients also exhibit a fragmented 24-hour sleep-wake pattern in the form of partial or complete reversal of the sleep-wake schedule, with increased wakefulness at night and somnolence during the daytime (Chokroverty, 1996).

Parkinsonism is a group of neurological disorders characterized by resting tremor, akinesia (reduced spontaneous movement), postural rigidity, and bradykinesia (slowness of movement). Sleep disturbance is reported by 60–90% of patients with Parkinson's disease (PD), and it tends to gradually worsen with disease progression. Insomnia is the most common complaint in these patients. The inability to get out of or turn over in bed, nocturia, painful leg cramps, back pain, limb jerks, central or obstructive sleep apnea, and medication sleep effects can all cause insomnia, sometimes with concomitant daytime sleepiness (Aldrich, 1994, ASDA, 1997; Partinen, 1997).

Characteristic polysomnographic abnormalities in PD patients include increased sleep latency, Stage 1 sleep, and the number and duration of nocturnal awakenings, as well as reduced amounts of REM and slow-wave sleep. Sleep disordered breathing (various forms of sleep apnea), REM sleep behavior disorder (RBD), and periodic limb movement disorder (PLMS) are prevalent in PD patients and can further disrupt their sleep or produce daytime sleepiness. Levodopa treatment of Parkinsonism can improve sleep disturbance due to such symptoms of the disease as rigidity or bradykinesia, but it may at the same time cause new symptoms (e.g., insomnia, vivid dreaming, nocturnal vocalizations, myoclonic movements, dyskinesias). Depression, which is a common comorbid illness in PD patients, can also contribute to sleep disturbance (Chokroverty, 1996).

**Sleep-Related Epilepsy.** Sleep-related epilepsy is associated with either abrupt awakenings, unexplained urinary incontinence, or abnormal muscle activity during sleep. To be considered sleep-related epilepsy, 75% or more of the seizures must occur during sleep and at least two other features must be present: automatisms, specific limb movements, or tongue biting (ASDA, 1997). Individuals suspected of this disorder usually undergo daytime EEG monitoring, nocturnal polysomnography with video monitoring, and possibly CT or MRI scanning.

**Sleep-Related Headaches.** Cluster or migraine headaches that occur during sleep are related to REM sleep. Breathing disturbances during sleep or alcohol ingestion may bring on cluster headaches. High levels of daytime stress, weather change, or other events may precipitate migraine headaches during sleep. Individuals typically awaken from sleep, usually late in the sleeping period and out of a REM period, aware of the presence of the headache.

## Sleep Disorders Associated with Medical Disorders

A broad range of physical illnesses affects sleep. Our discussion is selective and focuses on respiratory disorders, nocturnal cardiac ischemia, chronic pain, fibromyalgia, and AIDS.

**Respiratory Disorders.** Respiratory disorders that affect sleep include disorders of respiratory control, disorders of the respiratory musculature, and disease of the airways and lung parenchyma. Respiratory disorders often worsen during sleep and cause sleep disturbances. The severity of sleep disturbances correlates with the progression of the underlying pulmonary disease. Chronic obstructive pulmonary disease (COPD) and asthma are the respiratory disorders that frequently lead to sleep complaints.

COPD is characterized by a chronic reduction in airflow, with symptoms of dyspnea and cough are most common. Hypoxemia, hypoventilation, and impaired lung function are the physiological consequences. A high percentage of patients with COPD experience difficulty in initiating and maintaining sleep (Douglas, 2000). Shortness of breath in the recumbent position and frequent episodes of coughing keep COPD patients from falling asleep. Severe sleep fragmentation, again due to respiratory symptoms, often leads to a unrefreshed feeling upon awakening and to excessive daytime sleepiness. Polysomnographic features include decreased total sleep time, the amount of slow-wave and REM sleep, frequent sleep-stage changes, and increased number of arousals and awakenings. COPD patients become more hypoxemic during sleep, especially in REM sleep, than during resting wakefulness, because of hypoventilation, worsening ventilation perfusion mismatch, the loss of accessory muscles, and the medicines used to treat COPD; the xanthine derivatives particularly such as theophylline can also contribute to sleep disturbance (ASDA, 1997; Douglas, 1998).

Patients with asthma have a reversible reduction in airflow. The reduction can be abrupt and dramatic, triggering acute attacks of wheezing, shortness of breath, coughing, and chest tightness. In general, asthmatic individuals have hyperreactive airways. Exposure to allergens or irritating stimuli produces airway obstruction, secondary to spasm of the bronchial muscles, as well as increased secretion and, if exposures are recurrent, bronchial mucus hyperplasia.

Bronchodilators, such as beta agonists (albuterol, solmeterol) or theophylline compounds ameliorate asthma symptoms but may cause increased wake time during sleep. Many asthmatics patients have symptoms at night; in studies of these patients, 61–74% report nighttime awakenings due to asthmatic attacks. Unrestorative sleep and daytime fatigue are also common complaints of asthmatics. Polysomnographic studies reveal that nocturnal asthma attacks rarely occur in slow-wave sleep and tend to cluster in the later part of the sleep period, perhaps as the bronchodilating effects of medicine taken before bed declines. Hypoxemia with attacks is rarely severe (ASDA, 1997; D'Ambrosio & Mohsenin, 1998). Compared to the sleep of controls, asthmatics patients have less total sleep time, lower sleep efficiency, and more awakenings (Montplaisir et al., 1982).

**Nocturnal Cardiac Ischemia.** The relationship between sleep and cardiac ischemia is controversial because the factors that precipitate nocturnal cardiac ischemia are not clear. It may occur as the result of increased myocardial oxygen demand, decreased cardiac perfusion, or increased filling of the left ventricle from lying in a recumbent position (Motta & Guilleminault, 1985).

Symptoms of nocturnal cardiac ischemia include the feeling of pressure during sleep that is often described as a "clenched fist." Pain often radiates to the left arm and upward into the neck or jaw (ASDA, 1997). These symptoms may be present during waking hours but result from activity.

The prevalence of nocturnal cardiac ischemia is unknown. However, patients with obstructive sleep apnea may experience severe oxygen desaturation and have a higher incidence of cardiac ischemia than the general population (Burack, 1984). Ischemia can also cause severe sleep fragmentation in the absence of sleep apnea (Schafer, Koehler, Ploch, & Peter, 1997). Electrocardiographic changes that occur in the early morning hours are typically associated with REM sleep, and changes that occur at the beginning of sleep are typically associated with a fall in blood pressure and heart rate.

The presence of ischemia on an electrocardiogram is indicative of coronary artery disease. Other possible precipitating factors of nocturnal ischemia include hypertension, elevated blood cholesterol and low-density lipoprotein, cigarette smoking, obesity, and sleep-induced hypoxemia (ASDA, 1997).

**Chronic Pain.** Chronic pain is a common cause of sleep complaints, especially in the elderly. Rheumatological disorders such as osteoarthritis, a degenerative joint disease, tend to be frequent causes of insomnia. During the day, the joints are kept mobile which helps to maintain flexibility and reduce pain. These joints become stiff at night and sleep may be disturbed by sudden pain when the individual moves or attempts to turn over in bed (Morgan, 1987). Adequate dosage of anti-arthritic medication before bedtime can greatly alleviate the problem.

Other chronic pain conditions that may precipitate complaints of insomnia include burning foot pain from diabetes and chest and epigastric pain due to angina, reflux, esophagitis, or peptic ulcer disease. Cancer patients often exhibit more severely disturbed sleep patterns than either normals or other patients with medical conditions. Complaints of insomnia are often reported with feelings of anxiety or depression rather than pain which has led to the suggestion that antianxiety drugs may help improve sleep (Anch et al., 1988).

**Fibromyalgia.** Fibromyalgia (FMS) is a central nervous system disorder of unknown etiology. Its main symptom is widespread musculoskeletal pain with tenderness in at least eleven of eighteen specific anatomic sites. In addition, symptoms of fibromyalgia include fatigue and dyssomnia, unrefreshing sleep, and a higher than average prevalence of alpha sleep (Moldofsky et al., 1975; Ware, Russell, & Campos, 1986) in which an alpha EEG frequency wave occurs simultaneously with slower EEG waves. Compared with controls, fibromyalgia patients have less delta (0.5–3.5 Hz) and theta (3.5–8 Hz) and more alpha (8–12 Hz) and sigma (12–14.5 Hz) in all stages of sleep, but especially so during NREM sleep (Drewes et al., 1995).

It has been proposed that alpha sleep may cause the musculoskeletal symptoms of fibromyalgia (Moldofsky & Scarisbrick, 1976) and that it may be involved more generally in disorders that affect the immune system. Not surprisingly, there is a strong association between the severity of fibromyalgia, based on clinical examination, as well as on average daily self-rating of pain, and disturbed sleep, as indicated by lower sleep efficiencies and greater morning difficulties (Manber et al., 1998).

**Acquired Immune Deficiency Disorder (AIDS).** Approximately one-third of asymptomatic HIV-seropositive individuals report sleep onset or maintenance difficulties (Rothenberg et al., 1990). These differences are not attributable to those taking zidovudine (AZT) (Moeller, Wiegand, Oechsner, Krieg, Holsboer, & Emminger, 1992). Polysomnographic studies of asymptomatic individuals have often, but not always, found increased sleep fragmentation, increased amounts of slow-wave sleep, slow-wave sleep distributed throughout the night, and an alpha sleep pattern (Norman et al., 1992; Wiegand et al., 1991). Abnormal sleep architecture was evident at a 1-year follow-up (Norman, Chediak, Kiel, Gazeroglu, & Mendez, 1990).

# Conclusion

As indicated throughout this chapter, understanding sleep and sleepiness is crucial to understanding all behavior, including psychopathology. Sleep is a sensitive barometer of the quality of our lives. It is affected by, and in turn affects, developmental, physiological, psychological, and sociocultural processes. To understand sleep disorders, research must continue to be pursued as a multidisciplinary enterprise. This chapter indicates that there have been substantial advances in our understanding of the etiology and treatment of sleep disorders. This has included advances in the neurophysiology and pharmacology of sleep, our understanding of the sleep-wake circadian rhythm, and behavioral treatments for sleep disorders. But this is a field in its infancy, and we eagerly anticipate the advances still to come.

# References

Adair, R., Zuckerman, B., Bauchner, H., Philipp, B., & Levenson, S. (1992). Reducing night waking in infancy: A primary care intervention. *Pediatrics, 89,* 585–588.

Adamson, J., & Burdick, J. A. (1973). Sleep of dry alcoholics. *Archives of General Psychiatry, 28,* 146–149.

Akerstedt, T. (1985). Adjustment of physiological circadian rhythms and the sleep-wake cycle to shift work. In S. Folkard & T. H. Monk (Eds.), *Hours of work: Temporal factors in work scheduling* (pp. 199–210). New York: Wiley.

Akerstedt, T., Torsvall, L., & Gillsberg, M. (1982). Sleepiness and shiftwork: Field studies. *Sleep, 5,* 95–106.

Akpinar, S. (1987). Restless legs syndrome treatment with dopaminergic drugs. *Clinical Neuropharmacology, 10,* 69–79.

Aldrich, M. S. (1994). Parkinsonism. In M. H. Kryger, T. Roth, & W. C. Dement (Eds.), *Principles and practice of sleep medicine* (2nd ed., pp. 783–789). Philadelphia: W.B. Saunders.

Aldrich, M. S. (2000a). Cardinal manifestations of sleep disorders. In M. H. Kryger, T. Roth, & W. C. Dement (Eds.), *Principles and practice of sleep medicine* (3rd ed., pp. 526–533). Philadelphia: W.B. Saunders.

Aldrich, M. S. (2000b). Parkinsonism. In M. H. Kryger, T. Roth, & W. C. Dement (Eds.), *Principles and practice of sleep medicine* (3rd ed., pp. 1051–1057). Philadelphia: W.B. Saunders.

Aldrich, M. S., Chervin, R. D., & Malow, B. A. (1997). Value of the multiple sleep latency test (MSLT) for the diagnosis of narcolepsy. *Sleep, 20,* 620–629.

Allen. R. P. (1991). Early morning awakening insomnia: Bright-light treatment. In P. J. Hauri (Ed.), *Case studies in insomnia* (pp. 207–220). New York: Plenum.

Allen, R., Rosenthal, N., Joseph-Vanderpool, J., Nadean, J., Kelly, K., Schultz, P., & Souetre, G. (1989). Delayed sleep phase syndrome: Polysomnographic characteristic. *Sleep Research, 18,* 133.

American Sleep Disorders Association. (1995a). Practice parameters for the use of polysomnography in the evaluation of insomnia. *Sleep, 18,* 55–57.

American Sleep Disorders Association. (1995b). Practice parameters for the use of actigraphy in the clinical assessment of sleep disorders. *Sleep, 18,* 285–287.

American Sleep Disorders Association [ASDA]. (1997). The international classification of sleep disorders, revised: Diagnostic and coding manual. Rochester, MN: Author.

Amlaner, C. J., Jr., & Ball, N. J. (1994). Avian sleep. In M. H. Kryger, T. Roth, & W. C. Dement (Eds.), *Principles and practice of sleep medicine* (2nd ed., pp. 81–94). Philadelphia: W.B. Saunders.

Anch, A. M., Browman, C. P., Mitler, M. M., & Walsh, J. K. (1988). *Sleep: A scientific perspective.* NJ: Prentice-Hall.

Anch, A. M., Saskin, P., & Moldofsky, H. (1989). Behaviorally signalled awakenings in normals and fibromyalgia patients. *Sleep Research, 18,* 327.

Ancoli-Israel, S. (1997). Sleep problems in older adults: Putting myths to bed. *Geriatrics, 52,* 20–30.

Ancoli-Israel, S., Kripke, D. F., Mason, W., & Massin, S. (1981). Comparisons of home sleep recordings and polysomnograms in older adults with sleep disorders. *Sleep, 10,* 45–56.

Andres, T. F., & Weinstein, P. (1972). Sleep and its disorders in infants and children: A review. *Pediatrics, 50,* 312–324.

Ariagno, R. I. (1987). Infant apnea and the sudden infant death syndrome: The NIH report. Paper presented at symposium on *Monitoring and Evaluation of Sleep/Wake Disorders in the Home and Work Environment,* San Francisco.

Arkin, A. (1978). Sleep talking. In A. Arkin, J. Antrobus, & S. Ellman (Eds.), *The mind in sleep: Psychology and psychophysiology.* New York: Erlbaum.

Ascoff, J. (1978). Features of circadian rhythms relevant for the design of shift schedules. *Ergonomics, 21,* 739–754.

Association of Professional Sleep Societies. (1986). Guidelines for the Multiple Sleep Latency Test (MSLT); A standard measure of sleepiness. *Sleep, 9,* 519–524.

Benca, R. M. (1994). Mood disorders. In M. H. Kryger, T. Roth, & W. C. Dement (Eds.), *Principles and practice of sleep medicine* (2nd ed., pp. 899–913). Philadelphia: W.B. Saunders.

Benca, R. M., Obermeyer, W. H., Thisted, R. A., & Gillin, J. C. (1992). Sleep and psychiatric disorders: A meta analysis. *Archives of General Psychiatry, 49*, 651–668.

Bishop, C., Rosenthal, L., Helmus, T., Roehrs, T., & Roth, T. (1996). The frequency of multiple sleep onset REM periods among subjects with no excessive daytime sleepiness. *Sleep, 19*, 727–730.

Bixler, E. O., Kales, A., Soldatos, C. R., Kales, J. D., & Healey, S. (1979). Prevalence of sleep disorders in the Los Angeles metropolitan area. *American Journal of Psychiatry, 136*, 1257–1262.

Bliwise, D. L. (2000a). Normal aging. In M. H. Kryger, T. Roth, & W. C. Dement (Eds.), *Principles and practice of sleep medicine* (3rd ed., pp. 26–42). Philadelphia: W.B. Saunders.

Bliwise, D. L. (2000b). Dementia. In M. H. Kryger, T. Roth, & W. C. Dement (Eds.), *Principles and practice of sleep medicine* (3rd ed., pp. 1058–1071). Philadelphia: W.B. Saunders.

Blum, K., Rebuffat, E., Levitt, S., Alexander, M., Grosswasser, J., & Muller, M. (1988). Polysomnographic studies in infants who subsequently died of sudden infant death syndrome. *Sleep Research, 17*, 196.

Bootzin, R. R. (1972). A stimulus control treatment for insomnia. *Proceedings of the American Psychological Association*, 395–396.

Bootzin, R. R. (1977). Effects of self-control procedures for insomnia. In R.B. Stuart (Ed.), *Behavioral self-management: Strategies and outcomes*. New York: Brunner/Mazel.

Bootzin, R. R., & Engle-Friedman, M. (1981). The assessment of insomnia. *Behavioral assessment, 3*, 107–126.

Bootzin, R. R., Epstein, D., & Wood, J. M. (1991). Stimulus control instructions. In P. Hauri (Ed.), *Case studies in insomnia*. New York: Plenum.

Bootzin, R. R., Manber, R., Perilis, M. L., Salvio, M. A., & Wyatt, J. K. (1993). Sleep disorders. In P. B. Sutker & H. E. Adams (Eds.), *Comprehensive handbook of psychopathology* (2nd ed., pp. 531–561). New York: Plenum.

Bootzin, R. R., & Nicassio, P. (1978). Behavioral treatments for insomnia. In M. Hersen, R. M. Eisler, & P. M. Miller (Eds.), *Progress in behavior modification*, Vol. 6. New York: Academic Press.

Bootzin, R. R., Quan, S. F., Bamford, C. R., & Wyatt, J. K. (1995). Sleep disorders. *Comprehensive Therapy, 21*, 401–406.

Bootzin, R. R., & Rider, S. (1997). Behavioral techniques and biofeedback for insomnia. In M. R. Pressman & W. C. Orr (Eds.), *Understanding sleep: The evaluation and treatment of sleep disorders*. Washington, DC: American Psychological Association.

Borkovec, T. D., Grayson, J. B., O'Brien, G. T., & Weerts, T. C. (1979). Relaxation treatment of pseudoinsomnia and idiopathic insomnia: An electroencephalographic evaluation. *Journal of Applied Behavior Analysis, 12*, 37–54.

Borkovec, T. D., & Weerts, T. C. (1976). Effects of progressive relaxation on sleep disturbance: An electroencephalographic evaluation. *Psychosomatic Medicine, 38*, 173–180.

Borbely, A. A., & Wirz-Justice, A. (1982). A two-process model of sleep regulation. II. Implications for depression. *Human Neurobiology, 1*, 205–210.

Brown, S. L., Salive, M. E., Pahor, M., Foley, D. J., Corti, C., Langlois, J. A., Wallace, R. B., & Harris, T. B. (1995). Occult caffeine as a source of sleep problems in an older population. *Journal of the American Geriatric Society, 43*, 860–864.

Brownman, C. P. Sampson, M. G., Yolles, S. F., et al. (1984). Obstructive sleep apnea and body weight. *Chest, 85*, 435–436.

Burack, B. (1984). Hypersomnia sleep apnea syndrome: Its recognition in clinical cardiology. *American Heart Journal, 107*, 543–548.

Busto, U., Sellers, E. M., Naranjo, C. A., Cappell, H., Sanches-Craig, M., & Sykora, K. (1986). Withdrawal from long-term therapeutic use of benzodiazepines. *New England Journal of Medicine, 315*, 854–859.

Buysse, D., Kupfer, D. J., Frank, E., Monk, T., Rittenour, A., & Ehlers, C. L. (1992). Electroencephalographic sleep studies in depressed patients treated with psychotherapy, I: Baseline studies in responders and nonresponders. *Psychiatry Research, 42*, 13–26.

Campbell, K., Bell, I., & Bastien, C. (1992). Evoked potential measures of information processing during natural sleep. In R. J. Broughton & R. D. Ogilvie (Eds.), *Sleep, arousal and performance* (pp. 88–116). Boston: Birkhauser.

Carskadon, M. A. (1994). Measuring daytime sleepiness. In M. H. Kryger, T. Roth, & W. C. Dement (Eds.), *Principles and practice of sleep medicine* (2nd ed., pp. 961–966). Philadelphia: W.B. Saunders.

Carskadon, M. A., & Dement, W. C. (1981). Cumulative effects of sleep restriction on daytime sleepiness. *Psychophysiology, 18*, 107–113.

Carskadon, M. A., & Dement, W. C. (1987). Sleepiness in the normal adolescent. In C. Guilleminault (Ed.), *Sleep and its disorders in children* (pp. 53–66). New York: Raven Press.

Carskadon, M. A., & Dement, W. C. (1994). Normal human sleep: An overview. In M. H. Kryger, T. Roth, & W. C. Dement (Eds.), *Principles and practice of sleep medicine* (2nd ed., pp. 16–25). Philadelphia: W.B. Saunders.

Carskadon, M. A., Dement, W. C., Mitler, M. M., et al. (1986). Guidelines for the Multiple Sleep Latency Test (MSLT): A standard measure of sleepiness. *Sleep, 9*, 519–524.

Carskadon, M. A., Dement, W. C., Mitler, M. M., Guilleminault, C., Zarcone, V. P., & Spiegel, R. (1976). Self-reports versus sleep laboratory findings in 122 drug-free subjects with complaints of chronic insomnia. *American Journal of Psychiatry, 133*, 1382–1388.

Carskadon, M. A., Littell, W. P., & Dement, W. C. (1985). Constant routine: Alertness, oral body temperature, and performance. *Sleep Research, 14*, 293.

Carskadon, M. A., Mancuso, J., & Rosekind, M. R. (1989). Impact of part-time employment on adolescent sleep patterns. *Sleep Research, 18*, 114.

Carskadon, M. A., van den Hoed, J., & Dement, W. C. (1980). Insomnia and sleep disturbances in the aged: Sleep and daytime sleepiness in the elderly. *Journal of Geriatric Psychiatry, 13*, 135–151.

Carskadon, M. A., Viera, C., & Acebo, C. (1993). Association between puberty and delayed phase preference. *Sleep, 16*, 258–262.

Cartwright, R. D. (1978). *A primer on sleep and dreaming*. Reading, MA: Addison-Wesley.

Cartwright, R. D., Lloyd, S., Lilie, J., & Kravitz, H. (1985). Sleep position training as treatment for sleep apnea syndrome: A preliminary study. *Sleep, 8*, 87–94.

Cashman, M. A., & McCann, B. S. (1988). Behavioral approaches to sleep/wake disorders in children and adolescents. In M. Hersen, R. M. Eisler, & P. M. Miller (Eds.), *Progress in behavior modification* (pp. 215–283). Newbury Park, CA: Sage.

Chan, J. K. W., Leung, R. C. C., & Lai, C. K. W. (1998). Diagnosis and treatment of obstructive sleep apnea. *Clinical Pulmonary Medicine, 5,* 60–68.

Chase, J. E., & Gidal, B. E. (1997). Melatonin: Therapeutic use in sleep disorders. *Annals of Pharmacotherapy, 31*(10), 1218–1226.

Chervin, R. D., & Guilleminault, C. (1996). Obstructive sleep apnea and related disorders. *Neurologic Clinics, 14,* 583–609.

Choo, K. L., & Guilleminault, C. (1998). Narcolepsy and idiopathic hypersomnolence. *Clinics in Chest Medicine, 19,* 169–181.

Chokroverty, S. (1996). Sleep and degenerative neurologic disorders. *Neurologic Clinics, 14,* 807–826.

Clarkson, S., Williams, S., & Silva, P. A. (1986). Sleep in middle childhood: A longitudinal study of sleep problems in a large sample of Dunedin children aged 5–9 years. *Australian Pediatric Journal, 22,* 31–35.

Conway, W., Fujita, S., Zorick, F., et al. (1985). Uvulopalatopharyngoplasty: A one-year followup. *Chest, 88,* 385–387.

Corbishley, M., Beutler, L., Quan, S., Bamford, C., Meredith, K., & Scogin, F. (1990). Rapid eye movement density and latency and dexamethasone suppression as predictors of treatment response in depressed older adults. *Current Therapy Research, 47,* 846–859.

Craske, M. G., & Rowe, M. K. (1997). Nocturnal panic. *Clinical Psychology: Research and Practice, 4,* 153–174.

Czeisler, C. A., Allan, J. S., Strogatz, S. H., Ronda, J. M., Sanchez, R., Rios, C. D., Frietag, W. O., Richardson, G. S., & Kronauer, R. E. (1986). Bright light resets the human circadian pacemaker independent of the timing of the sleep-wake cycle. *Science, 233,* 667.

Czeisler, C. A., Duffy, J. F., Shanahan, T. L., Brown, E. N., Mitchell, J. F., Rimmer, D. W., Ronda, J. M., Silva, E. J., Allan, J. S., Emens, J. S., Dijk, D.-J., & Kronauer, R. E. (1999). Stability, precision, and near-24-hour period of the human circadian pacemaker. *Science, 284,* 2177–2181.

Czeisler, C. A., Johnson, M. P., Duffy, J. F., Brown, E. N., Ronda, J. M., & Kronauer, R. E. (1990). The effect of scheduled exposure to bright light and darkness on reported daytime sleep duration in simulated night work. *Sleep Research, 19,* 391.

Czeisler, C. A., Kronauer, R. E., Allen, J. S., Duffy, J. F., Jewett, M. E., Brown, E. N., & Ronda, J. M. (1989). Bright light induction of strong (type 0) resetting of the human circadian pacemaker. *Science, 244,* 1328–1333.

Czeisler, C. A., Richardson, G. S., Coleman, R. M., Zimmerman, J. C., Moore-Ede, M. C., Dement, W. C., & Weitzman, E. D. (1981). Chronotherapy: Resetting the circadian clocks of patients with delayed sleep phase insomnia. *Sleep, 4,* 1–21.

Daan, S., & Lewy, A. J. (1984). Scheduled exposure to daylight: A potential strategy to reduce "jet lag" following transmeridian flight. *Psychopharmacology Bulletin, 20,* 566–568.

D'Ambrosio, C. M., & Mohsenin, V. (1998). Sleep in asthma. *Clinics in Chest Medicine, 19,* 127–137.

Dahl, R. E. (1992). The pharmacologic treatment of sleep disorder. *Psychiatric Clinics of North America, 1,* 161–178.

DeFazio, V. J., Rustin, S., & Diamond, A. (1975). Symptom development in Vietnam era veterans. *American Journal of Orthopsychiatry, 45,* 158–163.

Dement, W. C. (1955). Dream recall and eye movements during sleep in schizophrenics and normals. *Journal of Nervous and Mental Disease, 122*(3), 263–269.

Dement, W. C., Carskadon, M. A., & Richardson, G. S. (1978). Excessive daytime sleepiness in the sleep apnea syndrome. In C. Guilleminault & W. C. Dement (Eds.), *Sleep apnea syndromes* (pp. 23–46). New York: Alan R. Liss.

Dement, W. C., Miles, L. E., & Carskadon, M. A. (1982). "White paper" on sleep and aging. *Journal of the American Geriatrics Society, 30,* 25–50.

Dinges, D. F. (1992). Probing the limits of functional capability: The effects of sleep loss on short-duration tasks. In R. J. Broughton & R. D. Ogilvie (Eds.), *Sleep, arousal, and performance* (pp. 177–188). Boston: Birkhauser.

Dinges, D. F., Pack, F., Williams, K., Gillen, K. A., Powell, J. W., Ott, G. E., Aptowicz, C., & Pack, A. I. (1997). Cumulative sleepiness, mood disturbance, and psychomotor vigilance performance decrements during a week of sleep restricted to 4–5 hours per night. *Sleep, 29*(4): 267–277.

Dittmann, R. W., & Wolter, S. (1996). Primary nocturnal enuresis and desmopressin treatment: do psychosocial factors affect outcome? *European Child and Adolescent Psychiatry, 5*(2): 101–109.

Doghramji, K., Mitler, M. M., Sangal, R. B., Shapiro, C., Taylor, S., Walsleben, J., Belisle, C., Erman, M. K., Hayduk, R., Hosn, R., O'Malley, E. B., Sangal, J. M., Schutte, S. L., & Youakim, J. M. (1997). A normative study of the maintenance of wakefulness test (MWT). *Electroencephalography and Clinical Neurophysiology, 103,* 554–562.

Dorsey, C., & Bootzin, R. R. (1987). Subjective and psychophysiologic insomnia: Multiple sleep latency test, sleep tendency, and personality. *Sleep Research, 16,* 328.

Douglas, N. J. (1998). Sleep in patients with chronic obstructive pulmonary disease. *Clinics in Chest Medicine, 19,* 115–125.

Dougles, N. J. (2000). Chronic obstructive pulmonary disease. In M. H. Kryger, T. Roth, & W. C. Dement (Eds.), *Principles and practice of sleep medicine* (3rd ed., pp. 965–975). Philadelphia: W.B. Saunders.

Drewes, A. M., Gade, K., Nielsen, K. D., Bjerregard, K., Taagholt, S. J., & Svendsen, L. (1995). Clustering of sleep electroencephalographic patterns in patients with the fibromyalgia syndrome. *British Journal of Rheumatology, 34,* 1151–1156.

Durand, V. M., & Mindell, J. A. (1990). Behavioral treatment of multiple childhood sleep disorders. *Behavior Modification, 14,* 37–49.

Edinger, J. D., Morey, M. C., Sullivan, R. J., Higginbotham, M. B., Marsh, G. R., Dailey, D. S., & McCall, W. V. (1993). Aerobic fitness, acute exercise and sleep in older men. *Sleep, 16,* 351–359.

Ehlers, C. L., & Kupfer, D. J. (1997). Slow-wave sleep: Do young adult men and women age differently? *Journal of Sleep Research, 6,* 211–215.

Engleman, H. M., Martin, S. E., Deary, I. J., & Douglas, N. J. (1997). Effect of CPAP therapy on daytime function in patients with mild sleep apnoea/hypopnoea syndrome. *Thorax, 52,* 114–119.

Espie, C. A., Inglis, S. J., Tessier, S., & Harvey, L. (2001). The clinical effectiveness of cognitive behaviour therapy for chronic insomnia: Implementation and evaluation of a sleep clinic in general medical practice. *Behaviour Research and Therapy, 39,* 45–60.

Feinberg, I., Braun, M., Koresko, R. L., & Gottlieb, F. (1969). Stage 4 sleep in schizophrenia. *Archives of General Psychiatry, 21,* 262–266.

Feinberg, I., Koresko, R., & Heller, N. (1967). EEG sleep patterns as a function of normal and pathological aging in man. *Journal of Psychiatric Research, 5,* 107–144.

Feinberg, I., March, J. D., Floyd, T. C., Jimison, R., Bossom-Demitrach, L., & Katz, P. H. (1985). Homeostatic changes during postnap sleep maintain baseline levels of delta EEG. *Electroencephalography and Clinical Neurophysiology, 61,* 134–137.

Feldman, W. (1983). Nocturnal enuresis. *Canadian Medical Association Journal, 128,* 114–116.

Ferber, R. (1985). *Solve your child's sleep problems.* New York: Simon & Schuster.

Ferber, R. (1990). Sleep-schedule dependent causes of insomnia and sleepiness in middle childhood and adolescence. *Pediatrician, 17,* 13–20.

Ferber, R., & Boyle M. D. (1983). Delayed sleep phase syndrome versus motivated sleep phase delay in adolescents. *Sleep Research, 12,* 239.

Ferber, R., & Kryger, M. (Eds.). (1995). *Principles and practices of sleep medicine in the child.* Philadelphia: W. B. Saunders.

Franklin, J. (1981). The measurement of sleep onset latency in insomnia. *Behavioural Research and Therapy, 19,* 547–549.

Fredrickson, P. A., & Krueger, B. R. (1994). Insomnia associated with specific polysomnographic findings. In M. H. Kryger, T. Roth, & W. C. Dement (Eds.), *Principles and practice of sleep medicine* (2nd ed., pp. 523–534). Philadelphia: W.B. Saunders.

Fuller, K. H., Waters, W. F., Binks, P. G., & Anderson, T. (1997). Generalized sleep anxiety and sleep architecture: a polysomnographic investigation. *Sleep, 20*(5), 370–376.

Ganguli, R., Reynolds, C. F., III, & Kupfer, D. J. (1987). Electroencephalographic sleep in young, never-medicated schizophrenics. *Archives of General Psychiatry, 44,* 36–44.

Giles, D. E., Kupfer, D. J., & Roffwarg, H. P. (1990). EEG sleep before and after the first episode of depression. *Sleep Research, 19,* 161.

Gillin, J. C. (1994). Sleep and psychoactive drugs of abuse and dependence. In M. H. Kryger, T. Roth, & W. C. Dement (Eds.), *Principles and practice of sleep medicine* (2nd ed., pp. 934–942). Philadelphia: W.B. Saunders.

Gillin, J. C., Buchsbaum, M. S., Jacobs, L. S., Fram, D. H., Williams, R. B. J., Vaughan, T. B. J., Mellon, E., Snyder, F., & Wyatt, R. J. (1974). Partial REM sleep deprivation, schizophrenia, and field articulation. *Archives of General Psychiatry, 30,* 653–662.

Gillin, J. C., & Byerley, W. F. (1990). The diagnosis and management of insomnia. *New England Journal of Medicine, 322,* 239–248.

Gillin, J. C., Smith, T. L., Irwin, M., Butters, N., Demodena, A., & Schuckit, M. (1994). Increased pressure for rapid eye movement sleep at time of hospital admission predicts relapse in nondepressed patients with primary alcoholism at 3-month follow-up. *Archives of General Psychiatry, 51*(3), 189–197.

Graziano, A. M., Mooney, K. C., Huber, C., & Ignasiak, D. (1979). Self control instructions for children's fear-reduction. *Journal of Behaviour Therapy and Experimental Psychiatry, 10,* 221–227.

Greenberg, R., Pearlman, C. A., & Gampel, D. (1972). War neuroses and the adaptive function of REM sleep. *British Journal of Medical Psychology, 45,* 27–33.

Guilleminault, C. (1994a). Narcolepsy syndrome. In M. H. Kryger, T. Roth, & W. C. Dement (Eds.), *Principles and practice of sleep medicine* (2nd ed., pp. 549–561). Philadelphia: W.B. Saunders.

Guilleminault, C. (1994b). Clinical features and evaluation of obstructive sleep apnea. In M. H. Kryger, T. Roth, & W. C. Dement (Eds.), *Principles and practice of sleep medicine* (2nd ed., pp. 667–677). Philadelphia: W.B. Saunders.

Guilleminault, C., & Dement, W. C. (1988). Sleep apnea syndromes and related sleep disorders. In R. L. Williams, I. Karacan, & C. A. Moore (Eds.), *Sleep disorders: Diagnosis and treatment* (2nd ed., pp. 47–71). New York: Wiley.

Guilleminault, C., Mancuso, J., Salva, M. A. Q., Hayes, B., Mitler, M., Poirer, G., & Montplaisir, J. (1986). Viloxazine hydrochloride in narcolepsy: A preliminary report. *Sleep, 9,* 275–279.

Guilleminault, C., Moscovitch, A., & Leger, D. (1995). Forensic sleep medicine: Nocturnal wandering and violence. *Sleep, 18,* 740–748.

Guilleminault, C., & Robinson, A. (1996). Central sleep apnea. *Neurologic Clinics, 14,* 611–628.

Hansen, A. F., & Jorgensen, T. M. (1997). A possible explanation of wet and dry nights in enuretic children. *British Journal of Eurology, 80*(5), 809–811.

Harper, R. M., Leake B., Miyahara L., Mason, J. Hoppenbrouwers, T., Sterman, M. B., & Hodgman, J. (1981). Temporal sequencing in sleep and waking states during the first 6 months of life. *Experimental Neurology, 72,* 294–307.

Hartmann, E. (1966). Reserpine: Its effects on the sleep-dream cycle in man. *Psychopharmacologia, 9,* 242–247.

Hartmann, E., Russ, D., Oldfield, M., Sivan, I., & Cooper, S. (1987). Who has nightmares? *Archives of General Psychiatry, 44,* 49–56.

Hartse, K. M. (1994). Sleep in insects and nonmammalian vertebrates. In M. H. Kryger, T. Roth, & W. C. Dement (Eds.), *Principles and practice of sleep medicine* (2nd ed., pp. 95–104). Philadelphia: W.B. Saunders.

Haskell, E. H., Palca, J. W., Walker, J. M., Berger, R. J., & Heller, H. C. (1981). The effects of high and low ambient temperatures on human sleep stages. *Electroencephalography and Clinical Neurophysiology, 51,* 494–501.

Hauri, P. (1982). *Sleep disorders.* Kalamazoo, MI: Upjohn Company.

Hauri, P., Chernik, D., Hawkins, D., & Mendels, J. (1974). Sleep of depressed patients in remission. *Archives of General Psychiatry, 31,* 386–391.

Hauri, P., Friedman, M., & Ravaris, C. L. (1989). Sleep in patients with spontaneous panic attacks. *Sleep, 12*(4), 323–337.

Hauri, P., & Hawkins, D. R. (1973). Alpha-delta sleep. *Electroencephalography and Clinical Neurophysiology, 34,* 233–237.

Hauri, P., & Olmstead, E. (1980). Childhood onset insomnia. *Sleep, 3,* 59–65.

Henschel, A., & Lack, L. (1987). Do many adolescents sleep poorly or just too late? *Sleep Research, 16,* 354.

Hiatt, J. F., Floyd, T. C., Katz, P. H., & Feinberg, I. (1985). Further evidence of abnormal non-rapid-eye-movement sleep in schizophrenia. *Archives of General Psychiatry, 42,* 797–802.

Hinze-Selch, D., Mullington, J., Orth, A., Lauer, C. J., & Pollmächer, T. (1997). Effects of clozapine on sleep: A longitudinal study. *Biological Psychiatry, 42,* 260–266.

Hoddes E., Zarcone, V. Smythe, H. Phillips, R., & Dement, W. C. (1973). Quantification of sleepiness: A new approach. *Psychophysiology, 10,* 431–436.

Hoelscher, T. J., & Edinger, J. D. (1988). Treatment of sleep-maintenance insomnia in older adults: Sleep period reduction, sleep education, and modified stimulus control. *Psychology and Aging, 3,* 258–263.

Hohagen, F., Lis, S., Krieger, S., Winkelman, G., Riemann, D., Fritsch-Montero, R., Rey, E., Aldenhoff, J., & Berger, M. (1994). Sleep EEG of patients with obsessive-compulsive disorder. *European Archives of Psychiatry and Clinical Neuroscience, 243*(5), 273–278.

Honda, Y., Asaka, A., Tanimura, M., & Furusho, T. (1983). A genetic study of narcolepsy and excessive daytime sleepiness in 308 families with a narcolepsy of hypersomnia proband. In C. Guilleminault & E. Lugaresi (Eds.), *Sleep/wake disorders: Natural history, epidemiology and long term evolution* (pp. 187–199). New York: Raven Press.

Horne, J. (1988). *Why we sleep.* Oxford: Oxford University Press.

Hudson, J. I., Lipinski, J. F., Keck, P. E., Jr., Lukas, S. E., Dorsey, C. M., Rothschild, A. J., & Aizley, H. G. (1990). Sleep in mania versus unipolar depression. *Sleep Research, 19,* 166.

Hurwitz, T. (1986). Treatment of somnambulism and pavor nocturnus in adults with hypnosis. *Sleep Research, 15,* 131.

Hurwitz, T., & Mahowald, M. (1988). Further experience with hypnosis in the treatment of somnambulism and pavor nocturnus in adults. *Sleep Research, 17,* 190.

Insel, T. R., Gillin, C., Moore, A., Mendelson, W. B., Loewenstein, R. J., & Murphy, D. L. (1982). The sleep of patients with obsessive-compulsive disorder. *Archives of General Psychiatry, 39,* 1372–1377.

Issa, F., & Sullivan, C. (1982). Alcohol, snoring, and sleep apnea. *Journal of Neurology, Neurosurgery and Psychiatry, 42,* 353–359.

Jarret, R. T. B., Rush, A. J., Khatami, M., & Roffwarg, H. P. (1990). Does the pretreatment polysomnogram predict response to cognitive therapy in depression outpatients? A preliminary report. *Psychiatry Research, 33,* 285–299.

Johns, M. W. (1991). A new method for measuring daytime sleepiness: the Epworth Sleepiness Scale. *Sleep, 14,* 540–545.

Johns, M. W. (1994). Sleepiness in different situations measured by the Epworth Sleepiness Scale. *Sleep, 17,* 703–710.

Johnson, L. C. (1972). Sleep patterns in chronic alcoholics. In N. K. Mello & J. H. Mendelson (Eds.), *Recent advances in the studies of alcoholism.* Washington, DC: U.S. Government Printing Office.

Kales, A., & Kales, J. D. (1984). *Evaluation and treatment of insomnia.* New York: Oxford University Press.

Kales, A., Soldatos, C., Cadwell, A., Kales, J., Humphrey, F., Charney, D., & Schweitzer, P. (1980). Somnambulism: Clinical characteristics and personality patterns. *Archives of General Psychiatry, 37,* 1406–1410.

Kales, J. D., Soldatos, C. R., & Kales, A. (1980). Childhood sleep disorders. *Current Pediatric Therapy, 9,* 28–30.

Karacan, I. (1988). Parasomnias. In R. L. Williams, I. Karacan, & C. A. Moore (Eds.), *Sleep disorders: Diagnosis and treatment* (2nd ed.). New York: Wiley.

Karacan, I., Anch, M., Thornby, J. I., Okawa, M., & Williams, R. L. (1975). Longitudinal sleep patterns during pubertal growth: Four year follow-up. *Pediatric Research, 9,* 842–846.

Karacan, I., & Howell, J. W. (1988). Narcolepsy. In R. L. Williams, I. Karacan, & C. A. Moore (Eds.), *Sleep disorders: Diagnosis and treatment* (2nd ed., pp. 87–105). New York: Wiley.

Kauffman, C. D., Reist, C., Djenderedjian, A., et al. (1987). Biological markers of affective disorders and posttraumatic stress disorder: a pilot study with desipramine. *Journal of Clinical Psychiatry, 48,* 366–367.

Kay, D. C., & Samiuddin, Z. (1988). Sleep disorders associated with drug abuse and drug of abuse. In R. L. Williams, I. Karacan, & C. A. Moore (Eds.), *Sleep disorders: Diagnosis and treatment* (2nd ed., pp. 315–371). New York: Wiley.

Keshavan, M. S., Reynolds, C. F., III, Miewald, J. M., & Montrose, D. M. (1996). A longitudinal study of EEG sleep in schizophrenia. *Psychiatry Research, 59,* 203–211.

Keshavan, M. S., Reynolds, C. F., III, Miewald, J. M., Montrose, D. M., Sweeney, J. A., Vaski, R. C. Jr., & Kupfer, D. J. (1998). Delta sleep deficits in schizophrenia: Evidence from automated analyses of sleep data. *Archives of General Psychiatry, 55,* 443–448.

King, D. (1977). Pathological and therapeutic consequences of sleep loss: A review. *Journal of Clinical Psychiatry, 38*(11), 873–879.

Klackenberg, G. (1982). Sleep behavior studied longitudinally: Data from 4–16 years on duration, night-awakening and bed-sharing. *Acta Paediatrica Scandinavica, 71,* 501–506.

Klink, M., & Quan, S., (1987). Prevalence of reported sleep disturbances in a general adult population and their relationship to obstructive airways diseases. *Chest, 91,* 540–546.

Kribbs, N. B., & Dinges, D. (1994). Vigilance decrement and sleepiness. In J. Harsh, & R. D. Ogilvie (Eds.), *Sleep onset mechanisms* (pp. 113–125). Washington, DC: American Psychological Association.

Kribbs, N. B., Pack, A. I., Kline, L. R., et al. (1993). Objective measurement of patterns of nasal CPAP use by patients with obstructive sleep apnea. *American Review of Respiratory Diseases, 147,* 887–895.

Kripke, D. F., Ancoli-Israel, S., Klauber, M. R., Wingard, D. L., Mason, W. J., & Mullaney, D. J. (1997). Prevalence of sleep-disordered breathing in ages 40–60 years: A population-based survey. *Sleep, 20,* 65–76.

Kronholm, E., Hyyppä, M. T., Alanen, E., Halonen, J-P., & Partinen, M. (1995). What does the Multiple Sleep Latency Test measure in a community sample? *Sleep, 18,* 827–835.

Kryger, M. H., Roth, T., & Dement, W. C. (Eds.). (2000). *Principles and practice of sleep medicine* (3rd ed.). Philadelphia: W.B. Saunders.

Kupfer, D. J., & Reynolds, C. F., III (1997). Management of insomnia. *New England Journal of Medicine, 336,* 341–346.

Kupfer, D. J., Reynolds, C. F., III, Ulrich, R. F., & Grochocinski, V. J. (1986). Comparison of automated REM and slow-wave sleep analysis in young and middle-aged depressed subjects. *Biological Psychiatry, 21,* 189–200.

Kupfer, D. J., Wyatt, R. J., Scott, J., & Snyder, F. (1970). Sleep disturbance in acute schizophrenic patients. *American Journal of Psychiatry, 126*(9), 1213–1223.

Lack, L., & Wright, H. (1993). The effect of evening bright light in delaying the circadian rhythms and lengthening the sleep of early morning awakening insomniacs. *Sleep, 16,* 436–443.

Lahmeyer, H. W., Janicak, P., Easton, M., Smith, M., & Davis, J. M. (1989). ECT's effect on sleep in major depression. *Sleep Research, 18,* 346.

Lask, B. (1988). Novel and non-toxic treatment for night terrors. *British Medical Journal, 297,* 592.

Lavie, P., Hefez, A., Halperin, G., et al. (1979). Long-term effects of traumatic war-related events on sleep. *American Journal of Psychiatry, 136,* 175–178.

Lavigne, G. J., & Manzini, C. (2000). Bruxism. In M. H. Kryger, T. Roth, & W. C. Dement (Eds.), *Principles and practice of sleep medicine* (3rd ed., pp. 773–785). Philadelphia: W.B. Saunders.

Lin, L., Faraco, J., Li, R., Kadotani, H., Rogers, W., Lin, X., Qiu, X., de Jong, P., Nishino, S., & Mignot, E. (1999). The sleep disorder canine narcolepsy is caused by a mutation in the hypocretin (orexin) receptor 2 gene. *Cell, 98,* 365–376.

Lin, S., MaLaren, J., Harris, C., Holubar, J., Richardson, J., Erie, J., & Fredrickson P. (1990). Pupillometric findings in patients with symptoms of excessive daytime sleepiness and normals. *Sleep Research, 19,* 246.

Lingjaerde, O., Bratlid, T., & Hansen, T. (1985). *Acta Psychiatrica Scandinavica, 71,* 506–512.

Lobbezzo, F., Lavigne, G. J., Tanguay, R., & Montplaisir, J. Y. (1997). The effect of catecholamine precursor L-dopa on sleep bruxism: A controlled study. *Movement Disorders, 12*(1), 73–78.

Loewy, D. H., & Bootzin, R. R. (1998). Event-related potential measures of information processing in insomniacs at bedtime and during sleep. *Sleep, 21*(3 Suppl.), 98.

Lugaresi, E., Cirignotta, F., Mondini, S., Montagna, P., & Zucconi, M. (1988). Sleep in clinical neurology. In R. L. Williams, I. Karacan, & C. A. Moore (Ed.), *Sleep disorders: Diagnosis and treatment* (2nd ed., pp. 245–263). New York: Wiley.

Mahowald, M. W., & Schenck, C. H. (1994). REM sleep behavior disorder. In M. H. Kryger, T. Roth, & W. C. Dement (Eds.), *Principles and practice of sleep medicine* (2nd ed., pp. 574–588). Philadelphia: W.B. Saunders.

Mahowald, M. W., & Schenck, C. H. (1998). Parasomnias including the restless legs syndrome. *Clinic in Chest Medicine, 19,* 183–202.

Manber, R., & Armitage, R. (1999). Sex, steroids, and sleep: A review. *Sleep, 22,* 540–555.

Manber, R., Bootzin, R., Acebo, C., & Carskadon, M. (1996). Reducing daytime sleepiness by regularizing sleep-wake schedules of college students. *Sleep, 19,* 432–441.

Manber, R., Castro, W. L. M., & Hadjiannou, M. (1998). The relationships between sleep, pain, fatigue, and psychological factors in fibromyalgia patients. *Sleep, 21,* 55.

McClain, L. G. (1979). Childhood enuresis. *Current Problems In Pediatrics, 9,* 1–36.

Mellinger, G. D., Balter, M. B., & Uhlenhuth, E. H. (1985). Insomnia and its treatment. *Archives of General Psychiatry, 42,* 225–232.

Mellman, T., & Uhde, T. (1989a). Electroencephalographic sleep in panic disorder: A focus on sleep-related panic attacks. *Archives of General Psychiatry, 46*(2), 178–184.

Mellman, T., & Uhde, T. (1989b). Sleep panic attacks: New clinical findings and theoretical implications. *American Journal of Psychiatry, 146*(9), 1204–1207.

Mendelson, W. B. (1987). *Human sleep: Research and clinical care.* New York: Plenum.

Mignot, E. (1998). Genetics and familial aspects of narcolepsy. *Neurology, 50*(Suppl. 1), S16–S22.

Miles, L. E., & Dement, W. C. (1980). Sleep and aging. *Sleep, 3,* 119–120.

Miles, L. E., Raynal, D. M., & Wilson, M. A. (1977). Blind man living in normal society has circadian rhythm of 24.9 hours. *Science, 198,* 421–423.

Minde, K., Faucon, A., & Faulkner, S. (1994). Sleep problems in toddlers: Effects of treatment on their daytime behavior. *Journal of the American Academy of Child and Adolescent Psychiatry, 33,* 1114–1121.

Mindell, J. A. (1990). Treatment of night wakings in early childhood through generalization effects. *Sleep Research, 19,* 121.

Mitler, M. M., Gujavarty, K. S., & Browman, C. P. (1982). Maintenance of wakefulness test: A polysomnographic technique for evaluating treatment in patients with excessive somnolence. *Electroencephalography and Clinical Neurophysiology, 53,* 658–661.

Mitler, M. M., Nelson, S., & Hajdukovich, R. (1987). Narcolepsy: Diagnosis, treatment, and management. *Psychiatric Clinics of North America, 10,* 593–606.

Mitler, M. M., Browman, C. P., Gujavarty, K., Timms, R. M., & Menn, S. J. (1984). Nocturnal myoclonus: Treatment efficacy of clonazepam and temazepam. *Sleep Research, 13,* 58.

Mitler, M. M., Shafor, R., Hajdukovich, R. M., Timms, R. M., & Browman, C. P. (1986). Treatment of narcolepsy: Objective studies on methylphenidate, pemoline and protriptyline. *Sleep, 9,* 260–264.

Moeller, A. A., Wiegand, M., Oechsner, M., Krieg, J. C., Holsboer, F., & Emminger, C. (1992). Effects of zidovudine on EEG sleep in HIV-infected men [Letter]. *Journal of Acquired Immune Deficiency Syndrome, 5,* 636–637.

Moldofsky, H., Gilbert, R., Lue, F. A., & MacLean, A. W. (1995). Sleep-related violence. *Sleep, 18,* 731–739.

Moldofsky, H., & Scarisbrick, P. (1976). Induction of neurasthenic musculoskeletal pain syndrome by selective sleep stage deprivation. *Psychosomatic Medicine, 38,* 35–44.

Moldofsky, H., Scarisbrick, P., England, R., & Smythe, H. (1975). Musculoskeletal symptoms and non-REM sleep disturbance in patients with "fibrocitis syndrome" and healthy subjects. *Psychosomatic Medicine, 37,* 341–351.

Moldofsky, H., Tullis, C., Quance, G., & Lue, F.A. (1985). Nitrazepam for insomnia or excessive daytime somnolence associated with periodic movements in sleep (sleep-related myoclonus). *Sleep Research, 14,* 191.

Montplaisir, J., Walsh, J., & Malo, J. L. (1982). Nocturnal asthma: features of attacks, sleep and breathing patterns. *American Review of Respiratory Disease, 125,* 18–22.

Montplaisir, J., & Godbout, R., Boghen, D., DeChamplain, J., Young, S. N., & Laptierr, G. (1985). Familial restless legs with periodic movements in sleep: Electrophysiologic, biochemical, and pharmacologic study. *Neurology, 35,* 130–134.

Montplaisir, J., Nicolas, A., Godbout, R., & Walters, A. (2000). Restless legs syndrome and periodic limb movement disorders. In M. H. Kryger, T. Roth, & W. C. Dement (Eds.), *Principles and practice of sleep medicine* (3rd ed., pp. 742–752). Philadelphia: W.B. Saunders.

Moore, C. A., & Gurakar, A. (1988). Nocturnal myoclonus and restless legs syndrome. In R. L. Williams, I. Karacan, & C. A. Moore (Eds.), *Sleep disorders: Diagnosis and treatment* (2nd ed., pp. 73–86). New York: Wiley.

Moore-Ede, M. C., Sulzman, F. M., & Fuller, C. A. (1982). *The clocks that time us.* Cambridge, MA: Harvard University Press.

Morgan, K. (1987). *Sleep and aging: A research based guide to sleep in later life.* Baltimore: John Hopkins University Press.

Morin, C. M. (1993). *Insomnia: Psychological assessment and management*. New York: Guilford.

Morin, C. M., & Gramling, S. E. (1989). Sleep patterns and aging: Comparison of older adults with and without insomnia complaints. *Psychology and Aging, 4,* 290–294.

Morin, C. M., & Kwentus, J. A. (1988). Behavioral and pharmacological treatments for insomnia. *Annals of Behavioral Medicine, 10,* 91–100.

Morin, C. M., Culbert, J. P., & Schwartz, S. M. (1994). Nonpharmacological interventions for insomnia: A meta-analysis of treatment efficacy. *American Journal of Psychiatry, 151,* 1172–1180.

Morin, C. M., Stone, J., McDonald, K., & Jones, S. (1994). Psychological management of insomnia: A clinical replication series with 100 patients. *Behavior Therapy, 25,* 291–309.

Morin, C. M., Hauri, P. J., Espie, C., Spielman, A., Buysse, D. J., & Bootzin, R. R. (1999). Nonpharmacologic treatment of chronic insomnia: An American Academy of Sleep Medicine Review. *Sleep, 22,* 1–25.

Morris, A. M., So, Y., Lee, K. A., Lash, A. A., & Becker, C. E. (1992). The P300 event-related potential. The effects of sleep deprivation. *Journal of Occupational Medicine, 34*(12), 1143–1152.

Morrison, A. R. (1988). Paradoxical sleep without atonia. *Archives Italiennes de Biologie, 126,* 275–289.

Mosko, S., Richard, C., & McKenna, J. (1997). Maternal sleep and arousals during bedsharing with infants. *Sleep, 20,* 142–150.

Motta, J., & Guilleminault, C. (1985). Cardiac dysfunction during sleep. *Annals of Clinical Research, 17,* 190–198.

Muller, K., & Wood, J. M. (1991). Nightmare prevalence in a group of pre-adolescent and early-adolescent children. *Sleep Research, 20,* 304.

Murtagh, D. R. R., & Greenwood, K. M. (1995). Identifying effective psychological treatments for insomnia: A meta-analysis. *Journal of Consulting and Clinical Psychology, 63,* 79–89.

Norman, S. E., Chediak, A. D., Freeman, C., Kiel, M., Mendez, A., Duncan, R., Simoneau, J., & Nolan, B. (1992). Sleep disturbances in men with asymptomatic Human Immunodeficiency (HIV) infection. *Sleep, 15,* 150–155.

Norman, S. E., Chediak, M., Kiel, H., Gazeroglu, H., & Mendez, A. (1990). HIV infection and sleep: Follow up studies. *Sleep Research, 19,* 339.

Oaklander V. (1988). *Windows to our children*. Highland, NY: Gestalt Journal.

Okawa, M., Mishima, Y., Hishikawa, Y., Hozumi, S., Hori, H., & Takahashi, K. (1991). Circadian rhythm disorders in sleep-waking and body temperature in elderly patients with dementia and their treatment. *Sleep, 14,* 478–485.

Ollendick, T. H., Matson, J. L., & Helsel, W. J. (1985). Fears in children and adolescents: Normative data. *Behaviour Research and Therapy, 23,* 465–467.

Ollendick, T. H., & Cerny, J. A. (1981). *Clinical behavior therapy with children*. New York: Plenum.

Oosterhuis, A., & Klip, E. C. (1997). The treatment of insomnia through mass media: The results of a televised behavioural training programme. *Social Science and Medicine, 8,* 1223–1229.

Palm, L., Blennow, G., & Wetterberg, L. (1997). Long-term melatonin treatment in blind children and young adults with circadian sleep-wake disturbances. *Developmental Medicine and Child Neurology, 39,* 319–325.

Palm, L., Persson, E., Elmqvist, D., & Blennow, G. (1989). Sleep and wakefulness in normal preadolescent children. *Sleep, 12,* 299–308.

Partinen, M. (1997). Sleep disorder related to Parkinson's disease. *Journal of Neurology, 244,* S1–S6.

Partinen, M., & Guilleminault, C. (1990). Daytime sleepiness and vascular morbidity at seven-year follow-up in obstructive sleep apnea, *Chest, 97,* 27–32.

Penn, P. E., & Bootzin, R. R. (1990). Behavioural techniques for enhancing alertness and performance in shift work. *Work and Stress, 4,* 213–226.

Perlis, M. L. (1989). Prevalence of sleep disorders in college students. Unpublished data. University of Arizona.

Perlis, M. L., Giles, D. E., Buysse, D. J., Tu, X., & Kupfer, D. J. (1997). Self-reported sleep disturbance as a prodromal symptom in recurrent depression. *Journal of Affective Disorders, 42,* 209–212.

Perlis, M. L., Giles, D. E., Mendelson, W. B., Bootzin, R. R., & Wyatt, J. K. (1997). Psychophysiological insomnia: The behavioral model and a neurocognitive perspective. *Journal of Sleep Research, 6,* 179–188.

Pollak, C. P. (1997). How should the Multiple Sleep Latency Test be analyzed? *Sleep, 20,* 34–39.

Pressman, M., & Fry, J. (1989). Relationship of autonomic nervous system activity to daytime sleepiness and prior sleep. *Sleep, 12,* 239–245.

Price, V. A., Coates, T. J., Thoresen, C. E., & Grinstead, O. A. (1978). Prevalence and correlates of poor sleep among adolescents. *American Journal of the Disabled Child, 132,* 583–586.

Prinz, P. N (1995). Sleep and sleep disorders in older adults. *Journal of Clinical Neurophysiology, 12,* 130–146.

Prinz, P., Vitiello, M., Smallwood, R., Schoene, R., & Halter, J. (1984). Plasma norepinephrine in normal young and aged men: Relationship with sleep. *Journal of Gerontology, 39,* 561–567.

Rechtschaffen, A., & Kales, A. (Eds.). (1968). *A manual of standardized terminology, techniques and scoring system for sleep stages of human subjects*. Los Angeles: UCLA Brain Information Service/Brain Research institute.

Rediehs, M. H., Reis, J. S., & Creason, N. S. (1990). Sleep in old age: Focus on gender differences. *Sleep, 13,* 410–424.

Redline, S., & Strohl, K. (1998). Recognition and consequences of obstructive sleep apnea hyponea syndrome. *Clinics in Chest Medicine, 19,* 1–19.

Reinberg, A., Vieux, N., Ghata, J., Chaumont, A. J., & Laporte, A. (1978). Circadian rhythm amplitude and individual ability to adjust to shift work. *Ergonomics, 21,* 763–766.

Reynolds, C. F., III (1989). Sleep in affective disorders. In M. H. Kryger, T. Roth, & W. C. Dement (Eds.), *Principles and practice of sleep medicine* (pp. 413–415). Philadelphia: W.B. Saunders.

Reynolds, C. F., III, Shaw, D. H., Newton, T. F., Coble, P. A., & Kupfer, D. J. (1983). EEG sleep in outpatients with generalized anxiety. *Psychiatry Research, 8,* 81–89.

Reynolds, C. F., ***, Kupfer, D. J., & Taska, L. S. (1985). Slow wave sleep in elderly depressed, demented, and healthy subjects. *Sleep, 8,* 155–159.

Reynolds, C. F., III, Kupfer, D. J., Thase, M. E., Frank, E., Jarrett, D. B., Coble, P. A., Hoch, C. C., Buysse, D. J., & Houck, P. R. (1990). Sleep, sex, and depression: An analysis of gender effects on the electroencephalographic sleep of 302 depressed outpatients. *Sleep Research, 19,* 173.

Richardson, G. S., Carskadon, M. A., Flagg, W, van den Hoed, J., Dement, W. C., & Mitler, M. M. (1978). Excessive daytime sleepiness in man: Multiple sleep latency measurement in narcoleptic and control subjects. *Electroencephalography and Clinical Neurophysiology, 45,* 621–627.

Richardson, G. S., & Malin, H. V. (1996). Circadian rhythm sleep disorders: Pathophysiology and treatment. *Journal of Clinical Neurophysiology, 13,* 17–31.

Richman, N., Douglas, J., Hunt H., Lansdown, R., & Levere, R. (1985). Behavioral methods in the treatment of sleep disorders: A pilot study. *Journal of Child Psychology and Psychiatry, 26,* 581–590.

Rickles, K., Schweizer, E., Case, W. G., & Greenblatt, D. J. (1990). Long-term therapeutic use of benzodiazepines, I: Effects of abrupt discontinuation. *Archives of General Psychiatry, 47,* 899–907.

Robinson, R. W., & Zwillich, C. W. (1985). The effect of drugs on breathing during sleep. *Clinics in Chest Medicine, 6,* 603–614.

Roehrs, T., Zorick, F., & Roth, T. (1994). Transient insomnia and insomnias associated with circadian rhythm disorders. In M. H. Kryger, T. Roth, & W. C. Dement (Eds.), *Principles and practice of sleep medicine* (2nd ed., pp. 486–493). Philadelphia: W.B. Saunders.

Roehrs, T., Zorick, F., Wittig, R., Paxton, C., Sicklesteel, J., & Roth, T. (1986). Alerting effects of naps in patients with narcolepsy. *Sleep, 9,* 194–199.

Rosenthal, N. E., Joseph-Vanderpool, J. R., Levendosky, A. A., Johnston, S. H., Allen, R., Kelly, K. A., Souetre, E., Schultz, P. M., & Starz, K. E. (1990). Phase shifting effects of bright morning light as treatment for delayed sleep phase syndrome. *Sleep, 13,* 354–361.

Rosenthal, N. E., Sack, D. A., Gillin, J. C., et al. (1984). Seasonal affective disorder: A description of the syndrome and preliminary findings with light therapy. *Archives of General Psychiatry, 41,* 72–80.

Roth, T., Zorick, F., Wittig, R., McLenaghan, A., & Roers, T. (1982). The effects of doxepin HCl on sleep and depression. *Journal of Clinical Psychiatry, 43,* 366–368.

Rothenberg, S., Zozula, R., Funesti, J., & McAuliffe, V. (1990). Sleep habits in asymptomatic HIV-seropositive individuals. *Sleep Research, 19,* 342.

Roy-Byrne, P. P., Uhde, T. W., & Post, R. M. (1986). Effect of one night's sleep deprivation on mood and behavior in panic disorder. *Archives of General Psychiatry, 43,* 895–899.

Rush, A. J., Schlesser, M. A., Woffwarg, H. P., & Parker, C. R. (1982). Sleep EEG and DST findings in outpatients with unipolar major depressive disorder. *Biological Psychiatry, 17,* 327–340.

Sack, R. L., Hughes, R. J., Edgar, D. M., & Lewy, A. J. (1997). Sleep-promoting effects of melatonin: At what dose, in whom, under what conditions, and by what mechanisms? *Sleep, 20,* 908–915.

Sadeh, A. (1994). Assessment of intervention for infant night waking: Parental reports and activity-based home monitoring. *Journal of Consulting and Clinical Psychology, 62,* 63–98.

Sadeh, A., Alster, J. Urbach, D., & Lavie, P. (1989). Actigraphically based automatic bedtime sleep-wake scoring: Validity and clinical applications. *Journal of Ambulatory Monitoring, 2,* 209–216.

Sadeh, A., Lavie, P., Scher, A., Tirosh, E., & Epstein, R. (1991). Actigraphic home monitoring of sleep-disturbed and control infants and young children: A new methods of pediatric assessment of sleep-wake patterns. *Pediatrics, 87,* 494–499.

Salvio, M., Wood, J. M., & Schwartz, J. (1991). Nightmare prevalence in the healthy elderly. *Sleep Research, 20,* 318.

Sanchez, R., & Bootzin, R. R. (1985). A comparison of white noise and music: Effects of predictable and unpredictable sounds on sleep. *Sleep Research, 14,* 121.

Sangal, R. B., Thomas, L., & Mitler, M. M. (1992). Disorders of excessive sleepiness. Treatment improves ability to stay awake but does not reduce sleepiness. *Chest, 102,* 699–703.

Sasaki, M., Kurosaki, Y., Onda, M., Yamaguchi, O., Nishimura, H., Kashimura, K., & Graeber, R. C. (1989). Effects of bright light and circadian rhythmicity and sleep after transmeridian flight. *Sleep Research, 18,* 426.

Schafer, H., Koehler, U., Ploch, T., & Peter, J. H. (1997). Sleep-related myocardial ischemia and sleep structure in patients with obstructive sleep apnea and coronary heart disease. *Chest, 111*(2), 387–393.

Schenck, C., & Mahowald, M. (1990). Treatment outcome data for 52 patients with the REM sleep behavior disorder: Sustained clonazepam efficacy at 0.5–7 year follow-up in > 75% of patients. *Sleep Research, 19,* 283.

Schneider-Helmert, D. (1988). Why low-dose benzodiazepine-dependent insomniacs can't escape their sleeping pills. *Acta Psychiatrica Scandinavica, 78,* 706–711.

Schnelle, J. F., Cruise, P. A., Alessi, C. A., Ludlow, K., Al-Samarrai, N. R., & Ouslander, J. G. (1998). Sleep hygiene in physically dependent nursing home residents: Behavioral and environmental intervention implications. *Sleep, 21,* 515–523.

Schultz, H., Salzarulo, P., Fagioli, I., & Massetani R. (1983). REM latency: Development in the first year of life. *Electroencephalography and Clinical Neurophysiology, 56,* 316–322.

Schuman, M. J. (1981). Neuromuscular relaxation, a method for inducing sleep in young children. *Pediatric Nursing, 7,* 9–13.

Schweitzer, E., Rickels, K., Case, W. G., & Greenblatt, D. J. (1990). Long-term use of benzodiazepines. II: Effects of gradual taper. *Archives of General Psychiatry, 47,* 908–915.

Shoham-Salomon, V., & Rosenthal, R. (1987). Paradoxical interventions: A meta-analysis. *Journal of Consulting and Clinical Psychology, 55,* 22–28.

Smallwood, R., Vitiello, M., Giblin, E., & Prinz, P. (1983). Sleep apnea: Relation to age, sex, and Alzheimer's dementia. *Sleep, 6,* 16–22.

Smith, J. R., Karacan, I., & Yang, M. (1977). Ontogeny of delta activity during human sleep. *Electroencephalography and Clinical Neurophysiology, 43,* 299–237.

Spielman, A. J., Saskin, P., & Thorpy, M. J. (1987). Treatment of chronic insomnia by restriction of time in bed. *Sleep, 10,* 45–56.

Stepansky, E., Lamphere, J., Badia, P. Zorick, F. & Roth, T. (1984). Sleep fragmentation and daytime sleepiness. *Sleep, 7,* 18–26.

Stores, G. (1990). Sleep disorders in children. *British Medical Journal, 301,* 351–352.

Strauch, I., & Meier, B. (1988). Sleep need in adolescents: A longitudinal approach. *Sleep, 11,* 378–386.

Sullivan, C. E., Issa, F. G., Berthon-Jones, M., & Eves, L. (1981). Reversal of obstructive sleep apnea by continuous positive airway pressure applied through the nares. *Lancet, 1,* 862–865.

Taasan, V. C., Block, A. J., & Boysen, P. G. (1981). Alcohol increase sleep apnea and alcohol desaturation in asymptomatic men. *American Journal of Medicine, 71,* 240–245.

Terman, M. (1994). Light therapy. In M. H. Kryger, T. Roth, & W. C. Dement (Eds.), *Principles and practice of sleep medicine* (2nd ed., pp. 1012–1030). Philadelphia: W.B. Saunders.

Terzano, M. G., Mancia, D., Salati, M. R., Costani, G., Decembrino, A., & Parrino, L. (1985). The cyclic alternating pattern as a physiologic component of normal NREM sleep. *Sleep, 8,* 137–145.

Terzano, M. G., & Parrino, L. (1992). Evaluation of EEG cyclic alternating pattern during sleep in insomniacs and controls under placebo and acute treatment with zolpidem. *Sleep, 15,* 64–70.

Thase, M. E., Reynolds, C. F., III, Frank, E., Jennings, J. R., Nofzinger, E., Fasiczka, A. L., Garamoni, G. L., & Kupfer, D. J. (1994). Polysomnographic studies of unmedicated depressed men before and after treatment with cognitive therapy. *American Journal of Psychiatry, 151,* 1615–1621.

Thase, M. E., Simons, A. D., & Reynolds, C. F., III (1993). Psychobiological correlates of poor response to cognitive behavior therapy. *Psychopharmacology Bulletin, 29,* 293–301.

Thorpy, M., & Glovinsky, P. (1987). Parasomnias. *The Psychiatric Clinics of North America, 10,* 623–639.

Thorpy, M. J., Korman, E., Spielman A. J., & Glovinsky P. B. (1988). Delayed sleep phase syndrome in adolescents. In W. P. Koella , F. Obal, H. Schulz, & P. Visser (Eds.), *Sleep '86* (pp. 425–426). New York: Gustav Fischer.

Troup, C., & Hodgson, N. (1971). Nocturnal functional bladder capacity in enuresis children. *Journal of Urology, 105,* 129–132.

Uhde, T. W., Roy-Byrne, P., Gillin, J. C., et al. (1985). The sleep of patients with panic disorder: A preliminary report. *Psychiatry Research, 12,* 251–259.

van der Kolk, B. A., Hartmann, E., Burr, A., et al. (1980). A survey of nightmare frequencies in a veterans' outpatient clinic. *Sleep Research, 9,* 229.

Vitiello, M. V. (1997). Sleep disorders and aging: Understanding the causes. *Journal of Gerontology: Medical Sciences, 52A(4),* M189–M191.

Vitiello, M. V., Schwartz, R. S., Davis, M. W., Ward, R. R., Ralph, D. D., & Prinz, P. N. (1992). Sleep quality and increased aerobic fitness in healthy aged men: Preliminary findings. *Journal of Sleep Research, 1*(Suppl.), 245.

Vogel, G. W., Buffenstein, A., Minter, K., & Hennessey, A. (1990). Drug REM sleep deprivation and drug antidepressant activity. *Sleep Research, 19,* 360.

Vogel, G. W. (1975). A review of REM sleep deprivation. *Archives of General Psychiatry, 32,* 749–761.

Vogel, G. W. (1981). The relationship between endogenous depression and REM sleep. *Psychiatry Annals, 11,* 423–428.

Wagner, D. R. (1996). Disorders of the circadian sleep-wake cycle. *Neurologic Clinics, 14,* 651–670.

Walsh, J. K., Muehlbach, M. J., & Schweitzer, P. K. (1984). Acute administration of triazolam for daytime sleep rotating shift workers. *Sleep, 7,* 223–229.

Ware, J., Russell, J., & Campos, E. (1986). Alpha intrusions into the sleep of depressed and fibromyalgia syndrome (fibromyalgia) patients. *Sleep Research, 15,* 210.

Webb, W. B. (1992). *Sleep: The gentle tyrant* (2nd ed.). Bolton, MA: Anker.

Webb, W. B., & Campbell, S. S. (1980). Awakenings and the return to sleep in an older population. *Sleep, 3,* 41–46.

Weitzman, E. D., Czeisler, C. A., Coleman, R. M., Spielman, A. J., Zimmerman, J. C., & Dement, W. C. (1981). Delayed sleep phase syndrome. A chronobiological disorder with sleep onset insomnia. *Archives of General Psychiatry, 38,* 737–746.

Weitzman, E. D., Moline, M. L., Czeisler, C. A., et al. (1982). Chronobiology of aging: Temperature, sleep-wake rhythms and entrainment. *Neurobiology of Aging, 3,* 299.

Wetter, D. W., Fiore, M. C., Baker, T. B., & Young, T. B. (1995). Tobacco withdrawal and nicotine replacement influence objective measures of sleep. *Journal of Consulting and Clinical Psychology, 63,* 58–67.

Whelton, C., Saskin, P., Salit, I., & Moldofsky, H. (1988). Postviral fatigue syndrome and sleep. *Sleep Research, 17,* 307.

White, D. P. (1994). Central sleep apnea. In M. H. Kryger, T. Roth, & W. C. Dement (Eds.), *Principles and practice of sleep medicine* (2nd ed., pp. 678–693). Philadelphia: W.B. Saunders.

White, L., Hahn, P. M., & Mitler, M. M. (1980). Sleep questionnaire in adolescents. *Sleep Research, 9,* 108.

Wiegand, M., Moeller, A. A., Schreiber, W., Krieg, J. C., Fuchs, D., Wachter, H., & Holsboer, F. (1991). Nocturnal sleep EEG in patients with HIV infection. *European Archives of Psychiatry and Clinical Neuroscience, 240,* 153–158.

Williams, R. L., Karacan, I., & Hursch, C. J. (1974). *EEG of human sleep: Clinical applications.* New York: Wiley.

Williams, R. L., Karacan, I., & Moore, C. A. (1988). *Sleep disorders: Diagnosis and treatment* (2nd ed.). New York: Wiley.

Wood, J. M., & Bootzin, R. R. (1990). The prevalence of nightmares and their independence from anxiety. *Journal of Abnormal Psychology, 99,* 64–68.

Yoss, R. E., Moyer, N., & Ogle, K. (1969). The pupillogram and narcolepsy. *Neurology, 19,* 921–928.

Young, T., Evans, L., Finn, L., & Palta, M. (1997). Estimation of the clinically diagnosed proportion of sleep apnea syndrome in middle-aged men and women. *Sleep, 20,* 705–706.

Young, T., Palta, M., Dempsey, J., Skatrud, J., Weber, S., & Badr, S. (1993). The occurrence of sleep-disordered breathing among middle-aged adults. *New England Journal of Medicine, 328,* 1230–1235.

Youngstedt, S. D., O'Connor, P. J., & Dishman, R. K. (1997). The effects of acute exercise on sleep: A quantitative synthesis. *Sleep, 20,* 203–214.

Zarcone, V. P. (1988). Sleep and schizophrenia. In R. L. Williams, I. Karacan, & C. A. Moore (Eds.), *Sleep disorders: Diagnosis and treatment* (2nd ed., pp. 165–188). New York: Wiley.

Zarcone, V. P. (1994). Sleep hygiene. In M.H. Kryger, T. Roth & W.C. Dement (Eds.), *Principles and practice of sleep medicine* (2nd ed., pp. 542–546). Philadelphia: W.B. Saunders.

Zarcone, V. P., Gulevich, G., Pivik, T., Azumi, K., & Dement, W. C. (1969). REM deprivation and schizophrenia. *Biological Psychiatry, 1,* 179–184.

Zarcone, V. P., Benson, K. L., & Berger, P. A. (1987). Abnormal rapid eye movement latencies in schizophrenia. *Archives of General Psychiatry, 44,* 45–48.

Zepelin, H. (1994). Mammalian sleep. In M. H. Kryger, T. Roth, & W. C. Dement (Eds.), *Principles and practice of sleep medicine* (2nd ed., pp. 69–80). Philadelphia: W.B. Saunders.

# CHAPTER 25

# Sexual Dysfunctions

## Victor J. Malatesta and Henry E. Adams

## Introduction

Human sexuality is diverse and encompasses a complex and multifaceted set of biological, psychological, and sociocultural variables. An individual's sexuality includes everything ranging from one's sex organs, hormones, and basic sex drive, to sexual response, gender identity, and body image. This array of biopsychosocial factors interacts within a framework composed of individual cognition (thoughts and fantasies), behavior, and emotions that occur in response to sexual stimulation. In addition, unlike many forms of human behavior, one's sexuality and sexual activity are expressed in a relational and intimate interpersonal context. The interactive nature of human sexual behavior introduces an additional set of variables, including partner satisfaction, reproduction and (in)fertility, communication, and the ability to negotiate intimate relationships. Individual sexuality is also enmeshed with developmental and learning history, in addition to personality, mood state, and the culture in which one lives. Thus, human sexual behavior is subject to the influences of family of origin, moral and religious teachings, anxiety and power, and societal rules that govern the expression of sexuality.

Not surprisingly, the complexity of human sexuality poses unique challenges for the study and understanding of sexual health and normal sexual behavior. In addition, the field is challenged by an ambivalent society that is, on the one hand, preoccupied and titillated with issues of sexual expression, and—at the same time—inhibited and avoidant regarding discussion of sexuality. Tragedies associated with autoimmune disorder (AIDS) and our increased knowledge about the profound effects of sexual victimization have complicated these matters. A similar ambivalence is displayed by the academic and scientific community. On the one hand, the field is blessed with many outstanding clinical researchers and scholar-practitioners. Their work has defined this important field. At the same time, there is an unusual dearth of courses and practicums in human sexuality and sexual disorders offered by clinical psychology and psychiatry residency programs. This paucity comes at a time when issues of sexual health and sexual dysfunction have gained new importance as we enter the new millennium.

This chapter begins with a historical perspective and traces the study and treatment of sexual dysfunctions to the present. Highlighting important developments and recent trends, the chapter provides an overview of the description, diagnosis, etiology, assessment, and treatment of sexual dysfunctions. The emphasis of the chapter assumes a heterosexual orientation. However, we believe that more research on sexual minorities is needed—even while it is argued that because overlap is considerable between heterosexual and homosexual behavior and dysfunctions, general research is applicable (Sadock, 1995). For additional study, the reader is referred to Behrendt and

Victor J. Malatesta • Pennsylvania Hospital and University of Pennsylvania School of Medicine.   Henry E. Adams • Department of Psychology, University of Georgia, Athens, Georgia 30602-3013.

*Comprehensive Handbook of Psychopathology* (Third Edition), edited by Patricia B. Sutker and Henry E. Adams. Kluwer Academic / Plenum Publishers, New York, 2001.

George (1995) and MacDonald (1998). Finally, as clinicians, we affirm the importance of a keen understanding of normal sexuality as a prerequisite for studying, evaluating, and treating sexual dysfunctions.

## A Historical Perspective

Emphasizing the case study approach, Havlock Ellis (1933/1966), Richard von Krafft-Ebing (1899), and Sigmund Freud (1943) focused their pioneering work on human sexuality and on abnormal sexual behavior in particular. From the beginning of the twentieth century until the late 1960s, sexual disorders—like other forms of psychopathology—were typically understood within the context of psychoanalytic theory. From this perspective, sexual problems were viewed as "symptoms" of underlying psychopathology, originating from unresolved parent–child conflicts, basic attachment difficulties, or trauma. Consequently, sexual disorders were viewed as part of a neurotic or personality disorder. Later formulations emphasized more the interpersonal dynamics of sexual disorders. At the same time, powerful scientific and social changes were occurring.

Beginning in the 1920s and culminating in the work of Kinsey in the 1940s and 1950s, a tradition of social bookkeeping began focusing on the sexual behavior of relatively normal persons. Methodologically such studies moved away from the case study and from populations who were defined as criminal or neurotic. At the same time, general social changes were occurring that were directly affecting the rates and directions of sexual conduct in the society. The work of Alfred Kinsey charted these changes and in turn influenced public attitudes, public policy, and research interests during the 1950s and 1960s. (Gagnon, 1975, p. 111)

Kinsey's research challenged Freudian control-repression and drive models of sexuality and legitimized sex as an area of scientific pursuit. Clinicians were already applying learning principles to the treatment of sexual problems (Lazarus, 1963; Wolpe, 1958). However, it was Masters and Johnson (1966) who revolutionized the field with the landmark volume, *Human Sexual Response*.

Masters and Johnson's initial goal was to develop a physiological understanding of human sexual response from their extensive laboratory observational studies. Based on careful testing of 382 women and 312 men in more than 10,000 episodes of sexual activity, Masters and Johnson gathered an unprecedented array of information about the physical processes and manifestations of sexual arousal and orgasm during various types of sexual stimulation. Their discoveries included (1) the essential similarity of male and female sexual response, (2) the nature of vaginal lubrication, (3) the notion of ejaculatory inevitability and the male refractory period, (4) the finding that women were potentially multiorgasmic, and (5) the finding of continued sexual capacity in older adults. Masters and Johnson also devised an empirical model of normal sexual behavior to describe these physiological changes.

Having developed a model of normal sexual "function," Masters and Johnson (1970) logically extended their work to develop a treatment approach for male and female sexual "dysfunction" in their second landmark volume, *Human Sexual Inadequacy*. In contrast to intrapsychic factors, their approach emphasized learning deficits and performance anxiety in the etiology and maintenance of sexual dysfunctions. Intervention comprised a relatively brief, problem-focused and directive approach that was largely behavioral in technique. Treatment objectives consisted of (re)educating clients regarding sexuality, skill building, and alleviating performance anxiety.

Great enthusiasm was associated with Masters and Johnson's sex therapy because of its optimistic and sexually affirmative approach. Remarkably high rates of success were being reported. Overall, their failure rate was only 20% for all sexual dysfunctions combined. Certain dysfunctions, such as premature ejaculation, were successfully treated 100% of the time. The success and enthusiasm were also fueled by important demographic and sociocultural factors, that is, the majority of men and women who sought help tended to be under 40 years of age, well educated, and members of the "60s generation." Recall that the 1960s had ushered in an era of increased sexual freedom, experimentation, and relaxed sexual inhibitions. Women were exercising their recently found sexual rights and the freedoms afforded by the contraceptive revolution, the women's movement, and Masters and Johnson's work. Their scientific findings had showed that, in contrast to men, women were not restricted by a refractory period and were physiologically capable of multiple orgasms. Thus, although male sexual prowess was challenged for the first time, a brief, nonperjorative, and effective sex therapy was available.

In the wake of Masters and Johnson, Helen

Kaplan (1974) introduced her version of the "new" sex therapy that was geared more toward practitioners. Representing a blending of psychoanalytic and more contemporary behavioral approaches, her model also emphasized an initial focus on sexual symptoms. More psychological in nature, Kaplan's model provided a therapeutic alternative if a problem-focused treatment met with "resistance" or failure. A modified psychodynamic approach then emphasized underlying intrapsychic or interpersonal factors that purportedly maintained sexual dysfunction. Thus, Kaplan's sequential approach indicated an initial symptom-focused treatment, followed by a more dynamic intervention if the first approach failed.

Kaplan's clinical approach aroused the enthusiasm of psychiatry and clinical psychology. Her treatment was an outpatient approach that could be applied easily in the office. In conjunction with Masters and Johnson's scientific foundation, many clinicians began practicing sex therapy with relatively good outcome. More successfully treated problems, such as anorgasmia in women and premature ejaculation, were the prominent sexual dysfunctions presented to clinicians in the "early days" of modern sex therapy (Rosen & Leiblum, 1995a). Moreover, many of the clients of the 1970s benefitted greatly from simple education, permission-giving, and directed relaxation of negative sexual attitudes and behaviors. As a result, treatment outcome was favorable, and optimism about the efficacy of sex therapy dominated the field. Finally, the mass media communicated this optimism by providing education and self-help about a range of sexual topics.

As a result of these developments, less complex cases that early therapists saw became scarce (Schover & Leiblum, 1994). Clinical researchers were also having difficulty replicating the impressive treatment outcomes of the Masters and Johnson approach. Reviews of the clinical literature demonstrated that the majority of research in the area of sexual dysfunction consisted of clinical reports, psychometric descriptions, and poorly controlled outcome studies (e.g., Kilmann, 1978). There was also a preoccupation with treatment techniques at the expense of more basic issues such as etiology, classification, and case formulation (Malatesta & Adams, 1986, 1993). The optimism and enthusiasm that accompanied Masters and Johnson's work abated, and even they became a focus for criticism (Zilbergeld & Evans, 1980). On the positive side, sex research became more sophisticated and addressed a more complex interplay of physiological, behavioral, and cognitive variables (Beck & Barlow, 1984).

These changes were accompanied by the modern discovery of the concept of "sexual desire" and its more treatment-resistant manifestations (Kaplan, 1979). A disorder described as "inhibited sexual desire" was officially recognized in 1980 by the American Psychiatric Association. Although it addressed an important clinical problem, the study and treatment of sexual desire opened a Pandora's box. Because of the biopsychosocial complexity of sexual desire, therapists struggled with issues of treatment intervention, theoretical controversy was stimulated, and a range of clinical and empirical challenges was unleashed (e.g., Schover & LoPiccolo, 1982). Sex therapy was becoming broader, less symptom-focused, and addressed necessarily a wider range of individual, relational, and developmental factors.

The 1980s also ushered in increased awareness of the important role of biological factors in sexual dysfunction (e.g., Spark, White, & Connolly, 1980). This phenomenon occurred within the context of new developments in urology, behavioral endocrinology, and penile implant surgery (Tiefer, Pedersen, & Melman, 1988). Medicine had found a new area of specialty in the era of managed care that was embraced with a "gold-rush-like enthusiasm" (Stief & Jonas, 1998). Sexual psychophysiology displayed comparable development and became a subspecialty within urology as it pertained to the differential diagnosis of erectile problems (Rosen & Beck, 1988). In addition, a greater emphasis on the sexual aspects of disease and disability occurred (Schover & Jensen, 1988). Similar emphasis was focused on the sexuality of older adults—whether partnered, single, or living within a nursing home (Malatesta, 1989). Consequently, "medicalization" of the field occurred, and some began to lament the stagnation of psychological conceptualizations of sexual dysfunctions (Schover & Leiblum, 1994). In a critical appraisal of the state of theory in sex therapy, Wiederman (1998) quoted an eminent sexual scientist on his assessment of the field:

Sex research today lives in a conceptual ghetto, theoretically poverty stricken, and lacking in consensus. It is still mired in the organic versus psychogenic dilemma, its own version of the long-obsolete nature/nurture dichotomy. For the most part, it still follows the experimental design of classical physics and celestial mechanics, and searches for univariate cause and effect, whereas the phenomena of sex research are, virtually without exception, multivariately determined. (John Money, 1988, p. 14)

As we entered the 1990s, Money's stinging appraisal of the field gave way to the development of multivariate conceptualizations of sexual dysfunction for men and women alike (e.g., Cranston-Cuebas & Barlow, 1990; Palace, 1995).

In the 1990s the reality was also accepted that the client base for sexual dysfunctions and sex therapy had changed dramatically. Increasing focus was directed at individuals who were often older and who presented with more pervasive, chronic, and biologically influenced sexual problems (Fisher, Swingen, & O'Donohue, 1997). The medicalization of sex therapy attracted a diverse audience that was interested in pharmacological and surgical treatments for erectile disorders. Clinical psychology developed a complementary role in the multicomponent assessment of these problems (Ackerman & Carey, 1995). Some of these individuals also sought psychological help to improve their relationships. Although treatment of sexual addiction and sexual compulsivity was popularized in the 1990s, less attention was focused on issues of classification and diagnosis (Malatesta & Robinson, 1995). More importantly, confronted by the AIDS tragedy and the reality of sexual abuse, an emerging traditionalism in long-term relationships occurred. Reluctant to seek sexual gratification outside of marriage, a growing number of individuals in distressed marriages sought couples therapy to negotiate the complexities of intimate relationships (Gottman, 1999).

The 1990s also witnessed several appraisals of the field with respect to the treatment of sexual dysfunction (Hawton, 1995; Rosen & Leiblum, 1995a), women's sexuality (Andersen & Cyranowski, 1995), and hypoactive sexual desire disorder (Beck, 1995). It was also concluded that only a few empirically supported treatments existed for sexual dysfunctions (Baucom, Shoham, Mueser, Daluto, & Stickle, 1998). Perhaps in a search for new impetus and bold ideas in the conceptualization of sexual dysfunction, the field revisited the psychological case study approach (Rosen & Leiblum, 1995b).

As we enter the new millennium, issues of sexual health and sexual functioning have taken on a new urgency because of at least five major developments. First, the aging "baby boom genera-

tion"—for whom sexual expression was part and parcel of the 60s and 70s—remains committed to maintaining active sexuality. Second, wide access to the Internet has caused unprecedented availability of information about sexuality (see Cooper, 1998). Again, people are better informed about a wide range of sexual matters. Third, the heightened power of women, minorities, and the disabled has called attention to the need for more sexuality research with respect to these populations. Fourth, the introduction and widespread use of sildenafil (Viagra) and similar medications has produced what may be the next "sexual revolution." In addition to providing a relatively inexpensive and effective treatment for erectile disorder, Viagra and its mass marketing have reduced the stigma associated with having a sexual dysfunction, have encouraged many men and women to seek help who might not otherwise, and have spurred needed emphasis on women's sexuality (e.g., Kaplan et al., 1999). Finally, not since the publication of the Kinsey Reports of a half-century ago have we had access to large-scale scientific information about the widespread sexual problems of men and women. This research has shown that four out of ten women and nearly one-third of men suffer from some type of sexual dysfunction (Laumann, Paik, & Rosen, 1999). In addition to raising consciousness, this work has indicated that sexual dysfunctions are a major public health problem that deserve increased study, understanding, and treatment.

## Models of Sexual Response

Human sexual behavior has been viewed as the most sensitive of the biological response systems because it is functionally responsive to an array of physiological, cognitive-behavioral, and psychosocial variables (Adams, 1981). Several clinical researchers have attempted to describe this biopsychosocial complexity by developing models of sexual behavior. This section will describe the major models of sexual behavior to provide a foundation for examining the various types of sexual dysfunction. Although an understanding of the anatomical and neurophysiological underpinnings of sexual behavior represents an important prerequisite to working with the sexual disorders, this section will highlight only these components. More detailed information on these biological

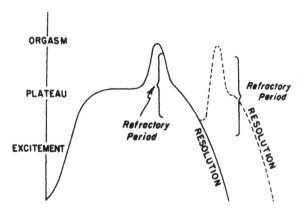

**Figure 1.** The male sexual response cycle. From W. H. Masters and V. E. Johnson (1966), *Human Sexual Response* (p. 5). Copyright 1966 by Little, Brown & Company. Reprinted with permission.

aspects of sexual response is provided in Rowland (1995), Sadock (1995), and Schover and Jensen (1988).

### Masters and Johnson's Sexual Response Cycle

As noted earlier, Masters and Johnson (1966, 1970) developed the first empirical model of human sexual response which paved the way for our understanding of human sexual function and dysfunction. Even today, their model of the sexual response cycle continues to provide the basis for much of our thinking about sexual function. The model will be described in some detail. As shown in Figures 1 and 2, the four successive phases of the sexual response cycle are (a) excitement, (b) plateau, (c) orgasm, and (d) resolution. According to Masters and Johnson, the excitement phase commences in response to any form of cognitive, sensory-motor, or emotional stimulation that produces erotic feelings and sensations. In both men and women, an important physiological response to this erotic stimulation is an increase in muscle tension throughout the body (myotonia) and engorgement of the blood vessels (vasocongestion), particularly in the genital region. In men, this engorgement leads to tumescence of the penis;

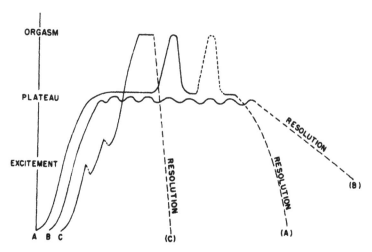

**Figure 2.** The female sexual response cycle. From W. H. Masters and V. E. Johnson (1966), *Human Sexual Response* (p. 5). Copyright 1966 by Little, Brown & Company. Reprinted with permission.

### Table 1. Human Sexual Response Cycle: Genital Reactions

| Male | Female |
|---|---|
| *Excitement phase* | |
| Penile erection (3 to 8 seconds) as phase is prolonged | Vaginal lubrication (5 to 15 seconds) as phase is prolonged |
| Thickening, flattening, and elevation of the scrotum | Thickening of vaginal walls, flattening and elevation of labia majora as phase is prolonged |
| Moderate testicular elevation and size increase | Expansion of inner ⅔ vaginal barrel and elevation of cervix and body of the uterus |
| *Plateau phase* | |
| Increase in penile coronal circumference and testicular tumescence (½ to 1 × enlarged) | Orgasmic platform in outer ⅓ of vagina |
| Full testicular elevation and rotation (30–35°) | Full inner ⅔ vaginal expansion, uterine, and cervical elevation |
| Purple cast to corona of penis (inconsistent, even if orgasm is to ensue) | "Sex-skin" discoloration of labia minora (constant, if orgasm is to ensue) |
| Mucoid-like emission from Cowper's gland | Mucoid-like emission from Bartholin's gland |
| *Organism phase* | |
| Ejaculation | Pelvic response |
| 1. Contraction of accessory organs of reproduction<br> a. Vas deferens<br> b. Seminal vesicles<br> c. Ejaculatory duct<br> Prostate | 1. Contractions of uterus from fundus toward lower uterine segment |
| 2. Relaxation of external bladder sphincter | 2. Minimal relaxation of external cervical os |
| 3. Contractions of penile urethra at 0.8 s intervals for 2 to 3 contractions (slowing thereafter for 2 to 4 more contractions) | 3. Contraction of vagina orgasmic platform at 0.8 s intervals for 4 to 8 contractions (slowing thereafter for 2 to 4 more contractions) |
| 4. External rectal sphincter contractions (2 to 4 contractions at 0.8 s intervals) | 4. External rectal sphincter contractions (2 to 4 contractions at 0.8 s intervals)<br>External urethral sphincter contractions (2 to 3 contractions at irregular intervals) |
| *Resolution phase* | |
| 1. Refractory period with rapid loss of pelvic vasocongestion | 1. Ready return to orgasm with retarded loss of pelvic vasocongestion |
| 2. Loss of penile erection in primary (rapid) and secondary (slow) stages | 2. Loss of "sex-skin" color and orgasmic platform in primary (rapid) stage<br>Remainder of pelvic vasocongestion as secondary (slow) stage |

in women, it leads to vasocongestion in the pelvis and clitoris, along with vaginal lubrication and swelling of the external genitalia (see Table 1).

As sexual stimulation continues, a number of other physiological changes occur that, in general, become more pronounced during the plateau stage (e.g., increased heart rate, respiration, and blood pressure; testicular elevation; breast enlargement). These physiological changes associated with the excitement phase are subject to disruption by extraneous stimuli, cessation of erotic stimulation, or negative mood or cognitive states. In the normal situation, however, sexual excitement may be regained by resuming stimulation and maintaining a conducive sexual environment.

The plateau phase is characterized by (a) an intensification of physiological and muscular changes if erotic stimuli are maintained and (b) a leveling off or plateau in these changes, indicating the high degree of sexual arousal necessary to trigger orgasm. The duration of this phase varies widely and may be particularly brief for early ejaculators or overly extended for women who experience difficulty in reaching orgasm.

The orgasmic phase represents a pervasive physiological response of the entire body in which vasocongestion and myotonia reach their maximum and are discharged through orgasm. Orgasm commences in both men and women with involuntary contractions of the internal genital organs, followed by ejaculation in the male and a wide variability of response in the female. For example, some women display the capacity for extended or multiple orgasms and can experience a number of orgasms without falling below the plateau phase. Masters and Johnson indicated that men do not share the capacity for multiple orgasms, because immediately following orgasm, the male enters a resolution or refractory period during which further orgasm is impossible. This refractory period varies considerably for men (e.g., as a function of age) and is reflected in a gradual return to preexcitement-phase levels. For the woman, this return occurs more slowly and may be altered by reinstituting effective sexual stimulation. Controversy surrounds the existence of a female ejaculate and the Grafenberg spot—the vaginal site whose stimulation is associated with heightened pleasure (see Davidson, Darling, & Conway-Welch, 1989). Similarly, the strength of the circumvaginal musculature and its relationship to female orgasm reflect equivocal research findings (Trudel & Saint-Laurent, 1983).

Because their goal was to develop an objective and measurable framework, Masters and Johnson focused their model exclusively on the role of peripheral physiology in describing sexual response (e.g., genital vasocongestive processes and other autonomic changes). Thus, their work was guided by the fact that penile and vaginal vasocongestion are the only physiological responses that are specific to sexual arousal and are generally insensitive to other emotional states (Zuckerman, 1971). Consequently, however, their model has been criticized for ignoring important cognitive and affective processes, as well as the interaction of physiological, cognitive, and affective components. On a related level, Masters and Johnson's model of sexual response has been criticized because a sexual desire phase was not included within their framework. Also implicit in their model was the male tradition of focusing on orgasm as the culmination of sexual arousal. Although they recognized the need for an objective measure of sexual outlet (i.e., orgasm), this focus has tended to overshadow other aspects of sexual response (see Tiefer, 1991).

## Models Incorporating a Sexual Desire Phase

Noting the absence of a cognitive-affective-motivational dimension in the Masters and Johnson model, Lief (1977) and Kaplan (1977) independently described the need for a sexual desire-phase component to conceptualize the sexual response cycle best. Sexual desire is a multiply determined, subjective feeling state characterized by the inclination and motivation to be sexual. Lief and Kaplan indicated that in clinical practice, individuals presenting with desire-phase difficulties represented a substantial portion of patients who sought sex therapy. Whereas Lief (1977) argued for a five-state model, Kaplan conceptualized a triphasic model that consisted of three components: desire, excitement, and orgasm. Though postulating that the sexual desire phase was mediated by limbic system activation, her concept of sexual desire was more akin to the traditional idea of libido and was derived largely from a psychodynamic perspective. Consequently, neither Kaplan nor Leif offered an operationalized definition of sexual desire, and, other than anecdotal clinical data, they did not provide empirical support for their models. Nevertheless, the Kaplan (1977) triphasic model has had a great impact on the classification of sexual dysfunctions, and a growing body of research supports its importance (Beck, 1995).

## Interactive Models

The basic assumption of interactive models is that the interrelationships among various dimensions of sexual arousal are critical in defining a sexual experience. These dimensions of sexual arousal include physiological, cognitive, and af-

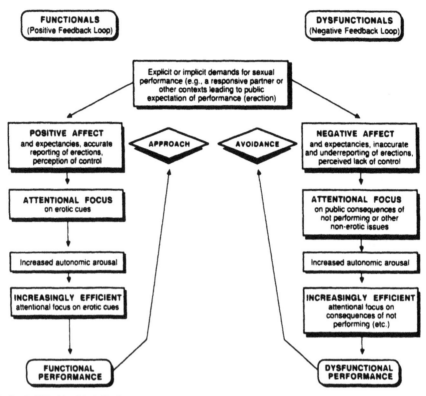

**Figure 3.** Barlow's "Working Model" of inhibited sexual excitement. From D. H. Barlow (1986), "Cases of Sexual Dysfunction: The Role of Anxiety and Cognitive Interference," *Journal of Consulting and Clinical Psychology*, *54*, 140–148. Copyright 1986 by the American Psychological Association Reprinted by permission.

fective components. From this perspective, "sexual arousal cannot be defined adequately without highlighting the critical role of cognitive labeling and subjective experience in determining the response to a given stimulus as sexual" (Rosen & Beck, 1988, p. 28). Thus, although they maintain an emphasis on the traditional peripheral physiology of sexual response, these models (which borrow from the cognitive arousal theory of emotion) can address a range of interactive phenomena in sexual function and dysfunction. For instance, the significant rates of discordance between physiological and subjective dimensions of sexual response reported in the experimental literature highlight the need for multidimensional models of sexual behavior (Palace, 1995; Rosen & Beck, 1988).

A number of theorists have developed interactional models of sexual response (see Cranston-Cuebas & Barlow, 1990). A feature common to each of these models is the emphasis on cognitive-affective processes in mediating sexual arousal.

Special emphasis is also placed on the perception of physiological activation (or deactivation) and the processing of erotic and nonerotic cues. Barlow's (1986) model of sexual dysfunction has been developed and refined in experimental literature. As shown in Figure 3, Barlow postulated a sequence of interactive processes that leads to either functional or dysfunction sexual response. In the case of sexual dysfunction, the sexual situation is perceived by the individual as threatening and uncontrollable, and there are expectations of anxiety and performance difficulty. The individual responds emotionally to these perceptions with a negative affective evaluation. According to Barlow, at this point a critical shift in attention occurs from a focus on erotic cues (e.g., the partner) to a more internal, self-evaluative focus. The affective response also triggers autonomic arousal, which, according to experimental findings, further sharpens attentional focus. Patients at this point may become negatively distracted and have an intense and narrow focus on negative affective stimuli.

Impaired performance occurs, which eventually leads to sexual avoidance. Growing support for this model has been derived from a number of experimental studies that involved women and men, functional and dysfunction samples, and novel feedback manipulations (see Back, Brown, & Barlow, 1999; Palace, 1995). These studies suggest that low self-efficacy expectations—more than negative affect, anxiety, or low subjective arousal—may result in decreased physiological arousal.

Although Barlow's model represents an important step in developing multidimensional, interactive models of sexual response, its clinical application has not been realized. However, an exciting development regarding this model is recent work that addresses the sexual responses of functional and sexually dysfunctional women and their differential responses to distraction and performance feedback (see Elliott & O'Donohue, 1997).

## DSM-IV Sexual Response Cycle

The *Diagnostic and Statistical Manual of Mental Disorders* (DSM-IV; American Psychiatric Association [APA], 1994) continues to borrow heavily from the work of Masters and Johnson (1966, 1970) and Kaplan (1974, 1979). DSM-IV utilizes a four-stage model consisting of the following phases:

1. Desire: This phase consists of fantasies and thoughts about sexual activity and an interest or inclination to be sexual.
2. Excitement: This phase reflects both a subjective sense of pleasure and the accompanying physiological changes associated with sexual arousal. The DSM-IV excitement phase represents a combination of Masters and Johnson's excitement and plateau phases.
3. Orgasm: This reflects a peaking of sexual pleasure and is synonymous with the orgasmic phase described by Masters and Johnson.
4. Resolution: This phase reflects a sense of general relaxation, well-being, and muscular relaxation. The typical refractory period (which differs for men and women) is also included within this resolution phase.

The DSM-IV notes that "disorders of sexual response" can occur at any one or more of the four phases, although dysfunction in the resolution phase is rarely of primary clinical significance.

The DSM-IV also states that more than one sexual dysfunction may be present, reflecting the clinical reality that dysfunction at one phase (e.g., orgasm) may adversely affect functioning at another phase (e.g., desire). Thus, the sexual dysfunction classified by the DSM-IV are divided into the following categories: Sexual Desire Disorders, Sexual Arousal Disorders, Orgasmic Disorders, Sexual Pain Disorders, and Sexual Dysfunction Not Otherwise Specified. Unlike its predecessors, the DSM-IV also includes categories for Sexual Dysfunction Due to a General Medical Condition and Substance-Induced Sexual Dysfunction. These diagnoses are appropriate if the dysfunction can be attributed entirely either to a biological disorder or to the adverse effects of substance use or medication. Note that the DSM-IV uses a binary classification system to diagnose either the presence or absence of a sexual dysfunction. Although a binary system has limitations (Malatesta & Adams, 1993), other approaches to classification have not been widely accepted (e.g., Schover, Friedman, Weiler, Heiman, & LoPiccolo, 1982; Trudel, Ravart, & Matte, 1993).

For accurate diagnosis, the DSM-IV requires both an impairment in desire or objective performance and an indication that the disturbance causes "marked distress or interpersonal difficulty." Therefore, it is possible that an individual may have impairment in a phase of sexual response (e.g., desire), but not be distressed by it—personally or interpersonally. In this case, the individual would not meet full diagnostic criteria for a sexual dysfunction. Finally, the DSM-IV states that all of the sexual dysfunctions may be classified additionally as Lifelong or Acquired (i.e., developing after a period of normal functioning), Generalized or Situational (i.e., limited to certain types of stimulation, situations, or partners), and/or Due to Psychological Factors or Due to Combined Factors (i.e., psychological factors and a general medical condition).

## Definition, Description, and Diagnosis

**Sexual Desire Disorders.** There has been an evolution in the description and classification of sexual desire disorders. Freud defined sexual desire within the concept of libido, which he viewed as an instinctive, biological urge for sexual expression. Later definitions emphasized the psychological aspects of libido as more a function of developmental and environmental influences. The modern description of a disorder of sexual desire was offered independently by Lief (1977) and Kaplan (1977). They argued that individuals with this condition could not be diagnosed adequately by using the four categories outlined by Masters and Johnson.

Although the third edition of the DSM (DSM-III; APA, 1980) introduced a more subjective and mentalistic aspect to diagnostic models of sexual functioning (see Money, 1988), it responded to this clinical development by including, for the first time, sexual desire problems as an independent diagnostic entity. Labeled as "Inhibited Sexual Desire" in the DSM-III, this entity's definition included "persistent and pervasive inhibition of sexual desire" (APA, 1980, p. 278). Because difficulty was inherent in attempting to measure inhibited sexual desire, some diagnostic confusion and theoretical controversy resulted.

Following the publication of the DSM-III, however, sexual desire-phase disorders began to attract significant clinical and investigative attention (Rosen & Leiblum, 1987). Research studies confirmed the commonality of desire-phase disorders in clinical practice (Kilmann, Boland, Norton, Davidson, & Caid, 1986). Others wrestled with the clinical complexity in conceptualizing and treating such problems (Kaplan, 1979; Schover & LoPiccolo, 1982) and the theoretical challenge posed by desire-phase disorders (Levine, 1984, 1988; Singer & Toates, 1987). In this regard, Levine (1988) reported that sexual desire can be conceptualized as incorporating at least three critical dimensions: (1) a biological-drive component based on neuroendocrine mechanisms and evidenced by "endogenous or spontaneous manifestations of genital excitement" (p. 24); (2) a cognitive or attitudinal component that reflects the inclination or "wish" to be sexual; and (3) an affective or interpersonal component, characterized by a willingness to engage in sex. More recent conceptualizations continue this tradition by emphasizing the multidimensional nature of sexual desire and its disorders (see Beck, 1995).

The DSM-III-R (APA, 1987) elaborated on the DSM-III's initial classification of desire-phase disorders by including two distinct categories: hypoactive sexual desire disorder and sexual aversion disorder. The term "inhibited" was dropped from the DSM-III-R to avoid a more conflict-based conceptualization, in favor of the atheoretical term, "hypoactive." The DSM-IV follows the same tradition regarding description and classification of sexual desire disorders.

### Hypoactive Sexual Desire Disorder (302.71).

A. Persistently or recurrently deficient (or absent) sexual fantasies and desire for sexual activity. The judgment of deficiency or absence is made by the clinician, taking into account factors that affect sexual functioning, such as age and the context of the person's life.
B. The disturbance causes marked distress or interpersonal difficulty.
C. The sexual dysfunction is not better accounted for by another Axis I disorder (except another Sexual Dysfunction), and is not due exclusively to the direct physiological effects of a substance (e.g., a drug of abuse, a medication) or a general medical condition. (APA, 1994, p. 498)

The DSM-IV definition of hypoactive sexual desire disorder (HSDD) includes both a cognitive ("fantasies") and a more affective-motivational ("desire for sexual activity") referent. Thus, HSDD can reflect a lack of, or a deficiency in, erotic cognition, interest, and/or sexual goal-seeking behaviors (e.g., sexual initiation with a partner). The presence of sexual activity, however, does not rule out the possibility of HSDD because people may engage in sexual behavior for a number of reasons other than desire (Malatesta & Robinson, 1995).

Conversely, HSDD can also reflect a lack of sexual responsiveness to a partner's initiation. As noted by Rosen and Leiblum (1989), this distinction is influenced by gender biases, and failure to initiate is more commonly associated with male desire problems and a lack of sexual responsivity often associated with female desire disorders. We have witnessed a blurring of this distinction in recent years because of emphasis on the commonalities of women and men in the expression of sexual desire disorders.

Hypoactive sexual desire disorders can be generalized or situational. Thus, in its most extreme form, generalized HSDD would include a complete absence of erotic thoughts, fantasies, and activity. Situational HSDD may reflect problems with a specific partner or activity. The presence of a desire-phase disorder exclusively during the course of another psychiatric condition (e.g., major depression) would not warrant a diagnosis of HSDD. The diagnosis of HSDD would be made only if the loss of sexual desire persisted after the psychiatric condition was resolved.

As noted by Rosen and Leiblum (1989), the current diagnostic classification does not permit an analysis of a frequent sexual complaint presented by couples—desire discrepancies. Individual differences in sexual interest may be a source of relationship conflict, and this situation often results in a couple presenting for sex therapy. Some clinicians have reconceptualized HSDD in interactional terms (Zilbergeld & Evans, 1980), and others have argued that disparate levels of sexual interest are common and should not be formalized with a diagnosis: "... no matter how loving and caring a relationship might be, the two individuals in it are not going to have absolute synchrony in their sexual appetites any more than they would always be hungry or thirsty or sleepy at exactly the same time" (Masters et al., 1994, p. 84).

From another perspective, converging evidence supports the view that complaints of low or absent sexual desire are one of the most common sexual dysfunctions in clinical and nonclinical populations alike. Although earlier studies reflected prevalence estimates that ranged from 15–55% (see Beck, 1995), a recent comprehensive study indicated a 22% prevalence rate of low sexual desire in a large sample of normal women (Laumann, Paik, & Rosen, 1999). Large clinical studies have indicated that 65% of individuals with sexual dysfunction present with a primary diagnosis of HSDD (Segraves & Segraves, 1991).

*Sexual Aversion Disorder (302.79).*

A. Persistent or recurrent extreme aversion to, and avoidance of, all (or almost all) genital sexual contact with a sexual partner.
B. The disturbance causes marked distress or interpersonal difficulty.
C. The sexual dysfunction is not better accounted for by another Axis I disorder (other than a Sexual Dysfunction). (APA, 1994, p. 500)

Sexual aversion disorder (SAD) is a relatively new diagnostic category that appeared for the first time in the DSM-III-R (APA, 1987). SAD goes beyond the simple avoidance of sexual activity to include sexual panic, sexual repugnance, and sexual phobia. Kaplan (1987) drew attention to this class of disorders with her emphasis on sexual panic states and their integrated treatment using pharmacotherapy, insight-oriented psychotherapy, and behavioral exercises. Schover and LoPiccolo (1982) conceptualized sexual avoidance as lying on a continuum, where HSDD is at the mild extreme and sexual aversions and sexual phobias are at the most severe end point. As Kaplan (1987) noted, however, some of these patients may experience normal sexual desire and interest, and can enjoy sexual fantasy and autoerotic activity, but when confronted with an interpersonal sexual situation, they may experience aversion to partner touch or to contact with the partner's genitalia. Conversely, in some cases it may be appropriate to diagnose both HSDD and SAD in the same individual (Sadock, 1995).

Very little is known about the prevalence and etiology of SAD. Masters et al. (1994) reported that SAD involves women two to three times more frequently in its clinical presentation than men. This estimate is consistent with that of other clinical researchers (Rosen & Leiblum, 1989; Schover & LoPiccolo, 1982). As noted by Masters et al., however, it is unclear whether this actually reflects a sex difference or is a function of other factors.

**Sexual Arousal Disorders.** As discussed in the Models section, sexual arousal remains a complex term. On one hand it denotes a range of physiological responses to erotic stimulation and, on the other hand, it reflects an individual's cognitive and emotional reaction to these changes or lack thereof. These aspects of sexual arousal are not necessarily concordant. For example, some middle-aged male patients may present with adequate erections in response to sexual stimulation but report negative feeling and judge the experience as unpleasurable because the erection "is not hard enough." Certain female patients may react to physical sensations of sexual arousal with fears and self-statements about being out of control.

In the DSM-IV, the definition of sexual arousal disorder avoids subjective and affective criteria and focuses instead on physiological arousal. The sexual arousal disorders are divided into (1) Female Sexual Arousal Disorder, which is characterized by the absence or deficiency in vaginal lubrication-swelling in response to adequate sexual stimulation; and (2) male erectile disorder, which reflects an inability to attain and maintain an adequate erection to complete sexual activity. The diagnoses assume that the focus, intensity, and duration of sexual stimulation are adequate to maintain the vasocongestive response in the typical case. Remarkable progress has been made in the biomedical and psychophysiological evaluation of male erectile disorder (e.g., Ackerman & Carey, 1995; Melman & Gingell, 1999), but our knowledge of female sexual arousal and its disorders lags behind. Recent psychophysiological and multivariate studies are advancing our understanding of the interplay of female physiology, emotion, and subjective response as it relates to effective as well as deficient sexual arousal in women (Andersen & Cyranowski, 1995; Elliot & O'Donohue, 1997; Laan & Everaerd, 1995; Meston & Gorzalka, 1996).

*Female Sexual Arousal Disorder (302.72).*

A. Persistent or recurrent inability to attain, or to maintain until completion of the sexual activity, an adequate lubrication-swelling response of sexual excitement.
B. The disturbance causes marked distress or interpersonal difficulty.
C. The sexual dysfunction is not better accounted for by another Axis I disorder (except another Sexual Dysfunction) and is not due exclusively to the direct physiological effects of a substance (e.g., a drug of abuse, a medication) or a general medical condition. (APA, 1994, p.502)

Female sexual arousal disorder (FSAD), referred to in the DSM-III as "inhibited sexual excitement," replaces the antiquated and highly perjorative term "frigidity" once used to describe all forms of female sexual dysfunction (ranging from lack of desire and low arousal to varying degrees of orgasmic dysfunction). FSAD reflects a deficiency or absence in the vasocongestive response to sexual stimulation. This definition emphasizes physiological arousal, but it has been argued that subjective arousal may be a more salient and meaningful criterion in defining a disorder of sexual arousal for women (see Rosen & Leiblum, 1995a). In making the diagnosis, the clinician should assess this aspect and take into account important moderating factors such as the woman's age, sexual experience, and comorbid problems, including other sexual dysfunction (e.g., HSDD). Distinguishing the latter from an arousal disorder may be difficult, as is ruling out an arousal disorder from a primary orgasmic disorder (Sadock, 1995; Segraves & Segraves, 1991).

Perhaps for these reasons, earlier studies showed variability and inconsistency in the prevalence of FSAD. In their review, Spector and Carey (1990) cited community estimates of FSAD that ranged from 11–48%. An early clinical study reported that 57% of women who sought therapy experienced arousal difficulties (Frank, Anderson, & Kupfer, 1976). A recent community study found that 19–27% of women complained of difficulty with lubrication. The range depended on the age, education, marital status, and ethnicity of the woman (Laumann et al., 1999). Finally, in a gynecology clinic sample, lubrication difficulties were reported by 13.6% of women; this rose to 44.2% in postmenopausal women (Rosen, Taylor, Leiblum, & Bachman, 1993).

*Male Erectile Disorder (302.72).*

A. Persistent or recurrent inability to attain, or to maintain until completion of the sexual activity, an adequate erection.
B. The disturbance causes marked distress or interpersonal difficulty.
C. The erectile dysfunction is not better accounted for by another Axis I disorder (other than a Sexual Dysfunction) and is not due exclusively to the direct physiological effects of a substance (e.g., a drug of abuse, a medication) or a general medical condition. (APA, 1994, p. 504)

Male erectile disorder (MED) is also referred to as "erectile dysfunction" and by the more generic term "impotence." Male erectile disorder reflects considerable variability among men. Some individuals experience firm erections during foreplay and/or oral sex but then detumesce on penetration. Other men achieve only a partial erection (insufficient for intromission) throughout sexual activity, whereas some will experience situational erectile difficulty under certain conditions (e.g., with a new partner). In most cases of MED due to psychological factors, there is usually minimal difficulty in attaining an erection during self-stimulation; rather, the problem seems to be restricted to attempts at intercourse. The DSM-IV definition of MED does not indicate that intercourse is necessarily part of the "sexual activity" to make the diagnosis.

The frequency of erectile disorder is strongly related to age, chronic illness, and/or other factors (e.g., use of medication). Data from the Massachusetts Male Aging Study showed that the overall incidence of mild to complete erectile difficulty was 52% in men between the ages of 40 and 70 (Feldman, Goldstein, Hatzichristou, Krane, & McKinlay, 1994). The prevalence of complete erectile difficulty during intercourse was 9.6%, which tripled from 5 to 15% between the ages of 40 and 70 for these healthy men. Focusing on a younger community sample, Spector and Carey (1990) estimated that 4–9% of men experienced erectile disorder. This estimate compares with recent figures which showed that 7–18% of men between the ages of 18 and 59 complained of trouble maintaining or achieving erection (Laumann et al., 1999).

**Orgasmic Disorders.** Female and male orgasmic disorder is a lack of, or marked delay in the orgasmic response following a normal excitement phase. Women and men who can experience orgasm with noncoital clitoral or penile stimulation but cannot achieve orgasm during intercourse (in the absence of manual stimulation) are not necessarily categorized as anorgasmic. Premature ejaculation is also classified within the orgasmic disorders, and refers to male orgasm before, on, or shortly after vaginal penetration, but before the person desires it. In making a diagnosis of an orgasmic disorder, the clinician must make judgements as to (1) the presence of a normal excitement phase, (2) the adequacy and duration of stimulation, and (3) normal situational factors that may exacerbate an orgasmic problem (e.g., premature ejaculation with a new partner).

### Female Orgasmic Disorder (302.73).

A. Persistent or recurrent delay in, or absence of, orgasm following a normal sexual excitement phase. Women exhibit wide variability in the type or intensity of stimulation that triggers orgasm. The diagnosis of Female Orgasmic Disorder should be based on the clinician's judgement that the woman's orgasmic capacity is less than would be reasonable for her age, sexual experience, and the adequacy of sexual stimulation she receives.
B. The disturbance causes marked distress or interpersonal difficulty.
C. The orgasmic dysfunction is not better accounted for by another Axis I disorder (except another Sexual Dysfunction) and is not due exclusively to the direct physiological effects of a substance (e.g., a drug of abuse, a medication) or a general medical condition. (APA, 1994, pp. 506–507)

Female patterns of reaching orgasm can be conceptualized as varying along a continuum that ranges from occasional difficulty in achieving climax under certain conditions to complete inability to reach orgasm through any means. By definition, however, female orgasmic disorder (FOD) is a "persistent or recurrent delay in, or absence of" orgasm despite sufficient sexual stimulation and a normal excitement phase. Thus, whereas occasional difficulties in achieving orgasm may be fairly common for most individuals, the diagnosis of FOD is typically reserved for those women who experience either significant problems in reaching climax or complete inability to experience orgasm.

Physiologically, a woman with FOD (unlike the female suffering from an excitement-phase disorder) may show vaginal lubrication and swelling and may experience subjective arousal in response to various sexual activities (e.g., foreplay and penile intromission). Similarly, in contrast to desire-phase disorders, a woman who is anorgasmic may report (at least initially) adequate sexual desire,

may seek out sexual experiences, and may report erotic thoughts and fantasies. Although FOD is by definition an orgasmic-phase disorder, it is common to find desire-phase and/or excitement-phase problems developing in women who complained initially of FOD dysfunction or vice versa.

Not surprisingly, there has been controversy regarding criteria for diagnosing FOD, and in response, clinical researchers have identified subtypes of FOD (see Andersen & Cyranowski, 1995; Fisher & Barak, 1989; Wakefield, 1987). Kaplan (1974), for instance, presented an early distinction based on "absolute" versus "situational" types of female orgasmic dysfunction. Absolute dysfunction was defined as the inability to experience orgasm under any circumstances; this definition is comparable to that of generalized orgasmic disorder. The term "preorgasmic" was also applied to this group, connoting a positive prognosis and the belief that the experience of orgasm is a learnable activity (Barbach, 1975). The ability to attain orgasm primarily under specified conditions (e.g., only through self-masturbation while alone) was referred to as situational orgasmic dysfunction. Similarly, secondary orgasmic dysfunction has been used to refer to women who are orgasmic but express concern about the frequency and circumstances of the occurrence of orgasm. Andersen and Cyranowski (1995) argued that this pattern represents a normal variation in sexual response for many women and is usually not a diagnostic entity.

FOD prevalence data derived from early community and clinic samples reflected variability that ranged from 5–20% (Spector & Carey, 1990). More recently, only 29% of women in a large nonclinical sample of women reported that they always had an orgasm with their regular partner during sex and 24% reported an inability to have orgasm (Laumann, Gagnon, Michael, & Michaels, 1994). Laumann et al. (1999) reported that 18–32% of women reported being unable to achieve orgasm during the past 12 months. Percentage differences were a function of age, education, marital status, and ethnicity.

### Male Orgasmic Disorder (302.74).

A. Persistent or recurrent delay in, or absence of, orgasm following a normal sexual excitement phase during sexual activity that the clinician, taking into account the person's age, judges to be adequate in focus, intensity, and duration. This failure to achieve orgasm is usually restricted to an inability to reach orgasm in the vagina, with orgasm possible with other types of stimulation, such as masturbation.

B. The disturbance causes marked distress or interpersonal difficulty.

C. The orgasmic dysfunction is not better accounted for by another Axis I disorder (except another Sexual Dysfunction) and is not due exclusively to the direct physiological effects of a substance (e.g., a drug of abuse, a medication) or a general medical condition. (APA, 1994, p. 509)

Although male orgasmic disorder (MOD) represents the male counterpart of female orgasmic disorder, there are several important distinctions. First, clinically speaking, MOD is a relatively rare disorder, compared to the commonality of FOD. Spector and Carey (1990) reported that MOD was the least common male sexual dysfunction whose occurrence is less than 4–10% in the general population. Laumann et al. (1999) reported that 7–11% of men between the ages of 18 and 59 complained of inability to achieve orgasm during the past year. Although MOD may be relatively more common in the general population, individuals who have such difficulties are not likely to come into treatment. It has been noted that the major reason these individuals do seek treatment is because of partner demands for impregnation through intravaginal ejaculation (Apfelbaum, 1989). Thus, a second contrast with FOD is that a major focus of MOD is the male's inability to experience vaginal or coital orgasm. For women, more flexibility is afforded in describing FOD, in that lack of coital orgasm may not be an indication of a disorder. Third, though a biomedical condition may be associated with MOD (Rosen, 1991), this appears less commonly for FOD. Finally, MOD has been called inhibited male orgasm (APA, 1987) and "retarded or delayed ejaculation" which suggests a slowness to ejaculate during intercourse. In psychogenic cases, however, the clinical research suggests that such individuals cannot usually experience orgasm with a partner and may reflect psychopathology (Sadock, 1995).

For these reasons, Apfelbaum (1989) reconceptualized MOD and introduced the term "partner anorgasmia" to call attention to the fact that the primary difficulty in the male who has MOD is reaching any kind of orgasm with any partner. Autoerotic activities, such as masturbation, may be unimpaired. Thus, Apfelbaum argued that MOD may represent one end of a continuum that ranges from those who strongly prefer stimulation by a partner to those who, like the individual with MOD, are more responsive to their own stimulation. There also is, however, a small group of men who (like the women with primary orgasmic dysfunction) have difficulty reaching orgasm under any conditions. Thus, clinical researchers have presented case studies that have spanned a continuum of male orgasmic dysfunction—ranging from total lifelong inability to experience orgasm by any means to ejaculation that is restricted to highly circumscribed situations and methods (Munjack & Kanno, 1979; Sadock, 1995).

### Premature Ejaculation (302.75).

A. Persistent or recurrent ejaculation with minimal sexual stimulation or before, on, or shortly after penetration and before the person wishes it. The clinician must take into account factors that affect duration of the excitement phase, such as age, novelty or the sexual partner or situation, and recent frequency of sexual activity. (APA, 1994, p. 511)

B. The disturbance causes marked distress or interpersonal difficulty.

C. The premature ejaculation is not due exclusively to the direct effects of a substance (e.g., withdrawal from opiates).

Although premature ejaculation is the most prevalent male sexual dysfunction (Laumann et al., 1999; Spector & Carey, 1990), the concept of premature ejaculation (PE) is deceptively simple and subject to misconception. The term "early ejaculation" was introduced a decade ago (McCarthy, 1989) to provide a less perjorative term and to focus description on the role of orgasmic control. However, efforts to generate a precise clinical definition have illuminated the complexity of PE (Metz et al., 1997; St. Lawrence & Madakasira, 1992). Some have argued that PE may not be considered a dysfunction except in extreme cases (Wincze & Carey, 1991), and others have stated that PE is potentially debilitating and often is a precursor to other dysfunctions (McCarthy, 1989).

Part of the definitional difficulty is related to the fact that, for many individuals, premature ejaculation is defined as a problem on the basis of the partner's response. In other words, the latency of male ejaculation is usually viewed within the context of the partner's sexual response cycle. Thus, if the man's early ejaculation consistently limits his partner's sexual satisfaction, a problem has been defined. For some couples, however, abbreviated ejaculatory latencies may not restrict or prevent a partner's satisfaction; this is particularly the case if the woman's excitement phase has been extended through foreplay and/or other sexual behaviors (e.g., cunnilingus) and if she finds these activities highly pleasurable and arousing.

In spite of these difficulties, premature ejaculation has been defined arbitrarily as the inability of the male to control ejaculation for a length of time sufficient to satisfy his partner in at least 50% of their coital encounters, provided there is no female sexual dysfunction evident (Masters & Johnson, 1970). In contrast, Kaplan (1974) focused greater attention on the male's self-regulation or pacing of his excitement phase by defining prematurity as the absence of voluntary control over the ejaculatory reflex. Finally, Masters et al. (1994) state, "While experts have long debated over the precise definition of premature ejaculation, almost every man with this problem knows he's got it: Splitting fine semantic hairs doesn't add much to our understanding" (p. 102).

In the light of the previous discussion, the DSM-IV definition of premature ejaculation emphasizes both temporal and self-evaluative criteria. This definition provides enough flexibility to address normative differences in ejaculatory control associated with age, context (e.g., with a new partner, or following sexual abstinence), and primary versus secondary or situational PE (Cooper, Cernovsky, & Colussi, 1993; Spiess, Geer, & O'Donohue, 1984). Finally, in past decades, it was believed that men with more education displayed greater concerns about partner satisfaction and thus greater concern about PE. Recent data, however, show that men of varying educational backgrounds and ethnicity express similar concerns about climaxing "too early" (Laumann et al., 1999). Contrary to clinical lore, older men expressed as much concern about PE as younger men.

**Sexual Pain Disorders.** Dyspareunia is recurrent and persistent pain during intercourse in either women or men. In men, it is relatively rare (Bancroft, 1989; Sadock, 1995). In women, it is a highly prevalent condition that occurs at 10–21% in community samples and particularly in younger women (Laumann et al., 1999); Rosen, Taylor, Leiblum, & Bachman, 1993). Dyspareunia is a common presenting complaint in gynecologic clinics but is less frequently encountered in mental health settings. Female dyspareunia may be related to biomedical problems (e.g., anatomical defect, infection, surgical scar tissue). In other cases, female dyspareunia may reflect insufficient lubrication or postmenopausal hormonal insufficiency, which affects both vaginal lubrication and the elasticity of the vaginal lining (Masters et al., 1994; Meana & Binik, 1994). If the dyspareunia is caused exclusively by a biological disorder, then the appropriate diagnosis would be Dyspareunia Due to a Medical Condition. Psychological and/or relational factors may be implicated in many cases of dyspareunia (Lazarus, 1989; Sadock, 1995). Vaginismus—an involuntary spasm of the vaginal musculature that interferes with coitus—may be more often associated with psychological variables (Wincze & Carey, 1991), even though biomedical factors may be implicated in the genesis of this disorder. For instance, a medical condition that produces pain during intercourse may precipitate conditioning of vaginal musculature and result in vaginismus, even after the physical cause has been resolved (Kolodny et al., 1979). Similarly, even in its less severe forms, vaginismus often exacerbates dyspareunia because a woman tenses her circumvaginal muscles in anticipation of painful intercourse (Carey & Gordon, 1995; Tollison & Adams, 1979). In either case, however, sexual pain disorders may exist to a far greater degree than reported because individuals with these disorders may avoid sexual activity and/or intimate relationships.

*Dyspareunia (302.76).*

A. Recurrent or persistent genital pain associated with sexual intercourse in either a male or a female.
B. The disturbance causes marked distress or interpersonal difficulty.
C. The disturbance is not caused exclusively by Vaginismus or lack of lubrication, is not better accounted for by another Axis I disorder (except another Sexual Dysfunction), and is not due exclusively to the direct physiological effects of a substance (e.g., a drug of abuse, a medication) or a general medical condition. (APA, 1994, p. 513)

Dyspareunia may be expressed by a variety of pain phenomena that range from postcoital vaginal irritation to severe discomfort with intromission and penile thrusting. Persistent dyspareunia may lead to other sexual dysfunctions, such as vaginismus, desire-, and/or excitement-phase disorders. Dyspareunia in men, though rare, is often associated with a medical condition and may be expressed as a postejaculatory pain disorder (Sadock, 1995).

*Vaginismus (306.51).*

A. Recurrent or persistent involuntary spasm of the musculature of the outer third of the vagina that interferes with sexual intercourse.
B. The disturbance causes marked distress or interpersonal difficulty.
C. The disturbance is not better accounted for by another Axis I disorder (e.g., Somatization Disorder) and is not due exclu-

sively to the direct physiological effects of a general medical condition. (APA, 1994, p. 515)

Vaginismus can range from severe cases where penile insertion into the vagina is impossible because of the spasm, constriction, and consequent pain, to situations where intercourse is possible but only with considerable discomfort. Partial and situational vaginismus may also occur, but these individuals are not inclined generally to seek treatment (Leiblum et al., 1989; Masters et al., 1994). In the generalized type of vaginismus, the woman may be unable to tolerate tampon or finger insertion or pelvic examination (which may need to be performed under general anesthesia). In some cases, a significant phobic element (e.g., fear of penetration by a foreign body) may occur, and sexual encounters are avoided. The presence of a clear avoidance of pain or vaginal penetration *per se* distinguishes vaginismus from a sexual aversion disorder.

Vaginismus can result in desire- or excitement-phase difficulties. However, it may be more common to find that this condition does not interfere with sexual responsiveness, arousal, and orgasmic capability (Kolodny et al., 1979; Masters et al., 1994). In fact, oral-genital sex and other noncoital sexual activities may be quite pleasurable and sexually satisfying to these women. This may be one reason many of these women do not seek treatment. Leiblum et al. (1989) state that in these cases, "often, it is the desire to have children that ultimately propels the couple to seek assistance" (p. 114). At the same time, women presenting with either vaginismus or dyspareunia should be assessed for prior sexual trauma, even though research is inconclusive (Carey & Gordon, 1995).

# Etiology of Sexual Dysfunction

A multivariate perspective is crucial in appreciating the causal complexity and variability of problems in sexuality. Why does one woman with a history of childhood sexual abuse suffer from desire-phase difficulties and avoid all sexual encounters, whereas a second woman with a similar history is sexually active but complains of orgasmic difficulties and a general lack of pleasure? Similarly, why is obsessive anxiety associated with premature ejaculation in one man and with erectile dysfunction in another? Why is a third person able to perform without difficulty even though he displays greater anxiety than the first

two men? To understand the causes of sexual dysfunction and appreciate that sexual function occurs in the face of psychological adversity (McCarthy, 1998; Sarrell & Masters, 1982) is a complex issue that is only beginning to be unraveled. This section begins with a clinical model of etiological factors in sexual dysfunction.

## A Clinical Model of Etiology

During the last 20 years, an important development in the field has been the recognition that sexual dysfunctions in general are caused by a unique interplay of biological, psychological, and interpersonal factors. In the area of erectile disorder, for instance, etiological emphasis has been placed upon vascular, hormonal, and neurological variables (Melman & Gingell, 1999), as well as cognitive-affective and information-processing factors (Bach et al., 1999). Conceptualization of premature ejaculation—which focused initially upon a hypersensitivity to penile stimulation—has proven more complicated (Grenier & Byers, 1995; Rowland, Cooper, Slob, & Houtsmuller, 1997). Female desire-phase difficulties have emphasized hormonal and relational-marital factors (Beck, 1995), whereas sexual trauma has been associated with a range of sexual problems in many women and men (Bartoi & Kinder, 1998; Backer, 1989; Laumann et al., 1999).

Wincze and Barlow's (1997) "Balancing Scale" is an initial approach to conceptualization of these etiological factors. The Balancing Scale shown in Figure 4 is useful as a clinical heuristic and teaching tool for clients. In the left column, the figure lists nine positive psychological factors and nine positive physical factors. In general, these positive factors have been associated with intact sexual functioning and overall sexual enjoyment. In the right column, the Scale also lists nine negative psychological and nine negative physical factors that have been associated with an increased likelihood of sexual dysfunction and distress. However, it is the number of negative risk factors that will "tilt the balance" toward development of a sexual dysfunction. In addition, it is also assumed that the interaction and individual processing of many of these factors are critical in determining whether they lead to sexual dysfunction. For example, an individual who possesses a flexible attitude toward sex (positive psychological factor) may be better able to cope with and actively manage the negative sexual side effects of antihypertensive

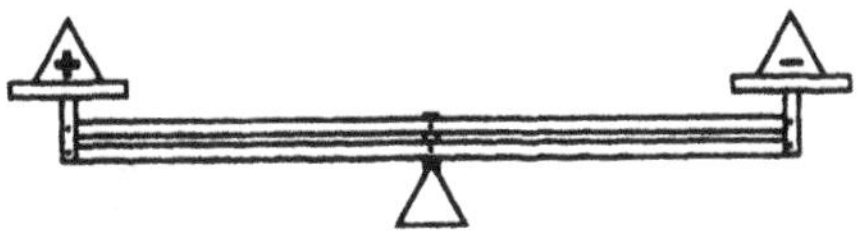

|  | Successful Sexual Functioning | Dysfunctional Sexual Functioning |
|---|---|---|
| Psychological Factors | Good emotional health<br>Attraction toward partner<br>Positive attitude toward partner<br>Positive sex attitude<br>Focus on pleasure<br>Newness<br>Good self-esteem<br>Comfortable environment for sex<br>Flexible attitude toward sex | Depression or PTSD<br>Lack of partner attraction<br>Negative attitude toward partner<br>Negative attitude toward sex<br>Focus on performance<br>Routine, habit<br>Poor self-esteem<br>Uncomfortable environment for sex<br>Rigid, narrow attitude toward sex |
| Physical Factors | No smoking<br>No excess alcohol<br>No medications that affect sex<br>Good physical health<br>Regular, appropriate exercise<br>Good nutrition | Smoking<br>Too much alcohol<br>Antihypertensive medication (heart)/Drugs<br>Poor physical health<br>Heart and blood-flow problems<br>Diabetes |

**Figure 4.** Wincze and Barlow's Balancing Scale: Positive and negative factors that affect secual functioning. From *Enhancing Sexuality: A Problem-Solving Approach* Copyright 1997 by Graywind Publications. Reproduced by permission of publisher, The Psychological Corporation. All rights reserved.

medication (negative physical factor). Similarly, an isolated episode of erectile failure associated with excessive alcohol intake (negative physical factor) may pose minimal difficulty to an emotionally healthy individual (positive psychological factor), but it represents a traumatic event that leads to future erectile problems for an anxious individual who is cognitively focused on his performance (negative psychological factor).

Thus, the mere presence of a negative etiological factor may not necessarily result in sexual dysfunction. Instead, the interaction of an environmental event, biological integrity, interpersonal support, and individual psychological makeup will determine whether a sexual dysfunction develops in a given individual. Although a relatively simple model, the Balancing Scale reflects the multivariate process of conceptualizing etiological factors in sexual dysfunction. Moreover, it is similar to the medical approach of identifying an individual's behavioral and biological "risk" factors versus "health" factors to determine the likelihood of developing medical disorders related to life-style such as heart disease.

## Biological Risk Factors

**Disease and Illness.** Sexual dysfunctions are often related to biomedical illness, which may operate by differential interaction of physical and secondary factors. These problems range from a predominant physical causation (as in the case of prostate or cervical cancer) to a medical etiology with indirect but significant psychological sequelae. For example, for 50% of female gynecologic cancer survivors, posttreatment sexual difficulties do not resolve—even though improvement occurs in other life areas, including mood and social adjustment (see Andersen, Andersen, & deProsse, 1989). Sexual problems have included arousal difficulties, orgasmic disorder, and dyspareunia (Andersen, 1985). For these women, research has shown that a psychological factor, "sexual self-schema," accounts for variance comparable to that of two physical factors (the extent of cancer treatment and menopausal symptoms) in predicting current sexual behavior and responsiveness (Andersen, Woods, & Copeland, 1997).

Although any major organ-system dysfunction (renal, pulmonary, cardiac, or hepatic) may cause sexual dysfunction, psychological factors may aggravate the case, for example, where transient and remitting sexual disturbance is an early disease symptom (e.g., in diabetes). In these cases, the onset of illness-induced sexual dysfunction may be characterized by etiological uncertainty and misattribution. In other cases (as in the postcoronary male), the sexual situation often reflects misinformation, anxiety, and fear of the "coital coronary." As an adjunctive problem, certain surgical procedures and classes of medication can also exert negative influences on sexual interest and functioning (Galyer, Conaglen, Hare, & Conaglen, 1999).

During the last decade, clinical researchers have directed greater investigative attention to the sexual needs and problems of women and men who suffer from chronic illness and physically disabling conditions. In the past, disability status often carried the stigma of asexuality. Moreover, less attention was focused on the sexual lives of women with disability. Today, a number of clinical researchers active in this area display a sophistication in psychological issues related to illness and sexuality and also keen understanding of the medical, physiological, and pharmacological variables within this complex area (e.g., Andersen et al., 1997; McCormick, 1996; Schover & Jensen, 1988). Work has addressed the spectrum of disease and illness that ranges from life-threatening crises (e.g., cardiovascular disease, cancer, end-stage renal disease) to insidious illnesses (e.g., diabetes, chronic obstructive pulmonary disease). Similar studies have addressed sexual and relationship dysfunction in multiple sclerosis patients (McCabe et al., 1996; Schover, Thomas, Lakin, Montague, & Fischer, 1988) and sexual rehabilitation in cancer patients (Schover, Evans, & von Eschenbach, 1987). Others have focused on sex problems and therapy issues for patients with spinal cord injury (Whipple, Gerdes, & Komisaruk, 1996). Diabetes and sexual dysfunction in men and women is an active area of research (Jensen, 1986; Lipshultz & Kim, 1999; Prather, 1988; Weinhardt & Carey, 1996). Finally, studies are addressing the unique sexual problems of women with chronic pain, interstitial cystitis, and types of spinal cord injury (Schlesinger, 1996; Spiski, Alexander, & Rosen, 1999; Webster, 1996).

For additional study of the topic of physical illness/chronic disease and sexuality, see Table 2, which presents a brief listing of relevant literature (see also the journal *Sexuality and Disability*).

**Aging.** The later years, once synonymous with impairment and eventual loss of sexual desire and activity, now reflect more accurately both a variability and stability in sexual expression (Adams & Turner, 1985; Butler & Lewis, 1993; Fisher, Swingen, & O'Donohue, 1997; Malatesta, 1989). Many studies that address older adult sexuality use cross-sectional designs that confound the effects of age and cohort. Consequently, these studies

**Table 2. Selective Listing of Additional Sources Relevant to Physical Illness and Chronic Disease and Sexual Dysfunction**

| Illness or disease | Source |
|---|---|
| General reviews | Farber (1985) |
|  | Schover (1989) |
|  | Schover & Jensen (1988) |
| Women and disability | Krotoski, Nosek, & Turk (1996) |
|  | McCormick (1996) |
|  | Monga (1995) |
| Brain injury | Blackerby (1990) |
|  | Griffith & Lemberg (1993) |
| Cancer | Schover and Randers-Pehrson (1988a,b) |
| Developmental disabilities | Monat-Haller (1992) |
| Heart disease | Kinchla & Weiss (1985) |
|  | Papadopoulos et al. (1986) |
| Multiple sclerosis | McCabe et al. (1996) |
| Scleroderma | Saad & Behrendt (1996) |
| Spinal cord injury/ paralysis | Ducharme & Gill (1997) |

present a deceptively pessimistic picture that shows a precipitous "age-related" decline in sexual desire and activity. In reality, cross-sectional studies only tell us about age differences (i.e., differences between age groups) while telling us little about age changes (i.e., changes in the same age group during a period of time). Longitudinal data have shown that although advancing age *per se* may be related to quantitative but not qualitative changes in sexual activity (George & Weiler, 1981; Pfeiffer, 1977), a host of variables that accompanies aging may exert significantly adverse effects on sexual behavior and interest: (1) physical debility; (2) chronic disease; (3) increased use of medication; (4) age-related emotional problems; (5) interpersonal logistics (e.g., widowhood, lack of privacy, nursing home); (6) societal, family, and personal expectations; and (7) a previous life-style of low sexual activity (Butler & Lewis, 1993; Malatesta, Chambless, Pollack, & Cantor, 1988; Martin, 1981; Weizman & Hart, 1987).

For healthy women, aging is not associated with decreased sexual desire or a decreased capacity for orgasm (Masters & Johnson, 1966). The most frequently encountered problems (atrophy of the vaginal mucosa and decreased vaginal lubrication) usually become apparent with postmenopausal hormone deficiencies and may cause dyspareunia, which is treatable by vaginal lubricating agents and/or estrogen replacement therapy (Masters et al., 1994; Sherwin, 1991).

The normal pattern of sexual aging in older men is qualitatively different from that in women. In contrast to the female aging process, there is usually not as dramatic a decrease in sex-steroid hormone levels, although a gradual reduction in the circulating levels of testosterone is usually evident after age 60 (see Butler & Lewis, 1993; Masters et al., 1994). Considerable variability exists, but male aging is typically associated with (1) increased latency to erection, (2) greater need for longer tactile stimulation to produce erection, (3) mild but noticeable changes in penile tumescence, (4) decreased ejaculatory intensity and decreased urgency to reach orgasm, and (5) an increased refractory period (Butler & Lewis, 1993; Masters & Johnson, 1966). Not surprisingly, these age-related sexual changes may be misinterpreted by both the uninformed male and his partner, who may then attribute his "difficulties" to loss of masculinity or partner attractiveness, or to any number of variables. Clearly, the availability of age-relevant sexual information is crucial for handling these sexual alterations associated with aging.

It is important to emphasize that individual sexual patterns established early in life tend to be maintained in middle and old age and that complicating factors such as physical illness, partner availability, and societal expectations are the greatest causes of sexual problems among older adults. The issue of prolonged celibacy or sexual abstinence as a cause of sexual problems in older adults remains a controversial and generally unsubstantiated finding (Schover & Jensen, 1988). It has been argued and generally assumed that extended periods of sexual abstinence may exert a "physiological handicap" for the elderly who wish to resume sexual activity at a later time. There are minimal data to substantiate this claim, and this belief may represent another myth associated with sexuality and older adults.

The sexual problems of older adults may not significantly differ from those of younger individuals, but greater sensitivity must be paid to the impact of biological and psychological factors (Fisher, Swingen, & O'Donohue, 1997; Leiblum

& Segraves, 1989). Any therapeutic intervention should reflect a respect for the continuity of one's sexual life-style and a readiness to explore alternative methods of meeting the sexual and affectional needs of older adults who remain interested in their sexuality but who are disabled, without partners, or live within a restricted environment (Malatesta, 1989).

**Pharmacological Influences.** Multiple studies show that a vast array of drugs can interfere with any phase of sexual response. A number of sources provide comprehensive information on drug actions with specific reference to sexual side effects (Ashton, Hamer, & Rosen, 1997; Gitlin, 1994; Sadock, 1995). Work has also addressed the sexual side effects of psychotropic drugs on women (see Crenshaw & Goldberg, 1996; Jani & Wise, 1988; Riley & Riley, 1993; Segraves, 1988).

Some of the more popular medications associated with sexual dysfunction are (1) selective serotonin re-uptake inhibitors (SSRIs); (2) heterocyclic antidepressants (e.g., anticholinergic agents) and monoamine oxidase inhibitors (MAOIs); (3) dopamine-blocking agents (e.g., haloperidol and the phenothiazines); (4) antihypertensive drugs (e.g., beta-blockers and diuretics); (5) antiandrogenic compounds (e.g., estrogen and progesterone); and (6) narcotics and sedative hypnotics, which decrease CNS cortical activity.

Alcohol, another CNS depressant, has received attention in studies that address its effects on sexual functioning among individuals who display either moderate or addictive drinking patterns (Crowe & George, 1989; Rosen, 1991; Schover & Jensen, 1988; Wilsnack, 1991). It has been shown empirically that acute alcohol intoxication in nonalcoholic samples of men and women affects sexual arousal (Briddell & Wilson, 1976; Wilson & Lawson, 1978) and orgasm (Malatesta, Pollack, Crotty, & Peacock, 1982; Malatesta, Pollack, Wilbanks, & Adams, 1979). Other studies have addressed the detrimental effects of alcohol intoxication and cognitive distractors on male sexual arousal (Wilson, Niaura, & Adler, 1985).

Similar findings have been reported for male alcohol abusers (Wilson, Lawson, & Abrams, 1978), and sexual detriments tend to last well after alcohol intake stops (Schiavi, 1990). A study of 116 male alcoholic inpatients revealed that at least one sexual problem was reported by 75% of the sample: erectile dysfunction in 42%, premature ejaculation in 43%, low sexual desire in 46%, and delayed orgasm in 23% (Fahrner, 1987). Female alcoholics report a range of dysfunctions, including heightened premenstrual dysphoria, reduced sexual desire and arousal, anorgasmia, dyspareunia, and vaginismus (Wilsnack, 1984, 1991). Moreover, heavy drinking may block ovulation and cause other hormonal abnormalities in some healthy women (Mendelson & Mello, 1988).

A range of complex and interactive etiological factors may account for the disruptive effects of chronic alcohol abuse and alcoholism on sexual function (Goldman & Roehrich, 1991; Wilsnack, 1980). These include (1) the acute depressant effects of alcohol on sexual response, (2) the disruption of gonadal hormone metabolism secondary to liver damage, (3) reduced sexual sensation as a result of alcohol-induced neuropathy, (4) organic brain damage that causes impairment of both interpersonal and sexual interest, and (5) concomitant medical and psychological problems associated with alcoholism (e.g., hypertension, psychopathology).

## Psychosocial Risk Factors

Our knowledge of the complex role of psychosocial risk factors reflects a range of data sources, including clinical impression, observational studies, correlational designs with clinical and nonclinical samples, and more formal experimental research. There are inherent difficulties in studying psychological causes of sexual dysfunction. Moreover, compared with many areas, there is a dearth in funding opportunities for basic sex research. As a consequence, there has been less emphasis on hypothesis testing, theory research, and more rigorous experimental methods. Still, the contribution of laboratory research, including theory-driven approaches, cannot be underestimated (e.g., Bach et al., 1999; Palace, 1995; Rowland, 1999).

**Predisposing Factors.**    Based upon their extensive clinical observation, Masters and Johnson (1970) indicated that a rigid religious orthodoxy was the greatest single cause of sexual dysfunction. Obviously a complex issue (Davidson, Darling, & Norton, 1995; Rundel, 1998), negative sexual learning that involves religious themes has been associated with the range of sexual dysfunctions, including low sexual desire (LoPiccolo & Friedman, 1988), arousal and orgasmic problems (Kaplan, 1974; Masters et al., 1994), and vaginismus (Silverstein, 1989). "In these cases, it is

not the religious teachings per se that are the problem, but the often-associated family attitudes that are imparted to the child that sex is dirty and sinful" (Masters et al., 1994, pp. 140–141). Similarly, it is assumed that an early childhood sexual environment characterized by negative attitudes and misinformation is not conducive to healthy sexual learning; instead, it can be expected to result in sexual inhibitions, fears, and negative attitudes about sexual expression. Deficits in sexual knowledge or experience may be expected to exert a similar influence, as would early-learned negative sexual sanctions (Leight, 1990).

Sexual trauma has been consistently related to the development of sexual dysfunction in both women and men (Bartoi & Kinder, 1998; Becker & Kaplan, 1991; Laumann et al., 1999). Note, however, that "Sexual trauma is a multicausal, multidimensional phenomenon with variable outcomes and vast individual differences" (McCarthy, 1998, p. 91). Traumatic experiences such as sexual abuse/assault, incest, and other illicit sexual activity have been associated with a range of difficulties, including intimacy and trust issues, sexual avoidance, arousal disorders, and negative conditioning, including dyspareunia. In a retrospective study of 372 sexual assault survivors, Becker and her colleagues reported that 58% of these women experienced sexual dysfunctions, compared to 17% of a control group without a history of sexual assault (see Becker & Kaplan, 1991). The most common sexual dysfunctions involved fear of sex, arousal dysfunctions, and desire problems. Several authors have noted that women who have a history of incest may present with vaginismus as part of their sexual dysfunction (LoPiccolo & Stock, 1987; Carey & Gordon, 1995). Finally, male victims of adult–child contact are three times as likely to experience erectile dysfunction and twice as likely to experience low sexual desire and premature ejaculation (Laumann et al., 1999).

Although empirical data are lacking, early negative conditioning events have been associated with sexual dysfunction (Masters et al., 1994; Tollison & Adams, 1979). In particular, one explanation of premature ejaculation has focused on the conditioning of rapid orgasm engendered by early sexual experiences (Ruff & St. Lawrence, 1985). These experiences might include, for example, masturbation, intercourse with prostitutes who encourage rapid ejaculation, and intercourse in semiprivate situations where a related fear of detection is conducive to rapid orgasm. Fear of pregnancy and fear of detection represent important anxiety-conditioning factors to female sexual dysfunction, and vaginismus can be a reactive or self-protective conditioning event secondary to traumatic sexual experiences or other unwanted sexual contacts (see Carey & Gordon, 1995).

Relationship difficulties are obviously an important risk factor in the development of various sexual dysfunctions, including desire, arousal, and orgasmic disorders. Conflict, intimacy and control problems, stress, and poor communication and technique have been noted most frequently (see Beck, 1995; LoPiccolo & Friedman, 1988; Morokoff & Gillilland, 1993; Rosen & Leiblum, 1995a). Unresolved partner differences in sexual desire may also be precursors of a couple's sexual problems (Zilbergeld & Ellison, 1980). Sexual boredom or habituation, though sometimes reflecting a couple's lack of creativity and innovation, often predates sexual dysfunction in the middle and later years (Butler & Lewis, 1993). Finally, there is need for clinical research to address the unique stresses and challenges associated with couples who are coping with infertility and its effects on individual and couple sexuality (Lasker & Borg, 1995).

**Precipitating and Maintaining Factors.** Precipitating factors have a close temporal relationship to the onset of sexual dysfunction and are assumed to have instigated it. Maintaining factors, in contrast, perpetuate dysfunctional activity. In many cases, a discrete precipitating factor cannot be identified, but an array of variables, including stress and emotional problems (Laumann et al., 1999), have been hypothesized to precipitate sexual failure, distress, and avoidance. Predisposing factors discussed before may also function as precipitating and/or maintaining factors. Early formulations, relying on data suggesting that penile erection and vaginal lubrication/swelling are predominantly parasympathetic functions, emphasized increased sympathetic nervous activity as one construct to explain sexual failure in men and women (Masters & Johnson, 1970; Wolpe, 1982). There are any number of variables that increase sympathetic activity that could be relevant to sexual dysfunction. Negative mood states, especially anxiety, were implicated in this process. In particular, anxiety arising from performance demands, perceived inadequacy of sexual performance, or fear of performance failure was believed to be the most important precipitating (as well as maintaining) factor in sexual dysfunction (Kaplan, 1974; Masters & Johnson, 1970).

Because sexual arousal is mediated by both parasympathetic and sympathetic activation (see Rowland, 1995), anxiety *per se* is inadequate to explain the range of clinical phenomena in sexual dysfunctions. Beck and Barlow (1984) described a number of very different studies showing that elevated anxiety can actually increase sexual response under certain conditions. A growing number of studies also illustrates the complex relationships among anxiety and mood state, cognitive factors, and affective response in mediating sexual arousal and dysfunction (see Bach et al., 1999; Meston & Gorzalka, 1996; Palace, 1995). These studies show that sexually dysfunctional and sexually functional men and women respond quite differently to anxiety, distraction, and performance-related feedback (Mitchell, DiBartolo, Brown, & Barlow, 1998).

Although sexual dysfunction may represent a common final outcome of a sexual problem, the critical issue is this: Almost everyone has had at least one sexual episode that has resulted in distress and/or failure. Why do some people develop sexual dysfunction as a result, whereas others do not? If one responds to an initial failure with alarm and distress and attempts to cognitively "check" oneself in the next encounter, another failure is more likely. Masters and Johnson (1970) described this cognitive response as "spectatoring," that is, an individual's self-monitoring of sexual response during an encounter that reduces sexual pleasure, interferes with attention and response to more relevant sexual cues, and heightens anxiety level when the desired response is not achieved. This experience is likely to condition and solidify the dysfunctional pattern (Masters & Johnson, 1970). Experimental studies described earlier help to articulate this process. In addition, research has shown that sexually functional men tend to ignore or do not attend to declines in physiological arousal (Mitchell et al., 1998). These studies imply that if one can maintain a positive sexual self-efficacy in the face of impaired performance, then sexual dysfunction is less likely to develop (Bach et al., 1999). This has been described as "resistance to the dysfunctional mentality" (see Barlow, Chorpita, & Turovsky, 1996). Relatedly, based on experimental studies, it has been suggested that for sexually dysfunctional women, attempts to increase autonomic responsivity (perhaps through physical activity) may facilitate genital response and positive sexual learning and promote more rapid extinction of conditioned negative response patterns (Palace, 1995).

**The Role of Psychopathology.** Traditionally, psychopathology has been associated with sexual problems. Early psychoanalytic thinkers, for instance, equated female orgasmic dysfunction with psychological maladjustment (Fenichel, 1945), and even Freud referred to his early work as a sexual theory of neuroses. To date, however, a direct cause and effect relationship between psychopathology and sexual dysfunction has been difficult to establish. Still, even with the limited data available from clinical and correlational studies, two important conclusions can be drawn: (1) Many individuals (as well as their partners) who seek treatment for sexual dysfunction have diagnosable psychiatric disorders and (2) many individuals who seek treatment for psychiatric problems also display significant sexual dysfunction or distress (Derogatis, Meyer, & King, 1981; Rosenheim & Neuman, 1981; Schreiner-Engel & Schiavi, 1986; Sadock, 1995).

Psychopathology may be a cause, a consequence, or a concomitant of sexual dysfunction. In the first case, psychopathology, it can be hypothesized, operates as a predisposing, precipitating, and/or maintaining factor. For instance, work has addressed the conceptual relationship between panic disorder and sexual dysfunction (Sbrocco, Weisberg, Barlow, & Carter, 1997). Other studies have focused on the role of obsessive-compulsive disorder in relation to the degree of sexual distress and dysfunction (e.g., Freund & Steketee, 1989; Staebler, Pollard, & Merkel, 1993). Studies have also addressed the well-known association between depression and diminished sexual desire (Schreiner-Engel & Schiavi, 1986). In this case, however, it is unclear whether depression is exerting its influence on sexual desire via biochemical substrates, lowered self-esteem, loss of pleasure and sensual awareness, or other undisclosed variables. Note that sexual desire and arousal problems are a common response to depression, and other sexual dysfunctions occur considerably less often (Masters et al., 1994). Finally, the challenge of untangling etiological factors is exemplified in the association between eating disorders and sexual dysfunction (Renshaw, 1990; Wiederman,

1996). The etiology of sexual dysfunction in individuals with eating disorders includes biomedical factors, possible sexual abuse history, body-image distortion, maturational fears, and sexual phobia (Werlinger, King, Clark, Pera, & Wincze, 1997).

# Comprehensive Assessment of Sexual Dysfunction

The assessment of sexual dysfunction, particularly the investigation of its psychophysiological correlates, continues to develop (Ackerman & Carey, 1995; Rowland, 1999). The assessment of sexual dysfunction should include biobehavioral, cognitive, and interpersonal components, even though the nature of the relationships among these components is not yet fully understood.

## Sexual Assessment

The hallmarks of adequate sexual assessment can be classified into three major areas. First, the assessment of sexual dysfunction requires systematic investigation across three components of response: verbal or self-report (cognitive-subjective), behavioral indexes, and physiological measurement. This tripartite assessment approach is sensitive to the intricacies of sexual response and provides important data regarding response congruences and discrepancies that are of value in hypothesis testing and treatment planning.

Second, sexual assessment should attend to four distinct but ultimately related systems of sexuality: (1) biological/medical/health status; (2) the phases of sexual response (e.g., desire, arousal, orgasm); (3) individual psychological makeup, including personality, developmental liabilities, mood-state variables, and psychopathology; and (4) interpersonal issues, relationship status, and partner variables. Although each of these systems is important to an individual's sexuality, different system combinations will predominate in a given case.

Third, comprehensive assessment involves two essential processes that should be used in all cases: preintervention assessment (the composite of procedures to arrive at a final formulation and treatment plan) and continuous assessment (the ongoing monitoring of selected components and systems throughout the treatment and follow-up phases). This continuous assessment is a constant check on the accuracy of one's formulation, provides a system of feedback for treatment progress, and offers a method of outcome evaluation.

### Self-Report Techniques

**Clinical Interview.** The interview remains the most common and useful assessment technique for obtaining relevant data and for developing an initial problem formulation. This format can be optimized by imposing a systematic (but sensitive) interview strategy that, in addition to relevant assessment areas, considers the level of sexual knowledge and the comfort of the couple in talking about their sexual habits and beliefs. The clinical interview represents the first important step in conducting a sexual assessment. This first formal contact with the patient will determine whether sufficient data are available to proceed with an objective assessment and whether the clinician has engendered sufficient trust, professional respect, and therapeutic hope to allow the patient or couple to participate actively in an assessment process. Clinical interviewing for sexual problems is a highly sensitive area that demands judgment, flexibility, and common sense.

In addition to the goal of problem specification and analysis, the aims of the initial interview are (1) to establish a therapeutic alliance that emphasizes comfortable communication between patient and therapist about sexual matters in particular; (2) to generate hypotheses about the development and maintenance of the sexual disorder; (3) to address factors that would make sexual assessment inappropriate at this time (e.g., medical problems, other psychopathology, severe marital conflict); (4) to arrive at a tentative formulation about the case; and (5) to develop a plan for the more formalized, objective assessment of the individual and his or her partner.

Specific guidelines and formats for sexual interviewing can be found in Carey and Gordon (1995), Sadock (1995), and Wincze and Barlow (1997). Catania (1999) provides a state-of-the-art review of sexual assessment, including issues related to reporting bias. Similarly, several semistructured interviews are available for either broad-based or problem-focused sexual assessment (see Ackerman & Carey, 1995; Derogatis, 1997).

**Self-Administered Questionnaires and Inventories.** Pencil-and-paper assessment tools that provide more detailed and somewhat more objective data continue to be developed. These instruments play an important role in sexual assessment and treatment evaluation, particularly in view of the expense and specific difficulties in obtaining valid and reliable physiological measures. The variety and range of questionnaires and inventories are too numerous to discuss separately, but the *Handbook of sexuality-related measures* provides a complete listing and analysis of scales and inventories for various areas of sexuality (Davis, Yarber, Bauserman, Schreer, & Davis, 1998). Many of these instruments have been subjected to psychometric analysis and test development procedures. Table 3 provides a brief listing of current scales and the areas of sexuality that they assess. Some provide an individual profile analysis of various aspects of sexual function and dysfunction (Derogatis, 1978, 1997), whereas others focus on sexual preferences and specific patient populations (Brockway & Steger, 1980; Purnine, Carey, & Jorgensen, 1996; White, 1982). Although all suffer the weaknesses and threats to validity that are common to most self-report instruments, their judicious use offers a range of information sometimes unavailable in the standard interview, allows quantifying the assessment data, and some instruments provide a method of continuous assessment of pre–post–therapy changes.

**Self-Monitoring and Other Recording Techniques.** Self-monitoring is a well-known behaviorally oriented technique (Bornstein, Hamilton, & Bornstein, 1986). Writing methods and other recording techniques can be used in both assessment and treatment (e.g., Apfelbaum, 1995). Within the area of sexual dysfunction, the typical format requires the couple to record individually and sometimes to evaluate their intimate and sexual activity, including the level of sexual desire and arousal, affectional behaviors, sexual initiation responses, quality and frequency of orgasmic experience, pleasure, and perceived partner satisfaction. Cognitive, emotional, or more qualitative data may also be collected. Besides providing a level of external validity, the flexibility of these procedures permits specific hypothesis testing, as well as a quantifiable means of measuring treatment progress. Conte (1986) describes the most popular sexually oriented self-monitoring procedures, and Apfelbaum (1995) provides an interesting example of writing assignments within the context of couple treatment for low sexual desire.

Table 3. Questionnaires and Inventories Used in Sexual Assessment

| Assessment area | Questionnaire |
|---|---|
| Sexual knowledge and attitudes | Sexual Knowledge Inventory (Casselman & Durham, 1979); Aging Sexuality Knowledge/Attitude Scale (White, 1982); Sexual Opinion Inventory (Gilbert & Gamache, 1984); Sexual Attitudes Scale (Hendrick & Hendrick, 1987) |
| Sexual arousal, anxiety, and preferences | Sexual Arousability Inventory—Expanded Version (SAI-E; Chambless & Lifshitz, 1984); Sex Anxiety Inventory (Janda & O'Grady, 1980); Sexual Aversion Scale (Katz, Gipson, Kearl, & Kirskovick, 1989); Inventory of Dyadic Heterosexual Preferences (Purnine, Carey, & Jorgensen, 1996); Intimacy Scale (Waring & Reddon, 1983) |
| Sexual dysfunction and satisfaction | Derogatis Interview for Sexual Functioning—Self-Report (Derogatis, 1997); Derogatis Sexual Functioning Inventory (Derogatis, 1978); Marital Satisfaction Inventory—Revised (Snyder, 1997); Sexual Dysfunction Scale (McCabe, 1997); Inventory of Sexual Satisfaction (Rust & Golombok, 1986); Pinney Sexual Satisfaction Inventory (Pinney, Gerrard, & Denny, 1987); Sexual Interaction Inventory (LoPiccolo & Steger, 1974); Index of Sexual Satisfaction (Hudson, Harrison, & Crosscup, 1981) |

## Direct Behavioral Observation

In the light of the serious ethical and legal problems associated with the direct observation of a patient's sexual activity, such measures do not represent a viable clinical assessment option. Although the pioneering work of Masters and Johnson (1966) illustrates an exception to this rule, others received much negative criticism for their questionable assessment practices (Hartmann & Fithian, 1974). The use of sexual surrogates, initiated but later abandoned by Masters and Johnson, is similarly frowned upon (Apfelbaum, 1977) and fraught with potential legal, moral, and interpersonal tangles. However, the direct observation of nonsexual but related behavior and interaction patterns (e.g., communication skills, expression of intimacy) can provide important assessment data that may lend indirect support to hypothesized sexual problem areas (see Larson, Anderson, Holman, & Niemann, 1998; McCabe, 1997; Purnine & Carey, 1997).

## Biomedical and Psychophysiological Methods

**Biomedical Assessment.** From multiple perspectives (ethical, evaluative, and therapeutic), a case of sexual dysfunction is outside the domain of the mental health professional until biomedical factors have been addressed by medical personnel. The medical workup represents an essential prerequisite for formal psychological assessment of sexual dysfunction and also reflects the need for a working relationship with a specialist physician (urologist, gynecologist) (see Perelman, 1994). Moreover, the biomedical evaluation has become increasingly important as the issue of sexuality has interfaced to a greater extent with those of advancing age, illness and disability, medication and drug use, and our increased biological understanding of arousal disorders (Laan & Everaerd, 1995; Melman & Gingell, 1999). This emphasis has mirrored a growing sophistication in the biomedical assessment of erectile dysfunction and the availability of "urology-based evaluation centers" that specialize in the comprehensive assessment and multidisciplinary treatment of these disorders (Tiefer & Melman, 1989).

The medical data base is typically derived from four subareas of assessment: (1) a thorough medical and health history; (2) physical examination; (3) laboratory evaluation; and where indicated, (4) specialized clinical laboratory testing. These procedures have been outlined and described by a number of clinicians (Kolodny et al., 1979; Schover & Jensen, 1988; Tiefer & Melman, 1989). It is also recommended that each partner undergo the complete medical workup, including endocrine testing (e.g., plasma testosterone, serum estrogens, pituitary function) (see Sadock, 1995). Specialized laboratory evaluations have focused on penile response assessments, including vascular testing (e.g., penile arterial pressure, doppler sonography and cavernosography, or penile venous outflow), neurological testing (e.g., nerve conductivity), and nocturnal penile tumescence/rigidity testing (see Rowland & Slob, 1995).

**Psychophysiological Assessment.** Although focused initially on basic sex research, quantitative measurement of the psychophysiological aspects of arousal and orgasm is an increasingly active domain of sexual assessment. This complex area continues to receive considerable investigative attention, and several methodological and nontechnical reviews have appeared in the literature (Ackerman & Carey, 1995; Rosen & Beck, 1988; Rowland, 1999). Psychophysiological assessment of female sexual dysfunction continues to lag behind, even though promising developments have occurred (Andersen & Cyranowski, 1995; Laan & Everaerd, 1995; Rosen & Beck, 1988).

There is also a growing understanding that a simple dichotomy between biogenic and psychogenic arousal disorders is artificial, misleading, and inadequate in addressing actual clinical cases. This view has been replaced by a biopsychosocial approach that incorporates a multivariate perspective. In addition, there is greater clarity that male arousal disorders result from the culmination of various interacting vascular, hormonal, neurobehavioral, cognitive-affective, and life-style factors (National Institutes of Health, 1993). Therefore, to delineate etiology, "state of the science assessment" requires input from several disciplines (see Ackerman & Carey, 1995). Clinical psychophysiology has developed an important role in this process.

The most commonly used psychophysiological procedure in diagnosing erectile disorder is nocturnal penile testing (NPT) during the sleep cycle. NPT is based upon the rationale that naturally occurring REM-related erectile responses will be exhibited during sleep, particularly because interfering psychological phenomena (e.g., performance demands, interpersonal and emotional conflict) should be inoperative at that time. Those cases with a substantial organic basis typically exhibit impaired or absent erections. Typically, two to three consecutive nights of NPT assessment are required. This evaluation also includes regular sleep-laboratory evaluation to document REM periods and sleep architecture. A less costly but more experimental procedure is that of NPT monitoring during naps (Gordon & Carey, 1995). If portable NPT monitors, "snap gauges," and stamp-ring

testing (which do not verify sleep stages) are used, they should be viewed only as screening devices (Rosen & Beck, 1988). One exception is the "RigiScan Diagnostic Monitor," a computerized device that measures erectile rigidity, tumescence, and duration throughout the sleep cycle (Levine & Caroll, 1994). It is a popular alternative to sleep-laboratory NPT. Related developments include comparing these NPT procedures with visual sexual stimulation and/or with vasoactive penile injections (see Ackerman & Carey, 1995). Overall, however, NPT is best regarded as one component in the comprehensive assessment of erectile dysfunction.

### Case Formulation

An important goal of assessment is development of an individual and/or couple "case formulation" (Meyer & Turkat, 1979). Sometimes confused with diagnosis and functional analysis, the case formulation is an attempt to identify and describe the major biological, psychological, and interpersonal components in a case. The formulation should (1) explain the relationship of all of the patient's or couple's problems (sexual and otherwise) to one another, (2) delineate why and how these problems developed and are maintained, and (3) provide specific predictions of the patient's and couple's behavior in the treatment process (Carey, Flasher, Maisto, & Turkat, 1984; Meyer & Turkat, 1979). In essence, the case formulation, based on integrating assessment and historical data, should posit a discrete explanation statement or hypothesis that can be tested clinically and that will then govern the treatment selection, planning, and the treatment process. Difficulties such as noncompliance, symptom fluctuation and relapse, and barriers to a collaborative therapist–patient relationship are anticipated, and one hopes minimized, by relying on this formulation (AuBuchon & Malatesta, 1998). Even though good clinicians from varying orientations formulate their cases at least on an intuitive level (see Rosen & Leiblum, 1995b; Perry, Cooper, & Michels, 1987), it is good clinical practice and a fruitful clinical discipline to actually record one's case formulation in a written format. Examples of cognitive and behavioral formulations can be found in Bruch and Bond (1998), Persons (1989), and Turkat (1985). Psychodynamic, systems, and ego analytic case formulations are discussed in Rosen and Leiblum (1995b).

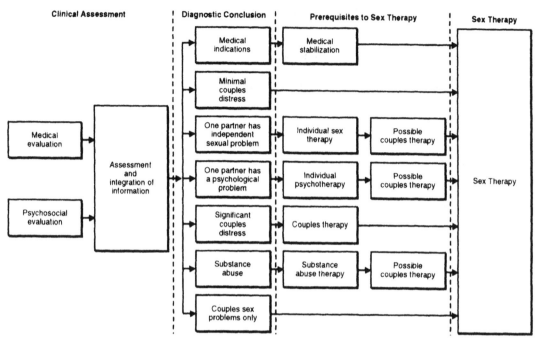

**Figure 5.** A flow chart depicting "Seven Critical Pathways" or sequences of clinical events based on assessment, diagnosis, and case formulation. From *Enhancing Sexuality: A Problem-Solving Approach.* Copyright 1997 by Graywind Publications. Reproduced by permission of publisher, The Psychological Corporation. All rights reserved.

The case formulation is used in two major ways: (1) to guide treatment selection and/or (2) to orchestrate and pace the process of psychological treatment. With respect to general treatment selection, Wincze and Barlow (1997) offer a useful flow chart, described as "Seven Critical Pathways," which outlines different sequences of clinical events that depend on diagnosis and case formulation. As shown in Figure 5, the flow chart assumes that—in addition to sexual assessment findings—the clinician has detailed assessment data regarding the medical status of the patient and his or her partner, the quality of the couple's relationship, and a psychological understanding of the client and his or her partner. As illustrated, the treatment pathways will differ as a function of (1) whether a medical basis for the problem is identified, (2) the presence or absence of substance abuse, (3) the degree of concomitant individual psychopathology, and (4) the degree of couple distress.

In the second situation, the case formulation is used to guide, pace, and organize psychological treatment, which eventually, may include sex therapy *per se.* In this way, the formulation assists the clinician in focusing first on more central or keystone problem areas, as well as anticipating resistances and potential areas of noncompliance. For example, the formulation in the case of an anxious woman who displays primary orgasmic disorder in addition to other problem areas (e.g., high anxiety about self-disclosure and avoidance of nonsexual intimacy) might indicate a general fear of relaxing personal control. This general fear may relate to a developmental history showing rigid and perfectionistic parents who discouraged and punished even minor displays of relaxing personal control (e.g., laughing, sharing personal information). In this case, then, the patient would be overwhelmed by and resist behavioral prescriptions for masturbation training to promote orgasmic responding. Instead, therapeutic emphasis might need to focus first upon (1) the therapist–patient relationship, helping the individual to begin to trust and relax personal control within that context and (2) ways to encourage and teach the individual to relax personal control in other nonsexual situations (e.g., dancing, receiving massage, relaxation training). Only then might this individual be ready for sex therapy *per se* (see AuBuchon & Malatesta, 1998; Bruch & Bond, 1998).

Other case formulations will span the range of etiologies. At one end of the continuum, a primary biological formulation for a case of secondary erectile disorder in a severely diabetic male with peripheral neuropathology who has been nonresponsive to oral and penile injection pharmacotherapy might necessitate penile implantation and couples sex therapy of a primarily educational and supportive nature. At the other end of the continuum, a case of low sexual desire in an individual who survived childhood sexual trauma might require initial treatment for posttraumatic stress disorder and/or a more exploratory psychotherapy within the context of a trusting therapeutic relationship (Golden, 1988). This particular treatment sequence, however, may not be indicated in another case of childhood sexual trauma (McCarthy, 1998). The process of case formulation within the area of sexual dysfunction is still within its infancy. The work of Rosen and Leiblum (1995b) provides examples of this important clinical skill.

# Treatment of Sexual Dysfunction

## Overview

As a semantic label, sex therapy is a general term for a variously defined group of educational, behavioral, cognitive, and other psychotherapeutic procedures for (1) improving sexual knowledge, communication, and sexual attitudes; (2) decreasing inhibitions, fears, and skill deficits associated with sexual activity; (3) improving the range of sexual response, including sexual desire, arousal, and orgasm, as well as the biobehavioral, cognitive, and affective components of this experience; and (4) enhancing sexual satisfaction, pleasure, and general intimacy in both the patient and his or her partner.

In actuality, sex therapy encompasses a variety of psychotherapeutic methods and procedures ranging from more directive approaches to skill-building and couples therapy. In fact, there has been a general blending and integration of sex therapy procedures with marital therapy techniques (Baucom et al., 1998; Weeks & Hof, 1987). Although the multidetermined nature of human sexuality, however, affords therapeutic contributions from a number of disciplines and approaches, it

also makes it impossible to encompass sex therapy under a single theoretical umbrella. As a consequence, the sex-therapy literature reveals a multiplicity of labels for similar therapeutic activities and a scientific orientation that ranges from atheoretical to multitheoretical (Rosen & Leiblum, 1995a,b). A "mixed model pragmatic approach" is currently popular (Segraves, 1998), and the move toward empirically supported treatments has helped to delineate the most effective interventions for sexual dysfunction (Baucom et al., 1998). This section provides a brief overview of the most common sex-therapy interventions.

## General Components of Sex Therapy

**Education.** The first component of sex therapy is providing accurate and sensitive information about individual and couple sexuality. With few exceptions, an effective sex-therapy plan should ascertain that the presenting couple or individual adequately understands human sexual response, especially with regard to the presenting complaint. It is not uncommon to find well-educated men and women who are misinformed about a variety of sexual issues—including, for example, age changes in sexual function, gender differences in sexual arousal patterns, and the competing influences of drugs, mood states, and couples conflict on sexual desire and responsiveness. Education also helps to challenge negative beliefs about sex and sexuality and may represent a starting point for cognitive interventions (Carey & Gordon, 1995).

Psychoeducation also helps to prepare the couple for active participation in the treatment process. Providing sexual information may also function as an initial step in attitude change, in permission giving (e.g., for sexual experimentation), and in helping the individual or couple to understand the problem. Therefore, psychoeducation is limited only by the therapist's creativity and the resources available and may reflect any format combination, including books (Heiman & LoPiccolo, 1988; McCarthy & McCarthy, 1998; van Lankveld, 1998), shared readings, and films (see Winks & Semans, 1997). Finally, note that education is a component of each of the empirically supported interventions described by Baucom et al. (1998).

**Communication, Intimacy, and Relationship Skills Training.** In the past, issues of communication and intimacy were often underemphasized in sex-therapy literature. In actuality,

Masters and Johnson's (1970) treatment approach emphasized interventions that improved couple communication and nongenital physical intimacy. The commonality of desire disorders also necessitated a greater therapeutic focus on communication and other relationship issues. Thus, because the strength of the relationship is ultimately tied to the couple's motivation to participate actively in treatment, most sex-therapy programs routinely include systematic attention to issues of communication, intimacy, and general relationship skills (Baucom et al., 1998; Beck, 1995; Heiman, 1986; Rosen & Leiblum, 1995a,b).

Built on the education component of sex therapy, communication skills and relationship therapy ranges from training in assertiveness and problem solving to negotiation and conflict management skills. More fundamentally, from the beginning of assessment and throughout the treatment process, "the therapist should serve as a model of good communication by active listening, display of empathy, asking clients to express themselves clearly, and other such social and communication skills" (Carey & Gordon, 1995, p. 191). Where necessary, interventions may extend to more general relationship issues (e.g., life-style, power and control). Finally, training in general intimacy skills may be indicated where individuals and/or couples are focused excessively on genital sexual expression at the expense of other kinds of intimacy (Malatesta, 1989).

**Structured Behavioral Activities.** Popularized by Masters and Johnson (1970), the prescription of a systematized plan of structured sexual activities remains an integral feature of sex therapy. Much as a desensitization hierarchy does, the activities typically represent a graduated series of sexual tasks that may begin with individual body-awareness exercises or masturbation, progress to mutual nongenital touching, and finally culminate in partner-guided sexual intercourse. The term *sensate focus* was used by Masters and Johnson (1970) to describe a set of behavioral exercises designed to help a couple develop sensual awareness and focus on sexual sensations, rather than sexual performance. The goal in this case may be to improve body image and response, to minimize and control anxieties and distractions associated with sexual activity, and to help the couple gradually to shape and redevelop their sexual relationship. This is why, for example, a ban on attempting intercourse and genital touching may be suggested to some couples who present with sexual dysfunction. This approach allows a couple to begin focusing on and enjoying other aspects of sexuality that are often ignored (e.g., sensual communication, nongenital touch, and massage) without anxiously wondering whether or not erection or lubrication—and thus intercourse—is forthcoming.

In other cases, the initial behavioral prescription may involve graduated masturbation training to facilitate orgasmic responding or to improve ejaculatory control (Baucom et al., 1998; LoPiccolo & Stock, 1986; Masters et al., 1994). Interventions may be individual, partner-assisted, or couples-based. In cases of sexual aversion, phobia, and sexual pain disorders, the structured behavioral exercises may most closely resemble a traditional desensitization or *in vivo* exposure and mastery hierarchy (see Wincze & Barlow, 1997).

Another aspect of behavioral prescriptions concerns the extent to which couples can (1) disengage from extraneous stimuli, such as work or children; (2) promote an interesting and creative atmosphere for sexual expression; and (3) focus on individual and partner sexuality. In some cases, activity scheduling is needed to encourage "intimacy time" when the partners are not fatigued or preoccupied with other matters. Environmental issues may also reflect ways to help couples expand and enhance their repertoire of sexual stimuli, including exposure to sensitive erotica (Robinson, Manthei, Scheltema, Rich, & Koznar, 1999).

**Biomedical Treatments.** Although biomedical approaches are not necessarily under the guise of sex therapy *per se*, they have acquired an important role in treating sexual dysfunctions that reflect either a primary organic or mixed etiology. Pharmacotherapy and surgical interventions have been two major treatments. Oral pharmacotherapy for sexual dysfunctions has developed dramatically and has focused primarily on treating erectile disorders (Marks, Duda, Dorey, Macairan, & Santos, 1999), premature ejaculation (Kim & Seo, 1998), and mixed female sexual dysfunctions (Kaplan et al., 1999). Before the development of oral medications such as Viagra, the self-injection of vasoactive substances (e.g., papaverine and phentolamine) directly into the intracavernous area of the penis to induce erection was heralded as a breakthrough in treating men with organic, mixed, and even chronic psychogenic erectile disorder (Kiely, Williams, & Goldie, 1987). Whether this therapy was administered by the patient or a physician, however, it has significant problems (Lehmann, Casella, Blochlinger, & Gasser, 1999). Treatment dropout rate may range up to 60%, side effects may be significant (e.g., prolonged erection, liver function abnormalities), success is variable, and self-injection poses a formidable challenge for the patient (e.g., injections need to be self-administered before sex; Althof et al., 1989; Sexton, Benedict, & Jarow, 1998). Recent work includes study of alternative delivery systems for the vasoactive substance (Segraves, 1998).

A range of SSRI and heterocyclic antidepressant medications has been investigated in treating sexual dysfunction (Riley & Riley, 1993; Strassberg, Brazao, Rowland, Tan, & Slob, 1999). In addition, androgen-replacement and estrogen-replacement therapies are increasingly helpful to postmenopausal women, and there is increasing agreement that androgens play a key role in female sexuality (Davis, 1998).

Surgical treatments of erectile dysfunction represent a reasonable alternative when pharmacotherapy fails (Shabsigh, 1998). This treatment usually involves surgical implantation of one of three types of penile prostheses: (1) the semirigid, which results in the penis being permanently erect, (2) the adjustable, which also causes a permanent erection but allows for the penis to be placed in different positions for sexual intercourse, and (3) the inflatable, which contains an implanted pump for controlling the erection by inflating a storage reservoir located in the penis. Although patients may derive benefit from these surgical treatments (Sexton et al., 1998; Tiefer, Pederson, & Melman, 1988), much of the evaluative research has employed global measures of patient satisfaction and has not addressed partner satisfaction and psychosexual adjustment (see Lehmann et al., 1999). In this regard, psychosocial factors may interfere with successful postoperative adjustment, and these procedures have potentially serious side effects (Kaufman, Kaufman, & Borges, 1998).

Taken together, developments in biomedical treatment provide sex therapists with unprecedented opportunities for educating women and men about the importance of psychosocial factors in evaluating and treating sexual dysfunction (Perelman, 1998). In addition, much work needs to be done to determine (1) predictors of success for medical treatments, (2) the interactive and sequential roles of biological and psychosocial interven-

tions, and (3) the positive and negative "psychosocial side effects" of pharmacological treatments (Segraves, 1998; Wise, 1999).

## Summary and Concluding Comments

Sexual dysfunctions have been recognized as a major public health problem that deserves increased study, evaluation, and intervention. Developments in biological understanding and treating sexual dysfunction have spurred what may be the next sexual revolution by attracting a huge and more diverse population of men and women who seek help for sexual problems. Changes in age demographics have contributed to this diversity because older adults, who are more likely to be coping with chronic health problems and taking medication, are presenting with more complex and multifaceted sexual dysfunctions. In addition, the increased focus on the sexuality of women and physically challenged individuals must remain a priority. Similar attention must be devoted to the unique sexual needs and problems associated with ethnicity and homosexuality.

To meet these challenges, a range of important developments has occurred in the field of sexual dysfunction. Multivariate approaches hold promise for the future, and assessment of sexuality, including psychophysiological methods, will continue to represent an important clinical function. Increased understanding of psychosocial etiology and developments in empirically supported treatments of sexual dysfunction will help to maintain the importance of psychosocial interventions. On the other hand, because there has been a "marked decline in the number of studies evaluating psychological, as opposed to medical or surgical approaches to treatment" (Rosen & Leiblum, 1995a, p. 885), some have questioned if sex therapy research has "withered on the vine" (Hawton, 1992). Funding for psychosocial outcome research will continue to be a challenge, but developments in biomedical treatment and increased focus on relationship interventions offer sex therapists a range of new opportunities in basic and clinical sex research. Thus, sex therapists have a responsibility to contribute to the vitality of the field. Sex therapists also have a responsibility to respect the continuity of their patients' sexual life-styles and to be ready to explore methods of meeting the sexual needs of diverse individuals and couples. Finally, sex therapists have an ethical and professional responsibility to maintain firm knowledge of basic and clinical research in sexuality and an empirical openness to scrutinize and alter their treatments where appropriate.

# References

Ackerman, M. D., & Carey, M. P. (1995). Psychology's role in the assessment of erectile dysfunction: Historical precedents, current knowledge, and methods. *Journal of Consulting and Clinical Psychology, 63*, 862–876.

Adams, C. G., & Turner, B. F. (1985). Reported change in sexuality from young adulthood to old age. *Journal of Sex Research, 21*, 126–141.

Adams, H. E. (1981). *Abnormal psychology*. Dubuque, IA: Brown.

Althof, S. E., Turner, L. A., Levine, S. B., Risen, C., Kursh, E., Bodner, D., & Resnick, M. (1989). Why do so many people drop out from auto-injection therapy for impotence? *Journal of Sex and Marital Therapy, 15*, 121–129.

American Psychiatric Association. (1980). *Diagnostic and statistical manual of mental disorders* (3rd ed.). Washington, DC: Author.

American Psychiatric Association. (1987). *Diagnostic and statistical manual of mental disorders* (3rd ed., rev.). Washington, DC: Author.

American Psychiatric Association. (1994). *Diagnostic and statistical manual of mental disorders* (4th ed.). Washington, DC: Author.

Andersen, B. L. (1983). Primary orgasmic dysfunction: Diagnostic considerations and review of treatment. *Psychological Bulletin, 93*, 105–136.

Andersen, B. L. (1985). Sexual functioning morbidity among cancer survivors: Present status and future research directions. *Cancer, 55*, 1835–1842.

Andersen, B. L., Andersen, B., & deProsse, C. (1989). Controlled prospective longitudinal study of women with cancer: II. Psychological outcomes. *Journal of Consulting and Clinical Psychology, 57*, 692–697.

Andersen, B. L., & Cyranowski, J. M. (1995). Women's sexuality: Behaviors, responses, and individual differences. *Journal of Consulting and Clinical Psychology, 63*, 891–906.

Andersen, B. L., Woods, X. A., & Copeland, L. J. (1997). Sexual self-schema and sexual morbidity among gynecologic cancer survivors. *Journal of Consulting and Clinical Psychology, 65*, 221–229.

Apfelbaum, B. (1977). The myth of the surrogate. *Journal of Sex Research, 13*, 238–249.

Apfelbaum, B. (1989). Retarded ejaculation: A much-misunderstood syndrome. In S. R. Leiblum & R. C. Rosen (Eds.), *Principles and practice of sex therapy*, 2nd ed. (pp. 168–206). New York: Guilford.

Apfelbaum, B. (1995). Masters and Johnson revisited: A case of desire disparity. In R. C. Rosen & S. R. Leiblum (Eds.), *Case studies in sex therapy* (pp. 23–45). New York: Guilford.

Ashton, A. K., Hamer, R., & Rosen, R. C. (1997). Serotonin reuptake inhibitor-induced sexual dysfunction and its treatment: A large-scale retrospective study of 596 psychiatric outpatients. *Journal of Sex and Marital Therapy, 23*, 165–175.

AuBuchon, P. G., & Malatesta, V. J. (1998). Managing the therapeutic relationship in behavior therapy: The need for a case formulation. In M. Bruch & F. W. Bond (Eds.), *Beyond diagnosis: Case formulation approaches in cognitive-behavior therapy*. London: Wiley.

Bach, A. K., Brown, T. A., & Barlow, D. H. (1999). The effects of false negative feedback on efficacy expectancies and sexual arousal in sexually functional males. *Behavior Therapy, 30*, 79–95.

Bancroft, J. (1989). *Human sexuality and its problems*. New York: Churchill Livingstone.

Barbach, L. (1975). *For yourself: The fulfillment of female sexuality*. New York: Doubleday.

Barlow, D. H. (1986). Causes of sexual dysfunction: The role of anxiety and cognitive interference. *Journal of Consulting and Clinical Psychology, 54*, 140–148.

Barlow, D. H. (1988). *Anxiety and its disorders*. New York: Guilford.

Barlow, D. H., Chorpita, B. F., & Turovsky, J. (1996). Fear, panic, anxiety, and disorders of emotion. In D. A. Hope (Ed.), *Perspectives on anxiety, panic, and fear* (pp. 251–328). Lincoln: University of Nebraska Press.

Bartoi, M. G., & Kinder, B. N. (1998). Effects of child and adult sexual abuse on adult sexuality. *Journal of Sex and Marital Therapy, 24*, 75–90.

Baucom, D. H., Shoham, V., Mueser, K. T., Daiuto, A. D., & Stickle, T. R. (1998). Empirically supported couple and family interventions for marital distress and adult mental health problems. *Journal of Consulting and Clinical Psychology, 66*, 53–88.

Beck, J. G. (1995). Hypoactive sexual desire disorder: An overview. *Journal of Consulting and Clinical Psychology, 63*, 919–927.

Beck, J. G., & Barlow, D. H. (1984). Current conceptualizations of sexual dysfunction: A review and an alternative perspective. *Clinical Psychology Review, 4*, 363–378.

Beck, J. G., Barlow, D. H., & Sakheim, D. K. (1983). The effects of attentional focus and partner arousal on sexual responding in functional and dysfunctional men. *Behaviour Research and Therapy, 21*, 1–8.

Becker, J. V. (1989). Impact of sexual abuse on sexual functioning. In S. R. Leiblum & R. C. Rosen (Eds.), *Principles and practice of sex therapy*, 2nd ed. (pp. 298–318). New York: Guilford.

Becker, J. V., & Kaplan, M. S. (1991). Rape victims: Issues, theories, and treatment. *Annual Review of Sex Research, 2*, 267–292.

Behrendt, A. E., & George, K. D. (1995). Sex therapy for gay and bisexual men. In L. Diamant & R. D. McAnulty (Eds.), *The psychology of sexual orientation, behavior, and identity: A handbook* (pp. 220–236). Westport, CT: Greenwood Press.

Blackerby, W. F. (Ed.). (1990). Sexuality and head injury [Special issue]. *Journal of Head Trauma Rehabilitation, 5*(2).

Bornstein, P. H., Hamilton, S. B., & Bornstein, M. T. (1986). Self-monitoring procedures. In A. R. Ciminero, K. S. Calhoun, & H. E. Adams (Eds.), *Handbook of behavioral assessment*, 2nd ed. (pp. 176–122). New York: Wiley.

Briddell, D. W., & Wilson, G. T. (1976). The effects of alcohol and expectancy set on male sexual arousal. *Journal of Abnormal Psychology, 85*, 225–234.

Brockway, J. A., & Steger, J. C. (1980). Sexual attitude and information questionnaire: Reliability and validity in a spinal cord injured population. *Sexuality and Disability, 3*, 49–60.

Bruch, M., & Bond, F. W. (1998). *Beyond diagnosis: Case formulation approaches in cognitive-behavior therapy*. London: Wiley.

Butler, R. N., & Lewis, M. I. (1993). *Sex after sixty: A guide for men and women for their later years*. New York: Harper & Row.

Carey, M. P., Flasher, L. V., Maisto, S. A., & Turkat, I. D. (1984). The a priori approach to psychological assessment. *Professional Psychology: Research and Practice, 15*, 515–527.

Carey, M. P., & Gordon, C. M. (1995). Sexual dysfunction among heterosexual adults: Description, epidemiology, assessment, and treatment. In L. Diamant & R. D. McAnulty (Eds.), *The psychology of sexual orientation, behavior, and identity* (pp. 165–191). Westport, CT: Greenwood Press.

Casselman, D., & Durham, R. L. (1979). Demographic differences for sexual knowledge and attitudes. *Journal of Sex Education and Therapy, 1*, 29–36.

Catania, J. A. (1999). Methods of inquiry about sex: New advances [special issue]. *Journal of Sex Research, 36*(2).

Chambless, D. L., & Lifshitz, J. L. (1984). Self-reported sexual anxiety and arousal: The expanded sexual arousability inventory. *Journal of Sex Research, 20*, 241–254.

Conte, H. R. (1986). Multivariate assessment of sexual dysfunction. *Journal of Consulting and Clinical Psychology, 54*, 149–157.

Cooper, A. (1998). Sexuality and the Internet: Surfing into the new millennium. *CyberPsychology and Behavior, 1*, 181–187.

Cooper, A. J., Cernovsky, Z. Z., & Colussi, K. (1993). Some clinical and psychometric characteristics of primary and secondary premature ejaculators. *Journal of Sex and Marital Therapy, 19*, 276–288.

Cranston-Cuebas, M. A., & Barlow, D. H. (1990). Cognitive and affective contributions to sexual functioning. *Annual Review of Sex Research, 1*, 119–161.

Crenshaw, T. L., & Goldberg, J. P. (1996). *Sexual pharmacology: Drugs that affect sexual function*. New York: W.W. Norton.

Crowe, L. C., & George, W. H. (1989). Alcohol and human sexuality: Review and integration. *Psychological Bulletin, 105*, 374–386.

Davidson, J. K., Darling, C. A., & Conway-Welch, C. (1989). The role of the Grafenberg spot and female ejaculation in the female orgasmic response: An empirical analysis. *Journal of Sex and Marital Therapy, 15*, 102–120.

Davidson, J. K., Darling, C. A., & Norton, L. (1995). Religiosity and the sexuality of women: Sexual behavior and sexual satisfaction revisited. *Journal of Sex Research, 32*, 235–243.

Davis, C. M., Yarber, W. L., Bauserman, R., Schreer, G., & Davis, S. L. (1998). *Handbook of sexually-related measures*. Thousand Oaks, CA: Sage.

Davis, S. (1998). The clinical use of androgens in female sexual disorders. *Journal of Sex and Marital Therapy, 24*, 153–163.

Derogatis, L. R. (1978). *Derogatis sexual functioning inventory*, rev. ed. Baltimore: Clinical Psychometrics Research.

Derogatis, L. R. (1997). The Derogatis interview for sexual functioning (DISF/DISF-SR): An introductory report. *Journal of Sex and Marital Therapy, 23*, 291–304.

Derogatis, L. R., Meyer, J. K., & King, K. M. (1981). Psychopathology in individuals with sexual dysfunction. *American Journal of Psychiatry, 138*, 757–763.

Ducharme, S. H., & Gill, K. M. (1997). *Sexuality after spinal cord injury: Answers to your questions*. Baltimore: Paul H. Brookes.

Elliott, A. N., & O'Donohue, W. T. (1997). The effects of anxiety and distraction on sexual arousal in a nonclinical sample of heterosexual women. *Archives of Sexual Behavior, 26*, 607–624.

Ellis, H. (1933/1966). *Psychology of sex*, 2nd ed. New York: Harcourt Brace Jovanovich.

Fahrner, E. M. (1987). Sexual dysfunction of male alcohol addicts: Prevalence and treatment. *Archives of Sexual Behavior, 16*, 247–257.

Farber, M. (Ed.). (1985). *Human sexuality: Psychosexual effects of disease*. New York: Macmillan.

Feldman, H. A., Goldstein, I., Hatzichristou, G., Krane, R. J., & McKinlay, J. B. (1994). Impotence and its medical and psychosocial correlates: Results of the Massachusetts male aging study. *Journal of Urology, 151*, 54–61.

Fenichel, O. (1945). *A psychoanalytic theory of neurosis*. New York: W.W. Norton.

Fisher, W. A., & Barak, A. (1989). Bias and fairness in the diagnosis of primary orgasmic dysfunction in women. *American Psychologist, 44*, 1080–1081.

Fisher, J. E., Swingen, D. N., & O'Donohue, W. (1997). Behavioral interventions for sexual dysfunction in the elderly. *Behavior Therapy, 28*, 65–82.

Frank, E., Anderson, C., & Kupfer, D. (1976). Profiles of couples seeking sex therapy and marital therapy. *American Journal of Psychiatry, 133*, 559–652.

Freud, S. (1943). *General introduction to psychoanalysis*. Garden City, NY: Garden City Publishers.

Freund, B., & Steketee, G. (1989). Sexual history, attitudes and functioning of obsessive-compulsive patients. *Journal of Sex and Marital Therapy, 15*, 31–41.

Gagnon, J. H. (1975). Sex research and social change. *Archives of Sexual Behavior, 4*, 111–141.

Galyer, K. T., Conaglen, H. M., Hare, A., & Conaglen, J. V. (1999). The effect of gynecological surgery on sexual desire. *Journal of Sex and Marital Therapy, 25*, 81–88.

George, L. K., & Weiler, S. J. (1981). Sexuality in middle and late life: The effects of age, cohort, and gender. *Archives of Sexual Behavior, 38*, 919–923.

Gilbert, F. S., & Gamache, M. P. (1984). The sexual opinion survey: Structure and use. *Journal of Sex Research, 20*, 293–309.

Gitlin, M. (1994). Psychotropic medications and their effects on sexual function: Diagnosis, biology and treatment approaches. *Journal of Clinical Psychiatry, 55*, 406–413.

Gold, M. S., & Roehrich. (1991). Alcohol, expectancies and sexuality. *Alcohol Health and Research World, 15*, 126–132.

Golden, J. (1988). A second look at a case of inhibited sexual desire. *Journal of Sex Research, 25*, 304–306.

Gottman, J. M. (1999). *The marriage clinic: A scientifically based marital therapy*. New York: W.W. Norton.

Grenier, G., & Byers, E. S. (1995). Rapid ejaculation: A review of conceptual, etiological and treatment issues. *Archives of Sexual Behavior, 24*, 447–472.

Griffith, E. R., & Lemberg, S. (1993). *Sexuality and the person with traumatic brain injury: A guide for families*. Philadelphia: Davis.

Hartmann, W. E., & Fithian, M. A. (1974). *Treatment of sexual dysfunction: A biopsychosocial approach.* New York: Jason Aronson.

Hawton, K. (1992). Sex therapy research: Has it withered on the vine? *Annual Review of Sex Research, 3,* 49–72.

Hawton, K. (1995). Treatment of sexual dysfunctions by sex therapy and other approaches. *British Journal of Psychiatry, 17,* 307–314.

Heiman, J. R. (1986). Treating maritally distressed sexual relationships. In N. S. Jacobson & A. S. Gurman (Eds.), *Clinical handbook of marital therapy* (pp. 261–284). New York: Guilford.

Heiman, J. R., & LoPiccolo, J. (1988). *Becoming orgasmic: A sexual and personal growth program for women,* rev. ed. New York: Prentice-Hall.

Hendrick, S., & Hendrick, S. (1987). Multidimensionality of sexual attitudes. *Journal of Sex Research, 23,* 502–526.

Hudson, W. W., Harrison, D. F., & Crosscup, P. C. (1981). A short-term scale to measure sexual discord in dyadic relationships. *Journal of Sex Research, 17,* 157–174.

Janda, L. H., & O'Grady, K. E. (1980). Development of a sex anxiety inventory. *Journal of Consulting and Clinical Psychology, 48,* 169–175.

Jani, N. N., & Wise, T. N. (1988). Antidepressants and inhibited female orgasm. *Journal of Sex and Marital Therapy, 14,* 279–284.

Jensen, S. B. (1984). Sexual dysfunction in younger married alcoholics: A comparative study. *Acta Psychiatrica Scandinavica, 69,* 543–559.

Jensen, S. B. (1986). Sexual dysfunction and diabetes mellitus: A six-year follow-up study. *Archives of Sexual Behavior, 15,* 271–284.

Kaplan, H. S. (1974). *The new sex therapy: Active treatment of sexual dysfunctions.* New York: Brunner/Mazel.

Kaplan, H. S. (1977). Hypoactive sexual desire. *Journal of Sex and Marital Therapy, 3,* 3–9.

Kaplan, H. S. (1979). *Disorders of sexual desire.* New York: Simon & Schuster.

Kaplan, H. S. (1987). *Sexual aversion, sexual phobias, and panic disorder.* New York: Brunner/Mazel.

Kaplan, S. A., Reis, R. B., Kohn, I. J., Ikeguchi, E. F., Laor, E., Te, A. E., & Martins, A. C. P. (1999). Safety and efficacy of sildenafil in postmenopausal women with sexual dysfunction. *Urology, 53,* 481–485.

Katz, R. C., Gipson, M. T., Kearl, A., & Kriskovick, M. (1989). Assessing sexual aversion in college students: The Sexual Aversion Scale. *Journal of Sex and Marital Therapy, 15,* 135–140.

Kaufman, J. M., Kaufman, J. L., & Borges, F. D. (1997). Immediate salvage procedure for infected penile prothesis. *Journal of Urology, 159,* 816–818.

Kiely, E., Williams, G., & Goldie, L. (1987). Assessment of the immediate and long-term effects of pharmacologically induced penile erections in the treatment of psychogenic and organic impotence. *British Journal of Urology, 59,* 164–169.

Kilmann, P. R. (1978). The treatment of primary and secondary orgasmic dysfunction: A methodological review of the literature since 1970. *Journal of Sex and Marital Therapy, 4,* 155–176.

Kilmann, P. R., Boland, J. P., Norton, S. P., Davidson, E., & Caid, C. (1986). Perspectives of sex therapy outcome: A survey of AASECT providers. *Journal of Sex and Marital Therapy, 12,* 116–138.

Kim, S. C., & Seo, K. K. (1998). Efficacy and safety of fluoxetine, sertraline and clomipramine in patients with premature ejaculation: A double-blind, placebo controlled study. *Journal of Urology, 159,* 425–427.

Kinchla, J., & Weiss, T. (1985). Psychologic and social outcomes following coronary artery bypass surgery. *Journal of Cardiopulmonary Rehabilitation, 5,* 274–283.

Kolodny, R. C., Masters, W. H., & Johnson, V. E. (1979). *Textbook of sexual medicine.* Boston: Little, Brown.

Kriss, R. T., & Kraemer, H. C. (1986). Efficacy of group therapy for problems with postmastectomy self-perception, body image, and sexuality. *Journal of Sex Research, 22,* 438–451.

Krotoski, D. M., Noesek, M. A., & Turk, M. A. (Eds.). (1996). *Women with physical disabilities: Achieving and maintaining health and well-being.* Baltimore: Paul H. Brookes.

Laan, E., & Everaerd, W. (1995). Determinants of female sexual arousal: Psychophysiological theory and data. *Annual Review of Sex Research, 6,* 32–76.

Larson, J. H., Anderson, S. M., Holman, T. B., & Niemann, B. K. (1998). A longitudinal study of the effects of premarital communication, relationship stability, and self esteem on sexual satisfaction in the first year of marriage. *Journal of Sex and Marital Therapy, 24,* 193–206.

Lasker, J. N., & Borg, S. (1995). *In search of parenthood: Coping with infertility and high-tech conception.* Philadelphia: Temple University Press.

Laumann, E. O., Paik, A., & Rosen, R. C. (1999). Sexual dysfunction in the United States: Prevalence and predictors. *Journal of the American Medical Association, 281,* 537–544.

Laumann, E. O., Gagnon, J. H., Michael, R. T., & Michaels, S. (1994). *The social organization of sexuality.* Chicago: University of Chicago Press.

Lazarus, A. A. (1963). The treatment of chronic frigidity by systematic desensitization. *Journal of Nervous and Mental Disease, 63,* 272–278.

Lazarus, A. A. (1989). Dyspareunia: A multimodal psychotherapeutic perspective. In S. R. Leiblum & R. C. Rosen (Eds.), *Principles and practice of sex therapy* (pp. 89–112). New York: Guilford.

Lehmann, R., Casella, R., Blochlinger, A., & Gasser, T. C. (1999). Reasons for discontinuing intracavernous injection therapy with prostaglandin E (Alprostadil). *Urology, 53,* 397–400.

Leiblum, S. R., Pervin, L. A., & Campbell, E. H. (1989). The treatment of vaginismus: Success and failure. In S. R. Leiblum & R. C. Rosen (Eds.), *Principles and practice of sex therapy,* 2nd ed. (pp. 113–138). New York: Guilford.

Leiblum, S. R., & Rosen, R. C. (Eds.). (1988). *Sexual desire disorders.* New York: Guilford.

Leiblum, S. R., & Rosen, R. C. (Eds.). (1989). *Principles and practice of sex therapy,* 2nd ed. New York: Guilford.

Leiblum, S. R., & Segraves, R. T. (1989). Sex therapy with aging adults. In S. R. Leiblum & R. C. Rosen (Eds.), *Principles and practice of sex therapy,* 2nd ed. (pp. 352–381). New York: Guilford.

Leight, L. (1990). *Raising sexually healthy children.* New York: Avon.

Levine, L., & Carroll, R. (1994). Nocturnal penile tumescence and rigidity in men without complaints of erectile dysfunction using a new quantitative analysis software. *Journal of Urology, 152,* 1103–1107.

Levine, S. B. (1984). An essay on the nature of sexual desire. *Journal of Sex and Marital Therapy, 10,* 83–96.

Levine, S. B. (1988). Intrapsychic and individual aspects of sexual desire. In S. R. Leiblum & R. C. Rosen (Eds.), *Sexual desire disorders* (pp. 21–44). New York: Guilford.

Lief, H. I. (1977). Inhibited sexual desire. *Medical Aspects of Human Sexuality, 7,* 94–95.

Lipshultz, L. I., & Kim, E. D. (1999). Treatment of erectile dysfunction in men with diabetes. *Journal of the American Medical Association, 281,* 465–466.

LoPiccolo, J., & Friedman, J. M. (1988). Broad-spectrum treatment of low sexual desire: Integration of cognitive, behavioral, and systemic therapy. In S. R. Leiblum & R. C. Rosen (Eds.), *Sexual desire disorders* (pp. 107–144). New York: Guilford.

LoPiccolo, J., & Steger, J. C. (1974). The sexual interaction inventory: A new instrument for assessment of sexual dysfunction. *Archives of Sexual Behavior, 2,* 585–595.

LoPiccolo, J., & Stock, W. E. (1986). Treatment of sexual dysfunction. *Journal of Consulting and Clinical Psychology, 54,* 158–167.

LoPiccolo, J., & Stock, W. E. (1987). Sexual counseling in gynecological practice. In Z. Rosenwaks, F. Benjamin, & M. Stone (Eds.), *Basic gynecology.* New York: Macmillan.

MacDonald, B. J. (1998). Issues in therapy with gay and lesbian couples. *24,* 165–190.

Malatesta, V. J. (1989). Sexuality and the older adult: An overview with guidelines for the health care professional. *Journal of Women and Aging, 1,* 93–118.

Malatesta, V. J., & Adams, H. E. (1993). The sexual dysfunctions. In P. B. Sutker & H. E. Adams (Eds.), *Comprehensive handbook of psychopathology,* 2nd ed. (pp. 725–775). New York: Plenum.

Malatesta, V. J., & Adams, H. E. (1986). Assessment of sexual behavior. In A. R. Ciminero, K. S. Calhoun, & H. E. Adams (Eds.), *Handbook of behavioral assessment,* 2nd ed. (pp. 496–525). New York: Wiley.

Malatesta, V. J., Chambless, D. L., Pollack, M., & Cantor, A. (1988). Widowhood, sexuality, and aging: A life-span analysis. *Journal of Sex and Marital Therapy, 14,* 49–62.

Malatesta, V. J., Pollack, R. H., Crotty, T. D., & Peacock, L. J. (1982). Acute alcohol intoxication and female orgasmic response. *Journal of Sex Research, 18,* 1–17.

Malatesta, V. J., Pollack, R. H., Wilbanks, W. A., & Adams, H. E. (1979). Alcohol effects on the orgasmic-ejaculatory response in human males. *Journal of Sex Research, 15,* 101–107.

Malatesta, V. J., & Robinson, M. S. (1995). Hypersexuality and impulsive sexual behaviors. In I. Diamant & R. D. McAnulty (Eds.), *The psychology of sexual orientation, behavior, and identity* (pp. 307–326). Westport, CT: Greenwood Pres.

Malatesta, V. J., & Turkat, I. D. (1988). Psychodynamic and behavioral case formulation [letter to the editor]. *American Journal of Psychiatry, 145,* 770.

Marks, L. S., Duda, C., Dorey, F. J., Macairan, M. L., & Santos, P. B. (1999). Treatment of erectile dysfunction with sildenafil. *Urology, 53,* 19–24.

Martin, C. E. (1981). Factors affecting sexual functioning in 60- to 79-year-old married males. *Archives of Sexual Behavior, 10,* 399–420.

Masters, W. H., & Johnson, V. E. (1966). *Human sexual response.* Boston: Little, Brown.

Masters, W. H., & Johnson, V. E. (1970). *Human sexual inadequacy.* Boston: Little, Brown.

Masters, W. H., Johnson, V. E., & Kolodny, R. C. (1994). *Heterosexuality.* New York: Gramercy.

McCabe, M. P. (1997). Intimacy and quality of life among sexually dysfunctional men and women. *Journal of Sex and Marital Therapy, 23,* 276–290.

McCabe, M. P., McDonald, E., Deeks, A. A., Vowels, L. M., & Cobain, M. J. (1996). The impact of multiple sclerosis on sexuality and relationships. *Journal of Sex Research, 33,* 241–248.

McCarthy, B. (1988). *Male sexual awareness.* New York: Carroll and Graf.

McCarthy, B. (1989). Cognitive-behavioral strategies and techniques in the treatment of early ejaculation. In S. R. Leiblum & R. C. Rosen (Eds.), *Principles and practice of sex therapy,* 2nd ed. (pp. 141–167). New York: Guilford.

McCarthy, B. (1998). Commentary: Effects of sexual trauma on adult sexuality. *Journal of Sex and Marital Therapy, 24,* 91–92.

McCarthy, B., & McCarthy, E. (1998). *Couple sexual awareness.* New York: Carroll and Graf.

McCormick, N. B. (1996). Bodies besieged: The impact of chronic and serious physical illness on sexuality, passion, and desire [special issue]. *Journal of Sex Research, 33*(3).

Meana, M., & Binik, Y. M. (1994). Painful coitus: A review of female dyspareunia. *Journal of Nervous and Mental Disease, 182,* 264–272.

Melman, A., & Gingell, J. C. (1999). The epidemiology and pathophysiology of erectile dysfunction. *Journal of Urology, 161,* 5–11.

Mendelson, J. H., & Mello, N. K. (1988). Chronic alcohol effects on anterior pituitary and ovarian hormones in healthy women. *Journal of Pharmacology and Experimental Therapeutics, 245,* 407–412.

Meston, C. M., & Gorzalka, B. B. (1996). Differential effects of sympathetic activation on sexual arousal in sexually dysfunctional and functional women. *Journal of Abnormal Psychology, 105,* 582–591.

Metz, M. E., Pryor, J. L., Nesvacil, L. J., Abuzzahab, F., & Koznar, J. (1997). Premature ejaculation: A psychophysiological review. *Journal of Sex and Marital Therapy, 23,* 3–23.

Meyer, V., & Turkat, I. D. (1979). Behavioral analysis of clinical cases. *Journal of Behavioral Assessment, 1,* 259–270.

Mitchell, W. B., DiBartolo, P. M., Brown, T. A., & Barlow, D. H. (1998). Effects of positive and negative mood on sexual arousal in sexually dysfunctional and functional males. *Archives of Sexual Behavior, 27,* 197–207.

Monat-Haller, R. K. (1992). *Understanding and expressing sexuality: Responsible choices for individuals with developmental disabilities.* Baltimore: Paul H. Brooks.

Money, J. (1988). Commentary: Current status of sex research. *Journal of Psychology and Human Sexuality, 1,* 5–15.

Monga, T. N. (Ed.). (1995). *Physical medicine and rehabilitation state of the arts review: Sexuality and disability.* Philadelphia: Hanley and Belfus.

Morokoff, P. J., & Gillilland, R. (1993). Stress, sexual functioning, and marital satisfaction. *Journal of Sex Research, 30,* 43–53.

Munjack, D. J., & Kanno, P. H. (1979). Retarded ejaculation: A review. *Archives of Sexual Behavior, 8,* 139–150.

National Institutes of Health. (1993). Consensus development panel on impotence. *Journal of the American Medical Association, 270,* 83–90.

Palace, E. M. (1995). A cognitive-physiological process model of sexual arousal and response. *Clinical Psychology: Science and Practice, 2,* 370–384.

Papadopoulos, C., Shelley, S. I., Piccolo, M., Beaumont, C., & Barnett, L. (1986). Sexual activity after coronary bypass surgery. *Chest, 90,* 681–685.

Perelman, M. A. (1994). The urologist and cognitive behavioral sex therapist. *Contemporary Urology, 6,* 27–33.

Perelman, M. A. (1998). Commentary: Pharmacological agents for erectile dysfunction and the human sexual response cycle. *Journal of Sex and Marital Therapy, 24,* 309–312.

Perry, S., Cooper, A. M., & Michels, R. (1987). The psychodynamic formulation: Its purpose, structure, and clinical application. *American Journal of Psychiatry, 144,* 543–550.

Persons, J. B. (1989). *Cognitive therapy in practice: A case formulation approach.* New York: W.W. Norton.

Pfeiffer, E. (1974). Sexuality in the aging individual. *Journal of the American Geriatric Society, 22,* 481–484.

Pfeiffer, E. (1977). Sexual behavior in old age. In E. G. Busse & E. Pfeiffer (Eds.), *Behavior and adaptation in late life,* 2nd ed. (pp. 130–141). Boston: Little, Brown.

Pinney, E. M., Gerrard, M., & Denny, N. W. (1987). The Pinney Sexual Satisfaction Inventory. *Journal of Sex Research, 23,* 233–251.

Prather, R. C. (1988). Sexual dysfunction in the diabetic female: A review. *Archives of Sexual Behavior, 17,* 277–284.

Purnine, D. M., & Carey, M. P. (1997). Interpersonal communication and sexual adjustment: The roles of understanding and agreement. *Journal of Consulting and Clinical Psychology, 65,* 1017–1025.

Purnine, D. M., Carey, M. P., & Jorgensen, R. S. (1996). Inventory of Dyadic Heterosexual Preferences: Development and psychometric evaluation. *Behaviour Research and Therapy, 34,* 375–387.

Renshaw, D. (1990). Sex and eating disorders. *Medical Aspects of Human Sexuality, 24,* 68–77.

Riley, A. J., & Riley, E. J. (1993). Pharmacotherapy for sexual dysfunction: Current status. In A. J. Riley, M. Peet, & C. Wilson (Eds.), *Sexual pharmacology* (pp. 211–226). Oxford: Clarendon Press.

Robinson, B. E., Manthei, R., Scheltema, K., Rich, R., & Koznar, J. (1999). Therapeutic uses of sexually explicit materials in the United States and the Czech and Slovak Republics: A qualitative study. *Journal of Sex and Marital Therapy, 25,* 103–119.

Rosen, R. C. (1991). Alcohol and drug effects on sexual response: Human experimental and clinical studies. *Annual Review of Sex Research, 2,* 119–180.

Rosen, R. C., & Beck, J. G. (1988). *Patterns of sexual arousal: Psychophysiological processes and clinical application.* New York: Guilford.

Rosen, R. C., & Leiblum, S. R. (1987). Current approaches to the evaluation of sexual desire disorders. *Journal of Sex Research, 23,* 141–162.

Rosen, R. C., & Leiblum, S. R. (1989). Assessment and treatment of desire disorders. In S. R. Leiblum & R. C. Rosen (Eds.), *Principles and practice of sex therapy,* 2nd ed. (pp. 19–47). New York: Guilford.

Rosen, R. C., & Leiblum, S. R. (1995a). Treatment of sexual disorders in the 1990s: An integrated approach. *Journal of Consulting and Clinical Psychology, 63,* 877–890.

Rosen, R. C., & Leiblum, S. R. (Eds.). (1995b). *Case studies in sex therapy.* New York: Guilford.

Rosen, R. C., Taylor, J. F., Leiblum, S. R., & Bachman, G. A.

(1993). Prevalence of sexual dysfunction in women: Results of a survey study of 329 women in an outpatient gynecological clinic. *Journal of Sex and Marital Therapy, 19,* 171–188.

Rosenheim, E., & Neuman, M. (1981). Personality characteristics of sexually dysfunctional males and their wives. *Journal of Sex Research, 17,* 124–138.

Rowland, D. L. (1995). The psychobiology of sexual arousal and behavior. In L. Diamant & R. D. McAnulty (Eds.), *The psychology of sexual orientation, behavior, and identity* (pp. 19–42). Westport, CT: Greenwood Press.

Rowland, D. L. (1999). Issues in the laboratory study of human sexual response: A synthesis for the nontechnical sexologist. *Journal of Sex Research, 36,* 3–15.

Rowland, D. L., Cooper, S. E., Slob, A. K., & Houtsmuller, E. J. (1997). The study of ejaculatory response in men in the psychophysiological laboratory. *Journal of Sex Research, 34,* 161–166.

Rowland, D. L., & Slob, A. K. (1995). Understanding and diagnosing sexual dysfunction: Recent progress through psychophysiological methods. *Neuroscience and Biobehavioral Reviews, 19,* 201–209.

Ruff, G. A., & St. Lawrence, J. S. (1985). Premature ejaculation: Past research progress, future directions. *Clinical Psychology Review, 5,* 627–639.

Rundel, G. (1998). Sexual morality of Christianity. *Journal of Sex and Marital Therapy, 24,* 103–122.

Russell, L. (1990). Sex and couples therapy: A method of treatment to enhance physical and emotional intimacy. *Journal of Sex and Marital Therapy, 16,* 111–120.

Rust, J., & Golombok, S. (1986). The GRISS: A psychometric instrument for the assessment of sexual dysfunction. *Archives of Sexual Behavior, 15,* 157–165.

Saad, S. C., & Behrendt, A. E. (1996). Scleroderma and sexuality. *Journal of Sex Research, 33,* 215–220.

Sadock, V. A. (1995). Normal human sexuality and sexual and gender identity disorders. In H. I. Kaplan & B. J. Benjamin (Eds.), *Comprehensive textbook of psychiatry,* 6th ed. (pp. 1295–1321). Baltimore: Williams & Wilkins.

Sarrel, D. M., & Masters, W. H. (1982). Sexual molestation of men by women. *Archives of Sexual Behavior, 11,* 117–131.

Sbrocco, T., Weisberg, R. B., Barlow, D. H., & Carter, M. M. (1997). The conceptual relationship between panic disorder and male erectile dysfunction. *Journal of Sex and Marital Therapy, 23,* 212–220.

Schiavi, R. C. (1990). Chronic alcoholism and male sexual dysfunction. *Journal of Sex and Marital Therapy, 16,* 23–33.

Schlesinger, L. (1996). Chronic pain, intimacy, and sexuality: A qualitative study of women who live with pain. *Journal of Sex Research, 33,* 249–256.

Schover, L. R. (1989). Sexual problems in chronic illness. In S. R. Leiblum & R. C. Rosen (Eds.), *Principles and practice of sex therapy: Update for the 1990s* (pp. 319–351). New York: Guilford.

Schover, L. R., Evans, R. B., & von Eschenbach, A. C. (1987). Sexual rehabilitation in a cancer center: Diagnosis and outcome in 384 consultations. *Archives of Sexual Behavior, 16,* 445–461.

Schover, L. R., Friedman, J. M., Weiler, S. J., Heiman, J. R., & LoPiccolo, J. (1982). Multiaxial problem-oriented system for sexual dysfunctions. *Archives of General Psychiatry, 39,* 614–619.

Schover, L. R., & Jensen, S. B. (1988). *Sexuality and chronic illness: A comprehensive approach.* New York: Guilford.

Schover, L. R., & Leiblum, S. R. (1994). Commentary: The

stagnation of sex therapy. *Journal of Psychology and Human Sexuality, 6,* 5–30.

Schover, L. R., & LoPiccolo, J. (1982). Treatment effectiveness for dysfunctions of sexual desire. *Journal of Sex and Marital Therapy, 8,* 179–197.

Schover, L. R., & Randers-Pehrson, M. (1988a). *Sexuality and cancer: For the man who has cancer, and his partner* (Publication No. 4657). New York: American Cancer Society.

Schover, L. R., & Randers-Pehrson, M. (1988b). *Sexuality and cancer: For the woman who has cancer, and her partner* (Publication No. 4657). New York: American Cancer Society.

Schover, L. R., Thomas, A. J., Lakin, M. M., Montague, D. K., & Fischer, J. (1988). Orgasm-phase dysfunction in multiple sclerosis. *Journal of Sex Research, 25,* 548–554.

Schreiner-Engel, P., & Schiavi, R. C. (1986). Life-time psychopathology in individuals with low sexual desire. *Journal of Nervous and Mental Disease, 174,* 646–651.

Schuster, C. L. (1988). *Alcohol and sexuality.* New York: Praeger.

Segraves, K. A., & Segraves, R. T. (1991). Hypoactive sexual desire disorder: Prevalence and comorbidity in 906 subjects. *Journal of Sex and Marital Therapy, 17,* 55–58.

Segraves, K. A., Segraves, R. T., & Schoenberg, H. W. (1987). Use of sexual history to differentiate organic from psychogenic impotence. *Archives of Sexual Behavior, 16,* 125–137.

Segraves, R. T. (1988). Psychiatric drugs and inhibited female orgasm. *Journal of Sex and Marital Therapy, 14,* 202–207.

Segraves, R. T. (1998). Editorial: Pharmacological era in the treatment of sexual disorders. *Journal of Sex and Marital Therapy, 24,* 67–68.

Sexton, W. J., Benedict, J. F., & Jarow, J. P. (1998). Comparison of long-term outcomes of penile prostheses and intracavernosal injection therapy. *Journal of Urology, 159,* 811–815.

Shabsigh, R. (1998). Editorial: Penile prostheses toward the end of the millennium. *Journal of Urology, 159,* 819.

Sherwin, B. B. (1991). The psychoendocrinology of aging and female sexuality. *Annual Review of Sex Research, 2,* 181–198.

Silverstein, J. L. (1989). Origins of psychogenic vaginismus. *Psychotherapy and Psychosomatics, 52,* 197–204.

Singer, B., & Toates, F. M. (1987). Sexual motivation. *Journal of Sex Research, 23,* 455–460.

Sipski, M. L., Alexander, C. J., & Rosen, R. C. (1999). Sexual response in women with spinal cord injuries: Implications for our understanding of the able bodied. *Journal of Sex and Marital Therapy, 25,* 11–22.

Snyder, D. K. (1997). *Marital satisfaction inventory, revised.* Los Angeles: Western Psychological Services.

Spark, R., White, R., & Connolly, P. (1980). Impotence is not always psychogenic. *Journal of the American Medical Association, 243,* 750–755.

Spector, I. P., & Carey, M. P. (1990). Incidence and prevalence of the sexual dysfunctions: A critical review of the literature. *Archives of Sexual Behavior, 19,* 389–408.

Spiess, W. F. J., Geer, J. H., & O'Donohue, W. T. (1984). Premature ejaculation: Investigation of factors in ejaculatory latency. *Journal of Abnormal Psychology, 93,* 242–245.

St. Lawrence, J. S., & Madakasira, S. (1992). Evaluation and treatment of premature ejaculation: A critical review. *International Journal of Psychiatry in Medicine, 22,* 77–97.

Staebler, C. R., Pollard, C. A., & Merkel, W. T. (1993). Sexual history and quality of current relationships in patients with obsessive compulsive disorder: A comparison with two other psychiatric samples. *Journal of Sex and Marital Therapy, 19,* 147–153.

Stief, C. G., & Jonas, U. (1998). Editorial: After the gold rush—advancing research based care for patients with erectile dysfunction. *Journal of Urology, 159,* 120–121.

Strassberg, D. S., Gouveia de Brazao, C. A., Rowland, D. L., Tan, P., & Slob, K. (1999). Clomipramine in the treatment of rapid (premature) ejaculation. *Journal of Sex and Marital Therapy, 25,* 89–101.

Strassberg, D. S., Kelly, M. P., Carroll, C., & Kircher, J. C. (1987). The psychophysiological nature of premature ejaculation. *Archives of Sexual Behavior, 16,* 327–336.

Tiefer, L. (1991). Historical, scientific, clinical and feminist criticisms of "the human sexual response cycle" model. *Annual Review of Sex Research, 2,* 1–23.

Tiefer, L., & Melman, A. (1989). Comprehensive evaluation of erectile dysfunction and medical treatments. In S. R. Leiblum & R. C. Rosen (Eds.), *Principles and practice of sex therapy,* 2nd ed. (pp. 207–236). New York: Guilford.

Tiefer, L., Pedersen, B., & Melman, A. (1988). Psychosocial follow-up of penile prosthesis implant patient and partners. *Journal of Sex and Marital Therapy, 14,* 184–201.

Tollison, C. D., & Adams, H. E. (1979). *Sexual disorders: Treatment, theory, and research.* New York: Gardner.

Trudel, G., Ravart, M., & Matte, B. (1993). The use of the multiaxial diagnostic system for sexual dysfunctions in the assessment of hypoactive sexual desire. *Journal of Sex and Marital Therapy, 19,* 123–130.

Trudel, G., & Saint-Laurent, S. (1983). A comparison between the effects of Kegel's exercises and a combination of sexual awareness relaxation and breathing on situational orgasmic dysfunction in women. *Journal of Sex and Marital Therapy, 9,* 204–209.

Turkat, I. D. (Ed.). (1985). *Behavioral case formulation.* New York: Plenum.

van Lankveld, J. J. D. M. (1998). Bibliotherapy in the treatment of sexual dysfunctions: A meta-analysis. *Journal of Consulting and Clinical Psychology, 66,* 702–708.

von Krafft-Ebing, R. (1899/1969). *Psychopathia sexualis.* Philadelphia: Davis (Reprinted: New York: G.P. Putnam).

Wakefield, J. C. (1987). Sex bias in the diagnosis of primary orgasmic dysfunction. *American Psychologist, 42,* 464–471.

Waring, E. M., & Reddon, J. R. (1983). The measurement of intimacy in marriage: The Waring Intimacy Questionnaire. *Journal of Clinical Psychology, 39,* 53–57.

Webster, D. C. (1996). Sex, lies, and stereotypes: Women and interstitial cystitis. *Journal of Sex Research, 33,* 197–203.

Weeks, G. R., & Hof, L. (1987). *Integrating sex and marital therapy: A clinical guide.* New York: Brunner/Mazel.

Weinhardt, L. S., & Carey, M. P. (1996). Prevalence of erectile disorder among men with diabetes mellitus: Comprehensive review, methodological critique, and suggestions for future research. *Journal of Sex Research, 33,* 205–214.

Weizman, R., & Hart, J. (1987). Sexual behavior in healthy married elderly men. *Archives of Sexual Behavior, 16,* 39–44.

Werlinger, K., King, T. K., Clark, M. M., Pera, V., & Wincze, J. P. (1997). Perceived changes in sexual functioning and body image following weight loss in an obese female population: A pilot study. *Journal of Sex and Marital Therapy, 23,* 74–78.

Whipple, B., Gerdes, C. A., & Komisaruk, B. R. (1996). Sexual response to self-stimulation in women with complete spinal cord injury. *Journal of Sex Research, 33,* 231–240.

White, C. B. (1982). A scale for the assessment of attitudes and knowledge regarding sexuality in the aged. *Archives of Sexual Behavior, 11,* 491–502.

Wiederman, M. W. (1996). Women, sex, and food: Review of

research on eating disorders and sexuality. *Journal of Sex Research, 33,* 301–311.

Wiederman, M. W. (1998). The state of theory in sex therapy. *Journal of Sex Research, 35,* 88–99.

Wilsnack, S. C. (1980). Alcohol, sexuality, and reproductive dysfunction in women. In E. L. Abel (Ed.), *Fetal alcohol syndrome: Human studies,* Vol. 2. Boca Raton, FL: CRC.

Wilsnack, S. C. (1984). Drinking, sexuality and sexual dysfunction in women. In S. C. Wilsnack & L. J. Beckman (Eds.), *Alcohol problems in women: Antecedents, consequences and interventions* (pp. 189–227). New York: Guilford.

Wilsnack, S. C. (1991). Sexuality and women's drinking: Findings from a U.S. national study. *Alcohol Health and Research World, 15,* 147; 150.

Wilson, G. T., & Lawson, D. M. (1978). Expectancies, alcohol, and sexual arousal in women. *Journal of Abnormal Psychology, 87,* 358–367.

Wilson, G. T., Lawson, D. M., & Abrams, D. B. (1978). Effects of alcohol on sexual arousal in male alcoholics. *Journal of Abnormal Psychology, 87,* 609–616.

Wilson, G. T., Niaura, R. S., & Adler, J. A. (1985). Alcohol, selective attention and sexual arousal in men. *Journal of Studies on Alcohol, 46,* 107–115.

Wincze, J. P., & Barlow, D. (1997). *Enhancing sexuality: A problem-solving approach* [Therapist Guide]. San Antonio: Psychological Corporation.

Wincze, J. P., & Carey, M. P. (1991). *Sexual dysfunction: A guide for assessment and treatment.* New York: Guilford.

Winks, C., & Semans, A. (1997). *The new Good Vibrations guide to sex,* 2nd ed. San Francisco, CA: Cleis Press.

Wise, T. N. (1999). Psychosocial side effects of sildenafil therapy for erectile dysfunction. *Journal of Sex and Marital Therapy, 25,* 145–150.

Wolpe, J. (1958). *Psychotherapy by reciprocal inhibition.* Stanford, CA: Stanford University Press.

Wolpe, J. (1982). *The practice of behavior therapy,* 3rd ed. New York: Pergamon Press.

Zilbergeld, B., & Ellison, C. R. (1980). Desire discrepancies and arousal problems in sex therapy. In S. R. Leiblum & A. Pervin (Eds.), *Principles and practices of sex therapy* (pp. 65–101). New York: Guilford.

Zilbergeld, B., & Evans, M. (1980). The inadequacy of Masters and Johnson. *Psychology Today, 14,* 29–43.

Zuckerman, M. (1971). Physiological measures of sexual arousal in the human. *Psychological Bulletin, 75,* 297–329.

# CHAPTER 26

# Sexual Deviation: Paraphilias

## Richard D. McAnulty, Henry E. Adams, and Joel Dillon

## Introduction

Sexuality has always been viewed as a force that must be tightly controlled and regulated. Sexual behavior has been considered a legitimate topic of scientific inquiry only for the past 50 years, beginning with Alfred Kinsey's landmark surveys (Bullough, 1998). Before that time, sexuality and its problems were to be regulated by the church, the government, or medicine. Accordingly, sexual behavior that deviated from the established norm, however it was defined at the time, was declared sinful, criminal, or sick. Deviant behavior, then, called for penitence, punishment, or a cure. This historical heritage still influences our thinking about sexual deviation. Do persons with sexual deviation suffer from an evil nature, a criminal/psychopathic disposition, or a mental illness?

We do not presume to answer such a question because, like most questions relating to sexual behavior, it hinges on personal values and beliefs. There are currently no universal and objective criteria for evaluating the adaptive value of sexual attitudes and practices. Outside of sexual homicide, no sexual behavior is universally deemed dysfunctional. Although most definitions of sex-

ual disorders emphasize that the associated patterns of sexual arousal deviate from normative patterns (hence the term *sexual deviations*), there are presently no clear criteria for defining normal sexual arousal or behavior. Definitions of what is entailed under the heading of "normal" vary over time and across cultures. Sexual norms change, as illustrated by the shift in professional and societal attitudes toward homosexuality. Whereas homosexuality was classified as a sexual deviation in the 2nd ed. of the *Diagnostic and Statistical Manual of Mental Disorders* (DSM-II; American Psychiatric Association [APA], 1968), it has been omitted from the most recent versions of the official psychiatric nomenclature (APA, 1987, 1994). The rationale for excluding homosexuality from the category of sexual deviation category was apparently the lack of evidence that homosexuality *per se* is a harmful dysfunction (Wakefield, 1992). Curiously, the same line of reasoning has not been applied to other "disorders" such as fetishism and consensual sadomasochism. We agree with Laws and O'Donohue (1997) that such conditions are not inherently harmful and their inclusion in this category reflects an inconsistency in classification.

The topic of sexual deviation has the distinction of being one of the most controversial in clinical psychology and related fields. Few disorders elicit as much curiosity and outrage as sexual deviations, or *paraphilias*, as they are officially known (APA, 1994). Numerous cases of sexual offenses and the ensuing sensational media coverage have rekindled the public's fascination and alarm. Studies of victims (Koss, Gidycz, & Wisniewski,

Richard D. McAnulty and Joel Dillon • Department of Psychology, University of North Carolina, Charlotte, North Carolina 28223. Henry E. Adams • Department of Psychology, University of Georgia, Athens, Georgia 30602-3013.

*Comprehensive Handbook of Psychopathology* (Third Edition), edited by Patricia B. Sutker and Henry E. Adams. Kluwer Academic / Plenum Publishers, New York, 2001.

1987) and perpetrators (Abel et al., 1987) reveal that the prevalence of sexual offending is higher than previously believed. Finally, international computer network services that have sexually explicit sites, chat rooms, and special interest groups have brought sexual deviation out of the closet and into cultural awareness. Themes of sexual deviation are evident in several mainstream films, and they are regular features in televised talk shows and documentaries.

Unfortunately, there remains a great amount of undocumented information and often misinformation about paraphiliac disorders. More than ever before, there is a need for sound research on sexual deviation. There are many unanswered questions about the features, etiologies, and effective treatments of the DSM-IV paraphilias. As we reviewed the research literature to update this chapter, we were surprised and disappointed that few advances have occurred in our understanding of most sexual deviations. Most research in the area has concerned nonconsenting paraphiliacs, namely, child molesters and rapists. The attention to these problems is clearly warranted, but we still have much to learn about other paraphilias that may be even more prevalent. Additionally, these other sexual deviations may sometimes be associated with sexual violence and coercion, which renders them equally legitimate and important topics of study.

The objective of this chapter is to provide an overview of paraphiliac disorders. This presentation begins with a discussion of issues related to classifying and assessing these disorders. The empirical literature pertinent to specific paraphilias is subsequently presented with an overview of etiological theories. Treatment strategies will be briefly covered, followed by a summary of legal and professional issues.

## Definitions and Classification

The diagnostic criteria of paraphilias have changed considerably during the past 30 years. In the original DSM (APA, 1952), these disorders were subsumed under the heading of "sociopathic personality disturbance." The following edition of the official psychiatric nomenclature, the DSM-II (APA, 1968), defined sexual deviations as a type of personality disorder, though they were no longer classified under sociopathic personality disorders. Specific subtypes (e.g., pedophilia, fetishism) were introduced in the DSM-II. In both early clas-

sification schemes, the diagnosis was based on inferred personality dynamics, in accord with the prevailing psychoanalytic formulations of these disorders.

Historically, psychoanalytic writers favored the term *perversions* (Freud, 1953; Stoller, 1975a), but this term has been relegated to the vernacular in recent years. Sexual deviations were renamed *paraphilias* and were classified in a separate category of *psychosexual disorders*, along with sexual dysfunctions, in the 3rd ed. of the DSM (APA, 1980). This revision paralleled the shift toward an atheoretical nosology. The term *paraphilia* was borrowed from Karpman (1954) and was adopted because it was more descriptive (specifying the aberration, *para-*, to which the person is attracted, *-philia*) than previous labels. The new classification schemes, including the DSM-III-R and DSM-IV (APA, 1987,1994), do not assume that the deviant sexual interests necessarily pervade the individual's entire range of interpersonal functioning or personality. The defining features of the disorder may be limited to the individual's sexual behavior and causes minimal impairment in other areas of functioning. A noteworthy change in the DSM-III-R from the previous edition is the removal of the criterion specifying that the given paraphilia is the *preferred* or *exclusive* means of attaining sexual pleasure. Therefore, individuals may prefer "normal" heterosexual intercourse but receive paraphiliac diagnoses if they have fantasized about or actually exposed their genitals in public on occasion during the previous 6 months (or longer).

According to the DSM-IV, paraphilias entail arousal that often interferes with "the capacity for reciprocal, affectionate sexual activity" (APA, 1994, p. 524). The preferred sexual stimulus is typically highly specific, and it may be necessary for sexual functioning and, thus, may become a major focus in the individual's life. The diagnosis requires that individuals have acted on their deviant urges or are distressed by them and that the pattern of arousal is evident for a minimum of 6 months. In this nosology, paraphilias are characterized by intense, recurring sexual urges and fantasies related to (1) nonhuman objects (e.g., womens' undergarments), (2) suffering or humiliation of oneself or one's partner in a manner that is not merely simulated (e.g., bondage), or (3) children or other nonconsenting partners. Paraphilias are almost exclusively seen in males. The specific types of paraphilias are listed in Table 1.

## Table 1. DSM-IV Paraphilias

| Disorder | Sexual fantasies, urges, and/or activities |
|---|---|
| Exhibitionism | Exposing to an unsuspecting stranger |
| Fetishism | Use of a nonliving object (not limited to cross-dressing) |
| Frotteurism | Touching or rubbing against a nonconsenting person |
| Pedophilia | Sexual activity with a prepubescent child |
| Sexual masochism | Being humiliated, beaten, bound, or otherwise made to suffer |
| Sexual sadism | Inflicting psychological or physical suffering |
| Transvestic fetishism | Cross-dressing |
| Voyeurism | Observing an unsuspecting person is who disrobing or having sex |

| Paraphilia Not Otherwise Specified | |
|---|---|
| Telephone scatologia | Making obscene phone calls |
| Necrophilia | Sexual activity with corpses |
| Partialism | Exclusive sexual focus on part of the body |
| Zoophilia | Bestiality or sex with animals |
| Coprophilia | Sexual arousal to feces |
| Klismaphilia | Sexual arousal to enemas |
| Urophilia | Sexual arousal to urine |

Gender identity disorders, formerly known as *transsexualism*, are no longer classified as sexual disorders. For historical reasons, these disorders are included in the same section as sexual dysfunctions and paraphilias in the DSM-IV. The essential feature of gender identity disorder involves incongruence between one's biological sex and gender identity (the individual's subjective experience of his or her sex), combined with persistent discomfort with one's biological sex. Consistent with the DSM-IV, we provide an overview of gender identity disorder in this chapter.

### Issues in Classifications

Though the DSM-III-R and DSM-IV classification schemes represent significant improvements over previous nosologies, they are not uniformly accepted by experts on paraphilia. For example, Money (1984, 1986) argued that there are more than thirty subtypes of paraphilias; the majority of them would be classified as "paraphilia not otherwise specified" in the DSM-IV. Other criticisms involve the lack of information provided by some diagnostic labels and the false impression of homogeneity implied by diagnostic categories.

Several other controversies exist in the classification of paraphilias. As previously mentioned, homosexuality is no longer classified as a sexual deviation, although some specialized books continue to include sections on homosexuality (e.g., McConaghy, 1993). As evident in Table 1, the paraphilia category includes a heterogeneous group of conditions. We question the validity of including such disparate conditions as fetishism and pedophilia in the same category. Although both are socially unacceptable to most people, pedophilia involves nonconsenting and harmful sexual behavior, whereas fetishism is usually victimless (unless the person steals the fetish from an unsuspecting person). We believe that the etiologies of these conditions are also very different. These are empirical questions that merit attention and scrutiny.

An important distinction should be made between sexual behavior and preference. Sexual activity is not always indicative of sexual preference; some homosexual males may engage in heterosexual intercourse, although they clearly prefer male sexual partners (and may resort to homosexual fantasy during encounters with females). As previously noted, sexual preference is no longer required as a diagnostic criterion for paraphilia. Sexual preferences, values, and behavior may be incongruent, as evidenced by the observation that some paraphiliacs find their erotic interests despicable. Yet, they regularly engage in these "immoral" acts. Hence, overt sexual behavior is not perfectly correlated with sexual preference or arousal. Subjective distress over erotic preferences, however, is clearly not a sufficient criterion for defining paraphiliac arousal (i.e., some paraphiliacs resent interference by social agencies and view their behavior as enjoyable and normal). This view is recognized in the DSM-IV because subjective distress is not a requisite for a diagnosis of paraphilia.

Other issues center on such questions as whether rape is a sexual offense or exclusively an act of aggression. Though some feminists have emphasized the aggressive component of rape, there is clearly a sexual element in at least some forms of rape. The term *rape* is at best ambiguous because the legal and political aspects of this concept have hindered a neutral, scientific definition of this behavior. The vast majority of researchers and clinicians who work with rapists tend to classify rape as a paraphilia (Freund, 1990; Laws & O'Donohue, 1997). Abel and Rouleau (1990) also criticized the exclusion of rape from the DSM because they believe that rapists display "recurrent, repetitive, and compulsive urges and fantasies to commit rapes" (p. 18), thereby qualifying it as a paraphilia.

Another issue pertains to the relationship between incest and pedophilia. There are some significant differences between these categories; for example, in pedophilia, a prepubertal partner is often involved, which may not be the case in incest. Finally, controversy continues to exist over the occurrence of multiple deviations. Although a number of authorities argue that the presence of multiple paraphilias in one person is not uncommon (e.g., Abel et al., 1987; Langevin, 1983), such a view is not unanimously accepted. Money (1984) argued that it is rare "for a person to have more than one paraphilia, or to change from one to another" (p. 166). Based on clinical experience, McConaghy (1993) also concluded that most paraphiliacs have a single preferred deviation, although they may occasionally experiment with others. This issue remains unresolved. Furthermore, the belief that all or most paraphiliacs progress from minor disorders (such as exposing their genitals) to major disorders (such as child molestation or rape) is not well documented and is controversial. These issues will be addressed in more detail in the discussions of the specific disorders.

## Assessment of Paraphiliac Disorders

Although a detailed overview of assessment strategies with this population is beyond the scope of this discussion, a brief summary is essential. Assessment, or measurement, is the technological implementation of a classification system (Adams & Haber, 1984). In paraphilia, there are four major areas to be assessed: (1) sexual arousal (to deviant and normal stimuli); (2) heterosexual skills, including sexual knowledge, experience, and cognitive distortions; (3) heterosocial skills (e.g., dating skills, assertiveness); and (4) gender identity and behavior. A comprehensive evaluation of these areas is essential for classification, treatment selection, and implementation (Malatesta & Adams, 1986; McAnulty & Adams, 1992). Assessment results should facilitate the determination of the person's ability to engage in reciprocal affectionate activity with a partner and the nature of sexual urges, fantasies, and erotic preferences.

The most common methods include interviews, questionnaires and other self-report measures, and penile plethysmography. Though useful information may be obtained via self-report measures, these methods suffer from a number of problems. Self-report measures are notoriously sensitive to the patient's response set, biases, and motivation. As has been widely documented, paraphiliacs frequently tend to minimize, and even deny, their deviant sexual interests and behaviors (Haywood & Grossman, 1994; Rosen & Kopel, 1977). Second, such instruments as the Minnesota Multiphasic Personality Inventory (MMPI) are notoriously insensitive to the vagaries of paraphilias (Erickson, Luxenberg, Walbek, & Seely, 1987; McAnulty, Adams, & Wright, 1994). Other psychometric tests for evaluating paraphiliacs such as the Clarke Sexual History Questionnaire (Paitich, Langevin, Freeman, Mann, & Handy, 1977) and the Multiphasic Sex Inventory (Nichols & Molinder, 1984) are available but all are transparent and prone to response biases such as social desirability.

Among the various measures of sexual arousal, penile plethysmography (entailing the direct measurement of erectile responses to explicit sexual stimuli), is the most useful (Barbaree & Seto, 1997; Freund & Blanchard, 1989; Rosen & Beck, 1988). As applied to the measurement of deviant sexual arousal, the procedure entails exposing the person to a variety of deviant and nondeviant stimuli to assess sexual responsiveness to these cues. The technique has been used successfully to differentiate heterosexual arousal from homosexuality (Freund, 1963; Tollison, Adams, & Tollison, 1979), pedophilia (Abel, Becker, Murphy, & Flanagan, 1981; Avery-Clark & Laws, 1984), and rape (Quinsey, Chaplin, & Upfold, 1984). For a discussion of the applications and limitations of penile plethysmography, the reader is referred to Murphy and Barbaree (1994) and O'Dohonue and Letourneau (1992).

The Abel Screening Test for Sexual Deviation (Abel, Lawry, Karlstrom, Osborn, & Gillespie, 1994) consists of a visual reaction time (VRT) and a subjective rating of sexual interest in a series of slides of both black and white adult males and females, adolescent males and females, very young males and females (2 to 4 years old), young males and females (ages 8 to 10 years), and various types of sexual activities. An Abel Questionnaire that inquires about various types of sexual history items is usually given in conjunction with the Abel Screen. This questionnaire also has a Social Desirability scale, a cognition distortion scale that measures the individual's attempt to justify child sexual abuse, a risk of recidivism scale and a scale for determining the type of deviant sexual activities that the individual admits. The Abel Screen is a comprehensive, cognitive measure of objective (reaction time) and subjective (ratings) sexual interest and preferences, compared to the physiological measure of sexual arousal obtained by the penile plethysmograph. It has several advantages compared to the penile plethysmograph. First, the people shown in the slides are clothed, eliminating concerns about showing pornography to the patient, although nude slides would probably increase its discriminant validity (Wright & Adams, 1991). Second, it does not have invalid protocols if administered properly, compared to the penile plethysmograph where a significant number of patients show "flat lines" or no response. Further, it has been shown that it has good reliability and validity similar to the penile plethysmograph (Abel, Huffman, Warberg, & Holland, 1998). It is a very useful tool, but more research is needed. When used with the penile plethysmograph (they provide similar results), clinicians' confidence in their opinions is greatly enhanced because cognitive and physiological measures indicate similar conclusions.

## Characteristics of Paraphilias

The term "sexual deviation" conjures many images that are largely without empirical support. The existing literature suggests that paraphiliac disorders consist of a fairly heterogeneous group with respect to psychosocial adjustment, sexual history, erotic preference, criminal charges, and scores on psychometric tests. The empirical data for some subtypes of this disorder are limited, whereas significant progress in understanding others has been accomplished. This is largely attributable to the fact that most paraphiliacs come to the attention of clinicians only when coerced by the family or the courts. Furthermore, some types of these disorders are apparently quite rare. Hence, many generalizations about these paraphilias are tentative and need further investigation.

### Exhibitionism

The diagnostic criteria of *exhibitionism* in the DSM-IV consist of recurrent, intense urges and fantasies of genital exposure that are enacted or are subjectively distressing. The urges and fantasies center on exposing oneself to an unsuspecting female for sexual excitement. Exhibitionism, or "indecent exposure," it is estimated, accounts for one-third of all sexual offenses in England, Wales, Canada, and the United States (Rooth, 1973; Smukler & Schiebel, 1975). Community and college student surveys reveal that 32–44% of women have been victims of exhibitionists (Cox & MacMahon, 1978; Gittelson, Eacott, & Mehta, 1978). Exposers typically have a large number of victims. Abel et al. (1987) found that their sample of 142 exhibitionists reported having a mean of 514 victims (median: 34); thus, a relatively small number of offenders may account for many victims.

The exhibitionist often experiences an erection and may masturbate during exposure, although this is not always the case. Contrary to popular belief, exhibitionists do not typically seek to shock or frighten their victims. Most exposers report that they hope the victim will derive enjoyment and sexual arousal from the sight of the exposed penis (Lang, Langevin, Checkley, & Pugh, 1987; Langevin et al., 1979). The desire for sexual intercourse with the victim apparently plays a secondary role because less than one-third of exposers claim that they desire sexual relations with the victim (Langevin et al., 1979). In terms of the nature of the act, Abel, Levis, and Clancy (1970) noted that the individual tends to engage in a relatively prolonged sequence of behaviors including (1) reviewing stimulating memories from previous exposures, (2) going to the site of exposure, (3) locating a victim, (4) mentally rehearsing and anticipating the act, (5) exposing himself, and (6) masturbating or achieving orgasm passively in some cases. Most exposers tend to have preferred settings for exposing (e.g., libraries, bus stations) that may relate to the availability of potential victims and decreased chances of being apprehended.

In their review of the characteristics of exhibitionists, Blair and Lanyon (1981) reported that the age of onset is usually in the early to mid-twenties, although it is commonly assumed that the activity begins in adolescence. One study found that the deviant sexual interest developed before age eighteen in half of the cases (Abel & Rouleau, 1990). The onset is correlated with interpersonal difficulties and is related to a variety of situations. Exhibitionistic behavior declines after age forty, suggesting a "burn out" process like that documented in psychopathic men (Hare, 1998). This decline, however, does not occur in every case, and the authors (R. M. and H. A.) have treated exhibitionists who had exposed well into their sixties. By definition, exhibitionism is limited to males. A few cases of female exhibitionism have been reported; most involve women who are retarded or mentally ill (Hollender, Brown, & Roback, 1977). Females who engage in genital exposure as nude models or striptease should not be labeled exhibitionists because their behavior is not associated with sexual arousal. As Skipper and McCaghy (1970) noted, these women appear nude for financial rather than sexual reasons (McAnulty, Satterwhite, & Gullick, 1995). Therefore, striptease and topless dancers would not have sexual urges and fantasies of exposing themselves to strangers.

One-half to two-thirds of exposers are married, although marital and sexual adjustment is marginal. Intelligence, educational level, and vocational interests do not differentiate them from the general population (Murphy, 1997). In terms of criminal history, including sexual and nonsexual offenses, exhibitionists have a greater than average number of convictions. The majority of them (72%) are for sexual offenses. Blair and Lanyon (1981) stated that most studies were consistent in reporting that exhibitionists suffered from inferiority feelings and were viewed as timid and unassertive, socially inept, and had problems expressing hostility. Other studies (e.g., Langevin et al., 1979), however, have found that exposers are unremarkable in terms of personality functioning. Gender identity is typically masculine, and narcissistic features may be noted in some cases (Lang et al., 1987; Langevin, 1983).

The sexual history of exhibitionists is characterized by a reliance on masturbation during adolescence and adulthood. This is apparently more common in unmarried exposers (Blair & Lanyon, 1981). Sexual dysfunctions such as erectile failure and premature ejaculation are reportedly uncommon (Lang et al., 1987). Although some authors believe that the presence of other sexual deviations is uncommon, several studies reveal that exhibitionism may be associated with voyeurism (Langevin, 1983; Langevin et al., 1979; Rooth, 1973); 50% of the exposers studied by Lang et al. (1987) had been voyeurs, as were 32% of the 241 exhibitionists described by Freund (1990). Exhibitionism may also be associated with frotteurism and obscene telephone calling (Freund & Watson, 1993). Lang et al. (1987) found that 41% of their sample of exposers had engaged in transvestic fetishism. It has been reported that exposers frequently choose children as victims, and it is estimated that between one-fifth and one-third of victims are female children (MacDonald, 1973; Mohr, Turner, & Jerry, 1964). This observation has led some to postulate a relationship between exposing and pedophilia (e.g. Rooth, 1973). However, studies using penile measures of arousal reveal that exhibitionists respond most to adult females and respond minimally to children (Langevin et al., 1979). Furthermore, in pedophilia, the victim is usually known to the offender, close bodily proximity and physical contact are sought, and the incident tends to occur in a private rather than a public setting. The choice of prepubertal victims by some exhibitionists may relate to the fact that children are less likely to report the incident to the police; hence, they are safer victims. We should note, however, that men who expose predominantly to children and adolescents may actually be pedophiles.

A number of theories of exhibitionism have been formulated. The biological theories postulate an association between epilepsy, especially excess neural discharges in the limbic system, and exposing; however, there is little or no support for this view (Blair & Lanyon, 1981). The psychoanalytic explanations have centered on the concepts of castration anxiety and oedipal conflicts. According to Fenichel (1945), for the exposer, the victims' reactions are reassurances against castration fears. Other psychoanalytic themes include sadistic impulses directed at women and masochistic needs to be caught and punished. As Kline (1987) noted, "it is disappointing to find that the often elaborate and fantastical psychoanalytic theories of sexual deviance are so lacking in objective support" (p. 173).

Behavioral models of exhibitionism emphasize the importance of conditioning experiences. McGuire, Carlisle, and Young (1965) suggested that deviant sexual behavior is often based on one-trial learning from crucial, often incidental, sexual experiences. These experiences are subsequently incorporated into masturbatory fantasy; the pairing of these fantasies with orgasm strengthens their sexually arousing properties. Several case studies provide some support for this view. In two cases reported by McGuire et al. (1965), the male was surprised by an attractive female while urinating in a semipublic place. The encounter was subsequently included in masturbatory fantasies, which thereafter inclined the males to repeat the act. In support of this theory, Zechnich (1971) noted a striking amount of nudity among family members in the history of exhibitionists. More recently, Marshall, Eccles, and Barbaree (1991) hypothesized that assertiveness deficits, problems with adult intimacy, and perfectionism are characteristic of exhibitionists. These predictions await independent replication.

## Voyeurism

The essential feature of *voyeurism* is a pattern of repeatedly observing an unsuspecting person who is nude, disrobing, or engaged in sexual activity (APA, 1994). By definition, "peeping" is done to attain sexual gratification, and no sexual activity with the unsuspecting victim is sought. The sample of voyeurs studied by Abel et al. (1987) reported a mean of 430 victims (median: 8.5). As is the case for exposing, the sexual act does not typically involve physical contact with the victim. Sagarin (1973) and Yalom (1960) emphasized the importance of the lack of victim consent, which distinguishes voyeurism from viewing pornography and striptease acts. Gebhard, Gagnon, Pomeroy, and Christenson (1965) stressed the importance of distinguishing between individuals who take advantage of an opportunity to observe a person disrobing, thereby exhibiting poor judgment, from the peeper, who repeatedly seeks such situations.

Empirical literature on voyeurism is extremely limited. Langevin, Paitich, and Russon (1985b) found no exclusive cases of voyeurism in a sample of more than 600 paraphiliacs. Voyeurism was associated with a number of other paraphilias but never existed as an exclusive sexual deviation. In fact, Langevin (Langevin, 1983; Langevin, Paitich, & Russon, 1985b) questions the existence of voyeurism as a discrete clinical entity. The dearth of clinical evidence for the disorder may stem from the covert nature of voyeuristic activity, as opposed to exhibitionism. One study of male college students found that 42% had engaged in voyeuristic behaviors (Templeman & Stinnett, 1991). Abel (1989) reported that 13% of adults who sought treatment at his clinic for sexual deviation were voyeurs. Voyeurism, it has been found, coexists with several other paraphilias, including frotteurism, pedophilia, and exhibitionism (Abel & Rouleau, 1990; Langevin, Paitich, & Russon, 1985b; Rooth, 1973; Yalom, 1960). According to Abel and Rouleau (1990), one-third of the voyeurs they studied had committed rape. The belief that peepers are prone to violence, including rape, has received mixed support; some individuals who are accused of voyeurism and rape are probably more accurately described as rapists who engaged in surveillance of their prospective victims.

As a group, peepers frequently report disturbed relationships with their parents during their development and are less likely to identify with either parent than normal and other deviant groups (Langevin, Paitich, & Russon, 1985b). Their early home environment is described as hostile and emotionally distant. In terms of sexual history and functioning, contrary to expectations, voyeurs tend to have a greater than average amount of sexual experiences with adult females. Approximately one-third to one-half are married, but these men often have heterosexual fears and deficits (Kaplan & Krueger, 1997).

According to psychoanalytic theory, a voyeur seeks to observe a woman's "castrated" genitals while reassuring himself through masturbation that he has a penis (Meyer, 1995). The late psychoanalyst Robert Stoller (1975a) proposed that voyeurism, like all paraphilias, stemmed from unconscious hostility. Paraphiliacs attempt to harm or humiliate their victims in retaliation for their own feelings of having been humiliated. Overall, voyeurism remains one of the least studied sexual deviations.

## Pedophilia

According to the DSM-IV, *pedophilia* (literally, *love of children*) consists of (1) recurrent and intense sexual urges and fantasies that involve sexual activity with a prepubertal child (usually 13 years old or younger) and (2) an age discrepancy of at least 5 years. To receive the diagnosis, the person must be at least 16, and it is specified that a relationship between an older adolescent and a 12- to 13-year-old would not qualify as pedophilia (APA, 1994). Although the terms "pedophile" and "child molester" are often used interchangeably, we believe that there are important differences (see also, Barbaree & Seto, 1997). Pedophilia is reserved for those individuals who evidence a marked preference for children. Child molestation may be motivated by the unavailability of an adult partner (Freund, McKnight, Langevin, & Cibiri, 1972), due to cognitive deficits such as mental retardation or dementia, or due to disinhibitory influences such as substance dependence or psychopathy (Dorr, 1998). In other words, pedophilia is but one of several possible motives behind child molestation. Such a distinction in terms is not simply a matter of semantics but has important implications for treatment selection.

An important aspect of the current nosology is the provision for specifying preferred victim gender (male, female, or both), relationship to the victim (incestuous vs. nonincestuous), and whether the pattern is exclusive (i.e., the pedophile is attracted only to children) or nonexclusive. The distinction between homosexual, bisexual, and heterosexual pedophilia is well established (Langevin, 1983; Lanyon, 1986). Heterosexual pedophilia is more common than the homosexual variant, whereas the bisexual subtype is uncommon. Homosexual pedophiles, however, tend to have a larger number of victims than heterosexual pedophiles. For example, Abel et al. (1987) found that their sample of heterosexual child molesters (nonincestuous) reported an average of 20 victims, compared to 150 for homosexual pedophiles (nonincestuous). Incestuous offenders in the same study (Abel et al., 1987) admitted to an average of 1.8 female victims and 1.7 male victims. As with nonincestuous child molestation, most incestuous pedophiles chose female victims. In contrast to homosexual pedophilia, heterosexual child molesters are more likely to be married (Langevin, Hucker, Handy et al., 1985). Contrary to popular belief, pedophiles are not "dirty old men"; as most incarcerated pedophiles are in their mid-twenties to mid-thirties (Groth & Birnbaum, 1978; Langevin, Hucker, Handy et al., 1985). By defini-

tion, the victims in both groups are prepubertal; the average victim's age is approximately 10 years (Groth & Birnbaum, 1978). Approximately 25% of victims are less than 6 years of age, another 25% are between 6 and 10 years old, and roughly 50% are between 11 and 13 years of age (Erickson, Walbek, & Seely, 1988).

The type of sexual activity with the victim ranges from fondling to oral-genital contact and actual penetration (Erickson et al., 1988). Among heterosexual pedophiles, fondling of the victim is by far most common (54%), although vaginal contact (41.5%) and cunnilingus (19%) are not rare. For homosexual offenders, fondling of the victim is also most common (43%), followed by the performance of fellatio on the victim (41%). Anal contact in the latter group occurs in one-third of cases. In cases involving younger children, actual anal or vaginal penetration is uncommon; contact usually entails rubbing the penis against the orifice or between the thighs (Erickson et al., 1988; Langevin, Hucker, Handy et al., 1985). In cases of intrafamilial incest, there tends to be a progression from masturbation and fondling to actual attempts at intercourse over time. Aggressive and sadistic sexual activity occurs in less than 20% of cases (Groth & Birnbaum, 1978). Methods of obtaining victim compliance include enticement via bribery, seduction, appeal to curiosity, and intimidation and threats in some cases. The majority of pedophiles is at least acquainted with their victims. Incestuous pedophiles commonly molest biological, adoptive, or stepchildren, whereas the victims of nonincestuous offenders may include neighbors, relatives, and acquaintances.

With respect to criminal histories, a significant proportion of pedophiles has prior criminal convictions for sexual and nonsexual offenses; however, they tend to display fewer antisocial features than rapists (Bard et al., 1987). Of possible etiological significance is the finding that more than 50% of child molesters report having been the victim of sexual abuse during childhood (Bard et al., 1987). Pedophiles typically have facilitating cognitions regarding sexual contact with children (Hanson, Gizzarelli, & Scott, 1994; Ward, Hudson, Johnston, & Marshall, 1997). Specifically, they tend to believe in beneficial effects for the child from adult sexual contacts, assume less responsibility on the adult's part, and perceive greater child complicity in the sexual activity than rapists and normal subjects (Stermac & Segal, 1989).

A useful typology of pedophiles is the distinction between preferential and situational pedophilia (Lanyon, 1986). This typology is similar to the exclusive-versus-nonexclusive dichotomy of the DSM-IV and to the fixated-versus-regressed classification proposed by Cohen, Seghorn, and Calmas (1969) and Groth and Birnbaum (1978). *Preferential* or *fixated* pedophiles are primarily interested in children as sexual partners and tend to be unmarried. Homosexual pedophiles are usually preferential molesters. Their sexual experiences with adults tend to be very limited; they commonly have experienced lifelong difficulties in relating to adults, and their sexual development is described as fixated. Most encounters with children are premeditated rather than impulsive. These individuals tend to be more comfortable socially and sexually with children. The *situational* or *regressed* pedophiles tend primarily to be heterosexual child molesters. Incestuous offenders would generally be classified as situational offenders. These individuals are more likely to be married and to have more extensive sexual experience with adult partners than preferential pedophiles. A common pattern is an apparently normal development with adequate social and heterosexual skills. As the person enters adulthood, however, his social, occupational, and marital adjustment become tenuous and marginal. The pedophilic acts are typically precipitated by direct confrontation with a female or a threat to the person's masculinity. These individuals' sexual encounters with children are more impulsive, usually with older but prepubescent females, and tend to occur intermittently rather than continuously (Lanyon, 1986). A major question is whether these individuals have always had some sexual arousal to children as well as to adults. It is important to note that some degree of heterogeneity is evident within both of these categories (Fischer & McDonald, 1998).

A final category includes the *aggressive* pedophile (Cohen et al., 1969) or sadistic child molester. Boys are typically the preferred victims, and the sexual activity is clearly vicious and cruel. Sexual activity may include the mutilation of the victim's genitalia and insertion of foreign objects into bodily orifices. In some cases, forcible anal intercourse (with resultant rectal lacerations) may occur. Avery-Clark and Laws (1984) identified a group of aggressive pedophiles who were equally aroused by depictions of consenting intercourse with a child and graphic descriptions of aggressive assault of a child. Penile measures of arousal suggested that these pedophiles were sexually aroused or at least not sexually inhibited by sexual aggression and violence directed at children. Although these individuals are fairly rare, the results of their deviant sexual arousal are tragic; these offenders may be involved in serial molestation and murder of boys.

As a group, pedophiles have been characterized as shy, unassertive, and passive (Langevin, 1983). Additionally, they have been described as introverted and socially withdrawn (Bard et al., 1987; Langevin, Hucker, Ben-Aron, Purins, & Hook, 1985). However, no single personality profile is consistently observed among pedophiles (Levin & Stava, 1987; Okami & Goldberg, 1992). Pedophiles tend to be concerned with negative evaluations by females, to view themselves as unassertive, and to hold very conservative stereotypes of women (Overholser & Beck, 1986). In interactions with adult females, they rate their performance more poorly than rapists (Segal & Marshall, 1985). In terms of additional diagnoses, pedophiles most frequently receive a personality disorder diagnosis (Langevin, Hucker, Handy et al., 1985). Depending on the sample and measures used, 8–30% of child molesters meet the diagnostic criteria for antisocial personality disorder and/or psychopathy (Quinsey, Harris, & Rice, 1995; Serin, Malcolm, Khanna, & Barbaree, 1994; for a review, see Dorr, 1998). Alcohol abuse is one of the most commonly reported problems among child molesters (Marshall, 1997). Paradoxically, some pedophiles are moralistic, conservative individuals in other aspects of their lives (Marshall & McKnight, 1975).

The sexual arousal of pedophiles has been extensively studied with penile plethysmography. As a group, nonincestuous child molesters exhibit as much or more penile erection in response to stimuli involving children than to stimuli involving adults (Freund, 1967; Marshall, Barbaree, & Butt, 1988; Quinsey, Steinman, Bergersen, & Holmes, 1975). These findings are consistent with the notion of an erotic preference for prepubertal partners. Incestuous pedophiles, however, tend to be more like nonoffenders in measured sexual preference (Marshall, Barbaree, & Christophe, 1986; Quinsey, Chaplin, & Carrigan, 1979). Some incest offenders respond most to adult females, which has led some authors (e.g., Quinsey, 1977) to speculate about nonsexual motives in incest. Barbaree and Marshall (1989) discovered five separate sexual preference profiles among child molesters. Two profiles were indicative of pedophilic arousal, one suggested a normal adult heterosexual orientation, one revealed a preference for adolescents, and the last involved indiscriminate arousal. In sum, child molesters, including pedophiles, represent a heterogeneous group with respect to psychopathology, personality style, and sexual preference.

Psychoanalytic theories emphasize that pedophiles choose children as partners because they elicit less castration anxiety than adults (Fenichel, 1945). Others have hypothesized an aversion to adult females and an association with homosexuality. The experimental evidence, however, does not support these theoretical views (Langevin, 1983; Langevin, Hucker, Ben-Aron et al., 1985). The behavioral or social learning theories stress the importance of early conditioning, direct reinforcement, or modeling experiences, such as the presence of sexual abuse in the offender's past or an initial or early sexual experience with a younger child (McGuire et al., 1965). The single most popular factor theory of pedophilia is the "abused-abuser hypothesis" which postulates that individuals who were sexually abused in childhood are predisposed to developing pedophilia. As Garland and Dougher (1990) commented, despite the popularity of this view, there is surprisingly little empirical support. There are at least three theoretical problems with this hypothesis: (1) most victims of child sexual abuse are females, but the vast majority of pedophiles is male; (2) fewer than half of all child molesters have personal histories of sexual victimization by an adult in childhood (Garland & Dougher, 1990; Weeks & Widom, 1998), and (3) some pedophiles allege having been sexually abused in childhood as a ploy to reduce their perceived responsibility for their sexual offenses (Freund, Watson, & Dickey, 1990). Thus, the majority of individuals who were sexually molested as children do *not* develop pedophilia (Hansen & Slater, 1988).

Araji and Finkelhor (1985) advanced a four-factor model of pedophilia. According to them, pedophilia may be understood in terms of (1) *emotional congruence*, or the emotional need to relate to children (e.g., faulty development, inadequacy); (2) *blockage*, or the inability to attain alternative sources of gratification (e.g., skills deficits, heterosocial fears); (3) *disinhibition*, the failure to be deterred from socially disapproved sexual behavior (e.g., alcoholism, sociopathy); and (4) *sexual arousal* to prepubertal partners. Araji and Finkelhor (1985) noted that most existing theories of pedophilia include one or more of these factors. This proposed model is promising because it stresses the multidetermined aspect of the disorder, but empirical tests are needed.

In their review of incest, Dixen and Jenkins (1981) outlined five factors that appear important in initiating incest:

1. The occurrence of incest in either parent's family.
2. Unsatisfactory marital sexual relationships in which the wife is sexually inaccessible to the husband.
3. Frequent absence of the mother, especially in the evening.
4. Any condition that reduces impulse control, such as alcoholism, sociopathy, or subnormal intelligence.
5. The oldest daughter having been coerced into adult responsibilities, with a role-reversal between mother and daughter.

Psychoanalytic theories of incest state that the victim experiences oral deprivation in the preoedipal stage; the incestuous relationship occurs as a revenge against the mother and as a form of oral gratification. Several other theories stress the importance of a dysfunctional family system. In such views, incest represents a maladaptive attempt to maintain family homeostasis (Dixen & Jenkins, 1981; see Long, 1995).

One of the newest and most elaborate multifactorial theories of sexual offending was proposed by Marshall and colleagues (Marshall, 1989; Marshall, Hudson, & Hodkinson, 1993). In this formulation, a lack of intimacy in adulthood and the resulting experience of loneliness predispose some individuals to sexually aggressive behavior (Garlick, Marshall, & Thornton, 1996; Seidman, Marshall, Hudson, & Robertson, 1994). This deficiency in adult intimacy may interact with sociocultural influences, precocious sexualization, conditioning events, and biological factors in the development and maintenance of deviant sexuality (Marshall & Eccles, 1993). According to the model, the developmental history of sex offenders renders them vulnerable to various influences and events; this proposed developmental vulnerability is attributed to inadequate parent–child attachment early in life (Smallbone & Dadds, 1998; Weeks & Widom, 1998). Consequently, the child lacks the skills and self-confidence necessary to master the challenges in the transition to adolescence. The vulnerable male experiences pubertal development and emerging sexual urges and feels socially inept, especially with female peers. Thus, the individual is believed to be especially susceptible to nondemanding and nonthreatening sexual scripts (Marshall & Eccles, 1993). Examples of nonthreatening scripts for a socially incompetent male might include child molestation, voyeurism, and fetishism. Likewise, for a male who fears intimacy, nonconsenting sexual activity, including rape, may be less threatening. These individuals may also be attracted to cultural messages that perpetuate gender role stereotypes, such as the view that males are naturally aggressive and women are inherently passive. It is further postulated that if the individual incorporates these nonthreatening and distorted fantasies into masturbating practices, this may strengthen the conditioning process (McGuire et al., 1965). Any disinhibiting influences, including drug abuse and brain damage, may further increase the risk of enacting any existing deviant urges.

### Sexual Sadism and Sexual Masochism

*Sexual sadism*, as defined in the DSM-IV, consists of sexual urges and fantasies centering on the actual (not simulated) infliction of psychological and physical suffering on a victim. The victims' involvement in these activities may range from fully consenting (in the case of a sadomasochistic relationship) to a complete lack of consent (as might occur in sadistic rape). The sadistic fantasies and acts may range from verbal humiliation to bondage, forceful restraint, spanking, and in extreme cases, torture, mutilation, and killing. *Sexual masochism* entails recurrent sexual urges and fantasies of being actually humiliated, beaten, bound, or made to suffer. An extreme form of masochism is known as "asphyxiophilia" or "autoerotic strangulation," which entails derivation of sexual pleasure and intensification of orgasm via oxygen deprivation (Garos, 1994). Although apparently rare, the latter condition is sometimes publicized after the person's escape mechanism from the self-strangulation contraption fails (Resnik, 1972). In such cases, the dead individual is found by an unsuspecting spouse or relative,

and the incident may be erroneously explained as suicide.

The majority of sadists and masochists are heterosexual, although both disorders occur among homosexuals (Gosselin, 1987; Kamel, 1980). Although many sadists and masochists tend to favor their respective roles, some role reversal does occur, suggesting that these disorders may coexist in some cases (Gosselin, 1987). Masochism is believed to be one of the few paraphilias found in women (Levitt, Moser, & Jamison, 1994). In the vast majority of instances, sadomasochistic sexual interactions are consensual (Stoller, 1991). Gosselin (1987) described the "sadomasochistic contract" which governs the sexual scripts of sadists and their masochistic partners. With few exceptions, sadists do not derive pleasure from inflicting more harm than is desired by their partners (Gosselin & Wilson, 1984). In fact, most sadists seek a partner who is sexually excited by suffering or humiliation rather than one who would not enjoy these practices (Gosselin, 1987; McConaghy, 1993). Masochists have very specific preferences for the type of pain or humiliation they seek; as Stoller commented, "no sadomasochists like all kinds of pain" (1991, p. 16). According to Weinberg (1995), control rather than pain is at the core of sadomasochism. Thus, most sadists and masochists are interested in consensual sexual activities that include elements of mental or physical control, and some individuals alternate between giving and receiving the suffering or humiliation (Stoller, 1991).

According to Gosselin (1987), who has extensively studied sadomasochism, three aspects are characteristic:

*Beatings* that may vary drastically in intensity and duration (up to 200 strokes in some cases). The stereotypical whip is reportedly seldom used because of difficulties in controlling its impact.

*Bondage* that is ritualistic and often associated with beatings. Common forms include mouth gags, hoods, blindfolds, immobilization, and rope or leather restraints, sometimes to the point of partial asphyxiation.

*Humiliation* that may range from bootlicking and crawling to the use of urine, feces, and enemas.

Sexual sadism is distinct from psychopathy by virtue of the fact that sadists are highly sensitive to their partners' emotions and delight in controlling their display (Gosselin, 1987). Furthermore, in sadomasochistic relationships, the sexual encounters are governed by explicit rules and agreements about the boundaries of acceptable behavior. Although empirical data are limited, sadomasochism (or S & M) is not rare, as evidenced by the availability of S & M handbooks (e.g., Masters' and Mistresses' Handbooks), magazines, clubs, online computer sites, and societies.

Rape is not included in the DSM-III-R nosology for two apparent reasons: (1) Many rapists are not considered paraphiliacs, and (2) there was concern that paraphiliac rape might be used as a legal defense to avoid prosecution. Curiously, this latter line of reasoning was not applied to pedophilia or other paraphilias. According to the DSM-III-R, approximately 10% of rapists meet diagnostic criteria for sexual sadism. Sadistic rapists and lust murderers who seek nonconsenting victims meet the DSM-IV criteria for *severe* sadism. However, we have serious reservations about grouping such extreme and rare individuals in the same category as couples who enjoy consenting sadomasochistic interactions.

Among the various classification schemes of rapists (e.g., Rada, 1978), several subtypes have been consistently proposed. According to Knight and colleagues (Knight & Prentky, 1990; Knight, Rosenberg, & Schneider, 1985; Prentky, Knight, & Rosenberg, 1987), the following subtypes have some empirical support:

1. *Opportunistic* rapists use force to obtain victim compliance. For these individuals, rape is just one aspect of a predatory life-style. According to Rada (1978), 30–40% of rapists fall into this category. The majority of these individuals have antisocial and/or psychopathic personalities.
2. *Pervasively angry* rapists evidence undifferentiated anger and tend to be very aggressive. This is a very uncommon type of rapist (Barbaree, Seto, Serin, Amos, & Preston, 1994).
3. *Vindictive* rapists are primarily motivated by aggression; rape is an expression of rage and anger that is specifically directed at women. The rape is intended to punish and degrade the victim.
4. *Sexual sadistic* rapists evidence sexual-aggressive erotic fantasies. The infliction of pain and suffering is sexually arousing for these individuals who meet the DSM-IV criteria for severe sexual sadism.

5. *Sexual nonsadistic* rapists are those for whom aggression is instrumental in securing sexual compliance, and the rape is associated with nonsadistic sexual fantasies.

According to Prentky et al. (1987), victim injury varies across rapist types, although it is often difficult to determine the true intent of a perpetrator: Was the aggression solely instrumental or gratuitous? The authors noted that the dimensions of social competence and life-style impulsivity may further enhance the classification of rapists. Blader and Marshall (1989) noted that sadistic rapists consistently evidence an erotic preference for nonconsenting and aggressive sexual activity with women, as documented by tumescence studies of rapists. The other subtypes may appear normal on tumescence measures of arousal by responding most to consensual sexual activity but may fail to inhibit arousal to a partner's resistance or suffering (as in the case of normal males). In most other respects, incarcerated rapists resemble the general inmate population in criminal history, psychosocial adjustment, comorbidity, and social competence (Polaschek, Ward, & Hudson, 1997).

The phenomenon of *acquaintance* or *date rape* has been a topic of interest in recent years. Estimates of the prevalence of date rape range from 5–54% of female college students (Koss, 1989). According to Muehlenhard and Linton (1987), the following risk factors for date rape have been identified:

1. The male initiates and takes a dominant role in the date.
2. Miscommunication regarding sex.
3. Heavy alcohol or drug use.
4. Going to a secluded area, or "parking."
5. Male acceptance of traditional gender roles, interpersonal violence, antagonism toward relationships, and rape myths.

Malamuth and colleagues (1989, 1993) found that several variables, including hostility toward women, antisocial features, and sexual arousal to rape cues, were predictive of the propensity of male college students to engage in forceful sexual activity. According to them, two separate pathways, hostile masculinity and sexual promiscuity, lead to sexual aggression. It remains unclear how these persons who commit acquaintance rape fit into the classification scheme of rapists. It seems likely that some of these individuals who engage in date rape may progress into a recurrent pattern of opportunistic or sexual nonsadistic rape. More research is needed to understand males who perpetrate date and other types of rape. Particularly significant is the role of force and victim suffering in instigating or failing to inhibit sexual arousal. Cues indicative of a victim's suffering and fear do not inhibit sexual arousal in sexually coercive male college students (Lohr, Adams, & Davis, 1997).

## Frotteurism

Previously classified as an "atypical paraphilia," frotteurism (from the French *frotter*, "to rub") remains a full-fledged category in the DSM-IV. The criteria for frotteurism include intense urges, fantasies, or behaviors centering on touching and rubbing (frottage) against a nonconsenting female. The criteria emphasize that the act of rubbing, rather than the coercive element, is the arousing stimulus. Experts on paraphilia tend to distinguish frotteurism from "toucherism" (arousal by touching a stranger's body), although the DSM-IV makes no such distinction. Individuals who engage in frottage typically engage in this activity by boarding crowded public transportation vehicles and positioning themselves next to an attractive female. The individual takes advantage of the proximity afforded by the crowding and swaying of the vehicle to rub his genitals against the victim's thighs, buttocks, or crotch. The individual typically fantasizes that he is having a consenting sexual encounter with the victim. The frequent stops of subways and buses allow escape should the victim become aware of the activity and protest.

There are very few accounts of frotteurism in the clinical literature; either the condition is uncommon or, more likely, frotteurs are rarely seen in clinical settings. In their large-scale study of paraphilias, Abel et al. (1987) examined sixty-two self-proclaimed frotteurs. The mean number of victims was 901 (median: 29.5). After exhibitionists, frotteurs accounted for the greatest percentage (18.1%) of total paraphiliac acts in the sample of 561 admitted paraphiliacs. Freund (1990) reported that 61% of the 119 frotteurs he studied had also engaged in exhibitionism. More than 30% admitted to voyeuristic acts, and 22% admitted to having raped a woman.

Money (1986) claims that the impersonal nature of the sexual contact is essential to the frotteur. Others argue that frotteuristic patterns can be seen as a distortion of the normal sexual or erotic tactile interaction phase (Freund & Watson, 1993). According to Langevin (1983), frotteurism can be classified as a form of sexual aggression on the basis of the lack of consent that characterizes the sexual activity.

## Fetishism

In the DSM-IV, the essential features of fetishism include intense sexual urges, fantasies, or behaviors that involve the use of nonliving objects; these items may be used with a partner who wears the item during sexual activity to facilitate the fetishist's sexual arousal. It is specified that female clothing items used for cross-dressing purposes are criteria for transvestic fetishism rather than simple fetishism. Docter (1988) differentiated fetishism from fetishistic transvestism on the basis of the extent of cross-dressing and gender identity: fetishists occasionally wear the fetish but do not seek to appear as women, and gender identity is masculine. Blanchard (1991) argued that specific features of female clothing items may differentiate fetishism from transvestic fetishism: In the former, the preferred item (e.g., panties) has been previously worn by a female instead of being purchased new in a store. In some cases, the fetish is necessary for sexual arousal, and erectile failure may occur in its absence (Gosselin & Wilson, 1984). Arousal to a specific nonsexual body part (e.g., feet or hair) was previously labeled fetishism, although the preferred term among experts in the area is "partialism." In the DSM-IV, partialism is categorized as a Paraphilia Not Otherwise Specified. The separation of partialism and fetishism has generated some debate because the majority of researchers believes that these conditions are related (Bancroft, 1989; De Silva, 1993).

In their study of fetishists, Chalkley and Powell (1983) found that approximately 60% preferred clothing items (e.g., panties, stockings, raincoats), 23% were aroused by rubber items, 15% chose footwear, and 15% preferred body parts (i.e., partialism), whereas the remainder was excited by stimuli ranging from leather to nylon garments. In this sample, 44% preferred to wear the item, 23% enjoyed seeing the item worn by another person, and 37.5% regularly stole the preferred fetish. According to McConaghy (1993), fetishists most commonly receive professional attention only after being apprehended for theft.

According to Money (1984, 1986), fetishes may

be categorized according to texture, such as silk or nylon, or smell, usually associated body parts (as with soiled undergarments). Rubber and leather combine both texture and smell. Bancroft (1989) suggested that virtually all fetishes are directly or symbolically associated with the body. Weinberg, Williams, and Calhan (1994) investigated the fetishistic preference and sexual behavior of 262 homosexual or bisexual males who expressed sexual interest in male feet or footwear. Participants were recruited through an organization for foot fetishists. Sixty percent of the respondents found clean feet sexually arousing, followed by boots (52%), shoes (49%), sneakers (47%), and smelly socks (45%). Other fetishistic objects were sexually arousing; almost half of the respondents were also aroused by clothes and leather. In addition, the respondents expressed great specificity in their shoe fetishes: wing-tips, penny loafers, etc. Almost three-fourths of the respondents said they were very particular in the type of footwear that aroused them, and 60% were equally specific in the type of feet they found sexually arousing. For the reasons that the respondents were aroused by feet and footwear, 50% made a direct reference to sensual aspects of the fetish object (taste, touch, smell etc.), 30% emphasized symbolic themes, and 20% were unable to explain their attraction. When asked about the importance of the fetish object in their sexual fantasies, 83% of the respondents masturbated at least once a week while fantasizing about feet or footwear. Finally, a third of the respondents was currently involved in an intimate relationship, and almost 80% of these reported engaging in "foot play" with their partners. Furthermore, nearly 60% evaluated foot/footwear activities as an important part of their sex lives with their steady partners.

In a large-scale study of fetishists, transvestites, and sadomasochists, Wilson and Gosselin (1980) found significant overlap among sexual fantasies and activities. Eighty-eight percent of their fetishists, it was found, engaged in sadomasochism and/or transvestism. In terms of personality functioning, all three groups were described as introverted, shy, mildly anxious, and depressed. Weinberg, Williams, and Calhan (1995), however, found that fewer than one in four men in their nonclinical sample of foot fetishists endorsed psychological problems. This finding suggests that clinical samples of fetishists may not be representative of the larger population of fetishists. Approximately 60–

70% of the participants in Wilson and Gosselin's (1980) survey had steady sex partners, and the modal age for all groups was around 40–50 years. In their cross-sectional survey in the United States, Janus and Janus (1993) found that 11% of men and 6% of women had personal experiences with fetishes. The authors did not specify the extent of the women's involvement, but it appears that it involved having a male partner with a fetishistic preference. This finding would be consistent with reports that this paraphilia is rare in women.

Epstein (1969) argued that the etiology of fetishism involves increased orgasmic excitability, which he viewed as indicative of cerebral pathophysiology. According to this theory, fetishism is associated with epilepsy and temporal lobe dysfunction (Langevin, 1983); however, this claim has not been substantiated by others (e.g., Landsdell, 1971). Pesta (1993), using classic Freudian theory, considered early childhood events and trauma as developing factors in adult fetishism. Most psychodynamic formulations of fetishism postulate that it stems from castration anxiety and the fantasy of the phallic woman (Bak, 1968). The fetish symbolizes the penis from this perspective.

A classic study by Rachman (1966) illustrated a conditioning paradigm for acquiring fetishistic arousal. In a laboratory setting, photographs of women's boots were paired with slides of nude adult females. After a number of conditioning trials, the participants (seven psychology graduate students), it was found, exhibited increased erectile responses to the boots alone. Furthermore, some generalization to other types of women's shoes was reported. Although the conditioning model received support, a number of questions remain unanswered: What predisposes an individual to develop this pattern of arousal? Why do some evidence this type of sexual response (apparently an uncommon condition in clinical settings), whereas others do not? Are those former students still "turned on" by women's boots?

## Transvestic Fetishism

The term *transvestic fetishism* replaces the former DSM-III category of *transvestism*. The diagnostic criteria for transvestic fetishism in the DSM-IV include (1) for at least 6 months, recurrent sexual urges, fantasies, or behaviors in a heterosexual male that involve cross-dressing; (2) the urges have been enacted or are subjectively distressing; and (3) the person does not meet the criteria for a gender identity disorder. Thus, the diagnosis precludes conditions in which a homosexual male (a "drag queen") cross-dresses, as well as disorders that involve a subjective sense of discomfort and incongruence between one's biological sex and gender identity, such as in transsexualism. An important differentiation between these disorders is that cross-dressing is sexually arousing in transvestic fetishism but not in the other conditions (Docter, 1988). According to Docter (1988), there are five essential characteristics that identify transvestic fetishism: heterosexual orientation, sexual arousal to cross-dressing, the cross-dressing is periodic, no desire for surgical or hormonal gender reassignment, and gender identity is masculine except when cross-dressed. In cases where the sexual arousal in response to cross-dressing declines over time, the diagnosis may be revised to a gender identity disorder. Some evidence suggests that a number of transvestites eventually develop transsexualism (see Blanchard, 1993; Langevin, 1985).

Some sadomasochists also cross-dress (Wilson & Gosselin, 1980); however, it is unclear if this is associated with fetishistic arousal or with humiliation rituals. Langevin, Paitich, and Russon (1985a) found, surprisingly, that up to one-fourth of the rapists they studied engaged in cross-dressing. In transvestism, gender identity is masculine, although many report experiencing a feminine side while cross-dressed. Therefore, it appears that cross-dressing entails a fairly heterogeneous group of individuals. As defined by the DSM-IV, the fetishistic component in a heterosexual male is essential.

In a replication study of Prince and Bentler's (1972) classic survey of 504 transvestites, Docter and Prince (1997) investigated various demographic, sexual, and cross-gender variables among 1032 self-defined periodic cross-dressers. With few exceptions, the second survey findings closely mirrored those of the first survey. As expected, the vast majority of respondents (87% to 89%) was heterosexual although nearly one-third in both samples had some prior homosexual experience. The initiation of cross-dressing began before the age of ten for 54–66% of respondents. In both samples, nearly two-thirds of the transvestites were married, and the vast majority also had children. The majority of wives was aware of their husbands' cross-dressing; the most common reac-

tion was ambivalence; fewer than one-third was accepting. Most cross-dressers preferred to cross-dress in full costume (85–93%). Nearly three-fourths of transvestites had appeared in a public setting while cross-dressed, but only one-quarter reported going to highly visible or crowded places such as public transportation, restaurants, or shopping centers where they might be recognized. With regard to the participants' "view of self when cross-dressed," 80% reported that cross-dressing represented an "expression of a different part of myself." Nearly 75% of respondents agreed that cross-dressing elicited sexual arousal at least occasionally.

According to Fenichel (1945), transvestism incorporates the homosexual's identification with the mother with the fetishist's denial that the female has no penis. Castration anxiety and the oedipal complex have figured prominently in psychoanalytic interpretations of transvestism (Wise & Meyer, 1980). Learning theories emphasize the importance of conditioning experiences in the development of the disorder. For example, being cross-dressed as a child (e.g., "petticoat punishment") or praised for feminine appearance may reinforce these behaviors; incorporating these activities and fantasies into masturbatory activity may further strengthen the sexually arousing properties of cross-dressing (McGuire et al., 1965).

Money (1974) proposed that the disorder develops as a product of "postnatal programming." According to him, gender role is developed by identification with the same-sex parent and is reinforced by the complementary actions of the opposite-sex parental figure. Transvestism, in Money's view, arises because of faulty identification and inappropriate family reinforcement phenomena. Interestingly, boys who display cross-gender (i.e., effeminate) behaviors tend to develop into adult homosexuals instead of transvestites or transsexuals. Zucker and Blanchard (1997) noted that mother–son conflict, characterized by anger, hostility, and rejection, is characteristic of the childhood of most transvestites. Hostility toward females may play a role in the development of transvestic fetishism.

## Gender Identity Disorder

Gender identity disorder is characterized by incongruence between the individual's biological sex and gender identity. Gender identity disturbance, or *gender dysphoria*, is relatively rare and is usually evident during childhood. The DSM-IV criteria for gender identity disorder, or *transsexualism* as it was formerly known, include (1) strong and cross-gender identification (not merely a desire for any cultural advantage of being the other sex), (2) persistent discomfort with one's sex or a sense of inappropriateness in the gender role of that sex, and (3) the absence of any physical intersex condition such as androgen insensitivity syndrome. The disorder involves a preoccupation with getting rid of primary and secondary sex characteristics and/or the conviction that the person was born the wrong sex. The primary goal for transsexuals is to pass successfully in society as a member of the other sex on a full-time basis (Pauly, 1990). Children with gender identity disorder frequently voice their desire to be the other sex, may cross-dress, and prefer playing with peers of the other sex. They typically identity with the other sex gender role. Children and adolescents with gender identity disorder have deficits in same-sex skills and in peer interactions (Bradley & Zucker, 1997). Gender identity disorder is more prevalent among males.

Sexual orientation may be asexual, heterosexual, homosexual, or unspecified. In biological female transsexuals, only the homosexual subtype has been reported (Zucker & Bradley, 1995). These individuals describe themselves as males trapped in women's bodies, and they are erotically attracted to females. In males, heterosexual transsexualism consists of the subjective conviction of being a female, and attraction is to females. Conversely, homosexual transsexualism in males also involves a feminine gender identity and sexual preference for males (Zucker & Bradley 1995). The confusion in terminology may be clarified if one understands that the specified sexual orientation refers to the individual's *biological* partner preference: a homosexual transsexual prefers a partner of the same biological gender, whereas the heterosexual variant involves a preference for an opposite-sex partner. Homosexual transsexualism is considered the most common form of the disorder in males and is the exclusive type in females (Blanchard, 1989, 1990). In one study of the sexual orientation of gender dysphoric patients, one of seventy-two females was attracted to men (Blanchard, Clemmensen, & Steiner, 1987).

The distinction between transvestism and male transsexualism is based on several differences: (1) Transvestites cross-dress for purposes of sexual excitement, whereas transsexuals' cross-dressing is associated with gender dysphoria; (2) transsexuals, in contrast to transvestites, desire to rid themselves of their masculine anatomy; and (3) transsexualism is associated with feminine gender identity. Congruent with the male transsexuals' belief that they are not genuine males, they reportedly tend to avoid using their penises during sexual encounters (Langevin, 1985).

In their study of homosexual transsexual males who requested sex-reassignment surgery, Freund, Langevin, Zajac, Steiner, and Zajac (1974) found that a major goal for the sex-change operation was the ability to attract heterosexual male partners. During sexual intercourse with another male, homosexual transsexuals tend to fantasize that they are a female engaged in sexual activity with a male. Male transsexuals have a more pronounced feminine gender identity than nontranssexual homosexuals, and there is minimal overlap between these groups (Freund, Nagler, Langevin, Zajac, & Steiner, 1974). Although homosexual transsexuals are attracted to members of the same biological gender, they resent being labeled "gay" because they perceive themselves as women; hence, their attraction to males is seen as equivalent to heterosexuality.

Some transsexuals assume a cross-gender role by cross-dressing permanently and establishing themselves as members of the opposite sex in the community. In some cases, homosexual transsexuals may initiate hormone intake (estrogens for males and testosterone for females) to acquire some cross-gender secondary sex characteristics. In a biological male, regular estrogen intake leads to a redistribution of body fat, a reduction in facial and body hair, and mild to moderate breast enlargement (Steiner, 1985). A percentage of transsexuals will seek sex reassignment surgery (some extreme cases of autocastration have been reported in transsexuals). Surgical sex reassignment is generally more effective for males than for females. The creation of an artificial penis is difficult and often unsatisfactory (see Steiner, 1985). For males, surgery entails removing the penis and testes and creating a vagina and breast augmentation. In his review of the literature on reassignment surgery outcome, Blanchard (1985a) concluded that the majority of transsexuals who have undergone surgery are satisfied with the outcome, although the level of satisfaction is variable. The level of postsurgical adjustment is highly correlated with presurgical adjustment and the effectiveness of the operation (Kuiper & Cohen-Kettenis, 1988). Transsexuals who present evidence of co-existing psychopathology are less likely to benefit from surgical sex reassignment (Bodlund & Kullgren, 1996; Midence & Hargreaves, 1997). Additionally, female-to-male transsexuals tend to have more favorable outcomes than male-to-female counterparts. Postsurgical complications, such as excessive scarring and collapse of the neovagina, also influence the individual's satisfaction with the procedure (Ross & Need, 1989). Regarding the relationship of orgasm to sexual and general satisfaction in postsurgical transsexuals, Lief and Hubschman (1993) found a decrease in orgasmic capacity in male-to-female patients and an increase in female-to-male patients. However, despite the decrease in the ability to experience orgasm in male-to-female patients, satisfaction with the quality of sexual activity and general satisfaction with the results of surgery were high in both groups of patients. Although the majority of transsexuals is satisfied with the outcome of sex reassignment surgery, prospective candidates must be carefully evaluated because up to 10% later regret undergoing the procedure. Additionally, a few cases experience severe distress and commit suicide (Pauly, 1990). Therefore, postoperative psychotherapy may be advisable (Rehman, Lazer, Benet, Schaefer, & Melman, 1999).

Clinicians and researchers in gender dysphoria have recognized that this disorder is far more complex than previously assumed (Bradley et al., 1991; Pauly, 1990). There is no scientific consensus on the determinants of gender dysphoria. From their review, Bradley and Zucker (1997) concluded that prenatal exposure to maternal sex hormones is probably implicated in the etiology of this disorder (see Money, 1974; Pillard & Weinrich, 1987). Hoenig (1985) noted that hormonal and antigen abnormalities, cerebral dysfunction, and genetic factors were likely to be important in the etiology of gender dysphoric behavior. However, other researchers contend that there is insufficient evidence of a biological determinant of this disorder (Coleman, Gooren, & Ross, 1989; Gooren, 1987). Stoller (1975b) proposed that psychoanalytic formulations can be applied to this disorder and that oedipal complex and castration fears play key roles. Green (1974, 1987) argued that environmental factors are critical in determining gender dysphoria. According to him, as children, male transsexuals tend to be treated as girls in dress, are overprotected by the mother, prefer female friends,

and experience an absence of male role models. Pauly (1974, 1990) emphasized family dynamics in the etiology of gender identity disorder. In support of these views, Bradley and Zucker (1997) observed that many of the mothers of boys with gender identity disorder had experienced major disappointment over not having a girl. Consequently, such parents are less likely to discourage gender nonconformity, and they may actually reinforce such behavior in their children.

## Paraphilia Not Otherwise Specified

Paraphiliac disorders that do not meet criteria for any of the specific sexual deviations previously discussed are classified as paraphilia not otherwise specified (NOS). The DSM-IV provides a list of seven paraphilia NOS, although this listing is by no means all-inclusive (for a review, see Milner & Dopke, 1997). The empirical data on these disorders are limited and consist mostly of descriptive case studies:

1. *Telephone scatologia* or lewdness entails sexual arousal associated with exposing a victim to obscene language over the telephone. The condition may be functionally related to exhibitionism, where auditory exposure is the equivalent of visual exposure. The individual may masturbate while talking to the victim; in support of this view, Alford, Webster, and Sanders (1980) demonstrated that obscene phone calling and genital exposure were functionally related in one subject. Heavy breathing may also be a type of voyeurism, where listening is similar to looking. Approximately one-third of female college students and 11% of male have received obscene phone calls (Matek, 1988; Murray & Beran, 1968).

2. *Necrophilia* involves sexual activity with a corpse. Access to a morgue or funeral parlor is essential for a person with this erotic preference (Money, 1986). In some extreme cases, necrophilia may be linked with severe sexual sadism; in such cases, the individual may murder the victim for sexual access (Rosman & Resnick, 1989). Access to a nonresistant and nonrejecting sexual partner is a prime motive of necrophiliacs.

3. *Partialism* is considered by many experts to be a form of fetishism. By definition, it consists of exclusive arousal to a specific body

part, usually not associated with sexual activity. This may include feet, hair, or legs.

4. *Zoophilia* entails sexual arousal in response to animals. The preferred animal is often one to which the person has been exposed during childhood, such as a household pet or farm animal. Although some males raised on a farm may experiment in sexual activity with livestock, this probably does not constitute a paraphilia unless intense urges and fantasies are involved and the pattern is repetitive. There are, however, cases of males who describe a lifelong sexual attraction to an animal.

5. *Coprophilia* involves the derivation of sexual excitement from feces. This pattern of arousal may be incorporated in sadomasochistic rituals in some cases. There are few empirical findings on this disorder which is rarely seen in clinical settings.

6. *Urophilia* is the equivalent of coprophilia with urine. It usually consists of a desire to be urinated upon by a partner; vernacular terms for this activity include "water sports" and "golden showers." Like coprophilia, this paraphilia may be associated with sadomasochistic practices.

7. *Klismaphilia* involves sexual arousal associated with administering or receiving enemas. It may be an adjunct to rubber fetishism or sadomasochism. Although homosexual males may use enemas before anal intercourse, this does not entail klismaphilia because it is a sanitary rather than erotic practice. The majority of practitioners are heterosexual men (Arndt, 1991).

## Treatment of Paraphilias

A multitude of interventions for modifying deviant sexual arousal have been proposed over the years. In the majority of cases, however, the effectiveness of these treatments has not been established. Group and insight-oriented psychotherapies, for example, are commonly used with sex offenders despite the absence of evidence for their effectiveness.

Two general approaches to modifying deviant sexual arousal have been empirically evaluated: pharmacological approaches and cognitive behavior therapy. The pharmacological approaches entail administering agents that reduce or eliminate the individual's sex drive. Dubbed "chemical castration," it has been shown that the use of anti-androgen drugs (medroxyprogesterone acetate and cyproterone acetate) lowers sexual urges, fantasies, and behaviors in sex offenders (Gijs & Gooren, 1996; Money, 1987; Robinson & Valcour, 1995). Although these treatments do not alter the offenders' deviant sexual interests, they generally reduce rates of both normal and deviant sexual behavior. Hall (1995) concluded that pharmacological approaches reduce revicidivism rates although they have not been shown superior to cognitive behavioral approaches. A number of problems are associated with pharmacological approaches, including noncompliance, side effects (such as weight gain, testicular atrophy, and hypertension), and high relapse rates upon discontinuation. Furthermore, the long-term effects of these medications remain unknown. More recently, anecdotal reports and case studies suggest that selective serotonin re-uptake inhibitors (SSRIs) may be promising agents for selectively lowering deviant sexual urges. Galli and colleagues (1998), for example, reported successfully treating a male with multiple paraphilias by using fluoxetine (Prozac). Abouesh and Clayton (1999) administered another SSRI, Paroxetine, to a voyeur and an exhibitionist and reported reductions in paraphiliac urges. However, pharmacological interventions are not a panacea, and they should only be used in combination with other interventions as part of a multicomponent treatment plan.

Cognitive behavioral interventions are designed to decreased deviant sexual arousal, to eliminate facilitating cognitive distortions, and to build skills that will facilitate the formation of normal intimate relationships. Additionally, relapse prevention has become an integral component of treatment (Laws, 1989). A problem inherent in many treatment outcome studies is the lack of adequate follow-up data. It has been documented that recidivism rates increase over time; therefore, extended follow-up periods are necessary (Furby, Weinrott, & Blackshaw, 1989). Contrary to popular belief, not all sex offenders relapse. A recent review suggests that sex offender recidivism rates are near 55%, which is comparable to recidivism rates for nonsexual criminals (Heilbrun, Nezu, Keeney, Chung, & Wasserman, 1998). Hall (1995) concluded that pharmacological and cognitive behavioral treatments produced a 30% decrease in recidivism.

Early cognitive behavioral treatments relied on

aversive conditioning. A study by Quinsey and colleagues (1980) supports the effectiveness of electrical aversion in reducing pedophilic arousal. Other studies, however, have produced equivocal results (Rice, Quinsey, & Harris, 1991). Olfactory aversion is a variation that is less controversial; aversive odors can be self-administered in the natural environment by motivated clients. Another procedure, known as masturbatory satiation, requires prolonged masturbation to deviant fantasy to pair paraphiliac fantasy with boredom (Laws & Marshall, 1991). Maletzky described the use of covert sensitization with large samples of paraphiliacs, and his reported success rates are impressive (Maletzky, 1991). Vicarious sensitization is a variation that involves exposing offenders via films to aversive consequences for deviant sexual behavior (see Maltezky, 1997). Cognitive interventions are designed to challenge and modify distorted beliefs relevant to deviant urges and practices. Additionally, cognitive interventions may be used for empathy training. The strategies of relapse prevention entail (1) teaching individuals to recognize high risk situations; (2) learning strategies to avoid these situations that may lead to relapse; and (3) teaching coping strategies, such as assertiveness training and anger management, that will help lower relapse risk (Pithers, 1990). Accountability and supervision are common components of relapse prevention.

Although cognitive behavioral treatments reduce recidivism rates among sex offenders (Hall, 1995; Heilbrun et al., 1998), the exact mechanism by which they achieve such change remains unclear. Their efficacy seems to involve more than a simple conditioning process, and therefore, a self-control model may be more accurate in explaining the effectiveness of cognitive behavioral and pharmacological interventions for paraphilias. Along these lines, the relapse prevention model of change emphasizes self-management rather than a cure.

# Professional, Legal, and Research Issues

The assessment and treatment of paraphiliacs poses unique ethical, legal, and professional issues. Because most paraphiliacs enter treatment under coercion, their motivation to change is typically low. Therefore, the validity of their self-reports is questionable. In summary, this population is considered difficult and challenging.

Increasingly, clinicians are serving as expert witnesses in the courtroom and other legal situations (e.g., parole hearings) in cases involving sex crimes. This role places the professional in a relatively foreign situation, namely, in an adversarial process. It imperative that clinicians be aware of the limits of their expertise (Blau, 1985). All findings presented in this context must be data-based, which requires a thorough knowledge of the properties (including the limitations) of assessment instruments. Additionally, expert consultants must possess a comprehensive understanding of the research findings, theories, and issues pertaining to sexual deviations. The expert witness must understand that any information presented in court may be entered in evidence (Weiner, 1985). As experts, clinicians must maintain a neutral and objective stand, which may be challenging in view of the reprehensible nature of some paraphiliac practices.

Clinicians are increasingly being asked to provide a risk assessment, a prediction of an individual's likelihood of perpetrating future offenses. Overall, psychometric instruments have limited predictive validity in this respect. Static factors such as criminal history are moderately effective predictors. Dynamic predictors such as deviant sexual arousal and psychopathy may also be useful (Hanson, 1998; Hanson & Bussiere, 1996; Quinsey, Harris, & Rice, 1995). Risk assessment is a critical process that requires aggressive empirical investigation. The consequences of inaccurate risk assessment can be costly to the offenders who may face unnecessarily prolonged incarceration and to society in terms of sexual victimization. Clinicians and researchers bear a heavy responsibility in keeping abreast of developments in this area.

Therapists in every state are required to report evidence of sexual abuse. Mandatory reporting represents one exception to confidentiality and privileged communication, which may drastically alter the therapeutic relationship. Clinicians involved in the assessment, treatment, or research of paraphilias need a thorough understanding of state and local laws in these matters.

Because of the continuing misinformation about sexual deviation among the public and professionals alike, there is a critical need for sound clinical research. There is an urgent need for treatment outcome research, prospective studies of risk factors in paraphilia, and controlled descriptive studies using homogeneous samples. Although major advances in our understanding of paraphilias have occurred in the past several decades, many unanswered questions remain.

# References

Abel, G. G. (1989). Paraphilias. In H. I. Kalpan & B. J. Saddock (Eds.), *Comprehensive textbook of psychiatry* (pp. 1069–1085). Baltimore: Williams & Wilkins.

Abel, G. G., Becker, J. V., Mittelman, M., Cunningham-Rathner, J., Rouleau, J. L., & Murphy, W. D. (1987). Self-reported sex crimes of nonincarcerated paraphiliacs. *Journal of Interpersonal Violence, 2,* 3–25.

Abel, G. G., Becker, J. V., Murphy, W. D., & Flanagan, B. (1981). Identifying dangerous child molesters. In R. B. Stuart (Ed.), *Violent behavior: Social learning approaches to prediction, management, and treatment* (pp. 116–137). New York: Brunner/Mazel.

Abel, G. G., Huffman, J., Warberg, B., & Holland, C. L. (1998) Visual reaction time and plethysmography as measures of sexual interest in child molesters. *Sexual Abuse: A Journal of Research and Treatment, 10,* 81–95.

Abel, G. G., Lawry, S. S., Karlstrom, E. M., Osborn, C. A., & Gillespie, C. F. (1994). Screening tests for pedophilia. *Criminal Justice and Behavior, 21,* 115–131.

Abel, G. G., Levis, D., & Clancy, J. (1970). Aversion therapy applied to taped sequences of deviant behavior in exhibitionists and other sexual deviations: Preliminary report. *Journal of Behavior Therapy and Experimental Psychiatry, 1,* 59–60.

Abel, G. G., & Rouleau, J. L. (1990). The nature and extent of sexual assault. In W. L. Marshall, D. R. Laws, & H. E. Barbaree (Eds.), *Handbook of sexual assault: Issues, theories, and treatment of the offender* (pp. 9–21). New York: Plenum.

Abouesh, A., & Clayton, A. (1999). Compulsive voyeurism and exhibitionism: A clinical response to paroxetine. *Archives of Sexual Behavior, 28,* 23–30.

Adams, H. E., & Haber, J. (1984). The classification of behavior. In H. E. Adams & P. B. Sutker (Eds.), *Comprehensive handbook of psychopathology* (pp. 3–26). New York: Plenum.

Alford, G. S., Webster, J. S., & Sanders, J. H. (1980). Covert aversion of two interrelated deviant sexual practices: Obscene phone calling and exhibitionism. A single case analysis. *Behavior Therapy, 11,* 15–25.

American Psychiatric Association. (1952). *Diagnostic and statistical manual of mental disorders.* Washington, DC: Author.

American Psychiatric Association. (1968). *Diagnostic and statistical manual of mental disorders* (2nd ed.). Washington, DC: Author.

American Psychiatric Association. (1980). *Diagnostic and statistical manual of mental disorders* (3rd ed.). Washington, DC: Author.

American Psychiatric Association. (1987). *Diagnostic and statistical manual of mental disorders* (3rd ed., rev.). Washington, DC: Author.

American Psychiatric Association. (1994). *Diagnostic and statistical manual of mental disorders* (4th ed.). Washington, DC: Author.

Araji, S., & Finkelhor, D. (1985). Explanation of pedophilia: Review of empirical research. *Bulletin of the American Academy of Psychiatry and Law, 13,* 17–37.

Arndt, W. B., Jr. (1991). *Gender disorders and the paraphilias.* Madison, CT: International Universities Press.

Avery-Clark, C. A., & Laws, D. R. (1984). Differential erection response patterns of sexual child abusers to stimuli describing activities with children. *Behavior Therapy, 15,* 71–83.

Bak, R. C. (1968). The phallic woman: The ubiquitous fantasy in perversions. *Psychoanalytic Study of the Child, 23,* 15–36.

Bancroft, J. (1989). *Human sexuality and its problems,* 2nd. ed. Edinburgh: Churchill Livingstone.

Barbaree, H. E., & Seto, M. C. (1997). Pedophilia: Assessment and treatment. In D. R. Laws, & W. O'Donohue (Eds.), *Sexual deviance: Theory, assessment, and treatment* (pp. 175–193). New York: Guilford.

Barbaree, H. E., Seto, M. C., Serin, R. C., Amos, N. L., & Preston, D. L. (1994). Comparisons between sexual and nonsexual rapist subtypes: Sexual arousal to rape, offense precursors, and offense characteristics. *Criminal Justice and Behavior, 21,* 95–114.

Barbaree, H. E., & Marshall, W. L. (1989). Erectile responses among heterosexual child molesters, father–daughter incest offenders and matched nonoffenders: Five distinct age preference profiles. *Canadian Journal of Behavioral Science, 21,* 70–82.

Bard, L. A., Carter, D. L., Cerce, D. D., Knight, R. A., Rosenberg, R., & Schneider, B. (1987). A descriptive study of rapists and child molesters: Developmental, clinical, and criminal characteristics. *Behavioral Sciences and the Law, 5,* 203–220.

Blader, J. C., & Marshall, W. L. (1989). Is assessment of sexual arousal in rapists worthwhile? A critique of current methods and the development of a response compatibility approach. *Clinical Psychology Review, 9,* 569–587.

Blair, C. D., & Lanyon, R. I. (1981). Exhibitionism: Etiology and treatment. *Psychological Bulletin, 89,* 439–463.

Blanchard, R. (1985a). Gender dysphoria and gender reorientation. In B. W. Steiner (Ed.), *Gender dysphoria: Development, research, management* (pp. 365–392). New York: Plenum.

Blanchard, R. (1985b). Research methods for the typological study of gender disorders in males. In B. W. Steiner (Ed.), *Gender dysphoria: Development, research, management* (pp. 227–258). New York: Plenum.

Blanchard, R. (1989). The classification and labeling of nonhomosexual gender dysphorias. *Archives of Sexual Behavior, 18,* 315–334.

Blanchard, R. (1990). Gender identity disorders in adult men. In Blanchard, R. & B. W. Steiner (Eds.), *Clinical management of gender identity disorder in children and adults* (pp. 47–76). Washington, DC: American Psychiatric Press.

Blanchard, R. (1991). Clinical observations and systematic studies of autogynephilia. *Journal of Sex and Marital Therapy, 17,* 235–251.

Blanchard, R. (1993). Varieties of autogynephilia and their relationship to gender dysphoria. *Archives of Sexual Behavior, 22,* 241–251.

Blanchard, R., Clemmensen, L. H., & Steiner, B. S. (1987). Heterosexual and homosexual gender dysphoria. *Archives of Sexual Behavior, 16,* 139–152.

Blau, T. H. (1985). The psychologist as expert in the courts. *Clinical Psychologist, 38,* 76–78.

Bodlund, O., & Kullgren, G. (1996). Transsexualism—General outcome and prognostic factors: A five-year follow-up of nineteen transsexuals in the process of changing sex. *Archives of Sexual Behavior, 25,* 303–316.

Bradley, S. J., & Zucker, K. J. (1997). Gender identity disorder: A review of the past 10 years. *Journal of the American Academy of Child and Adolescent Psychiatry, 36,* 872–880.

Bradley, S., Blanchard, R., Coates, S., Green, R., Levine, S., Meyer-Bahlburg, H. F. L., Pauly, I., & Zucker, K. (1991). Interim report of the DSM-IV subcommittee on gender identity disorders. *Archives of Sexual Behavior, 20,* 333–343.

Bullough, V. L. (1998). Alfred Kinsey and the Kinsey Report: Historical overview and lasting contributions. *Journal of Sex Research, 35,* 127–131.

Chalkley, A. J., & Powell, G. E. (1983). The clinical description of forty-eight cases of sexual fetishism. *British Journal of Psychiatry, 142,* 292–295.

Cohen, M. L., Seghorn, T., & Calmas, W. (1969). Sociometric study of the sex offender. *Journal of Abnormal Psychology, 74,* 249–255.

Coleman, E., Gooren, L., & Ross, M. (1989). Theories of gender transpositions: A critique and suggestions for further research. *Journal of Sex Research, 26,* 525–538.

Cox, D. J., & MacMahon, H. (1978). Incidence of male exhibitionism in the United States as reported by victimized female college students. *National Journal of Law and Psychiatry, 1,* 453–457.

De Silva, P. (1993). Fetishism and sexual dysfunction: Clinical presentation and management. *Sexual and Marital Therapy, 8,* 147–155.

Dixen, J., & Jenkins, J. O. (1981). Incestuous child sexual abuse: A review of treatment strategies. *Clinical Psychology Review, 1,* 211–222.

Docter, R. F. (1988). *Transvestites and transsexuals: Toward a theory of cross-gender behavior.* New York: Plenum.

Docter, R. F., & Prince, V. (1997). Transvestism: A survey of 1032 cross-dressers. *Archives of Sexual Behavior, 26,* 589–605.

Dorr, D. (1998). Psychopathy in the pedophile. In T. Millon, E. Simonsen, M. Birket-Smith, & R. D. Davis (Eds.), *Psychopathy: Antisocial, criminal, and violent behavior* (pp. 304–320). New York: Guilford.

Epstein, A. W. (1969). Fetishism: A study of its psychopathology with particular reference to a proposed disorder in brain mechanisms as an etiological factor. *Journal of Nervous and Mental Disorders, 130,* 107–119.

Erickson, W. D., Luxenberg, M. G., Walbek, N. H., & Seely, R. K. (1987). Frequency of MMPI two-point code types among sex offenders. *Journal of Consulting and Clinical Psychology, 55,* 566–570.

Erickson, W. D., Walbek, N. H., & Seely, R. K. (1988). Behavior patterns of child molesters. *Archives of Sexual Behavior, 17,* 77–86.

Fenichel, O. (1945). *The psychoanalytic theory of neurosis.* New York: W.W. Norton.

Fischer, D. G., & McDonald, W. L. (1998). Characteristics of intrafamilial and extrafamilial child sexual abuse. *Child Abuse and Neglect, 22,* 915–929.

Freud, S. (1953). Three essays on the theory of sexuality. In J. Strachey (Ed. and Trans.), *The standard edition of the complete psychological works of Sigmund Freud,* Vol. 7 (pp. 123–246). London: Hogarth. (Original work published 1905.)

Freund, K. (1963). A laboratory method for diagnosing predominance of homo- and heteroerotic interests in the male. *Behaviour Research and Therapy, 1,* 85–93.

Freund, K. (1967). Erotic preference in pedophilia. *Behaviour Research and Therapy, 5,* 339–348.

Freund, K. (1990). Courtship disorders. In W. L. Marshall, D. R. Laws, & H. E. Barbaree (Eds.), *Handbook of sexual assault: Issues, theories, and treatment of the offender* (pp. 195–207). New York: Plenum.

Freund, K., & Blanchard, R. (1989). Phallometric diagnosis of pedophilia. *Journal of Consulting and Clinical Psychology, 57,* 100–105.

Freund, K., Langevin, R., Zajac, Y., Steiner, B., & Zajac, A. (1974). The transsexual syndrome in homosexual males. *Journal of Nervous and Mental Diseases, 158,* 145–153.

Freund, K., McKnight, C. K., Langevin, R., & Cibiri, S. (1972). The female child as a surrogate object. *Archives of Sexual Behavior, 2,* 119–133.

Freund, K., Nagler, E., Langevin, R., Zajac, A., & Steiner, B. (1974). Measuring feminine gender identity in homosexual males. *Archives of Sexual Behavior, 3,* 249–260.

Freund, K., Scher, H., & Hucker, S. (1983). The courtship disorders. *Archives of Sexual Behavior, 12,* 369–379.

Freund, K. & Watson, R. J. (1993). Gender identity disorder and courtship disorder. *Archives of Sexual Behavior, 22,* 13–21.

Freund, K., Watson, R., & Dickey, R. (1990). Does sexual abuse in childhood cause pedophilia: An exploratory study. *Archives of Sexual Behavior, 19,* 557–568.

Furby, L., Weinrott, M. R., & Blackshaw, L. (1989). Sex offender recidivism: A review. *Psychological Bulletin, 105,* 3–30.

Galli, V., Raute, N. J., McConville, B. J., & McElroy, S. L. (1998). An adolescent male with multiple paraphilias successfully treated with fluoxetine. *Journal of Child and Adolescent Psychopharmacology, 8,* 195–197.

Garland, R. J., & Dougher, M. J. (1990). The abused/abuser hypothesis of child sexual abuse: A critical review of theory and research. In J. R. Feierman (Ed.), *Pedophilia: Biosocial dimensions* (pp. 488–509). New York: Springer Verlag.

Garlick, Y., Marshall, W. L., & Thornton, D. (1996). Intimacy deficits and attribution of blame among sexual offenders. *Legal and Criminological Psychology, 1,* 251–288.

Garos, S. (1993–1994). Autoerotic asphyxiation: A challenge to death educators and counselors. *Omega, 28,* 85–99.

Gebhard, P. H., Gagnon, J. H., Pomeroy, W. B., & Christenson, C. V. (1965). *Sex offenders.* New York: Harper & Row.

Gijs, L., & Gooren, L. (1996). Hormonal and psychopharmacological interventions in the treatment of paraphilias: An update. *Journal of Sex Research, 33,* 273–290.

Gittelson, N. L., Eacott, S. E., & Mehta, B. M. (1978). Victims of indecent exposure. *British Journal of Psychiatry, 132,* 61–66.

Gooren, L. J. G. (1987). Reversal of the LH response to estrogen administration after orchidectomy in a male subject with androgen insensitivity syndrome. *Hormonal Versus Metabolic Research, 19,* 138.

Gosselin, C. C. (1987). The sadomasochistic contract. In G. D. Wilson (Ed.), *Variant sexuality: Research and theory* (pp. 229–257). Baltimore: Johns Hopkins University Press.

Gosselin, C., & Wilson, G. (1984). Fetishism, sadomasochism and related behaviors. In Howells, K. (Ed.), *The psychology of sexual diversity* (pp. 89–110). Oxford, England: Basil Blackwell.

Green, R. (1974). *Sexual identity conflicts in children and adults.* New York: Basic Books.

Green, R. (1987). *The "sissy boy syndrome" and the development of homosexuality.* New Haven, CT: Yale University Press.

Groth, N. A., & Birnbaum, H. J. (1978). Adult sexual orientation and attraction to underage persons. *Archives of Sexual Behavior, 7,* 175–181.

Hall, G. C. N. (1995). Sexual offender recidivism revisited: A meta-analysis of recent treatment studies. *Journal of Consulting and Clinical Psychology, 63,* 802–809.

Hall, G. C. N., Maiuro, R. D., Vitaliano, P. P., & Proctor, W. C. (1986). The utility of the MMPI with men who have sexually assaulted children. *Journal of Consulting and Clinical Psychology, 54,* 493–496.

Hanson, R. K. (1998). What do we know about sex offender risk assessment? *Psychology, Public Policy, and Law, 4,* 50–72.

Hanson, R. K., & Bussiere, M. T. (1996). *Predictors of sexual offender recidivism: A meta-analysis.* Ottawa: Solicitor General Canada.

Hanson, R. K., & Slater, S. (1988). Sexual victimization in the history of sexual abusers: A review. *Annals of Sex Research, 1,* 485–499.

Hanson, R. K., Gizzarelli, R., & Scott, H. (1994). The attitudes of incest offenders: Sexual entitlement and the acceptance of sex with children. *Criminal Justice and Behavior, 21,* 187–202.

Hare, R. (1998). Psychopaths and their nature: Implications for the mental health and criminal justice systems. In T. Millon, E. Simonsen, M. Birket-Smith, & R. D. Davis (Eds.), *Psychopathy: Antisocial, criminal, and violent behavior* (pp. 188–212). New York: Guilford.

Haywood, T. W., & Grossman, L. S. (1994). Denial of deviant sexual arousal and psychopathology in child molesters. *Behavior Therapy, 25,* 327–341.

Heilbrun, K., Nezu, C. M., Keeney, M., Chung, S., & Wasserman, A. L. (1998). Sexual offending: Linking assessment, intervention, and decision making. *Psychology, Public Policy, and Law, 4,* 138–174.

Heim, N. (1981). Sexual behavior of castrated sex offenders. *Archives of Sexual Behavior, 10,* 11–19.

Hoenig, J. (1985). Etiology of transsexualism. In B. W. Steiner (Ed.), *Gender dysphoria: Development, research, management* (pp. 33–73). New York: Plenum.

Hollender, M. H., Brown, C. W., & Roback, H. B. (1977). Genital exhibitionism in women. *American Journal of Psychiatry, 134,* 436–438.

Hunt, D. D., & Hampson, J. L. (1980). Follow-up of 17 biologic male transsexuals after sex reassignment surgery. *American Journal of Psychiatry, 137,* 432–438.

Janus, S. S., & Janus, C. L. (1993). *The Janus report on sexual behavior.* New York: Wiley.

Kamel, G. W. L. (1980). The leather career: On becoming a sadomasochist. *Deviant Behavior: An Interdisciplinary Journal, 1,* 171–191.

Kaplan, M. S., & Krueger, R. B. (1997). Voyeurism: Psychopathology and theory. In D. R. Laws & W. O'Donohue (Eds.), *Sexual deviance: Theory, assessment, and treatment* (pp. 297–331). New York: Guilford.

Karpman, B. (1954). *The sexual offender and his offenses.* New York: Julian.

Keller, L. O. (1992). Addiction as a form of perversion. *Menninger Clinic, 56,* 221–231.

Kline, P. (1987). Sexual deviation: Psychoanalytic research and theory. In G. D. Wilson (Ed.), *Variant sexuality: Research*

and theory (pp. 150–173). Baltimore: Johns Hopkins University Press.

Knight, R. A., & Prentky, R. A. (1990). Classifying sexual offenders: The development and corroboration of taxonomic models. In W. L. Marshall, D. R. Laws, & H. E. Barbaree (Eds.), *Handbook of sexual assault: Issues, theories, and treatment of the offender* (pp. 23–52). New York: Plenum.

Knight, R. A., Rosenberg, R., & Schneider, B. A. (1985). Classification of sexual offenders: Perspectives, methods, and validation. In A. W. Burgess (Ed.), *Rape and sexual assault: A research handbook* (pp. 222–293). New York: Garland.

Koss, M. P. (1989). Hidden rape: Sexual aggression and victimization in a national sample of students in higher education. In M. A. Pirog-Good & J. E. Stets (Eds.), *Violence in dating relationships* (pp. 145–168). New York: Praeger.

Koss, M. P., Gidycz, C. J., & Wisniewski, N. R. (1987). The scope of rape: Incidence and prevalence of sexual aggression and victimization in a national sample of students in higher education. *Journal of Consulting and Clinical Psychology, 55,* 162–170.

Kuiper, B., & Cohen-Kettenis, P. (1988). Sex reassignment surgery: A study of 141 Dutch transsexuals. *Archives of Sexual Behavior, 17,* 439–457.

Landsdell, H. C. (1971). A general intellectual factor affected by temporal lobe dysfunction. *Journal of Clinical Psychology, 27,* 182–184.

Lang, R. A., Langevin, R., Checkley, K. L., & Pugh, G. (1987). Genital exhibitionism: Courtship disorder or narcissism? *Canadian Journal of Behavioral Science, 19,* 216–232.

Langevin, R. (1983). *Sexual strands: Understanding and treating sexual anomalies in men.* Hillsdale, NJ: Erlbaum.

Langevin, R. (1985). The meanings of cross-dressing. In B. W. Steiner (Ed.), *Gender dysphoria: Development, research, management* (pp. 207–225). New York: Plenum.

Langevin, R., Hucker, S. J., Ben-Aron, M. H., Purins, J. E., & Hook, H. J. (1985). Why are pedophiles attracted to children? Further studies of erotic preference in heterosexual pedophilia. In R. Langevin (Ed.), *Erotic preference, gender identity, and aggression in men: New research studies* (pp. 181–210). Hillsdale, NJ: Erlbaum.

Langevin, R., Hucker, S. J., Handy, L., Purins, J., Russon, A. E., & Hook, H. J. (1985). Erotic preference and aggression in pedophilia: A comparison of heterosexual, homosexual, and bisexual types. In R. Langevin (Ed.), *Erotic preference, gender identity, and aggression in men: New research studies* (pp. 137–160). Hillsdale, NJ: Erlbaum.

Langevin, R., Paitich, D., Ramsay, G., Anderson, C., Kamrad, J., Pope, S., Geller, G., Pearl, L., & Newman, S. (1979). Experimental studies of the etiology of genital exhibitionism. *Archives of Sexual Behavior, 8,* 307–331.

Langevin, R., Paitich, D., & Russon, A. E. (1985a). Are rapists sexually anomalous, aggressive, or both? In R. Langevin (Ed.), *Erotic preference, gender identity, and aggression in men: New research studies* (pp. 17–38). Hillsdale, NJ: Erlbaum.

Langevin, R., Paitich, D., & Russon, A. E. (1985b). Voyeurism: Does it predict sexual aggression or violence in general? In R. Langevin (Ed.), *Erotic preference, gender identity, and aggression in men: New research studies* (pp. 77–98). Hillsdale, NJ: Erlbaum.

Lanyon, R. I. (1986). Theory and treatment in child molestation. *Journal of Consulting and Clinical Psychology, 54,* 176–182.

Laws, D. R. (Ed.). (1989). *Relapse prevention with sex offenders.* New York: Guilford.

Laws, D. R., & Marshall, W. L. (1991). Masturbatory reconditioning with sexual deviates: An evaluative review. *Advances in Behavior Research and Therapy, 13,* 13–25.

Laws, D. R., & O'Donohue, W. (1997). Introduction: Fundamental issues in sexual deviance. In D. R. Laws & W. O'Donohue (Eds.), *Sexual deviance: Theory, assessment, and treatment* (pp. 1–21). New York: Guilford.

Levin, S. M., & Stava, L. (1987). Personality characteristics of sex offenders: A review. *Archives of Sexual Behavior, 16,* 57–79.

Levitt, E. E., Moser, C., & Jamison, K. V. (1994). The prevalence and some attributes of females in the sadomasochistic subculture: A second report. *Archives of Sexual Behavior, 32,* 465–473.

Lief, H., & Hubschman, L. (1993). Orgasm in the postoperative transsexual. *Archives of Sexual Behavior, 22,* 145–155.

Lohr, B. A., Adams, H. E., & Davis, J. M. (1997). Sexual arousal to erotic and aggressive stimuli in sexually coercive and noncoercive men. *Journal of Abnormal Psychology, 106,* 230–242.

Long, P. J. (1995). Perpetrators of incest. In L. Diamant & R. D. McAnulty (Eds.), *The psychology of sexual orientation, identity, and behavior: A handbook* (pp. 282–306). Westport, CT: Greenwood Press.

MacDonald, J. (1973). *Indecent exposure.* Springfield, IL: Charles C. Thomas.

Malamuth, N. M. (1989). Predictors of naturalistic sexual aggression. In M. A. Pirog-Good & J. E. Stets (Eds.), *Violence in dating relationships* (pp. 219–240). New York: Praeger.

Malamuth, N. M., Heavey, C. L., & Linz, D. (1993). Predicting men's antisocial behavior against women: The interaction model of sexual aggression. In G. C. N. Hall, R. Hirschman, J. R. Graham, & M. S. Zaragoza (Eds.), *Sexual aggression: Issues in etiology, assessment and treatment* (pp. 63–97). Washington, DC: Taylor and Francis.

Malatesta, V., & Adams, H. E. (1986). Assessment of sexual behavior. In A. R. Ciminero, K. S. Calhoun, & H. E. Adams (Eds.), *Handbook of behavioral assessment,* 2nd ed. (pp. 496–525). New York: Wiley.

Maletzky, B. M. (1991). *Treating the sexual offender.* Newbury Park, CA: Sage.

Maletzky, B. M. (1997). Exhibitionism: Assessment and treatment. In D. R. Laws & W. O'Donohue (Eds.), *Sexual deviance: Theory, assessment, and treatment* (pp. 40–74). New York: Guilford.

Marshall, W. L. (1989). Intimacy, loneliness, and sexual offenders. *Behaviour Research and Therapy, 27,* 491–503.

Marshall, W. L. (1997). Pedophilia: Psychopathology and theory. In D. R. Laws & W. O'Donohue (Eds.), *Sexual deviance: Theory, assessment, and treatment* (pp. 152–174). New York: Guilford.

Marshall, W. L., & Barbaree, H. E. (1988). The long-term evaluation of a behavioral treatment program for child molesters. *Behaviour Research and Therapy, 6,* 499–511.

Marshall, W. L., Barbaree, H. E., & Butt, J. (1988). Sexual offenders against male children: Sexual preferences. *Behaviour Research and Therapy, 26,* 383–391.

Marshall, W. L., Barbaree, H. E., & Christophe, D. (1986). Sexual offenders against female children: Sexual preferences for age of victims and type of behaviour. *Canadian Journal of Behavioral Science, 18,* 424–439.

Marshall, W. L., & Eccles, A. (1993). Pavlovian conditioning

processes in adolescent sex offenders. In H. E. Barbaree, W. L. Marshall, & S. M. Hudson (Eds.), *The juvenile sex offender* (pp. 118–142). New York: Guilford.

Marshall, W. L., Eccles, A., & Barbaree, H. E. (1991). The treatment of exhibitionists: A focus on sexual deviance versus cognitive and relationship features. *Behaviour Research and Therapy, 29,* 129–135.

Marshall, W. L., Hudson, S. M., & Hodkinson, S. (1993). The importance of attachment bonds in the development of juvenile sex offending. In H. E. Barbaree, W. L. Marshall, & S. M. Hudson (Eds.), *The juvenile sex offender* (pp. 164–181). New York: Guilford.

Marshall, W. L., & McKnight, R. D. (1975). An integrated treatment program for sexual offenders. *Canadian Psychiatric Association Journal, 20,* 133–138.

Matek, O. (1988). Obscene phone callers. *Journal of Social Work and Human Sexuality, 7,* 113–130.

McAnulty, R. D., & Adams, H. E. (1992). Behavior therapy with paraphiliac disorders. In S. M. Turner, K. S. Calhoun, & H. E. Adams (Eds.), *Handbook of clinical behavior therapy,* 2nd ed. (pp. 175–201). New York: Wiley.

McAnulty, R. D., Adams, H. E., & Wright, L. W. (1994). Relationship between MMPI and penile plethysmograph in accused child molesters. *Journal of Sex Research, 31,* 179–184.

McAnulty, R. D., Satterwhite, R., & Gullick, E. G. (1995, March). Topless dancers: Personality and background. Paper presented at the *Meeting of the Southeastern Psychological Association,* Savannah, GA.

McConaghy, N. (1993). *Sexual behavior: Problems and management.* New York: Plenum.

McGuire, R. J., Carlisle, J. M., & Young, B. G. (1965). Sexual deviations as conditioned behaviour: A hypothesis. *Behaviour Research and Therapy, 2,* 185–190.

Meyer, J. K. (1995). Paraphilias. In H. I. Kaplan & B. J. Sadock (Eds.), *Comprehensive textbook of psychiatry VI,* Vol. 1, 6th ed. (pp. 1334–1347). Baltimore: Williams & Wilkins.

Midence, K. & Hargreaves, I. (1997). Psychosocial adjustment in male-to-female transsexuals: An overview of the research evidence. *Journal of Psychology, 131,* 602–614.

Milner, J. S., & Dopke, C. A. (1997). Paraphilia not otherwise specified: Psychopathology and theory. In D. R. Laws & W. O'Donohue (Eds.), *Sexual deviance: Theory, assessment, and treatment* (pp. 394–423). New York: Guilford.

Mohr, J. W., Turner, R. E., & Jerry, M. B. (1964). *Pedophilia and exhibitionism.* Toronto: University of Toronto Press.

Money, J. (1974). Two names, two wardrobes, two personalities. *Journal of Homosexuality, 1,* 65–70.

Money, J. (1984). Paraphilias: Phenomenology and classification. *American Journal of Psychotherapy, 38,* 164–179.

Money, J. (1986). *Love maps: Clinical concepts of sexual/erotic health and pathology, paraphilia, and gender transposition in childhood, adolescence, and maturity.* New York: Irvington.

Money, J. (1987). Treatment guidelines: Antiandrogen and counseling of paraphiliac sex offenders. *Journal of Sex and Marital Therapy, 13,* 219–223.

Muehlenhard, C. L., & Linton, M. A. (1987). Date rape and sexual aggression in dating situations: Incidence and risk factors. *Journal of Counseling Psychology, 34,* 186–196.

Murphy, W. D. (1997). Exhibitionism: Psychopathology and theory. In D. R. Laws & W. O'Donohue (Eds.), *Sexual deviance: Theory, assessment, and treatment* (pp. 22–39). New York: Guilford.

Murphy, W. D., & Barbaree, H. E. (1994). *Assessments of sex offenders by measures of erectile response: Psychometric properties and decision making*. Brandon, VT: Safer Society.

Murray, F. S., & Beran, L. C. (1968). A survey of nuisance telephone calls received by males and females. *Psychological Record, 18*, 107–109.

Nichols, H. R., & Molinder, I. (1984). *Multiphasic sex inventory manual* (available from the authors, 437 Bowes Drive, Tacoma, WA, 98466).

O'Donohue, W., & Letourneau, E. (1992). The psychometric properties of the penile tumescence assessment of child molesters. *Journal of Psychopathology and Behavioral Assessment, 14*, 123–174.

Okami, P., & Goldberg, A. (1992). Personality correlates of pedophilia: Are they reliable indicators? *Journal of Sex Research, 29*, 297–328.

Overholser, J. C., & Beck, S. (1986). Multimethod assessment of rapists, child molesters, and three control groups on behavioral and psychological measures. *Journal of Consulting and Clinical Psychology, 54*, 682–687.

Paitich, D., Langevin, R., Freeman, R., Mann, K., & Handy, L. (1977). The Clarke SHQ: A clinical sex history questionnaire for males. *Archives of Sexual Behavior, 6*, 421–435.

Pauly, I. (1974). Female transsexualism, Parts I & II. *Archives of Sexual Behavior, 3*, 487–525.

Pauly, I. B. (1990). Gender identity disorders: Evaluation and treatment. *Journal of Sex Education and Therapy, 16*, 2–24.

Pesta, T. (1993). Fetishism. *Zeitschrift fur Psychoanalytische Theorie und Praxis, 8*, 342–360.

Pillard, R. C., & Weinrich, J. D. (1987). The periodic table of the gender transpositions: A theory based on masculinization and feminization of the brain. *Journal of Sex Research, 23*, 425–454.

Pithers, W. D. (1990). Relapse prevention with sexual aggressors: A method for maintaining therapeutic gains and enhancing external supervision. In W. L. Marshall, D. R. Laws, & H. E. Barbaree (Eds.), *Handbook of sexual assault: Issues, theories, and treatment of the offender* (pp. 343–362). New York: Plenum.

Polaschek, D. L. L., Ward, T., & Hudson, S. M. (1997). Rape and rapists: Theory and treatment. *Clinical Psychology Review, 17*, 117–144.

Prentky, R. A., Knight, R. A., & Rosenberg, R. (1987). Validation analyses on a taxonomic system for rapists: Disconfirmation and reconceptualization. *Annals of the New York Academy of Sciences, 528*, 21–40.

Prince, V., & Bentler, P. M. (1972). Survey of 504 cases of transvestism. *Psychological Reports, 31*, 903–917.

Quinsey, V. L. (1977). The assessment and treatment of child molesters: A review. *Canadian Psychological Review, 18*, 204–220.

Quinsey, V. L., Chaplin, T. C., & Carrigan, W. F. (1979). Sexual preferences among incestuous and nonincestuous child molesters. *Behavior Therapy, 10*, 562–565.

Quinsey, V. L., Chaplin, T. C., & Carrigan, W. F. (1980). Biofeedback and signaled punishment in the modification of inappropriate sexual age preferences. *Behavior Therapy, 11*, 576–576.

Quinsey, V. L., Chaplin, T. C., & Upfold, D. (1984). Sexual arousal to nonsexual violence and sadomasochistic themes among rapists and non-sex offenders. *Journal of Consulting and Clinical Psychology, 52*, 651–657.

Quinsey, V. L., Harris, G. T., & Rice, M. E. (1995). Actuarial prediction of sexual recidivism. *Journal of Interpersonal Violence, 10*, 85–105.

Quinsey, V. L., Steinman, C. M., Bergersen, S. G., & Holmes, T. F. (1975). Penile circumference, skin conductance, and ranking responses of child molesters and "normals" to sexual and nonsexual visual stimuli. *Behavior Therapy, 6*, 213–219.

Rachman, S. (1966). Sexual fetishism: An experimental analogue. *Psychological Record, 16*, 293–296.

Rada, R. T. (1978). *Clinical aspects of the rapist*. New York: Grune & Stratton.

Rehman, J., Lazer, S., Benet, A. E., Schaefer, L. C., & Melman, A. (1999). The reported sex and surgery satisfaction of 28 postoperative male-to-female transsexual patients. *Archives of Sexual Behavior, 28*, 71–89.

Resnik, H. L. P. (1972). Erotized repetitive hanging: A form of self-destructive behavior. *American Journal of Psychotherapy, 26*, 4–21.

Rice, M. E., Quinsey, V. L., & Harris, G. T. (1991). Sexual recidivism among child molesters released from a maximum security psychiatric institution. *Journal of Consulting and Clinical Psychology, 59*, 381–386.

Robinson, T., & Valcour, F. (1998). The use of depo-provera in the treatment of child molesters and sexually compulsive males. *Sexual Addiction and Compulsivity, 2*, 277–294.

Rooth, G. (1973). Exhibitionism, sexual violence and pedophilia. *British Journal of Psychiatry, 122*, 705–710.

Rosen, R. C., & Beck, G. (1988). *Patterns of sexual arousal: Psychophysiology processes and clinical applications*. New York: Guilford.

Rosen, R. C., & Kopel, S. A. (1977). Penile plethysmography and biofeedback in the treatment of a transvestite-exhibitionist. *Journal of Consulting and Clinical Psychology, 45*, 908–916.

Rosman, J. P., & Resnick, P. J. (1989). Sexual attraction to corpses: A psychiatric review of necrophilia. *Bulletin of the American Academy of Psychiatry and the Law, 17*, 153–163.

Ross, M. W., & Need, J. A. (1989). Effects of adequacy of gender reassignment surgery on psychological adjustment: A follow-up of fourteen male-to-female patients. *Archives of Sexual Behavior, 18*, 145–153.

Russell, D. E. H. (1983). The incidence and prevalence of intrafamilial and extrafamilial sexual abuse of female children. *Child Abuse and Neglect, 7*, 133–146.

Sagarin, E. (1973). Power to the peephole. *Sexual Behavior, 3*, 2–7.

Segal, Z. V., & Marshall, W. L. (1985). Heterosexual social skills in a population of rapists and child molesters. *Journal of Consulting and Clinical Psychology, 53*, 55–63.

Seidman, B. T., Marshall, W. L., Hudson, S. M., & Robertson, P. J. (1994). An examination of intimacy and loneliness in sex offenders. *Journal of Interpersonal Violence, 9*, 518–534.

Serin, R. C., Malcolm, P. B., Khanna, A., & Barbaree, H. E. (1994). Psychopathy and deviant sexual arousal in incarcerated sexual offenders. *Journal of Interpersonal Violence, 9*, 3–11.

Skipper, J. K., & McCaghy, C. H. (1970). Stripteasers: The anatomy and career contingencies of a deviant occupation. *Social Problems, 17*, 391–405.

Smallbone, S. W., & Dadds, M. R. (1998). Childhood attachment and adult attachment in incarcerated adult male sex offenders. *Journal of Interpersonal Violence, 13*, 555–573.

Smukler, A. J., & Schiebel, D. (1975). Personality characteristics of exhibitionists. *Diseases of the Nervous System, 36,* 600–603.

Steiner, B. W. (1985). The management of patients with gender disorders. In B. W. Steiner (Ed.), *Gender dysphoria: Development, research, management* (pp. 325–350). New York: Plenum.

Steiner, B. W., Blanchard, R., & Zucker, K. J. (1985). Introduction. In B. W. Steiner (Ed.), *Gender dysphoria: Development, research, management* (pp. 1–10). New York: Plenum.

Stermac, L. E., & Segal, Z. V. (1989). Adult sexual contact with children: An examination of cognitive factors. *Behavior Therapy, 20,* 573–584.

Stoller, R. J. (1975a). *Perversion: The erotic form of hatred.* New York: Pantheon Books.

Stoller, R. J. (1975b). *Sex and gender.* Vol. II: *The transsexual experiment.* New York: Jason Aronson.

Stoller, R. J. (1991). *Pain and passion: A psychoanalyst explores the world of S&M.* New York: Plenum.

Templeman, T. L., & Stinnett, R. D. (1991). Patterns of sexual arousal and history in a "normal" sample of young men. *Archives of Sexual Behavior, 20,* 137–150.

Tollison, C. D., Adams, H. E., & Tollison, J. W. (1979). Cognitive and physiological indices of sexual arousal in homosexual, bisexual, and heterosexual males. *Journal of Behavioral Assessment, 1,* 305–314.

Wakefield, J. C. (1992). The concept of mental disorder: On the boundary between biological facts and social values. *American Psychologist, 47,* 373–388.

Ward, R., Hudson, S. M., Johnston, L., & W. L. Marshall (1997). Cognitive distortions in sex offenders: An integrative review. *Clinical Psychology Review, 17,* 479–507.

Weeks, R., & Widom, C. S. (1998). Self-reports of early childhood victimization among incarcerated adult male felons. *Journal of Interpersonal Violence, 13,* 346–361.

Weinberg, M. S., Williams, C. J., & Calhan, C. (1994). Homosexual foot fetishism. *Archives of Sexual Behavior, 23,* 611–626.

Weinberg, M. S., Williams, C. J., & Calhan, C. (1995). "If the shoe fits": Exploring male homosexual foot fetishism. *Journal of Sex Research, 32,* 17–27.

Weinberg, T. S. (Ed.). (1995). *S&M: Studies in dominance and submission.* Amherst, NY: Prometheus.

Weiner, I. B. (1985). Preparing forensic reports and testimony. *Clinical Psychologist, 38,* 78–80.

Wilson, G. D., & Gosselin, C. (1980). Personality characteristics of fetishists, transvestites, and sadomasochists. *Personality and Individual Differences, 1,* 289–295.

Wise, T. N., & Meyer, J. K. (1980). Transvestism: Previous findings and new areas of inquiry. *Journal of Sex and Marital Therapy, 6,* 116–128.

Wright, L. W., Jr., & Adams, H. E. (1991) The effects of varying levels of sexually arousing stimuli on cognitive processes. *Journal of Sex Research.*

Yalom, I. (1960). Aggression and forbiddenness in voyeurism. *Archives of General Psychiatry, 3,* 305–319.

Zechnich, R. (1971). Exhibitionism: Genesis, dynamics, and treatment. *Psychiatric Quarterly, 45,* 70–75.

Zucker, K. J., & Blanchard, R. (1997). Transvestic fetishism: Psychopathology and theory. In D. R. Laws & W. O'Donohue (Eds), *Sexual deviance: Theory, assessment, and treatment* (pp. 253–279). New York: Guilford.

Zucker, K. J., & Bradley, S. J. (1995). *Gender identity disorder and psychosexual problems in children and adolescents.* New York: Guilford.

# PART V

# Disorders Associated with Physical Trauma and Medical Illness

# CHAPTER 27

# Psychobiology of Health and Disease

## Phillip J. Brantley and Steven C. Ames

### Introduction

For centuries, philosophers and scientists have remained interested in psychological processes believed to influence health. As early as the fifth century B.C., Hippocrates posited that the workings of the brain were related to bodily processes and illness (Pattishall, 1989; Watson & Evans, 1991). Although his theory of bodily humors was later falsified, his notion that health can be realized by maintaining a balance with the physical world is consistent with contemporary theories.

Interest in psychological factors and illness waned when the seventeenth-century philosopher Rene Descartes popularized the concept of mind and body as distinct entities with entirely different governing principles. Cartesian dualism had a lasting impact on science such that interest in psychological factors as determinants of health did not resurface as a prominent area of investigation until the nineteenth century and the advent of psychoanalytic theory (Levy, 1989; Pattishall, 1989).

Psychosomatic medicine developed as a result of this renewed interest in the influence of psycho-logical processes on health and was initially concerned with psychoanalytic explanations of personality and the subsequent development of particular types of disease. Early psychoanalytically based psychosomatic theories considered that particular diseases result from unconsciously displaced expressions of conflict and age regression to early childhood. Childhood was viewed as a time when emotions are expressed as bodily activities. Such thinking gave rise to "specificity theories" of illness. Collectively, these theories attempted to explain physical illness in terms of common features of individuals who experience a particular illness. Although specificity theories persist, they are currently considered less credible due to equivocal research findings (Levy, 1989; Suls & Rittenhouse, 1987).

Since the 1950s, investigators have emphasized psychological factors such as the impact of stress common to nearly all diseases. In particular, the approaches formulated by Selye (1956, 1976) and Holmes and Rahe (1967), which propose how stressful life events impact health and illness, have remained influential. Current research is focusing on the association of life stress and physiological processes believed to underlie diseases. Health behavior is another common psychological factor in illness. Empirical support has been found for a strong association between common high-risk health behaviors (e.g., smoking sedentary lifestyle, poor diet) and a variety of diseases. Determining how high-risk behaviors are acquired and maintained will hopefully provide insight into

Phillip J. Brantley • Pennington Biomedical Research Center, Louisiana State University, Baton Rouge, Louisiana 70805. Steven C. Ames • Nicotine Research Center, Mayo Clinic, Rochester, Minnesota 55905.

*Comprehensive Handbook of Psychopathology* (Third Edition), edited by Patricia B. Sutker and Henry E. Adams. Kluwer Academic / Plenum Publishers, New York, 2001.

ways that these behaviors can be reduced. Further, as a result of the growing influence of behavioral psychology since the 1950s and the advent of the medical behavioral science model (i.e., psychobiological model), researchers continue to remain interested in the role that learning plays in the expression of physical illness.

This chapter will review psychobiological models of health and disease. Initially, the reader will be introduced to early specificity theories and modern advancements of these theories. Second, the impact of stress on illness will be examined. Third, the nature of chronic illness will be explored, and chronic pain syndromes will be discussed from a psychobiological perspective. Fourth, the acquisition of illness behavior and failure to change high-risk health behavior will be discussed in the context of behavior models. Throughout the chapter, a psychobiological approach will be emphasized to highlight the biological mechanisms by which behavioral factors influence health outcome.

## Specificity Theories of Illness

Early psychodynamic formulations of "specificity theory" can be traced to Dunbar's (1935) use of the term "personality profile" to refer to the personality traits of individuals who experience the same physical ailments. Alexander (1950) later expanded upon this work and became an influential proponent of specificity theory by proposing that underlying unconscious conflicts predisposed an individual to illness. Alexander's theory rested on the notion that persons with particular personality profiles, specific underlying unconscious conflicts, and preexisting organ vulnerability had an increased likelihood of developing a specific illness when situations arose that activated the conflict. Alexander believed that this conflict then led to autonomic, neural, or hormonal activation that caused the physiological changes associated with the disease.

Somewhat later, Alexander and his colleagues (Alexander, French, & Pollack, 1968) proposed that seven distinct types of illness existed that, it was hypothesized, result from particular identifiable unconscious conflicts. However, Alexander's theory emphasized that the underlying unconscious conflicts could occur within a wide variety of individuals with different personalities. The seven psychosomatic diseases included bronchial asthma, essential hypertension, neurodermatitis,

peptic ulcer, rheumatoid arthritis, thyroid toxicosis, and ulcerative colitis.

For example, Alexander and his colleagues posited that bronchial asthma resulted from conflicts that were associated with attachment to a mother figure. A child's attempts to gain the mother figure's attention by crying aroused anxiety associated with the potential for maternal rejection. Thus, Alexander and his colleagues proposed that "asthmatic attacks could be understood as an inhibition of the expiratory act for communication, either by crying or confession" (Alexander et al., 1968, p. 12). Similarly, conflicts associated with neurodermatitis were believed to include unconscious themes of exhibitionism, guilt, masochism, and a strong desire for affection. Alexander and colleagues commented that neurodermatitis is "precipitated after the patient achieves some form of exhibitionistic victory. The victory arouses guilt and creates a need for suffering in the precise part of the body that is involved in the exhibitionistic success" (Alexander et al., 1968, p. 14).

As noted earlier, specificity theory has been considered less credible in recent years. Research that examined Alexander's (1950) unconscious conflict hypothesis has proven inconsistent. Research conducted in the 1950s and 1960s concluded that Alexander's approach offered little explanatory or predictive power in understanding the role of personality variables in physical disease (Suls & Rittenhouse, 1987). However, the hypothesis that underlying conflicts play a role in physical illness and specificity theories in general remained influential in clinical practice and psychosomatic research in the 1940s and 1950s. Although interest in the specificity theories of illness declined after the 1950s, the lasting influence of these theories can be seen by their impact on the 2nd ed. of the *Diagnostic and Statistical Manual of Mental Disorders* (American Psychiatric Association [APA], 1968).

The 1980s saw renewed interest in the personality–health relationship. Researchers attempted to address the limitations of earlier work by trying to define personality variables more precisely and to examine the biomechanical mechanisms that linked psychological variables to disease (Holroyd & Coyne, 1987). Interest in the relationship of personality variables and health in the 1990s has largely focused on the Type A behavior pattern and its relationship to coronary artery disease. Research focusing on the relationship between personality variables and health has merged with research that examines the relationship between stress and illness. This merging of trait and more behavioral approaches arises from efforts to develop more comprehensive and meaningful explanations of the way psychological factors affect physical processes. This merger of approaches is well characterized by the current state of the Type A behavior pattern literature.

## Type A Behavior Pattern (TABP)

Most of the research that has focused on the relationship between personality and coronary heart disease (CHD) has centered around TABP. The TABP was described by Rosenman (1986) as a behavior pattern consisting of competitive striving for achievement, time urgency, impatience, aggressiveness, and easily aroused hostility. It is worth noting that TABP does not simply refer to individuals who are considered to have very high levels of involvement in their jobs (Shapiro, 1996). Glass (1977) asserted that a strong desire to control the environment was inherent in individuals with TABP, and Rosenman (1986) argued that those with TABP exhibit limited insight into their disorder. Related to these hypotheses, it is interesting to note that much earlier in the century, Alexander (1939) proposed a hypothesis suggesting that excessive and inhibited hostile impulses were central to developing cardiovascular disease (i.e., essential hypertension).

Based on the results of the Western Collaborative Group Study (Rosenman et al., 1975) and the Framington Heart Study (Haynes, Feinlieb, & Kannel, 1980), it was found that TABP is associated with the incidence of CHD. Specifically, after statistically controlling for all other known risk factors, the presence of TABP was associated with approximately twice as many incidents of CHD than in those who did not test positive for this set of characteristics (Type Bs). These studies and subsequent research led an expert review panel convened by the National Institutes of Health to conclude that TABP is an independent risk factor for developing CHD, as significant as other risk factors such as elevated blood cholesterol, hypertension, or smoking (National Heart, Lung, and Blood Institute, 1981).

Subsequently, studies began to yield negative results suggesting that the National Heart, Lung, and Blood Institute's conclusion was premature (for reviews see Myrtek, 1995; Siegman, 1994a). Arguably, the largest study yet done to date, the

Multiple Risk Factor Intervention Trial, followed 12,700 men free of CHD at baseline for an average of 7 years (Shekelle et al., 1985). The results of this study revealed that TABP is unrelated to the incidence of CHD. Similarly, in the Aspirin Myocardial Infarction Study, which examined survivors of a first myocardial infarction, men with TABP, it was found, did not have a greater risk of a second myocardial infarction or death related to CHD, compared to those without TABP (Ruberman, Weinblatt, Goldberg, & Chaudhury, 1984). Likewise, a recent review of ten studies by Cohen, Ardjoen, & Sewpersad (1997) failed to find an association between TABP and the risk of death or cardiac morbidity following a myocardial infarction, compared to those without this behavior pattern. The literature regarding TABP led Eysenck (1990) to comment that "Both the positive and negative results are neatly balanced to show that as a predictor Type A behaviour is of doubtful value, and may be quite useless. Weighting the results by numbers of participants, it is doubtful if the total can be regarded as significant in a socially meaningful rather than a statistical sense" (p. 26).

Investigators have more recently proposed that mixed findings regarding TABP result from the fact that only particular components of the TABP are related to CHD. Recently, research focused predominantly on the component of hostility after a number of studies suggested that this construct is the primary toxic element related to CHD (Dembroski & Costa, 1988; Dembroski, MacDougall, Costa, & Grandits, 1989; Hecker, Chesney, Black, & Frautschi, 1988). Siegman (1994a) insists that the negative findings (Dembroski, MacDougall, Williams, Haney, & Blumenthal, 1985; Hearn, Murray, & Luepker, 1989; Helmer, Ragland, & Syme, 1991; Leon, Finn, Murray, & Bailey, 1988) for the association between hostility and CHD may result from a failure to appropriately conceptualize hostility as a multidimensional construct. Furthermore, he notes that only some of the dimensions of hostility may be related to CHD. For example, research suggests that it may be the expression of hostility and not simply its experience that may be related to CHD (Siegman, 1994b).

The mechanism by which hostility may influence coronary morbidity has prompted the development of a number of theoretical models. Williams, Barefoot, and Shekelle (1985) proposed a psychophysiological model. This model suggests that individuals high in hostility have greater reactivity in blood pressure, heart rate, and stress hormone release in response to stressors. Over time, this exaggerated reactivity may initiate and speed the development of CHD or other illnesses. Alternatively, Smith and Frohm (1985) proposed the psychosocial vulnerability model. This model argues that hostile individuals simply have a more difficult interpersonal environment, which leads to deleterious effects on their health. A third model, the transactional model, proposes that hostile individuals themselves create more frequent and severe contacts with stressors and maintain a high level of interpersonal conflict in their lives (Smith & Pope, 1990). Thus, negative health impacts are seen as caused by both increased reactivity to everyday stressors and also by additional irritants caused by a hostile style of interaction. A fourth model, proposed by Leiker and Hailey (1988) asserts that hostile people have an increased risk of illness because they have poor health habits. Finally, the constitutional vulnerability model (Krantz & Durel, 1983) suggests a biological diathesis (i.e., a genetic and/or acquired physiological predisposition is combined with exposure to critical environmental factors). Some degree of evidence exists for each of these models, and the mechanisms outlined in each of these models might complement those of the other models; that is, these models may not be mutually exclusive. A thorough review of the literature addressing the mechanisms that links hostility to health is beyond the scope of this chapter. The interested reader is referred to Smith (1992) for a review.

In summary, despite recent evidence of an association between hostility and CHD (Lahad, Heckbert, Koepsell, Psaty, & Patrick, 1997; for a review, see Miller, Smith, Turner, Guijarro, & Hallet, 1996), the status of the literature is currently equivocal. Future research needs to isolate which components of hostility are related to CHD and how these components can be measured in a standardized manner (Helmers, Posluszny, & Krantz, 1994). In addition, researchers need to continue to delineate the mechanisms by which hostility impacts illness.

## Stress and Illness

Interest in the concept of stress can be traced to the early work of Claude Bernard, Walter Cannon, and Hans Selye. Bernard (1865/1961) asserted that the survival of an organism depends on maintaining the internal environment of the organism constant, regardless of changing external environmental conditions. Out of this viewpoint arose the notion that challenges to the integrity of the organism provoke responses designed to counteract those threats. Cannon's (1935) work can be seen as building on that of Bernard and is concerned with the *stimulus* properties of physical or emotional stress in disrupting internal homeostatic mechanisms. Somewhat later, Selye (1956, 1976) became interested in the way that stress produced a *response* in organisms. The confusion inherent in these two seemingly opposing approaches has persisted in the stress literature and influenced study panels both at the Institute of Medicine and the National Academy of Sciences. These panels concluded in 1979 that, "after thirty-five years, no one has formulated a definition of stress that satisfies even a majority of stress researchers" (Elliot & Eisdorfer, 1982, p. 11). This situation remains largely unchanged today, twenty-two years after the initial report by the panel.

Presently there are three primary means of conceptualizing stress. Stress may be viewed (1) as a response, in accordance to Selye's notions; (2) as a stimulus, similar to Cannon's notion; or (3) as an interaction or relationship between environmental events and appraisal by the individual (see Figure 1). Although many researchers retain an allegiance to one of these three viewpoints, some commentators have argued that the concept of stress has become so arbitrary as to be meaningless (see Engel, 1985).

The early work of Selye stands out as principal among the response theorists. Essentially, Selye (1976) thought that it was the body's pattern of physiological responses that defined stress. Additionally, Selye asserted that a variety of stressors (e.g., emotional arousal, pain, injury, positive events) could produce stress. Thus, both cognitive and emotional factors, as well as physical stressors, could evoke stress. Finally, Selye was careful to note that stress is not inherently a negative experience. Rather, he proposed that stressors might also be experienced as positive events and labeled the response associated with positive stressors, *eustress* (Selye, 1974). Alternatively, *distress* resulted from the harmful effects of demands.

Selye (1976) formulated the idea that stress is manifested by a triphasic pattern of adaptive responses. Either a sufficient number or intensity of stressors results in a general response, which Selye

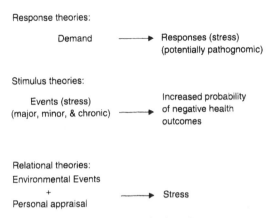

**Figure 1.** Conceptualization of stress.

**Table 1. Physiological Responses in the General Adaptation Syndrome**[a]

Alarm stage
  Adrenal medullary stimulation
  ACTH release
  Cortisol release
  Growth hormone release
  Prolactin release
  Increased thyroid activity
  Gonadotropin activity increased
Resistance stage
  Reduction in adrenal cortical activity
  Reduction in sympathetic nervous system activity
  Homeostatic mechanisms engaged
Exhaustion phase
  Enlargement of lymphatic structures
  Target organ disease/dysfunction manifest
  Increased vulnerability to opportunistic disease
  Psychological exhaustion: depression
  Physiological exhaustion: disease → death?

[a]From G. E. Everly, Jr. (1989). *A Clinical Guide to the Treatment of Human Stress Response*. New York: Plenum. Printed with permission of Plenum Press.

labeled the *general adaptation syndrome* (GAS). The first phase, the *alarm reaction*, consists of a relatively short-lived period during which the body's physiological defenses are alerted. Note that the alarm reaction phase is generally considered equivalent to the fight or flight response. The underlying physiological responses of the alarm reaction include arousal of the sympathetic nervous system (SNS), neuroendocrine stimulation of the adrenal medulla, and the release of hormones by the anterior pituitary (Cotton, 1990).

Continued exposure to the stressor leads to the second phase of the GAS, the stage of *resistance*, in which the most appropriate bodily defenses against a given stressor are determined. During this stage, there is an increased secretion of cortisol, which results in heightened metabolism, increased muscle strength, decreases in swelling and inflammation, and decreased immunity (Cotton, 1990). Thus, although the organism is attempting to provide maximum resistance to the identified stressor, it is susceptible to other stressors. Additionally, because Selye's model of stress postulates a closed system, continued activation of this stage depletes the organism's resources, and unless the stress is resolved, the organism's defenses will ultimately weaken.

Once prolonged exposure to the stressor has depleted the organism's adaptation energy, the third and final stage occurs, the stage of *exhaustion*. Once this stage is attained, adaptation no longer prevails, and the effects of high levels of cortisol begin to exert pronounced negative effects (Cotton, 1990). During this stage, shock, decreased resistance to infection, tissue damage, and, in the most extreme cases, death results. Table 1 presents a summary of the physiological events associated with the GAS.

Despite the fact that Selye's work was the impetus for much of the later stress research, his theory has not stood without criticism. Researchers have criticized Selye's theory for three major reasons (for a review see Steptoe, 1991). First, research has called into question Selye's emphasis on the nonspecificity of the response. Second, the hypothesis that the physiological stress response is adapted to enhance the organism's biological defenses appears in conflict with the anti-inflammatory response and immunosuppression. Third, Selye's view that peripheral physiological changes result from central nervous system activation has been called into question by evidence suggesting bidirectional traffic between the two. Despite the criticisms that have been leveled against it, Selye's model provided the first systematic theoretical notion of potential changes in physiological functioning resulting from psychological stimuli. The proposed physiological changes posited by Selye would later be an important means of investigating the relationship between stress and illness.

Cannon's (1935) early work led to the development of another tradition within the field of stress research, that of conceptualizing stress as a stimulus linked to environmental events (Dohronwend & Dohronwend, 1974). Thus, stress was defined and measured in terms of exposure to stressful life events (Brantley & Jones, 1993). Much of the early research that examined the role of life events as stressors was conducted by Holmes and Rahe (1967) and involved examining the link between major life events and subsequent physical illness. Examples of major life events include stress associated with marriage, the birth of a child, or the death of a loved one and reportedly significantly increase the likelihood of developing a variety of physical disorders (Holmes & Rahe, 1967). The occurrence of life events is currently believed to be a risk factor for a variety of adverse health outcomes.

More recently, investigators interested in the relationship between stress and illness have focused their attention on "daily minor stressors," also referred to as "small life events" or "hassles" (Eckenrode & Bolger, 1995). Examples of minor stressors include having automobile trouble, running out of pocket money, getting stuck in traffic, or performing poorly on a task. Compared to life events, minor stressors occur more frequently, possibly daily, and are perceived as less intense (Brantley & Jones, 1989). Interestingly, a number of studies that assessed both life events and minor stressors have suggested that minor stressors may be better predictors of health outcomes than major stressors (Brantley, Waggoner, Jones, & Rappaport, 1987; Delongis, Coyne, Dakof, Folkman, & Lazarus, 1982; Garrett, Brantley, Jones, & McKnight, 1991; Holahan & Holahan, 1987; Kanner, Coyne, Schaefer, and Lazarus, 1981; Monroe, 1983; Weinberger, Hiner, & Tierney, 1987). Despite this, most investigations of stress continue to measure both major and minor life events in an attempt to obtain a comprehensive assessment of stress.

Along with life events and daily minor stressors, investigations have examined the impact of chronic stressors on health and disease (Cohen et al., 1998). "Chronic stressors are usually conceived of as discrete events and conditions, or constellations of related events and conditions, that persist over time" (Lepore, 1995, p. 103). Examples of chronic stressors include overcrowding, environmental pollution (e.g., noise pollution, air pollution), un-

employment, or inability to afford the basic necessities of living, such as food or clothing. More recently, measures of minor stress have been used to address the extent to which daily events comprise the elements of the experience of chronic stress (Eckenrode & Bolger, 1995). There is evidence that chronic stressors may be more important in the stress-illness relationship than acute stressors (Cohen et al., 1998).

Lepore has suggested that investigating chronic stressors may be important for a number of reasons. First, he asserts that it is theoretically more plausible to link diseases that have a long-term period of development to persistent stressors, in contrast to those that are acute and time-limited. Second, Lepore notes that emerging evidence has suggested that humans do not always habituate to chronic stressors and that these stressors may enhance the negative impact of acute stressors (see Brown & Harris, 1978; Hebert & Cohen, 1993; McGonagle & Kessler, 1990). Third, attempts to cope with chronic stressors may create psychological or physical fatigue and may lead to decreased mental performance, psychological distress, or disregulation of neuroendocrine or immunologic functioning. Fourth, Lepore asserts that some chronic stressors may cause individuals to become socially avoidant and decrease their social support resources that might enhance health. Finally, Scarinci, Ames, and Brantley (1999) have found a limited amount of evidence to suggest that individuals may perceive chronic stressors as more intense than minor stressors.

A final approach to conceptualizing stress involves examining the interaction or relationship between potentially stressful stimuli (e.g., environmental events) and personal appraisal (e.g., perceived threat). Lazarus and Folkman (1984) noted that relational theorists argue that an event alone is not sufficient to produce illness and criticize the stimulus and response theories as overly simplistic and at times tautological. Instead, relational theorists assert that a diathesis in the organism is a necessary condition for disease to become manifest. According to this approach, "stress is a particular response between the person and environment that is appraised by the person as taxing or exceeding his or her resources and endangering his or her well-being" (Lazarus & Folkman, 1984, p. 21). Thus, relational theorists focus on determining factors that increase vulnerability to environmental events. In sum, these theorists view both individual (e.g., cognitive appraisal, coping skills) and environmental variables (e.g., predictability or ambiguity of the event) as important influences in susceptibility to stress (for a review see Lazarus & Folkman, 1984).

### The Link Between Stress and Illness

Evidence that associates stress with physical and psychological illness has emerged from a variety of research studies (Steptoe, 1991). Investigations of the relationship between stress and illness have examined a wide spectrum of factors, ranging from investigations of autonomic, endocrine, and immunologic mechanisms to epidemiological studies that have examined the role of psychosocial factors and health. The relationship between stress and illness is particularly relevant to the 4th ed. of the *Diagnostic and Statistical Manual of Mental Disorders* (DSM-IV; APA, 1994) diagnostic category of "psychological factors affecting medical condition." Diagnostic criteria for this disorder require "the presence of one or more specific psychological or behavioral factors that adversely affect a general medical condition" (APA, 1994, p. 675). Further, the DSM-IV notes that physiological reactions to environmental or social stressors may affect a medical condition in a variety of ways, including "development or exacerbation of, or delayed recovery from the medical condition" (APA, 1994, p. 675). As noted before, although evidence is accumulating that stress affects health, not everyone who experiences stress becomes physically ill, nor have scientists identified the precise mechanisms by which stress influences health. Finally, scientists have recognized that different individuals respond to stressors in different ways (Lovallo, 1997). Additionally, it is also recognized that the same stressor, experienced on different occasions or under different circumstances, may also produce very different consequences.

Some stress researchers argue that alterations in physiological functioning that occur secondary to exposure to stressors increase the likelihood of disease or illness. After exposure to prolonged or intense stimuli that elicit a stress response, changes that occur in the functioning of the autonomic nervous system, neuromuscular system, neurotransmitter integrity, endocrine, or immunologic function increase the probability that an illness will develop. In addition to the direct effects on physiological function that stressors may have, stressors might also have more indirect effects on health. Specifically, an increase in behavioral risk factors for illness (e.g., increased smoking or alcohol consumption, decreased sleep) may accompany increased levels of psychological stress (Cohen, Kessler, & Gordon, 1995).

Another group of investigators argues that stress may trigger a host of psychoneuroimmunologic processes that may reduce the organism's resistance to disease and predispose it to later illness (for a review, see Cohen & Hebert, 1996). Psychoneuroimmunology is the investigation of the interrelationships between the immune system and the central nervous system. Because it is assumed that the relationships between the nervous system and immune system are bidirectional, the term interrelationships is used. Accumulating evidence suggests that both laboratory and naturalistic stressors may compromise the integrity of the immune system and may lead to future susceptibility to a variety of illnesses (Cohen & Hebert, 1996). Specifically, researchers have discovered data suggesting that life events, minor (i.e., daily) stressors, and chronic stressors have immunologic consequences. Further, although it is still in the early stages of development, research also suggests that psychological factors may play a role in autoimmune diseases such rheumatoid arthritis and cancer.

Although some researchers have found a relationship between stress and immunologic function, a number of important questions remain unanswered. First, as Steptoe (1991) indicates, despite evidence that relates stress to illness, the specific mechanisms through which stress responses increase susceptibility to illness continue to remain poorly understood. Second, Steptoe asserts that the reasons for individual differences in illness susceptibility are also poorly understood and remain a concern which can only be resolved once the mechanisms by which stress affects illness are better understood. Third, Cohen and Hebert (1996) note that the literature is missing strong evidence that the relationships between psychological factors and illness are attributable to changes in immune function, rather than to changes in health behavior (e.g., adherence to medical regimen, smoking). Even many recent studies fail to adequately measure and control such variables. Fourth, Cohen and Hebert indicate that the question of whether stress reduction interventions can help alleviate immune deficits, assuming that stress is reliably associated with immune change, has yet to be adequately addressed. In sum, these authors indicate that the few existing studies that have examined this issue fail to provide convincing evidence.

Another hypothesis that has recently received a great deal of attention in the stress–illness relationship is the psychophysiological hyperreactivity hypothesis. "Psychophysiological hyperreactivity is the tendency to respond to behavioural stress with abnormally large autonomic or neuroendocrine reactions, or to display delayed recovery following termination of the stressful encounter" (Steptoe, 1991, pp. 639–640). Psychophysiological hyperreactivity result from physiological diatheses or learned response patterns and may be restricted to particular organ systems. Although, currently, the literature that examines this hypothesis is equivocal, support for the psychophysiological hyperreactivity hypothesis has been found in the hypertension and CHD literature (Carroll, Harris, & Cross, 1991; Everson, Lovallo, Sausen, & Wilson, 1992; Manuck, Kasprowicz, & Muldoon, 1990; for a review, see Blascovich & Katkin, 1993). Related to the psychophysiological hyperactivity hypothesis, some researchers argue that intense physiological reactions to stressors may act through an additional mechanism termed the disease stability process (Steptoe, 1991). Central to this hypothesis is the notion that physiological responses to stressors may affect the progression or stability of an illness.

Still other researchers assert that stress may affect health when an individual's ability to cope effectively with the stressor is exceeded (Steptoe, 1991). Important variables in this relationship include current psychosocial demands; the intensity, chronicity, and complexity of the stressor, and the stressor's novelty, predictability, and foreseeable controllability. Additionally, the coping resources that the individual has available are also important. Such factors as prior experience with threatening situations, optimism, hardiness, and the presence of social support may modulate the ability of the individual to cope with the situation. Steptoe adds that, although a number of different coping resources have been identified, currently researchers are trying to better understand which coping responses are most adaptive in different situations. Figure 2 graphically presents the models of stress and illness reviewed before.

Although the theories reviewed help assess hypotheses about the relationship of stress and illness, currently no definitive model exists that shows how stress may cause or increase an individual's vulnerability to illness. Additionally, none of the hypotheses reviewed earlier are mutually exclusive. Thus, the current status of the literature suggests a need for a comprehensive model of stress. Further, this model needs to incorporate multiple variables to adequately explain the stress–illness relationship.

## Illness as Learned Behavior

Individuals display a wide variety of reactions to illness. Although, several patients may have a similar illness in terms of laboratory indexes, they may each present with very different symptom profiles. Likewise, some individuals may present as being fairly indifferent to their symptoms continue to go about their daily routines in the same manner as they did before contracting their illness, and complain only when they are very ill. On the other hand, other individuals may complain at the slightest perception of pain or discomfort. Overall, responses to illness are difficult to explain if solely pathophysiological changes in the body are relied upon (Dworkin & Wilson, 1993). Prior learning experiences can be an important source of variance in accounting for the divergent ways that different individuals experience the same physical illness. Specifically, previous learning may be one factor that might account for the reasons that some individuals readily accept the "sick role" and arrange much of their lives around their illness, whereas others resist changing their daily routine. Prior learning experiences may also help account for the reason that some individuals seek medical attention for minor ailments, whereas others are reluctant to seek medical care for potentially life-threatening problems. According to a number of conceptualizations of illness as a learned behavior, operant and classical conditioning factors may help to explain these differences.

As a concept, *illness behavior* represents an attempt to explain the way individuals monitor their bodies, interpret and define their symptoms, and seek and use medical care in an attempt to relieve their symptoms (Mechanic, 1962, 1966, 1982). Illness behavior can be considered adaptive and appropriate when an individual's behavior is

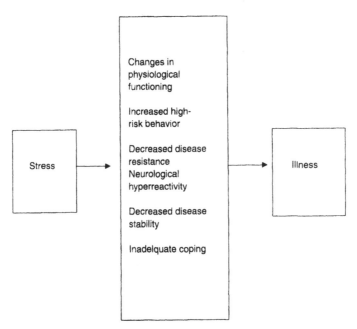

**Figure 2.** Models of stress and illness.

viewed as acceptable by the social reference group and results in an acceptable method of intervention (Schwartz, Gramling, & Mancini, 1994). However, illness behavior can also be viewed as maladaptive in the case of Somatoform Disorders. Other researchers (e.g., Blackwell, Wooley, & Whitehead, 1974) have referred to a syndrome of behavior, including disability disproportionate to the illness, a life-style centered on illness, and a continual search for medical care, as *chronic illness behavior*. Naturally, when a patient's illness behavior is perceived by a physician as maladaptive or when the patient's symptoms remain continually disproportionate to the illness, mutual frustration and dissatisfaction on the part of the doctor and patient alike often results (Dworkin, 1991). Consequently, patients who exhibit excessive illness or maladaptive behaviors often come to the attention of psychologists who work in medical settings.

Inherent in the concept of illness behavior is the notion that illness results from an interaction of biological, psychological, and sociological influences (Dworkin, 1991). In his review, Dworkin discusses two additional fundamental premises that define the concept of illness behavior: (1) the *disease-illness distinction* and (2) the *sick role*

concept. Dworkin asserts that particular dangers exist when providing treatment as if the dimensions of disease and illness are equivalent. Disease can be defined as a physiological event resulting from a disruption of a body structure or system due to physiological change. In contrast, illness may be defined as the subjective experience of physical discomfort, alterations in emotion, behavioral limitations, and psychosocial disruption. Thus, disease and illness may require different interventions, for though bodily systems may become diseased, individuals manifest illness behavior based on the subjective knowledge that a disease is present.

The second fundamental premise in the concept of illness behavior is the concept of a sick role. The concept of a sick role incorporates the notion that illness experience is shaped by prior learning, cultural definition, social climate, personal needs, and pathophysiological change (Dworkin, 1991; Mechanic, 1992). The sick role is viewed as appropriate only when the individual recognizes that it is a generally undesirable role that consists of an obligation to cooperate with medical professionals to restore health and return to the role of an adequately functioning member of society.

The DSM-IV (APA, 1994) diagnostic category

of Pain Disorder is the disorder where it can be most clearly seen that the concept of illness behavior has a significant role. As indicated in the DSM-IV, an essential feature of Pain Disorder is that, "psychological factors are judged to play a significant role in the onset, severity, exacerbation, or maintenance of the pain" (APA, 1994, p. 458). Similarly, models of chronic pain have relied heavily on environmental influences on overt pain behaviors (e.g., pain complaints, posturing, requests for medication) to account for the maintenance of subjective pain in the absence of medically verifiable pain-producing stimuli (Fordyce, 1976). Additionally, a body of evidence suggests that a number of other environmental and psychological factors may have important roles. Specifically, these factors include social learning, operant learning, respondent conditioning, beliefs about pain, beliefs about controllability of pain, self-efficacy, coping skills, and mood (see Turk, 1996 for a review). Other environmental contingencies may also influence behavior associated with Pain Disorder and more generally Hypochondriasis and Conversion Disorder. Environmental reinforcers such as disability payments, attention from caregivers, and escape from anxiety provoking or unpleasant situations (e.g., work, school) may have a role in maintaining behaviors associated with somatoform disorders (Maldonado, 1989; Turk, 1996).

## Acquisition of Illness Behavior

Evidence suggests that prior learning is an important determinant of illness behavior. As noted earlier, different individuals vary widely in their responses to illness. Further, researchers have discovered that individuals vary in their desire to seek medical care when suffering from the same symptoms, and in their response to identical treatments (Turk, 1996). Ethnic group membership also influences the way individuals perceive, label, respond to, and communicate physical symptoms, as well as how and from whom care is sought (Mechanic, 1978; Segall, 1988; Weidman, 1988). Social learning may influence the way different groups interact with those who are ill, and it may also influence the relationship that a patient has with the health care provider (Turk, 1996). Researchers have attempted to account for these individual and cultural differences by examining the ways that social learning, operant conditioning, and classical conditioning impact the acquisition of illness behavior.

Illness behavior may be acquired through social learning which includes both observational learning and modeling processes. Thus, individuals may acquire new behaviors by observing others who respond in similar ways. According to Bandura's social learning theory, vicarious learning occurs after observing behavior completed by another individual (Bandura, 1969). Behaviors that are reinforced are more likely to be performed again in the future by the observer. A number of studies have demonstrated that adulthood health care utilization and the frequency of somatic symptoms are associated with modeled sick role behavior during childhood (Jamison & Walker, 1992; Whitehead et al., 1994).

Operant approaches to illness behavior focus on the way the consequences of a behavior may lead to future occurrences of that behavior (Fordyce, 1976), that is, the operant conditioning model proposes that reinforced behaviors are more likely to occur than behaviors that have been punished. Thus, direct reinforcement of illness behaviors increase the likelihood that these behaviors will be performed again in the future. In support of this notion, a number of studies have discovered a positive relationship between pain behaviors and positive reinforcement provided by a family member, as would be predicted by the operant conditioning model (Turk & Okifuji, 1997). Additionally, illness behavior may be maintained by negative reinforcement because it increases the likelihood that an individual can escape from noxious stimulation by using drugs or rest or by avoiding undesirable activities such as work (Turk, 1996). Third, normal behavior may not be adequately reinforced, and as a result the more rewarding illness behavior may be maintained. Because the consequences of behavior maintain the occurrence of certain future behaviors, the operant model explains why illness behaviors tend to persist long after the illness is over.

Health care professionals and family members may help maintain these behaviors at a high level of frequency by shaping or reinforcement. For example, an individual who sustained a back injury as a result of an automobile accident may originally have had a recognized pathophysiological mechanism for the experience of pain. The pain initially experienced as a result of the back injury is viewed as respondent pain, that is, pain that results from physiological injury caused by the accident (Fordyce, 1976). As a direct result of the pain the individual is experiencing, he is allowed to avoid an aversive job and household chores, while receiving a high level of care and attention from his spouse. Over time, behaviors associated with expression of pain are seen as coming under the control of environmental contingencies. Illness behaviors that are now associated with positive consequences or that have been negatively reinforced as a result begin to occur more frequently. These pain behaviors that are now being maintained by their positive consequences are what Fordyce (1976) labeled operant pain. As a result of operant conditioning, operant pain can persist over time without an existing pathophysiological mechanism.

Classical (respondent) conditioning is the third approach that has been used to explain the way illness behaviors are acquired. According to this model, a previously benign stimulus repeatedly paired with an unconditioned stimulus elicits a conditioned response. When this model is applied to illness behaviors, it predicts that a previously neutral experience can elicit discomfort associated with a given disorder. For example, an individual who is suffering from chronic back pain may experience an exacerbation in pain (unconditioned response) as a result of being seated in a chair (unconditioned stimulus) all day at work. Over time, the sight of a chair, preparing for work, or even thinking about going to work (conditioned stimulus) may result in the onset of back pain (conditioned response). Interestingly, classical conditioning has been shown capable of modifying immune responses in animals (Ader & Cohen, 1993).

In sum, learning is viewed as an important determinant of illness behavior. However, the degree to which learning processes influence illness behavior may vary between different individuals and across different disorders. Some behaviors may be influenced more by one type of learning, or multiple types of conditioning may be interacting. Although conditioning influences may vary across different individuals in their impact on symptom acquisition and maintenance, it is important to acknowledge that learning processes may be influencing illness behavior when assessing patients presenting with somatic complaints.

## Health Behavior

The ultimate efficacy of any medical intervention is based on the willingness of the individual to perform the necessary behaviors (e.g., taking medication) or abstain from injurious activities (e.g., cigarette smoking) (Becker, 1990). Unfortunately, research reveals that individuals frequently fail to comply with professional advice whenever some form of discretionary action or self-administration is required. Further, the therapeutic benefits of medical treatment are often compromised by chronically ill individuals because they do not consistently adhere to prescribed medical regimens (Dunbar-Jacob, Burke, & Puczynski, 1995; German, 1988). Sackett (1976) estimated that half of medical patients do not take prescription medications as instructed. Other estimates indicate that 20–80% of patients drop out of long-term treatment and that as many as 20–50% of medical appointments are missed (Becker, 1985; Sackett, 1976). Health behavior is an issue that is important to every patient because as many as 80% of patients may be at least partially nonadherent to their medical regimen at some time during treatment (Dunbar-Jacob et al., 1995).

Interest in the study of health behavior is based on two fundamental assumptions. First, it is assumed that in industrialized nations a significant proportion of mortality from the leading causes of death is due to particular patterns of behavior (Stroebe & Stroebe, 1995, cited in Conner & Norman, 1995). Second, the study of health behavior assumes that these behaviors, once identified, are modifiable. As it becomes more widely recognized that health behavior (e.g., diet, exercise, cigarette smoking) is an important and modifiable factor in preventing disease, more research continues to be generated. Recently, research has focused on identifying the processes that underlie health behavior and conversely, on identifying the processes that inhibit choosing healthy ways of behaving. Out of this interest, a number of models of illness behavior and health behavior have been constructed in an attempt to account for these factors.

### Obstacles to Healthy Behavior

Numerous factors can inhibit one's ability to discontinue unhealthy behaviors or adopt healthier ways of living. The term *compliance* has been defined in a number of different ways in the literature. Haynes' (1979) classic definition defines compliance as "the extent to which a person's behavior (in terms of taking medications, following diets, or executing lifestyle changes) coincides with medical or health advice" (pp. 2–3). Al-

## Table 2. Factors Affecting Adherence

Type of treatment
  Curative vs. preventive
  Length of treatment
  Life-style change required
  Complexity of regimen
Illness variables
  Symptomatic vs. asymptomatic
  Concern about physical condition
Provider–patient relationship
  Patient satisfaction with care
  Consistency of care
Cognitive variables
  Knowledge of treatment regimen
  Coping skills
  Beliefs
  Motivation
  Self-concept
  Intelligence
  Locus of control
Biological variables
  Side effects of medication
  Side effects of nonmedication treatments
  Interference of health behaviors with biological reinforcers
  Physical or cognitive deficits
  Absence or misinterpretation of biological cues
  Substance abuse
Environmental variables
  Social support
  Stress
  Cultural influences

toward the patient influences patient cooperation, as discussed later, for the purposes of this review, the terms *compliance* and *adherence* will be used interchangeably. Potential influences on adherence are listed in Table 2.

A number of techniques have been identified that have been successful in increasing patient adherence (see Becker, 1990, for a review). Additionally, Becker notes that these factors might influence treatment adherence when used by any member of a health care team (e.g., physician, nurse, social worker). In a review of the compliance literature, Leventhal and Cameron (1987) suggest that an integrated, multidimensional approach may be the best model of nonadherence, that is, an integration of models that focuses on health beliefs, learning theory, and self-regulation may help explain how multiple factors (i.e., cognitive, affective, and behavioral variables) interact to influence compliance. However, to date, relatively few investigators have conducted comprehensive studies that examined the interaction of multiple determinants of adherence (Kaplan De-Nour, 1986).

Although differences in adherence rates may be partially attributable to the characteristics of both setting and subject, recent reviews indicate that a number of factors may influence treatment adherence (Becker, 1990; German, 1988; Grunberg & Lord, 1990; Joos & Hickam, 1990). First, higher rates of noncompliance are typically found for prophylactic as opposed to curative treatments. Further, if the individual is asymptomatic or has difficulty identifying signs of improved health, individuals will be less likely to adhere to their medical regimen than if it produced a noticeable improvement in their symptoms (e.g., rid them of an infection). Second, individuals show high nonadherence rates when medical regimens require significant life-style changes (e.g., smoking or dietary changes). Prior estimates have indicated that as many as 80% of individuals discontinue treatments that require significant life-style changes (Dunbar & Stunkard, 1979). Medical regimens that are complicated or have a greater duration also consistently have higher rates of nonadherence (Agras, 1989; Goodall & Halford, 1991). Because longer term treatment regimens are required for those with chronic disorders (e.g., diabetes) and have poor adherence, individuals with chronic medical conditions may have an increased risk of developing side effects from nonadherence.

The relationships that patients have with their

though Haynes' definition is very general and allows a great deal of variability in assessing compliance, some theorists have objected to it because they feel it implies that the patient assumes full responsibility for complying with a medical regimen. Originating from this position, some believe that the term compliance denotes a passive, subservient state of agreement with an authoritarian health care provider (Turk, Salovey, & Litt, 1986). In contrast, *adherence* implies a collaborative approach, where the patient and the health care provider share joint responsibility for compliance (Gerber, 1986). Finally, Barofsky (1978) suggested using the term *therapeutic alliance* to highlight the fact that an interactive or reciprocal relationship exists. Although it has been shown that the behavior that the health care provider displays health-care providers may also have an impact on adherence. Investigators have discovered associations between adherence and patient satisfaction with the visit, the therapist, or the clinic. A patient's satisfaction with the clinic typically includes variables such as convenience, waiting times, and consistency of care (Becker, 1990). The literature suggests that, in general, adherence is greater when patients perceive that their expectations have been met, when the health-care provider elicits and respects patients' concerns and provides information about their conditions and progress, and when sincere concern and sympathy are shown.

Knowledge of the treatment regimen, it has been shown, influences the likelihood of patient adherence. Svarstad (1979, cited in Becker, 1990) found that 50% of low-income patients at a neighborhood health center could not correctly report how long they were to take their medications. Seventeen percent could not report how often they were to take their medications, 16% felt that their medications marked "prn" were to be taken regularly, and 23% could not identify the purpose of each medication they were taking. Further, 73% of those who could correctly identify their physician's instructions adhered to their prescribed regimen, and 16% of those who made one or more errors about their physicians' instructions adhered to their regimen. Simple and succinct instructions, repetition of instructions, patient repetition of instructions with correction by the health-care provider, telephone calls or mailed reminders of future appointments, and conveying instructions in both written and oral form have a positive impact on adherence (Becker, 1990; Joos & Hickman, 1990).

A number of other cognitive variables such as coping skills, illness attitudes and beliefs, self-concept, intelligence, and locus of control may also impact patient adherence. However, generally speaking, researchers agree much less on the impact of these variables than those previously discussed.

Biological variables may effect the cognitive abilities of the patient (Grunberg & Lord, 1990). For example, a patient's dementia may interfere with the exchange of information between the health care provider and the patient. Unpleasant medication side effects (e.g., impaired sexual functioning), side effects of nonmedication treatment (e.g., skeletal muscle pain resulting from physical therapy), or interference of health behav-iors with biological pleasures (e.g., restrictive diets) may also reduce adherence rates. Finally, substances that have reinforcing biological effects (e.g., opiods, nicotine, alcohol) may interfere with adherence as a result of either physiological or psychological dependence, or may reduce competence or motivation to comply with prescribed health behaviors.

Evidence is accumulating that social support, support of one's family, cultural variables, and environmental stressors are also important factors that influence adherence (Becker, 1990; German, 1988). Social support, it has been found, is associated with keeping appointments, taking medication, and making life-style changes (German, 1988). Social support is especially important when treatment plans require the patient to maintain long-term, continuous behavioral changes (Becker, 1990). Other researchers have found that living in a family setting and garnering assistance from one's spouse may impact treatment adherence positively (Hartman & Becker, 1978; O'Brien, 1980).

Environmental stressors may also negatively influence adherence. Daily, minor stressors, it has been found, are related to noncompliant behavior as measured by intersession weight gain in hemodialysis patients (Everett et al., 1993). However, the incidence of daily stress, it was found, is related to measures of depression. These results suggest that stressors may directly or indirectly affect treatment adherence. Further research is required to better examine how environmental stressors may impact treatment adherence.

## Models of Health Behavior

A number of models have been proposed to account for the mechanisms that influence health behavior change or account for factors that maintain health behavior, such as abstinence (Schwarzer, 1992). However, these two lines of research originate from separate traditions. Some models have been created to explain and predict the intention of behavior change, and other models have originated from a desire to better explain why individuals fail to maintain health behaviors that they have already initiated (i.e., explain why they relapse). Currently, the literature is missing a unifying theory that accounts for all aspects of health behavior. Although a comprehensive review of all existing health behavior models is outside the scope of this chapter, four of the most well-known models will be highlighted. These include the health belief model, the social cognitive model, the transtheoretical (stages of change) model, and the relapse model. For reviews of other models, the reader is referred to Clark & Becker (1998) and Rogers & Prentice-Dunn, (1997).

Of all the models of health behavior, the *health belief model* has received the most research attention (Becker, 1990). The original version of this model was developed by psychologists who worked at the U.S. Public Health Service (Rosenstock, 1974). The health belief model rests on the notion that individuals base their health behavior on (1) a desire to avoid illness and (2) the belief that a given health behavior will lead to that goal (Becker, 1974; Maiman & Becker, 1974; Rosenstock, 1974). According to this model, an individual's *perceived susceptibility to illness* (i.e., subjective perception of contracting an illness) in addition to their *perceived severity of the illness* results in a *perceived threat of disease* (Becker, 1990). Additionally, this relationship can be modified by individual differences in demographic (e.g., age, gender, race) and sociopsychological variables (e.g., social support, personality). The individual's perceived threat of disease may also be modified by *cues to action*, including mass media campaigns, advice from others, reminders to schedule doctor's appointments, illness of family members or friends, etc. Thus, an individual's *likelihood of action* is determined by the individual's perceived threat of disease, in addition to a subjective rationale analysis that weighs the perceived benefits of preventive action against the perceived barriers to this action.

Investigations have found that this model can account for considerable variance in initiating preventive health behavior, desire to seek diagnoses, and adherence to a medical regimen. However, this model has been criticized on a number of theoretical grounds (see Schwarzer, 1992).

The social cognitive model is based on Bandura's social cognitive theory which in turn relies heavily on the concept of self-efficacy. Self-efficacy (i.e., a perceived sense of personal control), it has been found, is related to better health, higher achievement, and better social integration (see Schwarzer, 1992; Schwarzer & Fuchs, 1995, for reviews). Further, evidence suggests that individuals' ability to change undesirable behavior is related to their perception of the self-efficacy of the behavior in question. According to Bandura's (1977, 1986, 1991, 1992) social cognitive theory,

behavior is governed by incentives and expectancies. Expectancies can be subdivided into three categories: (1) *situation-outcome expectancies*, in which consequences will occur without personal action; (2) *action-outcome expectancies*, in which outcomes occur as result of personal action; and (3) *perceived self-efficacy*, which is one's own perception of one's capability of performing a behavior to attain a desired outcome (Schwarzer, 1992; Schwarzer & Fuchs, 1995). Therefore, the likelihood that an individual will discontinue a harmful habit or adopt a healthy behavior depends on three types of cognitions: (1) the expectancy that one's health is at risk, (2) the expectancy that behavior change will reduce this risk, and (3) the expectancy that one is capable of adopting a healthy behavior or abstaining from an unhealthy one.

Before a new behavior change occurs, individuals first form an intention to change and then attempt to execute the change (i.e., action phase). Although outcome expectancies are important determinants in forming intentions to change behavior, they are generally viewed as less important in the action phase. However, self-efficacy is viewed as having an important impact on both stages because it represents the individuals' view that they serve as active agents of change and possess the skills necessary to initiate and maintain change and to regain control should relapse occur.

The transtheoretical model originated from the work of Prochaska and DiClemente (1982, 1984). This model represents an attempt to integrate several previous models of behavior change. It was developed from a desire to present a comprehensive model of the process of behavior change that would be useful to health professionals in their attempts to motivate their patients. Using this approach, motivation is viewed as an individual's current state of readiness for change. Thus, the transtheoretical model is based on the notion that motivation is an internal state that can be influenced by external factors.

The model proposes that individuals pass through discrete *stages of change* as they alter their behavior. In the *precontemplation* stage, individuals have not yet made a personal commitment to change given behaviors. Rather, they may feel coerced by the legal system or by significant others (e.g., their physician wants them to quit smoking, but they are currently not interested in quitting). In the *contemplation* stage, individuals are aware that distressing life situations exist and are interested in determining whether their problems are resolvable and whether treatment would benefit them. In the determination or *preparation* stage, individuals attempt to understand the parameters of the problem area and they typically make commitments to change. In the *action stage*, the individual engages in actual behaviors intended to bring about a change. Finally, in the *maintenance* stage, the challenge is to sustain the behavior change accomplished by prior action and to avoid relapse.

The transtheoretical model also outlines specific *processes of change* that may be used to alter behavior. One is of these processes is *consciousness-raising* which may involve educating an individual about the causes, course, and consequences of a behavior. Another process of change is *counterconditioning* that consists of learning new behaviors to substitute for undesirable behaviors (e.g., learning assertiveness to refuse your mom's offer of another serving of dessert). The transtheoretical model proposes that processes of change need to be matched to appropriate stages of change to assure success. For example, an individual in precontemplation to stop smoking is highly unlikely to benefit from efforts to teach them to restrict their smoking to only a few locations or times of day (i.e., process of *stimulus control*). Instead treatment efforts that involve the process of consciousness-raising are likely to be most helpful in moving the individual to the next stage of the change process. Behavioral medicine professionals are often called upon to assess patients' readiness for change and to make treatment recommendations.

Research on the stages of change has established that they provide a reliable method of measuring change in both clinical and nonclinical populations (Procahaska & DiClemente, 1982; McConnaughy, DiClemente, Prochaska, & Velicer, 1989; Prochaska, DiClemente, & Norcross, 1992). Research generally supports the notion that when individuals change, they do so predictably from one stage to the next. However, there is some evidence that individuals can be involved in attitudes and behaviors characteristic of more than one stage at the same time (McConnaughy et al., 1989).

The first three models focus on attempts to change behavior, but the last model provides a structure for understanding relapse. Based on the work of Marlatt and his associates (Marlatt, 1978; Marlatt & George, 1998), this model postulates that individuals who have made a desirable health behavior change (e.g., stopped smoking) experience a sense of control that grows stronger the longer they are compliant. This sense of control is threatened, however, when the individual encounters a high-risk situation. In their analysis of potential high-risk situations, Marlatt and colleagues identified three major categories most likely to produce relapse. These include negative emotional states, interpersonal conflict, and social pressure. This model suggests that any behavior change effort that desires long-term change must address attitudes, beliefs, and behaviors associated with potential high-risk situations. This model proposes a wide variety of treatment strategies that can be categorized into three areas: (1) *skills training* in behavioral and cognitive coping strategies, (2) *cognitive reframing* to lessen the impact of high-risk situations and minor relapses, and (3) *life-style rebalancing* strategies such as relaxation training and meditation. Research that examined components of this model and their ability to predict relapse is promising (Marlatt and George, 1998).

## Summary

Researchers have proposed a number of models to account for the way psychological factors impact health. Based on Freudian theory, early personality theorists attempted to explain illness in terms of specific traits, attitudes, or conflicts. Although these early specificity theories are no longer considered adequate to account for the development of illness, interest in the role of personality in illness has continued. Modern investigation of the relationship between personality and health has focused on examining factors that are believed to contribute to the incidence of cardiovascular disease. Although this remains a controversial area of interest, research on TABP, and more recently trait hostility, typifies modern research on personality and illness.

A second area in which the impact of psychological factors that affect illness has been examined involves the impact of stress on health. Models that account for a stress–illness relationship have focused primarily on physiological changes that accompany stress, the effects of stress on immunity and vulnerability to disease, and the role of coping. Although no single model of stress and illness currently predominates, research suggests that the effects of stress on health may be complex and multiply determined. A third approach to explaining the role of psychological factors in health focuses on the role of learning or conditioning variables. Investigators have proposed that social learning, classical conditioning, and operant conditioning models may partially determine health outcome.

Finally, the ultimate efficacy of a given medical intervention rests on the individual participating in recommended health behaviors. A number of biopsychosocial factors have been discovered that impact adherence, or the likelihood that an individual will perform the necessary health behaviors. Additionally, models have been developed to account for factors that lead to initiating positive health behavior changes or that account for factors that influence discontinuation of unhealthy habits.

Each of the psychosocial or psychobiological models of illness reviewed in this chapter makes significant contributions to understanding how psychological factors may influence health or illness. However, no one model is superior or adequate to account for the impact of psychological factors on health. Further, the models presented are not mutually exclusive; numerous factors may interact to increase the likelihood that illness will develop. Evidence that a multitude of variables is at least partially involved in the development of illness suggests that a comprehensive model that incorporates personality influences, biological variables, life-style factors, the effects of stress, and learning influences will be required to adequately explain the effects of biopsychosocial factors on health.

# References

Ader, R., & Cohen, N. (1993). Psychoneuroimmunology: Conditioning and stress. *Annual Review of Psychology, 44*, 53–85.

Agras, S. (1989). Understanding compliance with the medical regimen: The scope of the problem and a theoretical perspective. *Arthritis Care and Research, 2*, S2–S7.

Alexander, F. (1939). Emotional factors in essential hypertension. *Psychosomatic Medicine, 1*, 173–179.

Alexander, F. (1950). *Psychosomatic medicine.* New York: W.W. Norton.

Alexander, F., French, T. M., & Pollack, G. H. (1968). *Psychosomatic specificity.* Chicago: University of Chicago Press.

American Psychiatric Association. (1968). *Diagnostic and statistical manual of mental disorders* (2nd ed.). Washington, DC: Author.

American Psychiatric Association. (1994). *Diagnostic and statistical manual of mental disorders* (4th ed.). Washington, DC: Author.

Bandura, A. (1969). *Principles of behavior modification.* New York: Holt, Rinehart & Winston.

Bandura, A. (1977). Self-efficacy: Toward a unifying theory of behavioral change. *Psychological Review, 84*, 191–215.

Bandura, A. (1986). *Social foundations of thought and action.* Englewood Cliffs, NJ: Prentice-Hall.

Bandura, A. (1991). Self-efficacy conception of anxiety. In R. Schwarzer & R. A. Wicklund (Eds.), *Anxiety and self-focused attention* (pp. 89–110). New York: Harwood.

Bandura, A. (1992). Self-efficacy mechanism in psychobiologic functioning. In R. Schwarzer (Ed.), *Self-efficacy: Thought control of action* (pp. 355–394). Washington, DC: Hemisphere.

Barofsky, I. (1978). Compliance, adherence, and the therapeutic alliance: Steps in the development of self-care. *Social Science and Medicine, 12*, 369–376.

Becker, M. H. (1974). The health belief model and sick role behavior. *Health Education Monographs, 2*, 409–419.

Becker, M. H. (1985). Patient adherence to prescribed therapies. *Medical Care, 23*, 539–555.

Becker, M. H. (1990). Theoretical models of adherence and strategies for improving adherence. In S. A. Shumaker, E. B. Schron, J. K. Ockene, C. T. Parker, J. L. Probstfield, & J. M. Wolle (Eds.), *The handbook of health behavior change* (pp. 5–43). New York: Springer.

Bernard, C. (1961). *An introduction to the study of experimental medicine* (H. C. Greene, Trans.). New York: Collier. (Original work published 1865.)

Blackwell, B., Wooley, S., & Whitehead, W. E. (1974). Psychosomatic illness: A new treatment approach. *Journal of the Cincinnati Academy of Medicine, 55*, 95–98.

Blascovich, J., & Katkin, E. S. (Eds.). (1993). *Cardiovascular reactivity to psychological stress and disease.* Washington, DC: American Psychological Association.

Brantley, P. J., & Jones, G. N. (1989). *Daily Stress Inventory: Professional manual.* Odessa, FL: Psychological Assessment Resources.

Brantley, P. J., & Jones, G. N. (1993). Daily stress and stress-related disorders. *Annals of Behavioral Medicine, 15*, 17–25.

Brantley, P. J., Waggoner, C. D., Jones, G. N., & Rappaport, N. B. (1987). A daily stress inventory: Development, reliability, and validity. *Journal of Behavioral Medicine, 10*, 61–74.

Brown, G. W., & Harris, T. W. (1978). *The social origins of depression: A study of psychiatric disorders in women.* New York: The Free Press.

Cannon, W. B. (1935). Organization for physiological homeostasis. *Physiological Reviews, 9*, 399–431.

Carroll, D., Harris, M. G., & Cross, G. (1991). Hemodynamic adjustments to mental stress in normotensives and subjects with mildly elevated blood pressure. *Psychophysiology, 28*, 438–446.

Clark, N. M., & Becker, M. H. (1998). Theoretical models and strategies for improving adherence and disease management. In S. A. Shumakers, E. B. Schron, J. K. Ockene, & W. L. McBee (Eds.), *The handbook of health behavior change* (2nd ed., pp. 5–32). New York: Springer.

Cohen, L., Ardjoen, R. C., & Sewpersad, K. S. M. (1997). Type

A behavior pattern as a risk factor after myocardial infarction: A review. *Psychology and Health, 12,* 619–632.

Cohen, S., Frank, E., Doyle, W. J., Skoner, D. P., Rabin, B. S., & Gwaltney, J. M. Jr. (1998). Types of stressors that increase susceptibility to the common cold in healthy adults. *Health Psychology, 17,* 214–223.

Cohen, S., & Hebert, T. B. (1996). Health psychology: Psychological factors and physical disease from the perspective of human psychoneuroimmunology. *Annual Review of Psychology, 47,* 113–142.

Cohen, S., Kessler, R. C., & Gordon, L. U. (1995). Strategies for measuring stress in studies of psychiatric and physical disorders. In S. Cohen, R. C. Kessler, & L. U. Gordon (Eds.), *Measuring stress: A guide for health and social scientists* (pp. 80–101). New York: Oxford University Press.

Conner, M., & Norman, P. (1995). The role of social cognition in health behaviours. In M. Conner & P. Norman (Eds.), *Predicting health behaviour: Research and practice with social cognition models* (pp. 1–21). Buckingham, England: Open University Press.

Cotton, D. H. (1990). *Stress management: An integrated approach to therapy.* New York: Brunner/Mazel.

Delongis, A., Coyne, J. C., Dakof, G., Folkman, S., & Lazarus, R. S. (1982). Relationship of daily hassles, uplifts, and major life events to health status. *Health Psychology, 1,* 119–136.

Dembroski, T. M., & Costa, P. T. (1988). Assessment of coronary-prone behavior: A current overview. *Annals of Behavioral Medicine, 10,* 60–63.

Dembroski, T. M., MacDougall, J. M., Costa, P. T., & Grandits, G. A. (1989). Components of hostility as predictors of sudden death and myocardial infarction in the Multiple Risk Factor Intervention Trial. *Psychosomatic Medicine, 51,* 514–522.

Dembroski, T. M., MacDougall, J. M., Williams, R. B., Jr., Haney, T. L., & Blumenthal, J. A. (1985). Components of Type A, hostility, and anger in: Relationship to angiographic findings. *Psychosomatic Medicine, 47,* 219–233.

Dohrenwend, B. S., & Dohrenwend, B. P. (1974). A brief historical introduction to research on stressful life events. In B. S. Dohrenwend & B. P. Dohrenwend (Eds.), *Stressful life events: Their nature and effects* (pp. 1–5). New York: Wiley.

Dunbar, H. F. (1935). *Emotions and bodily changes.* New York: Columbia University Press.

Dunbar, J., & Stunkard, A. (1979). Adherence to diet and drug regimen. In R. Levy, B. Rifkin, & N. Ernst (Eds.), *Nutrition: Lipids and coronary heart disease* (pp. 391–423). New York: Raven Press.

Dunbar-Jacob, J., Burke, L. E., & Puczynski, S. (1995). Clinical assessment and management of adherence to medical regimens. In P. M. Nicassio & T. W. Smith (Eds.), *Managing chronic illness: A biopsychosocial perspective* (pp. 313–349). Washington, DC: American Psychological Association.

Dworkin, S. F. (1991). Illness behavior and dysfunction: Review of concepts and application to chronic pain. *Canadian Journal of Physiology and Pharmacology, 69,* 662–671.

Dworkin, S. F., & Wilson, L. (1993). Measurement of illness behavior: A review of concepts and common measures. In P. M. Conn (Ed.), *Methods in neurosciences: Vol. 14. Paradigms for the study of behavior* (pp. 329–342). San Diego, CA: Academic Press.

Eckenrode, J., & Bolger, N. (1995). Daily and within-day event measurement. In S. Cohen, R. C. Kessler, & L. U. Gordon

(Eds.), *Measuring stress: A guide for health and social scientists* (pp. 80–101). New York: Oxford University Press.

Elliot, G. R., & Eisdorfer, C. (1982). *Stress and human health: Analysis and implications of research.* New York: Springer.

Engel, B. T. (1985). Stress is a noun! No, a verb! No, an adjective! In T. M. Field, P. M. McCabe, & N. Schneiderman (Eds.), *Stress and coping* (pp. 3–12). Hillsdale, NJ: Erlbaum.

Everett, K. D., Sletton, C., Carmack, C. L., Brantley, P. J., Jones, G. N., & McKnight, G. T. (1993). Predicting noncompliance to fluid restrictions in hemodialysis patients. *Dialysis and Transplantation, 22(10),* 614–622.

Everson, S. A., Lovallo, W. R., Sausen, K. P., & Wilson, M. F. (1992). Hemodynamic characteristics of young men at risk for hypertension at rest and during laboratory stressors. *Health Psychology, 11,* 24–31.

Eysenck, H. J. (1990). Type A behaviour and coronary heart disease: The third stage. *Journal of Social Behavior and Personality, 5,* 25–44.

Fordyce, W. E. (1976). *Behavioral methods for chronic pain and illness.* St. Louis: Mosby.

Garrett, V. D., Brantley, P. J., Jones, G. N., & McKnight, G. T. (1991). The relation between daily stress and Crohn's disease. *Journal of Behavioral Medicine, 14,* 87–96.

Gerber, K. E. (1986). Compliance in the chronically ill: An introduction to the problem. In K. E. Gerber & A. M. Nehemkis (Eds.), *Compliance: The dilemma of the chronically ill* (pp. 12–23). New York: Springer.

German, P. (1988). Compliance and chronic disease. *Hypertension, 11,* 56–60.

Glass, D. C. (1977). *Behavior patterns, stress, and coronary disease.* Hillsdale, NJ: Erlbaum.

Goodall, T. A., & Halford, W. K. (1991). Self-management of diabetes mellitus: A critical review. *Health Psychology, 10,* 1–8.

Grunberg, N. E., & Lord, D. (1990). Biological barriers to adoption and maintenance of health-promoting behaviors. In S. A. Shumaker, E. B. Schron, J. K. Ockene, C. T. Parker, J. L. Probstfield, & J. M. Wolle (Eds.), *The handbook of health behavior change* (pp. 221–229). New York: Springer Verlag.

Hartman, P. E., & Becker, M. H. (1978). Noncompliance with prescribed regimen among chronic hemodialysis patients: A method of prediction and educational diagnosis. *Dialysis and Transplantation, 7,* 978–989.

Haynes, R. B. (1979). Strategies to improve compliance with referrals, appointments, and prescribed medical regimens. In R. B. Haynes, D. W. Taylor, & D. L. Sackett (Eds.), *Compliance in health care* (pp. 49–62). Baltimore: Johns Hopkins University Press.

Haynes, S. G., Feinlieb, M., & Kannel, W. B. (1980). The relationship of psychosocial factors to coronary heart disease in the Framingham study: III. Eight-year incidence of coronary heart disease. *American Journal of Epidemiology, 111,* 37–58.

Hearn, M. D., Murray, D. M., & Luepker, R. V. (1989). Hostility, coronary heart disease, and total mortality: A 33-year follow-up study of university students. *Journal of Behavioral Medicine, 12,* 105–121.

Hebert, T., & Cohen, S. (1993). Stress and immunity in humans: A meta-analytic review. *Psychosomatic Medicine, 55,* 364–379.

Hecker, M., Chesney, M. A., Black, G. W., & Frautschi, N. (1988). Coronary-prone behaviors in the Western Collaborative Group Study. *Psychosomatic Medicine, 50,* 153–164.

Helmer, D. C., Ragland, D. R., & Syme, S. L. (1991). Hostility and coronary artery disease. *American Journal of Epidemiology, 133*, 112–122.

Helmers, K. F., Posluszny, D. M., & Krantz, D. S. (1994). Associations of hostility and coronary artery disease: A review of studies. In A. W. Siegman & T. W. Smith (Eds.), *Anger, hostility, and the heart* (pp. 1–21). Hillsdale, NJ: Erlbaum.

Holahan, C. K., & Holahan, C. J. (1987). Life stress, hassles, and self-efficacy in aging: A replication and extension. *Journal of Applied Social Psychology, 17*, 574–592.

Holmes, T. H., & Rahe, R. H. (1967). The social readjustment rating scale. *Journal of Psychosomatic Research, 11*, 213–218.

Holroyd, K. A., & Coyne, J. (1987). Personality and health in the 1980s: Psychosomatic medicine revisited? *Journal of Personality, 55*, 359–375.

Jamison, R. N., & Walker, L. S. (1992). Illness behavior in children of chronic pain patients. *International Journal of Psychiatry in Medicine, 22*, 329–342.

Joos, S. K., & Hickam, D. H. (1990) How health professionals influence health behavior: Patient-provider interaction and health care outcomes. In K. Glanz, F. M. Lewis, & B. K. Rimer (Eds.), *Health behavior and health education: Theory, research, and practice* (pp. 216–241). San Francisco, CA: Jossey-Bass.

Kanner, A. D., Coyne, J. C., Schaefer, C., & Lazarus, R. S. (1981). Comparison of two modes of stress measurement: Daily hassles and uplifts versus major life events. *Journal of Behavioral Medicine, 4*, 1–39.

Kaplan De-Nour, A. (1986). Foreword. In K. E. Gerber & A. M. Nehemkis (Eds.), *Compliance: The dilemma of the chronically ill* (pp. xi–xiii). New York: Springer.

Krantz, D. S., & Durel, L. A. (1983). Psychobiological substrates of the Type A behavior pattern. *Health Psychology, 2*, 393–411.

Lahad, A., Heckbert, S. R., Koepsell, T. D., Psaty, B. M., & Patrick, D. L. (1997). Hostility, aggression and the risk of nonfatal myocardial infarction in postmenopausal women. *Journal of Psychosomatic Research, 43*, 183–195.

Lazarus, R. S., & Folkman, S. (1984). *Stress, appraisal, and coping.* New York: Springer Verlag.

Leiker, M., & Hailey, B. J. (1988). A link between hostility and disease: Poor health habits? *Behavioral Medicine, 3*, 129–133.

Leon, G. R., Finn, S. E., Murray, D., & Bailey, J. M. (1988). The inability to predict cardiovascular disease from hostility scores of MMPI items related to Type A behavior. *Journal of Consulting and Clinical Psychology, 56*, 597–600.

Lepore, S. J. (1995). Measurement of chronic stressors. In S. Cohen, R. C. Kessler, & L. U. Gordon (Eds.), *Measuring stress: A guide for health and social scientists* (pp. 80–101). New York: Oxford University Press.

Leventhal, H., & Cameron, L. (1987). Behavioral theories and the problem of compliance. *Patient Education and Counseling, 10*, 117–138.

Levy, N. B. (1989). Psychosomatic medicine and consultation-liaison psychiatry: Past, present, and future. *Hospital and Community Psychiatry, 40*, 1049–1056.

Lovallo, W. R. (1997). *Stress and health: Biological and psychological interactions.* Thousand Oaks, CA: Sage.

Maiman, L. A., & Becker, M. H. (1974). The health belief model: Origins and correlates in psychological theory. *Health Education Monographs, 2*, 336–353.

Maldonado, L. (1989). Behavioral concepts, methods and approaches to pain management. *Psychotherapy in Private Practice, 7*, 17–29.

Manuck, S. B., Kasprowicz, A. L., & Muldoon, M. F. (1990). Behaviorally-evoked cardiovascular reactivity and hypertension: Conceptual issues and potential association. *Annals of Behavioral Medicine, 12*, 17–29.

Marlatt, G. A. (1978). Craving for alcohol, loss of control and relapse: A cognitive behavioral analysis. In P. E. Nathan, G. A. Marlatt, & T. Loberg (Eds.), *Alcoholism: New directions in behavioral research and treatment* (pp. 271–314). New York: Plenum.

Marlatt, G. A., & George, W. H. (1998). Relapse prevention and the maintenance of optimal health. In S. A. Shumaker, E. B. Schron, J. K. Ockene, & W. L. McBee (Eds.), *The handbook of health behavior change* (2nd ed., pp. 33–58). New York: Springer.

McConnaughy, E. A., DiClemente, C. C., Prochaska, J. O., & Velicer, W. F. (1989). Stages of change in psychotherapy: A follow-up report. *Psychotherapy, 26*, 494–503.

McGonagle, K. A., & Kessler, R. C. (1990). Chronic stress, acute stress, and depressive symptoms. *American Journal of Community Psychology, 18*, 681–706.

Mechanic, D. (1962). The concept of illness behavior. *Journal of Chronic Disease, 15*, 189–194.

Mechanic, D. (1966). Response factors in illness: The study of illness behavior. *Social Psychiatry, 1*, 11–20.

Mechanic, D. (1978). Effects of psychological distress on perceptions of physical health and use of medical and psychiatric facilities. *Journal of Human Stress, 4*, 26–32.

Mechanic, D. (1982). The epidemiology of illness behavior and its relationship to physical and psychological distress. In D. Mechanic (Ed.), *Symptoms, illness behavior, and help seeking* (pp. 1–24). New York: Prodist.

Mechanic, D. (1992). Health and illness behavior and patient-practitioner relationships. *Social Science and Medicine, 12*, 1345–1350.

Miller, T. Q., Smith, T. W., Turner, C. W., Guijarro, M. L., & Hallet, A. J. (1996). A meta-analytic review of research on hostility and physical health. *Psychological Bulletin, 119*, 322–348.

Monroe, S. M. (1983). Major and minor life events as predictors of psychological distress: Further issues and findings. *Journal of Behavioral Medicine, 6*, 189–205.

Myrtek, M. (1995). Type A behavior pattern, personality factors, disease, and physiological reactivity: A meta-analytic update. *Personality and Individual Differences, 18*, 491–502.

National Heart, Lung, and Blood Institute. (1981). Coronary-prone behavior and coronary heart disease: A critical review. *Circulation, 63*, 1199–1215.

O'Brien, M. E. (1980). Hemodialysis regimen compliance and social environment: A panel analysis. *Nursing Research, 29*, 250.

Pattishall, E. G. (1989). The development of behavioral medicine: Historical models. *Annals of Behavioral Medicine, 11*, 43–48.

Prochaska, J. O., & DiClemente, C. C. (1982). Transtheoretical therapy: Toward a more integrative model of change. *Psychotherapy: Theory, Research and Practice, 19*, 276–288.

Prochaska, J. O., & DiClemente, C. C. (1984). *The transtheoretical approach: Crossing traditional boundaries of therapy.* Homewood, IL: Dow Jones/Irwin.

Prochaska, J. O., DiClemente, C. C., & Norcross, J. C. (1992). In search of how people change: Applications to addictive behaviors. *American Psychologist, 47*, 1102–1114.

Rogers, R. W., & Prentice-Dunn, S. (1997). Protection motivation theory. In D. S. Gochman (Ed.), *Handbook of health behavior research I: Personal and social determinants* (pp. 113–132). New York: Plenum.

Rosenman, R. H. (1986). Current and past history of Type A behavior pattern. In T. H. Schmidt, T. M. Dembroski, & G. Blumchen (Eds.), *Biological and psychological factors in cardiovascular disease* (pp. 15–40). New York: Springer Verlag.

Rosenman, R. H., Brand, R. J., Jenkins, D., Friedman, M., Straus, R., & Wurm, M. (1975). Coronary heart disease in the Western Collaborative Group Study: Final follow-up experiences of 8½ years. *Journal of the American Medical Association, 233*, 872–877.

Rosenstock, I. M. (1974). Historical origins of the health belief model. *Health Education Monographs, 2*, 328–335.

Ruberman, W., Weinblatt, E., Goldberg, J., & Chaudhury, B. (1984). Psychosocial influences on mortality after myocardial infarction. *New England Journal of Medicine, 311*, 552–559.

Sackett, D. L. (1976). The magnitude of compliance and noncompliance. In D. L. Sackett & R. B. Haynes (Eds.), *Compliance with therapeutic regimens* (pp. 9–25). Baltimore: Johns Hopkins University Press.

Scarinci, I. C., Ames, S. C., & Brantley, P. J. (1999). Chronic minor stressors and major life events experienced by low-income patients attending primary care clinics: A longitudinal examination. *Journal of Behavioral Medicine, 22*, 143–156.

Schwartz, S. M., Gramling, S. E., & Mancini, T. (1994). The influence of life stress, personality, and learning history on illness behavior. *Journal of Behavior Therapy and Experimental Psychiatry, 25*, 135–142.

Schwarzer, R. (1992). Self-efficacy in the adoption and maintenance of health behaviors: Theoretical approaches and a new model. In R. Schwarzer (Ed.), *Self-efficacy: Thought control of action* (pp. 217–243). Washington, DC: Hemisphere.

Schwarzer, R., & Fuchs, R. (1995). Self-efficacy and health behaviours. In M. Conner & P. Norman (Eds.), *Predicting health behaviour: Research and practice with social cognition models* (pp. 163–196). Buckingham: Open University Press.

Segall, A. (1988). Cultural factors in sick-role expectations. In D. S. Gochman (Ed.), *Health behavior: Emerging research perspectives* (pp. 249–260). New York: Plenum.

Selye, H. (1956). *The stress of life*. New York: McGraw-Hill.

Selye, H. (1974). *Stress without distress*. Philadelphia: Lippincott.

Selye, H. (1976). *The stress of life* (rev. ed.). New York: McGraw-Hill.

Shapiro, P. A. (1996). Psychiatric aspects of cardiovascular disease. *Consultation-Liaison Psychiatry, 19*, 613–629.

Shekelle, R. B., Hulley, S., Neaton, J. D., Billings, J. H., Borhani, N. O., Gerace, T. A., Jacobs, D. R., Lasser, N. L., Mittlemark, M. B., & Stamler, J. (1985). The MRFIT behavior pattern study: II. Type A behavior pattern and incidence of coronary heart disease. *American Journal of Epidemiology, 122*, 559–570.

Siegman, A. W. (1994a). From Type A to hostility and anger: Reflection on the history of coronary-prone behavior. In A. W. Siegman & T. W. Smith (Eds.), *Anger, hostility, and the heart* (pp. 1–21). Hillsdale, NJ: Erlbaum.

Siegman, A. W. (1994b). Cardiovascular consequences of expressing and repressing anger. In A. W. Siegman & T. W. Smith (Eds.), *Anger, hostility, and the heart* (pp. 173–197). Hillsdale, NJ: Erlbaum.

Smith, T. W. (1992). Hostility and health: Current status of the psychosomatic hypothesis. *Health Psychology, 11*, 139–150.

Smith, T. W., & Frohm, K. D. (1985). What's so unhealthy about hostility? Construct validity and psychosocial correlates of the Cook and Medley Ho scale. *Health Psychology, 4*, 503–520.

Smith, T. W., & Pope, M. K. (1990). Cynical hostility as a health risk: Current status and future directions. *Journal of Social Behavior and Personality, 5*, 77–88.

Steptoe, A. (1991). The links between stress and illness. *Journal of Psychosomatic Research, 35*, 633–644.

Stroebe, W., & Stroebe, M. S. (1995). *Social psychology and health*. Buckingham: Open University Press.

Suls, J., & Rittenhouse, J. D. (1987). Personality and physical health: An introduction. *Journal of Personality, 55*, 155–167.

Turk, D. C. (1996). Biopsychosocial perspective on chronic pain. In R. J. Gatchel & D. C. Turk (Eds.), *Psychological approaches to pain management: A practitioner's handbook* (pp. 3–32). New York: Guilford.

Turk, D. C., & Okifuji, A. (1997). Evaluating the role of physical, operant, cognitive, and affective factors in the pain behaviors of chronic pain patients. *Behavior Modification, 21*, 259–280.

Turk, D. C., Salovey, P., & Litt, M. D. (1986). Adherence: A cognitive-behavioral perspective. In K. E. Gerber & A. M. Nehemkis (Eds.), *Compliance: The dilemma of the chronically ill* (pp. 44–72). New York: Springer.

Watson, R. I., & Evans, R. B. (1991). *The great psychologists: A history of psychological thought* (5th ed.). New York: HarperCollins.

Weidman, H. H. (1988). A transcultural perspective on health behavior. In D. S. Gochman (Ed.), *Health behavior: Emerging research perspectives* (pp. 261–280). New York: Plenum.

Weinberger, M., Hiner, S. L., & Tierney, W. M. (1987). In support of hassles as a measure of stress in predicting health outcomes. *Journal of Behavioral Medicine, 10*, 19–31.

Whitehead, W. E., Crowell, M. D., Heller, B. R., Robinson, J. C., Schuster, M. M., & Horn, S. (1994). Modeling and reinforcement of the sick role during childhood predicts adult illness behavior. *Psychosomatic Medicine, 56*, 541–550.

Williams, R. B., Barefoot, J. C., & Shekelle, R. B. (1985). The health consequences of hostility. In M. A. Chesney & R. H. Rosenman (Eds.), *Anger and hostility in cardiovascular and behavioral disorders* (pp. 173–185). Washington, DC: Hemisphere.

# CHAPTER 28

# Emotional Disorders and Medical Illness

## Richard L. Gibson and Earl A. Burch

## Introduction

The emotional reactions to illness may be more troublesome than the illness itself, particularly if the illness is chronic and results in significant lifestyle changes. These emotional reactions are distressing to the person but do not always meet the criteria set out in the *Diagnostic and Statistical Manual of Mental Disorders*, 4th ed. (DSM-IV; American Psychiatric Association, 1994) or the *International Classification of Diseases*, 10th ed. (ICD-10; World Health Organization, 1992) for a specific disorder. In this chapter, we are particularly concerned with chronic medical illness, but much of what is reviewed also applies to acute illness.

It is undisputed that medical illness, especially chronic illness, is stressful and may be associated with emotional disorders. However, the nature of the association, particularly with regard to causal relationships and proper classification, remains unclear. Both the DSM-IV and the ICD-10 classify reactions to stress into three principle groups: (1) acute reactions, in DSM-IV called acute stress disorder; (2) adjustment disorder, classified in

Richard L. Gibson • Mississippi State Hospital, Whitfield, Mississippi 39193. Earl A. Burch • William Jennings Bryan Dorn Veterans Hospital, Columbia, South Carolina 29201.

*Comprehensive Handbook of Psychopathology* (Third Edition), edited by Patricia B. Sutker and Henry E. Adams. Kluwer Academic / Plenum Publishers, New York, 2001.

both the ICD-10 and the DSM-IV according to predominant symptoms, such as with depression, with mixed anxiety and depression, with disturbance of conduct, and with disturbance of emotions and conduct; (3) posttraumatic stress disorder (PTSD), an abnormal response to a severe stressor with symptoms that involve intrusive recollection, emotional numbing or avoidance, and arousal. Although PTSD and Acute Stress reactions are seldom diagnosed in connection with medical illness, adjustment disorders certainly are, and in patients with cancer, the prevalence may be nearly 50% (Spiegel, 1996).

Coexisting symptoms of anxiety and depression are prominent among the emotional responses in ill patients that are difficult to classify. It has been known for years that these symptoms are commonly present in medically ill patients and are difficult to separate (Lewis, 1956). The ICD-10 has a category called "mixed anxiety and depressive disorder" which is used when symptoms are not severe enough to meet criteria for a specific disorder and where the association with a stressor is not close enough to warrant a diagnosis of adjustment disorder. The DSM-IV has no such diagnosis, but the appendix includes both "mixed anxiety and depressive disorder" and "minor depressive disorder," either of which could be applicable. The DSM-IV suggests that at present there is insufficient empirical evidence to support including these conditions in the classification. In the *Oxford Textbook of Psychiatry*, 3rd ed. (Gelder, Guth, Mayon, & Cowen, 1996) these symptoms are called "minor affective disorders," and the clinical picture includes anxiety, depression, insomnia, fatigue, irritability, and poor concentration. Such somatic symptoms due, it is thought, to psychological factors, were present in 52% of patients presenting to a primary care practice. However, in such a group of patients, one should not assume that the symptoms are due to psychological factors, and the etiology must be investigated.

Classification is not simple; neither is cause and effect. Notions of cause and effect abound, but they are seldom evidence-based. In the case of psychiatric disorders, three major theoretical constructs relate stress and illness, (although there are many variations) all described by Dohrenwend and Dohrenwend (1981). The first is the *innocent victim* model, in which there is exposure to some stressful circumstance. If the stressor is severe enough or if there is special susceptibility, illness occurs. This model accounts well for PTSD and adjustment disorders, but is otherwise lacking. Building on the first model, the *vulnerability hypothesis* says that stress triggers illness in those already predisposed to develop psychiatric illnesses; and the source of the vulnerability can include genetics, social relationships, or early childhood experiences. This model is popular and invoked often for many illnesses, including depression. The third model builds on the first two and is called the *interactive model*, which postulates that deficient coping skills result in the inability to prevent undesirable events and perhaps even cause undesirable events, which then result in illness.

Having introduced the notion of coping, we will now examine it in some detail, because at least a basic understanding of coping is necessary to work effectively with people who are ill. Traditional psychiatric views of coping and especially defense mechanisms stem from the theoretical work of Sigmund Freud and his followers, and a hierarchical developmental system is usually employed to classify defensive strategies as either mature/healthy (usually called coping strategies and including such things as humor and suppression) or immature/not so healthy (such as projective identification, psychotic denial, and splitting). George Vaillant has described this system very well (Vaillant, 1977, 1992).

Coping can also be viewed as a process, rather than a hierarchy based at least in part on preconceived notions of health and illness. This approach

has been reviewed by Lazarus (1993) who divides coping strategies into adaptive and maladaptive. Adaptive strategies may be further divided into problem solving strategies, which modify some adverse circumstance so as to reduce stress, and emotion-reducing strategies, which enhance one's ability to deal with stress.

Examples of problem solving include obtaining advice or help, making a plan to deal with the problem, or confronting someone about behavior.

Examples of emotion-reducing strategies include ventilation (expressing emotion), avoidance (not thinking about or dealing with a problem right away), accepting or rejecting responsibility for a problem, and reframing the experience so that it is viewed in a positive light.

In our culture, problem solving strategies are often valued more highly than emotion-reducing strategies, but both may be equally effective.

Horowitz (1997) combined elements of process and hierarchy into a unique scheme for looking at response to stress on an individual in terms of *controls* that are used to regulate emotional reaction to a stressful life event. Controls maintain an emotional state or mind-set and may also be responsible for the transition from one state to another. The scheme includes controls of mental set, concepts of self and others, and information flow. Table 1, dealing with control of self-concept is reproduced here to illustrate the method.

As an illustration of the advantage of using a process approach to evaluate coping, consider denial, which is a relatively primitive or immature way of coping in a hierarchical defensive system; yet, research clearly shows that denial can be adaptive in some circumstances, and use of denial may actually improve prognosis (Levenson et al., 1994; Ness & Ende, 1994). Note that Vaillant continues to generate data supporting the use of a hierarchical system (Soldz & Vaillant, 1998). The terminology used to describe hierarchical defenses is widely known and will be briefly reviewed.

In Freudian theory, defense mechanisms are considered unconscious processes, that is, they are not employed deliberately, and the person who uses them is unaware of doing so. Common defense mechanisms include

- Regression, or a return to behavior appropriate to an earlier stage of development.
- Reaction formation, or behaving in a way that reflects the opposite of one's true feelings.

## Table 1. Controls of Self-Concept[a]

| | Sample outcomes | | |
| Processes | Coping | Defense | Succumbing to stress |
|---|---|---|---|
| Altering self-schema that are activated self-concepts | Heightened sense of identity by using the most competent self-concept in the subject's repertoire of self-views | Omnipotent denial of personal vulnerability, "as-if" concepts, regressions to earlier self-concepts | Depersonalization, chaotic lapse of identity, annihilation anxiety |
| Altering dominance hierarchy of available role relationship models and scripts | Seeking help, sublimation | Dissociations and splitting passive-dependent expectations | Sensation of helplessness, separation anxiety |
| Altering dominance hierarchcy of available world views | Increased sense of unity or ideological commitment, altruism, increased sense of reality, sublimation | Altruistic surrender, increased self-centeredness | Sense of meaninglessness or derealization |

[a]*Stress responses syndrome: PTSD, grief, and adjustment disorders*, (p. 106), by M. J. Horowitz, 1997, Northvale, NJ: Jason Aronson Inc. Modified with permission.

- Repression, probably the only defense mechanism described by Sigmund Freud, is the exclusion from consciousness of memories or emotions that would be distressing.
- Denial, mentioned before, is inferred when a person behaves as though unaware of something that should be known. For example, a person told of having a terminal illness may act as if unaware of the diagnosis and may continue normal activities; and as mentioned previously, sometimes this may be adaptive. Denial is frequently inferred in evaluating patients with suspected substance use disorder, and at least in some cases the observed behavior may be due to neurological deficits, not a psychodynamic process (Duffy, 1995).
- Rationalization, unconsciously providing an acceptable explanation for behavior that actually has some other cause.
- Displacement, the transfer of emotion from one person, object, or situation to another (presumably less threatening) person, object, or situation.
- Projection, the attribution to someone else of thoughts or feelings similar to one's own thoughts or feelings.
- Identification, unconsciously adopting the characteristics or activities of another.

- Sublimation, the unconscious diversion of unacceptable impulses into acceptable outlets. For example, turning a need to dominate into organizing a drive for charity.
- Suppression, a *conscious* decision to remove something troubling from immediate awareness until a later date. Because this is a *conscious* decision, some would argue that it is not a defense mechanism but rather a coping skill. The result is the same. Table 2 shows some defense mechanisms arranged hierarchically.

There is no doubt that such mental phenomena occur and can be identified in clinical practice. However, interrater reliability in identifying defense mechanisms is quite poor even when precise definitions are provided (Perry & Cooper, 1989).

How often do emotional disorders occur in patients with medical illness? Superficially, this may seem a simple question but it is fraught with problems of definition. How does one define "emotional disorder?" Rates may differ among acute medical illness, chronic medical illness, *terminal* medical illness, painful illness, disfiguring illness, or combinations. Are we to exclude emotional disorders caused by treating the medical illness or include them? Rate, or the occurrence of cases in a

**Table 2. Hierarchical Classification of Defense Mechanisms (Level)**

| Adaptive level | |
| --- | --- |
| Humor | Anticipation |
| Suppression | Self-assertion |
| Sublimation | Denial[a] |

| Compromise (neurotic) level | |
| --- | --- |
| Repression | Undoing |
| Intellectualization | Reaction formation |
| Displacement | Denial[a] |

| Primitive level | |
| --- | --- |
| Acting out | Projection |
| Passive aggression | Dissociation |
| Hypochondriasis | Denial[a] |

| Very primitive level | |
| --- | --- |
| Splitting | Projective identification |
| Omnipotence | Denial[a] |
| Distortion | |

[a]Denial is placed at all levels to indicate (1) denial can be understood in different ways; (2) the basic problem of a hierarchical system—preconceived notions of whether or not a mental operation is healthy.

population, is the basis of epidemiology. In the case of emotional disorders and medical illness, it has been impossible to define "case" or "population" rigorously, so we are left with estimates. It has been said that "the most conspicuous feature of the emotional response of most people to serious physical illness is their resilience" (Gelder et al., 1996, p. 358), that is, psychiatric disorder does not occur in most people with serious medical illness, but it may occur in 30% or more of those who have serious illness, especially progressive illness that results in a changed life-style.

In addition to psychological reactions to illness and hospitalization, emotional symptoms can represent the direct effects of the physical illness or the treatment process (e.g., drug-induced confusion). In fact, the first step in evaluating a medically ill patient is to consider organic etiologies first and purely psychological reactions second. This is supported by data from large series of consecutive consultations in general hospitals. Knights and Folstein (1977) reported that 37% of general medical ward patients with cognitive impairment went undiagnosed by ward physicians. Additionally, nurses failed to identify 55%, and

medical students overlooked 46%. DePaulo and Folstein (1978) examined thirty-three patients with cognitive impairment on a neurological inpatient ward and found that 30% were not diagnosed by the attending neurologists. Folks and Ford (1985) evaluated 195 patients (60-years old or older) at the request of their primary care physicians. An organic mental disorder was diagnosed in 42%, but in 62% of these cases, the physicians who requested the consultations had not recognized the presence of cognitive dysfunction.

A survey of 118 male veteran patients examined by a psychiatric consultation team diagnosed cognitive dysfunction at a significantly higher rate in older than in younger male patients. Using the Mini-Mental State Exam (MMSE; Folstein, Folstein, & McHugh, 1975), 49.3% of seventy-five male patients 55-years old or older scored abnormally low as compared to 11.6% of forty-three men younger than age 55 (MMSE mean score = 21.4 vs. 27.4; normal: 24–30; paired t-test: $p <$ .0001; Chiarello & Burch, 1989).

As a general guideline, sudden changes in "personality" in an adult with no previous psychiatric history should alert the clinician to the possibility of a nonpsychiatric illness. Some case examples will be used to illustrate this point.

**Case 1.** Mr. A was a 57-year-old white man who was brought to the emergency room (ER) because of increased agitation, anorexia, tearfulness, and suicidal ideation. The patient stated that his change in mood occurred 2 weeks before admission when he tried to get into his car to drive. He had difficulty remembering how to use his keys to unlock the car door and once in the car, could not remember how to drive. His family had interpreted this as a driving phobia. On examination, Mr. A was anxious and tearful, with decreased concentration, short-term memory problems, suicidal ideation, and paranoia. He demonstrated components of expressive and receptive aphasia, with limb and ideational apraxias. His MMSE score was 15 out of 30. Because he had undergone a radical neck dissection for squamous cell cancer 1 year previously, a CT scan of the brain was ordered to rule out metastasis. The CT revealed multiple cystic metastatic lesions in the frontal lobes, with widespread edema. Treatment with radiation and steroids improved his mood, and his MMSE score increased to 24.

**Case 2.** Mr. B was a 49-year-old white man with no previous medical or psychiatric treatment who came to the ER complaining of the acute onset of slurred speech and lethargy during the previous 24 hours. He was overweight and hypertensive (blood pressure = 168/110 mmHg). He had mild ankle edema and an irregular pulse. A neurological exam was normal except for the slurred speech (drug or alcohol intoxication was suspected); a CT of the brain was read as normal. He was admitted to the medical service for treatment of his hypertension and heart failure. Psychiatry was consulted to evaluate Mr. B's depression. It was noted that he had decreased verbal output and was lethargic and disheveled (he was not shaving, combing his hair, or brushing his teeth). Although he did look and sound depressed, his MMSE score was 22, with deficits in calculating ability, short-term recall, spontaneous writing, and design copying. More detailed testing yielded the diagnostic impression of aphasic syndrome with buccofacial and limb apraxias. A repeat CT scan of the brain revealed a small hypodense area in the region of the caudate nucleus (subcortical stroke).

This patient's depressive symptoms improved spontaneously as his aphasia and apraxias resolved. However, it has been reported that 30–60% of acutely and chronically ill poststroke patients have significant levels of depression (Lipsey, Spencer, Rabins, & Robinson, 1986). Because about half of the depressions fulfill the criteria for major depression and last more than 6 months (Lipsey et al., 1986), treatment is important in reducing chronic disability. This is especially true given that poststroke depression is responsive to antidepressant intervention (Lipsey, Robinson, Pearlson, Rao, & Price, 1984).

**Case 3.** Mr. C was a 27-year-old Black female who became anxious when she discovered that her husband was seeing another woman. When her husband asked for a legal separation, the patient went to live with her parents in another state. But Ms. C became increasingly anxious, prompting her family to take her to their medical doctor. The physician referred her to a mental health center, where she was diagnosed with paranoid schizophrenia and treated with 400 mg per day of chlorpromazine. She continued to worsen, with increased agitation and paranoia. The family took her again to the family physician who performed a physical exam and noted an enlarged and palpable thyroid. Thyroxine (T4) level was "too high to measure," and Ms. C was treated with a thyroid-blocking medication and chlorpromazine. Once

the thyroid function normalized, her mental status returned to normal, and she underwent a subtotal thyroidectomy. She was able to become employed, live in the community, and did not require psychiatric drugs.

**Case 4.** Mr. D was a 64-year-old Black man who was brought to the ER by his wife because of a 3-week personality change. Just before Mr. D's personality began changing, he had an argument with his daughter over finances, and she stated that she never wanted to see him again. Mr. D became withdrawn and depressed, had crying spells, and would sit motionless in his chair each day. One week before the hospital visit, it was noted that he was more talkative, animated, and hyperreligious, believing that he was "the Messiah." On examination, he was pacing, hyperactive, and talkative. His speech was pressured, and he demanded that everyone bow down because he was the Messiah. His affect was labile, and he would intermittently become agitated and aggressive. Because he had an history of chronic obstructive pulmonary disease, mitral valve disease, cardiac arrhythmias, and congestive heart failure, he was admitted to the medicine service. The psychiatry consultant medicated him with intramuscular haloperidol so that he could be given a physical exam. Once it was determined that his medical status was stable, he was transferred to the inpatient psychiatry service and placed on oral haloperidol. A CT scan of the brain revealed multiple infarcts, including an apparently recent right occipital infarct. Interestingly, the neurological exam was "nonfocal"; the diagnostic impression was organic mood disorder secondary to cerebral embolization. During the next year, Mr. D developed signs of multi-infarct dementia.

**Case 5.** Mr. E was a 58-year-old man with a long history of hypertension who had been recently discharged from the hospital with congestive heart failure. His blood pressure regimen was changed to methyl dopa, and his wife reported that he had developed a personality change since his discharge. He was lethargic, exhibited little interest, and suffered crying spells. He had begun to consider that life was not worth living but was too religious to commit suicide. On examination, Mr. E was tearful and depressed, and he showed psychomotor retardation. His MMSE score was 20. He had no previous psychiatric history. A tentative diagnosis of drug-induced depression was proposed, and it was recommended that his antihypertensive drug be changed to atenolol (he had tolerated this in the past, and it may cause less depression than methyl dopa) (Henningsen & Mattiasson, 1979). Two weeks after the medicine change, Mr. E was no longer depressed. Thus, his hypertension could be controlled with atenolol while avoiding the drug-induced depression associated with methyl dopa. Likewise, by correctly diagnosing a drug-induced depression (organic mood disorder), Mr. E was spared treatment with an antidepressant medication that would have exposed him to additional side effects.

**Case 6.** Mr. G was a 30-year-old Black male who was HIV positive and was admitted to the coronary care unit for monitoring because of an arrhythmia. Psychiatry was consulted because the patient was highly anxious and agitated over being diagnosed HIV positive. He stated that when he told his girlfriend, she started screaming and told him that she never wanted to see him again. Likewise, his male friends called him a homosexual, which he fervently denied. He also denied drug use and could not understand how this could have happened. He said that he knew it was a "death sentence" because every time he read the newspapers the headlines would say, "No Cure for AIDS." Because of the diagnosis, he felt that his sex life was over, he felt overwhelmed and could not sleep. He was glad to have someone to talk with after so many rejections. Treated with lorazepam, his anxiety symptoms and insomnia improved.

In view of the current AIDS pandemic, it is particularly important to consider the multitude of emotional reactions associated with the diagnosis of HIV infection. The mental health consultant should keep in mind that HIV infection has a predilection for the brain (Gabuzda & Hirsch, 1987) and that invasion of the brain by this virus can cause a variety of changes in personality and mental status, including cognitive and psychotic alterations (Femandez & Ruiz, 1989).

## Psychodiagnosis and Psychological Testing

Psychodiagnosis improved dramatically in reliability with the introduction of the American Psychiatric Association's *Diagnostic and Statistical Manual of Mental Disorders*, 3rd ed. (DSM-III; 1980). The manual is periodically revised and the current edition is the DSM-IV. To achieve interrater reliability, specific and explicit criteria are set forth for each disorder using a polythetic scheme (criteria for different disorders overlap). The *kappa statistic*, proposed in 1960 (Cohen, 1960) as a way of measuring agreement among clinicians, was used in the DSM-III and subsequent DSM editions to assess reliability. Reliability is considered poor if kappa is less than .40, fair if between .40 and .59, good if between .60 and .74, and excellent at or above .75 (Fieiss, 1981; Perry, 1992).

It is generally agreed that acceptable reliability in diagnosing Axis I disorders was achieved by publication of the DSM-III (Grove, 1981, 1987). However, a few disagree (Kutchins & Kirk, 1986).

Unweighted kappa coefficients in phase one and two of the DSM-III field trials were 0.68 and 0.72, respectively, for Axis I disorders in adults, and 0.56 and 0.64, respectively, for Axis II disorders in adults (American Psychiatric Association, 1980, pp. 470–471). Considerably lower kappa coefficients have been reported when diagnosing personality disorder. For instance in one study, clinicians first determined if a personality disorder was present or not; kappa for that was 0.41. For diagnosis of specific personality disorders, kappa was still lower; for example, for borderline personality disorder, it was only 0.29 (Mellsop, Varghese, Joshua, & Hicks, 1982).

Achieving reliability in diagnosis depends largely on adherence to diagnostic criteria. However, there is abundant evidence that clinicians frequently do not apply criteria strictly when making diagnoses, and therefore reliability suffers (Davis, Blashfield, & McEllroy, 1993; Morey & Ochon, 1989). Although it may sound simple, the most important element of making a reliable diagnosis is strict adherence to the diagnostic criteria. Does psychological testing add something if diagnostic criteria are strictly applied? For projective tests, probably not (Garb, 1998). For objective tests such as the MMPI-II, perhaps; in the authors' opinion, the best use of psychological testing is to improve the database used in determining whether criteria are met. For example, neuropsychological testing will determine whether memory loss or visuospatial defects are present in a person suspected of having early dementia, and intelligence testing assists in diagnosing mental retardation.

Garb (1998) suggests several other factors that will improve diagnostic accuracy, such as attention to research; awareness of cultural bias; description of patients' strengths as well as weaknesses; a systematic, comprehensive approach; use of specific strategies to reduce bias; and being very cautious when attempting difficult diagnostic tasks such as predicting violence or making judgments about personality in a depressed patient.

## Evaluating Depression

In a general hospital, "evaluate for depression" is a frequent request to mental health specialists who consult on the medically ill. Of 118 consultations to the New Orleans VA psychiatric consultation service, more than one-third (36%) were for suspected depression (Chiarello & Burch, 1989). The Beck Depression Inventory (BDI); (Beck, 1967) continues to be used to screen for depression among the medically ill; using a BDI cutoff score of 14, Moffic and Paykel (1975) reported that 28.7% of the medically ill they surveyed met the criteria for depression. But would all these patients be classified depressed by the DSM-IV criteria? Probably not, because the BDI is weighted with somatic items and the underlying physical illness must be considered when interpreting the score. Between 50 and 80% of medically ill patients report psychomotor retardation, work inhibition, fatigue, appetite disturbance, weight loss, sleep disturbances, and somatic distress (Cavanaugh, 1984). Complicating further the picture of depression in the medically ill, Cavanaugh, Clark, and Gibbons (1983) reported the presence of a common emotional response in about one-third of medical inpatients that consisted of irritability, sadness, crying, mild dissatisfaction, mild discouragement with the future, and mild indecisiveness. No somatic symptoms were found that were valid, consistent discriminators of medically ill depressed from nonmedically ill depressed patients. These authors, however, concluded that the presence of four affective/cognitive symptoms were important in identifying depression in the medically ill: sense of failure, loss of social interest, sense of punishment, and suicidal ideation.

Craven, Rodin, Johnson, and Kennedy (1987) studied a group of renal dialysis patients using the Diagnostic Interview Schedule (Robins, Helzer, Croughan, Williams, & Spitzer, 1981) and applying the DSM-III criteria. Eight percent of the sample met criteria for major depression, and half of

these had histories of major depressive episodes. Compared to patients without current major depression, patients with major depression were distinguished by the following criteria: depressed mood or loss of interest, feelings of worthlessness or excessive guilt, anorexia or weight loss, and slowed or mixed up thought. Somatic symptoms did not differ in depressed and nondepressed patients. Rapp and Vrana (1989) also used nonsomatic symptoms to diagnose depression in a group of 150 elderly male medical inpatients. The four symptoms they used, tearfulness/depressed appearance, social withdrawal/decreased talkativeness, brooding/self-pity/pessimism, and lack of reactivity to environmental events, were significantly more accurate in diagnosing depression than somatic symptoms.

## Evaluating Substance Use Disorders

Currently, research into the biology of addictions is proceeding at an explosive rate; but for decades, observers have studied the psychology of addictions, and there are important insights from those studies that should not be neglected. For example, Kohut proposed that drugs act as a replacement for some defect in the psychic structure, thereby enabling addicts to cope with rage, shame, hurt, and loneliness (Kohut, 1971). Cognitive behaviorists take the view that alcoholism and drug dependence are maladaptive coping mechanisms that can be changed by learning new ways of coping and new problem solving skills (Beck, 1993). Although such insights are valuable in understanding and treating addicted persons, it is clear that there indeed is a biological foundation of addiction. The psychodynamic theorist George Vaillant studied alcoholism prospectively for 30 years and refuted the idea of an addictive personality (Vaillant, 1983); and catecholamine depletion in the central nervous system, it has been shown, is associated with the desire to reuse drugs, making ego-deficits and unhappy childhoods irrelevant in many cases (Koob & Bloom, 1980).

Diagnosis of substance use disorders requires familiarity with the DSM-IV, which divides substance-related disorders into use disorders (further divided into dependence and abuse syndromes) and induced disorders, which include intoxication, withdrawal, mood disorder, anxiety disorder, delirium, dementia, and others.

Therefore, the differential diagnosis is broad, and diagnosis is often confounded by the fact that patients and families may distort, deny, minimize, or lie about substance use and related problems. A high degree of suspicion about drug use is required, and permission should be sought to obtain collateral data from family members and other sources. Common presentations include insomnia, chronic pain, mood disorder, and anxiety. Psychotic symptoms also occur, as do many others.

The term dual diagnosis generally is applied to persons with comorbid psychiatric and addictive disorders and is clearly one of the major problems within the mental health field currently (Committee on Training & Education in Addiction Psychiatry, 1994). Rates of comorbid disorders range from 15–40% (Regier, 1990; Kessler et al., 1994). At least one reason for the high rate of comorbid disorders is that those who have comorbid psychological and drug problems (alcohol in this study) are more likely to seek help (Helzer & Pryzbeck, 1988). Helzer and Pryzbeck also emphasized that prematurely labeling a psychiatric syndrome of depression, anxiety, or psychosis as major depressive disorder, panic disorder, or schizophrenia can delay treating the actual problem. It is amply demonstrated that the course of a substance-induced psychiatric syndrome is different from the course of a psychiatric disorder not induced by a substance; symptoms are not disorders (Weingold et al., 1968; Brown & Schuckit, 1988; Shuckit et al., 1990; Anthenelli, 1993).

Correct diagnosis is made more difficult because individuals who have primary psychiatric disorders such as schizophrenia or bipolar disorder are at much higher risk of a substance use disorder than nonmentally ill persons. For instance, more than 50% of bipolar patients have substance use disorders at some time in their lives (Regier, 1990; Anthenelli, 1994).

Important aids to accurate diagnosis include

1. Maintain a high index of suspicion for drug use.
2. Use collateral data.
3. Distinguish psychiatric symptoms from psychiatric disorders.
4. Follow the patient and remain flexible.
5. Consider drug screens.

Treatment of addicted patients, especially patients with comorbid psychiatric addictive disorders, is not easy. The authors believe that there is a biological basis underlying the addictive use of substances and that patients are more likely to accept treatment when the diagnosis is couched in terms of illness rather than moral failure (Clark, 1981).

However, broad knowledge of psychology is essential preparation for treating addicted patients who almost universally manifest various defense mechanisms such as denial, rationalization, minimalization, and projection. These psychological mechanisms must be recognized and strategies developed for undermining or supporting the defense, whichever is more appropriate.

Outcome studies do not allow making definitive statements about treatment programs, but in general a multidisciplinary approach seems important (Fox, 1968), as does regular and prolonged outpatient care (Pittman & Tate, 1969; Vannicelli, 1978).

The role, length, and need for inpatient hospitalization versus outpatient treatment remains controversial (Adelman & Weiss, 1989; Cole et al., 1981; Stein et al., 1975). The cost-effectiveness of treating alcoholism is not a settled question either, although the authors believe that the weight of the evidence is solidly on the side that treatment is cost-effective (Rundell & Pardees, 1979; Holder & Hallan, 1986; National Association of Addiction Treatment Providers, 1991).

## Psychopharmacology

The following section is a brief review of psychopharmacology that emphasizes the patient who has both medical and psychiatric illness. It is not intended to be comprehensive or exhaustive, and the reader is referred to other sources for more information, including material on psychotropic drug use in pregnancy, which is not covered here.

### Antipsychotics

Antipsychotic drugs are also called neuroleptics and major tranquilizers. Neuroleptic refers to side effects, and the term major tranquilizer can mislead as to the principal use of the drug; so antipsychotic is used here. A large number of antipsychotic drugs are available, and many are listed in

## Table 3. Generic and Trade Names of Psychotropic Medications Discussed

| Generic name | Trade name | Generic name | Trade name |
|---|---|---|---|
| Antipsychotics | | Benzodiazepines | |
| Chlorpromazine | Thorazine | Alprazolam | Xanax |
| Droperidol | Inapsine | Chlordiazepoxide | Librium |
| Haloperidol | Haldol | Clonazepam | Klonopin |
| Loxapine | Loxitane | Diazepam | Valium |
| Mesoridazine | Serentil | Flurazepam | Dalmane |
| Molindone | Moban | Lorazepam | Ativan |
| Pimozide | Orap | Oxazepam | Serax |
| Thioridazine | Mellaril | Triazolam | Halcion |
| Thiothixine | Navane | | |
| Antidepressants | | | |
| Atypical agents | | Amitriptyline | Elavil |
| Clozapine | Clozaril | Buproprion | Wellbutrin |
| Olanzapin | Zyprexa | Desipramine | Norpramine |
| Quetiapine | Seroquel | Doxepin | Sinequan |
| Risperidone | Risperdal | Fluoxetine | Prozac |
| | | Fluvoxamine | Luvox |
| Mood stabilizers | | Imipramine | Tofranil |
| Carbamazepine | Tegretol | Mirtazapine | Remaron |
| Lithium carbonate | Eskalith | Nefazodone | Serzone |
| | Lithobid | Nortriptyline | Pamelor |
| | Lithane | Trazodone | Desyrel |
| Sodium valproate | Depakote | Venlafaxine | Effexor |
| | Depakene | | |
| Miscellaneous | | | |
| Zolpidem | Ambien | | |

Table 3. The table distinguishes newer, so called "atypical" antipsychotic drugs; the reason for this is that these newer agents have assumed great importance in treating psychotic illness because they are effective in improving the negative symptoms of schizophrenia (anhedonia, alogia, apathy, blunt affect), whereas the older drugs are not. The newer agents are also less likely to cause extrapyramidal (neuroleptic) side effects. The first of the newer agents to become available, clozapine, it was shown in controlled studies, results in improvement in up to 50% of patients who were not helped by other drugs (Kane et al., 1988). Unfortunately, there is a significant risk of agranulocytosis (1–2%), which can be fatal and which requires regular hematologic monitoring. The newer atypical antipsychotics, risperidone, olanzapine, and quetiapine, have some of the benefits of clozapine without the risk of agranulocytosis. They are all too new to make specific recommendations about their use, but certainly they should be tried if older antipsychotics have failed and should be considered drugs of choice for a patients with significant negative symptoms.

All antipsychotics have in common an ability to block dopamine receptors, which may account for the therapeutic effect, although this is still being investigated. Most antipsychotic drugs, especially the older ones, bind strongly to the dopamine D2 receptor, and this appears to account for both antipsychotic action and the development of move-ment disorders. Clozapine, one of the newer agents, has a relatively weak affinity for D2 recep-tors, and the antipsychotic effect may be due to blockade of multiple receptors, including dop-amine D4 and serotonin 5-HT receptors (Coward, 1992). Movement disorders are unlikely to occur with clozapine.

**Side Effects.** Detailed side effects of individual drugs can be found in any standard clinical phar-macology reference, which should be consulted before prescribing any agent. Here we review only a few major areas. *Extrapyramidal effects*: The effects result from dopamine blockade and can be divided into four major categories: *Acute dystonia* occurs soon after treatment begins, especially in young men. It is prevented by using low doses of antipsychotics and can be treated by anticho-linergic agents (benztropine mesylate) or anti-histaminic drugs (diphenhydramine). Acute dys-tonia involves spasm of large muscle groups, particularly in the upper body and neck and may need to be treated with IM or IV drug if severe, and especially if there is respiratory distress because of laryngeal spasm. *Akathisia* is a very unpleasant sensation of restlessness, resulting in an inability to stay still. It is treated with dose reduction, anti-cholinergic drugs, or beta-blockers. *Parkinsonism* is characterized by akinesia, rigidity, tremor, ex-pressionless face, stooped posture, and occa-sionally festinating gait. It is treated with anti-Parkinson drugs, but usually not L-dopa for fear the psychosis will worsen. *Tardive dyskinesia* is characterized by involuntary movements of the mouth and tongue which may resemble chewing, grimacing, or sucking, by choreoathetoid move-ments of the upper extremities, and by truncal ataxia in severe cases. It may not reverse when the drugs are stopped, and there is no effective treat-ment, so this is a particularly serious problem. The older antipsychotics are more likely to cause these problems than the newer ones, hence the increas-ing popularity of the newer agents.

## Which Drug to Choose?

It is a general rule of psychotropic drug use that if a patient is doing well on a particular drug or has done well on it in the past, use that drug. If nega-tive symptoms are present, use a newer "atypical" drug. The authors now start most new patients on olanzapine or risperidone. Risperidone is quite useful in low doses in elderly patients who may be prone to extrapyramidal effects and who may be oversedated with olanzapine or quetiapine.

Chlorpromazine, droperidol, and haloperidol may all be given IM to produce rapid calming (IM chlorpromazine is quite painful). It is also com-mon practice to combine haloperidol with lorazepam (a benzodiazepine) as an IM mixture to produce rapid calming. At this time, the newer atypical agents are not available for IM or IV use. Halo-peridol can be given IV, and there is considerable experience with it, but it is an "off label use," one that is not approved by the FDA; the prescriber should be aware that, although such use is per-fectly legal, there is added responsibility to inform the patient or the patient's surrogate.

## Antidepressants

Depressive disorders are common in the medi-cally ill, although not so common as popularly believed. For instance, Silverstone found that only 27% in a group of 313 medically ill patients met criteria for any DSM-IV disorder and about 5% had major depressive disorder (Silverstone, 1996). The rate of any depressive disorder may be higher in patients with chronic medical illness such as cancer (Spiegel, 1996). Studies have consistently shown that in a primary care setting, depression is both underrecognized and undertreated. Depres-sion does have substantial morbidity and even mortality, and therefore recognition and adequate treatment are important. Serotonin specific re-uptake inhibitors (SSRIs) have become the most popular first-line treatment for depression because they are easy to use (not much dose adjustment is necessary) and they have few side effects. Practi-tioners develop preferences for one SSRI over another based (probably) on episodic successful use (a form of intermittent reinforcement). There actually is little data to suggest that one is better than another. There are questions about the efficacy of SSRIs in treating severe depression (Rudorfer & Potter, 1989). For severe depression not respon-sive to an SSRI, the addition of a tricyclic (TCA) or another agent may enhance the antidepressant response. Some newer agents that deserve men-tion are venlafaxine, nefazodone, buproprion, and mirtazapine. Venlafaxine (Effexor) blocks se-rotonin and norepinephrine re-uptake and has little in the way of sedative or anticholinergic side effects (Feighner, 1994). Nefazodone (Serzone), is related to trazodone but is not as sedating. Buproprion (Wellbutrin) was introduced in the United States in the mid-1980s, withdrawn because of an association with seizures, and then reintroduced in 1989. It is effective, seizure incidence is not alarming if the dose is not too high, and it has no sexual side effects. Mirtazapine (Remeron) is the newest antidepressant drug available at this time. It is structurally different from any other antidepressant available in the United States and enhances both noradrenergic and serotonergic transmission, probably its mechanism of action.

In the decade from 1988 (Prozac introduced) to 1998, there has been a paradigm shift in antidepressant prescribing patterns. The drugs mentioned earlier are used almost exclusively to treat depression and various other disorders for which antidepressants may be indicated; drugs in use before 1988, the TCAs and the monoamine oxidase inhibitors (MAOIs), are infrequently used now. As mentioned, the reasons for this shift are that the newer agents have few side effects, dose-response relationships are simple, and they are generally effective. TCAs and MAOIs have multiple side effects, and dosing is difficult, but they are very effective if adequate doses are given.

## Which Drug to Use?

The authors recommend an SSRI as the first-line treatment for depression; venlafaxine or mirtazapine can be used for patients with a history of SSRI nonresponsiveness, and buproprion may be helpful if sexual side effects are a problem. TCAs and MAOIs still have a place but probably should be used only by experts. The combination of a TCA plus an SSRI is effective, but care must be taken to ensure that the TCA blood level does not reach the toxic range (Bell & Cole, 1988; Kahn, 1990; Vaughn, 1988). In particular patients, antidepressant choice may be influenced by potential drug interactions related to the cytochrome P450 system, especially among the medically ill (Nemeroff et al., 1996).

### Anxiolytics

Antidepressants, especially SSRIs and TCAs, may be useful in treating anxiety. Both SSRIs and TCAs are effective in blocking panic attacks;

TCAs are effective in generalized anxiety disorder, and MAOIs may be effective in both but are difficult to use.

Antihistamines are sometimes used to treat anxiety when prescribers are concerned about benzodiazepine (BZ) abuse. Although clearly less effective than BZs, they may be indicated for some patients. Hydroxyzine is most commonly used but is anticholinergic and should be used with caution, especially for the elderly.

Barbiturates are less effective than BZs, less safe, and more likely to be abused. They should no longer be used to treat anxiety.

Buspirone (Buspar) is chemically different from the BZs. It does not impair arousal or reaction time and has no abuse potential. It is effective for generalized anxiety disorder, although less effective for individuals previously treated with BZs. It has many characteristics of an ideal antianxiety drug but has been somewhat disappointing in clinical practice for reasons not entirely clear. It is not effective at all in treating panic disorder. Buspar does have mild antidepressant actions at doses higher than its anxiolytic dosage (Fabre, 1990).

### Mood Stablilizers

Lithium carbonate has been used for decades to treat acute mania, but valproate is becoming a favored alternative. Lithium is inexpensive, and most clinicians are familiar with it, but it can be toxic to the kidneys, and renal function must be monitored during its use. A further limitation in medically ill patients is that diuretics, nonsteroidal anti-inflammatory agents, and several other drugs, can raise lithium levels. Levels should be monitored to prevent toxicity. Lithium may have neurotoxic effects, even at therapeutic levels, and patients with preexisting brain disease (e.g., stroke or dementia) are more sensitive to these effects, which include headache, decreased memory, poor concentration, muscle weakness, and tremor.

Valproic acid has been used to treat seizures since the 1960s. In 1995, divalproex sodium, an enteric-coated equimolar combination of valproic acid and sodium valproate, was approved for treating acute mania (Bowden, Brugger, & Swan, 1994). It may be started in fairly small divided doses (250 mg, two to three times a day), and the doses are gradually increased, or a loading dose of 20 mg/kg may be started and continued until levels are between 50 and 125 mg/mL. The response may be very rapid if loading doses are used (McElroy et al., 1996).

Carbamazepine (CBZ), structurally related to the TCAs, is generally considered effective in treating acute mania and may prevent recurrence of bipolar illness, but firm proof is lacking. CBZ may be used with lithium, valproate, a neuroleptic, or as mono therapy. If used with another agent, especially valproate, levels of each agent should be monitored. CBZ induces its own metabolism, making it necessary to adjust dosage to maintain an effective level. It may also cause cardiac conduction abnormalities, thus limiting its usefulness in patients with heart disease.

Lamotrigine (Lamictal), another anticonvulsant drug, may have antidepressant and mood stabilizing effects, but it has not been well studied.

# Particular Stresses on Health Care Providers

## Burnout

Burnout has been much talked about and has been actually studied fairly well. There are several definitions of the term and the authors prefer the one derived by Pines and Aronson (1988) which is that burnout is "a state of physical, emotional, and mental exhaustion caused by long term involvement in emotionally demanding situations." It has been studied specifically in mental health workers where high levels of burnout were found that resulted in low morale, high absenteeism, and high job turnover (Pines & Maslach, 1978).

Burnout occurs when people who are highly invested in their work, usually demanding work, do not achieve what they expect. People want their work to be significant, to mean something, and if they think they have failed, burnout occurs.

**Case Example.** A psychiatrist was consulted by the head nurse of a medical unit to assist in resolving a crisis among the nursing staff who worked on the unit. A meeting was scheduled for the nurses, and they described the following scenario. A nursing colleague they all knew and loved had been hospitalized on their unit (at their request). This nurse was dying of chronic hepatitis that she contracted while working in the hospital. She was being treated by the most respected liver specialist in the community (this was in the days before liver transplantation). But the nurses were angry and

frustrated about the care this physician was providing: "He's not doing enough for her. She's deteriorating every day. There's got to be more that can be done!" At this point, all the nurses were crying. They understood that their friend was dying, but emotionally, they identified with her: "It could be any of us lying there suffering." In this tragic situation, they felt they had failed and also displaced part of the blame for this failure onto the physician. When confronted, they admitted they could not think of anything else that could be done. They acknowledged that their attempts to provide physical and psychological support to their friend were helping her be more comfortable but that the emotional energies devoted to their friend were not leaving time or energy to care for the other patients.

Several things were accomplished with this consultation. First, the nurses were able to admit that everything was being done that was medically available and that their interventions were appreciated by the patient. Furthermore, their interventions had led to a greater level of comfort for the patient. Acknowledging that having their friend on the unit was overwhelming, they agreed to transfer her to another ward. Because this was the consultant's decision, the nurses did not feel guilty for abandoning their friend, which they might otherwise have done. There was a sense of relief after the transfer occurred.

Dealing with burnout requires understanding *coping*, introduced earlier in this chapter. Coping can also be understood as an effort to overcome challenges or threats of harm when an automatic response is not available (Monat & Lazarus, 1985). Coping does not imply success in dealing with a stressful situation, only that an effort is made. It is the link between stress and adaptation; four categories of coping have been identified in studies of burnout:

1. active, direct (e.g., confront and alter the stress)
2. inactive, direct (e.g., ignore or leave the stressful situation)
3. active, indirect (e.g., talk about the stress with a supportive person)
4. inactive, indirect (e.g., use alcohol or drugs).

The active strategies tend to work best and successful coping requires four things:

1. awareness of the problem

2. taking responsibilities for dealing with the problem
3. clarifying what can possibly be changed and what probably cannot
4. improving existing coping skills & developing new ones (Pines & Kafry, 1981; Pines & Aronson, 1988; Pines, 1993).

## Malpractice

A claim of malpractice is particularly stressful for health care workers because it calls their professional competency into question. The process is unfamiliar to most health care workers and is controlled by lawyers and judges, so that the accused health care worker feels powerless, and "failure" is certainly implied. This is true whether or not a malpractice claim has merit. If indeed there has been some degree of negligence, an element of guilt is added which contributes to the feelings of failure and may accelerate burnout (Ely et al., 1995). Malpractice suits commonly involve physicians, but all other health care workers are subject to suit as well, and this sometimes leads to conflicts among health care workers as one worker tries to place blame for an incident on another. Although not well studied, in the authors' experience, it is not uncommon for physicians being sued to present for treatment with significant symptoms, including depression, sleeplessness, anxiety, and substance use problems.

## HIV Infection

The AIDS epidemic has taken a staggering toll. In 1998, the World Health Organization reported there had been 130,000 adult deaths in the United States and 2.3 million worldwide; 2.5 million people in the United States are HIV positive and more than 30 million are positive worldwide (WHO, 1998). The disease is transmittable, not curable, and working with infected patients has added tremendous stress on the health care profession. Wallack (1989) conducted a survey of house staff (resident physicians) and nurses at a New York City hospital in 1985 regarding attitudes and beliefs about AIDS. Sixty-five percent of the house staff and 63% of the nursing staff felt that they were at risk of contracting HIV infection, even if they followed the hospital's infection control policies. Eighty-seven percent of those surveyed admitted to experiencing greater anxiety when car-

ing for AIDS patients, compared to other patients. These attitudes can affect the kind of care that is delivered. Avoidance of entering an AIDS patient's room can lead to isolation when the patient needs psychological support. On the other hand, transmission of the incurable viral infection through needle sticks or via blood splashing in the eye or into a cut is a daily reality for health care providers.

AIDS is an incurable disease that affects mainly young patients, and overidentification can add to the emotional responses among health care providers.

## Dying Patients

There is an extensive and rapidly growing literature on the way to deal with patients who are dying, including advice on responding to requests for assistance in dying, how to manage pain, and what to do about other physical or emotional problems. There is little data, however, about the effects on caregivers of dealing with dying patients. Block and Andrews have written about many aspects of working with dying patients, and they believe (as do the authors) that "for many physicians a dying patient represents a personal failure" and that the responses of caregivers to working with dying patients may include depression, avoidance, anger, denial, and guilt (Block & Billings, 1998). The mental health consultant may be asked to deal with these problems in caregivers and may have to suggest tactfully that the caregiver's response is the problem that needs to be addressed because the problem may not be recognized by those dealing with the patient, as illustrated by the case example in this section.

## References

Adelman, S. A., & Weiss, R. D. (1989). What is therapeutic about inpatient alcoholism treatment? *Hospital and Community Psychiatry, 40*, 515–519.

American Psychiatric Association. (1980). *Diagnostic and statistical manual of mental disorders*, 3rd ed. (pp. 470–471). Washington, DC: Author.

American Psychiatric Association. (1994). *Diagnostic and statistical manual of mental disorders* (4th ed.). Washington, DC: Author.

Anthenelli, R. M. (1994). The initial evaluation of the dual diagnosis patient. *Psychiatric Annals, 24*, 407–411.

Anthenelli, R. M., & Schuckit, M. A. (1993). Affective and anxiety disorders and alcohol and drug dependence: Diagnosis and treatment. *Journal of Addictive Disorders, 12*, 73–87.

Beck, A. T. (1967). *Depression: Clinical, experimental and theoretical aspects.* New York: Hoeber.

Beck, A. T., Wright, F. D., Newman, C. F., & Liese, B. S. (1993). *Cognitive therapy of substance abuse.* New York: Guilford.

Bell, J. R., & Cole, J. O. (1988). Fluoxetine induces elevation of desipramine level and exacerbation of geriatric nonpsychotic depression. *Journal of Psychopharmacology, 8,* 447–448.

Block, S. D., & Billings, J. A. (1998). Evaluating patient requests for euthanasia and assisted suicide in terminal illness: The role of the psychiatrist. In M. D. Steinberg & S. J. Younger (Eds.), *End-of-life decisions.* Washington, DC: American Psychiatric Press.

Bowden, C. L., Brugger, A. M., & Swann, A. C. (1994). Efficacy of divalproex versus lithium and placebo in the treatment of mania. *Journal of the American Medical Association, 271,* 918–924.

Brown, S. A., & Schuckit, M. A. (1988). Changes in depression among abstinent alcoholics. *Journal of Studies on Alcohol, 49,* 412–417.

Cavanaugh, S. V. A. (1984). Diagnosing depression in the hospitalized patient with chronic medical illness. *Journal of Clinical Psychiatry, 45,* 13–16.

Cavanaugh, S. V. A., Clark, D. C., & Gibbons, R. D. (1983). Diagnosing depression in the hospitalized medically ill. *Psychosomatics, 24,* 809–815.

Chiarello, N., & Burch, E. A., Jr. (1989). Recognition and treatment of psychiatric disorders in the hospitalized medically ill elderly (abstract). *Southern Medical Journal, 8,* 138.

Clark, W. B. (1981). Alcoholism: Blocks to diagnosis and treatment. *American Journal of Medicine, 71,* 275–286.

Cohen, J. (1960). A coefficient of agreement for nominal scales. *Educational and Psychological Measurement, 20,* 37–46.

Cole, S. G., Lehman, W. E., & Cole, E. A. (1981). Inpatient versus outpatient treatment of alcohol and drug abusers. *American Journal of Drug and Alcohol Abuse, 8,* 329–345.

Committee on Training and Education in Addiction Psychiatry. (1994). Position statement on the need for improved training for treatment of patients with combined substance use and other psychiatric disorders. *American Journal of Psychiatry, 151,* 795–796.

Coward, D. (1992). General pharmacology of clozapine. *British Journal of Psychiatry, 160*(Suppl. 17), 5–11.

Craven, I. L., Rodin, G. M., Johnson, L., & Kennedy, S. H. (1987). The diagnosis of major depression in renal dialysis patients. *Psychosomatic Medicine, 49,* 482–492.

Davis, R. T., Blashfield, R. U., & McElroy, R. A. (1993). Weighing criteria in the diagnosis of a personality disorder. A demonstration. *Journal of American Psychology, 102,* 319–322.

DePaulo, J. R., & Folstein, M. E. (1978). Psychiatric disturbances in neurological patients: Detection, recognition, and hospital course. *Annals of Neurology, 4,* 225–228.

Dohrenwend, B. S., & Dohrenwend, B. P. (1981). Life stress and illness: Formulation of the issues. In B. S. Dohrenwend & B. P. Dohrenwend (Eds.), *Stressful life events and their contexts.* New York: Watson.

Duffy, J. D. (1995). The neurology of alcoholic denial: Implication for assessment and treatment. *Canadian Journal of Psychiatry—Revue Canadienne de Psychiatrie, 40,* 257–263.

Ely, J. W., Levinson, W., Elder, N. C., Mainous, A. G., & Vinson, D. C. (1995). Perceived causes of family physicians' errors. *Journal of Family Practice, 40*(4), 337–344.

Fabre, L. F. (1990). Buspirone in the management of major depression: A placebo-controlled comparison. *Journal of Clinical Psychiatry, 51*(9 Suppl.), 55–61.

Feighner, J. P. (1994). The role of venlafaxine in rational antidepressant therapy. *Journal of Clinical Psychiatry, 59*(9 Suppl. A), 62–68.

Fernandez, E., & Ruiz, R. (1989). Psychiatric aspects in HIV disease. *Southern Medical Journal, 78,* 239–241.

Fleiss, J. L. (1981). *Statistical methods for rates and proportions,* 2nd ed. New York: Wiley.

Folks, D. B., & Ford, C. V. (1985). Psychiatric disorders in geriatric medical/surgical patients. Part 1: Report of 195 consecutive consultations. *Southern Medical Journal, 78,* 239–241.

Folstein, M. E., Folstein, S. E., & McHugh, P. R. (1975). "Minimental state": A practical method for grading the cognitive state of patients for the clinician. *Journal of Psychiatric Research, 12,* 189–198.

Fox, R. (1968). A multidisciplinary approach to the treatment of alcoholism. *International Journal of Psychiatry, 1,* 34–44.

Freudenberger, H. J. (1974). Staff burnout. *Journal of Social Issues, 30,* 159–165.

Gabuzda, D. H., & Hirsch, M. S. (1987). Neurologic manifestations of infection with human immunodeficiency virus: Clinical features and pathogenesis. *Annals of Internal Medicine, 107,* 383–391.

Garb, H. N. (1998). *Studying the clinician. Judgment research and psychological assessment* (p. 233). Washington, DC: American Psychological Association.

Gelder, M., Guth, D., Mayon, R., & Cowen, P. (1996). *Oxford textbook of psychiatry,* 3rd ed. (p. 358). New York: Oxford University Press.

Grove, W. M. (1987). The reliability of psychiatric diagnosis. In C. G. Last & M. Hersen (Eds.), *Issues in diagnostic research* (pp. 99–119). New York: Plenum.

Grove, W. M., Andreasen, N. C., McDonald-Scott, P., Keller, M. B., & Shapiro, R. W. (1981). Reliability studies of psychiatric diagnosis. *Archives of General Psychiatry, 38,* 408–413.

Helzer, J. E., & Przybeck, T. R. (1988). The co-occurrence of alcoholism with other psychiatric disorders in the general population and its impact on treatment. *Journal of Studies in Alcohol, 49,* 219–224.

Henningsen, N. C., & Mattiasson, I. (1979). Long-term clinical experience with atenolol—a new selective beta-I-blocker with few side effects from the central nervous system. *Acta Medica Scandinavica, 205,* 61–66.

Holder, H. D., & Hullan, J. B. (1986). Impact of alcoholism treatment on total healthcare costs: A six year study. *Advances in Alcohol and Substance Abuse, 6,* 1–15.

Horowitz, M. (1997). *Stress response syndromes: PTSD, grief and adjustment disorders,* 3rd ed. Northvale, NJ: Jason Aronson.

Kahn, D. G. (1990). Increased plasma nortriptyline concentration in a patient treated with fluoxetine. *Journal of Clinical Psychiatry, 51,* 36.

Kane, J., Honigfeld, G., Singer, J., & Meltzer, H. (1988). Clozapine for the treatment-resistant schizophrenic: A double blind comparison with chlorpromazine. *Archives of General Psychiatry, 45,* 789–796.

Kessler, R. C., McGonagle, K. A., & Zhao, S. (1994). Lifetime and 12-month prevalence of DSM-III-R psychiatric disorders in the United States: Results from the National Comorbidity Survey. *Archives of General Psychiatry, 51,* 8–19.

Knights, E. B., & Folstein, M. E. (1977). Unsuspected emotional and cognitive disturbances in medical patients. *Annals of Internal Medicine, 87*, 723–724.

Kohut, H. (1971). *The analysis of the self*. New York: International Universities Press.

Koob, G. F., & Bloom, F. E. (1980). Cellular and molecular mechanisms of drug dependence. *Science, 242*, 715–723.

Kutchins, H., & Kirk, S. A. (1986). The reliability of DSM-III: A critical review. *Social Work Research and Abstracts, 22*, 3–12.

Lazarus, R. S. (1993). Coping theory and research: Past, present, and future. *Psychosomatic Medicine, 55*, 234–247.

Levenson, J. L., Mishra, A., Hamer, R. M., & Hastillo, A. (1994). Denial and medical outcome in unstable angina. *Psychosomatic Medicine, 51*, 27–35.

Lewis, A. J. (1956). Psychological medicine. In D. Hunter (Ed.), *Price's textbook of the practice of medicine*, 9th ed. London: Oxford University Press.

Lipsey, J. R., Robinson, R. G., Pearlson, G. D., Rao, K., & Price, T. R. (1984). Nortriptyline for post-stroke depression: A double blind study. *Lancet, 1*, 297–300.

Lipsey, J. R., Spencer, W. C., Rabins, P. V., & Robinson, R. G. (1986). Phenomenological comparison of poststroke depression and functional depression. *American Journal of Psychiatry, 143*, 527–529.

Maslach, C. (1976). Burned out. *Human Behavior, 5*, 16–22.

McElroy, S. L., Kech, P. L., Stanton, S. P., Tugrul, K. C., Bennett, J. A., & Strukowski, S. M. (1996). A randomized comparison of divalproex oral loading versus haloperidol in the initial treatment of acute psychotic mania. *Journal of Clinical Psychiatry, 57*, 142–146.

Mellsop, G., Varghese, F., Joshua, S., & Hicks, A. (1982). The reliability of Axis II of DSM-III. *American Journal of Psychiatry, 139*, 1360–1361.

Moffic, H. S., & Paykel, E. S. (1975). Depression in medical inpatients. *British Journal of Psychiatry, 126*, 346–353.

Monat, A., & Lazarus, R. S. (1985). *Stress and coping*. New York: Columbia University Press.

Morey, L. C., & Ochon, E. S. (1989). An investigation of adherence to diagnostic criteria: Clinical diagnosis of the DSM-III personality disorders. *Journal of Personality Disorders, 3*, 180–187.

National Association of Addiction Treatment Providers. (1991). *Treatment is the answer: A white paper on the cost effectiveness of alcoholism and drug dependency treatment*. Laguna Hills, CA: Author.

Nemeroff, C. B., DeVane, C. L., & Pollock, B. G. (1996). Newer antidepressants and the cytochrome P450 system. *American Journal of Psychiatry, 153*, 311–320.

Ness, D. E., & Ende, J. (1994). Denial in the medical interview: Recognition and management. *Journal of the American Medical Association, 272*, 1777–1781.

Perry, J. C., & Cooper, S. H. (1989). An empirical study of defense mechanisms: Clinical interview and life vignette ratings. *Archives of General Psychiatry, 46*, 444–452.

Perry, J. C. (1992). Problems and considerations in the valid assessment of personality disorders. *American Journal of Psychiatry, 149*, 1645–1653.

Pines, A., & Aronson, E. (1988). *Career burnout: Causes and cures*, 2nd ed. New York: The Free Press.

Pines, A., & Kafry, D. (1981). Coping with burnout. In J. Jones (Ed.), *The burnout syndrome*. Parkridge, IL: London House Press.

Pines, A., & Maslach, C. (1978). Characteristics of staff burnout in mental health settings. *Hospital and Community Psychiatry, 29*, 233–237.

Pines, A M. (1993). Burnout. In L. Goldberger & S. Bresnitz (Eds.), *Handbook of stress: Theoretical and clinical aspects*. New York: The Free Press.

Pittman, D. J., & Tate, R. I. (1969). A comparison of two treatment programs for alcoholics. *Quarterly Journal of Studies on Alcoholism, 30*, 888–899.

Rapp, S. R., & Vrana, S. (1989). Substituting nonsomatic for somatic symptoms in the diagnosis of depression in elderly male medical patients. *American Journal of Psychiatry, 146*, 1197–1120.

Regier, D. A., Farmer, M. E., & Rae, D. S. (1990). Comorbidity of mental disorders with alcohol and other drug abuse—results from the Epidemiologic Catchment Area (ECA) study. *Journal of the American Medical Association, 264*, 2511–2518.

Robins, L. N., Helzer, J. E., Croughan, J., Williams, I. B. W., & Spitzer, R. L. (1981). The NIMH Diagnostic Interview Schedule: Version III (DHHS Publication ADM T-42-3). Washington, DC: U.S. Government Printing Office.

Rudorfer, M. V., & Potter, W. Z. (1989). Anti-depressants: A comparative review of the clinical pharmacology and therapeutic use of the "newer" versus the older drugs. *Drugs, 37*, 713–738.

Rundell, O. H., & Pardee, A. (1979). Benefit-cost methodology in the evaluation of therapeutic services for alcoholism. *Alcohol Clinical and Experimental Research, 3*, 324–333.

Shuckit, M. A., Irwin, M., & Brown, S. A. (1990). The history of anxiety symptoms among 171 primary alcoholics. *Journal of Studies in Alcohol, 49*, 412–417.

Silverstone, P. H. (1996). Prevalence of psychiatric disorders in medical inpatients. *Journal of Nervous and Mental Disease, 184*, 43–51.

Soldz, S., & Vaillant, G. E. (1998). A 50-year longitudinal study of defense use among inner city men: A validation of the DSM-IV defense axis. *Journal of Nervous and Mental Diseases, 186*, 104–111.

Spiegel, D. (1996). Cancer and depression. *British Journal of Psychiatry, 30*(Suppl.), 109–116.

Stein, L. F., Newton, J. R., & Bowman, R. S. (1975). Duration of hospitalization for alcoholism. *Archives of General Psychiatry, 32*, 247–252.

Vaillant, G. E. (1977). *Adaptation to life*. Boston: Little, Brown.

Vaillant, G. E. (1983). *The natural history of alcoholism: Causes, patterns, and paths to recovery*. Cambridge, MA: Harvard University Press.

Vaillant, G. E. (1992). *Ego mechanisms of defense*. Washington, DC: American Psychiatric Press.

Vannicelli, M. (1978). Impact of aftercare in the treatment of alcoholics: A cross-legged panel analysis. *Journal of Studies in Alcohol, 39*, 1875–1886.

Vaughn, D. A. (1988). Interaction of fluoxetine with tricyclic antidepressants. *American Journal of Psychiatry, 145*, 1478.

Wallack, J. J. (1989). AIDS anxiety among health care professionals. *Hospital and Community Psychiatry, 40*, 507–510.

Weingold, J. P., Luchlin, J. M., Bell, H., & Coxe, R. C. (1968). Depression as a symptom of alcoholism: Search for a phenomenon. *Journal of Abnormal Psychology, 73*, 195–197.

# CHAPTER 29

# Behavioral Disorders Associated with Central Nervous System Dysfunction

## Steven A. Castellon, Charles H. Hinkin, and Paul Satz

## Introduction

In this chapter, we introduce some of the behavioral disturbances that are associated with acquired insult or injury to the central nervous system (CNS). Because the CNS ultimately mediates all aspects of human behavior, neurological disorder, regardless of etiology, can produce changes in cognition, perception, emotion, affect, and/or personality. In this chapter, we have chosen to focus our attention on the changes in emotion, affect, and personality that accompany neurological disease/disorder.

Study of the behavioral expression of neurological disorder has been a contribution of the fields of neuropsychology, neuropsychiatry, and behavioral neurology. The cognitive/intellectual deficits associated with specific neurological conditions have been well characterized elsewhere (e.g. Kolb & Wishaw, 1995; Lezak, 1995) and in this chapter, we only briefly address these changes.

Instead we devote most of our attention to the less thoroughly studied realm of *psychiatric* morbidity in neurological conditions. This chapter, after providing some basic background information, provides an overview of the main classes of psychiatric symptoms and signs that may occur in diseases and disorders of the CNS. Then, we examine several specific neurological conditions with particular regard to the types of psychopathology seen in each.

### Background Considerations

Much of what we know about the functioning of the brain has been learned by studying individuals who have suffered some form of brain pathology. The behavioral consequences of brain insult or injury vary extraordinarily depending on multiple factors, including age, gender, and the affected individual's previous level of intellectual function. Perhaps more important is the type of injury or insult incurred. Lesion size and location often have reliable and predictable effects on the behavioral disturbances noticed. It is well beyond the scope of this chapter to detail the neuroanatomy and behavioral geography of the human brain, but we will briefly introduce a few key concepts. **Organization of the Human Brain.** Providing any but the most basic neuroanatomy of the

Steven A. Castellon, Charles Hinkin, and Paul Satz • Department of Psychiatry and Biobehavioral Sciences, UCLA School of Medicine, Los Angeles, California 90024.

*Comprehensive Handbook of Psychopathology* (Third Edition), edited by Patricia B. Sutker and Henry E. Adams. Kluwer Academic / Plenum Publishers, New York, 2001.

brain is well beyond the scope of this chapter. Where possible and practical, we will attempt to provide basic background information necessary to understand the more relevant concepts. The human brain can be very roughly divided along three organizational planes: lateral, longitudinal, and vertical. *Lateralization* refers to differences between the right and left hemispheres of the brain, which for the most part are mirror images of one another. The primary sensory and motor areas of the brain are positioned in both hemispheres, and with few exceptions, these centers in each cerebral hemisphere predominate in mediating the activities of the contralateral half of the body. In general, in the vast majority of individuals, the left hemisphere plays a dominant role in verbal, symbolic, and analytic function, whereas the right hemisphere is crucial in nonverbal and spatial processing. As we will detail later, there are some important differences in the types of emotional and personality disturbances seen following left- versus right-sided lesions. Longitudinally, the brain can be roughly divided into *anterior* and *posterior* regions. Although a vast oversimplification, the anterior portion of the brain mediates motor response and executive function (the initiation, coordination, execution, and oversight of purposeful behavior), and the posterior portion of the brain is related to sensory and perceptual function. Vertical organization refers to differences between cortical and subcortical areas, which we describe in greater detail later.

Finally, two prominent fissures on the surface of the brain, as well as visually prominent sulci, divide the brain into four lobes—frontal, parietal, temporal, and occipital. Note that these lobes are defined solely on the basis of surface markings, rather than more functional characteristics. In terms of the way these different brain regions relate to behavior, there is a rich and extensive history of theory about brain–behavior relations. Theories of localization implied that specific mental operations/functions resided in specific areas in the brain, and lateralization theories suggested that some functions were predominately mediated by one hemisphere or the other. A more integrative and widely accepted theory is that of parallel distributed processing (PDP). PDP implies the existence of integrated neuronal circuits that are widely distributed in the brain and can be modified (within limits) by learning. Any point in the circuit may interconnect with other circuits; hence, there

can be multiple potential effects from a single lesion. It follows then that similar effects could emerge from lesions at different points within the same circuit. Note that a PDP model of brain behavior relationships is not inconsistent with the assertion that certain brain structures or regions are intimately tied to certain types of behavioral outputs.

**History and Terminology: Functional versus Organic.** A long history of classifying behavioral disorders as "functional" or "organic" is giving way to a conceptualization of behavior that sees both psychiatric and cognitive behaviors as dual-pronged manifestations of CNS activity. The term "idiopathic" to describe those symptoms or syndromes that have no known or likely neurological precipitant and "neuropsychiatric" to describe those that do is a more useful way of viewing psychiatric symptoms/signs. Another useful classification scheme is *primary* versus *secondary* disorders. Primary disorders are those that are idiopathic, whereas secondary disorders are those that are known, or at least it is thought, have a neurological, systemic, or pharmacological cause. Many of the disorders described in earlier chapters (e.g., schizophrenia, unipolar and bipolar depression), which have traditionally been labeled as "functional" disorders, involve dramatically altered neurochemistry and response to "organic" interventions (e.g., pharmacological manipulation of brain neurotransmitter levels).

In general, any type of behavior observed in idiopathic (i.e., primary) psychiatric syndromes can occur in association with a neurological disorder. For this reason, it is often hard to differentiate primary psychiatric disorders from secondary neuropsychiatric disorders. Late-onset disorders are likely to be related to brain disease, but neuropsychiatric disorders are not limited to the elderly. Patients with neuropsychiatric illnesses often lack the premorbid psychiatric or personality alterations that occur in many idiopathic psychiatric disorders. Also, they often lack the family history of psychiatric disability common in those with idiopathic psychiatric disorders (an exception is hereditary neurological illnesses such as Huntington's disease).

While changes in mood, affect, personality, and cognition may be direct effects of CNS insult, many individuals will suffer indirect or reactive changes in these domains. Often, CNS injury leads to losses of important capacities or functions such as physical mobility or intellectual acuity. Clearly, the often chronic frustration and life-style changes that accompany such losses can trigger profound mood and personality changes that are not primary consequences of the CNS injury. In reality, it is difficult to state conclusively whether a mood or personality alteration is the direct effect of CNS injury or a secondary reaction to the injury. Most likely, a complex and dynamic interaction of primary and secondary factors is at work when psychopathological conditions are noted following CNS disturbance.

**Prevalence of CNS Disorders in the United States.** Behavioral disorders, ranging from subtle personality change to full blown dementia, are common following insult or injury to the CNS. Estimates of the prevalence of CNS disorders vary dramatically, depending on the criteria used to define "disorder." It is challenging to accurately estimate the number of individuals in the United States who have some degree of acquired CNS dysfunction because not all affected individuals will present to health care professionals. For example, many of the elderly who might meet criteria for a CNS degenerative disorder such as Alzheimer's disease may function with the help of family members and do not seek treatment. Many CNS diseases, such as neurodegenerative conditions like Alzheimer's and Parkinson's disease, also have long latency periods that precede symptom onset. As will be discussed in more detail later, CNS disease/disorder can affect individuals of any age, although increasing age is a primary risk factor for many CNS diseases, such as stroke, Alzheimer's disease, and Parkinson's disease (Aronson et al., 1991; Cummings, 1992; Jorm & Jolley, 1998). On the other hand, brain tumors, HIV/AIDS-associated dementia, and head injury are CNS disorders that are at least as likely to affect individuals in younger age groups (i.e., <50) as they are to affect the elderly. Estimates of the number of individuals suffering from CNS disorders in the United States are shown in Table 1.

## Neuropsychiatric Symptoms Following CNS Injury

### Introduction

It has long been noted that insult or injury to certain brain regions can produce relatively selec-

**Table 1. Estimated Prevalence of Persons in the United States with Diseases and/or Disorders of the CNS**

| Disease or disorder | Estimated number of cases |
|---|---|
| Alzheimer's disease | 2,500,000–4,000,000 |
| Frontotemporal degeneration | 750,000–1,000,000 |
| Parkinson's disease | 500,000–600,000 |
| Huntington's disease | 20,000–50,000 |
| Cerebrovascular event (stroke) | 3,000,000[a] |
| Head injury | 1,000,000–2,500,000 |

[a]This number represents an estimate of the number of individuals living in the United States who have suffered and/or still suffer disability (physical, cognitive, and/or emotional) due to stroke. Approximately 500,000 persons are disabled to some extent due to stroke each year.

tive deficits in behavior. More than 100 years ago, surgeon Paul Broca observed that damage to the anterior part of the left side of the brain led to an inability to produce speech but spared the ability to comprehend speech. Considerable brain–behavior specificity exists with regard to the genesis of sensorimotor deficits and, to a lesser degree, cognitive deficits. For example, ablation of the left precentral gyrus will inevitably give rise to a right-sided hemiparesis. No such anatomic specificity is present for the neuroanatomic underpinnings of emotion. Nonetheless, damage to certain brain structures, most notably prefrontal cortex and/or temporal-limbic region structures such as the amygdala, are far more likely to result in neuropsychiatric disturbance.

**The Frontal Lobes and Frontal-Subcortical Circuits.** The frontal lobes comprise approximately one-third of the total cortical surface area of the brain and are by far the largest of the four lobes. In terms of our phylogenetic history, they represent the latest evolutionary addition. The frontal lobes play an important role in mediating complex human behavior. Frontal cortical areas subserve *executive functions*, those behaviors that allow us to organize, coordinate, initiate, and execute purposeful behavior. Social and goal-directed cognition, behavior, and emotion are intimately associated with and depend on the frontal lobes (Damasio & Anderson, 1993).

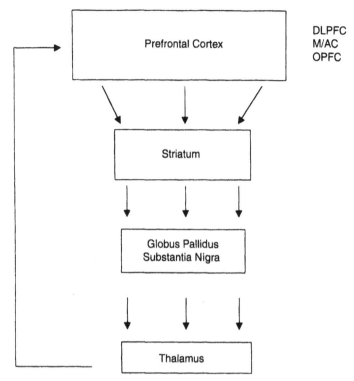

**Figure 1.** General organization of the frontal-subcortical-thalamic circuits. Three circuits are most closely associated with behavioral disturbance in CNS disease/disorder. Note: DLPFC, dorsolateral prefrontal cortex; M/AC, mesial frontal–anterior cingulate; OPFC, orbitofrontal prefrontal cortex. Adapted from Cummings (1993).

Alexander and colleagues (1986) introduced the concept of parallel but segregated frontal-subcortical circuits that have important behavioral functions. Cummings (1993) identified three major behavioral syndromes associated with the pathology of different prefrontal regions or the circuit connecting those regions with subcortical and thalamic structures. It is important to note that disruption anywhere along the circuit can lead to similar behavioral deficits, which mean that subcortical pathology can produce the same constellation of symptoms as prefrontal lesions. The three prefrontal regions are the dorsolateral area (i.e., the outer convexity of the frontal lobe), the orbitofrontal area (the parts of the frontal lobe resting above the orbital bone), and the mesial-frontal/cingulate area (middle, deeper portions) of the frontal lobes. Figure 1 shows a schematic representation of the frontal-subcortical circuits. As diagramed in Figure 1, three specific circuits, each with prefrontal, subcortical, and thalamic connections, have been identified. In general, lesions to the prefrontal cortex produce more distinct behavioral syndromes than similarly-sized lesions to the smaller subcortical-thalamic structures. In other words, when the site of pathology is subcortical, there is a greater chance of disrupting more than one circuit and thereby, seeing neuropsychiatric phenomena from more than one frontal-subcortical syndrome.

The dorsolateral prefrontal cortex (DLPFC) is that area of the frontal lobe on the outer convexity of the frontal lobe. Patients with damage to the DLPFC or connected subcortical structures often show deficits in planning and organizing behavior. These individuals may be unusually dependent on environmental cues and less able than neurologically normal persons to adapt to an ever changing, novel environment. Many times these patients will seem unable to use environmental cues effectively or to profit maximally from experience. It is not uncommon for patients with damage anywhere along the DLPFC circuit to show perseverative behavior, in which they repeat an act unwittingly and often involuntarily. Mood changes are common with dorsolateral prefrontal lesions. A large number of individuals with DLPFC lesions have depressive symptoms, and approximately half of these meet criteria for Major Depression.

The orbitofrontal syndrome leads to the most dramatic behavioral disturbances of the frontal lobe syndromes. This area of the prefrontal cortex is especially vulnerable to injury during motor vehicle accidents or other causes of head injuries because it rests above the bony orbital roof. Frequently, individuals with previously normal behavior, who have suffered injury to orbitofrontal structures or circuits, are entirely transformed (as illustrated later in the Personality Alterations section where we discuss the case of Phineas Gage). Typically these individuals show deficits in empathic, civil, and socially appropriate behavior and display prominent *disinhibition* and an obvious lack of behavioral restraint (Duffy & Campbell, 1994). Individuals with this syndrome ignore social conventions and exhibit undue familiarity by talking to strangers and touching or fondling others without permission. They are often tactless in conversation and may make uncivil or lewd remarks. Many times, these individuals are extremely impulsive and respond immediately (and unpredictably) to changing environmental circumstances. They lack conscientiousness and fail to complete assigned tasks. A salient characteristic of their behavior is that they seem unconcerned about the consequences of their behavior and may in fact engage in activities that endanger themselves or others. Risk assessment is typically impaired in these individuals (Cummings, 1993). Mood alterations often accompany the orbitofrontal syndrome. Lability and irritability, both of which are discussed in detail later, are the most common changes. Patients with orbitofrontal damage may rapidly shift from happiness or an empty euphoria to anger and/or sadness. Mood changes are only rarely sustained, and anger often dissipates as the individual's attention is drawn to some new activity or stimulus. Hypomania and mania may accompany orbitofrontal dysfunction (Duffy & Campbell, 1994).

Apathy, anergia, indifference, and emotional withdrawal characterize the mesial prefrontal/cingulate syndrome. Many patients with disturbance of this circuit appear depressed, but they often lack the dysphoria seen in depression (Cummings, 1993). Both motor and information-processing slowing is often evident among individuals with cingulate pathology or disruption somewhere along this circuit. Decreased creativity and spontaneity are common (Chow & Cummings, 1999). At times, the apathy and indifference is so profound as to leave patients unresponsive to their environments. Interestingly, many of these profoundly apathetic patients deny distress, although they are aware that they have undergone personality change.

## Mood and Affective Disorders

Disturbances of mood and affect are among the most common behavioral concomitants of CNS disturbance. *Mood* can be defined as a pervasive and sustained (even if only briefly) emotion that is subjectively experienced and reported by the individual. *Affect* is the observed outward behavioral expression of emotion. Typically, mood and affect are consistent with one another (i.e., someone who says that they are sad typically looks sad), but this is not always the case. For example, we will briefly discuss later a syndrome known as pseudobulbar affect in which patients often show a dramatic disconnection between mood and affect. Patients with this disorder often have episodes of laughing or crying without being aware of feeling either happy or sad. This condition is typically thought of as involving a disturbance in affect (i.e., it is disconnected from mood), but diseases or disorders that lead to disturbance of both mood and affect are much more common. Several types of mood disorder may occur following damage to the CNS. We will focus on three of the most common varieties of mood disturbance: depression, mania, and increased anxiety.

**Depression.** Depression is an alteration of mood that involves either prominent sadness and/or *anhedonia*, a term used to describe the experience of diminished interest in or pleasure from daily activities. A constellation of cognitive symptoms (e.g., pessimism regarding the future, guilty feelings, self-reproach) often accompanies sad mood and/or anhedonia. Additionally, somatic symptoms and signs, such as sleep and appetite disturbance, fatigue, and diminished libido, are often part of a depressive syndrome. As detailed in Chapter 11, according to the *Diagnostic and Statistical Manual of Mental Disorders*, 4th edition

(DSM-IV; American Psychiatric Association [APA], 1994), the clinical syndrome of Major Depression exists when a constellation of at least five of these symptoms (one of which must be either depressed mood or anhedonia) is present and prominent for at least 2 weeks. For a diagnosis of Major Depression according to the DSM-IV, an important criterion is that the depressive symptoms and signs are not better accounted for by a systemic/medical illness, that is, they have an idiopathic etiology. When depressive symptomatology appears to be secondary to a CNS disturbance (e.g., stroke) and/or medical condition (e.g., hypothyroidism), the DSM labels this diagnostic category "Mood Disorder Due to a General Medical Condition." Finally, specifiers such as "with depressive features" or "with major depressive-like episode" qualify the intensity of the observed depressive syndrome.

Idiopathic (i.e., primary) and secondary depression share certain characteristics. Both have been shown to be consistently associated with decreased serotonin levels (McAllister-Williams, Ferrier, & Young, 1998), and both respond well to antidepressant medications. Functional neuroimaging such as positron emission tomography (PET) or single photon emission computerized tomography (SPECT) consistently demonstrate the involvement of both frontal and subcortical structures (especially caudate) and circuits in both primary and secondary depression (Mayberg, Mahurin, & Brannan, 1998). Information-processing slowing, retrieval deficits, attentional disruption, and difficulty with executive functioning characterize the pattern of cognitive deficits seen among a subset of individuals with depression, whether of idiopathic or neurological etiology. That this pattern emerges in both primary and secondary depression implies that each may be a consequence of disturbance of frontal-subcortical regions that subserve both affect and cognition.

As suggested earlier, there is no obligatory relationship between the site of CNS pathology and mood disorder. However, insult or injury to certain regions/structures/circuits increases the likelihood that significant depressive features will emerge. For example, depression is a fairly common consequence of neurological disorders that affect the left prefrontal cortex (Cummings, 1994; Royall, 1999). Functional neuroimaging studies have shown greater involvement of left frontal than of

right frontal regions in depressed neurological patients and some have suggested that the intensity/severity of depression seen in neurological disease is associated with the distance of the lesion from the left frontal pole (Buchsbaum et al., 1984; Robinson & Starkstein, 1990). Among patients who have suffered a stroke, depression is far more common when the site of the infarct is anterior rather than posterior and is on the left rather than the right; left prefrontal infarcts then are the most likely to lead to a major depressive episode (Cummings, 1994; Robinson & Price, 1982).

Depression is an extremely common consequence of cerebrovascular disease (Robinson & Starkstein, 1997). Estimates of the prevalence of depression vary (largely based on sampling techniques and/or the definition of depression that is used), but anywhere from 30–50% of patients experience prominent depression following a stroke. Astrom and colleagues (1993) conducted a 3-year longitudinal study of stroke patients and reported that approximately 40% had some sort of clinical depression (either major depression or minor depression/dysthymia). Additionally, the phenomenology of depression associated with cerebrovascular disease is quite similar to that seen in patients with primary (idiopathic) depressive disorders (Robinson & Starkstein, 1997).

Another secondary cause of depression is disorders that involve the endocrine system. Both hyper- and hypothyroidism involve endocrine system dysfunction and have depression prevalence rates exceeding those found in the general population. Hypothyroidism often leads to a constellation of symptoms, including depression, lethargy, and concentration difficulty (Lezak, 1995) that can often be effectively treated with thyroid replacement therapy. Table 2 lists some of the CNS diseases and disorders in which depression often occurs.

Depression is a common consequence of CNS disturbance, but measuring it is not always straightforward. Often, individuals with neurological (or other medical) disorders, which may give rise to mood disturbance, also have somatic complaints (e.g., insomnia, appetite loss, preoccupation with physical status) that are diagnostically ambiguous. Clearly, such complaints among physically healthy individuals with evidence of depression are best conceptualized as part of a depressive syndrome. However, such complaints among those with medical illness usually do not indicate mood disorder

**Table 2. Neurological and Systemic Disorders Associated with Depression**

| Neurologic disorders |
| --- |

Diffuse degenerative diseases
    Alzheimer's disease[a]
    Frontotemporal degeneration[a]
    Multiple sclerosis
Regional degenerative disorders
    Parkinson's disease[a]
    Huntington's disease[a]
    Pick's disease
    Fahr's disease
    Progressive supranuclear palsy
    Wilson's disease
Focal lesions
    Stroke (frontal, basal ganglia)[a]
    Tumor
    Surgical ablation
    Epilepsy (temporal, frontal, cingulate)
Miscellaneous
    Carbon monoxide exposure

| Systemic disorders |
| --- |

Endocrine
    Hypothyroidism and hyperthyroidism
    Adrenal disease (Cushing's disease)
Inflammatory/infectious
    Lupus
    Neurosyphilis
    AIDS
    Tuberculosis
    Chronic fatigue syndrome

[a]Discussed in detail in the current chapter.

in the absence of prominent cognitive/affective mood disturbance. Instead, complaints of weight loss, diminished appetite, and insomnia are not unexpected correlates of being physically ill.

**Mania.** Mania refers to an affective syndrome that features an elevated, expansive, and/or irritable mood. In addition, other symptoms and signs are often present, including a sense of grandiosity, decreased need for sleep, increased talkativeness or pressured speech, flight of ideas, psychomotor agitation, heightened distractibility, and excessive involvement in pleasurable and/or high-risk behavior. When these symptoms or signs arise secondary to a neurological disorder or a toxic/ metabolic process, they are commonly termed secondary mania (Krauthammer & Klerman, 1978). As noted in Chapter 11, according to the DSM-IV (APA, 1994), a primary manic episode is diagnosed only when a constellation of these symptoms is present for at least 1 week and *is not* due to the effects of a substance (street drug or prescribed medication) or a medical (i.e., neurological) condition. Secondary manic episodes are referred to in the DSM-IV as "Mood Disorder Due to a General Medical Condition." Then, they are labeled "with manic features" if primarily euphoric, elated, or irritable symptoms predominate, or "with mixed features" if both manic and depressed symptoms are present.

There is compelling evidence that at least some individuals with primary (i.e., idiopathic) mania have brain irregularities. For example, Dupont and colleagues (1995) found that patients with bipolar disorder but no evidence of current or past neurologic illness had subcortical brain abnormalities, as measured by MRI. A study using functional neuroimaging techniques found that some, but not all, of the primary manic individuals had blood flow irregularities, especially in the right hemisphere (El-Hilu et al., 1998). More specifically, among five patients with primary mania, SPECT scanning revealed significantly lower blood flow in the basal portion of the right temporal lobe, compared to matched non-manic controls (Migliorelli, Starkstein, Teson, & de Quiros, 1993). Individuals with a history of primary mania may have subtle neuroanatomical and/or neurochemical irregularities, but it has been suggested that they are generally less likely to be cognitively impaired than patients with secondary mania (Hoff, Shukla, Cook, & Aronson, 1988).

Secondary mania has been observed in a wide variety of neurologic conditions. Nearly all lesions and/or neurologic conditions that produce mania involve the right hemisphere and/or the frontal lobes. As noted before, pathology in the orbitofrontal cortex, caudate nuclei, and/or temporal limbic structures often produces mania. In Huntington's disease (discussed in detail later), a disorder that involves pathology of the caudate nuclei, mania is commonly observed in a subset of affected patients. In fact, manic symptomatology may antedate the appearance of either movement disorder or cognitive deterioration in this disease (Folstein, Brandt, & Folstein, 1990). Additionally, heightened rates of aggressive outbursts and sexual promiscuity, both characteristic manic phenomena, are not uncommon in this disease (Maricle, 1989). Mania is much more common among head-injured patients with prominent orbitofrontal and/or temporal limbic damage than in the general population (Shukla et al., 1987). Starkstein and colleagues (1990) used positron emission tomography to explore cerebral metabolism in eight brain-injured patients who had developed a secondary manic syndrome and found that right-sided metabolic abnormalities were evident in all eight patients. Euphoria and prolonged manic periods have been observed in a subset of individuals with multiple sclerosis who also show prominent involvement of prefrontal white matter (Filley, 1994; Pine, Douglas, Charles, & Davies, 1995). Finally, in conditions where full-blown manic episodes are rare but prominent euphoria is not, there is again evidence of frontal dysfunction. Alzheimer's disease patients with pronounced euphoria were more likely to show metabolic abnormalities in prefrontal regions and neuropsychological impairment suggestive of frontal dysfunction than Alzheimer's patients without prominent euphoria (Lebert, Pasquier, Danel, & Steinling, 1994).

In addition to neurological conditions, secondary mania may also arise from substance-induced and systemic disorders. Prominent manic symptoms, including full-blown manic episodes are not uncommon effects of intoxication by stimulants including cocaine and methamphetamine (Miller, Mena, Giombetti, & Villanueva-Meyer, 1992; Waters & Lapierre, 1981). Mania may occur as a side effect of prescription drugs, including those used to treat neurological conditions such as Parkinson's disease. Systemic disorders such as uremia, hyperthyroidism, or vitamin $B_{12}$ deficiency (Goggans, 1983; Jack et al., 1983), and post-partum states also lead to mania in a subset of individuals affected by these conditions

## Alterations in Personality

"Gage was no longer Gage." This quote, well known to students of neuropsychiatry, captures the aftermath of a head injury suffered by a Mr. Phineas Gage in 1848. A hard working, temperate, conscientious gentleman, Gage was a worker on a railroad crew charged with dynamiting rock before laying track. While tamping down a load of

dynamite, a spark accidentally flew, igniting a charge which propelled Gage's tamping rod (which weighed 13 pounds and was more than 3½ feet long and 1½ inches in diameter at its widest) into his cheekbone, up through his frontal lobes, and out the top of his head, ultimately landing over 100 feet away. Surprisingly, chroniclers of this event report that he barely lost consciousness, if at all. However, he did lose his old personality. He became disinhibited, vulgar, puerile, childish, and impulsive, a drinker, and a fighter. In short, the complete opposite of his former self.

This tragic tale is repeated daily among many patients who suffer damage to the frontal lobes. In addition to stroke, tumor, and frontal lobe dementia, the most common cause of frontal personality disorder is closed head injury such as that sometimes sustained in an automobile accident. The orbitofrontal region of the brain lies directly behind the bony protuberances where the eyes rest in the skull. Damage to this area of the brain frequently gives rise to disinhibited, inappropriate behavior. This is particularly true when the damage is to the right orbitofrontal lobe. Damage to the left orbitofrontal cortex has been associated with a radically different constellation of behavioral changes, including withdrawal, apathy, inertia, and depression.

It has long been recognized that disturbance in brain structure, physiology, or chemistry can lead to prominent changes in personality, but it has not always been easy to codify these changes. The three most recent editions of the DSM give increasingly more attention to the concept of personality alteration as an important sequelae of brain insult or injury. The DSM-III (APA, 1980) describes an "Organic Personality Syndrome" that is characterized by emotional lability and pronounced impulsivity. As we will make evident later, this characterization does not do justice to the wide variety of personality alterations that may accompany CNS disease/disorder. The revision of the 3rd edition of the DSM (APA, 1987) left the term "Organic Personality Syndrome" in place but added several additional behavioral descriptors as potential symptoms and signs. These additions included suspiciousness or paranoid ideation, marked apathy and indifference, affective instability (e.g., marked shifts from normal mood to depression, irritability, or anxiety) and recurrent aggressive outbursts. The DSM-IV (APA, 1994) uses the term "Personality Change Due to A General Medical Condition" and has added five specific subtypes of personality change. These subtypes are as follows: Labile (e.g., affective lability), Disinhibited (e.g., poor impulse control), Aggressive, Apathetic (e.g., marked apathy or indifference), and Paranoid. Mixed types are probably more common than not. We describe here two of the more common personality alterations that occur secondary to CNS disturbance.

**Apathy/Indifference.** Apathy is a reduction in goal-related thoughts, emotions, and behavioral responses and occurs secondary to reduced or absent motivation (Marin, 1991). Apathy is a behavioral domain that significantly overlaps with, but can be reliably discriminated from, depression, as it has been in several CNS diseases/disorders (Castellon, Hinkin, Wood, Yarema, 1998; Levy et al., 1998; Marin, Firinciogullari, & Biedrzycki, 1994). As noted earlier, apathy is a common neuropsychiatric consequence of disruption to the mesial-cingulate prefrontal circuit. In subcortical conditions such as Parkinson's disease and HIV-1 infection, apathy has been associated with other indicators of CNS disturbance such as cognitive impairment, especially executive dysfunction (Castellon et al., 1998; Castellon, Hinkin, & Myers, 2000; Starkstein et al., 1992). In several of the CNS disorders discussed here, including stroke and Alzheimer's disease, the presence of apathy was associated with prefrontal and temporal reduced blood flow and hypometabolism (Craig et al., 1996; Duffy & Kant, 1997; Okada et al., 1997; Ott, Noto, & Fogel, 1996).

**Aggressive/Irritable/Agitated.** There is significant evidence for the role of serotonergic dysregulation in impulsive aggression. A decrease in serotonin is found in the brain stems of aggressive rats that spontaneously kill mice introduced into their cages, and the introduction of tryptophan (the precursor of serotonin) reduces or abolishes this violence (Sabrie, 1986). Prefrontal and temporal limbic structures have been implicated in the neuroanatomy of agitation/irritability. Two recent studies of patients with temporal lobe epilepsy (TLE) have implicated both prefrontal cortex and the amygdala as crucial regions associated with violent and/or aggressive outbursts (Woermann et al., 2000; van Elst et al., 2000). Limbic system tumors, infections, and blood vessel abnormalities have been associated with violence (Cherkasky and Hollander, 1997). The prefrontal cortex modulates limbic and hypothalamic activity and, it is

thought, is associated with the social and judgmental aspects of aggression. The coordination of timing social cues, often before the expression of associated emotions, is among the myriad responsibilities of the prefrontal cortex (Cherkasky & Hollander, 1997). Patients with violent behavior have a high frequency of frontal lobe lesions (Kandel & Freed, 1989). Some have proposed that prefrontal damage may cause aggression by a secondary process that involves lack of inhibition of the limbic area.

Finally, it should be noted that Axis II diagnostic categories such as Antisocial and Borderline Personality Disorder clearly have biological underpinnings (also see Chapters 15 and 16 of this volume) for at least a subset of individuals so diagnosed. A recent study by De la Fuente and colleagues (1997) of patients diagnosed with Borderline Personality Disorder found cerebral metabolic abnormalities in the cingulate cortex and in parts of the caudate and thalamus by using positron emission tomography. EEG and other brain abnormalities have also been observed in patients diagnosed with antisocial personality disorder (Deckel, Hesselbrock, & Bauer, 1996; Finn, Ramsey, & Earlywine, 2000).

### Psychotic-Spectrum Disorders

Neurological disease can give rise to a wide array of psychotic symptomatology, including hallucinations and delusions. A *hallucination* is a false sensory perception not associated with real external stimuli. Hallucinations may occur in any sensory modality and may or may not be associated with a delusional interpretation of the false perceptual experience. A *delusion* is a firmly held false belief based on an incorrect inference about external reality that is not consistent with the individual's level of intelligence and cultural background. As mentioned in Chapters 13 and 14 of this volume, these symptoms are key elements of psychotic-spectrum disorders such as schizophrenia or schizoaffective disorder. As with the mood disorders, when these symptoms are a prominent and enduring part of the symptom picture and arise secondarily to a neurological condition, DSM-IV states that they are *not* considered schizophrenia. Rather, when delusions or hallucinations follow CNS insult, they should be labeled "Psychotic Disorder Due to General Medical Condition." An exception to this coding would be if the psychotic

### Table 3. Different Types of Delusions

| | |
|---|---|
| Persecution | False belief that one is being harassed, cheated, or persecuted |
| Grandeur | Exaggerated conception of one's own importance, power, or identity |
| Reference | False belief that the behavior of others refers to oneself; that events, objects or others have a particular and unusual significance |
| Control | One's will, thoughts, or feelings are being controlled by external forces |
|    Thought withdrawal | One's thoughts are being removed from individual's mind by another person or force |
|    Thought insertion | Thoughts are being implanted in one's mind by another person or force |
|    Thought broadcasting | False belief that one's thoughts can be heard by others as though they were being broadcast into the air |
|    Thought control | Delusional belief that one's thoughts are being controlled by other persons or forces |
| Erotomanic | Delusional belief that someone is deeply in love with the individual |
| Othello | Delusional belief that the individual's spouse is unfaithful |
| Parasitosis | False belief that the individual is infested with insects, worms, lice, or other vermin |

phenomenology is observed secondarily to a disease process such as Alzheimer's disease, in which case the proper diagnostic label would be "Dementia of the Alzheimer's Type, With Delusions." In any event, all cases of delusions or hallucinations secondary to CNS disturbance are typically called secondary psychosis.

Although secondary psychoses triggered by central nervous system disease/insult share considerable phenomenological overlap with primary or idiopathic psychosis, there are several ways in which the two classes of psychosis can be distinguished. First, secondary psychoses tend to have a later age of onset. For example, schizophrenia typically has an onset in the late teens and twenties, whereas secondary psychoses are more common in older individuals. Second, patients with a primary psychosis are more likely to have a family history of psychosis. Third, there tends to be a correlation among patients with secondary psychoses between degree of intellectual impairment and how well elaborated their delusions and hallucinations are. Finally, secondary psychoses tend to be more ego-dystonic.

**Delusions.** Delusions can be seen in a wide variety of neurological diseases, including Alzheimer's disease, vascular dementia, closed head injury, cerebral neoplasm, multiple sclerosis, and Huntington's disease (Table 3). They are more common in diseases that affect subcortical rather than cortical brain structures, particularly diseases that affect the limbic system and medial temporal lobes or their projections to basal ganglia, thalamus, and rostral brain stem structures. It has been estimated that up to one-half of all patients with Alzheimer's disease will manifest delusional thinking at some point in their disease. Members of our group (Sultzer et al., 1995) have found that frontal hypometabolism among patients with Alzheimer's disease, as indexed by positron emission tomography, is linked to delusions as well as hallucinations. This finding converges with evidence using structural imaging that has reported heightened rates of frontal white matter lesions in Alzheimer's and vascular dementia patients with prominent delusions (Binetti, Padovani, Magni, & Bianchetti, 1995). Excessive dopamine is also known to play an important role in psychotic phenomenology. Two prominent dopamine systems in which disruption is known to lead to psychotic symptomatology are the mesocortico-limbic and nigrostriatal dopamine systems.

Clarke and colleagues (1998) relate a case study of a patient with multiple sclerosis (MS), a disease that affects subcortical structures and white matter, who repeatedly stabbed himself in the stomach due to self-loathing and persecutory delusions. Although delusions are not a typical presentation of this disease, they are seen more commonly among MS patients, who may suffer from psychotic depression, than in the general population (Clarke et al., 1998).

Although virtually every type of delusion can be seen among patients with CNS disease, Schneiderian first-rank delusions such as thought insertion, withdrawal, and broadcasting tend to be uncommon. Demented patients, instead, commonly present with persecutory delusions or delusions of jealousy. One can speculate that such delusions may at least in part reflect a rational response to their cognitive decline. The individual with severe short-term memory impairment who cannot remember that his wife has only momentarily run out to the store may instead believe she has run off with another. The patient who cannot recall where she has left her keys may conclude that somebody has stolen them.

Several types of delusions tend to be overrepresented in patients with dementing disorders. One such delusion is the *phantom boarder delusion*, in which patients will contend that a stranger is living in their homes against their wishes. *Capgras syndrome* is the delusional belief that members of one's own family or friends have been replaced with identically-appearing impostors. Capgras syndrome is more common among patients who have suffered damage to the right as opposed to the left hemisphere (Singer, 1992). A related delusion if the *Fregoli syndrome* in which patients believe that their persecutor can mimic the appearance of others.

Delusional jealousy, also known as the "*Othello syndrome*," is the delusional belief that one's spouse or partner has been unfaithful. The delusional belief that a famous individual is actually secretly in love with you is termed erotomania, or more colorfully, *De Clarambault* syndrome. Somatic delusions are also common in CNS dysfunction. Among the more florid delusions are *lycanthropy*—the belief that you are a werewolf, and delusions of infestation or *parasitophobia*—the delusional belief that one's body has been invaded by insects, parasites, worms, etc. Delusions of infestation are particularly common in metabolic/toxic psychoses and deficiency syndromes (e.g., $B_{12}$ deficiency). Heutoscopy, or the *Doppelganger syndrome*, is the delusional belief in the existence of an exact duplicate of oneself. This needs be distinguished from *autoscopy*—a visual hallucination of oneself which the individual realizes is illusory.

Among the most fascinating delusional syndromes is *anosognosia* which is the unawareness of a deficit. Most commonly seen in patients who have suffered right parietal stroke, anosognosia has also been seen in patients with left parietal lesions, frontal lobe damage, especially secondary to closed head injury and anterior subcortical structures, as well as in progressive dementias such as Alzheimer's disease and frontotemporal

dementia. The anosognosic patient may deny even the most dramatic impairment. For example, a patient who is hemiplegic following a right middle cerebral artery stroke may claim that there is nothing wrong with the paralyzed arm. Another example is the patient with *Anton's syndrome* who is cortically blind after suffering bilateral occipital lobe damage but nonetheless claims to be able to see. For a thorough review of anosognosia, the interested reader is directed to the work of McGlynn & Schacter (1997).

**Hallucinations.** Hallucinations are not uncommon among patients with CNS disease. Patients with secondary hallucinations tend to recognize that their hallucinations are not real, a degree of insight not always shared by psychiatric patients. Such patients may react to their hallucinations with a range of emotions ranging from bemused fascination to terror. Unlike the functional psychoses like schizophrenia in which the frequency of auditory hallucinations far outweighs visual hallucinations, visual hallucinations tend to be the most common among patients with secondary hallucinations. Visual hallucinations can range from the most mundane, such as unformed flashes of light, to the bizarre and outlandish. Patients may hallucinate copies of themselves (*autoscopy*). Objects in their visual field may appear very small (*Lilliputian hallucinations*) or very large (*Brobdignagian hallucinations*). This alteration in the size of objects needs be distinguished from *micropsia* and *macropsia* in which the entire visual field is altered in size. *Psychedelic hallucinations* such as repetitive geometric shapes, lattice work, etc., may occur as can *palinopsia*—the persistence of a visual image after its removal, a benign form of which can be triggered in normals by a camera flashbulb. Visual hallucinations also need to be distinguished from *illusions* in which patients misinterpret actual visual stimuli.

Visual hallucinations of animals (zoopsia) are also common among patients with secondary psychosis. Among patients with structural lesions who hallucinate, right hemisphere lesions are more likely than left to give rise to visual hallucinations. The more posterior the lesion (i.e., occipital lobes), the more poorly formed the hallucination.

Patients with seizure disorders frequently report hallucinatory experiences as part of the peri-ictal experiences. Such "auras" can be auditory, visual, tactile, olfactory, and even gustatory. Substance intoxication and withdrawal stages also give rise to hallucinations. The "pink elephants" seen in alcohol hallucinosis and delirium tremens are well chronicled. Stimulant intoxication has been linked to delusions (particularly paranoid), as well as to hallucinations. One specific type of stimulant-induced hallucination is tactile hallucinations in which patients feel that insects are crawling on or under their skin. This condition is known as formication or "the cocaine bugs." Patients in the midst of deliriums, or acute confusional state, are at high risk for delusions and hallucinations, as well as agitation. Sensory deprivation, common in older patients with visual impairments such as cataracts or hearing loss, can also give rise to hallucinations and delusions.

## Specific Neurological Conditions and Their Behavioral Sequelae

### Degenerative Disorders of the CNS

Several disease processes involve progressive deterioration of brain tissue and behavior. Some of these conditions are relatively commonplace, whereas others are quite rare. The prevalence of dementia in individuals over the age of 65 in North America is approximately 6–10% (Hendrie, 1998), although this is a dramatic underestimate if milder cases of dementia are included. As our population continues to age and medical technology enables us to live longer, the number of patients with degenerative diseases will grow dramatically. Of these diseases, Alzheimer's disease is by far the most prevalent and accounts for nearly two-thirds of all cases of dementia. Following, we discuss several degenerative diseases of the CNS in some detail. We start with the most common and some would say, the prototypical degenerative disorder, Alzheimer's disease, before turning to frontotemporal degeneration and two of the more common subcortical degenerative disorders, Parkinson's and Huntington's diseases.

### Alzheimer's Disease

**Introduction.** Alzheimer's disease (AD) is a progressive neurological disorder that primarily affects cortical neurons. Most typically, AD is a disorder of later life and onset rarely occurs before age 45. There is currently no diagnostic test for AD, and a definite diagnosis can be made only by autopsy or biopsy of the brain. As mentioned before, it is far and away the most common form of degenerative dementia (Cummings and Benson, 1992; Hendrie, 1998; LaRue, 1992) and currently afflicts roughly 4 million U.S. citizens. It is estimated that approximately 10% of all individuals over the age of 65 are affected by AD (LaRue, 1992).

The cardinal neuropathological sign of AD is the presence of senile *plaques, neurofibrillary tangles*, and amyloid angiopathy. Plaques are caused by neuronal degeneration and can be found in all areas of the cerebral cortex but are often most common in the parietal lobe and hippocampal and amygdaloid regions. Neurofibrillary tangles are tangled bundles of fine fibers within the cell bodies of neurons that occur throughout the brain but particularly around the hippocampus. Autopsies indicate that 50–60% of clinically demented individuals have brain changes that are consistent with diagnoses of Alzheimer's disease and another 10–20% show AD-consistent changes in combination with other neuropathology (Katzman, 1986). The most common neuroanatomical changes seen in the brains of individuals with AD include prominent atrophy in the gyri of the associative areas of the cerebral cortex, with the primary motor and sensory areas of the cortex relatively unaffected (Katzman, 1986). In Alzheimer's, multiple neurotransmitter abnormalities have been documented, but the most reliable and striking changes occur in the cholinergic system (La Rue, 1992).

There are several risk factors for developing AD; advancing age is the most robust. A Finnish study found that approximately 2% of their sample between the ages of 65 and 74 had AD, whereas 6% of those between 75 and 84 and 15% of those over 85 had the disease (Sulkava et al., 1985). Other studies that examined more restricted populations reported somewhat higher rates, especially for the older age categories (Evans et al., 1989; Pfeffer, Afifi, & Chance, 1987). Women may be at slightly greater risk for developing AD than men (Amaducci, Rocca, & Schoenberg, 1986; Sulkava et al., 1985), and there is some evidence that individuals with prior histories of head injury have a greater risk of developing AD (Mortimer, French, Hutton, & Schuman, 1985). A family history of AD also confers higher risk (Cummings & Benson, 1992; Kay, 1989), although the magnitude of the risk is unclear. This strongly implicates a genetic component of the disease. Another relatively recently discovered risk factor for AD is the presence of a particular form of the ApoE gene, the ε4 allele ApoE (apolipoprotein E) is a cholesterol-transporting protein that is produced mainly in the liver and the CNS. Individuals who inherit two copies of the ApoE 4 allele have a risk of developing AD that is eight times higher, where those with one ε4 allele have approximately three times the risk (Lopez et al., 1997). The exact role of ApoE in the pathogenesis of AD is currently unclear.

**Cognitive Changes Associated with Alzheimer's Disease.** AD is known primarily for the profound cognitive and intellectual impairments that follow diagnosis. Consistent with the known sites of neuropathology (parietal and temporal association cortex, limbic structures), the earliest signs of the disease are typically memory and visuospatial impairment. The pattern of memory disturbance seen in AD involves short-term memory deficits characterized by both impaired encoding and retrieval; patients with AD are unable to recall or learn new material effectively. Verbal spontaneity in the AD patient is often deficient because word-finding compromise may impact the flow of speech. The cognitive/intellectual deficits seen in AD and the steadily progressive course of deterioration have been well described elsewhere (see Zec, 1993). For the purposes of this chapter, we wish to point out that the profound cognitive changes that accompany AD, in particular the devastation of short-term memory, often contribute to the psychiatric picture of an affected individual.

**Psychiatric Changes Associated with Alzheimer's Disease.** The psychiatric changes that accompany AD vary widely from one patient to another. Prominent mood disturbance, including increased rates of depression, irritability, and anxiety, and personality alterations such as apathy, heightened agitation and hostility are common in patients with AD. Inappropriate behavior (e.g., sexual, aggressive), sleep and appetite disturbance, and psychotic symptoms are also commonly observed in the patient with AD.

Estimates of the rate of depression among patients with AD vary considerably, in part due to the dramatically different depression criteria used across studies. Clearly, however, AD patients have higher rates of depression than seen among individuals of similar age without neurological compromise. Major Depression is less common than more minor variants of depressive syndromes (e.g., dysthymia, minor depression). A prospective longitudinal study by Starkstein and colleagues (1997) showed that 19% of sixty-two patients with probable AD diagnoses suffered a Major Depression, whereas 34% had evidence of a milder mood syndrome. Of note, a majority of those patients with Major Depression at study entry still met criteria for this syndrome at follow-up (1 to 2 years later), whereas only 28% of those with a minor mood syndrome at study entry showed any evidence of mood disturbance at follow-up. Another recent study of 109 patients with probable AD found roughly similar rates of Major Depression (22%) and Minor Depression (27%) in a cross-sectional investigation (Lyketsos et al., 1997). A potential problem with compiling prevalence figures of mood disturbance from direct interviews of AD patients is that they tend to underreport mood disturbance, compared to clinicians or caregivers (Weiner, Svetlik, & Risser, 1997).

Though some suggest that prominent changes in mood and personality are not typical of the earliest stages of AD (Cummings and Benson, 1992), these changes do occur fairly early for some affected individuals. A retrospective study of the course of psychiatric symptoms among 100 individuals with autopsy-confirmed diagnoses of AD reported that psychiatric symptoms often occurred in the year before the patients were diagnosed with AD (Jost and Grossberg, 1996). Clearly, as the disease progresses, pronounced changes in personality become evident. For example, it is not at all uncommon for AD patients to display little interest in self-care, work or household tasks, social or family activities, and/or the emotional needs of other individuals. This apathy often occurs without evidence of prominent depression (Reichman, Coyne, Amirneni, Molino, & Egan, 1996) and often precedes the development of disinhibited, agitated, and aggressive behaviors (Cummings & Benson, 1992). Negative symptoms such as apathy, anhedonia, and avolition are correlated with dementia severity in AD and show an inverse relationship to functional capacity (Reichman et al., 1996).

Delusions and hallucinations occur with regularity in AD. Cummings and Benson (1992) estimate that approximately 50% of patients with AD exhibit delusional beliefs at some point following diagnosis. For some individuals, psychotic symptoms/signs may be the presenting manifestation of the disease. As mentioned earlier, the delusions typically seen in schizophrenia (e.g., thought broadcasting, thought withdrawal) are not common in AD. Instead, delusions are often persecutory and involve theft of property or infidelity of the spouse. A fascinating delusional belief that is not uncommon in AD is Capgras syndrome, the belief that a familiar person, often the spouse, has been replaced by an impostor (Rubin, Drevets, & Burke, 1988). Two recent studies have shown that psychotic symptoms are fairly common and that delusions are more prevalent than hallucinations. One study of fifty-eight patients diagnosed with probable AD reported that 53% had prominent delusions and 35% had experienced hallucinations (Klatka, Louis, & Schiffer, 1996). Another recent study reported that 34% of the 70 subjects examined had delusions in the previous month and 11% had suffered hallucinations (Gormley & Rizwan, 1998). The latter study found that men experienced more psychotic symptoms than women and that these symptoms were not associated with age at illness onset, dementia severity, or scores on a depression rating scale. A recent interesting study using SPECT found that AD patients with delusions had decreased cerebral blood flow in the left prefrontal region, whereas patients with hallucinations had right parietal hypoperfusion (Kotrla, Chacko, Harper, Jhingran, & Doody, 1995).

Ramachandran and colleagues (1996) reported that both depression and psychosis were three times as prevalent in AD patients who had at least one copy of the ApoE 4 allele, compared to AD patients without this allele. They concluded that the phenotype of AD associated with the $\epsilon$4 allele is more likely to include psychiatric manifestations. However, a recent study by Lopez and colleagues (1997) failed to find such a connection. They examined psychiatric symptomatology in 194 patients with AD (115 of whom had at least one copy of the $\epsilon$4 allele) and found that the allele was associated with earlier onset of AD but appeared unrelated to the expression of psychiatric disturbance. Finally, our group (Sultzer et al., 1995) has shown that psychiatric symptomatology is a fundamental expression of the cortical dysfunction seen in AD. Using functional neuroimaging

(PET), significant associations between agitation/disinhibition and cerebral metabolism in the frontal and temporal regions and psychosis and frontal metabolism were observed among twenty-one patients with probable AD.

## Frontotemporal Dementia

**Introduction.** Frontotemporal dementias (FTD) are neurodegenerative diseases that produce disproportionate atrophy and/or neuropathology of the frontal and/or temporal lobes (unlike AD, where the medial temporal lobes and the associative cortex of the parietal and temporal lobes are initially affected). Often there is asymmetric degeneration of these regions, and many cases of FTD show either predominantly right- or predominantly left-sided involvement of the frontal and/or temporal lobes (Miller et al., 1991). However, in most FTD patients, both hemispheres are somewhat involved (Lezak, 1995). There are multiple types of FTD distinguished by subtle neurohistological differences (see Neary & Snowden, 1996), but these different subtypes share enough similarities to permit generalizations about FTD.

As mentioned before, the frontal lobes are the primary sites of the earliest degenerative changes in FTD, and the anterior portions of the temporal lobes are also affected early. The parietal and occipital lobes and the posterior portions of the superior temporal gyrus remain relatively unaffected (Neary & Snowden, 1996). The age of onset for FTD is typically between 50 and 70 years of age, and it may be inherited as an autosomal-dominant disorder in a minority of individuals (Cummings & Benson, 1992). The mean duration of illness for FTD is about 8 years, although there is considerable variability in survival time; many FTD patients survive for 12–15 years after diagnosis (Neary & Snowden, 1996).

**Behavioral Characteristics of FTD.** Relative to other degenerative disorders, FTD is much more likely to have prominent psychiatric symptoms that predate obvious cognitive or intellectual impairment (Cummings & Benson, 1992; Miller et al., 1991). The most salient and pervasive feature throughout the course of FTD disease is profound alteration in social conduct and personality (Neary & Snowden, 1996). Cognitive/intellectual deterioration inevitably occurs with FTD, but it is overshadowed initially by the often dramatic changes in mood, affect, personality, and behavior. Table 4

**Table 4. Behavioral and Affective Symptoms of Frontotemporal Dementia as Outlined by the Research Groups in Lund, Sweden, and Manchester, England**

Insidious onset and slow progression

Early loss of personal and social awareness

Early loss of insight

Early signs of disinhibition (e.g., unrestrained sexuality, violent behavior, inappropriate jocularity, restless pacing)

Mental rigidity and inflexibility

Stereotyped and perseverative behavior (e.g., wandering, clapping, singing, hoarding of objects, rituals involving dressing or hygiene)

Hyperorality (e.g., dietary changes, overeating, food fads, excessive smoking and/or alcohol consumption, oral exploration of objects)

Distractibility, impulsivity, and impersistence

Utilization behavior (e.g., unrestrained exploration/use of objects in the environment)

Depression, anxiety, excessive sentimentality

Bizarre somatic preoccupation

Emotional unconcern and remoteness; lack of empathy

Inertia, apathy, lack of spontaneity

lists the most typical behavioral and affective symptoms/signs of FTD, as outlined by the research groups from Lund, Sweden, and Manchester, England (Brun et al., 1994).

Typically, signs of disinhibition appear early in the course of the disease and include physical restlessness, impulsivity, irritability, aggressiveness, and excessive sentimentality (Brun & Gustafson, 1999). Some patients with FTD will crave affection and sexual contact and may become easily and frequently provoked when these needs are not met. A lack of empathy for the feelings and concerns of others, including family members and significant others, often makes FTD patients difficult to manage. The presence of stereotyped behavior often develops early in the course of FTD and occasionally manifests in hoarding behavior or habitual shopping. Self-care is almost inevitably affected in FTD; patients become less concerned with their personal appearance (Brun & Gustafson, 1999).

The personality disruption observed in FTD is not uniform; some individuals become restless, agitated, disinhibited, and overly jocular, and

others become apathetic and inert and lack drive, motivation, and initiative. Most patients diagnosed with FTD have relatively normal premorbid personality and the neuropsychiatric features of FTD are typically much more strongly associated with the distribution of cerebral dysfunction than with premorbid personality characteristics (Lebert, Pasquier, & Petit, 1995; Miller et al., 1993). One of the most striking behavioral syndromes associated with FTD is the Kluver–Bucy syndrome. In this syndrome, which was originally seen in monkeys with ablated amygdalae, emotional blunting with loss of fear and affective response, altered dietary preferences, mandatory oral exploration of novel environmental stimuli, and hypersexuality are observed. FTD does not inevitably lead to Kluver–Bucy, but many of these behavioral manifestations will be present in a subset of affected individuals.

Typically, FTD is easily distinguished from the early stages of AD. A study that compared the neuropsychiatric symptom profile of FTD with that of patients with AD found that, as a group, patients with FTD had significantly higher levels of disinhibition, apathy, euphoria, and aberrant motor behavior (stereotyped movements, motor tics), and lower levels of depression and anxiety than early stage AD patients (Levy, Miller, Cummings, Fairbanks, & Craig, 1996). However, as AD progresses and begins to involve more anterior cortical regions (i.e., the prefrontal cortex) the two disorders may look more similar from a neuropsychiatric perspective; at this point, the AD patient will often show much more profound cognitive/intellectual deficits than the FTD individual.

## Subcortical Disorders/Diseases

**Subcortical Versus Cortical Dementia.** Whereas syndromes such as AD and FTD involve pathology that, at least initially, affects cortical regions of the brain, other syndromes cause prominent behavioral disturbances that first affect subcortical structures and circuits. Two of the most common of the subcortical disorders, Parkinson's disease (PD) and Huntington's disease (HD), can first appear without prominent cognitive disruption. When intellectual deterioration (i.e., dementia) is present in individuals with PD and HD, one of the most prominent neurocognitive deficits is pronounced slowing of information-processing speed. Additionally, disturbances of attention and concentration, memory problems characterized by retrieval deficits, and executive dysfunction are typical sequelae of these subcortical syndromes (Lezak, 1995). Below we examine two of the most common forms of subcortical degenerative disorders here.

### Parkinson's Disease

**Introduction.** Parkinson's disease (PD) is a movement disorder that can, and often does, lead to prominent changes in cognitive function and psychological status. It has been estimated that from 20–40% of all patients with PD eventually develop a dementia syndrome (Brown & Mardsen, 1984; Lerner et al., 1997; Mayeux et al., 1988; Rajput, 1992). The rate of progression of PD symptoms varies, but it is generally accepted that most individuals with PD will show significant physical disability within 10–15 years of diagnosis (Freedman, 1990). The likelihood of intellectual and psychological deterioration increases as the illness progresses (Lerner et al., 1997).

It is important to clarify the difference between *Parkinsonism* and Parkinson's disease. Parkinsonism is a generic term used to describe a cluster of motor symptoms that includes difficulty in initiating movement and bradykinesia (slowness of movement), in addition to tremor, rigidity, gait disturbance (e.g., shuffling gait with many rapid, small steps), and postural changes (i.e., stooped posture). These symptoms and signs can result from a variety of specific illnesses (e.g., viral encephalitis) and/or toxin exposure (e.g., manganese poisoning) and are often seen as side effects of long-term use of antipsychotic medications (La Rue, 1992). Parkinson's Disease (PD) is the occurrence of this constellation of symptoms with a gradual onset and progressive course without a specific cause or etiology. Lezak (1995) has suggested that approximately 80% of all cases that involve prominent Parkinsonism are idiopathic.

The most common neuropathological features of PD are neuron loss in the substantia nigra and other pigmented brain-stem nuclei (Gibb, 1989). The substantia nigra is a principal site of dopaminergic neurons, and cell death in this region produces a deficiency in dopamine in associated brain regions, including the striatum and prefrontal regions. This dopaminergic disruption, it is thought, is responsible for the motor disturbances seen in PD.

PD is primarily a disease of late middle age and beyond. According to La Rue (1992), the average age at onset of PD ranges from 59–62 years. PD is quite uncommon before age 40, after which incidence rates increase sharply to the ages of 70–79 years (Marttila, 1987). PD affects approximately 1 million individuals in North America (Lerner et al., 1997). It has been suggested that PD is more common in men than in women (Diamond et al., 1990); this is not consistently borne out by epidemiological studies, some of which have found similar prevalence rates for both sexes (Marttila, 1987). There are few clear risk factors for developing PD other than advancing age and a family history of dementia. Note that although nearly one-third of all cases of idiopathic PD are familial, relative to other diseases (e.g., AD, Huntington's disease), genetics are not strongly implicated in this disorder (Payami & Zareparsi, 1998; Vieregge, Schiffke, Friedrich, & Muller, 1992).

**Cognitive and Motor Changes Associated with Parkinson's Disease.** As noted earlier, many patients with PD show cognitive impairment, although often not severe enough to warrant a label of dementia. Only a small minority of patients present with dementia as the first sign of PD (Hedera et al., 1994). Slowed cognition (bradyphrenia) is the most common cognitive change. Forgetfulness and executive dysfunction, such as difficulty in planning, sequencing, and problem solving are also relatively common in PD. For excellent reviews of the cognitive deficits associated with PD, see Lezak (1995) and La Rue (1992). The motor signs of PD are typically easily identified and include the posture and gait abnormalities mentioned before, resting tremor, and speech irregularities such as hypophonia (reduced voice volume) and dysarthria (difficulty producing speech).

**Psychiatric Characteristics of Parkinson's Disease.** Tremor and other motor disturbances are typically the most common presenting signs of PD, but depression or other psychiatric problems may predate obvious motor abnormalities in a small minority of cases (Mayeux, 1987). As mentioned before, depression is a very common feature of PD. Cummings (1992) suggested that it is the most common neuropsychiatric feature of this disease, and approximately 40–50% of all PD patients experience prominent depression at some time during their illness. Based on two longitudinal studies of depression in PD, Cummings noted that there is some degree of mood stability over the course of PD; those who are depressed at study entry tended to be depressed at follow-up, and those who were not depressed at study entry tended to remain unaffected. Though mood disturbance may occur in reaction to the losses and stressors that accompany PD, evidence suggests that the majority of depression in PD results directly from CNS disturbance. Depression, for example, is not associated with the degree of disability in PD, a finding that runs counter to a reactive depression hypothesis (Troster et al., 1995). In contrast, depression is associated with other markers of frontal-subcortical pathology in PD (Kostic et al., 1994; Mayberg et al., 1990; Wertmann et al., 1993).

Some have suggested that depression is more common among patients with early-onset PD and is especially likely to be associated with neurocognitive impairment in this group (Kostic et al., 1994; Starkstein et al., 1989). However, others have found no differences in age of onset in depression (Dubois et al., 1990; Ludin & Ludin, 1989). Brain imaging of depressed PD patients suggests that metabolic activity in the caudate and orbital regions of the frontal lobes is reduced relative to age and disability-matched nondepressed PD patients (Mayberg et al., 1990). The literature on gender differences in rates of depression in PD is mixed. Some investigators have found higher rates of depression among women with PD than among men (Brown and MacCarthy, 1990; Gotham, Brown, & Mardsen, 1986), but this finding has not always been confirmed (Mayeux et al., 1984).

PD patients with depression often show a profile of depressive symptoms that differs in important ways from patients with idiopathic depressive disorders. Depressed PD patients were less likely to complain of feelings of guilt, failure, or self-reproach but are instead more likely to manifest irritability, anxiety, sad mood, and pessimism regarding their future (Cummings, 1992). A recent study has also suggested that a subset of PD patients show deficits in processing and interpreting materials with emotional content (Benke, Boesch, & Andree, 1998). Mixed results have emerged from studies that examined whether depression is associated with cognitive deficits in PD; clearly, however, such an association does exist among the more severely depressed PD patients (Boller, Marcie, Starkstein, & Traykov, 1998).

Psychotic-spectrum symptoms occur in PD but are less prevalent than in AD. However, hallucinations are not uncommon consequences of long term *treatment* of PD (Factor, Molho, Podskalny, & Brown, 1995). These hallucinations are typically vivid, visual hallucinations that occur with well-preserved orientation and awareness. A recent study found that approximately 15% of a sample of twenty-six autopsy-confirmed PD patients showed evidence of delusions, compared to 53% of all AD patients (Klatka et al., 1996).

## Huntington's Disease

**Introduction.** Huntington's disease (HD) is a genetically transmitted, progressive, degenerative disorder whose clinical manifestations typically first become obvious between the ages of 30 and 50. Three features characterize this degenerative disorder: movement disorder, dementia, and familial transmission. The earliest manifestations of the movement disorder in HD involve brief, irregular, jerking movements (choreoform), along with slower, snake-like, writhing motions that tend to occur when action is initiated. Early in the course of HD, these movement irregularities can occasionally be suppressed or minimized to a certain extent. In the later stages of the illness, movements become far less controllable, and almost constant grimacing, nodding, head bobbing, and a "dancing" gait are seen (Lerner, Strauss, & Whitehouse, 1997). It is not uncommon for psychiatric disturbance to precede the onset of movement disorder in HD. We do not spend much time discussing the typical neurocognitive profile of HD (see Lezak, 1995 for more thorough coverage), other than to mention that executive functions, psychomotor speed, short-term episodic memory retrieval (not encoding), visuospatial skills, and procedural memory are often affected to varying degrees.

The average age of onset is between 35 and 40 years of age, but a juvenile onset variant of the disease occurs in 3–10% of all diagnosed cases of HD (Lerner et al., 1997). HD gradually progresses over many years and ends in death an average of 12–17 years after onset, although a high number of completed suicides obviously shorten group life expectancy post-diagnosis (Mendez, 1994). The main types of neuropathology in HD are atrophy and neuronal loss in the striatum, which begins in the medial caudate nucleus and progresses laterally to involve other areas of the caudate and putamen (Folstein, Brandt, & Folstein, 1990). HD is transmitted as an autosomal dominant trait with complete lifetime penetrance, which means that children of an individual with HD have a 50% probability of developing the disease. Men and women are equally likely to be affected by HD, and, though estimates of the prevalence of HD vary considerably by population, it is believed that somewhere between forty to seventy persons per million population are affected (Cummings & Benson, 1992). CT and MRI scans often reveal enlarged ventricles in structural brain images in HD ("box-car ventricles") as a result of the degeneration of the caudate nucleus and prominent atrophy in the frontal lobes. Functional imaging such as positron emission or single photon computerized tomography typically reveals decreased glucose metabolism in caudate and other basal ganglia structures, whereas cortical metabolism remains roughly normal (Bamford et al., 1989; Nagel et al., 1988).

**Psychiatric Characteristics of Huntington's Disease.** Individuals with HD often undergo significant personality changes that can precede the appearance of movement disorder and/or cognitive deficits (Folstein et al., 1990). As noted by Lerner and colleagues (1997), George Huntington, from whom HD takes its name, described one of three cardinal features as "insanity with a tendency to suicide" and, indeed, studies have documented increased rates of completed suicide in HD (Folstein et al., 1990). Several studies have suggested that as many as half of all patients ultimately diagnosed with HD first present with psychiatric symptoms and anywhere from 35–50% of HD patients have psychiatric disorders (Cummings, 1995).

Depression, the most common psychiatric disorder, affects an estimated 38–60% of all HD patients at some time, and 20% suffer chronic depression (Cummings, 1995). The depression seen in HD can be conceptualized as an understandable reaction to a terrible disease, but several lines of evidence suggest that depressive disorders are not solely reactive to diagnosis. Mood disturbances tend to be episodic and not closely associated with the degree of physical or cognitive deterioration (Zappacosta et al., 1996). A significant minority of HD patients also show evidence of a bipolar mood disorder with prominent and frequent manic episodes (Folstein et al., 1990). Perhaps the most convincing line of evidence can be found in studies of HD patients who were adopted and thus are unaware that they were at risk of developing the disease. These individuals have a significantly higher rate of psychiatric disorder, including suicide, *before* the onset of the motor symptoms of HD, and thus before they knew they were at risk of the disease, indicating that a reactive-depression hypothesis can be discarded.

There is an elevated incidence of pronounced irritability and "intermittent explosive disorder" among patients with HD. Studies summarized by S. E. Folstein (1989) suggested that 31% of 186 patients surveyed met criteria for the DSM-III diagnostic category of Intermittent Explosive Disorder. Shiwach (1994) reported that significant personality alterations were noted in 72% of a sample of 110 HD patients, and irritability and hostility were quite common. A recent study of neuropsychiatric symptomatology among patients with HD found that in twenty-nine patients with agitation, irritability and anxiety were among the most common and salient symptoms (Litvan, Paulsen, Mega, & Cummings, 1998). These personality changes, which often include increased hostility, aggression, and/or irritability, may be harbingers of the onset of HD in individuals known to be at risk for the disease. Baxter and colleagues (1992) reported that among fifty-two at-risk subjects, those determined most likely to develop HD (based on genetic marker studies and functional neuroimaging) had higher anger/hostility ratings on a semistructured mood inventory than at-risk subjects determined less likely to develop HD. Clinical lore and retrospective review of the history of those with HD suggest that increased irritability or hostility is often triggered by events that previously never provoked such a reaction. Increased rates of sexual aggression, promiscuity, exhibitionism, and pedophilia have been noted among individuals with HD (Cummings, 1995). As noted by Lerner et al. (1997), these types of personality changes often go unreported by the HD patient, making it of utmost importance that other informants (e.g., caregiver, spouse) be queried regarding the patient's psychiatric status. A recent literature review by DeMarchi and Mennela (2000) concluded that the precise characterization of both the psychiatric status of the HD patients showing psychopathological changes and of their families might help to identify or delineate different subtypes of HD.

In addition to prominent mood disturbance, HD patients may present with psychotic symptoms such as delusions and/or hallucinations (Folstein et al., 1990; Brooks, Murphy, Janota, & Lishman, 1987). Maricle (1989) points out that the bizarre kinds of hallucinations and delusions that are first-rank symptoms of schizophrenia are rare. Instead, HD patients are more likely to be jealous, suspicious, or obsessional. Prominent psychotic-spectrum symptoms are typically first noted after motor and cognitive irregularities are obvious, but this is not always the case (e.g., Lovestone, Hodgson, Sham, Differ, & Levy, 1996).

Because HD is a familial disease and offspring of infected individuals are at heightened risk of developing the disease themselves, there is considerable interest in the psychiatric status of "at-risk" individuals. Some studies have found that psychiatric symptoms/disorders are more common among these individuals (Baxter et al., 1992), and others have found no differences between their psychiatric functioning and that of controls (Jensen et al., 1993; Shiwach & Norbury, 1994).

## Stroke

**Introduction.** Although the incidence of stroke is declining, most likely due to advances in the treatment of hypertension among elderly adults, nonetheless, it is one of the leading causes of mortality and morbidity in the United States. It is the third leading cause of death in the United States (Robinson & Starkstein, 1997). Stroke has been defined as a "focal neurological disorder of abrupt development due to a pathological process in blood vessels" (Walton, 1994); the mechanism of pathology is disruption of the supply of oxygen (and nutrients such as glucose) to the brain as a result of disrupted blood flow. Without oxygen and glucose, brain tissue dies or is damaged. These areas of tissue damage are termed *infarcts*. The two main classes of strokes are the obstructive and hemorrhagic types; each has slightly different behavioral sequelae, as discussed later. Obstructive strokes represent roughly 75–85% of all strokes (see Powers, 1990; Robinson & Starkstein, 1997) and occur when the buildup of materials in the arterial walls prevents blood from traveling freely and bringing oxygen and nutrients to brain tissue. Hemorrhagic strokes often result from hypertension that causes weakening and eventual rupturing of brain blood vessels but may also occur secondarily to aneurysms. Hypertensive hemorrhagic strokes are considerably more common among elderly individuals, whereas younger persons are more likely to suffer ruptured aneurysms (Lezak, 1995).

**Psychiatric Changes Associated with Stroke.** Stroke can lead to a wide range of cognitive, emotional, and personality changes that at least partially depend on the location and nature of the pathology. Depressive symptomatology is the most common neuropsychiatric disturbance associated with stroke. Estimates of the prevalence of depression following stroke vary, but an estimate of 40–50% is reasonable. One reason for the tremendous variability in estimates of depression prevalence among studies is that very different criteria for defining depression are used (e.g., structured diagnostic criteria versus self-report rating scales). The 4th edition of the DSM (APA, 1994) labels a pronounced mood syndrome following a stroke, "Mood disorder due to stroke with major depressive-like episode," and less severe symptoms, "Mood disorder due to stroke with depressive features" (p. 370). Often, however, studies of poststroke depression use rating scales, rather than structured diagnostic interviews, to assess depressive symptomatology. As we discuss later, high scores on these scales do not necessarily indicate the presence of a clinical syndrome.

Depression is a far more likely occurrence following left-hemisphere strokes, especially when the site of pathology is anterior (i.e., frontal). Several studies have suggested that the distance of the lesion (or infarction) from the left frontal pole is inversely correlated with the severity of depression (Morris, Robinson, & Raphael, 1992; Robinson & Szetela, 1981). Members of our group conducted a longitudinal study to investigate emotional change following stroke at acute, 2-month, and 6-month intervals (Nelson, Cicchetti, Satz, & Stern, 1993). Indifference and depression were both significantly more common among patients who had suffered a left-hemisphere infarction, and these symptoms often persisted throughout the follow-up period. Clearly then, depression is often not merely an acute reaction to stroke but rather a lasting problem. Robinson and Starkstein (1997) reported that nearly one-third of a sample of patients who were not depressed immediately fol-

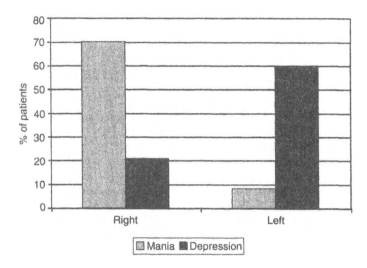

**Figure 2.** Percentages of individuals with mania or major depression following stroke, divided by lesion location as visualized with computerized tomography scan. Adapted from Robinson *et al.* (1988).

lowing their stroke became depressed sometime following discharge from the hospital. Similarly, Astrom and colleagues (1993) found that twenty-seven of their 80 patients had developed major depressive syndromes either in the hospital or by 3-months after hospital discharge and that twelve of these patients (15% of the original sample) continued to show prominent depression 3 years following the stroke. Note that depression is not limited to left-hemisphere stroke as studies have shown that right posterior strokes (especially in the parietal white matter) can lead to elevated rates of depression (e.g., Finset, 1988).

The caregivers of patients who suffered a left-hemisphere stroke reported high rates of blunted emotional expression among their affected relatives and highlighted the need to consider apathy as well as depression when evaluating the psychiatric sequelae of stroke (Nelson, Cicchetti, Satz, & Stern, 1993). As mentioned before, apathy is not uncommon following a stroke and may exist independently of depression in a subset of stroke patients (Starkstein et al., 1993). Patients who had suffered lesions that involved the posterior limb of the internal capsule were most likely to be apathetic but not depressed.

Manic syndromes may occur poststroke, but they are much less common than depression (Cummings & Mendez, 1984). When secondary mania does occur, it is often phenomenologically indistinguishable from primary mania (Starkstein, Boston, & Robinson, 1988). Poststroke mania is most commonly seen when right-sided lesions, especially in limbic-related areas, are present. Although lesions to the right limbic areas are more likely to produce secondary mania, they clearly do not in the majority of patients with such lesions. Figure 2 adapted from Robinson and colleagues (1988), captures the right/left differences seen in depression versus mania. Robinson and Starkstein (1997) suggested that a risk factor for secondary mania may be a family history of mood disorder, implicating a genetic predisposition.

Secondary psychotic symptoms are relatively rare following stroke, but they can occur. When present, they are most often associated with right-sided lesions that involve frontal and parietal areas. There is some preliminary evidence to suggest that subcortical pathology in the context of right frontal-parietal or temporal-parietal lesions may be most likely to produce poststroke psychosis (Robinson & Starkstein, 1997). An interesting behavioral disturbance that may emerge following stroke is pronounced emotional lability characterized by rapid alternation of the patient between laughter and crying. In most emotionally labile patients, the affective outburst is mood-congruent (that is, crying will accompany a sad mood) and inappropriate only in its intensity and seemingly uncontrollable nature. However, affect and mood in some individuals are disconnected, and these patients inappropriately burst into episodes of laughing or crying that seemingly have no context. The term emotional incontinence has been used to describe this inability to modulate emotional expression.

## Traumatic Brain Injury

**Introduction.** Traumatic brain injury (TBI) is among the most common precipitants of brain damage. In fact, disorders arising from TBI are more common than any other neurological disease, except headaches (Kurtzke, 1984). Each year several million persons in the United States sustain some degree of head trauma; many of these are from motor vehicle accidents or falls (Satz et al., 1997). The range of severity among individuals who do not die from TBI is dramatic; some show no discernible adverse cognitive or psychiatric effects, whereas others are left profoundly and permanently disabled, both cognitively and psychologically.

There are several mechanisms by which brain damage can occur following TBI; contusions and diffuse axonal injury are the most common primary mechanisms of neuronal damage. *Contusions* affect specific areas of the brain and usually occur as a result of low-velocity injury such as falls or blunt blows to the head. *Diffuse axonal injury* refers to the mechanical or chemical damage to the axons in cerebral white matter that commonly occurs during acceleration or deceleration injuries. Due to the way the brain sits in the skull, shearing or laceration often take place on the bony prominences that surround the orbital, frontal, and temporal areas along the base of the skull. In addition to these primary mechanisms of neuroanatomical and/or neurochemical alterations, secondary effects such as hematomas (subdural, epidural), cerebral edema (i.e., swelling), and increased intracranial pressure may lead to behavioral changes by altering brain function. In addition to the type of head injury incurred, several factors influence the degree to which an individual will show cognitive and/or psychiatric sequelae secondary to TBI.

**Mediating Factors.** Several studies have shown the people most likely to suffer from brain injury due to head trauma are those in the 15- to 24-year-old age group (Frankowski, Annegers, & Whitman, 1985; Goldstein & Levin, 1990), although

head injury is also more common in the first 5 years of life and in the elderly. One of the best predictors of the likelihood of showing changes in cognition and psychiatric functioning is the severity of the injury, which is often qualified by factors such as the length of loss of consciousness, posttraumatic amnesia, and the need for hospitalization. Obviously, those with more severe head trauma are more likely to show changes in cognitive and psychiatric function.

**Psychiatric Disturbance Following TBI.** Emotional and personality changes are among the most problematic sequelae of TBI. The case of Mr. Phineas Gage, which we described earlier, is a classic example of TBI that produces profound and socially incapacitating changes in the absence of obvious cognitive deterioration. The family members and caregivers of patients who have suffered significant head injury often report that changes in this domain are more problematic than either the physical or the cognitive/intellectual changes that accompany the injury. Unlike in primary psychiatric disorders, where symptom onset is often gradual, the mood, emotional, and personality changes that follow TBI frequently begin suddenly and are pronounced. Many times, changes in mood and personalitiy secondary to TBI remit with time (e.g., with the reduction of cerebral edema), but in some patients, persistent or even permanent deficits in these domains are observed (Silver, Hales, & Yudofsky, 1997). Among the neuropsychiatric disorders, depression is perhaps the most common following TBI. Prevalence rates of depression are clearly elevated following TBI, although estimates vary dramatically depending on the way depression is defined and on the severity of the head injury surveyed (Bornstein, Miller, & van Schoor, 1989; Satz et al., 1998).

The neuropsychiatric consequences of TBI are not dissimilar to those from stroke in terms of the effects of the lesion site. For example, depression is much more common following left frontal injury, whereas mania is more commonly seen when right frontal or right temporal injury is incurred. Historically, the term pseudopsychopathic has been used to describe the patient who shows extreme irritability, facetiousness, impulsivity, sexual disinhibition, inappropriate social and personal behavior, and lack of concern for others. As mentioned earlier, this behavioral profile often occurs following damage to the orbitofrontal cortex and may be especially likely following right-sided orbitofrontal pathology (Cummings, 1993). Manic episodes and bipolar disorders have been reported following TBI, but they are much less common than depression (Bamrah & Johnson, 1991; Burstein, 1993). Right-sided damage, particularly to the basal region of the temporal lobe and the orbitofrontal cortex, was most common among secondary manic patients with TBI (Starkstein et al., 1990). Psychosis is relatively rare as an acute reaction following TBI, but previously head-injured patients are typically vastly overrepresented among those with psychotic-spectrum disorders such as schizophrenia (Buckley et al., 1993).

## Recent Developments in the Clinical Assessment of Neurobehavioral Disorders

This chapter has provided a brief review of some of the major neurobehavioral disorders and their putative neural substrates. We have attempted to highlight some of the key symptoms and signs that are often associated with these disorders, which, in turn, may aid in the differential diagnosis of an underlying CNS versus psychiatric disorder. As noted in this review, a number of neurological disorders can present with psychiatric/psychological symptoms. Frontal lobe lesions, temporal lobe epilepsy, limbic system damage, Alzheimer's disease, Parkinson's disease, Huntington's disease, stroke, and traumatic brain injury are some of the many neurological conditions that can give rise to neuropsychiatric phenomena. Because of the apparent similarity in clinical presentation among many neurobehavioral and psychiatric disorders, the risk of misdiagnosis and mistreatment is high. This state of affairs has been fostered in part by over reliance on assessment instruments that have been standardized and validated on patients with primary (i.e. idiopathic) psychiatric disorders (although, as we have attempted to point out, mounting evidence shows that these disorders have a neuroanatomic and/or neurochemical substrate). As noted by Nelson et al. (1989), these methods have included personality questionnaires (e.g., MMPI-2, MCMI-III), symptom checklists (SCL-90), and clinician-administered rating scales (e.g., Hamilton Depression Rating Scale). Unfortunately, such assessment instruments were not designed with specific knowledge of brain–behavior relationships in

mind and thus have had little direct applicability to neurological disorders. Although recent efforts have been made to modify existing measures such as the MMPI-2 to improve their ability to detect subtle emotional changes associated with brain injury (Gass, 1991; Satz et al., in press), the risk of misdiagnosis is still high, given their historical psychometric roots in personality theory. An additional concern with some of the personality instruments is their reliance on self-report, which restricts their application to patients whose brain insult may compromise awareness of deficits (anosognosia), energy level, and cognitive capacity. A final concern with traditional psychological instruments has been their failure to account for change, pre- to post-injury. Comparing premorbid with present levels of functioning is crucial to understanding the impact of acquired brain insult.

Following, we describe some recent assessment approaches that have addressed these issues so as to familiarize the reader with the tests and their potential application in clinical and research activity.

1. *Neurobehavioral Rating Scale (NRS: Levin et al., 1987).* This scale was developed from the Brief Psychiatric Rating Scale (Overall & Gorham, 1962) to focus on neurobehavioral sequelae of traumatic brain injury, rather than on general psychiatric disorders (see Spreen & Strauss, 1998, for a review). A clinician or other informant familiar with the patient completes seven-point ratings on twenty-seven items that represent four factors: cognition/energy (e.g., disorientation, emotional withdrawal, conceptual disorganization, fatigability, blunted affect), metacognition (e.g., inaccurate insight and self-appraisal), somatic/anxiety (e.g., somatic concerns, anxiety), and language function (e.g., comprehension deficits, expressive language deficits). It has been shown that the NRS has adequate psychometric properties (i.e., reliability and validity). Despite the appear of this instrument for use with brain-injured patients, the NRS does require substantial examiner administration and observation time to ensure appropriate reliability and validity. The NRS also provides no preinjury/postinjury comparison of items to control for potential preinjury risk factors. According to Spreen and Strauss (1998), there are no normative data available because "normal healthy subjects" are not expected to show elevations on any of these scales except for "minor elevations in the somatic-anxiety factor area." The scale authors

also note that women who have sustained TBI score slightly higher on depression items, but otherwise sex differences are negligible on the NRS. Presently, no commercial source exists for this instrument.

2. *Neuropsychology Behavior and Affect Profile (NBAP: Nelson et al., 1989)*. This instrument was developed and standardized in the late 1980s by a group of neuropsychologists at UCLA to measure perceived changes in affect and behavior following trauma or suspected brain injury. The instrument consists of 106 items on which explicit behaviors and emotions are rated dichotomously (present or absent) at each of two times (preinjury and postinjury). Both observer and self-rated versions are available, though initial research has focused on using the observer-rated form. Typically, the "observer" is a family member, significant other long-time friend, or caregiver who has known the brain-injured patient well. Five clinical scales were developed on the basis of previous research on patients with neurobehavioral disorders. The items purport to measure the following five constructs, which were constructed on an a priori basis and were subjected to content validation by expert sortings: (1) *indifference* (anosognosia or a tendency to minimize disability, apathy), (2) *inappropriateness* (unusual or bizarre behavior), (3) *pragnosia* (defect in pragmatics of communication), (4) *depression* (sadness, anhedonia), and (5) *mania* (elevated, expansive mood, euphoria, heightened activity level). Several validation studies have been published by the test authors on populations with closed head injury and Alzheimer's and Downs syndrome (see Spreen & Strauss, 1998, for a review).

Despite the reasonable support found for the NBAP's discriminant validity, there are potential problems with any observer-rated instrument, and the NBAP is no exception. Such potential confounds as halo effects, leniency or severity bias, and central tendency or restriction effects should always be considered when an observer rates another individual with an instrument. For this reason, several steps were taken to reduce potential rater inaccuracies and biases. Items were written at a reading level appropriate for the general population; all item wording was specific, concrete, and descriptive. Neutral items (i.e., written without a negative emotional valence) were also added to assess overendorsing tendencies. Some items were also developed to serve as internal consis-

tency checks, and item wording was either almost identical or opposite in meaning to other items. Because of the potential observer bias in cases of litigation, four validity scales were developed for the NBAP that have shown promising discriminant validity (Satz et al., 1996). Finally, to control for undersampling (i.e., insufficient rater knowledge of the subject's behaviors), the NBAP used only informants with sufficient knowledge of the patient's behaviors both pre- and postinjury.

The NBAP, including norms, manual, and scoring instructions, is available for review from the test's publisher, Mind Garden, located in Palo Alto, California.

3. *Neuropsychiatric Inventory (NPI: Cummings et al., 1994)*. The NPI is a tool designed for assessing psychopathology among patients with dementia and other neurological disorders. It is a brief, clinician-administered interview that obtains information about the patient's behavior across twelve neuropsychiatric symptom domains (e.g., delusions, agitation, depression, anxiety, apathy, etc.). NPI items are typically administered to a person intimately familiar with the patient's behavior, such as a family member, significant other, or paid caregiver. The format of NPI dictates that a screening question is asked first (in each of the twelve domains) and is followed up with more specific queries if the response to the screening question suggests disturbance in that particular domain. After administering the specific queries in any domain, informant is asked to rate the frequency and severity of disturbance as well as the degree of distress caused them by the patient's behavior in this domain. A key feature of the NPI is that it is interested in *behavioral change* since the onset of the neurological disease/disorder. For example, patients who were mildly depressed before they received a diagnosis of Alzheimer's disease and remain depressed would be coded only if their depression had changed (i.e., intensified). The behavioral domains sampled by the NPI include depression, anxiety, delusions, hallucinations, agitation, disinhibition, euphoria/elation, apathy/indifference, irritability, aberrant motor behavior, sleep functioning, and appetite/eating change.

It has been shown that scores on the NPI are only minimally influenced by the normal aging process; the vast majority of healthy, normal elderly controls obtains scores of zero on the majority of symptom domains; when symptom domains are positively endorsed among the normal elderly, they tend to be depression, irritability, and disinhibition (Cummings et al., 1994). The validity and reliability of the NPI symptom scales, as well as the caregiver distress scale, have been demonstrated (Cummings, 1997; Kaufer et al., 1998).

The NPI is similar to both the NBAP and the NRS and recognizes the importance of obtaining information regarding behavioral changes from sources other than the affected patient who may be a less than reliable informant due to cognitive limitations. However, our group has used a modification of the apathy and irritability subscales from the NPI for *direct* administration to relatively high-functioning individuals with CNS diseases such as HIV/AIDS who maintain the ability to accurately report on these symptoms. Using direct administration, we have found interesting relationships between neurocognitive, neurophysiological, and neuropsychiatric variables (Castellon et al., 1998).

These three measurement instruments have in common that they attempt to integrate theory and clinical practice in assessing psychopathology among individuals with CNS disorders. Although they represent significant advances over instruments constructed (and validated) for use with primary psychiatric populations, additional research will be required to continue to integrate neuropsychological empiricism with psychometrically sound measurement theory. This stated, however, it should be noted that many psychopathology instruments initially constructed for use in primary psychiatric/ psychological populations, nonetheless, can provide useful information about the symptom profile of brain-injured individuals. When using such instruments, we caution the user to realize that many of the sequelae of CNS insult or injury can be confused with symptoms of psychiatric disorder (e.g., sleep disturbance, fatigue, somatic concerns). To the extent that this occurs, the symptoms of neurological or physical illness might be mistakenly attributed to psychiatric disorder.

## Conclusion

We hope that this chapter has conveyed the fact that many of the psychiatric symptoms, signs, and syndromes described in earlier chapters of this text commonly appear following CNS disturbance. Likewise, many of the most prevalent neurological disorders have important psychiatric se-

quelae. Freud, in his *Project for a scientific psychology*, speculated that in the future we would find that "behind every crooked thought lies a crooked neuron," recognizing the intimate relationship between psychological phenomenon and neurophysiology. Fortunately, the Cartesian dualism, which has artificially dichotomized disorders of the mind and disorders of the brain, has faded considerably during the last decade. With the continued advances in neuropsychology and kindred disciplines, especially neuroimaging, Freud's prediction again appears prescient.

## References

Alexander, G. E., DeLong, M. R., & Strick, P. L. (1986). Parallel organization of functionally segregated circuits linking basal ganglia and cortex. *Annual Review of Neuroscience, 9,* 357–381.

Amaducci, L. A., Rocca, W. A., & Schoenberg, B. (1986). Origin of the distinction between Alzheimer's disease and senile dementia: How history can clarify nosology. *Neurology, 36,* 1497–1499.

American Psychiatric Association. (1980). *Diagnostic and statistical manual of mental disorders* (3rd ed.). Washington, DC: Author.

American Psychiatric Association. (1987). *Diagnostic and statistical manual of mental disorders* (3rd ed., rev.). Washington, DC: Author.

American Psychiatric Association. (1994). *Diagnostic and statistical manual of mental disorders* (4th ed.). Washington, DC: Author.

Aronson, M. K., Ooi, W. L., Geva, D. L., Masur, D., Blau, A., & Frishman, W. (1991). Dementia. Age-dependent incidence, prevalence, and mortality in the old old. *Archives of Internal Medicine, 151,* 989–992.

Astrom, M., Adolfsson, R., & Asplund, K. (1993). Major depression in stroke patients: A 3-year longitudinal study. *Stroke, 24,* 976–982.

Bamford, K., Caine, E., Kido, D. K., Plassche, W. M., & Shoulson, I. (1989). Clinical-pathologic correlation in Huntington's disease: A neuropsychological and computed tomography study. *Neurology, 39,* 796–801.

Bamrah, J. S., & Johnson, J. (1991). Bipolar affective disorder following head injury. *British Journal of Psychiatry, 158,* 117–119.

Baxter, L., Mazziotta, J., Pahl, J. et al. (1992). Psychiatric, genetic, and positron emission tomographic evaluation of persons at risk for Huntington's disease. *Archives of General Psychiatry, 49,* 148–154.

Benke, T., Boesch, S., & Andree, B. (1998). A study of emotional processing in Parkinson's disease. *Brain and Cognition, 38,* 36–52.

Binetti, G., Padovani, A., Magni, E., & Bianchetti, A. (1995). Delusions and dementia: Clinical and CT correlates. *Acta Neurologica Scandinavica, 91,* 271–275.

Boller, F., Marcie, P., Starkstein, S. E., & Traykov, L. (1998). Memory and depression in Parkinson's disease. *European Journal of Neurology, 5,* 291–295.

Bornstein, R. A., Miller, H. B., & van Schoor, J. T. (1989). Neuropsychological deficit and emotional disturbance in head-injured patients. *Journal of Neurosurgery, 70,* 509–513.

Brooks, D. S., Murphy, D., Janota, I., & Lishman, W. A. (1987). Early onset Huntington's Chorea: Diagnostic clue. *British Journal of Psychiatry, 151,* 850–853.

Brown, R. G., & MacCarthy, B. (1990). Psychiatric morbidity in patients with Parkinson's disease. *Psychological Medicine, 20,* 77–87.

Brown, R. G., & Mardsen, C. D. (1984). How common is dementia in Parkinson's disease? *Lancet, 2,* 1262–1265.

Brun, A., & Gustafson, L. (1999). Clinical and pathological aspects of frontotemporal dementia. In B. L. Miller & J. L. Cummings (Eds.), *The human frontal lobes: Functions and disorders.* New York: Guilford.

Brun, A., Englund, B., Gustafson, L., Passant, U., Mann, D. M. A., Neary, D., & Snowden, J. (1994). Clinical and neuro-pathological criteria for frontotemporal dementia. *Journal of Neurology, Neurosurgery, and Psychiatry, 57,* 416–418.

Buchsbaum, M. S., Cappelletti, J., Ball, R., Hazlett, E., King, A. C., Johnson, J., Wu, J., & deLisi, L. E. (1984). Positron emission tomographic image measurement in schizophrenia and affective disorders. *Annals of Neurology, 15*(Suppl.), S157–S165.

Buckley, P., Stack, J. P., Madigan, C., O'Callaghan, E., Larkin, C., Redmond, O., Ennis, J. T., & Waddington, J. L. (1993). Magnetic resonance imaging of schizophrenia-like psychoses associated with cerebral trauma: Clinicopathological correlates. *American Journal of Psychiatry, 150,* 146–148.

Burstein, A. (1993). Bipolar and pure mania disorders precipitated by head trauma. *Psychosomatics, 34,* 194–195.

Castellon, S. A., Hinkin, C. H., Wood, S., & Yarema, K. (1998). Apathy, depression, and cognitive performance in HIV-1 infection. *Journal of Neuropsychiatry and Clinical Neurosciences, 10,* 320–329.

Castellon, S. A., Hinkin, C. H., & Myers, H. F. (2000). Neuropsychiatric disturbance is associated with executive dysfunction in HIV-1 infection. *Journal of the International Neuropsychological Society, 6,* 373–379.

Cherkasky, S., & Hollander, E. (1997). Neuropsychiatric aspects of impulsivity and aggression. In S. C. Yudofsky & R. E. Hales (Eds.), *The American Psychiatric Press textbook of neuropsychiatry.* Washington, DC: American Psychiatric Press.

Chow, T., & Cummings, J. L. (1999). Frontal-subcortical circuits. In B. L. Miller & J. L. Cummings (Eds.), *The human frontal lobes: Functions and disorders.* New York: Guilford.

Clarke, T., Wadhwa, U., & Leroi, I. (1998). Psychotic depression: An atypical initial presentation of multiple sclerosis. *Psychosomatics, 39,* 72–75.

Craig, A. H., Cummings, J. L., Fairbanks, L., Itti, L., Miller, B. L., Li, J., & Mena, I. (1996). Cerebral blood flow correlates of apathy in Alzheimer's disease. *Archives of Neurology, 53,* 1116.

Cummings, J. L. (1997). The Neuropsychiatric Inventory: Assessing psychopathology in dementia patients. *Neurology, 48*(Suppl. 6), S10–S16.

Cummings, J. L. (1995). Behavioral and psychiatric symptoms associated with Huntington's disease. *Advances in Neurology, 65,* 179–186.

Cummings, J. L. (1994). Depression in neurologic disease. *Psychiatric Annals, 24,* 525–531.

Cummings, J. L. (1993). Frontal-subcortical circuits and human behavior. *Archives of Neurology, 50,* 873–880.

Cummings, J. L. (1992). Depression and Parkinson's disease: A review. *American Journal of Psychiatry, 149,* 443–454.

Cummings, J. L., Mega, M., Gray, K., Rosenberg-Thompson, S., Carusi, D. A., & Gornbein, J. (1994). The Neuropsychiatric Inventory: Comprehensive assessment of psychopathology in dementia. *Neurology, 44,* 2308–2314.

Cummings, J. L., & Benson, D. F. (1992). *Dementia: A clinical approach* (2nd ed.). Boston, MA: Butterworth.

Cummings, J. L., & Mendez, M. F. (1984). Secondary mania with focal cerebrovascular lesions. *American Journal of Psychiatry, 141,* 1084–1087.

Damasio, A. R., & Anderson, S. W. (1993). The frontal lobes. In K. M. Heilman & E. Valenstein (Eds.) *Clinical neuropsychology* (3rd ed, pp. 409–460). New York: Oxford University Press.

De la Fuente, J. M., Goldman, S., Stanus, E., Vizuete, C., Morlan, I., Bobes, J., & Mendlewicz, J. (1997). Brain glucose metabolism in borderline personality disorder. *Journal of Psychiatric Research, 31,* 531–541.

De Marchi, N., & Mennella, R. (2000). Huntington's disease and its association with psychopathology. *Harvard Review of Psychiatry, 7,* 278–289.

Deckel, W. A., Hesselbrock, V., & Bauer, L. (1996). Antisocial personality disorder, childhood delinquency, and frontal brain functioning: EEG and neuropsychological findings. *Journal of Clinical Psychology, 52,* 639–650.

Diamond, S. G., Markham, C. H., Hoehn, M. M., et al. (1990). An examination of male-female differences in progression and mortality of Parkinson's disease. *Neurology, 40,* 763–766.

Dubois, B., Pillon, B., Sternic, N., Lhermitte, F., & Agid, Y. (1990). Age-induced cognitive disturbances in Parkinson's disease. *Neurology, 40,* 38–41.

Duffy, J. D., & Kant, R. (1997). Apathy secondary to neurologic disease. *Psychiatric Annals, 27,* 39–43.

Duffy, J. D., & Campbell, J. J. (1994). The regional prefrontal syndromes: A theoretical and clinical overview. *Journal of Neuropsychiatry and Clinical Neurosciences, 6,* 379–387.

Dupont, R. M., Jernigan, T. L., Heindel, W., & Butters, N. (1995). Magnetic resonance imaging and mood disorders: Localization of white matter and other subcortical abnormalities. *Archives of General Psychiatry, 52,* 747–755.

El-Hilu, S. M., Abdel-Dayem, H. M., Sehweil, A., Almoktar, N., Simdonov, S., Tuli, M., Jahan, S., Higazi, E., Salhat, M., & Almohannadi, S. (1998). Regional cerebral blood flow in drug-naive patients with depression and mania using Tc-99m HMPAO single photon emission computerized tomography. *European Journal of Psychiatry, 12,* 119–127.

Evans, D. A., Funkenstein, H. H., Albert, M. S., Scherr, P. A., Cook, N. R., Chown, M. J., Hebert, L., Hennekens, C. H., & Taylor, J. O. (1989). Prevalence of Alzheimer's disease in a community population of older persons. *Journal of the American Medical Association, 262,* 2551–2556.

Factor, S. A., Molho, E. S., Podskalny, G. D., & Brown, D. (1995). Parkinson's disease: Drug induced psychiatric states. *Advances in Neurology, 65,* 115–138.

Filley, C. M. (1994). Neurobehavioral aspects of cerebral white matter disorders. In B. S. Fogel, R. S. Schiffer, & S. M. Rao (Eds.), *Neuropsychiatry: A comprehensive textbook.* Baltimore: Williams & Wilkins.

Finn, P. R., Farnsey, S. E., & Earlywine, M. (2000). Frontal EEG response to threat, aggressive traits and a family history of alcoholism: A preliminary study. *Journal of Studies on Alcohol, 61,* 38–45.

Finset, A. (1988). Depressed mood and reduced emotionality

after right hemisphere brain damage. In M. Kinsbourne (Ed.), *Cerebral hemisphere function in depression*. Washington, DC: American Psychiatric Press.

Folstein, S. E. (1989). *Huntington's disease: A disorder of families*. Baltimore: Johns Hopkins University Press.

Folstein, S. E., Brandt, J., & Folstein, M. F. (1990). Huntington's disease. In J. L. Cummings (Ed.), *Subcortical dementia* (pp. 87–107). New York: Oxford University Press.

Frankowski, R. F., Annegers, J. F., & Whitman, S. (1985). The descriptive epidemiology of head trauma in the United States. In D. P. Becker & J. T. Povlishock (Eds.), *Central nervous system trauma: Status report, 1985*. Bethesda, MD: National Institutes of Health.

Freedman, M. (1990). Parkinson's disease. In J. L. Cummings (Ed.). *Subcortical dementia* (pp. 108–122), New York: Oxford University Press.

Gass, C. S. (1991). MMPI-2 interpretation and closed head injury: A correction factor. *Psychological Assessment, 3*, 27–31.

Gibb, W. R. G. (1989). Dementia and Parkinson's disease. *British Journal of Psychiatry, 154*, 596–614.

Goggans, F. C. (1983). A case of mania secondary to vitamin B$_{12}$ deficiency. *American Journal of Psychiatry, 141*, 300–301.

Goldstein, F. C., & Levin, H. S. (1990). Epidemiology of traumatic brain injury: Incidence, clinical characteristics, and risk factors. In E. D. Bigler (Ed.), *Traumatic brain injury*. Austin, TX: Pro-ed.

Gormley, N., & Rizwan, M. R. (1998). Prevalence and clinical correlates of psychiatric symptoms in Alzheimer's disease. *International Journal of Geriatric Psychiatry, 13*, 410–414.

Gotham, A. M., Brown, R. G., & Mardsen, C. D. (1986). Depression in Parkinson's disease: A quantitative and qualitative analysis. *Journal of Neurology, Neurosurgery, and Psychiatry, 49*, 381–389.

Hedera, P., Cohen, M. L., Lerner, A. J., et al. (1994). Dementia preceding motor symptoms in Parkinson's disease: A case study. *Neuropsychiatry, Neuropsychology, and Behavioral Neurology, 7*, 67–72.

Hendrie, H. C. (1998). Epidemiology of dementia and Alzheimer's disease. *American Journal of Geriatric Psychiatry, 6*(Suppl): S3–18.

Hoff, A. L., Shukla, S., Cook, B. L., & Aronson, T. A. (1988). Cognitive function in manics with associated neurologic features. *Journal of Affective Disorders, 14*, 251–255.

Jack, R. A., Rivers-Bulkeley, N. T., & Robin, P. L. (1983). Secondary mania as a presentation of progressive dialysis encephalopathy. *Journal of Nervous and Mental Disease, 171*, 193–195.

Jensen, P., Sorensen, S. A., Fenger, K., & Bolwig, T. G. (1993). A study of psychiatric morbidity in patients with Huntington's disease, their relatives, and controls: Admissions to psychiatric hospitals in Denmark from 1969 to 1991. *British Journal of Psychiatry, 163*, 790–797.

Jorm, A. F., & Jolley, D. (1998). The incidence of dementia: A meta-analysis. *Neurology, 51*, 728–733.

Jost, B. C., & Grossberg, G. T. (1996). The evolution of psychiatric symptoms in Alzheimer's disease: A natural history study. *Journal of the American Geriatrics Society, 44*, 1078–1081.

Kandel, E., & Freed, D. (1989). Frontal-lobe dysfunction and antisocial behavior: A review. *Journal of Clinical Psychology, 45*, 404–413.

Katzman, R. (1986). Alzheimer's disease. *New England Journal of Medicine, 314*, 964–973.

Kaufer, D. I., Cummings, J. L., Christine, D., Bray, T., Castellon, S. A., Masterman, D., MacMillan, A., Ketchel, P., & DeKosky, S. T. (1998). Assessing the impact of neuropsychiatric symptoms in Alzheimer's disease: The Neuropsychiatric Inventory Caregiver Distress Scale. *Journal of the American Geriatrics Society, 46*, 210–215.

Kay, D. W. K. (1989). Genetics, Alzheimer's disease and senile dementia. *British Journal of Psychiatry, 154*, 311–320.

Klatka, L. A., Louis, E. D., & Schiffer, R. B. (1996). Psychiatric features in diffuse Lewy body disease: A clincopathologic study using Alzheimer's disease and Parkinson's disease comparison groups. *Neurology, 47*, 1148–1152.

Kolb, B., & Whishaw, I. Q. (1990). *Fundamentals of human neuropsychology* (3rd ed.). New York: W.H. Freeman.

Kostic, V. S., Filipovic, S. R., Lecic, D., Momcilovic, D., Sokic, D., & Sternic, N. (1994). Effect of age at onset on frequency of depression in Parkinson's disease. *Journal of Neurology, Neurosurgery, and Psychiatry, 57*, 1265–1267.

Kotrla, K. J., Chacko, R. C., Harper, R. G., Jhingran, S., & Doody, R. (1995). SPECT findings on psychosis in Alzheimer's disease. *American Journal of Psychiatry, 152*, 1470–1475.

Krauthammer, C., & Klerman, G. L. (1978). Secondary mania. *Archives of General Psychiatry, 35*, 1333–1339.

Kurtzke, J. F. (1984). Neuroepidemiology. *Annals of Neurology, 16*, 265–277.

La Rue, A. (1992). *Aging and neuropsychological assessment*. New York: Plenum.

Lebert, F., Pasquier, F., Danel, T., & Steinling, M. (1994). Psychiatric, neuropsychologic, and SPECT evidence of elated mood in dementia of the Alzheimer's type. *Neuropsychiatry, Neuropsychology, and Behavioral Neurology, 7*, 299–302.

Lebert, F., Pasquier, F., & Petit, H. (1995). Personality traits and frontal lobe dementia. *International Journal of Geriatric Psychiatry, 10*, 1046–1049.

Lerner, A. J., Strauss, M. E., & Whitehouse, P. J. (1997). Neuropsychiatric aspects of degenerative dementias associated with motor dysfunction. In S. C. Yudofsky & R. E. Hales (Eds.), *The American Psychiatric Press textbook of neuropsychiatry*. Washington, DC: American Psychiatric Press.

Levin, H. S., High, W. M., Goethe, K. E., Sisson, R. A., Overall, J. E., Rhoades, H. M., Eisenberg, H. M., Kalisky, Z., & Gary, H. E. (1987). The neurobehavioral rating scale: Assessment of the behavioral sequelae of head injury by the clinician. *Journal of Neurology, Neurosurgery, and Psychiatry, 50*, 183–193.

Levy, M. S., Miller, B. L., Cummings, J. L., Fairbanks, L. A., & Craig, A. (1996). Alzheimer's disease and frontotemporal dementias. *Archives of Neurology, 53*, 687–690.

Lezak, M. D. (1995). *Neuropsychological assessment* (3rd ed.). New York: Oxford University Press.

Litvan, I., Paulsen, J. S., Mega, M. S., & Cummings, J. L. (1998). Neuropsychiatric assessment of patients with hyperkinetic and hypokinetic movement disorders. *Archives of Neurology, 55*, 1313–1319.

Lopez, O. L., Kamboh, M. I., Becker, J. T., Kaufer, D. I., & DeKosky, S. T. (1997). The apolipoprotein E epsilon 4 allele is not associated with psychiatric symptoms or extrapyramidal signs in probable Alzheimer's disease. *Neurology, 49*, 794–797.

Lovestone, S., Hodgson, S., Sham, P., Differ, A. M., & Levy, R. (1996). Familial psychiatric presentation of Huntington's disease. *Journal of Medical Genetics, 33*, 128–131.

Ludin, S. M., & Ludin, H. P. (1989). Is Parkinson's disease of early onset a separate disease entity? *Journal of Neurology, 236*, 203–207.

Lyketsos, C. G., Steele, C., Baker, L., Galik, E., Kopunek, S., Steinberg, M., & Warren, A. (1997) Major and minor depression in Alzheimer's disease: Prevalence and impact. *Journal of Neuropsychiatry and Clinical Neurosciences, 9*, 556–561.

Maricle, R. A. (1989). Common psychiatric problems associated with Huntington's disease. *Genetics Northwest, 6*, 5–7.

Marin, R. S., Firinciogullari, S., & Biedrzycki, R. C. (1994). Group differences in the relationship between apathy and depression. *Journal of Nervous and Mental Disease, 182*, 235–239.

Marin, R. S. (1991). Apathy: A neuropsychiatric syndrome. *Journal of Neuropsychiatry and Clinical Neurosciences, 3*, 243–254.

Marttila, R. J. (1987). Epidemiology. In W. D. Keller (Ed.), *Handbook of Parkinson's disease* (pp. 35–50). New York: Marcel Dekker.

Mayberg, H. S., Mahurin, R. K., & Brannan, S. K. (1997). Neuropsychiatric aspects of mood and affective disorders. In S. C. Yudofsky & R. E. Hales (Eds.), *The American Psychiatric Press textbook of neuropsychiatry*. Washington, DC: American Psychiatric Press.

Mayberg, H. S., Starkstein, S. E., Peyser, C. E., et al. (1990). Selective hypometabolism in the inferior frontal lobe in depressed patients with Parkinson's disease. *Annals of Neurology, 28*, 57–64.

Mayeux, R. (1987). Mental state. In W. D. Keller (Ed.), *Handbook of Parkinson's disease* (pp. 127–144). New York: Marcel Dekker.

Mayeux, R., Stern, Y., Cote, C., & Williams, J. B. (1984). Altered serotonin metabolism in depressed patients with Parkinson's disease. *Neurology, 34*, 642–646.

Mayeux, R., Stern, Y., Rosenstein, R., Marder, K., Hauser, A., Cote, L., & Fahn, S. (1988). An estimate of the prevalence of dementia in idiopathic Parkinson's disease. *Archives of Neurology, 45*, 260–262.

McAllister-Williams, R. H., Ferrier, I. N., & Young, A. H. (1998). Mood and neuropsychological function in depression: The role of corticosteriods and serotonin. *Psychological Medicine, 28*, 573–584.

McGlynn, S. M., & Schacter, D. L. (1997). The neuropsychology of insight: Impaired awareness of deficits in a psychiatric context. *Psychiatric Annals, 27*, 806–811.

Mendez, M. F. (1994). Huntington's disease: Update and review of neuropsychiatric aspects. *International Journal of Psychiatric Medicine, 24*, 189–208.

Migliorelli, R., Starkstein, S. E., Teson, A., & de Quiros, G. (1993). SPECT findings in patients with primary mania. *Journal of Neuropsychiatry and Clinical Neurosciences, 5*, 379–383.

Miller, B. L., Chang, L., Mena, I., Boone, K., & Lesser, I. M. (1993). Progressive right frontotemporal degeneration: Clinical, neuropsychological and SPECT characteristics. *Dementia, 4*, 204–213.

Miller, B. L., Mena, I., Giombetti, R., & Villanueva-Meyer, J. (1992). Neuropsychiatric effects of cocaine: SPECT measurements. *Journal of Addictive Diseases, 11*, 47–58.

Miller, B. L., Cummings, J. L., Villanueva-Meyer, J., Boone, K., Mehringer, C. M., Lesser, I., & Mena, I. (1991). Frontal lobe degeneration: Clinical, neuropsychological and SPECT characteristics. *Neurology, 41*, 1374–1382.

Morris, P. L. P., Robinson, R. G., & Raphael, B. (1992). Lesion location and depression in hospitalized stroke patients: Evidence supporting a specific relationship in the left hemisphere. *Neuropsychiatry, Neuropsychology, and Behavioral Neurology, 3*, 75–82.

Mortimer, J. A., French, L. R., Hutton, J. T., & Schuman, L. M. (1985). Head injury as a risk factor for Alzheimer's disease. *Neurology, 35*, 264–267.

Nagel, J. S., Johnson, K. A., Ichise, M., English, R. J., Walshe, T. M., Morris, J. H., & Holman, B. I. (1988). Decreased iodine-123 IMP caudate nucleus uptake in patients with Huntington's disease. *Clinical Nuclear Medicine, 13*, 486–490.

Neary, D., & Snowden, J. (1996). Fronto-temporal dementia: Nosology, neuropsychology, and neuropathology. *Brain and Cognition, 31*, 176–187.

Nelson, L. D., Cicchetti, D., Satz, P., & Stern, S. (1993). Emotional sequelae of stroke. *Neuropsychology, 7*, 553–560.

Nelson, L. D., Satz, P., Mitrushina, M., van Gorp, W., Cicchetti, D., Lewis, R., & van Lancker, D. (1989). Development and validation of the Neuropsychology Behavior and Affect Profile. *Psychological Assessment, 1*, 266–272.

Okada, K., Kobayashi, S., Yamagata, S., Takahashi, K., & Yamaguchi, S. (1997). Poststroke apathy and regional cerebral blood flow. *Stroke, 28*, 2437–2441.

Ott, B. R., Noto, R. B., & Fogel, B. S. (1996). Apathy and loss of insight in Alzheimer's disease: A SPECT imaging study. *Journal of Neuropsychiatry and Clinical Neurosciences, 8*, 41–46.

Overall, J. E., & Gorham, D. R. (1962). The Brief Psychiatric Rating Scale. *Psychological Reports, 10*, 799–812.

Payami, H., & Zareparsi, S. (1998). Genetic epidemiology of Parkinson's disease. *Journal of Geriatric Psychiatry and Neurology, 11*, 98–106.

Pfeffer, R. I., Afifi, A. A., & Chance, J. M. (1987). Prevalence of Alzheimer's disease in a retirement community. *American Journal of Epidemiology, 125*, 420–436.

Pine, D. S., Douglas, C. J., Charles, E., & Davies, M. (1995). Patients with multiple sclerosis presenting to psychiatric hospitals. *Journal of Clinical Psychiatry, 56*, 297–306.

Powers, W. J. (1990). Stroke. In A. L. Pearlman & R. C. Collins (Eds.), *Neurobiology of disease*. New York: Oxford University Press.

Rajput, A. H. (1992). Prevalence of dementia in Parkinson's disease. In S. J. Huber & J. L. Cummings (Eds.), *Parkinson's disease: Neurobehavioral aspects*. New York: Oxford University Press.

Ramachandran, G., Marder, K., Tang, M., Schofield, P. W., Chun, M. R., Devanand, D. P., Stern, Y., & Mayeux, R. (1996). A preliminary study of apolipoprotein E genotype and psychiatric manifestations of Alzheimer's disease. *Neurology, 47*, 256–259.

Reichman, W. E., Coyne, A. C., Amirneni, S., Molino, B., & Egan, S. (1996). Negative symptoms in Alzheimer's disease. *American Journal of Psychiatry, 153*, 424–426.

Robinson, R. G., & Price, T. R. (1982). Post-stroke depressive disorders: A follow-up study of 103 patients. *Stroke, 13*, 635–641.

Robinson, R. G., & Starkstein, S. E. (1990). Current research in affective disorders following stroke. *Journal of Neuropsychiatry and Clinical Neurosciences, 2*, 1–14.

Robinson, R. G., & Starkstein, S. E. (1997). Neuropsychiatric aspects of cerebrovascular disorders. In S. C. Yudofsky & R. E. Hales (Eds.), *The American Psychiatric Press textbook of neuropsychiatry.* Washington, DC: American Psychiatric Press.

Robinson, R. G., & Szetela, B. (1981). Mood change following left hemispheric brain injury. *Annals of Neurology, 9,* 477–453.

Robinson, R. G., Boston, J. D., Starkstein, S. E., & Price, T. R. (1988). Comparison of mania and depression after brain injury: Causal factors. *American Journal of Psychiatry, 145,* 172–178.

Royall, D. R. (1999). Frontal systems impairment in major depression. *Seminars in Clinical Neuropsychiatry, 4,* 13–23.

Rubin, R. T., & Harris, G. J. (1999). Obsessive-compulsive disorder and the frontal lobes. In B. L. Miller & J. L. Cummings (Eds.), *The human frontal lobes: Functions and disorders.* New York: Guilford.

Rubin, E. H., Drevets, W. C., & Burke, W. J. (1988). The nature of psychotic symptoms in senile dementia of the Alzheimer type. *Journal of Geriatric Psychiatry and Neurology, 1,* 16–20.

Sabrie, P. (1986). Reconciling the role of central serotonin neurons in human and animal behavior. *Behavioral and Brain Sciences, 9,* 319–364.

Satz, P., Alfano, M. S., Light, R., Morgenstern, H., Zaucha, K., & Asarnow, R. F. (in press). Persistent post-concussive syndrome: A proposed methodology and literature review to determine the effects, if any, of mild head and other bodily injury. *Journal of Clinical and Experimental Neuropsychology.*

Satz, P., Forney, D. L., Zaucha, K., Asarnow, R., Light, R., McCleary, C., Levin, H., Kelly, D., Bergsneider, M., Hovda, D., Martin, N., Namerow, N., & Becker, D. (1998). Depression, cognition, and functional correlates of recovery outcome after traumatic brain injury. *Brain Injury, 12,* 537–553.

Satz, P., Holston, S. G., Uchiyama, C. L., Shimahara, G., Mitrushina, M., et al. (1996). Development and evaluation of validity scales for the Neuropsychology Behavior and Affect Profile: A dissembling study. *Psychological Assessment, 8,* 115–124.

Satz, P., Zaucha, K., McCleary, C., Light, R., Asarnow, R., & Becker, D. (1997). Mild head injury in children and adolescents: A review of studies (1970–1995). *Psychological Bulletin, 122,* 107–131.

Shiwach, R. S. (1994). Psychopathology in Huntington's disease patients. *Acta Psychiatrica Scandinavica, 90,* 241–246.

Shiwach, R. S., & Norbury, C. G. (1994). A controlled psychiatric study of individuals at risk for Huntington's disease. *British Journal of Psychiatry, 165,* 500–505.

Shukla, S., Cook, B. L., Mukheree, S., et al. (1987). Mania following head trauma. *American Journal of Psychiatry, 144,* 93–96.

Silver, J. M., Hales, R. E., & Yudofsky, S. C. (1997). Neuropsychiatric aspects of traumatic brain injury. In S. C. Yudofsky & R. E. Hales (Eds.), *The American Psychiatric Press textbook of neuropsychiatry.* Washington, DC: American Psychiatric Press.

Singer, S. F. (1992). Capgras symptom and delusions of reduplication in neurologic disorders. *Neuropsychiatry, Neuropsychology, & Behavioral Neurology, 5,* 138–143.

Spreen, O., & Strauss, E. (1998). *A compendium of neuropsychological tests* (2nd ed.). New York: Oxford University Press.

Starkstein, S. E. Chemerinski, E., Sabe, L., Kuzis, G., Petracca, G., Tesaon, A., & Leiguarda, R. (1997). Prospective longitudinal study of depression and anosognosia in Alzheimer's disease. *British Journal of Psychiatry, 171,* 47–52.

Starkstein, S. E., Fedoroff, J. P., Price, T. R., Leiguarda, R., & Robinson, R. G. (1993). Apathy following cerebrovascular lesions. *Stroke, 24,* 1625–1630.

Starkstein, S. E., Mayberg, H. S., Preziosi, T. J., Andrezejewski, P., Leiguarda, R., & Robinson, R. G. (1992). Reliability, validity, and clinical correlates of apathy in Parkinson's disease., *Journal of Neuropsychiatry and Clinical Neurosciences, 4,* 134–139.

Starkstein, S. E., Mayberg, H. S., Berthier, M. L., & Federoff, J. (1990). Mania after brain injury: Neuroradiological and metabolic findings. *Annals of Neurology, 27,* 652–659.

Starkstein, S. E., Berthier, M. L., Bolduc, P. L., Preziosi, T. J., & Robinson, R. G. (1989). Depression in patients with early versus late onset of Parkinson's disease. *Neurology, 39,* 1441–1445.

Starkstein, S. E., Boston, J. D., & Robinson, R. G. (1988). Mechanisms of mania after brain injury: 12 case reports and review of the literature. *Journal of Nervous and Mental Disease, 176,* 87–100.

Sulkava, R., Wikstrom, J., Aromaa, A., Raitasalo, R., Lehtenen, V., Lehtela, K., & Palo, J. (1985). Prevalence of severe dementia in Finland. *Neurology, 35,* 1025–1029.

Sultzer, D. L., Mahler, M. E., Mandelkern, M. A., Cummings, J. L., van Gorp, W., Hinkin, C. H., & Beresford, M. A. (1995). The relationship between psychiatric symptoms and regional cortical metabolism in Alzheimer's disease. *Journal of Neuropsychiatry and Clinical Neurosciences, 7,* 476–484.

Troster, A. I., Stalp, L. D., Paolo, A. M., Fields, J. A., & Koller, W. C. (1995). Neuropsychological impairment in Parkinson's disease with and without depression. *Archives of Neurology, 52,* 1164–1169.

van Elst, L. T., Woermann, F. G., Lemieux, L., Thompson, P. J., & Trimble, M. (2000). Affective aggression in patients with temporal lobe epilepsy: A quantitative MRI study of the amygdala. *Brain, 123,* 234–243.

Vieregge, P., Schiffke, K. A., Friedrich, H. J., & Muller, B. (1992). Parkinson's disease in twins. *Neurology, 42,* 1453–1461.

Walton, J. N. (1994). *Brain diseases of the nervous system* (10th ed.). Oxford: Oxford University Press.

Waters, B. G. H., & Lapierre, Y. D. (1981). Secondary mania associated with sympathomimetic drug use. *American Journal of Psychiatry, 138,* 837–838.

Weiner, M. F., Svetlik, D., & Risser, R. C. (1997). What depressive symptoms are reported in Alzheimer's patients? *International Journal of Geriatric Psychiatry, 12,* 648–652.

Wertmann, E., Speedie, L., Shemesh, Z., et al. (1993). Cognitive disturbances in Parkinsonian patients with depression. *Neuropsychiatry, Neuropsychology, and Behavioral Neurology, 6,* 31–37.

Woermann, F., van Elst, L., Koepp, M. J., Free, S. L., Thompson, P. J., Trimble, M., & Duncan, J. S. (2000). Reduction of frontal neocortical grey matter association with affective aggression in patients with temporal lobe epilepsy: An objective voxel by voxel analysis of automatically segmented MRI. *Journal of Neurology, Neurosurgery and Psychiatry, 68,* 162–169.

Zappacosta, B., Monza, D., Meoni, C., Austoni, L., Soliveri, P., Gellera, C., Alberti, R., Mantero, M., Penati, G., Caraceni, T., & Girotti, F. (1996). Psychiatric symptoms do not correlate with cognitive decline, motor symptoms, or CAG repeat length in Huntington's disease. *Archives of Neurology, 53,* 493–497.

Zec, R. F. (1993). Neuropsychological functioning in Alzheimer's disease. In R. W. Parks, R. F. Zec, & R. S. Wilson (Eds.), *Neuropsychology of Alzheimer's disease and other dementias.* New York: Oxford University Press.

# CHAPTER 30

# Cognitive Approaches to the Memory Disorders of Demented Patients

## William C. Heindel and David P. Salmon

## Introduction

Dementia is primarily (but not solely) an affliction of the elderly, and the prevalence increases dramatically with age to include almost a third of the population over 85 (Mahandra, 1984). Because of the change in population demographics that has been brought about by increases in life expectancy, in recent years dementia has been elevated from an issue of relative obscurity and neglect to one of the utmost interest and importance. Although this increased attention may create the impression that the study of dementia is of relatively recent origin, interest in this topic in fact dates back to antiquity. The term "dementia" was probably coined in the first century A.D., but for the next millennium or so was generally quite ill-defined and often used (along with delirium) to refer to insanity in general (Lipowski, 1981; Mahandra, 1984). It is also likely that no real distinction was made between dementia and the changes in cognitive function associated with normal aging (Mahandra, 1984).

William C. Heindel • Department of Psychology, Brown University, Providence, Rhode Island 02912.    David P. Salmon • Department of Neurosciences, University of California, San Diego, San Diego, California 92093-0948.

*Comprehensive Handbook of Psychopathology* (Third Edition), edited by Patricia B. Sutker and Henry E. Adams. Kluwer Academic/Plenum Publishers, New York, 2001.

Early in this century, the term "organic psycho-syndrome" was used by Bleuler to refer to a set of behavioral manifestations of chronic diffuse cortical damage. The behavioral manifestations involved decrements in memory, judgment, perceptual discrimination and attention, emotional lability, and defective impulse control (Lipowski, 1981). This was essentially the classification adopted by the American Psychiatric Association (APA) in the early editions of its *Diagnostic and Statistical Manual of Mental Disorders* (DSM-I and DSM-II; APA, 1952, 1968). Specifically, the DSM-II defined "organic brain syndrome" as a "basic mental condition characteristically resulting from diffuse impairment of brain tissue function from whatever cause," and manifested behaviorally as an impairment in orientation, memory, intellectual functions, judgment, and affect (Lipowski, 1981). In this classification, brain dysfunction resulted in a single behavioral syndrome, regardless of the etiology and site of neuropathology (Lipowski, 1981).

Partly in response to the inadequacy of the simple "organic brain syndrome" classification, the more recent versions of the *Diagnostic Manual* (DSM-III-R and DSM-IV; APA, 1987, 1994) recognize many separate categories of psychopathological syndromes; two of them (Delirium and Dementia) are characterized by relatively global cognitive impairment. Delirium is distinguished from dementia primarily by the clouding of consciousness in delirium, but not in dementia, and by the fluctuating nature of the symptoms in delirium versus the relatively stable symptoms in dementia. According to the DSM-IV,

The essential feature of Dementia is the development of multiple cognitive deficits that include memory impairment and at least one of the following cognitive disturbances: aphasia, apraxia, agnosia, or a disturbance of executive functioning. The cognitive deficits must be sufficiently severe to cause impairment in occupational or social functioning and must represent a decline from a previously higher level of functioning. The diagnosis of dementia should not be made if the cognitive deficits occur exclusively during the course of a delirium. However, a dementia and a delirium may both be diagnosed if the dementia is present at times when the delirium is not present. (APA, 1994, pp. 134)

The diagnostic criteria for dementia also require that a specific organic factor (or factors) can be either demonstrated or presumed (through the exclusion of all "functional" mental disorders) to be etiologically related to the disturbance. Dementing disorders that share a common symptom presentation but differ in etiology are distinguished in the DSM-IV. For example, the DSM-IV includes, among others, disorders such as Dementia of the Alzheimer Type, Vascular Dementia, Dementia Due to HIV Disease, Dementia Due to Head Trauma, Dementia Due to Parkinson's Disease, and Dementia Due to Huntington's Disease.

Although it has long been acknowledged that dementia can be associated with a wide range of neuropathology, it has only been relatively recently that clinicians have recognized that dementias can manifest themselves *behaviorally* in different ways as well (Bayles & Kaszniak, 1987). Now, there is increasing awareness that (1) Demented patients do *not* possess a global disorder of intellectual impairment, but instead show areas of relatively *preserved* intellectual ability and (2) The *pattern* of preserved and impaired abilities can *vary* depending on the etiology and neuropathology of the dementia.

One of the major catalysts for this change in awareness has been the proposed distinction between "cortical" and "subcortical" dementias. Albert and his colleagues (Albert, Feldman, & Willis, 1974) referred to the pattern of cognitive dysfunction observed in patients with progressive supranuclear palsy as a subcortical dementia characterized by (1) forgetfulness, (2) slowness of thought processes, (3) altered personality with apathy or depression, and (4) impaired ability to manipulate acquired knowledge. At about the same time, McHugh and Folstein (1975) described similar cognitive changes in patients with Huntington's disease and contrasted this pattern of impairment with the aphasic, apraxic, and agnostic disturbances observed in demented patients with primary cortical dysfunction (e.g., Alzheimer's disease). Subsequent studies further delineated the qualitative differences in the cognitive deficits associated with so-called "cortical" and "subcortical" dementing disorders (Brandt, Folstein, & Folstein, 1988; Huber, Shuttleworth, Paulson, Bellchambers, & Clapp, 1986; Salmon, Kwo-on-Yuen, Heindel, Butters, & Thal, 1989), which led a number of researchers to suggest that cortical and subcortical dementias should be recognized as distinct clinical syndromes (for reviews, see Cummings, 1990; Cummings & Benson, 1984). Although criticized on a number of grounds (Brown & Marsden, 1988; Whitehouse, 1986), the cortical–subcortical distinction has descriptive and heuristic value and has proven useful for guiding research that compares the cognitive deficits of different dementing disorders. The distinction, however, is somewhat simplistic and artificial, and a more preferable investigative strategy may be to try to relate specific cognitive impairments with specific dementing disorders.

# Descriptions of Different Dementing Illnesses

## Dementia of the Alzheimer Type

Dementia of the Alzheimer type is the most common form of dementia in the elderly and accounts for roughly 50% of all reported cases (Cummings & Benson, 1992; Katzman, 1986). A large-scale study that sampled elderly individuals who lived in the geographically defined community of East Boston, Massachusetts (Evans et al., 1989) found an overall Alzheimer's disease prevalence estimate of 10.3% among those over age 65 and almost a 50% prevalence rate among those 85 years and over.

Although the cause of Alzheimer's disease (AD) remains unknown, a number of risk factors have been identified. Age is considered the single most important risk factor, given that the prevalence and incidence of AD double approximately every 5 years between the ages of 65 and 85. It is estimated that new cases of AD will be diagnosed each year in approximately 0.5% of individuals between the ages of 65 and 69, 0.75% of those between the ages of 70 and 74, 1.5% of those between the ages of 75 and 79, 2.5% of those between the ages of 80 and 84, and 4.5% of those age 85 and over (Katzman & Kawas, 1994).

The risk of developing AD is increased approximately fourfold by a family history of the disease in a first-degree relative, and there is little question that this familial association is genetically based. Mutations on three genes have been identified in large families that display an autosomal dominant inheritance pattern of an early-onset form of the disease (i.e., onset generally before the age of 60): the amyloid precursor protein gene on chromosome 21, the presenilin 1 gene on chromosome 14, and the presenilin 2 gene on chromosome 1 (for a review, see Bird, 1999). These forms of familial Alzheimer's disease are rare and account for only about 1–2% of all cases of the disease. A far more common genetic risk factor for sporadic, late-onset Alzheimer's disease is the type $\varepsilon 4$ allele of the gene for apolipoprotein E (APOE), a low-density lipoprotein cholesterol carrier. Located on chromosome 19, the APOE $\varepsilon 4$ allele has been found in 50–60% of patients with AD (compared to 20–25% of healthy older adults), regardless of whether or not they have a family history of dementia (Strittmatter et al., 1993). Unlike the genes associated with early-onset familial AD, the APOE $\varepsilon 4$ allele is not deterministic, but it confers an approximately threefold risk of developing AD if one copy of the $\varepsilon 4$ allele is present and an eightfold risk if two copies are present (Katzman & Kawas, 1994).

A number of other risk factors for AD have been identified (Katzman & Kawas, 1994), but they have only a weak association with the disease (generally a twofold risk or less). Women have a slightly greater risk of AD than men; however, this may be attributable, in part, to differential survival after the onset of dementia due to their longer life expectancy. A previous head injury that led to loss of consciousness or hospitalization has been identified as a risk factor for AD, particularly (and perhaps exclusively) in conjunction with the presence of the $\epsilon 4$ allele of the gene for APOE. Several epidemiological studies have shown that lack of education and/or low occupational attainment may be an important risk factor for AD, perhaps because these variables are a surrogate for a brain or cognitive reserve that helps to delay the onset of the usual clinical manifestations of the disorder.

Although a distinction has traditionally been made between AD in the presenium (i.e., before

age 65) and senile dementia of the Alzheimer type, the general lack of any observed bimodality in the distribution of age-specific incidence rates argues against this distinction (Rocca, Amaducci, & Schoenberg, 1986). A study by Huff, Growdon, Corkin, and Rosen (1987), however, did obtain a bimodal distribution of age at onset with a division at about age 65 and also found that the rate of progression of dementia was more rapid in the senile than in the presenile cases. There have also been reports of greater left-hemisphere (i.e., language) vulnerability in early-onset cases and greater right-hemisphere (i.e., visuospatial) vulnerability in late-onset cases (Filley, Kelly, & Heaton, 1986; Seltzer & Sherwin, 1983). Becker, Huff, Nebes, Holland, & Boller (1986) further suggested that, within the language domain, severity of syntactic but not lexical/semantic impairments are related to age at onset.

The primary clinical manifestation of AD is a profound global dementia characterized by severe amnesia with additional deficits in language, "executive" functions, attention, and visuospatial and constructional abilities (Bayler & Kaszniak, 1987; Cummings & Benson, 1992). Alzheimer's disease is characterized neuropathologically by neocortical atrophy and neuronal loss (Terry, Peck, DeTeresa, Schechter, & Horoupian, 1981) and by the presence of neurofibrillary tangles and neuritic plaques (Tomlinson, 1977; Terry & Katzman, 1983a). Plaques and tangles are most extensive in the associative cortices, particularly in the parietal and temporal regions, and primary sensory cortical areas are relatively spared (Brun, 1983). The presence of both plaques and tangles correlates significantly with the presence of dementia (Blessed, Tomlinson, & Roth, 1968; Tomlinson, Blessed, & Roth, 1970; Wilcock & Esiri, 1982). Studies using the synaptic vesicle-associated protein synaptophysin have also found that patients with AD demonstrate an extensive loss of synaptic density (Masliah, Terry, DeTeresa, & Hansen, 1989) and that severity of dementia correlates better with synaptic density than with plaques and tangles (Terry et al., 1991). These results have led Terry et al. (1991) to speculate that synaptic loss may be the primary determinant of the dementia of AD. In terms of subcortical neuropathology, patients with AD reportedly have neuronal loss in the nucleus basalis of Meynert and the nucleus locus coeruleus, along with a corresponding decrement in neocortical levels of cholinergic and noradrenergic markers, respectively (Bondareff, Moutjoy,

& Roth, 1982; Mann, Yates, & Marcyniuk, 1984; Whitehouse, Price, Struble, Clark, Coyle, & De-Long, 1982).

Because there are no known peripheral biological markers for AD, the disease can be definitively diagnosed only by histopathological verification of the presence of the characteristic neurodegenerative abnormalities (i.e., neuritic plaques and neurofibrillary tangles) in the brain. However, documentation of the presence of dementia and the exclusion of all other known potential causes allows clinical diagnosis of dementia of the Alzheimer type during life with some certainty. To aid in this process and to standardize the diagnosis to some degree, criteria for the clinical diagnosis of probable and possible AD were developed by the Work Group on the Diagnosis of Alzheimer's Disease established by the National Institute of Neurological and Communicative Disorders and Stroke and the Alzheimer's Disease and Related Disorders Association (NINCHS-ADRDA; McKhann et al., 1984). Probable AD is indicated when dementia is documented, other causes are excluded, and the disorder aligns with the typical presentation and course. Possible AD refers to those cases of documented dementia in which AD is suspected but the disorder has an atypical onset, presentation, or clinical course, or a second disorder capable of producing dementia (e.g., alcohol abuse) is present, although it is not considered the primary source of cognitive dysfunction. When tested against autopsy verification of AD or one of its variants (i.e., the Lewy body variant of AD, mixed AD, and vascular disease), the accuracy of clinical diagnoses made using the NINCDS-ADRDA criteria ranges from 85–100%, even with the clinical diagnosis is made in the early stages of the disorder.

## Vascular Dementia

Vascular dementia is a cumulative decline in cognitive function secondary to multiple or strategically placed infarctions, ischemic injury, or hemorrhagic lesions. Criteria for vascular dementia outlined in the DSM-IV require the presence of multiple cognitive deficits, significant impairment and decline in either social or occupational functioning, and that the deficits not occur exclusively during the course of a delirium. Furthermore, there must be focal neurological signs and symptoms or laboratory (e.g., CT or MRI scan)

evidence indicative of cerebrovascular disease, that are considered etiologically related to the cognitive impairment.

A relationship between dementia and cerebrovascular disease is often indicated if the onset of dementia occurs within several months of a recognized stroke, if there is an abrupt deterioration in cognitive functioning, or if the course of cognitive deterioration is fluctuating or stepwise. Vascular dementia will also sometimes be accompanied by gait disturbances and a history of unsteadiness and frequent falls, urinary disturbances not related to urologic disease, psuedobulbar palsy, and mood and personality changes (e.g., depression, emotional incontinence) (Cummings & Benson, 1992).

The most widely studied form of vascular dementia, Multi-Infarct Dementia (MID), arises primarily from multiple medium or large vessel cortical infarcts. Although epidemiological data on MID is scarce, it is estimated that roughly 18% of the elderly dementia cases are attributable to MID, and another 10% are due to the combination of Alzheimer's disease and MID (Terry & Katzman, 1983b; Tomlinson et al., 1970). In a study of 175 patients with MID, Meyer and his colleagues (Meyer, McClintic, Rogers, Sims, & Mortel, 1988) confirmed previous reports of greater prevalence in males (61%) than in females. Meyer et al. also found that MID was strongly associated with risk factors for stroke (particularly hypertension and heart disease) and that the most frequently occurring lesions were multiple lacunar infarctions (seen alone in 43% of cases and with other lesions in an additional 21% of the cases).

To clinically differentiate MID from primary degenerative dementia (i.e., Alzheimer's disease), Hachinski and his colleagues (Hackinski et al., 1975) developed an "Ischemic Score" based on the distinguishing characteristics and associated risk factors of MID. A higher score reflects an increased probability of MID. Hachinski et al. (1975) found that the Ischemic Scores of twenty-four patients with comparable levels of dementia fell cleanly into two nonoverlapping groups and classified patients with scores of 4 or less as having primary degenerative dementia and patients with scores of 7 or more as having MID. Subsequent studies with pathological verification have confirmed that the Ischemic Score can correctly classify more than 70% of MID patients and almost 90% of AD patients (Molsa, Palijarvi, Rinne,

Rinne, & Sako, 1985; Rosen, Terry, Fuld, Katzman, & Peck, 1980).

If an adequate history is not available to determine a patient's Ischemic Score, however, differentiation between AD and MID can be extremely difficult. Several studies have shown that a significantly greater proportion of MID than normal controls has increased white matter lucency in the cerebral hemispheres on CT scan, but up to 55% of AD patients also demonstrate increased lucency (Aharon-Peretz, Cummings, & Hill, 1988; Erkinjuntti, Ketonen, Sulkava, Sipponen, Vuorialho, & Iivanainen, 1987; Steingart et al., 1987). Cerebral grey matter blood flow (CBF) is decreased bilaterally in both MID and AD patients, but this decrement is more regional in MID patients and more diffuse in AD patients (Tachibana, Meyer, Kitagawa, Rogers, Okayasu, & Mortel, 1984; Yamaguchi, Meyer, Yamamoto, Sakai, & Shaw, 1980). Meyer and his colleagues (Meyer, Rogers, Judd, Mortel, & Sims, 1988) also found that, although reductions in CBF correlate with the severity of dementia in both MID and AD patients, cognition and CBF fluctuate longitudinally more in MID patients than in AD patients.

Behaviorally, MID and AD patients are primarily distinguishable by their speech and language impairments (Bayles & Kaszniak, 1987). Powell, Cummings, Hills, and Benson (1988) found that AD patients were worse than MID patients in linguistic features (i.e., information content of spontaneous speech and confrontation naming), whereas MID patients were worse than AD patients in mechanical aspects of speech (i.e., pitch, melody, articulation, and rate). A stepwise discriminant function analysis revealed that information content and speech melody were the most effective distinguishing characteristics and correctly classified about 90% of the patients as either MID or AD.

Because the Hachinski Ischemia Scale was directed primarily toward vascular dementia from one cause (i.e., medium or large vessel cortical infarcts), specific research criteria for the diagnosis of broadly defined vascular dementia were recently proposed by an international workgroup supported by the Neuroepidemiology Branch of the National Institute of Neurological Disorders and Stroke (NINDS) and the Association Internationale pour la Recherche et l'Enseignement en Neurosciences (AIREN) (Roman et al., 1993; see Chui, Victoroff, Margolin, Jagust, Shankle, &

Katzman, 1992, for similar diagnostic criteria). These criteria are intended to encompass dementia from all vascular causes, including infarction, ischemia, and hemorrhagic brain lesions. The NINDS-AIREN criteria include diagnoses of probable, possible, and definite vascular dementia, as well as a subcategorization of the specific types of vascular lesions (as determined by clinical, radiological, and neuropathological features). As with the NINCDS-ADRDA criteria for AD, the diagnosis of definite vascular dementia requires histopathological evidence of cerebrovascular disease. In addition, this evidence must occur in the absence of neurofibrillary tangles and neuritic plaques exceeding those expected for age and without clinical evidence of any other disorder capable of producing dementia (e.g., Pick's disease, diffuse Lewy bodies, etc.). Note also that the NINDS-AIREN criteria specify that the term "Alzheimer's disease with cerebrovascular disease" should be used to classify patients who meet the NINCDS-ADRDA criteria for possible AD and who also show clinical and/or brain imaging evidence of relevant cerebrovascular disease.

## Huntington's Disease

Huntington's disease (HD) is an inherited, autosomal dominant disorder with clinical onset in the fourth or fifth decades of life and with an average duration of 17 years (Bruyn, 1968; Folstein, 1989; Hayden, 1981). A rare form of juvenile HD has also been noted, whose onset is before the age of 20 and has a shorter duration of illness than the adult form (Hayden, 1981). The genetic determinant of HD has been identified as an unstable expansion of trinucleotide repeats (cytosine-adenine-guanine; CAG) in the IT15 gene located on chromosome 4 (Huntington's Disease Collaborative Research Group, 1993). The prevalence of HD is much lower than that of AD; it occurs in roughly thirty–seventy individuals per million of the population (Hayden, 1981). Neuropathologically, the disease is characterized primarily by a progressive degeneration of the neostriatum (caudate nucleus and putamen), a selective loss of the small spiny neurons, and a relative sparing of aspiny interneurons (Bruyn, Bots, & Dom, 1979; Vonsattel, Myers, Stevens, Ferrante, Bird, & Richardson, 1985).

The onset of HD often begins with subtle changes in personality such as increased irritability and moodiness, as well as with complaints of incoordination and clumsiness (Folstein, 1989; Hayden, 1981). As the disease progresses, most patients develop severe chorea and dysarthria (Folstein, 1989; Hayden, 1981; Petit & Milbled, 1973) and a dementia characterized by a moderate memory disturbance, attentional dysfunction, problem solving deficits, visuoperceptual and constructional deficits, and a deficiency in performing arithmetic (Brandt & Butters, 1986; Butters, Sax, Montgomery, & Tarlow, 1978). In this stage of the disease, little or no aphasia is apparent, although patients may be dysarthric due to the motor dysfunction inherent in the disease. Some patients may also develop gait and oculomotor disturbances. In the later stages, patients with HD become impaired in most tests of cognitive and memory ability, but still retain relatively intact naming ability (Butters et al., 1978).

## Parkinson's Disease

Idiopathic Parkinson's disease (PD) is a neurodegenerative disorder characterized neuropathologically by a loss of pigmented cells in the substantia nigra pars compacta (Jellinger, 1987) and behaviorally by the classic motor symptom triad of resting tremor, rigidity, and bradykinesia (Jankovic, 1987). Alzheimer-like changes in the cerebral cortex, basal forebrain, and locus coeruleus have also been reported (Cash, Dennis, L'Heureux, Raisman, Javoy-Agid, & Scatton, 1987; Gaspar & Gray, 1984; Hakim & Mathieson, 1979; Perry et al., 1985; Whitehouse, Hedreen, White, & Price, 1983). The prevalence ratio of PD in the United States is roughly 150 per 100,000 (Marttila, 1987). The mean age at onset is around 60 years, and the disease rarely occurs before age 40.

Although not included in James Parkinson's original description of the disorder, dementia has been found more frequently than would be expected in a general population of the same age. Estimates of the prevalence of dementia in PD have ranged from less than 10% to more than 80% (see Brown & Marsden, 1984, for a review). This wide disparity of estimates is most likely due to differences in both the patient sampling methods and in the criteria used to diagnose dementia. More recent studies have found a roughly 30% prevalence rate of dementia in PD (Mindham, Ahmed, & Clough, 1982; Stroka, Elizan, Yahr,

Burger, & Mendoza, 1981). Thus, unlike AD and HD, dementia is *not* always associated with the presence of PD.

Despite the general agreement that dementia can be associated with PD, there is still considerable controversy concerning the underlying nature of this dementia. First, consensus has yet to be reached on which, if any, specific cognitive deficits are invariably seen in all PD patients, regardless of the presence or absence of dementia. Although visuospatial deficits have commonly been reported in patients with PD, these findings may be related more to their motoric and set-shifting difficulties than to impaired visuospatial processing *per se* (Brown & Marsden, 1986; Stelmach, Philips, & Chau, 1989).

Stronger support is found for a fundamental impairment in attentional mechanisms in PD patients. Wright and his colleagues (Wright, Burns, Geffen, & Geffen, 1990) have suggested that PD patients may be impaired in maintaining attention due to an increased tendency to disengage from the current object of focus. Such an attentional deficit may be involved in PD patients' set-shifting difficulties. Flowers and Robertson (1985) found that PD patients' impairment in an Odd-Man-Out test were due to an inability to *maintain* a cognitive set, rather than to increased *perseverative* behavior. Furthermore, Mayeux, Stern, Sano, Cote, & Williams (1987) suggest that impairments in attention and vigilance may also underlie the bradyphrenia (i.e., a slowing of mental processing) that has been observed in PD patients (Wilson Kaszniak, Klawans, & Garron, 1980).

Although demented patients with PD do display more *pervasive* cognitive impairments than their nondemented counterparts, their most *severe* impairments are in the same cognitive domains that are also impaired in nondemented patients. In characterizing the nature of the dementia seen in PD, several investigators (Albert, 1978; Huber et al., 1986; Mayeux, Stern, Rosen, & Benson, 1981) have stressed the features (e.g., preserved language) that it shares with the dementia of HD and other subcortical dementias. In contrast, other investigators (Alvord, Forno, Kusske, Kauffman, Rhodes, & Goetowski, 1974; Boller, Mizutani, Roessmann, & Gambetti, 1980) suggested that the dementia of PD may result from superimposition of Alzheimer-type changes on the primary subcortical pathology. Most likely, both groups are right:

The dementia of PD may reflect the coexistence of both cortical and subcortical features within the same disease.

**Dementia with Lewy Bodies.** A number of investigators recently described a neuropathological condition in demented patients that is characterized by typical subcortical changes in the substantia nigra, locus coeruleus, and dorsal vagal nucleus of PD; the typical cortical distribution of senile plaques and neurofibrillary tangles of AD; and in addition, Lewy bodies that are diffusely distributed throughout the neocortex (Hansen et al., 1990; Kosaka, Yoshimura, Ikeda, & Budka, 1984; Dickson et al., 1987; Gibb, Esiri, & Lees, 1985; Perry, Irving, Blessed, Fairbairn, & Perry, 1990; Lennox, Lowe, Landon, Byrne, Mayer, & Godwin-Austen, 1989). This neuropathological condition, designated the Lewy body variant (LBV) of AD by Hansen and colleagues (1990), is not rare and may occur in approximately 25% of all demented patients. The condition has been reported under a number of different names (e.g., senile dementia of the Lewy body type, diffuse Lewy body disease), and recently the more inclusive designation of Dementia with Lewy Bodies (DLB) has been proposed.

The clinical manifestation of DLB is similar to that of AD in many respects, and these patients are often diagnosed with probable or possible AD during life. This is not surprising, given that DLB often initially produces insidious and progressive cognitive decline without other significant neurological abnormalities. Patients with DLB do not always present with memory impairment as the earliest and most prominent feature, but this aspect of cognition is often affected early in the disorder's course. As in AD, the cognitive deficits that occur in DLB are widespread and progressive and have a significant impact on the patient's ability to engage in the normal activities of daily living. Patients with DLB often manifest a pattern of cognitive deficits similar to that of AD, and disproportionately severe deficits occur in verbal fluency, attention, and visuospatial abilities (Salmon & Galasko, 1996).

Despite the similarities in the clinical presentations of the two disorders, retrospective studies indicate that DLB may be clinically distinguishable from AD. Hansen and colleagues (1990), for example, found that DLB patients differed from patients with "pure" AD in that a greater propor-

tion had mild Parkinsonian or extrapyramidal motor findings (e.g., bradykinesia, rigidity, masked facies, but without a resting tremor). McKeith and colleagues (McKeith, Perry, Fairbairn, Jabeen, & Perry, 1992) also found that patients with DLB were significantly more likely than "pure" AD patients to manifest extrapyramidal motor features at some point during the course of the disease, as well as an increased likelihood of fluctuating cognitive impairment, visual or auditory hallucinations, and unexplained falls. In another study, Galasko and colleagues (Galasko, Katzman, Salmon, Thal, & Hansen, 1996) compared clinical and neuropathological features in thirty-eight autopsy-confirmed DLB and thirty-eight autopsy-confirmed "pure" AD patients. Significantly more DLB patients than AD patients exhibited rigidity, bradykinesia, masked facies, and Parkinsonian gait, and a significantly greater percentage of DLB (32%) than AD (11%) patients reported visual hallucinations. These general findings led to the recent development of clinical criteria for diagnosing DLB (McKeith et al., 1996) that include dementia, spontaneous motor features of Parkinsonism, recurrent and well-formed visual hallucinations, and fluctuating cognition with pronounced variations in attention or alertness. Probable DLB is diagnosed if two of these three features are present; possible DLB if only one is present. A recent examination of the performance of these consensus guidelines against autopsy verification of DLB demonstrated 83% sensitivity and 92% specificity. This was comparable to the 78% sensitivity and 87% specificity for AD (using NINCDS-ADRDA criteria) that was obtained in the same study (Ince, Jaros, Ballard, McKeith, & Perry, in press).

# Memory Impairments in Dementia

Memory impairment is one of the earliest and most prominent symptoms of dementia. In fact, the DSM-IV (1992) requires that an impairment in memory be evident before the diagnosis of dementia can be made. Given the large significance attached to memory functions in identifying demented patients, the rather primitive nature of most clinical memory tests is quite remarkable. Standardized memory tests have traditionally been constructed without any underlying theoretical rationale and often yield only a single score. Such tests may be useful in identifying the presence of a memory deficit but are notoriously ineffective in characterizing the underlying nature of the impairment. In contrast, experimental neuropsychological studies designed within the theoretical paradigms of cognitive psychology have yielded substantial insights into the processes involved in the memory deficits of different dementing illnesses. In the light of these successes, newer standardized memory tests such as the California Verbal Learning Test (Delis, Kramer, Kalan, & Ober, 1987) and, to some degree, the Wechsler Memory Scale-Revised (WMS-R; Wechsler, 1987) have been designed in terms of current cognitive models of memory.

In the next section, experimental neuropsychological investigations into the processes that underlie the memory deficits of patients with different dementing illnesses will be reviewed. Although the vast majority of these studies has been concerned with dementia of the Alzheimer type, several studies allow direct comparisons between patients with AD and patients with more "subcortical" dementias such as HD. As will be seen, two patient groups that superficially display equivalent memory impairments according to a standardized test can in fact have strikingly different processing deficits underlying their impairments. When possible, an effort will be made to illustrate how currently available standardized memory tests can be used to identify these distinct processing deficits. To make the distinction between AD and HD patients more intelligible, we shall also compare these patients' memory impairments to those found in patients with circumscribed amnesic syndromes, particularly patients with alcoholic Korsakoff's syndrome (Butters & Cermak, 1980). This comparison is particularly useful because the impairments seen for some aspects of memory in AD patients are strikingly similar to those seen in alcoholic Korsakoff patients.

## A Taxonomy of Memory

One of the major contributions of cognitive psychology to the neuropsychology of memory is the recognition that memory is not a single, homogeneous entity (Butters, 1984). Rather, memory seems to be comprised of several distinct yet mutually interacting systems and subsystems; each differs either in the type of information stored, the processes acting on that information, or both. Investigations of memory in impaired patient populations have validated this viewpoint and also helped to identify the neuroanatomical structures of different memory systems (Figure 1). Based on these studies, neuropsychological models of memory have been developed that provide a powerful conceptual framework for the clinical assessment and classification of the distinctive patterns of memory impairment observed in different neuropsychiatric disorders.

Within the taxonomy of memory that has emerged from this research, a fundamental distinction has been made between explicit (or declarative) memory and implicit (or nondeclarative) memory (Graf & Schacter, 1985; Squire, 1987). Explicit memory requires the conscious recollection of information acquired during prior study episodes, whereas implicit memory represents an unconscious change in task performance that is attributable simply to exposure to information during a previous study episode (Schacter, 1987). Classic tests of explicit memory include recall or recognition of a previously presented paragraph or list of words that a subject was told to try to remember. In tests of implicit memory, in contrast, subjects are never asked to remember a previous episode but instead are simply asked to perform a particular task that could be influenced by prior exposure to information. For example, classical conditioning, motor skill learning, and priming (i.e., a phenomenon in which the presentation of a stimulus influences subsequent processing of either the same or a related stimulus) all involve implicit memory.

Studies of patients with circumscribed amnesic syndromes suggest that explicit and implicit memory are mediated by distinct neuroanatomical substrates. Amnesic patients, it has been found, exhibit profound impairments in tests of explicit memory, yet generally show normal performance in tests of implicit memory (Cohen & Squire, 1980; Gardner, Boller, Moreines, & Butters, 1973; Graf, Squire, & Mandler, 1984; Warrington & Weiskrantz, 1970). These studies indicate that explicit, but not implicit, memory depends critically on the medial temporal and diencephalic brain regions that are damaged in amnesia. Implicit memory, in contrast, does not depend on a single neuroanatomical system. Rather, implicit memory reflects changes within the specific processing

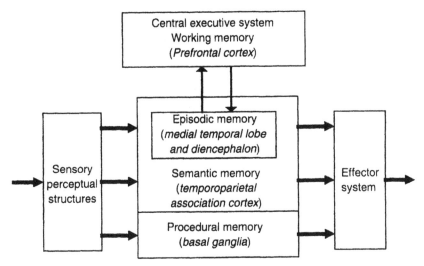

**Figure 1.** A schematic diagram showing the different forms of memory and their proposed neural substrates that are affected in various dementing disorders.

structures that are involved in performing different tasks. For example, skill learning may depend critically on a corticostriatal system involved in programming motor sequences, classical conditioning may involve changes within the cerebellum, and verbal priming may depend on the temporary activation of semantic representations stored in neocortical associative areas.

Explicit memory can be further subdivided into short-term or working memory, episodic memory, and semantic memory. Working memory (Baddeley, 1986) is viewed as a limited capacity system in which information is quickly (i.e., within 20 to 30 seconds) lost unless continuously rehearsed. With rehearsal, however, information can be maintained in working memory indefinitely. The capacities of patients' working memories are most frequently assessed using a digit span task in which subjects are asked to recall progressively longer sequences of numbers. Normal subjects can retain between five and nine digits in working memory with continual rehearsal (Miller, 1956). In contrast, long-term memory can essentially be considered virtually unlimited in capacity and can store experiences, factual knowledge, and skills over an entire lifetime (Klatzky, 1980).

Working memory can be thought of as the information that one is immediately attending to, or "working" on, and impairments in working memory capacity have been associated with underlying deficits in attentional processes. The working memory model postulates a primary central executive system that is aided by two subsidiary buffer systems: a visuospatial scratch pad, responsible for holding visuospatial information and a phonological loop, responsible for holding speech-based information (such as the series of digits in the digit span test). The working memory system (in particular the central executive system) is critically responsible for the planning, organization, and other strategic aspects of memory that facilitate both encoding and retrieving information in long-term memory. Although the anatomical substrates of working memory are not fully known, recent evidence suggests that the frontal associative cortices are important for the normal functioning of this aspect of memory.

Episodic memory encompasses memories for personal experiences and events that depend on temporal and/or spatial cues to retrieve them (Tulving, 1983). For example, remembering what you had for breakfast this morning or when you last saw a physician would require retrieval from episodic memory. Most of the traditional verbal learning and memory techniques (e.g., list learning, paired-associate learning) used in cognitive psychology involve retrieval from episodic memory. For instance, when subjects are given a list of words and later asked to recall them, they must retrieve the words from a specific temporal (one minute previously) and spatial (same examining room) context. Recalling any list of words encountered during their lifetimes would not be appropriate or correct.

Semantic memory, on the other hand, refers to memories of generic facts that are completely independent of contextual cues for retrieving them (Tulving, 1983). Knowledge of the meanings of words, the ability to name common objects, or to recollect well-known geographical, historical, and arithmetical facts are examples of semantic memory. In each case, the specific information can be retrieved without recalling the particular episode in which that information was acquired. It has been proposed that semantic information exists as a representation of knowledge based on an organized network of interrelated categories, concepts, and attributes.

As with the distinction between explicit and implicit memory, episodic and semantic memory can be neurobiologically and neuropsychologically distinguished by the differential impairment of these two forms of memory in patients with circumscribed amnesia. Patients with neurologically based amnesic syndromes are especially impaired in their attempts to acquire new episodic information (i.e., anterograde amnesia), whereas their semantic memory is relatively intact (for a review, see Squire, 1987). For instance, amnesic patients who cannot remember their physician's names for more than a few seconds or minutes usually retain knowledge of arithmetical, geographical, and historical facts. This pattern of spared and impaired abilities is consistent with the notion that episodic memory, but not semantic memory, critically depends on the medial temporal lobe and diencephalic structures that are damaged in amnesic patients. Semantic memory, in contrast, is likely to be mediated by the associative cortices in the temporal, frontal, and parietal lobes that are intact in patients with circumscribed amnesia.

The ability to remember autobiographical information from the distant past (i.e., remote memory) does not neatly fit into the episodic-semantic distinction but probably relies on both types of memory. Retrograde amnesia (i.e., a deficit in recalling information that was acquired before the onset of a memory deficit) is a common component of the amnesic syndrome, and in many cases, it is temporally graded with information from the distant past that is better recalled than information from the more recent past (Butters & Cermak, 1980). One explanation for this temporal gradient is that information from the very remote past has passed from episodic to semantic memory, whereas events from the recent past remain in episodic memory (Butters & Cermak, 1986; Cermak, 1984). The elegance of this explanation is that it allows ready application of the episodic-semantic model to both of the major features (anterograde and retrograde amnesia) of the amnesic syndrome.

## Working Memory

A number of recent studies indicate that damage to the prefrontal cortex can produce working memory impairments that are distinguishable from the episodic memory deficits classically observed following medial temporal lobe damage (Shimamura, Janowsky, & Squire, 1990). Patients with circumscribed amnesia are characterized by an inability to acquire and retain new episodic information; patients with frontal lobe damage can store new episodic information normally but have difficulty manipulating both new and old episodic memories in a strategic manner. Thus, like amnesics, frontal patients are impaired in free recall tests of memory for items previously presented. However, unlike amnesics, they can actually perform normally when tested by using a recognition memory format that places minimal demands on retrieval processes. Moreover, frontal patients display selective impairments in other strategic aspects of memory such as the ability to remember the temporal order in which items were previously presented, to make metamemory judgments about their ability to successfully identify items on a subsequent recognition test, and to remember where and when items were actually presented to them.

Despite their severe learning impairments, alcoholic Korsakoff patients demonstrate normal digit span performance (Butters & Cermak, 1980). Patients with AD have also exhibited normal digit span performance in some studies (Huber et al., 1986), but not in all (Kaszniak, Garron, & Fox, 1979; Kopelman, 1985). These discrepancies probably reflect differences in the severity of dementia of the AD patient groups used in the various studies (Berg et al., 1984). In contrast, digit span performance has been consistently impaired in all but the very earliest stages of HD (Butters et al., 1978; Caine, Ebert, & Weingartner, 1977), suggesting that unlike patients with Korsakoff syndrome or AD, these patients suffer early deficits in working memory.

Studies using the revised version of the WMS-R further document the usefulness of attentional or working memory measures for differentiating AD from HD patients in both the early and middle stages of the diseases (Butters et al., 1988; Troster, Jacobs, Butters, Cullum, & Salmon, 1989). The WMS-R includes an Attention/Concentration Index that is derived from performance on tests of digit span (forward and backward), visual memory span (forward and backward), and mental control. Butters and colleagues (Butters et al., 1988; Troster et al., 1989) showed that mildly demented patients with AD earned near-normal scores on the Attention/Concentration Index, whereas equally demented patients with HD were impaired and performed significantly more poorly than the AD patients. As the disease progressed, Attention/Concentration scores declined in both groups, but HD patients continued to perform more poorly than their counterparts with AD (Troster et al., 1989). Similar clinical differentiation between AD and HD patients has been observed with the attention items of both the Mini-Mental State Exam (MMSE; Brandt et al., 1988; Folstein, Folstein, & McHugh, 1975) and the Dementia Rating Scale (DRS; Mattis, 1976; Salmon et al., 1989). The particularly severe attentional deficits exhibited by patients with HD are not surprising, given the extensive damage that the disease produces to frontostriatal circuits (for a review, see Cummings, 1990).

Although not as severe as in patients with HD, patients with AD do display progressive impairment to different components of working memory as the severity of the disease increases (Collette, Van der Linden, Bechet, & Salmon, 1999). Mildly demented AD patients primarily suffer disruption to the central executive along with relative sparing of the intact phonological loop. This results in a relatively intact span (i.e., working memory capacity) in the face of increased sensitivity to distraction. More severely demented patients, in contrast, have an additional impairment of the phonological loop itself which results in a diminished span and an actual decrease in working memory capacity.

Although alcoholic Korsakoff patients demonstrate normal working memory capacity when they are allowed to maintain information through rehearsal, their performance deteriorates rapidly if

even a few seconds of distractor activity intervenes between presentation and recall (i.e., the Brown-Peterson paradigm; Peterson & Peterson, 1959). For example, if Korsakoff patients are presented with three words (e.g., apple, bird, roof), and then are required to count backward from 100 by threes to prevent rehearsal (a distractor task), they will be impaired in recalling the three words after only 9 or 18 seconds of such counting activity (Butters & Cermak, 1980). Similar increased sensitivity to distraction has also been observed in patients with AD (Kopelman, 1985), HD (Butters et al., 1978; Caine et al., 1977), and PD (Tweedy, Langer, & McDowell, 1982).

## Episodic Memory

The earliest demonstrations of selective impairment of only certain aspects of memory were provided by studies of episodic memory in patients with amnesia that arose from damage to the medial temporal lobe and related diencephalic brain structures. Despite preserved general intelligence, relatively normal performance in other cognitive domains, and intact semantic knowledge, these patients exhibit a strikingly severe inability to acquire new verbal and nonverbal episodic information (i.e., anterograde amnesia). Such long-term episodic memory deficits are exemplified experimentally by the poor performance these patients display in list learning tasks, paragraph recall tests, and tests of verbal paired-associate learning (for a review, see Squire, 1987).

Over the years, numerous studies with amnesic patients confirmed that acquiring and retaining episodic memories depend critically on the medial temporal lobe and midline diencephalic regions that are damaged in these patients (Squire, 1987). Although the actual episodic memory representations, it is thought, are stored within the neocortex, the medial temporal lobe system is responsible for consolidating the episodic memories within the neocortex by gradually binding together the multiple cortical regions that, together, store the memory for a particular event. This binding or integration is achieved through the reciprocal pathways that connect the hippocampus, via the entorhinal cortex, to the neocortex.

Experimental and clinical neuropsychological studies of memory in patients with various dementing disorders indicate that episodic memory impairment is also a ubiquitous feature of dementia.

However, the processes that underlie the episodic memory impairment associated with the various dementing disorders is quite variable and depends on the etiology and neuropathology of the particular disorder. In one of the first studies to directly compare the episodic memory deficit engendered by different amnesic and dementing disorders, Delis and colleagues examined the performance of patients with alcoholic Korsakoff syndrome, AD, and HD in a rigorous list-learning task, the California Verbal Learning Test (CVLT; Delis et al., 1987; Delis, Massman, Butters, Salmon, Cermak, & Kramer, 1991).

The CVLT is a standardized memory test that was developed to assess a variety of memory processes identified through cognitive psychological studies of normal memory. The CVLT assesses the rate of learning, retention after short- and long-delay intervals, semantic encoding ability, recognition (i.e., discriminability), intrusion and perseverative errors, and response biases. In the test, subjects are given five presentations/free recall trials for a list (List A) of sixteen items (four items in each of four semantic categories) and then are given a single interference trial using a second, different list (List B) of sixteen items. Immediately after the List B trial, subjects are given a free-recall and then a cued-recall (using the names of the four categories) test for the items on the initial list (List A). Twenty minutes later, the free-recall and cued-recall tests are repeated for List A, followed by a yes-no recognition test consisting of the sixteen List A items and twenty-eight randomly interspersed distractor items.

The results of the study by Delis and Colleagues (1991) showed that patients with AD, HD, and Korsakoff's syndrome were similarly impaired (compared to age- and gender-corrected normative data) on most measures from the CVLT, including the number of items recalled on the first and the fifth recall trials, the rate of learning across the five initial trials, and the number of items recalled on the free and cued long-delay recall trials. The groups did differ, however, in several crucial aspects of their performance.

One major difference was that patients with AD and Korsakoff's syndrome were just as impaired in the recognition discriminability trial as they were in the immediate and delayed-recall trials of the CVLT, whereas patients with HD were less impaired in the recognition discriminability trial than in the various recall trials. Furthermore, the HD patients were significantly less impaired in the recognition discriminability trial than the AD and KS patients. Delis and colleagues viewed this result as evidence that the episodic memory impairments exhibited by patients with AD and HD may reflect different underlying deficits. The significant improvement shown by the HD patients when memory was tested with a recognition procedure rather than with a free-recall procedure suggests that deficient retrieval mechanisms may contribute significantly to their memory impairment (but see Brandt, Corwin, & Krafft, 1992). When the need for effortful retrieval was reduced by using a recognition format, the HD patients' memory impairment was somewhat ameliorated (also see Butters, Wolfe, Martone, Granholm, & Cermak, 1985). On the other hand, the failure of a recognition format to reduce the degree of episodic memory impairment exhibited by the AD and Korsakoff's syndrome patients suggests that these patients have a defect at the level of consolidation or storage (Butters, 1984; Delis et al., 1991; Martin, Brouwers, Cox, & Fedio, 1985). Regardless of the degree of retrieval support provided by the task, patients with AD and Korsakoff's syndrome could not effectively recall or recognize the items from the CVLT.

Further evidence that the episodic memory deficit of the AD patients reflects ineffective consolidation (or storage) was provided by the second major finding from the study by Delis and colleagues (1991). Patients with AD and Korsakoff's syndrome forgot information significantly faster during the 20-minute delay interval than the patients with HD. This difference was evident when savings scores were calculated that took into account the amount of information initially acquired (trial 5 List A recall) and the amount retained after the delay (long-delay, free-recall trial). Patients with HD retained approximately 72% of the initially acquired information during the delay interval, but patients with AD and Korsakoff's syndrome retained only 17 and 15%, respectively (see Figure 2).

A number of recent studies have shown that indexes of rapid forgetting have important clinical utility for early detection and differential diagnosis of AD (e.g., Butters et al., 1988; Locascio, Growdon, & Corkin, 1995; Welsh, Butters, Hughes, Mohs, & Heyman, 1991; but see Robinson-Whelan & Storandt, 1992). Welsh and colleagues (Welsh

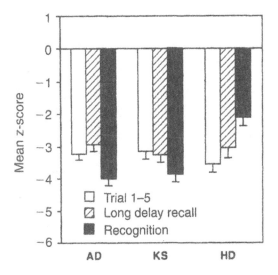

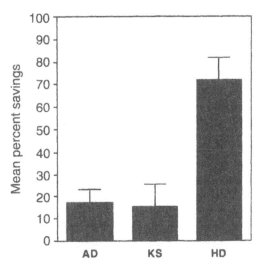

**Figure 2.** The mean z-scores achieved by patients with Alzheimer's disease (AD), amnesia due to Korsakoff's syndrome (KS), and Huntington's disease (HD) in key measures from the California Verbal Learning Test (left panel). The mean percentage of information retained over the 20-minute delay interval by each patient group is also shown (right panel). Adapted from Delis et al., 1991.

et al., 1991), for example, found that the amount of information recalled after a 10-minute delay differentiated very early AD patients from healthy elderly controls with better than 90% accuracy. This measure was superior in this regard to a number of other verbal memory measures such as immediate recall on each of three learning trials, recognition memory, and the number of intrusion errors produced throughout the test. A savings score (i.e., amount recalled after the delay divided by the amount recalled on the third learning trial) was the only measure that approached delayed recall in discriminative power, and it may have been less effective because analyses of savings were restricted to individuals who successfully learned two or more words by the third learning trial, thus eliminating the most severely amnesic individuals.

Butters and colleagues (1988) similarly found that delayed-recall scores and savings scores on the Logical Memory and Visual Reproduction tests of the WMS-R effectively differentiated between mildly demented patients with AD and normal elderly individuals. Furthermore, patients with AD had significantly lower scores on these measures than patients with HD who were similar in overall level of dementia. Thus, the patients with AD forgot verbal and figural materials more

quickly than the HD patients. Troster and colleagues (1993) examined the sensitivity and specificity of these savings scores for differentiating among AD patients, HD patients, and their respective age-matched normal control groups. Discriminant function analyses (DFAs) using Logical Memory and Visual Reproduction savings scores produced satisfactory to excellent overall classification accuracy with 94% of AD patients versus elderly control subjects correctly classified, 81% of HD patients versus middle-aged control subjects correctly classified, and 82% of AD patients versus HD patients correctly classified.

The particularly severe episodic memory deficit exhibited by patients with AD is not surprising, given the extensive evidence suggesting that neuropathological changes in the hippocampus and entorhinal cortex are the first and most severe to occur in the disease (Braak & Braak, 1991; Hyman, Van Hoesen, Damasio, & Barnes, 1984). Both human and animal studies have shown that these medial temporal lobe brain structures are critical for acquiring and retaining new information (for a review, see Squire, 1992), and a number of recent studies using magnetic resonance imaging (MRI) have confirmed a relationship between the degree of structural abnormality in these structures and the severity of episodic memory impairment in patients with AD (Cahn et al., 1998; De-weer et al., 1995; Fama et al., 1997; Kohler et al., 1998; Pantel et al., 1997; Scheltens et al., 1992; Stout, Bondi, Jernigan, Archibald, Delis, & Salmon, 1999; Stout, Jernigan, Archibald, & Salmon, 1996; Wilson, Sullivan, deToledo-Morrell, Stebbins, Bennet, & Morrell, 1996).

Another prominent feature of the performance of patients with AD on episodic memory tests is the frequent occurrence of intrusion errors (i.e., when previously learned information is produced during the attempt to recall new material; Delis et al., 1991; Fuld, 1983; Fuld, Katzman, Davies, & Terry, 1982). Butters and colleagues, for example, found that when patients with AD were asked to recall a series of four short stories, facts from the first story intruded into their attempts to recall the second, third, and fourth stories (Butters, Granholm, Salmon, Grant, & Wolfe, 1987). In subsequent studies, Delis and colleagues found that patients with AD and amnesic patients with Korsakoff's syndrome produced significantly more intrusion errors than patients with HD in the various components of the CVLT (Delis et al., 1991). For example, nearly 70% of the total responses in the cued-recall condition were intrusion errors for both the AD and amnesic patient groups, whereas only 20% were intrusion errors for the HD group. Jacobs and colleagues (Jacobs, Troster, Butters, Salmon, & Cermak, 1990; Jacobs, Salmon, Troster, & Butters, 1990) obtained similar results when they compared the intrusion errors produced by patients with AD and patients with HD in the Visual Reproduction test from the WMS or WMS-R. Like normal control subjects, patients with HD only occasionally intruded components of a prior figure into their drawing of a subsequent figure. Patients with AD were much more likely to make these intrusion errors and produced significantly more than HD patients or normal control subjects.

Patients with AD and HD also exhibit strikingly different patterns of performance in memory tasks that employ an encoding specificity paradigm (Thomson & Tulving, 1970). In a study by Granholm and Butters (1988), patients with AD, like patients with alcoholic Korsakoff's syndrome (Cermak, Uhly, & Reale, 1980), performed better in a cued-recall task when strongly-related cues were present at retrieval, regardless of whether the same cue was present at encoding, than when a weakly related cue was present at both encoding and retrieval. This result indicates that patients

with AD are impaired in their ability to encode the semantic relationship between the two works during the study phase or cannot use the product of encoding at the time of retrieval. Patients with HD, in contrast, performed like control subjects (although their memory performance was impaired overall) by exhibiting better performance when the cue was identical during encoding and retrieval, regardless of the strength of its relationship to the target word, than when the cues differed at study and test. This result suggests that patients with HD could successfully encode the relationship between the cue and target words, but were generally impaired on the memory tasks due to an inability to initiate systematic retrieval strategies.

Although the studies described before indicate that different processing deficits underlie the episodic memory impairments of patients with AD, a "cortical" dementia, and patients with HD, a "subcortical" dementia, additional evidence indicates that not all so-called "subcortical" dementing disorders produce identical episodic memory deficits. Massman and colleagues (Massman, Delis, Butters, Leaven, & Salmon, 1990) directly compared the performance of PD and HD patients on the CVLT. Although these two groups performed similarly on many of the variables that distinguished HD from alcoholic Korsakoff's syndrome and AD patients (i.e., retention of information over delay periods, intrusion rates, and delayed recognition ability), there were also marked differences between the two groups. Specifically, the HD patients demonstrated a slower rate of acquisition, a larger regency effect, a higher preservation rate, and poorer free- and cued-recall performance than patients with PD. These differences between HD and PD patients suggest that somewhat different processing deficits may mediate the episodic memory impairments of these two patient groups and attests to the deficiencies of the cortical-subcortical distinction, even when it is used for heuristic purposes.

## Semantic Memory

The studies described in the previous section indicate that the episodic memory capabilities of alcoholic Korsakoff patients are strikingly similar to those of AD patients, but quite different from those of patients with HD. The situation is somewhat reversed for semantic memory. Of the three patient groups, only patients with AD have a marked disruption in the organization of semantic memory. In contrast, the performance of alcoholic Korsakoff and HD patients both reflect the superimposition of other cognitive deficits on an otherwise relatively intact semantic memory network.

The presence of an intact semantic memory in alcoholic Korsakoff patients is evidenced by their preserved ability to remember the meaning of words, the rules of syntax, and basic arithmetic skills (Kinsbourne & Wood, 1975), as well as by their normal performance in tests of verbal fluency. Weingartner and his colleagues (Weingartner, Grafman, Boutelle, Kaye, & Martin, 1983) demonstrated that, despite equivalent and severe episodic memory deficits, only patients with progressive degenerative dementia (presumably AD), *not* alcoholic Korsakoff patients, were impaired relative to normal controls in several tests of semantic memory, including verbal fluency. These results suggest that the demented patients possess an impairment in accessing knowledge in semantic memory that is not present in Korsakof patients. Impaired verbal fluency has also been observed in both early and advanced HD patients (Butters et al., 1978, 1987), but the relatively normal confrontation naming ability of these patients suggests that their fluency deficit is not due to a general language dysfunction. Rather, the fluency deficit of patients with HD reflects their difficulty in retrieving information from long-term memory.

Butters et al. (1987) directly compared the performance of patients with alcoholic Korsakoff's syndrome, AD, and HD in letter and category verbal fluency tasks. In the letter fluency task (Benton, 1968; Borkowski, Benton, & Spreen, 1967), subjects were asked to generate orally as many words as possible that begin with the letters "F," "A," or "S." Subjects were allowed 60 seconds for each letter. In the category fluency task, subjects were allowed 60 seconds to generate orally as many animals as possible.

The HD patients were severely impaired in both the letter and category fluency tasks and produced fewer correct responses than any other subject group. The alcoholic Korsakoff's syndrome patients showed a mild-to-moderate impairment in both fluency tasks, and like the patients with HD, the severity of their fluency deficit was not related to the linguistic constraints (i.e., letter vs. category fluency) of the semantic memory task. The performance of the patients with AD, in contrast, was directly related to the linguistic demands of the

two fluency tests: AD patients performed normally in the letter fluency task but were severely impaired in the category fluency task.

Similar results were reported by Monsch and colleagues (Monsch et al., 1994) when comparing larger groups of AD and HD patients than in the study by Butters and colleagues (Butters et al., 1987). When the performances of the patient groups were expressed as fluency scores normalized to their respective normal control group scores, patients with AD were impaired in both tasks but demonstrated much greater impairment in the category fluency task than in the letter fluency task. Patients with HD, in contrast, were severely and equally impaired in both fluency tasks (see Figure 3).

The results of these studies support the notion that qualitatively different processes underlie the verbal fluency deficits of AD and HD patients. The greater impairment exhibited by patients with AD in the category than in the letter fluency tasks is consistent with the notion that they suffer a loss or breakdown in organizing semantic memory, rather than a general inability to retrieve or access semantic knowledge. Normal individuals can use their knowledge of the attributes, exemplars, and organization that define a particular semantic category to generate words efficiently from a small and highly related set of exemplars. The letter fluency task does not place great demands on the organization of semantic memory because it can be performed by using phonemic cues to search a very extensive set of appropriate exemplars within the lexicon. Therefore, a loss of semantic knowledge or a breakdown in the organization of semantic memory impacts performance in this task less than performance in the category fluency task. The fact that patients with AD are more impaired in the fluency task that places greater demands on the integrity of semantic memory suggests that they have deficient semantic knowledge.

Patients with HD, on the other hand, were equally impaired in the letter and category fluency tasks which suggests that their impairment reflects a general retrieval deficit rather than semantic memory dysfunction (Butters et al., 1985; Caine et al., 1978). Regardless of the demands that the fluency task placed on the semantic network, these patients had difficulty in retrieving successfully stored information. This interpretation is consistent with the general retrieval deficit that, it was postulated, underlies the impairment in episodic

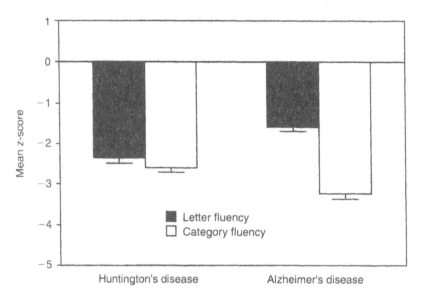

**Figure 3.** The mean z-scores of patients with Alzheimer's disease and Huntington's disease in the letter and category verbal fluency tasks. Patients with Alzheimer's disease were significantly more impaired in the category than in the letter fluency task, whereas patients with Huntington's disease were equally impaired in both tasks. Adapted from Monsch et al., 1994.

memory exhibited by patients with HD in recall and recognition memory tests (Butters et al., 1985, 1986; Delis et al., 1991).

Further evidence for a deterioration of the semantic network in patients with AD was provided by a recent study that examined the temporal dynamics of retrieval from semantic memory during verbal fluency tasks (Rohrer, Wixted, Salmon, & Butters, 1995). This study employed a mathematical model of exponential decline in retrieval from semantic memory as a function of time. The model assumed that the retrieval cue provided during the fluency task (e.g., farm animals) delimits a mental search set that contains the relevant exemplars (e.g., cow, horse, pig, etc.). According to well-known random search models (McGill, 1963), the exemplars are randomly sampled one at a time, at a constant rate, and each item has the same probability of being sampled. Each sampled exemplar is recognized as either a not-yet-sampled item (and reported) or as a previously-sampled item (and not reported). As the number of not-yet-sampled items decreases, the number of items retrieved correspondingly declines throughout the recall period and produces the exponential function. Thus, mean response latency (the average of the time intervals between the production of each response

and the onset of the recall period) increases when either the size of the search set increases or the duration of each sampling increases.

When applied to the verbal fluency performance of patients with AD, the measure of mean latency provides a direct test of the two proposed mechanisms of semantic memory deficits in these patients. If the set size for a particular semantic category is reduced in AD patients due to a loss of semantic knowledge, mean latency should *decrease* and be lower than normal. On the other hand, if the semantic set size remains intact but retrieval is slowed, mean latency should *increase* and be higher than normal. The results of this study showed that the mean response latency of patients with AD was significantly lower than that of the control subjects in the semantic category fluency task, but not in the letter fluency task. These results are consistent with the view that patients with AD suffer a true loss of semantic knowledge.

A subsequent study (Rohrer, Salmon, Wixted, & Paulsen, 1999) compared the mean response latencies of patients with HD in the semantic category fluency task to those produced by patients with AD in the previous study. The results revealed an opposite pattern of performance in the two groups. Patients with HD exhibited a higher than normal mean response latency which is consistent with the view that the disease results in disrupting retrieval processes. As mentioned earlier, patients with AD exhibited a lower than normal mean latency consistent with a loss of semantic knowledge.

An examination of the qualitative nature of AD patients' performance in both an object naming and supermarket fluency test (Martin & Fedio, 1983) provide further support for the notion that these patients' verbal fluency deficits result from a disruption of the hierarchical organization of semantic memory. The supermarket fluency test is a component of the DRS and requires the subject to orally generate in 60 seconds as many items as possible that could be found in a supermarket. Martin and Fedio (1983) found that, despite normal performance on the Vocabulary and Similarities subtests of the WAIS-R, moderately demented AD patients were impaired both in the number of items correctly identified in the naming task and in the total number of words produced in the supermarket fluency task. In addition, the impairment in these two tasks were highly correlated with each other ($r = .80$).

Of more interest were the *types* of responses of AD patients in the naming and fluency tests. The AD patients' errors in the object naming task were primarily language-related rather than perceptual. A similar result was subsequently reported by Hodges and colleagues (Hodges, Salmon, & Butters, 1991) who found that patients with AD produced primarily semantically based errors (e.g., superordinate errors such as calling a "camel" an "animal") in an object naming task (also see, Huff, Corkin, & Growdon, 1986), whereas patients with HD tended predominantly to make perceptual errors (e.g., calling a "pretzel" a "snake"). In the supermarket fluency task, the AD patients produced significantly fewer specific items (e.g., "bananas") per general category (e.g., "fruits"), as well as a significantly larger ratio of category names to total words produced than normal control subjects.

These findings have been interpreted as reflecting a disruption in the organization of AD patients' semantic knowledge that is best characterized as a loss of specific attributes along with a relative preservation of general categories (Martin, 1987; Martin & Fedio, 1983), that is, if verbal representations of objects and categories are orga-

nized hierarchically with the most general aspects at the top and with more specific physical and functional features at the bottom, then the AD patients demonstrate a progressive *bottom-up* deterioration of the semantic network. Thus, AD patients may experience a loss of the defining attributes and exemplars of objects and categories but still retain general features and categories.

Troster and his colleagues (Troster, Salmon, McCullough, & Butters, 1989) extended the findings of Martin and Fedio (1983) by comparing the supermarket fluency performances of mildly and moderately demented patients with AD and HD. As expected, the moderately demented AD patients demonstrated a marked reduction in the number of specific exemplars generated per category and in addition, produced an increased percentage of category labels. The qualitatively similar (although less severe) pattern of performance that was also observed in the mildly demented patients with AD indicated that semantic knowledge is disrupted, even in the very early stages of the disease.

Surprisingly, the HD patients also exhibited a reduction in the number of exemplars generated per category that was similar to that of the mild AD patients, and this reduction worsened as the severity of the dementia increased (Troster et al., 1989). These results suggested that, in addition to their retrieval deficits, patients with HD may experience some disruption of the structure of semantic memory. A similar pattern of performance was observed in demented patients with PD (Troster, Heindel, Salmon, & Butters, 1989), that is, demented, but not nondemented, PD patients demonstrated both a decrease in the total number of words produced and in the number of exemplars per category label in the supermarket fluency test. Again, these results, along with those that demonstrated mild category naming impairments in patients with PD (Bayles & Tomoeda, 1983), indicate that these patients may also possess some semantic memory dysfunction.

Additional evidence for differences in the semantic memory deficits associated with various dementing disorders comes from a series of studies that addressed the issue within the framework of current cognitive psychological models of semantic memory (e.g., Collins & Loftus, 1975) that propose that our representations of knowledge are organized as a network of interrelated categories, concepts, and attributes (for a review, see

Salmon & Chan, 1994). In several recent studies, Chan and colleagues (Chan, Butters, Paulsen, Salmon, Swenson, & Maloney, 1993; Chan, Butters, Salmon, Johnson, Paulsen, & Swenson, 1995; Chan, Butters, Salmon, & McGuire, 1993) attempted to model the organization of semantic memory in AD and HD patients by using clustering and multidimensional scaling techniques (Romney, Shepard, & Nerlove, 1972; Shepard, Romney, & Nerlove, 1972; Tversky & Hutchinson, 1986). Multidimensional scaling provides a method for generating a spatial representation of the degree of association between concepts in semantic memory. The spatial representation, or cognitive map, generated in this manner clusters concepts along one or more dimensions according to their proximity, or degree of relatedness, in the patient's semantic network. The distance between concepts in the cognitive map reflects the strength of their association.

One study in this series compared the cognitive maps of AD, HD, and age-matched normal control subjects. The strength of association between concepts, or their proximity, was estimated using a triadic comparison task in which subjects chose, from among three concepts (i.e., among three animals), the two that are most alike. Every possible combination of three animals, from a total sample of twelve animals, was presented. This procedure produced a proximity score reflecting the strength of association for each pair of animals in relation to all other animal names, that is, how often those two animals were chosen as most alike. The proximity data derived in this manner for the three subject groups were subjected to multidimensional scaling analysis.

The results of this study showed that, although the semantic networks of both the AD and elderly control subjects generated in this analysis were best represented by three dimensions (domesticity, predation, and size), they differed significantly in a number of ways. First, AD patients focused primarily on concrete perceptual information (i.e., size) in categorizing animals, whereas control subjects stressed abstract conceptual knowledge (i.e., domesticity). Second, a number of animals that were highly associated and clustered together for control subjects were not strongly associated for patients with AD. Third, AD patients were less consistent than control subjects in using the various attributes of animals in categorization.

In contrast to the AD patients, the semantic networks of HD patients and their age-matched control subjects were best represented by two dimensions (domesticity and size). The cognitive maps of these two groups were virtually identical, and domesticity for both groups was the most salient dimension for categorizing animals. Furthermore, HD patients and their controls did not differ in the importance applied to the various dimensions or in their reliance on a particular dimension for categorization.

The results from these multidimensional scaling studies are consistent with the notion that AD patients suffer a breakdown in the structure and organization of semantic memory. Because of this semantic deterioration, AD patients tend to rely heavily on a concrete perceptual dimension (i.e., size) in categorizing animals rather than the more semantically demanding abstract conceptual dimension (i.e., domesticity) used by control subjects and patients with HD.

Converging evidence from studies of brain-damaged patients (e.g., McCarthy & Warrington, 1988; Warrington & McCarthy, 1987; Warrington & Shallice, 1984) and functional imaging in normal individuals (e.g., Demonet et al., 1992; Martin, Haxby, Lalonde, Wiggs, & Ungerleider, 1995; Martin, Wiggs, Ungerleider, & Haxby, 1996; Tulving, Markowitsch, Kapur, Habib, & Houle, 1994) suggests that semantic memory is mediated to a large extent by associative areas of the lateral and inferior temporal lobe cortex. These cortical regions are prominent sites of the neuropathological changes associated with AD (Terry & Katzman, 1983a,b). As the pathology of AD progressively spreads throughout the temporal lobe associative cortices, it is likely that the concepts and associations that comprise the semantic network gradually deteriorate and semantic knowledge is lost.

Consistent with this notion, several studies have provided evidence that semantic memory is actually lost relatively early in the course of AD and that this loss of semantic knowledge worsens as the disease progresses. Chertkow and Bub (1990), for example, found that patients with AD were significantly impaired in a wide variety of measures of semantic memory, regardless of the method of access or output required by the task, and showed remarkable item-to-item consistency across tasks. These investigators administered a picture naming test and a word-to-picture matching test, each comprised of the same 150 pictorial stimuli, to patients with AD who were carefully screened to ensure that they had no visual perceptual deficits. In the matching test, subjects were shown each target with four distractor pictures from the same semantic category and were asked to point to the picture that corresponded to the verbal label. Alzheimer's disease patients were markedly impaired in the naming test (correctly identified only 72% of the pictures) and failed to derive any additional benefit in this test from semantic cueing (i.e., only 13% of the unnamed pictures were correctly named after presentation of the semantic cue). The patients with AD were also significantly impaired in the matching test, and showed remarkable consistency between the items failed in the matching test and the picture naming test, that is, 85% of the items correctly identified in the matching test were also correctly named, whereas only 21% of items incorrectly identified in the matching test were named correctly. Hodges and colleagues reported similar item-to-item consistency in the performance of patients with AD across various semantic memory tasks (Hodges, Salmon, & Butters, 1992).

The progressive loss of semantic knowledge by patients with AD has been demonstrated in several recent longitudinal studies. For example, when Chan, Butters, and Salmon (1997) examined the degree of deterioration of the semantic networks of patients with AD across time, they found that the semantic network for "animals" became more and more distorted as the disease progressed and that the patients focused less and less on the abstract dimension of domesticity when classifying animals. In another study, Norton and colleagues (Norton, Bondi, Salmon, & Goodglass, 1997) found that the performance of patients with AD in the Number Information Test (NIT; Goodglass, Biber, & Freedman, 1984), a test designed to assess generic semantic knowledge in a way that minimizes language demands, declined over three annual evaluations. Furthermore, the patients were highly consistent across evaluations in the individual items they missed. Finally, Salmon and colleagues (Salmon, Heindel, & Lange, 1999) found that the performance of patients with AD declined over four annual evaluations in both letter (i.e., FAS) and category fluency tasks, but the rate of decline was faster in the category than in the letter fluency task. Examination of individual responses across the annual evaluations revealed that when patients with AD failed to generate a

particular response in the category fluency task in a given year, they were unlikely to produce that item in a subsequent year. Taken together, the results of these studies are consistent with the notion that patients with AD suffer a gradual deterioration of the organization and content of semantic memory as the disease progresses.

## Remote Memory

In addition to their severely impaired ability to learn and retain new information (i.e., anterograde amnesia), patients with AD exhibit a pronounced deficit in the ability to recollect information that was known before the onset of their dementing disorder (i.e., retrograde amnesia; Beatty, Salmon, Butters, Heindel, & Granholm, 1988; Hodges, Salmon, & Butters, 1993; Kopelman, 1989; Sagar, Cohen, Sullivan, Corkin, & Growdon, 1988; Wilson, Kaszniak, & Fox, 1981). This deficit was clearly demonstrated by Beatty and colleagues (Beatty et al., 1988) who found that even mildly demented patients with AD were strikingly impaired in Famous Faces and Public Events tests (Albert, Butters, & Levin, 1979) that required subjects to identify individuals or events that were widely known during the past decades of their life. Interestingly, the remote memory loss exhibited by the AD patients was temporally graded in that they recalled significantly more information from the 1940s and 1950s than from the 1960s, 1970s, or 1980s.

The temporal gradient in the remote memory loss of patients with AD is similar to the pattern of loss exhibited by patients with circumscribed amnesia associated with selective medial temporal lobe brain damage (Salmon, Lasker, Butters, & Beatty, 1988; Squire, Haist, & Shimamura, 1989) or diencephalic damage associated with Korsakoff's syndrome (Albert et al., 1979). These patients often have severe retrograde amnesia characterized by poorer memory for the more recent past (i.e., late adulthood) than for the more distant past (i.e., childhood and early adulthood). This gradient has been attributed to the interruption of a long-term consolidation process that depends critically on the hippocampal-diencephalic memory system (see Zola-Morgan & Squire, 1990 for a discussion of the role of consolidation and medial temporal lobe brain structures in temporally graded retrograde amnesia). When this process is interrupted by disease or trauma that affects the hippocampal system, older remote memories that have been more fully consolidated are better retained than more recent remote memories that have not been fully consolidated. In one version of this notion, Cermak (1984) suggested that consolidation may reflect the transfer of information from a time-limited, context-dependent form (i.e., episodic memory) to a relatively permanent, context-free form (i.e., semantic memory). According to this view, information that remains fully in episodic memory is lost when hippocampal damage occurs, and information that has become part of the diffusely distributed semantic knowledge system is retained.

To explore the possibility that the retrograde amnesia of AD is due to a retrieval deficit rather than an inability to adequately consolidate information over time, Hodges and colleagues (Hodges et al., 1993) examined the performance of patients with AD on an updated version of the Famous Faces test that employed recognition and cueing formats. These latter conditions allowed assessing remote memory across decades and greatly reduced the retrieval demands of the task. Patients were first shown four faces simultaneously and were asked simply to point out the one who was a famous person. Then, they were asked to name the person, then to identify the persons if they could not name them, and then to name the persons following the presentation of a semantic (e.g., an actor) or a phonemic (e.g., the person's initials) cue. The results demonstrated that patients with AD were impaired in the Famous Faces test, even when retrieval demands were minimized by using a recognition procedure. Furthermore, the retrograde amnesia that was evident in the recognition and phonemic cueing formats was temporally graded with information from the distant past that was retained better than information from the more recent past.

The severe, temporally graded retrograde amnesia exhibited by patients with AD is not a general feature of all dementia syndromes. In the study described before, Beatty and colleagues (1988) found that patients with HD exhibited a mild retrograde amnesia that was equally severe across all decades (also see, Albert, Butters, & Brandt, 1981). This divergent pattern was evident, even though the HD and AD patients were matched for overall severity of dementia, as measured by the DRS (see Figure 4).

A similar pattern of results was obtained when

patients with AD and patients with HD were compared in a test that assessed geographical knowledge for regions of the country in which subjects lived early and late in their lives (Beatty & Salmon, 1991). In this test, subjects were shown outline maps of regions of the country and had to identify the approximate locations of a number of cities or geographic features. Beatty (1988) had previously shown that the ability to perform this task is related to whether and how long an individual had lived in the targeted region. Subjects were tested with maps of regions in which they had spent their early lives and where they currently resided, and groups were carefully matched for the amount of time they had lived in each region. The results showed that both AD and HD patients were impaired, relative to their control subjects, in locating features in both regions. However, the AD patients, but not the HD patients, showed a temporally graded remote memory loss for this geographic knowledge, that is, their memory for the region of more recent residence was more impaired than their memory for the region of past residence.

When considered together, the results of the studies described suggest that the retrograde amnesia associated with various dementing disorders is likely to be mediated by different underlying abnormal processes. The severe, temporally graded retrograde amnesia of AD most likely arises from a loss of remote knowledge due to a consolidation deficit mediated by medial temporal lobe damage. The retrograde amnesia may be particularly severe, even for information from the distant past, because remote knowledge that has already been consolidated as semantic knowledge may also be lost as the structure and organization of semantic memory deteriorates. In contrast, the relatively mild and time-independent retrograde amnesia of HD may be another reflection of the general retrieval deficit that equally affects information from any decade of their lives.

## Implicit Memory

As mentioned earlier, tests of explicit memory require the conscious recollection of previously learned information, whereas tests of implicit memory do not. Instead, implicit memory is manifested indirectly through changes in performance that can be attributed simply to previous exposure to the stimuli or procedures used in a particular

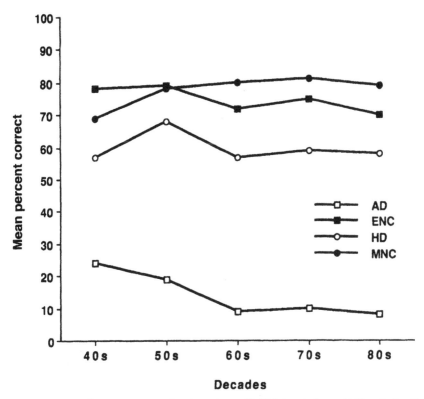

**Figure 4.** The mean percentage of correct responses given by patients with Alzheimer's disease (AD), patients with Huntington's disease (HD), elderly normal control (ENC) subjects, and middle-age normal control (NC) subjects in the remote memory battery (cues condition). Adapted from Beatty et al., 1988.

task. Despite their profound explicit memory impairments, amnesic patients often demonstrate essentially normal performance on implicit memory tests that involve priming and skill learning (for a review, see Squire, 1987). These findings have been instrumental in demonstrating that implicit memory does not depend critically on the medial temporal and diencephalic brain regions that, it is thought, mediate explicit memory, but they have shed little light on the neurological substrates that actually underlie implicit memory.

Unlike patients with circumscribed amnesia, demented patients often exhibit impaired performance in tests of implicit memory. What is more intriguing, however, are the results of studies that indicate that demented patients are not globally impaired in all implicit memory tests; rather, they evidence selective impairments in a subset of related tests, and different demented patient populations display distinct patterns of preserved and impaired ability across a variety of implicit tests.

These findings provide strong support for the notion that implicit memory is *not* a single entity, but instead a collection of independent systems mediated by distinct neuroanatomic structures. These results also suggest that implicit memory tests may ultimately have some diagnostic utility in distinguishing very mildly demented patients from both amnesic patients and neurologically intact subjects.

**Skill Learning.** One form of implicit memory that is preserved in amnesic patients is the ability to acquire and retain rule-based motor and cognitive skills. Specifically, alcoholic Korsakoff patients demonstrate normal learning on visuomotor tasks such as tracing two-dimensional line drawings while viewing the drawing as a mirror reflection (i.e., a mirror tracing task) and maintaining contact between a handheld stylus and a rotating metallic disk (i.e., a pursuit rotor task) (Brooks & Baddeley, 1976; Cermak, Lewis, Butters, & Goodglass, 1973). In addition, alcoholic Korsakoff patients have exhibited preserved learning ability in more cognitively loaded skills such as reading words that have been mirror-reversed (Cohen & Squire, 1980). In this task, amnesic patients could learn to read mirror-reversed words and retained this ability normally during a 3-month period, even though their ability to remember either the test sessions or the specific words read was significantly impaired.

Now, a number of studies indicate that demented patient populations can be differentiated by their performance in skill learning tasks that are performed normally by amnesic patients. Martone and her colleagues (Martone, Butters, Payne, Becker, & Sax, 1984) found that the ability of patients with HD to acquire the mirror reading skill in the task developed by Cohen and Squire was impaired (1980). On the other hand, Eslinger and Damasio (1986) reported that patients with AD demonstrate normal acquisition of the motor skills underlying a pursuit rotor task. Considered together, the results of these two studies provide evidence that the neostriatum (damaged in HD but preserved in the early stages of AD) may be critically involved in the acquisition of some visuomotor skills.

This possibility was further examined in studies by Heindel and colleagues (Heindel, Butters, & Salmon, 1988; Heindel, Salmon, Shults, Walicke, & Butters, 1989) that directly compared the motor skill learning ability of amnesic patients, patients with AD, patients with HD, and both demented and nondemented PD patients. These investigations employed a pursuit rotor task in which subjects were required to maintain contact between a handheld stylus and a rotating metallic disk. The amount of time the stylus was kept in contact with the disk on each 20-second trial was measured across blocks of trials. To ensure that any observed group differences in skill acquisition could not be attributable to ceiling or floor effects, the initial levels of performance among the groups was equated by manipulating the difficulty (i.e., speed of rotation of the disk) of the task.

The results of these studies showed that AD patients and amnesic patients demonstrated systematic and extensive motor learning across trials that was equivalent to that of normal control subjects. The preserved motor learning of these groups has been replicated (Bondi, Kaszniak, Bayles, & Vance, 1993) and extended to the learning of the visuomotor skills necessary to trace a pattern seen in a mirror-reversed view (Gabrieli, Corkin, Mickel, & Growdon, 1993), and it provides further evidence that this form of implicit memory is not mediated by the medial temporal lobe structures damaged in these two patient populations. Patients with HD, in contrast, were impaired in learning the motor skill underlying pursuit rotor task performance, and the little learning they did exhibit was significantly correlated with their overall level of dementia (as measured by the DRS) but not with the severity of their choreiform movements. Based on these findings, Heindel et al. (1989) concluded that HD patients have a true motor learning deficit that may be an integral part of their dementia, rather than simply a reflection of their primary motor impairment. In conjunction with the findings of Martone et al. (1984) and Eslinger and Damasio (1986), these results also support the notion that the neostriatum is indeed involved in the acquisition of motor skills and particularly in the acquisition and generation of motor programs (see Figure 5).

The analysis of human performance in tracking tasks suggests that the motor system is hierarchically organized into different levels of motor control (Pew, 1974; Summers, 1981). In learning a motor skill, a performer must combine the appropriate movements into both the correct serial order and the correct temporal pattern within that order. The awkward performance seen in the early stages of learning a motor task can be adequately described by an elementary closed-loop negative feedback system that relies directly on visually perceived errors to generate new motor commands. However, the smoother, more coordinated movements seen after much practice are due to the acquisition and modification of motor programs that allow the performer to organize a sequence of movements in advance of their performance. Skill learning, then, involves the development of increasingly more accurate motor programs.

From this point of view, the impaired performance of the patients with HD in the pursuit rotor task may be attributable to their reliance on the visual error-correction mode of motor performance. Although these patients could demonstrate some improvement during the first few blocks of trials by improving their error-correction strategy, their inability to generate new motor programs would prevent them from adopting the more effective, predictive mode of performance used by patients with AD, amnesic patients, and control subjects.

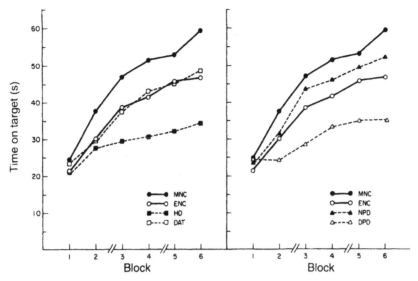

**Figure 5.** Performance of Huntington's disease (HD) patients, demented (DPD) and nondemented (NPD) Parkinson's disease patients, with dementia of the Alzheimer type (DAT), and middle-aged (MNC) and elderly (ENC) normal control subjects in the pursuit rotor motor learning task. From Heindel et al., 1989.

Heindel et al. (1989) also found that, although nondemented patients with PD exhibited normal learning on the pursuit rotor task, the learning of the demented PD patients was as impaired as that of the HD patients (see Figure 5). Similarly, the residual motor skill learning ability of the patients with PD was significantly correlated with their overall level of dementia but not with the severity of their motor symptoms (i.e., tremor, rigidity, bradykinesia). Although early studies (e.g., Flowers, 1978) initially suggested that nondemented PD patients may have open-loop motor control deficits, the results of the study by Heindel and colleagues are consistent with subsequent studies (Bloxham, Mindel, & Frith, 1984; Bondi & Kaszniak, 1991; Day, Dick, & Marsden, 1984) that showed that nondemented PD patients can in fact employ predictive motor strategies in tracking tasks. These studies and others that demonstrate the ability of PD patients to use advance information effectively in preparing for movement (Rafal, Inhoff, Friedman, & Bernstein, 1987; Stelmach, Worringham, & Strand, 1986) suggest that motor programs are intact in nondemented PD patients. This is not the case for demented PD patients, however, because they exhibit a motor learning deficit, perhaps due to the presence of greater corticostriatal damage in these patients than in

their nondemented counterparts (Agid, Ruberg, Dubois, & Pillon, 1987).

To examine more directly whether HD patients' skill learning impairments are related to a motor programming deficit, Heindel, Salmon, and Butters (1991) administered a modification of Helson's (1948) classic adaptation-level task, which involves biasing weight judgments, to HD patients, AD patients, and control subjects. In this task, subjects first lift a series of weights and judge whether each weight is heavier or lighter than the immediately preceding weight. Twenty minutes later, these subjects are asked to judge the heaviness of a standard set of ten weights on a nine-point scale. Benzing and Squire (1989) previously found that both amnesic patients and control subjects tended to rate the standard set of weights heavier, when they had been exposed initially to a relatively light series of weights (light bias condition), and lighter when they had initially been exposed to a relatively heavy set of weights (heavy bias condition). In the case of the amnesic patients, this effect occurred despite impaired recall for the earlier biasing session.

The weight biasing task, like motor skill learning, may involve modifying programmed movement parameters. A number of studies (see Jones, 1986, for a review) indicate that weight perception is normally mediated by centrally generated motor commands and that sensations of heaviness can be influenced by discrepancies between the intended, or programmed, force, and the actual force needed to lift objects. Prior experience with relatively heavy or light weights during the initial biasing trials may result in an increase or decrease in the amount of force programmed for lifting the weights, which would then lead to an illusory decrease or increase in the perceived heaviness of the standard set of weights. Because the task requires little overt movement, a demonstration that HD patients are less likely than patients with AD to manifest normal weight biasing would further strengthen the probability that their motor learning deficits are due to a failure in skill acquisition, not to some basic motor dysfunction.

The results of the study by Heindel et al. (1991) showed that AD and HD patients did indeed differ in the extent to which their judgments of heaviness were biased by prior experience. Although unable to explicitly remember the initial biasing trials, both mildly and moderately demented patients with AD, like normal control subjects, perceived that the standard set of weights was heavier after previous exposure to the series of light weights than after previous exposure to the series of heavy weights. In contrast, only mildly demented patients with HD exhibited the same biasing effect. Moderately demented patients with HD showed no evidence that their ratings of the standard weights were influenced by the prior biasing trials. This difference in performance in the weight biasing task occurred despite the fact that both patient groups could discriminate easily among the different weights, indicating that the weight judgments were not limited by any sensory or motor deficit.

A related study compared the performance of AD and HD patients in a task that assessed their ability to develop a new perceptual-motor response required by the use of laterally displaced vision (Paulsen, Butters, Salmon, Heindel, & Swenson, 1993). In this task, subjects were required to point to a target while wearing distorting prisms that shifted the perceived location of objects 20° to the right or left. The groups demonstrated comparable ability to perform the basic pointing task, as assessed by baseline pointing accuracy without prisms or visual feedback regarding accuracy. After thirty trials of training while wearing the prisms, patients with AD displayed a new perceptual-motor response that al-

lowed them to point accurately to the target with laterally displaced vision. In addition, the AD patients displayed normal negative aftereffects in the pointing task, when the prisms were removed. Patients with HD, in contrast, failed to exhibit normal adaptation or negative aftereffects in this task. Given that perceptual-motor adaptation to this lateral spatial distortion, it is thought, is mediated by the modification of central motor programs through visual feedback regarding the accuracy of intended movements, these results are consistent with motor skill learning deficits displayed by HD patients in the pursuit rotor and weight biasing tasks.

The results from the pursuit rotor, weight biasing, and prism adaptation studies, in conjunction with studies showing that patients with HD (Knopman & Nissen, 1991; Willingham & Koroshetz, 1993) or PD (Ferraro, Balota, & Connor, 1993; Pascual-Leone et al., 1993) but not patients with AD (Knopman & Nissen, 1987; Grafman et al., 1990; but see Ferraro et al., 1993) have deficits in implicitly learning sequences of movements in a serial reaction task (Nissen & Bullemer, 1987), suggest that the motor learning deficits of patients with HD may result from an inability to generate central motor programs. Such of a programming deficit is certainly consistent with the neuropathology of the disease. A number of studies (for a review, see Alexander, DeLong, & Strick, 1986) demonstrated the presence of several anatomically and functionally distinct circuits that link the cortex and basal ganglia. One such circuit, dubbed the motor circuit by Alexander et al., is critically involved in programming movements. The motor circuit consists of inputs to the putamen from the motor, premotor, and sensorimotor cortical regions. This information is subsequently integrated through the pallidum and thalamus and is returned to the supplementary motor area (SMA). A number of studies provided evidence that this circuit is critically involved in programming and executing motor movements. For example, DeLong and colleagues (DeLong, Alexander, Georgopoulos, Mitchell, & Richardson, 1984) demonstrated that cells in the basal ganglia respond to the direction, amplitude, and amount of force required by a movement. Neurons in the SMA it has been shown, discharge during actual limb movement and during preparation for limb movement (Brinkman & Porter, 1979; Tanji, Taniguchi, & Saga, 1980). Regional cerebral blood flow studies have shown that the SMA is activated when a subject rehearses and prepares for complex limb movements (Orgogozo & Larsen, 1979; Roland, 1984; Roland, Larsen, Lassen, & Skinhoj, 1980). It has been found that lesions to the SMA (Watson, Fleet, Gonzalez-Rothi, & Heilman, 1986) or basal ganglia (De Renzi, Faglioni, Scarpa, & Crisi, 1986) cause apraxia (i.e., an impairment in executing skilled movements). Taken together, these studies suggest that damage to the motor circuit in patients with HD creates a motor programming deficit that most likely mediates the deficits in motor skill learning, weight biasing, and prism adaptation displayed by these patients.

Alexander et al. (1986) described several other corticostriatal loops that pass through the basal ganglia and follow the same general pattern of organization as in the "motor" circuit. In each of these "complex" circuits, inputs from functionally related cortical associative areas project primarily to the caudate nucleus and ultimately project back to a specific region of the prefrontal cortex. Given the parallel organization of these circuits, it is likely that they are all performing similar operations, even though the information transmitted through individual circuits might differ considerably. In particular, if the "motor" circuit is involved in programming external actions (i.e., movements), then it is possible that the "complex" circuits may be involved in programming internal actions (i.e., cognitive processes). Because these "complex" loops are compromised in HD and PD, they may represent the neurological substrate that underlies the reported deficits of these patients in acquiring the visuomotor skills necessary to read mirror-reversed text (Martone et al., 1984), in acquiring the cognitive skills necessary to solve complex puzzles efficiently (Butters et al., 1985; Saint-Cyr, Taylor, & Lang, 1988), and the inability to acquire the cognitive skill necessary to perform a probabilistic classification task (Knowlton, Mangels, & Squire, 1996). In addition, these complex loops might also be associated with the retrieval deficits that patients with Huntington's disease exhibit in tests of explicit memory (Butters et al., 1985; Caine et al., 1978).

**Priming.** In addition to normal skill learning, patients with circumscribed amnesia perform normally in a wide variety of priming tasks that involve temporary and unconscious facilitation of performance simply from prior exposure to stimuli (Shimamura, 1986). For example, amnesic patients and normal control subjects have an equivalently strong tendency (relative to chance) to complete three-letter word stems (e.g., MOT) with previously presented words (e.g., MOTEL), despite the failure of the amnesic patients to recall or recognize these words in standard memory tests (Graf et al., 1984; Warrington & Weiskrantz, 1968, 1970). Similar normal priming effects have been reported in severely amnesic patients with alcoholic Korsakoff's syndrome in tasks that require generating exemplars from particular semantic categories (Gardner et al., 1973; Shimamura & Squire, 1984), identifying words flashed for very short durations (e.g., 35 ms) on a computer screen (Cermak, Talbot, Chandler, & Wolbarst, 1985), or identifying incomplete (i.e., "fragmented") line drawings of animate and inanimate objects (Warrington & Weiskrantz, 1968, 1970).

Although the effects of previous exposure to stimuli (i.e., priming) can arise from a variety of processes, some investigators have made a theoretical distinction between perceptual (or data-driven) priming and conceptual priming (Blaxton, 1989; Roediger & Blaxton, 1987). Perceptual priming, it is thought, involves processes that operate at the level of the visual or auditory form of a target stimulus, and it is not affected by the particular meaning or content of the stimulus. It can, however, be influenced by manipulations of the surface features of the stimulus (e.g., changes in modality or typeface). Conceptual priming, in contrast, it is thought, involves processes that operate at the level of the meaning or content of a target stimulus, and it is influenced by manipulations of the depth of conceptual analysis of the stimulus.

Gabrieli and colleagues recently suggested that the distinction between perceptual and conceptual priming may have a neurological as well as a psychological basis (Fleishman et al., 1995; Gabrieli, Fleischman, Keane, Reminger, & Morrell, 1995). It is important to point out, however, that tasks used to assess priming often do not exclusively engage either conceptual or perceptual processes. Rather, both types of processing may contribute to normal priming performance, and the relative contribution of each depends on the specific features of the task. Priming effects in normal individuals and in amnesic patients in the widely used word-stem completion task, for example, are greater following elaborative processing of a semantic, rather than a physical, feature of the stim-

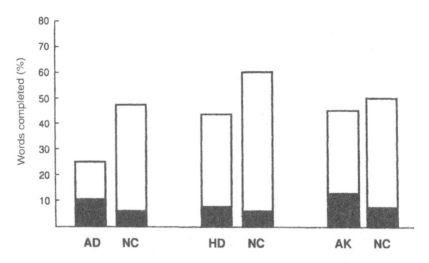

**Figure 6.** Percentage of word stems completed with previously presented words in the lexical priming task by alzheimer's disease (AD), Huntington's disease (HD), alcoholic Korsakoff (AK) patients, and their age-matched normal control (NC) subjects. The shaded portion of the bar indicated the baseline guessing rate for each subject group. Adapted from Salmon et al., 1988.

ulus during study (indicating a conceptual processing component) and also as well as when the stimulus is presented in the same modality, rather than in different modalities, in study and test (indicating a perceptual processing component) (Carlesimo, 1994).

Some of the first studies to examine conceptual priming in patients with dementia (Salmon, Shimamura, Butters, & Smith, 1988; Shimamura, Salmon, Squire, & Butters, 1987) compared the performance of AD, HD, and alcoholic Korsakoff's syndrome patients in the word-stem completion task previously used by Graf et al. (1984). In this task, subjects were shown ten words (e.g., MOTEL, ABSTAIN), one at a time, and were asked to rate how much they liked each word on a five-point scale. Following these presentation trials, the subject were shown twenty three-letter word stems (e.g., MOT, ABS) and were asked to complete each stem with the first word that came to mind. Ten of the stems could be completed using study words, and the other ten stems were used to assess baseline guessing rates.

As expected, the alcoholic Korsakoff patients and control subjects displayed equivalent and significant increases (relative to baseline guessing rates) in the number of stems completed with previously presented words, despite the profound explicit memory impairments of the alcoholic Korsakoff patients. Although both groups of de-

mented patients were also severely impaired in explicit memory and did not differ in baseline guessing rates, they performed quite differently on the priming test. Patients with HD, like the alcoholic Korsakoff patients, displayed normal lexical priming, whereas the patients with AD showed little tendency to complete the word stems with the previously presented words (see Figure 6). This deficit in the stem-completion priming performance of AD patients has now been replicated in numerous studies (Heindel et al., 1989; Keane et al., 1991; Randolph, 1991; Bondi & Kaszniak, 1991; Perani et al., 1993; but see Deweer et al., 1994; Huberman, Moscovitch, & Freedman, 1994).

Subsequent studies examined the stem-completion priming performance of patients with PD. Heindel et al. (1989) and Bondi and Kaszniak (1991) observed normal stem-completion priming effects in nondemented patients with PD. However, demented patients with PD, like patients with AD, exhibited impaired priming in this task (Heindel et al., 1989).

Another study that examined conceptual priming in demented patients (Salmon et al., 1988) compared the performance of AD, HD, and control subjects in a semantic priming task that employed a paired-associate procedure. In this task, subjects were asked to judge categorically or functionally related word pairs (e.g., BIRD-ROBIN, NEEDLE-THREAD) and later to say the first word that came to mind when presented with the first word (e.g., BIRD, NEEDLE) of a pair. The subjects' semantic priming abilities are reflected by their tendencies to produce the second word of the functionally or categorically related word pairs. As in the lexical priming task, HD patients demonstrated normal levels of semantic priming. Patients with AD, in contrast, primed significantly less than HD patients and control subjects and actually failed to prime above baseline guessing rates. Using a somewhat different free-association procedure, Brandt et al. (1988) also found significantly impaired priming in patients with AD.

The deficits exhibited by patients with AD in conceptually based priming tasks has been extended in several studies to priming of meaningful pictorial stimuli (Bondi & Kaszniak, 1991; Bondi, Kaszniak, Rapcsak, & Butters, 1993; Corkin, 1982; Heindel, Salmon, & Butters, 1990; but see Gabrieli et al., 1994). Heindel et al. (1990), for example, developed a picture priming task that was designed to be directly comparable to the stem-completion test of verbal priming. In this task, subjects were first shown complete, realistic line drawings of common animate and inanimate objects (e.g., tree, bicycle) and were simply asked to name the object depicted. Then, subjects were given the pictorial priming test in which they were asked to say the first thing they thought of when shown incompletely drawn (i.e., fragmented) pictures, half of which were previously shown to the subject in the naming task. Priming effects were reflected in the enhanced identification of objects previously seen in the naming task relative to the novel objects. Although all subjects performed well in the initial naming task, patients with AD exhibited significantly less facilitation in identifying fragmented pictures from this prior exposure than the HD patients or control subjects. The patients with HD were not impaired in this pictorial priming task, and they actually demonstrated significantly greater facilitation than the control subjects.

Although the pictorial priming task appears, at first glance, to evoke perceptually based processes, some investigators suggest that pictures and words simply have differential access to different features within a common semantic store (Nelson, Reed, & McEvoy, 1977), that is, pictures may access the semantic features of a concept more directly than words, whereas words may access phonemic features more directly than pictures. To the extent that words and pictures are indeed represented by a single, shared semantic representation, a common conceptual processing deficit could underlie the impaired performance of patients with AD on the stem-completion, paired-associates, and pictorial priming tasks.

One possible explanation of AD patients' deficits in the various conceptual priming tasks is rooted in their previously described deficiencies in semantic knowledge, that is, the hierarchic associative network that forms the skeletal structure of semantic knowledge may have deteriorated sufficiently to greatly limit the capacity of available cues to activate traces of previously presented stimuli. For example, the cue BIRD may not have evoked an unconscious activation of the categorical associate ROBIN in the semantic priming task because the association between the two words has been greatly weakened. Similarly, the association in semantic memory between the word stem MOT and the word MOTEL in the lexical priming task may have been sufficiently disrupted to negate the facilitating effect of the word's presentation. In the pictorial priming tasks, the initial presentation of the intact picture of an object may not have sufficiently activated the semantic representation of that object to aid in identifying it, when it was presented in a fragmented form.

In contrast to the studies described before, some studies indicate that patients with AD can, under certain conditions, demonstrate intact long-term semantic priming. One such study examined verbal priming in AD patients using a homophone spelling bias task (Fennema-Notestine, Butters, Heindel, & Salmon, 1994). In this study, subjects were asked to spell series of homophonic words (to establish the initial spelling preference) and then to spell these words again a few minutes later after they had been biased against their preference by presenting the homophone within a semantic context. For example, depending on whether subjects' preferred spelling had initially been either "son" or "sun," they were then asked in the second phase to spell this word immediately after having heard either "moon and stars" or "father and daughter," respectively. After the biasing trials, AD patients and normal control subjects displayed comparable and significant increases in their tendency to shift to their nonpreferred spelling of the target words.

In a similar study, patients with AD displayed a normal biasing effect of verbal labels on memory for ambiguous figures (Ostergaard, Heindel, & Paulsen, 1995). In this task, ambiguous figures were presented to the subjects along with a verbal label corresponding to one of two possible interpretations of the figure. Biasing was reflected in a subject's tendency to produce responses and response latencies on a subsequent recognition test that were consistent with these verbal labels. Alzheimer's disease patients displayed a normal biasing effect despite their chance performance on the recognition test.

The normal priming exhibited by patients with AD in these two semantic biasing tasks casts some doubt on the notion that these patients' priming impairments can be attributed simply to a disruption in the organization of their semantic memory. It is still possible, however, to accommodate these findings within the semantic memory framework by assuming that different verbal priming tasks place different demands on the capacity of AD patients' compromised semantic structure. In this view, prior exposure to stimulus may be sufficient to activate the general contextual or superordinate semantic information that remains relatively intact in patients with AD to a level that can support normal priming in the homophone and ambiguous figures biasing tasks. However, prior exposure may not prove sufficient to activate the specific semantic associates or exemplars that are particularly disrupted in patients with AD, and this leads to impaired priming in the stem-completion, paired-associates, and pictorial priming tasks.

In contrast to their impairments in more conceptually driven priming tasks, patients with AD consistently perform normally in more perceptually driven priming tasks, including lexical decision (Ober & Shenalt, 1988), simple reading (Balota & Duchek, 1991), reading geometrically transformed script (Deweer, Pillon, Michon, & Dubois, 1993; Grober, Ausubel, Sliwinski, & Growdon, 1992; Moscovitch, Winocur, & MacLachlan, 1986), and identifying briefly presented words and nonwords (Keane et al., 1991, 1994; but see Ostergaard, 1994). A recent study (Heindel, Salmon, Fennema-Notestine, & Chan, 1998) examined the repetition priming ability of AD patients using novel, nonverbal stimuli that do not have preexisting lexical or semantic representations. In this task, subjects discriminated perceptually between geometric designs that had either a continuous ("closed") or discontinuous ("open") perimeter. With the open

stimuli, AD patients and control subjects displayed significant and equivalent levels of priming after immediate repetition of the stimuli.

This demonstration provides strong support for the claim that perceptual priming is normal in patients with AD and suggests that this form of priming is mediated by brain regions different from those that support conceptual priming and that are damaged in AD. Consistent with this suggestion, Gabrieli and colleagues (Fleischman et al., 1995; Gabrieli et al., 1995) presented evidence that perceptual priming may be mediated by a putative visual memory mechanism in the right occipital cortex, a brain area not prominently affected by AD. These investigators examined explicit memory and perceptual identification priming in a patient (M.S.) with a left homonymous hemianopsia due to a right-hemisphere temporal lobectomy performed as treatment for pharmacologically intractable epilepsy. Despite normal performance in a visually based explicit recognition memory test, patient M.S. was impaired in a perceptual identification priming test.

Although the pattern of impaired conceptual priming and intact perceptual priming exhibited by patients with AD is consistent with the possibility that their priming deficit is mediated by deterioration of semantic memory, other evidence suggests that a more general factor may be at fault. Several studies, for example, demonstrated that patients with AD exhibit normal priming of semantic relationships when on-line tasks that require very short-term effects are employed. In one study, for example, Nebes and colleagues (Nebes, Martin, & Horn, 1984) tested patients with AD in a task in which a given word was preceded (by approximately 500 ms) either by a semantically related word (primed trials) or by an unrelated word (unprimed trials), and priming was measured by the difference in naming latencies between primed and unprimed trials. Patients with AD and control subjects displayed a slight and equivalent facilitation in naming latency when a word was preceded by a semantic associate (i.e., semantic priming). From these and similar results, Nebes et al. (1984) concluded that semantic memory is unimpaired in patients with AD when it is assessed by techniques that rely solely on automatic information processing. According to Nebes and colleagues, the deficits that these patients display on other implicit and explicit tests of semantic memory are due to the heavy attentional demands of these tasks, rather than to an impairment in semantic memory *per se*. Ober, Shenaut, Jagust, and Stillman (1991) reached a similar conclusion.

Another general factor that may contribute to the priming deficit of patients with AD is a deficiency in the level of steady-state cortical activation, or "cortical tonus" (Sara, 1985), that modulates the efficiency of cortical information processing (Salmon & Heindel, 1992). This steady-state cortical activation, it is thought, is maintained by the noradrenergic projection system (i.e., the locus coeruleus; Sara, 1985) that is often damaged in patients with AD (Bondareff et al., 1982). It may be that poor cortical tonus leads to insufficient levels of activation or inadequate maintenance of activation of representations required to support long-term priming. Representations may still be sufficiently activated, however, to manifest intact priming over the very short (e.g., 500 ms) delay intervals used in the Nebes et al. (1984) paradigm. This explanation might also account for the observations that, though patients with AD display intact immediate priming in the homophone (Fennema-Notestine et al., 1994) and nonverbal perceptual (Heindel et al., 1998) priming tasks, they also display abnormally rapid dissipation of the priming effect in both tasks. Although these explanations remain tentative, future investigations into the processes that underlie the priming deficits of patients with AD should provide information about the necessary and sufficient conditions for priming phenomena and about the nature of the neuropsychological deficits of the disease.

## Summary

The goals of this chapter have been twofold: (1) to demonstrate the diagnostic, theoretical, and neurological value of applying concepts derived from cognitive psychology to the severe memory impairments of demented patients and (2) to stress the heterogeneity of the memory and underlying cognitive disorders of different types of dementia.

It is evident that, though patients with so-called "cortical" and "subcortical" dementias may generate quantitatively similar scores in some standardized tests of memory and mental status, the cognitive processes that underlie their performance are often quite distinct. Patients with AD

(i.e., a "cortical" dementia) cannot store new information, are highly sensitive to proactive interference, and rapidly forget what little information they can acquire initially. Qualitative analyses of AD patients' performance in semantic memory tasks indicate that they have endured some breakdown of the hierarchical structure of semantic knowledge. In tests of implicit memory, AD patients have an intact ability to acquire and retain motor and visuomotor skills but their ability to manifest lexical, semantic, and pictorial priming is often severely impaired. Although the role of semantic, perceptual, attentional, and arousal factors in these priming deficits remains uncertain, the available evidence suggests that the association cortices are involved in mediating this type of implicit memory task.

When similar analyses are applied to the memory disorder associated with HD (i.e., a "subcortical" dementia), a different profile of cognitive deficiencies becomes apparent. Huntington's disease patients' episodic and semantic memory impairments are characterized by an inability to initiate retrieval of stored information. In comparison to AD patients, patients with HD demonstrate less sensitivity to proactive interference and better retention of information over time. In tests of implicit memory, the pattern of impairments is the opposite of that seen in patients with AD. Although HD patients exhibit normal lexical, semantic, and pictorial priming, their learning of motor skills is severely impaired, and they perform poorly in other tasks that require the acquisition of central motor programs. Given these data and existing neuroanatomical knowledge, the notion that motor skill learning depends on the integrity of the striatum and complex corticostriatal circuits has substantial support.

Finally, it is important to stress that not all forms of dementia can be assumed under an *Alzheimer-type* or *Huntington-type* profile of memory and cognitive deficits. Studies with demented PD patients, for example, suggest that their memory deficiencies may reflect a combination of the features associated with AD and HD. Rather, the investigations reviewed in this chapter should be seen as prototypical analyses that can provide novel insights into the nature of the memory disorders of *all* forms of dementia and perhaps even contribute new clues to the neurological bases of various memory systems.

ACKNOWLEDGMENTS.. The preparation of this chapter was supported, in part, by NIH grants AG15375 to Brown University and AG05131 to the University of California, San Diego.

# References

Agid, Y., Ruberg, M., Dubois, B., & Pillon, B. (1987). Anatomoclinical and biochemical concepts of subcortical dementia. In S. M. Stahl, S. D. Iverson, & E. C. Goodman (Eds.), *Cognitive neurochemistry* (pp. 248–271). Oxford: Oxford University Press.

Aharon-Peretz, J., Cummings, J. L., & Hill, M. A. (1988). Vascular dementia and dementia of the Alzheimer type. Cognition, ventricular size, and leuko-araiosis. *Archives of Neurology, 45,* 719–721.

Albert, M. L. (1978). Subcortical dementia. In R. Katzman, R. D. Terry, & K. L. Bick (Eds.), *Alzheimer's disease: Senile dementia and related disorders* (pp. 173–179). New York: Raven Press.

Albert, M. L., Feldman, R. G., & Willis, A. L. (1974). The 'subcortical dementia' of progressive supranuclear palsy. *Journal of Neurology, Neurosurgery, and Psychiatry, 37,* 121–130.

Albert, M. S., Butters, N., & Brandt, J. (1981). Development of remote memory loss in patients with Huntington's disease. *Journal of Clinical and Experimental Neuropsychology, 3,* 1–12.

Albert, M. S., Butters, N., & Levin, J. (1979). Temporal gradients in the retrograde amnesia of patients with alcoholic Korsakoff disease. *Archives of Neurology, 36,* 211–216.

Alexander, G. E., DeLong, M. R., & Strick, P. L. (1986). Parallel organization of functionally segregated circuits linking basal ganglia and cortex. *Annual Review of Neuroscience, 9,* 357–381.

Alvord, E. C., Forno, L. S., Kusske, J. A., Kauffman, R. J., Rhodes, J. S., & Goetowski, C. R. (1974). The pathology of Parkinsonism: A comparison of degeneration in cerebral cortex and brainstem. In F. McDowell & A. Barbeau (Eds.), *Advances in neurology,* Vol. 5: *Second Canadian-American Conference on Parkinson's disease* (pp. 175–193). New York: Raven Press.

American Psychiatric Association. (1952). *Diagnostic and statistical manual of mental disorders.* Washington, DC: Author.

American Psychiatric Association. (1968). *Diagnostic and statistical manual of mental disorders* (2nd ed.). Washington, DC: Author.

American Psychiatric Association. (1987). *Diagnostic and statistical manual of mental disorders* (3rd ed., rev. ed.). Washington, DC: Author.

American Psychiatric Association. (1994). *Diagnostic and statistical manual of mental disorders* (4th ed.). Washington, DC: Author.

Baddeley, A. A. (1986). *Working memory.* Oxford: Clarendon Press.

Balota, D. A., & Duchek, J. M. (1991). Semantic priming effects, lexical repetition effects, and contextual disambiguation effects in healthy aged individuals and individuals

with senile dementia of the Alzheimer's type. *Brain and Language, 40,* 181–201.

Bayles, K. A., & Kaszniak, A. W. (1987). *Communication and cognition in normal aging and dementia.* Boston: College Hill Press.

Bayles, K. A., & Tomoeda, C. K. (1983). Confrontation naming impairment in dementia. *Brain and Language, 19,* 98–114.

Beatty, W. W. (1988). The Fargo Map Test: A standardized method of assessing remote memory for visuospatial information. *Journal of Clinical Psychology, 44,* 61–67.

Beatty, W. W., & Salmon, D. P. (1991). Remote memory for visuospatial information in patients with Alzheimer's disease. *Journal of Geriatric Psychiatry and Neurology, 4,* 14–17.

Beatty, W. W., Salmon, D. P., Butters, N., Heindel, W. C., & Granholm, E. L. (1988). Retrograde amnesia in patients with Alzheimer's disease or Huntington's disease. *Neurobiology of Aging, 9,* 181–186.

Becker, J. T., Huff, F. J., Nebes, R. D., Holland, A., & Boller, F. (1988). Neuropsychological function in Alzheimer's disease: Pattern of impairment and rates of progression. *Archives of Neurology, 45,* 263–268.

Benton, A. L. (1968). Differential behavioral effects in frontal lobe disease. *Neuropsychologia, 6,* 53–60.

Benzing, W. C., & Squire, L. R. (1989). Preserved learning and memory in amnesia: Intact adaptation-level effects and learning of stereoscopic depth. *Behavioral Neuroscience, 103,* 538–547.

Berg, L., Danziger, W. L., Storandt, M., Coben, L. A., Gado, M., Hughes, C. P., Knesevich, J. W., & Botwinick, J. (1984). Predictive features in mild senile dementia of the Alzheimer type. *Neurology, 34,* 563–569.

Bird, T. D. (1999). Clinical genetics of familial Alzheimer's disease. In R. D. Terry, R. Katzman, K. L. Bick, & S. S. Sisodia (Eds.), *Alzheimer disease* (pp. 57–66). Philadelphia: Lippincott Williams & Wilkens.

Blaxton, T. A. (1989). Investigating dissociations among memory measures: Support for a transfer-appropriate processing framework. *Journal of Experimental Psychology: Learning, Memory, and Cognition, 15,* 657–668.

Blessed, G., Tomlinson, B. E., & Roth, M. (1968). The association between quantitative measures of dementia and of senile change in the cerebral grey matter of elderly subjects. *British Journal of Psychiatry, 114,* 797–811.

Bloxham, C. A., Mindel, T. A., & Frith, C. D. (1984). Initiation and execution of predictable and unpredictable movements in Parkinson's disease. *Brain, 107,* 371–384.

Boller, F., Mizutani, T., Roessmann, U., & Gambetti, P. (1980). Parkinson disease, dementia, and Alzheimer disease: Clinicopathological correlations. *Annals of Neurology, 7,* 329–335.

Bondareff, W., Mountjoy, C. Q., & Roth, M. (1982). Loss of neurons of origin of the adrenergic projection to cerebral cortex (nucleus locus ceruleus) in senile dementia. *Neurology, 32,* 164–167.

Bondi, M. W., & Kaszniak, A. W. (1991). Implicit and explicit memory in Alzheimer's disease and Parkinson's disease. *Journal of Clinical and Experimental Neuropsychology, 13,* 339–358.

Bondi, M. W., Kaszniak, A. W., Bayles, K. A., & Vance, K. T. (1993). Contributions of frontal system dysfunction to memory and perceptual abilities in Parkinson's disease. *Neuropsychology, 7,* 89–102.

Bondi, M. W., Kaszniak, A. W., Rapcsak, S. Z., & Butters, M. A. (1993). Implicit and explicit memory following anterior communicating artery aneurysm rupture. *Brain and Cognition, 22*(2), 213–229.

Borkowski, J. G., Benton, A. L., & Spreen, O. (1967). Word fluency and brain damage. *Neuropsychologia, 5,* 135–140.

Braak, H., & Braak, E. (1991). Neuropathological staging of Alzheimer-related changes. *Acta Neuropathologica, 82,* 239–259.

Brandt, J., & Butters, N. (1986). The neuropsychology of Huntington's disease. *Trends in Neuroscience, 9,* 118–120.

Brandt, J., Corwin, J., & Krafft, L. (1992). Is verbal recognition memory really different in Huntington's and Alzheimer's disease? *Journal of Clinical and Experimental Neuropsychology, 14,* 773–784.

Brandt, J., Folstein, S. E., & Folstein, M. F. (1988). Differential cognitive impairment in Alzheimer's and Huntington's disease. *Annals of Neurology, 23,* 555–561.

Brandt, J., Spencer, M., McSorley, P., & Folstein, M. F. (1988). Semantic activation and implicit memory in Alzheimer disease. *Alzheimer Disease and Associated Disorders, 2,* 112–119.

Brinkman, C., & Porter, R. (1979). Supplementary motor area in the monkey: Activity of neurons during performance of a learned motor task. *Journal of Neurophysiology, 42,* 681–709.

Brooks, D. N., & Baddeley, A. D. (1976). What can amnesic patients learn? *Neuropsychologia, 14,* 111–122.

Brown, R. G., & Marsden, C. D. (1984). How common is dementia in Parkinson's disease? *The Lancet, 2*(8414), 1262–1265.

Brown, R. G., & Marsden, C. D. (1986). Visuospatial function in Parkinson's disease. *Brain, 109,* 987–1002.

Brown, R. G., & Marsden, C. D. (1988). 'Subcortical dementia': The neuropsychological evidence. *Neuroscience, 25,* 363–387.

Brun, A. (1983). An overview of light and electron microscopic changes. In B. Reisberg (Ed.), *Alzheimer's disease* (pp. 37–47). New York: The Free Press.

Bruyn, G. W. (1968). Huntington's chorea: Historical, clinical and laboratory synopsis. In P. J. Vinken & G. W. Bruyn (Eds.), *Handbook of clinical neurology, Vol. 6: Diseases of the basal ganglia* (pp. 83–94). New York: Raven Press.

Bruyn, G. W., Bots, G., & Dom, R. (1979). Huntington's chorea: Current neuropathological status. In T. Chase, N. Wexler, & A. Barbeau (Es.), *Advances in neurology, Vol. 23: Huntington's disease* (pp. 83–94). New York: Raven Press.

Butters, N. (1984). The clinical aspects of memory disorders: Contributions from experimental studies of amnesia and dementia. *Journal of Clinical and Experimental Neuropsychology, 9,* 479–497.

Butters, N., & Cermak, L. S. (1980). *Alcoholic Korsakoff's syndrome: An information-processing approach to amnesia.* New York: Academic Press.

Butters, N., & Cermak, L. S. (1986). A case study of the forgetting of autobiographical knowledge: Implications for the study of retrograde amnesia. In D. Rubin (Ed.), *Autobiographical memory* (pp. 253–272). New York: Cambridge University Press.

Butters, N., Granholm, E., Salmon, D. P., Grant, I., & Wolfe, J. (1987). Episodic and semantic memory: A comparison of amnesic and demented patients. *Journal of Clinical and Experimental Neuropsychology, 9,* 479–497.

Butters, N., Heindel, W. C., & Salmon, D. P. (1990). Dissociation of implicit memory in dementia: Neurological implications. *Bulletin of the Psychonomic Society, 28,* 359–366.

Butters, N., Salmon, D. P., Cullum, C. M., Cairns, P., Troster, A. I., Jacobs, D., Moss, M., & Cermak, L. S. (1988). Differentiation of amnesic and demented patients with the Wechsler memory scale-revised. *The Clinical Neuropsychologist, 2,* 133–148.

Butters, N., Sax, D. S., Montgomery, K., & Tarlow, S. (1978). Comparison of the neuropsychological deficits associated with early and advanced Huntington's disease. *Archives of Neurology, 35,* 585–589.

Butters, N., Wolfe, J., Martone, M., Granholm, E., & Cermak, L. S. (1985). Memory disorders associated with Huntington's disease: Verbal recall, verbal recognition and procedural memory. *Neuropsychologia, 23,* 729–743.

Butters, N., Wolfe, J., Granholm, E., & Martone, M. (1986). An assessment of verbal recall, recognition and fluency abilities in patients with Huntington's disease. *Cortex, 22,* 11–32.

Cahn, D. A., Sullivan, E. V., Shear, P. K., Marsh, L., Fama, R., Lim, K. O., Yesavage, J. A., Tinklenberg, J. R., & Pfefferbaum, A. (1998). Structural MRI correlates of recognition memory in Alzheimer's disease. *Journals of the International Neuropsychological Society, 4,* 106–114.

Caine, E. D., Ebert, M. H., & Weingartner, H. (1977). An outline for the analysis of dementia: The memory disorder of Huntington's disease. *Neurology, 27,* 1087–1092.

Caine, E. D., Hunt, R., Weingartner, H., & Ebert, M. (1978). Huntington's dementia: Clinical and neuropsychological features. *Archives of General Psychiatry, 35,* 377–384.

Carlesimo, G. A. (1994). Perceptual and conceptual priming in amnesic and alcoholic patients. *Neuropsychologia, 32,* 903–921.

Cash, R., Dennis, T., L'Heureux, R., Raisman, R., Javoy-Agid, F., & Scatton, B. (1987). Parkinson's disease and dementia: Norepinephrine and dopamine in locus ceruleus. *Neurology, 37,* 42–46.

Cermak, L. S. (1984). The episodic-semantic distinction in amnesia. In L. R. Squire & N. Butters (Eds.), *Neuropsychology of memory* (pp. 55–62). New York: Guilford.

Cermak, L. S., Lewis, R., Butters, N., & Goodglass, H. (1973). Role of verbal mediation in performance of motor tasks by Korsakoff patients. *Perceptual and Motor Skills, 37,* 259–262.

Cermak, L. S., Talbot, N., Chandler, K., & Wolbarst, L. R. (1985). The perceptual priming phenomenon in amnesia. *Neuropsychologia, 23,* 615–622.

Cermak, L. S., Uhly, B., & Reale, L. (1980). Encoding specificity in the alcoholic Korsakoff patient. *Brain and Language, 11,* 119–127.

Chan, A. S., Butters, N., Paulsen, J. S., Salmon, D. P., Swenson, M. R., & Maloney, L. T. (1993). An assessment of the semantic network in patients with Alzheimer's disease. *Journal of Cognitive Neuroscience, 5,* 254–261.

Chan, A., Butters, N., & Salmon, D. P. (1997). The deterioration of semantic networks in patients with Alzheimer's disease: A cross-sectional study. *Neuropsychologia, 35,* 241–248.

Chan, A. S., Butters, N., Salmon, D. P., Johnson, S. A., Paulsen, J. S., & Swenson, M. R. (1995). Comparison of the semantic networks in patients with dementia and amnesia. *Neuropsychology, 9,* 177–186.

Chan, A. S., Butters, N., Salmon, D. P., & McGurie, K. A. (1993). Dimensionality and clustering in the semantic network of patients with Alzheimer's disease. *Psychology and Aging, 8,* 411–419.

Chertkow, H., & Bub, D. (1990). Semantic memory loss in dementia of the Alzheimer's type: What do various measures measure? *Brain, 113,* 397–417.

Chui, H. C., Victoroff, J. I., Margolin, D., Jagust, W., Shankle, R., & Katzman, R. (1992). Criteria for the diagnosis of ischemic vascular dementia proposed by the State of California Alzheimer's Disease Diagnostic and Treatment Centers. *Neurology, 42,* 473–480.

Cohen, N., & Squire, L. R. (1980). Preserved learning and retention of pattern analyzing skills in amnesia: Dissociation of knowing how and knowing that. *Science, 210,* 207–210.

Collette, F., Van der Linden, M., Bechet, S., & Salmon, E. (1999). Phonological loop and central executive functioning in Alzheimer's disease. *Neuropsychologia, 37,* 905–918.

Collins, A. M., & Loftus, E. F. (1975). A spreading activation theory of semantic processing. *Psychological Review, 82,* 407–428.

Corkin, S. (1982). Some relationships between global amnesias and the memory impairments in Alzheimer's disease. In S. Corkin, K. L. Davis, J. H. Growdon, & E. Usdin (Eds.), *Alzheimer's disease: A report of progress in research* (pp. 149–164). New York: Raven Press.

Cummings, J. L. (1990). *Subcortical dementia.* New York: Oxford University Press.

Cummings, J. L., & Benson, D. F. (1984). Subcortical dementia: Review of an emerging concept. *Archives of Neurology, 41,* 874–879.

Cummings, J. L., & Benson, D. F. (1992). *Dementia: A clinical approach* (2nd ed.). Boston: Butterworth-Heinemann.

Day, B. L., Dick, J. P. R., & Marsden, C. D. (1984). Patients with Parkinson's disease can employ a predictive motor strategy. *Journal of Neurology, Neurosurgery, and Psychiatry, 47,* 1299–1306.

Delis, D. C., Kramer, J. H., Kaplan, E., & Ober, B. A. (1987). *The California Verbal Learning Test.* New York: The Psychological Corporation.

Delis, D. C., Massman, P. J., Butters, N., Salmon, D. P., Cermak, L. S., & Kramer, J. H. (1991). Profiles of demented and amnesic patients on the California verbal learning test: Implications for the assessment of memory disorders. *Psychological Assessment, 3,* 19–26.

DeLong, M. R., Alexander, G. E., Georgopoulous, M. D., Mitchell, S. J., & Richardson, R. T. (1984). Role of basal ganglia in limb movements. *Human Neurobiology, 2,* 235–244.

Demonet, J. F., Chollet, F., Ramsay, S., Chardebat, D., Nespoulos, J. L., Wise, R., Rascol, A., & Frackowiak, R. (1992). The anatomy of phonological and semantic processing in normal subjects. *Brain, 115,* 1753–1768.

De Renzi, E., Faglioni, P., Scarpa, M., & Crisi, G. (1986). Limb apraxia in patients with damage confined to the left basal ganglia and thalamus. *Journal of Neurology, Neurosurgery, and Psychiatry, 49,* 1030–1038.

Deweer, B., Ergis, A. M., Fossati, P., Pillon, B., Boller, F., Agid, Y., & Dubois, B. (1994). Explicit memory, procedural learning and lexical priming in Alzheimer's disease. *Cortex, 30,* 113–126.

Deweer, B., Lehericy, S., Pillon, B., Baulac, M., Chiras, J., Marsault, C., Agid, Y., & Dubois, B. (1995). Memory disorders in probable Alzheimer's disease: The role of hippocampal atrophy as shown with MRI. *Journal of Neurology, Neurosurgery and Psychiatry, 58,* 590–597.

Deweer, B., Pillon, B., Michon, A., & Dubois, B. (1993). Mirror reading in Alzheimer's disease: Normal skill learning and acquisition of item-specific information. *Journal of Clinical and Experimental Neuropsychology, 15,* 789–804.

Dickson, D. W., Davies, P., Mayeux, R., Crystal, H., Horopian, D. S., Thompson, A., & Goldman, J. E. (1987). Diffuse Lewy body disease: Neuropathological and biochemical studies of six patients. *Acta Neuropathologica, 75,* 8–15.

Erkinjuntti, T., Ketonen, L., Sulkava, R., Sipponen, J., Vuorialho, M., & Iivanainen, M. (1987). Do white matter changes on MRI and CT differentiate vascular dementia from Alzheimer's disease? *Journal of Neurology, Neurosurgery and Psychiatry, 50,* 37–42.

Eslinger, P. J., & Damasio, A. R. (1986). Preserved motor learning in Alzheimer's disease: Implications for anatomy and behavior. *Journal of Neuroscience, 6,* 3006–3009.

Evans, D. A., Funkenstein, H. H., Albert, M. S., Scherr, P. A., Cook, N. R., Chown, M. J., Hebert, L. E., Hennekens, C. H., & Taylor, J. O. (1989). Prevalence of Alzheimer's disease in a community population of older persons: Higher than previously reported. *Journal of the American Medical Association, 262,* 2551–2556.

Fama, R., Sullivan, E. V., Shear, P. K., Marsh, L., Yesavage, J. A., Tinklenberg, J. R., Lim, K. O., & Pfefferbaum, A. (1997). Selective cortical and hippocampal volume correlates of Mattis Dementia Rating Scale in Alzheimer's disease. *Archives of Neurology, 54,* 719–728.

Fennema-Notestine, C., Butters, N., Heindel, W. C., & Salmon, D. P. (1994). Semantic homophone priming in patient with dementia of the Alzheimer type. *Neuropsychology, 8,* 579–587.

Ferraro, F. R., Balota, D. A., & Connor, L. T. (1993). Implicit memory and the formation of new associations in nondemented Parkinson's disease individuals and individuals with senile dementia of the Alzheimer type: A serial reaction time (SRT) investigation. *Brain and Cognition, 21,* 163–180.

Filley, C. M., Kelly, J., & Heaton, R. K. (1986). Neuropsychologic features of early- and late-onset Alzheimer's disease. *Archives of Neurology, 43,* 574–576.

Fleischman, D. A., Gabrieli, J. D. E., Reminger, S., Rinaldi, J., Morrell, F., & Wilson, R. (1995). Conceptual priming in perceptual identification for patients with Alzheimer's disease and a patients with right occipital lobectomy. *Neuropsychology, 9,* 187–197.

Flowers, K. (1978). Lack of prediction in the motor behaviour of Parkinsonism. *Brain, 101,* 35–52.

Flowers, K. A., & Robertson, C. (1985). The effect of Parkinson's disease on the ability to maintain a mental set. *Journal of Neurology, Neurosurgery, and Psychiatry, 48,* 517–529.

Folstein, S. E. (1989). *Huntington's disease: A disorder of families.* Baltimore: Johns Hopkins University Press.

Folstein, M. F., Folstein, S. E., & McHugh, P. R. (1975). "Mini-Mental State: A practical method for grading the cognitive state of patients for the clinician. *Journal of Psychiatric Research, 12,* 189–198.

Fuld, P. A. (1983). Word intrusions as a diagnostic sign of Alzheimer's disease. *Geriatric Medicine Today, 2,* 33–41.

Fuld, P. A., Katzman, R., Davies, P., & Terry, R. D. (1982). Intrusions as a sign of Alzheimer dementia: Chemical and pathological verification. *Annals of Neurology, 11,* 155–159.

Gabrieli, J. D. E., Corkin, S., Mickel, S. F., & Growdon, J. H. (1993). Intact acquisition and long-term retention of mirror-tracing skill in Alzheimer's disease and global amnesia. *Behavioral Neuroscience, 107,* 899–910.

Gabrieli, J. D. E., Fleischman, D. A., Keane, M. M., Reminger, S. L., & Morrell, F. (1995). Double dissociation between memory systems underlying explicit and implicit memory in the human brain. *Psychological Science, 6*, 76–82.

Gabrieli, J. D. E., Keane, M. M., Stanger, B. Z., Kjelgaard, M. M., Corkin, S., & Growdon, J. H. (1994). Dissociations among structural-perceptual, lexical-semantic, and event-fact memory systems in Alzheimer, amnesic, and normal subjects. *Cortex, 30*, 75–103.

Galasko, D., Katzman, R., Salmon, D. P., Thal, L. J., & Hansen, L. (1996). Clinical and neuropathological findings in Lewy body dementias. *Brain and Cognition, 31*, 166–175.

Gardner, H., Boller, F., Moreines, J., & Butters, N. (1973). Retrieving information from Korsakoff patients: Effects of categorical cues and reference to the task. *Cortex, 9*, 165–175.

Gaspar, P., & Gary, F. (1984). Dementia in idiopathic Parkinson's disease: A neuropathological study of 32 cases. *Acta Neuropathologica, 64*, 43–52.

Gibb, W. R. G., Esiri, M. M., & Lees, A. J. (1985). Clinical and pathological features of diffuse cortical Lewy body disease (Lewy body dementia). *Brain, 110*, 1131–1153.

Goodglass, H., Biber, C., & Freedman, M. (1984). Memory factors in naming disorders in aphasics and Alzheimer patients. Paper presented at the *Annual Conference of the International Neuropsychological Society*, Houston, TX.

Graf, P., & Schacter, D. (1985). Implicit and explicit memory for new associations in normal and amnesic subjects. *Journal of Experimental Psychology: Learning, Memory, and Cognition, 11*, 501–518.

Graf, P., Squire, L. R., & Mandler, G. (1984). The information that amnesic patients do not forget. *Journal of Experimental Psychology: Learning, Memory, and Cognition, 10*, 164–178.

Grafman, J., Weingartner, H., Newhouse, P. A., Thompson, K., Lalonde, F., Litvan, I., Molchan, S., & Sunderland, T. (1991). Implicit learning in patients with Alzheimer's disease. *Pharmacopsychiatry, 23*, 94–101.

Granholm, E., & Butters, N. (1988). Associative encoding and retrieval in Alzheimer's and Huntington's disease. *Brain and Cognition, 7*, 335–347.

Grober, E., Ausubel, R., Sliwinski, M., & Gordon, B. (1992). Skill learning and repetition priming in Alzheimer's disease. *Neuropsychologia, 30*, 849–858.

Hachinski, V. C., Iliff, L. D., Zilhka, E., Du Boulay, G. H., McAllister, V. L., Marshall, J., Russell, R. W. R., & Symon, L. (1975). Cerebral blood flow in dementia. *Archives of Neurology, 32*, 632–637.

Hakim, A. M., & Mathieson, M. B. (1979). Dementia in Parkinson disease: A neuropathologic study. *Neurology, 29*, 1209–1214.

Hansen, L., Salmon, D., Galasko, D., Masliah, E., Katzman, R., DeTeresa, R., Thal, L., Pay, M., Hofstetter, R., Klauber, M., Rice, V., Butters, N., & Alford, M. (1990). The Lewy body variant of Alzheimer's disease: A clinical and pathologic entity. *Neurology, 40*, 1–8.

Hayden, M. R. (1981). *Huntington's chorea*. Berlin: Springer Verlag.

Heindel, W., Butters, N., & Salmon, D. (1988). Impaired learning of a motor skill in patients with Huntington's disease. *Behavioral Neuroscience, 102*, 141–147.

Heindel, W. C., Salmon, D. P., & Butters, N. (1990). Pictorial priming and cued recall in Alzheimer's and Huntington's disease. *Brain and Cognition, 13*, 282–295.

Heindel, W. C., Salmon, D. P., & Butters, N. (1991). The

biasing of weight judgments in Alzheimer's and Huntington's disease: A priming or programming phenomenon? *Journal of Clinical and Experimental Neuropsychology, 13*, 189–203.

Heindel, W. C., Salmon, D. P., Fennema-Notestine, C., & Chan, A. S. (1998). Repetition priming with non-verbal stimuli in patients with dementia of the Alzheimer type. *Neuropsychology, 12*, 43–51.

Heindel, W. C., Salmon, D. P., Shults, C. W., Walicke, P. A., & Butters, N. (1989). Neuropsychological evidence for multiple implicit memory systems: A comparison of Alzheimer's, Huntington's, and Parkinson's disease patients. *Journal of Neuroscience, 9*, 582–587.

Helson, H. (1948). Adaptation-level as a basis for a quantitative theory of frames of reference. *Psychological Review, 55*, 297–313.

Hodges, J. R., Salmon, D. P., & Butters, N. (1991). The nature of the naming of deficit in Alzheimer's and Huntington's disease. *Brain, 114*, 1547–1558.

Hodges, J. R., Salmon, D. P., & Butters, N. (1992). Semantic memory impairment in Alzheimer's disease: Failure of access or degraded knowledge? *Neuropsychologia, 30*, 301–314.

Hodges, J. R., Salmon, D. P., & Butters, N. (1993). Recognition and naming of famous faces in Alzheimer's disease: A cognitive analysis. *Neuropsychologia, 31*, 775–788.

Huber, S. J., Shuttleworth, E. C., Paulson, G. W., Bellchambers, M. J. G., & Clapp, L. E. (1986). Cortical vs subcortical dementia: Neuropsychological differences. *Archives of Neurology, 43*, 392–394.

Huberman, M., Moscovitch, M., & Freedman, M. (1994). Comparison of patients with Alzheimer's and Parkinson's disease on different explicit and implicit tests of memory. *Neuropsychiatry, Neuropsychology, and Behavioral Neurology, 7*, 185–193.

Huff, F. J., Corkin, S., & Growdon, J. H. (1986). Semantic impairment and anomia in Alzheimer's disease. *Brain and Language, 28*, 235–249.

Huff, F. J., Growdon, J. H., Corkin, S., & Rosen, T. J. (1987). Age at onset and rate of progression of Alzheimer's disease. *Journal of the American Geriatrics Society, 35*, 27–30.

Huntington's Disease Collaborative Research Group. (1993). A novel gene containing a trinucleotide repeat that is expanded and unstable on Huntington's disease chromosomes. *Cell, 71*, 971–983.

Hyman, B. T., Van Hoesen, G. W., Damasio, A., & Barnes, C. (1984). Alzheimer's disease: Cell-specific pathology isolates the hippocampal formation. *Science, 225*, 1168–1170.

Ince, P. G., Jaros, E., Ballard, C., McKeith, I. G., & Perry, R. H. (in press). Prospective evaluation of consensus diagnosis criteria for dementia with Lewy bodies. *Neuropathology and Applied Neurobiology*.

Jacobs, D., Salmon, D. P., Troster, A. I., & Butters, N. (1990). Intrusion errors in the figural memory of patients with Alzheimer's and Huntington's disease. *Archives of Clinical Neuropsychology, 5*, 49–57.

Jacobs, D., Troster, A. I., Butters, N., Salmon, D. P., & Cermak, L. S. (1990). Intrusion errors on the visual reproduction test of the Wechsler Memory Scale and Wechsler Memory Scale-revised: An analysis of demented and amnesic patients. *The Clinical Neuropsychologist, 4*, 177–191.

Jankovic, J. (1987). Pathophysiology and clinical assessment of motor symptoms in Parkinson's disease. In W. C. Koller

(Ed.), *Handbook of Parkinson's disease* (pp. 99–126). New York: Marcel Dekker.

Jellinger, K. (1987). The pathology of Parkinsonism. In C. D. Marsden & S. Fahn (Eds.), *Movement disorders 2. Neurology*, Vol. 7 (pp. 124–165). London: Butterworth.

Jones, L. A. (1986). Perception of force and weight: Theory and research. *Psychological Bulletin, 100*, 29–42.

Kaszniak, A., Garron, D., & Fox, J. (1979). Differential effects of age and cerebral atrophy upon span of immediate recall and paired-associate learning in older patients suspected of dementia. *Cortex, 15*, 285–295.

Katzman, R. (1986). Alzheimer's disease. *New England Journal of Medicine, 314*, 964–973.

Katzman, R., & Kawas, C. (1994). The epidemiology of dementia and Alzheimer disease. In R. D. Terry, R. Katzman, & K. L. Bick (Eds.), *Alzheimer disease* (pp. 105–122). New York: Raven Press.

Keane, M. M., Gabrieli, J. D. E., Fennema, A. C., Growdon, J. H., & Corkin, S. (1991). Evidence for a dissociation between perceptual and conceptual priming in Alzheimer's disease. *Behavioral Neuroscience, 105*, 326–342.

Keane, M. M., Gabrieli, J. D. E., Growdon, J. H., & Corkin, S. (1994). Priming in perceptual identification of pseudowords is normal in Alzheimer's disease. *Neuropsychologia, 32*, 343–356.

Kinsbourne, M., & Wood, F. (1975). Short-term memory processes and the amnesic syndrome. In D. Deutsch & J. A. Deutsch (Eds.), *Short-term memory*. New York: Academic Press.

Klatzky, R. L. (1980). *Human memory: Structures and processes*. San Francisco: W. H. Freeman.

Knopman, D. S., & Nissen, M. J. (1987). Implicit learning in patients with probable Alzheimer's disease. *Neurology, 37*, 784–788.

Knopman, D. S., & Nissen, M. J. (1991). Procedural learning is impaired in Huntington's disease: Evidence from the serial reaction time test. *Neuropsychologia, 29*, 245–254.

Knowlton, B. J., Mangels, J. A., & Squire, L. R. (1996). A neostriatal habit learning system in humans. *Science, 273*, 1399–1402.

Kohler, S., Black, S. E., Sinden, M., Szekely, C., Kidron, D., Parker, J. L., Foster, J. K., Moscovitch, M., Winocur, G., Szalai, J. P., & Bronskill, M. J. (1998). Memory impairments associated with hippocampal versus parahippocampal gyrus atrophy: An MR volumetry study in Alzheimer's disease. *Neuropsychologia, 36*, 901–914.

Kopelman, M. D. (1985). Rates of forgetting in Alzheimer-type dementia and Korsakoff's syndrome. *Neuropsychologia, 23*, 623–638.

Kopelman, M. D. (1989). Remote and autobiographical memory, temporal context memory and frontal atrophy in Korsakoff and Alzheimer patients. *Neuropsychologia, 27*, 437–460.

Kosaka, K., Yoshimura, M., Ikeda, K., & Budka, H. (1984). Diffuse type of Lewy body disease: Progressive dementia with abundant cortical Lewy bodies and senile changes of varying degree: A new disease? *Clinical Neuropathology, 3*, 185–192.

Lennox, G., Lowe, J., Landon, M., Byrne, E. J., Mayer, R. J., & Godwin-Austen, R. B. (1989). Diffuse Lewy body disease: Correlative neuropathology using anti-ubiquitin immunocytochemistry. *Journal of Neurology, Neurosurgery, and Psychiatry, 52*, 1236–1247.

Lipowski, Z. J. (1981). Organic mental disorders: Their history and classification with special reference to DSM-III. In N. E. Miller & G. D. Cohen (Eds.), *Clinical aspects of Alzheimer's disease and senile dementia. Aging*, Vol. 15 (pp. 37–45). New York: Raven Press.

Locascio, J. J., Growdon, J. H., & Corkin, S. (1995). Cognitive test performance in detecting, staging, and tracking Alzheimer's disease. *Archives of Neurology, 52*, 1087–1099.

Mahandra, B. (1984). *Dementia: A survey of the syndrome of dementia*. Lancaster, England: MTP Press.

Mann, D. M. A., Yates, P. O., & Marcyniuk, B. (1984). A comparison of changes in the nucleus basalis and locus coeruleus in Alzheimer's disease. *Journal of Neurology, Neurosurgery, and Psychiatry, 47*, 201–203.

Martin, A. (1987). Representation of semantic and spatial knowledge in Alzheimer's patients: Implications for models of preserved learning in amnesia. *Journal of Clinical and Experimental Neuropsychology, 9*, 191–224.

Martin, A., Brouwers, P., Cox, C., & Fedio, P. (1985). On the nature of the verbal memory deficit in Alzheimer's disease. *Brain and Language, 25*, 323–341.

Martin, A., & Fedio, P. (1983). Word production and comprehension in Alzheimer's disease: The breakdown of semantic knowledge. *Brain and Language, 19*, 124–141.

Martin, A., Haxby, J. V., Lalonde, F. M., Wiggs, C. L., & Ungerleider, L. G. (1995). Discrete cortical regions associated with knowledge of color and knowledge of action. *Science, 270*, 102–105.

Martin, A., Wiggs, C. L., Ungerleider, L. G., & Haxby, J. V. (1996). Neural correlates of category-specific knowledge. *Nature, 379*, 649–652.

Martone, M., Butters, N., Payne, M., Becker, J., & Sax, D. S. (1984). Dissociations between skill learning and verbal recognition in amnesia and dementia. *Archives of Neurology, 41*, 965–970.

Marttila, R. J. (1987). Epidemiology. In W. C. Koller (Ed.), *Handbook of Parkinson's disease* (pp. 35–50). New York: Marcel Dekker.

Masliah, E., Terry, R. D., DeTeresa, R. M., & Hansen, L. A. (1989). Immuno-histochemical quantification of the synapse-related protein synaptophysin in Alzheimer disease. *Neuroscience Letters, 103*, 234–239.

Massman, P. J., Delis, D. C., Butters, N., Levin, B. E., & Salmon, D. P. (1990). Are all subcortical dementias alike?: Verbal learning and memory in Parkinson's and Huntington's disease patients. *Journal of Clinical and Experimental Neuropsychology, 12*, 736–751.

Mattis, S. (1976). Mental status examination for organic mental syndrome in the elderly patient. In L. Bellak & T. B. Karasu (Eds.), *Geriatric psychiatry: A handbook for psychiatrists and primary care physicians* (pp. 77–121). New York: Grune & Stratton.

Mayeux, R., Stern, Y., Rosen, J., & Benson, D. F. (1981). Subcortical dementia: A recognizable clinical entity. *Transactions of the American Neurological Society, 106*, 313–316.

Mayeux, R., Stern, Y., Sano, M., Cote, L., & Williams, D. S. W. (1987). Clinicao and biochemical correlates of bradyphrenia in Parkinson's disease. *Neurology, 37*, 1130–1134.

McCarthy, R. A., & Warrington, E. K. (1988). Evidence for modality-specific meaning systems in the brain. *Nature, 334*, 428–430.

McGill, W. J. (1963). Stochastic latency mechanisms. In R. D. Luce, R. R. Brush, & E. Galanter (Eds.), *Handbook of mathematical psychology*, Vol. 1 (pp. 309–360). New York: Wiley.

McHugh, P. R., & Folstein, M. F. (1975). Psychiatric symptoms of Huntington's chorea: A clinical and phenomenologic study. In D. F. Benson & D. Blumer (Eds.), *Psychiatric aspects of neurological disease* (pp. 267–285). New York: Raven Press.

McKeith, I., Galasko, D., Kosaka, K., Perry, E., Dickson, D., Hansen, L., Salmon, D., Lowe, J., Mirra, S., Byrne, E., Quinn, N., Edwardson, J., Ince, P., Bergeron, C., Burns, A., Miller, B., Lovestone, S., Collerton, D., Jansen, E., deVos, R., Wilcock, G., Jellinger, K., & Perry, R. (1996). Clinical and pathological diagnosis of dementia with Lewy bodies (DLB): Report of the Consortium on Dementia with Lewy Bodies (CDLB) International Workgroup. *Neurology, 47*, 1113–1124.

McKeith, I. G., Perry, R. H., Fairbairn, A. F., Jabeen, S., & Perry, E. K. (1992). Operational criteria for senile dementia of Lewy body type (SDLT). *Psychological Medicine, 22*, 911–922.

McKhann, G., Drachman, D., Folstein, M., Katzman, R., Price, D., & Stadlin, E. M. (1984). Clinical diagnosis of Alzheimer's disease: Report of the NINCDS-ADRDA work group under the auspices of the Department of Health and Human Services Task Force on Alzheimer's Disease. *Neurology, 34*, 939–944.

Meyer, J. S., McClintic, K. L., Rogers, R. L., Sims, P., & Mortel, K. F. (1988). Aetiological considerations and risk factors for multi-infarct dementia. *Journal of Neurology, Neurosurgery and Psychiatry, 51*, 1489–1497.

Meyer, J. S., Rogers, R. L., Judd, B. W., Mortel, K. F., & Sims, P. (1988). Cognition and cerebral blood flow fluctuate together in multi-infarct dementia. *Stroke, 19*, 163–169.

Miller, G. A. (1956). The magical number seven, plus or minus two: Some limits on our capacity for processing information. *Psychological Review, 63*, 81–97.

Mindham, R. H. S., Ahmed, S. W. A., & Clough, C. G. (1982). A controlled study of dementia in Parkinson's disease. *Journal of Neurology, Neurosurgery, and Psychiatry, 45*, 969–974.

Molsa, P. K., Palijarvi, L., Rinne, J. O., Rinne, U. K., & Sako, E. (1985). Validity of clinical diagnosis in dementia: A prospective clinicopathological study. *Journal of Neurology, Neurosurgery, and Psychiatry, 48*, 1085–1090.

Monsch, A. U., Bondi, M. W., Butters, N., Paulsen, J. S., Salmon, D. P., Brugger, P., & Swenson, M. (1994). A comparison of category and letter fluency in Alzheimer's disease and Huntington's disease. *Neuropsychology, 8*, 25–30.

Moscovitch, M., Winocur, G., & McLachlan, D. (1986). Memory as assessed by recognition and reading time in normal and memory-impaired people with Alzheimer's disease and other neurological disorders. *Journal of Experimental Psychology: General, 115*, 331–347.

Nebes, R. D., Martin, D., & Horn, L. (1984). Sparing of semantic memory in Alzheimer's disease. *Journal of Abnormal Psychology, 93*, 321–330.

Nelson, D. L., Reed, V. S., & McEvoy, C. L. (1977). Learning to order pictures and words: A model of sensory and semantic encoding. *Journal of Experimental Psychology: Human Learning and Memory, 3*, 485–497.

Nissen, M. J., & Bullemer, P. (1987). Attentional requirements of learning: Evidence from performance measures. *Cognitive Psychology, 19*, 1–32.

Norton, L. E., Bondi, M. W., Salmon, D. P., & Goodglass, H. (1997). Deterioration of generic knowledge in patients with Alzheimer's disease: Evidence from the Number Information Test. *Journal of Clinical and Experimental Neuropsychology, 19*, 857–866.

Ober, B. A., & Shenaut, G. K. (1988). Lexical decision and priming in Alzheimer's disease. *Neuropsychologia, 26*, 273–286.

Ober, B. A., Shenaut, G. K., Jagust, W. J., & Stillman, R. C. (1991). Automatic semantic priming with various category relations in Alzheimer's disease and normal aging. *Psychology and Aging, 6*, 647–660.

Orgogozo, J. M., & Larsen, B. (1979). Activation of the supplementary motor area during voluntary movement in man suggests it works as a supramotor area. *Science, 206*, 847–850.

Ostergaard, A. L. (1994). Dissociations between word priming effects in normal subjects and patients with memory disorders: Multiple memory systems or retrieval? *Quarterly Journal of Experimental Psychology, 47A*, 331–364.

Ostergaard, A. L., Heindel, W. C., & Paulsen, J. S. (1995). The biasing effect of verbal labels on memory for ambiguous figures in patients with progressive dementia. *Journal of the International Neuropsychological Society, 1*, 271–280.

Pantel, J., Schroder, J., Schad, L. R., Friedlinger, M., Knopp, M. V., Schmitt, R., Geissler, M., Bluml, S., Essig, M., & Sauer, H. (1997). Quantitative magnetic resonance imaging and neuropsychological functions in dementia of the Alzheimer type. *Psychological Medicine, 27*, 221–229.

Pascual-Leone, A., Grafman, J., Clark, K., Stewart, M., Massaquoi, S., Lou, J., & Hallett, M. (1993). Procedural learning in Parkinson's disease and cerebellar degeneration. *Annals of Neurology, 34*, 594–602.

Paulsen, J. S., Butters, N., Salmon, D. P., Heindel, W. C., & Swenson, M. R. (1993). Prism adaptation in Alzheimer's and Huntington's disease. *Neuropsychology, 7*, 73–81.

Perani, D., Bressi, S., Cappa, S. F., Vallar, G., Alberoni, M., Grassi, F., Caltagirone, C., Cipolotti, L., Franceschi, M., Lenzi, G. L., & Fazio, F. (1993). Evidence of multiple memory systems in the human brain. *Brain, 116*, 903–919.

Perry, E. K., Curtis, M., Dick, D. J., Candy, J. M., Atack, J. R., Bloxham, C. A., Blessed, G., Fairbairn, A., Tomlinson, B. E., & Perry, R. H. (1985). Cholinergic correlates of cognitive impairment in Parkinson's disease: Comparisons with Alzheimer's disease. *Journal of Neurology, Neurosurgery, and Psychiatry, 48*, 413–421.

Perry, R. H., Irving, D., Blessed, G., Fairbairn, A., & Perry, E. K. (1990). Senile dementia of the Lewy body type: A clinically and neuropathologically distinct form of Lewy body dementia in the elderly. *Journal of Neurological Sciences, 95*, 119–139.

Peterson, L. R., & Peterson, M. J. (1959). Short-term retention of individual verbal items. *Journal of Experimental Psychology, 58*, 193–198.

Petit, H., & Milbled, G. (1973). Anomalies of conjugate ocular movements in Huntington's chorea: Application to early detection. In A. Barbeau, T. N. Chase, & G. W. Paulson (Eds.), *Advances in neurology*, Vol. 1: *Huntington's chorea, 1872–1972* (pp. 287–294). New York: Raven Press.

Pew, R. W. (1974). Levels of analysis in motor control. *Brain Research, 71*, 393–400.

Powell, A. L., Cummings, J. L., Hill, M. A., & Benson, D. F. (1988). Speech and language alterations in multi-infarct dementia. *Neurology, 38*, 717–719.

Rafal, R. D., Inhoff, A. W., Friedman, J. H., & Bernstein, E. (1987). Programming and execution of sequential movements in Parkinson's disease. *Journal of Neurology, Neurosurgery, and Psychiatry, 50,* 1267–1273.

Randolph, C. (1991). Implicit, explicit and semantic memory functions in Alzheimer's disease and Huntington's disease. *Journal of Clinical and Experimental Neuropsychology, 13,* 479–494.

Robinson-Whelan, S., & Storandt, M. (1992). Immediate and delayed prose recall among normal and demented adults. *Archives of Neurology, 49,* 32–34.

Rocca, W. A., Amaducci, L. A., & Schoenberg, B. S. (1986). Epidemiology of clinically diagnosed Alzheimer's disease. *Annals of Neurology, 19,* 415–424.

Roediger, H. L., & Blaxton, T. A. (1987). Effects of varying modality, surface features, and retention interval on priming in word fragment completion. *Memory and Cognition, 15,* 379–388.

Rohrer, D., Salmon, D. P., Wixted, J. T., & Paulsen, J. S. (1999). The disparate effects of Alzheimer's disease and Huntington's disease on the recall from semantic memory. *Neuropsychology, 13,* 381–388.

Rohrer, D., Wixted, J. T., Salmon, D. P., & Butters, N. (1995). Retrieval from semantic memory and its implications for Alzheimer's disease. *Journal of Experimental Psychology: Learning, Memory and Cognition, 21,* 1–13.

Roland, P. E. (1984). Organization of motor control by the normal human brain. *Human Neurobiology, 2,* 205–216.

Roland, P. E., Larsen, B., Lassen, N. A., & Skinhof, E. (1980). Supplementary motor area and other cortical areas in organization of voluntary movements in man. *Journal of Neurophysiology, 43,* 118–136.

Roman, G. C., Tatemichi, T. K., Erkinjuntti, T., Cummings, J. L., Masdeu, J. C., Garcia, J. H., Amaducci, L., Orgogozo, J. M., Brun, A., Hofman, A., Moody, D. M., O'Brien, M. D., Yamaguchi, T., Grafman, J., Drayer, B. P., Bennett, D. A., Fisher, M., Ogata, J., Kokmen, E., Bermejo, F., Wolf, P. A., Gorelick, P. B., Bick, K. L., Pajeau, A. K., Bell, M. A., DeCarli, C., Culebras, A., Korczyn, A. D., Bogousslavsky, J., Hartmann, A., & Scheinberg, P. (1993). Vascular dementia: Diagnostic criteria for research studies. Report of the NINDS-AIREN International Workshop. *Neurology, 43,* 250–260.

Romney, A. K., Shepard, R. N., & Nerlove, S. B. (1972). *Multidimensional scaling: Theory and applications in the behavioral sciences,* Vol. II. New York: Seminar Press.

Rosen, W. G., Terry, R. D., Fuld, P. A., Katzman, R., & Peck, A. (1980). Pathological verification of ischemic score in differentiation of dementias. *Annals of Neurology, 7,* 486–488.

Sagar, J. J., Cohen, N. J., Sullivan, E. V., Corkin, S., & Growdon, J. H. (1988). Remote memory function in Alzheimer's disease and Parkinson's disease. *Brain, 111,* 525–539.

Saint-Cyr, J. A., Taylor, A. E., & Lang, A. E. (1988). Procedural learning and neostriatal dysfunction in man. *Brain, 111,* 941–959.

Salmon, D. P., & Chan, A. S. (1994). Semantic memory deficits associated with Alzheimer's disease. In L. S. Cermak (Ed.), *Neuropsychological explorations of memory and cognition: Essays in honor of Nelson Butters* (pp. 61–76). New York: Plenum.

Salmon, D. P., & Galasko, D. (1996). Neuropsychological aspects of Lewy body dementia. In R. Perry, I. McKeith, &

E. Perry (Eds.), *Dementia with Lewy bodies* (pp. 99–113). Cambridge: Cambridge University Press.

Salmon, D. P., & Heindel, W. C. (1992). Impaired priming in Alzheimer's disease: Neuropsychological implications. In L. R. Squire & N. Butters (Eds.), *Neuropsychology of memory* (2nd ed.). (pp. 179–187). New York: Guilford.

Salmon, D. P., Heindel, W. C., & Lange, K. L. (1999). Differential decline in word generation from phonemic and semantic categories during the course of Alzheimer's disease: Implications for the integrity of semantic memory. *Journal of the International Neuropsychological Society, 5,* 692–703.

Salmon, D. P., Kwo-on-Yuen, P. F., Heindel, W. C., Butters, N., & Thal, L. J. (1989). Differentiation of Alzheimer's disease and Huntington's disease with the Dementia Rating Scale. *Archives of Neurology, 46,* 1204–1208.

Salmon, D. P., Lasker, B. R., Butters, N., & Beatty, W. W. (1988). Remote memory in a patient with amnesia due to hypoxia. *Brain and Cognition, 7,* 201–211.

Salmon, D. P., Shimamura, A. P., Butters, N., & Smith, S. (1988). Lexical and semantic priming deficits in patients with Alzheimer's disease. *Journal of Clinical and Experimental Neuropsychology, 10,* 477–494.

Sara, S. (1985). The locus coeruleus and cognitive function: Attempts to relate noradrenergic enhancement of signal/noise in the brain to behavior. *Physiological Psychology, 13,* 151–162.

Schacter, D. L. (1987). Implicit memory: History and current status. *Journal of Experimental Psychology: Learning, Memory, and Cognition, 13,* 501–517.

Scheltens, P. H., Leys, D., Barkhof, F., Huglo, D., Weinstein, H. C., Vermersch, P., Kuiper, M., Steinling, M., Wolters, E. C., & Valk, J. (1992). Atrophy of medial temporal lobes on MRI in 'probable' Alzheimer's disease and normal ageing: Diagnostic value and neuropsychological correlates. *Journal of Neurology, Neurosurgery and Psychiatry, 55,* 967–972.

Seltzer, B., & Sherwin, I. (1983). A comparison of clinical features in early- and late-onset primary degenerative dementia: One entity or two? *Archives of Neurology, 40,* 143–146.

Shepard, R. N., Romney, A. K., & Nerlove, S. B. (1972). *Multidimensional scaling: Theory and applications in the behavioral sciences,* Vol. I. New York: Seminar Press.

Shimamura, A. (1986). Priming effects in amnesia: Evidence for a dissociable memory function. *Quarterly Journal of Experimental Psychology [A], 38,* 619–644.

Shimamura, A. P., Janowsky, J. S., & Squire, L. R. (1990). Memory for the temporal order of events in patients with frontal lobe lesions and amnesic patients. *Neuropsychologia, 28,* 803–813.

Shimamura, A. P., Salmon, D. P., Squire, L. R., & Butters, N. (1987). Memory dysfunction and word priming in dementia an amnesia. *Behavioral Neuroscience, 101,* 347–351.

Shimamura, A., & Squire, L. R. (1984). Paired-associate learning and priming effects in amnesia: A neuropsychological study. *Journal of Experimental Psychology: General, 113,* 556–570.

Squire, L. R. (1987). *Memory and brain.* New York: Oxford University Press.

Squire, L. R. (1992). Memory and the hippocampus: A synthesis from findings with rats, monkeys and humans. *Psychological Review, 99,* 195–231.

Squire, L. R., Haist, F., & Shimamura, A. P. (1989). The neurology of memory: Quantitative assessment of retrograde amnesia in two groups of amnesic patients. *Journal of Neuroscience, 9* 828–839.

Steingart, A., Hachinski, V. C., Lau, C., Fox, A. J., Fox, H., Lee, D., Inzitari, D., & Merskey, H. (1987). Cognitive and neurologic findings in demented patients with diffuse white matter lucencies on computer tomographic scan (leukoaraiosis). *Archives of Neurology, 44,* 36–39.

Stelmach, G. E., Phillips, J. G., & Chau, A. W. (1989). Visuospatial processing in Parkinsonians. *Neuropsychologia, 27,* 485–493.

Stelmach, G. E., Worringham, C. J., & Strand, E. A. (1986). Movement preparation in Parkinson's disease: The use of advance information. *Brain, 109,* 1179–1194.

Stout, J. C., Bondi, M. W., Jernigan, T. L., Archibald, S. L., Delis, D. C., & Salmon, D. P. (1999). Regional cerebral volume loss associated with verbal learning and memory in dementia of the Alzheimer type. *Neuropsychology, 13,* 188–197.

Stout, J. C., Jernigan, T. L., Archibald, S. L., & Salmon, D. P. (1996). Association of dementia severity with grey matter hyperintensities in dementia of the Alzheimer type. *Archives of Neurology, 53,* 742–749.

Strittmatter, W. J., Saunders, A. M., Schmechel, D., Pericak-Vance, M., Enghild, J., Salvesen, G. S., & Roses, A. D. (1993). Apolipoprotein-E–High-avidity binding to B-amyloid and increased frequency of type 4 allele in late-onset familiar Alzheimer disease. *Proceedings of the National Academy of Sciences USA, 90,* 9649–9653.

Stroka, H., Elizan, T. S., Yahr, M. D., Burger, A., & Mendoza, M. R. (1981). Organic mental syndrome and confusional states in Parkinson's disease: Relationship to computerized tomographic signs of cerebral atrophy. *Archives of Neurology, 38,* 339–342.

Summers, J. J. (1981). Motor programs. In D. Holding (Ed.), *Human skills* (pp. 41–64). New York: Wiley.

Tachibana, H., Meyer, J. S., Kitagawa, Y., Rogers, R. L., Okayasu, H., & Mortel, K. F. (1984). Effects of aging on cerebral blood flow in dementia. *Journal of the American Geriatric Society, 32,* 114–119.

Tanji, J., Taniguchi, K., & Saga, T. (1980). Supplementary motor area: Neuronal response to motor instructions. *Journal of Neurophysiology, 43,* 60–68.

Terry, R. D., & Katzman, R. (1983a). Senile dementia of the Alzheimer type. *Annals of Neurology, 14,* 497–506.

Terry, R. D., & Katzman, R. (1983b). Senile dementia of the Alzheimer type: Defining a disease. In R. Katzman & R. D. Terry (Eds.), *The neurology of aging* (pp. 51–84). Philadelphia: Davis.

Terry, R. D., Masliah, E., Salmon, D. P., Butters, N., DeTeresa, R., Hill, R., Hansen, L. A., & Katzman, R. (1991). Physical basis of cognitive alterations in Alzheimer's disease: Synapse loss is the major correlate of cognitive impairment. *Annals of Neurology, 30,* 572–580.

Terry, R. D., Peck, A., DeTeresa, R., Schechter, R., & Horoupian, D. S. (1981). Some morphometric aspects of the brain in senile dementia of the Alzheimer type. *Annals of Neurology, 10,* 184–192.

Thomson, D. M., & Tulving, E. (1970). Associative encoding and retrieval: Weak and strong cues. *Journal of Experimental Psychology, 86,* 255–262.

Tomlinson, B. E. (1977). The pathology of dementia. In C. E. Wells (Ed.), *Dementia* (2nd ed.). (pp. 113–153). Philadelphia: Davis.

Tomlinson, B. E., Blessed, G., & Roth, M. (1970). Observations of the brains of demented old people. *Journal of Neurological Science, 11,* 205–242.

Troster, A. I., Butters, N., Salmon, D. P., Cullum, C. M., Jacobs, D., Brandt, J., & White, R. F. (1993). The diagnostic utility of savings scores: Differentiating Alzheimer's and Huntington's diseases with the logical memory and visual reproduction tests. *Journal of Clinical and Experimental Neuropsychology, 15,* 773–788.

Troster, A. I., Heindel, W. C., Salmon, D. P., & Butters, N. (1989). *Category fluency performance in Parkinson's disease with and without dementia.* Paper presented at the *Meeting of the American Psychological Association,* New York.

Troster, A. I., Jacobs, D., Butters, N., Cullum, C. M., & Salmon, D. P. (1989). Differentiating Alzheimer's disease from Huntington's disease with the Wechsler memory scale-revised. *Clinics in Geriatric Medicine, 5,* 611–632.

Troster, A. I., Salmon, D., McCullough, D., & Butters, N. (1989). A comparison of the category fluency deficits associated with Alzheimer's and Huntington's disease. *Brain and Language, 37,* 500–513.

Tulving, E. (1983). *Elements of episodic memory.* New York: Oxford University Press.

Tulving, E., Markowitsch, H. J., Kapur, S., Habib, R., & Houle, S. (1994). Novelty encoding networks in the human brain: Positron emission tomography data. *Neuroreport, 5,* 2525–2528.

Tversky, A., & Hutchinson, J. W. (1986). Nearest neighbor analysis of psychological spaces. *Psychological Review, 93,* 3–22.

Tweedy, J. R., Langer, K. G., & McDowell, F. H. (1982). The effect of semantic relations on the memory deficit associated with Parkinson's disease. *Journal of Clinical Neuropsychology, 4,* 235–247.

Vonsattel, J.-P., Myers, R. H., Stevens, T. J., Ferrante, R. J., Bird, E. D., & Richardson, E. P. (1985). Neuropathological classification of Huntington's disease. *Journal of Neuropathology and Experimental Neurology, 44,* 559–577.

Warrington, E., & McCarthy, R. A. (1987). Categories of knowledge: Further fractionations and an attempted integration. *Brain, 110,* 1273–1296.

Warrington, E., & Shallice, T. (1984). Category specific semantic impairments. *Brain, 107,* 829–854.

Warrington, E. K., & Weiskrantz, L. (1968). New method of testing long-term retention with special reference to amnesic patients. *Nature, 217,* 972–974.

Warrington, E. K., & Weiskrantz, L. (1970). Amnesic syndrome: Consolidation or retrieval? *Nature, 228,* 628–630.

Watson, R. T., Fleet, W., Gonzalez-Rothi, L., & Heilman, K. M. (1986). Apraxia and the supplementary motor area. *Archives of Neurology, 43,* 787–792.

Wechsler, D. (1987). *Wechsler memory scale-revised.* New York: Psychological Corporation.

Weingartner, H., Grafman, J., Boutelle, W., Kaye, W., & Martin, P. R. (1983). Forms of memory failure. *Science, 221,* 380–382.

Welsh, K., Butters, N., Hughes, J., Mohs, R., & Heyman, A. (1991). Detection of abnormal memory decline in mild cases of Alzheimer's disease using CERAD neuropsychological measures. *Archives of Neurology, 48,* 278–281.

Whitehouse, P. J. (1986). The concept of subcortical and cortical dementia: Another look. *Annals of Neurology, 19,* 1–6.

Whitehouse, P. J., Hedreen, J. C., White, C. L., & Price, D. L. (1983). Basal forebrain neurons in the dementia of Parkinson disease. *Annals of Neurology, 13*, 243–248.

Whitehouse, P. J., Price, D. L., Struble, R. G., Clark, A. W., Coyle, J. T., & DeLong, M. R. (1982). Alzheimer's disease and senile dementia: Loss of neurons in the basal forebrain. *Science, 215*, 1237–1239.

Wilcock, G. K., & Esiri, M. M. (1982). Placques, tangles and dementia. A quantitative study. *Journal of Neurological Science, 56*, 343–356.

Willingham, D. B., & Koroshetz, W. J. (1993). Evidence for dissociable motor skills in Huntington's disease patients. *Psychobiology, 21*, 173–182.

Wilson, R. S., Kaszniak, A. W., & Fox, J. H. (1981). Remote memory in senile dementia. *Cortex, 17*, 41–48.

Wilson, R. S., Kaszniak, A. W., Klawans, H. L., & Garron, D. C. (1980). High speed memory scanning in Parkinsonism. *Cortex, 16*, 67–72.

Wilson, R. S., Sullivan, M., deToledo-Morrell, L., Stebbins, G. T., Bennett, D. A., & Morrell, F. (1996). Association of memory and cognition in Alzheimer's disease with volumetric estimates of temporal lobe structures. *Neuropsychology, 10*, 459–463.

Wright, M. J., Burns, R. J., Geffen, G. M., & Geffen, L. B. (1990). Covert orientation of visual attention in Parkinson's disease: An impairment in the maintenance of attention. *Neuropsychologia, 28*, 151–159.

Yamaguchi, F., Meyer, J. S., Yamamoto, M., Sakai, F., & Shaw, T. (1980). Non-invasive regional cerebral blood flow measurements in dementia. *Archives of Neurology, 37*, 410–418.

Zola-Morgan, S., & Squire, L. R. (1990). The primate hippocampal formation: Evidence for a time-limited role in memory storage. *Science, 250*, 288–290.

# PART VI

# Disorders Arising in Specific Life Stages

CHAPTER 31

# Psychopathology in Children

## Paul J. Frick and Persephanie Silverthorn

## Introduction

A significant number of children and adolescents are affected by psychopathological conditions. Prevalence estimates vary widely, depending on the age group, type of disorder, and method of assessment. However, epidemiological studies conducted in the United States (Cohen et al., 1993; Costello, 1989; Costello et al., 1988, 1996, 1997; Kashani et al., 1987; Lewinsohn et al., 1993; Shaffer et al., 1996; Simonoff et al., 1997), New Zealand (Anderson, Williams, McGee, & Silva, 1987; McGee, Feehan, Williams, & Anderson, 1992), Canada (Offord et al., 1987), Puerto Rico (Bird et al., 1988; Shaffer et al., 1996), and the Netherlands (Verhulst et al., 1997) suggest that from 9–22% of children and from 18–22% of adolescents have significant emotional or behavioral problems at any given time. Rates of disorders in preschoolers have been less extensively studied, although a similar range of problems (9–21%) has been found in this age group (Lavigne et al., 1996).

These overall rates of childhood disorders obscure important differences in boys and girls. Regardless of the specific diagnosis, in preschool age children, boys are diagnosed with disorders at a greater rate than girls (e.g., Lavigne et al., 1996). During childhood, this pattern is maintained, and

Paul J. Frick and Persephanie Silverthorn • Department of Psychology, University of New Orleans, New Orleans, Louisiana 70148.

*Comprehensive Handbook of Psychopathology* (Third Edition), edited by Patricia B. Sutker and Henry E. Adams. Kluwer Academic / Plenum Publishers, New York, 2001.

most studies indicate that boys are more often diagnosed with disorders than girls (e.g., Anderson et al., 1987; Cohen et al., 1993; Costello et al., 1996, 1997; McGee et al., 1992). In adolescence, the male predominance for most forms of psychopathology disappears; some studies find that boys and girls are equally diagnosed (e.g., Simonoff et al., 1997; Verhulst et al., 1997), and other studies find that girls are more often diagnosed than boys (e.g., Cohen et al., 1993; Lewinsohn et al., 1993; McGee et al., 1992). These changes in prevalence rates for boys and girls are more pronounced for some forms of psychopathology (e.g., depression, conduct disorders) than for others, and these diagnosis-specific changes are discussed in more detail later in the chapter.

When classifying and studying childhood disorders, two major paradigms have generally been used. The first paradigm has been variously labeled as the multivariate, empirical, or psychometric approach. There are two key aspects to this approach. First, this approach typically relies on statistical techniques (e.g., factor analyses) to isolate interrelated patterns of behavior that are usually assessed by using standardized behavior rating scales (Achenbach, 1995; Quay, 1986). Reviews of studies that use such multivariate techniques have consistently identified two major dimensions of psychopathology (Achenbach, 1995; Achenbach & Edelbrock, 1978; Quay, 1986). One dimension has been labeled undercontrolled or externalizing and includes various acting out, disruptive, delinquent, hyperactive, and aggressive behaviors. The second broad dimension of childhood behavior problems has been labeled overcontrolled or internalizing and includes such behaviors as social withdrawal, anxiety, and depression. Second, this approach to classification views emotional and behavior problems as a continuum from normal to deviant. Abnormality or "psychopathology" is defined by comparing a child's functioning to those of children in a normative sample. For example, children are considered to have disorders when their behavior exceeds some set level of deviance from the general population (e.g., the 95th percentile).

The second major paradigm for conceptualizing childhood psychopathology is the clinical paradigm, and it is exemplified by the 4th edition of the *Diagnostic and Statistical Manual of Mental Disorders* (DSM-IV), the classification system promulgated by the American Psychiatric Association (1994). Rather than relying solely on multivariate statistical approaches to define psychopathology, this approach places a greater emphasis on clinical observations of disordered individuals or on theoretical models of abnormal behavior to define psychopathological conditions. Although there is less emphasis on patterns of behavioral covariation that result from multivariate analyses, such patterns are often considered in defining a psychopathological category in this approach (e.g., Carlson, Lahey, & Frick, 1997). A more dramatic point of divergence between these two approaches, however, is the focus of the clinical paradigm on functional impairment to define breaks with normality, rather than a focus on deviations from a normative sample, that is, clinical approaches to defining psychopathology, such as the DSM-IV, focus on behaviors that lead to significant levels of impairment in a child or adolescent's everyday functioning as at home, at school, or with peers (see Lahey et al., 1994, for an example). This determination is made whether or not the level or severity of symptomatology is rare in the general population.

Despite the strong opinions concerning the value of one method of classifying psychopathological conditions over another (e.g., Achenbach, 1995), there is often great correspondence with respect to which children are identified as having psychopathological conditions using these two approaches (see Jensen et al., 1996). Furthermore, for most clinical and research applications, it is unnecessary to "choose" one approach over another. The two approaches simply provide different perspectives from which to understand a child or adolescent's behavior. Assessments that inte-

grate both types of information typically provide the best way to understand a child's psychosocial functioning (Kamphaus & Frick, 1996). Due to the large-scale use of the DSM-IV for both research and clinical practice, the organization and terminology of this chapter are heavily guided by this classification system. However, we do not limit the discussion only to this view of psychopathological conditions, especially when there is clear evidence to support alternative ways of conceptualizing a specific disorder.

## Attention Deficit Hyperactivity Disorder

### Overview

ADHD is one of the most common reasons in the United States for referring children to mental health clinics, it accounts for as many as 50% of all child referrals to outpatient mental health clinics (Cantwell, 1996). The essential features of this disorder focus on two symptom clusters: developmentally inappropriate degrees of inattention-disorganization (e.g., difficulty sustaining attention, failure to finish tasks, difficulty organizing tasks) and developmentally inappropriate degrees of impulsivity-overactivity (e.g., difficulty sitting still, talking excessively, difficulty awaiting a turn). Although the hyperactive child syndrome has long been recognized as a psychopathological condition, there has been great debate over the core symptoms of the disorder. Some authors emphasize the importance of deficits in attention and impulse control (Douglas, 1972; Douglas & Peters, 1979) and others focus on motor hyperactivity (Porrino, Rapoport, Behar, Sceery, Ismond, & Bunney, 1983). However, the DSM-IV decision to define ADHD along the two symptom domains was based on a substantial amount of research that showed that factor analyses in both clinical and community samples have consistently isolated these two correlated dimensions of behavior (Carlson et al., 1997; Frick & Lahey, 1991).

ADHD is generally considered a lifelong disorder that is not solely a function of a single environmental stressor. As a result, the DSM-IV specifies that the ADHD symptoms must be present early in childhood, must continue for a extensive period of time, and must be displayed in more than one setting (American Psychiatric Association, 1994). Also critical in the classification of ADHD is the presence of several subtypes. Based on the two core symptom clusters, the DSM-IV defines three subtypes of ADHD: a primarily hyperactive-impulsive type (approximately 18% of ADHD children), a primarily inattentive type (approximately 27%), and a combined type (approximately 55%) (Lahey et al., 1994). There is little research on the primarily hyperactive-impulsive subtype of ADHD. However, rather extensive research documents important differences between the primarily inattentive subtype (which was formerly called Attention Deficit Disorder without Hyperactivity, American Psychiatric Association, 1980) and the combined subtype. Specifically, those children with the problems of inattention without high rates of impulsivity and hyperactivity (i.e., the primarily inattentive subtype) tend to show fewer conduct problems, less peer rejection, and are more anxious and shy than those children who are also impulsive and hyperactive (see Carlson et al., 1997; Frick & Lahey, 1991 for reviews). The two subtypes may also show differences in the types of attentional processes that are deficient (Barkley, DuPaul, & McMurray, 1991; Carlson et al., 1997; Pliska, 1998), and the inattentive type shows a different response curve to stimulant medication (Barkley et al., 1991). These latter two findings clearly illustrate both the theoretical and clinical importance of distinguishing between these two subtypes of ADHD.

## Epidemiology

The DSM-IV reported estimates that ADHD is present in from 3–5% of school-age children (American Psychiatric Association, 1994), and recent epidemiological studies reported prevalence rates from 2–9% in childhood (Anderson et al., 1987; Cohen et al., 1993; Costello et al., 1996, 1997; Offord et al., 1989; Verhulst et al., 1997) and from 2–4.5% in adolescence (Kashani et al., 1987; Lewinsohn et al., 1993; McGee et al., 1990). In general, ADHD affects more boys than girls; ratios range from 4:1 in community samples and are as high as 9:1 in clinical samples (American Psychiatric Association, 1994; Cantwell, 1996).

Although there is a clear and dramatic difference in the prevalence of ADHD in boys and girls, whether there are other gender-specific manifestations of the disorder is less conclusive. Recent data

from the DSM-IV field trials showed that girls are more likely to have ADHD Primarily Inattentive Type (Lahey et al., 1994). Some early studies also reported that girls with ADHD had more severe cognitive deficits (Berry et al., 1985; Brown et al., 1991), more language deficits (Brown et al., 1991; James & Taylor, 1990), and a higher rate of ADHD in their relatives (James & Taylor, 1990; Mannuzza & Gittelman, 1984) than boys. However, more recent studies using more stringent criteria to diagnose ADHD failed to find such differences between boys and girls with ADHD (Farone et al., 1991; Silverthorn et al., 1996) or have found that girls with ADHD had *fewer* cognitive and executive functioning deficits than boys with ADHD (Seidman et al., 1997).

## Comorbid Disorders

In addition to the primary symptoms of ADHD, children with this disorder often show other adjustment problems. One such problem is poor school performance: ADHD children are at risk of grade retention, being placed in special education classes, and dropping out of school (Barkley, 1981; Semrud-Clikeman et al., 1992; Weiss & Hechtman, 1993). Furthermore, about a third to a half of children with ADHD meet criteria for a learning disability (Frick et al., 1991; Jensen et al., 1997; Pliska, 1998; Semrud-Clikeman et al., 1992). There is no conclusive evidence that any of the subtypes of ADHD are more strongly associated with learning disabilities (Carlson et al. 1997). It is also not clear what accounts for this correlation between academic difficulties and ADHD (Hinshaw, 1992). It may be that the symptoms of ADHD (i.e., inattention, impulsivity, and overactivity) impair children's abilities to learn up to their potentials. It is also possible that the same mechanisms that cause ADHD also place children at risk for having a learning disability.

Children with ADHD are also likely to have peer difficulties; children with ADHD Combined Type are more likely to be unpopular or rejected by peers, and those with ADHD Primarily Inattentive Type are more likely to be shy and withdrawn (Cantwell & Baker, 1992; Carlson, Lahey, & Neeper, 1986; Lahey et al., 1984, 1987). Children with ADHD also have high rates of emotional disorders. As many as 20–50% of ADHD children have comorbid anxiety disorder, and from 9–38% have comorbid depressive disorder (Jensen et al., 1997; Pliska, 1998). Children with ADHD Primarily Inattentive Type are more likely to exhibit depression and anxiety than children with the Combined Type (Pliska, 1998).

The most significant correlate of ADHD is conduct problems/aggression; estimates of children that have a codiagnosis of ADHD and Conduct Disorder range from 30–90% (Hinshaw, 1987; Loney & Milich, 1982; Sandberg, Weiselberg, & Shaffer, 1980; Stewart, Cummings, Singer, & de-Blois, 1981). In the past, this high degree of overlap led to considerable debate whether these two behavior domains were in fact separate entities (see Hinshaw, 1987; Quay, 1986; Rutter, 1983). However, there is now substantial evidence that these disorders are separate conditions. For example, a seminal review of the literature by Hinshaw (1987) showed several lines of evidence to support the distinction between these two disorders, including factor analytic support and findings of different correlates to the two disorders. Studies show that conduct disorder, but not ADHD, is related to low self-esteem (SES)(Loney, Langhome, & Paternite, 1978), parental psychopathology (Frick, Lahey, Christ, Loeber, & Green, 1991; Lahey, Piacentini et al., 1988; Lahey, Russo, Walker, & Piacentini, 1989; Stewart, deBlois, & Cummings, 1980), dysfunctional parenting practices (Frick, 1994), and marital instability (August & Stewart, 1983). All of these studies suggest that ADHD and conduct disorder are correlated but meaningfully distinct syndromes.

## Etiology

Most current causal theories of the etiology of ADHD focus on neurobiological mechanisms (see Zametkin & Liotta, 1998, for a review). In support of this biological focus, several studies using magnetic resonance imaging (MRI) have found abnormalities in the basal ganglia (the caudate nucleus and putamen, globus pallidus, and substantia nigra) and corpus callosum of children with ADHD (Hynd et al., 1993; Lou et al., 1984, 1989; Tannock, 1998). In addition, studies using positron emission tomography (PET) have also implicated the basal ganglia (McCracken, 1998; Zametkin et al., 1990, 1993). Investigations into potential neurochemical correlates to ADHD have been less conclusive (Barkley, 1998; Zametkin & Liotta, 1998), although the potential role of catecholamines in the etiology of ADHD has been proposed (Zametkin & Rapoport, 1986).

A number of other possible etiologies have been

proposed for ADHD, such as exposure to environmental toxins (e.g., lead exposure) and dietary factors (e.g., food allergies, increased sugar sensitivity). However, most of the research into these factors suggest that they could account for only a very small percentage of children with ADHD, if any at all (e.g., Wolraich et al., 1994). Although children with ADHD often come from families in which parents use less than optimal child-rearing techniques, it also appears that this is largely due to difficulties and stressors involved in raising a child with ADHD (Barkley, 1998). Although these familial factors do not play a causal role in the development of ADHD symptoms, they can increase the severity of the ADHD symptoms and they can lead to the development of conduct problems in children with ADHD (Frick, 1994), both of which can affect the severity and course of the disorder.

Despite the focus on neurobiological mechanisms in the causes of ADHD, it is not clear what leads to the neurological deficits exhibited by ADHD children. There is evidence that both genetic factors and environmental trauma (e.g., pre- and perinatal traumas) could play a role (Pliska, 1998). As a result, the same neurological deficit can result from multiple causal pathways. It is also unclear what the core deficit is that results from the neurological dysfunction and underlies the behavioral symptomatology associated with ADHD. In one of the best articulated theories to date, Barkley (1997) posits that ADHD Combined Type is the result of deficits in behavioral inhibition. Impairments in delayed response lead to difficulties with self-regulation, which lead to the symptoms of hyperactivity, impulsivity, distractibility, and secondary symptoms of inattention and executive dysfunctions. In addition, Barkley (1997) contends that ADHD Primarily Hyperactive-Impulsive Type is the preschool and early elementary school version of ADHD Combined Type and that accompanying symptoms of inattention emerge only later in school. In contrast, ADHD Primarily Inattentive is considered a completely separate disorder that is less related to response inhibition and more related to primary problems in regulating attention (Barkley, 1998).

## Prognosis and Treatment

The outcome of children with ADHD has been the focus of several follow-up studies that have largely dispelled the myth that children with

ADHD outgrow their disorder in adolescence and adulthood. Initial studies suggested that approximately 31% of hyperactive children continue to show the full syndrome as adolescents (Gittelman, Mannuzza, Shenker, & Bonegura, 1985). However, more recent research suggests that as many as 50–80% of children diagnosed with ADHD in childhood will continue to show symptoms into adolescence and 30–50% will show symptoms into adulthood (Barkley, 1998; Biederman, 1998). It has been argued that the primary symptoms of ADHD tend to become less debilitating in adolescence and that overt hyperactivity becomes manifested as an internal sense of restlessness (Barkley, 1990; Cantwell, 1996). However, more recent studies have shown that children and adolescents referred to clinics present with similar symptom profiles (Biederman et al., 1998). In addition, Barkley (1998) argues that the apparent decrease of symptomatology and the reduced prevalence of ADHD in adolescence may be related to problems with the diagnostic criteria, rather than to actual changes in the prevalence of the disorder.

Regardless of whether the actual symptomatology decreases or changes over development, several studies have shown that adolescents and adults with ADHD continue to exhibit a number of adjustment problems (Hechtman, 1996), including academic and occupational difficulties, difficulties in relationships, low self-esteem, and higher rates of psychopathology (Weiss & Hechtman, 1993). Antisocial and delinquent behavior is one type of adjustment problem that is especially prevalent in adolescents and young adults with ADHD; from 23–45% are diagnosed with antisocial personality disorder (Gittelman et al., 1985; Loney et al., 1983; Weiss, Hechtman, Milroy, & Perlman, 1985), and 40% have been arrested (Mannuzza et al., 1989). There is some evidence that the risk for antisocial behaviors in adolescence and adulthood may be more related to the frequent presence of conduct problems or aggressiveness in these children (August, Stewart, & Holmes, 1983; Hechtman, 1996; Gittelman et al., 1985; Loney et al., 1978).

The most common form of intervention for children with ADHD is the use of medication, typically a central nervous system (CNS) stimulant such as methylphenidate (Ritalin), dextroamphetamine (Dexedrine), Pemoline (Cylert), methamphetamine (Desoxyn), or amphetamine salts (Adderall) (Pelham, 1987, Sallee & Gill, 1998). These drugs decrease the rate of many of the disruptive behaviors associated with ADHD; positive effects are most marked in measures of attention and activity and, to a lesser extent, in conduct problems (Barkley & Cunningham, 1979; Sallee & Gill, 1998; Solanto & Conners, 1982). Furthermore, stimulants increase in-task classroom behavior, improve peer status, and improve performance in academic tasks in some children with ADHD (Pelham, Bender, Caddell, Booth, & Moorer, 1985; Whalen et al., 1989). Stimulants show an immediate beneficial response in approximately 70% of ADHD children. However, they have not proven effective in altering the long-term prognosis of ADHD children (Conners & Werry, 1979; Findling & Dogin, 1998; Pelham et al., 1998; Riddle & Rapoport, 1976).

In addition to stimulant medication, clinical researchers have investigated several psychosocial treatments for ADHD. One of the most promising of these treatments is behavioral parent training and classroom behavior management (see Pelham et al., 1998). These programs focus on helping parents and teachers design and implement very structured and consistent behavioral management programs that (1) set clear behavioral goals for the child, (2) have a clear monitoring system to assess progress toward these goals, and (3) have a structured set of consequences designed to encourage behavioral goals and discourage negative behaviors (e.g., Barkley, 1997; Pfiffner & O'Leary, 1993). Cognitive-behavioral techniques have also been tested as treatment for children with ADHD, based on the assumption that ADHD children have failed to develop age-appropriate cognitive strategies that help to regulate their behavior. Unfortunately, controlled outcome studies on the effects of cognitive-behavioral techniques with ADHD children have found significant effects on laboratory measures of attention and impulsivity but little generalization to either home or school behavior (Abikoff, 1985; Richters et al., 1995).

Although both stimulant medication and behavioral programs have proven effective in treating ADHD, a multimodal treatment approach combining treatment approaches may be the most effective approach to intervention. Several investigators have shown that children with ADHD who receive multimodal treatment strategies do not differ from normal classmates following treatments (Gittelman-Klein et al., 1980), require lower doses of psychostimulants (Horn & Ialongo, 1988), and may show a lower rate of teenage arrest than those treated only with medication (Satterfield,

Satterfield, & Schell, 1987). However, more data are needed on the potential synergistic effects of different treatments for ADHD to determine the optimal combination of treatment approaches (Arnold et al., 1997; Richters et al., 1995).

# Disruptive Behavior Disorders

## Overview

Antisocial and aggressive behavior is another common reason that children and adolescents are referred to mental health clinics (Kazdin, Siegel, & Bass, 1990). One of the most critical aspects to understanding these behaviors is the recognition that children who show these behaviors can differ dramatically in the causes, course, and response to treatment. As a result, a significant amount of research has focused on defining meaningful subgroups of children with Disruptive Behavior Disorders. One of the main distinctions made in the DSM-IV is between Oppositional Defiant Disorder (ODD) and Conduct Disorder (CD) (American Psychiatric Association, 1994). ODD is defined as a pattern of negativistic, hostile, and defiant behavior, whereas CD is a persistent pattern of behavior in which the basic rights of others and/or major societal norms or rules are violated. These CD symptoms fall into four categories: aggression to people or animals, destruction of property, deceitfulness or theft, and serious violation of rules.

The distinction between ODD and CD is not based simply on severity, but there is also a developmental and hierarchical relation between these disorders, that is, ODD symptoms often precede the development of CD in prepubertal boys. For example, in a 4-year longitudinal study of boys (ages 6 to 13) who developed CD, the vast majority (82%) had a diagnosis of ODD in the previous year (Lahey et al., 1995). Importantly, there is an asymmetry to this relation. Although most children who develop CD show ODD in previous years, less than half of children with ODD (47%) progress to the more serious CD (Lahey et al., 1995). The link between ODD and CD also holds only for children who develop CD prior to adolescence; those who show a later onset to their CD are less likely to show this progression of conduct problems from ODD to CD (Hinshaw, Lahey, & Hart, 1993).

This difference in development progression between childhood and adolescent-onset patterns of CD was a major consideration in the adoption of a further subtyping of CD by the DSM-IV. The DSM-IV recognizes a childhood-onset type of CD in which the serious symptoms of CD onset before age 10, usually as a culmination of a process that began early in life in which the child progresses into more and more severe types of conduct problems over time (Lahey & Loeber, 1994). The adolescent-onset type of CD, in contrast, is defined by a later development of CD symptoms (on or after age 10) without clear signs of dysfunction before puberty.

In addition to the DSM-IV approach, there have been several other methods for dividing children with CD into more homogeneous subtypes. For example, a distinction has been made based on whether the child (1) can sustain social relationships and tends to commit antisocial behavior with other deviant peers (socialized or group type) or (2) cannot sustain social relationships and commits antisocial acts alone (undersocialized or solitary type) (Quay, 1986). Distinctions have also been made as to whether the child shows primarily aggressive or primarily nonaggressive symptoms of CD (Hinshaw et al., 1993). Some approaches to subtyping children with CD also have been based on the co-occurrence of other disorders. For example, Lynam (1996) suggested that the presence of ADHD with CD results in a distinct subtype of CD, and others have suggested that the presence or absence of anxiety disorders may designate important subtypes of children with CD (McBurnett et al., 1991; Walker et al., 1991).

Another promising approach to dividing children with CD into subtypes is based on the presence of a callous and unemotional interpersonal style that has been used to designate psychopathy in adults. Psychopathic traits are characterized by pathological egocentricity, an absence of empathy, an absence of guilt, superficial charm, shallow emotions, an absence of anxiety, and the inability to form and sustain lasting and meaningful relationships (Cleckley, 1976; Hare, 1994; McCord & McCord, 1964). These traits are only moderately correlated with ODD and CD symptoms in children (Frick, O'Brien, Wootton, & McBurnett, 1994), and more importantly, designate a very severely disordered group of children within the childhood-onset type of CD. For example, children with CD and callous and unemotional traits tend to show a greater number and variety of antisocial behaviors (including aggression), they have a higher rate of police contacts at a young age, and they have a stronger family history of criminal and antisocial behavior than other children with CD (Christian, Frick, Hill, Tyler, & Frazer, 1997). Furthermore, the most severe and violent juvenile offenders (i.e., violent sex offenders) tend to show high rates of these callous and unemotional traits (Caputo, Frick, & Brodsky, in press).

## Epidemiology

The prevalence of antisocial and aggressive behavior depends on a number of factors, including the number and severity of problem behaviors, the age group studied, and the sex of the child. To illustrate the relation with severity, a longitudinal study conducted in Dunnedin, New Zealand, reported that almost all (94%) of the adolescents who participated in the study admitted engaging in some illegal behavior (e.g., underage drinking, using fake ID's), but only 6% showed severe enough antisocial behavior to be arrested by the police, and only about 7.3% met criteria for a disruptive behavior disorder (McGee et al., 1992; Moffitt, 1993).

To illustrate changes across different age groups, it has been estimated that the prevalence of serious oppositional conduct problems in preschoolers is from 4–9% (Cohen et al., 1987). In elementary school-aged children, the prevalence of ODD is within a similar range of 6–12% (Anderson et al., 1987; Bird et al., 1988; Cohen et al., 1993; Costello et al., 1988; Shaffer et al., 1996), but it is estimated that more severe conduct disorders are present in only about 2–4% of school-age children (Anderson et al., 1987; Costello et al., 1988; Shaffer et al., 1996). In adolescence, the rates of both ODD and CD show a dramatic rise; estimated rates of ODD are as high as 15% (Cohen et al., 1993), and the rate of CD is estimated at from 6–12% (McGee et al., 1992).

The final factor that influences the prevalence of these disorders is gender. Overall, boys tend to show more conduct problems than girls. However, this is moderated somewhat by age. For example, school-age boys outnumber girls with CD at a ratio of about 4:1 (Anderson et al., 1987; Cohen et al., 1993; Offord et al., 1987). Estimates in adolescent samples also show male predominance, but the ratio drops to about 2:1 (Cohen et al., 1993; Offord, Adler, & Boyle, 1986). Some studies have even found an equal sex ratio of CD in adolescence (McGee et al., 1992). It is also clear that the male predominance of CD is much greater for aggressive and violent antisocial behavior and much less for nonaggressive behaviors (McGee et al., 1992) or for relational aggressive behaviors (e.g., excluding children from play groups, spreading rumors about children so that they are rejected by others) (Crick & Grotpeter, 1995).

## Comorbid Disorders

ADHD is by far the most common comorbid diagnosis for children with ODD or CD; rates of ADHD range from 65% (Stewart, Cummings, Singer, & deBlois, 1981; Trites & Laprade, 1983) to 90% (Abikoff & Klein, 1992) for clinic-referred children diagnosed with these disorders. Although there is no widely accepted explanation to account for this overlap between these disorders, their comorbidity is quite important for several reasons. First, the presence of ADHD in children with ODD or CD leads to more severe behavior problems. Children with CD who also show ADHD have a greater number of conduct problem symptoms, have an earlier age of onset of severe conduct problems, show more aggressive conduct problems, and show earlier and greater substance use than children with CD who do not have ADHD (Loeber, Brinthaupt, & Green, 1990; Thompson, Riggs, Mikulich, & Crowley, 1996; Walker, Lahey, Hynd, & Frame, 1987). Second, the presence of ADHD in children with CD predicts greater risk of poor adjustment in adolescence and adulthood. Specifically, children with CD and ADHD carry out a greater variety of delinquent acts in adolescence, show more severe aggression in adolescence, and show more violent offending in adulthood than children with CD but without ADHD (Klinteberg, Andersen, Magnusson, & Stattin, 1993; Loeber et al., 1990; Moffitt, 1993).

Learning disabilities are another frequent comorbidity in children with severe conduct problems (Cantwell & Baker, 1992; Rutter, Tizard, Yule, Graham, & Whitmore, 1976). There are many explanations for this link, and there is some evidence that the learning problems are more related to the ADHD which is frequently comorbid with conduct problems, rather than to the conduct problems themselves (Frick et al., 1991; Maughan,

Pickles, Hagell, Rutter, & Yule, 1996). However, this explanation applies largely to children in the childhood-onset group; some children with learning disabilities develop conduct problems in adolescence without an early history of ADHD or other behavior problems (Hinshaw, 1992).

Children with severe conduct problems also show high rates of emotional disorders, such as depression and anxiety. From 15–31% of children with CD have comorbid depression and from 22–33% of children in community samples and between 60–75% in clinic samples have comorbid anxiety disorder (Russo & Biedel, 1994; Zoccolillo, 1993). One important issue in this comorbidity between conduct problems and emotional disorders is that children with CD and depression are at increased risk of suicidal ideation. For example, in a community sample of seventh and eighth grade students, 31% of the children with CD and depression reported suicidal ideation compared to only 12% of the students with CD only (Capaldi, 1992). Also, for many children with CD, the presence of anxiety and depression largely results from interpersonal conflicts (e.g., with peers, teachers, and police) and other stressors (e.g., family dysfunction, school failure) that are often experienced by children with CD (Capaldi, 1992; Panak & Garber, 1992). As a result, the anxiety and depression experienced by these children is often best conceptualized as emotional distress or negative affectivity that results from their impaired psychosocial functioning (Frick, 1998a).

CD is also associated with alcohol and drug use. The comorbidity between CD and substance abuse is important because, when children with CD also abuse substances, they tend to show an early onset of substance use and they are more likely to abuse multiple substances (Lynskey & Fergusson, 1995). Although most of the research on the association between CD and substance abuse before adulthood has been conducted with adolescents, the association between conduct problems and substance use may begin very early in development. In an urban community sample (n = 2573) of children in the first, fourth, and seventh grades, substance use was fairly rare in first and fourth grade children (Van Kammen, Loeber, & Stouthamer-Loeber, 1991). When it did occur in these early grades, however, it was usually associated with the presence of significant conduct problems. In the seventh grade, substance use became more common, especially the use of milder substances like alcohol. However, the use of harder drugs and the use of multiple drugs were associated with CD. Therefore, CD is associated with *nonnormative substance use* throughout childhood and adolescence.

## Etiology

A number of different factors, both within children and within their psychosocial contexts, have been associated with conduct problems in research (see Frick, 1998b for a review). For example, several aspects of a child's family environment have been consistently associated with CD and ODD (see Frick, 1994; Loeber & Stouthamer-Loeber, 1986 for reviews). These include higher rates of parental psychopathology, especially substance abuse and antisocial disorders, higher rates of divorce and marital conflict, and dysfunctional parenting practices (e.g., low parental involvement, poor monitoring and supervision, and harsh or inconsistent discipline practices). Children with CD also tend to be rejected and isolated by peers (Coie, Dodge, & Kupersmidt, 1990). As a result of this peer rejection, the child does not experience the socialization of prosocial peers in developing nonaggressive and nonaversive means of interacting with others. It also places a child at risk of associating with other antisocial and rejected peers (Keenan, Loeber, Zhang, Stouthamer-Loeber, & Van Kammen, 1995). Another aspect of a child's psychosocial context that has been related to conduct problems is living in economically impoverished circumstances that limit a child's chances of advancing educationally, occupationally, or socially (Wilson, 1987).

In addition to these aspects of a child's psychosocial context, there are individual vulnerabilities within the child that have been associated with ODD and CD. For example, research has documented a number of neurological correlates to CD. Antisocial children have lower levels of serotonin (Kreusi et al., 1990), lower levels of epinephrine (Magnusson, 1988; Olweus, Mattesson, Schalling, & Low, 1988), and higher levels of testosterone (Olweus et al., 1988; Scerbo & Kolko, 1994) than other children. In addition, studies have found abnormalities in the central nervous system functioning of children with CD by using skin conductance measures (Schmidt, Solanto, & Bridget, 1985), heart rate measures (Raine, Venables, &

Williams, 1990), and event-related electroencephalographic potentials (Raine et al., 1990). In their summary of this literature, Lahey, McBurnett, Loeber, and Hart (1995) concluded that most of these biological correlates are interrelated and may reflect a small number of physiological processes related to abnormalities in the sympathetic arm of the autonomic nervous system.

These autonomic irregularities may underlie some of the unique temperamental features found in children with conduct problems. As already mentioned, children with ODD and CD are more likely to have significant problems in impulse control and response inhibition, as reflected by the high rate of ADHD. They also are more likely to show a preference for thrill- and adventure-seeking activities (Frick et al., 1994) and to show a reward-dominant response style in which their behavior is more responsive to cues of reward than to punishment (O'Brien & Frick, 1996; O'Brien, Frick, & Lyman, 1994). Children with CD are also more likely to show a number of neurocognitive deficits, including lowered overall IQ and other more specific cognitive deficits, such as deficits in their verbal abilities and in their executive functioning (Lynam, 1996; Moffitt, 1993). Finally, children and adolescents with severe conduct problems often show social information-processing deficits that make them more likely to respond aggressively in interpersonal contexts. Social information processing is the sequential steps that are involved in interpreting social information and choosing appropriate responses based on this interpretation (see Crick & Dodge, 1996; Dodge & Frame, 1982).

In much of the past research, there has been little attempt to go beyond the documentation of these many factors in children and in their psychosocial environments that are associated with ODD and CD. The most common model for viewing these correlates has been from a "cumulative risk" perspective in which the development of ODD and CD is seen as a function of the number of risk factors to which a child is exposed. In recent years, however, there has been an attempt to develop more sophisticated developmental models for the causes of ODD and CD that consider the potential for different causal pathways underlying these disorders. For example, research has illustrated that childhood-onset and adolescent-onset patterns of CD have very different correlates that could suggest the operation of different causal

mechanisms (see Frick, 1998b; Moffitt, 1993). Specifically, the childhood-onset group exhibits higher rates of cognitive and neuropsychological dysfunction and family dysfunction than the adolescent-onset group. As a result, the childhood-onset group has a more characterological disorder that involves the "juxtaposition of a vulnerable and difficult infant with an adverse rearing context that initiates ... a transactional process in which the challenge of coping with a difficult child evokes a chain of failed parent-child encounters" (Moffitt, 1993, p. 682). In contrast, the adolescent-onset group is viewed as more of an exaggeration of the normative developmental process of separation and individuation that characterizes adolescence (Moffitt, 1993).

There is evidence to suggest that there may even be another pathway that can be identified within the childhood-onset category, based on the presence or absence of callous and unemotional traits (see Frick, 1998b for a review), that is, children with callous and unemotional traits show a more severe pattern of behavior, as mentioned previously, and they also show several other characteristics that differentiate them from other children with CD. For example, children in this group are more likely to show autonomic irregularities (Lahey et al., 1991), a thrill- and adventure-seeking or fearless temperament (Frick et al., 1994), and a reward-dominant response style (O'Brien & Frick, 1996) than other children with CD. However, they are *less* likely to be impaired intellectually (Christian et al., 1997), and their behavior is less strongly associated with dysfunctional parenting practices (Wootton et al., 1997). Therefore, this group shows a temperament defined by low behavioral inhibition that is characterized physiologically by a higher threshold of reactivity in their autonomic nervous system functioning and behaviorally by low fearfulness to novel or threatening situations and poor responsiveness to cues to punishment (Kagan & Snidman, 1991; Rothbart, 1989). This temperament can influence the development of guilt and empathy in children (see Kochanska, 1993, for seven different theories to account for this link) and may make these children less susceptible to parental attempts at socialization.

Using callous and unemotional traits to designate a distinct group of children with conduct disorders could explain some of the diversity within the childhood-onset pattern of conduct disorders. However, all of these models have substantial limitations when attempting to account for the development of severe antisocial behavior in girls (Silverthorn & Frick, 1999). As was evident from the age and sex trends in the prevalence of CD, girls with CD often show an adolescent-onset to their antisocial behavior, as reflected by the decrease in the male predominance of the disorder in adolescence. However, despite the later onset, girls with CD have many characteristics that make them similar to boys with childhood-onset CD, such as a chronic course with poor adult outcomes, high rates of neuropsychological and cognitive deficits, and high rates of family dysfunction. As a result, Silverthorn and Frick (1999) described the developmental pattern in girls as a "delayed-onset" trajectory to illustrate that these girls are likely to show temperamental and environmental vulnerabilities throughout most of their lives, but they do not manifest overt antisocial and aggressive behavior until adolescence.

## Prognosis and Treatment

Recently, Frick and Loney (in press) reviewed twenty-one prospective longitudinal studies that documented both the short term (n = 12; more than 8 months to 6 years) and long term (n = 9; 7 to 30 years) stability of CD in children and adolescents. From these studies, there is evidence for substantial stability across many types of samples, many different definitions of CD, and many different methods for estimating stability. For example, during a 4-year period, from 45–50% of children with CD can be rediagnosed with the disorder (Lahey et al., 1995; Offord et al., 1992). Longitudinal studies that followed children with CD into adulthood found that from 43–64% of boys and approximately 17% of girls with CD were arrested for criminal behavior by adulthood and about 31% of boys and 17% of girls were diagnosed with antisocial personalities as adults (Krazter & Hodgins, 1997; Robins, 1966).

Frick and Loney (in press) provided evidence that even these substantial stability estimates may underestimate the true level of stability of severe conduct problems due to a number of methodological factors, such as a failure to use measures that capture varying manifestations of CD across development, reliance on single follow-up assessments that do not capture the fluctuating severity of symptoms over time, and failure to control for measurement error in the estimates of

stability. More importantly, a substantial degree of stability is accounted for by a small proportion of childhood CD. For example, about 5% of the most persistent juvenile offenders account for about 50% of reported crimes (Farrington, Ohlin, & Wilson, 1986), and the stability of CD is dramatically reduced when the most persistent 5% of children with CD are excluded from the estimates (Moffitt, 1993). Variables that predict persistence in children with CD are displaying a large number and multiple types of CD symptoms in multiple settings, developing CD symptoms at an early age (prior to adolescence), and having a comorbid diagnosis of ADHD (Frick & Loney, in press).

Given the stability of CD, the development of effective prevention and treatment programs becomes quite important. Four interventions have proven effective in treating children with ODD and CD in controlled outcome studies (Frick, 1998b). These include structured contingency management programs based on operant principles, parent management training (PMT) programs that teach parents how to develop and implement very structured contingency management programs in the home and that teach them how to change other family processes (e.g., poor supervision) related to conduct problems, and cognitive-behavioral interventions that help children with CD to overcome deficits in social cognition and deficits in social problem-solving that can lead to their behavior problems. In addition, because a substantial proportion of clinic-referred children with CD also show ADHD and because the impulsivity associated with ADHD may directly lead to some of the aggressive and other poorly regulated behaviors of children with CD, the use of stimulant medication in reducing the ADHD symptoms also leads to a reduction in the rate and severity of conduct problems in children with both ADHD and CD (Hinshaw, 1991; Hinshaw, Heller, & McHale, 1992; Pelham et al., 1993).

Although each of the four treatment approaches has proven effective in controlled outcome studies, research has also documented substantial limitations in their effectiveness for older children, who have more severe conduct problems and are from more dysfunctional family environments (Frick, 1998b). Furthermore, the treatment gains made by these interventions have not always been sustained over time. As a result, some of the more promising approaches to treatment use more comprehensive interventions that simultaneously target multiple processes that could lead to conduct disorders, such as the Families and Schools Together (FAST Track) Program (Conduct Problems Prevention Research Group, 1992). Many of these comprehensive approaches, such as Multi-Systemic Therapy (MST) (Henggeler & Borduin, 1990), are also designed to be flexible in their implementation, in which the comprehensive intervention is tailored to the needs of the individual children and their families. The success of MST (see Borduin et al., 1995; Henggeler, Melton, & Smith, 1992; Henggeler, Schoenwald, & Pickrel, 1995) illustrates that successful treatment of CD does not involve simply selecting one "best" intervention and implementing it for all children and adolescents with the disorder. Rather, it illustrates that successful intervention must address the various factors that contribute to the child's antisocial behavior and it must be tailored to the needs of the individual child (see Frick, 1998b, for a general intervention framework).

## Anxiety Disorders

### Overview

The DSM-IV (American Psychiatric Association, 1994) has child-specific criteria for only one anxiety disorder, Separation Anxiety Disorder. Several other anxiety disorders are frequently diagnosed in childhood and adolescence, including Generalized Anxiety Disorder, Social Phobia, Specific Phobia, Obsessive-Compulsive Disorder, Panic Disorder, Agoraphobia, Posttraumatic Stress Disorder, and Acute Stress Disorder. However, children are diagnosed for these disorders using the same criteria as those used for adults. This is a major change from past versions of the DSM (DSM-III and DSM-III-R; American Psychiatric Association, 1980, 1987) in which there were two additional anxiety disorders with child-specific criteria. The first was Avoidant Disorder which focused on excessive shrinking from contact with unfamiliar persons or extreme shyness. The second diagnosis was Overanxious Disorder which focused on a chronic and generalized pattern of anxious behavior across a number of situations. These diagnoses were eliminated because it was thought that the constructs were adequately captured by the adult Social Phobia criteria (Avoidant Disorder) and the criteria for Generalized Anxiety

Disorder (Overanxious Disorder) (American Psychiatric Association, 1994).

Separation Anxiety Disorder (SAD), the one anxiety disorder with child-specific criteria, is characterized by anxiety for at least 2 weeks over separation from a major attachment figure. During the course of development, there are changes in the way this anxiety is expressed. For example, Francis, Last, and Strauss (1987) found that young children (ages 5–8) with SAD were more likely to report nightmares that involved separation, worry about attachment figures, and worry about calamitous events happening to themselves. Older children (ages 9–12) with SAD were more likely to report excessive distress upon separation from major attachment figures, including withdrawal, apathy, sadness, and poor concentration. Adolescents (ages 12–19) with SAD often presented with refusal to attend school and physical symptoms when confronted with separation.

From this description of the symptoms of SAD, it is evident that some children and adolescents with SAD can express their concerns about separation through refusal to attend school. For these children, the refusal to attend school is precipitated by fear of leaving the caretaker or home. Other children with school phobia refuse to attend school because of an actual fear of school or some aspect of the school situation. In both cases, the child or adolescent expresses specific or vague fears associated with school or presents with somatic complaints as an explanation for avoiding school (Kearney, 1995). However, when children who refuse to attend school as a result of SAD are compared to children who refuse to attend school due to a school phobia, those with SAD tend to be younger, female, from lower socioeconomic families, from single parent families, have another comorbid disorder, and have mothers with a history of an anxiety or affective disorder (Last, Francis, Hersen, Kazdin, & Strauss, 1987; Last & Strauss, 1990).

Unlike SAD in which the anxiety is somewhat circumscribed around a common theme (e.g., separation from a major attachment figure), Generalized Anxiety Disorder (GAD) is characterized by anxiety around a large number of different events, such as worry about future events (e.g., upcoming tests), anxiety about being criticized or making mistakes, worry about social activities, and worry about school performance (Last, Francis, & Strauss, 1989). Children with GAD are also perfectionistic and self-conscious and report a high rate of somatic complaints (e.g., heart palpitations, feelings of shakiness) (Biedel, Christ, & Long, 1991). Given the diversity of anxiety symptoms that they exhibit, it is not surprising that one-half of the children with GAD also exhibit another anxiety disorder (Last, Hersen, Kazdin, Finkelstein, & Strauss, 1987).

Social Phobia is another common anxiety disorder in children that is characterized by extreme performance anxiety or evaluative anxiety in social situations. Children with Social Phobia fear that they will be humiliated or embarrassed in these situations. In recent years, it has been recognized that children with Social Phobia can have more generalized forms of social anxiety in which their anxiety is shown in most social situations or more circumscribed social fears are displayed only in discrete situations (e.g., at parties) (American Psychiatric Association, 1994). Like children with GAD, children with Social Phobia often also have somatic complaints. In fact, Biedel et al. (1991) reported that 50% of their sample of children (ages 6–13) with School Phobia endorsed feelings of nausea, shakiness, heart palpitations, sweating, flushes and chills, and feelings of going crazy.

As the name implies, Specific Phobia refers to a discrete fear focused on a specific stimulus. For example, the DSM-IV recognizes five types of specific phobias that involve (1) fears of animals; (2) environmental fears (e.g., heights, storms, darkness, water); (3) fears of blood, shots, or bodily injury; (4) fears that involve specific situations (e.g., airplanes, cars, elevators); and (5) miscellaneous fears (e.g., loud noises, costumed figures). An important consideration in viewing phobias in children is that mild fears are relatively common in childhood years. In fact, most children experience some fears (Campbell, 1986; Muris, Meesters, Merckelbach, Sermon, & Zwakhalen, 1998), and the most common types of fears change over development in a predictable manner related to the tasks of a given developmental stage (Bauer, 1976). However, phobias, which by definition have to be severe enough to cause significant impairments for the child, are not normative in children and can be quite stable over time (Ollendick & King, 1994).

There has recently been increased awareness that children may respond acutely to exposure to traumatic and life-threatening events, similar to adults who experience Acute Stress Disorder

(ASD) or Posttraumatic Stress Disorder (PTSD; Eth & Pynoos, 1985). For example, one study investigated elementary school-age children's reaction to a sniper attack on their school yard in which a child and passerby were killed and 13 other children were injured (Pynoos et al., 1987). These authors reported finding three classes of responses exhibited by children. One (intrusiveness/numbing/avoidance) involved intrusive thoughts, a wish to avoid feelings and anhedonia; a second (fear/anxiety) involved fears of reoccurrence and being jumpy or easily startled; and a third class (disturbances in sleep/concentration) involved bad dreams, difficulty paying attention, and sleep disturbance. The most significant variable that influenced the occurrence of a posttraumatic stress reaction was the level of exposure to the traumatic event (e.g., being in the school yard at the time of the shooting vs. being home from school and hearing about the shooting). Knowledge of the victims was also associated with a stress reaction, whereas sex, age, ethnicity, exposure to recent previous trauma, and worry about a sibling were not significantly associated with the severity of the reaction.

## Epidemiology

Silverman and Ginsburg (1998) provide an excellent review of the prevalence of anxiety disorders in children across ten epidemiological studies conducted from 1987–1993. Overall, rates of anxiety disorders ranged from 6–18% across the samples; the most common disorders were SAD (3–12%) and GAD (3–12%). Interestingly, there is little evidence for consistent relations between anxiety disorders and sociodemographic variables, such as socioeconomic status, ethnicity, and gender. To illustrate the inconsistency of the findings, Cohen et al. (1993) found an almost equal gender ratio in the prevalence of SAD and GAD in a large community sample of children, whereas Anderson, Williams, McGee, and Silva (1987) found a female predominance for SAD (0.4:1) but a male predominance for GAD (1.7:1). The failure to find consistent gender differences is still somewhat striking, however, given the clear female predominance of anxiety disorders in adults.

## Comorbidity

In the previous sections, we reviewed the literature on the comorbidity between anxiety disorders and ADHD and between anxiety disorders and

CD/ODD. Similar to the high rates of comorbidity between the externalizing disorders (i.e., ADHD, CD, and ODD), there is also a high rate of comorbidity within the internalizing disorders of anxiety and depression. Studies of clinic-referred children have reported that between one-third and one-half of children diagnosed with an anxiety disorder also have a depressive disorder (Bernstein & Garfinkel, 1986; Strauss, Last, Hersen, & Kazdin, 1988). As for externalizing disorders, this high rate of comorbidity has led some researchers to question the utility of distinguishing between these emotional disorders and to consider the possibility of a single category of "negative affectivity" or internalizing disorders (see Finch, Lipovosky, & Casat, 1989). Also similar to the research on the comorbidity among externalizing disorders, there are some important differences in children with both anxiety and depression: these children tend to be older, tend to exhibit a more severe disturbance, and tend to be more socially impaired than children with anxiety disorders alone (Mitchell, McCauley, Burke, & Moss, 1988; Strauss, Last et al., 1988).

Anxious children may have difficulties in two other areas, school achievement and social interactions. For example, Strauss, Frame, and Forehand (1987) reported that teachers rated children with anxiety disorders as having more deficits in performance than nonanxious children, and Reeves, Werry, Elkind, and Zametkin (1987) reported that children with anxiety disorders were somewhat more likely to underachieve on achievement test scores (20–29%), compared to nonanxious controls (5–10%). Anxious children are also neglected by their peers, signifying difficulties in their ability to make friends (Strauss, Lahey, Frick, Frame, & Hynd, 1988), and are described by parents and teachers as lonely, lacking appropriate social skills, shy, and socially withdrawn (Strauss, Lease, Kazdin, Dulcan, & Last, 1989).

### Etiology

For many decades, behavioral and social learning conceptualizations dominated etiological theories of anxiety disorders (see Menzies and Clark, 1995 for a review). Many of these theories were developed from basic classical conditioning paradigms that focused on a child who acquires a feared response to a stimulus that is consistently paired with a noxious and aversive event. Many of these basic paradigms were extended to consider cognitive expectancies involved in the pairing of an unconditioned stimulus to a noxious event (e.g., a child expects a stimulus to lead to an aversive outcome) (see Reiss, 1991) and to consider the reinforcing aspects of avoiding the anxiety-producing stimulus to enhance and maintain the anxious behavior (Mowrer, 1939). In addition to models based on classical conditioning, other models focused on operant conditioning have been proposed and are supported by research that shows that parents often deliver positive reinforcement for anxious behavior, such as providing special considerations for their children's anxious behavior, that could serve to maintain this maladaptive behavior (Ayllon, Smith, & Rogers, 1970; Kennedy, 1965). Finally, social learning theorists have provided evidence that modeling can be a powerful influence in developing and maintaining anxious behavior (Bandura & Menlove, 1968).

Although these social learning theories remain influential in explaining the development of anxiety disorders, more recent models have begun to integrate genetic/biological and cognitive factors. The role of heredity has been supported by a number of family history studies that show that mothers of children with anxiety disorders also tend to have histories of anxiety disorders (Last, Hersen, Kazdin, Francis, & Grubb, 1987; Reeves et al., 1987). Although these studies do not indicate whether the transmission across generations is by genetic or environmental mechanisms, some evidence from behavioral genetic studies indicates that there is a heritable component in at least the more severe types of anxiety disorders in children (Rutter, 1976). This leads to the logical question of how this transmission takes place.

The work of Kagan and colleagues on the temperamental style called "behavioral inhibition to the unfamiliar" could provide some clues to this transmission (Kagan, Reznick, Clarke, Snidman, & Garcia-Coll, 1984). These authors found that children as young as 21 months could be classified as either behaviorally inhibited or behaviorally uninhibited; inhibited children show a tendency to avoid novel and unfamiliar stimuli and situations (e.g., new toys, new children, strange adults). This is the opposite end of the continuum of the thrill- and adventure-seeking tendencies or behaviorally *uninhibited* styles of the callous and unemotional children with CD, described previously. Importantly, this behaviorally inhibited temperament has been associated with distinct biological markers related to a lower threshold of response or higher "reactivity" of the sympathetic arm of the autonomic nervous system (Kagan, Reznick, & Snidman, 1987), and these physiological markers can be identified as early as 2 months of age (Kagan & Snidman, 1991).

Theoretically, this temperamental style could explain why some children are more easily "conditioned" to anxiety than others. Specifically, behaviorally inhibited children could become aroused to more stimuli and become more strongly aroused to these stimuli than other children, making them more likely to develop conditioned anxiety responses and making the avoidance of anxiety-producing stimuli more reinforcing. It also could explain the mechanism that is passed from parent to child in family history studies. In support of both these possibilities, children that are behaviorally inhibited to the unfamiliar during three assessment periods are at a higher risk of an anxiety disorder (Hirshfeld et al., 1992) and children of parents with anxiety disorders are at higher risk of being behaviorally inhibited (Rosenbaum et al., 1988).

The second trend for explaining anxiety disorders in children is to focus on cognitive factors that can relate to the development and maintenance of anxious behavior. For example, anxious children in general tend to interpret ambiguous information as threatening, are more likely to express avoidant plans when confronted with ambiguity, and show a tendency to assign higher probabilities to the potential occurrence of threatening events (Chorpita, Albano, & Barlow, 1996). Taken together, these findings suggest that anxious children tend to show a bias for interpreting events as threatening. Anxious children also use less positive self-statements in a large number of situations (Treadwell & Kendall, 1996). Many of these anxiety-related cognitive styles specifically relate to anxiety-producing stimuli, for example, test-anxious children anticipate more negative performance outcomes in testing situations (Prins, Groot, & Hanewald, 1994), and social phobic children are more likely to view social situations as threatening (Bell-Dolan, 1995). Although these negative cognitive styles are often viewed as predisposing a child to act anxiously to certain situations, the correlational nature of these studies make it impossible to determine the direction of influence. Therefore, it is also possible that these cognitive styles result from the child's anxiety. It also appears that these cognitive styles can be influenced by processes within the family that encourage biased ways of processing information (Dadds, Barrett, Rapee, & Ryan, 1996).

## Prognosis and Treatment

In discussing the prognosis of children with anxiety disorders, it is important to note that there is not nearly the same amount of longitudinal research conducted with anxious children as there has been for children with externalizing disorders like ADHD and CD. In addition, when follow-up studies are conducted, typically they do not provide stability estimates that are separate for anxiety and depression but provide estimates for internalizing behaviors in general (e.g., Verhulst & Ende, 1992) or for emotional disorders that combine both anxiety and depression (Offord et al., 1992). The follow-up periods for these disorders also tend to be relatively short; virtually no data are available on the adult outcome of children with anxiety disorders. Therefore, conclusions about the stability of anxiety disorders must be quite tentative (see Ollendick & King, 1998). However, the limited evidence available suggests that anxiety disorders may be more chronic than was once thought (Agras, Chapin, & Oliveau, 1972; Kohlberg, LaCrosse, & Ricks, 1972; Rutter, 1976).

This contention is based on several research findings. First, retrospective reports of adults with anxiety disorders suggest that many of these adults report an onset of their anxiety in childhood (Last et al., 1987). Second, although Verhulst, Koot, and Berden (1990) reported the stability coefficients only for internalizing behaviors or for a combined anxiety/depression scale for a 4-year period, they did report that the most stable symptom within these broader composites was the symptom, "Acts nervous or high strung." Third, in the few studies that did report stability estimates for anxiety disorders separate from other emotional disturbances, the disorders tend to be fairly stable, especially for more generalized anxiety disorders like GAD. For example, in a sample of 151 children (ages 2–15) referred to a speech and hearing clinic, 50% of those children with a GAD diagnosis at initial testing were rediagnosed during a 4- to 5-year follow-up period. Similarly, Cohen, Cohen, and Brook (1993) reported that 47% of the children with GAD in a community sample of 734 children (ages 9–18) were rediagnosed with the disorder during a 2½-year follow-up period. Therefore, although these stability estimates are based on a limited amount of research, they suggest that anxiety disorders, especially GAD, are not as transient as was once thought.

A recent review of the literature on published treatment outcome studies of children with anxiety disorders reported that the most successful treatments tended to be those based on behavioral and social learning conceptualizations of anxiety (Ollendick & King, 1998). Specifically, use of participant modeling and reinforced practice, use of *in vivo* and imaginal desensitization procedures, and use of various types of modeling approaches have proven effective for treating a large number of children with anxiety disorders. Unfortunately, these techniques have proven most effective in treating discrete forms of anxiety such as fears and phobias (Ollendick & King, 1998). One approach to enhancing the treatment for more generalized anxiety disorders has been the use of anxioloytic and other pharmacological medications. However, except for the treatment of childhood OCD (see Allen, Leonard, & Swedo, 1995), literature on the effectiveness of these treatments consists largely of uncontrolled clinical reports that make firm conclusions about the effectiveness of these interventions impossible.

One promising approach to the treatment of GAD is the cognitive-behavioral approach tested by Kendall and colleagues in two controlled outcome studies (Kendall, 1994; Kendall et al., 1997). The treatment specifically addresses the cognitive distortions that are often displayed by children with anxiety disorders combined with an exposure-based component that addresses the avoidance behavior that often maintains and reinforces anxious behavior. Specifically, the first sessions involve establishing a hierarchy of anxiety-producing events for the child and teaching the child a relaxation technique to use when exposed to these events. The next several sessions focus on teaching the child to recognize anxious feelings and somatic reactions to anxiety, to recognize cognitions leading to anxiety, to develop methods for modifying anxious self-statements (e.g., "I am going to fail this test"), to develop ways of evaluating performance in anxiety-producing situations, and to administer self-reinforcement for adaptive coping. Finally, both imaginal and *in vivo* exposure trials are conducted with the child, beginning with low anxiety-producing situations and progressing to high anxiety-producing situations, and the child is encouraged to use the skills taught in early sessions. In the two studies that tested the effectiveness of this intervention, 53–66% of the children (ages 9–13) did not meet criteria for a diagnosis of their pretreatment anxiety disorder at the end of the program, and these gains were maintained at a 1-year follow-up (Kendall et al., 1997).

These gains are impressive, given the past difficulties in treating generalized anxiety in children, but it is obvious that there is room to improve the effectiveness of this intervention. As mentioned previously, there is evidence that parents can play a role in reinforcing children's anxious behavior and in maintaining an anxious cognitive processing style. As a result, Dadds and colleagues attempted to enhance a cognitive-behavioral approach to treatment by adding a family component to the intervention that includes teaching parents (1) child management skills, (2) anxiety management skills, and (3) communication/problem-solving skills (Barrett, Dadds, & Rapee, 1996). These authors reported that a larger percentage of children who received the family intervention combined with the cognitive-behavioral intervention were free from an anxiety disorder at posttreatment (84 versus 57%) and at a 1-year posttreatment follow-up (96 versus 70%). A later study suggested that the critical component of this family intervention was the parent training in anxiety management techniques (Cobham, Dadds, & Spence, 1998).

## Depressive Disorders

### Overview

Today, there is little debate that clinical depression can be manifested in prepubertal children in ways similar to those of adults (Cantwell, 1983a; Quay, Routh, & Shapiro, 1987). However, this is a relatively new consensus (e.g., Lefkowitz & Burton, 1978; Rie, 1966). The DSM-IV (American Psychiatric Association, 1994) includes two types of major affective disorders, major depression and bipolar disorder. Because bipolar disorder rarely has onsets before puberty and because this disorder was discussed elsewhere in this book, our focus will be on Major Depression. In the DSM-IV, major depression is defined as a change from previous functioning that lasts at least 2 weeks and is characterized by either depressed mood (or irritable mood in children and adolescents) or anhedonia (loss of interest in usual activities) and at least four other vegetative symptoms (e.g., change in appetite, change in sleep patterns, psychomotor agitation or retardation, fatigue, feelings of worthlessness, diminished ability to concentrate, and suicidal ideation). In addition to episodic major depression, the DSM-IV also specifies a chronic mood disturbance labeled Dysthymic Disorder and a category of adjustment disorder with depressed mood in which there is a reaction to an identifiable psychosocial stressor(s) and the primary manifestation is in the form of depressed mood, tearfulness, and feelings of hopelessness.

Despite the use of the adult criteria to diagnose depression in children and adolescents, there are some unique features of depression in youth. For example, depressed prepubertal children are more likely to show somatic complaints, psychomotor retardation, and depressive hallucinations, whereas depressed adolescents are more likely to show high levels of hopelessness, hypersomnia, and weight changes (Birmaher et al., 1996; Ryan et al., 1987). The overlap between anxiety and depression that was discussed previously is also greater for children than for adolescents and adults (e.g., Cole, Truglio, & Peeke, 1997; Hinden, Compas, Howell, & Achenbach, 1997).

Despite these developmental variations, the symptomatology exhibited by depressed children and adolescents is quite similar to that of adults with major depression. For example, in a study of ninety-five prepubertal children and ninety-two postpubertal adolescents with major depression, the most common symptoms for both groups were depressed mood (97%), anhedonia/lack of interest (88%), decreased concentration (86%), irritability and anger (83%), fatigue (81%), negative self-esteem (79%), insomnia (74%), social withdrawal (68%), psychomotor retardation (65%), suicidal ideation (60%), excessive or inappropriate guilt (52%), and anorexia (51%) (Ryan et al., 1987). Although it is quite rare, there are reports of depressive disorders in preschool children, and the symptomatology in this group is also relative consistent with that found in depressed adults. For example, in a small study of eight children ages 2–6 years diagnosed with major depression or dysthymic disorder, the most common symptoms were sadness/irritability (100%), concentration problems (100%), poor appetite (87.5%), low self-esteem (87.5%), sleep problems (75%), and fatigue (75%) (Kashani, Allen, Beck, Bledsoe, & Reid, 1997).

## Epidemiology

Although changes in manifesting major depression are somewhat minor across development, there are dramatic changes in the prevalence of depressive disorders from preschoolers to adoles-

cents (Quay et al., 1987). Prevalence rates in community samples of preschool children are reportedly below 1%, whereas the rates in elementary school age children range from 2–4% (Anderson et al., 1987; Angold & Costello, 1993; Costello et al., 1997; McGee et al., 1992; Verhulst et al., 1997). In contrast, the prevalence of depressive disorders increases dramatically in adolescence to a rate of about 7% (Angold & Costello, 1993; McGee et al., 1992).

In addition to this clear jump in prevalence in depressive disorders in adolescence, there are two additional trends in the epidemiology of depressive disorders. First, there is considerable evidence of a cohort effect that operates for both adults and children; persons born more recently are significantly more likely to experience major depression than persons in older cohorts (Lewinsohn, Rohde, Seeley, & Fischer, 1993). Second, there are dramatic changes in the sex ratio of depressive disorders that coincide with the onset of puberty. In childhood, boys experience more depression than girls at about a 2:1 ratio (Angold & Costello, 1993; Angold, Costello, & Worthman, 1998; Rutter, 1990). In adolescence, however, this sex ratio changes; more girls report depression than boys at about a 2:1 ratio, and this ratio continues into adulthood. The shift in prevalence is due to an increased rate of depression in girls once they reach mid-puberty (Tanner stage 3) and a decreased rate of depression in boys once they reach puberty (Angold et al., 1998). One explanation for this change in the sex ratio of depression at adolescence suggests that girls have predisposing characteristics and risk factors that make them vulnerable to developing depression, and after the onset of puberty, depression develops in vulnerable individuals (Nolen-Hoeksema & Girgus, 1994).

## Comorbidity

Like other childhood disorders, childhood depression tends to co-occur with other forms of psychological disturbance (Hammen & Compas, 1994), most often with anxiety disorders and conduct disorder. From 37–75% of children with depression also exhibit an anxiety disorder (Angold & Costello, 1993), although some estimates have been as high as 100% (Mitchell et al., 1988; PuigAntich, Blau, Marx, Greenhill, & Chambers, 1978; Ryan et al., 1987). Similarly, from 22–84% of children with depression also exhibit ODD or

CD (Angold & Costello, 1993). These rates of comorbidity depend somewhat on the type of depressive disorder. For example, children diagnosed with adjustment disorder with depressed mood show the least amount of overlap with other diagnostic groups; only 45% have an additional diagnosis (Kovacs, Feinberg, Crouse-Novak, Paulauskas, & Finkelstein, 1984a,b). In contrast, 79% of children with major depression had an additional diagnosis (38% with dysthymia, 33% with an anxiety disorder, and 7% with conduct disorder), and 93% of children with dysthymia had an additional diagnosis (57% with major depression, 36% with an anxiety disorder, 14% with an attention-deficit disorder, and 11% with conduct disorder).

## Etiology

Evidence is strong that genetic factors play an important etiological role in primary affective disorders in adults (Cantwell, 1983b). However, this has not been well studied for childhood depression, and most of this research has relied on family history studies. For example, children with major depression are more likely to have higher rates of major depression, alcoholism, and other psychiatric disorders (mostly anxiety disorders) in both first- and second-degree relatives compared to control children (Puig-Antich et al., 1989). Although it is possible that the link between parent and child depression is through a genetic predisposition, it is also possible that the link is mediated by other forms of familial dysfunction (Puig-Antich et al., 1978). In addition, children of depressed parents have higher rates of many types of emotional and behavior disturbances (e.g., anxiety, conduct problems), suggesting that the link may be through a "nonspecific" vulnerability to problems in adjustment, not through a mechanism that is specific to depression (Birmaher et al., 1996).

The search for biological correlates to childhood and adolescent depression have typically yielded negative or inconclusive results. For example, there are often reports that depressed children and adolescents have higher rates of sleep problems and various neurochemical abnormalities than other children (e.g., Ryan et al., 1987). However, these neurochemical abnormalities are not consistently found across studies (see Birmaher et al., 1996 and Emslie, Weinberg, & Kowatch, 1998

for reviews). One of the more promising avenues of biological research focuses on differences in the brain activity of infants of depressed mothers. These infants show abnormalities in their frontal lobe activation which could underlie problems in their ability to regulate emotion and predispose them to affective disorders (e.g., Dawson, Frey, Panagiotides, Osterling, & Hessl, 1997).

One of the more consistent psychosocial correlates to depression in children is the presence of a high number of stressful life events ranging from severe stressors, such as parental death or divorce or the suicide of a friend, to milder stressful events such as a poor grade on a test, an argument with a parent or teacher, or a broken date (Birmaher et al., 1996). Although the presence of more stressful events are consistently found in depressed children, the reason for this association is not clear. It is possible that children who experience chronic uncontrollable stressors or who at least perceive that the stressors are uncontrollable, develop a "learned helplessness" attributional style that leads to depression (Seligman, 1975). This is a compelling model for explaining the correlation between stressful life events and depression, but it is also still possible that, possibly due to their problems in emotional regulation, depressed children put themselves at risk of experiencing more stressful life events than other children (Garber, Braafladt, & Zeman, 1991).

As in adult depression, however, many models to explain the development of depression in children focus on cognitive factors. Children who develop depression often show a negative cognitive style that involves low self-esteem, cognitive distortions (e.g., perfectionistic standards), a negative attributional style (e.g., attributing failures to internal, global, and stable factors), hopelessness, and excessive self-criticism (Dixon & Ahrens, 1992). However, there are two important issues that involve the association between these cognitive factors and depression in children. First, rather than leading directly to depression in children, these cognitions may form a predisposing way of interpreting information (i.e., a cognitive diathesis) that makes a child less likely to cope competently with life stressors (Garber, 1992). Second, the cognitive diathesis may not emerge until later childhood and adolescence, and therefore, it may not play as prominent a role in the development of depression in younger children (Turner & Cole, 1994).

## Prognosis and Treatment

Despite early views that childhood depression is a transitory developmental phenomenon, current research suggests that major depressive disorders in children are as chronic as adult depression. For example, studies have shown that the average length of a major depressive episode in prepubertal children is 7–9 months, and it is approximately 2 years before 90% of children can expect to have complete remission of their symptoms (Kovacs et al., 1984a; Kovacs, Feinberg, Crouse-Novak, Paulauskas, Pollock, & Finkelstein, 1984b). In addition, the likelihood of a relapse is high; 40% of children relapse within 2 years, and 70% relapse within 5 years (Flemming et al., 1993; Lewinsohn et al., 1994). As one would expect, Dysthymic Disorder is even more chronic; the average duration is 3 years, and 69% of children develop a superimposed major depressive episode within a 5-year period (Kovacs et al., 1984a,b). Children with an adjustment disorder have the best prognosis; 90% recover within 9 months, and none develop a major depressive episode within a 5-year period (Kovacs et al., 1984a,b). Unfortunately, given this chronicity over a short period of time, data on the long-term outcome of children with a depressive disorder are limited.

Because pharmacological intervention for adult depression has had well-documented effectiveness, it is not surprising that this has been the focus of initial attempts to treat childhood depression. The most common treatment for children with major depression has been the use of tricyclic antidepressants and, more recently, selective serotonin re-uptake inhibitors (SSRI) (Emslie et al., 1998). Despite this widespread practice, most well-controlled studies have failed to find that either form of medication is more effective than placebo in double-blind medication trials (Puig-Antich et al., 1987). For example, a recent meta-analysis of all available placebo-controlled trials showed that the effectiveness of tricyclic antidepressant medications was too low to be clinically significant (Emslie et al., 1998), and similar results were reported for the newer SSRIs (Simeon et al., 1995). Much of the failure to document medication effectiveness in these controlled studies has not been due to the fact that children treated with medication do not show symptomatic improvement; it is more due to the fact that children in the placebo condition also show dramatic improvement although they are not on an active dose of medication (Emslie et al., 1997).

These findings suggest that expectancies for treatment success may play a major role in the treatment of childhood depression which has led to the development of cognitive-behavioral interventions that attempt to increase positive expectancies in depressed children and adolescents. For example, most of the psychosocial interventions focus on increasing the positive events experienced by children, directly altering negative cognitive styles, and teaching the children skills necessary to increase positive events in their lives (see Kaslow & Thompson, 1998). As an example of an intervention that combines all of these components, Lewinsohn, Clarke, Hops, and Andrews (1990) reported on a fourteen-session cognitive behavioral intervention for adolescents that involved increasing pleasant activities, training in relaxation exercises to cope with stressors, controlling depressive thoughts, improving social interactions, and developing conflict resolution skills.

All of these cognitive-behavioral interventions appear promising in that they have brought about positive changes in children's depressive symptomatology that have been maintained at follow-up intervals of 1–2 years (Kaslow & Thompson, 1998). However, most studies were conducted with nonreferred children and adolescents. Therefore, their effectiveness with clinic-referred children who are likely to experience more severe disturbances remains untested. Furthermore, there have been few studies comparing the effectiveness of interventions to determine the *relative* efficacy of various treatment approaches to childhood depression or whether a combination of treatments (e.g., medication combined with cognitive-behavioral interventions) lead to even greater treatment success than either intervention alone.

# Autistic Disorder and Other Pervasive Developmental Disorders

## Overview

Autistic disorder is a pervasive, stable disorder whose onset is prior to age 3 and is characterized by conspicuously abnormal or impaired social interactions, marked deficits in or absence of communication skills, and participation in an extremely restricted and repetitive range of activities and interests (American Psychiatric Association, 1994). Impaired development in social interest is characterized by severe deficits in reciprocal social interactions, including failure to use nonverbal behaviors (e.g., eye-to-eye gaze), failure to establish developmentally appropriate peer relationships, an inability to share experiences verbally or nonverbally (e.g., pointing to show an object), and a lack of reciprocal social or emotional interactions. Communication deficits include abnormal speech (e.g., echolalia, pronoun reversal), an inability to initiate or sustain conversations, or complete lack of communicative speech. Restrictive patterns of behaviors or interests include preoccupation with certain interests or activities, stereotypical motor movements (hand flapping), and rigid adherence to routines (American Psychiatric Association, 1994). In the DSM-IV, Autistic Disorder is one of five diagnoses listed under the heading of Pervasive Developmental Disorders. The others include Rhett's Disorder, Asperger's Disorder, Childhood Disintegration Disorder, and Pervasive Developmental Disorder Not Otherwise Specified.

Autism was first described in 1943 by Kanner who differentiated children with childhood-onset schizophrenia (Mesibov, Adams, & Klinger, 1997). One of the critical distinctions between autism and schizophrenia is the very early onset of autism; some studies show evidence of the disorder as early as 12 months (Osterling & Dawson, 1994) to 18 months of age (Baron-Cohen et al., 1996), and clear impairments are evident in the third year of life (Mesibov et al., 1997). Children with autism are often significantly impaired in many aspects of functioning; up to 77% of autistic children have IQ scores in the mentally retarded range of intellectual functioning (Gillberg, 1984), and proportionally more females than males are in the lowest range of intellectual functioning (American Psychiatric Association, 1994; Eme, 1992; Lord & Schopler, 1987). Children with autism often have better developed visual-spatial skills compared to their verbal skills (Mesibov et al., 1997). In fact, up to 50% of children with autism never develop communicative speech or language skills (Werry, 1996b). Both the general cognitive delay and the delay in verbal abilities are the key points in differentiating between Autistic Disorder and Asperger's Disorder which first appeared in the DSM-IV. Asperger's Disorders are defined by the presence of significant social impairments and a se-verely restricted range of activities and interests, but no delay in language or cognitive development (American Psychiatric Association, 1994).

Other associated characteristics of autism include a variety of externalizing behaviors, such as aggressiveness, self-injurious behaviors, temper tantrums, hyperactivity, attention deficits, and impulsive behaviors (Mesibov et al., 1997). In addition, children with autism often exhibit sleep disturbances, eating problems, and severe anxiety to common household items, such as vacuum cleaners and blenders (Klinger & Dawson, 1996). Furthermore, sensory abnormalities, including overresponsiveness to some sounds and an intolerance to some tactile stimuli but extreme tolerance to pain, are also evident in many children diagnosed with autism (Schreibman & Charlop-Christy, 1998). Finally, approximately 20–30% of children eventually develop seizure disorders, typically in adolescence (Gillberg, 1991; Werry, 1996b).

In addition to Autistic Disorder and Asperger's Disorder, the DSM-IV lists three other pervasive developmental disorders. Considerable argument exists whether all of these disorders should be considered different diagnoses or variants of an autistic spectrum (e.g., Szatmari, 1997). As mentioned previously, Autistic Disorder and Asperger Disorders share many features that could support a relationship based on the severity of impairment between the two disorders. However, the other pervasive developmental disorders show quite distinct characteristics. For example, Rhett's Disorder is found only in females and is characterized by normal development for the first 5 months, followed by significant deterioration of previously acquired skills (language skills, hand movements, trunk movements), deceleration of head growth beginning between the ages of 5 and 48 months, and subsequent development of stereotypical hand movements (American Psychiatric Association, 1994). Childhood Disintegration Disorder, or Heller's Disorder, is characterized by normal development for the first 2 years of life, followed by a significant loss of skills before age 10 in at least two of five areas: language, social skills, elimination functions, play, and/or motor skills (American Psychiatric Association, 1994). Therefore, unlike Autistic Disorder, both Rhett's Disorder and Childhood Disintegration Disorder occur after a clear period of normal development (Mesibov et al., 1997; Volkmar & Rutter, 1995). The remaining disorder in this category, Pervasive Developmental Disorder Not Otherwise Specified, is an ill-defined category that captures children with pervasive developmental delays who do not fall into any of the other four diagnostic categories.

## Epidemiology

Given the relative recent division of the Pervasive Developmental Disorders into more discrete categories, most of what we know about the epidemiology and etiology of these disorders has focused on children with autism, some of whom were high functioning intellectually and who would, as a result, most likely meet current criteria for Asperger's Disorder. Even with the broader definition of autism, it is still quite a rare form of psychopathology, and estimates of prevalence range from 2–5 per 10,000 (American Psychiatric Association, 1994) up to 11.6 per 10,000 (Gillberg et al., 1991). Recent estimates have yielded higher prevalence rates of autism, in part due to improved methods of identifying the disorder. However, more accurate diagnosis does not fully account for the increase in prevalence. It is possible that the increased survival rate of children with severe perinatal complications (Ornitz, 1989), coupled with the fact that higher functioning autistic individuals marry and have children (Ciaranello, 1995) also contributes to the increased rate of autistic disorder (Mesibov et al., 1997).

Epidemiological studies also suggest that more males than females are diagnosed with autism; ratios are 3:1 to 4:1 (Eme, 1992; Lord & Schopler, 1987). Early reports suggested that children with Autistic Disorder were more likely to come from high SES homes (Volkmar et al., 1996). However, several studies have shown that the apparent high SES level found for children with autism is based on patterns of referral, not on the disorder itself (Tsai, Stewart, Faust, & Shook, 1982; Wing, 1980). In addition, most studies that found more autistic children in higher social classes were conducted before 1970, and few SES differences have been found in studies conducted after that (Mesibov et al., 1997; Tsai et al., 1982).

## Etiology

Several biological factors have been linked to autism, including genetic, neurochemical, and neuroanatomical factors. Numerous studies have found strong evidence that genetic factors are

likely to play a role in the development of autism. For example, siblings of autistic children are at increased risk of autism and other developmental disorders (Smalley, Asarnow, & Spence, 1988; Szatmari et al., 1993). Studies have found a high rate of concordance for autism in monozygotic twins that ranges from 36–91%, whereas the same studies failed to find any significant concordance in dizygotic twins (Klinger & Dawson, 1996; Mesibov et al., 1997). In addition, other developmental problems, including learning disabilities, language delays, and mental retardation, have been found in up to 25% of siblings of autistic children; this suggests that Autistic Disorder may be on a continuum with other cognitive deficits (Klinger & Dawson, 1996; Schreibman & Charlop-Christy, 1998).

There is also evidence that the genetic causes of autism may be varied and complex. For example, certain single gene abnormalities are found in a subset (10–20%) of autistic individuals (Mesibov et al., 1997; Smalley, Levitt, & Bauman, 1998). It is also estimated that 5% of autistic males have Fragile X Syndrome and that 1–3% of individuals with autism have tuberous sclerosis (Smalley et al., 1998). In addition to genetic factors, prenatal and perinatal complications have been implicated in the development of autism, including maternal bleeding after the first trimester and an excessive gestational period (Mesibov et al., 1997). There is also evidence to suggest that immune factors, such as maternal viral infections, may play a role in the development of Autistic Disorder in some children (Smalley et al., 1998).

The focus on genetic factors and early types of neurological trauma illustrates the current view of Autistic Disorder as a neurobiological disorder. This conceptualization is supported by a number of studies that documented several neurochemical abnormalities associated with Autistic Disorder. For example, more than twenty-five published investigations have found elevated platelet serotonin (5-HT) levels in individuals with Autistic Disorder, compared to nonautistic individuals (McBride et al., 1998), although this may be present in only 33% of autistic individuals (Smalley et al., 1998; Volkmar et al., 1996). Other investigators have attempted to implicate other neurochemicals, including opioid system functions, noradrenergic functions, and dopaminergic functions, but the results of these studies are less consistent (Smalley et al., 1998). Neuroanatomical abnormalities have also been found in children with autism, most often in the areas of the cerebellum, limbic system, cerebral cortex (parietal lobe, frontal lobe), and overall brain size (see Mesibov et al., 1997, for a review).

## Prognosis and Treatment

In general, individuals with Autistic Disorder have poor outcomes, and the vast majority continue to manifest significant impairments into adulthood. Less than 10% of children with Autistic Disorder recover from their symptoms, and more than 90% exhibit social and intellectual deficits over their life-spans (Werry, 1996b). Worse prognosis is associated with lower IQ (<50) and/or lack of communication skills at age 5. Therefore, children with Asperger's Disorder may have better prognoses than other children with autism (Gillberg, 1991; Werry, 1996b). Nevertheless, even these individuals without cognitive and language impairments often show a number of social deficits and interpersonal rigidity throughout their lives that can significantly impair their educations and occupational and social functioning (Werry, 1996b; Wing, 1981).

Given the view of Autistic Disorder as a neurobiological disorder, it is not surprising that a number of medications have been used to treat children with this disorder. Unfortunately, none of the medications that have been tested in controlled outcome studies have proven very effective, although some of the SSRI's (clomipramine, fluoxetine, fluvaoxamine) have led to a reduction of the stereotypies and aggression in children with autism (Smalley et al., 1998).

Given the poor response to medication, behavioral treatments have also been developed for treating Autistic Disorder. In general, these behavioral interventions usually fall within one of two broad categories: focal treatments directed toward ameliorating specific symptoms and comprehensive programs directed toward an overall increase in functioning (Rogers, 1998). Examples of comprehensive programs include Division TEACCH (e.g., Mesibov, 1997) and the Lovaas approach (Lovaas, 1987). The Lovaas (1987) approach is based on operant training techniques that include positive reinforcement and punishment to help a child develop more appropriate social and adaptive skills. Early results provided by Lovaas (1987) suggested that intensive, one-on-one training for 30–40 hours per week resulted in significant gains in IQ and reductions in symptomatology for many children with autism (Rogers, 1998). Interventions such as Division TEACCH are based on cognitive-behavioral principles and are designed to help the child with autism understand expectations and relationships in the environment (see Mesibov et al., 1997). For example, through structured teaching, the environment of the autistic child is simplified, schedules and routines are used to enhance predictability, and work systems are developed so that the child knows the length of time required to complete a task.

# Childhood Schizophrenia

## Overview

The typical onset to schizophrenia is in late adolescence or early adulthood, but there is a growing consensus that, while quite rare, prepubertal onset of schizophrenia does occur (Werry, 1997). In addition, there is considerable evidence that schizophrenia which has onsets in childhood is similar to the adult form of the disorder (e.g., Jacobsen & Rapoport, 1998; Volkmar, 1996; Werry, 1996a; Werry & McClellan, 1992). For example, the DSM-IV uses the same criteria for diagnosing schizophrenia in both adults and children. This diagnosis requires the presence of at least two of five characteristic symptoms, including delusions, hallucinations, disorganized speech, disorganized or catatonic behavior, and/or negative symptoms (flat affect, alogia), for at least 1 month, some signs of the disorder for at least 6 months, and the symptoms must significantly interfere with social or occupational functioning (American Psychiatric Association, 1994).

Although the criteria presented for a diagnosis of schizophrenia appear appropriate for both children and adults, children are more likely to experience some symptoms of schizophrenia in the course of other disorders (e.g., hallucinations as part of a mood disorder) and are less likely than adults to experience certain symptoms during the course of schizophrenia (e.g., poverty of thinking, well-formed delusions) (Werry, 1997). When these factors are combined with the low base rate of the disorder, it makes the diagnosis of schizophrenia much more difficult in children. Thus, it is not surprising that the validity and reliability of childhood-onset schizophrenia is often low (Werry, 1996a). Upon reassessment, children diagnosed with schizophrenia often receive different diagnoses, including psychotic depression, bipolar disorder, schizoaffective disorder, and personality disorders (Jacobsen & Rapoport, 1998; Werry & McClellan, 1992; Werry, 1996a).

## Epidemiology

Actual estimates of prevalence of childhood-onset schizophrenia are difficult to obtain, given its low prevalence. However, it is estimated that the onset of schizophrenia before age 13 occurs with less frequency than autism (Volkmar, 1996). In adulthood, schizophrenia is generally considered to affect males and females equally, particularly when community-based estimates are used (American Psychiatric Association, 1994). However, several investigations of early-onset schizophrenia suggested that the disorder was found more commonly in males than females (Asarnow & Asarnow, 1996; Green et al., 1984, 1992), although this is not a consistent finding (Galdos et al., 1993).

## Etiology

Like the presence of schizophrenia in adults, genetic factors, it is thought, influence childhood-onset schizophrenia. In fact, it has been noted that the earlier the age of onset, the more likely that family members have the disorder (Asarnow & Asarnow, 1996; Werry, 1996a). Also consistent with research on adults, a number of studies have suggested that neurological abnormalities are associated with childhood schizophrenia (Rapoport et al., 1997). For example, studies have found differences between schizophrenic children and normal controls in measures of autonomic activity and reactivity (Zahn et al., 1997), cerebral and ventricle volume (Rapoport et al., 1997), and basal ganglia structures (Rapoport et al., 1997). The temporal and frontal lobes of the cerebral cortex are other structural areas that may be involved in childhood schizophrenia (Werry, 1996a). Neurotransmitters implicated include dopamine, noradrenaline, and serotonin, although recent research suggests that negative symptoms and cognitive deficits are less related to dopamine than positive symptoms (Asarnow & Karatekin, 1998).

## Prognosis and Treatment

Early-onset schizophrenia generally has an insidious or gradual onset which is associated with a worse prognosis, so it is not surprising that the course of the disorder is often chronic and stable when its onset is in childhood (Jacobsen & Rapoport, 1998). More than half of children who receive a diagnosis of schizophrenia continue to show significant symptomatology during follow-up assessments, regardless of the time elapsed from diagnosis to follow-up (Gillberg, Hellgren, & Gillberg, 1993; Green et al., 1992; Jacobsen & Rapoport, 1998; Werry et al., 1991). Even those who are not diagnosed at follow-up often show significant symptomatology. For example, only 13% (Gillberg et al., 1993) to 17% (Werry et al., 1991) of children with schizophrenia had full recoveries. Jacobsen and Rapoport (1998) reported that, similarly to adults, children show intellectual declines after the onset of schizophrenia. However, unlike adults, children continued to show declines nearly 2 years after the onset of their symptoms.

The primary treatment for adult-onset schizophrenia is neuroleptic treatment, and similar medications have been used with children. Double-blind studies have found that haloperidol is more effective than placebo, particularly for positive symptoms, although there were significant adverse side effects associated with the medication, including extrapyramidal symptoms (Spencer et al., 1992). A recent double-blind study revealed that clozapine is superior to haloperidol for treating both positive and negative symptoms in children. However, the side effects of clozapine were even more significant, and 38% of children required discontinuation of treatment (Kumra et al., 1997).

Psychosocial treatments are often advocated in combination with medication. However, none of these treatments has been subjected to controlled trials in children, and the utility of these treatments for enhancing the effects of medication has not been conclusively shown. Generally, behavioral family treatment that emphasizes having a parent teach their children communication skills, problem-solving skills, and social skills through intensive instruction and practice is recommended (Asarnow & Asarnow, 1996). Many of these interventions also support parents in coping with a child with a severe and impairing psychiatric disorder, and they help parents to obtain needed educational and rehabilitation services (Asarnow & Asarnow, 1996).

## Learning Disorders

### Overview

A learning disorder, or learning disability, is a disorder in one or more of the basic psychological processes involved in understanding or in using language (spoken and written) that may manifest itself in an impaired ability to listen, speak, read, write, spell, or perform mathematical calculations. Although there is general agreement about this definition of learning disorders, there is a great deal of confusion how best to classify children using it (Beitchman & Young, 1997; Culbertson, 1998). For example, some definitions of learning disorders classify children according to the cognitive processes that interfere with acquiring basic academic skills. Using this approach, a broad distinction can be made between language-based or verbal disorders and perceptual-organizational or nonverbal disorders. However, many other distinctions can be made, depending on the cognitive processes assessed (Beitchman & Young, 1997; Swanson, Carson, & Saches-Lee, 1996). In contrast, other classification systems, like the DSM-IV, focus on the academic skills that are deficient in a child. The DSM-IV recognizes four learning disorders: Reading Disorder, Mathematics Disorder, Disorder of Written Expression, and Learning Disorder Not Otherwise Specified (American Psychiatric Association, 1994). These two different approaches to classification identify very different children because different processing deficits (e.g., visual-perceptual deficit or deficient verbal comprehension) can lead to delays in the same academic subject (e.g., reading) (Beitchman & Young, 1997).

Another difficulty involved in classifying learning disorders is the practice in many school systems of using a significant discrepancy between a child's intellectual abilities and academic achievement to diagnose a learning disorder. The rationale for this method is that the child's intelligence test score represents the child's "academic potential," and performance on a standardized test of achievement below this potential reveals the presence of a learning disorder. However, this method is flawed

for a number of reasons (See Culbertson, 1998; Kamphaus, Frick, & Lahey, 1991). First, it assumes that the child's score on an intelligence test would not be influenced by the processing deficit that caused the learning disorder and thereby provides a "pure" measure of the child's academic potential. Intelligence tests are designed to assess cognitive processes, so this assumption is tenuous. For example, a child with a verbal processing deficit is likely to have a lower score on an intelligence test due to this processing weakness. Second, scores on intelligence tests are correlated with scores on achievement tests. As a result, there are regressive effects at more extreme levels of intelligence that make larger discrepancies less meaningful at higher intelligence levels than at lower levels of intelligence and make smaller discrepancies more meaningful at lower intellectual levels. As a result of this, corrections have been developed to calculate differences between intelligence test scores and academic achievement to adjust for these regressive effects (e.g., Kamphaus et al., 1991).

### Epidemiology

These conceptual issues are critical for interpreting all of the research on learning disorders because the way learning disorders are defined can affect prevalence rates, comorbid disorders, and the causes of the disorder. This confusion is the reason that estimates of learning disorders range from 2–10% (American Psychiatric Association, 1994; Beitchman & Young, 1997), and some estimates are as high as 15% (Gaddes & Edgell, 1993). Although boys exhibit a higher incidence of learning disabilities than girls, this difference could be due to the fact that boys with learning disorders are more likely to exhibit comorbid behavior problems, which increases the likelihood that they will be referred for evaluation and treatment (Beitchman & Young, 1997; Culbertson, 1998).

### Comorbid Disorders

Several psychological disorders occur at higher rates in children with learning disorders than in normal children; these include hyperactivity, depression, social withdrawal, anxiety, language disorders, and somatic complaints (Beitchman & Young, 1997; Culbertson, 1998; Frick et al., 1991; Fuerst, Fisk, & Rourke, 1989; Porter & Rourke,

1985). For example, from 20–30% of children with learning disorders also have ADHD and between 10–50% of children with ADHD have learning disabilities (Hinshaw, 1992). However, it is important to note that a large number of children with learning disabilities (30–55%) do not show significant emotional or behavioral problems and there is no specific pattern of behavioral or emotional disturbance that is distinctive for children with learning disabilities (Fuerst, Fisk, & Rourke, 1989; Porter & Rourke, 1985; Speece, McKinney, & Appelbaum, 1995). One possible exception is the finding that children with nonverbal learning disabilities often have more social problems and difficulties interpreting social cues than children with language-based learning disorders (Rourke, 1988).

## Etiology

It is clear that learning disorders run in families. In a review of the literature, Pennington (1990; Pennington & Smith, 1988) found that from 35–40% of sons of learning-disordered parents were affected; the risk to daughters was approximately 18%. There is also mounting evidence of a genetic component in this transmission, at least for certain types of learning disorders. For example, twin and adoption studies in combination with genetic linkage studies have suggested that deficits in phonological awareness leading to one type of reading disability may be linked to chromosome 6 and deficits with single-word reading may be linked to chromosomee 15 (Pennington, 1990).

One of the most popular etiological theories for learning disorders is the neuropsychological approach which proposes that learning disorders result from neuroanatomical and/or neurofunctional deficits. The location of the dysfunction determines the specific cognitive processing problems that affect a child's abilities to learn (e.g., visual-perceptual problems, perceptual-motor problems, sequencing deficits) (Beitchman & Young, 1997; Hynd & Willis, 1988). A second common theory views learning disorders as a consequence of deficits in psycholinguistic functioning (e.g., impaired phonological processing skills or deficits in manipulating individual speech sounds) (e.g., Torgesen, 1986). However, advances in our understanding of learning disorders have been limited by the lack of agreement on classifying children with these disorders.

## Prognosis and Treatment

In general, learning disorders persist though late adolescence and adulthood (Maughan & Hagell, 1996). Specific academic deficits, such as deficits in reading comprehension, word recognition skills, phonological coding, and reading speed, continue to be present for a number of adults previously diagnosed as learning disordered (see Beitchman & Young, 1997, for a review). In addition, there is some evidence that psychosocial functioning may also be impaired in adulthood; learning disordered individuals are at risk of educational failure, poorer occupational achievement, and emotional disturbances (e.g., anxiety and depression) (Spreen, 1988). A summary of these longitudinal studies estimated that about one-third of individuals who experienced reading disorders as children experience adult psychosocial problems and those affected as adults often had the most severe forms of learning disorders (Beitchman & Young, 1997; Maughan & Hagell, 1996). Unfortunately, these longitudinal studies have yet to document any consistent relationship between intervention for the learning disorder in childhood and improved adult outcome.

Intervention strategies for children with learning disabilities vary greatly and heavily depend on the way these disorders are conceptualized (Ingersol & Goldstein, 1993). For example, treatment strategies that originate from neuropsychological theories advocate using instruction designed to emphasize intact processing capabilities to bypass processing weaknesses. Treatment approaches based on the psycholinguistic model of learning disabilities involve including a language-based curriculum that teaches children specific linguistic skills that are components of general reading skills (e.g., analyzing phonological structure of words, use of sound-symbol relations; Lyon & Moats, 1988; Torgesen, 1986). A recent meta-analysis by Swanson et al. (1996) found that cognitive interventions (e.g., problem-solving skills, solution strategies, self-monitoring) show some of the greatest effects of treatment ($d = 1.07$) for children with learning disorders, followed by direct instruction (e.g., structured learning, corrective feedback; $d = .91$) and remedial instruction (e.g., phonic, letter-sound associations; $d = .68$) (see also Lloyd, Hallahan, Kaufmann, & Keller, 1998, for a description of other treatment options).

# Elimination Disorders

## Enuresis

Enuresis is urinary incontinence that occurs in a child after an age at which urinary control is typically attained and in the absence of organic pathology. The DSM-IV requires repeated voiding of urine at least twice a week for at least three months in children age 5 years or older for a diagnosis (American Psychiatric Association, 1994). Enuresis can be diurnal, which is daytime wetting, or the more common nocturnal form, which is wetting the bed at night. Reviews of the literature indicate that approximately 15–20% of 5-year-olds, 7–15% of 7-year-olds, 5–7% of 9- to 10-year-olds, and 2–4% of 12- to 14-year-olds suffer from nocturnal enuresis (Costello et al., 1996; Doleys, 1977; Shaffer et al., 1996; Walker, Milling, & Bonner, 1988). In contrast, diurnal enuresis is much less prevalent; approximately 6% of 6-year-olds and 1% of children between the ages of 7–17 show this type of enuresis (Walker et al., 1988). A distinction is also made between primary enuresis, in which a significant period of bladder control has never been achieved, and secondary enuresis, in which urinary incontinence occurs after a period of bladder control. Primary enuresis accounts for approximately 85% of all cases of enuresis (de Jonge, 1973). In general, boys suffer from enuresis approximately twice as often as girls (Costello et al., 1997; Mellon & Stern, 1998).

A number of organic factors, such as neurological pathology, structural abnormalities, urinary or bladder infections, and diabetes can cause urinary incontinence (Walker et al., 1988; Werry, 1986). For this reason, children with enuresis, especially secondary diurnal enuresis, should have a physical evaluation to rule out physical causes for the incontinence. By definition, however, enuresis occurs in the absence of such an organic dysfunction. Nevertheless, there is a fairly strong genetic component in enuresis (Bakwin, 1973), and this may be related to a smaller functional bladder capacity that is transmitted across generations (Muellner, 1960). Although some have speculated that children with enuresis may have differences in their sleep patterns such as "heavy sleeping" that lead them to miss bodily cues to use the bathroom, research has not consistently shown differences in the sleep architecture of enuretic children (Ondersma & Walker, 1998).

In addition to biological theories of enuresis, some authors have focused on learning mechanisms such as the failure of the child to learn to control the urination reflex adequately and to discriminate cues necessary to inhibit urination to reach the bathroom (Walker et al., 1988). One psychological theory that has not been supported by research is the role of an emotional disturbance in causing enuresis. Well-controlled studies have indicated that, although enuretic children show a higher rate of anxiety, family disruption, and other stressful events than nonenuretic children, the vast majority of enuretic children do not suffer from emotional disturbance (Ondersma & Walker, 1998; Walker et al., 1988; Werry, 1986).

Although approximately 15% of untreated enuretic children attain bladder control each year (de Jong, 1973; Forsyth & Redmond, 1974; Lyman, Schierberl, & Roberts, 1992), a large proportion of children with this problem continues to exhibit enuresis for extended periods of time, and they experience increasing impairment in social functioning as they get older. Several psychopharmacological interventions have been tested with children; the most common is the tricyclic antidepressant, imipramine. Controlled studies suggest that 85% of enuretic children treated with imipramine improve within 2 weeks. Unfortunately, there are a number of side effects, and there is a very high relapse rate after discontinuing the medication (Ondersma & Walker, 1998).

Given the potential for side effects and the high relapse rate with medication, behavioral interventions have been very popular for treating enuresis. The urine alarm technique, introduced by Mowrer and Mowrer (1938), involves using a urine sensitive pad, placed in the child's bed or sewn into his or her pajamas, that activates an alarm or buzzer when wet. When the alarm is activated, the child is awakened and is instructed to go to the bathroom to finish voiding. Over time, the child begins to awaken before wetting and before activating the alarm. The urine alarm has an effectiveness rate that ranges from 60–90%, and although the initial relapse rate is rather high (41%), a short reintroduction of the alarm leads to rapid and sustained remission of the enuresis (Ondersma & Walker, 1998). A controlled study that compared treatment with imipramine to treatment with the urine alarm reported that use of the urine alarm produced a larger percentage of children who reached the cure criterion (e.g., fourteen dry nights), showed beneficial effects sooner, and resulted in children who were less likely to relapse (Wagner, Johnson, Walker, Carter, & Witmer, 1982).

## Encopresis

Encopresis is the second elimination disorder found in children. This is defined as fecal incontinence in a child past the age at which bowel control is expected and where no organic pathology can be found. According to the DSM-IV, a child age 4 years or older must show fecal incontinence at least once a month for at least three months to meet the criteria for encopresis (American Psychiatric Association, 1994). Like enuresis, encopresis can be diurnal or nocturnal and primary (continuous) or secondary (discontinuous). For encopresis, however, nocturnal soiling appears to be much less common than diurnal encopresis (Levine, 1975).

Research suggests that there are at least three major types of encopresis (Schroder & Gordon, 1991; Walker et al., 1988). Manipulative soiling involves a pattern of soiling that results in successful manipulation of the environment, such as avoiding school, avoiding parental punishment, or expressing anger. Irritable bowel syndrome involves expulsion of feces diarrhetically as a reaction to stress and emotional upset. Retentive encopresis, the third category, accounts for the vast majority of cases of encopresis (80–95%). In such cases, children become constipated for some reason (e.g., poor learning of toileting skills, poor diet, previous painful bowel movement, toilet phobia), and fecal material becomes impacted in the intestine, preventing full evacuation of fecal material. Fluid material from stomach and intestine seep around the blockage out of the anus leaving a stain in the child's clothing. Because of the extension of the intestine by the impacted fecal material, the child typically is unaware of the need to defecate.

It is estimated that encopresis occurs in approximately 0.3–0.8% of children (Costello et al., 1996; Lyman et al., 1992; Walker et al., 1989). The proportion of child referrals to psychiatric clinics who are encopretic ranges from 6–10% (Walker et al., 1988), whereas approximately 3% of referrals to pediatric clinics (Abrahamiam & Lloyd-Still, 1984; Levine, 1975) and 25% of referrals to pediatric gastroenterology clinics (Taitz, Wales, Urwin, & Molnar, 1986) are for encopresis. Males are predominant in encopretic samples, and male to female ratios range from 2:1 to 5:1 (Abrahamian & Lloyd-Still, 1984; American Psychiatric Association, 1994; Costello et al., 1996; Levine, 1975).

Early studies based on referrals to psychiatric clinics suggested that children with encopresis tended to show a typical personality style characterized by immaturity, excessive dependence, spitefulness, vindictiveness, and lack of creativity, and had families with an overcontrolling and rejecting mother and a weak, uninvolved, and ineffective father (Bemporad, Pfeifer, Gibbs, Cortner, & Bloom, 1971). Such characteristics are related to the fact that these were referrals to psychiatric clinics. Studies of children referred to general pediatric clinics have failed to find a typical personality style related to encopresis (Abrahamian & Lloyd-Still, 1984; Levine, 1975). These studies reported that only 20–30% of encopretic children show significant psychological disturbance. Thus, the general conclusion is that the data do not support a causal relationship between psychological disturbance and encopresis for many children (Walker et al., 1988).

In contrast to the large literature of well-controlled studies that document the effective treatment of enuresis, there are few such studies that tested the treatment of encopresis. This is unfortunate, given the very distressful circumstances confronting the encopretic child. Appropriate treatment for encopresis depends on the type of encopresis exhibited, which necessitates a thorough assessment of the child and family. Manipulative soiling is best treated by teaching parents how to eliminate reinforcers to the soiling, to reinforce appropriate toileting, and to teach the child more appropriate ways of controlling his or her environment (Walker et al., 1988). Irritable bowel syndrome or chronic diarrhea is related to stress and anxiety experienced by the child, and so treatment should focus on altering environmental sources of stress or teaching the child anxiety-reduction techniques (Walker et al., 1988). The most promising treatment for retentive encopresis is a combination of medical and behavioral approaches. Fireman and Koplewicz (1992) and Wright and Walker (1976) reported successful results using a two-stage treatment; stage one involves evacuating the impacted colon by using cathartics. In stage two, the child relearns control over bowel movements and appropriate toileting through the use of reinforcement and punishment. A complete program using such a two-stage approach can be found in Walker et al. (1988) and Schroder and Gordon (1991).

## Tic Disorders

Tics are involuntary, sudden, rapid, repetitive, nonrhythmic, unexpected, and purposeless muscular movements or vocal utterances (Evans, King, & Lechman, 1996). Tics can often be suppressed for brief periods and may be exacerbated by stress and fatigue (Evans et al., 1996). Tic disorders are commonly divided into four general categories: Tourette's Disorder, Chronic Motor or Vocal Tic Disorder, Transient Tic Disorder, and Tic Disorder Not Otherwise Specified (DSM-IV; American Psychiatric Association, 1994). Current research suggests that all four tic disorders can best be considered as a continuum, where Transient Tic Disorder is on the mild end and Tourette's Disorder is at the more severe end (Leckman & Cohen, 1991). Estimates of the prevalence of tic disorders suggest that from 2.9–5.9 per 10,000 individuals are affected (Apter et al., 1993; Burd, Kerbeshian, Wikenheiser, & Fisher, 1986; Caine et al., 1988); the male to female sex ratio is approximately 9:1 (Burd et al., 1986), and a typical onset is between the ages of 5 and 7 years (Leckman et al., 1987; Rapoport & Ismond, 1996).

Transient Tic Disorder is defined by the DSM-IV as single or multiple motor and/or vocal tics that occur many times a day, nearly every day, for at least 4 weeks, but for no longer than 12 consecutive months. In general, transient tics are the most common of all tic disorders. Fortunately, they also are the most benign of all tic disorders; they have a high rate of spontaneous remission, and little association is found with learning and behavioral disorders (Lerer, 1987). Chronic Motor or Vocal Tic Disorder is distinguished from Transient Tic Disorder primarily by its chronicity, that is, Chronic Tic Disorder is defined as either a motor or vocal tic, but not both, that occurs either continuously or intermittently throughout a period of more than 1 year (American Psychiatric Association, 1994).

Tourette's Disorder, the most severe of the tic disorders, is characterized by the presence of both motor and vocal tics with a course that lasts at least 1 year. Often, Tourette's Disorder begins with a single facial tic, usually eye blinking or eye rolling, between the ages of 5 to 9 years (Leckman et al., 1987), that later becomes complex and involves multiple muscle groups of the torso or legs (Lerer, 1987; Shapiro et al., 1988). Motor tics may involve echokinesis (imitation of movement of others) and copropraxia (vulgar or obscene gesturing). Vocal tics typically develop later than motor tics, between the ages of 9 and 12, and commonly include grunting, sniffing, snorting, barking, whistling, coughing, throat clearing, and humming (Bruun, 1988). More complex vocal tics, including coprolalia (involuntary utterances of obscene words), echolalia (repetition of others' words or phrases), and palilalia (repetition of one's own words or phrases), occur much less frequently; echolalia and palalia occur in less than 17% of children with Tourette's Disorder (Leckman et al., 1987). Coprolalia, one of the most commonly recognized symptoms of Tourette's Disorder and often the most disruptive symptom for the child, occurs even less frequently, and typically does not emerge until early adolescence (Shapiro et al., 1988; Shapiro & Shapiro, 1982).

Reviews of the literature on Tourette's Disorder have indicated that approximately half of the children with this disorder experience other emotional or behavioral difficulties such as Obsessive-Compulsive Disorder, Attention Deficit Hyperactivity Disorder, and learning disabilities (Bruun, 1984; Lerer, 1987; Pennington & Smith, 1988). Often children are referred for treatment due to the comorbid disorder rather than for the Tourette's Disorder itself, and this may lead to increased estimates of comorbidity in clinic samples (Apter et al., 1993). For example, a community-based sample of children with Tourette's Disorder found that only 12% of nonreferred children met the criteria for ADHD, compared to 50% in clinic-referred samples (Apter et al., 1993). Conversely, from 30–40% of children with Tourette's disorder are diagnosed with Obsessive-Compulsive Disorder in both clinic-referred and community samples (Apter et al., 1993; Peterson, Leckman, & Cohen, 1995).

The exact pathogenesis of Tourette's disorder is unknown. It is generally accepted, however, that the disorder requires a genetic predisposition and this may be a shared predisposition with Obsessive Compulsive Disorder (e.g., Sallee & Spratt, 1998). There is also evidence for neurochemical abnormalities in children with Tourette's Disorder, specifically in the dopaminergic pathways. Therefore, it is not surprising that the most effective treatments for Tourette's Disorder are dopamine angonists (e.g., haloperidol and pimozide) (Towbin & Cohen, 1996). Use of these medications results in a significant reduction in symptoms for the vast majority of patients (70–80%) (Shapiro, Shapiro, Young, & Feinberg, 1988). However, these medications do not completely eliminate symptoms, and there are numerous side effects associated with dopamine anatogonists even at low doses, including tardive-dyskinesia and extrapyramidal symptoms, which can affect from 34–42% of treated children (Sallee & Spratt, 1998).

Due to the side effects of most medications used in treating tic disorders and due to the continued presence of symptoms even under the best medical management, it is not surprising that psychosocial interventions are often advocated in combination with medication. Self-monitoring is frequently used to determine the frequency and severity of tics, and this procedure may result in some reductions in symptomatology (Thomas, Abrams, & Johnson, 1971). Other behavioral techniques that have been recommended for reducing tics include massed negative practice, contingency management, relaxation training, and habit reversal (Teichman & Eliahu, 1986; Walter & Carter, 1997). Schroder and Gordon (1991) present a comprehensive treatment protocol for treating tic disorders that includes many of these individual components, including self-monitoring, competing-response training, relaxation training, and contingency management.

## Selective Mutism

Selective mutism is characterized by the consistent failure of a child to speak in one or more social situations (American Psychiatric Association, 1994). In the DSM-IV-R, this disorder was termed elective mutism, and the definition included a "persistent refusal" to speak (American Psychiatric Association, 1987). However, in the change to the DSM-IV, the emphasis was changed to a "consistent failure" to speak, which is consistent with the current conceptualization that selective mutism is a disorder that originates from fear or anxiety, as opposed to a voluntary, oppositional disorder (Rapoport & Ismond, 1996).

In general, few empirical studies have investigated selectively mute children. However, two studies have found that school is the most common place for a child to be mute; nearly all children (88–89%) are selectively mute at school (Steinhausen & Juzi 1996; Wilkins, 1985). In addition, almost all selectively mute children were mute with adult strangers (89%), whereas less than half were mute with general groups of other children (42%), specific other children (34%), or family members (13%) (Steinhausen & Juzi, 1996). The typical onset of selective mutism is from 4–5 years of age, and boys tend to have a somewhat earlier onset than girls (Rapoport & Ismond, 1996; Steinhausen & Juzi, 1996).

Although a transient form of mutism is not uncommon in children, particularly when a child starts school (Brown & Lloyd, 1975), more persistent forms of selective mutism are quite rare, and estimates are as low as 0.8 per 1,000 (Fundudis, Kolvin, & Garside, 1979). Unlike most other behavioral disturbances in childhood, selectively mute girls outnumber boys at a ratio of approximately 1.6:1. Steinhausen and Juzi (1996) and Wilkins (1985) found several typical factors in selectively mute children. For example, approximately one-third of mute children evidenced premorbid speech and language disorders, and one-third to one-half were also diagnosed with separation anxiety disorder. In fact, comorbid internalizing problems are typically found with selectively mute children, and 85% are reportedly shy, 66% are reportedly anxious, and 36% are reportedly depressed (Steinhausen & Juzi, 1996).

Given the limited research on this form of psychopathology, it is not surprising that little is known about the clinical course and treatment of selective mutism. Kolvin and Fundudis (1981) found that a substantial proportion (approximately 42%) of their sample of selectively mute children showed significant improvement before the age of 10. Children who remain selectively mute after age 10 tend to have a very poor prognosis, and relatively few children improve with (Dummitt, Klein, Tancer, Asche, & Martin, 1996) or without treatment (Wilkins, 1985).

In general, the most common form of treatment is psychotherapy; psychotherapy as an intervention is offered to 42% of selectively mute children (Steinhausen & Juzi, 1996). Recently, fluoxetine has been used in clinical trials with some efficacy; however, the efficacy varied by age (Dummitt et al., 1996). Specifically, 93% of children under age 10 improved, whereas only 33% of children over age 10 improved, again suggesting that prognosis is much worse for selectively mute children over the age of 10. Past research has also shown the efficacy of operant procedures in treating children with selective mutism (Kratochwill, 1981; Lahey, 1973).

## Summary

In this chapter, we tried to provide an overview of some of the more common forms of childhood psychopathology. For some disorders, such as ADHD and Disruptive Behavior Disorders, there is a fairly substantial literature on the phenomenology, etiology, course, and treatment of the disorder. For other disorders, such as childhood depression, there is much less research. Generally, externalizing disorders have been the focus of more research than internalizing disorders because children with externalizing disorders are much more disruptive to those around them which leads to their more frequent referral to child mental health clinics. However, it is becoming increasingly clear that internalizing disorders, such as anxiety and depression, are more chronic and impairing in children than was once thought, making research on these disorders an important goal of child psychologists.

Another important issue that has become clear from research on childhood psychopathology is that comorbidity is the rule rather than the exception. Children who show significant emotional, behavioral, social, or learning disturbances are quite likely to have problems in multiple domains. This suggests that factors that make a child vulnerable to one type of disturbance also make a child vulnerable to other difficulties. However, some authors have suggested that the high degree of comorbidity among disorders could be an artifact of our imperfect methods of classifying psychopathology that create artificial boundaries among disorders (Lilienfeld, Waldman, & Israel, 1994). Whatever the reason for the high degree of comorbidity among the various forms of psychopathology, it is clear from our review of the research that comorbid conditions can greatly affect the presentation, course, and treatment of the primary disorder.

Another theme that emerged from this review is the fact that research is beginning to recognize the importance of classification for guiding advances in causal theories and for guiding advances in treating childhood psychopathology. Specifically, it has become increasingly clear that many disorders are not homogenous conditions with single causal pathways that lead to the disorder (e.g., Frick, 1998a,b). Instead, many disorders result from multiple causal pathways; each involves a distinct constellation of causal processes. As research begins to uncover more homogenous groups within the various childhood disorders, causal theories can be developed to explain the different causal mechanisms that underlie the behavior of the different subgroups, and treatments can be developed that are more specifically focused on the needs of children within a diagnostic category.

Finally, and perhaps most importantly, in summarizing the research on childhood psychopathology, it is clear that it is critical to embed theoretical models within a developmental context. Many disorders of childhood share common features with related disorders found in adults. However, throughout this chapter, we attempted to highlight important developmental differences in the way the disorders are manifested in children. Most of these differences can be understood within the context of the developmental challenges and tasks that children and adolescents face that lead to variations in presenting the disorders across development. Furthermore, advances in our causal theories of these conditions are likely to come from integrating our knowledge of normal developmental processes into our theories of the way these processes can deviate and lead to psychopathological conditions. Such a developmental perspective for understanding childhood psychopathology is critical for guiding future research in this area and for providing a sound scientific basis to develop more effective prevention and treatment programs for all of the childhood disorders.

## References

Abikoff, H. (1985). Efficacy of cognitive training interventions in hyperactive children: A critical review. *Clinical Psychology Review, 5,* 479–512.

Abikoff, H., & Klein, R. G. (1992). Attention-deficit hyperactivity disorder and conduct disorder: Comorbidity and implications for treatment. *Journal of Consulting and Clinical Psychology, 60,* 881–892.

Abrahamian, F. P., & Lloyd-Still, I. D. (1984). Chronic constipation in childhood: A longitudinal study of 186 patients. *Journal of Pediatric Gastroenterology and Nutrition, 3,* 460–467.

Achenbach, T. M. (1995). Empirically based assessment and taxonomy: Applications to clinical research. *Psychological Assessment, 7,* 261–274.

Achenbach, T. M., & Edelbrock, C. S. (1978). The classification of child psychopathology: A review and analysis of empirical efforts. *Psychological Bulletin, 85,* 1275–1301.

Agras, W. S., Chapin, H. N., & Oliveau, D. C. (1972). The natural history of phobias: Course and prognosis. *Archives of General Psychiatry, 26,* 315–317.

Allen, A. J., Leonard, H., & Swedo, S. E. (1995). Current knowledge of medications for the treatment of childhood anxiety disorders. *Journal of the American Academy of Child and Adolescent Psychiatry, 34,* 976–986.

American Psychiatric Association. (1980). *Diagnostic and statistical manual of mental disorders* (3rd ed.). Washington, DC: Author.

American Psychiatric Association. (1987). *Diagnostic and statistical manual of mental disorders* (3rd ed., rev.). Washington, DC: Author.

American Psychiatric Association. (1994). *Diagnostic and statistical manual of mental disorders* (4th ed.). Washington, DC: Author.

Anderson, J. C., Williams, S., McGee, R., & Silva, P. (1987). DSM-III disorders in preadolescent children. *Archives of General Psychiatry, 44,* 69–76.

Angold, A., & Costello, E. J. (1993). Depressive comorbidity in children and adolescents: Empirical, theoretical, and methodological issues. *American Journal of Psychiatry, 150,* 1779–1791.

Angold, A., Costello, E. J., & Worthman, C. M. (1998). Puberty and depression: The roles of age, pubertal status and pubertal timing. *Psychological Medicine, 28,* 51–61.

Applegate, B., Lahey, B. B., Hart, E. J., Biederman, J., Hynd, G. W., Barkley, R. A., Ollendick, T., Frick, P. J., Greenhill, L., McBurnett, K., Newcorn, J., Kerdyk, L., Garfinkel, B., Waldman, I., & Schaffer, D. (1994). Validity of the age-of-onset criterion for ADHD: A report from the DSM-IV field trials. *Journal of the American Academy of Child and Adolescent Psychiatry, 36,* 1211–1221.

Apter, A., Pauls, D. L., Bleich, A., Zohar, A. H., Kron, S., Ratzoni, G., Dycian, A., Kotrel, M., Wizman, A., Gadot, N., & Cohen, D. J. (1993). An epidemiologic study of Gilles de la Tourette's syndrome in Israel. *Archives of General Psychiatry, 50,* 734–738.

Arnold, L. E., Abikoff, H. B., Cantwell, D. P., Conners, C. K., Elliot, G., Greenhill, L. L., Hechtman, L., Hinshaw, S. P., Hoza, B., Jensen, P. S., Kraemer, H. C., March, J. S., Newcorn, J. H., Pelham, W. E., Richters, J. E., Schiller, E., Severe, J. B., Swanson, J. M., Vereen, D., & Wells, K. C. (1997). National institute of mental health collaborative multimodal treatment study of children with ADHD (the MTA). *Archives of General Psychiatry, 54,* 865–870.

Asarnow, J. R., & Asarnow, R. F. (1996). Childhood-onset schizophrenia. In E. J. Mash & R. A. Barkley (Eds.), *Childhood psychopathology* (pp. 340–361). New York: Guilford.

Asarnow, R., & Karatekin, C. (1998). Childhood-onset schizophrenia. In C. E. Coffey & R. A. Brumback (Eds.), *Textbook of pediatric neuropsychiatry* (pp. 617–646). Washington, DC: American Psychiatric Association.

August, G. J., & Stewart, M. A. (1983). Familial subtypes of childhood hyperactivity. *Journal of Nervous and Mental Disease, 171,* 362–368.

August, G. J., Stewart, M. A., & Holmes, C. S. (1983). A four year follow-up of hyperactive boys with and without conduct disorder. *British Journal of Psychiatry, 143,* 192–198.

Ayllon, T., Smith, D., & Rogers, M. (1970). Behavioral management of a school phobia. *Journal of Behavior Therapy and Experimental Psychiatry, 1,* 125–128.

Bakwin, H. (1973). The genetics of enuresis. In I. Kolvin, R. C. MacKeith, & R. Meadow (Eds.), *Bladder control and enuresis.* Philadelphia: W. B. Saunders.

Bandura, A., & Menlove, F. L. (1968). Factors determining vicarious extinction of avoidance behavior through symbolic modeling. *Journal of Personality and Social Psychology, 8,* 99–108.

Barkley, R. A. (1981). *Hyperactive children: A handbook for diagnosis and treatment.* New York: Guilford.

Barkley, R. A. (1990). Attention Deficit Disorders: History, definition, and diagnosis. In M. Lewis and S. M. Miller (Eds.), *Handbook of developmental psychopathology* (pp. 65–75). New York: Plenum.

Barkley, R. A. (1997). Behavioral inhibition, sustained attention and executive functions: Constructing a unifying theory of ADHD. *Psychological Bulletin, 121,* 65–94.

Barkley, R. A. (1998). Attention-deficit/hyperactivity disorder. In E. J. Mash & R. A. Barkley (Eds). *Child psychopathology* (pp. 63–112). New York: Guilford.

Barkley, R. A., & Cunningham, C. E. (1979). The effects of methylphenidate on the mother–child interactions of hyperactive children. *Archives of General Psychiatry, 36,* 201–208.

Barkley, R. A., DuPaul, G. J., & McMurray, M. B. (1991). Attention deficit disorder with and without hyperactivity: Clinical response to three dose levels of methylphenidate. *Pediatrics, 87,* 519–531.

Baron-Cohen, S., Cox, A., Baird, G., Swettenham, J., Nightengale, N., Morgan, K., Drew, A., & Charman, T. (1996). Psychological markers in the detection of autism in infancy in a large population. *British Journal of Psychiatry, 168,* 158–163.

Barrett, P. M., Dadds, M. R., & Rapee, R. M. (1996). Family treatment of childhood anxiety: A controlled trial. *Journal of Consulting and Clinical Psychology, 64,* 333–342.

Bauer, D. H. (1976). An exploratory study of developmental changes in children's fears. *Journal of Child Psychology and Psychiatry, 17,* 69–74.

Beitchman, J. H., & Young, A. R. (1997). Learning disorders with a special emphasis on reading disorders: A review of the past 10 years. *Journal of the American Academy of Child and Adolescent Psychiatry, 36,* 1020–1032.

Bell-Dolan, D. J. (1995). Social cue interpretation of anxious children. *Journal of Clinical Child Psychology, 24,* 1–10.

Bemporad, J. R., Pfeifer, C. M., Gibbs, L., Cortner, R. H., & Bloom, W. (1971). Characteristics of encopretic patients and their families. *Journal of the American Academy of Child Psychiatry, 10,* 272–292.

Bernstein, G. A., & Garfinkel, B. D. (1986). School phobia: The overlap of affective and anxiety disorders. *Journal of the American Academy of Child Psychiatry, 25,* 235–241.

Berry, C. A., Shaywitz, S. E., & Shaywitz, B. A. (1985). Girls with Attention Deficit Disorder: A silent minority? A report on behavioral and cognitive characteristics. *Pediatrics, 76,* 801–809.

Biedel, D. C., Christ, M. A. G., & Long, P. J. (1991). Somatic complaints in anxious children. *Journal of Abnormal Child Psychology, 19,* 659–670.

Biederman, J. (1998). Attention-deficit/hyperactivity disorder: A lifespan perspective. *Journal of Clinical Psychiatry, 59* (Suppl. 7), 4–16.

Biederman, J., Faraone, S. V., Taylor, A., Sienna, M., Williamson, S., & Fine, C. (1998). Diagnostic continuity between child and adolescent ADHD: Findings from a longitudinal clinical sample. *Journal of the American Academy of Child and Adolescent Psychiatry, 37,* 305–313.

Bird, H. R., Canino, G., Rubio-Stipec, M., Gould, M. S., Ribera, J., Sesman, M., Woodbury, M., Huertas-Goldman, S., Pagan, A., Sanchez-Lacay, A., & Moscoso, M. (1988). Estimates of the prevalence of childhood maladjustment in a community survey in Puerto Rico. *Archives of General Psychiatry, 45,* 1120–1126.

Birmaher, B., Ryan, N. D., Williamson, D. E., Brent, D. A., Kaufman, J., Dahl, R. E., Perel, J., & Nelson, B. (1996). Childhood and adolescent depression: A review of the past 10 years. Part I. *Journal of the American Academy of Child and Adolescent Psychiatry, 35,* 1427–1439.

Borduin, C. M., Mann, B. J., Cone, L. T., Henggeler, S. W., Fucci, B. R., Blaske, D. M., & Williams, R. A. (1995). Multisystemic treatment of serious juvenile offenders: Long term prevention of criminality and violence. *Journal of Consulting and Clinical Psychology, 63,* 569–578.

Brown, B. J., & Lloyd, H. (1975). A controlled study of children not speaking in school. *Journal of the Association of Workers with Maladjusted Children, 3,* 49–63.

Brown, R. T., Madan-Swain, A., & Baldwin, K. (1991). Gender differences in a clinic-referred sample of attention-deficit disordered children. *Child Psychiatry and Human Development, 22,* 111–128.

Bruun, R. D. (1984). Gilles de la Tourette's syndrome: An overview of clinical experience. *Journal of the American Academy of Child Psychiatry, 23,* 126–133.

Burd, L., Kerbeshian, J., Wikenheiser, M., & Fisher, W. (1986). A prevalence study of Gilles de la Tourette syndrome in North Dakota school-age children. *Journal of the American Academy of Child Psychiatry, 25,* 552–553.

Caine, E. O., McBride, M. C., Chiverton, P., Bamford, K. A., Rediess, S., & Shiao, J. (1988). Tourette's syndrome in Monroe County school children. *Neurology, 38,* 472–475.

Campbell, S. B. (1986). Developmental issues in childhood anxiety. In R. Gittelman (Ed.), *Anxiety disorders of childhood* (pp. 24–57). New York: Guilford.

Cantwell, D. P. (1983a). Depression in childhood: Clinical picture and diagnostic criteria. In D. R. Cantwell & G. A. Carlson (Eds.), *Affective disorders in childhood and adolescence—an update* (pp. 3–18). New York: Spectrum.

Cantwell, D. P. (1983b). Overview of etiological factors. In D. P. Cantwell & G. A. Carlson (Eds.), *Affective disorders in childhood and adolescence—an update* (pp. 206–210). New York: Spectrum.

Cantwell, D. P. (1996). Attention Deficit Disorder: A review of the past 10 years. *Journal of American Academy of Child and Adolescent Psychiatry, 35,* 978–987.

Cantwell, D. P., & Baker, L. (1992). Attention deficit disorder with and without hyperactivity: A review and comparison of matched groups. *Journal of the American Academy of Child Psychiatry, 31,* 432–438.

Capaldi, D. M. (1992). Co-occurrence of conduct problems and depressive symptoms in early adolescent boys: II. A 2-year follow-up at Grade 8. *Development and Psychopathology, 4,* 125–144.

Caputo, A. A., Frick, P. J., Brodsky, S. L. (in press). Family violence and juvenile sex offending: Potential mediating roles of psychopathic traits and negative attitudes toward women. *Criminal Justice and Behavior.*

Carlson, C. L., Lahey, B. B., & Frick, P. J. (1997). Attention deficit disorders: A review of research relevant to diagnostic classification. In T. A. Widiger, A. J. Frances, H. A. Pincus, R. Ross, M. B. First, & W. Davis (Eds.), *DSM-IV sourcebook,* Vol. 3 (pp. 163–188). Washington, DC: American Psychiatric Association.

Carlson, C. L., Lahey, B. B., & Neeper, R. (1986). Direct assessment of cognitive correlates of attention deficit disorders with and without hyperactivity. *Journal of Psychopathology and Behavioral Assessment, 8,* 69–86.

Chorpita, B. F., Albano, A. M., & Barlow, D. H. (1998). The structure of negative emotions in a clinical sample of children and adolescents. *Journal of Abnormal Psychology, 107,* 74–85.

Christian, R., Frick, P. J., Hill, N., Tyler, L. A., & Frazer, D. (1997). Psychopathy and conduct problems in children: II. Subtyping children with conduct problems based on their interpersonal and affective style. *Journal of the American Academy of Child and Adolescent Psychiatry, 36,* 233–241.

Ciaranello, A. L. & Ciaranello, R. D. (1995). The neurobiology of infantile autism. *Annual Review of Neuroscience, 18,* 101–128.

Cleckley, H. (1976). *The mask of sanity* (5th ed.). St. Louis, MO: Mosby.

Cobham, V. E., Dadds, M. R., & Spence, S. H. (1998). The role of parental anxiety in the treatment of childhood anxiety. *Journal of Consulting and Clinical Psychology, 66,* 893–905.

Cohen, P., Cohen, J., & Brook, J. (1993). An epidemiological study of disorders in late childhood and adolescence-II. Persistence of disorders. *Journal of Child Psychology and Psychiatry, 34,* 869–877.

Cohen, P., Cohen, J., Kasen, S., Velez, C. N., Hartmark, C., Johnson, J., Rojas, M., Brook, J., & Streuning, E. L. (1993). An epidemiological study of disorders in late childhood and adolescence-I. Age- and gender-specific prevalence. *Journal of Child Psychology and Psychiatry, 34,* 851–867.

Cohen, P., Velez, C. N., Kohn, M., Schwab-Stone, M., & Johnson, J. (1987). Child psychiatric diagnosis by computer algorithm: Theoretical issues and empirical tests. *Journal of the American Academy of Child and Adolescent Psychiatry, 26,* 631–638.

Coie, J. D., Dodge, K. A., & Kupersmidt, J. B. (1990). Peer group behavior and social status. In S. R. Asher & J. D. Coie (Eds.), *Peer rejection in childhood: Cambridge studies in social and emotional development* (pp. 17–59). New York: Cambridge University Press.

Cole, D. A., Truglio, R., & Peeke, L. (1997). Relation between symptoms of anxiety and depression in children: A multitrait-multimethod-multigroup assessment. *Journal of Consulting and Clinical Psychology, 65,* 110–119.

Conduct Problems Prevention Research Group. (1992). A developmental and clinical model for the prevention of conduct disorder: The FAST Track Program. *Development and Psychopathology, 4,* 509–527.

Conners, C. K., & Werry, J. S. (1979). Pharmacotherapy. In H. C. Quay & J. S. Werry (Eds.), *Psychopathological disorders of childhood,* (2nd ed.) New York: Wiley.

Costello, E. (1989). Developments in child psychiatry epidemiology. *Journal of the American Academy of Child Psychiatry, 28,* 836–841.

Costello, E. J., Angold, A., Burns, B. J., Stangl, D. K., Tweed, D. L., Erkanli, A., & Worthman, C. M. (1996). The Great Smoky Mountains Study of Youth: Goals, design, methods, and the prevalence of DSM-III-R disorders. *Archives of General Psychiatry, 53*, 1129–1136.

Costello, E. J., Costello, A. J., Edelbrock, C., Burns, B. B., Dulcan, M. K., Brent, D., & Janiszewski, S. (1999). Psychiatric disorders in pediatric primary care. *Archives of General Psychiatry, 45*, 1107–1116.

Costello, E. J., Farmer, E. M., Angold, A., Burns, B. J., & Erkanli, A. (1997). Psychiatric disorders among American Indian and white youth in Appalachia: The Great Smoky Mountains Study. *American Journal of Public Health, 87*, 827–832.

Crick, N. R., & Dodge, K. A. (1996). Social information processing mechanisms in reactive and proactive aggression. *Child Development, 67*, 993–1002.

Crick, N. R., & Grotpeter, J. K. (1995). Relational aggression, gender, and social-psychological adjustment. *Child Development, 66*, 710–722.

Culbertson, J. L. (1998). Learning disabilities. In T. H. Ollendick & M. Hersen (Eds.), *Handbook of child psychopathology*, 3rd ed. (pp. 117–156). New York: Plenum.

Dadds, M. R., Barrett, P. M., Rapee, R. M., & Ryan, S. (1996). Family process and child anxiety and aggression: An observational analysis. *Journal of Abnormal Child Psychology, 24*, 715–734.

Dawson, G., Frey, K., Panagiotides, H., Osterling, J., & Hessl, D. (1997). Infants of depressed mothers exhibit atypical frontal brain activity: A replication and extension of previous findings. *Journal of Child Psychology and Psychiatry, 38*, 179–186.

de Jonge, G. A. (1973). Epidemiology of enuresis: A survey of the literature. In I. Kolvin, R. C. MacKeith, & S. R. Meadow (Eds.), *Bladder control and enuresis*. Philadelphia: Lippincott.

Dixon, J. F., & Ahrens, A. H. (1992). Stress and attributional style as predictors of self-reported depression in children. *Cognitive Therapy and Research, 16*, 623–634.

Dodge, K. A., & Frame, C. L. (1982). Social cognitive biases and deficits in aggressive boys. *Child Development, 53*, 620–635.

Doleys, M. (1977). Behavioral treatments for nocturnal enuresis in children: A review of the recent literature. *Psychological Bulletin, 84*, 30–54.

Douglas, V. I. (1972). Stop, look, and listen: The problem of sustained attention and impulse control in hyperactive and normal children. *Canadian Journal of Behavioral Sciences, 4*, 259–282.

Douglas, V. I., & Peters, K. G. (1979). Toward a clear definition of the attention deficit in hyperactive children. In G. A. Hale & M. Lewis (Eds.), *Attention and cognitive development*. New York: Plenum.

Dummitt, E. S., Klein, R. G., Tancer, N. K., Asche, B., & Martin, J. (1996). Fluoxetine treatment of children with selective mutism: An open trial. *Journal of the American Academy of Child and Adolescent Psychiatry, 35*, 615–621.

Eme, R. F. (1992). Selective female affliction in the developmental disorders of childhood: A literature review. *Journal of Child Clinical Psychology, 21*, 354–364.

Emslie, G. J., Rush, J., Weinberg, W. A., Kowatch, R. A., Hughes, C. W., Carmody, T., & Rintelmann, J. (1997). A double-blind, randomized, placebo-controlled trial of fluox-etine in children and adolescents with depression. *Archives of General Psychiatry, 54*, 1031–1037.

Emslie, G. J., Weinberg, W. A., & Kowatch, R. A. (1998). Mood disorders. In C. E. Coffey & R. A. Brumback (Eds.), *Textbook of pediatric neuropsychiatry* (pp. 359–392). Washington, DC: American Psychiatric Association.

Eth, S., & Pynoos, R. S. (1985). *Posttraumatic stress disorder in children*. Washington, DC: American Psychiatric Press.

Evans, E. W., King, R. A., & Lechman, J. F. (1996). Tic Disorders. In Mash & Barkley (Eds.), *Child psychopathology* (pp. 436–454). New York: Guilford.

Farrington, D. P., Ohlin, L., & Wilson, J. Q. (1986). *Understanding and controlling crime*. Berlin: Springer-Verlag.

Finch, A. J., Lipovsky, J. A., & Casat, C. D. (1989). Anxiety and depression in children and adolescents: Negative affectivity or separate constructs? In P. C. Kendall & D. Watson (Eds.), *Anxiety and depression: Distinctive and overlapping features* (pp. 171–196). San Diego, CA: Academic Press.

Findling, R. L., & Dogin, J. W. (1998). Psychopharmacology of ADHD: Children and adolescents. *Journal of Clinical Psychiatry, 59 (Suppl. 7)*, 42–49.

Fireman, G., & Koplewicz, H. S. (1992). Short-term treatment of children with encopresis. *Journal of Psychotherapy Practice and Research, 1*, 64–71.

Flemming, J. E., Offord, D. R., & Boyle, M. H. (1993). Prevalence of childhood and adolescent depression in the community: Ontario Child Health Study. *Child and Adolescent Psychiatric Clinics of North America, 1*, 129–167.

Forsyth, W. L., & Redmond, A. (1974). Enuresis and spontaneous cure rate: Study of 1129 enuretics. *Archives of Disease in Childhood, 49*, 259–263.

Francis, G., Last, C. G., & Strauss, C. C. (1987). Expression of separation anxiety disorder: The roles of age and gender. *Child Psychiatry and Human Development, 18*, 82–89.

Frick, P. J. (1994). Family dysfunction and the disruptive behavior disorders: A review of recent empirical findings. In T. H. Ollendick & R. J. Prinz (Eds.), *Advances in clinical child psychology*, Vol. 16 (pp. 203–226). New York: Plenum.

Frick, P. J. (1998a). Callous-unemotional traits and conduct problems: Applying the two-factor model of psychopathy to children. In D. J. Cooke, A. Forth, & R. Hare, (Eds.), *Psychopathy: Theory, research, and implications for society* (pp. 161–188). Dordrecht, Netherlands: Kluwer Academic.

Frick, P. J., & Lahey, B. B. (1991). The nature and characteristics of attention deficit hyperactivity disorder. *School Psychology Review, 20*, 163–173.

Frick, P. J. (1998b). *Conduct disorders and severe antisocial behavior*. New York: Plenum.

Frick, P. J., & Loney, B. R. (1999). Outcomes of children and adolescents with oppositional defiant disorder and Conduct Disorder. In H. C. Quay & A. E. Hogan (Eds.), *Handbook of disruptive behavior disorders* (pp. 507–524). New York: Plenum.

Frick, P. J., Kamphaus, R. W., Lahey, B. B., Loeber, R., Christ, M. G., Hart, E. L., & Tannenbaum, L. E. (1991). Academic underachievement and the disruptive behavior disorders. *Journal of Consulting and Clinical Psychology, 59*, 289–294.

Frick, P. J., Lahey, B. B., Christ, M. A. G., Loeber, R., & Green, S. (1991). History of childhood behaviors problems in biological relatives of boys with Attention-Deficit Hyperactivity Disorder and Conduct Disorder. *Journal of Child Clinical Psychology, 20*, 445–451.

Frick, P. J., O'Brien, B. S., Wootton, J., & McBurnett, K. (1994). Psychopathy and conduct problems in children. *Journal of Abnormal Psychology, 103,* 700–707.

Fuerst, D. R., Fisk, J. L., & Rourke, B. P. (1989). Psychosocial functioning of learning-disabled children: Replicability of statistically derived subtypes. *Journal of Consulting and Clinical Psychology, 57,* 275–280.

Fundudis, T., Kolvin, I., & Garside, R. (1979). *Speech retarded and deaf children: Their psychological development.* London: Academic Press.

Gaddes, W. H., & Edgell, D. (1993). *Learning disabilities and brain function,* 3rd ed. New York: Springer Verlag.

Galdos, P. M., Van Os, J. J., & Murray, R. M. (1993). Puberty and onset of psychosis. *Schizophrenia Research, 10,* 7–14.

Garber, J. (1992). Cognitive models of depression: A developmental perspective. *Psychological Inquiry, 3,* 235–240.

Garber, J., Braafladt, N., & Zeman, J. (1991). The regulation of sad affect: An information-processing perspective. In J. Garger & K. Dodge (Eds.), *The development of emotional regulation and dysregulation* (pp. 208–240). New York: Cambridge University Press.

Gillberg, C. (1984). Infantile autism and other childhood psychoses in a Swedish urban region: Epidemiological aspects. *Journal of Child Psychology and Psychiatry, 25,* 35–43.

Gillberg, C. (1991). The treatment of epilepsy in autism. *Journal of Autism and Developmental Disorders, 21,* 61–77.

Gillberg, I. C., Hellgren, L., & Gillberg, C. (1993). Psychotic disorders diagnosed in adolescence. Outcome at age 30 years. *Journal of Child Psychology and Psychiatry, 34,* 1173–1185.

Gillberg, C., Steffenburg, S., & Schaumann, H. (1991). Is autism more common now than ten years ago? *British Journal of Psychiatry, 158,* 403–409.

Gittelman, R., Mannuzza, S., Shenker, R., & Bonegura, N. (1985). Hyperactive boys almost grown up. *Archives of General Psychiatry, 42,* 937–947.

Gittelman-Klein, R., Abikoff, H., Pollack, E., Klein, D. F., Katz, S., & Mattes, J. (1980). A controlled trial of behavior modification and methylphenidate in hyperactive children. In C. Whalen & B. Henker (Eds.), *Hyperactive children: The social ecology of identification and treatment.* New York: Academic Press.

Green, W. H., Campbell, M., Hardesty, A. S., Grega, D. M., Padron-Gayol, M., Shell, J., & Erlenmeyer-Kimling, L. (1984). A comparison of schizophrenic and autistic children. *Journal of the American Academy of Child Psychiatry, 23,* 399–409.

Green, W. H., Padron-Gayol, M., Hardesty, A. S., & Bassiri, M. (1992). Schizophrenia with childhood onset: A phenomenological study of 38 cases. *Journal of the American Academy of Child and Adolescent Psychiatry, 31,* 968–976.

Hammen, C., & Compas, B. E. (1994). Unmasking unmasked depression in children and adolescence: The problem of comorbidity. *Clinical Psychology Review, 14,* 585–603.

Hare, R. D. (1994). *Without conscience: The disturbing world of psychopaths among us.* New York: Simon & Schuster.

Hechtman, L. (1996). Attention-deficit/hyperactivity disorder. In L. Hechtman (Ed.), *Do they grow out of it? Long-term outcomes of childhood disorders* (pp. 17–38). Washington, DC: American Psychiatric Association.

Henggeler, S. W., & Borduin, C. M. (1990). *Family therapy and beyond: A multisystemic approach to teaching the behavior problems of children and adolescents.* Pacific Grove, CA: Brooks/Cole.

Henggeler, S. W., Melton, G. B., & Smith, L. A. (1992). Family preservation using multisystemic therapy: An effective alternative to incarcerating juvenile offenders. *Journal of Consulting and Clinical Psychology, 60,* 953–961.

Henggeler, S. W., Schoenwald, S. K., & Pickrel, S. G. (1995). Multisystemic therapy: Bridging the gap between university- and community-based treatment. *Journal of Consulting and Clinical Psychology, 63,* 709–718.

Hinden, B. R., Compas, B. E., Howell, D. C., & Achenbach, T. M. (1997). Covariation of the anxious-depressed syndrome during adolescence: Separating fact from artifact. *Journal of Consulting and Clinical Psychology, 65,* 6–14.

Hinshaw, S. P. (1987). On the distinction between attentional deficits/hyperactivity and conduct problems/aggression in child psychopathology. *Psychological Bulletin, 101,* 443–463.

Hinshaw, S. P. (1991). Stimulant medication and the treatment of aggression in children with attention deficits. *Journal of Clinical Child Psychology, 20,* 301–312.

Hinshaw, S. P. (1992). Externalizing behavior problems and academic underachievement in childhood and adolescence: Causal relationships and underlying mechanisms. *Psychological Bulletin, 111,* 127–155.

Hinshaw, S. P., Heller, T., & McHale, J. P. (1992). Covert antisocial behavior in boys with attention-deficit hyperactivity disorder: External validation and effects of methylphenidate. *Journal of Consulting and Clinical Psychology, 60,* 274–281.

Hinshaw, S. P., Lahey, B. B., & Hart, E. L. (1993). Issues of taxonomy and comorbidity in the development of Conduct Disorder. *Development and Psychopathology, 5,* 31–49.

Hirshfeld, D. R., Rosenbaum, J. F., Biederman, J., Bolduc, E. A., Fararone, S. V., Snidman, N., Reznick, J. S., & Kagan, J. (1992). Stable behavioral inhibition and its association with anxiety disorder. *Journal of the American Academy of Child and Adolescent Psychiatry, 31,* 103–111.

Horn, W. E., & Ialongo, N. (1988). Multimodal treatment of attention deficit hyperactivity disorder in children. In H. E. Fitzgerald, B. M. Lester, & M. W. Yogman (Eds.), *Theory and research in behavioral pediatrics,* Vol. 4 (pp. 175–220). New York: Plenum.

Hynd, G. W., & Willis, W. G. (1988). *Pediatric neuropsychology.* New York: Grune & Stratton.

Hynd, G. W., Hern, K. L., Novey, E. S., Eliopulos, D., Marshall, R., Gonzales, J. J., & Voeller, K. K. (1993). Attention-deficit hyperactivity disorder and asymmetry of the caudate nucleus. *Journal of Child Neurology, 8,* 339–347.

Ingersol, B. D., & Goldstein, S. (1993). *Attention deficit disorder and learning disabilities: Realities, myths, and controversial treatments.* New York: Main Street Books, Doubleday.

Jacobsen, L. K., & Rapoport, J. L. (1998). Childhood-onset schizophrenia: Implications of clinical and neurobiological research. *Journal of Child Psychology and Psychiatry, 39,* 101–112.

James, A., & Taylor, E. (1990). Sex differences in the hyperkinetic syndrome of childhood. *Journal of Child Psychology and Psychiatry, 31,* 437–446.

Jensen, P. S., Martin, D., & Cantwell, D. P. (1997). Comorbidity in ADHD: Implications for research, practice, and DSM-V. *Journal of the American Academy of Child and Adolescent Psychiatry, 36,* 1065–1079.

Jensen, P. S., Wanatabe, H. K., Richters, J. E., Roper, M., Hibbs, E. D., Salzberg, A. D., & Liu, S. (1996). Scales, diagnoses, and child psychopathology: II. Comparing the CBCL and the DISC against external validators. *Journal of Abnormal Child Psychology, 24*, 151-168.

Kagan, J., & Snidman, N. (1991). Temperamental factors in human development. *American Psychologist, 46*, 856-862.

Kagan, J., Reznick, J. S., & Snidman, N. (1987). The physiology and psychology of behavioral inhibition in children. *Child Development, 58*, 1459-1473.

Kagan, J., Reznick, J. S., Clarke, C., Snidman, N., & Garcia-Coll, C. (1984). Behavioral inhibition to the unfamiliar. *Child Development, 55*, 2212-2225.

Kamphaus, R. W., & Frick, P. J. (1996). *The clinical assessment of children's emotion, behavior, and personality.* Boston: Allyn & Bacon.

Kamphaus, R. W., Frick, P. J., & Lahey, B. B. (1991). Methodological issues and learning disabilities diagnosis in clinical populations. *Journal of Learning Disabilities, 24*, 613-618.

Kashani, J. H., Allen, W. D., Beck, N. C., Bledsoe, Y., & Reid, J. C. (1997). Dysthymic disorder in clinically referred preschool children. *Journal of the American Academy of Child Psychiatry, 36*, 1426-1433.

Kashani, J. H., Beck, N. C., Hoeper, E. W., Fallahi, C., Corcoran, C. M., MacAllister, J. A., Rosenberg, T. K., & Reid, J. C. (1987). Psychiatric disorders in a community sample of adolescents. *American Journal of Psychiatry, 144*, 584-589.

Kaslow, N. J., & Thompson, M. P. (1998). Applying the criteria for empirically supported treatments to studies of psychosocial interventions for child and adolescent depression. *Journal of Clinical Child Psychology, 27*, 146-155.

Kazdin, A. E., Siegel, T. C., & Bass, D. (1990). Drawing on clinical practice to inform research on child and adolescent psychotherapy: Survey of practitioners. *Professional Psychology: Research and Practice, 21*, 189-198.

Kearney, C. A. (1995). School refusal behavior. In A. R. Eisen, C. A. Kearney, & C. A. Schaefer (Eds.), *Clinical handbook of anxiety disorders in children and adolescents* (pp. 251-281). Northvale, NJ: Jason Aronson.

Keenan, K., Loeber, R., Zhang, Q., Stouthamer-Loeber, M., & Van Kammen, W. B. (1995). The influence of deviant peers on the development of boys' disruptive and delinquent behavior: A temporal analysis. *Development and Psychopathology, 7*, 715-726.

Kendall, P. C., (1994). Treating anxiety disorders in children: A controlled trial. *Journal of Consulting and Clinical Psychology, 62*, 100-110.

Kendall, P. C., Flannery-Schroeder, E., Panichelli-Mindel, S. M., Southam-Gerow, M., Henin, A., & Warren, M. (1997). Therapy for youths with anxiety disorders: A second randomized clinical trial. *Journal of Consulting and Clinical Psychology, 65*, 366-380.

Kennedy, W. A. (1965). School phobia: Rapid treatment of fifty cases. *Journal of Abnormal Psychology, 70*, 285-289.

Klinger, L. G., & Dawson, G. (1996). Autistic disorder. In E. J. Mash & R. A. Barkley (Eds). *Child psychopathology* (pp. 311-339). New York: Guilford.

Klinteberg, B. A., Andersson, T., Magnusson, D., & Stattin, H. (1993). Hyperactive behavior childhood as related to subsequent alcohol problems and violent offending: A longitudinal study of male subjects. *Personality and Individual Differences, 15*, 381-388.

Kochanska, G. (1993). Toward a synthesis of parental socialization and child temperament in early development of conscience. *Child Development, 64*, 325-347.

Kohlberg, L., LaCrosse, J., & Ricks, D. (1972). The predictability of adult mental health from childhood behavior. In B. B. Wolman (Ed.), *Manual of child psychopathology.* New York: McGraw-Hill.

Kolvin, I., & Fundudis, I. (1981). Elective mute children: Psychological development and background factors. *Journal of Child Psychology and Psychiatry, 22*, 219-232.

Kovacs, M., Feinberg, T. L., Crouse-Novak, M. A., Paulauskas, S. L., & Finkelstein, R. (1984a). Depressive disorders in childhood: I. A longitudinal prospective study of characteristics and recovery. *Archives of General Psychiatry, 41*, 229-237.

Kovacs, M., Feinberg, T. L., Crouse-Novak, M. A., Paulauskas, S. L., Pollock, M., & Finkelstein, R. (1984b). Depressive disorders in childhood: II. A longitudinal study of the risk for a subsequent major depression. *Archives of General Psychiatry, 41*, 643-649.

Kratochwill, T. R. (1981). *Selective mutism: Implications for research and treatment.* Hillsdale, NJ: Erlbaum.

Kratzer, L., & Hodgins, S. (1997). Adult outcomes of child conduct problems: A cohort study. *Journal of Abnormal Child Psychology, 25*, 65-81.

Kreusi, M. J. P., Rappaport, J. L., Hamburger, S., Hibbs, E., Potter, W. Z., Lenane, M., & Brown, G. L. (1990). Cerebrospinal fluid monamine metabolites, aggression, and impulsivity in disruptive behavior disorders of children and adolescents. *Archives of General Psychiatry, 47*, 419-426.

Kumra, S., Frazier, J. A., Jacobsen, L., McKenna, K., Gordon, C. T., Lenane, M. C., Hamburger, S. D., Smith, A. K., Albus, K. E., Alaghband-Rad, J., & Rapoport, J. L. (1997). Childhood-onset schizophrenia: A double-blind clozapine-haloperidol comparison. *Archives of General Psychiatry, 53*, 1090-1097.

Lahey, B. B. (1973). *The modification of language behavior.* Springfield, IL: Charles C. Thomas.

Lahey, B. B., & Loeber, R. (1997). Attention-deficit/hyperactivity disorder, oppositional defiant disorder, and adult antisocial behavior: A life span perspective. In D. M. Stoff, J. Breiling, & D. Maser (Eds.), *Handbook of antisocial behavior* (pp. 51-59). New York: Wiley.

Lahey, B. B., Strauss, C. C., & Frame, C. L. (1984). Are attention deficit disorders with and without hyperactivity similar or dissimilar disorders? *Journal of the American Academy of Child and Adolescent Psychiatry, 23*, 302-309.

Lahey, B. B., Schaughency, E. A., Hynd, G. W., Carlson, C. L., & Nieves, N. (1987). Attention deficit disorder with and without hyperactivity: Comparison of behavioral characteristics of clinic-referred children. *Journal of the American Academy of Child and Adolescent Psychiatry, 26*, 718-723.

Lahey, B. B., Piacentini, J. C., McBurnett, K., Stone, P., Hartdagen, S. E., & Hynd, G. (1988). Psychopathology and antisocial behavior in the parents of children with conduct disorder and hyperactivity. *Journal of the American Academy of Child and Adolescent Psychiatry, 27*, 163-170.

Lahey, B. B., Russo, M. E., Walker, J. L., & Piacentini, J. C. (1989). Personality characteristics of the mothers of children with disruptive behavior disorders. *Journal of Consulting and Clinical Psychology, 57*, 512-515.

Lahey, B. B., Applegate, B., McBurnett, K., Biederman, J., Greenhill, L., Hynd, G. W., Barkley, R. A., Newcorn, J.,

Jensen, P., Richters, J., Garfinkel, B., Kerdyk, L., Frick, P. J., Ollendick, T., Perzez, D., Hart, E. J., Waldman, I., & Schaffer, D. (1994). DSM-IV field trials for attention deficit hyperactivity disorder in children and adolescents. *American Journal of Psychiatry, 151,* 1673–1685.

Lahey, B. B., Loeber, R., Hart, E. L., Frick, P. J., Applegate, B., Zhang, Q., Green, S. M., & Russo, M. F. (1995). Four-year longitudinal study of conduct disorder in boys: Patterns and predictors of persistence. *Journal of Abnormal Psychology, 104,* 83–93.

Lahey, B. B., McBurnett, K., Loeber, R., & Hart, E. L. (1995). Psychobiology of conduct disorder. In G. P. Sholevar (Ed.), *Conduct disorders in children and adolescents: Assessments and interventions* (pp. 27–44). Washington, DC: American Psychiatric Press.

Lahey, B. B., Loeber, R., Quay, H. C., Frick, P. J., & Grimm, J. (1997). Oppositional defiant disorder and conduct disorder. In T. A. Widiger, A. J. Francis, H. A. Pincus, R. Ross, M. B. First, & W. Davis (Eds.), *DSM-IV sourcebook* Vol. 3 (pp. 189–209). Washington, DC: American Psychiatric Association.

Lahey, B. B., Pelham, W. E., Stein, M. A., Loney, J., Trapani, C., Nugent, K., Kipp, H., Schmidt, E., Lee, S., Cale, M., Gold, E., Hartung, C. M., Willcott, E., & Baumann, B. (1988). Validity of DSM-IV attention deficit/hyperactivity disorder for younger children. *Journal of the American Academy of Child and Adolescent Psychiatry, 37,* 695–702.

Last, C. G., & Strauss, C. C. (1990). School refusal in anxiety-disordered children and adolescents. *Journal of the American Academy of Child and Adolescent Psychiatry, 29,* 31–35.

Last, C. G., Francis, G., Hersen, M., Kazdin, A. E., & Strauss, C. C. (1987). Separation anxiety and school phobia: A comparison using DSM-III criteria. *American Journal of Psychiatry, 144,* 653–657.

Last, C. G., Hersen, M., Kazdin, A. E., Finkelstein, R., & Strauss, C. C. (1987). Comparison of the DSM-III separation anxiety and overanxious disorder: Demographic characteristics and patterns of comorbidity. *Journal of the American Academy of Child and Adolescent Psychiatry, 26,* 527–531.

Last, C. G., Hersen, M., Kazdin, A. E., Francis, G., & Grubb, H. J. (1987). Psychiatric illness in the mothers of anxious children. *American Journal of Psychiatry, 144,* 1580–1583.

Last, C. G., Francis, G., & Strauss, C. C. (1989). Assessing fears in anxiety-disordered children with the Revised Fear Survey Schedule for Children (FSSC-R). *Journal of Clinical Child Psychology, 18,* 137–141.

Lavigne, J. V., Gibbons, R. D., Christoffel, K. K., Arend, R., Rosenbaum, D., Binns, H., Dawson, N., Sobel, H., & Isaacs, C. (1996). Prevalence rates and correlates of psychiatric disorders among preschool children. *Journal of the American Academy of Child and Adolescent Psychiatry, 35,* 204–214.

Leckman, J. F., & Cohen, D. J. (1991). Clonidine treatment of Gilles de la Tourette's syndrome. *Archives of General Psychiatry, 48,* 324–328.

Leckman, J. F., Walkup, J. T., Riddle, M. A., & Cohen, D. J. (1987). Tic disorders. In H. Y. Meltzer, W. Bunney, J. Coyle, J. David, I. Kopin, C. Schuster, R. Shader, & G. Simpson (Eds.), *Psychopharmacology, the third generation of progress* (pp. 1239–1246). New York: Raven Press.

Lefkowitz, M. M., & Burton, N. (1978). Childhood depression: A critique of the concept. *Psychological Bulletin, 85,* 716–726.

Lerer, R. J. (1987). Motor tics, Tourette syndrome, and learning disabilities. *Journal of Learning Disabilities, 20,* 266–267.

Levine, M. D. (1975). Children with encopresis: A descriptive analysis. *Pediatrics, 56,* 412–416.

Lewinsohn, P. M., Clarke, G. N., Hops, H., & Andrews, J. (1990). Cognitive-behavioral treatment for depressed adolescents. *Behavior Therapy, 21,* 385–401.

Lewinsohn, P. M., Hops, H., Roberts, R. E., Seeley, J. R., & Andrews, J. A. (1993). Adolescent psychopathology: I. Prevalence and incidence of depression and other DSM-III-R disorders in high school students. *Journal of Abnormal Psychology, 102,* 133–144.

Lewinsohn, P. M., Rohde, P., Seeley, J. R., & Fischer, S. A. (1993). Age-cohort changes in the lifetime occurrence of depression and other mental disorders. *Journal of Abnormal Psychology, 102,* 110–120.

Lewinsohn, P. M., Clarke, G. N., Selley, J. R., & Rohde, P. (1994). Major depression in community adolescents: Age at onset, episode duration, and time to recurrence. *Journal of the American Academy of Child and Adolescent Psychiatry, 36,* 809–818.

Lilienfeld, S. O., Waldman, I. D., & Israel, A. C. (1994). A critical examination of the use of the term and concept of comorbidity in psychopathology research. *Clinical Psychology: Science and Practice, 1,* 71–99.

Lloyd, J. W., Hallahan, D. P., Kauffman, J. M., & Keller, C. E. (1998). Academic problems. In R. J. Morris & T. R. Kratochwill (Eds.), *The practice of child therapy,* (3rd ed., pp. 167–198). Boston: Allyn & Bacon.

Loeber, R., Brinthaupt, V. P., & Green, S. M. (1990). Attention deficits, impulsivity, and hyperactivity with or without conduct problems: Relationships to delinquency and unique contextual factors. In R. J. McMahon & R. D.V. Peters (Eds.), *Behavior disorders of adolescence: Research, intervention, and policy in clinical and school setting* (pp. 39–61). New York: Plenum.

Loeber, R., & Stouthamer-Loeber, M. (1986). Family factors as correlates and predictors of juvenile conduct problems and delinquency. In M. Tonry & N. Morris (Eds.), *Crime and justice,* Vol. 7. Chicago: University of Chicago Press.

Loney, J., Langhorne, J. E., & Paternite, C. E. (1978). An empirical basis for subgrouping the hyperkinetic/minimal brain dysfunction syndrome. *Journal of Abnormal Psychology, 87,* 431–444.

Loney, J., & Milich, R. (1982). Hyperactivity, inattention, and aggression in clinical practice. In M. Woolraich & D. Routh (Eds.), *Advances in developmental and behavioral pediatrics,* Vol. 3. Greenwich, CT: JAI.

Lord, C., & Schopler, E. (1987). Neurobiological implications of sex differences in autism. In E. Schopler & G. B. Mesibov (Eds.), *Neurobiological issues in autism* (pp. 191–211). New York: Plenum.

Lou, H. C., Henriksen, L., & Bruhn, P. (1984). Focal cerebral hypoperfusion in children with dysphasia and/or attention deficit disorder. *Archives of Neurology, 41,* 825–829.

Lou, H. C., Henriksen, L., Bruhn, P., Borner, H., & Neilsen, J. B. (1989). Striatal dysfunction in attention deficit and hyperkinetic disorder. *Archives of Neurology, 46,* 48–52.

Lovaas, O. I. (1987). Behavioral treatment and normal educational and intellectual functioning in young autistic children. *Journal of Consulting and Clinical Psychology, 55,* 3–9.

Lyman, R. D., Schierberl, J. P., & Roberts, M. C. (1992). Enuresis and encopresis. In J. L. Matson (Ed.), *Handbook of treatment approaches in childhood psychopathology* (pp. 397–428). New York: Plenum.

Lynam, D. R. (1996). Early identification of chronic offenders: Who is the fledgling psychopath? *Psychological Bulletin, 120,* 209–234.

Lynsky, M. T., & Fergusson, D. M. (1995). Childhood conduct problems, attention deficit behaviors, and adolescent alcohol, tobacco, and illicit drug use. *Journal of Abnormal Child Psychology, 23,* 281–302.

Lyon, G. R., & Moats, L. C. (1988). Critical issues in the instruction of the learning disabled. *Journal of Consulting and Clinical Psychology, 56,* 830–835.

Magnusson, D. (1988). Aggressiveness, hyperactivity, and autonomic activity/reactivity in the development of social maladjustment. In D. Magnusson (Ed.), *Individual development from an interactional perspective: A longitudinal study* (pp. 152–172). Hillsdale, NJ: Erlbaum.

Mannuzza, S., & Gittelman, R. (1984). The adolescent outcome of hyperactive girls. *Psychiatry Research, 13,* 19–29.

Mannuzza, S., Klein, R. G., Konig, P. H., & Giampino, T. L. (1989). Hyperactive boys almost grown up: IV. Criminality and its relationship to psychiatric status. *Archives of General Psychiatry, 46,* 1073–1079.

Maughan, B., & Hagell, A. (1996). Poor readers in adulthood: Psychosocial functioning. *Development and Psychopathology, 8,* 457–476.

Maughan, B., Pickles, A., Hagell, A., Rutter, M., & Yule, W. (1996). Reading problems and antisocial behaviour: Developmental trends in comorbidity. *Journal of Child Psychology and Psychiatry, 37,* 405–418.

McBride, P. A., Anderson, G. M., Hertzig, M. E., Snow, M. E., Thompson, S. M., Khait, V. D., Shapiro, T., & Cohen, D. J. (1998). Effects of diagnosis, race, and puberty on platelet serotonin levels in autism and mental retardation. *Journal of the American Academy of Child and Adolescent Psychiatry, 37,* 767–776.

McBurnett, K., Lahey, B. B., Frick, P. J., Risch, C., Loeber, R., Hart, E. L., Christ, M. A. G., & Hanson, K. S. (1991). Anxiety, inhibition, and conduct disorder in children: I. Relation to salivary cortisol. *Journal of the American Academy of Child and Adolescent Psychiatry, 30,* 192–196.

McCord, W., & McCord, J. (1964). *The psychopath: An essay on the criminal mind.* Princeton, NJ: Van Nostrand.

McCracken, J. T. (1998). Attention-deficit/hyperactivity disorder II: Neuropsychiatric aspects. In C. E. Coffey & R. A. Brumback (Eds.), *Textbook of pediatric neuropsychiatry* (pp. 483–501). Washington, DC: American Psychiatric Association.

McGee, R., et al. (1990). DSM-III disorders in a large sample of adolescents. *Journal of the American Academy of Child and Adolescent Psychiatry, 29,* 611–619.

McGee, R., Feehan, M., Williams, S., & Anderson, J. (1992). DSM-III disorders from age 11 to age 15 years. *Journal of the American Academy of Child and Adolescent Psychiatry, 31,* 50–59.

Mellon, M. W., & Stern, H. P. (1998). Elimination disorders. In R. T. Ammerman & J. V. Campo (Eds.), *Handbook of pediatric psychology and psychiatry: Vol. 1. Psychological and psychiatric issues in the pediatric setting* (pp. 182–198). Boston: Allyn & Bacon.

Menzies, R. G., & Clarke, J. C. (1995). The etiology of phobia: A nonassociative account. *Journal of the American Academy of Child and Adolescent Psychiatry, 29,* 50–59.

Mesibov, G. B. (1997). Formal and informal measures on the effectiveness of the TEACCH program. *Autism, 1,* 25–35.

Mesibov, G. B., Adams, L. W., & Kinger, L. G. (1997). *Autism: Understanding the disorder.* New York: Plenum.

Mitchell, J., McCauley, E., Burke, R. M., & Moss, S. J. (1988). Phenomenology of depression in children and adolescents. *Journal of the American Academy of Child and Adolescent Psychiatry, 27,* 12–20.

Moffitt, T. E. (1993). Adolescence-limited and life-course-persistent antisocial behavioral: A developmental taxonomy. *Psychological Review, 100,* 674–701.

Mowrer, O. H. (1939). A stimulus-response theory of anxiety and its role as reinforcing agent. *Psychological Review, 46,* 553–565.

Mowrer, O. H., & Mowrer, W. M. (1938). Enuresis: A method for its study and treatment. *American Journal of Orthopsychiatry, 8,* 436–459.

Muellner, S. R. (1960). Development of urinary control in children. *Journal of the American Medical Association, 172,* 714–716.

Muris, P., Meesters, C., Merckelbach, H., Sermon, A., & Zwakhalen, S. (1998). Worry in normal children. *Journal of the American Academy of Child and Adolescent Psychiatry, 37,* 703–710.

Nolen-Hoeksema, S., & Girgus, J. S. (1994). The emergence of gender differences in depression and adolescence. *Psychological Bulletin, 115,* 424–443.

O'Brien, B. S., & Frick, P. J. (1996). Reward dominance: Associations with anxiety, conduct problems, and psychopathy in children. *Journal of Abnormal Child Psychology, 24,* 223–240.

O'Brien, B. S., Frick, P. J., & Lyman, R. D. (1994). Reward dominance among children with disruptive behavior disorders. *Journal of Psychopathology and Behavioral Assessment, 16,* 131–145.

Offord, D. R., Adler, R. J. M., & Boyle, M. H. (1986). Prevalence of sociodemographic correlates of conduct disorder. *The American Journal of Social Psychiatry, 6,* 272–278.

Offord, D. R., Boyle, M. H., Szatmari, P., Rae-Grant, N. I., Links, P. S., Cadman, D. R., Byles, I. A., Crawford, I. W., Blum, H. M., Byrne, C., Thomas, H., & Woodward, C. A. (1987). Ontario child health study. *Archives of General Psychiatry, 44,* 832–836.

Offord, D. R., Boyle, M. H., & Racine, Y. (1989). Ontario child health study: Correlates of disorder. *Journal of the American Academy of Child and Adolescent Psychiatry, 28,* 856–860.

Offord, D. R., Boyle, M. H., Racine, Y. A., Fleming, J. E., Cadman, D. T., Blum, H. M., Byrne, C., Links, P. S., Lipman, E. L., MacMillan, H. L., Grant, N. I. R., Sanford, M. N., Szatmari, P., Thoms, H., & Woodward, C. (1992). Outcome, prognosis, and risk in a longitudinal follow-up study. *Journal of the American Academy of Child and Adolescent Psychiatry, 31,* 916–923.

Ollendick, T. H., & King, N. J. (1998). Empirically supported treatments for children with phobic and anxiety disorders: Current status. *Journal of Clinical Child Psychology, 27,* 156–167.

Olweus, D., Mattesson, A., Schalling, D., & Low, H. (1988). Circulating testosterone levels and aggression in adolescent males: A causal analysis. *Psychosomatic Medicine, 50,* 261–272.

Ondersma, S. J., & Walker, C. E. (1998). Elimination disorders. In T. H. Ollendick & M. Hersen (Eds.) *Handbook of child psychopathology* (3rd ed., pp. 355–378). New York: Plenum.

Ornitz, E. M. (1989). Autism. In C. G. Last & M. Hersen (Eds.)., *Handbook of child psychiatric diagnosis* (pp. 233–278). New York: Wiley.

Osterling, J., & Dawson, G. (1994). Early recognition of children with autism: A study of the first birthday home videotapes. *Journal of Autism and Developmental Disorders, 24,* 247–257.

Panak, W. F., & Garber, J. (1992). Role of aggression, rejection, and attributions in the prediction of depression in children. *Development and Psychopathology, 4,* 145–166.

Pelham, W. E. (1987). What do we know about the use and effects of CNS stimulants in the treatment of ADD? In J. Loney (Ed.), *The young hyperactive child: Answers to questions about diagnosis, prognosis, and treatment.* New York: Haworth.

Pelham, W. E., Bender, M. E., Caddell, J., Booth, S., & Moorer, S. H. (1985). Methylphenidate and children with attention deficit disorder: Dose effects on classroom academic and social behavior. *Archives of General Psychiatry, 42,* 948–952.

Pelham, W. E., Walker, J. L., Sturges, J., & Hoya, J. (1989). Comparative effects of methylphenidate in ADD girls and ADD boys. *Journal of the American Academy of Child and Adolescent Psychiatry, 28,* 773–776.

Pelham, W. E., Carlson, C., Sams, S. E., Vallan, G., Dixon, M. J., & Hoza, B. (1993). Separate and combined effects of methylphenidate and behavior modification on boys with attention deficit-hyperactivity disorder in the classroom. *Journal of Consulting and Clinical Psychology, 61,* 506–515.

Pelham, W. E., Wheeler, T., & Chronis, A. (1998). Empirically supported psychosocial treatments for attention deficit hyperactivity disorder. *Journal of Clinical Child Psychology, 27,* 190–205.

Pennington, B. F. (1990). The genetics of dyslexia. *Journal of Child Psychology and Psychiatry, 31,* 193–201.

Pennington, B. E., & Smith, S. D. (1988). Genetic influences on learning disabilities: An update. *Journal of Consulting and Clinical Psychology, 56,* 817–823.

Peterson, B. D., Leckman, J. F., & Cohen, D. J. (1995). Tourette's syndrome: A genetically predisposed and an environmentally specified developmental psychopathology. In D. Cicchetti & D. J. Cohen (Eds.), *Developmental psychopathology,* Vol. 2: *Risk, disorder and adaptation* (pp. 213–242). New York: Wiley.

Pfiffner, L. J., & O'Leary, S. G. (1993). School-based psychological treatments. In J. L. Mattson (Ed.), *Handbook of hyperactivity in children* (pp. 234–245). Boston: Allyn & Bacon.

Pliska, S. R. (1998). Comorbidity of attention-deficit/hyperactivity disorder with psychiatric disorder: An overview. *Journal of Clinical Psychiatry, 59*(Suppl. 7), 50–58.

Porrino, L., I., Rapoport, J. L., Behar, D., Sceery, W., Ismond, D. R., & Bunney, W. E. (1983). A naturalistic assessment of the motor activity of hyperactive boys. *Archives of General Psychiatry, 40,* 681–687.

Porter, J., & Rourke, B. P. (1985). Socio-emotional functioning of learning disabled children: A subtypal analysis of personality patterns. In B. P. Rourke (Ed.), *Neuropsychology of learning disabilities: Essentials of subtype analysis* (pp. 257–279). New York: Guilford.

Prins, P. J. M., Groot, M. J. M., & Hanewald, G. J. F. P. (1994). Cognition in test-anxious children: The role of on-task and coping cognition reconsidered. *Journal of Consulting and Clinical Psychology, 62,* 404–409.

Puig-Antich, J., Blau, S., Marx, N., Greenhill, L. L., & Chambers, W. (1978). Prepubertal major depressive disorder. *Journal of the American Academy of Child Psychiatry, 78,* 695–707.

Puig-Antich, J., Goetz, D., Davies, M., Kaplan, T., Davies, S., Ostrow, L., Asnis, L., Twomey, J., Iyengar, S., & Ryan, N. D. (1989). A controlled family history study of prepubertal major depressive disorder. *Archives of General Psychiatry, 46,* 406–418.

Puig-Antich, J., Perel, I. M., Lupatkin, W., Chambers, W. J., Tabrizi, M. A., King, J., Goetz, R., Davies, M., & Stiller, R. L. (1987). Imipramine in prepubertal major depressive disorders. *Archives of General Psychiatry, 44,* 81–89.

Pynoos, R. S., Frederick, C., Nader, K., Arroyo, W., Steinberg, A., Eth, S., Nunez, F., & Fairbanks, L. (1987). Life threatening and posttraumatic stress in school-age children. *Archives of General Psychiatry, 44,* 1057–1063.

Quay, H. C. (1986). Classification. In H. C. Quay & J. S. Werry (Eds.), *Psychopathological disorders of childhood,* 3rd ed. (pp. 1–34). New York: Wiley.

Quay, H. C., Routh, A. K., & Shapiro, S. K. (1987). Psychopathology of childhood: From description to validation. *Annual Reviews in Psychology, 38,* 491–532.

Raine, A., Venables, P. H., & Williams, M. (1990). Relationships between central and autonomic measures of arousal at age 15 and criminality at age 24 years. *Archives of General Psychiatry, 47,* 1003–1007.

Rapoport, J. L., Giedd, J., Kumra, S., Jacobsen, L., Smith, A., Lee, P., Nelson, J., & Hamburger, S. (1997). Childhood-onset schizophrenia: Progressive ventricular change during adolescence. *Archives of General Psychiatry, 54,* 897–903.

Rapoport, J. L., & Ismond, D. R. (1996). *DSM-IV training guide for diagnosis of childhood disorders.* New York: Brunner/Mazel.

Reeves, J. C., Werry, J. S., Elkind, G. S., & Zametkin, A. (1987). Attention deficit, conduct, oppositional, and anxiety disorders in children: Clinical characteristics. *Journal of the American Academy of Child and Adolescent Psychiatry, 26,* 144–155.

Reid, A. H. (1983). Psychiatry of mental handicap. *Journal of the Royal Society of Medicine, 76,* 587–592.

Reiss, S. (1991). Expectancy model of fear, anxiety, and panic. *Clinical Psychology Review, 11,* 141–154.

Richters, J. E., Arnold, L. E., Jensen, P. S., Abikoff, H. B., Conners, C. K., Greenhill, L. L., Hechtman, L., Hinshaw, S. P., Pelham, W. E., & Swanson, J. M. (1995). NIMH collaborative multisite multimodal treatment study of children with ADHD: I. Background and rational. *Journal of the American Academy of Child and Adolescent Psychiatry, 34,* 987–1000.

Riddle, K. D,. & Rapoport, J. L. (1976). A two-year follow-up of 72 hyperactive boys. *Journal of Nervous and Mental Disease, 162,* 126–134.

Rie, H. E. (1966). Depression in childhood: A survey of some pertinent contributors. *Journal of the American Academy of Child Psychiatry, 5,* 653–685.

Robins, L. N. (1966). *Deviant children grown up.* Baltimore: Williams & Wilkins.

Rogers, S. J. (1998). Empirically supported comprehensive treatments for young children with autism. *Journal of Clinical Child Psychology, 27,* 168–179.

Rosenbaum, J. F., Biederman, J., Gersten, M., Hirshfeld, D. R., Meminger, S. R., Herman, J. B., Kagan, J., Reznick, J. S.,

Snidman, N. (1988). Behavioral inhibition in children of parents with panic disorder and agoraphobia: A controlled study. *Archives of General Psychiatry, 45*, 463–470.

Rothbart, M. K. (1989). Temperament in childhood: A framework. In G. A. Kohnstamm, J. A. Bates, & M. K. Rothbart (Eds.), *Temperament in childhood* (pp. 59–73). New York: Wiley.

Rourke, B. P. (1988). Socioemotional disturbances of learning disabled children. *Journal of Consulting and Clinical Psychology, 56*, 801–810.

Russo, M. F., & Biedel, D. C. (1994). Comorbidity of childhood anxiety and externalizing disorders: Prevalence, associated characteristics, and validation issues. *Clinical Psychology Review, 14*, 199–221.

Rutter, M. (1976). *Helping troubled children*. New York: Plenum.

Rutter, M. (1983). Behavioral studies: Questions and findings on the concept of a distinctive syndrome. In M. Rutter (Ed.), *Developmental neuropsychiatry* (pp. 259–279). New York: Guilford.

Rutter, M. (1990). Changing patterns of psychiatric disorders during adolescence. In J. Bancroft & J. M. Reinisch (Eds.), *Adolescence and puberty* (pp. 124–145). New York: Oxford University Press.

Rutter, M., Graham, P., Chadwick, O., & Yule, W. (1976). Adolescent turmoil: Fact or fiction. *Journal of Child Psychology and Psychiatry, 17*, 35–56.

Ryan, N. D., Puig-Antich, J., Ambrosini, R., Rabinovich, H., Robinson, A., Nelson, B., Iyengar, S., & Tworney, J. (1987). The clinical picture of major depression in children and adolescents. *Archives of General Psychiatry, 44*, 854–861.

Sallee, F. R., & Gill, H. S. (1998). Neuropsychopharmacology III: Psychostimulants. In C. E. Coffey & R. A. Brumback (Eds.), *Textbook of pediatric neuropsychiatry* (pp. 393–428). Washington, DC: American Psychiatric Association.

Sallee, F. R., & Spratt, E. G. (1998). Tics and Tourette's disorder. In T. H. Ollendick & M. Hersen (Eds.), *Handbook of child psychopathology*, 3rd ed. (pp. 337–353). New York: Plenum.

Sandberg, S. T., Weiselberg, M., & Shaffer, D. (1980). Hyperkinetic and conduct problem children in a primary school population: Some epidemiological considerations. *Journal of Child Psychology and Psychiatry, 21*, 293–312.

Satterfield, J. H., Satterfield, B. T., & Schell, A. M. (1987). Therapeutic interventions to prevent delinquency in hyperactive boys. *Journal of the American Academy of Child and Adolescent Psychiatry, 26*, 56–64.

Scerbo, A., & Kolko, D. J. (1994). Salivary testosterone and cortisol in disruptive children: Relationship to aggressive, hyperactive, and internalizing behavior. *Journal of the American Academy of Child and Adolescent Psychiatry, 33*, 1174–1184.

Schmidt, K., Solant, M. V., & Bridget, W. H. (1985). Electrodermal activity of undersocialized aggressive children: A pilot study. *Journal of Child Psychology and Psychiatry, 25*, 653–660.

Schreibman, L., & Charlop-Christy, M. H. (1998). Autistic disorder. In T. H. Ollendick & M. Hersen (Eds.), *Handbook of child psychopathology*, 3rd ed. (pp. 157–179). New York: Plenum.

Schroder, C. S., & Gordon, B. N. (1991). *Assessment and treatment of childhood problems*. New York: Guilford.

Seidman, L. J., Biederman, J., Farone, S. V., Weber, W., Mennin, D., & Jones, J. (1997). A pilot study of neuropsychological functioning in girls with ADHD. *Journal of the American Academy of Child and Adolescent Psychiatry, 36*, 366–373.

Seligman, M. (1975). *Helplessness: On depression, development, and death*. San Francisco: W. H. Freeman.

Semrud-Clikeman, M., Biederman, J., Sprich-Buckminster, S., Lehman, B. K., Farone, S. V., & Norman, D. (1992). Comorbidity between ADDH and learning disability: A review and report in a clinically referred sample. *Journal of the American Academy of Child and Adolescent Psychiatry, 31*, 439–448.

Shaffer, D., Fisher, P., Dulcan, M. K., Davies, M., Piacentini, J., Schwab-Stone, M. E., Lahey, B. B., Bourdon, K., Jensen, P. S., Bird, H. R., Canino, G., & Regier, D. A. (1996). The NIMH diagnostic interview schedule for children version 2.3 (DISC-2.3): Description, acceptability, prevalence rates, and performance in the MECA study. *Journal of the American Academy of Child and Adolescent Psychiatry, 35*, 865–877.

Shapiro, A. K., & Shapiro, E. (1982). An update in Tourette's syndrome. *American Journal of Psychiatry, 36*, 379–389.

Shapiro, E., Shapiro, A. K., Young, J. G., & Feinberg, T. E. (1988). *Gilles de la Tourette's syndrome*. New York: Raven Press.

Siassi, I. (1982). Lithium treatment of impulsive behavior in children. *Journal of Psychiatry, 43*, 341–356.

Silverman, W. K., & Ginsburg, G. S. (1998). Anxiety disorders. In T. H. Ollendick (Ed.), *Handbook of child psychopathology* (pp. 239–268). New York: Plenum.

Silverthorn, P., & Frick, P. J. (1999). Developmental pathways to antisocial behavior: The delayed-onset pathways in girls. *Development and Psychopathology, 11*, 101–126.

Silverthorn, P., Frick, P. J., Kuper, K., & Ott, J. (1996). Attention deficit hyperactivity disorder and sex: A test of two etiological models to explain the male predominance. *Journal of Clinical Child Psychology, 25*, 52–59.

Simeon, J. E., Dinicola, V. F., Ferguson, H. B., & Copping, W. (1995). Adolescent depression: A placebo-controlled fluoxetine study and follow up. *Progress in Neuropsychopharmacology and Biological Psychiatry, 14*, 791–795.

Simonoff, E., Pickles, A., Meyer, J. M., Silberg, J. L., Maes, H. H., Loeber, R., Rutter, M., Hewitt, J. K., & Eaves, L. J. (1997). The Virginia twin study of adolescent behavioral development: Influences of age, sex, and impairment of rates of disorders. *Archives of General Psychiatry, 54*, 801–808.

Smalley, S. L., Asarnow, R. F., & Spence, A. (1988). Autism and genetics: A decade of research. *Archives of General Psychiatry, 45*, 953–961.

Smalley, S. L., Levitt, J., & Bauman, M. (1998). Autism. In C. E. Coffey & R. A. Brumback (Eds.), *Textbook of pediatric neuropsychiatry* (pp. 393–428). Washington, DC: American Psychiatric Association.

Solanto, M. V., & Conners, C. K. (1982). A dose-response and time-action analysis of autonomic and behavioral effects of methylphenidate in attention deficit disorder with hyperactivity. *Psychophysiology, 19*, 657–658.

Speece, D. L., McKinney, J. D., & Appelbaum, M. I. (1985). Classification and validation of behavioral subtypes of learning-disabled children. *Journal of Educational Psychology, 77*, 67–77.

Spencer, E. K., Kafantaris, V., Padron-Gayol, M. V., & Rosenberg, C. R. (1992). Haloperidol in schizophrenic children:

Early findings from a study in progress. *Psychopharmacology Bulletin, 28*, 183–186.

Spreen, O. (1988). Prognosis of learning disability. *Journal of Consulting and Clinical Psychology, 56*, 836–842.

Steinhausen, H., & Juzi, C. (1996). Elective mutism: An analysis of 100 cases. *Journal of the American Academy of Child and Adolescent Psychiatry, 35*, 606–614.

Stewart, M. A., Cummings, C., Singer, S., & deBlois, C. S. (1981) The overlap between hyperactive and unsocialized aggressive children. *Journal of Child Psychology and Psychiatry, 22*, 35–45.

Stewart, M. A., deBlois, C. S., & Cummings, C. (1980). Psychiatric disorder in the parents of hyperactive boys and those with conduct disorder. *Journal of Child Psychology and Psychiatry, 21*, 283–292.

Strauss, C. C., Frame, C. L., & Forehand, R. (1987). Psychosocial impairment associated with anxiety in children. *Journal of Clinical Child Psychology, 16*, 235–239.

Strauss, C. C., Lahey, B. B., Frick, P. J., Frame, C. L., & Hynd, G. W. (1988). Peer social status of children with anxiety disorders. *Journal of Consulting and Clinical Psychology, 56*, 137–141.

Strauss, C. C., Last, C. G., Hersen, M., & Kazdin, A. E. (1988). Association between anxiety and depression in children and adolescents with anxiety disorders. *Journal of Abnormal Child Psychology, 16*, 57–68.

Strauss, C. C., Lease, C. A., Last, C. G., & Francis, G. (1988). Overanxious disorder: An examination of developmental differences. *Journal of Abnormal Child Psychology, 16*, 433–443.

Strauss, C. C., Lease, C. A., Kazdin, A. E., Dulcan, M. K., & Last, C. G. (1989). Multimethod assessment of the social competence of children with anxiety disorders. *Journal of Consulting and Clinical Psychology, 18*, 184–189.

Swanson, H. L., Carson, C., & Saches-Lee, C. M. (1996). A selective synthesis of intervention research for students with learning disabilities. *School Psychology Review, 25*, 370–391.

Szatmari, P. (1997). Pervasive developmental disorder not otherwise specified. In T. A. Widiger, A. J. Francis, H. A. Pincus, R. Ross, M. B. First, & W. Davis (Eds.), *DSM-IV sourcebook*, Vol. 3 (pp. 43–55). Washington, DC: American Psychiatric Association.

Szatmari, P., Jones, M. B., Tuff, L., Bartolucci, G., Fishman, S., & Mahoney, W. (1993). Lack of cognitive impairment in first-degree relatives of children with pervasive developmental disorders. *Journal of the American Academy of Child and Adolescent Psychiatry, 32*, 1264–1273.

Taitz, L. S., Wales, J. K. H., Urwin, O. M., & Molnar, D. (1986). Factors associated with outcome in management of defecation disorders. *Archives of Disease in Childhood, 61*, 472–477.

Tannock, R. (1998). Attention deficit hyperactivity disorder: Advances in cognitive, neurobiological, and genetic research. *Journal of Child Psychology and Psychiatry, 29*, 65–99.

Teichman, Y., & Eliahu, D. (1986). A combination of structural family therapy and behavioral techniques in treating a patient with two tics. *Journal of Clinical Child Psychology, 15*, 311–316.

Thomas, E. J., Abrams, K. S., & Johnson, J. B. (1971). Self-monitoring and reciprocal inhibition in the modification of multiple tics in Gilles de la Tourette's syndrome. *Journal of Behavior Therapy and Experimental Psychiatry, 2*, 159–171.

Thompson, L. L., Riggs, P. D., Mikulich, S. K., & Crowley, T. J. (1996). Contribution of ADHD symptoms to substance problems and delinquency in conduct-disordered adolescents. *Journal of Abnormal Child Psychology, 24*, 325–348.

Torgesen, J. K. (1986). Learning disabilities theory: Its current state and future prospects. *Journal of Learning Disabilities, 19*, 399–407.

Towbin, K. E., & Cohen, D. J. (1996). Tic disorders. In J. M. Weiner (Ed.), *Diagnosis and psychopharmacology of childhood and adolescent disorders*, 2nd ed. New York: Wiley.

Treadwell, K. R., & Kendall, P. C. (1996). Self-talk in youth with anxiety disorders: States of mind, content specificity, and treatment outcome. *Journal of Consulting and Clinical Psychology, 64*, 941–950.

Tsai, L. Y., Stewart, M. A., Faust, M., & Shook, S. (1982). Social class distribution of fathers of children enrolled in the Iowa Autism Program. *Journal of Autism and Developmental Disorders, 12*, 211–221.

Turner, J. E., & Cole, D. A. (1994). Developmental differences in cognitive diatheses for child depression. *Journal of Abnormal Child Psychology, 22*, 15–32.

Van Kammen, W. B., Loeber, R., & Stouthamer-Loeber, M. (1991). Substance use and its relationship to conduct problems and delinquency in young boys. *Journal of Youth and Adolescence, 20*, 399–413.

Verhulst, F. C., & Endhe, J. V. D. (1992). Six-year developmental course of internalizing and externalizing problem behaviors. *Journal of the American Academy of Child and Adolescent Psychiatry, 31*, 924–931.

Verhulst, F. C., Koot, H. M., & Berden, G. F. M. G. (1990). Four-year follow-up of an epidemiological sample. *Journal of the American Academy of Child and Adolescent Psychiatry, 29*, 440–448.

Verhulst, F. C., Ende, J. V. D., Ferdinand, R. F., & Kasius, M. C. (1997). The prevalence of DSM-III-R diagnoses in a national sample of Dutch adolescents. *Archives of General Psychiatry, 54*, 329–336.

Volkmar, F. R. (1996). Childhood and adolescent psychosis: A review of the past 10 years. *Journal of the American Academy of Child and Adolescent Psychiatry, 35*, 843–851.

Volkmar, F. R., Klin, A., Marans, W. D., & McDougle, C. J. (1996). Autistic disorder. In F. R. Volkmar (Ed.), *Psychoses and pervasive developmental disorders in childhood and adolescence* (pp. 129–190). Washington, DC: American Psychiatric Association.

Volkmar, F. R., & Rutter, M. (1995). Childhood disintegrative disorder: Results of the DSM-IV autism field trial. *Journal of the American Academy of Child and Adolescent Psychiatry, 34*, 1092–1095.

Wagner, W., Johnson, S. B., Walker, D., Carter, R., & Witmer, J. (1982). A controlled comparison of two treatments for nocturnal enuresis. *Journal of Pediatrics, 101*, 302–307.

Walker, C. E., Milling, L. S., & Bonner, B. L. (1988). Incontinence disorders: Enuresis and encopresis. In D. K. Routh (Ed.), *Handbook of pediatric psychology* (pp. 363–398). New York: Guilford.

Walker, J. L., Lahey, B. B., Hynd, G. W., & Frame, C. L. (1987). Comparison of specific patterns of antisocial behavior in children with conduct disorder with or without coexisting hyperactivity. *Journal of Consulting and Clinical Psychology, 55*, 910–913.

Walker, J. L., Lahey, B. B., Russo, M. F., Frick, P. J., Christ, M.

A. G., McBurnett, K., Loeber, R., Stouthamer-Loeber, M., & Green, S. M. (1991). Anxiety, inhibition and conduct disorder in children: I. Relations to social impairment. *Journal of the American Academy of Child and Adolescent Psychiatry, 30*, 187–191.

Walter, A. L., & Carter, A. S. (1997). Gilles de la Tourette's syndrome in childhood: A guide for school professionals. *School Psychology Review, 26*, 28–46.

Weiss, G., & Hechtman, L. (1993). *Hyperactive children grown up*, 2nd ed. New York: Guilford.

Weiss, G., Hechtman, L., Milroy, T., & Perlman, T. (1985). Psychiatric status of hyperactives as adults: A controlled prospective 15-year follow-up of 63 hyperactive children. *Journal of the American Academy of Child Psychiatry, 24*, 211–220.

Werry, J. S. (1986). Physical illness, symptoms, and allied disorders. In H. C. Quay & J. S. Werry (Eds.), *Psychopathological disorders of childhood*, 3rd ed. (pp. 232–293). New York: Wiley.

Werry, J. S. (1996a). Childhood schizophrenia. In F. R. Volkmar (Ed.), *Psychoses and pervasive developmental disorders in childhood and adolescence* (pp. 1–48). Washington, DC: American Psychiatric Association.

Werry, J. S. (1996b). Pervasive development, psychotic, and allied disorders. In L. Hechtman (Ed.), *Do they grow out of it? Long-term outcomes of childhood disorders* (pp. 195–223). Washington, DC: American Psychiatric Association.

Werry, J. S. (1997). Early-onset schizophrenia. In T. A. Widiger, A. J. Francis, H. A. Pincus, R. Ross, M. B. First, & W. Davis (Eds.), *DSM-IV sourcebook*, Vol. 3 (pp. 55–66). Washington, DC: American Psychiatric Association.

Werry, J. S., & McClellan, J. M. (1992). Predicting outcome in child and adolescent (early onset) schizophrenia and bipolar disorder. *Journal of the American Academy of Child and Adolescent Psychiatry, 31*, 147–150.

Werry, J. S., McClellan, M. J., & Chard, L. (1991). Childhood and adolescent schizophrenic, bipolar, and schizoaffective disorders: A clinical and outcome study. *Journal of the American Academy of Child and Adolescent Psychiatry, 30*, 457–465.

Whalen, C. K., Henker, B., Buhrmester, D., Hinshaw, S. P., Huber, A., & Laski, K. (1989). Does stimulant medication improve the peer status of hyperactive children? *Journal of Consulting and Clinical Psychology, 57*, 545–549.

Wilkins, R. (1985). A comparison of elective mutism and emotional disorders in children. *British Journal of Psychiatry, 146*, 198–203.

Wilson, W. J. (1987). *The truly disadvantaged: The inner city, the underclass, and public policy.* Chicago: University of Chicago Press.

Wing, L. (1980). Childhood autism and social class: A question of selection? *British Journal of Psychiatry, 137*, 410–417.

Wing, L. (1981). Asperger's syndrome: A clinical account. *Psychological Medicine, 11*, 115–129.

Wolraich, M. L., Lindgren, S. D., Stumbo, P. J., Stegink, L. D., Appelbaum, M. I., Kiritsy, M. C. (1994). Effects of diets high in sucrose and aspartame on the behavior and cognitive performance of children. *New England Journal of Medicine, 323*, 1361–1366.

Wootton, J. M., Frick, P. J., Shelton, K. K., & Silverthorn, P. (1997). Ineffective parenting and childhood conduct problems: The moderating role of callous-unemotional traits. *Journal of Consulting and Clinical Psychology, 65*, 301–308.

Wright, L., & Walker, C. E. (1976). Behavioral treatment of encopresis. *Journal of Pediatric Psychology, 1*, 35–37.

Zahn, T. P., Jacobsen, L., Gordon, C. T., McKenna, K., Frazier, J. A., & Rapoport, J. L. (1997). Autonomic nervous system markers of psychopathology in childhood-onset schizophrenia. *Archives of General Psychiatry, 54*, 904–912.

Zametkin, A. J., & Liotta, W. (1998). The neurobiology of attention-deficit/hyperactivity disorder. *Journal of Clinical Psychiatry, 59* (Suppl. 7), 17–23.

Zametkin, A. J., & Rapoport, J. L. (1986). The pathophysiology of attention deficit disorder with hyperactivity. In B. B. Lahey & A. E. Kazdin (Eds.), *Advances in clinical child psychology*, Vol. 9. New York: Plenum.

Zametkin, A. J., Nordahl, T. E., Gross, M., King, A. C., Semple, W. E., Rumsey, J., Hamburger, S., & Cohen, R. (1990). Cerebral glucose metabolism in adults with hyperactivity of childhood onset. *New England Journal of Medicine, 323*, 1361–1366.

Zametkin, A. J., Liebenauer, L. L., Fitzgerald, G. A., King, A. C., Minkunas, D. V., Herscovitch, P., Yamada, E. M., & Cohen, R. M. (1993). Brain metabolism in teenagers with attention deficit hyperactivity disorder. *Archives of General Psychiatry, 50*, 333–340.

Zoccolillo, M. (1993). Gender and the development of Conduct Disorder. *Development and Psychopathology, 5*, 65–78.

# CHAPTER 32

# Psychopathology in the Aged

## Jane E. Fisher, Antonette M. Zeiss, and Laura L. Carstensen

## Introduction

Our understanding of the influence of aging on psychopathology has undergone significant revision in the past few decades. Early negative stereotypes about increased rates of problems that occur in old age have been challenged by empirical accounts of reduced incidence and prevalence rates of many psychological problems in elderly cohorts or a nonlinear relationship between age and psychological problems (Dick & Gallagher-Thompson, 1996; Gatz, Kasl-Godley, & Karel, 1996; Kessler, Foster, Webster, & House, 1992; Kessler et al., 1994; Vaillant, 1996). In general, recent research on psychological functioning in old age suggests that, despite exposure to increasing numbers of uncontrollable changes and losses associated with aging such as health problems (Aldwin, 1995; Zeiss, Lewinsohn, Rohde, & Seeley, 1996) and bereavement (Zisook & Schuchter, 1991), the majority of older adults report greater levels of contentment that at any point in the life-span. These findings suggest that a lifetime of exposure to the inevitable stresses of life results in enhanced coping abilities and adaptation, not in

cumulative negative effects (Brandstedter, Wentura, & Greve, 1993). These recent findings present challenges for the field of clinical gerontology. As negative stereotypes of aging are debunked by empirical findings, new theoretical accounts of psychological functioning across the life-span will be needed.

In this chapter, we examine the theoretical assumptions and empirical status of research on psychopathology in old age. In studying the relationship between psychopathology and aging, the topic must be examined from several positions: (1) disorders may develop for the first time in old age; (2) disorders first evident earlier in adulthood may continue in old age and remain basically unaltered by the aging process; (3) disorders that begin in early or middle adulthood may continue into old age but be significantly altered by the aging process; (4) and disorders that begin in early or middle adulthood may remit in old age. As we examine the effects of aging on psychological problems, we will find that each of these positions is reflected in the literature across a variety of problems.

The study of psychopathology in old age is complicated by several methodological problems such as the confounding of age and cohort effects, the lack of standardized measures normed on an elderly population, and nonrepresentative sampling associated with selective dropout and differential mortality. For each of the disorders we examine in the chapter, we have attempted to address the relevance of these problems. Before reviewing research on the prevalence, etiology, and assessment of specific disorders, we attempt to provide a

Jane E. Fisher • Department of Psychology, University of Nevada-Reno, Reno, Nevada 89557.    Antonette M. Zeiss • VA Palo Alto Health Care System, Palo Alto, California 94304. Laura L. Carstensen • Department of Psychology, Stanford University, Stanford, California 94305.

*Comprehensive Handbook of Psychopathology* (Third Edition), edited by Patricia B. Sutker and Henry E. Adams. Kluwer Academic/Plenum Publishers, New York, 2001.

general orientation by examining some major issues relevant to this field of study.

## Composition of the Older Adult Population

The phrase "the graying of America" aptly reflects the fact that changes in the age composition of the U.S. population will be quite considerable during the next 30 years. As a group, the elderly are the fastest growing segment of the population. Changes in the age composition of the population are expected to have profound economic, medical, and social impact.

Gerontologists divide the 65-and-over age group into three groups: early old age (65–74 years), middle old age (75–84 years), and advanced old age (85 and above). In 1900, individuals over the age of 65 made up only 4% of the population; now, in the United States, persons age 65 and over comprise 12% of the population. Not only is the population over 65 increasing, but the number of persons who are 85 and over will double in the next 10 years. The age group over 85, sometimes referred to as the "old old," is the fastest-growing segment of our entire population. Between 1960 and 1990 the population of individuals over the age of 85 increased by 237%. Between 2000 and 2010, the segment of the population aged 75 to 84 will increase by 57%, and the number of those age 85 and over will grow by 91% (U.S. Bureau of the Census, 1990). The fastest growing population in most countries is persons 80 and over (World Health Organization, 1998). By the year 2030, it is expected that the elderly will comprise approximately 21% of the population.

There are gender and ethnic differences in the aging trends, at least in the United States. In terms of gender, differential longevity continues to occur, and women outlive men. The average lifespan for men was 72 in 1993 and for women 79, up by almost 30 years since 1900. For those who have managed to make it to age 65, the figures are even more promising: men of 65 can expect to live, on average, to age 77; women can expect to live, on average, to age 81. Ethnic minority elderly account for a significant proportion of the overall increase in older adults; their rates of growth are expected to exceed those of Whites during the next 50 years. For example, the percentage of minority group elderly is projected to increase from 10.2% in 1990 to 15.3% in 2020, and to 21.3% in 2050 (Angel &

Hogan, 1994). Demographic trends suggest that the number of African-Americans over age 65 is increasing, and the largest shift will occur in persons 85 years of age and older (U.S. Bureau of the Census, 1996).

Contrary to stereotypes about dependency in old age, the vast majority of the elderly reside in the community. Only about 5% of the elderly reside in nursing homes or convalescent centers at any time, although the lifetime probability of placement in a nursing home is 25–30%. As people age, the risk of nursing-home placement increases from 1 in 20 to 1 in 7 after the age of 80; in other words, 15% of the people over 80 years old reside in nursing homes (AARP, 1998). With advancing age comes an increased likelihood of dependence on government programs as safety nets for income and health care. The proposed projections of a dramatic increase in the proportion of the "oldest old" during the next 30 years is driving increased concern regarding the adequacy of current public policies for assisting older adults because benefits to this group already account for 40% of federal expenditures (Binstock, 1999).

# Methodological Issues in the Study of Aging and Psychopathology

A limitation of many epidemiological studies is that they place all subjects over the age of 65 into one group, whereas subjects age 18–64 are typically categorized into three to four separate age groups. For many disorders, this approach to age categorization presents an overly simplistic or distorted view of the relationship between aging and psychopathology (Kessler et al., 1994). Several inconsistencies have been identified in the methodology of studies of psychopathology in different age groups. Studies of elderly nursing-home residents, for example, may aggregate subjects ranging in age from 55 to 100. Feinson (1985) suggested that this practice indicates that age distinctions are viewed as important for young and middle-aged adults but not for older adults. Feinson and Thoits (1986) reviewed epidemiological studies of mental health problems among older adults and found prevalence rates of any psychopathology that varied from 6–37%, depending on the specific old age category. According to these authors, cross-sectional studies reported either positive, negative, or no association, depending on the methods and measures used.

## Cross-Sectional Versus Longitudinal Studies

Research on aging and psychopathology has typically relied on cross-sectional studies. In a cross-sectional study, samples of individuals of different ages are observed for the variables of interest at a single measurement time. A limitation of this approach is that it does not allow one to rule out the effects of cohort or time-of-measurement effects. For example, a researcher interested in the effects of aging on depression may find a sudden decline in mood at age 65. Although this finding may be "age-related," it may also be a reaction to an event such as retirement or an announcement that the government is reducing Medicare benefits. In these examples, the effects of age and history are confounded. Other cohort related factors that may impact psychological functioning in old age include differences in divorce rates, lifetime exposure to violence, gender-based employment opportunities, and exposure to risk factors from substance use and sexually transmitted diseases.

Another example of the limitations of cross-sectional designs is seen in the conclusions that were drawn from early research on intellectual functioning in old age. In the 1930s, 1940s, and 1950s, numerous investigators administered intelligence tests to individuals of different age groups. The results led investigators to conclude that intelligence increases up to early adulthood, reaches a plateau in the person's 30s, and begins to decline progressively around the age of 40. These conclusions went unchallenged until the appearance of the first longitudinal studies. In a longitudinal study, the variable(s) of interest are observed for the same individuals at two or more measurement times. Longitudinal studies found that different intellectual domains showed different rates of decline (e.g., Baltes & Schaie, 1976; Schaie, 1994, 1996; Schaie & Labouvie-Vief, 1974; Schaie & Stone, 1982); on measures of vocabulary and other skills associated with educational experience, for example, individuals maintained their levels of functioning into their 60s and 70s. Longitudinal studies also showed evidence for individual differences. Many people show no significant intellec-

tual decline into the eighth decade (Field, Schaie, & Leino, 1988), and the patterns of decline also vary across individuals (Schaie, 1989, 1990); few showed decline in all areas. Indeed, some individuals continue to show increases in intellectual abilities into old age (Field et al., 1988). One major reason that longitudinal results were so different is that cross-sectional studies of intelligence did not control for effects of cohort (e.g., education; for thorough reviews of methodological issues in developmental research, see Schaie, 1994, 1996).

When studying changes in psychopathology during the life-span, it also is important to consider the role of age-associated selection biases. Differential mortality is particularly problematic when sampling from the population of individuals in advanced old age (75 and older). There is good reason to assume that those who survive into advanced old age were previously more psychologically vigorous and/or physically healthy than the members of their cohort who died. Studying these individuals can result in overly optimistic inferences about age-related remission in psychopathology. This problem is especially relevant for studying behaviors that can have a direct impact on physical health (e.g., alcohol abuse, eating disorders, sexual behavior).

Selective dropout is another source of sampling bias that impacts research on psychopathology and aging. This problem is particularly relevant for longitudinal research. Subjects who die, move, or withdraw from the research are more likely in lower class populations and produce increased bias toward middle class samples during the course of a longitudinal study. Given that certain problems (e.g., schizophrenia, polysubstance abuse) occur at higher rates in lower classes (Susser & Wanderling, 1994), longitudinal research is particularly difficult to carry out for these disorders.

## Problems in Measurement

One of the most pervasive problems in studying psychopathology in old age is the lack of standardized instruments that have been normed on an elderly sample. Differences in the reliability, validity, and cutoff scores of assessment instruments normed on younger groups should be considered when they are applied to the elderly. Reliability, for example, may be affected by changes in memory. Further, although an assessment instrument may be reliable and valid for this population, the cutoff scores for elders may differ from those for younger adults. These issues will be explored more specifically in examining assessment procedures for each of the disorders discussed in the following sections.

## Mood Disorders

### Prevalence

Controversy has surrounded the study of the prevalence of depression among the elderly. Findings from recent reviews of epidemiological studies of depression in the aged (Kessler et al., 1994; Newman, 1989) suggest that the relationship of age to depression depends, in part, on the screening instrument used to measure depression. Most depression inventories include items that assess somatic symptoms of depression. Many of the somatic symptoms of depression, though, are changes that occur naturally in old age. These include increased fatigue, decreased appetite, and decreases in sleep. When somatic symptoms are included in surveys of depression in the elderly, the result may be an overestimate of prevalence because of the confounding of physical health status and emotional distress (Aldwin, Spiro, Levenson, & Bosse, 1989; Roberts, Kaplan, Shema, & Strawbridge, 1997). When clinical diagnostic criteria are used to estimate prevalence rates (e.g., Myers et al., 1984; Roberts, Kaplan, Shema, & Strawbridge, 1997; Weissmann et al., 1985) the rates of depression are lower in old age (see Newman, 1989, and Kessler, 1995, for critical reviews of this issue).

Depression-spectrum disorders, including subclinical depression, dysthymia, and adjustment disorder with depressed mood, may account for reports of increased rates of depression when *symptoms* of depression rather than diagnostic criteria are used to estimate prevalence rates. These disorders are more prevalent than major depression among the elderly (Lasser, Siegel, & Sunderland, 1998; Lyness, King, Cox, Yoediono, & Caine, 1999).

In considering the course of depression across the life-span, Lewinsohn, Zeiss, and Duncan (1989) found that the probability of relapse following recovery from a first episode of depression is equal for individuals who are over 40 and those under 40 at the time of the first episode of depres-

sion. The likelihood of experiencing a first episode of major depression in old age is very low. In studying the age distribution for first episodes of unipolar depression, Lewinsohn et al. (1986) found a peak between 45 and 55 years, followed by a decrease with increasing age to a risk of zero at 80 years or older.

Studies of lifetime prevalence rates of major depression indicate the operation of a cohort effect. In reviewing ten epidemiological studies, Klerman and Weissman (1989) noted that all of the studies found an increase in lifetime rates of major depression in younger age cohorts (i.e., those born after 1940) and a decrease in the lifetime prevalence in older cohorts.

Although overall rates of major depression are lower in the elderly, the rate of depression among nursing-home residents is much higher than the rate for the community-residing elderly (Futterman et al., 1995; Robins et al., 1984). Among the elderly who receive residential care, increases in clinical depression have been predictive of death (Parmelee, Katz, & Lawton, 1991).

The seriousness of geriatric depression becomes salient when one examines the disproportionately high rates of suicide in this age group. Suicide rates increase with age and are the highest among adults aged 65 and older (Center for Disease Control, 1999). The suicide rate for the general population is 12.4/100,000, but rates in 80- to 84-year-olds are 26.5/100,000. Suicide is particularly a problem for White men over the age of 85 who as a group have the highest suicide rates in the United States, 65.3/100,000. Risk factors for suicide among the elderly differ from those of younger adults. Leading risk factors for suicide in older adults include social isolation and physical illness.

### Bipolar Disorder

Bipolar disorder in older adults has not been studied extensively, presumably because of its very low base rate in this population. Results from NIMH catchment area studies indicated a prevalence rate for manic episodes of zero for the 65-plus age group. It has been suggested, however, that this disorder is often misdiagnosed in adults over the age of 60 and that its prevalence is underestimated. Young & Klenman (1992) reported that individuals who develop late-onset bipolar disorder have more frequent episodes than those with early onset. Research further suggests a poorer prognosis for older patients relative to younger adults with bipolar disorder due to more extensive neurological and cognitive deficits (Shulman, Tohen, Satlin, Mallya, & Kalunian, 1992).

## Theories of Etiology of Depression in the Elderly

Etiological theories of geriatric depression should address three areas: (1) the finding of decreased incidence of depression in old age; (2) the causes of depression in old age; and (3) the factors associated with maintaining depression throughout adulthood in certain individuals. For the most part, etiological theories of geriatric depression have been based on the assumption that the prevalence of depression actually decreases in old age (Dick & Gallagher-Thompson, 1996; Klerman & Weissman, 1989), it is apparent that new etiological theories of depression in old age are needed.

**Medical Illness and Depression.** Recent research has provided new insight into the relationship between health and depression in old age. When one compares the prevalence rates of depression and physical illness, it is clear that the majority of physically ill elderly does not develop major depression.

Reich, Zautra, and Guamaccia (1989) studied disabled elderly subjects and found that they exhibited significantly higher distress and lower levels of well-being compared with recently bereaved subjects and nonbereaved healthy subjects matched in age, socioeconomic status, and gender. Follow-up assessment conducted 13 to 16 months later revealed almost full recovery of the bereaved subjects and an absence of significant improvement in mental health for the disabled subjects. More recently, Zeiss and colleagues (Zeiss, Lewinsohn, Rohde, & Seeley, 1996) showed that medical illness *per se* is not a risk factor for depression in community-dwelling older adults, but that loss of function did increase the risk of becoming depressed. Illness may be the imminent cause of functional loss, so in a statistical sense, medical illness is likely to be associated with depression, but when illness and functional loss are examined separately, functional loss is the key factor. It is likely that this functional loss leads to depression through its psychological impact, particularly as functional changes limit valued activities and/or change an older adult's roles and opportunities.

It has also been suggested that major depression in the aged may result in greater morbidity and mortality from medical causes (Parmelee et al., 1991). The relationship between depression and medical illness in the aged is clearly complex and warrants further attention.

**Psychological Theories of Depression in Old Age.** *Psychodynamic Theories.* Psychodynamic theories of late-life depression typically focus on a combination of two factors: stress (particularly that associated with loss) and age-associated rigidity or lack of adaptability. Freud did not focus much attention on old age in his writings but generally viewed this period of life as one of ego rigidity and diminished cognitive ability. In discussing the applicability of psychoanalysis in advanced adulthood, he wrote,

Near and above the fifties the elasticity of the mental processes on which the treatment depends is lacking. Old people are no longer educable and on the other hand the mass of material to be dealt with would prolong the duration of treatment indefinitely. (Freud, 1924, p. 228)

Freud viewed grieving as a painful process involving the withdrawal of ties to the "love object"; this process is termed decathexis. The ego resists this withdrawal through denial by becoming preoccupied with the deceased and through loss of interest in the outside world. Eventually, mourners review memories and expectations of the deceased and gradually detach themselves from the lost love object. The grieving process ends when the individual is able to "cathect" or invert emotional energy in other relationships (Freud, 1917/1957). According to Freud, some individuals do not pass through the grieving process in this way, but instead develop a melancholic depression that may last for an extended period. This melancholic depression resembles normal grieving in many respects. According to Freud (1917/1957), there is one striking difference: Whereas normal mourning is limited to the loss of an external object, melancholia is associated with an internal loss and a sense of personal worthlessness. According to Freud, the elderly encounter the losses of old age with a fixed character structure. Characteristically, later psychoanalysts disagreed with Freud. Kaufman (1940) stated that the psychoses and neuroses of later age were definitely of a pregenital type. In discussing the treatment of depression in old age, he referred to an "inverted Oedipus complex" that makes dependent elderly individuals regard their children as they once regarded their parents. According to Kaufman (1940), this phenomenon results in much confusion when elderly individuals attempt to interact with their children. Grotjahn (1951) described aging as a narcissistic trauma that represents and repeats a castration threat. Therefore, depressive neuroses in old age represent a defense against castration anxiety. Hamilton (1942) suggested that the change from a mature to an aging personality is characterized by regression to the earlier life stages (i.e., childhood and adolescence). In the beginning of senescence, there is a weakening of unconscious urges that may be brought about by retirement and inactivity. The demands made by the ego, coupled with a reduced ability to cope with the instinctual urges of the id, result in feelings of inferiority, insecurity, guilt, and feelings of hostility toward younger people. Hamilton suggested that the preexisting and chronically unresolved conflicts of childhood that were repressed during maturity become reactivated in old age and lead to neurotic behavior. Several psychodynamically oriented theorists have suggested that regression plays a role in the development of psychological disturbance in old age (Modell, 1970; Zarsky & Blau, 1970). According to Modell (1970), the term regression can refer to a variety of processes, including the reemergence of earlier developmental stages and the emergence of more primitive defense mechanisms. It has been suggested that regression may be an adaptive response to the losses and stress of old age (Newton, Bauer, Gutmann, & Grunes, 1986). Regression is considered a pathological phenomenon if unconscious material is dominated by unresolved problems that originated in childhood and defenses developed in adulthood do not have sufficient integrity to be effective in protecting the elderly individual against primitive drives (Newton et al., 1986). Psychodynamic theories of depression in old age have not been adequately tested and therefore should be judged with the considerable skepticism due such speculative statements. It is also noteworthy that the dynamic theories generally predict an increased prevalence of depression with old age, whereas the opposite is actually true.

*Behavioral and Cognitive Theories.* Behavioral researchers have focused on age-associated changes in reinforcement frequency and magnitude to understand depression and other problems in old age. In contrast to the psychoanalytic conceptualiza-

tion of psychological problems, behavioral approaches are based on empirical evidence of behavioral plasticity in old age (Hussian, 1983; O'Donohue, Fisher, & Krasner, 1986). Reductions in reinforcement frequency associated with the loss of roles (e.g., because of retirement, relocation, or the death of significant others) and reductions in the magnitude of reinforcement stemming from sensory losses (e.g., taste, visual, and hearing deficits), it has been suggested all contribute to the development of depression in the elderly (Teri & Lewinsohn, 1986). Support for the role of reduced reinforcement in geriatric depression is seen in the findings of research on depression and bereavement (Gallagher, Breckenridge, Thompson, & Peterson, 1983) and studies of treatment that have involved increasing rates of reinforcement to reduce depression in the elderly (Hussian, 1983; Gallagher-Thompson, et al., 2000). It is unclear whether such reductions in reinforcement are actually relatively rare and result in the low prevalence of depression or whether elders use more effective coping strategies than younger adults when placed in low-reinforcement environments. Behavioral theorists have just begun to grapple with these issues (e.g., Lewinsohn, Zeiss, & Duncan, 1989). The applicability of the reformulated learned helplessness model (Abramson, Seligman, & Teasdale, 1978) to depression in old age has been partially supported by recent research (Hybels & Miller, 1987). The theory predicts that certain patterns of attributions regarding negative and positive events develop in those who have experienced noncontingent reinforcement and are depressed. In studying eighty-four nonpsychotic, non-demented elderly women, Hybels and Miller (1987) operationalized uncontrollable stress as physical impairment. In examining the relationship between attribution style and depression, they found that clinically depressed subjects made more external attributions for good events and more internal and global attributions for bad events than nondepressed subjects. This relationship held only for severely depressed subjects; when mildly depressed subjects were included, only the globality of attributions for negative outcomes remained significant. The authors suggested that, as in other research on the reformulated model of learned helplessness, their measure of attributional style may have been sensitive only to the extreme ends of the continuum. Research on the efficacy of cognitive therapy for depression in the aged indicates that a cognitive model of depression has some validity and utility for understanding depression in this population. Gallagher and Thompson (1983) described several cognitive distortions that are commonly held by the elderly. These include the beliefs "I'm too old to change," "If only X would change, I wouldn't be depressed," and "If only I had done X or Y earlier in my life, I wouldn't be depressed now" (p. 177). Cognitive theories will be more compelling, however, when they also begin to explore which cognitions may help protect most elders from becoming depressed in the face of losses, chronic illness, reduced reinforcement schedules, and so forth. Thus, a complete theory would identify effective coping strategies of typical elders and the factors that lead to the breakdown of cognitive coping in the minority of elders who become clinically depressed.

**Depression and Bereavement.** Bereavement is a common experience in old age. Depression and bereavement often coincide. Gilewski, Farberow, Gallagher, and Thompson (1988) found that 28.7% of bereaved elderly subjects scored in the depressed range of the Beck Depression Inventory (BDI) one month after the spouse's death. The reasons for individual differences in response to spousal bereavement are unclear. Factors that have been investigated in attempting to explain individual differences in response to spousal bereavement include gender (Farberow, Gallagher-Thompson, Gilewski, & Thompson, 1992; Hays, Kasl, & Jacobs, 1994; Nolen-Hoeksema, Parker, & Larson, 1994), differential social support (Feld & George, 1994; Harlow, Goldberg, & Comstock, 1991; Prigerson, Frank, Reynolds, George, & Kupfer, 1993), marital satisfaction before bereavement (Futterman, Gallagher, Thompson, Lovett, & Gilewski, 1990; Zisook & Shuchter, 1991), coping style (Herth, 1990; Nolen-Hoeksema et al., 1994), the suddenness of death (Byrne & Raphael, 1994; Carey, 1977; Lundin, 1984), and the age of the survivor (Zisook & Shuchter, 1991).

In considering age differences in responses to bereavement, recent research suggests that exposure to grief-related stimuli may have a significant impact on long-term response to bereavement. It is reasonable to expect that widows and widowers would attempt to avoid feelings of depression associated with bereavement. Further, such avoidance is often culturally sanctioned in the United States. Hayes (1994) writes "... it is not uncommon for a person facing the sadness associated with a death in the family to be told to think about something else, to get on with life, to focus on the positive things, to try to pour themselves into work, or to otherwise avoid the aversive properties of an inherently aversive event." (p. 15). Such advice advocates the denial of grief and decreases "... the ability of the individual to be present with their psychological reactions in difficult circumstances." (Hayes, p. 15). In considering the impact of avoiding grief, the possibility emerges that individual differences in adapting to bereavement may be related to variation in the willingness to confront the emotional correlates of loss. Experiential avoidance functions to help the individual escape aversive or anxiety-provoking internal stimuli result in a reduction in distress. This reduction in distress then strengthens the avoidance response through negative reinforcement.

It has been argued that experiential avoidance has long-term negative consequences for individuals who rely on it as a coping strategy (Hayes, Wilson, Gifford, Strosahl, & Follette, 1999). Avoidance, like thought suppression, produces a rebound effect in which individuals may successfully suppress their emotional experience until they return to the context in which suppression occurred. When presented with stimuli associated with suppression, classical conditioning leads to a recurrence of the suppressed private experience potentially at even more intense levels (Hayes et al., 1999). Therefore, individuals do not truly escape the experience that they attempted to avoid and may actually magnify the feared aspects of the experience.

Support for the detrimental effects of experiential avoidance following loss can be found in the bereavement literature. Research indicates that individuals whose primary coping strategies involve experiential avoidance have greater psychological distress, compared to individuals who rely on alternate strategies. Herth (1987) examined the relationship between eight different coping styles and grief resolution in an elderly sample. Grief resolution was measured by the Grief Resolution Index (Remondet & Hansson, 1987) which was designed to assess psychological distress and adjustment to the environment without the deceased. Remondet and Hansson (1987) defined the resolution of grief "... as psychological and physiological reactions to the loss and a degree of social reintegration ..." (p. 31). Sample items on the Grief Resolution

Index include "Accepted the death of my husband" and "Was able to think through what my husband's death meant to me." (p. 32). Items on this scale are rated on a five-point scale ranging from "1-very poorly" to "5-very well" (p. 32). The eight coping styles examined in this study were as follows: (1) evasive style-evasive and avoidant activities; (2) fatalistic style-pessimistic approach; (3) emotive style-expressive emotion; (4) confrontational style-constructive problem solving; (5) optimistic style-positive outlook; (6) palliative style-stress reducing methods; (7) self-reliant coping style-self-initiated activities; and (8) supportive style-reliance on supportive systems. Reliance on each of these coping styles was measured by the revised Jalowiec Coping Scale (Jalowiec, 1987, cited in Herth, 1987), a self-report questionnaire.

The results of the Herth (1987) study indicated that evasive, fatalistic, and emotive coping styles were significantly negatively correlated with grief resolution, whereas the remaining five coping styles were significantly positively correlated with successful grief resolution. The implication of these findings is that individuals who rely on confrontational rather than evasive coping techniques are more successful in resolving grief. These findings support the hypothesis that experiential avoidance is detrimental to return to preloss functioning.

Nolen-Hoeksema et al. (1994) studied the impact of ruminative coping styles in 253 individuals (aged 20–86) who had experienced the loss of a family member. Ruminative coping was defined as a passive focus on one's negative emotions and the meaning of these emotions. Rumination can be conceptualized as a form of emotional avoidance where the bereaved individuals focus predominantly or exclusively on a single aspect of the grief experience (e.g., perseveration around feelings of guilt), thus suppressing other aspects of their private experience of the loss (e.g., depression and loneliness). A self-report measure, the Response Styles Questionnaire (Nolen-Hoeksema & Morrow, 1991) was used to measure ruminative coping. This questionnaire was designed to assess responses to depression that are self-focused (e.g., "Why do I react this way?"), symptom-focused (e.g., "I think about how hard it is to concentrate"), or focused on possible consequences of their mood (e.g., "I think I won't be able to do my job if I don't snap out of this") (Nolen-Hoeksema et al., 1994). Nolen-Hoeksema and her colleagues found that people with poorer social support, more concurrent stressors, and higher levels of postloss depression reported more rumination than people with better social support, fewer stressors, and lower levels of initial depression. Further, rumination was significantly associated with depression at both 1 and 6 months following loss. Unfortunately, because this study was correlational, the direction of influence between depression and rumination is unknown. However, the finding of a significant correlation indicates that rumination is likely to be detrimental to recovery and is consistent with the thought suppression literature.

Gass (1987) studied the relationship between coping strategies and psychological and physical health in 100 widows ages 65–81. Subjects in this study had lost their husbands between 1 and 12 months before data collection and were not remarried. Gass defined coping as "cognitive and behavioral efforts made to master, minimize, alleviate, or reduce external and internal demands" (p. 30). Coping was measured with the Ways of Coping Checklist developed by Folkman and Lazarus (cited in Gass, 1987) to assess a broad range of behavioral and cognitive coping styles that a person uses in a specific stressful situation. Physical and psychological health were measured using the Sickness Impact Profile developed by Gibson et al. (1978; cited in Gass, 1987). The results of the Gass (1987) study indicated that widows evaluated a variety of avoidance activities that they had tried as ineffective coping strategies. These strategies included consumption of medications or alcohol, sleeping more, blaming oneself, and avoiding or getting mad at people. Conversely, 23% of the sample reported that the avoidant strategy of forgetting (e.g., getting rid of their husband's belongings shortly after death) helped them cope. However, Gass reported that widows who attempted to forget were in more psychological turmoil and, in general, had poorer physical and psychological health than widows who fostered memories.

Further support for the hypothesis that exposure affects grief involves the age of the survivor. Psychological symptoms of grief are more severe among young widows and widowers, compared to elderly survivors of spousal bereavement. Zisook and Shuchter (1991) reported that the average age of bereaved individuals with depression was significantly lower than those without depression. Further, widows and widowers older than 65 were significantly less likely to be depressed than younger individuals. Differences between age groups in reaction to the loss of a spouse may be due to increased exposure to grief and related facilitated acceptance of grief in elderly populations.

There are several reasons to believe that the elderly have more exposure to grief than younger populations. First, as a result of their advanced age, there is an increased chance that the elderly have experienced the loss of parents and friends. Second, older individuals are more likely to have anticipated the death of their spouse than younger individuals. As discussed earlier, anticipation may provide the opportunity for exposure and acceptance before bereavement and may lead to better postloss adjustment. Third, Thorson and Powell (1988) reported that the elderly had less fear of dying than younger populations. Because exposure is a vital component in treating anxiety, it is possible that the lower level of anxiety about death in the elderly reflects increased exposure. However, lower levels of fear related to death may also reflect a cohort effect unrelated to exposure.

A methodological limitation of the extant research investigating response to bereavement is that it is largely cross-sectional (Feld & George, 1994). The longitudinal studies have recruited subjects just before the death of a significant other and followed the sample for up to two years. Recruiting subjects immediately before the death of a loved one is problematic because it precludes gathering information about an individual's psychological functioning and methods of coping before the stressful experience of the loss or the receipt of information regarding impending death.

## Assessment of Mood Disorders

Depression in the elderly often presents a different symptomatic picture than that observed in younger groups. The task of the evaluator frequently involves determining whether complaints involve natural concomitants of aging, an underlying physical disorder, or symptoms of depression (Radloff & Teri, 1986; Gaylord & Zung, 1987). Several screening instruments that have been used with the elderly are reviewed later. The Beck Depression Inventory (Beck, 1967) has been studied extensively with the elderly. Because the format of the BDI makes administering it to cognitively impaired elderly rather cumbersome and because the large number of somatic items may inflate de-

pression scores for medically ill elderly, there has been some skepticism regarding its utility. It has worked out well in practice, as the following studies demonstrate. Gallagher et al. (1982) examined the test–retest reliability and internal consistency of the BDI with clinical and nonclinical samples of elderly subjects. Test–retest periods ranged from 6 to 21 days. The test–retest correlation for the entire sample was .90, the coefficient alpha was .91, and the split-half index was .84. These results indicate that the BDI has adequate reliability for use with the elderly. In an attempt to assess the concurrent validity of the BDI, Gallagher, Breckenridge, Steinmetz, and Thompson (1983) examined the relationship between BDI cutoff scores and selected diagnostic classifications of the Research Diagnostic Criteria (RDC; Spitzer, Endicott, & Robins, 1978) for a sample of 102 elderly persons who sought treatment for depression. Results indicated that the diagnosis for 91% of the subjects who scored 17 or greater on the BDI was that they were experiencing an episode of major depression disorder based on the Schedule for Affective Disorders and Schizophrenia (SADS; Endicott & Spitzer, 1978) and the RDC classification criteria. Further, 81% of the subjects who scored 10 or below did not meet criteria for any RDC depressive disorder. These findings were replicated in two other studies (Kilcourse, Gallagher, Thompson, Tanke, & Sheikh, 1988; Norris, Gallagher, Wilson, & Winograd, 1987). Norris et al. (1987) compared BDI cutoff scores with interview ratings based on the DSM-III criteria. They reported that 84% of the subjects who scored below 10 were correctly identified as not depressed and 84% of those with BDI scores greater than 17 were correctly identified. The Geriatric Depression Scale (GDS) (Yesavage et al., 1983) is a thirty-item questionnaire on which individuals respond "yes" or "no" to questions about the presence of depressive symptoms. Early validity studies involved comparing GDS ratings with those of other depression scales (e.g., Biggs, 1978; Hedlund & Viewig, 1979). Given the similarity of the items on the different depression scales, the significant correlations may be more accurately viewed as indicating the reliability rather than the convergent validity of the scale. More recently, Norris et al. (1987) reported that GDS ratings were consistent with RDC and DSM-III diagnoses for 84% and 77% of cases, respectively. Norris et al. suggest that, although BDI scores were slightly more consistent with RDC and DSM-III diagnoses than GDS scores, the simpler format and comparatively few (one vs. six) somatic items of the GDS may make it more useful for use with the medically ill and cognitively impaired elderly. A short version (fifteen items) of the GDS has also been developed. Sheikh and Yesavage (1986) reported that the short form correlates significantly ($r = .84$) with the long form and may be an attractive alternative to lengthier scales. The Zung Self-Rating Depression Scale (SDS; Zung, 1965) is one of the most widely used self-rating scales for assessing depression. Zung (1967) was the first to study the SDS in an elderly population. He assessed depressive symptomatology in normal subjects over the age of 65. When compared with younger groups, elderly subjects had significantly higher SDS scores. The higher scores of the elderly population were attributed to greater endorsement rates for somatic items; affective items were less likely to be endorsed in the elderly samples, compared with the younger groups. This response pattern has been found consistently is studies of the SDS. Zung and Zung (1986) reported that the findings of a number of studies indicate that starting at the age of 60, there is a linear increase in the mean SDS index from 43 to 49. The pattern of SDS scores suggests that it should be less valid for diagnosing depression in the elderly. In an effort to assess the concurrent validity of the SDS, Okimoto et al. (1982) compared SDS ratings with DSM-III diagnoses made by psychiatrists who were blind to the SDS results. The authors concluded that cutoff scores for the SDS vary, depending on the purpose of its application. Kitchell, Barnes, Veith, Okimoto, and Raskind (1982) attempted to evaluate the validity of the SDS by comparing Hamilton Depression Scale and SDS scores from forty-two elderly hospitalized medical patients. Both scales discriminated between depressed and nondepressed subjects diagnosed by the DSM-III criteria. The accuracy of the SDS for classification, however, was only 74%. Kitchell et al. (1982) suggested that readjusting scoring may produce higher sensitivities and improve the accuracy of classification of the SDS. Zung et al. (1974) used the SDS as a measure of treatment outcome and reported that it is sensitive to treatment effects. The SDS has also been studied with cognitively impaired elderly subjects. Heidell and Kidd (1975) measured depression levels in samples of cognitively impaired and healthy individuals over the age of 60. The results demonstrated that moderately cognitively impaired subjects scored significantly higher on the SDS than unimpaired subjects. These findings support the use of the SDS as a measure of treatment outcome for use with the cognitively impaired. In sum, research on depression scales used with the elderly provides support for the reliability and validity of several instruments. The Beck Depression Inventory currently enjoys the greatest support. Its use is recommended except for older populations known to have high cognitive impairment or serious chronic illness.

## Anxiety Disorders

### Prevalence

Epidemiological studies of anxiety present a complex picture of the prevalence and incidence of anxiety in advanced age. Recent epidemiological surveys have consistently found lower rates of anxiety in elderly cohorts and the highest rates among cohorts of young adults (Kessler et al., 1994; Robins & Regier, 1991). In the NIMH Epidemiological Catchment Area studies (Myers et al., 1984), the prevalence rates for all of the anxiety disorders were lowest for the 65-plus age group. In the ECA study, prevalence rates over a 6-month period for simple phobias averaged 3.3% for males older than age 65 and 7.0% for females older than age 65. The prevalence of agoraphobia averaged 1.6% for males and 3.0% for females older than age 65. The prevalence rates during a 6-month period for obsessive-compulsive disorder averaged 1.3% for males and 1.0% for females older than age 65. No males older than age 65 met the diagnostic criteria for panic disorder; the prevalence rates for panic in women older than age 65 averaged 0.2%. Assuming independence of disorders, this would be an overall total of 6.2% of men and 11.2% of women who reported an anxiety disorder. Feinson (1985) surveyed 313 randomly sampled older adults and found that anxiety was the only problem significantly associated with increased age. In this study, subjects older than age 85 reported higher rates of anxiety than individuals in the 65–84 age group. This finding is consistent with the age-associated differences in anxiety reported by Himmelfarb and Murrell (1984). It might at first appear to differ with the low prevalence rates found in the NIMH Epidemiological Catchment Area studies; however, recall that the ECA studies lumped together elders older than 65 into one age group, whereas the Feinson study presents a breakdown within that broad age range. Using a sophisticated sampling procedure, Himmelfarb and Murrell (1984) surveyed 713 males and 1338 females older than age 55 to assess the prevalence of anxiety symptoms among community-residing elderly. They found that 17.1% of males and 21.1% of females surveyed experienced sufficiently severe anxiety symptoms to warrant intervention. These investigators found several interesting interactions among anxiety and age, gender, and health. Anxiety scores decreased from ages 55–59 and reached a low point in the 65–69 age group; the scores increased in the 75–79 age group. These findings are consistent with the less detailed analyses presented by Feinson (1985). When gender was examined, it was found that never-married males had the highest anxiety scores among the males, whereas never-married women reported the lowest levels of anxiety within the female sample. Physical health and anxiety had the strongest association. High anxiety was significantly associated with the presence of several medical conditions, including hypertension, kidney or bladder disease, stomach ulcers, hardening of the arteries, stroke, and diabetes. Significant relationships were also found between anxiety and taking prescription medication; needing care from a doctor, hospital, home health agency, or mental health service; and not having medical needs met within the last 6 months. Wisocki (1988) surveyed ninety-four community-residing elderly to examine the prevalence of worrying. Respondents ranged in age from 60–90 and the mean age was 72. Wisocki found that few of the elderly (14%) in this sample reported significant levels of worrying. Worries concerning health were the only type that were correlated with age; marital status did not differentiate type or frequency of worrying. Respondents reporting the most worries were significantly more anxious and rated themselves in poorer health than the less worried respondents. The participants in this survey were sampled from senior citizen centers and meal sites and therefore may be representative of healthier elderly who are actively involved in the community. Because worry levels were not reported by age decades, precise comparability to earlier studies is also difficult. The overall level of worrying is comparable to the rates of anxiety reported in the general population older than 65 in the British (Ray, Beamish, & Roth, 1964) and American (Myers et al., 1984) epidemiological studies.

## Etiology of Anxiety

Etiological theories of anxiety and aging need to address (1) the decreased prevalence of anxiety in old age; (2) factors associated with increased vulnerability to developing anxiety in old age; and (3) environmental precipitants of anxiety in the aged. Systematic investigation of the prevalence and incidence of anxiety is needed before development of an adequate etiological theory. To date, there have been no longitudinal studies that investigated the natural history of anxiety or changes in worrying and coping across the life-span.

**Anxiety and Medical Illness.** Anxiety in older adults often occurs simultaneously with physical illness (Cohen, 1991; Himmelfarb & Murrell, 1984; Raj, 1993). The relationship between physical illness and anxiety in old age is not well understood. It is unclear, for example, whether the onset of the anxiety and the physical disorder occur simultaneously or whether one predates the other and has a possible causal influence. Physical disorders that are frequently accompanied by anxiety include angina, cerebral arteriosclerosis, epilepsy (particularly psychomotor), Parkinson's disease, hypoglycemia, hyperinsulinism, hypoxic states, hypothyroidism, and amine-secreting tumors. Hypothyroidism in the elderly, for example, may produce symptoms similar to those of anxiety, including sweating, tachycardia, cardiac arrhythmias, and restlessness. Detailed thyroid tests are necessary to rule out this condition.

In studying the effects of disability and bereavement, Reich et al. (1989) found that subjects recently disabled by an illness or accident reported higher levels of anxiety than both recently bereaved and nonbereaved healthy control subjects. All groups reported decreases in anxiety over time. The disabled subjects were found to have experienced significantly more health problems before the study, compared with either control group. These findings suggest that anxiety may occur simultaneously with or as a consequence of illness in the elderly. Because the psychological status of the disabled subjects before the onset of their disability was not known, however, the causal relationship between anxiety and illness cannot be determined.

**Anxiety and Cognitive Impairment.** The relationship between anxiety and cognitive impairment has not received much attention from researchers. Studies that have been reported have addressed either the relationship between anxiety and dementia or the impact of anxiety on the cognitive functioning of healthy older adults.

A difficulty associated with the study of anxiety in dementia patients involves the lack of validated measures of emotion for use with this population. When anxiety is reported, it is typically inferred from behavioral observations of agitation and/or escape behaviors. Swearer, Drachman, O'Donnell, & Mitchell (1988) found that 63% of caregivers of dementia patients who resided in the community reported that the patient exhibited one or more behavioral symptoms of anxiety, including general fearfulness, restlessness, pacing, a fear of specific objects of events, and worry over insignificant matters. In a study of forty-two Alzheimer's disease patients who resided in long-term care facilities, Fisher, Goy, Swingen, and Szymanski (1994) found that nurses described all of the patients who exhibited aggression as distressed before and during aggressive acts. In this sample, the aggressive behavior was consistently reported to be associated with an effort to escape from an aversive stimulus or with a high level of environmental stimulation. These findings suggest that aggressive behavior may function to terminate an anxiety-provoking stimulus for some dementia patients (see Fisher & Noll, 1996, for further discussion).

**Psychological Theories of Anxiety in Old Age.** *Psychodynamic Theories.* Psychodynamically oriented theorists have not addressed anxiety in old age to the extent that they have researched depression. In discussing anxiety in general, Freudian theorists have emphasized the role of intrapsychic forces in the form of forbidden instinctual drives that threaten to escape conscious control. Verwoerdt (1980) suggested that anxiety associated with the anticipation of loss of external resources may best characterize anxiety in old age. This form of anxiety is known as secondary or depletion anxiety and is distinguished from anxiety that results from an overpowering influx of stimuli or anxiety that is a response to unacceptable impulses. Anxiety from helplessness and dependency are cited as common examples of depletion anxiety. Although we could not locate any reports of direct empirical tests of Verwoerdt's assertions, indirect support might be found in the research on anxiety and medical illness described earlier.

*Behavioral Theories.* Learning theorists have presented several explanations of anxiety disorders. Mowrer (1948) and Dollard and Miller (1950) pro-

posed that anxiety develops through a two-stage process. The two-factor theory posits that in the course of an individual's experience, a neutral stimulus is paired with an aversive stimulus and through respondent conditioning arouses anxiety. The individual is motivated to reduce the fear and thus avoids the conditioned stimulus. This avoidance results in relief from anxiety and thus, through negative reinforcement, becomes habitual. Although this model has considerable clinical relevance because it suggests that behaviors that reduce fear are reinforcing, many studies suggest that it is insufficient as an explanation. For example, it has been found that fear continues even after avoidance responses have stopped (Riccio & Sylvestri, 1973). Further, fears are often acquired through modeling (Rachman, 1977). In an attempt to address the limitations of the two-factor theory, learning theorists have focused on the role of cognitive events in developing and maintaining anxiety. Cognitive theories of anxiety assume that the expectancy of harm mediates anxiety responses, that these expectancies are learned, and that the intensity of anxiety is a function of the perceived likelihood of anxiety. Chorpita & Barlow (1998), for example, in describing a model of the development of panic disorder, suggests that the psychological changes that accompany panic attacks become conditioned stimuli for further panic attacks. When these anxiety-associated psychological changes begin to occur, even for ordinary reasons, the individual begins to anticipate an attack. The fear of the attack intensifies the psychological response, and in a spiraling fashion, the fear and psychological reactions increase until an attack occurs.

It seems plausible that several age-associated changes in learning could affect anxiety in the aged. To date, learning theorists have not empirically investigated the effects of conditioning, psychological, and cognitive factors on anxiety in this population. A few researchers (Borkovec, 1988; Wisocki, 1988), however, have begun to speculate on the relationships between these age-associated changes and anxiety. In attempting to explain the low rates of worrying observed in a healthy sample of elderly, Wisocki (1988) offered some interesting hypotheses. She suggested that an age-associated biochemical change may result in a decline in cognitive acuity that may in turn reduce the impact of potentially worry-eliciting stimuli; she noted that now there is no clear evidence to support this hypothesis. Alternatively, Wisocki suggested that the elderly may develop effective coping strategies that allow them to adapt to environmental conditions. Borkovec (1988) suggested that if the latter is an accurate explanation of the frequency of worrying among the elderly, then their coping strategies should be investigated, as these may provide insight into better coping mechanisms for worry and anxiety in the general population. He suggests three mechanisms that might be operating: (1) long-term habituation that results in a lessening of the impact of stressful events; (2) development of realistic expectations regarding the probability of events and effective ways of coping with events as a result of experience; and (3) developmental changes in the attitudes and behaviors necessary to reduce worrying. Borkovec (1988) noted that these speculations rest on the assumption that the elderly do in fact worry less than younger age groups. Current data suggest this, but are not yet definitive.

### Assessment of Anxiety

As with other disorders, it is important to assess whether anxiety in an older person involves a continuation of a problem first seen in earlier adulthood or one that developed in old age. Anxiety symptoms with a rapid onset may be attributable to a physical disorder or to a toxic reaction to medication. The high consumption of prescription and nonprescription drugs and the prevalent practice of polypharmacy in the elderly makes it essential to assess the possibility of a toxic reaction as the precipitant of anxiety. There are very few anxiety-screening measures that have been normed on an elderly population. The State Trait Anxiety Inventory (Spielberger, 1983) includes norms for working males and females from ages 50–69. Spielberger (1983) compared data from norm studies of three age groups (19–39, 40–49, and 50–69) and found that although the mean anxiety scores for the two younger groups were quite similar, the scores for the oldest group were significantly lower. It should be noted, however, that these ratings were done with a group of relatively young, high-functioning, and healthy older adults.

## Psychotic Disorders in Late Life

The gerontological literature on psychotic disorders in later life has consistently reported an increase in the prevalence of psychotic symptoms in old age (Forsell & Henderson, 1998). Psychoses in later life may involve a continuation of a chronic disorder first evident earlier in adulthood or, more commonly, the development of psychotic symptoms associated with an underlying medical condition. The increase in psychotic *symptoms* is largely associated with underlying medical conditions such as delirium, dementia, and other neurological conditions (Ballard, Chithiramohan, Bannister, Handy, & Todd, 1991; Ballard & Oyebode, 1995; Forsell & Henderson, 1998). Older adults who experience neurological disorders may be at increased risk of psychotic symptoms when cognitive impairment is coupled with sensory deficits and social isolation (Thorpe, 1997).

The sparse literature on schizophrenia in old age reflects, in part, the long-held belief that this disorder follows a chronic deteriorating course. Until recently, many felt that the study of schizophrenia in old age would do little more than document an obvious pattern, namely, that deterioration continues until death. However, several longitudinal studies of psychiatric patients have provided evidence that calls into question previous thinking about psychopathology in old age (e.g., Ciompi, 1985; Harding, Brooks, Ashikaga, Strauss, & Breier, 1987; McGlashan, 1988). Contrary to expectations, evidence of stability and even improvement in some symptom patterns has been observed. Comparable gains in understanding have not have been made in the domain of late-life paranoia. Here, our knowledge base about age-specific characteristics remains quite limited. Clinical wisdom and case study continue to be our principal informants. In this section, we consider prevalence, etiology, and symptomatology separately for schizophrenic and delusional disorders. We caution the reader, however, that as a result of the poor diagnostic classification of psychosis in much of the geropsychiatric literature, there is a certain arbitrariness in the delineation.

### Schizophrenia

Virtually all clinical scientists believe that schizophrenia is a disease of the central nervous system (U. S. Department of Health and Human Services, 1988). It is considered a psychiatric disorder (as opposed to a medical disorder) because the manifestations are almost entirely cognitive or behavioral. Schizophrenia affects nearly every aspect of information processing and renders the afflicted individual impaired in the entire spectrum of mental processes from attentional abilities to speech generation and comprehension to eye-movement control. Thought content may be bizarre, marked by fixed delusional systems or simply faulty beliefs. Emotional response is often inappropriate, some times aberrant and exaggerated, but more often absent (i.e., flattened or subdued). Perceptual disturbances range from basic deficits in processing external information to visual and auditory hallucinations. Not surprisingly, schizophrenia typically results in serious impairment in social relationships. Symptoms of schizophrenia are typically subtyped as either positive or negative (Andreason, 1982; Carpenter, Heinrichs, & Wagman, 1988). Positive symptoms are florid symptoms such as hallucinations and delusions; negative symptoms, in contrast, refer to symptoms associated with the loss of normal functions, personal neglect, apathy, and slowed or absent movements (Strauss, Carpenter, & Bartko, 1974). It is difficult, if not impossible, to tease apart the effects of institutionalization, chronic use of major psychotropic medications, and aging *per* se on late-life symptomatology, but it appears that the aging process exerts a beneficial influence on positive symptoms of the disorder. In a study of patients hospitalized 28 years or more, Lawton (1972) found that patients were "less active, less agitated, less disorganized and more conforming" (p. 141) on follow-up than according to earlier records. Longitudinal research published during the past decade suggests that age in both hospitalized and nonhospitalized patients is related to reductions in the frequency and severity of positive symptomatology (Ciompi, 1985; Varner & Gaitz, 1982). General slowing and decreasing energy associated with normal aging may lead to the diminution of florid symptoms. Some researchers interpret these findings optimistically and even suggest that schizophrenia remits in old age (Harding, 1986), but others caution that such claims are premature (McGlashan, 1988). The exact processes that underlie decreases in positive symptoms also exacerbate negative symptoms and place older schizophrenics at risk of social isolation from friends and neglect by the mental health system. Among the elderly, just as in younger adults (Hooley, Richters, Weintraub, & Neale, 1987), negative symptoms (and not positive symptoms) predict social support and level of functioning (Meeks et al., 1990). Most of the current cohort of geropsychiatric patients experienced the radical changes in treatment that developed after the discovery of major tranquilizers in the 1950s. For many, it meant discharge from what would have been lifelong institutionalization. As this patient population aged, however, many patients faced a return to communities unprepared to meet their needs. And tardive dyskinisea, a serious motor disorder that stems from long-term use of antipsychotic medication, now afflicts a substantial proportion of older chronically mentally ill patients.

As in young people, the treatment for schizophrenia in old age is symptomatic. Psychotropic medication is considered the treatment of choice. Dosages, however, can be decreased; many times, they can be discontinued altogether.

**Prevalence.** The incidence of schizophrenia in the over-60 age group is slightly less than that in the general adult population. The decrease reflects the extremely low rate of new cases, coupled with a relatively high mortality rate among diagnosed schizophrenics largely the result of suicide and trauma (Post, 1980). In more than 90% of cases, onset occurs before the age of 40 (LaRue et al., 1985). Thus, most older schizophrenics are chronic patients grown old, not newly diagnosed schizophrenics. Rarely does schizophrenia appear for the first time in old age (Gurland & Cross, 1982). In fact, in the DSM-III, an initial onset of symptoms beyond age 45 precluded the diagnosis of schizophrenia. This criterion was disputed by some and dropped in the subsequent revision of the manual, but the fact that it was initially included speaks to the rarity of onset in late life. Studies of psychiatric hospitalizations show that the number of admissions attributable to schizophrenia is also relatively low in older age groups. Approximately 1% of first psychiatric admissions involve schizophrenia, less than half the number among younger psychiatric patients (Kastrop, 1985).

**Etiology.** It is widely accepted that genetic inheritance plays a causal role in the development of schizophrenia (Gottesman & Shields, 1972), even though the mode of transmission is indeterminate at present (Gottesman, McGuffin, & Farmer, 1987). Family, twin, and adoption studies have demonstrated that risk increases linearly with the degree of shared genetic inheritance with the afflicted proband (Gottesman & Shields, 1972). Just as widely accepted is the belief that environmental influence is essential to the onset of the disorder

(Stromgren, 1987). Most behavioral scientists subscribe to some variation of a diathesis-stress mode of transmission (e.g., Zubin & Spring, 1977). These models view genetic inheritance as a necessary but insufficient precursor to the disorder. Environmental stressors that serve as triggers for the onset of symptoms are also essential. The low incidence of initial-onset cases in old age may reflect the fact that, if one is vulnerable, one will have succumbed to the disease long before old age.

## Paranoia

As mentioned earlier, the most common form of psychosis in old age is paranoia. The term paranoia originated in Greek law; it referred to the deteriorated mental state in old men that allowed their sons to take over the management of their fathers' affairs (Post, 1987). The central feature of paranoia is an unshakable delusional belief system. These false beliefs may be limited to a circumscribed set of persons and circumstances or may be more elaborate and incorporate multiple people and multiple motives. It is important to note that we refer in this section only to the clinical syndrome of paranoia; paranoid symptoms that characterize early stages of Alzheimer's disease occur with considerable frequency in old age, but in such cases the cardinal feature is progressive cognitive decline. In paranoid psychosis, serious cognitive deterioration is not evident, and daily functioning is well preserved.

It is clear that paranoid delusions at any age seriously disrupt the ability to function and maintain social networks. For old people, especially those who require extended assistance from others, the consequences are potentially dire. Persecutory beliefs that target the very family members and professionals who are trying to help the patient can be so unsettling that assistance is discontinued. This usually leads to greater social isolation and an exacerbation of symptoms. Frequently, a central objective in treatment is reducing the anger and guilt that family members experience when their relative is suspicious of their motives.

There have been many attempts to establish classification systems for subtypes of paranoid disorders in old age, yet none has been widely accepted in the empirical literature. An unfortunate consequence has been an overabundance of terms in the literature that carry limited information about prevalence, course, or treatment. Examples of subtypes frequently used include senile paraphrenia, simple paranoia, paranoid hallucinosis, and transitional paranoid reaction, none of which appear in the DSM classification system.

Treatment for paranoia typically involves psychotropic medication. This course of treatment, however, is sometimes precluded by the patient's refusal to take medication. There is some evidence that behavioral interventions are also effective (Carstensen & Fremouw, 1981).

**Prevalence.** Paranoia is second only to depression in the frequency of occurrence among the elderly. It is considered the most common form of psychosis in the senium; unlike schizophrenia, new cases continue to appear well into old age. Accurate estimates of prevalence, however, are absent as a result of the classification problems referred to before. Some researchers, for example, differentiate paranoia from schizophrenia on the basis of late-life onset, whereas others attempt to differentiate one from the other on the basis of symptom patterns.

Using the DSM-III criteria for diagnosis, Varner and Gaitz (1982) estimated that 2% of outpatients and 4.6% of inpatients among the elderly suffer from paranoia. Still, quite commonly, paranoia fails to receive psychiatric attention; therefore, population estimates are assumed to be much higher.

**Etiology.** Most geriatric clinicians believe that interpersonal as well as biological loss play a role in the etiology of paranoia in old age. LaRue et al. (1985) cite several premorbid risk factors for late-onset paranoia, including never having married, being childless, being socially isolated, and suffering significant hearing loss. Impairment in hearing presents greater risk than vision impairment. A positive family history of schizophrenia and paranoid or schizoid premorbid personality also contributes to risk.

## Assessment of Psychosis

The troublesome lack of attention to (and agreement about) classification is central to the relative dearth of information about psychosis in old age. This limits the interpretation of many early studies. For example, numerous articles about paranoia consider cases of increased suspiciousness toward family members and cases involving complex delusional systems under the same rubric. Distinctions between schizophrenia of the paranoid type and paranoia are rarely made. There is no scientific justification for this pattern. Paranoid symptomatology in old age can indicate schizophrenia, dementia, or paranoid psychosis; the prevalence and prognosis are different for each.

Schizophrenics are no more likely than normals to develop dementia in old age (Ciompi, 1985). Even though the two disorders can co-occur, cognitive impairment usually indicates dementia rather than paranoia. Differentiation of drug-induced symptoms from psychotic symptoms is of paramount importance in assessment. Geriatric patients are more susceptible to toxic reactions from a wide range of prescription and nonprescription medications. It is essential to consider delirium whenever a new patient is assessed.

By and large, the same assessment instruments used with younger psychiatric patients are used with geropsychiatric populations. The Brief Psychiatric Rating Scale (BPRS), the SCL-90, and the Minnesota Multiphasic Personality Inventory (MMPI) are very commonly used. The Kincannon, a brief form of the MMPI, is sometimes preferred to the original form because it can be administered verbally.

## Summary

Psychotic disorders continue to appear in late life. Most geropsychiatric patients, however, are chronically mentally ill persons grown old. In some aspects, the long-term outlook for psychosis is good. Specifically, there is a muting of positive symptoms; because positive symptoms dampen or remit in advanced years, medications can frequently be reduced or discontinued. Remaining symptoms, however—particularly social withdrawal—place older patients at risk of an exacerbation of problems in the development of now-secondary problems because of the absence of adequate nutrition, insufficient medical care, and increasing social isolation. For this reason, it is essential to assess carefully and to treat negative symptoms, even when diminished positive symptoms suggest improvement.

## Psychoactive Substance Use Disorders

Prevalence surveys of psychoactive substance abuse have varied in sampling methods and in the definition of substance abuse. Most prevalence studies, for example, have sampled an urban population and have examined alcohol abuse rather than drug abuse. Bailey, Haberman, and Alksne (1965) surveyed households in Manhattan and found a bimodal peak prevalence for alcoholism. The peak prevalence for alcoholism occurred in the 45–54 age group (23 cases per 1000); prevalence declined to 17 per 1000 in the 55–65 age group, but it increased to 22 per 1000 in the 65–74 age group. This second peak was followed by a precipitous drop to 12 per 1000 for the 75-and-over age group. The highest rates were found among elderly widowers: 105 cases per 1000. These prevalence rates indicate that alcoholism is a serious problem for this particular group of elders, given that the prevalence rate for the entire population is 19 per 1000.

In a study of 1990 referrals to a geriatric outreach program, Reifler, Raskind, and Kethley (1982) found a 10% prevalence rate for substance abuse. The majority of the cases (82%) involved alcohol abuse rather than drug abuse. These authors reported a decline in alcohol and drug abuse between the ages of 60 and 90 or more years. For the age group of 60–69 years, the prevalence was 21%, whereas the prevalence rate after age 90 was 1%. These data are consistent with the findings of Daniel (1972) and Bailey et al. (1965) who also reported an age-associated decline in alcohol-related problems. Reifler et al. (1982) suggested that the observed decline may be attributable to the increased mortality associated with substance use disorders. Note that both Reifler et al. (1982) and Daniel (1972) sampled from elderly persons already involved in the mental health system; the prevalence rates reported by these investigators may be underestimated if elderly substance abusers do not find their way into the mental health system. This is highly possible, given that studies of patterns of mental health service utilization suggest that visits to mental health clinics by individuals older than 65 are rare (Shapiro et al., 1984). The prevalence may be overestimated, however, if substance abusers are more likely to develop problems that bring them to the attention of the health care system.

Medical care for the problems associated with long-term alcohol abuse is usually necessary for the elderly early-onset alcoholic. The prognosis for elderly alcoholics who began drinking in early adulthood is likely to be poorer. For those elderly who begin abusing alcohol in later life, the onset of the abuse is likely to be associated with a stressful event (Martin & Streissguth, 1982). Life events common in old age that may contribute to late-onset alcohol abuse include retirement, relocation, bereavement, and financial concerns. Stress associated with these circumstances may contribute to the development of anxiety or depression; the elderly individual may in turn attempt to obtain relief by self-medicating with alcohol. Valinis, Yeaworth, and Mullis (1988) surveyed bereaved and nonbereaved older adults and found, for example, that only 5.6% of bereaved males abstained from alcohol use, compared with 46% of nonbereaved males.

## Cognitive Impact of Alcohol Abuse in Old Age

Jones and Parsons (1971) suggested that the severe cognitive deficits typically seen in elderly alcoholics relative to younger alcoholics are attributable to the greater susceptibility of the aging brain to the effects of alcohol abuse. This is known as the increased susceptibility hypothesis. A second hypothesis, known as the premature aging hypothesis, developed from observations of the cognitive functioning of long-term alcohol abusers. It has been found that alcoholics can often perform tasks that require highly overlearned responses, but that they demonstrate severe deficits in tasks that require abstract reasoning, memory, learning, or visuoperceptual skills (Ryan, 1982). Ryan and Butters (1980) reported that in various learning and memory tasks, alcoholics typically perform at a level comparable to normal controls who are 10 years older. This relationship, it was found, held across the life-span. Noonberg, Goldstein, and Page (1985) suggested that a limitation of this research has been the disregard for whether the cognitive tests used are sensitive to both aging and the effects of alcohol. A study reported by Holden, McLaughlin, Reilly, and Overall (1988) provides support for the hypothesis that the effects of alcohol abuse on cognitive functioning are similar to the effects of aging. These investigators calculated mental age function from WAIS-scale score profiles for 164 alcoholics who ranged in age from 35–74. They found that the mean mental age for subjects in the alcoholic sample was approximately 7 years advanced aver age-matched controls.

Noonberg et al. (1985) suggested that a significant interaction between alcoholism and age is not necessary to support the premature aging hypothesis. These authors contend that the premature aging hypothesis predicts that the performance of alcoholics will be inferior to normal controls across the life-span. In contrast, the increased vulnerability hypothesis predicts that young alcoholics will not display significant decrements relative to normal controls. Furthermore, according to the increased susceptibility hypothesis, alcoholics should become susceptible to the effects of long-term alcohol abuse only in advanced old age (Holden et al., 1988). The increased susceptibility hypothesis developed from findings that there were no parallel relationships in the developmental curves of alcoholics and normal controls. Bertara and Parsons (1978), for example, found that alcoholics performed more poorly than normals in a scanning talk at all ages, but a relationship between age and performance was found only for the alcoholic group. Common findings of cognitive deficits observed in young alcoholics (e.g., Holden et al., 1988; Ryan & Butters, 1980) do not support this hypothesis. There is evidence, however, that recovery from the effects of alcohol abuse may be age-dependent. Reilly, Kelly, Pena, Overall, and Faillace (1983) reported that a deficit in visual evoked-potential latencies in newly detoxified alcoholics was reversible in younger alcoholics but progressively less so at older ages. At present, it is not clear whether recovery in cognitive functioning is also age-dependent. Zimberg (1987) developed a scale of alcohol abuse that he reports is useful in diagnosing alcohol abuse in the elderly and in measuring changes in the severity of abuse over time. He suggested that lower scores are indicative of abuse, compared to score levels for younger groups, because there is typically less evidence of addiction in the elderly and fewer physical sequelae. Unfortunately, he does not report any data that support the reliability and validity of the scale.

Zimberg (1987) suggested that classifying elderly alcoholics according to whether the problem drinking began early in life or whether the onset occurred in old age can have implications for treatment planning. Further, he noted that this approach to classification allows examining the effects of the stresses of aging that contribute to alcohol abuse. These factors can be compared with the characteristics of the early-onset alcoholic that are unrelated to the problems of aging. **Assessment.** Assessment of alcohol abuse in the elderly is hindered by an absence of standardized instruments with norms based on an elderly sample. It has been suggested that alcoholism in the elderly may be underidentified because elderly alcoholics typically drink relatively small amounts, compared to younger alcoholics (Willenbring, Christiansen, Spring, & Rasmussen, 1987). Elders who consume smaller amounts of alcohol are still considered alcohol abusers because they cannot metabolize alcohol as readily as younger adults (Saltman, Vander Kolk, & Shader, 1975). Older alcoholics are usually brought to the attention of the medical community because of the medical and cognitive complications that often accompany alcohol abuse in old age, rather than because of family or occupational difficulties, as is often the case with younger alcoholics. Willenbring et al. (1987) argued that the differences in symptomatology between older and younger alcoholics may limit the validity of screening instruments that have been normed on younger groups.

Willenbring et al. (1987) assessed the validity of four versions of the Michigan Alcoholism Screening Test (MAST) for elderly males. They reported that, using a cutoff score of 6 or more, the MAST correctly classified all cases and 90% of the controls. The brief versions of the MAST also have acceptable sensitivity and specificity for this population.

## Sexual Disorders

The film "Cocoon" exemplifies many of the myths and realities about aging and sexual dysfunction; a major goal of this section is to help clarify the realities and dispel some of the myths that the movie dramatizes. In this film, three older men (two married and one unmarried) are restored to youth, unknowingly, by swimming in a pool containing alien "cocoons" that are imbued with a mysterious "life force" by their alien rescuers. On their way home, all three share that each has a strong erection, the first in a long time. The two married men return home to initiate sex with their wives (who need no restoring "life force" to be eagerly receptive sexually). The unmarried man stops avoiding contact with an interested woman and becomes willing to date her and to begin a romance. The messages are clear, though implicit. First, and most positively, the film suggests that sex is not disgusting or inappropriate for elders; it is a joyful activity for both the men and the women

in the film. The other messages, however, are more problematic. The second message is that older men do not get spontaneous erections; only men "restored to youth" can do that. Third, only when men get spontaneous erections does sexual contact occur for couples. In fact, this expectation is so strong that the unmarried man avoids all personal, potentially intimate, social contact with women until he can get an erection. Fourth, older women are shown as dependent on their male partners' decisions to initiate or avoid sexual contact; they can accept but cannot make overtures.

### Prevalence

What does the literature suggest about the accuracy of these stereotypes of sexual functioning and dysfunction in elders? Unfortunately, well-designed epidemiological studies of functioning across a full range of healthy and ill elders of various ages and demographic characteristics are nonexistent; however, a patchwork of studies that examined various aspects of function is available.

The earliest studies to examine the prevalence of sexual problems in the elderly suggested that there was a general decline in sexual activity across the life-span. For example, Kinsey and his associates (Kinsey, Pomeroy, & Martin, 1949; Kinsey, Pomeroy, Martin, & Gebhard, 1953) found lower levels of sexual activity of all types with each increasing decade of age. They also reported a greater incidence of male dysfunction (particularly, difficulty obtaining or maintaining an erection) with each increasing decade of life, particularly starting around age 50. Similar findings have been reported by a number of investigators (e.g., Freeman, 1961; Newman & Nichols, 1960; Pfeiffer & Davis, 1972; Pfeiffer, Verwoerdt, & Davis, 1972; Pfeiffer, Verwoerdt, & Wang, 1969; Verwoerdt, Pfeiffer, & Wang, 1969a,b).

The major problem in all of this prior research has been the exclusive use of cross-sectional methodology. Thus, the effects of age have been confounded with cohort in these studies. In addition, when combining across individuals at each age, a smooth curve may be the picture of decline, when the actual longitudinal events may be more acute rather than gradual, that is, individuals may sustain a particular level of function throughout their lives without any decline until some dramatic event, such as the onset of a severe illness, changes the picture.

**Studies of Prevalence.** George and Weiler (1981) tested these possibilities using data from the Duke Longitudinal Study of Aging and followed 278 men and women, ages 46–71 and all married (though not necessarily to each other), for approximately 6 years. Using this longitudinal design, they found that "levels of sexual activity remain more stable over time than previously suggested" (George & Weiler, 1981, p. 918). They found that as people aged, the best predictor of their level of sexual behavior was their level of behavior when they were younger. For some couples during the period of study (8.3% of the men and 14.8% of the women), however, a dramatic decline in activity occurred. In most cases, the cause of this change was some physical change in the male partner that altered his interest in sex or his ability to be an active sexual partner (e.g., development of erectile failure attributable to medications). These authors concluded that "it is crucial to distinguish between aggregate trends and intraindividual change" (George & Weiler, 1981, p. 918), particularly when considering the clinical implications of these findings.

Since these findings have been reported, a handful of additional studies has become available. Among these is only one longitudinal study (Persson & Svanborg, 1992). These authors studied men in Sweden who were married and sexually active at age 70; men were again interviewed at age 75 regarding sexual activity. They found cessation of sexual activity among about half of the sample: 20 still had intercourse with their wives, whereas 21 did not. For men who had ceased sexual activity, cardiovascular causes were the most commonly cited reason. In addition, various life stresses, such as financial problems, were also typical of men who had ceased sexual activity. The authors further reported that there seemed to be additive effects of stress and cardiovascular disease, particularly hypertension. It is interesting to note that the authors of the study and, apparently, the men in the sample did not mention substituting other sexual activity when intercourse was no longer feasible. When the male partner had difficulty with erectile function, sexual activity of all kinds ceased.

Weizman and Hart (1987) reported maintenance of sexual interest and activity in healthy men ages 60–71. Similarly, Martin (1981) showed that individual differences in sexual functioning before middle age are likely to be maintained past middle age and to persist into old age. Laumann, Paik, and Rosen (1999) studied a large national probability study of men and women, but unfortunately covered only ages from 18–59. However, within this age range, they report the intriguing finding that the effects of age are different for men than for women. For women, increasing age led to a decreased prevalence of sexual problems across the spectrum of desire, orgasm, and pleasure experienced in sex. For men, the opposite was true: increasing age was associated with increased prevalence of difficulty, especially in relation to sexual desire and the experience of erection.

Bortz, Wallace, & Wiley (1999) surveyed men aged 58–94 to obtain information on sexual attitudes and activity. They found, as others have, that age was related to increased sexual dysfunction and decreased sexual activity. However, many of these men (along with those without difficulty) continued to engage actively in sexual behaviors and to report positive attitudes about sex. Health status was a major predictor of the presence or absence of dysfunction. Perceived partner responsiveness was also an important moderator of age effects.

Following on the importance of health status, two studies targeted physically healthy older adults. Bortz and Wallace (1999) obtained information from older men and women who attended the Fifty Plus Fitness Association, a group committed to an active life-style. They found that, in this select group, both male and female members had high levels of sexual activity and satisfaction. Sexual satisfaction was correlated with the degree of fitness. Steinke (1994) conducted studies, using the Aging Sexual Knowledge and Attitude Scale (White, 1982), of members of an older adults' wellness group and of a random sample of older adults. Both groups reported a moderate level of knowledge and permissive attitudes; there were no significant differences between men and women. There was a wide range of sexual activity, from 0 to 30 episodes of sexual activity per month. Surprisingly, there were no dramatic differences between the wellness group and the randomly selected older adults.

Socioeconomic status is another variable that appears to affect sexual attitudes and behavior in older age (Cogen & Steinman, 1990). In a study of older men (ages 61–84) who attended a VA geriatric clinic, these authors found that 59% of the men had erection difficulties that ranged from complete loss to frequent difficulty obtaining an erection significant for intercourse. Generally, these men were from lower socioeconomic backgrounds, and they reported infrequent use of manual or oral stimulation, even when intercourse was not possible. In fact, with one exception, all of the men who could not obtain erections adequate for intercourse ceased all sexual activity. This figure contrasts with the report from men of higher socioeconomic status of a high prevalence of using (up to 56%) alternative activities for sexual stimulation (Brecher, 1984; Starr & Weiner, 1981).

Unfortunately, the well-constructed NIMH Epidemiologic Catchment Area program (Regier et al., 1984) did not include questions about sexual function, so that there are still many unanswered questions regarding the prevalence of particular sexual dysfunctions in community-dwelling elders. There are some reports on the prevalence of sexual dysfunction in men (but unfortunately not in women) who have various medical problems (Slag et al., 1983).

**Medical Problems and Sexual Dysfunction.**
One influential study (Mulligan, Retchin, Chinchilli, & Bettinger, 1988) reported on 1180 men who received care in a Veterans Administration medical outpatient clinic; although the age range of the sample is not clearly reported, it is primarily an elderly sample judging by the mean ages for various groups (which ranged from 56.5 years old to 66.9 years old). In this group, which was preselected for medical problems and was likely to be using medications, 34% reported erectile dysfunction. Another study that examined medically ill elderly veterans (Mulligan et al., 1988) also reported high rates of inhibited sexual desire (31% in those ages 65–75 and 50% in those older than 75) and erectile dysfunction (27% in those ages 65–75 and 50% in those older than 75).

Much of this research supports the implication from earlier studies (e.g., George & Weiler, 1981; Persson & Skanborg, 1992) that it is not age *per se* but age-related physical illness that leads to sexual dysfunction in the elderly. It is also possible that normal age-related changes may contribute to dysfunction, however, that psychological attitudes may make ill elders more vulnerable to dysfunction, or that there may be complex interactions among normal age-related changes, medical conditions, psychological, and cultural factors in the etiology of sexual dysfunction in the elderly.

**Etiology and Assessment.** Masters and Johnson (1966) described the major age-related changes in physical response to sexual stimulation. Generally, these changes result in slowed and slightly diminished response to stimulation at every stage of the sexual arousal cycle, but at no stage of the cycle is responsiveness qualitatively changed, nor is the reduction in response great enough to prevent arousal, a wide range of sexual activity (including intercourse), or orgasm. Specifically, men need more direct penile stimulation to reach erection, and the erection may be 70–80% of the size and rigidity attained at a younger age. Longer, more intense stimulation is likely to be needed for orgasm (a boon to those who experienced premature ejaculation as young men), and a longer postorgasm refractory state will be experienced. For women, menopause results in reduced lubrication and vaginal elasticity, so that intercourse may be painful unless estrogen replacement or an artificial vaginal lubricant is used. Women may also need more intense stimulation to become fully aroused and to experience orgasm. Older women (like younger women) are potentially multiorgasmic and do not experience a refractory period. Underlying these changes are various endocrine, vascular, and metabolic changes; those best understood are the gradual decline of testosterone production in men (e.g., Davidson et al., 1983; Tsitouras, Martin, & Harman, 1982) and subclinical atherosclerotic changes that result in diminished genital vasocongestive capacity (e.g., Gewertz & Zarins, 1985; Kaiser et al., 1988).

In addition to these normal changes, a huge array of medical conditions and medications can physiologically disrupt various aspects of the sexual arousal cycle. An exhaustive description of all of them is far beyond the scope of this chapter; summaries can be obtained in Segraves and Schoenberg (1985), Schover and Jensen (1988), and Davis et al. (1985). The following, however, are worthy of special note.

Antihypertensives are a common cause of erectile difficulties (e.g., Segraves, Madsen, Carter, & Davis, 1985; Zeiss, Zeiss, & Dornbrand, 1989), and there is an age-related increase in hypertension and in the use of antihypertensive medication. A variety of neurological diseases, including multiple sclerosis, Parkinson's disease, stroke, and Alzheimer's disease, also affect sexual functioning (Coslett & Heilman, 1986; Mancall, Alonso, & Marlowe, 1985; Singer, Weiner, Sanchez-Ramos, & Ackerman, 1991; Zeiss, Davies, & Tinklenberg, 1990). Although some of this may be mediated by psychological distress about neurological symptoms (e.g., Zeiss, Davies, & Tinklenberg, 1990), sexual dysfunction usually increases for both males and females in direct proportion to the length and stage of disease (and thus is indirectly age-related).

It is also well-known that diabetes results in erectile difficulties in men in a large proportion of cases (often cited as 50%, although careful studies are lacking). Interestingly, problems with desire, ejaculation, or orgasm are almost never reported in men with diabetes, even when no erection can be obtained (e.g., Jensen, 1985). The degree of contribution of psychological factors is questionable (e.g., Jensen, 1986; Renshaw, 1985), but erectile problems do seem to be related to physiological indexes, particularly the presence of peripheral neuropathy. Recent research with female diabetics suggests that type II diabetes has negative effects on female sexual desire, orgasmic capacity, lubrication, sexual satisfaction, sexual activity, and relationship with the sexual partner (Schreiner-Engel, Schiavi, Vietorisz, & Smith, 1987) but that type I diabetes is not associated with dysfunction. Other research, however, suggests that psychological factors as well as physical factors may play an important mediating role in the impact of diabetes on sexual function in both men and women; acceptance of the disease and the presence of somatopsychological responses to the disease are important predictors of its impact on sexual function (Jensen, 1986; Newman & Bertelson, 1985).

Operations for prostatic problems are especially common in older males. A radical prostatectomy directly impacts sexual function because pubic nerves are severed during the surgery. Most surgery for enlarged prostates is now done via the transurethral resection of the prostate (TURP) procedure, which theoretically should have no direct negative physical consequences for erectile function (although retrograde ejaculation is often a physical consequence of the surgery). A series of studies by Libman and her associates, however, has demonstrated that older men are at elevated risk of developing sexual problems after a TURP, compared to men not undergoing surgery and to younger men undergoing TURPs (Libman et al., 1987). This elevated risk, however, seems to be most closely related to the man's sexual adjustment and couple satisfaction before surgery (Libman, Fichten, Jacobson, Creti, & Brender, 1986). In addition, older men who undergo inguinal hernia repair have negative consequences after surgery similar to those who undergo a TURP, so that the physical procedures involved in the TURP are less crucial than the negative physical and/or psychological impact of surgery *per se*.

Psychological factors involved in sexual dysfunction in the elderly include cultural stereotypes (which affect elders' expectations and their willingness to express sexual feelings), interpersonal issues (such as changes in couples' role relationships at retirement), and intra-personal factors (such as anxiety engendered by awareness of aging or failing health). A complete review of these factors is also outside the scope of this chapter, but reviews can be seen in Renshaw (1985), Schover (1986), and Weg (1983). The issues in psychosocial functioning are particularly well described by Renshaw (1985):

> Consider the woman whose 56-year-old husband has a partial erection for the first time. He panics and impotence might follow, not because he is aging but as a result of his anxiety. This is emotional impotence based on misperceptions that erections will be high and "instant" forever. If his wife has no greater knowledge, she may out of compassion avoid him sexually: "I would rather not be in bed with him. It upsets him because he cannot ..." The couple then has no loving contact at all, which may aggravate their distress and lead to physical as well as needless emotional distance. (P. 637)

This passage also illustrates the complex interaction of psychological factors (which lead to the loss of "instant" erections or full erections every time) and psychological factors (which compound the intrapsychic anxiety and the loss of the couple's closeness and result in a full-blown dysfunction).

The difficulty in talking about sexual experience by at least the current cohort of elders is another cultural factor that has psychological impact. At a younger age, the couple did not need to discuss sex, because their expectations for spontaneous arousal were physiologically supported by young, healthy bodies. As age-related normative changes and/or illnesses take their toll, however, the need to discuss concerns, engage in problem solving as a couple, and develop alternative strategies to enhance arousal and comfortable intercourse is essential. When the couple cannot discuss sex, this essential problem solving is impossible, and dysfunction results (Weg, 1983; Zeiss, Zeiss, & Dornbrand, 1989). Again, it is futile to argue whether this is essentially a psychologically caused problem (because the couple's mode of interpersonal functioning prevents finding an innovative solution) or a physical problem (because physical factors lead to the need for innovative problem solving).

## Implications

In reviewing the factors cited in the prevalence research at the start of this chapter, it is important to remember that the physical changes that lead to disruption of sexual functioning are those that affect the male partner's interest in sex and/or his ability to obtain an erection. This provides another example of the intricate interplay of physical and psychological factors in elders' sexual problems. It appears that the culturally induced emphasis on male sexual assertiveness and control underlies sexual problems for many elders. For example, both diabetic men and their partners could have mutually satisfying sexual activities resulting in orgasm for both, whether or not the man obtains an erection. Because the cultural expectation, however, is that the man's erection signals the start of sexual activity and is the defining basis of the most accepted activity, sexual intercourse, the loss of spontaneous erections all too often signals the loss of sexual intimacy and shared physical pleasure.

Numerous authors (e.g., Schiavi & Schreiner-Engel, 1988) have made similar points regarding the complex interplay of physical and psychosocial factors in the elderly. The developing consensus is well described in the following: "The data also strongly suggest that organogenic and psychogenic are not dichotomous categories and that a multi-faceted assessment of erectile potential, psychological factors, and the current social and interpersonal context of sexual behavior is necessary for successful medical or psychological treatment planning" (Sakheim, Barlow, Abrahamson, & Beck, 1987, p. 379).

It is instructive now to look back at the example from the movie "Cocoon" that began this section. What are the major lessons to be drawn from it? First, the film is quite correct in suggesting that older men do not get spontaneous erections, at least as often or as firmly as younger men; this probably has a physiological basis. It is also correct that an erect penis does seem to be the major criterion for active sexual participation in older couples; this emphasis is probably culturally mediated. Couples limit themselves because of their lack of knowledge regarding normal age-related changes and reversible medical problems or the effects of medication. They also limit themselves because of their difficulty in discussing sex and in planning effective solutions to minor problems. Finally, the double standard by which this cohort

of elders was raised, which dictated that only men should actively seek sexual activity and guide its expression, seems to cause problems. It leaves couples vulnerable to a shift from sustained sexual activity to a sudden cessation or sharp decline of sexual intimacy when major (or even minor) health problems affect the male partner's ability or willingness to sustain the burdens of that role.

## Eating Disorders

Eating disorders within the DSM-IV are classified under the heading of "disorders usually first evident in infancy, childhood, or adolescence." Stelnicki and Thompson (1989) suggested that this classification system may result in attributing disordered eating behaviors in the elderly to an underlying physical disorder. Consequently, the prevalence of eating disorders in this population may be underreported. The incidence of eating disorders in the elderly has not been studied systematically. Many cases reported in the literature involved individuals who displayed dysfunctional eating behaviors before reaching old age. It has been noted that the prevalence of eating disorders such as anorexia nervosa is much higher in younger cohorts (Stelnicki & Thompson, 1989). As these cohorts age, we may see an increased prevalence of such disorders in the elderly. Significant weight loss associated with anorexia, however, is already a common problem in old age. The problems of decreased food intake and malnutrition are considered of epidemic proportions among the institutionalized elderly in some areas (Morley & Silver, 1988). A survey of nursing homes in Florida, for example, indicated that up to 58% of residents experienced some degree of malnutrition (Pinchofsky-Devin & Kaminski, 1986). The majority of reports of eating disorders in the elderly are case studies. A review of the literature revealed no systematic prevalence surveys or group treatment studies with community-dwelling, noninstitutionalized populations. Price, Giannini, and Colella (1985) reported a case of anorexia nervosa in a 67-year-old widowed woman. The subject had lost 21 pounds during the course of a year, although she had no health problems. She reported that she was dieting and using laxatives and described herself as "fat and ungainly." She displayed no signs of a mood disorder. A behavioral treatment program that involved reinforcement contingent on weight gain was implemented; after approximately 1 year, she returned to her normal weight of 125 pounds.

Ronch (1985) described the case of an institutionalized 75-year-old man who displayed symptoms consistent with a diagnosis of anorexia nervosa. Assessment revealed a long history of disordered eating habits and several hospitalizations for treatment of malnutrition. He weighed 80 pounds, engaged in laxative abuse, and refused to eat sugars, fats, and carbohydrates. He also had several food phobias, frequently hoarded food, and occasionally induced vomiting after eating. A program of forced use of food supplements and intravenous feedings resulted in weight gain up to a high of 102 pounds, but treatment gains were not maintained. In an effort to improve treatment maintenance, a cognitive-behavioral program was implemented. The program focused on treating depression and nutrition reeducation. This resulted in a moderate weight gain (up to 92 pounds) and eliminated many of the anorexic behaviors. The subject continued to report "feeling fat" at treatment termination. Another reported case of bulimia nervosa involved a 70-year-old woman with a long history of fear of becoming obese (Kellett, Trimble, & Thorley, 1976). The subject gorged herself with fattening foods and then induced vomiting and used laxatives to purge herself. A few cases of pica in elderly individuals have also been reported (e.g., Nash, Broome, & Stone, 1987). All of these involved individuals with a diagnosis of mental retardation or dementia and therefore will not be reviewed here because these disorders are covered extensively in other chapters. Of interest is the finding that the prevalence of pica among the mentally retarded is highest on the group over the age of 71 (39% of cases). The groups ages 41–60 and 11–40 account for 14 and 29% of cases, respectively (Danford & Huber, 1982).

## Etiology

Several age-related physical changes may contribute to reduced calorie intake in the elderly. These include decreased demand as a result of lower metabolic rate and reduced activity; changes in taste, smell, and vision that occur with normal aging; teeth and denture problems; and decreased feeding drive, possibly related to alterations in neurotransmitters (especially endogenous opioids; Morley & Silver, 1988). Because it is a concomitant of normal aging, anorexia may also be associated with a variety of disease processes that are common in old age. These include conditions that cause pain on eating (e.g., abdominal ischemia) and recurrent infections (Morley & Silver, 1988). For example, it has been suggested that the anorexia-causing chemical cachetin (or tumornecrosis factor) is released during infection or cancer and may play a causative role in the excessive weight loss found in nursing-home patients who often experience repeated bouts of infection (Morley & Silver, 1988). Depression and dementia in the elderly are often associated with anorexia. Zung (1967) reported that decreased appetite is one of the most common symptoms seen in depressed elderly. A Finnish study (Kivela et al., 1986) found that a significant proportion of elderly depressed men reported problems that interfered with eating. These included a history of diarrhea (20%), constipation (36%), stomach pains (37%), nausea (17%), vomiting (10%), and loss of appetite (22%).

It has been suggested that deficiency of norepinephrine (NE) may play a role in anorexia associated with depression. As mentioned earlier, several studies demonstrated a significant age-related reduction in NE (Veith & Raskind, 1988). This age-related reduction in NE, coupled with NE deficits associated with depression, may account for the high prevalence of decreased appetite in geriatric depression. Corticotropin-releasing hormone (CRF), it has also been suggested plays a role in the anorexia of elderly depressives. Morley and Silver (1988) reasoned that because NE inhibits the release of CRF, NE reduction should be associated with an increased release of CRF. These authors noted that CRF acts within the central nervous system as a potent inhibitor of food intake, and thus excess CRF probably functions in anorexia associated with depression. Furthermore, it has been suggested that CRF plays a role in the development of anorexia nervosa (Morley, Silver, Fiatarone, & Mooradian, 1986). Dementia is commonly associated with significant weight loss and malnutrition. The causes of anorexia in individuals suffering from a dementing disorder may include reduced interest in eating, forgetting to eat, and impaired judgment that results in failure to recognize the need to eat (Sandman, Adolfsson, Nygren, Hallmanns, & Winblad, 1987).

Problems associated with eating have serious consequences for individuals with a dementing disorder. For example, Chenoweth and Spencer

(1986) found that among caregivers of demented individuals who resided in the community, behavior problems such as the inability to self-feed accounted for 18% of the reasons given for deciding to institutionalize. Several studies have found that the nutritional status of demented individuals is often seriously deficient. Sandman et al. (1987) found energy and/or protein malnutrition in 50% of demented subjects examined; the mean reference weight of subjects was 82% of ideal body weight. Patients with dementing disorders also have lower levels of zinc, vitamin B12, and serum iron (Greer, McBride, & Shenkin, 1986). These findings suggest that the nutritional status and self-feeding behaviors of individuals with dementing disorders warrant careful attention because they are at serious risk of malnutrition. At present, little is known about the role of neurotransmitter abnormalities and anorexia in dementia. The neuropathological changes associated with dementing disorders, coupled with the resulting behavioral deficits, present complex questions for researchers in attempting to understand and reduce nutritional deficits in this population.

## Conclusions

In this chapter, we reviewed the literature on psychopathology and aging. It is clear that early research and theory assumed that the incidence of psychological disorder increased with age. This was attributable, in part, to negative societal attitudes about the aging process and the methodological limitations of early research strategies.

In recent years, we witnessed improvement of sampling methods in epidemiological research and increased use of longitudinal designs. These methodological changes have dispelled some of the myths about aging and old age. Unfortunately, changes in theory have not kept pace with empirical findings. New etiological theories of depression, for example, are needed to account for the consistent finding of decreased incidence of depression in late adulthood. The knowledge base has increased significantly, and researchers are now faced with the challenge of identifying the relevant mechanisms. Although information about normal and pathological aging is developing at a significant pace, our understanding of the aging process is still in its infancy.

## References

AARP(1998). *A profile of older Americans: 1998.* Washington, D.C.: Author

Abraham, S., Carroll, M. D., & Dresser, C. M. (1977). Dietary intake of persons 1–74 years of age in the United States (Vital and Health Statistics of the National Center for Health Statistics, No. 6). Rockville, MD: Health Resources Administration, Public Health.

Abramson, L. Y., Seligman, M. E. P., & Teasdale, J. D. (1978). Learned helplessness in humans: Critique and reformulation. *Journal of Abnormal Psychology, 87,* 49–74.

Aldwin, C. (1995). The role of stressing aging and adult development. *Adult Development and Aging, 23,* 1–16.

Aldwin, C. M., Spiro, A., Levenson, M. R., & Bosse, R. (1989). Longitudinal findings from the Normative Aging Study: I. Does mental health change with age? *Psychology and Aging, 4,* 295–306.

Andreason, N. C. (1982). Negative symptoms in schizophrenia: Definition and reliability. *Archives of General Psychiatry, 39,* 784–788.

Angel, J. L., & Hogan, D. P. (1991). The demography of minority aging populations. In *Minority elders: Longevity, economics, and health* (pp 1–13). Washington, D.C.: Gerontological Society of America.

Avery, D., & Winokur, G. (1976). Mortality in depressed patients treated with electroconvulsive therapy and antidepressants. *Archives of General Psychiatry, 33,* 1029–1037.

Bailey, M. B., Haberman, P. W., & Alksne, H. (1965). The epidemiology of alcoholism in an urban residential area. *Quarterly Journal of Studies on Alcohol, 26,* 19–41.

Ballard, C. G., Chithiramohan, R. N., Bannister, C., Handy, S., & Todd, N. (1991). Paranoid features in the elderly with dementia. *International Journal of Geriatric Psychiatry, 6,* 155–157.

Ballard, C., & Oyebode, F. (1995). Psychotic symptoms in patients with dementia. *International Journal of Geriatric Psychiatry, 10,* 743–752.

Baltes, P. B., & Schaie, K. W. (1976). On the plasticity of intelligence in adulthood and old age: Where Horn and Donaldson fail. *American Psychologist, 31,* 720–725.

Barlow, D. H. (1988). *Anxiety and its disorders: The nature and treatment of anxiety and panic.* New York: Guilford.

Beck, A. T. (1967). *Depression: Clinical experimental, and theoretical aspects.* New York: Harper & Row.

Beck, A. T. (1978). *Depression inventory.* Philadelphia: Center for Cognitive Therapy.

Beller, S. A., & Overall, J. E. (1984). The Brief Psychiatric Rating Scale (BPRS) in geropsychiatric research: II. Representative profile patterns. *Journal of Gerontology, 39,* 194–200.

Bertera, J. H., & Parsons, O. A. (1978). Impaired visual search in alcoholics. *Alcoholism: Clinical and Experimental Research, 2,* 9–14.

Biggs, J. T., Wylie, L. T., & Ziegler, V. E. (1978). Validity of the Zung Self-Rating Depression Scale. *British Journal of Psychiatry, 132,* 381–385.

Binstock, R. H. (1999). Challenges to United States policies on aging in the millenium. *Hallym International Journal of Aging, 1,* 3–13.

Blazer, D. (1982). The epidemiology of psychiatric disorder in the elderly population. In L. Grinspoon (Ed.), *Psychiatry update,* Vol. 2. Washington, DC: American Psychiatric Association.

Borkovec, T. D. (1988). Comments on "Worry as a phenomenon relevant to the elderly." *Behavior Therapy, 19,* 381–383.

Bornstein, P., Clayton, P., Halikas, J., Maurice, W., & Robins, E. (1973). The depression of widowhood after thirteen months. *British Journal of Psychiatry, 122,* 561–566.

Bortz, W. M., & Wallace, D. H. (1999). Physical fitness, aging, and sexuality. *Western Journal of Medicine, 170,* 167–169.

Bortz, W. M., Wallace, D. H., & Wiley, D. (1999). Sexual function in 1,202 aging males: Differentiating aspects. *Journals of Gerontology A: Biological Sciences & Medical Sciences, 54,* M237–241.

Brandstadter, J., Wentura, D., & Greve, W. (1993). Adaptive resources of the aging self: Outlines of an emergent perspective. *International Journal of Behavioral Development, 16,* 323–350.

Brecher, E. M. (1984). *Love, sex, and aging.* Boston: Little, Brown.

Butler, R. N., & Lewis, M. I. (1983). *Aging and mental health.* St. Louis: Mosby.

Carey, R. (1977). The widowed: A year later. *Journal of Counseling Psychology, 24,* 125–131.

Carstensen, L. L., & Fremouw, W. (1981). The demonstration of a behavioral intervention for late life paranoia. *Gerontologist, 3,* 329–332.

Carpenter, W. T., Heinrichs, D. W., & Wagman, A. M. I. (1988). Deficit and nondeficit forms of schizophrenia: The concept. *American Journal of Psychiatry, 145,* 578–583.

Charney, D. S., & Heninger, G. R. (1986). Abnormal regulation of noradrenergic function in panic disorders. *Archives of General Psychiatry, 43,* 1042–1054.

Chenoweth, B., & Spencer, B. (1986). Dementia: The experience of family caregivers. *Gerontologist, 26,* 267–272.

Chorpita, B. F., & Barlow, D. H. (1998). The development of anxiety: The role of control in the early environment. *Psychological Bulletin, 124,* 3–21.

Ciompi, L. (1985). Aging and schizophrenic psychosis. *Acta Psychiatrica Scandinavica, 71,* 93–105.

Clayton, F. J., Halikas, J. A., & Maurice, W. L. (1972). The depression of widowhood. *British Journal of Psychiatry, 120,* 71–78.

Cogen, R., & Steinman, W. (1990). Sexual function and practice in elderly men of lower socioeconomic status. *The Journal of Family Practice, 31,* 162–166.

Cohen, G. D. (1991). Anxiety and general medical conditions. In C. Salzman & B. D. Lebowitz (Eds.), *Anxiety in the elderly.* New York: Springer.

Coslett, H. B., & Heilman, K. M. (1986). Male sexual function: Impairment after right hemisphere stroke. *Archives of Neurology, 43,* 1036–1039.

Daniel, R. (1972). A five year study of 693 psychogeriatric admissions in Queensland. *Geriatrics, 27,* 132–158.

Danford, D. E., & Huber, A. M. (1982). Pica among mentally retarded adults. *American Journal of Mental Deficiency, 87*(2), 141–146.

Davidson, J. M., Chen, J. J., Crape, L., Gray, G. D., Greenleaf, W. J., & Catania, J. A. (1983). Hormonal changes and sexual function in aging men. *Journal of Clinical Endocrinology and Metabolism, 57,* 71–77.

Davis, S. S., Viosca, S., Gurainik, M., Windsor, C., Buttiglieri, M. W., Baker, M., & Korenman, S. E. (1985). Evaluation of impotence in older men. *Western Journal of Medicine, 142,* 499.

Dollard, J., & Miller, N. E. (1950). *Personality and psychotherapy.* New York: McGraw-Hill.

Eisdorfer, C. (1980). Paranoia and schizophrenic disorders in later life. In E. W. Busse & D. G. Blazer (Eds.), *Handbook of geriatric psychiatry* (pp. 329–337). New York: Van Nostrand Reinhold.

Endicott, J., & Spitzer, R. L. (1978). A diagnostic interview: The schedule for affective disorders and schizophrenia. *Archives of General Psychiatry, 35,* 837–844.

Feinson, M. C. (1985). Aging and mental health: Distinguishing myth from reality. *Research on Aging, 7,* 155–174.

Feinson, M. C., & Thoits, P. A. (1986). The distribution of distress among elders. *Journal of Gerontology, 41,* 225–233.

Field, D., Schaie, K. W., & Leino, E. V. (1988). Continuity in intellectual functioning: The role of self-reported health. *Psychology and Aging, 3,* 385–392.

Fisher, J. E., Goy, E. R., Swingen, D. N., & Szymanski, J. (1994). *Functional characteristics of behavioral disturbance in Alzheimer's disease.* Paper presented at the Annual Meeting of the Association for the Advancement of Behavior Therapy, San Diego.

Fitten, L. J., Morley, J. E., Gross, P. L., Petry, S. D., & Cole, K. D. (1989). Depression: UCLA geriatric grand rounds. *Journal of the American Geriatrics Society, 37,* 459–472.

Forsell, Y., & Henderson, A. S. (1998). Epidemiology of paranoid symptoms in an elderly population. *British Journal of Psychiatry, 172,* 429–432.

Freeman, J. T. (1961). Sexual capacities in the aging male. *Geriatrics, 16,* 37–43.

Freud, S. (1924). On psychotherapy. In *Collected papers,* Vol. I. London: Hogarth.

Freud, S. (1957). Mourning and melancholia. In J. Strachey (Ed.), *The standard edition of the complete psychological works of Sigmund Freud,* Vol. 14. London: Hogarth. (Originally published in 1917.)

Futterman, A., Thompson, L. W., Gallagher-Thompson, D., & Ferris, R. (1995). Depression in late life: Epidemiology, assessment, etiology, and treatment. In E. E. Beckham & W. R. Leber (Eds.), *Handbook of depression* (2nd ed., pp 495–525). New York: Guilford.

Gallagher, D. E., & Thompson, L. W. (1983). Cognitive therapy for depression in the elderly: A promising model for treatment and research. In D. Breslau & M. R. Haug (Eds.), *Depression and aging.* New York: Springer.

Gallagher, D. E., Nies, G., & Thompson, L. W. (1982). Reliability of the Beck Depression Inventory with older adults. *Journal of Consulting and Clinical Psychology, 50,* 152.

Gallagher, C. E., Breckenridge, J., Steinmetz, J., & Thompson, L. (1983). The Beck Depression Inventory and Research Diagnostic Criteria: Congruence in an older population. *Journal of Consulting and Clinical Psychology, 510,* 945.

Gallagher, D. E., Breckenridge, J. N., Thompson, L. W., Peterson, J. A. (1983). Effects of bereavement on indicators of mental health in elderly widows and widowers. *Journal of Gerontology, 38,* 565–571.

Gallagher-Thompson, D., & Thompson, L. (1996). Applying cognitive-behavioral therapy to the psychological problems of later life. In S. H. Zarit & B. G. Knight (Eds.), *A guide to psychotherapy and aging* (pp. 61–82). Washington, DC: American Psychological Association.

Gallagher-Thompson, D., Lovett, S., Rose, J., McKibbin, C., Coon, D., Futterman, A., Thompson, L. (2000). Impact of psychoeducational interventions on distressed family caregivers. *Journal of Clinical Geropsychology, 6*, 91–110.

Gass, K. A. (1987). Coping strategies of widows. *Journal of Gerontological Nursing, 13*, 29–33.

Gaylord, S. A., & Zung, W. W. K. (1987). Affective disorders among the aging. In L. L. Carstensen & B. A. Edelstein (Eds.), *Handbook of clinical gerontology*. New York: Pergamon Press.

George, L. K. (1981). Subjective well-being conceptual and methodological issues. In C. Eisdorfer (Ed.), *Annual review of gerontology and geriatrics*, Vol. 2. New York: Springer.

George, L. K., & Weiler, S. J. (1981). Sexuality in middle and late life: The effects of age, cohort, and gender. *Archives of General Psychiatry, 38*, 919–923.

Gewertz, B. L., & Zarins, C. K. (1985). Vasculogenic impotence. In R. T. Segraves & H. W. Schoenberg (Eds.), *Diagnosis and treatment of erectile disturbances* (pp. 105–114). New York: Plenum.

Gilewski, M. J., Farberow, N. L., Gallagher, D. E., & Thompson, L. W. (1988, November). Depression and bereavement in the elderly. Presented at the *Annual Meeting of the Gerontological Society of America*, San Francisco.

Gottesman, I., & Shields, J. (1972). *Schizophrenia and genetics: A twin study vantage point*. New York: Academic Press.

Gottesman, I., McGuffin, P., & Farmer, A. E. (1987). Clinical genetics as clues to the "real" genetics of schizophrenia (a decade of modest gains while playing for time). *Schizophrenia Bulletin, 13*, 23–47.

Gray, J. A. (1985). Issues in the neuropsychology of anxiety. In A. H. Tuma & J. D. Maser (Eds.), *Anxiety and the anxiety disorders*. Hillsdale, NJ: Erlbaum.

Greer, A., McBride, D. H., & Shenkin, A. (1986). Comparison of the nutritional state of new and long-term patients in a psychogeriatric unit. *British Journal of Psychiatry, 149*, 738–741.

Grotjahn, M. (1951). Some analytic observations about the process of growing old. In G. Roheim (Ed.), *Psychoanalysis and social science*, Vol. 3. New York: International Universities Press.

Gurland, B., & Cross, P. (1982). Epidemiology of psychopathology in old age. *Psychiatric Clinics of North America, 5*, 11–26.

Gurland, B., Dean, L., Cross, P., & Golden, R. (1980). The epidemiology of depression and dementia in the elderly: The use of multiple indicators of these conditions. In J. O. Cole & J. E. Barrett (Eds.), *Psychopathology in the aged*. New York: Raven Press.

Hamilton, G. V. (1942). Changes in personality and psychosexual phenomena with age. In E. V. Cowdry (Ed.), *Problems of aging*. Baltimore: Williams & Williams.

Harding, C. M. (1986). Speculations on the measurement of recovery from severe psychiatric disorder and the human condition. *Psychiatric Journal of the University of Ottawa, 11*, 199–204.

Harding, C. M., Brooks, G. W., Ashikaga, T., Strauss, J., & Breier, A. (1987). The Vermont longitudinal study of persons with severe mental illness: II. Long-term outcome of subjects who retrospectively met DSM-III criteria for schizophrenia. *American Journal of Psychiatry, 144*, 727–735.

Hedlund, J. L., & Vieweg, B. W. (1979). The Zung Self-Rating Depression Scale: A comprehensive review. *Journal of Operational Psychiatry, 10*, 51–64.

Heidell, E. D., & Kidd, A. H. (1975). Depression and senility. *Journal of Clinical Psychology, 31*, 643–645.

Herth, K. (1990). Relationship of hope, coping styles, concurrent losses, and setting to grief resolution in the elderly widow(er). *Research in Nursing & Health, 13*, 109–117.

Himmelfarb, S., & Murrell, S. A. (1984). The prevalence and correlates of anxiety symptoms in older adults. *Journal of Psychology, 116*, 159–167.

Holden, K. L., McLaughlin, E. J., Reilly, E. L., & Overall, J. E. (1988). Accelerated mental aging in alcoholic patients. *Journal of Clinical Psychology, 44*, 286–292.

Hooley, J. M., Richters, J. E., Weintraub, S., & Neale, J. M. (1987). Psychopathology and marital distress: The positive side of positive symptoms. *Journal of Abnormal Psychology, 1*, 27–33.

Hussian, R. A. (1983). A combination of operant and cognitive therapy with geriatric patients. *International Journal of Behavioral Geriatrics, 1*, 57–61.

Hussian, R. A., & Lawrence, P. S. (1981). Social reinforcement of activity and problem-solving training in the treatment of depressed institutionalized elderly patients. *Cognitive Therapy and Research, 1*, 57–69.

Hybels, D. C., & Miller, S. M. (1987, November). Depression in the elderly: Does the reformulated helplessness theory fit? Presented at the *Annual Convention for the Advancement of Behavior Therapy*, Boston.

Insel, T. R. (1986). The neurobiology of anxiety: A tale of two systems. In B. E. Shaw, Z. V. Segal, T. M. Vallis, & F. E. Cashman (Eds.), *Anxiety disorders: Psychological and biological perspectives*. New York: Plenum.

Jackson, J. S., Chatters, L. M., & Taylor, R. J. (1993). Roles and resources of the Black elderly. In J. S. Jackson, L. M. Chatters, & R. J. Taylor (Eds.), *Aging in Black America* (pp. 1–20). Newbury Park, CA: Sage.

Jarvik, L. E., & Perl, M. (1981). Overview of psychologic dysfunctions related to psychiatric problems in the elderly. In A. J. Levenson and R. C. W. Hall (Eds.), *Aging*, Vol. 14: *Neuropsychiatric manifestations of disease in the elderly*. New York: Raven Press.

Jensen, S. B. (1985). Sexual relationships in couples with a diabetic partner. *Journal of Sex and Mental Therapy, 12*, 259–270.

Jensen, S. B. (1986). Sexual dysfunction in insulin-treated diabetics: A six-year follow-up study of 101 patients. *Archives of Sexual Behavior, 15*, 271–283.

Jones, B. M., & Parsons, O. A. (1971). Impaired abstract ability in chronic alcoholics. *Archives of General Psychiatry, 24*, 71–75.

Kaiser, E. E., Viosca, S. P., Morley, J. E., Mooradian, A. D., Davis, S. S., & Korenman, S. G. (1988). Impotence and aging: Clinical and hormonal factors. *Journal of the American Geriatrics Society, 36*, 511–519.

Kastrop, M. (1985). Characteristics of a nationwide cohort of psychiatric patients—with special reference to the elderly and the chronically admitted. *Acta Psychiatrica Scandinavica, 71*, 107–115.

Kaufman, M. R. (1940). Old age and aging: The psychoanalytic point of view. *American Journal of Orthopsychiatry, 10*, 73–84.

Kay, D. W. K., Beamish, P., & Roth, M. (1964). Old age mental disorders in Newcastle-upon-Snee. *British Journal of Psychiatry, 110*, 146–158.

Kay, D. W. K., & Roth, M. (1961). Environmental and hereditary factors in the schizophrenias of old age ("late paraphrenia") and their bearing on the general problem of causation in schizophrenia. *Journal of Mental Science, 107,* 649–686.

Kellett, J., Trimble, M., & Thorley, A. (1976). Anorexia nervosa after the menopause. *British Medical Journal, 1,* 1770–1773.

Kessler, R. C. (1995). The interplay of research design strategies and data analysis procedures in evaluating the effects of stress on health. In S. Kasl & C. L. Cooper (Eds.) *Stress and health: Issues in research methodology.* Wiley series on studies in occupational stress, pp. 113–140. New York: John Wiley & Sons.

Kessler, R. C., Foster, C., Webster, P. S., & House, J. (1992). The relationship between age and depressive symptoms in two national surveys. *Psychology & Aging, 7,* 119–126.

Kessler, R. C., McGonagle, K. A., Zhao, S., Nelson, C. B., et al. (1994). Lifetime and 12-month prevalence of DSM-III-R psychiatric disorders in the United States: results form the national comorbidity study. *Archives of General Psychiatry, 51,* 8–19.

Kilcourse, J., Gallagher, D., Thompson, L., Tanke, E., & Sheikh, J. (1988). Can rating scales differentiate depression from anxiety in older adults? Paper presented at the *41st Annual Meeting of the Gerontological Society of America,* San Francisco.

Kinsey, A. C., Pomeroy, W. B., & Martin, C. E. (1949). *Sexual behavior in the human male.* Philadelphia: W. B. Saunders.

Kinsey, A. C., Pomeroy, W. B., Martin, C. E., & Gebhard, P. H. (1953). *Sexual behavior in the human female.* Philadelphia: W. B. Saunders.

Kitchell, M., Barbes, R., Veith, R., Okimoto, J., & Raskind, M. (1982). Screening for depression in hospitalized geriatric medical patients. *Journal of the American Geriatrics Society, 30,* 174–177.

Kivela, S. L., Nissin, A., Tuomilehto, J., Pekkanen, J., Punsar, S., Lammi, U., & Puska, P. (1986). Prevalence of depressive and other symptoms in elderly Finnish men. *Acta Psychiatrica Scandinavica, 73,* 93–100.

Klerman, G. L. (1983). Problems in the definition and diagnosis of depression in the elderly. In L. O. Breslau, & M. R. Haig (Eds.), *Depression and aging: Causes, care, and consequences.* New York: Van Nostrand Reinhold.

Klerman, G. L., & Barrett, J. E. (1973). The affective disorders: Clinical and epidemiological aspects. In S. Gershon & B. Shopsin (Eds.), *Lithium: Its role in psychiatric research and treatment.* New York: Plenum.

Klerman, G. L., & Weissman, M. M. (1989). Increasing rates of depression. *Journal of the American Medical Association, 261,* 2229–2235.

Kosloski, K. (1987). Isolating age, period, and cohort effects in developmental research. *Research on Aging, 8,* 460–479.

Lader, M. (1982). Differential diagnosis of anxiety in the elderly. *Journal of Clinical Psychology, 43,* 4–7.

LaRue, A., Dessonville, C., & Jarvik, L. (1985). Aging and mental disorders. In J. E. Birren & K. W. Schaie (Eds.) *Handbook of the psychology of aging* (pp. 664–702). New York: Van Nostrand Reinhold.

Lasser, R., Siegel, E., Dukoff, R., & Sunderland, T. (1998). Diagnosis and treatment of geriatric depression. *CNS Drugs, 9,* 17–30.

Laumann, E. O., Paik, A., Rosen, R. C. (1999). Sexual dysfunction in the United States: Prevalence and predictors. *Journal of the American Medical Association, 281,* 537–544.

Lawton, P. (1972). Schizophrenia forty-five years later. *Journal of Genetic Psychology, 121,* 133–143.

Lewinsohn, P. M., Duncan, E. M., Stanton, A. K., & Hautzinger, M. (1986). Age at first onset for nonbipolar depression. *Journal of Abnormal Psychology, 95,* 378–383.

Lewinsohn, P. M., Zeiss, A. M., & Duncan, E. M. (1989). Probability of relapse after recovery from an episode of depression. *Journal of Abnormal Psychology, 98,* 107–116.

Libman, E., Fichten, C. S., Jacobson, S., Creti, L., & Brender, W. (1986). Risk factors related to sexual impairment after transurethral prostatectomy. Paper presented at *20th Annual Association for the Advancement of Behavior Therapy Convention,* Chicago.

Libman, E., Fichten, C. S., Amsel, R., Creti, L., Weinstein, N., & Brender, W. (1987). Differential consequences of prostatectomy on sexual function in younger and older males. Paper presented at *21st Annual Association for the Advancement of Behavior Therapy Convention,* Boston.

Lowenthal, M. E. (1964). *Lives in distress: The paths of the elderly to the psychiatric ward.* New York: Basic Books.

Lyness, J. M., King, D. A., Cox, C., Yoediono, Z., & Caine, E. D. (1999). The importance of subsyndromal depression in older primary care patients: Prevalence and associated functional disability. *Journal of the American Geriatrics Society, 47,* 647–652.

Mancall, E. L., Alonso, R. J., & Marlowe, W. B. (1985). Sexual dysfunction in neurological disease. In R. T. Segraves & H. W. Schoenberg (Eds.), *Diagnosis and treatment of erectile disturbances* (pp. 65–86). New York: Plenum.

Mann, A. H., Wood, K., Cross, P., Gurland, B., Schieber, P., & Hafner, H. (1984). Institutional care of the elderly: A comparison of the cities of New York, London, and Mannheim. *Social Psychiatry, 19,* 97–102.

Manton, K. G., Blazer, D. G., & Woodbury, M. A. (1987). Suicide in middle age–later life: Sex and race specific life table and cohort analysis. *Journal of Gerontology, 42,* 219–227.

Martin, C. E. (1981). Factors affecting sexual functioning in 60- to 70-year-old married males. *Archives of Sexual Behavior, 10,* 399–420.

Martin, J. C., & Streissguth, A. P. (1982). Alcoholism and the elderly: An overview: In C. Eisdorfer & W. E. Fann (Eds.), *Treatment of psychopathology in the aging.* New York: Springer.

Masters, W. H., & Johnson, V. E. (1966). *Human sexual response.* Boston: Little, Brown.

McGlashan, T. H. (1988). A selective review of recent North American long-term follow-up studies of schizophrenia. *Schizophrenia Bulletin, 14,* 515–542.

McIntosh, J. L. (1985). Suicide among the elderly: Levels and trends. *American Journal of Orthopsychiatry, 55,* 188–193.

Meeks, S., Carstensen, L. L., Stafford, P., Brenner, L. L., Weathers, F., Welch, R., & Oltmanns, T. E. (1990). Mental health needs of the chronically mentally ill elderly. *Psychology and Aging, 5,* 163–171.

Modell, A. H. (1970). Aging and psychoanalytic theories of regression. *Journal of Geriatric Psychology, 3,* 139–146.

Morley, J. E., & Silver, A. J. (1988). Anorexia in the elderly. *Neurobiology of Aging, 9,* 9–16.

Morley, J. E., Silver, A., Fiatarone, M., & Mooradian, A. D. (1986). UCLA Grand Rounds: Nutrition and the elderly. *Journal of the American Geriatrics Society, 34,* 823–832.

Mowrer, O. H. (1948). Learning theory and the neurotic paradox. *American Journal of Orthopsychiatry, 18,* 571–610.

Mulligan, T., Retchin, S. M., Chinchilli, V. M., & Bettinger, C. B. (1988). The role of aging and chronic disease in sexual dysfunction. *Journal of the American Geriatrics Society, 36,* 520–524.

Myers, J. K., Weissman, M. M., Tischler, G. L., Holyer, C. E., Leaf, F. J., Orvaschel, H., Anthony, J. C., Boyd, J. H., Burke, J. D., Kramer, M., & Stolzman, R. (1984). Six-month prevalence of psychiatric disorders in three communities. *Archives of General Psychiatry, 41,* 959–967.

Nash, D. L., Broome, J., & Stone, S. (1987). Behavior modification of pica in a geriatric patient. *Journal of the American Geriatrics Society, 35,* 79–80.

Nemeroff, C. B., Widerlov, E., Bissette, G., Walleus, H., Karlsson, I., Eklund, K., Kilts, C. D., Loosen, I. T., & Yale, W. (1984). Elevated concentrations of CSF corticotropin-releasing factor-like immunoreactivity in depressed patients. *Science, 226,* 1342–1343.

Newman, A. S., & Bertelson, A. D. (1966). Sexual dysfunction in diabetic women. *Journal of Behavioral Medicine, 9,* 261–270.

Newman, G., & Nichols, C. R. (1960). Sexual activities and attitudes in older persons. *Journal of the American Medical Association, 173,* 117–119.

Newman, J. P. (1989). Aging and depression. *Psychology and Aging, 4,* 150–165.

Newton, N. A., Bauer, D., Gutmann, D. L., & Grunes, J. (1986). Psychodynamic therapy with the aged: A review. In T. L. Brink (Ed.), *Clinical gerontology: A guide to assessment and intervention.* New York: Haworth.

Nolen-Hoeksema, S., Parker, L. E., & Larson, J. (1994). Ruminative coping with depressed mood following loss. *Journal of Personality and Social Psychology, 67,* 92–104.

Noonberg, A., Goldstein, G., & Page, H. A. (1985). Premature aging in male alcoholics: "Accelerated aging" or "Increased vulnerability"? *Alcoholism: Clinical and Experimental Research, 9,* 334–338.

Norris, J. T., Gallagher, D., Wilson, A., & Winograd, C. H. (1987). Assessment of depression in geriatric medical outpatients: The validity of two screening measures. *Journal of the American Geriatrics Society, 35,* 989–995.

O'Donohue, W. T., Fisher, J. E., & Krasner, L. (1986). Behavior therapy and the elderly: A conceptual and ethical analysis. *International Journal of Aging and Human Development, 23,* 1–15.

Okimoto, J., Barnes, R., Veith, R. C., Raskind, M., Inui, T., & Carter, W. (1982). Screening for depression in geriatric medical patients. *American Journal of Psychiatry, 139,* 799–802.

Osgood, N. J. (1985). *Suicide in the elderly.* Rockville, MD: Aspen.

Overall, J. E., & Beller, S. A. (1984). The Brief Psychiatric Rating Scale (BPRS) in geropsychiatric research: I. Factor structure on an inpatients unit. *Journal of Gerontology, 39,* 187–193.

Ownby, R. L., & Seibel, H. P. (1990). Empirical clusters of disordered behavior among older psychiatric inpatients. *Journal of Gerontology, 45,* P28–P32.

Parmelee, P. A., Katz, I. R., & Lawton, M. P. (1991). The relations of pain to depression among institutionalized aged. *Journal of Gerontology: Psychological Sciences, 46,* P15–P21.

Persson, G., & Svanborg, A. (1992). Marital coital activity in men at the age of 75: Relation to somatic, psychiatric, and social factors at the age of 70. *Journal of the American Geriatrics Society, 40,* 439–444.

Pfeiffer, E. (1977). Psychopathology and social pathology. In J. E. Birren & K. W. Schaie (Eds.), *Handbook of the psychology of aging.* New York: Van Nostrand Reinhold.

Pfeiffer, E., & Busse, E. W. (1973). Affective disorders. In R. W. Busse & E. Pfeiffer (Eds.), *Mental illness in later life.* Washington, DC: American Psychiatric Association.

Pfeiffer, E., & Davis, G. C. (1972). Determinants of sexual behavior in middle and old age. *Journal of the American Geriatrics Society, 20,* 151–158.

Pfeiffer, E., Verwoerdt, A., & Davis, G. C. (1972). Sexual behavior in middle life. *American Journal of Psychiatry, 128,* 82–87.

Pfeiffer, E., Verwoerdt, A., & Wang, H. S. (1969). The natural history of sexual behavior in a biologically advantaged group of aged individuals. *Journal of Gerontology, 24,* 193–198.

Pinchofsky-Devin, G. D., & Kaminski, M. V. (1986). Correlation of pressure sores and nutritional status. *Journal of the American Geriatrics Society, 34,* 435–440.

Post, E. (1980). Paranoid, schizophrenia-like, and schizophrenic states in the aged. In J. E. Birren & R. B. Sloan (Eds.), *Handbook of mental health and aging* (pp. 591–615). Englewood Cliffs, NJ: Prentice-Hall.

Post, E. (1987). Paranoid and schizophrenic disorders among the aging. In L. L. Carstensen & B. A. Edelstein (Eds.), *Handbook of clinical gerontology* (pp. 43–56). New York: Pergamon Press.

President's Commission on Mental Health. (1979). Mental health and the elderly: Recommendations for action (Report No. OHDS 80-20960). Washington, DC: U.S. Government Printing Office.

Price, W. A., Giannini, A. J., & Colella, J. (1985). Anorexia nervosa in the elderly. *Journal of the American Geriatrics Society, 33,* 213–215.

Rachman, S. (1977). The conditioning theory of fear-acquisition: A critical examination. *Behaviour Research and Therapy, 15,* 375–384.

Radloff, L. S., & Teri, L. (1986). Use of Center for Epidemiologic Studies: Depression scale with older adults. *Clinical Gerontologist, 5,* 119–137.

Raj, B. A., Corvea, M. H., & Dagon, E. M. (1993). The clinical characteristics of panic disorder in the elderly: A retrospective study. *Journal of Clinical Psychiatry, 54,* 150–155.

Regier, D. A., Myers, J. K., Kramer, M., Robins, L. N., Blazer, D. G., Hough, R. L., Eaten, W. W., & Locke, B. Z. (1984). The NIMH Epidemiologic Catchment Area program. *Archives of General Psychiatry, 41,* 934–941.

Reich, J. W., Zautra, A. J., & Guamaccia, C. A. (1989). Effects of disability and bereavement on the mental health and recovery of older adults. *Psychology and Aging, 4,* 57–65.

Reifler, B., Raskind, M., & Kethley, A. (1982). Psychiatric diagnoses among geriatric patients seen in an outreach program. *Journal of the American Geriatrics Society, 30,* 530–533.

Reilly, E. L., Kelly, J. T., Pena, Y. M., Overall, J. E., & Faillace, L. A. (1983). Short latency brain stem and somatosensory evoked potentials on alcoholics. *Clinical Electroencephalography, 14,* 8–16.

Renshaw, D. (1985). Sex, age, and values. *Journal of the American Geriatrics Society, 33,* 635–643.

Riccio, D. C., & Sylvestri, R. (1973). Extinction of avoidance behavior and the problem of residual fear. *Behavior Research and Therapy, 11*, 1–9.

Roberts, R. E., Kaplan, G. A., Shema, S. J., & Strawbridge, W. J. (1997). Prevalence and correlates of depression in an aging cohort: The Alameda County Study. *Journals of Gerotology: Social Sciences, 52B*, S252–S258.

Robins, L. N., Helzer, J. E., Weissman, M. M., Orvaschel, H., Greenberg, E., Burke, J. D., & Regier, D. A. (1984). Lifetime prevalence of specific disorders in three sites. *Archives of General Psychiatry, 41*, 949–958.

Robins, L. N., & Regier, D. A. (Eds.). (1991). *Psychiatric disorders in America: The Epidemiological Catchment Area Study.* New York: The Free Press.

Ronch, J. (1985). Suspected anorexia nervosa in a 75 year old institutionalized male: Issues in diagnosis and intervention. *Clinical Gerontologist, 4*, 31–38.

Roth, M. (1955). The natural history of mental disorder in old age. *Journal of Mental Science, 101*, 281.

Roth, M., & Kay, D. W. K. (1956). Affective disorders arising in the senium: II. Physical disability as an etiologic factor. *Journal of Mental Science, 102*, 141.

Ryan, C., & Butters, N. (1980). Learning and memory impairments in young and old alcoholics: Evidence for premature aging hypothesis. *Alcoholism: Clinical and Experimental Research, 4*, 288–293.

Ryan, C. (1982). Alcoholism and premature aging: A neuropsychological perspective. *Alcoholism: Clinical and Experimental Research, 6*, 22–30.

Sakheim, D. K., Barlow, D. H., Abrahamson, D. J., & Beck, J. G. (1987). Distinguishing between organogenic and psychogenic erectile dysfunction. *Behaviour Research and Therapy, 25*, 379–390.

Saltman, C., Vander Kolk, B., & Shader, R. I. (1975). Psychopharmacology and the geriatric patient. In R. I. Shader (Ed.), *Manual of psychiatric therapeutics.* Boston: Little, Brown.

Sandman, P. O., Adolfsson, R., Nygren, C., Hallmanns, G., & Winblad, B. (1987). Nutritional status and dietary intake in institutionalized patients with Alzheimer's disease and multi-infarct dementia. *Journal of the American Geriatrics Society, 35*, 31–38.

Sauer, W. J., & Warland, R. (1982). Morale and life satisfaction. In D. J. Mangen & W. A. Peterson (Eds.), *Research instruments in social gerontology: Clinical and social psychology.* Minneapolis: University of Minnesota Press.

Schaie, K. W. (1989). The hazards of cognitive aging. *The Gerontologist, 29*, 484–493.

Schaie, K. W. (1977). Quasi-experimental designs in the psychology of aging. In J. E. Birren & K. W. Schaie (Eds.), *Handbook of the psychology of aging* (pp. 39–58). New York: Van Nostrand Reinhold.

Schaie, K. W. (1994). The course of adult intellectual development. *American Psychologist, 49*, 304–313.

Schaie, K. W. (1996). *Intellectual development in adulthood: The Seattle longitudinal study.* New York: Cambridge University Press.

Schaie, K. W., & Labouvie-Vief, G. (1974). Generational versus ontogenetic components of change in adult cognitive behavior: A fourteen-year cross-sequential study. *Developmental Psychology, 10*, 305–320.

Schaie, K. W., & Stone, V. (1982). Psychological assessment. *Annual Review of Gerontology and Geriatrics, 3*, 329–360.

Schaie, K. W., Campbell, R. T., Meredith, W., & Rawlings, S. C. (Eds.) (1988). *Methodological issues in aging research.* New York: Springer.

Schaie, W. (1990). Intellectual development in adulthood. In J. E. Birren & K. W. Schaie (Eds.), *Handbook of the psychology of aging,* (4th ed., pp. 266–286). San Diego, CA: Academic Press.

Schiavi, R. C., & Schreiner-Engel, P. (1988). Nocturnal penile tumescence in healthy aging men. *Journal of Gerontology, 43*, M146–M150.

Schover, L. R. (1986). Sexual problems. In L. Teri & P. M. Lewinsohn (Eds.), *Geropsychological assessment and treatment: Selected topics* (pp. 145–187). New York: Springer.

Schover, L. R., & Jensen, S. B. (1988). *Sexuality and chronic illness.* New York: Guilford.

Schreiner-Engel, P., Schiavi, R. C., Vietorisz, D., & Smith, H. (1987). The differential impact of diabetes type on female sexuality. *Journal of Psychosomatic Research, 31*, 23–33.

Segraves, R. T., Madsen, R., Carter, C. S., & Davis, J. M. (1985). Erectile dysfunction associated with pharmacological agents. In R. T. Segraves & H. W. Schoenberg (Eds.), *Diagnosis and treatment of erectile disturbances* (pp. 23–64). New York: Plenum.

Segraves, R. E., & Schoenberg, H. W. (Eds.) (1985). *Diagnosis and treatment of erectile dysfunction.* New York: Plenum.

Shader, R. I., & Greenblatt, D. J. (1982). Management of anxiety in the elderly: The balance between therapeutic and adverse effects. *Journal of Clinical Psychology, 43*, 8–18.

Shapiro, S., Skinner, E. A., Kessler, L. G., Von Korff, M., German, P. S., Tischler, G. L., Leaf, P. J., Benham, L., Cottler, L., Regier, D. A. (1984). Utilization of health and mental health services. *Archives of General Psychiatry, 41*, 971–982.

Sheikh, J. I., & Yesavage, J. A. (1986). Geriatric Depression Scale (GDS): Recent evidence and development of a shorter version. In T. L. Brink (Ed.), *Clinical gerontology: A guide to assessment and intervention.* New York: Haworth.

Shulman, K. I., Tohen, M., Satlin, A., Mallya, G., & Kalunian, D. (1992). Mania compared with unipolar depression in old age. *American Journal of Psychiatry, 149*, 341–345.

Singer, C., Weiner, W. J., Sanchez-Ramos, J., & Ackerman, M. (1991). Sexual function in patients with Parkinson's disease. *Journal of Neurology and Neurosurgery and Psychiatry, 10*, 942.

Sirrocco, A. (1988). Nursing and related care homes as reported from the 1986 inventory of long term care places. In U.S. Department of Health and Human Services, Advance data from vital and health statistics (No. 147, DHHS Pub. No. PHS 88-1250). Hyattsville, MD: Public Health Service.

Slag, M. E., Morley, J. E., Elson, M. K., Trence, D. L., Nelson, C. J., Nelson, A. E., Kinlaw, W. B., Beyer, H. S., Nuttall, E. Q., & Shafer, R. B. (1983). Impotence in medical clinic outpatients. *Journal of the American Medical Association, 249*, 1736–1740.

Spencer, G. (1989). Projections of population of the United States by age, sex, and race: 1988–2080. Current population reports, population estimates, and projections (Series P-25, No. 1018). Washington, DC: U.S. Department of Commerce, Bureau of the Census.

Spielberger, C. D. (1983). *Manual for the state-trait anxiety inventory.* Pale Alto, CA: Consulting Psychologists Press.

Spitzer, R. L., Endicott, J., & Robins, E. (1978). Research

Diagnostic Criteria: Rationale and reliability. *Archives of General Psychiatry, 35,* 773.

Starr, B. D., & Weiner, M. B. (1981). *Sex and sexuality in the mature years.* New York: McGraw-Hill.

Steinke, E. E. (1994). Knowledge and attitudes of older adults about sexuality in aging: A comparison of two studies. *Journal of Advanced Nursing,, 19,* 477–485.

Stelnicki, G., & Thompson, J. K. (1989). Eating disorders in the elderly. *Behavior Therapist, 12,* 7–9.

Strauss, J. S., Carpenter, W. T., & Bartko, J. J. (1974). The diagnosis and understanding of schizophrenia: Part II. Speculations on the processes that underlie schizophrenic symptoms and signs. *Schizophrenia Bulletin, 11,* 61–69.

Stremgren, E. (1987). Changes in the incidence of schizophrenia? *British Journal of Psychiatry, 150,* 1–7.

Susser, E., & Wanderling, J. (1994). Epidemiology of nonaffective acute remitting psychosis versus schizophrenia: Sex and sociocultural setting. *Archives of General Psychiatry, 53,* 294–301.

Swearer, J. M., Drachman, D. A., O'Donnell, B. F., & Mitchell, A. L. (1988). Troublesome and disruptive behavior in dementia: Relationships to diagnosis and disease severity. *Journal of the American Geriatrics Society, 36,* 784–790.

Taylor, M., & Abrams, R. (1973). Manic states: A genetic study of early and late onset affective disorders. *Archives of General Psychiatry, 28,* 656–658.

Teri, L., & Lewinsohn, P. M. (1986). *Gerontological assessment and treatment: Selected topics.* New York: Springer.

Thorpe, L. (1997). The treatment of psychotic disorders in late life. *Canadian Journal of Psychiatry, 42,* 19S–27S.

Thorson, J. A., & Powell, F. C. (1988). Elements of death anxiety and meanings of death. *Journal of Clinical Psychology, 44,* 691–701.

Tsitouras, P. D., Martin, C. E., & Harman, S. M. (1982). Relationship of serum testosterone to sexual activity in healthy elderly men. *Journal of Gerontology, 37,* 288–293.

Uhde, T. W., Roy-Byme, P. P., Vittone, B. J., Boulenger, J. P., & Post, R. M. (1985). Phenomenology and neurobiology of panic disorder. In A. H. Tuma & J. D. Laser (Eds.), *Anxiety and the anxiety disorders.* Hillsdale, NJ: Erlbaum.

Uhlenhuth, E. H., Baiter, M. B., Mellinger, G. D., Cisin, I. H., & Clinthorne, J. (1983). Symptom checklist syndromes in the general population. *Archives of General Psychiatry, 40,* 1167–1173.

U.S. Bureau of the Census. (1993). Population profile of the United States: 1990. Washington, D.C.: U.S. Government Printing Office.

U.S. Bureau of the Census. (1993). Population profile of the United States: 1996. Washington, D.C.: U.S. Government Printing Office.

U.S. Department of Health and Human Services. (1988). NIMH National Plan for Schizophrenia Research: Panel recommendations. *Schizophrenia Bulletin, 14,* 413–417.

Valanis, B., Yeaworth, R. C., & Mullis, M. R. (1988). Alcohol use among bereaved and nonbereaved older persons. *Journal of Gerontological Nursing, 13,* 26–32.

Vaillant, G. E. (1996). A long-term follow-up of male alcohol abuse. *Archives of General Psychiatry, 53,* 243–250.

Varner, R., & Gaitz, C. (1982). Schizophrenic and paranoid disorders of the aged. *Psychiatric Clinics of North America, 5,* 107–118.

Veith, R. C., & Borson, S. (1986). Does age make a difference? *Generations, 10,* 9–13.

Verwoerdt, A. (1980). Anxiety, dissociative and personality disorders in the elderly. In E. W. Busse & D. G. Blazer (Eds.), *Handbook of geriatric psychiatry.* New York: Van Nostrand Reinhold.

Verwoerdt, A., Pfeiffer, E., & Wang, H. S. (1969a). Sexual behavior in senescence: I. Changes in sexual activity and interest of aging men and women. *Journal of Geriatric Psychiatry, 2,* 163–180.

Verwoerdt, A., Pfeiffer, E., & Wang, H. S. (1969b). Sexual behavior in senescence: II. Patterns of sexual activity and interest. *Geriatrics, 24,* 137–154.

Weg, R. (1983). *Sexuality in the later years: Roles and behavior.* New York: Academic Press.

Weizman, R., & Hart, J. (1987). Sexual behavior in healthy married elderly men. *Archives of Sexual Behavior, 16,* 39–44.

White, C. B. (1982). A scale for the assessment of attitudes and knowledge regarding sexuality in the aged. *Archives of Sexual Behavior, 11,* 491–502.

Willenbring, M. L., Christiansen, K. J., Spring, W. D., & Rasmussen, R. (1987). Alcoholism screening in the elderly. *Journal of the American Geriatrics Society, 35,* 864–869.

Wisocki, P. A. (1988). Worry as a phenomenon relevant to the elderly. *Behavior Therapy, 19,* 369–379.

Wong, D. E., Wagner, H. N., Dannals, R. E., Links, J. M., Frost, J. J., Ravert, H. T., Wilson, A. A., Rosenbaum, A. E., Gjedde, A., Douglass, K. H., Pentronis, J. D., Folstein, M. E., Toung, J. K. T., Burns, H. D., & Kuhar, M. J. (1984). Effects of age on dopamine and serotonin receptors measured by positron tomography on the living human brain. *Science, 226,* 1395–1396.

World Health Organization. (1998). Life in the 21st Century—A Vision for All. Bulletin of the World Health Organization, *76,* 256.

Young, R. C., & Klerman, G. L. (1992). Mania in late life: Focus on age at onset. *American Journal of Psychiatry, 149,* 867–876.

Zarsky, E. L., & Blau, D. (1970). The understanding and management of narcissistic regression and dependency in an elderly woman observed over an extended period of time. *Journal of Geriatric Psychiatry, 3,* 160–176.

Zeiss, A. M., Davies, H., Wood, M., & Tinklenberg, J. (1990). The incidence and correlates of male erectile dysfunction in Alzheimer's disease patients. *Archives of Sexual Behavior, 19,* 325–331.

Zeiss, A. M., Lewinsohn, P. M., Rohde, P., & Seeley, J. R. (1996). Relationship of physical disease and functional impairment to depression in older people. *Psychology and Aging, 11,* 572–581.

Zeiss, A. M., Zeiss, R. A., & Dornbrand, L. (1989). Treating sexual problems in older adults: Predictors of outcome. Paper presented at 23rd Annual Association for the Advancement of Behavior Therapy convention, Washington, DC.

Zimberg, S. (1987). Alcohol abuse among the elderly. In L. L. Carstensen & B. A. Edelstein (Eds.), *Handbook of clinical gerontology.* New York: Pergamon Press.

Zimmer, J. G., Watson, N., & Treat, A. (1984). Behavioral problems among patients in skilled nursing facilities. *American Journal of Public Health, 74,* 1118–1121.

Zisook, S., & Shuchter, S. R. (1991). Early psychological reaction to the stress of widowhood. *Psychiatry, 54,* 320–333.

Zubin, J., & Spring, B. (1977). Vulnerability—a new view on schizophrenia. *Journal of Abnormal Psychology, 86,* 103–126.

Zung, W. W. K. (1965). A self-rating depression scale. *Archives of General Psychiatry, 12,* 63–70.

Zung, W. W. K. (1967). Depression in the normal aged. *Psychosomatics, 8,* 287–292.

Zung, W. W. K., Gianturaco, D., Pfeiffer, E., Wang, S., Whanger, A., Bridge, T., & Potkin, S. (1974). Pharmacology of depression in the aged: Evaluation of Gerovital H3 as an antidepressant. *Psychosomatics, 15,* 127–131.

Zung, W. W. K., & Zung, E. M. (1986). Use of the Zung Self-Rating Depression Scale in the elderly. In T. L. Brink (Ed.), *Clinical gerontology: A guide to assessment and intervention.* New York: Haworth.

# Index